Textbook of
Rheumatology

Textbook of Rheumatology

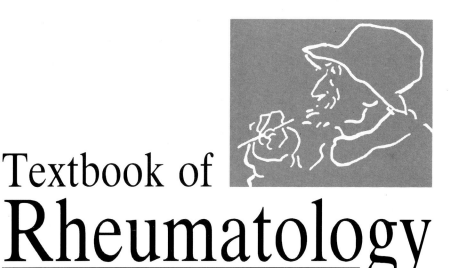

Fourth Edition   Volume 2

WILLIAM N. KELLEY, M.D.

Chief Executive Officer
University of Pennsylvania Medical Center
Executive Vice President and Robert G. Dunlop
  Professor of Medicine and Biochemistry and Biophysics
University of Pennsylvania
Dean, University of Pennsylvania School of Medicine
Philadelphia, Pennsylvania

EDWARD D. HARRIS, Jr., M.D.

Arthur L. Bloomfield Professor and Chairman
Department of Medicine
Stanford University School of Medicine
Stanford, California

SHAUN RUDDY, M.D.

Elam Toone Professor of Internal Medicine,
  Immunology, and Microbiology
Chairman
Division of Rheumatology, Allergy, and Immunology
Department of Internal Medicine
Medical College of Virginia
Virginia Commonwealth University
Richmond, Virginia

CLEMENT B. SLEDGE, M.D.

John B. and Buckminster Brown Professor of Orthopedic Surgery
Harvard Medical School
Chairman
Department of Orthopedic Surgery
Brigham and Women's Hospital
Boston, Massachusetts

W.B. SAUNDERS COMPANY
Harcourt Brace Jovanovich, Inc.
Philadelphia   London   Toronto   Montreal   Sydney   Tokyo

W.B. SAUNDERS COMPANY
Harcourt Brace Jovanovich, Inc.

The Curtis Center
Independence Square West
Philadelphia, Pennsylvania 19106

Library of Congress Cataloging-in-Publication Data

Textbook of rheumatology / William N. Kelley . . . [et al.].—
4th ed.

    p.   cm.

Includes bibliographical references and indexes.

ISBN 0–7216–3157–6 (set)

1. Rheumatology.   I. Kelley, William N., 1939–
    [DNLM: 1. Arthritis.   2. Rheumatic Diseases.
    WE 544 T355 1993]

RC927.T49 1993   616.7'23—dc20

DNLM/DLC
for Library of Congress   92–48331
                                 CIP

TEXTBOOK OF RHEUMATOLOGY, Fourth Edition   ISBN

                                      Volume I   0–7216–3155–X
                                        Volume II   0–7216–3156–8
                                        Two Volume Set 0–7216–3157–6

Printed in the United States of America.

Last digit is the print number: 9   8   7   6   5   4   3   2   1

We wish to dedicate this edition of the
Textbook of Rheumatology to our families.

Lois Kelley and children:
Paige Kelley Nath, Ginger Kelley Yost, Lori Kelley, and Mark Kelley.

Ned Harris, Tom Harris, and Chandler Harris.

Millicent Ruddy and children:
Christi Ruddy and Candace Ruddy Lau-Hansen.

Georgia Sledge and children:
Margaret Sledge Tracy, John Sledge, Matthew Sledge, and Claire Sledge.

Contributors

CAROLINE M. ALEXANDER, Ph.D.
Postdoctoral Fellow, University of California, San Francisco, School of Medicine, San Francisco, California
Proteinases and Matrix Degradation

ROY D. ALTMAN, M.D.
Professor of Medicine, Arthritis Division, University of Miami School of Medicine; Chief, Arthritis Section, Department of Veterans Affairs Medical Center; Staff Physician, University of Miami Hospital and Clinics; Staff Physician, Jackson Memorial Hospital, Miami, Florida
Hypertrophic Osteoarthropathy

WILLIAM P. AREND, M.D.
Professor of Medicine and Head, Division of Rheumatology, University of Colorado Health Sciences Center; Attending Physician, University Hospital, Denver, Colorado
Cytokines and Growth Factors

M. AMIN A. ARNAOUT, M.D.
Associate Professor of Medicine, Harvard Medical School, and Department of Medicine, Massachusetts General Hospital; Director, Leukocyte Biology and Inflammation Program, Associate Physician, Department of Medicine, Massachusetts General Hospital, Boston, Massachusetts
Cell Adhesion Molecules

WILLIAM J. ARNOLD, M.D.
Clinical Professor of Medicine, University of Chicago Pritzker School of Medicine, Chicago; Chairman, Department of Medicine, Lutheran General Hospital, Park Ridge, Illinois
Sarcoidosis

LLOYD AXELROD, M.D.
Associate Professor of Medicine, Harvard Medical School; Physician and Chief of the James Howard Means Firm, Massachusetts General Hospital, Boston, Massachusetts
Glucocorticoids

STANLEY P. BALLOU, M.D.
Associate Professor of Medicine, Case Western Reserve University; Director of Arthritis Clinic, MetroHealth Medical Center, Cleveland, Ohio
Laboratory Evaluation of Inflammation

ROBERT M. BENNETT, M.D., F.R.C.P.
Professor of Medicine and Chairman, Division of Arthritis and Rheumatic Diseases, The Oregon Health Sciences University, Portland, Oregon
The Fibromyalgia Syndrome: Myofascial Pain and the Chronic Fatigue Syndrome; Mixed Connective Tissue Disease and Other Overlap Syndromes

HÅKAN BERGSTRAND, Ph.D.
Professor, University of Lund; Assistant Director, Scientific Advisor, Pharmacology I, Astra Draco, Lund, Sweden
Neutrophils and Eosinophils

MARIE-JOSEÉ BERTHIAUME, M.D., F.R.C.P.S.
Musculoskeletal Radiologist and Associate Professor, Royal Victoria Hospital, McGill University Faculty of Medicine, Montreal, Quebec, Canada
Imaging

ALAN L. BISNO, M.D.
Professor, Department of Medicine, University of Miami School of Medicine; Chief, Medical Service, Miami Veterans Affairs Medical Center; Attending Physician, Veterans Affairs Medical Center and Jackson Memorial Hospital, Miami, Florida
Rheumatic Fever

ARTHUR L. BOLAND, M.D.
Assistant Clinical Professor of Orthopedic Surgery, Harvard Medical School; Visiting Orthopedic Surgeon, Massachusetts General Hospital, Brigham and Women's Hospital, New England Baptist Hospital, Boston, Massachusetts
Sports Medicine

KENNETH D. BRANDT, M.D.
Professor of Medicine and Head, Rheumatology Division, Indiana University School of Medicine; Attending Physician, Indiana University Hospital, Indianapolis, Indiana
Pathogenesis of Osteoarthritis; Management of Osteoarthritis

DOREEN B. BRETTLER, M.D.
Associate Professor, University of Massachusetts Medical School, Director, New England Hemophilia Center, Worcester, Massachusetts
Hemophilic Arthropathy

GREGORY W. BRICK, M.D.
Clinical Instructor in Orthopedic Surgery, Harvard Medical School; Orthopedic Surgeon at Brigham and Women's Hospital and West Roxbury Veterans Administration Hospital, Boston, Massachusetts
The Hip

REBECCA H. BUCKLEY, M.D.
J. Buren Sidbury Professor of Pediatrics, Professor of Immunology, Duke University School of Medicine; Chief, Division of Allergy and Immunology, Department of Pediatrics, Duke University Medical Center, Durham, North Carolina
Specific Immunodeficiency Diseases, Excluding AIDS

DAVID S. CALDWELL, M.D.
Associate Professor of Medicine, Division of Rheumatology and Immunology, Department of Medicine, Duke University; Attending Physician, Duke University Hospital, Durham, North Carolina
Musculoskeletal Syndromes Associated with Malignancy

DENNIS A. CARSON, M.D.
Professor of Medicine, University of California, San Diego; Director, The Sam and Rose Stein Institute for Research on Aging, University of California, San Diego, San Diego, California
Rheumatoid Factor

JAMES T. CASSIDY, M.D.
Professor, Division of Pediatric Rheumatology, University of Missouri–Columbia School of Medicine; Professor of Child Health, University of Missouri–Columbia School of Medicine, Columbia, Missouri
Juvenile Rheumatoid Arthritis; Systemic Lupus Erythematosus, Juvenile Dermatomyositis, Scleroderma, and Vasculitis

EDGAR S. CATHCART, M.D., D.Sc.
Professor of Medicine, Boston University School of Medicine, Boston; Chief of Staff, Edith Nourse Rogers Memorial Department of Veterans Affairs Medical Center, Bedford, Massachusetts
Amyloidosis

PHILIP J. CLEMENTS, M.D.
Professor of Medicine, University of California, Los Angeles, School of Medicine; Physician, Center for Health Sciences, University of California, Los Angeles, Los Angeles, California
Nonsteroidal Anti-inflammatory Drugs (NSAIDs)

DOYT L. CONN, M.D.
John F. Finn, Minnesota Arthritis Foundation Professor of Medicine, Mayo Medical School; Consultant in Rheumatology and Internal Medicine, Mayo Clinic, Rochester, Minnesota
Vasculitis and Related Disorders

RAMZI S. COTRAN, M.D.
F. B. Mallory Professor of Pathology, Harvard Medical School; Chairman, Department of Pathology, Brigham and Women's Hospital, Boston, Massachusetts
Endothelial Cells

JOE CRAFT, M.D.
Associate Professor of Medicine and Chief, Section of Rheumatology, Department of Medicine, Yale University School of Medicine; Attending, Yale–New Haven Hospital, New Haven, Connecticut
Antinuclear Antibodies

JODY A. DANTZIG
Department of Physiology, University of Pennsylvania School of Medicine; Research Specialist, Pennsylvania Muscle Institute, Philadelphia, Pennsylvania
Muscle

LAURIE S. DAVIS, Ph.D.
Assistant Professor, Department of Internal Medicine/Division of Rheumatology, University of Texas Southwestern Medical Center, Dallas, Texas
T Cells and B Cells

RICHARD O. DAY, M.B., M.D., F.R.A.C.P.
Professor of Clinical Pharmacology, University of New South Wales; Director of Clinical Pharmacology, St. Vincent's Hospital, Darlinghurst, Sydney, Australia
Aspirin and Salicylates; Sulfasalazine

JEAN-MICHEL DAYER, M.D.
Associate Professor of Medicine, Division of Immunology and Allergy, University of Geneva; Attending Physician, University Hospital, Geneva, Switzerland
Cytokines and Growth Factors

JONATHAN T. DELAND, M.D.
Assistant Professor of Orthopedic Surgery, Cornell University Medical College; Orthopedic Surgeon, Hospital for Special Surgery, New York, New York
Foot Pain; Sports Medicine

PENG THIM FAN, M.D.
Clinical Professor of Medicine, University of California, Los Angeles; Attending Physician, V. A. Wadsworth Medical Center, Los Angeles, California
Reiter's Syndrome

ANTHONY S. FAUCI, M.D.
Chief, Laboratory of Immunoregulation, and Director, National Institute of Allergy and Infectious Diseases, National Institutes of Health, Bethesda, Maryland
Immunoregulatory Agents

ANDREW P. FERRY, M.D.
Professor and Chairman, Department of Ophthalmology, and Professor of Pathology, Medical College of Virginia, Virginia Commonwealth University, Richmond, Virginia
The Eye and Rheumatic Diseases

IRVING H. FOX, M.D., C.M.
Vice-President, Medical Affairs, Biogen; Clinical Professor of Medicine, Harvard Medical School; Clinical Associate, Massachusetts General Hospital, Boston, Massachusetts
Antihyperuricemic Drugs

ROBERT I. FOX, M.D., Ph.D.
Associate Member, Department of Immunology, The Scripps Research Institute, Department of Rheumatology, Scripps Clinic and Research Foundation, La Jolla, California
Sjögren's Syndrome

ANDREW G. FRANKS, Jr., M.D.
Clinical Associate Professor of Dermatology, New York University School of Medicine; Attending Physician, Tisch Hospital, The University Hospital of NYU; Associate Rheumatologist, Hospital for Joint Diseases, New York University Medical Center, New York, New York
The Skin and Rheumatic Diseases

BRUCE FREUNDLICH, M.D.
Associate Professor of Medicine, University of Pennsylvania School of Medicine; Chief, Clinical Rheumatology Service, Hospital of the University of Pennsylvania, Philadelphia, Pennsylvania
Eosinophilia-Myalgia Syndrome

WILLIAM W. GINSBURG, M.D.

Associate Professor, Mayo Medical School, Rochester, Minnesota; Consultant, St. Luke's Hospital, Jacksonville, Florida
Multicentric Reticulohistiocytosis

DON L. GOLDENBERG, M.D.

Professor of Medicine, Tufts University School of Medicine, Boston; Chief of Rheumatology, Director, Arthritis-Fibromyalgia Center, Newton-Wellesley Hospital, Newton, Massachusetts
Bacterial Arthritis

YALE E. GOLDMAN, M.D., PH.D.

Professor, Department of Physiology, University of Pennsylvania School of Medicine; Director, Pennsylvania Muscle Institute, Philadelphia, Pennsylvania
Muscle

DUNCAN A. GORDON, M.D., F.P.C.P.C., F.A.C.P.

Professor of Medicine, University of Toronto Faculty of Medicine; Senior Rheumatologist, The Toronto Hospital Arthritis Centre, Toronto, Ontario, Canada
Gold Compounds in Rheumatic Diseases

BEVRA H. HAHN, M.D.

Professor of Medicine and Chief of Rheumatology, University of California, Los Angeles; Physician, Center for the Health Sciences, University of California, Los Angeles, Los Angeles, California
Management of Systemic Lupus Erythematosus

THEODORE J. HAHN, M.D.

Professor of Medicine, University of California, Los Angeles, School of Medicine; Chief, Geriatric Medicine, and Director, Geriatric Research, Education and Clinical Center, Veterans Administration Medical Center, West Los Angeles; Director, Osteoporosis and Metabolic Bone Disorders Center, UCLA Medical Center; Attending Physician, UCLA Medical Center, UCLA School of Medicine, Los Angeles, California
Metabolic Bone Disease

LENA HÅKANSSON, PH.D.

Associate Professor, University of Uppsala; Research Engineer, Department of Clinical Chemistry, University Hospital, Uppsala, Sweden
Neutrophils and Eosinophils

JOHN A. HARDIN, M.D.

Professor and Chairman, Department of Medicine, School of Medicine, Medical College of Georgia, Augusta, Georgia
Antinuclear Antibodies

EDWARD D. HARRIS, JR., M.D.

Arthur L. Bloomfield Professor and Chairman, Department of Medicine, Stanford University School of Medicine; Chief of Medical Services, Stanford University Hospital, Stanford, California
Etiology and Pathogenesis of Rheumatoid Arthritis; Clinical Features of Rheumatoid Arthritis; Treatment of Rheumatoid Arthritis

JEROME H. HERMAN, M.D.

Professor of Medicine, University of Cincinnati College of Medicine; Attending Physician, University Hospital and Holmes Division of the University of Cincinnati Medical Sciences Center; Consultant (Immunology/Rheumatology), Veterans Administration Hospital, Cincinnati, Ohio
Polychondritis

GARY S. HOFFMAN, M.S., M.D.

Head, Vasculitis and Related Diseases, National Institutes of Health, National Institute of Allergy and Infectious Diseases, Laboratory of Immunoregulation, Bethesda, Maryland
Mycobacterial and Fungal Infections

GENE G. HUNDER, M.D.

Professor of Medicine, Mayo Medical School; Chairman, Division of Rheumatology, Mayo Clinic, Rochester, Minnesota
Examination of the Joints; Vasculitis and Related Disorders; Giant Cell Arteritis and Polymyalgia Rheumatica

JOHN N. INSALL, M.D.

Clinical Professor of Orthopaedic Surgery, Mt. Sinai School of Medicine; Attending Orthopaedic Surgeon and Director of Insall Scott Kelly Institute for Orthopaedic and Sports Medicine, Beth Israel Medical Center–North Division, New York, New York
The Knee

SILVIU ITESCU, M.D., F.R.A.C.P.

Assistant Professor, Division of Autoimmune and Molecular Diseases, Columbia University College of Physicians and Surgeons; Attending Physician, Presbyterian Hospital, New York, New York
Rheumatologic Manifestations of HIV Infection

ISRAELI A. JAFFE, M.D.

Professor of Clinical Medicine, College of Physicians and Surgeons, Columbia University; Attending Physician, Presbyterian Hospital, New York, New York
Penicillamine

KENNETH A. JOHNSON, M.D.

Professor, Mayo Medical School; Consultant, Mayo Clinic Scottsdale, Scottsdale, Arizona
The Ankle and Foot

HO-IL KANG, M.D, PH.D.

Postdoctoral Fellow, Department of Immunology, The Scripps Research Institute, La Jolla, California
Sjögren's Syndrome

WILLIAM N. KELLEY, M.D., M.A.C.P.

Chief Executive Officer, University of Pennsylvania Medical Center; Executive Vice President and Robert G. Dunlop Professor of Medicine and Biochemistry and Biophysics, University of Pennsylvania; Dean, University of Pennsylvania School of Medicine, Philadelphia, Pennsylvania
Hyperuricemia; Gout

PAUL D. KEMP, PH.D.

Winchester, Massachusetts
Matrix Glycoproteins and Proteoglycans

JOEL M. KREMER, M.D.
Professor of Medicine, Albany Medical College;
Attending Physician, Albany Medical Center Hospital,
Albany, New York
Nutrition and Rheumatic Diseases

IRVING KUSHNER, M.D.
Professor of Medicine and Pathology, Case Western
Reserve University; Rheumatologist, MetroHealth Medical
Center, Cleveland, Ohio
Laboratory Evaluation of Inflammation

R. ELAINE LAMBERT, M.D.
Assistant Professor of Medicine, Division of Immunology
and Rheumatology, Stanford University School of
Medicine; Medical Staff, Stanford University Medical
Center, Stanford, California
*Iron Storage Disease; Arthropathies Associated with Endocrine
Disorders*

MATTHEW H. LIANG, M.D., M.P.H.
Associate Professor of Medicine, Harvard Medical School;
Lecturer in Health Policy and Management, Harvard
School of Public Health; Attending, Brigham and
Women's Hospital, Boston, Massachusetts
Psychosocial Management of Rheumatic Diseases

PETER E. LIPSKY, M.D.
Professor of Internal Medicine, University of Texas
Southwestern Medical Center of Dallas; Attending,
Parkland Memorial Hospital, Zale-Lipshy University
Hospital, Dallas, Texas
T Cells and B Cells; Monocytes and Macrophages

STEPHEN J. LIPSON, M.D.
Associate Professor of Orthopedic Surgery, Harvard
Medical School; Orthopedic Surgeon-in-Chief, Beth Israel
Hospital; Orthopedic Surgeon, Brigham and Women's
Hospital, Boston, Massachusetts
Low Back Pain; The Cervical Spine

CARLO L. MAINARDI, M.D.
Professor and Vice Chairman, Department of Medicine,
University of Tennessee; Chief, Medical Service, Veterans
Administration Medical Center, Memphis, Tennessee
Fibroblast Function and Fibrosis; Localized Fibrotic Disorders

HENRY J. MANKIN, M.D.
Edith M. Ashley Professor of Orthopedic Surgery,
Harvard Medical School; Chief of the Orthopedic Service,
Massachusetts General Hospital, Boston, Massachusetts
*Pathogenesis of Osteoarthritis; Clinical Features of
Osteoarthritis*

W. JOSEPH McCUNE, M.D.
Associate Professor, Department of Internal Medicine,
and Associate Chief for Clinical Activities, Division of
Rheumatology, University of Michigan Medical Center,
Ann Arbor, Michigan
Monarticular Arthritis

JAMES L. McGUIRE, M.D.
Associate Professor of Medicine, Associate Dean for
Clinical Affairs and Graduate Medical Education,

Stanford University School of Medicine; Chief of Staff,
Stanford University Hospital, Stanford, California
*Iron Storage Disease; Arthropathies Associated with Endocrine
Disorders*

KATHERYN MEEK, D.V.M.
Assistant Professor, Internal Medicine, University of
Texas Southwestern Medical Center, Dallas, Texas
T Cells and B Cells

JEFFERY L. MEIER, M.D.
Clinical Associate, Laboratory of Clinical Investigation,
National Institute of Allergy and Infectious Diseases; The
Warren G. Magnuson Clinical Center, National Institutes
of Health, Bethesda, Maryland
Mycobacterial and Fungal Infections

ROBERT W. METCALF, M.D.
Late Professor of Orthopedic Surgery, University of Utah
School of Medicine, Salt Lake City, Utah
Arthroscopy

CLEMENT J. MICHET, M.D., M.P.H.
Associate Professor of Medicine, Mayo Medical School;
Consultant in Rheumatology, Mayo Clinic Scottsdale,
Scottsdale, Arizona
Examination of the Joints; Psoriatic Arthritis

LEWIS H. MILLENDER, M.D.
Clinical Professor of Orthopedic Surgery, Tufts University
School of Medicine; Assistant Chief, Hand Surgery
Section, New England Baptist Hospital, Boston,
Massachusetts
The Hand

MARC L. MILLER, M.D.
Assistant Clinical Professor of Medicine, University of
Vermont College of Medicine, Burlington; Attending
Physician, Maine Medical Center, Portland, Maine
Weakness

B. F. MORREY, M.D.
Professor, Mayo Medical School; Chairman, Department
of Orthopedic Surgery, Mayo Clinic, Mayo Foundation,
Rochester, Minnesota
Reconstruction and Rehabilitation of the Elbow Joint

ROLAND W. MOSKOWITZ, M.D.
Professor of Medicine, Case Western Reserve University;
Director, Division of Rheumatic Diseases, University
Hospitals of Cleveland; Director, Northeast Ohio
Multipurpose Arthritis Center, Cleveland, Ohio
*Diseases Associated with the Deposition of Calcium
Pyrophosphate or Hydroxyapatite*

GEORGE MOXLEY, M.D.
Assistant Professor, Internal Medicine, Medical College of
Virginia, Virginia Commonwealth University, Richmond,
Virginia
Immune Complexes and Complement

KENNETH K. NAKANO, M.D., M.P.H., S.M.,
F.R.C.P.(C)
Medical Director, Straub Foundation, Honolulu, Hawaii
Neck Pain; Entrapment Neuropathies and Related Disorders

EDWARD A. NALEBUFF, M.D.
Clinical Professor of Orthopedic Surgery, Tufts University School of Medicine; Chief of Hand Surgery Section, New England Baptist Hospital, Boston, Massachusetts
The Hand

CHARLES S. NEER II, M.D.
Professor of Clinical Orthopaedic Surgery, Emeritus, and Special Lecturer in Orthopaedic Surgery, Columbia University College of Physicians and Surgeons; Consultant Orthopaedic Surgeon, Emeritus, New York Orthopaedic–Columbia–Presbyterian Medical Center, New York, New York
The Shoulder

BARBARA S. NEPOM, M.D.
Research Assistant Member, Virginia Mason Research Center, and Affiliate Assistant Professor, Division of Immunology/Rheumatology, Department of Pediatrics, University of Washington School of Medicine, Seattle, Washington
Immunogenetics and the Rheumatic Diseases

GERALD T. NEPOM, M.D., Ph.D.
Member and Director, Immunology Program, Virginia Mason Research Center, and Associate Professor (Affiliate), Department of Immunology, University of Washington School of Medicine, Seattle, Washington
Immunogenetics and the Rheumatic Diseases

ALAN P. NEWMAN, M.D.
Associate Professor of Orthopedic Surgery, University of Utah School of Medicine; Staff Orthopedic Surgeon, University Hospital, Salt Lake City, Utah
Synovectomy

JOHN J. NICHOLAS, M.D.
Professor and Chairman, Department of Physical Medicine and Rehabilitation, Rush Medical College; Senior Attending Physician, Rush–Presbyterian–St. Luke's Medical Center; Consulting Staff, Marianjoy Rehabilitation Center and Clinics, Chicago, Illinois
Rehabilitation of Patients with Rheumatic Diseases

J. DESMOND O'DUFFY, M.D.
Professor of Medicine, Mayo Medical School; Staff, Methodist Hospital, St. Mary's Hospital, Rochester, Minnesota
Vasculitis and Related Disorders; Multicentric Reticulohistiocytosis

DUNCAN S. OWEN, Jr., M.D.
Taliaferro/Scott Professor of Internal Medicine, Medical College of Virginia, Virginia Commonwealth University; Attending Physician, Medical College of Virginia Hospitals; Consultant, Hunter Holmes McGuire Department of Veterans Affairs Medical Center, Richmond, Virginia
Aspiration and Injection of Joints and Soft Tissues

HAROLD E. PAULUS, M.D.
Professor of Medicine, University of California, Los Angeles, School of Medicine; Attending Physician, Center for Health Sciences, University of California, Los Angeles, Los Angeles, California
Nonsteroidal Anti-inflammatory Drugs (NSAIDs)

ROBERT S. PINALS, M.D.
Professor of Medicine, University of Medicine and Dentistry of New Jersey–Robert Wood Johnson Medical School, New Brunswick; Chairman, Department of Medicine, The Medical Center at Princeton, Princeton, New Jersey
Felty's Syndrome

ROBERT POSS, M.D.
Professor of Orthopedic Surgery, Harvard Medical School; Vice Chairman, Department of Orthopedic Surgery, Brigham and Women's Hospital, Boston, Massachusetts
The Hip

DARWIN J. PROCKOP, M.D., Ph.D.
Chairman and Professor, Department of Biochemistry and Molecular Biology, Jefferson Medical College, Philadelphia, Pennsylvania
Collagen and Elastin

ERIC L. RADIN, M.D.
Clinical Professor of Orthopedic Surgery, University of Michigan, Ann Arbor; Director, Henry Ford Hospital Bone and Joint Center; Chairman of Orthopedic Surgery, Henry Ford Hospital, Detroit, Michigan
Biomechanics of Joints

DONALD RESNICK, M.D.
Professor of Radiology, University of California, San Diego, School of Medicine; Staff, University Hospital, Veterans Affairs Medical Center, San Diego, California
Imaging

ANDREW E. ROSENBERG, M.D.
Assistant Professor, Harvard Medical School; Assistant Pathologist, Massachusetts General Hospital, Boston, Massachusetts
Tumors and Tumor-Like Lesions of Joints and Related Structures

DAVID W. ROWE, M.D.
Professor of Pediatrics, Division of Endocrinology/ Diabetes, University of Connecticut Health Center School of Medicine, Farmington, Connecticut
Heritable Disorders of Structural Proteins

CLINTON T. RUBIN, Ph.D.
Director, Musculo-Skeletal Research Laboratory; Associate Professor, Department of Orthopaedics, School of Medicine, State University of New York at Stony Brook, Stony Brook, New York
Biology, Physiology, and Morphology of Bone

SHAUN RUDDY, M.D.
Elam Toone Professor of Internal Medicine; Chairman, Division of Rheumatology, Allergy, and Immunology, Department of Internal Medicine, Medical College of Virginia, Virginia Commonwealth University, Richmond, Virginia
Immune Complexes and Complement; Complement Deficiencies and Rheumatic Diseases

RICHARD I. RYNES, M.D.
Professor of Medicine and Head, Division of
Rheumatology, Albany Medical College; Attending
Physician, Albany Medical Center Hospital, Albany, New
York
Antimalarial Drugs

CHARLES L. SALTZMAN, M.D.
Assistant Professor, Department of Orthopaedic Surgery,
University of Iowa, Iowa City, Iowa
The Ankle and Foot

DAVID J. SARTORIS, M.D.
Associate Professor of Radiology, University of California,
San Diego, School of Medicine; Chief, Quantitative Bone
Densitometry, University of California, San Diego,
Medical Center, San Diego; Staff, Veterans
Administration Medical Center, San Diego; Scripps Clinic
and Research Foundation, La Jolla, California
Imaging

ALAN L. SCHILLER, M.D.
Irene Heinz Given and John LaPorte Given Professor of
Pathology, Mt. Sinai School of Medicine; Professor and
Chairman, Department of Pathology, Mt. Sinai Medical
Center, New York, New York
*Tumors and Tumor-Like Lesions of Joints and Related
Structures*

THOMAS J. SCHNITZER, M.D., PH.D.
Professor of Internal Medicine and Director, Sections of
Rheumatology and Geriatric Medicine, Rush Medical
College; Senior Attending, Rush–Presbyterian–St. Luke's
Medical Center; Medical Director, Johnston R. Bowman
Health Center for the Elderly, Chicago, Illinois
Viral Arthritis

H. RALPH SCHUMACHER, JR., M.D.
Professor of Medicine, University of Pennsylvania School
of Medicine; Director, Arthritis-Immunology Center,
Veterans Affairs Medical Center; Acting Chief, Division
of Rheumatology, University of Pennsylvania School of
Medicine and Hospital of the University of Pennsylvania,
Philadelphia, Pennsylvania
*Synovial Fluid Analysis and Synovial Biopsy; Gout;
Hemoglobinopathies and Arthritis*

PETER H. SCHUR, M.D.
Professor of Medicine, Harvard Medical School; Senior
Physician, Brigham and Women's Hospital, Boston,
Massachusetts
Clinical Features of SLE

LAWRENCE B. SCHWARTZ, M.D., PH.D.
Charles and Evelyn Thomas Professor of Medicine,
Medical College of Virginia, Virginia Commonwealth
University, Richmond, Virginia
The Mast Cell

RICHARD D. SCOTT, M.D.
Associate Clinical Professor of Orthopaedic Surgery,
Harvard Medical School; Surgeon, Brigham and Women's
Hospital, New England Baptist Hospital, Boston,
Massachusetts
Surgical Management of Juvenile Rheumatoid Arthritis

JAMES R. SEIBOLD, M.D.
Director, Clinical Research Center, and Director, Program
in Clinical Pharmacology, University of Medicine and
Dentistry of New Jersey–Robert Wood Johnson Medical
School; Chief, Clinical Pharmacology, Attending in
Medicine/Rheumatology, Robert Wood Johnson
University Hospital, New Brunswick, New Jersey
Scleroderma

JOHN S. SERGENT, M.D.
Professor of Medicine, Vanderbilt University School of
Medicine; Chief of Medicine, St. Thomas Hospital,
Nashville, Tennessee
Polyarticular Arthritis

JAY R. SHAPIRO, M.D.
Associate Professor and Program Director for the General
Clinical Research Center, The Johns Hopkins University
School of Medicine, Baltimore, Maryland
Heritable Disorders of Structural Proteins

BARRY P. SIMMONS, M.D.
Associate Professor of Orthopedic Surgery, Harvard
Medical School; Chief, Orthopedic Hand Surgery Service,
Brigham and Women's Hospital; Associate in Orthopedic
Surgery, Brigham and Women's Hospital; Associate in
Orthopedic Surgery, Children's Hospital Medical Center,
Boston, Massachusetts
The Hand

SHELDON R. SIMON, M.D.
Professor and Chief, Division of Orthopaedics, Ohio State
University; Attending Staff, Ohio State University
Hospital, and Children's Hospital, Columbus, Ohio
Biomechanics of Joints

CLEMENT B. SLEDGE, M.D.
John B. and Buckminster Brown Professor of Orthopedic
Surgery, Harvard Medical School; Chairman, Department
of Orthopedic Surgery, Brigham and Women's Hospital,
Boston, Massachusetts
*Biology of the Joint; Biology, Physiology, and Morphology of
Bone; Introduction to Surgical Management; Surgical
Management of Juvenile Rheumatoid Arthritis*

NICHOLAS A. SOTER, M.D.
Professor of Dermatology, New York University School of
Medicine; Medical Director, Charles C. Harris Skin and
Cancer Pavilion; Attending Physician, Tisch Hospital, The
University Hospital of NYU, New York, New York
The Skin and Rheumatic Diseases

ALLEN C. STEERE, M.D.
Professor of Medicine, Tufts University School of
Medicine; Chief, Rheumatology/Immunology, New
England Medical Center, Boston, Massachusetts
Lyme Disease

DAVID R. STEINBERG, M.D.
Assistant Professor, Department of Orthopaedics,
University of California, Davis, School of Medicine;
Attending Surgeon, Department of Orthopaedics,
University of California, Davis, Medical Center,
Sacramento, California
Osteonecrosis

MARVIN E. STEINBERG, M.D.
Professor and Vice Chairman, Department of Orthopaedic Surgery, University of Pennsylvania School of Medicine; Director, Hip Clinic and Joint Reconstruction Center, Hospital of the University of Pennsylvania, Philadelphia, Pennsylvania
Osteonecrosis

JERRY TENENBAUM, M.D., F.R.C.P.(C), F.A.C.P.
Associate Dean of Continuing Medical Education and Associate Professor of Medicine, University of Toronto; Staff Physician, Mt. Sinai Hospital; Staff Consultant (Rheumatology), Baycrest Geriatric Center, and Toronto Hospital, Toronto, Ontario, Canada
Hypertrophic Osteoarthropathy

RANJENY THOMAS, M.B.B.S., F.R.A.C.P.
Fellow in Rheumatology, University of Texas, Southwestern Medical Center at Dallas; Fellow, Parkland Memorial Hospital, Dallas, Texas
Monocytes and Macrophages

THOMAS S. THORNHILL, M.D.
Associate Clinical Professor of Orthopedics, Harvard Medical School; Staff, Brigham and Women's Hospital, New England Baptist Hospital, Boston, Massachusetts
Shoulder Pain

ROBERT L. TRELSTAD, M.D.
Professor and Chairman, Department of Pathology, University of Medicine and Dentistry of New Jersey– Robert Wood Johnson Medical School; Staff, Robert Wood Johnson University Hospital, New Brunswick, New Jersey
Matrix Glycoproteins and Proteoglycans

PAUL J. TSAHAKIS, M.D.
Director of Arthritis Research, Carolinas Medical Center; Orthopedic Surgeon, Miller Orthopedic Clinic, Charlotte, North Carolina
The Hip

KATHERINE S. UPCHURCH, M.D.
Associate Professor of Medicine, University of Massachusetts Medical School; Chief, Division of Rheumatology, Medical Center of Central Massachusetts, Worcester, Massachusetts
Hemophilic Arthropathy

FRANK H. VALONE, M.D.
Associate Professor of Medicine, Dartmouth Medical School, Hanover; Attending Physician, Dartmouth-Hitchcock Medical Center, Lebanon, New Hampshire
Platelets

PHILIPP VANDENBERG, M.D.
Research Associate, Thomas Jefferson University, Department of Biochemistry, Philadelphia, Pennsylvania
Collagen and Elastin

PER VENGE, M.D.
Professor, University of Uppsala; Head, Department of Clinical Chemistry, University Hospital, Uppsala, Sweden
Neutrophils and Eosinophils

MARY C. WACHOLTZ, M.D., PH.D.
Assistant Professor in Internal Medicine (Rheumatology), University of Texas Southwestern Medical Center at Dallas; Medical Staff, Parkland Memorial Hospital and Zale-Lipshy University Hospital in Dallas, Dallas, Texas
T Cells and B Cells

MICHAEL E. WEINBLATT, M.D.
Associate Professor of Medicine, Harvard Medical School; Vice Chairman of Clinical Affairs, Department of Rheumatology, Brigham and Women's Hospital, Boston, Massachusetts
Methotrexate

BARBARA N. WEISSMAN, M.D.
Associate Professor of Radiology, Harvard Medical School; Chief, Musculoskeletal Radiology Section, and Assistant Chairman of Radiology for Ambulatory Services, Brigham and Women's Hospital, Boston, Massachusetts
Radiographic Evaluation of Total Joint Replacement

ZENA WERB, PH.D.
Professor of Anatomy, Radiology, and Radiobiology, University of California, San Francisco, School of Medicine, San Francisco, California
Proteinases and Matrix Degradation

CHARLENE J. WILLIAMS, PH.D.
Research Assistant Professor, Thomas Jefferson University, Department of Biochemistry and Molecular Biology, Philadelphia, Pennsylvania
Collagen and Elastin

ROBERT J. WINCHESTER, M.D.
Professor of Pediatrics and Head, Division of Autoimmune and Molecular Diseases, Department of Pediatrics, Columbia University College of Physicians and Surgeons; Attending Physician, Presbyterian Hospital, New York, New York
Rheumatologic Manifestations of HIV Infection

RUSSELL E. WINDSOR, M.D.
Associate Professor of Surgery (Orthopaedics), Cornell University Medical College; Associate Chief, The Knee Service, Hospital for Special Surgery; Associate Attending Orthopaedic Surgeon, Hospital for Special Surgery, New York, New York
The Knee

FRANK A. WOLLHEIM, M.D., PH.D.
Professor of Rheumatology, University of Lund Medical School; Professor and Chairman, Department of Rheumatology, Lund University Hospital, Lund, Sweden
Ankylosing Spondylitis; Enteropathic Arthritis

BRUCE T. WOOD, D.P.M.
Associate in Orthopedics-Podiatry, Harvard Medical School, and Brigham and Women's Hospital; Staff Podiatrist, Massachusetts Institute of Technology, Cambridge, Massachusetts
Foot Pain

VIRGIL L. WOODS, JR., M.D.
Associate Professor of Medicine, University of California, San Diego; Attending Physician, University of California, San Diego, Medical Center, San Diego, California
Pathogenesis of Systemic Lupus Erythematosus

ROBERT L. WORTMANN, M.D.
Professor and Chairman, Department of Medicine, East
Carolina University School of Medicine; Chief of
Medicine, Pitt County Memorial Hospital, Greenville,
North Carolina
Inflammatory Diseases of Muscle

K. RANDALL YOUNG, JR., M.D.
Director, Division of Pulmonary and Critical Care
Medicine, Department of Medicine, University of
Alabama at Birmingham; Staff Physician, University of
Alabama Hospital, Birmingham, Alabama
Immunoregulatory Agents

DAVID TAK YAN YU, M.D.
Professor of Medicine, University of California, Los
Angeles, School of Medicine; Staff, University of
California, Los Angeles, Medical Center, Los Angeles,
California
Reiter's Syndrome

ROBERT B. ZURIER, M.D.
Professor of Medicine and Director, Division of
Rheumatology, University of Massachusetts Medical
School; Attending Physician, University of Massachusetts
Medical Center Hospital, Worcester, Massachusetts
Prostaglandins, Leukotrienes, and Related Compounds

Preface

The field of rheumatology continues to show remarkable progress. An impressive transition has occurred from the empirical approach of the nineteenth-century spas to today's multidisciplinary specialty ranging from the monumental advances in molecular biology, immunogenetics, and immunoregulation to the modern miracles of total joint replacement and the promise of gene therapy. There have been many critical contributions to this evolution. Pathologists and orthopedic surgeons such as Goldthwait, Smith-Peterson, and Wilson began important work early in the century. In the 1930s, internists such as Bauer, Cecil, Hench, Holbrooke, and Pemberton added their creative, scientific, and organizational skills to the embryonic discipline. Societies were created to stimulate the exchange of ideas, and an explosion of federal funding for research fostered expansion of essential scientific information.

Over the past three decades, consolidation of efforts in diverse disciplines has provided a truly scientific basis for rheumatology. The basic structure and function of immunoglobulins are now clarified at both the gene and the protein levels. Highly sophisticated techniques have allowed the careful study of specific lymphocyte subpopulations and their roles in controlling the immune response. Investigation of the inflammatory process has defined a multitude of effectors and their target cells. The details of how proteolytic enzymes destroy tissues in joints in inflammatory arthritis have been deciphered. The genes coding for these effectors are being cloned, as are the genes for the receptors themselves. These studies will allow not only improved understanding of their specific structure and function but also, eventually, the production of effectors, receptors, and their analogues in pharmacologic quantities or as substrates for gene therapy. The identification within the major histocompatibility complex of specific genetic polymorphisms associated with unusual predisposition to rheumatic disease represents a major breakthrough. Transgenic animals now provide critical animal models of disease. Advances in bioengineering, matched with sophisticated surgical approaches, have established metal and polymer prostheses as major components of therapy. Considering all these frontiers along which we are advancing, the outlook for a better understanding of and new effective treatments for rheumatic diseases has never been brighter.

In the First Edition, the principal goal was to include a complete spectrum of the information necessary for the understanding, differential diagnosis, and management of the patient with a rheumatic complaint. This led to the inclusion of chapters addressing areas not covered by existing reference books in rheumatology, such as the scientific basis of rheumatology, a large section on the general approach to the patient, a full evaluation of the diagnostic tests utilized in the evaluation of patients with rheumatic diseases, and extensive coverage of rehabilitation and reconstructive surgery as they relate to rheumatology. The Second and Third Editions were reorganized and revised extensively.

The Fourth Edition has been comprehensively revised beyond the improvements of the first three editions. There are new chapters in areas such as immunogenetics and the rheumatic diseases, cell adhesion molecules, fibroblast function in fibrosis, laboratory evaluation of inflammation, sulfasalazine, the eosinophilia-myalgia syndrome, rheumatologic manifestations of human immunodeficiency virus infection, and specific immunodeficiency diseases excluding acquired immunodeficiency syndrome. We have combined and consolidated a number of other chapters in order to enhance the flow of information. All of these chapters include not only the many major advances in basic science occurring during the past several years but also the discussion of their possible clinical implications.

The editors continue to believe that the quality of this textbook depends on the quality of its contributors. We also recognize the importance of regular replacement of contributors to ensure that even the best chapters will be extensively updated over a period of several editions. In the Fourth Edition, we have continued to follow this policy, with the inclusion of 53 new authors. This has allowed us to approach certain areas differently and to consolidate several areas to improve the flow of text. Even those chapters that do not have new authors were substantially updated and, when possible, improved in quality. The editors are highly pleased with the final product.

We wish to express our thanks to our teachers and to our students, from whom we have learned much, as well as to our colleagues for their patience and understanding of the time and energy the development of this textbook has required of us. Throughout the preparation of this edition, the expertise of the professionals at W.B. Saunders has continued to impress us. We benefited from the assistance of Mr. Richard Zorab, Senior Acquisitions Editor; Mr. Lawrence McGrew, Senior Developmental Editor; Mr. Peter Faber, Production Manager; Ms. Gina Scala, Senior Copy Editor; Ms. Maureen Sweeney, Designer, and Mr. Walt Verbitski, Illustrations Coordinator. Their help has been essential and is deeply appreciated. Finally, we wish to thank our editorial assistants and secretaries, including Rebecca Trumbull, Jodi Sarkisian, Mary Wisch, Carole Wonsiewicz, Jean Doran, Gloria Smith, Michelle Young, and Phyllis White. They have been of immeasurable assistance.

WILLIAM N. KELLEY, M.D.
EDWARD D. HARRIS, JR., M.D.
SHAUN RUDDY, M.D.
CLEMENT B. SLEDGE, M.D.

Contents

xviii   Contents

xxii   Contents

xxiv   Contents

Section X
CONNECTIVE TISSUE DISEASES
CHARACTERIZED BY FIBROSIS 1113

Chapter 66
Scleroderma 1113
James R. Seibold

Chapter 67
Localized Fibrotic Disorders 1144
Carlo L. Mainardi

Chapter 68
Eosinophilia-Myalgia Syndrome 1150
Bruce Freundlich

Section XI
INFLAMMATORY DISEASES OF MUSCLE 1159

Chapter 69
Inflammatory Diseases of Muscle 1159
Robert L. Wortmann

Section XII
RHEUMATIC DISEASES OF CHILDHOOD 1189

Chapter 70
Juvenile Rheumatoid Arthritis 1189
James T. Cassidy

Chapter 71
Rheumatic Fever 1209
Alan L. Bisno

Chapter 72
Systemic Lupus Erythematosus, Juvenile
Dermatomyositis, Scleroderma, and
Vasculitis 1224
James T. Cassidy

COLOR PLATES

PLATE XI

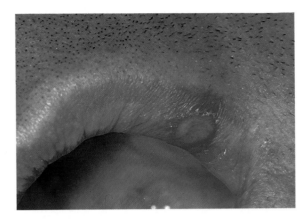

Figure 64–13. Painful oral aphtha of the upper lip; an erythematous border surrounds a necrotic yellow ulcer. (Courtesy of Dr. R. Rogers III.)

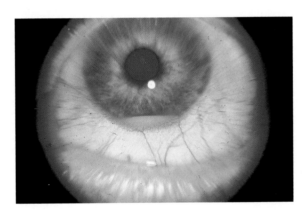

Figure 64–14. Hypopyon, or pus in the anterior chamber, is clearly shown as a yellow segment in front of the iris at 6 o'clock. Previously common in Behçet's disease, anterior uveitis of this severity is now uncommon. (Courtesy of Dr. Dennis Robertson.)

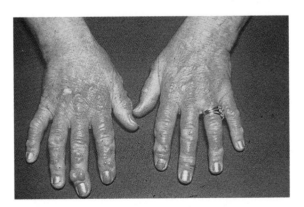

Figure 85–1. Reddish-brown nodules on dorsa of hands and around nailfolds.

Section VIII

Systemic Lupus Erythematosus and Related Syndromes

Chapter 60

Virgil L. Woods, Jr.

Pathogenesis of Systemic Lupus Erythematosus

ETIOLOGY OF SYSTEMIC LUPUS ERYTHEMATOSUS

Despite intensive efforts, no etiology has yet been found for systemic lupus erythematosus (SLE). Before ascribing this to a lack of insight or an insufficiency of current technology, it is important to consider other explanations. First, what we call SLE may be the expression of a common pathogenetic mechanism initiated by a variety of factors. Second, SLE may not be a single disease but rather a constellation of signs and symptoms produced by a variety of etiologic agents. Third, the etiology may be multifactorial. For instance, the development of SLE may require contact with a specific pathogen plus a particular predisposition of the host. A variety of factors have been proposed to be etiologic for SLE including viral, genetic, environmental, and hormonal influences. It is probable, however, that none of these factors operates independently in the production of clinical disease. Rather, the development of SLE probably requires a modification in the complex interrelationships between the host, the pathogen, and their environment. Any etiologic theory must explain the persistence and fluctuating severity of the disorder and the associated abnormalities of immunologic regulation.[1a]

Animal models of SLE have been influential in shaping our concepts of the etiology and pathogenesis of the human disease and are therefore considered in this review. The major strains of interest are the New Zealand black (NZB) mouse; the F1 hybrid of the NZB strain and the New Zealand white mouse (NZW), called the NZB/NZW; and the MRL/1 and BXSB mice. Two forms of disease develop in each mouse strain. Early in life the animals show multiple immunologic abnormalities; later each develops fatal immune complex nephritis and other features of human autoimmune diseases (Table 60–1). For instance, at an early age, female NZB/NZW mice acquire antinuclear and antinative DNA antibodies (dsDNA) and routinely die during the first year of an immune complex nephritis.[1] In the MRL/1 strain, both sexes get a massive nonmalignant lymphadenopathy and renal disease early (around the fourth month) in life. In the BXSB strain, only the males get a slowly progressive nephritis. The amount and type of antinuclear antibodies (ANA) vary among the strains. For instance, most serum samples from MRL mice react with the Sm antigen and contain rheumatoid factor, whereas NZB/NZW hybrids and BXSB lack these antibodies. BXSB mice make little anti-dsDNA antibody in contrast to MRL and NZB/NZW mice. Each mouse strain appears to have a genetic background that predisposes to autoimmune disease. Various superimposed factors then determine the time of appearance and severity of disease. Except for the BXSB, sex hormones function as accelerating factors. In the BXSB mouse, a gene linked to the Y chromosome exerts a major influence on the expression of disease, whereas in the MRL/1 strain, the *lpr* gene accelerates disease. Detailed genetic and virologic investigations have failed to demonstrate common denominators among the three strains, suggesting that murine lupus, perhaps like its human counterpart, is more a syndrome than a single disease.

Chronic Virus Infection

Enthusiasm for a viral etiology for SLE followed from the electron microscopic observations of un-

Table 60–1. IMMUNOLOGIC ABNORMALITIES IN AUTOIMMUNE MOUSE STRAINS

	NZB	NZB/NZW	BXSB	MRL/1
Quantitative Abnormalities				
B cells	↓	↓	↑	N
T cells	↓	↓	N	↑ ↑
Lymphoid hyperplasia	+	+	+ +	+ + +
Functional Abnormalities				
B lymphocytes				
Decreased tolerance, polyclonal activation	+, early	+, early	+	+, late
Effect of *xid* gene	Prevents disease	Prevents disease	Prevents disease	Retards disease
T lymphocytes				
Decreased tolerance	+	+	+	+
Helper T, suppressor	Lyt 23⁺ cells increased in aged animals, but decreased ability to generate new suppressors		?	Increased T cell help
Autoantibody production				
Anti-DNA	+	+ +	+ +	+ + +
Rheumatoid factor, anti-Sm	0	0	0	+
Sex Predilection	Female	Female	Male	Male, female
Accelerating Factors				
Sex hormone dependence	±	+	0	+
Genes	Multiple autosomal	Multiple autosomal	Multiple autosomal; Y chromosome– linked gene is major accelerator	Multiple autosomal; lpr gene is major accelerator
Virus infection	+	+	+	+

Symbols: ↑ = increased; ↓ = decreased; N = normal; 0 = absent; + = present; ? = not repeated.
Modified from Dixon, F. J.: Arthritis Rheum. 25:271, 1982; Steinberg, A. D., et al.: Ann. Intern. Med. 100:714, 1984; and Theofilopoulos, A. N., et al.: Springer Semin. Immunopathol. 9:121, 1986.

usual tubuloreticular inclusions in SLE tissues, which bear a superficial resemblance to the tubuloreticular structure and internal nucleoprotein core of paramyxoviruses, of which measles is an example. Work has shown that these structures are a nonspecific manifestation of cell injury induced by the action of elevated levels of alpha(α)-interferon in SLE patients. Serologic studies of serum antiviral antibodies in SLE reveal that although elevated levels are often found, they are directed at a number of apparently unrelated viruses including measles, rubella, parainfluenza, mumps, and Epstein-Barr virus. This result suggests that the antibodies may be the result of nonspecific B lymphocyte activation and not the result of heightened antigenic exposure. Gallo and co-workers have characterized a family of retroviruses, termed *human T lymphotrophic viruses* (HTLV), and their infectivity and pathogenic potential for humans has been established. Studies to date have failed to demonstrate antibodies to such viruses in patients with SLE.[2] Although the presence of viral antigens in tissues from SLE patients has been reported, direct virus isolation from SLE patients using either conventional or more sensitive co-cultivation techniques has been unrewarding. Ultrasensitive techniques for the detection of viral proteins or genomic material including the polymerase chain reaction (PCR) are now being used to examine SLE tissues for the presence of known and perhaps novel viruses. Even if viral material is detected with these techniques, it will remain to be shown that the virus expression is the cause rather than the result of SLE.

Part of the impetus for the study of type C retroviruses in human SLE derives from observations in NZW and other autoimmune mice. Throughout life all New Zealand strains have large concentrations of type C retrovirus particles and antigens in their tissues. These viruses appear to have a pathogenetic role in the nephritis of NZB/NZW hybrids because large amounts of antibody to virus-related antigens, especially viral envelope gp-70 antigen, can be identified in their glomerular deposits. There has been, however, no clear demonstration that the virus infection is responsible for the development of abnormalities of immunologic regulation or the perpetuation of the autoimmune process.

Genetics

Several lines of evidence indicate that genetic factors are critical in the development of SLE. Familial aggregation studies are based on the rationale that more cases of a genetically determined disorder will appear in the relatives of persons with a given disease than among the relatives of appropriately selected control subjects. Studies of the prevalence of SLE give different results depending on the geographic area studied, but approximate ten (range 2.9 to 400) affected persons per 100,000 of population.[3] SLE occurs in relatives of patients with the disease at increased frequency, between 0.4 and 5 percent, representing a several hundred–fold increase over that of the general population. Immunologic abnormalities are also found more often in family members of SLE patients than in controls.[4] There is a remarkable concordance of the presence of antinuclear antibodies (ANA), hypergammaglobulinemia, and disease expression between identical twins. On the other hand, the frequency of SLE in dizygotic twins is probably no different than in other first-degree relatives.[5–6a]

Certain ethnic groups have a high prevalence of SLE. African-Americans develop the disease three times more often than would be predicted by their representation in the general population.[6] Certain American Indian tribes have a much higher annual incidence of SLE than other tribes or control populations. Again, women make up a disproportionate number of those affected. Women of Asian and Polynesian ancestry appear to be at risk for more severe disease.

Histocompatibility antigens (HLA) have been extensively studied in patients with SLE, in an attempt to discover differences in susceptibility, serology, and outcome.[4] Normal persons who have HLA haplotypes containing HLA-B8/DR3 have evidence of immunologic hyper-responsiveness of both cellular and humoral immunity.[7] This hyper-responsiveness may be determined by HLA-coded polymorphisms in either the T cell, B cell, or antigen presenting cell immune response gene products. In SLE, there is only a weak genetic association with HLA-DR3 and DR2 (relative risk of three). Somewhat stronger associations have been found between particular HLA-DR specificities and production of certain autoantibodies in SLE than with the disease itself.[8] Given the strong genetic predisposition indicated by familial, twin, and ethnic comparisons, this result suggests that other genes located outside the major histocompatibility complex (MHC) also contribute to disease susceptibility.

Genes controlling the production of several complement components are located within the HLA region (class III MHC genes). Homozygous deficiencies of the early complement components, particularly C2 and C4, are frequently associated with SLE and discoid lupus erythematosus. Because the genes for these proteins are closely linked to and in linkage dysequilibrium with certain MHC immune response genes, it has been suspected that the association of SLE with deletions of these complement genes is largely coincidental, simply reflecting the presence or absence of linked pathogenetic HLA-DR immune response genes. An argument against this notion, however, is the observation that acquired deficiency of C2 and C4 as seen in hereditary angioedema also predisposes to the development of SLE and discoid lupus erythematosus. Further, studies of the role of complement genotypes in the susceptibility to SLE that were obtained from Mexican family studies indicate that genetically determined C4 deficiency, not associated with a particular HLA haplotype, confers disease susceptibility. Finally, approximately 45 percent of all Caucasian SLE patients have been found to have deletions of C4A from one or both chromosomes, and one half of DR3-positive SLE patients have a deleted C4A gene, making deletion of the C4A gene a very common genetic marker for disease susceptibility. These results suggest that the deficiency of C4A itself may confer susceptibility to the development of SLE and that some of the reported HLA-DR associations with SLE may be due to linked C4A null alleles.[8]

Several lines of evidence suggest that the erythrocyte complement receptor type 1 (CR1) plays an important role in humans in mediating the clearance of circulating immune complexes. Further, SLE patients show reduced numbers of CR1 on erythrocytes (see under "Pathogenesis"). There are two allelic forms of CR1, one correlating with high and the other with low expression of CR1. Restriction fragment length polymorphism (RFLP) analysis has demonstrated that the gene frequencies of these two alleles in SLE patients are not significantly different from those of normal subjects.[9] This result indicates that the reduction in erythrocyte CR1 seen in patients with SLE is an acquired abnormality and does not support the notion that any inherited variation in CR1 predisposes to SLE.

Logical candidates for the locus of disease predisposition are the genes coding for the various structures that make up the T cell antigen receptor. This receptor is composed of two chains, alpha (α) and beta (β), associated with the components of the CD3 complex. Studies using RFLP analysis reported that susceptibility to SLE is not genetically linked to variations in the β chain of the T cell antigen receptor.[10] Particular autoantibody specificities (anti-Ro) may be highly associated with certain forms of the T cell receptor β chain.[11] Whether polymorphisms in the other chains that constitute the T cell antigen receptor confer an increased susceptibility to SLE remains to be determined.

Analysis of murine lupus models cannot distinguish a single genetic basis for disease. The H2 genes of the various strains of mice that develop lupus are dissimilar.[1] Moreover, the H2d haplotype of NZB mice is shared by many strains that display no autoimmunity. When F1 hybrids are made by crossing MRL mice with NZB, NZW, or BXSB, they do not develop an accelerated disease, as do the offspring of the NZB by NZW matings. To date, in a variety of breedings between lupus mice and normal strains, no particular phenotypic feature appears to segregate with disease. For NZB/NZW mice, multiple unlinked genes appear to be responsible for disease manifestations, whereas in the MRL strains, a single gene has a major effect. The congenic MRL/Mp- +/+ mouse is genetically identical to the MRL/Mp-*lpr/lpr* (MRL/1) except for the absence of *lpr* genes. This animal has mild autoimmune disease and lacks the marked lymphoproliferation seen in the mice with the *lpr* gene. A single gene linked to the Y chromosome exerts a major effect on disease expression in the BXSB strain. Although RFLP studies indicate that the T cell antigen receptor β chain gene complex in NZW mice contains a large deletion, it is not clear if this deletion is associated with the development of autoimmunity.[12] This result suggests that genetically determined defects in the mouse T cell β chain may be involved in murine lupus.

Environmental Factors

Several pharmaceutical agents can induce a clinical syndrome with features similar to idiopathic SLE, termed *drug-induced SLE*. Although procainamide and hydralazine have proved to be the principal precipitating agents, many other drugs with this potential have been described. The mechanisms that underlie procainamide-induced and hydralazine-induced lupus remain unknown. It is no longer thought that particular hydralazine acetylator phenotypes are associated with a predisposition to SLE. The observation that lymphocytotoxic autoantibodies (a common occurrence in SLE) are present in more than a third of asymptomatic SLE relatives may implicate either genetic or contagious environmental factors.[13] Other factors are known to exacerbate preexisting SLE but not initiate disease. Ultraviolet light, a known precipitant of dermal and systemic manifestations in patients with existing SLE, is probably not an important risk factor for the development of SLE.

There has been an increased appreciation of the role of diet in SLE. Although probably not causal, nutritional factors may be able to modify the disease. In several strains of autoimmune mice, dietary caloric or fat restriction significantly delays the onset of immunoregulatory abnormalities, formation of immune complexes, and renal disease.[14] Mice fed a diet containing high fat show significantly accelerated immune deficiency and more severe cardiovascular and renal disease. Diets enriched in triglycerides containing eicosapentanoic acid appear to ameliorate immunoregulatory abnormalities and nephritis in autoimmune mice.[15] These differences may be due to alterations in the types of protaglandins synthesized on such a diet. Finally, a diet containing alfalfa sprouts has been shown to induce a disease very similar to SLE in monkeys. This property of alfalfa sprouts has been attributed to their nonprotein amino acid constituent, L-canavaline, which has been shown to induce in vitro immunoregulatory abnormalities in human lymphoid cells.[16] Reactivation of human SLE has been noted subsequent to the ingestion of alfalfa tablets.

Hormonal Influences

The marked propensity for women in their childbearing years to develop SLE has long been appreciated. This female predominance is not as evident in children or in the aged. SLE has been reported in males with the feminizing condition known as Klinefelter's syndrome (XXY karyotype), but the concurrence may be no more than that expected by chance association. Female SLE patients have been noted to excrete excessive amounts of material with high estrogenic activity and to have decreased levels of androgenic material when compared with other women.[17] Preliminary studies suggest that the severity of lupus decreases when women are treated with antigonadotropic drugs.[18]

Observations of important hormonal influences on the evolution or expression of SLE are paralleled by findings in NZB/NZW mice. Female NZB/NZW mice have a worse disease than males. It is characterized by an earlier appearance of antibodies to dsDNA and polyadenylic acid, greater severity of immune complex nephritis, and a decreased life span. Artificial manipulation of the hormonal environment by castration or drug treatment modifies the expression of autoimmunity. An overall increase in male hormones suppresses the disease, whereas female hormones accelerate the disease.[1] Androgens favorably influence survival, with the immune complex nephritis being less severe in female animals treated with male sex hormones. Hormonal influences are not paramount, however, because in other murine strains, like the MRL/1 mice, males and females develop a lupus-like disease at approximately the same age, and in the BXSB mouse, the disease is more severe in males, even though unrelated to sex hormones.

Autoimmunity

Immunity can be defined as a state of specific reactivity to a foreign substance resulting from prior exposure. Tolerance is a state of specific unresponsiveness to an antigen following exposure to that antigen. It is a learned response determined in part by the nature, dose, and route of administration of the antigen and the state of maturity of the immune system when the antigen is introduced. In general, the more immature the host, the easier it is to induce tolerance to a particular antigen. Tolerance can be induced and maintained at a number of different levels in the immune system, including both T and B cells.

The initial theories designed to explain autoimmunity suggested a failure in ontogeny to eliminate clones of autoreactive cells. Deletion or abortion of self-reactive T lymphocyte clones, especially those recognizing antigens of the MHC, occurs in the thymus, whereas autoreactive B lymphocytes appear to be eliminated at an early phase in their development before they emerge from the fetal liver or bone marrow. This process is not complete, as evidenced by the fact that B lymphocytes reactive with a number of autologous antigens, including thyroglobulin or DNA, can be detected in normal adult animals or humans. The existence of autoantibodies is by itself a cogent argument against the complete elimination of potentially responsive autoreactive B immunocytes. Thus, other mechanisms must be involved in preventing autoimmunity.

T lymphocytes can suppress antibody formation through an interaction with helper T lymphocytes or by a direct effect on the B lymphocyte. Certain serum factors, including antibody alone or complexed with antigen, can block antibody production. The factors responsible for upsetting this delicate immunologic homeostasis in SLE are not known, but a number of explanations have been proposed.

An immunologic profile of typical patients with SLE would include production of multiple autoantibodies, impaired T lymphocyte functions, and generally normal antibody responses to exogenous antigens. T lymphocytes recognize antigens on cell surfaces only when antigenic fragments are physically bound to and presented by membrane proteins coded by genes in the MHC. Thus, in the instance of antibody formation, helper T lymphocytes can respond to antigen only if it is associated with class II MHC molecules. These determinants have a limited distribution in the body. They are found mainly on macrophages; some lymphocytes, including B cells and activated T lymphocytes; vascular endothelium; and epidermal cells but are absent from most differentiated cells. It has been proposed that inappropriate class II MHC-protein expression on perturbed tissues may allow anomalous presentation of self-antigens to T cells in autoimmune disease.

Autoantibody formation can result from impaired B lymphocyte regulation. An augmentation of inappropriate T lymphocyte help or a failure to suppress B lymphocytes capable of making autoantibodies would have the same net effect. If a T lymphocyte can be induced to respond to a subregion of an autoantigen, it can provide help to pre-existing autoreactive B cells, resulting in a humoral response to other regions of the autoantigen. The host may lack T lymphocytes that recognize self-antigens, but if self-antigens become physically associated with foreign antigens, as when a virus attaches to an erythrocyte membrane, intermolecular T cell help can be provided by viral protein-reactive T cells, resulting in the production of antierythrocyte membrane autoantibodies. It has also been proposed that T cells directed primarily toward foreign microbial antigens may sufficiently cross-react with structurally related self-antigens as to provide help to autoreactive B cells, i.e., molecular mimicry.[19, 20] Alternatively, T cell reactivity toward a self-protein might result if the protein were physically altered. Incomplete enzymatic digestion of nucleoprotein or DNA, for instance, might result in ANA or anti-DNA antibodies, or the binding of an exogenously administered drug to self-proteins could induce antiprotein autoantibodies. Procainamide and hydralazine complex with nucleoprotein in vitro; this has been advanced as an explanation for their ability to induce ANA. Although indirect evidence indicates that T cells are involved

in autoantibody production in SLE,[21] the existence of autoantigen-reactive T cells has never been shown in human SLE.

An escape from tolerance accompanies nonspecific activation of T lymphocytes. In mice activation of T cells with adjuvants, mitogens or allogeneic cells cause the release of large amounts of cytokines and interleukins capable of nonspecifically activating "bystander" B cells. It has been suggested that antiidiotype antibodies might facilitate the development of autoimmunity by interfering with the tolerization of autoreactive B cells.[22] A remarkably SLE-like disease can be induced in several normal mouse strains by the injection of human monoclonal antibodies bearing the 16/6 idiotype common to many SLE autoantibodies (see under "Pathogenesis"), and disease manifestations in these mice can be modulated by sex hormone manipulation.[23]

Certain forms of chronic graft versus host (GVH) disease of humans and experimental animals have clinical and laboratory features similar to SLE. GVH disease develops following the introduction of allogeneic lymphocytes into a host that is incapable of eliminating the introduced lymphocytes. The donor's T lymphocytes respond to the host's transplantation antigens, primarily MHC structures. In mice, GVH disease is most easily produced by introducing parental lymphocytes into an F1 hybrid. Depending on the strain combinations and conditions, a variety of outcomes ensue, ranging from an acute, lethal runt disease to a chronic illness characterized by dermatitis, angiogenesis, extensive lymphadenopathy, and immune complex glomerulonephritis. Red blood cell, nucleoprotein, and dsDNA antibodies are all observed. T lymphocytes from the donor strain are required, but the autoantibodies are made by the B lymphocytes of the host, presumably stimulated by soluble products released by the activated T lymphocytes.[24]

Immunologic Abnormalities in Autoimmune Mice

Abnormalities have been found in virtually every aspect of the immune system of autoimmune mice and vary from strain to strain. It remains unclear which of these defects are primary and responsible for the initiation of autoimmune disease and which are secondary immunologic disorders produced by autoimmune attack on components of the immune system. Perhaps the best evidence for a primary B lymphocyte defect is in the NZB/NZW mouse.[1] B lymphocytes from these animals appear to be abnormally activated in that they produce exceptionally large amounts of gamma immunoglobulin M (IgM), are less readily rendered tolerant than normal B lymphocytes, and have cell-surface immunoglobulin phenotypes indicative of accelerated maturation. These abnormalities occur early in life, before the appearance of defects in other parts of the immune system and before the development of autoimmune disease. NZB mice depleted of immunocompetent T lymphocytes continue to manifest hyperreactivity and autoimmune disease. In NZB strains, B lymphocyte hyperactivity appears to be limited to a subpopulation of B lymphocytes responsible for certain thymus-independent responses. The CBA/N mouse bears a gene (the *xid* gene) that renders this particular subpopulation of B lymphocytes inactive. Introducing this gene into NZB mice causes B lymphocyte hyperactivity to disappear; autoantibodies are significantly reduced, and they do not develop immune complex disease. Much attention has focussed on a subpopulation of B cells bearing the human CD5 or murine equivalent Lyb 1 antigen. These cells constitute a large fraction of B cells in early development. They are committed to the production of relatively low affinity IgM antibodies that are able to bind to both self-antigens and foreign antigens, are found in high concentrations in the NZB autoimmune mouse strain, and are responsible for the production of a large number of the autoantibodies observed in these animals and patients with SLE. In SLE patients, however, there is no increase in CD5 bearing cells, and high-affinity anti-DNA antibodies are produced by CD5 negative B cells at high frequency. Both CD5 positive and CD5 negative B cells in human SLE produce anti-DNA autoantibodies, perhaps driven by differing mechanisms.[25]

T lymphocyte function is normal or increased early in the life of NZB animals.[1] This early T lymphocyte hyperactivity appears to be independent of B lymphocyte influences, since NZB animals bearing the *xid* gene, and therefore lacking B lymphocyte hyperactivity or autoantibody, continue to express the T lymphocyte abnormalities. With some assay systems, there is evidence of reduced T suppressor lymphocyte function in adult NZB/NZW mice; it has been proposed that autoantibodies specific for suppressor T lymphocytes mediate the decrease. This has not been confirmed with other assay systems.[26] Antiserum to murine lymphocyte membrane antigens can identify T lymphocyte subsets that perform different functions. For instance, helper T lymphocytes display the Lyt 1+ phenotype, whereas suppressor T lymphocytes are of the Lyt 23+ type. The number of Lyt 23+ (suppressor phenotype) T lymphocytes is increased in aged NZB and NZB/NZW animals, even though these animals are deficient in their ability to express suppressor function.

MRL/1 (lpr/lpr) mice have little evidence of a primary B lymphocyte defect, and B lymphocyte hyperactivity only develops late in the course of their autoimmune disease. The B lymphocyte subpopulation that produces anti-DNA antibody in this strain is different from the hyperactive subpopulation found in NZB mice. When the CBA/N *xid* gene is bred to MRL/1 mice, they continue to produce anti-DNA antibody. Additionally, the MRL/1 anti-DNA antibody is of the IgG type, suggesting that the responsible B lymphocytes are T lymphocyte dependent, not T independent as in the NZB mouse.

T lymphocyte defects probably account for the autoimmune disease in MRL/1 mice. MRL/1 mice develop massive lymphoid hyperplasia, and lymphocytes in these hyperplastic nodes are unusual in that each cell may express phenotypic markers of both T suppressor and helper T lymphocytes.[1] Functionally, however, they behave as helper T lymphocytes, for both polyclonal immunoglobulin production by B lymphocytes and spontaneous anti-DNA antibody production. Neonatal thymectomy of MRL/1 mice decreases the expression of lymphoid hyperplasia and autoantibodies, but when reconstituted with normal thymuses, these mice continue to express autoimmune disease, indicating that the defect resides in the lymphoid stem cell and not the thymus. MRL/1 T lymphocytes spontaneously produce a B lymphocyte differentiation factor that induces polyclonal IgG and IgM synthesis in lipopolysaccharide-activated B lymphocytes. T cells from lpr/lpr mice have been shown to have constitutive elevation of the c-myb oncogene, constitutive phosphorylation of CD3 and B220 proteins, and constitutive elevations in phospholipase A_2 activity.[27]

In the BXSB strain, polyclonal B lymphocyte activation is observed, associated with lymphoid proliferation and production of autoantibodies. The male BXSB mouse early in life displays a resistance to tolerance induction similar to that seen in other autoimmune strains, whereas the female BXSB is easily tolerized. If male bone marrow cells are transferred to irradiated female recipients along with either male or female thymuses, the resulting animal displays the male pattern of tolerance resistance. If female splenic T lymphocytes are transferred into the recipient at the same time as male bone marrow cells, the animal displays the female pattern of autoimmune disease, indicating that the abnormalities induced by male bone marrow cells can be suppressed by female splenic T lymphocytes.

Immunologic Abnormalities in Systemic Lupus Erythematosus

Practically every aspect of the immune system has been reported to be abnormal in patients with SLE. It remains unclear which of the multiplicity of immunologic defects are fundamental to the cause of lupus and which are secondarily induced. For example, the production of antilymphocyte autoantibodies in SLE is likely secondary to an abrogation of normal mechanisms of tolerance. Once produced there is abundant evidence that these antibodies can interact in vivo with subpopulations of lymphocytes, impairing their function. Some of these autoantibody-induced abnormalities may exacerbate the primary defect that initiated the autoantibody production. Under these circumstances, it is virtually impossible to discern which abnormality came first.

Humoral and Cellular Immunity

Studies of the in vivo humoral and cellular immune responses of patients with active SLE have produced conflicting results. Serum antibody responses to immunization are reported as either decreased or normal. When decreased, primary responses are generally diminished to a greater extent than secondary responses. There is evidence of overall heightened immunoglobulin production by patients with SLE, in that patients with active disease often have hypergammaglobulinemia. Reports of the delayed hypersensitivity responses in SLE patients challenged with antigens such as Candida, trichophyton, and streptokinase-streptodornase are conflicting. When patients with active SLE are purposely immunized with "new" antigens such as dinitrochlorobenzene or keyhole-limpet hemocyanin, they consistently fail to become sensitized. These observations suggest that the sensitization phase of the immune response is much more intact before the onset of SLE and that differences in preservation of premorbid immunologic memory may account for some of the variations seen in the response to in vivo challenge with environmental antigens. Lymphopenia is common in SLE, and the number of lymphocytes is related inversely to the activity of the disease. Although B lymphocytes are present in relatively normal numbers, peripheral blood T lymphocytes are decreased in number, and the decrease is often most marked in the T suppressor lymphocyte subpopulation.[28]

At the cellular level, abnormalities have been found in the manner in which lymphocytes from patients with active SLE interact with each other. The autologous mixed leukocyte reaction (AMLR) has been proposed to be a model system for studying immunoregulatory events that normally occur between T lymphocytes, B lymphocytes, and macrophages. In patients with active SLE, the AMLR is almost always deficient, whereas patients with inactive disease show near normal responses. The defective response in active disease is due to an impairment of both the stimulator (B lymphocytes, macrophages, or dendritic cells) and responder T lymphocyte populations, including helper T and suppressor T lymphocytes.[29] The marked abnormality of the AMLR in active SLE patients contrasts with the relatively normal responses seen when SLE lymphocytes are cultured with allogeneic lymphocytes. This difference in the perturbation of autoreactivity versus alloreactivity suggests that the cellular mechanisms responsible for these proliferative reactions may differ from each other.

B Lymphocyte Function

There is considerable evidence of B lymphocyte hyperactivity. Increased numbers of peripheral blood lymphocytes have cell-surface phenotypes indicative of abnormal B lymphocyte maturation and activation.

When cultured in vitro, SLE B lymphocytes produce abnormally large amounts of immunoglobulin in the absence of an exogenous stimulus, and the percentage of B lymphocytes spontaneously producing antibody is increased. In contrast, when cultured SLE B lymphocytes are challenged with mitogens, they are found to be markedly deficient in their ability to proliferate further or increase immunoglobulin synthesis, suggesting prior activation. Many of the antibodies spontaneously produced by SLE B lymphocytes appear to be the polyclonally produced products of unmutated germline-encoded immunoglobulin genes, some of the antibodies being reactive with self-constituents (autoantibodies) and others being reactive with non–self-antigens. Many autoantibodies in SLE, however, appear to undergo affinity maturation, the result of presumably antigen-driven clonal selection.[30, 31] It is likely that both polyclonal and antigen-specific B-cell stimulatory mechanisms occur and interact with each other in SLE.[32]

T Lymphocyte Function

There is also evidence of T lymphocyte hyperactivity. Patients with active SLE have increased numbers of circulating T lymphocytes bearing class II MHC antigens and other cell surface proteins associated with T lymphocyte activation. Additionally, there is a tenfold increase in the number of circulating T lymphocytes, which are found to be secreting soluble B cell stimulatory factors. This activation is reflected in increased T and B cell levels of mRNA coded for by certain proto-oncogenes (c-myc, c-myb, c-raf) in SLE.[33] Helper (CD4+) T cells appear to play a central role in the pathogenesis of murine lupus, and lupus patients have an increased percentage of CD29+ (4B4+) memory helper T cells in their blood.[34] These evidences of T cell activation should be contrasted with the observations that T cells in SLE are deficient in their production of interleukin-2 (IL-2)[35] and responsiveness to IL-2.[36]

Suppressor T lymphocyte function in SLE has been extensively studied in vitro.[37] When the disease is active, the T lymphocytes of SLE patients are almost always incapable of inhibiting mitogen-driven or spontaneous B lymphocyte proliferation and differentiation or the proliferative responses of other T lymphocytes. Patients with active lupus have a preferential loss of T cells (CD4+ CD45R+) with suppressor inducer function.[34, 38] It has been demonstrated that the defect results from an inability of their T lymphocytes to generate suppressive signals and not in the response of target cells to such signals. Suppressor cell defects have not been observed by all investigators, however, and other studies have documented decreased suppressor cell activity in clinically healthy family members of lupus patients.[34] It is possible that many of the observed suppressor cell defects are the result of the action of antilymphocyte antibody.

Natural Killer Cell Function

Natural killer (NK) cell activity is diminished in most patients with SLE. Interferon is normally an in vitro inducer of NK activity, and SLE NK cells seem hyporesponsive to the activating influences of interferon. SLE patients appear to have normal numbers of inactive NK cells but a deficiency of active, cytotoxic NK cells. Studies suggest that prolonged exposure to interferon-α impairs NK function[39] and that SLE patients have chronically elevated levels of interferon-α. This may have relevance to B cell hyperactivity because NK cells have been shown to be important regulators of B cell function.

Antilymphocyte Antibodies

Lymphocytotoxic antibodies are demonstrable in the serum of at least 80 per cent of patients with SLE, and they react with lymphocytes from most normal donors as well as with autologous lymphocytes. Although the role of these antibodies in vivo is unknown, many of the abnormalities of lymphocyte function seen in SLE can be produced by incubating SLE autoantibodies with normal lymphocytes. Some, primarily the cold-reactive IgM antibodies, are cytotoxic, whereas others, usually of the IgG class, interfere with in vitro lymphocyte functions. Absorption studies reveal that most SLE sera contain a mixture of T lymphocyte–specific and B lymphocyte–specific antibodies, in addition to cross-reactive antibodies specific for determinants present on both T and B lymphocytes. Antilymphocyte antibodies could perturb the immune system in a number of ways, either by effecting the removal of their target cells from the circulation or by binding to their surface and modifying their function.[40]

Defects in T suppressor function are one of the most constant findings in SLE; therefore it is of considerable interest that SLE antilymphocyte antibodies may show specific reactivity for and an ability to inactivate or kill suppressor T lymphocytes. Other antilymphocyte antibodies can specifically kill cell populations necessary for the generation of suppressor cells[38] or inhibit IL-2 production by lymphocytes.[41] Antibodies that react almost exclusively with helper (CD4) T cells have been described and appear to be responsible for the depletion of CD4 positive cells in patients with SLE.[42] Some antilymphocyte antibodies are specific for activated T lymphocytes and their secreted products, introducing the possibility that some autoantibodies interfere with the immune system by their interaction with activated, proliferating lymphocytes. Autoantibodies that are able to react with molecules needed for rapid proliferation, either interleukins or activation-dependent, cell-surface molecules, could inhibit clonal expansion and thus markedly disturb both the immune response and immunoregulatory events.

To understand these various possible pathoge-netic mechanisms fully, it will be necessary to define the nature of the cell-surface antigens on lymphoid cells that are recognized by antilymphocyte antibodies. Reactivities with histocompatibility-associated antigens, such as the HLA-A, B, and C molecular complexes, β_2-microglobulin, and Ia antigens have all been described (Table 60–2). Additionally, cross-reactivity has been reported between antilymphocyte cell-surface autoantibodies, constituents of the cell nucleus, and cell-surface antigens of central nervous system cell types. These later autoantibodies may be important in the pathogenesis of the central nervous system manifestations of SLE (discussed subsequently). Characterization of the cell-surface targets of antilymphocyte antibodies is a major area of SLE research and controversy.[40, 40a, 43–45]

Antinuclear Antibodies

The serologic hallmark of SLE is the production of high titer autoantibodies directed against a wide variety of nuclear components (ANAs; see later). The study of the fine specificity of these autoantibodies has contributed to a more precise classification of different subgroups of SLE and related autoimmune diseases. These ANAs have served as powerful tools with which to study the structure and function of their nuclear targets.[47] These targets have been found to include the nuclear membrane, where some of the autoantibodies are found to be specifically reactive with a major component of the nuclear membrane, lamin. Further, autoantibodies reactive with the various components of chromatin are found, including histones, high mobility group (HMG) proteins, and various forms of DNA. Finally, autoantibodies directed at a variety of ribonucleoprotein particles have

Table 60–2. SPECIFICITIES OF ANTILYMPHOCYTE ANTIBODIES IN SYSTEMIC LUPUS ERYTHEMATOSUS

Cell Membrane Antigens	Tissue Antigens
HLA	Nuclear antigens
Beta-2-microglobulin	Human brain tissue
HLA heavy-chain antigen	Trophoblastic antigens
Ia	Heat shock proteins
Non-HLA	
Unknown T and B lymphocyte surface antigens	
Lymphoid cell lines	
Chronic lymphocytic leukemia cells	
Cord erythrocyte i antigen	
Lymphoblasts	
T Lymphocyte Subsets	
CD4+	
CD8+	
Tu	
Autologous E rosette positive	

Modified from Searles, R. P., and Williams, R. C., Jr.: Antilymphocyte antibodies in the pathogenesis of SLE. Clin. Exp. Rheumatol. 4:175, 1986.

been described, which include small nuclear ribonucleoproteins (snRNPs), which reside in the nucleus. Examples of snRNP targets of SLE autoantibodies include the U1 through U5 snRNPs, which include the antigen targets of anti-Sm autoantibodies. It is now clear that snRNPs play major roles in the process by which introns are excised from heterogeneous nuclear RNA during its conversion into mature messenger RNA.[46] This processing function of snRNPs is referred to as splicing.

Although the ANAs found among patients with SLE and related disorders recognize many different cellular structures, Hardin[47] has emphasized that most patients with SLE exhibit a limited array of autoantibody specificities, and only a small group of SLE-associated autoantibodies—notably antihistone, anti-DNA, anti-U1 RNP, anti-Sm, and anti-Ro antibodies—are found repetitively and in high titer in the majority of patients with SLE. The patterns of ANAs produced in SLE correspond to the known compositions of three supramolecular structures, the nucleosome particle, the snRNP particles (of which U1 is the prime example), and the Ro particle. First, autoantibodies directed at nucleosome constituents include anti-DNA and antihistone autoantibodies. These autoantibodies appear to be directed at regions of DNA and histones (H1 and H2B), which are on the outside (exposed) regions of the folded nucleosome. Second, linked sets of antibodies appear to be directed at the components of snRNP particles. Anti-Sm autoantibodies are directed at one set of polypeptide constituents of snRNP particles, whereas anti-U1 RNP autoantibodies usually recognize another snRNP associated set of polypeptides, including the 68K, A, and C polypeptides. It is known that the production of anti-Sm autoantibodies in SLE is usually accompanied by the production of anti-U1 RNP antibodies. These findings suggest that in many SLE patients, the U1 snRNP particle behaves as an immunostimulatory unit. Finally, the common association of anti-Ro (also called SSA) autoantibodies with the production of anti-La (also called SS-B) autoantibodies may be due to the fact that both antigens may be (transiently) components of the same RNP particle.

Taken together, these results indicate that autoantibodies directed at the subcomponents of each of these particulate nuclear structures tend to be produced in concert, suggesting that in SLE patients, the immune system sees the structures in their relatively intact form. There must be a permissive factor in operation that allows these normally weak antigens to escape tolerance mechanisms.

PATHOGENESIS OF SYSTEMIC LUPUS ERYTHEMATOSUS

Immune Complex Disease

Although the etiology of SLE remains obscure, it is clear that much of the tissue damage, especially in blood vessels and kidney, is caused by the deposition of antigen-antibody complexes. Indeed, lupus is generally considered to be the prototype human immune complex disease. The interaction of antigen with antibody in the circulation results in the formation of soluble macromolecular complexes. These complexes localize in tissues for anatomic and physiologic reasons and not because of any immunologic specificity; therefore, their physical properties are of great importance. The size and solubility of the complexes, their concentration, their ability to engage and activate the complement system, and the duration of their presence in the circulation are all significant determinants.[48]

Rabbits given a single intravenous injection of a large quantity of foreign serum or plasma protein will, after several days, produce antibodies against the injected protein. As these antibodies are released into the circulation, they encounter an excess of antigen and form soluble complexes. With increasing antibody concentration, more and larger complexes are formed. Most are quickly removed from the circulation by the reticuloendothelial system, but some deposit in vascular endothelium and the renal glomerulus. Once deposited in tissue, the complexes interact with humoral and cellular elements of the host, causing characteristic biochemical, pharmacologic, and morphologic changes. Typical lesions can be found in the blood vessels, heart, and joints, but the best studied are in the glomerulus. Using fluorescein-labeled antibodies, the responsible antigen, host immunoglobulin, and complement components are detectable in a granular pattern along the glomerular basement membrane. This granular (lumpy, bumpy) appearance is the hallmark of immune complex disease. The remarkable inflammatory capacity of such complexes can be appreciated by the fact that only about 20 μg of antigen are present in both kidneys of animals with acute serum sickness and severe glomerulonephritis.

If foreign proteins are administered repeatedly, some rabbits respond by making amounts of antibody that lead to the formation of soluble complexes and the development of glomerulonephritis, whereas others make very large amounts of antibody, and neither complexes nor nephritis develop. Immunofluorescent staining of the kidney in rabbits that develop progressive, fatal glomerulonephritis reveals large granular deposits of antigen, host immunoglobulin, and C3 along the outer edge of the basement membrane. These correspond to dense granular deposits seen by electron microscopy. Typically, in chronic serum sickness, the deposits are on the epithelial side of the basement membrane, but they may be seen along the endothelium or within the mesangium. Initially, only minute amounts (0.04 percent) of the daily dose of antigen deposit in the glomeruli. After weeks of exposure to complexes, a compensatory mechanism is overwhelmed, allowing larger amounts (about 0.5 percent) of the daily dose to deposit in the glomerulus with concomitant severe functional abnormalities. These findings suggest that the mechanisms of injury in acute and chronic immune complex glomerulonephritis are different. An important component of the evanescent lesions of acute serum sickness is the release of pharmacologic agents, whereas the structural damage seen in the glomerulonephritis of chronic serum sickness is mediated by the complement system and polymorphonuclear leukocytes.

Multiple factors can influence the deposition of immune complexes. Any alteration of glomerular capillary permeability can enhance complex deposition. The release of vasoactive substances from mast cells and platelets or the administration of histamine or serotonin causes an increased endothelial deposition of colloidal carbon in mice and immune complexes in guinea pigs and rabbits. Antihistamines and antagonists of serotonin reduce the severity of acute serum sickness in rabbits, may benefit the spontaneous glomerulonephritis of New Zealand mice, and protect against human serum sickness. Blood pressure and hydrodynamic forces can also be influential. The toxic potential of immune complexes has been analyzed by infusing preformed complexes of known composition into experimental animals. Large complexes, formed near equivalence, are rapidly eliminated from the circulation and deposited in the mesangium and subendothelial regions of mouse glomeruli. Smaller, soluble complexes formed in antigen excess disappear from the circulation more slowly. Complexes smaller than 19S do not appear to be nephritogenic in rabbits with acute serum sickness, whereas larger complexes regularly deposit in the glomerulus and produce injury.

Immune complexes are normally removed from the blood by the mononuclear phagocytic system (MPS). The rate at which they are cleared is an important determinant of tissue injury. Phagocytosis of antibody-coated materials or antigen antibody complexes is preceded by binding to Fc or complement receptors on specialized mononuclear cells, such as the liver Kuppfer cells, alveolar macrophages, cells lining the splenic sinusoids, and circulating and tissue fixed macrophages. The function and expression of these receptors can be modulated by many agents, including lipopolysaccharide, lymphokines, interferons, glucocorticoids, and even antigen-antibody complexes. Phagocytic functions in the kidney are performed by the mesangium. Mesangial hypertrophy is an early response to localization of immune complexes. With continual exposure, the mesangial capacity appears to be compromised, leading to immune complex deposition in the glomerulus and overt functional impairment. Exposure of bound immune complexes containing C3b to fresh serum generates a C3b convertase (from the alternate pathway) that can disrupt the primary bonds between antigen and antibody, eventually leading to disaggregation of the complexes. Such "solubilized" complexes can no longer bind to receptors or efficiently activate complement through the classic pathway.

The strength of the bond between antigen and antibody is responsible for the stability of the complex. Low-affinity antibody binds less tightly or to a lesser number of sites on the antigen when compared with precipitating antibody. Antigens bound by low-affinity antibody are eliminated more slowly and theoretically have a greater opportunity to produce kidney damage. In experimental chronic glomerulonephritis, some rabbits develop renal lesions after many weeks of immunization, during which time little precipitating antibody is observed. Thus, the size, antigen to antibody ratio, and quality of the antibody are probably more important determinants of nephrotoxicity than the absolute quantity of circulating immune complex.[48]

The renal disease of autoimmune mice, especially the NZB/NZW strain, bears an amazing resemblance to lupus nephritis. Its immune complex pathogenesis and the responsible antigens have been extensively investigated.[49] When examined by the electron microscope, the glomerular basement membrane appears thickened, and there are dense deposits, initially in the mesangial region and then along the epithelial and to a lesser extent the endothelial margins. Immunofluorescence studies reveal granular deposits of mouse immunoglobulin and C3 in the mesangium, along the glomerular capillary wall, and in tubulointerstitial sites. Murine retroviral DNA can also be identified in an identical pattern to the mouse immunoglobulin deposits. Antibodies eluted from the kidney are primarily IgG, and much of their activity is directed at nuclear material, specifically nucleoprotein and DNA. The anti single-stranded (sDNA) and double-stranded (dsDNA) antibody activity of the eluates was many times greater than the serum antibody. Isoelectric focusing of the glomerular eluates from NZB/NZW and MRL/1 mice reveals a restricted population of anti-DNA antibodies (pI 8–9) in contrast to more heterogeneous DNA antibodies in the serum. Likewise, the eluates of renal lesions in the NZBxSWR model of lupus nephritis reveal a limited spectrum of cationic (positively charged) anti-DNA antibodies with restricted idiotypes.[47] This is consistent with other studies in experimental animals showing that cationic but not anionic immune complexes tend to localize in subepithelial and subendothelial sites in the glomerular basement membrane.[50]

The glomerular lesions in murine lupus nephritis regularly contain complement components, and predominantly complement fixing antibodies (IgG2a) are present in the eluates. Further, when complement-deficient (C5) A/J mice, which have anti-dsDNA antibodies, are injected with DNA, they do not develop severe glomerular disease.

Lupus Nephritis

SLE resembles immune complex–mediated, chronic experimental serum sickness. Antigen antibody complexes are demonstrable in renal glomeruli, blood vessels, skin, and the choroid plexus of the brain. The evidence that these complexes mediate the renal injury in SLE rests on a number of observations, including studies of the complement system, serial observations of antibodies and antigens during the course of the disease, measurements of immune complexes and cryoprecipitable proteins in the serum, immunofluorescent and electron microscopic examination of renal biopsies and kidneys obtained at autopsy, and identification of the immunoreactants eluted from kidneys.

Complement

Hemolytic complement activity is decreased in the serum of many patients with SLE at some time during their illness. The degree often relates to disease activity; the most marked hypocomplementemia occurs in patients with nephritis and less often in those with extensive skin or central nervous system disease. The greatest reduction is in those components that compose the classic complement system, i.e., C1, C4, and C3, in a pattern that suggests activation by immune complexes. C2 levels are less often depressed except in association with genetic defects. Static measurements of hemolytic activity or protein concentrations of complement components give an incomplete picture of activation of the complement system. Hypercatabolism can be masked by an increase in synthesis. Turnover studies using radiolabeled components or measurements of the breakdown products of components released from the native molecule during the activation process provide a truer picture. SLE patients with hypocomplementemia, especially those with active nephritis, display a higher fractional catabolic rate, an increased extravascular distribution of C3 and C5, and a reduction of C3 synthesis when compared with normal subjects.

A number of tests have been developed to measure by-products of complement activation. Breakdown products of C3 (C3d, C3c) and factor B are detected in relatively high concentration in plasma from patients with SLE. The level of these fragments is inversely related to the serum C3 concentration. Factor B and properdin concentrations are decreased, probably reflecting triggering of the C3b amplification loop or direct activation of the alternate complement pathway. The plasma concentrations of β1H globulin and the C3b inactivator, regulatory proteins of the alternate complement pathway, are also reduced. Most likely the observed activation of the complement system in SLE is a reflection of antigen binding to antibody based on the pattern of the complement profiles and the significant correlation between the increase of C3d plasma concentration and the serum levels of C1q binding activity.[51]

Serum Antigens and Antibodies

An enormous array of antibodies to cellular constituents is found in SLE serum. Many cross-react with bacterial and viral polynucleotides, suggesting that the immunogens could be exogenous rather than caused by native or altered tissue antigens. Antibodies to nucleohistone (the nucleoprotein complex formed between DNA and histone) were the first autoantibodies discovered in patients with SLE and were demonstrated to be responsible for the LE cell reaction. Subsequently, a multiplicity of nuclear and cytoplasmic antigens have been defined. The pathogenetic significance of many of them is questionable, but antibodies to DNA surely play a role in complex-mediated lesions.

Antibodies to native dsDNA are detected predominantly in the blood of patients with SLE. In contrast, antibodies reactive with single-stranded DNA (sDNA), although often found in SLE, are frequently demonstrated in other diseases. The antigens to which they react are a matter of considerable interest and debate. The availability of murine and human monoclonal anti-DNA antibodies has made possible an exquisite analysis of anti-DNA binding and demonstrated a diverse pattern of serologic reactivity not previously appreciated with serum anti-DNA antibodies.[52] Although some monoclonal anti-DNAs appear to bind to sequence-specific determinants, i.e., the base composition of polynucleotides, others recognize conformational determinants in DNA such as the sugar phosphate backbone. Anti-DNA antibodies can bind to a number of non-DNA epitopes, including phospholipids, proteoglycans, IgG, nuclear proteins, cytoskeletal elements, and bacterial and cell surface antigens. These results have led to consideration of a number of interesting possibilities: Perhaps anti-DNA antibody represents a response to an immunogen other than DNA; anti-DNA antibodies may be pathogenetic through interactions with antigens other than DNA—for instance, by binding to tissue components like basement membranes or by forming immune complexes with non-DNA material. Finally, since a single antibody to DNA can represent a number of autoantibody activities, such as antilymphocyte or antineuronal reactions, cardiolipin antibody, and the lupus anticoagulant, it is possible that the immune responses in SLE are more restricted than generally believed.[52] Still to be decided, however, is whether naturally occurring monoclonal antibodies with anti-DNA activity are truly representative of circulating SLE antibodies, and as a corollary, caution is indicated before extrapolating the results with them to explain the pathogenetic role of anti-DNA antibodies in SLE. More than 20 human anti-DNA antibody idiotypes have been identified, including the 16/6 idiotype, and most occur at increased levels in SLE patients.[53] The clinical consequences of the presence of DNA antibodies bearing these idiotypes, however, remain unclear.

Serial studies of some antinucleoprotein antibodies show a definite relationship between their concentration in serum and disease activity. Titers of anti-dsDNA antibody correlate best with hypocomplementemia and active nephritis in SLE patients. Both IgG and IgM antibodies to dsDNA are demonstrable in SLE serum, and there is some evidence that patients with IgM antibodies get nephritis less often. There are other important qualitative differences among anti-DNA antibodies with respect to the development of nephritis. For instance, patients whose antibodies both precipitate and bind to DNA are claimed to have a greater incidence of nephritis, whereas those whose sera precipitate DNA but do not form soluble complexes get nephritis only infrequently. Differences in avidity of anti-DNA antibodies have been reported, and low avidity antibodies are claimed to be more nephrotoxic. As is discussed subsequently, there are disagreements about such measurements, but it should be appreciated that antibodies present in serum may only be the residue after more avid antibody has deposited in the kidneys. The serum anti-DNA antibodies associated with nephritis are more likely to be of the complement fixing subclasses.

Mononuclear Phagocyte System Dysfunction

In experimental animals, defects in Fc receptors of the MPS can lead to a prolonged circulation of immune complexes and enhanced tissue deposition. The MPS has been less well studied in humans.[54] When IgG sensitized autologous erythrocytes are administered intravenously, they are rapidly cleared by the spleen in normal individuals. Clearance rates are markedly prolonged in patients with active SLE, especially those with active renal disease. Although these findings are interesting, it must be recognized that the disposal of most immune complexes occurs primarily in the liver, and a satisfactory system for measuring human hepatic Fc function is still not available. Moreover, when NZB/NZW mice were studied with artificial complexes that are preferentially removed by the liver, no defects were found.

Membrane associated C3 receptors (CR) participate in the clearance of immune complexes, which have activated the complement system and become coated with C3b. Three types of C3 receptors are recognized, but it is the CR type 1, termed the C3b/C4b receptor, which is most involved with removing complexes from the circulation.[55] Mast cells, glomerular podocytes, and most human peripheral blood cells have CR1 receptors, but because of the large numbers of red blood cells, more than 85 percent are erythrocyte associated. SLE red blood cells have a decrease in the number and function of CR1 receptors, either genetically determined or acquired as a consequence of the disease. A failure of these cells to bind circulating immune complexes could result in an enhanced delivery of complexes to the liver and spleen, causing MPS overload and dysfunction.

Immune Complexes and Cryoglobulins

Immune complexes have been demonstrated in the majority of patients with SLE. The many methods available for detecting immune complexes are described subsequently. In brief, some depend on the selective detection of a known antigen by discrimination between free and antibody-bound antigen in the complex. Others detect immune complexes independent of the nature of the antigen involved, taking advantage of the distinct properties of complexed immunoglobulin molecules when compared with free immunoglobulin molecules. These include the physical changes induced by complex formation or biologic activities of the immune complexes, such as complement fixation or binding to cell membranes. Cryoprecipitation and analytical ultracentrifugation are examples of the former, and C1q binding or reactions with Fc or C3 receptors on cultured lymphoblasts (Raji cells), mononuclear cells, or platelets are examples of the latter.

The nature of the antigens in SLE immune complexes is still a matter of disagreement, especially the important question of the relative involvement of the DNA–anti DNA system. Although it appears that small amounts of DNA–anti DNA are present in the circulation, their detection is confounded by the presence of free DNA in serum, the small size of the DNA antigens, and the vagaries of clearance. Other studies indicate that in lupus, DNA circulates complexed to histones.[56]

The quantity of cold precipitable proteins (cryoglobulins) in serum is closely associated with SLE disease activity and hypocomplementemia. The SLE cryoglobulins contained IgG; IgM; and C1q, C4, and C3. The IgM has rheumatoid factor activity, and isolated cryoproteins fix complement in vitro. If cryoprecipitates represent circulating immune complexes of pathogenetic significance, they should contain antigens and specific antibodies in amounts that are relatively enriched compared with their concentration in companion serum samples. Several different polynucleotide antibodies are found in SLE cryoglobulins. Some, such as the antibodies to dsDNA, sDNA, and n-RNP, are specifically concentrated. Certain cryoprecipitates contain anti-DNA antibodies, which are complexed with other autoantibodies that bind to anti-DNA antibodies and probably represent idiotype–anti-idiotype immune complexes.[57] SLE cryoglobulins appear to contain antigens from lymphocytes and neural tissues because immunization of rabbits with cryoprecipitates results in the production of antibodies that react with distinctive determinants on both SLE and normal lymphocytes and cultured neuronal and glial cells.[58]

Identification of Immunoreactants in Renal Tissues

Immunofluorescent studies of SLE nephritis indicate that immunoglobulins are deposited in the renal glomeruli in association with complement.[48] Three major patterns of localization are recognized: in a subendothelial or subepithelial position along the capillary wall or in the mesangium. The deposits are generally granular in appearance when located along the glomerular basement membrane. Mesangial immunofluorescence is characteristically irregular, with homogeneous strands lying between capillary loops, but may be granular (Fig. 60–1). Different immunoglobulin classes are observed in the glomeruli. Most commonly IgG is seen alone or in combination with IgM, but occasionally only IgM can be identified. Certain IgG subclasses may be selectively deposited.

Antibodies to nucleoproteins, sDNA and dsDNA, are present in glomerular eluates from most SLE cases of lupus glomerulonephritis, as are occasional anti-RNP and Sm antibodies. When the concentration of a particular antibody in the eluate is compared with its concentration in serum (based on relative IgG concentrations), the antibodies to dsDNA are dominant both in amount and in frequency, occasionally being found in eluates when no antibody is present in the serum. The avidity of the eluted antibody to dsDNA is significantly greater than the anti-dsDNA in the corresponding cryoprecipitates or serum. Immune complexes, identifiable by immunofluorescence or electron microscopy, are present in the tubular basement membrane and interstitium of 20 to 50 percent of patients with lupus nephritis. They are associated with conspicuous interstitial fibrosis and mononuclear cell infiltration as well as tubular cell damage, indicating their probable pathogenetic significance.

SLE renal lesions contain complement proteins of both the classic and alternative pathways. Indeed, even the terminal attack complex of late acting components (C5 to C9) responsible for membrane injury can be demonstrated at glomerular and tubular sites.[55] Because of their association with immunoglobulin, it is presumed that the complement proteins reside in the kidney bound to antigen and antibody. What is not known is whether the complexes arrive at the kidney with complement bound to them or if complement fixation occurs after their localization or independent of immunoglobulin.

Despite the general agreement that lupus renal disease is mediated by immune complexes, there is no ready explanation for why some patients get mild

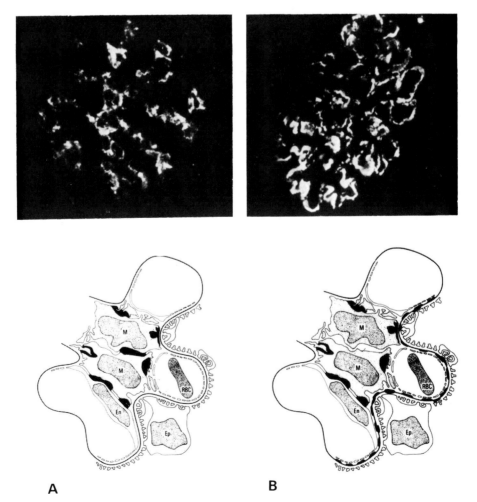

Figure 60–1. Schematic and immune fluorescent demonstration of immune complexes in various areas of the glomerulus. In *A*, the complexes are limited to the mesangial area. The specimen is a glomerulus from a patient with SLE showing minimal morphologic changes and mesangial deposits of IgG (upper left). The features demonstrated in *B* are seen in diffuse proliferative glomerulonephritis. Complexes are deposited in the mesangium and diffusely along the basement membrane, primarily in a subendothelial location. The glomerulus in the upper right is from a patient with diffuse proliferative lupus nephritis stained with a fluoresceinated antibody to IgG.

A   B

and others severe disease, or what accounts for the various types of SLE nephritis. The different patterns and locations of granular deposits and the variable immunoglobulin classes suggest a heterogeneity of complexes. No particular immunoglobulin class or subclass relates to severity of disease, although in the instance of proliferative lesions, the total amount of immunoglobulin deposited may be important. There is a broad correlation between the amount of immunoglobulin found in mesangium and the degree of proliferation seen by light microscopy, suggesting that proliferation is a secondary response to these deposits. Subendothelial deposits are rarely seen in the absence of mesangial deposits. The situation in membranous nephropathy is distinctively different; subepithelial deposits are unrelated to either subendothelial or mesangial deposits.

The reasons for the localization of complexes in one or another area of the glomerulus are becoming better understood.[48] Characteristics of the immunoreactants are undoubtedly important because only large lattice immune complexes deposit in the glomerulus. Anatomic features are also important. Glomerular endothelial cells are separated by tiny fenestrations. Intact immune complexes can pass through them and subsequently localize against the glomerular basement membrane, where they appear as subendothelial dense deposits. Whether macromolecular complexes can penetrate the basement membrane and deposit in the subepithelial region or if antigen and antibody pass individually and then combine is still conjecture. In animal experiments, the subepithelial site where the complexes lodge corresponds to the localization of polyanionic glomerular sialoprotein on epithelial cells and in filtration slits. This negatively charged material is thought to regulate the permeability of the glomerular capillary wall to circulating macromolecules. Manipulations that alter the charge of the sialoprotein or the antigen-antibody complex can enhance or decrease the localization of immune complexes.

A number of mechanisms have been proposed to explain the role of DNA antibody in the production of SLE renal disease.[60] Complexes of DNA–anti-DNA from the circulation may deposit directly into the kidney. Alternatively, anti-DNA antibodies may bind to DNA that has been "planted" in a critical area in the kidney.[61] DNA has an affinity for the positively charged collagen component of the glomerular basement membrane, and under certain circumstances free DNA can bind in vivo to glomeruli. Subsequent interaction with anti-DNA antibodies would lead to in situ immune complex formation. Alternatively, anti-DNA may bind directly to the glomerular basement membrane. A cross-reactivity between DNA antibodies and proteoglycan heparin sulfate, a normal constituent of glomerular basement membrane, is another mechanism for localizing immune injury. This is consistent with the idea that DNA antibodies are polyspecific and often react with epitopes unrelated to DNA.[62]

Skin

Immunoglobulins are present at the dermal-epidermal (D-E) junction in SLE skin lesions. Characteristically the immunofluorescence appears as a band of granular deposits along the D-E junction, hence the name lupus band test. Most (80 to 100 percent) of the skin biopsies show IgG, IgM, and components of the classic, alternative, and terminal complement components.[63] Similar abnormalities are present in the uninvolved skin of some SLE patients, most often in sun-exposed areas. Some disagreement exists concerning the relationship of the skin immunopathology to other aspects of the disease. Biopsies taken from lesional skin or from sun-exposed, noninvolved areas are of little prognostic value. When the results are compared with the findings in uninvolved, non–sun-exposed skin, however, most studies indicate that a positive band test correlates with more severe disease, the presence of nephritis, hypocomplementemia, and raised anti-DNA antibody levels, but it cannot predict the morphology of the glomerular lesions.

The reason for localization of complexes to this discrete area of the skin is not known. The D-E junction has no phagocytic cells analogous to the mesangium, but it is a vascular area in which the circulation is sluggish in the long horizontal segments that run parallel to the basement membrane. Sometimes immunofluorescent staining of blood vessel walls in the upper dermis is seen in combination with the subepidermal immunoglobulin deposits. Serologic abnormalities and hypocomplementemia have a rough correlation with granular deposits in noninvolved skin, which is an argument in favor of the localization of circulating complexes.

During keratinization of skin, the epidermal nuclei are broken down, and nucleoprotein and DNA are thought to back-diffuse into the dermis.[64] Normally, these substances would pass through the subepidermal region and enter the circulation, but in the presence of appropriate antibodies, precipitation might occur at the D-E junction. This is consistent with the positive association of ANA and anti-dsDNA antibodies with D-E immunoglobulin deposits in normal skin, the presence of ANA in eluates from uninvolved SLE skin, and the occasional demonstration of immunoglobulins fixed to the nuclei of epidermal cells in biopsy specimens examined by the direct fluorescent antibody technique.[65]

Immune complex deposition into skin is not likely to be the cause of all SLE dermal abnormalities. Early lupus skin lesions frequently show no immunoreactants, and those induced with exposure to monochromatic light may not develop demonstrable immunoglobulin and complement complexes for several months. Finally, it is difficult to envision a direct role for immune complexes when identical immunofluorescent and electron dense deposits are identified in normal, nonlesional skin from SLE patients. Of interest, however, is the finding that although

C1q and C3 are demonstrable in both lesional and nonlesional skin, only the abnormal skin shows the terminal membrane attack complex in association with immunoglobulin.[63]

A subset of lupus patients have a characteristic photosensitive nonscarring dermatitis, intermediate in severity between acute eruptions of SLE and the chronic lesions of discoid lupus erythematosus, termed *subacute cutaneous lupus erythematosus*. Similar lesions are seen in SLE patients with homozygous C2 deficiency. Both groups of patients also have in common the presence of antibodies to the Ro/SSA antigens. The relationship of these antibodies to the skin lesion has not been defined, but their potential pathogenicity is suggested by the finding that children born to mothers with Ro/SSA antibodies in their serum also develop similar-appearing skin lesions at birth or shortly thereafter on exposure to light.[66] The dermatitis clears as the factors transferred across the placenta are eliminated from the baby's circulation, but complete heart block and other cardiac abnormalities, which are also facets of the neonatal lupus syndrome, are irreversible lesions.[67]

Antibodies to Plasma Proteins and Constituents of Cell Membranes

SLE autoantibodies to normal plasma proteins and constituents of cell membranes are well known; autoimmune hemolytic anemia, red cell aplasia, defects in granulocyte number and function, and thrombocytopenia are all common in SLE and often associated with serum antibodies, which can bind to the surfaces of these cells.[68] SLE is also associated with perturbations of the coagulation and fibrinolytic systems, and both bleeding tendencies and a hypercoagulable state are recognized. Antibodies capable of directly binding to several different clotting factors including factor II (prothrombin) and factor VIII have been described.[69, 70] Additional autoantibodies termed the *lupus anticoagulant* are detected in at least 10 percent of SLE patients and have the property of simultaneously inhibiting the in vitro function of several phospholipid-dependent clotting factors in a manner that suggests that the autoantibodies are interfering with the ability of these clotting factors to bind to phospholipids. The term *lupus anticoagulant* is a misnomer because the antibodies seldom interfere in vivo with hemostasis and are found more often in individuals without SLE than in those with this diagnosis.

The classic lupus anticoagulant is an immunoglobulin that is thought to react in vitro with negatively charged phospholipids, causing an inhibition of the assembly clotting factors on the phospholipid surface to form the prothrombin activator complex, resulting in a prolongation of the partial thromboplastin time (PTT). It is a member of a family of related antiphospholipid antibodies, which include the reagenic antibody of treponemal infections and

anticardiolipin antibody. These antiphospholipid antibodies have been associated with a syndrome of venous and arterial thrombosis, fetal distress or death, livedo reticularis, and thrombocytopenia termed the *antiphospholipid syndrome*.[71] Only a fraction of SLE patients have antiphospholipid antibodies, perhaps 20 to 40 percent. More often they occur as an isolated event in otherwise healthy individuals or in association with other immunologic or myeloproliferative diseases. A number of hypotheses have been advanced to explain the pathogenicity of antiphospholipid antibodies. These theories have in common a concept of antibody binding to membrane phospholipids, especially vascular endothelial cell phospholipid, thereby interfering with the arachidonic acid pathway and the subsequent production of potent vasodilators, such as prostacyclin.[70] Thrombosis and fetal loss occur more often with high concentrations of IgG antiphospholipid antibodies and to be more successfully predicted by tests that measure the lupus anticoagulant, such as the Russell Viper venom time. Examination of the placenta in women who have had miscarriages associated with anticardiolipin antibodies reveals distinctive changes in the vascular endothelium similar to those seen in eclampsia.

As already noted, autoantibodies to lymphocyte membrane antigens may have profound effects on lymphocyte numbers and functions, both in vivo and in vitro. Antilymphocyte antibodies are more frequent and in higher titers in patients with active SLE. The IgM cold reactive lymphocytotoxic antibodies are associated with thrombocytopenia and central nervous system manifestations. Neurocytotoxic antibodies that cross-react with lymphocytes are reported in approximately 75 percent of serum samples from SLE patients. Their relationship to one another and to the neuropsychiatric manifestations of systemic lupus is detailed later.

Central Nervous System Manifestations of Systemic Lupus Erythematosus

Neurologic and psychiatric illnesses occur commonly in SLE, in perhaps a third of the patients, and are responsible for significant morbidity and mortality. Unlike lupus nephritis, little is known about the pathogenesis of central nervous system disease. The most likely explanation is a combination of microvascular injury and interference with normal cortical function as a result of autoantibodies reacting with membranes of neuronal cells.[71]

Postmortem examination of the brains of patients dying with SLE provides little information about pathogenesis. Some demonstrate degenerative and proliferative changes in small vessels, similar to those of hypertensive encephalopathy and thrombotic thrombocytopenic purpura. Microinfarcts and gliosis may be seen around small blood vessels. Affected arterioles show thickening of the intimal and medial coats and occasionally perivascular collections of mononuclear cells but no immunoglobulin or complement when studied with immunofluorescence. Inflammatory cell infiltrates and fibrinoid necrosis of the walls of small and medium-sized arteries typically seen in the lesions of SLE elsewhere in the body are only occasionally found in the brain. Although microvascular lesions may account for the clinical findings in some SLE patients, there is more often a remarkable lack of clinical-pathologic correlations. Patients with obvious lupus encephalopathy often show only minimal abnormalities at postmortem examination, suggesting that some features of central nervous system disease may be brought about by unique pathologic processes that do not appreciably perturb brain histology.

Autoantibodies reactive with brain tissue are potential mediators for such a process; for this reason, they have been the focus of a number of studies. The first clue came from the realization that SLE-related neuropsychiatric problems are found significantly more often in patients with increased serum lymphocytotoxic antibody titers and that more than 90 percent of the lymphocytotoxic activity in SLE sera is also reactive with antigenic determinants present in homogenized human brain and on cultured human neuronal and glial cells. Other central nervous system reactive autoantibodies that are not cross-reactive with antigenic determinants on lymphocytes may be specific for central nervous system cell subpopulations.

The potential pathogenicity of antibodies to brain constituents is supported by the observation that when injected into the ventricles or cerebral cortex of experimental animals they cause convulsions, meningitis, impaired memory, and motor dysfunction. Thus, brain-reactive autoantibodies could be responsible for certain forms of SLE central nervous system disease. Circulating antibodies, however, can cause neurologic disease only if they enter the central nervous system. To do this, they must escape the constraints of the blood–brain barrier. Evidence for exclusion of blood-borne autoantibodies is the finding that although most SLE patients have circulating neuron-reactive antibodies, neither the amount nor specificity of these antibodies predicts neuropsychiatric manifestations. Some investigators, however, have reported an association between active central nervous system disease and the amount of serum IgG antineuronal antibody.

Antibodies reactive with molecules on neuronal tissues can be detected within the nervous system. Most patients with active central nervous system lupus have antineuronal antibody in their cerebrospinal fluid. Those with more diffuse central nervous system manifestations, such as psychosis, organic brain syndrome, or generalized seizures, are more likely (90 percent) to have increased amounts of IgG antineuronal antibodies than are patients with anatomically localized lesions (25 percent). The manner by which antineuronal antibodies gain access to the central nervous system is still not clear.[73] Intrathecal production has been proposed based on a disproportionate increase in cerebrospinal fluid IgG levels relative to albumin. The paucity of immunocompetent cells in the brain tissues of patients dying with active SLE–central nervous system disease, however, speaks against local antibody production.

Circulating antibody might enter the central nervous system through two potential sites: either by passaging through the choroid plexus or by escaping the constraints of the tight gap junctions of the endothelial cells lining the small cerebral blood vessels. Choroidal deposits of immune complexes have been found to be a regular feature of SLE—with or without a history of central nervous system disease. These observations probably reflect the fact that the choroidal capillaries, like the vessels of the renal glomerulus, have open fenestrations, which allow immune complexes from the circulation to enter into the interstitium of the choroid plexus, where they are retained. Serum antineuronal antibodies might gain access to the central nervous system through the choroid plexus after it has been damaged by immune complexes.

Alternatively, immune-mediated injury to the small blood vessels of the brain might allow plasma antineuronal antibodies to enter the central nervous system. Circulating immune complexes could provide the vascular insult. Evidence favoring this idea is shown in Figure 60–2. Brain tissue was obtained

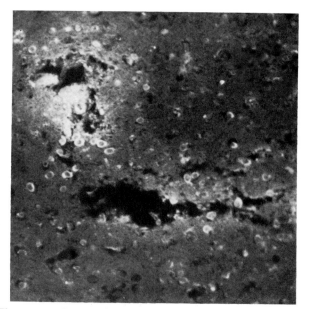

Figure 60–2. Immunofluorescent staining of cerebral cortex of a young woman who died with active SLE-related organic brain syndrome. This photomicrograph of anti-IgM immunofluorescence shows a ring pattern of staining of the neuronal cells clustered about a cerebral blood vessel. IgG staining (not shown) showed a similar ring pattern on cells throughout the field. Control proteins such as albumin and fibrinogen gave no staining. (From Zvaifler, N. J., and Bluestein, H. G.: The pathogenesis of central nervous system manifestations of systemic lupus erythematosus. Arthritis Rheum. 25:862, 1982.)

immediately after death from a young woman who had active systemic vasculitis and a severe SLE organic psychosis as part of her terminal illness. Tissue sections incubated with fluoresceinated rabbit antibodies to human proteins demonstrated that both human IgG and IgM but not fibrinogen were bound to neuronal cells. The intensity of the neuronal membrane immunofluorescence was proportional to the distance of the cells from the cerebral vessels, suggesting that the vessel was the exit site for the autoantibody.

Antibody capable of directly injuring cerebral blood vessels could provide another explanation for central nervous system manifestations. Both the lupus anticoagulant and anticardiolipin antibody (antiphospholipid antibodies) have been associated with arterial occlusions of the cerebral vasculature.[71, 74] Moderate reductions in platelet counts are a recognized correlate of central nervous system manifestations in lupus patients, and thrombocytopenia is a frequent accompaniment of antiphospholipid antibodies.[70] The interaction of antiphospholipid antibody with vascular endothelial cell phospholipid might be responsible for the noninflammatory lesions seen in the central nervous system, and a direct interaction of antiphospholipid antibodies and brain phospholipid has not been excluded.

The binding specificity of neuron-reactive antibodies in serum and cerebrospinal fluid is similar, but the actual molecules responsible for inducing these autoantibodies have not been identified. As noted earlier, a significant amount of antilymphocyte and antihuman brain cross-reactivity can be demonstrated by absorption experiments with SLE serum. The fact that rabbit antisera raised against lupus cryoglobulins frequently react with antigens on both lymphocytes and several cultured glial and neuronal lines also implies that there may be cell-surface molecules shared in common. Molecular characterization of cross-reactive neuronal membrane molecules has been accomplished by immunoprecipitation or immunoblotting of neuronal proteins with antibodies raised against human peripheral blood mononuclear cells and platelets.[69] These studies suggest that an interesting candidate for an important shared antigenic specificity are the family of molecules constituting the very late activation complex (CD29). These glycoproteins have been shown to be present on lymphocytes, cultured neuronal cells, and platelets and represent a subfamily of the integrin family of adhesion receptors.[75] Antiplatelet integrin autoantibodies frequently occur in chronic idiopathic thrombocytopenic purpura.[76] It remains to be seen whether very late activation molecules will serve as targets of an autoimmune response capable of invoking disease in the central nervous system.

References

1. Theofilopoulos, A. N., and Dixon, F. J.: Murine models of systemic lupus erythematosus. Adv. Immunol. 37:269, 1985.
1a. Steinberg, A. D.: Concepts of pathogenesis of systemic lupus erythematosus. Clin. Immunol. Immunopathol. 63(1):19, 1992.
2. McDougal, J. S., Kennedy, M. S., Kalyanaraman, V. S., et al.: Failure to demonstrate (cross-reacting) antibodies to human T lymphotrophic viruses in patients with rheumatic diseases. Arthritis Rheum. 28:1170, 1985.
3. Hochberg, M. C.: The incidence of systemic lupus erythematosus in Baltimore, Maryland, 1970–1977. Arthritis Rheum. 28:80, 1985.
4. Winchester, R. J., and Nunez-Roldon, A.: Some genetic aspects of systemic lupus erythematosus. Arthritis Rheum. 25:833, 1982.
5. Kaplan, D.: The onset of disease in twins and siblings with systemic lupus erythematosus. J. Rheumatol. 11:648, 1984.
6. Ballou, S. P., Kahn, M., and Kusher, A.: Clinical features of systemic lupus erythematosus. Differences related to race and age of onset. Arthritis Rheum. 25:55, 1982.
6a. Deapen, D., Escalante, A., Weinrib, L., et al.: A revised estimate of twin concordance in systemic lupus erythematosus. Arthritis Rheum. 35(3):311, 1992.
7. Kallenberg, C. G. M., Klaasen, R. J. L., Bellen, J. M., et al.: HLA-B8/DR3 phenotype and the primary immune responses. Clin. Immunol. Immunopathol. 34:135, 1985.
8. Reveille, J. D.: Molecular genetics of systemic lupus erythematosus and Sjögren's syndrome. Curr. Opin. Rheumatol. 2:733, 1990.
9. Tebib, J. G., Martinez, C., Granados, J., et al.: The frequency of complement receptor type 1 (CR1) gene polymorphisms in nine families with multiple cases of systemic lupus erythematosus. Arthritis Rheum. 32:1465, 1989.
10. Fronek, Z., Lentz, D., Berliner, N., et al.: Systemic lupus erythematosus is not genetically linked to the beta chain of the T cell receptor. Arthritis Rheum. 29:1023, 1986.
11. Frank, M. B., McArthur, R., and Harley, J. B.: Anti-Ro (SSA) autoantibodies are associated with T cell receptor β genes in systemic lupus erythematosus. J. Clin. Invest. 85:33, 1990.
12. Kotzin, B. L., Barr, V. L., and Palmer, E.: A large deletion within the T-cell receptor beta-chain gene complex in New Zealand white mice. Science 229:167, 1985.
13. DeHoratius, R. J., and Messner, R. P.: Lymphocytotoxic antibodies in family members of patients with systemic lupus erythematosus. J. Clin. Invest. 55:1254, 1975.
14. Diaz, A., Pope, R., Fischnach, M., et al.: Enhancement of circulating autoantibodies and immune complex levels in autoimmune prone mice by high dietary fat intake. Arthritis Rheum. 26:520, 1983.
15. Kelly, V. E., Ferretti, A., Izui, S., et al.: A fish oil diet rich in eicosapentanoic acid reduces cyclooxygenase metabolites, and suppresses lupus in MRL-lpr mice. J. Immunol. 134:1914, 1985.
16. Alcocer-Varela, J., Iglesias, A., Llorente, L., et al.: Effects of L-canavanine on T cells may explain the induction of systemic lupus erythematosus by alfalfa. Arthritis Rheum. 28:52, 1985.
17. Lahita, R. G., Bradlow, H. L., Ginzler, E., et al.: Low plasma androgens in women with systemic lupus erythematosus. Arthritis Rheum. 30:241, 1987.
18. Jungers, P., Kuttenn, F., Liote, F., et al.: Hormonal modulation in systemic lupus erythematosus. Arthritis Rheum. 28:1243, 1985.
19. Guldner, H. H., Netter, H. J., Szostecki, C., et al.: Human anti-p68 autoantibodies recognize a common epitope of U1 RNA containing small nuclear ribonucleoprotein and influenza B virus. J. Exp. Med. 171:819, 1990.
20. Kohsaka, H., Yamamoto, K., Fujii, H., et al.: Fine epitope mapping of the human SS-B/La protein. Identification of a distinct autoepitope homologous to a viral gag polyprotein. J. Clin. Invest. 85:1566, 1990.
21. Raveche, E. S., Novontny, E. A., Hansen, C. T., et al.: Genetic studies in NZB mice. V. Recombinant inbred lines demonstrate that separate genes control autoimmune phenotype. J. Exp. Med. 153:1187, 1981.
22. Klinman, D. M., and Steinberg, A. D.: Idiotypy and autoimmunity. Arthritis Rheum. 29:697, 1986.
23. Blank, M., Mendlovic, S., Fricke, H., et al.: Sex hormone involvement in the induction of experimental systemic lupus erythematosus by a pathogenic anti-DNA idiotype in naive mice. J. Rheumatol. 17:311, 1990.
24. Morris, S. C., Cheek, R. L., Cohen, P. L., et al.: Allotype-specific immunoregulation of autoantibody production by host B cells in chronic graft-versus-host disease. J. Immunol. 144:916, 1990.
25. Suzuki, N., Sakare, T., and Engelman, E.: Anti-DNA antibody production by CD5+ and CD5− B cells of patients with systemic lupus erythematosus. J. Clin. Invest. 85:238, 1990.
26. Knight, J. G., and Adams, D. D.: Failure of transferred thymus cells to suppress or prevent autoantibody production in NZB and NZBXNZW mice. J. Clin. Lab. Immunol. 1:151, 1978.
27. Tomita-Yamaguchi, M., Babich, J. F., Baker, R. C., et al.: Incorporation, distribution, and turnover of arachidonic acid within membrane phospholipids of B220+ T cells from autoimmune-prone MRL-lpr/lpr mice. J. Exp. Med. 171:787, 1990.
28. Morimoto, C., Reinherz, E. L., Distaso, J. A., et al.: Relationship between systemic lupus erythematosus T cell subsets, anti T cell antibodies and T cell functions. J. Clin. Invest. 73:689, 1984.

29. Riccardi, P. J., Hausman, P. B., Raff, H. V., et al.: The autologous mixed lymphocyte reaction in systemic lupus erythematosus. Arthritis Rheum. 25:820, 1982.

30. Reeves, W. H., Sthoeger, Z. M., and Lahita, R. G.: Role of antigen-selectivity in autoimmune responses to the Ku (p70/p80) antigen. J. Clin. Invest. 84:562, 1989.

31. St. Clair, E. W., Burch, J. A., Ward, M. M., et al.: Temporal correlation of antibody responses to different epitopes of the human La autoantigen. J. Clin. Invest. 85:515, 1990.

32. Steinberg, A. D., and Klinman, D. M.: Pathogenesis of systemic lupus erythematosus. Rheum. Dis. Clin. North Am. 14:25, 1988.

33. Boumpas, D. T., Tsokos, G. C., Mann, D. L., et al.: Increased proto-oncogene expression in peripheral blood lymphocytes from patients with systemic lupus erythematosus and other autoimmune diseases. Arthritis Rheum. 29:755, 1986.

34. Raziuddin, S., Nur, M. A., and Alwabel, A. A.: Selective loss of the CD4+ inducers of suppressor T cell subsets (2H4+) in active systemic lupus erythematosus. J. Rheumatol. 16:1315, 1989.

35. Sakane, T., Murakawa, Y., and Suzuki, N.: Familial occurrence of impaired interleukin-2 activity and increased peripheral blood B cells actively secreting immunoglobulins in systemic lupus erythematosus. Am. J. Med. 86:385, 1989.

36. Tanaka, T., Saiki, O., Negoro, S., et al.: Decreased expression of interleukin-2 binding molecules (p70/75) in T cells from patients with systemic lupus erythematosus. Arthritis Rheum. 32:552, 1989.

37. Handwerger, B. S.: Lymphocyte biology in lupus. Curr. Opin. Rheumatol. 2:749, 1990.

38. Tanaka, S., Matsuyama, T., Steinberg, A. D., et al.: Antilymphocyte antibodies against CD4+2H4+ cell populations in patients with systemic lupus erythematosus. Arthritis Rheum. 32:398, 1989.

39. Sibbitt, W. L., Gibbs, D. L., Kenny, C., et al.: Relationship between circulating interferon and anti-interferon antibodies and impaired natural killer cell activity in systemic lupus erythematosus. Arthritis Rheum. 28:624, 1985.

40. Winfield, J. B., Shaw, M., and Minota, S.: Modulation of IgM anti-lymphocyte antibody-reactive T cell surface antigens in systemic lupus erythematosus. J. Immunol. 136:3246, 1986.

40a. Winfield, J. B., and Mimura, T.: Pathogenetic significance of antilymphocyte autoantibodies in systemic lupus erythematosus. Clin. Immunol. Immunopathol. 63(1):13, 1992.

41. Miyagi, J., Minato, N., Sumiya, M., et al.: Two types of antibodies inhibiting interleukin-2 production by normal lymphocytes in patients with systemic lupus erythematosus. Arthritis Rheum. 32:1356, 1989.

42. Winfield, J. B., Shaw, M., Yamada, A., et al.: Subset specificity of antilymphocyte antibodies in systemic lupus erythematosus. Arthritis Rheum. 30:162, 1987.

43. Mimura, T., Fernsten, P., Shaw, M., et al.: Glycoprotein specificity of cold-reactive IgM antilymphocyte autoantibodies in systemic lupus erythematosus. Arthritis Rheum. 33:1226, 1990.

44. Mimura, T., Fernsten, P., Jarjour, W., et al.: Autoantibodies specific for different isoforms of CD45 in systemic lupus erythematosus. J. Exp. Med. 172:653, 1990.

45. Minota, S., Jarjour, W. N., Roubey, R. A., et al.: Reactivity of auto-antibodies and DNA/anti-DNA complexes with a novel 110-kilodalton phosphoprotein in systemic lupus erythematosus and other diseases. J. Immunol. 144:1263, 1990.

46. Luhrmann, R., Kastner, B., and Bach, M.: Structure of spliceosomal snRNPs and their role in pre-mRNA splicing. Biochem. Biophys. Acta 1087:265, 1990.

47. Hardin, J. A.: The structure, function and autoimmunogenic potential of the Sm snRNPs. Clin. Aspects Autoimmunity 3:16, 1989.

48. Wener, M. H., and Mannik, M.: Mechanisms of immune deposit formation in renal glomeruli. Springer Semin. Immunopathol. 9:219, 1986.

49. Theofilopoulos, A. N., Kofler, R., Noonan, D., et al.: Molecular aspects of murine systemic lupus erythematosus. Springer Semin. Immunopathol. 97:121, 1986.

50. Gavalchin, J., and Datta, S. K.: The NZBxSWR model of lupus nephritis. II. Autoantibodies deposited in renal lesions show a distinctive and restrictive idiotypic diversity. J. Immunol. 138:138, 1987.

51. Whaley, K., Schur, P. H., and Ruddy, S.: Relative importance of C3b inactivator and beta 1H globulin in the modulation of the properdin amplification loop in systemic lupus erythematosus. Clin. Exp. Immunol. 36:408, 1979.

52. Emlen, W., Pisetsky, D. S., and Taylor, R. P.: Antibodies to DNA. A perspective. Arthritis Rheum. 29:1417, 1986.

53. Isenberg, D. A.: Autoantibodies and their idiotypes. Curr. Opin. Rheumatol. 2:724, 1990.

54. Frank, M. M., Lawley, T. J., Hamburger, M. I., et al.: Immunoglobulin G Fc receptor mediated clearance in autoimmune disease. Ann. Intern. Med. 98:206, 1983.

55. Atkinson, J. P.: Complement activation and complement receptors in systemic lupus erythematosus. Springer Semin. Immunopathol. 9:179, 1986.

56. Rumore, P. M., and Steinman, C. R.: Endogenous circulating DNA in systemic lupus erythematosus. Occurrence as multimeric complexes bound to histone. J. Clin. Invest. 86:69, 1990.

57. Reeves, W., and Chiorazzi, N.: Interaction between anti-DNA and anti-DNA binding protein autoantibodies in cryoglobulins from sera of patients with systemic lupus erythematosus. J. Exp. Med. 164:1029, 1986.

58. Klippel, J. H., Bluestein, H. G., and Zvaifler, N. J.: Lymphocyte reactivity of antisera to cryoproteins in systemic lupus erythematosus. Clin. Immunol. Immunopathol. 12:52, 1979.

59. Biesecker, G., Katz, S., and Koffler, D.: Renal localization of the membrane attack complex in systemic lupus erythematosus nephritis. J. Exp. Med. 154:1779, 1981.

60. Waer, M.: The role of anti-DNA antibodies in lupus nephritis. Clin. Rheumatol. 9:111, 1990.

61. Raz, E., Brezis, M., Rosenmann, E., et al.: Anti-DNA antibodies bind directly to renal antigens and induce kidney dysfunction in the isolated perfused rat kidney. J. Immunol. 192:3076, 1989.

62. Eilat, D.: Cross-reactions of anti-DNA antibodies and the central dogma of lupus nephritis. Immunol. Today 6:123, 1985.

63. Biesecker, G., Lavin, L., Ziskind, M., et al.: Cutaneous localization of the membrane attack complex in discoid and systemic lupus erythematosus. N. Engl. J. Med. 306:264, 1982.

64. Gilliam, J. N.: The significance of cutaneous immunoglobulin deposits in lupus erythematosus and NZB/NZW F1 hybrid mice. J. Invest. Dermatol. 65:154, 1975.

65. Wells, J. V., Webb, J., VanDeventer, M., et al.: In vivo anti-nuclear antibodies in epithelial biopsies in SLE and other connective tissue diseases. Clin. Exp. Immunol. 38:424, 1979.

66. Watson, R. M., Lane, A. T., Barnett, N. K., et al.: Neonatal lupus erythematosus. A clinical, serologic, and immunogenetic study with review of the literature. Medicine 63:362, 1984.

67. Scott, J. S., Maddison, P. J., Taylor, P. V., et al.: Connective tissue disease, antibodies to ribonucleoprotein, and congenital heart block. N. Engl. J. Med. 309:209, 1983.

68. Laurence, J., and Nachman, R.: Hematologic aspects of systemic lupus erythematosus. In Lahita, R. G. (ed.): Systemic Lupus Erythematosus. New York, John Wiley & Sons, 1987.

69. S'anchez-Cuenca, J., Carmona, E., Villanueva, M. J., et al.: Immunological characterization of factor VIII inhibitors by a sensitive micro-ELISA method. Thromb. Res. 57:897, 1990.

70. Fleck, R. A., Rapaport, S. I., and Rao, L. V. M.: Anti-prothrombin antibodies and the lupus anticoagulant. Blood 72:512, 1988.

71. Lockshin, M. D.: Anticardiolipin antibodies and lupus anticoagulants. Curr. Opin. Rheumatol. 2:708, 1990.

72. Carreras, L. O., and Vermylen, J. G.: Lupus anticoagulant and thrombosis—possible role of inhibition of prostacyclin formation. Thromb. Haemost. (Stuttgart) 48:38, 1982.

73. Bluestein, H. G., Pischel, K. D., and Woods, V. L.: Immunopathogenesis of the neuropsychiatric manifestations of systemic lupus erythematosus. Springer Semin. Immunopathol. 9:237, 1986.

74. Asherson, R. A., Merry, P., Acheson, J. F., et al.: Antiphospholipid antibodies. A risk factor for occlusive ocular vascular disease in systemic lupus erthematosus and the "primary" antiphospholipid syndrome. Ann. Rheum. Dis. 48:358, 1989.

75. Pischel, K. D., Bluestein, H. G., and Woods, V. L.: Very late activation antigens (VLA) are human leukocyte-neuronal crossreactive cell surface antigens. J. Exp. Med. 164:393, 1986.

76. Woods, V. L., Jr., Oh, E. H., Mason, D., et al.: Autoantibodies against the platelet glycoprotein IIb/IIIa complex in patients with chronic ITP. Blood 63:368, 1984.

Clinical Features of SLE

GENERAL CONSIDERATIONS

Systemic lupus erythematosus (SLE) is a chronic inflammatory disease of unknown cause that may affect the skin, joints, kidneys, lungs, nervous system, serous membranes, and other organs of the body. Patients with SLE develop distinct immunologic abnormalities, especially antinuclear antibodies. The clinical course of SLE is characterized by periods of remission and chronic or acute relapses. Genetic and other (e.g., environmental) factors seem to play a role in its pathogenesis.

EPIDEMIOLOGY

The prevalence of SLE has been estimated to be between 4 and 250 cases per 100,000 population.[1] The wide range undoubtedly reflects varying criteria in different populations. SLE appears to be more common in urban than in rural areas.[2] The prevalence in the United States is higher among Asians (in Hawaii: 18–24 per 100,000) and black females (7.9–10.5 per 100,000) than in white females (4 per 100,000) or Puerto Rican females (1 per 100,000).[1, 3-5] In New Zealand, the prevalence was 14.6 in whites and 50.63 in Polynesians—with higher mortality rates for the latter.[6] The prevalence has been noted to be 1 per 1969 in San Francisco, 1 per 2400 in Minnesota,[3] 1 per 6780 in New Zealand,[7] 39 per 100,000 in Sweden,[8] 28 per 100,000 in Finland,[9] 16 per 100,000 in American Indians,[10] statistically comparable to rheumatoid arthritis in Jamaica, common in China and Southeast Asia,[12, 13] and seen infrequently in Africa,[14] especially in black Africans. In France, it is more common among immigrants from Spain, Portugal, North Africa, and Italy.[15] The prevalence is three times as great among black females as compared with all females, in San Francisco and Baltimore,[4] but not in Los Angeles or New York City.[16]

The increased frequency of SLE among females is thought to be due to unknown hormonal effect. However, some kindreds have been described that are mostly male.[17] In children, where sex hormonal effects are presumably minimal, the female:male ratio of SLE patients is 1.4 to 5.8:1,[16] in adults the female:male ratio ranges from 8:1 to 13:1,[15, 16] and it is 2:1 in "older" individuals.[16] Sixty-five percent of patients have an onset between ages 16 and 55,[15] 20 percent less than 16,[18] and 15 percent greater than age 55.[19] SLE in children tends to be symptomatically

more severe, with a high incidence of nephritis, pericarditis, hepatosplenomegaly, and hematologic abnormalities.[18] Males with lupus tend to have more thrombocytopenia and renal disease.[20] SLE in the elderly tends to be milder, with fewer renal and central nervous system manifestations and more serositis and musculoskeletal manifestations (i.e., presenting similarly to drug-induced lupus).[21] Blacks are more likely to have anti-Sm, anti-ribonucleoprotein (RNP), discoid skin lesions, proteinuria, psychosis, and serositis[22] and have a poorer prognosis than whites.[23] Clinical status is poorer in those with less education.[24]

The incidence of SLE and discoid LE is the same in Rochester, Minn. (25 per 100,000).[3]

Multiple independent segregating genes have been implicated in SLE. These genes could affect immune regulation, immune responses, complement, the reticuloendothelial system (including phagocytosis), immunoglobulins, and sex hormones. Four genes may be involved.[25] Evidence for these genes includes a high concordance rate (14–57 percent) of SLE in monozygotic twins;[26, 27] 5 to 12 percent of relatives of SLE patients also have SLE.[28] The genetic markers that have been observed more frequently in SLE patients than in the general population include HLA-B8,[29] HLA-DR2,[28, 29] HLA-DR3,[28-30] DQW1,[31] C2 deficiency (C2D),[32] C4 (especially C4A) deficiency (C4D),[30, 32] Gm,[33] and low levels of CR1.[34]

Although attempts to define subsets of SLE on purely clinical grounds have been largely unsuccessful, both subacute cutaneous and neonatal LE appear to be well-defined subsets. Both are associated with anti-Ro and HLA-DR3.[35]

Immune abnormalities frequently found in SLE patients may also be influenced by genetic factors. Autoantibodies are found more frequently in relatives of SLE patients than in the general population;[36] suppressor cell defects are found in relatives;[37] antibodies to DNA have been associated with DR3, DR7, and DR2;[29] antibodies to Sm have been associated with DR7[29] and DR4;[38] antibodies to La(SS-B) have been associated with DR3[39] and DQW2.3;[40] and antibodies to Ro(SS-A) with DR2, DR3, DQ1/DQ2, and C2D.[41]

CLINICAL FEATURES

General Symptomatology (Table 61–1)

Fatigue

Fatigue, the most common complaint and occasionally the most debilitating, occurs in 80 to 100

Table 61–1. FREQUENCY OF CLINICAL SYMPTOMS IN SLE AT ANY TIME

Symptoms	Percentage
Fatigue	80–100
Fever	>80
Weight loss	>60
Arthritis, arthralgia	95
Skin	>80
Butterfly rash	>50
Photosensitivity	<58
Mucous membrane lesion	27–41
Alopecia	<71
Raynaud's phenomenon	17–30
Purpura	15
Urticaria	8
Renal	50
Nephrosis	18
Gastrointestinal	38
Pulmonary	0.9–98
Pleurisy	45
Effusion	24
Pneumonia	29
Cardiac	46
Pericarditis	8–48
Murmurs	23
ECG changes	34–70
Lymphadenopathy	50
Splenomegaly	10–20
Hepatomegaly	25
Central nervous system	25–75
Functional	most
Psychosis	5–52
Convulsions	15–20

percent of patients, even when no other features of active disease are present. Fatigue is common to everyone; abnormal fatigue is operationally defined as more "bad" days than "good" ones. Fatigue in SLE is strongly associated with a diminished exercise tolerance test.[42] It is important to distinguish the fatigue due to lupus from that caused by other factors. An increased work load (job, children, school, house, marriage), sleep disturbances, depression, unhealthful habits (smoking, alcohol, fad diets, sedentary living, drug abuse), stress, deconditioning, anemia, use of certain medications (including prednisone), and any inflammatory disease all can cause fatigue. The association of onset of fatigue with other features or laboratory tests suggesting active lupus may mean that the fatigue is due to lupus. Fatigue in SLE patients has been reported to respond to prednisone[15] and to aerobic exercise training.[42]

Weight Changes

Weight loss often occurs *prior* to the diagnosis of SLE. Weight loss may be due to loss of appetite from medication side effects or gastrointestinal disease or may be the result of diuretics or a goal of the patient trying to lose weight.

Weight gain can also occur in the patient with active lupus, as a result of the water retention associated with the nephrotic syndrome or associated with the use of prednisone.

Fever

Fever is seen in over 80 percent of SLE patients. Episodic fever is more suggestive of SLE or infection. A sustained fever is more suggestive of central nervous system involvement,[15] a drug, or medication. In a study of 83 febrile episodes in 63 patients with SLE, 60 percent of the fevers were thought to be due to SLE, 23 percent due to infection, and 17 percent due to other causes.[43] Infectious complications develop in approximately one half of SLE patients, especially respiratory and urinary ones.[44] Opportunistic infections are a common cause of death.[45]

Other Symptoms

Aches and pains, swollen glands, nausea and vomiting, headaches, depression, easy bruising, hair loss, edema, and swelling may occur prior to the diagnosis of SLE or coincident with "major" symptoms of a flare.

Musculoskeletal Manifestations
(Table 61–2)

Arthralgia and arthritis have been noted in up to 95 percent of patients. These symptoms may precede the diagnosis of SLE by months or years or may be mistaken for another inflammatory arthritis. Complaints tend to be migratory, with symptoms in a particular joint often gone in 24 hours, and asymmetric with predilection to the knees, carpal joints, and the joints of the fingers, especially the proximal interphalangeal joint (PIP). The ankles, elbows, shoulders, and hips are less frequently involved. Morning stiffness is usually measured in minutes. The degree of pain often exceeds objective physical

Table 61–2. MUSCULOSKELETAL MANIFESTATIONS IN SLE

	SLE	RA
Arthralgia	Common	Common
Arthritis	Common	Deforming
Symmetry	Yes	Yes
Joints involved	PIP>MCP>wrist>knee	MCP>wrist>knee
Synovial hypertrophy	Rare	Common
Synovial membrane abnormality	Minimal	Proliferative
Synovial fluid	Transudate	Exudate
Subcutaneous nodules	Rare	35%
Erosions	Very rare	Common
Morning stiffness	Minutes	Hours
Myalgia	Common	Common
Myositis	Rare	Uncommon
Osteoporosis	Variable	Common
Avascular necrosis	5–50%	Uncommon
Deforming arthritis	Uncommon	Common
Swan neck	10%	Common
Ulnar deviation	5%	Common

MCP, Metacarpophalangeal joint; PIP, proximal interphalangeal joint.

findings. The presence of leukopenia and a positive antinuclear antibody (ANA) test in a patient with arthralgia/arthritis often facilitate the diagnosis of SLE.

Although the arthritis of lupus is generally considered to be nondeforming, flexion deformities, ulnar deviation, soft tissue laxity, and swan neck deformities have been noted in 15 to 50 percent of patients.[46, 47] These abnormalities tend to occur in patients with long-standing disease who take glucocorticoid medications. The deformities are usually easily reducible and are thought to be due to lax joint capsules, tendons, and ligaments, resulting in joint instability. Erosions in the hand are rare,[48] suggesting Jaccoud's arthritis.[49] Tenosynovitis has been noted in 10 to 13 percent of patients, including episodes of epicondylitis, rotator cuff tendinitis, Achilles tendinitis, posterior tibial tendinitis, and plantar fascitis.[15, 50] Infrapatellar and Achilles tendon ruptures are rare.[50a]

Synovial effusions are infrequent, usually small, and clear or slightly cloudy.[51] Fluids tend to have low protein levels and white blood cell counts. Antinuclear antibodies and LE cells have been observed in synovial fluids. The synovial histopathology tends to be nonspecific, with superficial fibrin-like material and local or diffuse lining cell proliferation. Vascular changes have included perivascular mononuclear cells, lumen obliteration, enlarged endothelial cells, and thrombi, but fibrinoid necrosis (i.e., vasculitis) is uncommon.[52]

Subcutaneous nodules have been noted in 5 to 7 percent of patients, generally in association with active disease.[46, 53] Pathology similar to rheumatoid nodules and a distinct pathology both have been noted.

Although patients with SLE are intrinsically immunosuppressed, and often additionally so with medication, septic arthritis is uncommon—but has been reported secondary to infections with *Salmonella*, gonococci, meningococci, and other organisms.[54]

Avascular necrosis occurs in 3 to 52 percent of patients, especially in the femoral head, although the humeral head, tibial plateau, and scaphoid navicular have also been affected.[46, 55] Involvement is usually bilateral and often asymptomatic, being detected by radionuclide scanning or magnetic resonance imaging (MRI). In a patient with groin pain and equivocal radiographs but a positive scan/MRI, an abnormal intraosseous phlebogram and an increased intramedullary pressure may be diagnostic. The mechanism of the avascular necrosis is initially interruption of the blood supply to the bone. Subsequently, the adjacent area becomes hyperemic, resulting in demineralization, trabecular thinning, and, if stressed, collapse.[50] SLE patients receiving steroids, especially higher doses for longer periods, are at greater risk for developing this complication; Raynaud's phenomenon and hyperlipidemia may also be risk factors.

Osteoporosis is a frequent complication following prolonged use of high doses of glucocorticoids. Trabecular bones (e.g., ribs, vertebrae) are more likely to be involved than are long cortical bones. There are no symptoms unless fractures occur. The risk of osteoporosis is increased in postmenopausal women (especially those with an early menopause—namely, early hysterectomy), those who are inactive, and those with a low intake of calcium or vitamin D.

Myalgia, muscle tenderness, and muscle weakness symptoms manifest themselves in up to 69 percent of patients[46, 56] and may be part of the initial symptoms. Severe muscle weakness, atrophy, or myositis is uncommon (7–15 percent).[46, 57] Pathologic examination of muscles has revealed perivascular and perifascicular mononuclear cell infiltrates in 25 percent of patients.[15]

Muscle weakness may also be due to medication (glucocorticoids, antimalarials).[56] Serum levels of creatine phosphokinase (CPK) and aldolase are usually normal, but lactate dehydrogenase (LDH) may be elevated.[58] Muscle biopsies generally reveal a picture of swollen sacrolemmal nuclei and prominent nuclei centrally located within the muscle fiber, within a vacuole.

Mucocutaneous Lesions

The skin and mucous membranes are symptomatically involved in over 80 percent of patients.[46, 57, 59, 60]

Photosensitivity

Society in the United States has been brainwashed by travel agents into thinking that a tan is healthy, but the lupus patient is told to think that "The Sun Is My Enemy." Photosensitivity occurs in up to 58 percent of SLE patients,[46] that is, they develop a rash after exposure to ultraviolet B (UVB) light (e.g., sunlight, fluorescent tanning lights). Some patients are also sensitive to UVA, and some may even be sensitive to the visible spectrum. Some patients also express vague feelings of being unwell while in the sun (although it is not clear that this represents photosensitivity). Glass will protect individuals sensitive to UVB but will only partially protect those sensitive to UVA. Blond, blue-eyed, fair-skinned individuals are much more photosensitive than are brunettes or individuals with pigmented skin.[61] Not all individuals with photosensitivity have lupus. Photosensitivity may vary in degree during a patient's illness. Acute, subacute, and discoid lesions as well as some bullous and urticarial lesions are photosensitive (Table 61–3). Patients with anti-Ro tend to be photosensitive.

The mechanism whereby UV light causes skin lesions is not clear. Some (or all) of the following UV effects may be responsible for the process:

1. UV light damages the DNA or proteins in the

Table 61–3. MUCOCUTANEOUS LESIONS

Photosensitivity
Acute, erythematous, edematous
Subacute
  Annular/polycyclic
  Psoriasiform
Discoid
Lupus profundus/panniculitis
Neonatal LE
Alopecia
Bullous lesions
Mucous membranes
Vascular lesion
  Periungual erythema
  Livedo reticularis
  Telangiectasia
  Raynaud's phenomenon
  Vasculitis
Urticaria/purpura
Atrophie blanche
Chilblain lupus
Steroid-induced ecchymoses

skin. The patient makes antibodies to these altered molecules, and the antigen-antibody reaction attracts other humoral factors (e.g., complement) and cells and causes a local inflammatory reaction (a rash).

2. UV light increases binding of anti-Ro, anti-La, and anti-RNP to keratinocytes.[62]

3. UV light causes significant alterations in cellular membrane phospholipid metabolism, which may affect inflammation.

4. UV light causes an increase in production and release of cytokines, including IL-1 (which can cause fever, local inflammation, increased antibody production) from cutaneous keratinocyte and Langerhans cells.

5. UV light stimulates the evolution of increased numbers of suppressor T cells.

The severity of cutaneous reaction will depend on the intensity of the UV source and the duration of exposure.

The *classic butterfly rash* (i.e., erythema over the cheeks and bridge of the nose) appears in approximately one half of patients (see Fig. 33–7) usually after UVB exposure. This symptom may precede other symptoms of lupus by months or even years. The involved skin feels warm and appears slightly edematous. Application of alcohol (found in many sunscreens) may actually increase the redness, owing to increased circulation to the skin. The rash may last for hours or days and often recurs. Any stress that naturally makes one feel "flushed" will accentuate the redness. The development of the rash may be accompanied by other symptoms and signs of acute SLE. Histopathologic examination is usually unimpressive, although basal layer abnormalities may be noted.[59, 60] Immunofluorescence may detect immunoglobulins and complement at the dermal-epidermal junction.

A lupus lesion may at times (21 percent) develop a maculopapular eruption with fine scaling.[46] This lesion will usually persist somewhat longer than other lesions. They generally heal without residue, although some hyperpigmentation may be noted. Lupus lesions appear on the face and elsewhere on the body in photoexposed areas and may be pruritic.

Discoid LE

Discoid lesions develop in up to 25 percent of patients with SLE[59, 60] but may also occur in the absence of any clinical or serologic feature of SLE (previously referred to as discoid LE; now referred to as the most common manifestation of cutaneous LE—as distinguished from systemic LE). Discoid lesions are characterized by discrete round, annular, erythematous, slightly infiltrated plaques covered by a well-formed adherent scale that extends into dilated hair follicles (see Fig. 33–5). Follicular plugging is prominent. Lesions generally expand slowly with active inflammation at the periphery, leaving depressed scars, telangiectasias, and depigmentation. Central scarring with atrophy is characteristic.[59] The outline of the lesions tends to be erythematous, sharp, and irregular. Lesions occur mostly on the face, neck, and scalp, but also on the ears and, infrequently, on the upper torso.

Some lesions may be hyperkeratotic and thus confused with psoriasis. This has therapeutic implications, since the latter is treated with UV light, which the lupus patient should avoid. A biopsy will often determine the correct diagnosis. Patients with discoid LE tend to have a milder form of SLE.[63] Patients with discoid LE without SLE (initially) have about a 10 percent risk of eventually developing (mild) SLE.

Pathologic examination of discoid skin lesions reveals hyperkeratosis, follicular plugging, and basal layer changes (e.g., loss of normal organization and orientation of basal cells, edema and vacuole formation, and mononuclear cell infiltration of the dermal-epidermal junction).[59] The mononuclear cell infiltrate, mostly of T cells, may appear in the dermis around blood vessels and appendages. Discoid lesions have more of a mononuclear cell infiltration than do the lesions of subacute cutaneous lupus erythematosus (SCLE) (see later). Immunofluorescence reveals immunoglobulin and complement components along the dermal-epidermal border in a granular pattern.[64]

Subacute Cutaneous Lupus Erythematosus (SCLE)

The character of the lesions of subacute cutaneous lupus erythematosus (SCLE) falls between those of the chronic discoid and the acute butterfly rash. Approximately 50 percent of patients with this type of skin lesion have (mild) SLE[59]—and about 10 percent of patients with SLE have this type of skin lesion.[59] SCLE lesions begin as small, erythematous, slightly scaly papules that evolve into either a psoriasiform (papulosquamous) or an annular form. The latter often coalesce to form polycyclic or figurate patterns. Lesions typically have erythematous edges. Follicular plugging, hyperkeratosis, dermal atrophy, permanent pigment changes, or scarring does not develop, although telangiectasia may develop. The most frequently affected areas are the shoulders, forearms, neck, and upper torso. The face is usually spared. There is a strong association with HLA-DR3 and antibodies to Ro(SS-A).[59, 60] The pathology of SCLE lesions is similar to that of discoid lesions, although basement membrane thickening is generally absent or minimal.[59]

Lupus profundus/panniculitis is a rare manifestation of LE. It represents a firm nodular lesion underneath a cutaneous lesion. When the nodules are present without skin lesions, it is called simply lupus panniculitis.[60] The nodules, often painful, may appear in the mid-dermal, deep dermal, or subcutaneous layer. They consist of perivascular infiltrates of mononuclear cells. The nodules may appear on the scalp, face, arms, chest, back, thighs, and buttocks. They usually resolve but may leave a depressed area. Ulcerations are uncommon. In addition to the perivascular lesions there is panniculitis (i.e., hyaline fat necrosis with mononuclear cell infiltration). Some patients with lupus panniculitis exhibit no other manifestations of SLE; thus, these patients may resemble those with Weber-Christian syndrome. However, in lupus there are usually immune deposits in the dermal basement membrane zone.

Bullous Lesions

Subepidermal bullae may be associated with any of the lupus skin lesions referred to before.[59, 60, 65] SLE is rarely associated with bullous pemphigoid, dermatitis herpetiformis, and epidermolysis bullosa. The diseases can usually be differentiated by their characteristic pathology, dermal immune deposits, and serum antibodies (which react with different parts of the dermis).

Neonatal Lupus

Neonatal lupus is a rare syndrome that represents a complication of maternal antibodies to Ro(SS-A) or La(SS-B) or both.[66] Infants develop typical discoid skin lesions shortly after birth and exposure to the UV light in the nursery. The rash clears within 6 months. Very few of these infants go on to develop SLE later in life. Some infants may also develop other transient complications of SLE, such as hemolytic anemia, thrombocytopenia, hepatosplenomegaly, and congenital heart block—which is rare but may be fatal.[60]

Alopecia

Hair loss occurs in up to 71 percent of SLE patients at some time during their illness.[46] Alopecia may involve the scalp, eyebrows, eyelashes, beard, or body hair.[60] Hair loss may precede other manifestations of SLE. When associated with scarring, as with discoid lesions of the scalp, the hair loss is usually permanent. Nonscarring alopecia has two major causes. The first is premature hair loss (telogen effluvium) characterized by a diffuse thinning of the scalp 3 months after a stressful event such as a severe illness (e.g., a flare of SLE), emotional upset, pregnancy, or the use of glucocorticoids.[60] The scalp hair has presumably been put into a resting (telogen) phase; normal hair usually grows back when the stress is alleviated. Second, lupus hair can cause alopecia.[67] This form of hair is generally seen during exacerbations of SLE and is characterized by thin, unruly hair that easily fractures. It usually occurs along the frontal hairline and grows back normally when disease activity subsides. Nail lesions, particularly pitting, ridging, and onycholysis, have been noted in 25 percent of SLE patients.[68]

Mucous Membranes

Mucous membrane involvement occurs in 27 to 41 percent of patients.[46, 57, 59, 60] Characteristic discoid lesions with erythema, atrophy, and depigmentation can occur on the lips. Irregularly shaped raised white plaques, silvery white scarred lesions, areas of erythema, and punched-out erosions or ulcers with erythema around them may appear on the soft or hard palate. These lesions are usually painful, may be the first sign of lupus, and are often not noted if not looked for. Oral lesions should be distinguished from those of lichen planus, candidiasis, aphthous stomatitis, bite marks, leukoplakia, and malignancy. The oral lesions of lupus demonstrate the typical histopathology of discoid lesions, including deposits of immunoglobulin and complement at the dermal-epidermal junction. These lesions tend to disappear quickly with glucocorticoid therapy. Gingivitis has also been noted, particularly in individuals with xerostomia.

Nasal ulcers have been noted in 20 percent of patients.[15] They are usually in the lower nasal septum, and tend to be bilateral. The appearance of nasal ulcers is likely to parallel other features of active SLE. Nasal perforation, possibly secondary to vasculitis, is rare.

Involvement of the mucosa of the upper airway may also occur and may cause hoarseness.[57]

Vascular Lesions

Skin lesions from vascular involvement including periungual erythema, livedo reticularis, telangiectasia, Raynaud's phenomenon, and various forms of vasculitis occur in approximately 50 percent of SLE patients.[59]

Periungual erythema is due to dilated tortuous loops of capillaries and a prominent subcapillary venous plexus along the base of the nail. Similar lesions have been noted in 12 percent of patients along the edges of the upper eyelid.[57]

Livedo reticularis is a reddish/cyanotic reticular pattern of the skin. It is seen on the arms, legs, and torso, particularly in cold environments. The syndrome is secondary to vasospasm of the dermal ascending arterioles.[60] The vasospasm results in a decreased blood supply to the superficial horizontal vascular plexus with a secondary increase in circulation to the remaining patent vessels. Pathologic examination of involved blood vessels reveals thickening of the walls of dermal capillaries with subsequent narrowing of the lumina. Livedo reticularis is associated with anticardiolipin antibodies and cerebrovascular disease.[69] Occlusion can result in ischemia and tissue infarction resulting in purpuric macules, cutaneous nodules, or painful ulcerations; this is often called lupus or livedo vasculitis. It usually occurs on the lower legs, about the ankles and the dorsa of the feet.

Telangiectasias are common findings in patients with lupus, typically appearing on the face. Telangiectasias consist of discrete dilated blood vessels and do not represent an active (inflammatory) lupus lesion. The blood vessels appear more prominent whenever there is an increased blood supply to the area, as when one blushes or is in a hot environment (e.g., shower), or takes vasodilators (e.g., alcohol). Histopathologic examination reveals dilated blood vessels without any feature suggesting inflammation. Telangiectasias are not specific for lupus and can be seen in association with solar damage, aging, hypertension, alcoholism, local pressure (e.g., glasses), diabetes, and other rheumatic diseases.

Raynaud's phenomenon occurs in approximately 17 to 30 percent of patients[15, 59] and is characterized by blanching of the nail beds, fingers, and toes (and occasionally ears, nose, and tongue), with accompanying pain. This phase is due to vasospasm of small to medium-sized arteries and is induced by exposure to cold, cigarette smoke, increased viscosity, low perfusion pressure, or stress. As the ischemia progresses, a bluish mottled cyanosis may ensue—or the vasospasm ends leaving a normal skin color. When ischemia persists, local anoxia develops with build-up of local carbon dioxide. As the level becomes critical, vasodilatation ensues with resultant pain and erythema. A rare outcome of persistent Raynaud's phenomenon is gangrene.

Vasculitis develops in at least 20 percent of SLE patients.[59, 60] Perhaps the most common (10–14 percent) form is urticaria. Urticaria is often a manifestation of an IgE-mediated allergic reaction lasting 4 to 6 hours and resolving without residue. Urticaria due to vasculitis results from fibrinoid necrosis of postcapillary venules. Lesions may persist for more than 24 hours and frequently have painful petechiae. They may heal with hyperpigmentation. Immune complexes form in the endothelial lining and cause fibrinoid necrosis. Complexes are cleared within a day or two. Lesions are infiltrated either with poly-morphonuclear leukocytes or with mononuclear cells. In the former situation, there are often associated cryoglobulins, elevated serum levels of immune complexes, and low levels of CH50, Clq, and C4, but normal levels of C3[70]; in the latter, these immune abnormalities are infrequent. SLE patients may also develop purpura as a manifestation of postvenule capillary vasculitis,[70] with a similar serologic picture.

The diagnosis of urticarial/purpuric vasculitis, in contrast with other forms of urticaria and purpura, lies in excluding thrombocytopenic purpura and performing a biopsy of the lesion.

Vasculitis may also affect small arteries, resulting in small microinfarcts of the tips of the fingers, toes, cuticles of the nailfolds (splinter hemorrhages), and extensor surface of the forearm—lesions are less uncommon on the palms of the hand, soles of the feet, or around the ankle.[15, 57] In the latter situation they may develop into painful punched-out ulcers and heal slowly. This form of vasculitis parallels general lupus activity and is usually associated with circulating immune complexes, low levels of serum complement, and elevated levels of anti-DNA antibodies. Pathologic examination of these lesions demonstrates fibrinoid necrosis and thrombosis, but a sparse cellular infiltrate—in contrast with the vasculitis discussed before. Serum antibodies to cardiolipin[71] and antibodies affecting endothelial cells and subsequently prostacyclin and platelet aggregation may play a pathogenic role.[72]

Painful, tender, erythematous, indurated lesions on the palms, especially on thenar eminences (Janeway spots) and the tips of the fingers (Osler's nodes), are uncommon and represent other manifestations of vasculitis. Sepsis should always be ruled out.

Atrophie blanche lesions have been noted in SLE.[60] They are ivory-white plaques with telangiectasia with surrounding hyperpigmentation. They begin as either erythematous papules or infiltrated lesions, or represent healed small ulcerations. The lesions may be the end result of various forms of vasculitis (not necessarily SLE). Immunoglobulins and complement have been noted in blood vessels in lesions.

Chilblain lupus (pernio) lesions are slightly tender, reddish blue nodules on the toes, fingers, heels, and calves that occur in cold weather.[60] The lesions have been noted in 10 percent of SLE patients and are thought to be secondary to chronic vasospasm.

Perhaps one of the most common cutaneous lesions of SLE patients is steroid-induced ecchymoses. These are noted in many patients. This condition results from the skin atrophy associated with long-term steroid therapy.

Pulmonary Manifestations

Involvement of the lung, its vasculature, the pleura, and the diaphragm, and breathing problems occur in 0.9 percent to 98 percent of patients.[73, 74]

Pleurisy, coughing, or dyspnea is often the first clue to either lung involvement or SLE itself. On the other hand, abnormal pulmonary function tests or abnormal chest radiographs may be accidentally detected in the absence of symptoms. Pulmonary abnormalities do not correlate with immune parameters.[75]

Chest pain on breathing occurs in approximately 50 percent of patients.[57, 76] In our experience, the most common source of chest pain is muscles, connective tissues, or the costochondral joints (costochondritis, Tietze's syndrome). Chest wall pain is characterized by painful deep breaths and is aggravated by motion and change of position (especially during sleep), and is elucidated by palpation of the painful area. The patient can be reassured that this specific pain does not represent lung involvement.

On the other hand, pleuritis, that is, inflammation of the pleura, may cause chest pain in the absence of a friction rub or radiographic pleural effusion. In this circumstance it is often difficult, if not impossible, to determine that the chest pain does, indeed, represent pleuritis. The presence of a rub, which is often very transient, facilitates the diagnosis. A pleural effusion, however, substantially enhances the probability of pleuritis. In one series of patients, 44 percent had pleurisy but only 20 percent had an effusion.[73] The effusion is usually small or moderate, although large effusions have been noted. Table 61–4 gives characteristics of pleural effusion in different conditions. Lymphocytes predominate in lupus effusions. Low complement levels characterize LE (and rheumatoid arthritis) effusions; the presence of rheumatoid factor suggests rheumatoid arthritis (RA). Pathologic examination of the pleura generally reveals some mononuclear cells.

Cough is often the only clue to pulmonary involvement. In our experience cough is usually due to an upper respiratory infection, usually viral. Infections are more prevalent in lupus patients per se and even more common in those taking glucocorticoid or immunosuppressive medications.[77]

Pulmonary edema may occur secondary to cardiac or renal failure or from fluid overload in a patient with mild renal insufficiency receiving glucocorticoids. The patient may have pleural effusions (usually bilateral) and confluent fluffy perihilar infiltrates.[76]

Acute lupus pneumonitis is an uncommon (5–12 percent) manifestation of SLE.[78] It is characterized by fever, cough (sometimes with hemoptysis), pleurisy, dyspnea, pulmonary infiltrates on radiograph (diffuse acinar infiltrates especially on the lower lungs), and significantly, no apparent infection (that is, a pathogen could not be cultured or isolated). The prognosis is poor, with a 50 percent short-term mortality rate; survivors have persistent pulmonary function abnormalities including severe restrictive ventilatory defects. Pathologic examination reveals acute alveolar wall injury, alveolar hemorrhage, alveolar edema, hyaline membrane formation, and immunoglobulin and complement deposition.[76] Some authors have doubted the existence of this syndrome, unless either interstitial fibrosis, vasculitis, hematoxylin bodies, interstitial pneumonitis, alveolitis, or pleuritis could be demonstrated.[79] Lupus pneumonitis may occur in the postpartum period, and has a poor prognosis.[76]

Chronic (fibrotic) lupus pneumonitis has been noted in 0 to 9 percent of series.[76] The syndrome is characterized by progressive dyspnea and diffuse interstitial infiltrates. Pulmonary function studies show a restricted pattern with reduction in lung volume and in carbon monoxide–diffusing capacity. This syndrome should be differentiated from pulmonary edema, adult respiratory distress syndrome, bilateral pneumonia, interstitial fibrosis, infection, malignancy, and granulomatous disease. Useful in this respect is a lung biopsy. Bronchoalveolar lavage findings of greater than 10 percent neutrophils are suggestive of chronic lupus pneumonitis rather than some of these other conditions. Nevertheless, the clinical and pathologic findings in this syndrome are quite similar to those of idiopathic pulmonary fibrosis. Generally other clinical and serologic features of SLE facilitate the diagnosis. The prognosis is poor.

Pulmonary hypertension is sometimes a compli-

Table 61–4. PLEURAL EFFUSIONS

	SLE	CHF	Infections	Malignancy	RA
Symptoms	Pleurisy	Dyspnea	Pleurisy	Varied	Pleurisy
Fluid					
Clarity	Clear	Clear	Cloudy	Variable	Variable
Protein	Low	Low	High	High	High
Glucose	Normal	Normal	Low	Normal >Low	Low
Red cells	0	0	±	+	0
White cells	3000–5000	<10,000	↑	↑	↑
Complement	↓↓↓	↓	Normal	Normal	↓↓
Immune complex	↑↑	Normal	Normal	Normal	↑↑
ANA	Positive	0	0	0	±
LDH	↑	Low	↑	↑↑	↑↑
RF	0	0	0	0	↑

CHF, Congestive heart failure; RF, rheumatoid factor.
Adapted from Lawrence, E. C.: Systemic lupus erythematosus and the lung. *In* Lahita, R. G. (ed.): Systemic Lupus Erythematosus. New York, John Wiley & Sons, 1987. Copyright © 1987 John Wiley & Sons, Inc. Reprinted by permission of John Wiley & Sons, Inc.

cation of SLE, although more frequently associated with scleroderma, mixed connective tissue disease (MCTD), or RA.[76] Patients are dyspneic, mildly hypoxemic, have clear chest radiographs, and demonstrate a restricted pattern and a reduced carbon dioxide–diffusing capacity. Diffusing abnormalities have been observed in 40 to 67 percent of patients without any symptomatology.[80] Raynaud's phenomenon commonly occurs. The clinical picture is suggestive of a fibrotic process and, therefore, not surprisingly resistant to treatment and associated with a poor prognosis.

The shrinking or vanishing lung syndrome has been noted in some patients. This syndrome is characterized by a progressive decrease in lung volume. The primary lesion appears to be a myositis or myopathy affecting both diaphragms, resulting in their elevation and poor function.[80] Pleural adhesions or basilar atelectasis may also play a role.[76] The syndrome should be suspected in individuals with dyspnea whose chest radiographs are clear.

Pulmonary hemorrhage, not necessarily with hemoptysis, has been noted.[81] Patients are acutely ill and have glomerulonephritis, dyspnea, cough, and bilateral pulmonary infiltrates. The prognosis is poor.

Cardiovascular Manifestations

Pericardial involvement is often suspected by the presence of ECG abnormalities or the detection of fluid on echocardiography.[82] The pericardial involvement may be asymptomatic. Pericarditis, manifesting itself either as an audible rub or as positional substernal chest pain, has been noted in 8 to 48 percent of large series of SLE patients.[83] Large effusions, suggestive of tamponade, are rare as is constrictive pericarditis.[15, 73, 83] Pericardial involvement has been noted in 80 percent of autopsy cases.[15] Pericardial fluid is a fibrinous exudate or transudate and has characteristics similar to those of pleural fluid (see Table 61–4). Immunologic abnormalities have been noted, including antinuclear antibodies, LE cells, low complement levels, and immune complexes. The pericardium may reveal foci of inflammatory lesions with immune complexes, but usually mononuclear cells predominate—or healed fibrous residua.

Myocarditis has been noted in 8 to 78 percent of large series.[83] Myocarditis should be suspected if there is resting tachycardia disproportionate to body temperature, ECG abnormalities (e.g., ST-T wave abnormalities), and unexplained cardiomegaly—the latter may result in symptoms and signs of congestive heart failure, conduction abnormalities, and arrhythmias. Acute myocarditis may accompany other manifestations of acute SLE, particularly pericarditis. Pathologically there is infiltration of the myocardium with mononuclear cells[83] resolving as fibrosis—but with continued cardiac dysfunction. Myocarditis has

been associated by some with antibodies to RNP and MCTD.[84]

Coronary artery disease has been recognized in 2 to 8 percent of large series of SLE cases.[57, 83, 85, 86] Rubin et al.[87] have pointed out the bimodal character of deaths due to SLE, noting that death in those with disease longer than 2.5 years was more likely to be due to myocardial infarction than to SLE. In the experience of this author and others,[15, 46] clinical coronary artery disease, with angina, myocardial infarction, and congestive heart failure, is becoming an increasing problem, particularly in the (young) patient with long-standing SLE, and especially in those maintained on glucocorticoids. Hypertension is often an accompanying problem. The mechanism for the premature atherosclerosis is not clear. It has been postulated, but rarely demonstrated,[88] that arteritis of the coronary arteries, with accompanying immune complex deposition, may predispose to atherosclerosis plaque formation, a process that may be aggravated by hypertension, glucocorticoid administration, and lipid abnormalities.[89]

Clinical valvular disease may be more common than previously appreciated.[90] Mitral valve prolapse has been observed in 25 percent of patients and 9 percent of controls.[91] Systolic murmurs have been noted in 16 to 44 percent of patients,[46, 57, 83] and may represent a response to anemia, fever, tachycardia, or cardiomegaly. On the other hand, diastolic murmurs have been noted in 1 to 3 percent of patients and often reflect aortic or mitral insufficiency.[46] Echocardiography is often useful in detecting Libman-Sacks (verrucous) endocarditis. The verrucae are usually near the edge of the valve and consist of accumulations of immune complexes, mononuclear cells, hematoxylin bodies, and fibrin and platelet thrombi. The most likely valves to be involved are the mitral, the aortic, and the tricuspid.[83] Healing usually leads to fibrosis, scarring, and even calcification. Some patients require valvular replacement because of heart failure. Bacterial endocarditis may develop on already damaged valves.[46, 57, 83] Therefore, the development of a fever and new murmur in a patient with SLE should warrant blood cultures and an echocardiogram to rule out an infectious endocarditis.

Thrombophlebitis is reported in about 10 percent of patients with SLE.[15] It generally involves the lower extremity but on occasion has been observed to affect the renal veins and inferior vena cava.[46] Pulmonary embolism is rare.[92] Thrombophlebitis may be due to antiphospholipid antibodies or the use of birth-control medications, particularly in association with smoking cigarettes.

Conduction defects have been noted in 34 to 70 percent of patients[46, 71] and may represent pericarditis or myocarditis. First-degree heart block is often transient, but higher degree heart block, or arrhythmias (e.g., atrial fibrillation), are unusual.[46, 57, 83] Autopsies have revealed focal inflammatory cells but more often fibrous scarring of the conduction system.[83] Congenital heart block may be part of the neonatal lupus syndrome. Many mothers of these infants have either SLE or Sjögren's syndrome, antibodies to Ro(SS-A) or La(SS-B), and are HLA-DR3.[66] The anti-Ro/La antibodies may prevent the normal development of the conduction fibers.

Hypertension develops in many patients. Hypertension may be due to the use of high doses of steroids for protracted periods and chronic renal disease. As renal disease is treated with glucocorticoids, a vicious cycle of nephritis, hypertension, and worsening of renal function may ensue. The sudden onset of hypertension may suggest a flare of nephritis. Interruption of this cycle by various means, including control of hypertension, will prolong (renal) survival.

Hematologic Considerations

Abnormalities of the formed elements of the blood and the clotting, fibrinolytic, and related systems are very common in lupus patients. Anemia may reflect inflammation, renal insufficiency, blood loss, dietary insufficiency, medications, immune mechanisms (hemolysis), or combinations thereof and occurs in approximately 50 percent of patients.[93, 94] The most frequent cause is suppressed erythropoiesis from chronic inflammation or uremia. The anemia is normocytic and normochromic; the reticulocyte count is relatively low for the degree of anemia; serum iron levels may be low, though bone marrow stores are more than adequate. Anemia may reflect acute or chronic blood loss from the gastrointestinal tract, usually secondary to medication, or may be due to excessive menstrual bleeding. Iron deficiency anemia is not uncommon, especially among teenagers or young women. Red cell aplasia has been observed, probably due to antibodies directed against erythroblasts.[138] Medications, including antimalarials and immunosuppressives, can cause bone marrow suppression.

Hemolytic anemia, characterized by an elevated reticulocyte count, low haptoglobin levels, and a positive direct Coombs' test has been noted in 10 to 40 percent of patients.[94] Presence of both immunoglobulin and complement on the red cell is usually associated with some degree of hemolysis, while the presence of only complement (e.g., C3 or C4) is often not associated with hemolysis.[93, 94] Antibodies are "warm," IgG, and are directed against Rh determinants. IgM-mediated cold agglutinin hemolysis is uncommon.

Leukopenia, that is, a white blood cell count of less than 4500, has been noted in 50 to 60 percent of patients,[93, 94] while leukopenia of less than 4000 (the ARA criterion) was observed in only 17 percent of patients.[15] Leukopenia can result from immune mechanisms, medications, and bone marrow dysfunctions. A greater deficiency of granulocytes than lymphocytes is usually found. Functional neutrophil defects have been noted but are thought to usually reflect serologic immune abnormalities (e.g., immune complexes, complement activation) or medications (e.g., glucocorticoids, immunosuppressives).[94–96] The number of basophils may also be decreased, particularly during active SLE.[97] Basophil degranulation with release of platelet activating factor (PAF) and other mediators may play a role in immune complex deposition and vascular permeability. Leukocytosis (mostly granulocytes) usually reflects infection or the use of glucocorticoids (in high doses), although it has occasionally been seen during acute exacerbations of SLE. A shift of granulocytes to more immature forms (a "left" shift) suggests infection.

Lymphocytopenia (i.e., a count of fewer than 1500 cells) of B cells and T cells (especially of suppressor T cells) has been observed in 84 percent of patients, particularly during active disease.[93, 94, 98] Lymphopenia is strongly associated with IgM, cold reactive, complement fixing, and presumably cytotoxic antilymphocyte antibodies. Some of these antibodies have specificities to T suppressor cells or to other antigen specificities—which may affect lymphocyte function.

Mild thrombocytopenia (platelet counts between 100,000 and 150,000 cells) has been noted in 25 to 50 percent of patients, while counts of fewer than 50,000 cells were noted in only 10 percent.[93] Thrombocytopenia may be due to myeloproliferative mechanisms (e.g., a megarkaryocyte defect, drugs), ineffective thrombopoiesis (e.g., megaloblastic anemia), abnormal platelet distribution (e.g., congestive splenomegaly), dilutional effects, and abnormal platelet destruction (consumptive as in disseminated intravascular coagulation [DIC], thrombotic thrombocytopenic purpura [TTP], and vasculitis; and immune mediated as in idiopathic thrombocytopenic purpura [ITP], infections, and drug induced). SLE may first manifest itself as ITP, followed by symptoms of SLE only many years later. SLE may develop after splenectomy for ITP, but there is no evidence that the splenectomy has any effect on the subsequent development of SLE as was suggested earlier. Most patients with both autoimmune thrombocytopenia and autoimmune hemolytic anemia (Evans' syndrome) have SLE. Thrombocytopenia in SLE is usually due to antiplatelet antibodies, causing them to be phagocytosed by macrophages through their Fc receptor in the spleen. The spleen is also a major site of antiplatelet antibody production. Clinically, platelet counts of fewer than 50,000 cells rarely cause more than a prolonged bleeding time, while counts of fewer than 20,000 cells may be associated with (and account for) petechiae, purpura, epistaxis, and gingival and other clinical bleeding.

Lymphadenopathy occurs in approximately 50 percent of patients. The nodes are typically soft, nontender, discrete, varying in size from 0.5 to several centimeters, and usually detected in the cervical, axillary, and inguinal areas. Lymphadenopathy is more frequently noted at the onset of disease or in association with an exacerbation. Biopsies reveal areas of follicular hyperplasia and necrosis. The (uncommon) appearance of hematoxylin bodies is highly suggestive of SLE. Hilar lymph node enlargement due to SLE is rare. Enlarged cervical nodes are also observed with upper respiratory tract infections, in the axilla in association with infections secondary to the use of antiperspirants, and in the inguinal region with pelvic inflammatory or infectious processes. When infections are present, the enlarged nodes are more likely to be tender. In the teenager experiencing fatigue and fever, infectious mononucleosis is often diagnosed (often with a positive test for antinuclear antibodies!). Enlarged nodes may represent a lymphoproliferative malignancy; when in doubt, biopsy.

Splenomegaly occurs in 10 to 20 percent of patients, particularly during active disease. Splenomegaly is not necessarily associated with hemolytic anemia. Patients who have had a splenectomy are particularly susceptible to pneumococcal sepsis—which has a high mortality rate. Pathologic examination of the spleen reveals an onion-skin appearance of the splenic arteries. This type of lesion is thought to represent healed vasculitis.

There is no apparent increase of lymphoproliferative or other malignancies in patients with SLE, although there is concern that (prolonged) therapy with immunosuppressive agents (e.g., cyclophosphamide) may favor the development of such malignancies.[93, 94]

Antibodies to a number of clotting factors, including factors VIII, IX, XI, XII, and XIII,[93, 94] have been noted in SLE patients. These antibodies not only may cause abnormalities of in vitro coagulation tests but also may cause bleeding. More common is the so-called lupus anticoagulant. This antibody is found in up to 25 percent of patients with SLE.[99] It is not associated with bleeding, except when thrombocytopenia is present. Patients with the lupus anticoagulant are more likely to be thrombocytopenic, have a positive Coombs' test, and have a false-positive test for syphilis. The lupus anticoagulant is usually recognized by a prolonged partial thromboplastin time (PTT), specifically when (diluted) patient plasma will prolong the PTT of a normal plasma, or a Russell's viper venom test. The lupus anticoagulant is found in individuals who also do not have SLE. The antibody (IgG or IgM) acts at the junction of the intrinsic and extrinsic coagulation pathways by blocking the activation of a prothrombin activator complex (consisting of factors Xa and V, calcium, and phospholipid—also known as platelet factor 3). The antibodies to this phospholipid cross-react with cardiolipin, accounting for the strong association between the presence of the circulating anticoagulant and false positive tests for syphilis. However, the lupus anticoagulant has not been observed in patients with syphilis. The name lupus anticoagulant is a misnomer, because it is associated with thrombotic disease. Because of the coagulation abnormalities it is often difficult to monitor therapeutic anticoagulant activity

in patients with this antibody. Antibodies to cardiolipin detected by solid phase immunoassay are found in up to 54 percent of SLE patients. There is a moderately strong association between IgG antibodies to cardiolipin and thrombocytopenia, arterial and venous thrombosis (including cerebrovascular accident), and midtrimester miscarriages.[99] Most SLE patients with antiphospholipid antibodies have an abnormal lupus anticoagulant and anticardiolipin antibody test; however, in approximately 10 percent of patients only one test will be (significantly) abnormal. Not all individuals with antibodies to phospholipid have lupus.[99, 100]

False-positive tests for syphilis have been noted in up to 25 percent of patients and may precede all other manifestations of SLE.[83] A false-positive test should be considered in an individual with a positive screening test who denies syphilis, for example, the Venereal Disease Research Laboratory test (VDRL), Hinton's test, and rapid plasma reagin test (RPR). The "false" nature of the test is confirmed when either a treponemal immobilization test (TPI) or a fluorescent treponemal antibody absorption test (FTA-ABS) is found to be negative. There are no indications for performing a test for syphilis in a patient with SLE, unless syphilis is suspected.

The erythrocyte sedimentation rate (ESR) is elevated in virtually all patients with SLE, particularly during active disease. The ESR has been noted to correlate with clinical activity by some but not by myself or others. On the other hand, a normal ESR speaks against active inflammation.

Genital-Renal-Urinary

Clinical lupus nephritis develops in approximately 50 percent of patients[101, 102] and is characterized by the presence of either urinary or functional (clearance) abnormalities. However, virtually all SLE patients exhibit histologic renal abnormalities by either immunofluorescence or electron microscopy, while not (necessarily) demonstrating any abnormalities on light microscopy. These immune abnormalities do not necessarily constitute nephritis.[43] Although lupus nephritis is often asymptomatic, its presence is cause for concern, for it can be associated with a poor prognosis. However, it is important to recognize that the spectra and severity of renal disease vary considerably from patient to patient—a fact that has both prognostic and therapeutic implications.

Proteinuria is the most common renal abnormality in patients, occurring at some time in 78 percent of patients.[15] In addition, 42 percent had hematuria or pyuria (i.e., more than five cells per high-powered field). Hyaline, granular, or cellular casts are noted in about 30 to 35 percent of patients. Most of the renal abnormalities were present during the first 6 to 36 months of illness after diagnosis.[103] Azotemia develops in approximately 30 percent of patients but is uncommon early in the disease. More refined definition of renal function can be ascertained by determining the amount of urinary protein excreted per 24 hours as well as determining the glomerular filtration rate.

Considerable attention has focused on the classification of renal pathology. The most common classification scheme is that promulgated by the World Health Organization (WHO) and modified slightly by Kent and Pollak[101] (Table 61–5). Approximately 24 percent of patients have either minimal or mesangial lupus nephritis. Those with minimal disease (type IIA) usually have immune deposits only in the mesangial area, which are detected by either electron microscopy or immunofluorescence, without any other light microscopic or renal function abnormalities. On the other hand, patients with mesangial nephritis (type IIB) will not only exhibit the immune deposits but demonstrate segmental or global, focal, or diffuse hypercellularity in the mesangial area. Occasional immune (of IgG or C3) deposits may be seen along the glomerular basement membrane or in the subendothelial area.

Focal proliferative nephritis is seen in approximately 15 percent of patients.[101] Fewer than 50 percent of the glomerular tufts are affected. There is usually segmental proliferation in glomerular tufts as well as proliferation in the mesangial area. Immunofluorescence and electron microscopy reveal immunoglobulins (especially IgG) and C3 in the mesangium as well as scattered granular deposits in the subendothelial, subepithelial, and intrabasement membrane areas.

Diffuse proliferative glomerulonephritis is seen in approximately 43 percent of patients.[101] Fifty percent or more of glomerular tufts are affected by hypercellularity, especially of mesangial cells, endothelial cells, monocytes, and neutrophils. Necrotizing changes and epithelial crescents of various sizes are common. Hyaline thrombi, consisting of IgG, IgM, perhaps complement, but especially fibrin, may be noted in capillary lumina of 50 percent of patients. Patients with these thrombi are particularly likely to develop glomerular sclerosis.[101] Tubular degenerative changes with interstitial accumulation of mononuclear cells are not uncommon. Immunofluorescence and electron microscopy reveal extensive granules and lumpy deposits of immunoglobulins and complement in the mesangial area but particularly along the glomerular basement membrane, especially on the endothelial side. These extensive endothelial and intramembranous deposits correspond to wire loops.

Both the Cincinnati[101] and National Institutes of Health (NIH)[104] groups have stressed the importance of determining whether the lesions represent active inflammation or inactive chronic lesions (Table 61–6), those findings being thought to have both prognostic and therapeutic implications. Glomerular thrombi and extensive subendothelial deposits herald progression to glomerular sclerosis and end-stage renal disease.

Membranous glomerulonephritis occurs in approximately 15 percent of patients.[101] There is very little if any cellular proliferation or infiltration. Rather, there is a diffuse, fairly uniform thickening of the glomerular basement membrane. Immunofluorescence and electron microscopy reveal immunoglobulins and complement components all along the

Table 61–5. LUPUS NEPHRITIS: SUMMARY OF CLINICAL FEATURES AND COURSE

	Focal Proliferative	Diffuse Proliferative (DPLN)	Membranous (MLN)	Mesangial (MesLN)
Onset	During 1st year SLE in about half	During 1st year SLE in the majority	During 1st year SLE in half	Perhaps characteristic of all SLE from onset
Clinical manifestations	Proteinuria in all, hematuria often. Nephrotic syndrome rare. Occasional mild renal insufficiency. Hypertension absent	Proteinuria and hematuria in all. Nephrotic syndrome at onset in over half, eventually in almost all. Renal insufficiency at onset in most; occasionally severe. Hypertension not common	Proteinuria in all at onset with rare exceptions. Nephrotic syndrome at onset in half, eventually in four fifths. Microscopic hematuria in half. Occasional hypertension and minimal renal insufficiency at onset	No clinical features of renal disease in some; minimal proteinuria and/or hematuria in others. Occasional mild renal insufficiency. Hypertension absent
Transition	Transitions to DPLN or MLN may occur	Transition to MesLN (with some glomerular sclerosis) or MLN may occur in association with remission	Rare transition to DPLN	Development of nephrotic syndrome with transition to DPLN or MLN may occur
Progression	Renal insufficiency does not develop	Progression to death within 2 years in half of the unremitted. Death due to uremia or of active SLE, often with infection. No progressive renal insufficiency during remission	Slowly progressive renal insufficiency during persistent nephrotic syndrome	No progression unless transition occurs; subsequent course then determined by the form of lupus nephritis that develops
Mortality	5-year mortality <10%	5-year mortality <25%	5-year mortality <25%	—
Pathology	Focal mild proliferative; IgG and C3 in mesangium	Cell proliferation; crescents. Lumpy bumpy Ig and C along GBM (subendothelial)	Thick GBM. Granular Ig and C on GBM (epithelial side)	Ig and C in mesangium

GBM, Glomerular basement membrane.

Table 61-6. PATHOLOGIC EVIDENCE OF INFLAMMATORY ACTIVITY IN RENAL LESION

Active Lesions	Inactive (Chronic) Lesions
Glomerulus	
Cellular proliferation	Basement thickening
Necrosis	Subepithelial deposits
Karyorrhexis	Sclerosis
Wire loops	Adhesions
Subendothelial deposits	Fibrous crescents
Hematoxyphil bodies	
Thrombi	
Epithelial crescents	
Tubulointerstitial	
Mononuclear cell infiltration	Interstitial fibrosis
Fibrinoid changes in	Tubular atrophy
arterioles	Arteriolar sclerosis

Data from Pollak and Kant[101] and Austin et al.[104]

glomerular basement membrane in a fine granular pattern, especially in the subendothelial region, beneath the fused foot processes. Intramembranous deposits are also common, as are mesangial deposits.

Tubulointerstitial disease and interstitial inflammation may be seen in 75 percent of patients and may cause tubular damage, fibrosis, and atrophy.[105] There is a predominance of mononuclear cell infiltration as well as immune deposits along the tubular basement membrane. In the majority of cases, the severity of the lesions parallels the degree of involvement of the glomerular lesion.

It is vital to remember that patients with SLE are infection-prone, a problem compounded by the use of medications that may decrease the host resistance to infections. Therefore, urinary tract infections are a frequent problem in SLE patients. Renal complications may also ensue with the use of nonsteroidal anti-inflammatory drugs (NSAIDs), which have on rare occasions been noted to cause either azotemia, proteinuria, or renal failure.[102]

Etiologic Considerations. There is considerable evidence that immune complexes cause mesangial, proliferative, and membranous nephritis. In the former two circumstances, immune complexes (consisting predominantly of IgG anti-DNA and complement) form in the circulation and deposit along the glomerular basement membrane. Complement activation causes the release of chemotactic factors that cause phagocytic cells to invade wherever the immune complexes have deposited, and during phagocytosis, to release enzymes that cause further tissue injury. In membranous nephritis, complexes appear to form in situ.[106] However, no cellular infiltrate ensues, despite the presence of complement in the lesions. Fibrin, its breakdown products, and other components of the clotting system may also contribute to glomerular damage. Patients with circulating anticoagulants may be more prone to develop renal thromboses.

Clinical-Laboratory-Pathologic Associations and the Question of Renal Biopsy. There has been considerable interest, and controversy, regarding the correlations between the pathologic findings, immune abnormalities, renal function, and prognosis.[43, 103, 107–109] Ultimately all of these factors have implications for therapy, whose goal is to maintain renal function. Table 61-7 represents a summary of the author's and others' experience regarding such correlations. The data in the table represent those patients with active nephritis, defined as either showing active inflammatory changes on biopsy[101] or demonstrating the recent onset of renal functional abnormalities.[107]

Patients with mild mesangial proliferation (type IIB) may have some proteinuria and sedimenturia, some decreases in total serum hemolytic complement (CH50) and complement 3 (C3) levels, and some increases in anti-DNA and immune complex levels. Tests of renal clearance are generally normal in these patients.

Patients with focal proliferative nephritis (type III), on the other hand, usually exhibit more severe abnormalities on urinalysis, as well as greater impairments in renal clearance and immune function.

Tests of renal and immune function are even more abnormal in patients with diffuse proliferative nephritis (type IV) (see Table 61-7). It is important to note, however, that some of the urinary and immune abnormalities (especially the derangements in complement and immune complex levels) are present only during active disease. In contrast, proteinuria or abnormal renal clearance may be present during both the active and inactive phases of the disease. Azotemia and creatinine clearances reflect the severity of pathologic lesions better than activity alone.[101] Hypertension and resultant cardiovascular problems as well as, possibly, symptoms of renal failure (i.e., uremia) are more likely to develop in patients with type IV nephritis. Although hypertension may develop in many patients with type III, IV, or V lupus nephritis, it is especially common in those with severe diffuse proliferative lesions, fibrosis, sclerosis, or arteriolar damage.

Patients with membranous nephritis (type V) typically present with the nephrotic syndrome, without abnormalities of urinary sediment, renal clearance, or immune function. Renal vein thrombosis has occurred in SLE patients and may mimic the nephrotic syndrome. Angiography may be required to distinguish the two. Patients with type V nephritis may develop late-onset hypertension and azotemia.

Patients with azotemia secondary to drugs (such as NSAIDs) are generally asymptomatic; renal failure develops only rarely in these patients.

Thus, the pathologic type of renal disease in an individual SLE patient can be predicted, with a reasonable degree of accuracy, by carefully analyzing clinical symptoms and tests of renal and immune function. Small amounts of proteinuria are consistent with type IIB, III, or IV nephritis, whereas proteinuria greater than 3.5 g per day suggests type IV or V

Table 61-7. CORRELATIONS BETWEEN CLINICAL AND LABORATORY FINDINGS AND PATHOLOGIC CLASSIFICATIONS IN LUPUS NEPHRITIS PATIENTS

	Mesangial IIA	Mesangial IIB	Focal Proliferative III	Diffuse Proliferative IV	Membranous V	Tubulo-interstitial	Infection	Drug-Induced
Symptoms	None	None	None	Renal failure Nephrotic syndrome	Nephrotic syndrome	None	Dysuria	Renal failure (rare)
Hypertension	None	None	±	Common	Late-onset	Late-onset	Late-onset	None
Proteinuria g/day	None	<1	<2	1–20	3.5–20	±	±	±
Hematuria RBCs/hpf	None	5–15	5–15	Many	None	±	±	None
Pyuria WBCs/hpf	None	5–15	5–15	Many	None	±	Many	None
Casts	None	±	±	None	None	None	None	None
GFR, ml/min	Nl	Nl	60–80	<60	Nl	Nl	Nl	Nl or ↓
CH50	Nl	↓	↓	↓↓	Nl	Nl	Nl	Nl
C3	Nl	↓	↓	↓↓	Nl	Nl	Nl	Nl
Anti-DNA	Nl	↑	↑	↑↑	Nl	Nl	Nl	Nl
Immune complexes	Nl	↑	↑	↑↑	Nl	Nl	Nl	Nl

RBC = red blood cell; hpf = high power field; WBC = white blood cell; GFR = glomerular filtration rate; CH50 = total serum hemolytic complement (expressed in 50% hemolytic units); C3 = complement 3; Nl = normal; ± = occasional, small amounts; ↑ = somewhat increased; ↑↑ = greatly increased; ↓ = somewhat decreased; ↓↓ = greatly decreased.

nephritis. Sediment (red or white blood cell or other casts) suggests active type IIA, III, or IV renal disease. Patients with hypertension and azotemia probably have type IV nephritis, or at least glomerular sclerosis or fibrosis.

In addition, the presence of certain abnormalities of immune function is suggestive of active renal disease. For example, patients with low CH50 and C3 levels and high anti-DNA and immune complex levels are more likely to have active renal disease than patients without these immune system abnormalities. The presence of active disease is even more likely if these parameters worsen over a few weeks or months, that is, if decreases in CH50 and C3 or increases in anti-DNA and immune complexes are observed.

The diagnosis of lupus nephritis per se obviously depends on the results of a renal biopsy. However, whether a biopsy is indicated in all patients is open to question.[43, 103, 104, 109, 110] My opinion is that SLE patients who exhibit urinary abnormalities (proteinuria, hematuria, casts) or renal clearance abnormalities, especially if coupled with depressed complement levels and elevated anti-DNA or immune complex levels, have lupus nephritis until proven otherwise. In these patients, therefore, a renal biopsy may not be necessary.

However, isolated pyuria, proteinuria, or poor renal clearance may stem from other etiologies, such as infection, glomerulonephritis, rapidly progressive glomerulonephritis, membranoproliferative glomerulonephritis, and drug nephrotoxicity. A renal biopsy may thus be helpful in differentiating lupus nephritis from these other causes.

A more important reason for performing a renal biopsy in patients with lupus nephritis is to determine therapy and assess prognosis.[104] Although diffuse proliferative nephritis (type IV) carries a poor prognosis, some patients with this type of disease have had good responses to pulse steroid therapy or cytotoxic agents.[102, 109] Therefore, knowing that a patient has type IV nephritis might lead the physician to advocate such aggressive therapy. A more important rationale for performing a renal biopsy is to determine whether lesions are acute or chronic and whether the disease is active or inactive. Proliferation of cells suggests activity, whereas atrophy, fibrosis, or sclerosis suggests chronicity.[95, 104] These distinctions may be useful in predicting therapeutic response, since the more acute the process, the more likely it can be at least partially reversed. A biopsy may be particularly helpful in determining whether patients with progressive renal dysfunction that proves unresponsive to conventional therapy should receive more aggressive therapy: a biopsy showing active proliferative lesions provides a rationale for using anti-inflammatory therapy, whereas a biopsy showing only fibrosis and sclerosis suggests that immunosuppressive therapy would likely be futile (see Table 61–6).

Although renal biopsy findings in most patients

with lupus nephritis are similar over months or years, repeat biopsies in some patients may show improvement or worsening.[102] However, these shifts may merely reflect differences in the tissue specimens obtained for biopsy, since lesions in different parts of the kidney may vary in severity.

Prognosis. The prognosis of patients with lupus nephritis has steadily improved in the last few years, probably as the result of better recognition and management. Whereas 20 years ago a patient with lupus nephritis might have survived 1 to 2 years, now more than 80 percent of patients survive for at least 10 years. Patients who have markedly elevated initial serum creatinine levels, who are young, male, who exhibit severe sclerosis and fibrosis on renal biopsy, who have prolonged depression of serum C3 levels (but not elevated anti-DNA levels), who have severe SLE, vasculitis, or hypertension are more likely to develop renal failure.[103, 108, 109] Patients with mesangial or membranous lupus nephritis rarely progress or develop renal failure.[101, 106, 111] In addition, hypertension, a high-protein, high-phosphate, high-lipid diet, and high blood cholesterol and triglycerides may predispose to progressive renal damage. SLE patients undergoing renal transplantation do as well as those with other diseases and have a 70 percent 5-year graft survival rate.[112]

Gastrointestinal Manifestations

Gastrointestinal manifestations occur in approximately 50 percent of patients.[113, 114] Many gastrointestinal symptoms are nonspecific for SLE and may frequently reflect SLE involvement of various organs of the gastrointestinal tract or the effects of medications. The involvement of other organs (namely, skin, joints, kidney, central nervous system, blood, immunologic) often tends to overshadow the gastrointestinal involvement. However, patients often have symptoms that stress the gastrointestinal tract and therefore warrant attention.

The esophagus is involved in 1.5 to 25 percent of patients.[113, 114] The most common complaint is difficulty swallowing. Symptoms are episodic and greatest during periods of stress. Visualization of the oropharynx either directly or by radiography rarely detects anything. Radiographic and manometric studies may reveal abnormalities, but they are generally less severe than those seen in patients with progressive systemic sclerosis (PSS). Patients with dysphagia are more likely to have Raynaud's phenomenon. Dysphagia may also result from gastric acid reflux, hiatus hernia, and esophageal candidiasis—but ulcers of the esophagus have rarely been noted.[83]

Dyspepsia has been noted in approximately 50 percent of patients, while peptic ulcers were present in 40 percent of these individuals.[46] Others have noted a lower incidence.[114] Gross (in contrast with microscopic) hemorrhage is uncommon (9 percent[115]) and perforation rare. Dyspepsia is common in patients taking glucocorticoids. Ulcers, particularly gastric, have been attributed by many authors to steroids,[46, 114] although other reports argue that SLE per se predisposes to ulcer formation. NSAIDs may also cause dyspepsia and aggravate the dyspepsia caused by steroids—indomethacin was the NSAID most likely to do this.

Abdominal pain accompanied by nausea and vomiting may occur in up to 30 percent of patients.[46] The etiology is often obscure, and various diagnostic procedures including blood tests and radiographs will reveal little. Medications should always be considered a cause, but in my experience the symptoms occasionally respond to steroids, suggesting an inflammatory mechanism (e.g., peritonitis).[57, 114] Autopsy studies have revealed frequent (50 percent) peritonitis.[57] Ascites is uncommon, and when present, infection or perforation should be excluded.

Of greater concern is mesenteric vasculitis.[114] Lower abdominal pain is generally insidious and intermittent for months prior to the development of an acute abdomen. During the earlier stages radiographic studies or arteriography may reveal segmental bowel dilatation, vasculitis, or ischemia of the small intestine or colon. Vasculitis generally involves small arteries. Perforations are rare, but catastrophic.

Pancreatitis occurs in about 8 percent of patients.[116] Symptoms include upper abdominal pain, nausea and vomiting, and an increase in serum amylase. It should be noted, however, that elevated levels of serum amylase have been detected in the absence of pancreatitis.[116] Pancreatitis is usually seen in the presence of active lupus elsewhere and may be due, at least in part, to vasculitis. Such cases have been described in patients not receiving steroids,[116] receiving steroids, and receiving azathioprine.

Hepatomegaly has been reported in up to 50 percent of patients,[15, 113, 114] although this generally refers to a palpable liver and may not in fact represent an enlarged liver. The liver is usually not tender to palpation. Jaundice is rare, and may in fact reflect hemolysis. On the other hand, liver chemistries (serum glutamic-oxaloacetic transaminase [SGOT], serum glutamic-pyruvic transaminase [SGPT], LDH, alkaline phosphatase) may be abnormal in patients with active lupus or in patients taking NSAIDs. Liver biopsies of patients with persistent liver chemistry abnormalities revealed cirrhosis, chronic active hepatitis, granulomatous hepatitis, cholestasis, centrilobular necrosis, chronic persistent hepatitis, primary biliary cirrhosis, steatosis, fatty liver, and drug toxicity, but no evidence for hepatitis B infection.[117] These studies suggest that liver disease may be due to lupus, coincident to lupus, or represent "lupoid hepatitis" (autoimmune chronic active hepatitis).

Neuropsychiatric Manifestations

Neuropsychiatric symptoms occur in anywhere from 25 to 80 percent of patients either prior to the diagnosis of LE or during the course of their illness.[15, 118–123] The symptoms are varied (Table 61–8). Of particular concern has been the difficulty in determining which symptoms are functional, which represent an organic abnormality, which are due to SLE, which are active (and inactive), and which have other causes. Unfortunately, to date, there remain only many descriptions (with few definitions of terms), no uniformly agreed on diagnostic criteria, a dearth of definitive laboratory or diagnostic tests, and the inability to study the brain anatomically or pathologically. Therefore, it becomes difficult to assign etiology or to be definitive regarding therapy. Given these limitations, we must assign probabilities regarding etiology and pathogenesis for each symptom. What I have tried to do here is describe the broad spectrum of neuropsychiatric aspects of lupus, from that which is usually functional to that which may be either functional or organic, and those aspects which are usually organic (see Table 61–8) and diagnostic maneuvers that may help differentiate functional from organic causes.

Functional Abnormalities

The most common symptom is depression. The depression is usually acute and represents a reaction to being ill and the realization that one may not ever be well again, enduring limitations placed on the things we take for granted in life (e.g., having children, the stamina necessary for raising them, enjoying a sunbath). Most patients recover within a year with the help of family, friends, physicians, or other professionals. Others may incorporate the depression into their personality, resulting in many concurrent (psycho)somatic complaints: insomnia, anorexia, constipation, myalgia, arthralgia, and fatigue. The depression can become "psychotic," with increasing despair, loss of hope, and even suicidal tendencies. Prompt intervention is essential.

Other patients may manifest symptoms of anxiety, either instead of or in addition to depression, often after the initial diagnosis or after an exacerba-

Table 61–8. NEUROPSYCHIATRIC MANIFESTATIONS

Generally Functional Etiology	Functional or Organic Etiology	Organic Etiology
Depression	Psychosis	Seizures 10–15%
Hypomania/ mania	Cognitive disorder	Neuropathy 10–15%
Anxiety	Dysesthesia	CVA/stroke/ paralysis 15%
Conversion reaction	Headache 10–35% have migrains	Movement disorders <5%
Affective disorder		Organic brain syndrome
Mood swing		Coma
Adjustment disorder		Transverse myelitis
		Meningitis

Data from references 118 through 122.

tion. The patient becomes anxious about disfigurement, disability, dependency, loss of a job, becoming isolated, or death. The anxiety may also manifest itself in (psycho)somatic ways, including palpitations, diarrhea, sweating, hyperventilation, dizzy spells, difficulty with speech, memory, or words, fear of "going crazy," and headaches. The anxious state may deteriorate into obsessive-compulsive behavior, phobias, hypochondriasis, and sleep disturbances.

Manic behavior characterized by a marked increase in energy, a hyper-rush of activity, irritability, and sleeplessness may on occasion be seen. Such behavior is usually due to usage of high doses of steroids.

Patients are often labeled as hysterical prior to the "diagnosis" of lupus, often presenting their symptoms in a dramatic manner, having incorporated the symptoms into their daily life. They may go from doctor to doctor seeking explanations, convinced that their symptoms cannot be explained by known biologic processes and hanging on to any positive laboratory test to confirm their suspicions. This pattern is often initiated and perpetuated by episodes of stress with which the patient cannot deal appropriately or adequately. Patients often (50–75 percent) report that psychologic stress precipitated the onset of their illness.[119] As stress may affect the immune system, stress may influence the development of immune abnormalities in SLE. On the other hand, many of the symptoms turn out to be the first signs of organic disease. Patients often relate (realistically) a long history of frustration in obtaining the proper diagnosis.[119] Unfortunately, physicians often dislike patients with symptoms and signs suggesting organic brain syndrome.[124]

These psychologic symptoms are thought to reflect functional disorders rather than representing organic disease. They are thought to represent the dynamic way an individual deals with the stresses of a chronic illness and the inner conflict and turmoil which that engenders. The specific psychologic pattern that ensues (depression, anxiety, mania, etc.) probably reflects that person's inner make-up rather than the specific disease process. Nevertheless, organic involvement, presumably by SLE, may manifest itself in these psychologic ways.[122] The evidence for organic involvement is based on abnormal results in tests of cognitive function, psychologic testing, computed tomography (CT) scans, radionuclide scans, single photon emission computerized tomography (SPECT) scans, evoked potentials, electroencephalograms (EEGs), cerebrospinal fluid (CSF) analysis, and a psychiatric interview.[122, 125] Of concern, diagnostically, are those individuals who have cognitive impairment recognized by neuropsychologic tests without other apparent neuropsychiatric symptoms. Cognitive impairment appears to be independent of psychologic distress and is common (80 percent).[122]

Organic (Neurologic Abnormalities)

Psychosis probably occurs in fewer than 24 percent of patients.[119] Psychosis is defined as a disturbance in mental functioning characterized by disordered, bizarre thinking, often including delusions and hallucinations. Psychosis will lead to increasing difficulty in coping with the demands of everyday living. Psychosis may present as "delirium," or as a "clouding of the consciousness."[121] Symptoms often fluctuate but are more likely to develop at night. Patients have poor attention span, are easily distracted, misinterpret their surroundings, may hallucinate, and may even become agitated and combative. Psychosis may also present as dementia, characterized by impaired memory and abstract thinking and difficulty in performing simple manual tasks. The patient may have difficulty in making decisions or controlling impulses. Psychosis may also present as an organic personality disorder, with a sudden marked change in personality. Symptoms may include apathy, indifference, emotional lability, sexual indiscretions, verbosity, religiosity, and aggressiveness.[121]

It is often difficult to determine whether the psychosis is due to SLE or to other causes. One should exclude functional disorders, renal failure (with uremic encephalopathy), hypertension (with multiple small infarcts), metabolic abnormalities, infection, and the use of medications with psychoactive effects (tranquilizers, antidepressants, narcotics, analgesics, β-blockers, NSAIDs, cimetidine, digoxin, α-methyldopa, and others). Of particular relevance has been the dilemma regarding glucocorticoids, which may cause psychosis, and ironically, are used to treat psychosis. Psychiatric disturbances may develop in SLE patients not receiving steroids or receiving low doses of steroids, or while the dose is being reduced. The psychosis frequently improves on high(er) doses of steroids. Steroids will not necessarily induce a psychosis similar to one previously experienced by the patient. There is no relationship between the dosage of steroids and the extent of psychopathology; psychosis often clears while the steroids are continued. The frequency of psychosis in SLE and other conditions treated with steroids is less than 5 percent.[119, 121] There is no apparent association between steroids and cognitive impairment.[122] Both azathioprine and ibuprofen can (rarely) cause an aseptic meningitis, and antimalarials have (rarely) caused headaches, auditory and visual hallucinations, involuntary movement disorders, mental confusion, toxic psychosis, seizures, or a neuromyopathy.

There is considerable evidence that antibodies to neuronal cells mediate the organic brain syndromes (reviewed by Bluestein[120]) but are not associated with cognitive defects.

Headaches are a frequent complaint of lupus patients. The most common is the tension, or muscle contraction, headache. It is usually triggered by stress, or holding the head in such a posture so as to chronically strain neck and head muscles. Patients usually complain of a dull ache, often as a vice encircling the head, and pain in the back of the neck, shoulders, and back of the head. Migraine headaches have been reported in 10 to 37 percent of patients.[15] Migraine headaches are not necessarily severe headaches, a common lay misinterpretation. Migraine headaches are often triggered by either hormonal changes, use of oral contraceptives, smoking, stress, alcohol, flashing lights, changes in the weather, or eating certain foods such as aged cheeses and chocolate. Visual or olfactory auras or numbness in a limb may precede the attack. The headache is usually sudden in onset, one-sided, mild to severe, often associated with nausea and vomiting, and often occurs in the presence of other aspects of active lupus. Migraines are thought to be due to localized vasospasm. Cluster headaches are rare. An organic basis for the headaches is suggested by their sudden development in someone previously free of headaches, associated double vision, minor seizures, or changes in personality. Those diagnostic procedures referred to earlier are often useful in differentiating functional from organic causes.

In dealing with headaches, one must consider such non-SLE causes as cold food, hangover, sexual orgasm, food with nitrites or monosodium glutamate (MSG), hunger, sinusitis, dental disease, eye diseases, and brain tumors.

Seizures are said to occur in approximately 15 to 20 percent of patients.[118] Grand mal convulsions are the most common, but petit mal, temporal lobe, focal, and Jacksonian convulsions all have been described. Seizures may antedate the onset of SLE, be among its first manifestations, or develop during the course of the illness. A lupus-like syndrome has been suspected in patients receiving either hydantoin, primidone, succinamide, or phenothiazines. However, many of these observations may be outdated, that is, made before the criteria for classification of SLE were developed; the seizures may simply have been the first symptoms of SLE. The cause for seizures may be varied, and may reflect either an acute inflammatory episode or be the result of old damage and a scar. Seizures can be due to metabolic imbalances, uremia, hypertension, infections, tumors, head trauma, or a vasculopathy. If the seizures develop concurrent with other aspects of organic brain involvement, it is relatively easy to ascribe the seizures to "central nervous system (CNS) lupus." CNS (lupus) vasculitis, in the absence of vasculitis or other manifestations of lupus elsewhere, is more an apocryphal story than a documented event.[126] Pathologic examination of autopsy brain specimens from SLE patients has revealed no vasculitis, but at most only vasculopathy and a few scattered microinfarcts.[127] The balanced view is that the development of focal seizures in the absence of other causes for seizures, and with negative angiograms (and CT, and MRI), may indeed be due to a local vasculopathy, vascular irritation, and leakage due to a local insult by circulating immune complexes.

Approximately 10 to 15 percent of patients develop either a cranial or peripheral neuropathy.[118, 120] Of the cranial neuropathies, the eye is most frequently involved. Depending on the localization of the neuropathy, symptoms may include diplopia, nystagmus, ptosis, visual field deficits, cortical blindness, or visual hallucinations. Trigeminal neuralgia, dysarthria, facial weakness, and vertigo have all been noted. Cranial neuropathy usually occurs at the same time as other manifestations of active lupus, in particular peripheral neuropathy. Peripheral neuropathy is usually asymmetric, is usually mild, may affect more than one nerve (mononeuritis multiplex), and affects sensory nerves more than motor nerves—but mixtures are common. Neuropathies are probably due to vasculopathy of small arteries supplying nerves.

Cerebrovascular accidents (CVAs) have been reported in 15 percent of patients with SLE.[128] The cause may be thrombosis of a major vessel in the neck or skull, detectable by angiography, or CVAs may be the result of an intracranial hemorrhage, detected by angiography or cerebrospinal fluid analysis. Patients with hypertension, thrombocytopenia, TTP, or antiphospholipid antibodies are at risk for the development of a stroke, resulting in hemiparesis, hemisensory loss, ocular field defects, aphasia, and so forth.

Movement disorders occur in fewer than 5 percent of patients. Symptoms may include ataxia, choreoathetosis, and hemiballismus. Symptoms are usually associated with other signs of active organic brain involvement. The movement abnormalities are thought to reflect lesions in the cerebellum or basal ganglia.

Transverse myelitis has been noted in patients presenting with the sudden onset of lower extremity weakness or sensory loss, and loss of rectal and urinary bladder sphincter control. The onset usually coincides with other signs of active SLE. The syndrome is thought to be due to arteritis with resultant ischemic necrosis of the spinal cord and may be associated with antiphospholipid antibodies.[129] An MRI may show localized edema.[130] The CSF has a high protein content and many cells. The mortality rate is high, and for those that survive, full recovery is rare.

Meningitis may develop due to infections (viral, bacterial, fungal, or tubercular), ibuprofen, or azathioprine.[120] In addition there are some lupus patients who develop an "aseptic" meningitis, with headache, nuchal rigidity, and a pleocytosis in the CSF, without any other apparent cause.

The eye may be involved. Eyelids may develop a lupus rash; conjunctivitis is usually infectious; keratoconjunctivitis may complicate the picture, but is usually mild. The most characteristic finding is cotton-wool exudates (cytoid bodies), which are usually near the disc and reflect microangiopathy of the retinal capillaries and localized microinfarction of the superficial nerve fiber layers of the retina; microaneurysms can be demonstrated by fluorescein dye angiography.[118] Older textbooks noted that cytoid bodies are found in 10 to 25 percent of patients, usually in association with other manifestations of active lupus, but their occurrence is rare in contemporary studies.[131]

Diagnostic Maneuvers

Laboratory tests and techniques are useful to determine (1) whether the patient has functional or organic involvement (or both); (2) whether the disorder is focal or diffuse; (3) the etiology or pathogenesis or pathomechanism of the disorder; and (4) whether the patient has an active process or the residue of previous insults. There are no specific tests. Patients with active CNS lupus usually, but not always, have active lupus elsewhere.

Serum levels of anti-DNA, complement, and immune complexes generally do not correlate with the activity of CNS lupus, but these and other tests can help confirm a diagnosis of SLE. Patients with antibodies to Sm may be more likely to have CNS lupus. Other studies have noted elevated levels of antilymphocyte antibodies (which may cross-react with brain cells), antiglycolipid, antiribosomal P protein, and antineuronal antibodies, and elevated levels of complement split products and α-interferon in some patients with CNS lupus.[132, 133] Antibodies to lymphocytes, and in particular antibodies to neuronal cells, correlate well with the presence of organic brain disease, but not focal disease.[120]

The cerebrospinal fluid (CSF) is usually normal. However, elevated levels of cells, protein, anti-DNA, IgG, immune complexes, and IL-6 and decreased hemolytic C4 and glucose have been reported to correlate somewhat with activity.[118, 120, 134]

Approximately 80 percent of patients with active CNS lupus will have an abnormal EEG.[125] Diffuse slow wave activity is the pattern most associated with organic brain syndromes, while focal changes are seen in patients with seizure disorders or focal neurologic problems. Evoked potentials may be more sensitive in detecting abnormalities. Abnormal EEGs have also been noted in patients without apparent CNS lupus. Radionuclide brain scanning has been of little help. Position emission tomography (PET) using radiolabeled oxygen to assess brain cell metabolism and radiolabeled CO_2 evaluation of cerebral vascular blood flow has demonstrated abnormalities.[135] CT scans are useful for detecting structural, focal abnormalities (CVA, tumors). Brain atrophy has been noted in some patients, which has been thought by some authors to reflect effects of steroid therapy.[120] MRI tests have revealed structural abnormalities with clinical improvement accompanied by test improvement.[136–138] Angiography is also useful to define local lesions (e.g., vasculopathy). SPECT scanning and psychometric testing have been useful in helping to differentiate functional from organic disease.[122, 125]

A note of caution regarding tests: when many tests are performed on a patient with some, or a suspicion of, psychoneurologic abnormalities, there is an increasing likelihood that at least one test will demonstrate an "abnormality." The significance of that abnormality must be assessed clinically.

Lupus, Menses, and Pregnancy

Some patients relate that their disease flares (especially skin and joint symptoms) just prior to or coincidental with their menses. It is often difficult to distinguish the symptoms of a mild flare of lupus from the symptoms (weight gain, myalgia, irritability) of the premenstrual syndrome (PMS). Some women complain of heavy, painful menses, and others have irregular scant menses, but it is unclear whether this frequency is any greater than in the general population. On the other hand, heavy menses may reflect thrombocytopenia or the use of NSAIDs, while a decreased flow, or an interruption of the normal menstrual cycle, may reflect disease activity or the use of glucocorticoid, while both heavy and scant menses are often seen premenopausally.

Patients with lupus, and their spouses, often raise the question of having children. Most couples elect to schedule having their children, making the immediate issue family planning and contraception. The use of oral contraceptives containing estrogen derivatives has been associated with an exacerbation of lupus[139] and should thus be avoided. Antibodies to estrogen, found in patients with SLE and oral contraceptive users,[140] may contribute to immune complex formation in women taking estrogens. Furthermore, such usage increases the likelihood of thrombophlebitis and strokes—in a population already vulnerable. On the other hand, oral contraceptives containing mostly progesterone[139] or low-dosage estrogens[141] may not be associated with adverse effects. Intrauterine devices are also associated with complications (hemorrhage, infections). When the time comes to consider pregnancy, the couple should be counseled regarding the increased demands of parenthood and, in particular, motherhood.

Although patients with SLE are as fertile as those in the general population, their pregnancies may be associated with unique problems; therefore they should be followed by an obstetrician knowledgeable in high-risk pregnancies.[142] In the past, exacerbations were observed in up to 50 percent of patients during pregnancy, occurring in all three trimesters in approximately equal frequency. In addition, exacerbations were frequently noted in the immediate postpartum period. However, the risk of exacerbation during pregnancy and post partum, especially in those in remission at the beginning of pregnancy, appears to have been progressively diminishing in the last 30 years,[15, 144] and many patients with active SLE carry to term. This improved outlook may reflect either better management, more use of steroids, increased use of abortion (in those who did flare), or just good luck. Pre-eclampsia is a frequent complication of pregnancy and has been noted in lupus patients.[145] Pre-eclampsia is often difficult to distinguish from a flare of lupus nephritis; but pre-eclampsia is much less likely to be associated with marked depressions of complement levels and elevated levels of immune complexes and anti-DNA.

Approximately 25 to 30 percent of pregnancies in lupus patients result in a miscarriage, overall fetal loss may approach 50 percent, and patients are more (three times) prone to premature delivery.[144, 145] Fetal death is more likely to occur in lupus patients with renal disease. Circulating anticoagulants or antibodies to cardiolipin are major factors in recurrent miscarriages and fetal death in the second trimester.[144] Of 737 non-LE pregnancies, 2 had circulating anticoagulants with midtrimester fetal loss; 12 had IgG anticardiolipin with 5 midtrimester losses.[145a] To date, the role of vasculitis or thrombotic events in the placenta remains inadequately studied.

Most infants born to lupus patients are normal, although often premature. Neonatal lupus occurs in approximately 5 percent of LE pregnancies, especially in women with anti-Ro antibodies[146] and HLA-B8, DR3.[147] Most have a rash, and fewer than one half have congenital heart block. Those with heart block have a high rate of mortality in the first few months of life. Patients with lupus having a child with neonatal lupus have a 25 percent likelihood of having a similar child in a subsequent pregnancy.[128]

Drug-Induced Lupus

It is not clear whether medications can exacerbate a pre-existing lupus condition, or even induce lupus in an individual predisposed to develop it. Earlier studies suggested that penicillin, sulfonamides, and anticonvulsants may be implicated.[148a] However, present opinion suggests that these patients had SLE and were receiving medication appropriate to their particular form of clinical exacerbation, or had an infection that caused an exacerbation. Oral contraceptives may cause a relapse of SLE.

More common, and well defined, is the syndrome of drug-induced lupus, which produces a clinical and immunologic syndrome quite similar to spontaneous SLE. Table 61–9 is a list of medications that have been incriminated.[148] The data are strongest for hydralazine and procainamide where large prospective studies have been reported. While isoniazid induces antinuclear antibodies in about 15 percent of individuals (presumably those with tuberculosis), mild SLE has rarely been noted. The clinical syndrome and the development of antinuclear antibodies are much more likely to develop, and develop sooner, in individuals who are slow acetylators.[149] HLA-DR4 has been associated with drug-induced lupus, particularly in respect to hydralazine and procainamide.[150] The frequency of acetylator fast and slow types is quite similar in normal subjects and in

Table 61–9. LUPUS-INDUCING DRUGS

Definite	Possible	Unlikely
Hydralazine	Dilantin	Griseofulvin
Procainamide	Penicillamine	Phenylbutazone
Isoniazid	Quinidine	Oral
Chlorpromazine	Sulfonamide	contraceptives
Methyldopa	Propylthiouracil	Gold salts
	Practolol	Penicillin
	Acebutolol	Hydrazine
	Lithium carbonate	L-Canaverine
	P-Aminosalicylate	
	Nitrofurantoin	
	Tartrazine	
	Atenolol	
	Metoprolol	
	Oxprenolol	
	Mephenytoin	
	Trimethadione	
	Ethosuximide	
	Methimazole	
	Captopril	

those with SLE. Other medications may possibly cause drug-induced lupus (see Table 61–9), but the data are scantier and no prospective studies or rechallenges have been reported. Many of the reports note the development of antinuclear antibodies and some arthralgia but rarely mention full-blown lupus. On the other hand, the development of lupus in patients taking the β-blocker practolol led to its withdrawal. Oral contraceptives may contribute to a relapse in patients with SLE but are unlikely to induce lupus. L-Canaverine, in the form of alfalfa sprouts, induced a lupus-like condition in monkeys.

The symptoms of drug-induced lupus are similar to those of SLE, but there are significant differences (Table 61–10). (1) Drug-induced lupus is reversible; when the drug is stopped, the symptoms gradually fade. (2) The symptoms tend to be mild in drug-induced lupus, with constitutional, joint, and pleuropericardial symptoms predominating. In that respect drug-induced lupus is similar to lupus in an older age group. Renal and central nervous system disease, leukopenia, mucocutaneous involvement, and anemia are uncommon. (3) The sex ratio is about equal for drug-induced lupus. (4) Drug-induced lupus is rare in blacks.[148]

The disease usually begins a few months after the medication is begun. The risk is higher in those who have ingested a total of 100 g of hydralazine or 1.25 g of procainamide.[151] About 14 percent of patients taking hydralazine develop antinuclear antibodies, while only 4 to 12 percent develop lupus.[151] About 50 to 100 percent of patients receiving procainamide develop antinuclear antibodies, but only about 25 percent of these individuals develop lupus. Therefore, the presence of a positive ANA test in individuals receiving these drugs indicates that they are at greater risk for developing drug-induced lupus but does not preclude use of this medication unless symptoms develop. N-Acetyl-procainamide, which is clinically as effective as procainamide, does not cause

Table 61–10. CLINICAL FEATURES OF DRUG-INDUCED LUPUS

	Spontaneous Lupus	Drug-Induced Lupus
Clinical Features		
Age	20–40	50
Sex (F:M)	9	1
Race	All	"No blacks"
Acetylation type	Slow-fast	Slow
Onset of symptoms	Gradual	Abrupt
Constitutional symptoms (fever, malaise, myalgia)	83%	50%
Arthralgia and arthritis	90%	95%
Pleuropericarditis	50%	50% (procainamide)
Hepatomegaly	25%	25%
Skin rash (all types)	74%	10–20%
Discoid lesions	20%	0%
Malar erythema	42%	2%
Renal disease	53%	5%
CNS disease	32%	0%
Hematologic disease	Common	Unusual
Immune Abnormalities		
ANA	95%	95%
LE cells	90%	90%
Anti-RNP	40–50%	20%
Anti-Sm	20–30%	Rare
Anti-DNA	80%	Rare
Antihistone	25%	90%
Complement	Reduced	Normal
Immune complexes	Elevated	Normal

drug-induced lupus, but it is not approved by the U.S. Food and Drug Administration (F.D.A.) for use in this country.

The differential between drug-induced lupus and spontaneous lupus is based on the clinical symptoms and immune profile (see Table 61–10). While both conditions are strongly associated with the presence of antinuclear antibodies, antibodies to double-stranded DNA and to Sm are rare in drug-induced lupus. Antibodies to histones are seen frequently in patients with drug-induced lupus but are also seen in at least 25 percent of patients with SLE. In the procainamide syndrome, the antihistone antibodies are mainly directed to the H2A-H2B complex, while the antibodies are directed to the H1 and H3-H4 complex in the hydralazine syndrome.[152] Serum complement and immune complex levels are generally normal in drug-induced lupus.

Precipitating Factors

The onset of SLE is infrequently attributed to a single clear-cut event although most physicians have seen patients in whom the disease began shortly following some event. Most patients try and identify a causal factor.

Exposure to the sun and other sources of UV light may cause exacerbations or induce the first sign of lupus. The usual relapse is limited to a rash, although other symptoms may also develop. Infec-tions can initiate lupus or cause a relapse. Stress has also been implicated in causing exacerbations particularly of mild disease.[15] Unfortunately, stress as an entity has never been clinically defined, except as it relates to its psychosomatic effects.[153] Stresses involving loss, such as the death of a loved one, divorce, financial disaster, or loss of a job, are difficult to cope with. Surgery can also cause exacerbation.[15] The mechanism in surgery is unclear but may relate to the release of nuclear and other antigens into the blood stream with resultant reaction with circulating antinuclear antibodies to form immune complexes. Pregnancy may cause an exacerbation, or even trigger the first symptoms of lupus; a relapse is more likely to develop in the postpartum period. Therapeutic abortion may also cause a relapse, perhaps through mechanisms related either to pregnancy or to the surgery itself.

Diagnosis of SLE—Differential Diagnosis

Lupus usually begins with either unexplained fever, fatigue, weight loss, anemia, photosensitive rash, arthralgia/arthritis, Raynaud's phenomenon, serositis, seizures, alopecia, phlebitis, recurrent abortion, psychosis, or nephritis. Lupus should also be suspected—especially in young women—with unexplained fever, purpura, easy bruising, diffuse adenopathy, hepatosplenomegaly, peripheral neuropathy, endocarditis, myocarditis, interstitial pneumonitis, peritonitis, or aseptic meningitis. A positive Coombs' test, low complement levels, and immune deposits at the dermal-epidermal junction are also suggestive of lupus. On first examination, patients are frequently misdiagnosed as having rheumatoid arthritis, rheumatic fever (especially children), juvenile rheumatoid arthritis, glomerulonephritis, scleroderma, Sjögren's syndrome, vasculitis, idiopathic thrombocytopenic purpura, Raynaud's phenomenon, lymphoma, anemia, subacute bacterial endocarditis, serum sickness, leukemia, TTP, secondary lues, sarcoidosis, bacterial sepsis, leprosy, infectious mononucleosis, polymyositis, urticaria, erythema multiforme, rosacea, lichen planus, epilepsy, multiple sclerosis, chronic active hepatitis (lupoid hepatitis), drug-induced lupus, mixed connective tissue disease, relapsing polychondritis, Weber-Christian disease, mixed cryoglobulinemia, Whipple's disease, periodic syndromes, neutropenia, chronic fatigue syndrome, or psychoneurosis.

Most physicians rely on the ARA revised Criteria for the Classification of SLE[154] (Table 61–11). It should be noted that these criteria were developed for the *classification* of SLE patients when SLE patients were compared with patients with other rheumatic diseases for study purposes. The diagnosis of SLE was made if four or more of the manifestations listed in Table 61–11 were present, either serially or simultaneously, during any interval of observations. However, most physicians rely on these criteria to diag-

Table 61–11. 1982 REVISED CRITERIA FOR CLASSIFICATION OF SYSTEMIC LUPUS ERYTHEMATOSUS

Criterion	Definition
1. Malar rash	Fixed erythema, flat or raised, over the malar eminences, tending to spare the nasolabial folds
2. Discoid rash	Erythematous raised patches with adherent keratotic scaling and follicular plugging; atrophic scarring may occur in older lesions
3. Photosensitivity	Skin rash as a result of unusual reaction to sunlight, by patient history or physician observation
4. Oral ulcers	Oral or nasopharyngeal ulceration, usually painless, observed by a physician
5. Arthritis	Nonerosive arthritis involving two or more peripheral joints, characterized by tenderness, swelling, or effusion
6. Serositis	a. Pleuritis—convincing history of pleuritic pain or rub heard by a physician or evidence of pleural effusion OR b. Pericarditis—documented by ECG or rub or evidence of pericardial effusion
7. Renal disorder	a. Persistent proteinuria greater than 0.5 g/day or greater than 3+ if quantitation not performed OR b. Cellular casts—may be red cell, hemoglobin, granular, tubular, or mixed
8. Neurologic disorder	a. Seizures—in the absence of offending drugs or known metabolic derangements; e.g., uremia, ketoacidosis, or electrolyte imbalance OR b. Psychosis—in the absence of offending drugs or known metabolic derangements, e.g., uremia, ketoacidosis, or electrolyte imbalance
9. Hematologic disorder	a. Hemolytic anemia—with reticulocytosis OR b. Leukopenia—less than 4000/mm total on 2 or more occasions OR c. Lymphopenia—less than 1500/mm on 2 or more occasions OR d. Thrombocytopenia—less than 100,000/mm in the absence of offending drugs
10. Immunologic disorder	a. Positive LE cell preparation OR b. Anti-DNA—antibody to native DNA in abnormal titer OR c. Anti-Sm—presence of antibody to Sm nuclear antigen OR d. False positive serologic test for syphilis known to be positive for at least 6 months and confirmed by *Treponema pallidum* immobilization or fluorescent treponemal antibody absorption test
11. Antinuclear antibody	An abnormal titer of antinuclear antibody by immunofluorescence or an equivalent assay at any point in time and in the absence of drugs known to be associated with drug-induced lupus syndrome

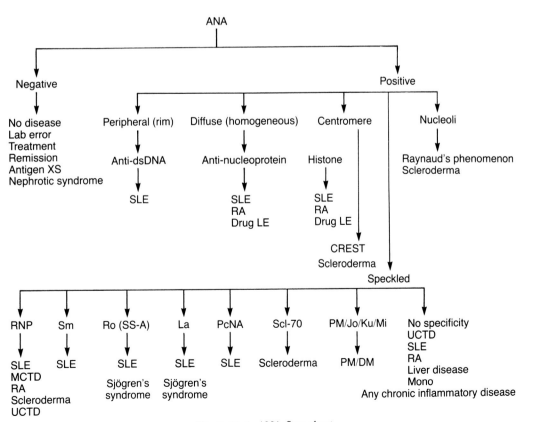

Figure 61–1. ANA flow sheet.

Table 61–12. SENSITIVITY VS. SPECIFICITY VS. PREDICTIVE VALUE

Antibody	SLE			Drug LE			RA			Scleroderma			PM/DM			Sjögren's		
	Sen	Spec	Pre	Sen	Spec	Pre	Sen	Spec	Pre	Sen	Spec	Pre	Sen	Spec	Pre	Sen	Spec	Pre
dsDNA	70%	95%	95%	—	1–5%	1–5%	—	1%	1%	—	<1%	<1%	—	<1%	<1%	—	1–5%	1–5%
ssDNA	80	50	50	80	50	50	mod	mod	mod		lo	lo		lo	lo	mod	mod	mod
Histone	30–80	mod	mod	95	hi	hi	lo	—	—	<1%	—	—	<1%	—	—	lo	lo	lo
Nucleo-protein	58	mod	mod	50	mod	mod	25	lo	lo	<1%	—	—	<1%	—	—	mod	mod	mod
Sm	25–30	99	97	1%	—	—	1%	—	—	<1%	—	—	<1%	—	—	1–5%	—	—
RNP	50	87–94	46–85				47			20						5–60		
Ro	25–35			lo			lo						lo			8–70	87	5–48
La	15			lo			lo						lo			14–60	94	26–41
PCNA	5	95	23	lo	0	0	lo	0	0	lo			lo					
Scl–70	0	0	0	0	0	0	0	0	0	20–60	hi	hi	30–50			5		
PM-1										lo								
Mi-1																		
Jo-1	lo			lo			lo			lo			30–50			lo		
Ku	lo																	
Nucleoli	26									54								
Centromere										12–30								

dsDNA, Double-stranded DNA; hi, high; lo, low; mod, moderate; Pre, predictive value; Sen, sensitivity; Spec, specificity; ssDNA, single-stranded DNA. Centromere = CREST; RNP = MCTD; Ro = SCLE; 1° biliary cirrhosis, vasculitis, CHB.

Table 61–13. QUESTIONNAIRE FOR THE DIAGNOSIS OF SLE

1. Have you ever had arthritis or rheumatism for more than 3 months?
2. Do your fingers become pale, numb, or uncomfortable in the cold?
3. Have you had any sores in your mouth for more than 2 weeks?
4. Have you been told that you have low blood counts (anemia, low WBC count, or low platelet count)?
5. Have you ever had a prominent rash on your cheeks for more than 1 month?
6. Does your skin break out after you have been in the sun (not sunburn)?
7. Has it ever been painful to take a deep breath for more than a few days (pleurisy)?
8. Have you ever been told that you have protein in your urine?
9. Have you ever had rapid loss of lots of hair?
10. Have you ever had a seizure, convulsion, or fit?

nose individual patients. When tested against other diseases, their sensitivity and specificity have been approximately 96 percent. Using the analogy of the ARA criteria for the diagnosis of RA, I suggest that patients be labeled as having classic SLE (many criteria), definite SLE (four or more criteria), probable SLE (three criteria), or possible SLE (two criteria). If patients with possible (or incomplete) lupus are followed long enough, few develop SLE; their symptoms may disappear or evolve into some other illness.[155] The ANA test is the best screening test for SLE. It is positive in virtually all patients with SLE and should be performed whenever SLE is suspected. If the ANA test is negative, the patient has a less than 0.14 percent probability of having SLE, while a positive ANA test has a 20 to 35 percent predictive value issue.[156–158] However, the test is also positive in 68 percent of patients with Sjögren's syndrome, 40 to 75 percent of patients with scleroderma (especially those with a speckled pattern of ANAs), 16 percent of patients with juvenile rheumatoid arthritis, and 25 to 50 percent of patients with rheumatoid arthritis (especially those with a diffuse pattern of ANAs). Antinuclear antibodies tend to be present in higher titer in patients with SLE than in patients with other disorders. Antibodies to double-stranded DNA and to Sm are highly diagnostic of SLE, although they are found in only about 75 percent and 25 percent of patients, respectively.

Antibodies to single-stranded DNA and nucleoprotein (NP) are frequently found in patients with SLE and RA; antibodies to RNP are frequently found in patients with SLE and scleroderma. Antibodies to Ro(SS-A) and La(SS-B) are frequently found in patients with SLE or Sjögren's syndrome. Figure 61–1 provides an outline for the differential diagnosis of an ANA test, and Table 61–12 provides the sensitivity and specificity and predictive value of specific ANA for SLE and related conditions. To help detect SLE and differentiate it from other conditions, ask the questions in Table 61–13. If three or more are answered positively, SLE is a possibility and an ANA test is indicated.

References

1. Lawrence, R. C., Hochberg, M. C., Kelsey, J. L., McDuffie, E. C., Medsger, T. A., Felts, W. R., and Shulman, L. E.: Estimates of the prevalence of selected arthritic and musculoskeletal diseases in the United States. J. Rheumatol. 14:427, 1989.
2. Waaler, E.: Connective tissue disorders and related conditions in Scandinavia. In Wagner, B. (ed.): The Connective Tissue. Baltimore, Williams & Wilkins, 1967.
3. Michet, C. J., McKenna, C. H., Elveback, L. R., Kaslow, R. A., and Kurland, L. T.: Epidemiology of systemic lupus erythematosus and other connective tissue disorders in Rochester, Minnesota, 1950 through 1979. Mayo Clin. Proc. 60:105, 1985.
4. Hochberg, M. C.: The incidence of systemic lupus erythematosus in Baltimore, Maryland, 1970–1977. Arthritis Rheum. 28:80, 1985.
5. Serdula, M. K., and Rhoads, G. G.: Frequency of systemic lupus erythematosus in different ethnic groups in Hawaii. Arthritis Rheum. 22:328, 1979.
6. Hart, H. H.: Ethnic difference in the prevalence of systemic lupus erythematosus. Ann. Rheum. Dis. 42:529, 1983.
7. Meddings, J., and Grennan, D. M.: The prevalence of systemic lupus erythematosus in Dunedin. N.Z. Med. J. 91:205, 1980.
8. Nived, O., Sturfelt, G., and Wollheim, F.: Systemic lupus erythematosus in an adult population in southern Sweden: Incidence, prevalence, and validity of ARA revised classification criteria. Br. J. Rheumatol. 24:147, 1985.
9. Helve, T.: Prevalence and mortality rates of systemic lupus erythematosus and causes of death in SLE patients in Finland. Scand. J. Rheumatol. 14:43, 1985.
10. Morton, R. O., Gershwin, M. E., Brady, C., et al.: The incidence of systemic lupus erythematosus in North American Indians. J. Rheumatol. 3:186, 1976.
11. Wilson, W. A., and Hughes, G. R.: Rheumatic diseases in Jamaica. Ann. Rheum. Dis. 38:320, 1979.
12. Feng, P. H., and Boey, M. L.: Systemic lupus erythematosus in Chinese: The Singapore experience. Rheumatol. Int. 2:151, 1982.
13. Engelman, E. P.: The current status of rheumatology in the People's Republic of China. Arthritis Rheum. 24:1324, 1981.
14. Lutalo, S. K.: Chronic inflammatory rheumatic diseases in black Zimbabweans. Ann. Rheum. Dis. 44:121, 1985.
15. Rothfield, N.: Clinical features of systemic lupus erythematosus. In Kelley, W. N., Harris, E. D., Ruddy, S., and Sledge, C. B. (eds.): Textbook of Rheumatology. Philadelphia, W. B. Saunders Company, 1981.
16. Wallace, D. J., and Dubois, E. L.: Definition, classification, and epidemiology of systemic lupus erythematosus. In Wallace, D. J. and Dubois, E. L. (eds.): Lupus Erythematosus. 3rd ed. Philadelphia, Lea and Febiger, 1987.
17. Lahita, R. G., Chiorazzi, N., Gibofsky, A., et al.: Familial systemic lupus erythematosus in males. Arthritis Rheum. 26:39, 1983.
18. Schaller, J.: Lupus in childhood. Clin. Rheumatol. Dis. 8:219, 1982.
19. Dallou, S. P., Khan, M. A., and Kushner, I.: Clinical features of systemic lupus erythematosus. Differences related to race and age of onset. Arthritis Rheum. 25:55, 1982.
20. Kaufman, I. D., Gomez-Reino, J. J., Heinicke, M. H., and Gorevic, P. D.: Male lupus: Retrospective analysis of the clinical and laboratory features of 52 patients, with a review of the literature. Semin. Arthritis Rheum. 18:189, 1989.
21. Ward, M. M., and Polisson, R. P.: A meta-analysis of the clinical manifestations of older-onset SLE. Arthritis Rheum. 32:1226, 1989.
22. Ward, M. M., and Studenski, S.: Clinical manifestations of systemic lupus erythematosus. Identification of racial and socioeconomic influences. Arch. Intern. Med. 150:849, 1990.
23. Reveille, J. D., Bartolucci, A., and Alarcon, G. S.: Prognosis in SLE. Negative impact of increasing age at onset, black race, and thrombocytopenia, as well as causes of death. Arthritis Rheum. 33:37, 1990.
24. Callahan, L. F., and Pincus, T.: Associations between clinical status questionnaire scores and formal educational levels in persons with systemic lupus erythematosus. Arthritis Rheum. 33:407, 1996.
25. Winchester, R. J.: Genetic aspects. In Schur, P. H. (ed.): The Clinical Management of Systemic Lupus Erythematosus. Orlando, Florida, Grune & Stratton, 1983.
26. Block, S. R., Winfield, J. B., Lockshin, M. D., et al.: Twin studies in systemic lupus erythematosus. A review of the literature and presentation of 12 additional sets. Am. J. Med. 59:533, 1975.
27. Deapen, D. M., Weinrib, L., Langholz, B., Horwitz, D. A., and Mack, T. M.: A revised estimate of twin concordance in SLE: A survey of 138 pairs. Arthritis Rheum. 29:S26, 1986.

28. Arnett, F. C., Reveill, J. D., Wilson, R. W., et al.: Systemic lupus erythematosus: Current state of the genetic hypothesis. Semin. Arthritis Rheum. 14:24, 1984.
29. Schur, P. H., Meyer, I., Garovoy, M., et al.: Associations between systemic lupus erythematosus and the major histocompatibility complex: Clinical and immunological considerations. Clin. Immunol. Immunopathol. 24:263, 1982.
30. Schur, P. H., Marcus-Bagley, D., Awdeh, Z., Yunis, E. J., and Alper, C. A.: The effect of ethnicity on major histocompatibility complex complement allotypes and extended haplotypes in patients with systemic lupus erythematosus. Arthritis Rheum. 33:985, 1990.
31. Fronek, Z., Timmerman, L. A., Alper, C. A., Hahn, B. H., Kalunian, K., Peterlin, B. M., and McDevitt, H. O.: Major histocompatibility complex genes and susceptibility to systemic lupus erythematosus. Arthritis Rheum. 37:1542, 1990.
32. Schur, P. H.: Inherited complement component abnormalities. Annu. Rev. Med. 37:333, 1986.
33. Schur, P. H., Pandey, J. P., and Fedrick, J. A.: Gm allotypes in white patients with SLE. Arthritis Rheum. 28:828, 1985.
34. Wilson, J. G., Wong, W. W., Schur, P. H., and Fearon, D. T.: Mode of inheritance of decreased C3b receptors on erythrocytes of patients with systemic lupus erythematosus. N. Engl. J. Med. 307:981, 1982.
35. Sontheimer, R. D., Stastny, P., and Gilliam, J. N.: Human leukocyte antigen associations in subacute cutaneous lupus erythematosus. J. Clin. Invest. 67:312, 1981.
36. Silvestris, F., Searles, R. P., Bankhurst, A. D., and Williams, R. C.: Family distribution of anti-F(ab')2 antibodies in relatives of patients with SLE. Clin. Exp. Immunol. 60:329, 1985.
37. Spencer-Green, G., Adams, L. E., Hurtibuse, P., et al.: Familial alterations of immunoregulation in SLE. J. Rheumatol. 12:498, 1985.
38. Smolen, J. S., Klippel, J. H., Penner, E., Reichlin, M., Steinberg, A. D., Chused, T. M., Scherak, O., Graninger, W., Hartler, E., Zielinski, C. C., Wolf, A., Davey, R. J., Mann, D. L., and Mayr, W. R.: HLA-DR antigens in systemic lupus erythematosus: Association with specificity of autoantibody responses to nuclear antigens. Ann. Rheum. Dis. 46:457, 1987.
39. Harley, J. B., Sestak, A. L., Willis, L. G., Fu, S. M., Hansen, J. A., and Reichlin, M.: A model for disease heterogeneity in systemic lupus erythematosus. Relationships between histocompatibility antigens, autoantibodies, and lymphopenia or renal disease. Arthritis Rheum. 32:826, 1989.
40. Reveille, J. D., Schrohenloher, R. E., Acton, R. T., and Barger, B. O.: DNA analysis of HLA-DR and DQ genes in American blacks with systemic lupus erythematosus. Arthritis Rheum. 32:1243, 1989.
41. Fujisaku, A., Frank, M. B., Neas, B., Reichlin, M., and Harley, J. B.: HLA-DQ gene complementation and other histocompatibility relationships in man with the Ro(SS-A) autoantibody response of systemic lupus erythematosus. J. Clin. Invest. 86:606, 1990.
42. Robb-Nicholson, L. C., Liang, M. H., Daltroy, L., Eaton, H., Gall, V., Schwartz, J., Wright, E., Faegenbaum, A., Hartley, L. H., and Schur, P. H.: Effects of aerobic conditioning in lupus fatigue: A pilot study. Br. J. Rheumatol. 28:500, 1989.
43. Stahl, J. I., Klippel, J. H., and Decker, J. L.: Fever in systemic lupus erythematosus. Am. J. Med. 67:933, 1979.
44. Nived, O., Sturfelt, G., and Wolheim, F.: Systemic lupus and infection: A controlled and prospective study including an epidemiologic group. Q. J. Med. 55:271, 1985.
45. Hellman, D. B., Petri, M., and Whiting-O'Keefe, Q.: Fatal infections in systemic lupus erythematosus: The role of opportunistic infections. Medicine 66:341, 1987.
46. Dubois, E. L., and Wallace, D. J.: Clinical and laboratory manifestations of SLE. In Wallace, D. J. and Dubois, E. L. (eds.): Lupus Erythematosus. Philadelphia, Lea & Febiger, 1987, pp. 317–449.
47. Alarcon-Segovia, D., Abud-Mendoza, C., Diaz-Jouanen, E., Iglesias, A., Delos Reyes, V., and Hernandez-Ortiz, J.: Deforming arthropathy of the hands in SLE. J. Rheumatol. 15:65, 1988.
48. Weissman, B. N., Rappoport, A. S., Sosman, J. L., and Schur, P. H.: Radiographic findings in the hands in patients with systemic lupus erythematosus. Radiology 126:313, 1978.
49. Esdaile, J. M., Danoff, D., Rosenthall, L., and Gutkowski, A.: Deforming arthritis in SLE. Ann. Rheum. Dis. 40:124, 1981.
50. Buyon, J. P., and Zuckerman, J. D.: Articular manifestations of systemic lupus erythematosus. In Lahita, R. G. (ed.): Systemic Lupus Erythematosus. New York, John Wiley & Sons, 1987.
50a. Morgan, J., and McCarty, D. J.: Tendon ruptures in patients with systemic lupus erythematosus treated with corticosteroids. Arthritis Rheum. 17:1033, 1974.
51. Pekin, T. J., Jr., and Zvaifler, N. J.: Synovial fluid findings in systemic lupus erythematosus. Arthritis Rheum. 13:777, 1970.
52. Labowitz, R., and Schumacher, H. R.: Articular manifestations of systemic lupus erythematosus. Ann. Intern. Med. 74:911, 1971.
53. Hahn, B. H., Yardley, J. H., and Stevens, M. B.: Rheumatoid nodules in systemic lupus erythematosus. Ann. Intern. Med. 72:49, 1970.
54. Schenfeld, L., Gray, R. G., Poppo, M. J., Gaylis, N. B., and Gottlieb, N. L.: Bacterial monoarthritis due to Weisseria meningitidis in systemic lupus erythematosus. J. Rheumatol. 8:145, 1981.
55. Zizic, T. M., Marcoux, C., Hungerford, D. S., and Stevens, M. B.: The early diagnosis of ischemic necrosis of bone. Arthritis Rheum. 29:1177, 1986.
56. Stevens, M. B.: Musculoskeletal manifestations. In Schur, P. H. (ed.): The Clinical Management of Systemic Lupus Erythematosus. Orlando, Florida, Grune & Stratton, 1983.
57. Ropes, M. W.: Systemic Lupus Erythematosus. Cambridge, Harvard University Press, 1976.
58. Kanayama, Y., Shiota, K., Horiguchi, I., Kato, N., Ohe, A., and Inove, T.: Correlation between steroid myopathy and serum lactic dehydrogenase in systemic lupus erythematosus. Arch. Intern. Med. 141:1176, 1981.
59. Gilliam, J. N.: Systemic lupus erythematosus and the skin. In Lahita, R. G. (ed.): Systemic Lupus Erythematosus. New York, John Wiley & Sons, 1987.
60. Provost, T. T., and Dore, N.: Cutaneous manifestations. In Schur, P. H. (ed.): The Clinical Management of Systemic Lupus Erythematosus. Orlando, Florida, Grune & Stratton, 1983.
61. Wurtman, R. J., Baum, M. J., and Potts, J. T., Jr.: The medical and biological effects of light. Ann. N.Y. Acad. Sci. 453:1, 1985.
62. Furukawa, F., Kashihara-Sawani, M., Lyons, M. B., and Norris, D. A.: Binding of antibodies to the extractable nuclear antigens SS-A/Ro and SS-B/La is induced on the surface of human keratinocytes by ultraviolet light (UVL): Implications for the pathogenesis of photosensitive cutaneous lupus. J. Invest. Dermatol. 94:77, 1990.
63. Prystowsky, S. D., and Gilliam, J. N.: Discoid lupus erythematosus as part of a larger disease spectrum: Correlation of clinical features with laboratory findings in lupus erythematosus. Arch. Dermatol. 111:1448, 1975.
64. Smith, C. D., Marino, C., and Rothfield, N. F.: The clinical utility of the lupus band test. Arthritis Rheum. 27:382, 1984.
65. Editorial. Bullous eruption of SLE. Ann. Intern. Med. 97:165, 1983.
66. Buyon, J. P., Ben-Chetrit, E., Karp, S., Roubey, R. A., Pompeo, L., Reeves, W. H., Tan, E. M., and Winchester, R.: Acquired congenital heart block. Pattern of maternal antibody response to biochemically defined antigens of the SSA/Ro-SSB/La system in neonatal lupus. J. Clin. Invest. 84:627, 1989.
67. Alarcon-Segovia, D., and Cetina, J. A.: Lupus hair. Am. J. Med. Sci. 267:241, 1974.
68. Urowitz, M. B., Gladman, D. D., Chalmers, A., and Ogryzlo, M. A.: Nail lesions in SLE. J. Rheumatol. 5:441, 1978.
69. Englert, H. J., Loizou, S., Derue, G. G. M., Walport, M. J., and Hughes, G. R. V.: Clinical and immunological features of livedo reticularis in lupus: A case-control study. Am. J. Med. 87:408, 1989.
70. Kammer, G. M., Soter, N. A., and Schur, P. H.: Circulating immune complexes in patients with necrotizing vasculitis. Clin. Immunol. Immunopathol. 15:658, 1980.
71. Greisman, S. G., Thayaparon, R. S., Goodwin, T. A., and Lockshin, M. D.: Occlusive vasculopathy in SLE: Association with anti-cardiolipin antibody. Arch. Intern. Med. 151:389, 1991.
72. Slater, D.: "Lupus" and prostacyclin formation. Lancet 1:383, 1981.
73. Rothfield, N. F.: Cardiopulmonary manifestations. In Schur, P. H. (ed.): The Clinical Management of Systemic Lupus Erythematosus. Orlando, Florida, Grune & Stratton, 1983.
74. Pines, A., Kaplinsky, N., Olchovsky, D., Rozenman, J., and Fankl, O.: Pleuro-pulmonary manifestations of systemic lupus erythematosus: Clinical features of its subgroups. Chest 88:129, 1985.
75. Silberstein, S. L., Barland, P., Grayzel, A. I., et al.: Pulmonary dysfunction in systemic lupus erythematosus: Prevalence classification and correlation with other organ involvement. J. Rheumatol. 7:187, 1980.
76. Lawrence, E. C.: Systemic lupus erythematosus and the lung. In Lahita, R. G. (ed.): Systemic Lupus Erythematosus. New York, John Wiley & Sons, 1987.
77. Ginzler, E., Diamond, H., Kaplan, D., Weiner, M., Schlesinger, M., and Seleznick, M.: Computer analysis of factors influencing frequency of infection in SLE. Arthritis Rheum. 21:37, 1978.
78. Matthay, R. A., Schwarz, M. I., Petty, T. L., et al.: Pulmonary manifestations of systemic lupus erythematosus: Review of twelve cases of acute lupus pneumonitis. Medicine 54:397, 1974.
79. Haupt, H. M., Moore, G. W., and Hutchins, G. M.: The lung in systemic lupus erythematosus: Analysis of the pathogenic changes in 120 patients. Am. J. Med. 71:791, 1981.
80. Rubin, L. A., and Urowitz, M. B.: Shrinking lung syndrome in SLE—A clinical pathologic study. J. Rheumatol. 10:973, 1983.
81. Eagen, J. W., Memoli, V. A., Roberts, J. L., Matthew, G. R., Schwartz, M. M., and Lewis, E. J.: Pulmonary hemorrhage in SLE. Medicine 57:545, 1978.
82. Klinkhoff, A. V., Thompson, C. R., Reid, G. D., and Tomlinson, C. W.: M-Mode and two-dimensional echocardiographic abnormalities in systemic lupus erythematosus. JAMA 253:3273, 1985.
83. Stevens, M. B.: Systemic lupus erythematosus and the cardiovascular

system. *In* Lahita, R. G. (ed.): Systemic Lupus Erythematosus. New York, John Wiley & Sons, 1987.

84. Hochberg, M. C., Dorsch, C. A., Feinglass, E. J., and Stevens, M. B.: Survivorship in systemic lupus erythematosus: Effect of antibody to extractable nuclear antigen. Arthritis Rheum. 24:54, 1981.

85. Estes, D., and Christian, C. L.: The natural history of SLE by prospective analysis. Medicine 50:85, 1971.

86. Rosner, S., Ginzler, E. M., Diamond, H. S., et al.: A multicenter study of outcome in systemic lupus erythematosus. Arthritis Rheum. 25:612, 1982.

87. Rubin, L. A., Urowitz, M. B., and Gladman, D. D.: Mortality in systemic lupus erythematosus—the bimodal pattern revisited. Q. J. Med. 55:87, 1985.

88. Cunningham, M. J., Rothenberg, P. L., Schatten, S., Schur, P. H., and Schoen, F. J.: Infected myocardial infarct with rupture in a young woman with systemic lupus erythematosus. Am. J. Cardiol. 59:488, 1987.

89. Ettinger, W. H., Goldberg, A. P., Applebaum-Bowden, D., and Hazzard, W. R.: Dyslipoproteinemia in SLE. Effect of corticosteroids. Am. J. Med. 83:503, 1987.

90. Straaton, K. V., Chatham, W. W., Reveille, J. D., Koopman, W. J., and Smith, S. H.: Clinically significant valvular heart disease in systemic lupus erythematosus. Am. J. Med. 85:645, 1988.

91. Barzizza, F., Venco, A., Grandi, M., and Finardi, G.: Mitral valve prolapse in systemic lupus erythematosus. Clin. Exp. Rheumatol. 5:59, 1987.

92. Gladman, D. D., and Urowitz, M. B.: Venous syndromes and pulmonary embolism in SLE. Ann. Rheum. Dis. 39:340, 1980.

93. Laurence, J., and Nachman, R.: Hematologic aspects of systemic lupus erythematosus. *In* Lahita, R. G. (ed.): Systemic Lupus Erythematosus. New York, John Wiley & Sons, 1986.

94. Shoenfeld, Y., and Schwartz, R. S.: Hematologic manifestations. *In* Schur, P. H. (ed.): The Clinical Management of Systemic Lupus Erythematosus. Orlando, Florida, Grune & Stratton, 1983.

95. Perez, H. D., Lipton, M., and Goldstein, I. M.: A specific inhibitor of complement (C5)-derived chemotactic activity in serum from patients with systemic lupus erythematosus. J. Clin. Invest. 62:29, 1978.

96. Abramson, S. B., Gren, W. P., Eddson, H. S., and Weissman, G.: Neutrophil aggregation induced by sera from patients with active systemic lupus erythematosus. Arthritis Rheum. 26:630, 1983.

97. Gamussi, G., Teffa, C., Coda, R., and Benveniste, J.: Release of platelet-activating factor in human pathology. Evidence for the occurrence of basophil degranulation and release of platelet-activating factor in systemic lupus erythematosus. Lab. Invest. 44:241, 1981.

98. Morimoto, C., Reinherz, E. L., Schlossman, S. F., et al.: Alterations in immunoregulating T cell subsets in active systemic lupus erythematosus. J. Clin. Invest. 66:1171, 1980.

99. Love, P. E., and Santoro, S. A.: Anti-phospholipid antibodies: Anti-cardiolipin and the lupus anticoagulant in systemic lupus erythematosus (SLE) and in non-SLE disorders. Prevalence and clinical significance. Ann. Intern. Med. 112:682, 1990.

100. Asherson, R. A., Khamashta, M. A., Ordi-Ros, J., Derksen, R. H. W. M., Machin, S. J., Barquinero, J., Outt, H-J., Harris, E. N., Vilardell-Torres, M., and Hughes, G. R. V.: The "primary" anti-phospholipid syndrome: Major clinical and serological features. Medicine 68:366, 1989.

101. Pollak, V. E., and Kant, K. S.: Systemic lupus erythematosus and the kidney. *In* Lahita, R. G. (ed.): Systemic Lupus Erythematosus. New York, John Wiley & Sons, 1987.

102. Rothfield, N. F.: Renal disease. *In* Schur, P. H. (ed.): The Clinical Management of Systemic Lupus Erythematosus. Orlando, Florida, Grune & Stratton, 1983.

103. Nossent, H. C., Henzen-Logmans, S. C., Vroom, T. M., Berden, J. H. M., and Swaak, T. J. G.: Contribution of renal biopsy data in predicting outcome in lupus nephritis. Analysis of 116 patients. Arthritis Rheum. 33:970, 1990.

104. Austin, H. A. III, Muenz, L. R., Joyce, K. M., et al.: Diffuse proliferative lupus nephritis: Identification of specific pathologic features affecting renal outcome. Kidney Int. 25:689, 1984.

105. Park, M. H., D'Agati, V., Appel, G. B., and Pirani, C. L.: Tubulointerstitial disease in lupus nephritis: Relationship to immune deposits, interstitial inflammation, glomerular changes, renal function, and prognosis. Nephron 44:309, 1986.

106. Couser, W. G., Salant, D. J., Madaio, M. P., et al.: Factors influencing glomerular and tubulointerstitial patterns of injury in SLE. Am. J. Kidney Dis. 2:126, 1982.

107. Lloyd, W., and Schur, P. H.: Immune complexes, complement and anti-DNA in exacerbations of systemic lupus erythematosus. Medicine 60:208, 1981.

108. Esdaile, J. M., Levinton, C., Federgreen, W., Hayslett, J. P., and Kashgarian, M.: The clinical and renal biopsy predictors of long-term outcome in lupus nephritis: A study of 87 patients and review of the literature. Q. J. Med. 269:779, 1989.

109. Pillemer, S. R., Austin, H. A., Tsokos, G. C., and Balow, J. E.: Lupus nephritis: Association between serology and renal biopsy measures. J. Rheumatol. 15:284, 1988.

110. Fries, J. F., Porta, J., and Liang, M. H.: Marginal benefit of renal biopsy in systemic lupus erythematosus. Arch. Intern. Med. 138:1386, 1978.

111. Appel, G. B., Cohen, D. J., Pirani, C. L., Meltzer, J. I., and Estes, D.: Long-term follow-up of patients with lupus nephritis. A study based on classification of the World Health Organization. Am. J. Med. 83:877, 1987.

112. Bumgardner, G. L., Mauer, S. M., Ascher, N. L., Payne, W. D., Dunn, D. L., Fryd, D. S., Sutherland, D. E., Simmons, R. L., and Narjarian, J. S.: Long-term outcome of renal transplantation in patients with systemic lupus erythematosus. Transplant. Proc. 21:2031, 1989.

113. Mayer, L. F.: Gastrointestinal manifestations of systemic lupus erythematosus. *In* Lahita, R. G. (ed.): Systemic Lupus Erythematosus. New York, John Wiley & Sons, 1987.

114. Zizic, T. M.: Gastrointestinal manifestations. *In* Schur, P. H. (ed.): The Clinical Management of Systemic Lupus Erythematosus. Orlando, Florida, Grune & Stratton, 1983.

115. Matolo, N. M., and Albo, D., Jr.: Gastrointestinal complications of collagen vascular diseases: Surgical implications. Am. J. Surg. 122:678, 1971.

116. Reynolds, J. C., Inman, R. D., Kimberly, R. P., et al.: Acute pancreatitis in systemic lupus erythematosus: Report of twenty cases and a review of the literature. Medicine 61:25, 1982.

117. Runyon, B. A., LaBreque, D. R., and Anuras, S.: The spectrum of liver disease in systemic lupus erythematosus. Report of 33 histologically-proved cases and review of the literature. Am. J. Med. 69:187, 1980.

118. Zvaifler, N. J.: Neurologic manifestations. *In* Schur, P. H. (ed.): The Clinical Management of Systemic Lupus Erythematosus. Orlando, Florida, Grune & Stratton, 1983.

119. Rogers, M. P.: Psychiatric aspects. *In* Schur, P. H. (ed.): The Clinical Management of Systemic Lupus Erythematosus. Orlando, Florida, Grune & Stratton, 1983.

120. Bluestein, H. G.: Neuropsychiatric disorders in systemic lupus erythematosis. *In* Lahita, R. G. (ed.): Systemic Lupus Erythematosus. New York, John Wiley & Sons, 1987.

121. Perry, S. W.: Psychiatric aspects of systemic lupus erythematosus. *In* Lahita, R. G. (ed.): Systemic Lupus Erythematosus. New York, John Wiley & Sons, 1987.

122. Carbotte, R. M., Denburg, S. D., and Denburg, J. A.: Prevalence of cognitive impairment in systemic lupus erythematosus. J. Nerv. Ment. Dis. 174:357, 1986.

123. Liang, M. H., Rogers, M. P., Larson, M., Eaton, H. M., Murawski, B. J., Taylor, J. E., Swafford, J., and Schur, P. H.: The psychological impact of SLE and RA. Arthritis Rheum. 27:13, 1984.

124. Goodwin, J. M., Goodwin, J. S., and Kellner, R.: Psychiatric symptoms in disliked medical patients. JAMA 241:1117, 1979.

125. Rogers, M. P., Liang, M. H., Waterhouse, E., Roberts, W. N., Stern, S., Fraser, P., Partridge, R., Murawski, B., Khoshbin, S., Nagel, J. S., and Schur, P. H.: Disturbed cognition and systemic lupus erythematosus: A subset of central nervous system lupus. Submitted for publication.

126. Bryant, G. L., Weinblatt, M. E., Rumbaugh, C., and Coblyn, J. S.: Cerebral vasculopathy: An analysis of sixteen cases. Semin. Arthritis Rheum. 15:297, 1986.

127. Johnson, R. T., and Richardson, E. P.: The neurologic manifestations of systemic lupus erythematosus: A clinical-pathological study of 24 cases and review of the literature. Medicine 47:337, 1968.

128. Futrell, N., and Millikan, C.: Frequency, etiology, and prevention of stroke in patients with systemic lupus erythematosus. Stroke 20:583, 1989.

129. Alarcon-Segovia, D.: Transverse myelitis: A manifestation of systemic lupus erythematosus strongly associated with antiphospholipid antibodies. J. Rheumatol. 17:34, 1990.

130. Boumpas, D. T., Patronas, N. J., Dalakas, M. C., Hakim, C. A., Klippel, J. H., and Balow, J. E.: Acute transverse myelitis in systemic lupus erythematosus: Magnetic resonance imaging and review of the literature. J. Rheumatol. 17:89, 1990.

131. Stafford-Brady, F. J., Urowitz, M. B., Gladman, D. D., and Easterbrook, M.: Lupus retinopathy. Patterns, associations, and prognosis. Arthritis Rheum. 31:1105, 1988.

132. Denburg, J. A., Carbotte, R. M., and Denburg, S. D.: Neuronal antibodies and cognitive function in SLE. Neurology 37:464, 1987.

133. Schneebaum, A. B., Singleton, J. D., West, S. G., Blodgett, J. K., Allen, L. G., Cheronis, J. C., and Kotzin, B. L.: Association of psychiatric manifestations with antibodies to ribosomal P protein in systemic lupus erythematosus. Am. J. Med. 90:54, 1991.

134. Hirohata, S., and Miyamoto, T.: Elevated levels of interleukin-6 in cerebrospinal fluid from patients with systemic lupus erythematosus. Arthritis Rheum. 33:644, 1990.

135. Pinching, A. J., Travers, R. L., Hughes, G. R. V., et al.: Oxygen-15 brain scanning for detection of cerebral involvement in systemic lupus erythematosus. Lancet I:898, 1978.

136. McCune, W. J., MacGuire, A., Aisen, A., and Gebarski, S.: Identification of brain lesions in NP-SLE by magnetic resonance scanning. Arthritis Rheum. 31:159, 1988.

137. Jacobs, L., Kinkel, P. R., Costello, P. B., Alukal, M. K., Kinkel, W. R., and Green, F. A.: Central nervous systemic lupus erythematosus: The value of magnetic resonance imaging. J. Rheumatol 15:601, 1988.

138. Griffey, R. H., Brown, M. S., Bankhurst, A. D., Sibbitt, R. R., and Sibbitt, W. L., Jr.: Depletion of high-energy phosphates in the central nervous system of patients with systemic lupus erythematosus as determined by ^{31}phosphorous nuclear magnetic resonance spectroscopy. Arthritis Rheum. 33:827, 1990.

139. Jungers, P., Dougados, M., Pelissier, C., et al.: Influence of oral contraceptive therapy on the activity of systemic lupus erythematosus. Arthritis Rheum. 25:618, 1982.

140. Bucala, R., Lahita, R. G., Fishman, J., Cerami, A.: Anti-estrogen antibodies in users of oral contraceptives and in patients with systemic lupus erythematosus. Clin. Exp. Immunol. 67:167, 1987.

141. Decker, J. L.: Management. In Schur, P. H. (ed.): The Clinical Management of Systemic Lupus Erythematosus. Orlando, Florida, Grune & Stratton, 1983.

142. Mintz, G., Niz, J., Gutierrez, G., Garcia-Alonso, A., and Karchmer, S.: Prospective study of pregnancy in systemic lupus erythematosus. Results of a multidisciplinary approach. J. Rheumatol. 13:4, 1986.

143. Estes, D., and Larson, D. L.: Systemic lupus erythematosus and pregnancy. Clin. Obstet. Gynecol. 8:307, 1965.

144. Lockshin, M. D.: Pregnancy does not cause SLE to worsen. Arthritis Rheum. 32:665, 1989.

145. Zurier, R. B.: Systemic lupus erythematosus and pregnancy. In Lahita, R. G. (ed.): Systemic Lupus Erythematosus. New York, John Wiley & Sons, 1987.

145a. Lockwood, C. J., Romero, R., Feinberg, R. F., Clyne, L. P., Coster, B., and Hobbins, J. C.: The prevalence and biologic significance of lupus anticoagulant and anticardiolipin antibodies in a general obstetric population. Am. J. Gynecol. 161:369, 1989.

146. Lockshin, M. D., Bonfa, E., Elkon, K., and Druzin, M. L.: Neonatal lupus risk to newborns of mothers with SLE. Arthritis Rheum. 31:697, 1988.

147. Arnaiz-Villena, A., Vazquez-Rodriquez, J. J., Vicario, J. L., Lavilla, P., Pascual, D., Morino, F., and Martinez-Laso, J.: Cogenital heart block immunogenetics. Evidence for an additional role of HLA class III antigens and independence of Ro antibodies. Arthritis Rheum. 32:1421, 1989.

148. McCune, A. B., Weston, W. L., and Lee, L. A.: Maternal and fetal outcome in neonatal lupus erythematosus. Ann. Intern. Med. 106:518, 1987.

148a. Hess, E. V.: Drug-related lupus: The same or different? In Lahita, R. G. (ed.): Systemic Lupus Erythematosus. New York, John Wiley & Sons, 1986.

149. Reidenberg, M. M., and Drayer, M. M.: Genetic regulation of drug metabolism and systemic lupus erythematosus. In Lahita, R. G. (ed.): Systemic Lupus Erythematosus. New York, John Wiley & Sons, 1986.

150. Batchelor, J. R., Welsh, K. I., Tinoco, R. M., et al.: Hydralazine-induced systemic lupus erythematosus: Influence of HLA-DR and sex on susceptibility. Lancet 1:1107, 1980.

151. Weinstein, A.: Lupus syndromes induced by drugs. In Schur, P. H. (ed.): The Clinical Management of Systemic Lupus Erythematosus. Orlando, Florida, Grune & Stratton, 1983.

152. Weinstein, A.: Laboratory diagnosis of drug-induced lupus. In Lahita, R. G. (ed.): Systemic Lupus Erythematosus. New York, John Wiley & Sons, 1986.

153. Schur, M.: Comments on the metapsychology of somatization. Psychoanal. Study Child 10:119, 1955.

154. Tan, E. M., Cohen, A. S., Fries, J. F., et al.: The 1982 revised criteria for the classification of systemic lupus erythematosus. Arthritis Rheum. 25:1271, 1982.

155. Greer, J. M., and Panush, R. S.: Incomplete lupus erythematosus. Arch. Intern. Med. 149:2473, 1989.

156. Griner, P. F., Mayewski, R. J., Mushlin, A. I., and Greenland, P.: Selection and interpretation of diagnostic tests and procedures. Ann. Intern. Med. 94:453, 1981.

157. Liang, M. H., Meenan, R. F., Cathcart, E. S., and Schur, P. H.: A screening strategy for population studies in systemic lupus erythematosus: Series design. Arthritis Rheum. 23:152, 1980.

158. Shiel, W. C., Jr., and Jason, M.: The diagnostic associations of patients with antinuclear antibodies referred to a community rheumatologist. J. Rheumatol. 16:782, 1989.

Management of Systemic Lupus Erythematosus

INTRODUCTION

Management of systemic lupus erythematosus (SLE) is a challenge because no interventions result in cure, exacerbations of disease can occur after months of stable maintenance treatment, and undesirable side effects of the therapies can be as troublesome as the disease. Careful and frequent monitoring of patients is important in selecting management plans, monitoring efficacy, and changing treatments.

INITIAL THERAPEUTIC DECISIONS

Because most therapeutic interventions in patients with SLE are associated with significant undesirable side effects, the physician must first decide whether a patient needs any treatment, and if so, whether conservative management is sufficient or whether aggressive immunosuppression is necessary. Figure 62–1 presents an algorithm for this decision making.

In general, patients with manifestations of SLE that are not life-threatening and are unlikely to be associated with organ damage should be managed conservatively. If quality of life is impaired very little, reassurance and careful follow-up may be adequate. If quality of life is impaired, it is appropriate to initiate strategies listed in Figure 62–1 as "Conservative Measures." On the other hand, if the disease is indeed life-threatening or major organ systems are at high risk for irreversible damage, aggressive intervention is mandatory. Aggressive therapy usually consists of immunosuppression. However, a few clinical subsets of SLE have been recognized in which either immunosuppression is not effective, or alternative therapies may be preferable. The best example is patients who experience recurring thrombosis as their sole or major manifestation of SLE. In the subsequent sections, conservative therapies, the approach to patients with life-threatening lupus, and therapies effective in different clinical subsets will be reviewed.

The pharmacology, mechanisms of action, benefits, and side effects of most of the drugs used in management of SLE are reviewed in Section V, "Clinical Pharmacology in Rheumatic Diseases." This chapter discusses the use of these agents in SLE.

CONSERVATIVE MANAGEMENT OF PATIENTS WITH SLE

Arthritis, Arthralgia, Myalgia

Arthritis, arthralgia, and myalgia are the most common manifestations of SLE. Severity ranges from mild to disabling. For patients with mild symptoms, administration of analgesics, nonsteroidal anti-inflammatory drugs (NSAIDs), or salicylates may provide adequate relief, although none are as effective

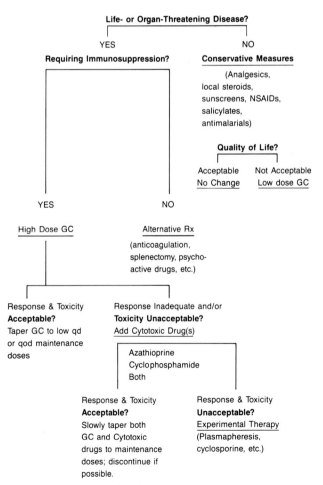

Figure 62–1. An algorithm for selecting management of patients with systemic lupus erythematosus.

as glucocorticoids.[1, 2] Nonacetylated salicylates are useful because they inhibit prostaglandin synthesis less than acetylated salicylates and NSAIDs and therefore are associated with a relatively low incidence of gastrointestinal symptoms and bleeding. They usually do not impair renal or platelet function. Therapeutic range (approximately 150–200 mg per dl) can be assessed by measuring serum salicylate levels. The use of NSAIDs requires special caution in patients with SLE. Several NSAIDs (ibuprofen, tolmetin, sulindac) can cause aseptic meningitis.[1, 2] Through their effects on renal prostaglandins, all NSAIDs can reduce glomerular filtration rates and renal blood flow, especially in patients who have clinical or subclinical nephritis, are taking diuretics, or have congestive heart failure or cirrhosis. Although sulindac is least likely to have this effect, it does occur; serum creatinine levels should be monitored after introduction of any salicylate or NSAID. Hyperkalemia and interstitial nephritis are uncommon side effects of NSAIDs. Salt retention secondary to NSAIDs may elevate blood pressure and cause pedal edema; NSAIDs may reduce the efficacy of furosemide and thiazide diuretics. Gastrointestinal toxicity with bleeding can develop at any time during therapy. Finally, patients with SLE have a higher incidence of hepatotoxicity than that of other patients taking NSAIDs[3]; this is usually manifested as transaminitis without permanent hepatic damage. In summary, SLE patients treated with NSAIDs should be monitored regularly for renal, gastrointestinal, and hepatic side effects.

Concomitant use of glucocorticoids increases the clearance of salicylates: lowering glucocorticoid doses may be accompanied by increases in serum salicylate levels.

In many SLE patients, musculoskeletal symptoms are not well controlled by salicylate or NSAID therapies. A trial of antimalarials may be useful in such individuals.[2, 4] Antimalarials are discussed in the subsequent section on treatment of cutaneous manifestations. Hydroxychloroquine is the preferred antimalarial in the United States (chloroquine may be more effective but has a higher incidence of retinal toxicity).[5] The usual dose of hydroxychloroquine for SLE patients with arthritis is 400 mg daily. If a response does not occur within 6 months, the patient may be considered a nonresponder, and the drug stopped. If hydroxychloroquine is used for more than 6 months, or chloroquine for more than 3 months, regular examinations by an ophthalmologist who can detect early evidence of damage to the retina are mandatory.[5] If antimalarials are effective, the maintenance dose should be reduced periodically, if possible, or withdrawn when a patient is doing well, since the retinal toxicity is cumulative.

Some patients with arthritis/arthralgia are not benefited by NSAIDs/salicylates with or without antimalarials. If quality of life is seriously impaired by pain—or by the deformities that develop in about 10 percent of individuals with lupus arthritis, the phy-

sician should consider institution of low-dose glucocorticoids—not to exceed 15 mg each morning. Rarely, patients may require high-dose glucocorticoids or, even, cytotoxic drugs. Such aggressive interventions should be avoided if possible.

Pain persisting in one or two joints may be due to ischemic necrosis of bone, or to septic arthritis; those conditions should be ruled out before such patients are treated for lupus arthritis.

Cutaneous Lupus

Recent data suggest that as many as 70 percent of all SLE patients are photosensitive.[6] Flares of SLE can be caused by ultraviolet light (usually UVB, sometimes UVA), infrared light, heat, or, rarely, fluorescent lights. Photosensitive patients should minimize their exposure by wearing protective clothing (including hats), using tinted glass in car windshields, avoiding direct exposure, and applying sunscreens. Most topical sunscreens are creams, oils, lotions, or gels that contain UV light–blocking chemicals such as para-aminobenzoic acid (PABA) and its esters, benzophenones, salicylates, anthralites, and cinnamates.[2, 7] All absorb UVB light; UVA is absorbed partially by benzophenones and anthranilates. The "sun protection factor" (SPF) is the ratio of time required to produce erythema when wearing sunscreen to the time required to produce the same degree of erythema in unprotected skin. SPFs range from 2 to 50; patients should use preparations with an SPF of 15 or higher. They should be reapplied after toweling or sweating. Table 62–1 lists some sunscreens currently available. They can be locally irritating (especially those containing PABA); patients may need to try several preparations to find one that is not irritating, drying, or staining and that stays on well.

Local glucocorticoids, including topical creams and ointments and injections into severe skin lesions, are also helpful in lupus dermatitis.[8] Patients with disfiguring (discoid) or extensive lesions should be seen by a dermatologist, since management of severe lupus dermatitis can be difficult. Fluorinated high-potency preparations, such as betamethasone dipropionate 0.05 percent and fluocinonide 0.05 percent, are among the most effective topical steroid ointments/creams but are also likely to cause atrophy, depigmentation, striae, acne, and folliculitis. They should probably not be used for more than 2 weeks (especially on face lesions), after which time less potent preparations (hydrocortisone, desonide) should be substituted for a brief period of time, or topical steroids stopped altogether. Skin lesions often worsen when topical therapies are discontinued, thus requiring additional strategies.

Antimalarials are useful in some patients with lupus dermatitis, whether the lesions are those of SLE, subacute cutaneous lupus, or discoid lupus.[2, 8] Antimalarials have multiple sun-blocking, anti-in-

Table 62–1. SUNSCREEN PREPARATIONS WITH SUN PROTECTION FACTOR (SPF) OF 15 OR GREATER

Product	SPF	Contents
Aramis SPF 20 Sun Protection	20	Padimate O, phenylbenzimidazole-5-sulfonic acid, benzophenone-3
Bain de Soleil, Ultra Sun Block 15	15	Padimate O, oxybenzone, dioxybenzone
Block Out Cream Lotion	15	Padimate O, dioxybenzone
Clinique SPF 19 Sun Block	19	Padimate O, octyl methoxycinnamate, benzophenone-3
Elizabeth Arden Sun Blocking Cream	15	Padimate O, oxybenzone
PreSun 15 and 39 Creams Lotions, Facial Preparation	15, 39	Octyl-dimethyl PABA, oxybenzone et al.
Sensitive Skin Preparations	15, 29	Octyl methoxycinnamate, oxybenzone, octyl salicylate et al.
Solbar PF 15 Liquid, Cream	15	Octyl methoxycinnamate, oxybenzone
Super Shade 15, Coppertone	15	Padimate O, oxybenzone
T1. Screen	15+	Ethylhexyl-p-methoxycinnamate, oxybenzone
Total Eclipse	15	Pamidate O, octylsalicylate, oxybenzone

Data from the Medical Letter 26:56, 1984; The Medical Letter 32:59, 1990; the Physician's Desk Reference 1990; Dubois, E. L., and Wallace, D. J.: Management of discoid and systemic lupus erythematosus. *In* Wallace, D. J., and Dubois, E. L. (eds.): Dubois' Lupus Erythematosus. 3rd ed. Philadelphia, Lea & Febiger, 1987.

flammatory, and immunosuppressive effects. They bind to deoxyribonucleic acid (DNA), cell membrane receptors, lysosomal membranes, and melanin.

A recent controlled trial[4] of hydroxychloroquine in patients with stable lupus showed that replacement of the antimalarial with placebo resulted in a significant increase in flare-ups, some of which were serious. In addition, multiple open studies of hundreds of patients with discoid LE, SLE, or subacute cutaneous LE have reported that 60 to 90 percent of patients with cutaneous lupus have good to excellent responses to antimalarials.[2, 8] Higher doses of each agent give earlier responses, and a larger proportion of patients improve. (However, higher doses are more toxic.) Responses to chloroquine and quinacrine are usually demonstrable within 4 to 16 weeks; responses to hydroxychloroquine may require 3 to 6 months. Antimalarials may be steroid sparing. Recommended initial doses of antimalarials are hydroxychloroquine 400 mg daily; chloroquine 500 mg daily; quinacrine 100 mg daily. Higher doses can be given for brief periods (a few weeks). Several months later, after disease is well controlled, the drugs can be slowly tapered. Daily doses can be reduced, or the drug can be given less frequently (e.g., 5 days a week, or every other day, or ultimately 2 days a week). The combination of hydroxychloroquine or chloroquine and atabrine is probably synergistic and may be used in patients refractory to single-drug therapy.

Toxicities of these agents are important but infrequent in comparison with those of other agents used to treat SLE. Retinal damage is the most important: in unmonitored patients it occurs in approximately 10 percent of individuals receiving chronic chloroquine therapy and in 3 to 4 percent of those receiving hydroxychloroquine.[5] Regular ophthalmologic examinations with appropriate special testing identifies retinal changes early. If changes occur, antimalarials should be stopped, or the daily dose decreased. This strategy substantially lowers the incidence of clinically important retinal toxicity. Retinopathy is rare in patients treated with quinacrine. Other significant toxic reactions include gastrointestinal disturbances, rashes, peripheral neuropathies, and myopathies of skeletal and cardiac muscles. Quinacrine is associated with aplastic anemia, especially in patients who develop an antecedent lichen-planus–like rash.[2] Pigment changes are common with quinacrine (usually a yellow discoloration of skin) and occur less frequently with chloroquine and hydroxychloroquine (depigmentation, hyperpigmentation, and blue-black discoloration of skin and mucous membranes). Development of neuropathies or myopathies requires discontinuation of the drugs; skin changes are usually tolerated by patients (in the case of quinacrine, any dermatitis other than pigment changes should cause the physician to discontinue treatment). The use of antimalarials during pregnancy is controversial, with conflicting reports of fetal damage and of good outcomes.[9] Use of antimalarials in lupus is reviewed in Table 62–2.

For individuals resistant to antimalarials and other conservative strategies, the physician must consider more aggressive approaches, including "experimental" therapies or systemic glucocorticoids. Dapsone has been used in discoid lupus, urticarial vasculitis, and bullous LE lesions with some success.[10] It has significant hematologic toxicities (including methemoglobinemia, sulfhemoglobinemia, and hemolytic anemia) and can occasionally worsen the rashes of LE. Etretinate has been beneficial in most patients with discoid LE and in some with subacute cutaneous or systemic lupus rashes.[11] The retinates are teratogenic, cause cheilitis in most patients, and elevate cholesterol and triglyceride levels in some.

Most lupus skin lesions of any type improve during systemic glucocorticoid therapy. There are steroid-resistant patients; some have improved when treated with cytotoxic drugs, such as azathioprine.[8]

Fatigue and Systemic Complaints

Fatigue is common in patients with SLE and may be the major disabling complaint.[12] Few strategies other than high-dose systemic glucocorticoid therapy improve fatigue. Less fatigue, weight loss, and fever

Table 62–2. USE OF ANTIMALARIALS AND EXPERIMENTAL REGIMENS TO TREAT CUTANEOUS LUPUS

Agent	Initial Dose	Maintenance Dose	Response	Toxicities
Hydroxychloroquine	400–600 mg daily	100–400 mg daily	Dermatitis (SLE, DLE, SCLE) Arthralgia Arthritis Oral ulcers Fatigue	Retinal damage Corneal deposit Skin pigmentation Rashes Alopecia Peripheral neuropathy Peripheral myopathy Cardiomyopathy Nausea, anorexia Diarrhea Psychosis ? Fetal abnormalities
Chloroquine	250–500 mg daily	125–500 mg daily	As for hydroxychloroquine Probably most effective for arthritis	As for hydroxychloroquine Probably most toxic for the retina
Quinacrine	100 mg daily	50–100 mg daily	Probably most effective for fatigue	Aplastic anemia (often preceded by lichen planus rash). Little or no retinal damage Yellow pigmentation of skin
Hydroxychloroquine or chloroquine plus quinacrine	As above	As above	Effects probably additive for dermatitis	Toxicities probably not additive
Experimental: Dapsone	25 mg twice daily	25 mg daily	Dermatitis (especially DLE, bullous LE)	Methemoglobinemia Sulfhemoglobinemia Hemolytic anemia GI intolerance
Etretinate	25 mg twice daily	10–25 mg daily	Dermatitis (especially DLE, SCLE)	Hyperlipidemia Cheilitis Fetal abnormalities

occur in some patients receiving antimalarials[2]; quinacrine may be best in this regard. Complaints of fatigue should be approached sympathetically with recommendations for increased rest periods and flexibility in working hours when possible. Fever and weight loss, if mild, can be managed with the conservative approaches outlined in the preceding paragraphs; when these side effects are severe, systemic glucocorticoid therapy is necessary.

Serositis

Episodes of chest and abdominal pain may be secondary to lupus serositis. In some patients, symptoms will respond to salicylate, NSAID (indomethacin may be best), or antimalarial therapies or to low doses of systemic glucocorticoids, such as 15 mg per day.[1] In other patients, systemic glucocorticoids must be given in high doses to achieve disease control.

AGGRESSIVE THERAPY FOR SYSTEMIC LUPUS ERYTHEMATOSUS

When Should Aggressive Therapy Be Used?

Aggressive therapy, beginning with high-dose glucocorticoids, should be used whenever a patient has life-threatening SLE that is likely to be steroid responsive. The serious manifestations of lupus that usually improve with glucocorticoid therapy are listed in Table 62–3. Some manifestations may not be steroid responsive (e.g., pure membranous glomerulonephritis, vascular occlusions). Other manifestations respond to therapy but may be mild enough that high doses of glucocorticoids are not necessary, for example, hemolytic anemia with hematocrits of 30 to 34 percent and no symptoms, thrombocytopenia of 50,000 to 120,000 cells per mm³ without bleeding, mesangial glomerulonephritis; mild cognitive dysfunction.

Infectious causes of the manifestations of "lupus" must be carefully excluded, especially in the presence of pulmonary infiltrates, confusion states, hematuria with pyuria, and fever. Finally, the physician must consider the presence of comorbid conditions that increase the risk of glucocorticoid therapy, such as infection, hypertension, diabetes mellitus, obesity, osteoporosis, and psychiatric disease. When all factors are carefully analyzed, and the decision is made to institute aggressive therapy, institution of high-dose glucocorticoids is the appropriate first step, sometimes with addition of cytotoxic drugs.

Efficacy of Daily High-Dose Glucocorticoid Therapy

Most of the randomized, prospective, controlled trials of glucocorticoid therapy in SLE have been

Table 62–3. SERIOUS AND LIFE-THREATENING MANIFESTATIONS OF SLE: RESPONSES TO GLUCOCORTICOIDS

Manifestations Usually Responsive to High-Dose Glucocorticoids
Vasculitis
Severe dermatitis of SCLE or SLE
Polyarthritis
Polyserositis—pericarditis, pleurisy, peritonitis
Myocarditis
Lupus pneumonitis*
Glomerulonephritis—proliferative forms
Hemolytic anemia
Thrombocytopenia
Organic brain syndromes*—coma, confusion, seizures
Myelopathies
Peripheral neuropathies
"Lupus crisis"*—high fever, prostration

Manifestations Not Often Responsive to Glucocorticoids
Thrombosis—includes strokes
Glomerulonephritis—scarred end-stage disease, pure membranous GN
Mild behavioral/cognitive disturbances
Resistant thrombocytopenia/hemolytic anemia—occurs in a minority of patients, consider splenectomy, danazol (see text)
Psychosis related to conditions other than SLE, such as glucocorticoid therapy

*Take special care to rule out infectious processes before instituting immunosuppressive therapies.

conducted in patients with life-threatening forms of lupus nephritis, with comparisons made between the efficacy of steroids and that of other interventions, which usually consist of steroids plus an additional drug. Therefore, guidelines for management of all serious disease come primarily from studies of patients with nephritis.

The most convincing evidence that high-dose glucocorticoids can be life-saving was provided by Pollak et al.[13, 14] in a retrospective study of patients with diffuse proliferative glomerulonephritis (DPGN). Figure 62–2 illustrates their outcomes. These data antedate the availability of dialysis and renal transplantation. Two years after renal biopsy, patients with DPGN treated with less than 40 mg of prednisone a day had a survival rate of zero; patients treated with 40 to 60 mg of prednisone for 4 to 6 months had a survival rate of 55 percent. The average doses were, in the low-dose group, 10 to 15 mg per day and, in the high-dose group, 47.5 mg per day for 6 months. These studies form the basis of current practice: patients with severe forms of lupus nephritis treated with single-drug therapy should receive at least 40 to 60 mg of prednisone daily for at least 4 months. Thereafter, the dose should be tapered as rapidly as the disease permits.

How Should Responses be Monitored?

Several problems arise when following these guidelines: (1) some patients fail to respond, (2) some patients respond initially but relapse when the dose

is tapered, and (3) toxic side effects of glucocorticoids are virtually universal. To minimize these problems the physician should set goals, including (1) establishing criteria for acceptable clinical responses and (2) setting time limits to achieve those responses. The criteria for response should include both clinical and laboratory parameters, when the laboratory parameters provide good measures of the clinical problem being addressed. For example, in patients with nephritis, levels of blood urea nitrogen and creatinine and of proteinuria usually *rise* during the first 1 to 2 weeks of steroid therapy but should improve thereafter. Serum levels of complement components begin to rise in 1 to 3 weeks, and antibodies to DNA fall. Proteinuria should diminish and renal function improve after 6 to 10 weeks of high-dose daily prednisone. In some patients, clinical improvement occurs without changes in autoantibody titers or serum complement levels. In contrast with nephritis, hemolysis and thrombocytopenia usually begin to improve within 5 to 15 days after steroid therapy is instituted. Manifestations of organic brain syndrome should improve within days. If the desired effect is not obtained within the appropriate time frame, the next decision must be whether to change the glucocorticoid dose, to introduce additional therapy, or to stop immunosuppression. Patients with renal insuf-

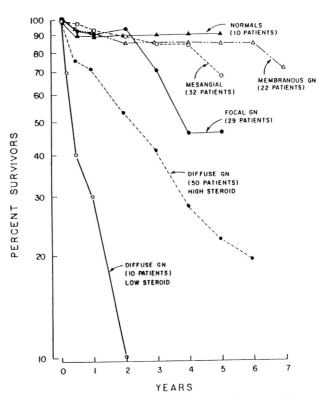

Figure 62–2. Survival in patients with systemic lupus erythematosus. Patients are classified according to the findings on initial renal biopsy, with survival calculated by life table analysis from the time at which the renal biopsy was done. (From Pollak, V. E., and Dosekun, A. K.: Evaluation of treatment in lupus nephritis: Effects of prednisone. Am. J. Kidney Dis. 2[Suppl. 1]:170, 1982, with permission.)

ficiency and high chronicity indices on renal biopsies are unlikely to improve. It is appropriate to plan for dialysis or renal transplantation in such patients. See the discussion later in this chapter in the section on outcomes in patients with SLE.

Intravenous Pulse Therapy and Alternate-Day Regimens

In an effort to increase response rates and the rapidity of responses, and to decrease side effects of daily high-dose glucocorticoid therapy, several experts have studied the efficacy of administering methylprednisolone (10–30 mg per kg: 500–1000 mg per dose) in single high intravenous doses for three to six doses, then maintaining responses with high doses of daily oral prednisone (40–60 mg), which are rapidly tapered.[15–21] Uncontrolled trials[15–17, 19] suggest that 75 per cent or more of lupus patients with severe active nephritis, central nervous system disease, pneumonitis, polyserositis, vasculitis, or thrombocytopenia improve within a few days. Some individuals who fail to improve while receiving 40 to 60 mg of prednisone daily respond to high-dose pulse therapy.[1] Patients with rapid increases in proteinuria and rapid increases in serum creatinine—i.e., those with active disease[15]—are most likely to respond. In a prospective, randomized controlled trial,[18] initial pulses followed by daily oral prednisone therapy improved renal function a mean of 12 weeks earlier than did standard daily therapy; the final inulin clearances were similar in both groups. Another controlled trial[20] compared 12 months of repeated pulses of intravenous methylprednisolone (given 3 sequential days each month and followed by high-dose daily prednisone, then tapered) with daily high-dose prednisone (then tapered) in patients with DPGN. After 1 year, renal function was significantly better, and the maintenance prednisone requirement was significantly lower in the group that received intravenous steroid pulses. A recent preliminary study[21] of patients with severe nephritis compared (1) one monthly dose of intravenous methylprednisolone (1 g per m²), (2) monthly intravenous cyclophosphamide, and (3) both. After 1 year, except for 2 of 18 patients in the intravenous steroid group who developed renal failure, patients in all groups improved, with most requiring low-dose daily or alternate-day glucocorticoids.

Overall, the incidence of adverse side effects is probably not increased when high-dose pulse therapy with glucocorticoids is compared with high-dose daily therapy. However, steroid withdrawal syndromes, acute psychosis, rapid increases in blood pressure, seizures, arrhythmias, and sudden death have been reported.[1]

In summary, many patients with severe, active SLE respond within days or a few weeks to intravenous pulses of methylprednisolone. The physician can administer 3 days of pulse therapy, then begin

40 to 60 mg of prednisone daily, then rapidly taper the dose to low levels of oral glucocorticoid maintenance therapy. Perhaps the taper can be faster if the initial therapy is pulse steroids rather than daily high oral doses. The author uses pulse glucocorticoid regimens in patients with severe SLE and rapid clinical deterioration. Repeating pulse glucocorticoid therapy monthly (1 to 3 days per month) may be an acceptable alternative to the addition of cytotoxic drugs. However, long-term results (10 years and more) are available for the regimens in which oral glucocorticoids are combined with cytotoxics, but only short-term (1 year) follow-up data are available for glucocorticoid intravenous pulse regimens.

With regard to treatment regimens employing alternate-day glucocorticoids, one study[22] reports response of five of seven patients with lupus nephritis treated initially with prednisone 100 to 120 mg every other day. However, the author has had little success with alternate-day therapy in patients with severe, active disease and cannot recommend it. It is desirable to taper the doses patients receive to maintenance regimens of a short-acting glucocorticoid (prednisone, prednisolone, methylprednisolone) given in the morning once every 48 hours. Such regimens, compared with daily glucocorticoid administration, are associated with significantly less suppression of the hypothalamic-pituitary axis, as well as less potassium and nitrogen wasting, hypertension, Cushingoid changes, and infection.[23] Disease must be well suppressed before such regimens are appropriate.

Summary of Glucocorticoid Use in Severe SLE

Glucocorticoid regimens are reviewed in Table 62–4. Most patients with severe active SLE improve substantially on glucocorticoid regimens. Initial therapy should be either high-dose daily glucocorticoids, 40 to 100 mg prednisone daily, or 1 to 1.5 mg per kg, given in divided doses, or high-dose intravenous methylprednisolone pulses followed by 40 to 60 mg of prednisone (or equivalent short-acting glucocorticoid) daily. Response of some manifestations may begin as early as 1 to 5 days; others require 3 to 10 weeks (especially nephritis). If the desired response is obtained within an appropriate time, tapering of daily glucocorticoid doses is initiated. Daily doses may be decreased by 5 to 10 percent weekly if flares do not occur. A substantial proportion of patients will experience steroid withdrawal during tapering (fever, joint pain, malaise, frank arthritis); such reactions should not last more than 3 days. There should be an attempt to reach a maintenance low daily or alternate-day glucocorticoid dose. In most cases, the disease flares during the taper; when this occurs, the dose should be increased and held at the level necessary to control severe disease. If the maintenance requirement is unacceptable because of side

Table 62–4. USE OF GLUCOCORTICOIDS IN SLE

Preparations	Dose	Advantages	Toxicities
Severe, Active SLE Regimen 1: Daily oral short-acting (prednisone, prednisolone, methylprednisolone)	1–2 mg/kg daily; begin in divided doses	Controls disease rapidly: 5–10 days for hematologic, CNS, serositis, vasculitis; 3–10 weeks for GN	High—INFECTIONS, sleeplessness, mood swings, hyperglycemia, psychosis, hypertension, weight gain, hypokalemia, fragile skin, bruising, osteoporosis, ischemic necrosis of bone, irregular menses, muscle cramps, sweats, acne, hirsutism, cataracts
	OR		
Regimen 2: Intravenous methylprednisolone	500–1000 mg every day for 3–5 days	Controls disease rapidly—may achieve results more rapidly than daily oral therapy	High—same as for daily except more rapid taper of daily maintenance steroid dose may be possible, leading to lower cumulative doses
	Then, 1–1.5 mg/kg/day of oral GC	A few nonresponders to Regimen 1 respond to Regimen 2	
	OR		

Regimen 3:
Combine Regimen 1 or 2 with a cytotoxic drug. See Table 62–5.

SLE Well Controlled by Therapy (Maintenance Regimens)
Regimen 1:
Continue daily oral glucocorticoid. Consolidate to a single morning dose. Then begin a slow taper of single daily dose; reduce by 5–15% every week if tolerated. When a dose of 30 mg daily is reached, reduce by 2.5 mg increments. When a dose of 10–15 mg daily is reached, reduce by 1 mg increments. If disease flares, increase to most recent effective dose and hold there for a few weeks.

Regimen 2:
Begin a taper to an alternate-day glucocorticoid regimen. Consolidate to single-dose daily therapy, then begin taper on alternate day. For example, 60 mg daily tapers to 60 mg alternating with 50 mg—work down to 60 mg every other day, then taper by 5–15% increments every 1–2 weeks.

Regimen 3:
To Regimen 1 or 2 add additional therapies that will optimize glucocorticoid taper, such as antimalarials for dermatitis/arthritis, NSAIDs for fever and arthritis and serositis.
If tapering to 15 mg daily or 30 mg every other day, or less, is achieved without disease flare, consider managing the disease with glucocorticoids alone. If maintenance doses are higher, consider adding a cytotoxic drug. See Table 62–5.

effects, institution of an additional agent is recommended.

Cytotoxic Drugs

Two groups of cytotoxic drugs have been used in large numbers of patients with severe SLE: purine antagonists and alkylating agents. The first such agent employed was nitrogen mustard,[24] which is still useful in patients who cannot tolerate other alkylating agents. The two drugs used most frequently are azathioprine (Imuran) and cyclophosphamide (Cytoxan). Of the two, cyclophosphamide is more effective and more toxic. Cyclophosphamide suppresses both humoral and cellular immune responses more effectively than does azathioprine and, in contrast with azathioprine, is not cell cycle depen-

dent. Doses of these drugs, their side effects, and guidelines to combination therapies are reviewed in Table 62–5.

Azathioprine. With regard to azathioprine, short-term studies (e.g., 1–2 years in duration) have failed to demonstrate a better outcome in patients with severe SLE treated with steroids plus azathioprine compared with those treated with steroids alone.[25, 26] However, in studies that follow patients for 5 to 15 years, individuals receiving combination therapy generally have (1) fewer chronic changes on renal biopsies, (2) better renal function, (3) fewer severe disease flares, and (4) lower glucocorticoid requirements.[27-29] Significant adverse side effects of chronic azathioprine therapy include increased rates of infection with opportunistic organisms (especially herpes zoster), ovarian failure, occasional bone marrow suppression (especially leukopenia), hepatic

Table 62–5. USE OF CYTOTOXIC DRUGS IN SLE (IN ADDITION TO GLUCOCORTICOIDS)

Drug	Initial Dose	Maintenance Dose	Advantages	Adverse Side Effects	Incidence (%)
Azathioprine	1–3 mg/kg/day	1–2 mg/kg/day (Requires 6–12 months to work well)	Probably reduces flares Reduces renal scarring Reduces GC dose reqt.	Bone marrow suppression Leukopenia Infections (*H. zoster*) Malignancies Infertility Menopause Hepatic damage Nausea	 <5 15 10 <5 15 10 <5 15
Cyclophosphamide	1–3 mg/kg/day oral OR 8–20 mg/kg intravenous once a mo. plus Mesna	0.5–2 mg/kg/day oral OR 8–20 mg/kg intravenous every 6–12 weeks plus Mesna OR daily Az (Requires 2–16 weeks to work well)	As for azathioprine Probably effective in higher proportion of patients	Bone marrow suppression Leukopenia Infections Malignancies Cystitis* Infertility Menopause Nausea Alopecia	<5 30 30 <5 15 50 50 20 20
Combination Therapy	Az: 1.5–2.5 mg/kg/day oral Cy: 1.5–2.5 mg/kg/day oral	Az: 1–2 mg/kg/day oral Cy: 1–2 mg/kg/day oral	Possibly more effective than one drug	Infections otherwise as above Cystitis*	40 15

*Hemorrhagic cystitis, urinary bladder sclerosis, and carcinoma of the urinary bladder are infrequent if cyclophosphamide is given intravenously, especially with Mesna.

Az = azathioprine; Cy = cyclophosphamide; mo = month; GC = glucocorticoids.

damage, and increased susceptibility to malignancies.[28–31] Some experts begin patients with severe SLE on daily or pulse glucocorticoid regimens and a cytotoxic drug (azathioprine in slowly progressive disease; cyclophosphamide in rapidly progressive disease). In general, the physician should allow 6 to 12 months for azathioprine to be effective. After disease is well controlled and glucocorticoid doses are tapered to the lowest possible maintenance levels, doses of azathioprine should be slowly tapered and discontinued if the disease is well controlled for a year or more.

Cyclophosphamide. Several studies have supported the efficacy of cyclophosphamide in management of severe SLE.[27, 28, 32, 32a, 33] In short-term trials (6–12 months) comparing cyclophosphamide plus glucocorticoids to glucocorticoids alone, the cyclophosphamide group had better laboratory parameters than those of the steroid groups. Levels of anti-DNA were lower, levels of complement were higher, and numbers of red cells in urine sediments were lower.[27, 32] In long-term trials (10 years or more of follow-up), the incidence of renal failure was significantly lower in the groups receiving cyclophosphamide, and progression of chronic changes on serial renal biopsies was less.[28, 32a] Cyclophosphamide is difficult to use without glucocorticoids, since steroids provide rapid control of extrarenal manifestations of SLE, and cyclophosphamide does not.

There are several regimens that combine cyclophosphamide and glucocorticoids. These are based partly on studies of the influences of cyclophospha-mide, azathioprine, and glucocorticoids on the nephritis of NZB/NZW F1 mice—an animal model of lupus.[28, 34, 35] In that model, all three drugs as single agents are effective in prolonging life (cyclophosphamide is best); combinations of any two are better than single-drug therapy, and combination of all three is most efficacious. Three different combination therapies have been studied in patients with lupus nephritis: glucocorticoids plus (1) daily oral cyclophosphamide, 2 to 3 mg per kg per day; (2) daily oral cyclophosphamide, 1.5 to 2.5 mg per kg per day plus daily oral azathioprine, 1.5 to 2.5 mg per kg per day; and (3) intermittent intravenous cyclophosphamide pulses given once every 4 to 12 weeks in doses of 8 to 20 mg per kg.[27, 28, 32, 32a] The oral regimens have the advantages of convenience and daily immunosuppression of severe disease. However, oral administration of cyclophosphamide carries a substantial risk of urinary bladder toxicity (hemorrhagic cystitis, sclerosing chronic cystitis, and carcinoma of the bladder). That risk is much lower with intravenous administration, especially if cyclophosphamide doses are accompanied by administration of mesna, which inactivates the oxazaphosphorine metabolite of cyclophosphamide that irritates the bladder.[36] (The author gives 1 mg of intravenous mesna for every 1 mg of intravenous cyclophosphamide, one half of the mesna just before and one half 2 hours after the cyclophosphamide infusion.) In one study[28] the patients with the best outcome with regard to renal function were those in the group that received intravenous cyclophosphamide once every 3 months compared with those who received a 2- or 3-drug daily oral regimen or those who received glucocorticoids alone. However, the numbers in the intravenous cyclophosphamide group were small. Nevertheless, subsequent studies[32, 33] have confirmed the short-term efficacy of monthly intravenous cyclophosphamide pulses in patients with lupus nephritis; thrombocytopenia also responded. It is the author's opinion that intravenous cyclophosphamide is effective in the majority of patients with severe disease, that daily oral administration is somewhat more effective than intermittent high-dose pulses (and more toxic), and that combination therapy of oral daily glucocorticoids plus azathioprine plus cyclophosphamide is the most effective regimen currently available (and also the most toxic).

Several questions regarding therapy with intravenous cyclophosphamide are unanswered; the minimal effective dose is unknown and probably varies from patient to patient. Some authorities recommend that the dose be increased each month until the leukocyte nadir 10 to 14 days later is fewer than 3500 cells per mm^3; it is not clear that such a nadir is required for clinical response. Another problem is when and how to stop this therapy. Most experts recommend treating monthly until maximal response is attained, then either decreasing the dose or increasing the interval between treatments, with treatment continuing for 1 to 2 years total. My approach is to give monthly doses of the highest cyclophosphamide dose tolerated (in terms both of nausea and of leukocyte nadir) until response is achieved, then increase intervals from 4 to 6 weeks, then to 8 weeks, then to 12 weeks, and to continue the treatments for a total of 2 years. Alternatively, if patients do not tolerate cyclophosphamide or the inconvenience of intravenous therapy, I maintain them on daily azathioprine after attaining improvement with cyclophosphamide, continuing the azathioprine for a total of 2 years of cytotoxic therapy. The methods of using cytotoxic drugs are reviewed in Table 62–5.

The majority of patients treated with cyclophosphamide develop adverse side effects.[28, 30, 31] As with azathioprine, the most important adverse side effect is disabling or life-threatening infections. The most common are herpes zoster, staphylococcal, gram-negative bacterial, or candidal sepsis, *Pneumocystis carinii*, and other opportunistic organisms.[30] These infections must be carefully sought if compatible symptoms are present, since (with the exception of herpes zoster) they are often fatal. Other toxicities include bone marrow suppression (especially leukopenia) and increased malignancies. Infertility is common in both men and women (consider banking sperm in men before instituting cyclophosphamide regimens) and may be reversible if it is detected early in young patients so that the drug can be stopped. Loss of ovarian function may also contribute to osteopenia and to accelerated arteriosclerotic disease in women receiving chronic glucocorticoid therapy. Hair loss is frequent, as are gastrointestinal side

effects including nausea, diarrhea, and dyspepsia. Some patients develop malaise and fatigue, which improve after discontinuing cytotoxic drugs. See Table 62–5 for a review of adverse side effects.

Several other cytotoxic drugs have been used in uncontrolled studies of patients with SLE. They include nitrogen mustard, chlorambucil, and methotrexate. The author has used nitrogen mustard or chlorambucil (with some success) in patients who are unresponsive to azathioprine and develop bladder toxicity from cyclophosphamide. In one study,[44] methotrexate diminished SLE arthritis, myositis, vasculitis, rash, serositis, and proteinuria in eight of ten patients; the author has had no success with this drug.

Summary of Use of Cytotoxic Drugs in SLE

Combination therapy with glucocorticoids and cytotoxic drugs is probably superior to glucocorticoids alone in controlling severe SLE, reducing irreversible tissue damage, and minimizing maintenance glucocorticoid requirements. Cyclophosphamide is more effective than azathioprine but is also more toxic. Triple therapy with glucocorticoids, azathioprine, and cyclophosphamide is also useful but is accompanied by a high incidence of adverse side effects. It is not clear that overall patient survival is improved by double or triple therapies compared with glucocorticoids alone.[28] All these therapies, whether glucocorticoids alone or glucocorticoids plus cytotoxics, require close patient follow-up with frequent monitoring for adverse side effects.

Methods of Maximizing Disease Control

The most important criteria of disease control are clinical outcomes. In most patients, an equilibrium is reached between mild, non–life-threatening disease activity and acceptable side effects of maintenance therapies. Complete long-term disease suppression may not be possible, especially in the absence of side effects. Acceptable clinical outcomes might include stable renal function (even though proteinuria is present), platelet and erythrocyte levels in ranges that are asymptomatic, arthralgias without arthritis, and mild skin lesions. The efficacy of treating to normalize serum levels of complement, antibodies to DNA (or other autoantibodies), and erythrocyte sedimentation rates is controversial. Although outcomes are usually better in patients with serum complement levels kept in the normal range,[37] there are patients with persistently low complement levels and high anti-DNA who have good outcomes,[38] and disease activity often does not correlate with serum levels of any autoantibodies.[39] It is useful to establish that, in each individual patient, changes in certain laboratory tests herald a disease flare; those tests may then be used to help guide therapy.

Methods of Minimizing Adverse Side Effects of Immunosuppressive Therapies

Several strategies are useful for minimizing adverse outcomes related to glucocorticoid and cytotoxic therapies[31, 40–43]; they are summarized in Table 62–6. Patients should be monitored frequently for signs of infection, and appropriate antimicrobial agents should be prescribed as soon as infection is suspected—then changed or discontinued as results of cultures become available. Infections with opportunistic organisms are common in immunosuppressed patients with SLE[30]; special procedures may be required to identify these organisms. For example, diagnosis of *Pneumocystis*, invasive *Candida*, aspergillosis, mycobacterial disease, and viruses such as

Table 62–6. STRATEGIES TO MINIMIZE THE ADVERSE EFFECTS OF TREATMENT WITH GLUCOCORTICOIDS OR CYTOTOXIC DRUGS IN PATIENTS WITH SLE

I. Methods of Using Drugs:
  A. Initiate use only in patients with life-threatening disease or severely impaired quality of life.
  B. Monitor at frequent intervals.
    1. Glucocorticoids: electrolytes, CBC, glucose levels, evidence of infection, blood pressure, intraocular pressure, formation of cataracts, evidence for osteoporosis
    2. Cytotoxic drugs: CBC, platelet count, liver function tests, evidence of infection, urinalysis for microscopic hematuria (with oral cyclophosphamide), signs of malignancy
  C. Reduce drug doses as frequently as possible.
II. Treatment and Prevention of Infections:
  A. Be aware of the high incidence of infections, both ordinary and opportunistic. The most frequent organisms are herpes zoster, urinary tract infections with gram-negative bacteria, staphylococcal infections, *Candida* (including sepsis), *Pneumocystis carinii*. Mycobacteria, fungi, and viruses such as CMV are not unusual. Monitor carefully for evidence of these.
  B. If you suspect infection, treat for the most likely organisms. Therapy can be discontinued or changed after culture information is available.
  C. Immunize to prevent infections. Annual influenza vaccine and one immunization with Pneumovax are recommended for all patients.
  D. Some recurring infections can be prevented, or their frequency diminished, by use of prophylactic antibiotics. Examples include: acyclovir for herpes, bactrim for urinary tract infections with susceptible organisms, bactrim for Pneumocystis.
III. Correct Manifestations of Glucocorticoid Toxicity:
  A. Control hypertension.
  B. Control hypokalemia.
  C. Control symptomatic hyperglycemia.
IV. Minimize osteoporosis
  A. Ensure daily calcium intake of 1000–1500 mg.
  B. If 24-hr urine calcium is <120 mg, consider adding vitamin D, 50,000 units 1 to 3 times weekly. This requires regular monitoring of serum and urine calcium levels.
  C. Consider hormone replacement therapy if menopause occurs, SLE is stable, and there are no contraindications.
  D. Consider additional preventive strategies that stabilize bone mass: calcitonin, biphosphonates.

cytomegalovirus may require biopsies of affected organs. Immunization of SLE patients with influenza and pneumococcal vaccines (and probably with most other vaccines) is safe and usually effective.[40, 41] Patients receiving high doses of immunosuppressive drugs may have inadequate protective antibody responses.

Careful attention to blood pressure control and correction of hypokalemia and symptomatic hyperglycemia are recommended for patients receiving glucocorticoids. Frequent monitoring for adverse effects on bone marrow, liver, and lung are recommended for patients receiving cytotoxic drugs.

Osteoporosis can be a serious problem in glucocorticoid-treated patients, especially in individuals who are Caucasian, postmenopausal, or over the age of 50. Several strategies help maintain bone mass in such individuals (none have been proven to reduce fracture rates).[43] These strategies include supplemental calcium to achieve a total daily intake of 1000 to 1500 g, vitamin D 50,000 units two to three times a week in patients with low urinary calcium (<120 mg in 24 hours), estrogen, progesterone, calcitonin, and bisphosphonates. Administration of estrogen to patients with SLE who become menopausal is controversial, since there is a theoretical possibility that disease might be aggravated by female sex hormones. However, in the author's experience, the intervention is usually safe.

Other Strategies

Some patients have disease manifestations that require management with interventions other than immunosuppression; these are discussed in the following paragraphs.

Patients with Thrombosis

Among the individuals with SLE who experience recurrent thrombosis as their sole or major disease manifestation (predominantly patients with antiphospholipid antibodies), anticoagulation is probably the therapy of choice. There are no controlled studies to support this view, but most experts recommend it,[45, 46] based on failure of immunosuppressive interventions to prevent clotting and generally favorable experiences with anticoagulation. Patients with venous clotting are usually managed successfully with long-term warfarin therapy. Patients with arterial clotting are more resistant to therapy, and their outcomes are generally worse. The author usually begins with daily low-dose aspirin; if clotting recurs, heparin or warfarin or even both can be added to aspirin. Such intervention is attended by high risk for bleeding and can only be used in settings that permit careful monitoring and good patient compliance. The lupus anticoagulant is usually steroid-responsive and will diminish if high-dose glucocorticoids are introduced. Antibodies to cardiolipin are more resistant; they may not be decreased by either glucocorticoids or cytotoxic drugs. Furthermore, it is not clear that hypercoagulability is related directly to titers of antiphospholipid antibodies, and therefore whether it is useful to try to lower titers of these antibodies. Immunosuppression has limited utility in these patients and is not recommended unless other manifestations of SLE require it.

Patients with Recurrent Fetal Loss

Since some women (with or without SLE) experience fetal loss as a consequence of antiphospholipid antibodies (a point of controversy), it seems appropriate to discuss management of these patients. In pregnant women with lupus anticoagulants or antibodies to cardiolipin who have experienced prior spontaneous fetal losses, there are several therapeutic choices. First, the physician can choose not to intervene; some pregnancies go well in these patients. However, the higher the number of prior fetal losses (especially if there are no live births), the lower the chance that subsequent pregnancies will have a good outcome.[47–49, 51] There are data suggesting that high-dose glucocorticoids, 40 to 60 mg of prednisone a day, plus low-dose aspirin, 80 mg daily, throughout pregnancy improve fetal survival[47, 48]; other data suggest this intervention *reduces* fetal survival.[49] Some authorities recommend low-dose daily aspirin as the sole treatment; such therapy is relatively safe and has the additional benefit of decreasing the risk of preeclampsia in women with nephritis.[50] Finally, at least one series has reported that women treated with full anticoagulating doses of subcutaneous heparin (average 20,000 units twice daily) from early pregnancy until delivery have improved fetal survival.[51] Frequent fetal and maternal monitoring are critical to good outcomes with any of these interventions: these high-risk pregnancies often require early delivery in response to clinical evidence of fetal distress.

Patients with Severe Cytopenias

Patients with the thrombocytopenia of SLE may benefit from several therapies in addition to immunosuppression. Most authorities recommend high-dose glucocorticoids (60–100 mg of prednisone daily) as the initial intervention in adults. Platelet counts begin to rise a few days after introduction of glucocorticoids; the increase is usually sustained. Administration of intravenous gamma globulin (400–1000 mg, or 6–15 mg per kg daily) for 4 to 7 days is usually followed by rapid increase in platelet count.[52, 53] A study[53] comparing (1) prednisone alone to (2) intravenous gamma globulin alone to (3) combination therapy in SLE patients with thrombocytopenia showed response appearing in a median of 5 days for each single-drug therapy and in 3 days for combination therapy. The mean times to reach peak counts were 9, 5, and 7 days. Relapse rates and the

percentage of patients requiring subsequent splenectomy were similar in the three groups.

Splenectomy[54–56] should be considered whenever glucocorticoids or intravenous gamma globulin therapies are ineffective, either initially or when tapered or discontinued. The objective of therapy is to maintain adequate levels of platelets (50,000 cells per mm^3 or higher). The efficacy of splenectomy in lupus cytopenias is somewhat controversial. If one uses the criterion of permanently sustained counts in the absence of any maintenance therapies, the response rate may be as low as 15 percent.[56] If one uses the criterion of adequate platelet counts with or without requirement for additional maintenance therapies, about 90 percent of patients have good initial responses and 65 to 70 percent have good sustained responses.[54, 55] Asplenic patients are at increased risk for infection with encapsulated microorganisms, particularly pneumococcus; patients should receive Pneumovax prior to splenectomy if possible. The author has had good short-term and long-term results with splenectomy in patients with steroid-resistant thrombocytopenia or hemolytic anemia and prefers it to cytotoxic drugs.

Danazol, an anabolic steroid, may be useful in some cases of SLE thrombocytopenia.[57, 58] The addition of danazol, 400 to 800 mg daily, to partially effective regimens may increase platelet counts to acceptable levels over a period of 2 to 12 weeks. Danazol has been effective in some patients who failed glucocorticoids, splenectomy, and cytotoxic drugs. Side effects of danazol include weight gain, lethargy, myalgia, mild virilization, menopausal symptoms, rash, pruritus, hepatic tumors, hepatitis, and pancreatitis.[58, 59]

Cytotoxic drugs, including cyclophosphamide (daily or intermittent intravenous pulses), azathioprine, and *Vinca* alkaloids are sometimes effective in patients with thrombocytopenia who are steroid and splenectomy resistant.[33] See the earlier discussion for dose and administration recommendations.

Hemolytic anemia of SLE, if severe, should also be treated initially with high-dose glucocorticoids. Splenectomy, danazol, and cytotoxic drugs are useful in some steroid-resistant individuals.[54] The leukopenia (usually lymphopenia) of SLE is rarely associated with important clinical sequelae. However, rare patients with granulocytopenia experience recurrent bacterial infections, which may resolve after the granulocyte count is increased with glucocorticoid therapy or splenectomy.

Patients with Central Nervous System Lupus

Individuals with central nervous system lupus should be divided into two groups for selection of the appropriate therapies: (1) those with strokes and (2) those with more diffuse central nervous system disease. Patients with strokes are likely to have hypercoagulable syndromes. It may be useful to consider anticoagulation rather than immunosuppression if strokes are the only central nervous system manifestations of lupus, especially if antibodies to phospholipids are present. On the other hand, if there are signs of diffuse cerebritis, especially with peripheral vasculitis, immunosuppression should be instituted. In patients with nonthrombotic diffuse central nervous system abnormalities, the nature of the manifestations may determine the best therapeutic choices. For example, seizures of various types are frequent in patients with SLE. If SLE is not active in other organ systems, treatment with anticonvulsants may be adequate therapy. Similarly, behavior disorders and psychosis may be manifestations of SLE or may be unrelated. Psychoactive drugs may be a safer initial intervention than immunosuppression. If patients improve, immunosuppression can be avoided. The author usually does not treat mild cognitive disorders with glucocorticoids, since their side effects are so great. More extensive central nervous system disease, such as severe organic brain syndromes, coma, and myelopathies, require immediate and aggressive intervention with high-dose glucocorticoids with or without cytotoxic drugs.

Patients with Pure Membranous Nephritis

Treatment of pure membranous lupus glomerulonephritis (GN) is different from treatment of proliferative GN. Renal biopsy is necessary to establish the diagnosis. These patients usually present with nephrotic syndrome; renal failure occurs but is less frequent and later than renal failure in proliferative GN.[13, 29] Lupus membranous GN often does not improve during glucocorticoid or cytotoxic therapies, using 24-hour protein excretion as the measure of response. The author usually treats this disease with high-dose daily or alternate-day glucocorticoids for 6 to 12 weeks. If proteinuria does not diminish, the therapy is discontinued. It is possible that long-term benefit would be obtained from 6 to 12 month administration of alternate-day glucocorticoids or glucocorticoids plus cytotoxics, as in nonlupus idiopathic membranous GN; no data are available in patients with SLE.

EXPERIMENTAL THERAPIES

Apheresis

Plasmapheresis, leukoplasmapheresis, and cryopheresis have all been used to treat patients with SLE.[60–62] It is not clear that these interventions are superior to standard approaches. Apheresis removes serum IgG and reduces levels of autoantibodies and immune complexes, which should result in rapid disease control. High levels of antibodies serve as negative feedback for B cells; a few days after autoantibody levels fall, they usually rebound in high quantities. Therefore, initiation of apheresis requires administration of a cytotoxic drug (usually cyclo-

phosphamide intravenously) on days 5 to 10 of the treatment. Apheresis is expensive and requires vascular access. Clotting factors are removed along with immunoglobulin; the plasma removed can be replaced initially with plasma substitutes, but substances (usually fresh frozen plasma) that contain clotting factors will have to be provided.

A controlled trial[62] compared plasmapheresis added to high-dose daily glucocorticoids plus daily cyclophosphamide to the two-drug therapy alone at initiation of treatment of severe proliferative lupus GN. There were no differences in outcome after 2 to 3 years of follow-up. Other investigators have reported good initial results and better long-term outcome in nephritic lupus patients who have received either initial or repeated courses of plasmapheresis.[60, 61] The author uses plasmapheresis in SLE patients with life-threatening disease who have not responded adequately over several days to pulse therapy with high-dose glucocorticoids and cyclophosphamide.

Cyclosporin A

Cyclosporin A and similar anti–T cell drugs are effective in suppressing nephritis in animal models of SLE, usually without affecting autoantibody levels.[63] Using low doses (e.g., 5 mg per kg per day) to minimize the nephrotoxicity of the drug, added to glucocorticoid therapy, some investigators have reported improvement in renal and extrarenal manifestations of SLE.[64, 65] Most individuals treated have developed transient rises in serum creatinine or hypertension. This drug should be considered for treatment of patients with severe, steroid-resistant SLE and bone marrow suppression, in whom cytotoxic drugs cannot be used. Additional undesirable side effects include hirsutism and tremor. Related drugs currently under development may be more useful if they are less nephrotoxic.

Manipulation of Sex Hormone Levels

Because estrogenic hormones have been implicated in the pathogenesis of SLE, several investigators have studied the efficacy of administering androgenic hormones or luteinizing hormone–blocking agents. Danazol is useful in some patients with thrombocytopenia,[57, 58] especially as adjunctive therapy (see prior discussion). Most data suggest that these agents are not effective in severe SLE; they may have mild steroid-sparing properties in some individuals with mild disease.[66]

Interventions that Regulate T-B Cell Interactions

Interventions that prevent B cell activation, by interrupting idiotypic circuits, by inactivating helper

T cells via antibody blockade of CD4, CD3, or interleukin-2 receptor, or by blocking recognition of antigen presented in class II MHC gene products on surfaces of antigen-presenting cells, all have been effective in preventing or suppressing nephritis in mouse models of SLE.[67–69] Treatment of patients with total lymph node irradiation inactivates both B and T lymphocytes over the short term, and some T cells are inactivated or deleted for several months. Patients with lupus nephritis have good outcomes at 3 to 4 years—similar to the outcomes with steroids plus cytotoxic drugs.[70] Studies of administration of antibodies to CD3 or subsets of helper T cells in patients with SLE are likely to be available within the next few years.

Administration of intravenous gamma globulin may have favorable effects on active SLE.[71] Such treatment may solubilize immune complexes, and provide anti-idiotypic down-regulation of autoantibody production, thus interfering with T-B cell signaling. In addition to the utility of this treatment in the management of lupus-induced thrombocytopenia,[53] there are reports of improvement in lupus nephritis.[72] Conversely, there are reports of this therapy worsening SLE rash and nephritis.[71]

OUTCOMES IN PATIENTS WITH SLE

In some patients with lupus nephritis, dialysis or renal transplantation are acceptable outcomes. Patients who present with serum creatinine levels greater than 3 mg per dl, in whom the creatinine has slowly risen over a period of a few years, often have irreversible kidney lesions. This can be confirmed by high chronicity scores and low activity scores on renal biopsies.[28] It is appropriate to plan for dialysis or transplant, rather than administer toxic immunosuppressive therapies to such patients. Two-year survival in SLE patients with renal transplants is 50 to 65 percent.[73] A recent study[74] reported renal graft survivals at 1 and 5 years of 68 percent and 54 percent, an overall patient survival after grafting of 87 percent at both time periods, and a decrease in disease activity scores and numbers of disease flares. Recurrence of lupus in the engrafted kidney occurred in 1 of 28 patients.

Death is caused most frequently by infection or severe nephritis.[30, 75, 76] Other manifestations of SLE that are frequently fatal include carditis, pneumonitis, pulmonary hypertension, cerebritis, stroke, myocardial infarction, intestinal perforations in areas of vasculitis, and extracranial arterial thromboses.

The prognosis of patients with SLE has improved considerably over the past 4 decades. In a series of patients reported by Ginzler et al. in 1983,[75] survival rates were: 1 year, 95 percent; 4 years, 88 percent; 10 years, 76 percent. These can be compared with a series reported by Harvey et al. in 1954,[77] in which survival rates were: 1 year, 78 percent; 4 years, 52 percent. At least some of this improvement should

be attributable to better management strategies. Nevertheless, current survival rates are not good enough—a fact that demands more effective approaches to the treatment of systemic lupus.

References

1. Kimberly, R. P.: Treatment. Corticosteroids and anti-inflammatory drugs. Rheum. Dis. Clin. North Am. 14:203, 1988.
2. Dubois, E. L., and Wallace, D. J.: Management of discoid and systemic lupus erythematosus. In Wallace, D. J., and Dubois, E. L. (eds.): Dubois' Lupus Erythematosus. Philadelphia, Lea & Febiger, 1987, p. 501.
3. Prescott, L. F.: Effect of non-narcotic analgesics on the liver. Drugs 32(Suppl. 4):129, 1986.
4. A randomized study of the effect of withdrawing hydroxychloroquine sulfate in systemic lupus erythematosus. The Canadian Hydroxychloroquine Study Group. N. Engl. J. Med. 324:150, 1991.
5. Bernstein, D. H. N.: Ophthalmologic considerations and testing in patients receiving long-term antimalarial therapy. Am. J. Med. 75:25, 1983.
6. Wysenbeek, A. J., Block, D. A., and Fries, J. F.: Prevalence and expression of photosensitivity in systemic lupus erythematosus. Ann. Rheum. Dis. 48:461, 1989.
7. Sunscreens. Medical Letter 30:61, 1988.
8. Callen, J. P.: Treatment of cutaneous lesions in patients with lupus erythematosus. Dermatol. Clin. 8:355, 1990.
9. Parke, A. L.: Antimalarial drugs, systemic lupus erythematosus and pregnancy. J. Rheumatol. 15:607, 1988.
10. Ruzicka, T., and Goerz, G.: Dapsone in the treatment of lupus erythematosus. Dramatic response to dapsone therapy. Ann. Intern. Med. 97:165, 1982.
11. Ruzicka, T., Meurer, M., and Braun-Falco, O.: Treatment of cutaneous lupus erythematosus with etretinate. Acta Derm. Venereol. (Stockholm) 65:324, 1985.
12. Krupp, L. B., LaRocca, N. G., Muir, J., et al.: A study of fatigue in SLE. J. Rheumatol. 17:1450, 1990.
13. Pollak, V. E., Pirani, C. L., and Kark, R. M.: Effect of large doses of prednisone on the renal lesions and life span of patients with lupus glomerulonephritis. J. Lab. Clin. Med. 57:495, 1961.
14. Pollak, V. E., and Dosekun, A. K.: Evaluation of treatment in lupus nephritis: Effects of prednisone. Am. J. Kidney Dis. 2(Suppl. 2):170, 1982.
15. Kimberly, R. P.: Steroid use in systemic lupus erythematosus. In Lahita, R. G. (ed.): Systemic Lupus Erythematosus. New York, John Wiley & Sons, 1987, p. 889.
16. Cathcart, E. S., Scheinberg, M. A., Idelson, B. A., et al.: Beneficial effects of methylprednisolone "pulse" therapy in diffuse proliferative lupus nephritis. Lancet 1:163, 1976.
17. Evanson, S., Passo, M. H., Aldo-Benson, M. A., et al.: Methylprednisolone pulse therapy for nonrenal lupus erythematosus. Ann. Rheum. Dis. 39:377, 1980.
18. Barron, K. S., Person, D. A., Brewer, E. J., Jr., et al.: Pulse methylprednisolone therapy in diffuse proliferative lupus nephritis. J. Pediatr. 101:137, 1982.
19. Isenberg, D. A., Morrow, W. J. W., and Snaith, M. L.: Methylprednisolone pulse therapy in the treatment of systemic lupus erythematosus. Ann. Rheum. Dis. 41:347, 1982.
20. Liebling, M. R., McLaughlin, K., Boonsue, S., et al.: Monthly pulses of methylprednisolone in SLE nephritis. J. Rheumatol. 9:543, 1982.
21. Scott, D. E., Lindahl, M., Gourley, M., et al.: Randomized trial of monthly methylprednisolone versus cyclophosphamide versus both in lupus nephritis (abstract). Arthritis Rheum. 33:S12, 1990.
22. Ackerman, G. L.: Alternate-day steroid therapy in lupus nephritis. Ann. Intern. Med. 72:511, 1970.
23. Fauci, A. S.: Alternate-day corticosteroid therapy. Am. J. Med. 64:729, 1978.
24. Dubois, E. L.: Nitrogen mustard in treatment of systemic lupus erythematosus. Arch. Intern. Med. 93:667, 1954.
25. Hahn, B. H., Kantor, O. S., and Osterland, C. K.: Azathioprine plus prednisone compared with prednisone alone in the treatment of systemic lupus erythematosus. Report of a prospective, controlled trial in 24 patients. Ann. Intern. Med. 85:597, 1975.
26. Donadio, J. V., Jr., Wagoner, R. D., McDuffie, F. C.: Treatment of lupus nephritis with prednisone and combined prednisone and azathioprine. Ann. Intern. Med. 77:829, 1972.
27. Donadio, J. F., Jr., Holley, K. E., Ferguson, R. H., et al.: Treatment of diffuse proliferative lupus nephritis with prednisone and combined prednisone and cyclophosphamide. N. Engl. J. Med. 299:1151, 1978.
28. Balow, J. E., Austin, H. A. III, Tsokos, G. C., et al.: Lupus nephritis. Ann. Intern. Med. 106:79, 1987.

29. Ginzler, E. M., Bollet, A. J., and Friedman, E. A.: The natural history and response to therapy of lupus nephritis. Annu. Rev. Med. 31:463, 1980.

30. Hellmann, D. B., Petri, M., and Whiting-O'Keefe, Q.: Fatal infections in systemic lupus erythematosus: The role of opportunistic organisms. Medicine 66:341, 1987.

31. Klippel, J. H.: Systemic lupus erythematosus. Treatment-related complications superimposed on chronic disease. J.A.M.A. 263:1812, 1990.

32. McCune, W. J., Golbus, J., Zeldes, W., et al.: Clinical and immunologic effects of monthly administration of intravenous cyclophosphamide in severe systemic lupus erythematosus. N. Engl. J. Med. 318:1423, 1988.

32a. Steinberg, A. D., and Steinberg, S. C.: Long-term preservation of renal function in patients with lupus nephritis receiving treatment that includes cyclophosphamide versus those treated with prednisone alone. Arthritis Rheum. 34:945, 1991.

33. Boumpas, D. T., Barez, S., Klippel, J.H ., et al.: Intermittent cyclophosphamide for the treatment of autoimmune thrombocytopenia in systemic lupus erythematosus. Ann. Intern. Med. 112:674, 1990.

34. Gelfand, M. C., Steinberg, A., Nagle, R., et al.: Therapeutic studies in NZB/W mice. I. Synergy of azathioprine, cyclophosphamide and methylprednisolone in combination. Arthritis Rheum. 15:239, 1972.

35. Hahn, B. H., Knotts, L., Ng, M., et al.: Influence of cyclophosphamide and other immunosuppressive drugs on immune disorders and neoplasia in NZB/NZW mice. Arthritis Rheum. 18:145, 1975.

36. deVries, C. R., Freiha, F. S.: Hemorrhagic cystitis: A review. J. Urol. 143:1, 1990.

37. Appel, A. E., Sablay, L. B., Golden, R. A., et al.: The effect of normalization of serum complement and anti-DNA antibody on the course of lupus nephritis. Am. J. Med. 64:274, 1978.

38. Gladman, D. D., Urowitz, M. B., and Keysone, E. C.: Serologically active clinically quiescent systemic lupus erythematosus. A discordance between clinical and serologic features. Am. J. Med. 66:210, 1979.

39. Isenberg, D. A., Shoenfeld, Y., and Schwartz, R. S.: Multiple serologic reactions and their relationship to clinical activity in systemic lupus erythematosus. Arthritis Rheum. 27:132, 1984.

40. Klippel, J. H., Karsh, J., Stahl, N. I., et al.: A controlled study of pneumococcal polysaccharide vaccine in systemic lupus erythematosus. Arthritis Rheum. 22:1321, 1979.

41. Herron, A., Dettleff, C., Hixon, B., et al.: Influenza vaccination in patients with rheumatic disease. Safety and efficacy. J.A.M.A. 242:53, 1979.

42. Hahn, B. H., and Hahn, T. J.: Methods for reducing undesirable side effects of glucocorticoids. In Avioli, L., et al. (eds.): Glucocorticoid Effects and Their Biological Consequences. New York, Plenum Publishing Co., 1984, p. 301.

43. Hahn, B. H.: Osteopenic bone disease. In McCarty, D. (ed.): Arthritis and Allied Conditions. 11th ed. Philadelphia, Lea & Febiger, 1989, p. 1812.

44. Rothenberg, R. I., Graziano, F. M., Grandone, J. T., et al.: The use of methotrexate in steroid-resistant systemic lupus erythematosus. Arthritis Rheum. 31:612, 1988.

45. Harris, E. N., Asherson, R. A., and Hughes, G. R.: Antiphospholipid antibodies—autoantibodies with a difference. Annu. Rev. Med. 39:261, 1988.

46. Rappaport, S. I., and Feinstein, S. I.: Lupus anticoagulant and other hemostatic problems. In Wallace, D. J., and Dubois, E. L. (eds.): Dubois' Lupus Erythematosus. 3rd ed. Philadelphia, Lea & Febiger, 1987, p. 271.

47. Branch, D. W., Scott, J. R., Kochenour, N. K., et al.: Obstetric complications associated with the lupus anticoagulant. N. Engl. J. Med. 313:1322, 1985.

48. Lubbe, W. F., Butler, W. S., Palmer, S. J., et al.: Fetal survival after prednisone suppression of maternal lupus-anticoagulant. Lancet 1:1361, 1983.

49. Lockshin, M. D., Druzin, M. L., and Qamar, M. A.: Prednisone does not prevent recurrent fetal death in women with antiphospholipid antibody. Am. J. Obstet. Gynecol. 169:439, 1989.

50. Lindheimer, M. D., and Katz, A. I.: Preeclampsia: Pathophysiology, diagnosis and management. Annu. Rev. Med. 40:233, 1989.

51. Rosove, M. Y., Tabsh, K., Wasserstrum, N., et al.: Heparin therapy for prevention of pregnancy complications in women with lupus anticoagulants or anticardiolipin antibodies. Obstet. Gynecol. 75:630, 1990.

52. Gordon, D. S.: Intravenous immunoglobulin therapy. New directions and unanswered questions. Am. J. Med. 83(Suppl. 4A):52, 1987.

53. Jacobs, P., and Wood, L.: The comparison of gamma globulin to steroids in treating adult immune thrombocytopenia. An interim analysis. Blut 59:92, 1989.

54. Coon, W. W.: Splenectomy for cytopenias associated with systemic lupus erythematosus. Am. J. Surg. 155:391, 1988.

55. Gruenberg, J. C., VanSlyck, E. J., and Abraham, J. P.: Splenectomy in systemic lupus erythematosus. Am. Surg. 52:366, 1986.

56. Hall, S., McCormick, J. L., Jr., Greipp, P. R., et al.: Splenectomy does not cure the thrombocytopenia of systemic lupus erythematosus. Ann. Intern. Med. 102:325, 1985.

57. West, S. G., and Johnson, S. C.: Danazol for the treatment of refractory autoimmune thrombocytopenia in systemic lupus erythematosus. Ann. Intern. Med. 108:703, 1988.

58. Ahn, Y. S., Rocha, R., Mylvaganam, R., et al.: Long-term danazol therapy in autoimmune thrombocytopenia: Unmaintained remission and age-dependent response in women. Ann. Intern. Med. 111:723, 1989.

59. Weill, B. J., Menkes, C. J., Cormier, C., et al.: Hepatocellular carcinoma after danazol therapy. J. Rheumatol. 15:1447, 1988.

60. Schroeder, J. O., Euler, H. H., and Loffler, H.: Synchronization of plasmapheresis and pulse cyclophosphamide in severe systemic lupus erythematosus. Ann. Intern. Med. 107:344, 1987.

61. Wallace, D. J., Goldfinger, D., Savage, G., et al.: Predictive value of clinical, laboratory, pathologic and treatment variables in steroid/immunosuppressive resistant lupus nephritis. J. Clin. Apheresis 4:30, 1988.

62. Schwartz, M. M., Lan, S. P., Bonsib, S. M., et al.: Clinical outcome of three discrete histologic patterns of injury in severe lupus glomerulonephritis. Am. J. Kidney Dis. 13:273, 1989.

63. Mountz, J. D., Smith, H. R., Wilder, R. L., et al.: CS-A therapy in MRL-lpr/lpr mice: Amelioration of immunopathology despite autoantibody production. J. Immunol. 138:157, 1987.

64. Feutren, G., Querin, S., Noel, L. H., et al.: Effects of cyclosporine in severe systemic lupus erythematosus. J. Pediatr. 111:1063, 1987.

65. Favre, H., Miescher, P. A., Huang, Y. P., et al.: Cyclosporin in the treatment of lupus nephritis. Am. J. Nephrol. 9:57, 1989.

66. Agnello, V., Pariser, K., Gell, J., et al.: Preliminary observations on danazol therapy of systemic lupus erythematosus: Effects on DNA antibodies, thrombocytopenia, and complement. J. Rheumatol. 10:682, 1983.

67. Klippel, J. H., Strober, S., and Wofsy, D.: New therapies for the rheumatic diseases. Bull. Rheum. Dis. 38:1, 1989.

68. Wofsy, D., and Seaman, W. E.: Reversal of advanced murine lupus in NZB/NZW F1 mice by in vivo treatment with anti-L3T4. J. Immunol. 138:2089, 1987.

69. Hahn, B. H., and Ebling, F. M.: Suppression of murine lupus nephritis by administration of an anti-idiotypic antibody to anti-DNA. J. Immunol. 132:187, 1984.

70. Strober, S., Farinas, M. C., Field, E. H., et al.: Treatment of lupus nephritis with total lymphoid irradiation. Observations during a 12–79 month follow-up. Arthritis Rheum. 31:850, 1988.

71. Jordan, S. C.: Intravenous gamma-globulin therapy in systemic lupus erythematosus and immune complex disease. Clin. Immunol. Immunopathol. 53:S164, 1989.

72. Lin, C. Y., Hsu, H. C., and Chaing, H.: Improvement of histological and immunological change in steroid and immunosuppressive drug-resistant lupus nephritis by high-dose intravenous gamma globulin. Nephron 53:303, 1989.

73. Jarrott, M. P., Santhanam, S., and DeGreco, F.: The clinical course of end-stage renal disease in systemic lupus erythematosus. Arch. Intern. Med. 153:1353, 1983.

74. Nossent, H. C., Swaak, T. J. G., Berden, J. H. M., et al.: Systemic lupus erythematosus after renal transplantation: patient and graft survival and disease activity. Ann. Intern. Med. 114:183, 1991.

75. Ginzler, E., Diamond, H. S., Weiner, M., et al.: A multi-center study of outcome in systemic lupus erythematosus. Arthritis Rheum. 25:605, 1982.

76. Ginzler, E. M., and Schorn, K.: Outcome and prognosis in systemic lupus erythematosus. Rheum. Dis. Clin. North Am. 14:67, 1988.

77. Harvey, A. M., Shulman, L. E., Tumulty, P. A., et al.: Systemic lupus erythematosus: Review of the literature and clinical analysis of 138 cases. Medicine (Baltimore) 33:291, 1954.

Mixed Connective Tissue Disease and Other Overlap Syndromes

Anyone who has seen half a dozen examples of common lupus and of lupus erythematosus is able with ease to distinguish one from the other . . . but let him wait a while and see more, and he will find before long that there are examples of mixed forms of the disease which it is impossible to denote concisely without employing hybrid names.[1]

This arcane clinical observation cited by Jonathan Hutchinson in 1880 is as relevant today as it was some 100 years ago.[1] According to current wisdom there are five classic connective tissue diseases: systemic lupus erythematosus (SLE), scleroderma (systemic sclerosis [SSC]), polymyositis (PM), dermatomyositis (DM), and rheumatoid arthritis (RA). Each of these may be associated with Sjögren's syndrome, which in its primary form may be the most common of the connective tissue diseases.[2]

The term "connective tissue disease" is somewhat of a misnomer and derives from the classic 1942 paper by Klemperer, Pollack, and Baehr,[3] who coined the term "collagen disease" to emphasize pathologic similarities between SLE, scleroderma, and PM. The classic descriptions of the diffuse connective tissue diseases (DCTDs) are well known, and patients late in the course of a well-differentiated disease are readily recognized without recourse to extensive investigations. However, as Hutchinson so aptly noted, it is not unusual to see the evolution over many years of features more commonly associated with another DCTDs. This propensity for evolution and transition between DCTDs has been said to occur in about 25 percent of patients.[4] Overlapping sometimes occurs concurrently, but more commonly it is the dimension of time that allows one syndrome to take on the features of another.

Over the past 2 decades there has been an intensive effort to link the fine specificity of antinuclear antibodies (ANAs) to distinctive clinical subsets of the DCTDs (see Chapter 9). One cannot invariably link a DCTD subset with a specific ANA specificity. In some instances, it is the absence of an antibody or antibodies that is the most distinctive feature. For example, patients with drug-induced lupus erythematosus and mixed connective tissue disease (MCTD) have ANAs to histones and U_1 ribonucleo-

protein (RNP), respectively, with a virtual absence of all other antibodies. Yet, histone antibodies are not diagnostic of drug-induced LE because they are also found in SLE, and RNP antibodies are not diagnostic of MCTD, having been described in SLE, SSC, PM, Sjögren's syndrome, and RA. ANA fine specificities are usually more closely associated with HLA profiles than with clinical correlates.[5]

SCLERODERMA OVERLAPS

Within the clinical spectrum of scleroderma, a logical distinction is between those patients who have systemic involvement (systemic sclerosis) and those who do not (sine scleroderma). Most scleroderma overlaps are seen with sine scleroderma and the CREST syndrome (calcinosis cutis, Raynaud's phenomenon, esophageal dysfunction, sclerodactyly, and telangiectasia). Tuffanelli and Winkelmann's review of 727 patients with scleroderma from the Mayo Clinic noted only two patients who had coexisting SLE.[6] Two patients with SLE that evolved into scleroderma at 5 and 10 years, respectively, were described by Tay.[7] Dubois and associates[8] described 14 patients with SLE, including one set of identical twins who developed a picture most consistent with scleroderma. These three reports antedate the description of detailed ANA profiles and, in particular, the association of MCTD with RNP antibodies in 1972.[9] Kahn and colleagues[10] have described four patients with sclerodactyly who later developed lupus nephritis; one patient developed anti-Sm and anti-ds DNA antibodies, the other three patients were negative for anti-RNP antibodies. An overlap between localized scleroderma (morphea) and linear scleroderma and discoid SLE has rarely been described.[11] The antibodies commonly found in scleroderma (topoisomerase-1, centromere, fibrillarin, ribonucleic acid [RNA] polymerase-1, 7–2 RNP, and PM-Scl) and those typical of SLE (double-stranded deoxyribonucleic acid [dsDNA], Sm, Ro, and histone) are seldom found in the same serum. The most common overlap between SLE and SSC is with the sine scleroderma variant. The reported prevalences are as follows:

Raynaud's phenomenon, 18 to 45 percent[12-15]; esophageal dysmotility, 10 to 25 percent[12, 16]; and pulmonary fibrosis, 1 to 6 percent.[17] It has been suggested that esophageal dysmotility in association with SLE is positively correlated with Raynaud's phenomenon[18]; a more recent study has found no such association.[19]

Approximately 60 percent of patients with scleroderma have obvious synovitis; 35 percent are positive for rheumatoid factor,[20] but a seropositive erosive arthritis has only rarely been described.[6, 21-23] A severe destructive arthritis has been occasionally noted,[24, 25] but in most patients radiographs are normal or show mild joint space narrowing and a few discrete erosions.[22, 26]

Scleroderma, Primary Biliary Cirrhosis, and Sjögren's Syndrome Overlap

The CREST syndrome, a limited form of scleroderma characterized by sclerodactyly, Raynaud's phenomenon, telangiectasia, esophageal dysmotility, and calcinosis, has a well-described but uncommon association with primary biliary cirrhosis (PBC).[27-31] Powell and colleagues[29] reviewed 558 patients with PBC and found that 22 (3.9 percent) had an associated CREST syndrome. The clinical features are shown in Fig. 63-1. Of particular interest was an association with Sjögren's syndrome in 91 percent. It is now apparent that about 20 percent of patients with PBC exhibit features of another autoimmune disease; this is often coupled with Sjögren's syndrome (Fig. 63-2).[32] In general, CREST features antedated PBC by a mean of 14 years (range, 1 to 28 years). The distinctive serologic feature of PBC is the finding of antimitochondrial antibodies; these have been found in 18 to 27 percent of patients with scleroderma, but only 4 percent had clinical evidence of PBC.[33, 34] Conversely anticentromere antibodies have been found in 10 to 29 percent of patients with PBC; approximately half developed some features of the

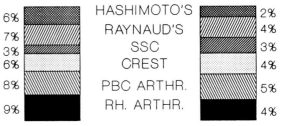

Figure 63–2. Primary biliary cirrhosis (PBC) is associated with another autoimmune disease in about 20 percent of cases. The prevalence of these associations is shown here; PBC has been described as having an associated arthritis that is thought to be distinct from its association with RA (PBC arthritis). These autoimmune associations often coexist with a secondary Sjögren's syndrome. (From Culp, K. S.: Autoimmune associations in primary biliary cirrhosis. Mayo Clin. Proc. 57:365, 1985, Used by permission.)

CREST syndrome.[21, 35] Thus, the serologic overlap between the two syndromes is more prevalent than the clinical overlap. Antimitochondrial antibodies commonly react with two proteins with molecular weights of 70 kilodaltons (kD) and 47 kD,[36] of which a component of the pyruvate dehydrogenase complex (E2) is the principal antigen.[37]

Environmental agents may trigger a scleroderma-like illness. These include epoxy resins, organic solvents such as trichlorethylene, vinyl chloride, silica dust, silicone implants, bleomycin, denatured rapeseed oil (toxic oil syndrome), and, most recently, a dimer of L-tryptophan.[38-45] An overlap of scleroderma, PBC, and Sjögren's syndrome has been described after breast augmentation with silicone prostheses.[46-48]

Sjögren's syndrome seems to be a common denominator in overlap with a second autoimmune disease. Patients who develop a chronic graft-versus-host disease following human bone marrow transplantation often develop features of scleroderma, PBC, and Sjögren's syndrome.[49-52] Minor salivary gland biopsies in scleroderma show lymphocytic infiltrates suggestive of Sjögren's syndrome in 15 to 20 percent of patients; approximately 50 percent have anti-Ro and/or La antibodies.[53] Necrotizing vasculitis is rare in scleroderma but may be found in some patients with a CREST–Sjögren's syndrome overlap in association with anti-Ro antibodies.[54]

Scleroderma-Polymyositis Overlap Syndrome

Scleroderma and DM were historically considered to be different clinical expressions of the same disease process.[55-57] From a population of 727 patients with scleroderma, 36 patients had overlapping features of both scleroderma and DM.[6] Low-grade muscle involvement occurs often in scleroderma, being described in 15 to 80 percent of patients,[58, 59] although

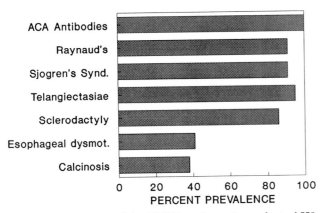

Figure 63–1. Features of the CREST syndrome in a subset of 558 patients with primary biliary cirrhosis (PBC); 22 (3.9 percent) had CREST. (From Powell, F. C., Schroeter, A. L., and Dickinson, E. R.: Primary biliary cirrhosis and the CREST syndrome: a report of 22 cases. Q. J. Med. 62:75, 1987, by permission of Oxford University Press.)

a clinically significant inflammatory myositis is less common. Mimori analyzed 240 Japanese patients with scleroderma and 105 patients with polymyositis-dermatomyositis (PM-DM); 27 patients fulfilled criteria for both diffuse scleroderma and PM-DM.[60] Seven of these 27 patients also fulfilled criteria for SLE. Sclerodermatous involvement was localized to the periphery but was generally more extensive than sclerodactyly (Fig. 63–3). Ku is an interesting nucleoprotein that binds to the ends of DNA strands in a nonsequence-specific interaction and was common in patients with scleroderma–PM–DM overlap. It is composed of two polypeptides (70 kD and 80 kD) and is thought to be involved in DNA repair or transposition.[61–63] Although its predominant location is in the nucleus, a recent study has described its association with cell membranes.[64] Anti-Ku is more common in Japanese patients and was found in only 16 percent of North American patients with autoimmune rheumatic diseases.[65] American patients with the SSC-PM overlap more commonly develop antibodies to the PM-Scl antigen.[66] This is found predominantly in the nucleolus and consists of 16 polypeptides ranging in molecular weight from 20 to 110 kD. The entire complex is precipitated by anti-PM–Scl sera, but immunoblotting has revealed that SSC-PM sera usually recognize a 110-kD protein.[67] Anti–PM–Scl antibodies have recently correlated with HLA-DR3.[68] Seventeen percent of 646 patients with SSC were found to have anti–PM-Scl; all these patients had a high prevalence of myositis and renal involvement.[69] Conversely, 8 percent of 168 patients with PM had PM-Scl antibodies; the prevalence of scleroderma features was as follows: Raynaud's phenomenon 55 percent; sclerodactyly, 40 percent; bibasilar pulmonary infiltrates, 35 percent; proximal scleroderma, 25 percent; and telangiectasia, 20 percent.[66] Fifty percent of PM-Scl–positive patients had no features of scleroderma.

In a study of 229 patients with SLE, scleroderma, MCTD, and other overlap syndromes, antibodies that precipitated U_2 RNA were found in eight patients.[70] All immunoblots contain antibodies to the A and B polypeptides associated with U_2 RNA; in four patients anti–U_1 RNP responses were linked to the anti–U_2 RNP response. There is accumulating evidence that antibodies to the 68-kD component of U_1 RNP constitute a common autoantibody profile in patients with an overlap of SLE–scleroderma–PM–MCTD (see later).

POLYMYOSITIS OVERLAPS

Polymyositis (PM) is an inflammatory disease of muscle. An association with an infiltration of CD8 T cells, the high prevalence of autoantibodies, and response to glucocorticoids provide persuasive evidence that autoimmunity is involved in its pathogenesis. Of all the classic DCTDs, PM has the most specific "end organ" response. Yet the same clinical picture and investigational findings may be found in patients with SLE, SSC, MCTD, and Sjögren's syndrome. If an inflammatory myopathy occurs as an isolated finding, it is usually designated as PM; if it occurs in association with a "named DCTD," it is considered secondary. When prominent inflammatory muscle disease develops in patients with scleroderma, there may be a distinctive antibody profile, as exemplified by the anti-Ku or anti–PM-Scl previously described. When an inflammatory myositis occurs in association with SLE, there are often clinical and serologic features to suggest a diagnosis of MCTD.

Some patients with PM develop an unusual but distinctive syndrome of Raynaud's phenomenon, inflammatory arthritis, and interstitial lung disease. This syndrome is associated with autoantibodies that

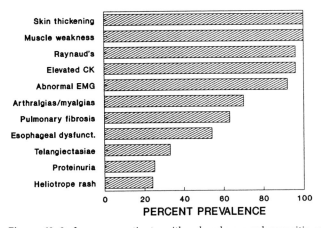

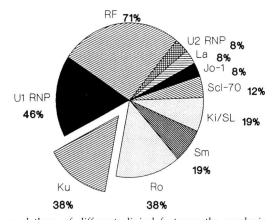

Figure 63–3. Japanese patients with scleroderma-polymyositis overlap have a plethora of different clinical features; the serologic associations are equally florid. The scleroderma skin changes were said to be more extensive than sclerodactyly. The Ku antibody, in particular, has been associated with this particular overlap. The high prevalence of anti-RNP antibodies may have led other investigators to classify some of these patients as having MCTD. (From Mimori, T.: Scleroderma-polymyositis overlap syndrome. Int. J. Dermatol. 26:419, 1987, used by permission.)

react with amino-acyl trRNA synthetases, a family of enzymes that catalyze the transfer of a specific amino acid to its cognate transfer RNA. The most common association is with anti–Jo-1 (histidine-trRNA synthetase). Other antibodies associated with this syndrome include anti–PL-7 (threonyl-trRNA synthetase), anti–Pl-12 (alanyl-trRNA synthetase), and "no name" antibodies to isoleucine-trRNA synthetase and glycine-trRNA synthetase.[71-75] The arthropathy associated with PM is characterized by deforming subluxations, particularly of the distal interphalangeal joints (DIPs) and thumbs, with only minor erosive changes (Fig. 63–4).[76-78] Interstitial lung disease may be an early feature of this group of patients and the major determinant of prognosis.[79, 80] Antibodies to the signal recognition particle (SRP) were recently noted in 4 percent of 265 sera from patients with SSC-PM; this antibody was associated with muscle disease of unusually severe and rapid onset in the *absence* of Raynaud's phenomenon, pulmonary fibrosis, or arthritis.[81]

LUPUS-SCLERODERMA-POLYMYOSITIS OVERLAP: MIXED CONNECTIVE TISSUE DISEASE

Within the sphere of overlap syndromes encompassing the classic DCTDs, an overlap syndrome of SLE, SSC, and PM has been recognized increasingly; this was named the "mixed connective tissue disease syndrome" by Sharp and colleagues in 1972.[9] This was the first overlap syndrome defined in terms of a specific autoantibody, antibodies to a ribonuclease-sensitive extractible nuclear antigen (ENA). In the

ensuing years, many studies looking at the clinical correlates of this antibody system (now called U_1 RNP) were undertaken; these were reviewed in the second edition of *Textbook of Rheumatology*.[82] Controversy arose as to whether MCTD was indeed a distinct entity or would be better defined as a subset of SLE[83, 84] or should be given another name, such as undifferentiated connective tissue disease (UCTD).[85] The reasons for these conflicting opinions are now becoming apparent as contemporary investigators elucidate the fine specificities of U_1 RNP and HLA associations.[86]

Diagnosis

The basic premise of the MCTD concept is that the presence of high titers of anti–U_1 RNP antibodies, as the major autoantibody system, modifies the expression of a DCTD in ways that are relevant to prognosis and treatment.[87-91] The first clue to diagnosing MCTD is usually a positive ANA with a high-titer speckled pattern. The titer is often greater than 1:1000 and sometimes greater than 1:10,000. This finding should prompt the measurement of antibodies of ENA by double immunodiffusion, immunoblotting, or enzyme-linked immunosorbent assay (ELISA)—using recombinant antigens now commercially available. Antibodies to dsDNA, Sm, and Ro are occasionally seen as a transient phenomenon in patients with MCTD, but when these are found consistently as the *predominant* antibody system the clinical picture is usually more consistent with classic SLE. Antibodies to the 68-kD antigen, and a unique epitope on the A' protein of U_1 RNP, are most closely

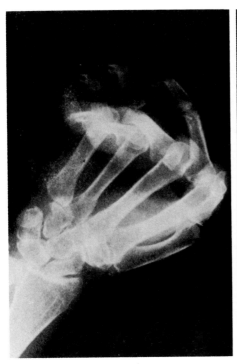
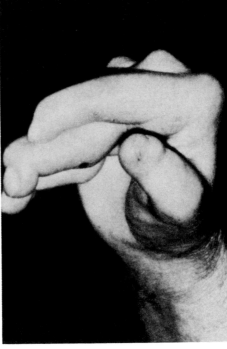

Figure 63–4. An example of joint involvement in a patient with anti–Jo-1 antibodies and polymyositis. Typically, such patients develop a deforming and mainly nonerosive arthropathy. Subluxations of the metacarpophalangeal (MCP) joints, proximal interphalangeal (PIP) joints, and, especially, the thumbs is the characteristic finding. Calcinosis is a frequent association. These patients often have an associated interstitial lung disease, which may be fatal. (From Oddis, C. V., Medsger, T. A., and Cooperstein, L. A.: A subluxing arthropathy associated with the anti–Jo-1 antibody in polymyositis/dermatomyositis. Arthritis Rheum. 33:1640, 1990, used by permission.)

associated with the clinical correlates that are considered characteristics of MCTD (Fig. 63–5).[88, 92–96]

The overlap features of MCTD seldom occur concurrently; it usually takes several years before enough overlapping features have appeared for the physician to be confident that MCTD is the most appropriate diagnosis.[87, 97] The most common clinical associations with U_1 RNP antibodies in the early phase of the disease are hand edema, arthritis, Raynaud's phenomenon, inflammatory muscle disease, and sclerodactyly.[9, 87, 89, 98–101] There have been several recent attempts to formulate useful criteria for diagnosing MCTD; one relatively simple set had 100 percent sensitivity and 99.6 percent specificity[100] (Table 63–1). Unfortunately, the criteria utilized an hemagglutination test to measure anti-RNP—this is seldom done routinely in laboratories.

General Features

The prevalence of MCTD in caucasians is not known. An epidemiologic study in Japan suggested a prevalence of 2.7 percent for MCTD, compared with 20.9 percent for SLE, 5.7 percent for SSC, and 4.9 percent for PM-DM.[102] The female-to-male ratio in this study was 16:1. The age at onset in MCTD is similar to those of the other DCTDs, with most cases presenting in the second or third decades. The syndrome of MCTD usually occurs as an isolated finding, but there are reports of a familial occurrence.[103, 104] Unlike the case with SLE, precipitation by sun or drug exposure has not been related to the onset of MCTD, although a transient appearance of anti-RNP antibodies has been seen at the initiation of procainamide therapy.[105] Unlike the case with SSC, in which a wide variety of environmental toxins and chemicals have been implicated in the pathogenesis, only vinyl chloride has so far been noted to have a possible association with MCTD.[106]

Table 63–1. SUGGESTED DIAGNOSTIC CRITERIA FOR MCTD

Serologic
Anti-RNP >1:600 (hemagglutination method)
Clinical
Hand edema
Synovitis ≥1 joint at any time
Myositis—biopsy or CK elevation
Raynaud's phenomenon
Acrosclerosis
Requirements for Diagnosing MCTD
Positive serology *plus:*
Three or more of the clinical criteria*

*The triad of hand edema, Raynaud's phenomenon, and acrosclerosis requires at least one of the other two criteria.

Data from Alarcon-Segovia, D., and Cardiel, M. H.: Comparison between three diagnostic criteria for mixed connective tissue disease. Study of 593 patients. J. Rheumatol. 16:328–334, 1989.

Early Symptoms

The assumption that a diagnosis of MCTD implies a *simultaneous* presence of features usually seen in SLE, SSC, and PM is erroneous. It is unusual to see such an overlap during the early course of MCTD; in time, the overlapping features usually occur sequentially. Early in the course of the disease most patients complain of easy fatiguability, poorly defined myalgias, arthralgias, and Raynaud's phenomenon; at this point, a diagnosis of RA, SLE, or UCTD seems most appropriate.[85, 97–99] If such a patient is found to have swollen hands, puffy fingers, or both (Fig. 63–6) in association with high-titer speckled pattern ANAs, he should be carefully followed for the evolution of overlap features. Less commonly there is an acute onset of MCTD, which gives little clue to the subsequent course; such presentations have included PM, acute arthritis, aseptic meningitis, digital gangrene, high fever, acute abdomen, and trigeminal neuropathy.

Fever may be a prominent feature of MCTD in the absence of an obvious cause.[97] Fever of unknown origin has been the initial presentation of MCTD; after careful evaluation, fever in MCTD can usually be traced to a coexistent myositis, aseptic meningitis, serositis, lymphadenopathy, or intercurrent infection (Fig. 63–7).

Joint pain and stiffness is an early symptom in nearly all patients who develop the MCTD syndrome. Joint involvement in MCTD is more common and more severe than that in classic SLE. About 60 percent of patients eventually develop an obvious arthritis, often with deformities commonly seen in RA, such as ulnar deviation, swan neck, and boutonnière changes.[107] Radiographs usually show a characteristic absence of severe erosive changes often resembling Jaccoud's arthropathy (Fig. 63–8). However, a destructive arthritis, including an arthritis mutilans, is a well-established association (Fig. 63–9).[107–111] Small marginal erosions, often with a well-demarcated edge, are the most characteristic radiologic feature in patients with severe joint

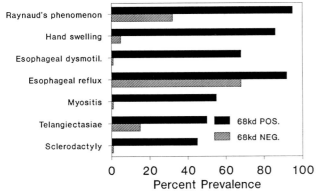

Figure 63–5. Patients with anti-RNP antibodies with a specificity for a 68-kD protein that is unique to U_1 RNA are most likely to present with clinical features suggestive of MCTD. (From Hoffman, R. W., Rettenmaier, I. J., et al.: Human autoantibodies against the 70-kD polypeptide of U1 small nuclear RNP are associated with HLA-DR4 among connective tissue disease patients. Arthritis Rheum. 33:666, 1990, used by permission.)

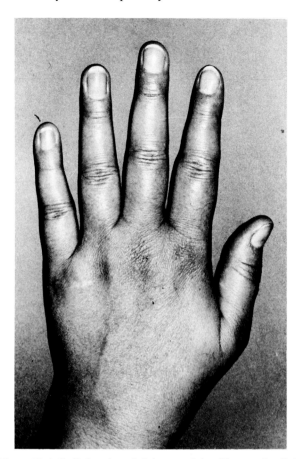

Figure 63–6. Puffy hands and tightness of the skin over the digits are characteristic in some patients with MCTD, but they are not exclusive to MCTD.

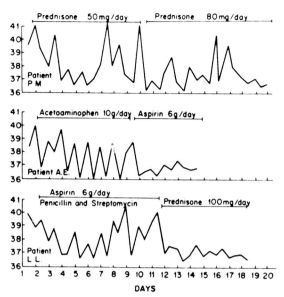

Figure 63–7. Fever patterns in three patients with MCTD. The top two patterns were associated with myositis; the bottom pattern was associated with aseptic meningitis. (From Bennett, R. M., and O'Connell, D. J.: Mixed connective tissue disease. A clinicopathological study of 20 cases. Semin. Arthritis Rheum. 10:25, 1980, used by permission.)

disease.[112, 113] Rib erosions may rarely be seen.[114, 115] Some patients develop a flexor tenosynovitis, which is an additional cause of hand deformities.[116] One case of acute-onset arthritis of the wrists and metacarpophalangeal and interphalangeal joints in a patient with MCTD was due to hydroxyapatite crystal deposition disease.[117] A positive rheumatoid factor is found in 50 to 70 percent of patients with MCTD; indeed, patients may be diagnosed as having RA and fulfill American College of Rheumatology (ACR) criteria for RA.[97, 99, 118] Piirainen[118] has noted that the occurrence of U_1 RNP antibodies and rheumatoid factor are predictive of articular erosions in MCTD and suggests that U_1 RNP antibodies should be sought in all patients presenting with an erosive polyarthritis. Rheumatoid-like nodules are occasionally seen in patients with MCTD.[109] The tendency to more severe arthritis in MCTD compared with classic SLE may be related to the strong association of U_1 RNP antibodies with the same HLA antigens that have been described in RA, namely HLA-DR4.[95, 119, 120]

Most patients with MCTD develop *mucocutaneous changes* sometime during the course of the syndrome. Raynaud's phenomenon is the most common problem and one of the earliest manifestations of MCTD.[9, 84, 89, 97, 98, 121, 122] It may be accompanied by puffy, swollen digits and, sometimes, total hand edema.[9,

[98, 99] It must be remembered that Raynaud's phenomenon is rare in RA. In some patients, skin changes commonly associated with classic SLE are prominent findings, particularly malar rash and discoid plaques.[97, 123, 124] Conversely, skin changes typical of DM rarely have been recorded. Mucous membrane lesions have included buccal ulceration,[97] sicca complex,[97, 125] orogenital ulceration,[126] and nasal septal perforation.[40, 127] Many of these associations may be the result of chance alone; the full spectrum of recorded changes is given in Table 63–2. Although sclerodactyly and calcinosis cutis occur as secondary accompaniments to the involvement of the digital arteries, truncal scleroderma is not a feature of MCTD. Immunofluorescence studies of skin biopsies in patients with MCTD have shown speckled intranuclear immunofluorescence of epidermal cells, suggesting that there may be in vivo cellular penetration of anti-RNP antibodies.[128–130] On the other hand, this observation may be artifactual—the result of biopsy sections being inadvertently exposed to MCTD plasma. The expression of differentiation and acti-

Table 63–2. MUCOCUTANEOUS PROBLEMS THAT HAVE BEEN ASSOCIATED WITH MCTD

Puffy hands	Calcinosis cutis
Raynaud's phenomenon	Skin ulceration
Alopecia	Subcutaneous nodules
Sclerodactyly	Heliotrope eyelids
Malar rash	Grotton's papules
Discoid LE	Erythema nodosum
Dyspigmentation	Lyell's disease
Telangiectasia	Buccal ulceration
Photosensitivity	Nasal septal perforation

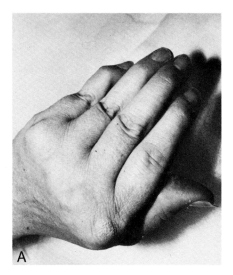

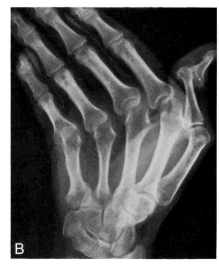

Figure 63–8. Patients with MCTD often have a severer form of arthritis than do patients with classic SLE. *A,* The patient seen here had several of the classic findings usually seen in RA: ulnar deviation, subluxed MCP joints, and swan neck deformities. *B,* The radiograph shows a relative paucity of erosive disease. (From Bennett, R. M., and O'Connell, D. J.: The arthritis of mixed connective tissue disease. Ann. Rheum. Dis. 37:397, 1978.)

vation antigens has been studied in punch biopsies from patients with discoid lupus erythematosus and MCTD; infiltrates were composed predominantly of T cells with a low CD4-CD8 ratio; compared with discoid LE, there was an increased expression of DR-positive cells.[131]

Myalgia is a common symptom in patients with the MCTD syndrome.[9, 97, 132, 133] In most patients, there is no demonstrable weakness, electromyographic abnormalities, or muscle enzyme changes. It is often unclear whether the symptom represents a low-grade myositis, physical deconditioning, a low-grade vasculitis, or an associated fibromyalgia syndrome. The inflammatory myopathy associated with MCTD is identical clinically and histologically to classic PM.[97, 134, 135] In most patients, myositis occurs as an acute flare-up against a background of general disease activity. Such patients usually respond well to a short course of high-dose glucocorticoid therapy, unlike patients with a low-grade inflammatory myopathy with an insidious onset. Some patients with PM associated with MCTD develop an impressive fever,[97]

other patients may give a history of febrile myalgias that have been diagnosed as "flu."

All three layers of the *heart* may be involved in MCTD. An abnormal electrocardiogram is noted in about 20 percent of patients.[136, 137] The most common electrocardiographic changes are right ventricular hypertrophy, right atrial enlargement, and interventricular conduction defects. Pericarditis is the most common clinical manifestation of cardiac involvement, being reported in 10 to 30 percent of patients.[9, 97, 136–141] Involvement of the myocardium is being appreciated with increasing frequency.[136, 137, 141–144] In some patients, myocardial involvement is secondary to pulmonary hypertension; this is often asymptomatic in its early stages. It should be suspected in any patient who has an unexplained tachycardia, a loud pulmonic component of the second heart sound, a fourth heart sound, or a gallop rhythm. Myocardial involvement is due to an inflammatory cell infiltrate and/or proliferative vasculopathy of the epicardial and intramural coronary arteries.[135, 137, 142, 145] This complication should be suspected in patients who

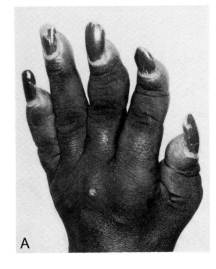

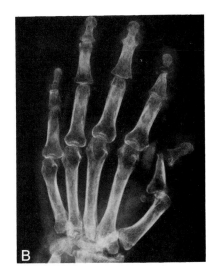

Figure 63–9. *A,* A few patients with MCTD develop a severe destructive form of arthritis (arthritis mutilans). *B,* The radiograph shows almost complete osteolysis of the carpal bones with focal osteolytic changes in several digits and bony fusion of the third distal interphalangeal joint (DIP) joint. (From Bennett, R. M., and O'Connell, D. J.: Mixed connective tissue disease. A clinicopathological study of 20 cases. Semin. Arthritis Rheum. 10:25, 1980, used by permission.)

have an unexplained resting tachycardia or dyspnea out of proportion to the lung involvement. Chest radiographs usually show cardiomegaly, and the electrocardiogram often shows premature ventricular beats and ST-T wave changes; some patients develop an elevated serum creatine kinase (CK)-MB fraction. Right heart catheterization has shown the changes of pulmonary hypertension in some asymptomatic patients.[136, 146] Conduction disturbances include bundle branch block and complete heart block.[97, 136, 137, 147, 148] An echocardiographic study of 17 patients with MCTD showed small pericardial effusions in two patients, pericardial thickening in two, mitral verrucous vegetations in two, and mild mitral regurgitation in one.[140] Mitral valve prolapse was noted in 26 percent of patients with MCTD, compared with 33 percent in patients with SLE, 29 percent in patients with SSC, and 10 percent in normal subjects.[149]

Pleuritic chest pain is common in patients with MCTD who have *pulmonary involvement*.[9, 97, 146, 150–152] Large pleural effusions are unusual but have been the presenting feature.[153] In contradistinction to the case with SLE,[154] significant respiratory muscle involvement is not seen in MCTD.[155] One prospective study reported that 85 percent of patients with MCTD had evidence of pulmonary involvement; in 73 percent of patients, this was asymptomatic.[146] As in scleroderma, the most discriminatory lung function test was the single breath diffusing capacity for carbon monoxide, which was abnormal in 72 percent of patients.[146] The most common radiographic pattern was small, irregular opacities involving the lower and middle lung fields. An increased uptake on gallium scanning was infrequent. A retrospective review of 81 adult patients with MCTD noted pleuropulmonary involvement in 25 percent.[151] The symptoms were dyspnea (16 percent), chest pain (7 percent), and cough (5 percent). Chest radiographs showed interstitial changes in 19 percent, pleural effusions in 6 percent, pneumonic infiltrates in 4 percent, and pleural thickening in 2 percent.[151] Pulmonary hemorrhage has occasionally been reported in MCTD.[156–158]

Pulmonary hypertension is the most common cause of death in MCTD (Fig. 63–10).[97, 146, 152, 159–170]

Unlike the case with SSC, in which pulmonary hypertension is usually secondary to an interstitial pulmonary fibrosis, pulmonary hypertension in MCTD is usually caused by a bland intimal proliferation and medial hypertrophy of pulmonary arterioles[135, 145, 146, 157, 159, 161] (Fig. 63–11). A similar picture is seen in the pulmonary hypertension of the CREST syndrome, but the medial hypertrophy is less evident. In patients with SLE who develop pulmonary hypertension, anticardiolipin antibodies have been noted in 68 percent, and anti-RNP antibodies in 21 percent.[171] There is one report of rapidly progressive fatal pulmonary hypertension in MCTD in association with a lupus anticoagulant.[164] It has been suggested that patients who have a nailfold capillary pattern similar to that seen in SSC are at a greater risk for developing pulmonary hypertension.[146] The response of this potentially fatal complication to glucocorticoids and cytotoxic agents has been variable.[146, 172]

In the initial description of MCTD, *renal involvement* was considered to be rare,[9] but 2 decades later it is evident that renal involvement occurs in about 25 percent of patients.[99, 170, 173] However, high titers of anti-U_1 RNP antibodies appear to be relatively protective against the development of diffuse proliferative glomerulonephritis, irrespective of whether they occur in a setting of classic SLE or MCTD.[97, 145, 174–179] When patients with MCTD do develop renal changes, they usually take the form of a membranous glomerulonephritis[169, 170, 173, 176, 180] (Fig. 63–12); often this is asymptomatic, but it may sometimes cause an overt nephrotic syndrome.[169, 170, 173] The development of diffuse proliferative glomerulonephritis or parenchymal interstitial disease has been rarely recorded in MCTD.[169, 170, 181–183] Immunofluorescence studies have shown granular deposits of IgG, C2, and C4 in glomeruli; electron microscopy has shown both intramembranous and subepithelial electron-dense deposits.[135, 169, 173, 176, 180] There have been descriptions of intimal proliferation of the renal vessels similar to that seen in the pulmonary vasculature. Some patients develop a renovascular hypertensive crisis similar to the scleroderma kidney,[184] or amyloidosis and azotemia.[185]

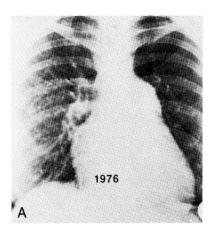

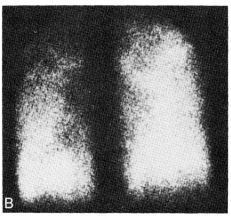

Figure 63–10. A 22-year-old woman with an 8-year history of MCTD, under apparent good control, suddenly went into respiratory and cardiac failure and died, within 2 weeks, of fulminant pulmonary hypertension. *A*, The chest radiograph shows cardiac dilation with enlargement of the pulmonary trunk and proximal pulmonary arteries. *B*, The lung scan shows multiple areas of ventilation-perfusion imbalance. (From Bennett, R. M., and O'Connell, D. J.: Mixed connective tissue disease. A clinicopathological study of 20 cases. Semin. Arthritis Rheum. 10:25, 1980, used by permission.)

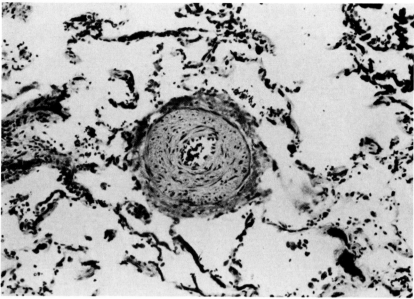

Figure 63–11. Intimal hyperplasia and smooth muscle hypertrophy without accompanying inflammation are the characteristic features of the vasculopathy of MCTD. When it occurs in the lung, as shown here, it may give rise to severe pulmonary hypertension (note absence of pulmonary fibrosis). (From Alpert, M. A., et al.: Cardiovascular manifestations of mixed connective tissue disease in adults. Circulation 6:1182, 1983, by permission of the American Heart Association, Inc.)

Gastrointestinal involvement is a major feature of the overlap with scleroderma, occurring in about 60 to 80 percent of patients.[39, 40, 177, 186] In a comparative study of 17 patients with MCTD and 14 patients with SLE, heartburn and regurgitation were found in 65 percent of patients with MCTD; 91 percent had manometric abnormalities.[187] Fifty-seven percent of the patients with SLE had similar symptoms, but abnormal manometric studies were found in only 20 percent.[187] A recent study of 61 patients with MCTD noted heartburn in 48 percent and dysphagia in 38 percent.[186] Seventeen percent had distal esophageal aperistalsis, and 43 percent had low-amplitude peristalsis. Upper esophageal sphincter hypotension was a common finding. Treatment with prednisone (average dose, 25 mg/day) in 10 patients followed for 67 weeks demonstrated a significant improvement in lower esophageal sphincter pressure and a trend toward improvement in proximal esophageal peristaltic waves.[186]

Abdominal pain in MCTD may result from bowel hypomotility, serositis, mesenteric vasculitis, colonic perforation, and pancreatitis. One patient with mesenteric vasculitis died of hemorrhage involving the small and large bowel.[188] Malabsorption syndrome can occur secondary to small bowel dilation, with bacterial overgrowth.[97] Liver involvement in the form of chronic active hepatitis and Budd-Chiari syndrome has been described.[186, 189–192] There are occasional reports of secretory diarrhea[193] and pancreatitis.[186] Pseudodiverticula, identical to those seen in SCC, may be seen along the antimesenteric border of the colon.[112, 194] Some patients have the radiographic findings of pneumatosis cystoides intestinalis.[112, 195, 196] Examples of these features are shown in Figure 63–13.

In keeping with Sharp's original description, *central neurologic* involvement has not been a conspicuous clinical feature in most patients with MCTD. The most common problem is a trigeminal neuropa-

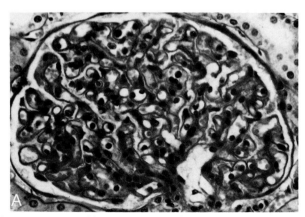
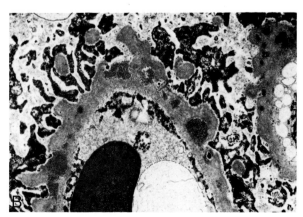

Figure 63–12. Renal biopsy specimens from a patient with MCTD and mild proteinuria. *A,* Light microscopy shows some enlargement of the glomerulus but no increase in cellularity. The capillary walls show irregular thickening. *B,* Electron microscopy shows thickening of the capillary basement membrane with prominent intramembranous electron-dense granular deposits.

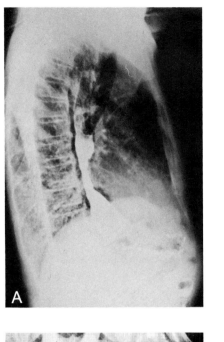
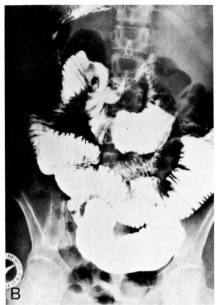
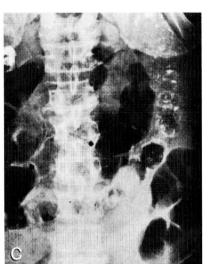
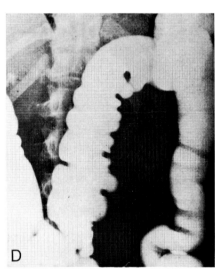

Figure 63–13. Four examples of gastrointestinal changes in patients with MCTD that resemble those seen in scleroderma. *A,* Reduced peristalsis in the lower two thirds of esophagus. *B,* Dilation of duodenal loop and proximal small bowel. *C,* Pneumatosis cystoides of the small bowel (arrows). *D,* Widemouthed pseudodiverticula in antimesenteric border of the colon. (From Bennett, R. M., and O'Connell, D. J.: Mixed connective tissue disease. A clinicopathological study of 20 cases. Semin. Arthritis Rheum. 10:25, 1980, and Br. J. Radiol. 50:620, 1977, used by permission.)

thy.[40, 99, 197, 198] Trigeminal involvement is relatively rare in classic SLE but is the most frequent manifestation of SSC. In a few instances, trigeminal neuropathy has been the presenting feature of MCTD.[97, 197–200] In contrast with central nervous system involvement in classic SLE, frank psychosis and convulsions have rarely been reported in MCTD.[9, 97, 197] Headaches are a relatively common symptom in MCTD; in the majority of patients, they are probably vascular in origin, with many of the components of classic migraine.[201] Some patients experience headaches that are accompanied by fever and sometimes myalgia, somewhat reminiscent of a viral syndrome.[97, 198] In a subset of these patients, signs of meningeal irritation develop, and examination of the cerebrospinal fluid reveals the changes of an aseptic meningitis.[198, 202] Aseptic meningitis has sometimes been described as a hypersensitivity reaction to nonsteroidal anti-inflammatory drugs (NSAIDs) (e.g., sulindac[202] and ibuprofen).[203] Spinal cord involvement in the form of

a cauda equina syndrome[124] and transverse myelitis[204] has been reported in isolated patients with MCTD. A propensity for cord involvement may be related to a concentration of RNP antigen in the anterior-horn cells.[205] Peripheral neuropathy[198, 206] and retinal vasculitis[207] have also been described in association with MCTD.

A bland intimal proliferation and medial hypertrophy affecting medium-sized and small vessels are the characteristic *vascular lesions* of MCTD.[135, 142, 145, 160, 208] A similar histologic picture is seen in the vasculopathy of SSC. These changes have been found in the lung and are the major cause of pulmonary hypertension in MCTD. Proliferative intimal changes have also been reported in the myocardium[142] and in the kidney.[184] This vascular lesion differs from the usual changes encountered in SLE, in which a perivascular inflammatory infiltrate and fibrinoid necrosis are more characteristic. An angiographic study of 13 patients with MCTD found that *all* patients had occlusions of digital arteries.[209] Complete obstruction was found in ulnar arteries in 60 percent, superficial palmar arches in 87 percent, and deep palmar arches in 13 percent (Fig. 63–14); no abnormalities were noted on renal angiography. Fingernail capillaroscopy indicated that 90 percent of patients with MCTD had the same pattern of capillary dilation and dropout as has been reported in SSC; the mean number of abnormal nailfolds per patient was 4.4.[209] In another study, all patients with MCTD had abnormal nailfold capillaroscopy with a pattern similar to that seen in SSC; in addition, a bushy pattern was noted in 73 percent.[210] It has been claimed that abnormal nailfold capillaroscopy has some prognostic significance in determining which patients may develop pulmonary hypertension.[146] It would appear that an SSC pattern on nailfold capillaroscopy is a distinctive feature of MCTD that is not seen in classic SLE[211] (Fig. 63–15). It is reasonable to postulate that the intimal proliferation is related to circulating factors that interact with endothelial cells. Meyer and associates[212] studied inhibition of in vitro vascular endothelial cell growth by sera from patients with various connective tissue diseases; cytotoxic effects were seen in MCTD (41 percent), SSC (23 percent), and SLE (15 percent). Anti–endothelial cell antibodies have been reported in 45 percent of patients with MCTD, correlating with pulmonary changes and spontaneous abortion.[213] Further support for endothelial cell injury in MCTD comes from a study of serum levels of factor VIII Rag; elevated levels were found in MCTD in 67 percent, in SSC in 62 percent, in SLE in 38 percent, and in primary Raynaud's phenomenon in 17 percent.[214]

Hematologic abnormalities are a common finding in MCTD. Anemia is found in 75 percent of patients, the usual profile is most consistent with the anemia of chronic inflammation.[97, 146, 175, 177, 215] A positive Coombs' test is found in about 60 percent of patients, but an overt hemolytic anemia is uncommon.[9, 97, 216]

As in SLE, a leukopenia affecting mainly the lymphocyte series is seen in about 75 percent of patients and tends to correlate with disease activity.[9, 97, 146, 174, 216] Less common associations have been thrombocytopenia,[9, 216] thrombotic thrombocytopenic purpura,[217, 218] and red cell aplasia.[219] The majority of patients with MCTD have hypergammaglobulinemia.[9, 97, 175, 177] One report estimates that up to 33 percent of the IgG molecules have an anti-RNP specificity.[220] Positive tests for rheumatoid factor have been found in about 50 percent of patients[97, 175, 177]; in general, this is associated with more severe degrees of arthritis.[109, 118] False-positive results of the Veneral Disease Research Laboratory (VDRL) test have been noted in about 10 percent of patients[9, 97]; studies of anticardiolipin antibodies or lupus anticoagulants have rarely been reported.[164] By definition, all patients with MCTD have anti–U_1 RNP antibodies. In general, there is not a close correlation with disease activity, but some patients who go into a sustained remission may become seronegative.[172, 221] Antibodies to single-stranded DNA occur in about 80 percent of patients with MCTD,[97, 122] but the occurrence of antibodies to double-stranded DNA is both rare and transient. In some instances, the finding of antibodies to double-stranded DNA may be a technical artifact resulting from single-stranded DNA antibodies reacting with double-stranded DNA contaminated with single-stranded regions.[222] Hypocomplementemia has been noted in several studies[9, 97, 138, 146, 177, 182]; it is not as prevalent as in classic SLE and has not been correlated with any particular clinical situation. Antilymphocytic antibodies are reported in about 20 percent of patients with MCTD[223–225]; this compares to a prevalence of about 93 percent in classic SLE. U_1 RNP immune complexes have been described in the sera of patients with MCTD and have been associated with disease activity.[226–230] Immune complex levels in patients with juvenile-onset RA, SLE, and MCTD have been correlated with IgG and IgM rheumatoid

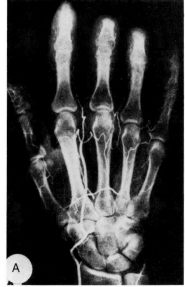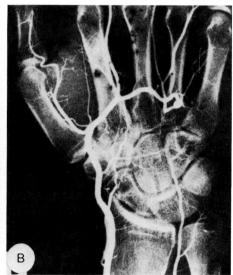

Figure 63–14. *A,* Digital angiogram showing multiple arterial occlusions with collateral formation. *B,* Digital angiogram showing ulnar artery occlusions. (From Peller, J. S., et al.: Angiographic findings in mixed connective tissue disease. Correlation with fingernail capillary photomicroscopy and digital photoplethysmography findings. Arthritis Rheum. 28:768, 1985, used by permission.)

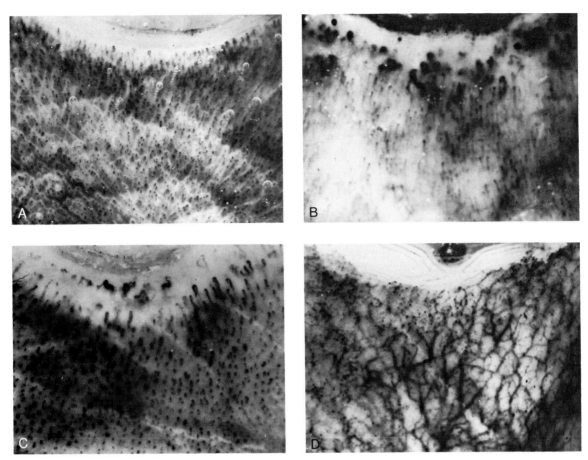

Figure 63–15. Different nail fold capillary patterns in health and disease. (All figures kindly provided by Dr. Maricq.) *A*, Normal pattern. (Courtesy of Microvascular Research.) *B*, Pattern in a patient with scleroderma. *C*, Pattern in a patient with MCTD (Courtesy of Clinics in Rheumatic Diseases). *D*, Pattern in a patient with acute SLE. (*B* and *D* from Maricq, H. R., et al.: Diagnostic potential of in vivo capillary microscopy in scleroderma and related disorders. Arthritis Rheum. 23:183, 1980, used by permission.)

factor.[231] Elevated levels of IgA antibodies to IgD have been found in MCTD (58 percent), SLE (27 percent), and RA (45 percent).[232] As most mature B cells possess IgD on their surface, it was suggested that cell surface antibodies may have a role as immune modulators in MCTD and other connective tissue diseases.

Pregnancy in MCTD

In a study of 31 patients with MCTD, 31 patients with SLE, and 51 control subjects, the fertility rates in both SLE and MCTD were unaltered, whereas parity and fetal wastage were increased in both SLE and MCTD.[233] Forty percent of patients exhibited an exacerbation of MCTD during pregnancy. In another analysis of pregnancy and MCTD, there were 38 live births of a total of 47 pregnancies. Disease exacerbations during pregnancy and the post partum period were not noted.[97] It is possible that premature birth in MCTD may be due to its strong association with Raynaud's phenomenon.[234]

The MCTD syndrome may first become apparent in childhood.[150, 235–240] From the reports to date, it

would seem that juvenile MCTD is associated with more morbidity than is the adult form. Significant myocarditis, glomerulonephritis, thrombocytopenia, seizures, and aseptic meningitis have been described.

Prognosis of MCTD

The original description of MCTD stressed two points, namely: ". . . a relatively good prognosis and an excellent response to corticosteroids."[9] With the benefit of two decades of hindsight, it is now apparent that both these claims need to be qualified. Patients with high titers of U$_1$ RNP antibodies have a low prevalence of serious renal disease and life-threatening neurologic problems; in this sense, MCTD can be favorably compared with classic SLE. In the follow-up study of the original 25 patients described by Sharp and colleagues,[241] eight had died by 1980 (Table 63–3).

It is now evident that not all patients with MCTD have a favorable prognosis and that death may occur from progressive pulmonary hypertension and its cardiac sequelae.[97, 146, 159–169] Pulmonary hypertension sometimes follows a rapidly accelerated course,

Table 63–3. REPORTED CAUSES OF DEATH IN MCTD

Pulmonary hypertension	Myocardial infarction*
Myocarditis	Gastrointestinal hemorrhage*
Mesenteric vasculitis	Ruptured aortic aneurysm*
Opportunistic infection	Ventricular fibrillation*
Pulmonary hemorrhage	Pulmonary embolism*
"Shock lung"	Cerebral hemorrhage*
Amyloidosis	Suicide
Budd-Chiari syndrome	

*Probably not a direct result of disease.

which can lead to death in a few weeks.[97] Primary myocardial involvement is another source of death. In contrast with SLE, in which the major cause of death is often related to secondary infections, nosocomial infections rarely have been described in patients with MCTD.[106, 170] Sharp describes a favorable course in 60 percent of his patients with MCTD; 36 percent required repeated courses of high doses of glucocorticoids.[172] In a Japanese study of 45 patients with MCTD the survival rate at 5 years was 90.5 percent, and at 10 years 82.1 percent. The corresponding figures for 274 patients with SLE were 90.2 percent and 79.6 percent.[242] In contrast, analysis of the MCTD data revealed that patients with predominant SSC-PM overlap had only a 33 percent 10-year survival.

Autoantibodies and HLA Associations

As is the case with all the classic DCTDs, there is a substantial body of evidence indicating an autoimmune etiology in MCTD (Table 63–4). Tan, Reichlin, and Sharp established the specificities of anti-Sm and anti-RNP antibodies for SLE and MCTD and also showed that Sm and RNP antigens were in some way physically associated.[122, 178, 246–249] Lerner and Steitz used the sera of patients to immunoprecipitate cell extracts labeled with phosphorus-32 (^{32}P) or sulfure-35 (^{35}S)-methionine.[250, 251] Studies using ^{32}P showed that anti-RNP antibodies precipitated a single species of RNA (U_1), whereas anti-Sm antibodies precipitated five different RNAs (U_1, U_2, U_4, U_5, and

Table 63–4. AUTOIMMUNE FEATURES OF MCTD

Immune Dysfunction	References
Hypergammaglobulinemia	9, 97, 215, 220
Circulating immune complexes	226, 227, 229–231, 243
Hypocomplementemia	9, 97, 146, 174, 182
Lymphocytotoxic antibodies	223–225
Lymphopenia	9, 97, 215, 224, 225
U_1 RNP antibodies	92–96, 250–252, 257
Positive rheumatoid factor	9, 97, 107–109, 118
Tissue infiltration by lymphocytes	97, 134, 141, 145, 181, 189, 199, 209, 228
Immune complex deposition	97, 169, 170, 173, 180, 228
Reticuloendothelial dysfunction	245
Microvascular changes	209–214

U_6); the "U" designation refers to the characteristically high uridine content of these RNAs, which are ubiquitous components of eukaryotic cells, highly conserved in evolution. They are called *small nuclear RNAs* (snRNAs) and are complexed with proteins that appear to be the site of immune reactivity for autoantibodies; these complexes are often referred to as "SNURPS" (snRNP). ^{35}S-methionine studies showed that anti-Sm antibodies precipitate five proteins with approximate molecular weights of 28 kD (B'B), 16 kD (D), 13 kD (E), 12 kD (F), and 11 kD (G); all five polypeptides are common to the U_1, U_2, U_4, U_5, and U_6 snRNAs. Anti-RNP antibodies precipitate three proteins with molecular weights of 68 kD, 33 kD (A'), and 22 kD (C); these polypeptides are *uniquely* associated with the U_1 snRNA. The clinical correlates considered distinctive for MCTD are associated with the 68-kD specificity.[88, 92–95, 252]

A major role of anti–U_1 RNP antibodies in the pathogenesis of MCTD seems unlikely, as the antibodies would have to gain entry into the cells. There is some evidence for this in vitro,[129] but whether this occurs in vivo is not known. The function of U_1, U_2, and U_6 snRNPs is to remove introns from premessenger RNA; a process referred to as "splicing." There is experimental evidence that U_1 RNP antibodies disrupt the function of this so-called spliceosome (U_1, U_2, plus U_6).[253] Fine specificity studies have determined the epitopes on the 68-kD polypeptide for both B and T cells.[88, 254–260] When these linear sequences are compared with other sequences in the gene bank, similarities have been described for epitopes on a murine retroviral p30 gag antigen and the human influenza B virus.[255, 261] Whether this represents an interesting chance association or whether these viruses are involved in stimulating autoimmunity by the mechanism of molecular mimicry is a matter for future research.

The 68-kD anti–U_1 RNP antibodies are associated with the HLA-DR4 phenotype in 66 percent of cases, compared with 28 percent of control subjects[95, 119, 120]; there is also a significant correlation with DRw35. There is no correlation with DR2 or DR3, as is seen in classic SLE, or HLA-A9, B8, DR3, and DR5, as have been noted in scleroderma.[262] There is also an association of anti-U_1 RNP with the IgG heavy chain phenotype Gm 1,3;5,21.[120] This association is strongest for anti–68-kD antibodies and may merely reflect the strong linkage disequilibrium of these antibodies with HLA-DR4. These findings are in distinct contrast with SLE, in which HLA-DR4 is under-represented compared with the normal population (Fig. 63–16). Predisposition to diffuse glomerulonephritis in SLE is strongly associated with HLA-DR2, DQw1, and, especially, DQB1.AZH[263]; the lack of severe renal involvement in MCTD may well turn out to be more closely related to fine HLA specificities, which, in turn, are associated with RNP antibodies. It may be that another gene with a strong linkage disequilibrium with HLA-DR4 or DRW35 is more closely related to the anti–68-kD autoantibody response. For

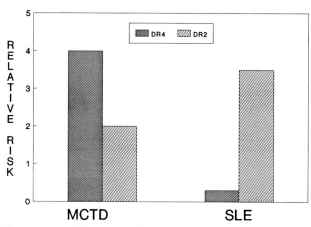

Figure 63–16. There is a close association with the HLA-DR4 haplotype and the presence of anti–68-kD antibodies and, hence, clinical features of MCTD. Conversely, the HLA-DR4 haplotype is under-represented in patients with classic SLE; they are more likely to have the HLA-DR2 haplotype. Diffuse proliferative glomerulonephritis in SLE is strongly related to HLA-DR2, DQw1, and especially DQB1.AZH. These associations may explain, in part, the "good renal prognosis" in MCTD. (Data taken from Hoffman et al.[95] and Fronek et al.[263])

instance, patients with RA have critical changes in amino acids in the third hypervariable region of both the *DR β1* and *DR β2* genes of the DR4 haplotype.[264, 265] Whether similar amino acid substitutions will be found in the HLA-DR4 genes associated with 68-kD activity may have a critical bearing on the immunopathogenesis of MCTD.

A second antibody system has been reported in MCTD,[266–268] anti-hnRNP. The antigenic moiety is complexed to the heterogeneous nuclear RNA (hnRNA), which is associated with the nuclear matrix. A recent study using recombinant hnRNP A1 in an ELISA assay found that it was a common target for autoimmunity in several rheumatic diseases: SLE (22 percent), SSC (10 percent), idiopathic Raynaud's phenomenon (10 percent), Sjögren's syndrome (5 percent), RA (50 percent), and MCTD (40 percent); the high prevalence in RA was possibly due to reactivity with the carbonyl-terminal region, which has some homology with keratin.[269]

Management

The rational management of MCTD is confounded by the absence of controlled trials. There is little disagreement that there is no cure for MCTD. Those features of the disease that are based on a scleroderma-like pathology usually possess an inexorable momentum that usually is unresponsive to current therapeutic modalities. It is now evident that some of the more severe problems, such as pulmonary hypertension and myocarditis, may be present for many years before they become symptomatic. In such patients, it would be reasonable to consider vigorous treatment with intravenous prostacycline[270] and angiotensin-converting enzyme (ACE) inhibi-

tors. Many of the problems causing morbidity in MCTD tend to be intermittent and responsive to glucocorticoids (e.g., aseptic meningitis, myositis, pleurisy, pericarditis, and myocarditis). On the other hand, nephrotic syndrome, Raynaud's phenomenon, deforming arthropathy, acrosclerosis, and peripheral neuropathies are usually steroid resistant. General guidelines for treating specific features of the MCTD spectrum are given in Table 63–5. Over the long term, concern usually mounts over the total glucocorticoid burden and the possibility of inducing an iatrogenic steroid myopathy, aseptic necrosis of

Table 63–5. GUIDELINES FOR MANAGING MCTD

Problems	Treatments
Fatigue, arthralgias, myalgias	NSAIDs, antimalarials, low-dose prednisone (≤10 mg/day)
Arthritis	NSAIDs, antimalarials, gold*, methotrexate
Pleurisy	NSAIDs, short course of prednisone, about 20 mg/day
Aseptic meningitis	Discontinue NSAIDs,† short course of high-dose prednisone, about 60 mg/day
Myositis	Acute onset/severe—prednisone, 60–100 mg/day Chronic/low grade—prednisone, 10–30 mg/day‡
Membranous glomerulonephropathy	Trial of prednisone, 15–60 mg/day
Nephrotic syndrome	Steroids seldom effective, may require dialysis/transplantation
Raynaud's phenomenon	Keep warm, avoid finger trauma. Nifedipine as tolerated. Pentoxifylline in cases of potential digital gangrene
Acute-onset digital gangrene	Intra-arterial prostacycline
Myocarditis	Trial of steroids and Cytoxan (cyclophosphamide); avoid digoxin§
Asymptomatic pulmonary hypertension	Trial of steroids and Cytoxan
Symptomatic pulmonary hypertension	Trial of intravenous prostacycline and angiotensin-converting enzyme inhibitors. Heart-lung transplantation
Vascular headache	Trial of propranolol or alternate-day aspirin, 350 mg
Dysphagia	Trial of prednisone, 15–30 mg/day
Heartburn	Raise head of bed, discontinue smoking, avoid caffeine H2 antagonists H⁺ proton pump blockers Metoclopramide
Trigeminal neuropathy	None

*Has been associated with frequent hypersensitivity reactions.[118]
†Sulindac and ibuprofen have been associated with a hypersensitivity aseptic meningitis.[202, 203]
‡Remain alert for steroid myopathy, aseptic necrosis of bone, and accelerated osteoporosis.
§Predisposes to ventricular arrhythmias.

bone, or accelerated osteoporosis. Unless contraindicated, all patients should take supplementary calcium (1 to 1.5 g per day) and vitamin D. Postmenopausal patients should be offered estrogen-progesterone replacement therapy unless there are specific contraindications; anecdotally, such therapy has not been associated with flare-ups of MCTD. Patients with severe hand deformities may be helped by soft tissue release operations and selected joint fusions.

There is often a tendency to assume that all patients with MCTD should be on long-term glucocorticoids; this mistake is compounded by the assumption that all medical problems in these patients are related to their underlying MCTD.

The initial claim of "its being characterized by an excellent response to corticosteroid therapy"[9] is now appreciated to be only partly correct. The management of patients with MCTD requires continuing reassessment of an ever-changing pattern of clinical problems and a constant alertness to the iatrogenic disease.

References

1. Hutchinson, J.: On lupus and its treatment. Br. Med. J. 650–652, 1880.
2. Hockberg, M. C.: Adult and juvenile rheumatoid arthritis: current epidemiologic perspectives. Epidemiol. Rev. 3:27, 1981.
3. Klemperer, P., Pollack, A., and Baehr, G.: Diffuse collagen disease: acute disseminated lupus erythematosus and diffuse scleroderma. J.A.M.A. 119:331, 1942.
4. Dubois, E. L., and Wallace, D. J.: Differential diagnosis. In Wallace, D. J., and Dubois, E. L. (eds.): Dubois' Lupus Erythematosus. Philadelphia, Lea & Febiger, 1987, p. 470.
5. Harley, J. B., Sestak, A. L., Willis, L. G., Fu, S. M., Hansen, J. A., and Reichlin, M.: A model for disease heterogeneity in systemic lupus erythematosus: relationships between histocompatibility antigens, autoantibodies, and lymphopenia or renal disease. Arthritis Rheum. 32:826, 1989.
6. Tuffanelli, D. L., and Winkelman, R. K.: Systemic scleroderma. A clinical study of 727 cases. Arch. Dermatol. (Chicago) 84:359, 1961.
7. Tay, C. H.: Cutaneous manifestations of systemic lupus erythematosus: a clinical study from Singapore. Aust. J. Dermatol. 11:30, 1970.
8. Dubois, E. L., Chandor, S., Friou, G. J., and Bischel, M.: Progressive systemic sclerosis (PSS) and localized scleroderma (morphea) with positive LE cell test and unusual systemic manifestations compatible with systemic lupus erythematous (SLE): presentation of 14 cases including one set of identical twins, one with scleroderma and the other with SLE. Review of the literature. Medicine (Baltimore) 50:199, 1971.
9. Sharp, G. C., Irvin, W. S., Tan, E. M., et al.: Mixed connective tissue disease: an apparently distinct rheumatic disease syndrome associated with a specific antibody to an extractable nuclear antigen (ENA). Am. J. Med. 52:148, 1972.
10. Kahn, M. F., Peltier, A. P., Degraeve, B., Mery, J. P., Morel-Maroger, L., de-Seze, S.: Successive connective tissue diseases: scleroderma, then lupus. Clinical and biological study of 4 cases. Ann. Intern. Med. 128:1, 1977.
11. Umbert, P., and Winkelmann, R. K.: Concurrent localized scleroderma and discoid lupus erythematosus: Cutaneous "mixed" or "overlap" syndrome. Arch. Dermatol. 114:1473, 1978.
12. Dubois, E. L., and Tuffanelli, D. L.: Clinical manifestations of systemic lupus erythematosus. J.A.M.A. 190:104, 1964.
13. Fries, J., and Holman, H.: Systemic Lupus Erythematosus: A clinical Analysis. Philadelphia, W. B. Saunders Co., 1975.
14. Haserick, J. R.: Modern concepts of systemic lupus erythematosus: review of 126 cases. J. Chronic Dis. 1:317, 1955.
15. Lee, P., Urowitz, M. B., Bookman, A. A. M., Koehler, B. E., Smythe, H. A., Gordon, D. A., and Ogryzlo, M. A.: Systemic lupus erythematosus: A review of 110 cases with reference to nephritis, the nervous system, infections, aseptic necrosis, and prognosis. Q. J. Med. 46:1, 1977.
16. Zizic, T. M.: Gastrointestinal manifestations. In Schur, P. (ed.): The Clinical Management of Systemic Lupus Erythematosus. New York, Grune & Stratton, 1983, p. 153.
17. Estes, D., and Christian, C. L.: The natural history of systemic lupus erythematosus by prospective analysis. Medicine 50:85, 1971.
18. Stevens, M. B., Hookman, P., Siegel, C. I., Esterly, J. R., Shulman, L. E., and Hendrix, T. R.: Aperistalsis of the esophagus in patients with connective tissue disorders and Raynaud's phenomenon. N. Engl. J. Med. 270:1218, 1964.
19. Clark, M., and Fountain, R. B.: Oesophageal motility in connective disease. Br. J. Dermatol. 33:449, 1967.
20. Clark, J. A., Winkelman, R. K., McDuffie, F. C., and Ward, L. E.: Synovial tissue changes and rheumatoid factor in scleroderma. Mayo Clin. Proc. 46:97, 1971.
21. Makinen, D., Fritzler, M., Davis, P., and Sherlock, S.: Anticentromere antibodies in primary cirrhosis. Arthritis Rheum. 26:914, 1983.
22. Rodnan, G. P., and Medsger, T. A.: The rheumatic manifestations of progressive systemic sclerosis. Clin. Orthop. 8:81, 1968.
23. Wild, W., and Beetham, W. P.: Erosive arthropathy in systemic scleroderma. J.A.M.A. 232:511, 1975.
24. Armstrong, R. D., and Gibson, T.: Scleroderma and erosive polyarthritis: a disease entity. Ann. Rheum. Dis. 41:141, 1982.
25. Baron, M., Srolovitz, H., Lander, P., and Kapusta, M.: The coexistence of rheumatoid arthritis and scleroderma: a case report and review of the literature. J. Rheumatol. 9:947, 1982.
26. Lovell, C. R., and Jayson, M. I. V.: Joint involvement in systemic sclerosis. Scand. J. Rheumatol. 8:154, 1989.
27. Epstein, O., Thomas, H. C., and Sherlock, S.: Primary biliary cirrhosis in a dry gland syndrome with features of chronic graft-versus-host disease. Lancet 1:1166, 1980.
28. Miller, F., Lane, B., Soterakis, J., and D'Angelo, W. A.: Primary biliary cirrhosis and scleroderma: the possibility of a common pathogenic mechanism. Arch. Pathol. Lab. Med. 103:505, 1979.
29. Powell, F. C., Schroeter, A. L., and Dickinson, E. R.: Primary biliary cirrhosis and the CREST syndrome: a report of 22 cases. Q. J. Med. 62:75, 1987.
30. O'Brien, S. T., Eddy, W. M., and Krawitt, E. L.: Primary biliary cirrhosis associated with scleroderma. Gastroenterology 62:118, 1972.
31. Reynolds, T. B., Denison, E. K., Frankl, H. D., Lieberman, F. L., and Peters, R. L.: Primary biliary cirrhosis with scleroderma, Raynaud's phenomenon, and telangiectasia. Am. J. Med. 50:302, 1971.
32. Culp, K. S.: Autoimmune associations in primary biliary cirrhosis. Mayo Clin. Proc. 57:365, 1985.
33. Barnett, A. J.: The systemic involvement in scleroderma. Med. J. Aust. 2:659, 1977.
34. Gupta, R. C., Siebold, J. R., Krishnan, M. R., and Steigerwald, J. C.: Mitochondrial antibodies in patients with systemic sclerosis (abstract). Clin. Res. 31:863A, 1983.
35. Bernstein, R. M., Callender, M. E., Neuberger, J. M., Hughes, G. R. V., and Williams, R.: Anticentromere antibody in primary biliary cirrhosis. Ann. Rheum. Dis. 41:612, 1982.
36. Alderuccio, F., Toh, B. H., Barnett, A. J., and Pedersen, J. S.: Identification and characterization of mitochondria autoantigens in progressive systemic sclerosis: identity with the 72,000-dalton autoantigen in primary biliary cirrhosis. J. Immunol. 137:1855, 1986.
37. Gershwin, E. G., Mackay, I. R., Sturgess, A., et al.: Identification and specificity of a cDNA encoding the 70-kd mitochondrial antigen recognized in primary biliary cirrhosis. J. Immunol. 138:3525, 1987.
38. Kumagai, Y., Shiokawa, Y., Medsger, T. A., et al.: Clinical spectrum of connective tissue disease after cosmetic surgery. Arthritis Rheum. 27:1, 1984.
39. Alonso-Ruiz, A., Zea-Mendoza, A. C., Salazar-Vallinas, J. M., et al.: Toxic oil syndrome: a syndrome with features overlapping those of various forms of scleroderma. Semin. Arthritis Rheum. 15:200, 1986.
40. Veltman, G., Lange, C. E., Juhe, S., et al.: Clinical manifestations and course of vinyl chloride disease. Ann. N.Y. Acad. Sci. 246:6, 1975.
41. Yamakage, A., Ishikawa, H., Saito, Y., et al.: Occupational scleroderma-like disorder occurring in men engaged in the polymerisation of epoxy resins. Dermatologica 161:33, 1980.
42. Flindt-Hansen, H., and Isager, H.: Scleroderma after occupational exposure to trichlorethylene and trichlorethane. Acta Derm. Venereol. (Stockh.) 67:263, 1987.
43. Owens, G. R., and Medsger, T. A.: Systemic sclerosis secondary to occupational exposure. Am. J. Med. 85:114, 1988.
44. Rodnan, G. P., Benedek, T. G., Medsger, T. A., et al.: The association of progressive systemic sclerosis (scleroderma) with coal-miners pneumoconiosis and other forms of silicosis. Ann. Intern. Med. 66:323, 1967.
45. Hertzman, P. A., Blevins, W. L., Mayer, J., Greenfield, B., Ting, M., and Gleich, G. J.: Association of the eosinophilia-myalgia syndrome with the ingestion of tryptophan. N. Engl. J. Med. 322:869, 1990.
46. Okano, Y., Nishikai, M., and Sato, A.: Scleroderma, primary biliary cirrhosis, and Sjögren's syndrome after cosmetic breast augmentation with silicone injection: a case report of possible human adjuvant disease. Ann. Rheum. Dis. 43:520, 1984.
47. Sahn, E. E., Garen, P. D., Silver, R. M., and Maize, J. C.: Scleroderma following augmentation mammoplasty: Report of a case and review of the literature. Arch. Dermatol. 126:1198, 1990.

48. Varga, J., and Jimenez, S. A.: Augmentation mammoplasty and scleroderma: Is there an association? Arch. Dermatol. 126:1220, 1990.
49. Shulman, H. M., Sale, G. E., Lerner, K. G., et al.: Chronic cutaneous graft-versus-host disease. Am. J. Pathol. 91:545, 1978.
50. Epstein, O.: Primary biliary cirrhosis and the CREST syndrome: new terminology. Hepatology 8:189, 1988.
51. Graham-Brown, R. A. C., and Sarkany, I.: Scleroderma-like changes due to chronic graft-versus-host disease. Clin. Exp. Dermatol. 8:531, 1983.
52. Hood, A. F., Soter, N. A., Rappeport, J., and Gigli, I.: Graft-versus-host reaction: cutaneous reactions following bone marrow transplantations. Arch. Dermatol. 113:1087, 1977.
53. Osial, T. A., Whiteside, T. L., Buckingham, R. B., Singh, B., Barnes, E. L., Pierce, J. M., and Rodnan, G. P.: Clinical and serological study of Sjögren's syndrome in patients with progressive systemic sclerosis. Arthritis Rheum. 26:500, 1983.
54. Oddis, C. V., Eisenbeis, C. H., Reidbord, H. E., Steen, V. D., and Medsger, T. A.: Vasculitis in systemic sclerosis: association with Sjögren's syndrome and the CREST syndrome variant. J. Rheumatol. 14:942, 1987.
55. Nixon, J. A.: Scleroderma and myositis. Lancet 1:79, 1907.
56. Oppenheim, H.: Zur Dermatomyositis. Berl. Klin. Wochenschr. 36:805, 1899.
57. Petjes, G., and Clejat, C.: Sclerose atrophique de la peau et myosite generalisee. Arch. Dermato-syphiligraphiques (Paris) 7:560, 1906.
58. Clements, P. J., Furst, D. E., Campion, D. S., Bohan, A., Harris, R., Levy, J., and Paulus, H.: Muscle disease in progressive systemic sclerosis: diagnostic and therapeutic considerations. Arthritis Rheum. 21:62, 1978.
59. Thompson, J. M., Bluestone, R., Bywaters, E. G. L., Dorling, J., and Johnson, M.: Skeletal muscle involvement in systemic sclerosis. Ann. Rheum. Dis. 28:281, 1969.
60. Mimori, T.: Scleroderma-polymyositis overlap syndrome. Int. J. Dermatol. 26:419, 1987.
61. Allaway, G. P., Vivino, A. A., Kohn, L. D., Notkins, A. L., and Prabhakar, B. S.: Characterization of the 70-kDa component of the human Ku autoantigen expressed in insect cell nuclei using a recombinant baculovirus vector. Biochem. Biophys. Res. Commun. 168:747, 1990.
62. Reeves, W. H., and Sthoeger, Z. M.: Molecular cloning of cDNA encoding the p70 (Ku) lupus autoantigen. J. Biol. Chem. 264:5047, 1989.
63. Yaneva, M., Wen, J., Ayala, A., and Cook, R.: cDNA-derived amino acid sequence of the 86-kDa subunit of the Ku antigen. J. Biol. Chem. 264:13407, 1989.
64. Prabhakar, B. S., Allaway, G. P., Srinivasappa, J., and Notkins, A. L.: Cell surface expression of the 70-kD component of Ku, a DNA-binding nuclear autoantigen. J. Clin. Invest. 86:1301, 1990.
65. Yaneva, M., and Arnett, F. C.: Antibodies against Ku protein in sera from patients with autoimmune diseases. Clin. Exp. Immunol. 76:366, 1989.
66. Reichlin, M., Maddison, P. J., Targoff, I., et al.: Antibodies to a nuclear/nucleolar antigen in patients with polymyositis overlap syndromes. J. Clin. Immunol. 4:40, 1984.
67. Gelpi, C., Alguero, A., Angeles Martinez M., Vidal, S., Juarez, C., and Rodriguez-Sanchez, J. L.: Identification of protein components reactive with anti-PM/Scl autoantibodies. Clin. Exp. Immunol. 81:59, 1990.
68. Genth, E., Mierau, R., Genetzky, P., von Mühlen, C. A., Kaufmann, S., von Wilmowsky, H., Meurer, M., Krieg, T., Pollmann, H. J., and Hartl, P. W.: Immunogenetic associations of scleroderma-related antinuclear antibodies. Arthritis Rheum. 33:657, 1990.
69. Reimer, G.: Autoantibodies against nuclear, nucleolar, and mitochondrial antigens in systemic sclerosis (scleroderma). Rheum. Dis. Clin. North Am. 16:169, 1990.
70. Mimori, T., Hinterberger, M., Pettersson, I., et al.: Autoantibodies to the U2 small nuclear ribonucleoprotein in a patient with scleroderma-polymyositis overlap syndrome. J. Biol. Chem. 259:560, 1984.
71. Mathews, M. B., and Bernstein, R. M.: Myositis autoantibody inhibits histidyl-tRNA synthetase: a model for autoimmunity. Nature 304:177, 1983.
72. Targoff, I. N., Arnett, F. C., and Reichlin, M.: Antibody to threonyl-transfer RNA synthetase in myositis sera. Arthritis Rheum. 31:515, 1988.
73. Mathews, M. B., Reichlin, M., Hughes, G. R. V., and Bernstein, R. M.: Anti-threonyl-tRNA synthetase, a second myositis-related autoantibody. J. Exp. Med. 160:420, 1984.
74. Bunn, C. C., Bernstein, R. M., and Mathews, M. B.: Autoantibodies against alanyl-tRNA synthetase and tRNAala coexist and are associated with myositis. J. Exp. Med. 163:1281, 1986.
75. Targoff, I. N.: Autoantibodies to aminoacyl-transfer RNA synthetases for isoleucine and glycine. Two additional synthetases are antigenic in myositis. J. Immunol. 144:1737, 1990.
76. Oddis, C. V., Medsger, T. A., and Cooperstein, L. A.: A subluxing

77. Schumacher, H. R., Schimmer, B., Gordon, G. C., Bookspan, M. A., Brogadir, S., and Dorwart, B. B.: Articular manifestations of polymyositis and dermatomyositis. Am. J. Med. 67:287, 1979.
78. Bunch, T. W., O'Duffy, J. D., and McLeod, R. A.: Deforming arthritis of the hands in polymyositis. Arthritis Rheum. 19:243, 1976.
79. Arsura, E. L., and Greenberg, A. S.: Adverse impact of interstitial pulmonary fibrosis on prognosis in polymyositis and dermatomyositis. Semin. Arthritis Rheum. 18:29, 1988.
80. Tazelaar, H. D., Viggiano, R. W., Pickersgill, J., and Colby, T. V.: Interstitial lung disease in polymyositis and dermatomyositis. Am. Rev. Respir. Dis. 141:727, 1990.
81. Targoff, I. N., Johnson, A. E., and Miller, F. W.: Antibody to signal recognition particle in polymyositis. Arthritis Rheum. 33:1361, 1990.
82. Bennett, R. M.: Mixed connective tissue disease and other overlap syndromes. In Kelley, W. N., Harris, E. D., Jr., Ruddy, S., and Sledge, C. B. (eds.): Textbook of Rheumatology. 3rd ed. Philadelphia, W. B. Saunders Co., 1985.
83. Lazaro, M. A., Cocco, J. A. M., Catoggio, L. J., Babini, S. M., Messina, O. D., and Morteo, O. G.: Clinical and serologic characteristics of patients with overlap syndrome: Is mixed connective tissue disease a distinct clinical entity? Medicine 68:58, 1989.
84. McHugh, N., James, I., and Maddison, P.: Clinical significance of antibodies to a 68-kDa U1RNP polypeptide in connective tissue disease. J. Rheumatol. 17:1320, 1990.
85. LeRoy, E. C., Maricq, H., and Kahaleh, M.: Undifferentiated connective tissue syndrome. Arthritis Rheum. 23:341, 1980.
86. Whittingham, S.: SLE or MCTD and the snurp in the splicing. J. Rheumatol. 17:1260, 1990.
87. Bennett, R. M.: Mixed connective tissue disease and other overlap syndromes. In Kelley, W. N., Harris, E. D. J., Ruddy, S. H., and Sledge, G. (eds.): Textbook of Rheumatology. 3rd ed. Philadelphia, W. B. Saunders, 1989, p. 1147.
88. Nyman, U., Lundberg, I., Hedfors, E., and Pettersson, I.: Recombinant 70-kD protein used for determination of autoantigenic epitopes recognized by anti-RNP sera. Clin. Exp. Immunol. 81:52, 1990.
89. Sharp, G. C., and Anderson, P. C.: Current concepts in the classification of connective tissue diseases. Overlap syndromes and mixed connective tissue disease (MCTD). J. Am. Acad. Dermatol. 2:269, 1980.
90. Bennett, R. M.: Mixed connective tissue disease. Compr. Ther. 8:11, 1982.
91. Bennett, R. M.: The differential diagnosis of mixed connective tissue disease. Intern. Med. 3:40, 1982.
92. Petterson, I., Wang, G., Smith, E., Wugzell, H., Hadfors, E., Horn, J., and Sharp, G. E.: Analysis of sera of patients with mixed connective tissue disease and systemic lupus erythematosus. A cross-sectional longitudinal study. Arthritis Rheum. 29:986, 1986.
93. Williams, D. G., Charles, P. J., and Maini, R. N.: Preparative isolation of p67, A, B, B' and D from nRNP/Sm and Sm antigens by reverse-phase chromatography. Use in a polypeptide-specific ELISA for independent quantitation of anti-nRNP and anti-Sm antibodies. J. Immunol. Methods 113:25, 1988.
94. Habets, W. J. A., Hoet, M. H., Sillekens, P. T. G., De Rooij, D. J. R. A. M., Van de Putte, L. B. A., and Van Venrooij, W. J.: Detection of autoantibodies in a quantitative immunoassay using recombinant ribonucleoprotein antigens. Clin. Exp. Immunol. 76:172, 1989.
95. Hoffman, R. W., Rettenmaier, L. J., Takeda, Y., Hewett, J. E., Pettersson, I., Nyman, U., Luger, A. M., and Sharp, G. C.: Human autoantibodies against the 70-kD polypeptide of U1 small nuclear RNP are associated with HLA-DR4 among connective tissue disease patients. Arthritis Rheum. 33:666, 1990.
96. Rettenmaier, L. J., Sharp, G. C., Takeda, Y., Luger, A. C., and Hoffman, R. W.: U1-68KD-positive mixed connective tissue disease appears genetically distinct, within HLA from systemic lupus erythematosus. Arthritis Rheum. 32:S39, 1989.
97. Bennett, R. M., and O'Connell, D.: Mixed connective tissue disease. A clinicopathological study of 20 cases. Semin. Arthritis Rheum. 10:25, 1980.
98. Rasmussen, E. K., Ullman, S., Hier-Madsen, M., Sorensen, S. F., and Halberg, P.: Clinical implications of ribonucleoprotein antibody. Arch. Dermatol. 123:601, 1987.
99. Kashiwazaki, S., Kondo, H., and Fukui, T.: Clinical features of anti-nRNP antibody–positive patients. In Kasukawa, R., and Sharp, G. (eds.): Mixed Connective Tissue Disease and Anti-nuclear Antibodies. Amsterdam, Excerpta Medica, 1987, pp. 261–266.
100. Alarcon-Segovia, D., and Cardiel, M. H.: Comparison between 3 diagnostic criteria for mixed connective tissue disease. Study of 593 patients. J. Rheumatol. 16:328, 1989.
101. Leibfarth, J. H., and Persellin, R. H.: Characteristics of patients with serum antibodies to extractable nuclear antigens. Arthritis Rheum. 19:851, 1976.
102. Nakae, K., Furusawa, F., Kasukawa, R., Tojo, T., Homma, M., and Aoki, K.: A nationwide epidemiological survey on diffuse collagen

arthropathy associated with the anti–Jo-1 antibody in polymyositis/dermatomyositis. Arthritis Rheum. 33:1640, 1990.

diseases: Estimation of prevalence rate in Japan. *In* Kasukawa, R., and Sharp, G. (eds.): Mixed Connective Tissue Disease and Anti-nuclear Antibodies. Amsterdam, Excerpta Medica, 1987, pp. 9–13.

103. Horn, J. R., Kapur, J. J., and Walker, S. E.: Mixed connective tissue disease in siblings. Arthritis Rheum. 21:709, 1978.

104. Ramos-Niembro, F., and Alarcon-Segovia, D.: Familial aspects of mixed connective tissue disease (MCTD). I. Occurrence of systemic lupus erythematosus in another member in two families and aggregation of MCTD in another family. J. Rheumatol. 5:433, 1978.

105. Winfield, J. B., Koffler, D., and Kunkel, H. G.: Development of antibodies to ribonucleoprotein following short-term therapy with procainamide. Arthritis Rheum. 18:531, 1975.

106. Kahn, M. F., Bourgeois, P., Aeschlimann, A., and De Truchis, P.: Mixed connective tissue disease after exposure to polyvinyl chloride. J. Rheumatol. 16:533, 1989.

107. Bennett, R. M., and O'Connell, D. J.: The arthritis of mixed connective tissue disease. Ann. Rheum. Dis. 37:397, 1978.

108. Halla, J. T., and Hardin, J. G.: Clinical features of the arthritis of mixed connective tissue disease. Arthritis Rheum. 21:497, 1978.

109. Ramos-Niembro, F., Alarcon-Segovia, D., and Hernandez-Ortiz, J.: Articular manifestations of mixed connective tissue disease. Arthritis Rheum. 22:43, 1979.

110. Okazaki, T., Saito, T., Izumiyama, T., and Hoshino, H.: RA-like features in MCTD: a controlled study. *In* Kasukawa, R., and Sharp, G. (eds.): Mixed Connective Tissue Disease and Anti-nuclear Antibodies. Amsterdam, Excerpta Medica, 1987, pp. 273–278.

111. Martinez-Cordero, E., and Lopez-Zepeda, J.: Resorptive arthropathy and rib erosions in mixed connective tissue disease. J. Rheumatol. 17:719, 1990.

112. O'Connell, D. J., and Bennett, R. M.: Mixed connective tissue disease—clinical and radiological aspects of 20 cases. Br. J. Radiol. 50:620, 1977.

113. Udoff, E. J., Genant, H. K., Kozin, F., and Ginsberg, M.: Mixed connective tissue disease: the spectrum of radiographic manifestations. Radiology 124:613, 1977.

114. Martinez-Cordero, E., and Lopez-Zepeda, J.: Resorptive arthropathy and rib erosions in mixed connective tissue disease. J. Rheumatol. 17:719, 1990.

115. Sargent, E. N., Turner, A. F., and Jacobson, G.: Superior marginal rib defects: an etiologic classification. Am. J. Roentgenol. 106:491, 1969.

116. Lewis, R. A., Adams, J. P., Gerber, N. L., Decker, J. L., and Parsons, D. B.: The hand in mixed connective tissue disease. J. Hand Surg. 3:217, 1978.

117. Hutton, C. W., Maddison, P. J., Collins, A. J., and Berriman, J. A.: Intra-articular apatite deposition in mixed connective tissue disease: crystallographic and technetium scanning characteristics. Ann. Rheum. Dis. 47:1027, 1988.

118. Piirainen, H. I.: Patients with arthritis and anti-U1-RNP antibodies: a 10-year follow-up. Br. J. Rheumatol. 29:345, 1990.

119. Black, C. M., Maddison, P. J., Welsh, K. I., Bernstein, R., Woodrow, J. C., and Pereira, R. S.: HLA and immunoglobulin allotypes in mixed connective tissue disease. Arthritis Rheum. 31:131, 1988.

120. Genth, E., Zarnowski, H., Mierau, R., Wohltmann, D., and Hartl, P. W.: HLA-DR4 and Gm(1,3;5,21) are associated with U1-nRNP antibody–positive connective tissue disease. Ann. Rheum. Dis. 46:189, 1987.

121. Ellman, M. H., Pachman, L., and Medof, M. E.: Raynaud's phenomenon and initially seronegative mixed connective tissue disease. J. Rheumatol. 8:632, 1981.

122. Sharp, G. C., Irvin, W. S., LaRoque, R. L., Velez, C., Daly, V., Kaiser, A. D., and Holman, H. R.: Association of autoantibodies to different nuclear antigens with clinical patterns of rheumatic disease and responsiveness to therapy. J. Clin. Invest. 50:350, 1971.

123. Gilliam, J. N., and Prystowsky, S. D.: Conversion of discoid lupus erythematosus to mixed connective tissue disease. J. Rheumatol. 4:165, 1977.

124. Kappes, J., and Bennett, R. M.: Cauda equina syndrome in a patient with high titer anti-RNP antibodies. Arthritis Rheum. 25:349, 1982.

125. Konttinen, Y. T., Tuominen, T. S., Piirainen, H. I., Kononen, M. H., Wolf, J. E., Hietanen, J. H., and Malstrom, M. J.: Signs and symptoms in the masticatory system in ten patients with mixed connective tissue disease. Scand. J. Rheumatol. 19:363, 1990.

126. Hamza, M.: Orogenital ulcerations in mixed connective tissue disease. J. Rheumatol. 12:636, 1985.

127. Willkens, R. F., Roth, G. J., Novak, A., and Walike, J. W.: Perforation of nasal septum in rheumatic diseases. Arthritis Rheum. 19:119, 1976.

128. Iwatsuki, K., Tagami, H., Imaizumi, S., Ginoza, M., and Yamada, M.: The speckled epidermal nuclear immunofluorescence of mixed connective tissue disease seems to develop as an in vitro phenomenon. Br. J. Dermatol. 107:653, 1982.

129. Alarcon-Segovia, D., Ruiz-Arguelles, A., and Fishbein, E.: Antibody penetration into living cells. I. Intranuclear immunoglobulin in peripheral blood mononuclear cells in mixed connective tissue disease and systemic lupus erythematosus. Clin. Exp. Immunol. 35:364, 1979.

130. Reimer, G., Huschka, U., Keller, J., Kammerer, R., and Horstein, O. P.: Immunofluorescence studies in scleroderma and mixed connective tissue disease. Br. J. Dermatol. 109:27, 1983.

131. Bergroth, V., Konttinen, Y. T., Piirainen, H., Johansson, E., Nordström, D., and Malmström, M.: Evaluation of lymphocyte activation in skin lesions of patients with mixed connective tissue disease and discoid lupus erythematodes. Arch. Dermatol. Res. 280:1, 1988.

132. McCain, G. A., Bell, D. A., Chodirker, W. B., and Komar, R. R.: Antibody to extractable nuclear antigen in the rheumatic diseases. J. Rheumatol. 5:399, 1978.

133. Leibfarth, J. H., and Persellin, R. H.: Characteristics of patients with serum antibodies to extractable nuclear antigens. Arthritis Rheum. 19:851, 1976.

134. Oxenhandler, R., Hart, M., Corman, L., Sharp, G., and Adelstein, E.: Pathology of skeletal muscle in mixed connective tissue disease. Arthritis Rheum. 20:985, 1977.

135. Hosoda, Y.: Review on pathology of mixed connective tissue disease. *In* Kasukawa, R., and Sharp, G. (eds.): Mixed Connective Tissue Disease and Anti-nuclear Antibodies. Amsterdam, Excerpta Medica, 1987, pp. 281–290.

136. Oetgen, W. J., Mutter, M. L., Lawless, O. J., and Davia, J. C.: Cardiac abnormalities in mixed connective tissue disease. Chest 83:185, 1983.

137. Alpert, M. A., Goldberg, S. H., Singsen, B. H., Durham, J. B., Sharp, G. C., Ahmad, M., Madigan, N. P., Hurst, P. P., and Sullivan, W. D.: Cardiovascular manifestations of mixed connective tissue disease in adults. Circulation 68:1182, 1983.

138. Grant, K. D., Adams, L. E., and Hess, E. V.: Mixed connective tissue disease—a subset with sequential clinical and laboratory features. J. Rheumatol. 8:587, 1981.

139. Leung, W.-H., Wong, K.-L., Lau, C.-P., and Wong, C.-K.: Purulent pericarditis and cardiac tamponade caused by *Nocardia asteroides* in mixed connective tissue disease. J. Rheumatol. 17:1237, 1990.

140. Leung, W. H., Wong, K. L., Lau, C. P., Wong, C. K., Cheng, C. H., and Tai, Y. T.: Echocardiographic identification of mitral valvular abnormalities in patients with mixed connective tissue disease. J. Rheumatol. 17:485, 1990.

141. Nunoda, S., Mifune, J., Ono, S., Nakayama, A., Hifumi, S., Shimizu, M., Takahashi, Y., and Tanaka, T.: An adult case of mixed connective tissue disease associated with perimyocarditis and massive pericardial effusion. Jpn. Heart J. 27:129, 1986.

142. Lash, A. D., Wittman, A. L., and Quismorio, F. P., Jr.: Myocarditis in mixed connective tissue disease: clinical and pathologic study of three cases and review of the literature. Semin. Arthritis Rheum. 15:288, 1986.

143. Przybojewski, J. Z., Mynhardt, J. H., van der Walt, J. J., and Tiedt, F. A.: Cardiac involvement in mixed connective tissue disease. A fatal case of scleroderma combined with systemic lupus erythematosus. S. Afr. Med. J. 68:680, 1985.

144. Whitlow, P. L., Gilliam, J. N., Chubick, A., and Ziff, M.: Myocarditis in mixed connective tissue disease. Association of myocarditis with antibody to nuclear ribonucleoprotein. Arthritis Rheum. 23:808, 1980.

145. Singsen, B. H., Swanson, V. L., Bernstein, B. H., Heuser, E. T., Hanson, V., and Landing, B. H.: A histologic evaluation of mixed connective tissue disease in childhood. Am. J. Med. 68:710, 1980.

146. Sullivan, W. D., Hurst, D. J., Harmon, C. E., Esther, J. H., Agia, G. A., Maltby, J. D., Lillard, S. B., Held, C. N., Wolfe, F., Sunderragan, E. V., Maricq, H. R., and Sharp, G. C.: A prospective evaluation emphasizing pulmonary involvement in patients with mixed connective tissue disease. Medicine 63:92, 1984.

147. Emlen, W.: Complete heart block in mixed connective tissue disease. Arthritis Rheum. 22:679, 1979.

148. Rakovec, P., Kenda, M. F., and Roxman, B.: Panconductional defect in mixed connective tissue disease. Association with Sjögren's syndrome. Chest 81:257, 1982.

149. Comens, S. M., Alpert, M. A., Sharp, G. C., Pressly, T. A., Kelly, D. L., Hazelwood, S. E., and Mukerji, V.: Frequency of mitral valve prolapse in systemic lupus erythematosus, progressive systemic sclerosis and mixed connective tissue disease. Am. J. Cardiol. 63:369, 1989.

150. Singsen, B. H., Bernstein, B. H., Kornreich, H. K., King, K. K., Hanson, V., and Tan, E. M.: MCTD in childhood. J. Pediatr. 90:893, 1977.

151. Udaya, B. S., and Prakash, M. D.: Intrathoracic manifestations in mixed connective tissue disease. Mayo Clin. Proc. 60:813, 1985.

152. Harmon, K. R., and Leatherman, J. W.: Respiratory manifestations of connective tissue disease. Semin. Respir. Infect. 3:258, 1988.

153. Hoogsteden, H. C., van Dongen, J. J., van der Kwast, T. H., Hooijkaas, H., and Hilvering, C.: Bilateral exudative pleuritis, an unusual pulmonary onset of mixed connective tissue disease. Respiration 48:164, 1985.

154. Gibson, G. J., Edmonds, J. P., and Hughes G. R. V.: Diaphragm function and lung involvement in systemic lupus erythematosus. Am. J. Med. 63:926, 1977.

155. Martens, J., and Demedts, M.: Diaphragm dysfunction in mixed

connective tissue disease. A case report. Scand. J. Rheumatol. 11:165, 1982.

156. Sanchez-Guerrero, J., Cesarman, G., and Alarcon-Segovia, D.: Massive pulmonary hemorrhage in mixed connective tissue diseases. J. Rheumatol. 16:1132, 1989.

157. Hosoda, Y., Suzuki, Y., Takano, M., Tojo, T., and Homma, M.: Mixed connective tissue disease with pulmonary hypertension: a clinical and pathological study. J. Rheumatol. 14:826, 1987.

158. Germain, M. J., and Davidman, M.: Pulmonary hemorrhage and acute renal failure in a patient with mixed connective tissue disease. Am. J. Kidney Dis. 3:420, 1984.

159. Jones, M. B., Osterholm, R. K., Wilson, R. B., Martin, F. H., Commers, J. R., and Bachmayer, J. D.: Fatal pulmonary hypertension and resolving immune-complex glomerulonephritis in mixed connective tissue disease. A case report and review of the literature. Am. J. Med. 65:855, 1978.

160. Rosenberg, A. M., Petty, R. E., Cumming, G. R., and Koehler, B. E.: Pulmonary hypertension in a child with mixed connective tissue disease. J. Rheumatol. 6:700, 1979.

161. Manthorpe, R., Elling, H., van der Meulen, J. T., and Sorensen, S. F.: Two fatal cases of mixed connective tissue disease. Description of case histories terminating as progressive systemic sclerosis. Scand. J. Rheumatol. 9:7, 1980.

162. Eulderink, F., and Cats, A.: Fatal primary pulmonary hypertension in mixed connective tissue disease. Z. Rheumatol. 40:25, 1981.

163. Kobayashi, H., Sano, T., Ii, K., Hizawa, K., Yamanoi, A., and Otsuka, T.: Mixed connective tissue disease with fatal pulmonary hypertension. Acta Pathol. Jpn. 32:1121, 1982.

164. Hainaut, P., Lavenne, E., Magy, J. M., and Lebacq, E. G.: Circulating lupus type anticoagulant and pulmonary hypertension associated with mixed connective tissue disease. Clin. Rheumatol. 5:96, 1986.

165. Ueda, N., Mimura, K., Maeda, H., Suyiyama, T., Kado, T., Kobayashi, K., and Fukuzaki, H.: Mixed connective tissue disease with fatal pulmonary hypertension and a review of the literature. Virchows Arch. 404:335, 1984.

166. Manthorpe, R., Elling, H., van der Meulen, J. T., and Sorensen, S.: Two fatal cases of mixed connective tissue disease. Scand. J. Rheumatol. 9:7, 1980.

167. Wiener-Kronish, J. P., Solinger, A. M., Warnock, M. S., Churg, A., Ordonez, N., and Golden, J. A.: Severe pulmonary involvement in mixed connective tissue disease. Am. Rev. Respir. Dis. 124:499, 1981.

168. Derderian, S. S., Tellis, C. J., Abbrecht, P. H., Welton, R. C., and Rjagopal, K. R.: Pulmonary involvement in mixed connective tissue disease. Chest 88:45, 1985.

169. Suzuki, T., and Shibata, T.: Clinical and microscopical study on renal involvement of patients with mixed connective tissue disease. In Kasukawa, R., and Sharp, G. (eds.): Mixed Connective Tissue Disease and Anti-nuclear Antibodies. Amsterdam, Excerpta Medica, 1987, pp. 303–308.

170. Kitridou, R. C., Akmal, M., Turkel, S. B., Ehresmann, G. R., Quismorio, F. P., Jr., and Massry, S. G.: Renal involvement in mixed connective tissue disease: a longitudinal clinicopathologic study. Semin. Arthritis Rheum. 16:135, 1986.

171. Asherson, R. A., Higenbottam, T. W., Dinh Xuan, A. T., Khamashta, M. A., and Hughes, G. R. V.: Pulmonary hypertension in a lupus clinic: Experience with twenty-four patients. J. Rheumatol. 17:1292, 1990.

172. Sharp, G. C.: Therapy and prognosis of MCTD. In Kasukawa, R., and Sharp, G. (eds.): Mixed Connective Tissue Disease and Anti-nuclear Antibodies. Amsterdam, Excerpta Medica, 1987, pp. 315–324.

173. Bennett, R. M., and Spargo, B. H.: Immune complex nephropathy in mixed connective tissue disease. Am. J. Med. 63:534, 1977.

174. Maddison, P. J., Mogovero, H., and Reichlin, M.: Patterns of clinical disease associated with antibodies to nuclear ribonucleoprotein. J. Rheumatol. 5:407, 1978.

175. Lemmer, J. P., Curry, N. H., Mallory, J. H., and Waller, M. V.: Clinical characteristics and course in patients with high titer anti-RNP antibodies. J. Rheumatol. 9:536, 1982.

176. Koboyashi, S., Nagase, M., Kimura, M., Ohyama, K., Ikeya, M., and Honda, N.: Renal involvement in mixed connective tissue disease. Am. J. Nephrol. 5:282, 1985.

177. Sharp, G. C., Irvin, W. S., May, C. M., Holman, H. R., McDuffie, F. C., Hess, E. V., and Schmid, F. R.: Association of antibodies to ribonucleoprotein and Sm antigens with mixed connective tissue disease, systemic lupus erythematosus and other rheumatic diseases. N. Engl. J. Med. 295:1149, 1976.

178. Reichlin, M., and Mattioli, M.: Correlation of a precipitin reaction to an RNA protein antigen and a low prevalence of nephritis in patients with systemic lupus erythematosus. N. Engl. J. Med. 286:908, 1972.

179. Jonsson, J., and Norberg, R.: Symptomatology and diagnosis in connective tissue disease. II. Evaluations and follow-up examinations in consequence of a speckled antinuclear immunofluorescence pattern. Scand. J. Rheumatol. 7:229, 1978.

180. Fuller, J. J., Richmann, A. V., Auerback, D., Alexander, R. W.,

181. Lottenberg, R., and Langley, S.: Immune complex nephritis in a patient with MCTD. Am. J. Med. 62:762, 1977.

181. Andrassy, K., Gebest, J., Tan, E., Thoenes, W., and Ritz, E.: Interstitial nephritis in a patient with atypical Sjögren's syndrome. Klin. Wochenschr. 58:563, 1980.

182. Palferman, T. G., McIntosh, C. S., and Kershaw, M.: Mixed connective tissue disease associated with glomerulonephritis and hypocomplementemia. Postgrad. Med. J. 56:177, 1980.

183. Cohen, I. M., Swerdlin, A. H., Steinberg, S. M., and Stone, R. A.: Mesangial proliferative glomerulonephritis in mixed connective tissue disease (MCTD). Clin. Nephrol. 13:93, 1980.

184. Crapper, R. M., Dowling, J. P., Mackay, I. R., and Whitworth, J. A.: Acute scleroderma in stable mixed connective tissue disease: treatment by plasmapheresis. Aust. N.Z. J. Med. 17:327, 1987.

185. Piirainen, H. I., Helve, A. T., Törnroth, T., and Pettersson, T. E.: Amyloidosis in mixed connective tissue disease. Scand. J. Rheumatol. 18:165, 1989.

186. Marshall, J. B., Kretschmar, J. M., Gerhardt, D. C., Winship, D. H., Winn, D., Treadwell, E. L., and Sharp, G. C.: Gastrointestinal manifestations of mixed connective tissue disease. Gastroenterology 98:1232, 1990.

187. Gutierrez, F., Valenzuela, J. E., Ehresmann, G. R., Quismorio, F. P., Kitridou, R. C.: Esophageal dysfunction in patients with mixed connective tissue diseases and systemic lupus erythematosus. Dig. Dis. Sci. 27:592, 1982.

188. Cooke, C. L., and Lurie, H. I.: Case report: fatal gastrointestinal hemorrhage in mixed connective tissue disease. Arthritis Rheum. 20:1421, 1977.

189. Maeda, M., Kanayama, M., Hasumura, Y., Takeuchi, J., and Uchida, T.: Case of mixed connective tissue disease associated with autoimmune hepatitis. Dig. Dis. Sci. 33:1487, 1988.

190. Marshall, J. B., Ravendhran, N., and Sharp, G. C.: Liver disease in mixed connective tissue disease. Arch. Intern. Med. 143:1817, 1983.

191. Rolny, P., Goobar, J., and Zettergren, L.: HBs Ag–negative chronic active hepatitis and mixed connective tissue disease syndrome. An unusual association observed in two patients. Acta Med. Scand. 216:391, 1984.

192. Cosnes, J., Levy, R. A., and Darnis, F.: Budd-Chiari syndrome in a patient with mixed connective tissue disease. Dig. Dis. Sci. 25:467, 1980.

193. Thiele, D. L., and Krejs, G. J.: Secretory diarrhoea in mixed connective tissue disease. Am. J. Gastroenterol. 80:107, 1985.

194. Feldman, F.: Mixed connective tissue disease. Radiol. Clin. North Am. 26:1235, 1988.

195. Samach, M., Brandt, L. J., and Bernstein, L. H.: Spontaneous pneumoperitoneum with Pneumatosis cystoides intestinalis in a patient with mixed connective tissue disease. Am. J. Gastroenterol. 69:494, 1978.

196. Lynn, J. T., Gossen, G., Miller, A., and Russell, I. J.: Pneumatosis intestinalis in mixed connective tissue disease: two case reports and literature review. Arthritis Rheum. 27:1186, 1984.

197. Bennett, R. M., Bong, D. M., and Spargo, B. H.: Neuropsychiatric problems in mixed connective tissue disease. Am. J. Med. 65:955, 1978.

198. Searles, R. P., Mladinich, E. K., and Messner, R. P.: Isolated trigeminal sensory neuropathy: early manifestation of mixed connective tissue disease. Neurology 28:1286, 1978.

199. Varga, E., Field, E. A., and Tyldesley, W. R.: Orofacial manifestations of mixed connective tissue disease. Br. Dent. J. 168:330, 1990.

200. Vincent, R. M., and Van Houzen, R. N.: Trigeminal sensory neuropathy and bilateral carpal tunnel syndrome: the initial manifestation of mixed connective tissue disease. J. Neurol. Neurosurg. Psychiatry 43:458, 1980.

201. Bronshvas, M. M., Prystowsky, S. D., and Traviesa, D. C.: Vascular headaches in mixed connective tissue disease. Headache 18:154, 1978.

202. Harris, G. J., Franson, T. R., and Ryan, L. M.: Recurrent aseptic meningitis as a manifestation of mixed connective tissue disease (MCTD). Wis. Med. J. 86:31, 1987.

203. Hoffman, M., and Gray, R. G.: Ibuprofen-induced meningitis in mixed connective tissue disease. Clin. Rheumatol. 1:128, 1982.

204. Weiss, T. D., Nelson, J. S., Woolsey, R. M., Zuckner, J., and Baldassare, A. R.: Transverse myelitis in mixed connective tissue disease. Arthritis Rheum. 21:982, 1978.

205. Saito, K., Sagawa, K., Nishimaki, T., Morito, T., Yoshida, H., and Kasukawa, R.: Localization of nRNP antigen in mammalian cells stained with peroxidase-labelled IgG fraction of anti-nRNP antibody obtained from a patient with mixed connective tissue disease (MCTD). Tohoku J. Exp. Med. 153:21, 1987.

206. Martyn, J. B., Wong, M. J., and Huang, S. H.: Pulmonary and neuromuscular complications of mixed connective tissue disease: a report and review of the literature. J. Rheumatol. 15:703, 1988.

207. Kraus, A., Guadulupe, C., Borojos, E., and Alarcon-Segovia, D.: Retinal vasculitis in mixed connective tissue disease. J. Rheumatol. 12:1122, 1985.

208. Tamai, S., Ishii, T., and Hosoda, Y.: Histopathology of esophageal lesions in mixed connective tissue disease. *In* Kasukawa, R., and Sharp, G. (eds.): Mixed Connective Tissue Disease and Anti-nuclear Antibodies. Amsterdam, Excerpta Medica, 1987, pp. 297–302.

209. Peller, J. S., Gabor, G. T., Porter, J. M., and Bennett, R. M.: Angiographic findings in mixed connective tissue disease. Correlation with fingernail capillary photomicroscopy and digital photoplethysmography findings. Arthritis Rheum. 28:768, 1985.

210. Granier, F., Vayssairat, M., Priollet, P., and Housset, E.: Nailfold capillary microscopy in mixed connective tissue disease. Comparison with systemic sclerosis and systemic lupus erythematosus. Arthritis Rheum. 29:189, 1986.

211. Maricq, H. R., LeRoy, E. C., D'Angelo, W. A., Medsger, T. A., Rodnan, G. P., Sharp, G. C., and Wolfe, J. F.: Diagnostic potential of in vivo capillary microscopy in scleroderma and related disorders. Arthritis Rheum. 23:183, 1980.

212. Meyer, O., Haim, T., Dryll, A., Lansaman, J., and Ryckewaert, A.: Vascular endothelial cell injury in progressive systemic sclerosis and other connective tissue diseases. Clin. Exp. Rheumatol. 1:29, 1983.

213. Bodolay, E., Bojan, F., Szegedi, G., Stenszky, V., and Farid, N. R.: Cytotoxic endothelial cell antibodies in mixed connective tissue disease. Immunol. Lett. 20:163, 1989.

214. James, J. P., Stevens, T. R., Hall, N. D., Maddison, P. J., Goulding, N. J., Silman, A., Holligan, S., and Black, C.: Factor VIII–related antigen in connective tissue disease patients and relatives. Br. J. Rheumatol. 29:6, 1990.

215. Prystowsky, D. F.: Mixed connective tissue disease. West. J. Med. 132:288, 1980.

216. Segond, P., Yeni, P., Jacquot, J. M., and Massias, P.: Severe autoimmune anemia and thrombopenia in mixed connective tissue disease. Arthritis Rheum. 21:995, 1978.

217. Ter Borg, E. J., Houtman, P. M., Kallenberg, C. G., Van Leeuwen, M. A., and van Ryswyk, M. H.: Thrombocytopenia and hemolytic anemia in a patient with mixed connective tissue disease due to thrombotic thrombocytopenic purpura. J. Rheumatol. 15:1174, 1988.

218. Paice, E. W., and Snaith, M. L.: Thrombotic thrombocytopenia purpura occurring in a patient with mixed connective tissue disease. Rheumatol. Int. 4:141, 1984.

219. Julkunen, H., Jantti, J., and Pettersson, T.: Pure red cell aplasia in mixed connective tissue disease. J. Rheumatol. 16:1385, 1989.

220. Maddison, P. J., and Reichlin, M.: Quantitation of precipitating antibodies to certain soluble nuclear antigens in SLE: their contribution to hypergammaglobulinemia. Arthritis Rheum. 20:819, 1977.

221. Pettersson, I., Wang, G., Smith, E. I., Wigzell, H., Hedfors, E., Horn, J., and Sharp, G. C.: The use of immunoblotting and immunoprecipitation of (U) small nuclear ribonucleoproteins in the analysis of sera of patients with mixed connective tissue disease and systemic lupus erythematosus. A cross-sectional, longitudinal study. Arthritis Rheum. 29:986, 1986.

222. Locker, J. D., Medof, M. E., Bennett, R. M., and Sukhupunyarksa, S.: Characterization of DNA used to assay sera for anti-DNA antibodies: determination of the specificities of anti-DNA antibodies in SLE and non-SLE rheumatic disease states. J. Immunol. 118:694, 1977.

223. Diaz-Jouanen, E., Llorente, L., Ramos-Niembro, F., and Alarcon-Segovia, D.: Cold-reactive lymphocytotoxic antibodies in mixed connective tissue disease. J. Rheumatol. 4:4, 1977.

224. Schocket, A. L., and Kohler, P. F.: Lymphocytotoxic antibodies in systemic lupus erythematosus and clinically related diseases. Arthritis Rheum. 22:1060, 1979.

225. Suginoshita, T.: Anti-lymphocyte antibodies in MCTD. *In* Kasukawa, R., and Sharp, G. (eds.): Mixed Connective Tissue Disease and Anti-nuclear Antibodies. Amsterdam, Excerpta Medica, 1987, pp. 201–206.

226. Fishbein, E., Ramos-Niembro, F., and Alarcon-Segovia, D.: Free serum ribonucleoprotein in mixed connective tissue disease and other connective tissue diseases. J. Rheumatol. 5:384, 1978.

227. Negoro, N., Kanayama, Y., Takeda, T., Koda, S., and Inoue, T.: A solid-phase radioimmunoassay for the detection of nRNP immune complexes. J. Immunol. Methods 91:83, 1986.

228. Negoro, X. I., Kanayama, Y., Yasuda, M., Okamura, M., Amatsu, K., Koda, S., Takeda, T., and Inoue, T.: Nuclear ribonucleoprotein immune complexes in pericardial fluid of a patient with mixed connective tissue disease. Arthritis Rheum. 30:97, 1987.

229. Halla, J. T., Volanakis, J. E., and Schronhenloker, R. E.: Circulating immune complexes in MCTD. Arthritis Rheum. 22:484, 1979.

230. Diez-Jovanen, E., Salazar, J. F., Abud-Mendoza, C., and Alarcon-Segovia, D.: Immune complexes in autoimmune disease. Differences in immune complexes detected by cellular receptor for complement and for Fc domains of IgG. Rev. Invest. Clin. (Mexico) 32:153, 1980.

231. Pope, R. M., Yoshinoya, S., and McDuffy, S. J.: Detection of immune complexes and their relationship to rheumatoid factor in a variety of autoimmune disorders. Clin. Exp. Rheumatol. 46:259, 1981.

232. Pope, R. M., Keightley, R., and McDuffy, S.: Circulating autoantibodies to IgD in rheumatic diseases. J. Immunol. 128:1860, 1982.

233. Kaufman, R. L., and Kitridou, R. C.: Pregnancy in mixed connective tissue disease: comparison with systemic lupus erythematosus. J. Rheumatol. 9:549, 1982.

234. Kahl, L. E., Blair, C., Ramsey-Goldman, R., and Steen, V. D.: Pregnancy outcomes in women with primary Raynaud's phenomenon. Arthritis Rheum. 33:1249, 1990.

235. Singsen, B. H., Kornreich, H. K., Koster-King, K., Brink, S. J., Bernstein, B. H., Hanson, V., and Tan, E. M.: Mixed connective tissue disease in children. Arthritis Rheum. 20:355, 1977.

236. Peskett, S. A., Ansell, B. M., Fizzman, P., and Howard, A.: Mixed connective tissue disease in children. Rheumatol. Rehab. 17:245, 1978.

237. Fraga, A., Gudino, J., Ramos-Niembro, E., and Alarcon-Segovia, D.: Mixed connective tissue disease in childhood. Relationship Sjögren's syndrome. Am. J. Dis. Child. 132:263, 1978.

238. Baldassare, A., Weiss, T., Auclair, R., and Zuckner, J.: Mixed connective tissue disease (MCTD) in children. Arthritis Rheum. 19:788, 1976.

239. Eberhardt, K., Svantesson, H., and Svensson, B.: Follow-up study of 6 children presenting with a MCTD-like syndrome. Scand. J. Rheumatol. 10:62, 1981.

240. De Rooij, D. J., Fiselier, T., Van de Putte, L. B., and Van Venrooij, W. J.: Juvenile-onset mixed connective tissue disease: Clinical, serological, and follow-up data. Scand. J. Rheumatol. 18:157, 1989.

241. Nimelstein, S. H., Brody, S., McShane, D., and Holman, H. R.: Mixed connective tissue disease: A subsequent evaluation of the original 25 patients. Medicine 59:239, 1980.

242. Miyawaki, S., and Onodera, H.: Clinical course and prognosis of patients with mixed connective tissue disease. *In* Kasukawa, R., and Sharpe, G. (eds.): Mixed Connective Tissue Disease and Anti-nuclear Antibodies. Amsterdam, Excerpta Medica, 1987, pp. 331–336.

243. Cunningham, P. H., Andrews, B. S., and Davis, J. S.: Immune complexes in progressive systemic sclerosis and mixed connective tissue disease. J. Rheumatol. 7:301, 1980.

244. Houtman, P. M., Kallenberg, C. G., Fidler, V., and Wouda, A. A.: Diagnostic significance of nailfold capillary patterns in patients with Raynaud's phenomenon. An analysis of patterns discriminating patients with and without connective tissue disease. J. Rheumatol. 13:556, 1986.

245. Hamburger, M. I., Lawley, T. J., Kimberly, R. P., Plotz, P. H., and Frank, M. M.: A serial study of splenic reticuloendothelial system Fc receptor functional activity in systemic lupus erythematosus. Arthritis Rheum. 25:48, 1982.

246. Tan, E. M.: Relationship of nuclear staining patterns with precipitating antibodies in systemic lupus erythematosus. J. Lab. Clin. Med. 70:800, 1967.

247. Tan, E. M., and Kunkel, H. G.: Characteristics of a soluble nuclear antigen precipitating with sera of patients with systemic lupus erythematosus. J. Immunol. 96:464, 1966.

248. Mattioli, M., and Reichlin, M.: Characterization of a soluble nuclear ribonucleoprotein antigen reactive with SLE sera. J. Immunol. 107:1281, 1971.

249. Mattioli, M., and Reichlin, M.: Physical association of two nuclear antigens and mutual occurrence of their antibodies: the relationship of the Sm and the RNA-protein (Mu) systems in SLE sera. J. Immunol. 110:1318, 1973.

250. Lerner, M. R., and Steitz, J. A.: Antibodies to small nuclear RNAs complexed with proteins are produced by patients with systemic lupus erythematosus. Proc. Natl. Acad. Sci. U.S.A. 76:5495, 1979.

251. Lerner, M. R., Boyle, J. A., Hardin, J. A., and Steitz, J. A.: Two novel classes of small ribonucleoproteins detected by antibodies associated with lupus erythematosus. Science 211:400, 1981.

252. Habets, W. J., Rooij, D. J., Hoet, M. H., Van de Putte, L. B., and van Verooij, W. J.: Quantitation of anti-RNP and anti-Sm antibodies in MCTD and SLE patients by immunoblotting. Clin. Exp. Immunol. 59:457, 1985.

253. Zieve, G. W., and Sauterer, R. A.: Cell biology of the snRNP particles. CRC Crit. Rev. Biochem. Mol. Biol. 25:1, 1990.

254. Netter, H. J., Guldner, H. H., Szostecki, C., and Will, H.: Major autoantigenic sites of the (U1) small nuclear ribonucleoprotein-specific 68-kDa protein. Scand. J. Immunol. 32:163, 1990.

255. Maul, G. G., Jimenez, S. A., Riggs, E., and Ziemnicka-Kotula, D.: Determination of an epitope of the diffuse systemic sclerosis marker antigen DNA topoisomerase. I: Sequence similarity with retroviral p30^{gag} protein suggests a possible cause for autoimmunity in systemic sclerosis. Proc. Natl. Acad. Sci. U.S.A. 86:8492, 1989.

256. Habets, W. J., Hoet, M. H., De Jong, B. A. W., Van der Kemp, A., and Van Venrooij, W. J.: Mapping of B cell epitopes on small nuclear ribonucleoproteins that react with human autoantibodies as well as with experimentally induced mouse monoclonal antibodies. J. Immunol. 143:2560, 1989.

257. Habets, W. J., Hoet, M. H., and Van Venrooij, W. J.: Epitope patterns of anti-RNP antibodies in rheumatic diseases: Evidence for an antigen-driven autoimmune response. Arthritis Rheum. 33:834, 1990.

258. Wolff-Vorbeck, G., Schlesier, M., Hackle, W., Luhrmann, R., and Peter, H. H.: A human T cell clone recognizing small nuclear ribonucleoproteins (UsnRNP). *In* Bautz, E. K. F., Kalden, J. R., Homma, M.,

and Tan, E. M. (eds.): Molecular and Cell Biology of Autoantibodies and Autoimmunity. Heidelberg, Springer-Verlag, 1989.

259. Guldner, H. H., Netter, H. J., Szostecki, C., Lakomek, H. J., and Will, H.: Epitope mapping with a recombinant human 68kDa (U1) ribonucleoprotein antigen reveals heterogeneous autoantibody profiles in human autoimmune sera. J. Immunol. 141:469, 1988.

260. Theissen, H., Etzerodt, M., Reuter, R., Schneider, C., Lottspeich, F., Argos, P., Luhrmann, R., and Philipson, L.: Cloning of the human cDNA for the U1 RNA–associated 70K protein. EMBO J. 5:3209, 1986.

261. Guldner, H. H., Netter, H. J., Szostecki, C., Jaeger, E., and Will, H.: Human anti-p68 autoantibodies recognize a common epitope of U1 RNA containing small nuclear ribonucleoprotein and influenza B virus. J. Exp. Med. 171:819, 1990.

262. Tiwari, J. L., and Terasaki, P. I.: Scleroderma, HLA, and Disease Associations. New York, Springer-Verlag, 1985.

263. Fronek, Z., Timmerman, L. A., Alper, C. A., Hahn, B. H., Kalunian, K., Peterlin, B. M., and McDevitt, H. O.: Major histocompatibility complex genes and susceptibility to systemic lupus erythematosus. Arthritis Rheum. 33:1542, 1990.

264. Nepom, G. T., Byers, P., Seyfried, C., Healey, L. A., Wilske, K. R., Stage, D., and Nepom, B. S.: HLA genes associated with rheumatoid arthritis: identification of susceptibility alleles using specific oligonucleotide probes. Arthritis Rheum. 32:15, 1989.

265. Merryman, P. F., Crapper, R. M., Lee, S., Gregersen, P. K., and Winchester, R. J.: Class II major histocompatibility complex gene sequences in rheumatoid arthritis: the third diversity region of both DR beta 1 and DR beta 2 genes in two DR1, DRw10-positive individuals specify the same inferred amino acid sequence as the DR beta 1 and DR beta 2 genes of a DR4 (Dw14) haplotype. Arthritis Rheum. 32:251, 1989.

266. Habets, W. J., Rooij, D. J., Salden, M. H., Verhagen, A. P., Van Eekelen, C. A., Van de Putte, L. B., and Von Venrooij, W. J.: Antibodies against distinct nuclear matrix proteins are characteristic for mixed connective tissue disease. Clin. Exp. Immunol. 54:265, 1983.

267. Fritzler, M. J., Ali, R., and Tan, E. M.: Antibodies from patients with mixed connective tissue disease react with heterogeneous nuclear ribonucleoprotein or ribonucleic acid (Rn RNP/RNA) of the nuclear matrix. J. Immunol. 132:1216, 1984.

268. Salden, M. H. L., Van Eekelen, C. A. G., Habets, W. J. A., Vierwinden, G., van de Putte, C. B. A., and Verooy, W. J.: Anti-nuclear matrix antibodies in mixed connective tissue disease. Eur. J. Immunol. 12:783, 1982.

269. Astaldi Ricotti, G. C. B., Bestagno, M., Cerino, A., Negri, C., Caporali, R., Cobianchi, F., Longhi, M., Montecucco, C. M.: Antibodies to hnRNP core protein A1 in connective tissue diseases. J. Cell. Biochem. 40:43, 1989.

270. Rubin, L. J., Mendoza, J., Hood, M., McGoon, M., Barst, R., Williams, W. B., Diehl, J. H., Crow, J., and Long, W.: Treatment of primary pulmonary hypertension with continuous intravenous prostacyclin (Epoprostenol). Results of a randomized trial. Ann. Intern. Med. 112:485, 1990.

Section IX

Vasculitic Syndromes

Chapter 64

Vasculitis and Related Disorders

Doyt L. Conn
Gene G. Hunder
J. Desmond O'Duffy

INTRODUCTION

Vasculitis is a clinical and pathologic process caused by inflammation of blood vessels. Inflammation may involve arteries of any size and the veins also. Many diseases may be associated with vascular inflammation. There is a group of diseases in which the vasculitis is the primary feature, and this is the group that will be discussed in detail. Vasculitis, as a disease entity, was first recognized in 1866 by Kussmaul and Maier when they reported a case of necrotizing arteritis and termed it periarteritis nodosa.[1] Their patient had widespread inflammation of the small and medium-sized arteries, and in some areas there were focal inflammatory exudations, which gave rise to palpable nodular excrescences along the course of the arteries. A number of different clinical and pathologic types of vasculitis have been described since then, and efforts have been made to classify these diseases. In the past, necrotizing vasculitis has been regarded as idiopathic, with no known cause. However, in recent years, it has been shown that some cases of the vasculitis are associated with hepatitis B surface antigen and human immunodeficiency virus (HIV), and there are undoubtedly other viruses and antigens yet to be found that can lead to vasculitis.

CLASSIFICATION

Although many classifications have been devised for the necrotizing vasculitides, none has been entirely satisfactory for the clinician. Zeek's classification, introduced in 1952,[2] was an early standard. It has five categories, which are based on clinical and pathologic findings and the size and type of vessel involvement. These are periarteritis nodosa, hyper-

sensitivity angiitis, allergic granulomatous angiitis, rheumatic arteritis, and temporal arteritis.

Not all cases of vasculitis fit nicely into Zeek's classification; consequently, many other classifications have been devised.[3-5, 7] From a clinical point of view, a classification based on the size of the vessel biopsied alone is not satisfactory for several reasons. Frequently, the size of the vessel examined is dependent on the tissue sampled or the technique used. For example, punch biopsy of the skin, needle biopsy of the kidney, and sural nerve biopsy sample only small vessels. Visceral arteriography reveals pathologic changes in medium-sized and larger vessels. Autopsy studies usually show an overlap in sizes of involved vessels in those cases thought to represent polyarteritis (periarteritis) nodosa or hypersensitivity angiitis. An example of variously sized vessel involvement is demonstrated in a case report of a patient with Churg-Strauss vasculitis and primary biliary cirrhosis. This patient initially had a small vessel vasculitis and later had larger artery involvement, including the temporal arteries.[6]

The type of pathologic change in the vessel wall can be helpful for classification in some situations, but it cannot be relied on exclusively. Granulomas and giant cell formation may be seen in arteritis of large arteries, including Takayasu's arteritis and giant cell arteritis (temporal arteritis). Extravascular granulomas may be found in Wegener's granulomatosis and allergic granulomatous vasculitis. Fibrinoid necrosis of the vessel wall is seen in polyarteritis nodosa and hypersensitivity angiitis. However, frequently these typical pathologic features may not be seen because of variability of sampling and the effects of time and treatment on the pathologic picture. The type of cellular infiltration may vary, depending on the stage of injury. Early in the course of vascular inflammation, polymorphonuclear leukocytes are fre-

1077

quently found, whereas later a chronic mononuclear cell infiltration is predominant.

It was thought that if the pathogenesis of the various vasculitides could be elucidated, this would provide a basis for establishing a rational classification. However, this has not been true thus far. For example, hepatitis B surface antigen appears to be related to the development of more than one type of vasculitis. No classification has been devised that is completely satisfactory.

Recently a subcommittee of the American College of Rheumatology developed criteria for the classification of seven forms of vasculitis by analysis of data from 1000 cases of vasculitis collected from 48 centers.[8-14] These seven types of vasculitis included polyarteritis nodosa, Churg-Strauss syndrome, Wegener's granulomatosis, hypersensitivity vasculitis, Henoch-Schönlein purpura, giant cell arteritis, and Takayasu's arteritis. The criteria for each were derived by comparing findings in patients with one form of vasculitis with those from patients with other forms of vasculitis as a group. Two statistical methods were used, one to derive criteria in the traditional format, and the second to develop a tree classification. Criteria for six of the seven forms of vasculitis in the traditional format are shown in Tables 64–1 and 64–3 through 64–7. Giant cell arteritis is discussed in a subsequent chapter. The criteria selected in these studies were those that both identify each vasculitis and separate it from others. As a result, the full spectrum of manifestations are not included in all instances, and the criteria are not appropriate for use in the diagnosis of individual patients. The criteria do provide a standard way of evaluating and describing patients with vasculitis in therapeutic, epidemiologic, and other studies, allowing comparisons of results found in different centers. The criteria should be used to describe patients in all studies on vasculitis. Data derived from the analysis of this large group of vasculitis patients also provide much information regarding the frequency of various clinical manifestations in each syndrome.

PATHOGENESIS

In the late 1930s and early 1940s, it was noted that necrotizing vasculitis sometimes appeared after injections of hyperimmune serum that were given in the treatment of pneumococcal pneumonia and after the administration of the newly discovered sulfonamides.[15] More recently, it has been shown that an immune complex–induced cutaneous vasculitis can develop as a result of serum sickness produced by horse antithymocyte globulin.[16] Hepatitis B surface antigen can cause vasculitis by an immune complex mechanism. In 1969, Gocke and coworkers[17] demonstrated hepatitis B surface antigen and IgM in an artery wall of a patient with polyarteritis. The findings of diminished serum complement, serum immune complexes, cryoglobulins, and viral particles

suggest that the arteritis is immune complex induced, with hepatitis B surface antigen as the inciting antigen.[18] Other viruses may be associated with vasculitis, including cytomegalovirus, hepatitis A, human T-cell lymphotropic virus-1 (HTLV-1), HIV, human parvovirus, and herpes zoster. The vasculitis associated with the herpes zoster virus is due to direct invasion of the arteries by the virus. This may account for the localized granulomatous vasculitis of the central nervous system that follows herpes zoster ophthalmicus. A vasculitic neuropathy may accompany Lyme disease. In this situation, as with the other viruses, the vasculitic mechanism may be either direct invasion of the arterial wall by the organism or deposition of immune complexes.[19]

Vasculitis has been reported in a wide variety of malignancies.[20] The cause of the vasculitis is not known in most cases, but in some cases it may be immune complex induced, triggered by a tumor antigen. Polyarteritis may complicate hairy cell leukemia. The mechanism of vasculitis may be immune complex induced, with cross-reacting antibodies to endothelial cells or hairy cells infiltrating the arterial wall.[21]

In most cases of vasculitis, there is indirect evidence of immune complex disease, although the inciting antigen is not found. In these patients, rheumatoid factor, diminished serum complement, and low levels of cryoglobulins have been found.[22] Frequently in polyarteritis and Wegener's granulomatosis, immunoglobulins and complement are not found in involved tissue, but only fibrin, leaving the role of immune complexes in these diseases uncertain.[23] Immune deposits may not always be found even if the lesion was initially immune complex induced. This is because immune complexes may be rapidly cleared after the induction of the lesion.[24] Consequently, the duration of the disease and the treatment will influence the immunopathologic findings.

Another factor influencing the pathogenicity of immune complexes is the ability of the reticuloendothelial system to clear immune complexes from the circulation. It is not known whether impairment of the reticuloendothelial system frequently occurs in human systemic vasculitis. There has been one report of patients with vasculitis with altered splenic reticuloendothelial function that was reversed by plasma exchange.[25] It is possible that abnormalities of the cellular complement receptors CR1, CR3, and CR4 or IgG F receptors may exist, impairing normal transport and removal of immune complexes. This exposes nonhepatic tissues to high concentrations of immune complexes, resulting in vascular inflammation.[26]

HLA typing for A and B locus antigens has not suggested an increased frequency of certain HLA antigens in patients with polyarteritis associated with hepatitis B antigenemia.[27] The association of HLA-B8 with Wegener's granulomatosis is debatable. There appears to be an increase in HLA-DR2 in Wegener's

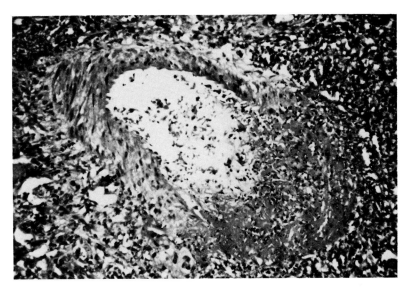

Figure 64–1. Polyarteritis. Right lower portion of arterial wall shows fibrinoid necrosis and formation of "microaneurysm." Intense infiltration of leukocytes is present in and about artery wall. (Hematoxylin & eosin, × 40.) (Courtesy of Dr. J. T. Lie.)

granulomatosis.[28] HLA-Bw52 has been associated with Takayasu's arteritis in Asians and with HLA-MB3 and HLA-DR4 in North Americans with this disease.[29] There appears to be some genetic predisposition to certain types of vascular inflammation.

The direct injury and resulting perturbation of the endothelial cells may trigger a series of pathologic events that may influence the clinical manifestations and outcome of the vasculitis. A direct effect of endothelial cell injury in vasculitis is the elevation of von Willebrand factor antigen and factor VIII in the blood of patients with systemic vasculitis.[30] The elevation of these factors is not specific for a particular type of vasculitis and can be elevated in noninflammatory vascular injury.

Coagulation abnormalities may occur in systemic vasculitis and could influence occlusive artery changes. Patients with active Takayasu's disease have evidence of hyperfibrinogenemia and hypofibrinolytic activity.[31] In active, early Kawasaki's disease, there is evidence of hyperfibrinogenemia, thrombocytosis, diminished fibrinolytic activity, and elevation of platelet-derived beta (β)-thromboglobulins in plasma (indicating increased platelet activation).[32] Examination of normal skin in cases of cutaneous vasculitis and systemic vasculitis has shown that endothelial cell release of tissue plasminogen activator is defective.[33] Studies of hemostasis in vasculitis have been limited, but the data available thus far show activation of the coagulation mechanism, frequently without the concomitant presence of inhibitory hemostatic factors. Studies of involved nerves in rheumatoid vasculitis have shown chronic occlusive arterial lesions to be associated with the deposition of fibrin.[34] Dominance of procoagulant activity would probably result in arterial occlusive changes.

POLYARTERITIS

Polyarteritis, also termed periarteritis nodosa and polyarteritis nodosa (PAN), is a disease of small and medium-sized arteries. Polyarteritis may affect any organ, but the skin, joints, peripheral nerves, gut, and kidney are most commonly involved. There is a spectrum of severity, from progressive fulminant disease to limited disease. Polyarteritis may also be a manifestation or complication of other diseases, such as rheumatoid arthritis, Sjögren's syndrome, and mixed cryoglobulinemia.

Epidemiology. Polyarteritis is an uncommon disease. Estimates of the annual incidence rate for PAN-type systemic vasculitis in a general population range from 4.6 per 1,000,000 in England, to 9.0 per 1,000,000 in Olmsted County, Minnesota, to 77 per 1,000,000 in a hepatitis B hyperendemic Alaskan Eskimo population. The estimated annual mortality rate for PAN in New York City in the 1950s was 1.2 to 1.5 per 1,000,000. The disease is more common in males, and the sex ratio is about 2 to 1. Polyarteritis is observed in children and the elderly, and the average age of diagnosis ranges from the mid-40s to the mid-60s. It is observed in all racial groups.[35]

Pathology. The pathology of polyarteritis consists of focal but panmural necrotizing inflammatory lesions in small and medium-sized muscular arteries, with a predilection for involvement at the vessel bifurcation. The lesions may occur in all parts of the body, but there is usually less involvement of the pulmonary and splenic arteries.[36] The inflammation is characterized by fibrinoid necrosis and pleomorphic cellular infiltration, with predominantly polymorphonuclear leukocytes and variable numbers of lymphocytes and eosinophils (Fig. 64–1). The normal architecture of the vessel wall, including the elastic laminae, is disrupted. There may be thrombosis or aneurysmal dilatation at the site of the lesion. Healed areas of arteritis show proliferation of fibrous tissue and endothelial cells, which may lead to vessel occlusion (Fig. 64–2). Lesions at all stages of progression and healing may be seen pathologically if sufficient tissue is available for study.

It is difficult to determine the frequency of in-

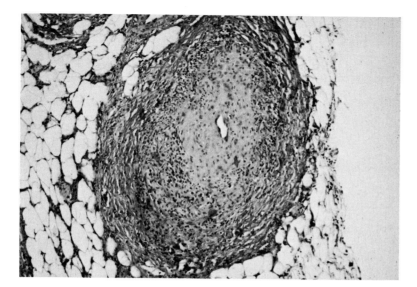

Figure 64–2. Mesenteric arteries involved with polyarteritis showing healed areas with intimal and smooth muscle proliferation and luminal occlusion.

volvement of various organs in polyarteritis because of the heterogeneity of patients included in most studies. In autopsy series, the kidneys and heart are involved in about 70 percent of cases, liver and gastrointestinal tract in 50 percent, peripheral nerves in 50 percent, mesentery and skeletal muscle in 30 percent, and central nervous system in 10 percent.[37] Cutaneous involvement varies from a few percentage points to 50 percent.[38]

Clinical Features. The disease may present in a variety of ways. There is a spectrum of severity from mild, limited disease to fulminating disease. Virtually any organ may be affected. Typically, the patient experiences constitutional features of fever, malaise, and weight loss along with manifestations of multisystem involvement, such as a skin rash, peripheral neuropathy, and asymmetric polyarthritis. Visceral involvement of the kidney or gut may present coincidentally with these features or may appear later. In other cases, single organ involvement may be present alone and may remain limited.[39]

Cutaneous lesions include palpable purpura, ulcerations, livedo reticularis, and ischemic changes of the distal digits (Figs. 64–3 and 64–4). Arthralgia or arthritis is present in polyarteritis in as many as 50 percent of patients.[40] An asymmetric, episodic, nondeforming polyarthritis involving the larger joints of the lower extremity may occur in 20 percent of cases and is common early in the course of the disease. Such symptoms may mimic those of rheumatoid arthritis, but as other manifestations appear, the polyarthritis usually subsides without residual joint damage. Synovial analysis is not diagnostic and shows evidence of mild inflammation, as indicated by a moderate increase in the leukocyte count.[22]

Peripheral neuropathy may occur in 50 to 70 percent of cases and may be the initial manifestation.[41] The upper and lower extremities are affected in about the same frequency. The onset may be sudden, with pain and paresthesias radiating in the distribution of a peripheral nerve, followed in hours

or days by a motor deficit of the same peripheral nerve. This may progress asymmetrically to involve other peripheral nerves and produce a mononeuritis multiplex. With addditional nerve damage, the final result may be a symmetric polyneuropathy involving all sensory modalities and motor function. The presence of mononeuritis multiplex in the setting of

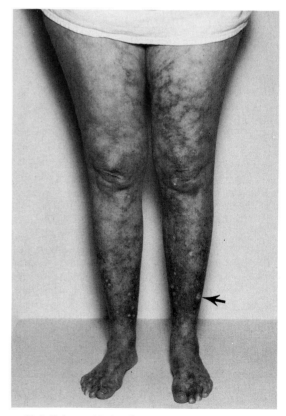

Figure 64–3. Polyarteritis involving skin of legs. Livedo reticularis is most prominent over left anterior region of thigh but is also visible over right thigh, legs below knees, and dorsa of feet. Petechiae and ulcers (*arrow*) are present on anterior and medial portions of lower legs.

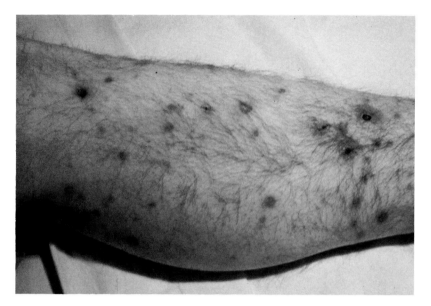

Figure 64–4. Polyarteritis involving skin. Sharply circumscribed skin infarcts are 1 to 1.5 cm in diameter and are in various stages of healing.

polyarteritis is, by itself, not associated with a poor prognosis.[40] Less commonly, a slowly evolving distal sensory neuropathy may occur. Brachial plexopathy has been reported. Clinical manifestations suggestive of central nervous system involvement are much less common than those of peripheral nerve involvement, but the two may appear together. Features suggestive of central nervous system involvement are seizures and hemiparesis.[42]

Clinical renal involvement occurs in about 70 percent of cases. Proteinuria is common, and, rarely, a nephrotic syndrome may develop. Equally common is a change in urinary sediment, with red blood cells and red blood cell casts suggestive of glomerular involvement. Acute renal failure has been reported but is distinctly unusual.[43] Hypertension may develop as a result of renal artery or glomerular involvement and is present in about 25 percent of cases.[40]

Abdominal pain is the most common gastrointestinal symptom and roughly correlates in location with the organ involved.[44] A patient may rarely present with abdominal pain owing to localized gallbladder or appendiceal involvement. In cases of diffuse abdominal pain, mesenteric thrombosis must be considered. Abdominal distention may indicate mesenteric thrombosis with or without peritonitis. Hematemesis and melena may be caused by vasculitis of the upper or lower gastrointestinal tract, respectively. Liver involvement, although common in autopsy studies, is rarely detected clinically except in those cases associated with HB_s antigen. The only abnormality reflecting liver involvement may be an elevated level of alkaline phosphatase without elevated bilirubin or transaminase levels. A needle biopsy may be normal despite hepatic vascular lesions. However, an open liver biopsy may help establish the diagnosis.

Cardiac involvement is common pathologically but is recognized less often clinically. Myocardial infarction, when it occurs, is usually silent.[45] Conges-

tive heart failure may develop as a result of coronary insufficiency or hypertension (or both). Tachycardia out of proportion to fever has been noted and may be unassociated with other cardiac findings.

Occasionally patients with polyarteritis have pulmonary involvement. Lung infiltrations may be diffuse and may precede the development of vascular involvement in other organs. In such cases, there is usually an underlying disease, such as Sjögren's syndrome. However, pulmonary lesions are more common in patients whose findings fit better with granulomatous vasculitis (see Wegener's granulomatosis and Churg-Strauss vasculitis).

Diffuse involvement of skeletal muscle arteries may cause pain and intermittent claudication. In the eye, polyarteritis may result in an exudative retinal detachment.[46] Toxic retinopathy with retinal hemorrhage or exudates is common. Scleritis rarely occurs in polyarteritis unassociated with granulomatous disease of the lung. Temporal artery involvement may occur in polyarteritis nodosa. It has not been recognized frequently and may be associated with jaw claudication. The pathologic picture in such cases reveals fibrinoid necrosis without giant cells.[47]

Polyarteritis occurring in childhood is rare and may take two forms.[48] The infantile form occurs in children younger than 2 years of age and may be similar to the mucocutaneous lymph node syndrome (Kawasaki's disease—see that section). Polyarteritis of older children is identical to adult polyarteritis. Children with the infantile form frequently have a limited number of organs involved and usually have some type of heart involvement.

The clinical and laboratory features in patients who have HB_s antigens are not different from those in patients who are antigen negative, except for variable hepatic dysfunction in some of the former patients. There is no constant temporal relationship between the onset of the polyarteritis and liver disease. The activity of the arteritis does not parallel the

Table 64–1. 1990 CRITERIA FOR THE CLASSIFICATION OF POLYARTERITIS NODOSA (TRADITIONAL FORMAT)*

Criterion	Definition
1. Weight loss ≥4 kg	Loss of 4 kg or more of body weight since illness began, not due to dieting or other factors
2. Livedo reticularis	Mottled reticular pattern over the skin of portions of the extremities or torso
3. Testicular pain or tenderness	Pain or tenderness of the testicles, not due to infection, trauma, or other causes
4. Myalgias, weakness, or leg tenderness	Diffuse myalgias (excluding shoulder and hip girdle) or weakness of muscles or tenderness of leg muscles
5. Mononeuropathy or polyneuropathy	Development of mononeuropathy, multiple mononeuropathies, or polyneuropathy
6. Diastolic BP >90 mm Hg	Development of hypertension with the diastolic BP higher than 90 mm Hg
7. Elevated BUN or creatinine	Elevation of BUN >40 mg/dl or creatinine >1.5 mg/dl, not due to dehydration or obstruction
8. Hepatitis B virus	Presence of hepatitis B surface antigen or antibody in serum
9. Arteriographic abnormality	Arteriogram showing aneurysms or occlusions of the visceral arteries, not due to arteriosclerosis, fibromuscular dysplasia, or other noninflammatory causes
10. Biopsy of small or medium-sized artery containing PMN	Histologic changes showing the presence of granulocytes or granulocytes and mononuclear leukocytes in the artery wall

*For classification purposes, a patient with vasculitis shall be said to have polyarteritis nodosa if at least 3 of these 10 criteria are present. The presence of any 3 or more criteria yields a sensitivity of 82.2% and a specificity of 86.6%. BP = blood pressure; BUN = blood urea nitrogen; PMN = polymorphonuclear neutrophils.

From Lightfoot, R. W., et al.: The American College of Rheumatology 1990 Criteria for the Classification of Polyarteritis Nodosa. Arthritis Rheum. 33:1088, 1990; with permission.

activity of the hepatitis.[49] There is a spectrum of vascular involvement in patients with associated HB$_s$ antigen, including polyarteritis, digital vasospasm, proliferative glomerulonephritis, and small vessel involvement with cryoglobulinemia.[50]

Laboratory Tests. Most tests are nonspecific and reflect the systemic inflammatory nature of the disease. An elevated erythrocyte sedimentation rate, normochromic anemia, and diminished levels of serum albumin are usually present. Neutrophilic leukocytosis, thrombocytosis, and elevation of serum globulins may be found. Eosinophilia is generally associated with pulmonary involvement, particularly in allergic angiitis and granulomatosis.

Diminished concentrations of serum whole complement and C3 and C4 components may be associated with active disease[22] and may be present in about 25 percent of the patients.[40] Such patients usually have diffuse cutaneous or renal disease. Rheumatoid factor may be present in individuals with hypocomplementemia.

HB$_s$ antigen has been found in 10 to 54 percent of patients, depending on the series.[22, 51] In some cases, the antigen is detected in the serum transiently, and serial determinations must be performed to detect it.

Immune complexes may be detected in patients with active polyarteritis by the monoclonal rheumatoid factor assay[52] and by polyethylene glycol precipitation.[53] It is not known whether these measurements are any more effective in following patients than the erythrocyte sedimentation rate. At present, they should be regarded as investigational tools.

Diagnosis. Because the symptoms in polyarteritis are so diverse, the diagnosis is often difficult and delayed (Table 64–1). Yet, making the diagnosis as early as possible is important because the disease may progress with time to involve vital organs. Polyarteritis should be suspected in a patient with findings such as fever, chills, weight loss, fatigue,

and multisystem involvement. A careful examination may reveal early cutaneous manifestations, a peripheral neuropathy, or renal involvement that might provide a clue to the diagnosis. The development of mononeuritis multiplex in a patient who has a systemic disease is highly suggestive of an underlying vasculitis. It must be remembered that the findings in patients with septicemia, infective endocarditis, malignancy, left atrial myxoma, and atherosclerosis with large-artery aneurysms and cholesterol embolization may resemble those of polyarteritis (Table 64–2). Patients with rheumatoid arthritis, Sjögren's syndrome, and certain malignancies may have a complicating necrotizing vasculitis similar to polyarteritis.

Evidence of vascular involvement should be established by biopsy or angiography. The likelihood of finding arteritis is greatest when clinically abnormal tissues are examined. The most accessible involved tissues are the skin, sural nerve, muscle, kidney, and testes. Biopsy of these tissues will sample small arteries. Small vessels in the dermis can be detected by a punch skin biopsy. Small-artery involvement in the subcutaneous tissue and muscle can be determined by an excisional biopsy. Muscle biopsy may be obtained when involved tissue is not easily identifiable or accessible. From 30 to 50 percent of "blind" muscle biopsies performed in cases of

Table 64–2. DISEASES SIMULATING SYSTEMIC VASCULITIS

Atrial myxoma
Septicemica (gonococcemia, meningococcemia, Rocky Mountain spotted fever)
Infective endocarditis
Lyme disease
Mycotic aneurysm and embolization
Malignancies—lymphoma
Cholesterol embolization from a large-artery aneurysm
Ergotism

polyarteritis may reveal evidence of arteritis.[22] The frequency of positive muscle biopsies may be higher if painful or tender muscles are biopsied. Involvement of the sural nerve can be verified by electromyography. A portion of the whole sural nerve must be sampled to provide arteries for analysis. In patients with abnormalities of urinary sediment or proteinuria, if no other accessible tissue is available, a kidney biopsy can be considered. It must be remembered that usually a segmental necrotizing glomerulonephritis will be found. This lesion can be seen commonly in all the vasculitides, and renal biopsy will not allow the differentiation of the type of vasculitis.[54] The renal biopsy may not sample a small vessel that might show vasculitis. If there is testicular pain, induration, or both, a testicular biopsy can be obtained.

Arteriography may be helpful diagnostically and may provide information on prognosis by defining the extent of disease. Positive findings include arterial saccular or fusiform aneurysms and narrowing or tapering of the arteries (Fig. 64–5).[55] This procedure is most appropriate when involved organs are not available for biopsy and in cases with evidence of intra-abdominal organ involvement. Aneurysms have been found most commonly in the kidney, followed by the liver, then the mesenteric arteries.[56] The lesions may disappear with improvement of the vasculitis.

It must be remembered that other conditions may be associated with an identical or a similar roentgenographic picture.[57] These conditions include Wegener's granulomatosis, acute angiitis and granulomatosis, systemic lupus erythematosus, thrombotic thrombocytopenic purpura, infective endocar-

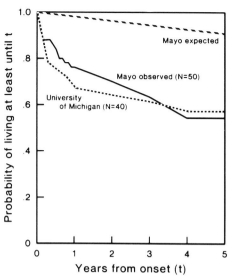

Figure 64–6. Graph showing five-year survival of patients with polyarteritis. (From Cohen, R. D., Conn, D. L., and Ilstrup, D. M.: Mayo Clin. Proc. 55:146, 1980; and Sack, M., Cassidy, J. T., and Bole, G. G.: J. Rheumatol. 2:411, 1975.)

ditis, atrial myxoma, metastatic malignancy involving the peritoneum, and spontaneous dissection of arteries.[58]

Prognosis. The outcome of polyarteritis is dependent on age and the presence and extent of visceral and central nervous system involvement. Most of the deaths occur within the first year of the disease (Fig. 64–6).[40] Deaths occurring within the first year are usually the result of uncontrolled vasculitis or infectious complications of treatment. Late deaths, occurring after 1 year of disease, are usually the result of complications of treatment or vascular deaths, such as myocardial infarction or stroke. The prognosis of untreated polyarteritis is poor, and the 5-year survival is less than 15 percent. Improved survivorship has occurred with the use of glucocorticoids, and most studies reveal a 5-year survival of between 50 and 60 percent. Recent studies indicate an even higher survival rate with the use of a combination of glucocorticoids and cytotoxic agents in selected cases.

Treatment. Glucocorticoids are the cornerstone of treatment in polyarteritis. Some retrospective studies have suggested an improved survival with the addition of cyclophosphamide or azathioprine.[59, 60] Other retrospective studies, however, have not clearly shown better results with cytotoxic drugs.[40, 61] Other modalities of treatment have been advocated in case reports for severe disease, including intravenous methylprednisolone,[62] and plasma exchange.[63]

Decisions regarding treatment of polyarteritis depend on the extent of disease, the organs involved, and the rate of progression of disease.

In patients with less severe involvement, prednisone alone, given orally in high divided doses, is usually sufficient. Such patients may have involve-

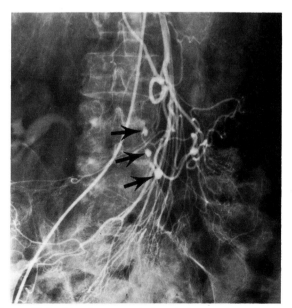

Figure 64–5. Superior mesenteric arteriogram in patient with polyarteritis. Several small aneurysms (arrows) are present in branches of superior mesenteric artery. (Courtesy of Dr. A. W. Stanson.)

ment of the skin, peripheral nerves, musculoskeletal system, and peripheral vascular system with milder visceral involvement, such as hematuria, red cell casts, and mild proteinuria without renal insufficiency. Patients with evidence of progressive renal, gastrointestinal, central nervous system, or heart involvement should also be treated with high doses of prednisone. The prednisone or its equivalent should be given in three or four divided doses a day and in total daily doses of from 60 to 100 mg. If this treatment does not result in early control of the disease, then one of several additional treatment modalities should be added: cyclophosphamide (2 mg per kg orally or intravenous pulse with approximately 500 mg per m² given monthly) or chlorambucil.

In some patients with polyarteritis whose conditions have been controlled with glucocorticoids, a cytotoxic agent may be added after weeks or months for the steroid-sparing effect. The side effects of these drugs must be monitored.

When the disease is controlled, the glucocorticoid dose should be tapered. This can be done by keeping the dose divided and gradually reducing each of the doses. An alternative tapering approach would be to double the dose given daily and administer it every other day in a single dose, and then gradually taper that dose. With the latter program, the potential exists for disease exacerbation. The reduction is dependent on the clinical status and the erythrocyte sedimentation rate. At times, the dose may need to be increased or stabilized for a period of time before reduction is again attempted. It should be the goal to reduce the prednisone dose to the lowest possible level that controls the inflammation.

Late complications and deaths associated with polyarteritis include renal vascular hypertension, cerebrovascular disease, and coronary artery disease.[40] These vascular occlusive complications may be the result of previous arterial inflammation plus the atherosclerosis-producing effects of the glucocorticoids. With inflammation of the arteries there is the potential for intimal proliferation and eventual luminal occlusion possibly augmented by glucocorticoids.[64] Treatment with antiplatelet drugs during treatment with glucocorticoids for polyarteritis should be considered as one way of possibly countering this effect.[65]

Despite good management, some patients with polyarteritis develop kidney failure. Kidney transplantation has been successful in some cases after the arteritis has become inactive. Patients with congestive heart failure should be managed with digoxin, and the hypertension should be vigorously controlled. Detailed attention should be given to fluid and electrolyte balance. Nonsteroidal anti-inflammatory drugs (NSAIDs) may be used, as necessary, for articular symptoms.

RHEUMATOID VASCULITIS

A small-vessel vasculitis is intimately associated with many of the clinical manifestations seen in rheumatoid arthritis. The early development of the rheumatoid nodule is associated with a small-vessel vasculitis. Small and medium-sized arteries in the extremities, peripheral nerves, and occasionally other organs may complicate rheumatoid arthritis. It is of note that patients with rheumatoid vasculitis have a higher frequency of HLA-DR4 than those with uncomplicated rheumatoid arthritis, suggesting an inherited susceptibility to this complication.[66]

Clinical Features. The superimposed systemic vasculitis complicating rheumatoid arthritis is uncommon. It usually occurs in rheumatoid patients who have had their disease for a number of years, usually for 10 years or more. However, rarely a systemic vasculitis occurs at the onset of rheumatoid arthritis, and in such cases the outcome is poor.[67] Males are afflicted as commonly as females. These patients have more severe rheumatoid arthritis with destructive joint disease, rheumatoid nodules, and a higher titer of rheumatoid factor.[66] Patients with Felty's syndrome are more likely to develop vasculitic complications. The rheumatoid synovitis may not be active at the time of the development of the clinical features of the systemic vasculitis. The clinical features include a variety of skin lesions: nailfold infarcts, leg ulcers, and digital gangrene (Fig. 64–7). The nailfold infarcts and leg ulcers are presumed to be due to involvement of small vessels. It should be noted that not all patients with nailfold infarcts and leg ulcers go on to systemic vasculitis. Distal sensory neuropathy is another manifestation seen in vasculitis that also may occur alone without progressing to widespread vascular involvement.

Patients with rheumatoid vasculitis may display constitutional features, including fever. The more ominous manifestations of vasculitis are the appearance of infarctions of the fingertips and a sensorimotor neuropathy.[68] If the rate of appearance of new areas of involvement is rapid, this indicates widespread arterial disease and a poorer outcome. In some patients the vasculitis may extend to involve mesenteric, coronary, and cerebral arteries.

The clinical picture of systemic rheumatoid vasculitis differs from that of polyarteritis. Rheumatoid vasculitis is not associated with significant renal involvement. Patients with rheumatoid vasculitis have a high titer of rheumatoid factor, a low level of serum complement, cryoglobulins, and immune complex material in their serum.[69] In addition, patients with rheumatoid vasculitis will usually have an elevated erythrocyte sedimentation rate, anemia, thrombocytosis, and a diminished serum albumin.

It has been thought by some that the widespread vasculitis complicating rheumatoid arthritis is caused by glucocorticoids. However, patients who have never received glucocorticoid therapy also may develop vasculitis. Wide fluctuations in glucocorticoid dose, such as those caused by abruptly stopping the drug, may allow an underlying vasculitis to progress rapidly.[70] Also, the long-standing use of glucocorticoids in rheumatoid arthritis predisposes to atherosclerosis and may permit an occlusive vasculopathy.[64]

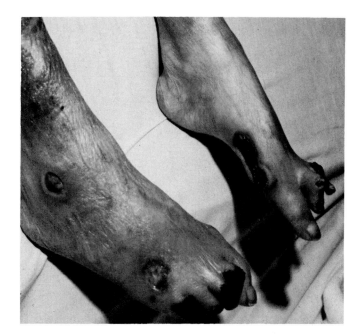

Figure 64–7. Gangrene of toes and ulcerations of feet due to rheumatoid vasculitis.

A study examining survival in rheumatoid vasculitis failed to show that any single clinical feature, such as the extent of peripheral neuropathy, was associated with a worse outcome.[71] Outcome is influenced by older age and the severity of involvement as indicated by the use of cytotoxic drugs. The cytotoxic agents may have contributed to the poor outcome.

Pathology. The study of involved vessels from patients with rheumatoid vasculitis reveals a pathologic picture identical to that seen in polyarteritis.[72] Small and medium-sized arteries are involved. In some cases the distribution of vascular lesions is like that in polyarteritis. Renal involvement, however, is rare. Arterial lesions may be found in various stages of inflammation and healing. Early lesions include fibrinoid necrosis of the wall, with an inflammatory cell infiltrate. Chronic changes with artery wall fibrosis, occlusion, and recanalization may be seen. One pathologic difference from polyarteritis is the finding of small and medium-sized arteries involved with an occlusive intimal proliferation without much inflammation.[73] The acute arterial lesions are immune complex induced, as indicated by the finding of immunoglobulins and complement in the involved arteries.[34] These immune deposits are not found in the more chronic lesions; rather, fibrinogen is found. The fibrin may stimulate the intimal proliferative response.

Treatment. The treatment of rheumatoid vasculitis depends on the type and the extent of the lesions. Nailfold infarcts, leg ulcers, and distal sensory neuropathy require local care and the usual program for rheumatoid arthritis, including nonsteroidal anti-inflammatory drugs and disease-modifying drugs. In these milder vasculitis cases, gold or another second-line drug should be considered, if it has not already been used previously. It is possible that methotrexate may accelerate nodulosis and pos-

sibly other vasculitic manifestations.[74] Patients with fingertip infarctions and a sensorimotor neuropathy whose disease is progressive should be treated with glucocorticoids, in doses described in the section on polyarteritis. Cyclophosphamide or chlorambucil should be started in most cases, to aid in the control of the disease and to allow smooth steroid tapering.[75] Plasma exchange can be considered for the patient resistant to the aforementioned drugs.[76]

VASCULITIS OF SMALL VESSELS (HYPERSENSITIVITY VASCULITIS)

This category includes a variety of conditions that are grouped together because involvement of small blood vessels of the skin is the most prominent clinical feature and a hypersensitivity mechanism is suspected in their pathogenesis. Leukocytoclastic vasculitis is the term used to describe the usual histopathology in which small blood vessels, especially postcapillary venules, are infiltrated with polymorphonuclear leukocytes. As the inflammatory process evolves, the leukocytes fragment and destruction of the vessel wall occurs. This picture was categorized by Zeek and colleagues[77] as hypersensitivity angiitis. The vasculitis in their cases occurred after an antigenic stimulus, such as the administration of horse serum. As might be expected in such a setting, all the lesions were in the same stage of development.[77] However, vasculitis with primary skin involvement and a leukocytoclastic pathologic picture can be seen in a number of conditions, including Henoch-Schönlein purpura, mixed cryoglobulinemia, a serum sickness–like reaction associated with drug hypersensitivity, hypocomplementemic vasculitis, vasculitis associated with certain connective tissue diseases such as Sjögren's syn-

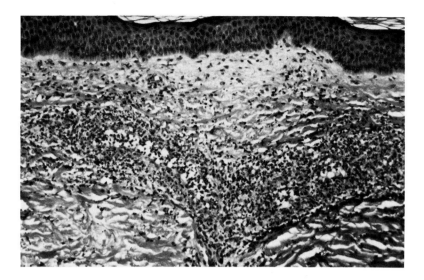

Figure 64–8. Cutaneous vasculitis. Dermal vessels, probably venules, are sectioned longitudinally. Intense infiltration of inflammatory cells (primarily polymorphonuclear leukocytes) has resulted in narrowing and occlusion of vessel lumen and in necrosis of wall. Fragments of degenerated leukocyte nuclei ("nuclear dust") are visible in perivascular areas. (Hematoxylin & eosin × 100.)

drome, vasculitis associated with other inflammatory conditions such as hypergammaglobulinemic purpura, chronic active hepatitis, ulcerative colitis, primary biliary cirrhosis, vasculitis associated with malignancies, and even polyarteritis nodosa and Wegener's syndrome.[78, 79] In most of these conditions, an inciting antigenic stimulus cannot be specifically identified. In addition, some variability of the histopathologic findings has been noted. Lymphocytes may at times be the most numerous infiltrating cells, especially during the healing phases.[80] The term "hypersensitivity vasculitis" is most appropriately used in cases in which the vasculitis develops after exposure to a sensitizing antigen or in cases in which such an agent is strongly suspected.

Pathogenesis. Many of these cases of vasculitis may be triggered by allergy to drugs, exposure to a number of bacterial, parasitic, and viral agents, and probably other yet-undefined antigens. Both immune complexes and cell-mediated reactions have been implicated in the development of necrotic vascular skin lesions.[81] Complement and immunoglobulins have been demonstrated in the walls of subepidermal small vessels obtained in biopsy specimens,[82] especially early lesions. Similarly sized vessels in other organs may be involved to varying extents, as described later. Immune reactants have been identified in the walls of vessels in the dermis of biopsy specimens taken from clinically normal skin that is within 2 to 3 cm of an active lesion. In some studies, immunoglobulins and complement have been found in vessels in normal skin in these cases after local injections of histamine, but not in vessels in normal uninjected skin.

In hypersensitivity vasculitis, the histopathologic appearance depends on the severity of the reaction and the age of the lesion.[83] In the acute phase, endothelial swelling is seen often, with occlusion of the vessel lumen. There is infiltration of the wall and perivascular areas by polymorphonuclear leukocytes, with leukocytoclasis and fragmentation of nuclei

("nuclear dust") (Fig. 64–8). Other features include necrosis of vessel walls, fibrinoid deposits, and extravasation of red blood cells. In later stages of a severe reaction, necrosis of much of the connective tissue of the dermis may be found, so that recognition of specific vessels is not possible.

Clinical Features. The manifestations usually appear abruptly with the appearance of maculopapular skin lesions. In cases that are drug induced, the symptoms usually appear within a few days of initiation of drug treatment. Many drugs have been implicated. The most common are penicillin and its derivatives and sulfa drugs. The fact that a patient has been receiving a drug for an extended time does not exclude that drug from consideration. Drug hypersensitivity is not time or dose dependent.[84]

The skin lesions appear as flat, erythematous, purpuric macules that progress to papules of "palpable purpura." The papular quality is an important feature, since it distinguishes these lesions from noninflammatory purpura. The eruption may occur on any part of the skin but is seen especially over the dependent areas, such as the lower extremities or back and gluteal regions of recumbent patients. Lesions are also commonly seen on the forearms and hands, but it is unusual to find lesions on the upper portion of the trunk or face.

Crops of cutaneous lesions may develop in episodes at irregular intervals. Individual lesions last from 1 to 4 weeks and leave hyperpigmented spots or sometimes atrophic scars. The size of the lesions varies from a millimeter to several centimeters when lesions coalesce. Vesicles and bullae containing bloody fluid may develop in more severe cases. Skin necrosis leads to ulceration. Smaller skin lesions rarely cause symptoms, but larger lesions are frequently painful. Edema of the lower part of the legs, ankles, and feet may develop.

Constitutional symptoms, including fever, frequently accompany the appearance of the skin lesions. Arthralgias are present in the majority of

Table 64–3. 1990 CRITERIA FOR THE CLASSIFICATION OF HYPERSENSITIVITY VASCULITIS
(TRADITIONAL FORMAT)*

Criterion	Definition
Age at disease onset >16 years	Development of symptoms after age 16
Medication at disease onset	Medication was taken at the onset of symptoms that may have been a precipitating factor
Palpable purpura	Slightly elevated purpuric rash over one or more areas of the skin; does not blanch with pressure and is not related to thrombocytopenia
Maculopapular rash	Flat and raised lesions of various sizes over one or more areas of the skin
Biopsy including arteriole and venule	Histologic changes showing granulocytes in a perivascular or extravascular location

*For purposes of classification, a patient with vasculitis shall be said to have hypersensitivity vasculitis if at least 3 of these 5 criteria are present. The presence of any 3 or more criteria yields a sensitivity of 71.0% and a specificity of 83.9%

From Calabrese, L. H., et al.: The American College of Rheumatology 1990 Criteria for the Classification of Hypersensitivity Vasculitis. Arthritis Rheum. 33:1088, 1990; with permission.

patients. Palpable synovitis is less common. Renal involvement is manifested by proteinuria, hematuria, and, occasionally, renal insufficiency. Abdominal pain and gastrointestinal bleeding can occur. Pulmonary infiltrations, either nodular or diffuse, may be seen on chest radiographs. Pleural effusions have been described. Neurologic findings include headaches, diplopia, and rarely, an organic brain syndrome. Other organ involvement is distinctly less common. A normochromic anemia and an increased erythrocyte sedimentation rate may be present during attacks and reflect the extent of the inflammatory process. Eosinophilia may be present. Classification criteria for hypersensitivity vasculitis are listed in Table 64–3.

Treatment. Any potential inciting drug or antigen should be discontinued or removed. In mild cases with a brief single episode of a few scattered purpuric areas without internal organ involvement, no specific treatment is needed. If systemic symptoms are present and skin lesions are diffuse, or if internal organ involvement is present, glucocorticoid treatment is usually necessary. The initial dosage can be varied, depending on the severity of the findings, and may range from 20 mg per day of prednisone, or the equivalent dose of another glucocorticoid, to 60 mg per day for multisystem involvement. When the clinical abnormalities have been suppressed, the dosage should be gradually reduced to the lowest amount necessary to control the symptoms and findings. Glucocorticoids are effective in most instances, but cytotoxic drugs may be considered when gluco-

corticoids have not been successful or if hypercortisonism has developed. However, cytotoxic drugs have not yet been clearly shown to be beneficial in most patients. In chronic cases with less well-defined precipitating factors, many forms of therapy have been tried, including dapsone, NSAIDs, and colchicine, with variable results.

Special Forms of Vasculitis of Small Vessels

Henoch-Schönlein purpura. The syndrome of Henoch-Schönlein purpura has become established as a distinct clinical condition. Persons of any age may be affected, but it occurs primarily in children, with a peak incidence between 4 and 11 years of age.[85] The syndrome is also referred to as anaphylactoid purpura and allergic purpura because of circumstantial evidence implicating hypersensitivity to bacteria or viruses as a possible cause. Classification criteria are shown in Table 64–4.

The cutaneous lesions and histopathology are as described previously. Immunofluorescence studies have shown immunoglobulins and complement deposits in cutaneous vessels and kidney, but serum complement levels are usually normal.[86] Immunoglobulin A is most abundant and sometimes the only immunoglobulin found in the skin and kidney lesions. Cases of Henoch-Schönlein purpura with the congenital absence of the second component of complement have been described.[87] This finding plus the observation of IgA deposits in involved tissues sug-

Table 64–4. 1990 CRITERIA FOR THE CLASSIFICATION OF HENOCH-SCHÖNLEIN PURPURA
(TRADITIONAL FORMAT)*

Criterion	Definition
1. Palpable purpura	Slightly raised "palpable" hemorrhagic skin lesions, not related to thrombocytopenia
2. Age ≤20 at disease onset	Patient 20 years or younger at onset of first symptoms
3. Bowel angina	Diffuse abdominal pain, worse after meals, or the diagnosis of bowel ischemia, usually including bloody diarrhea
4. Wall granulocytes on biopsy	Histologic changes showing granulocytes in the walls of arterioles or venules

*For purposes of classification, a patient with vasculitis shall be said to have Henoch-Schönlein purpura if at least 2 of these 4 criteria are present. The presence of any 2 or more criteria yields a sensitivity of 87.1% and a specificity of 87.7%.

From Mills, J. A., et al.: The American College of Rheumatology 1990 Criteria for the Classification of Henoch-Schönlein Purpura. Arthritis Rheum. 33:1114, 1990; with permission.

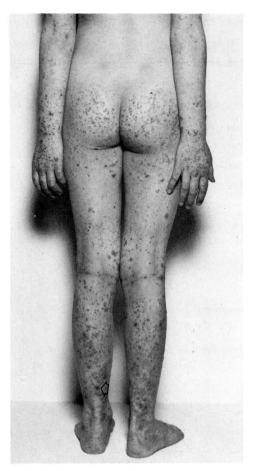

Figure 64–9. Cutaneous vasculitis—Schönlein-Henoch syndrome. Palpable purpura is most prominent over extensor surfaces of distal regions of upper and lower extremities and over buttocks. Some small skin infarcts are visible (*arrow*).

This disease is generally self-limited; its duration varies from 6 to 16 weeks. Between 5 and 10 percent of patients recover, only to relapse weeks or months later. Such patients with persistent or recurrent renal disease may suffer significant renal impairment. The prognosis is determined mainly by the extent of renal involvement. Allen and colleagues[90] found detectable renal impairment for at least 4 years in 28 percent of their patients.

Hypocomplementemic Vasculitis. McDuffie and coworkers[91] described hypocomplementemic vasculitis in 1973. The incidence is unknown, but the condition is uncommon. The patients described have been young adults, predominantly women. The cause is unknown, but lesional deposits of immunoglobulins and complement and the presence of serum factors that react with C1q and monoclonal rheumatoid factor suggest that the disease is an immune complex–induced process.[92]

Skin biopsies show leukocytoclastic vasculitis. In patients with renal involvement, renal biopsies show mild to moderate membranoproliferative glomerulonephritis, with IgG and complement deposited on the glomerular basement membranes in a lumpy, bumpy pattern.

The hallmark of this disease is an urticarial skin eruption. The eruption may occur on any part of the skin, but the face, upper extremities, and trunk are involved most commonly. Urticaria typically lasts 24 to 48 hours; it has a tendency to central clearing, and

gests that the alternative complement pathway rather than the classic pathway could be involved in the pathogenesis of this disease.

The disease occurs most often in the spring and often follows an upper respiratory tract infection. The classic triad that occurs in up to 80 percent of cases is that of palpable purpura, arthritis, and abdominal pain. Larger purpuric lesions tend to develop over the buttocks and lower extremities (Fig. 64–9). Edema of the feet and lower legs is common, and edema may also develop on the hands, scalp, and periorbital areas. The ankle and knee joints are affected most commonly and are swollen, warm, and tender. The arthritis is usually transient. Gastrointestinal lesions may cause severe cramping, abdominal pain, intussusception, hemorrhage, protein-losing enteropathy, or, rarely, perforation. Renal involvement occurs in approximately one half of the patients, and although such involvement is usually mild, persistent renal insufficiency can occur and is likely to be more severe in adults.[88]

For milder cases, supportive treatment alone may be adequate. In adults, glucocorticoids administered during the acute stage may control systemic features and prevent progression of renal disease.[89]

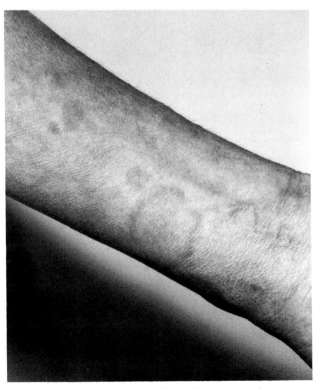

Figure 64–10. Cutaneous vasculitis with hypocomplementemia. Large resolving urticarial lesion on flexor surface of forearm shows central clearing.

it fades without leaving a residue (Fig. 64–10). The lesions may be several centimeters in diameter and are usually not pruritic. Some patients have persistent skin involvement, but others have episodes several times a year or more. Palpable purpura and vesicles may be seen.

Recurrent episodes of urticaria may be associated with fever, joint pain, and abdominal pain. Peripheral joint swelling may occur, and the pattern of joint involvement is similar to that in systemic lupus erythematosus, with symmetric involvement of the small joints but without any residual deformity. The abdominal pain may be accompanied by nausea, vomiting, and tenderness, but bowel sounds are usually normal and rectal bleeding has not been reported. Renal involvement is manifested by hematuria, proteinuria, and red blood cell casts. Chronic obstructive pulmonary disease has been found in almost half of these patients and is associated with heavy cigarette smoking.[93]

Reduced levels of both early- and late-reacting components of complement usually parallel the activity of the disease. Cryoglobulins are absent or present in only trace amounts. Sera in these patients do not contain significant titers of antinuclear antibodies or rheumatoid factor.

Patients may be treated satisfactorily with glucocorticoids. Cytotoxic agents may be used in selected instances in which the glucocorticoids are not effective or cannot be lowered to reasonable dosages. The disease appears to follow a chronic course. Renal involvement is not generally progressive. The associated chronic obstructive pulmonary disease may be the major cause of serious morbidity and mortality.

Mixed Cryoglobulinemia. The syndrome of purpura, arthralgia, weakness, and mixed cryoglobulinemia described by LoSpalluto and associates[94] and Meltzer and coworkers[95] also appears to be an uncommon but distinct clinical condition in which cutaneous vasculitis is a dominant feature. It affects middle-aged females most commonly. Immune deposits containing complement have been demonstrated in skin vessel walls and along the glomerular basement membrane. Cryoglobulins are present, but in small amounts, usually less than 100 mg per dl. They contain IgG and IgM, both of which are required for cryoprecipitation. Occasionally IgA is detected. Forty-eight hours or more at 0°C may be required for the demonstration of cryoprecipitation. The IgM component has anti-IgG (rheumatoid factor) activity. Two thirds of patients were found to be positive for HB$_s$ antigen or its antibody when both serum and cryoprecipitates were examined.[50] Moderate anemia, hyperglobulinemia, and hypocomplementemia are present.

Patients with this syndrome have recurrent episodes of palpable purpura, usually involving the lower extremities. Some may develop arthralgias, hepatosplenomegaly, lymphadenopathy, and mononeuritis multiplex. Diffuse glomerulonephritis may lead to terminal renal failure.[50]

The cutaneous and histologic pictures may be identical to those of Henoch-Schönlein purpura. However, the cryoglobulins, positive rheumatoid factor, and low levels of serum complement make distinguishing between these two conditions relatively simple. The absence of serum antibodies to double-stranded DNA helps separate it from systemic lupus erythematosus. Mixed cryoglobulinemia has also been seen in a number of other chronic autoimmune or infectious diseases.

Treatment of mixed cryoglobulinemia is dependent on the extent of involvement. Therapy in patients with disease limited to the skin may be tried with penicillamine. Patients with more extensive involvement are treated with high doses of prednisone, as described for polyarteritis. The addition of cytotoxic drugs, usually cyclophosphamide, may be required to control the disease and taper the prednisone to a reasonably low level. In some cases, plasma exchange may be used in combination with prednisone and cyclophosphamide or intravenous gamma globulin.[96]

ALLERGIC ANGIITIS AND GRANULOMATOSIS (CHURG-STRAUSS SYNDROME)

The association of asthma, eosinophilia, vasculitis, and extravascular granulomas was termed allergic angiitis and granulomatosis by Churg and Strauss in 1951.[97] These authors considered allergic factors to be important in the development of the disease.

Epidemiology. This form of vasculitis is rare, although no detailed epidemiologic analyses are available. Thirty patients with this condition were found over a 25-year period in one center.[98] In some studies, patients who have had Churg-Strauss syndrome have been grouped with patients with polyarteritis. In Rose and Spencer's analysis[3] of 111 patients with polyarteritis, some of the 32 patients with lung involvement had asthma and eosinophilia and probably had Churg-Strauss syndrome. The male-to-female ratio appears to be about 2 to 1. The age at onset varies from 15 to 70 years, with a mean of about 38.[99]

Pathology. The cause of allergic angiitis and granulomatosis is not known. Immunoglobulins and complement have been demonstrated in vessel walls, and fibrinogen alone has been found in extravascular granulomas.[100] No data have been reported regarding the role of immune complexes or cell-mediated mechanisms in this disease. Elevated serum IgE concentration has been noted in several cases and may indicate a response to an inciting antigen.[22] Alternatively, the increased IgE response may reflect a defect in cellular immunity.

The characteristic pathologic changes in this disease include small necrotizing granulomas as well as necrotizing vasculitis involving small arteries and venules. Granulomas are typically about 1 mm or more in diameter and are commonly located near small arteries or veins. They are composed of a central eosinophilic core surrounded radially by macrophages and epithelioid giant cells. Inflammatory cells are also present in the granulomas, with eosinophils predominating in the early stage of development and lesser numbers being present in the healing stages. Polymorphonucelar leukocytes and lymphocytes are found in varying but smaller numbers. Macrophages and giant cells predominate in the more chronic lesions. Necrotizing vasculitis of small arteries and veins is always seen in involved tissue. Extravascular granulomas and fibrinoid necrosis may be seen in about 50 percent.[98]

Renal biopsies may show a nonspecific focal glomerulonephritis.[98] Study of kidneys at autopsy may reveal more characteristic lesions with eosinophilic infiltration and eosinophilic granulomas. Cutaneous nodules usually show granulomas containing giant cells and eosinophils, often in a perivascular location. Vasculitis and granulomas may be found in the liver, spleen, lymph nodes, and urinary tract. Peripheral nerves show inflammation of epineural vessels and pathologic changes ranging from fibrinoid necrosis with an inflammatory cell infiltration to intimal proliferation and perivascular fibrosis similar to polyarteritis.[101]

Clinical Features. There may be three phases of disease. The prodromal period may last for years (more than 10 years) and consist of allergic manifestations of rhinitis, polyposis, and asthma. The second phase includes peripheral blood and tissue eosinophilia with Löffler's syndrome, eosinophilic pneumonia, or eosinophilic gastroenteritis. The third phase is the systemic vasculitis.[99] In fewer than 20 percent of cases, the phases may appear simultaneously. The development of fever and weight loss may herald the onset of systemic disease. At this time chest roentgenograms are abnormal in approximately half the cases and show changes ranging from patchy, shifting pneumonic infiltrates (Löffler's syndrome), through massive bilateral nodular infiltrates without cavitation, to diffuse interstitial lung disease. The symptoms of asthma often subside when the vasculitis emerges. Although the pneumonitis may be an eosinophilic pneumonia, the relationship of eosinophilic pneumonitis to Churg-Strauss vasculitis has not been definitely established.

Cutaneous lesions occur in approximately two thirds of the patients. Subcutaneous nodules are the most common skin manifestation. Petechiae, purpura, or skin infarctions may be seen. Peripheral neuropathy, usually mononeuritis multiplex, is found in the majority of patients. Cardiac involvement is common and may result in congestive heart failure. Abdominal symptoms occur in a small percentage of cases; these may be due to granulomatous vasculitis of vessels of the stomach or small bowel, which causes infarction, ulceration, or perforation. Bloody diarrhea, simulating chronic ulcerative colitis, may be caused by ischemia of the mucosa of the

large bowel. Granulomatous involvement of the bowel, liver, or omentum may produce a palpable mass.

Renal disease has been found to be frequent in some series and less common in others. Renal failure occurs infrequently.[99] Eosinophilic granulomatous involvement of the prostate and lower urinary tract is a unique feature of this disease. It occurs in only a small percentage of cases and may cause urinary retention. Polyarthralgias and arthritis are uncommon. Rarely, ulceration of the cornea or central nervous system manifestations, such as seizures, may occur.

Laboratory Tests. The characteristic laboratory abnormality is eosinophilia. In the original 13 patients of Churg and Strauss, the absolute counts ranged from 5000 to 10,000 eosinophils per mm³.[97] The eosinophilia often decreases as the patient improves or is treated. With active disease, anemia and an elevated erythrocyte sedimentation rate are found. Serum rheumatoid factor may be present in low titer.[98] In the few patients studied, an elevated serum IgE has been found, and the serum complement has been normal.[22, 99]

Diagnosis. The diagnosis of Churg-Strauss syndrome is made on the basis of both clinical and pathologic features (Table 64–5). As noted, the patient is usually middle-aged and has a history of asthma that has been present for several years. The appearance of a systemic illness in this setting should lead the clinician to consider this diagnosis. Diagnostically helpful features are noncavitary lung infiltrates, nodular skin lesions, heart failure, significant eosinophilia (usually accounting for 50 percent of the white blood cell count), and an elevated level of serum IgE. The diagnosis may be substantiated by biopsy of the involved tissues, usually the lung or the skin, which reveals the characteristic eosinophilic necrotizing extravascular granulomas and necrotizing small vessel vasculitis.

Treatment and Course. The treatment of choice is glucocorticoids, in a dosage sufficient to control the inflammatory manifestations of the disease. An initial dosage of 40 to 60 mg of prednisone a day, in divided doses, or the equivalent dosage of another glucocorticoid is usually sufficient to control the disease. Data concerning the use of cytotoxic agents in this condition are meager.

The outlook may be better than that observed in patients with typical polyarteritis. Rose and Spencer noted that patients who had polyarteritis nodosa with lung involvement had a less fulminating course and that approximately one third were living at the end of 1 year.[3] There were some deaths due to lung disease in this group, but fewer due to renal failure than in patients without lung involvement. In a study of 30 patients with allergic angiitis and granulomatosis, Chumbley and coworkers[98] noted a 90 percent 1-year survival rate and a 62 percent 5-year survival rate. In this series, the most common cause of death was myocardial infarction, followed by congestive

Table 64–5. 1990 CRITERIA FOR THE CLASSIFICATION OF CHURG-STRAUSS SYNDROME
(TRADITIONAL FORMAT)*

Criterion	Definition
Asthma	History of wheezing or diffuse high-pitched rales on expiration
Eosinophilia	Eosinophilia >10% on white blood cell differential count
Mononeuropathy or polyneuropathy	Development of mononeuropathy, multiple mononeuropathies, or polyneuropathy (i.e., glove/stocking distribution) attributable to a systemic vasculitis
Pulmonary infiltrates, non-fixed	Migratory or transitory pulmonary infiltrates on radiographs (not including fixed infiltrates), attributable to a systemic vasculitis
Paranasal sinus abnormality	History of acute or chronic paranasal sinus pain or tenderness or radiographic opacification of the paranasal sinuses
Extravascular eosinophils	Biopsy including artery, arteriole, or venule, showing accumulations of eosinophils in extravascular areas

*For classification purposes, a patient with vasculitis shall be said to have Churg-Strauss syndrome (CSS) if at least 4 of these 6 criteria are positive. The presence of any 4 or more of the 6 criteria yields a sensitivity of 85% and a specificity of 99.7%.

From Masi, A. T., et al.: The American College of Rheumatology 1990 Criteria for the Classification of Churg-Strauss Syndrome (Allergic Granulomatosis and Angiitis). Arthritis Rheum. 33:1094, 1990; with permission.

heart failure. Other causes of death were status asthmaticus, *Salmonella* septicemia, ruptured aneurysm, renal failure, pneumonia, and small bowel infarction. Some of these deaths were direct complications of the glucocorticoid treatment.

WEGENER'S GRANULOMATOSIS

Wegener's granulomatosis was initially described in the 1930s.[102, 103] It is characterized by necrotizing granulomatous lesions of the respiratory tract, glomerulonephritis, and, frequently, vasculitis involving other organs.[104] Less extensive, or limited, forms of this condition have been described in which some features of the disease may be absent.[105] Subclinical renal disease has been demonstrated by kidney biopsy in such cases.[106] Today, the disease is considered to be a continuum. It begins with limited organ involvement and may progress with variable speed to a generalized form with nose, lung, and kidney involvement.[107]

Epidemiology. The annual incidence of Wegener's granulomatosis in the general population is not known. A preliminary estimate from Rochester, Minnesota, was 0.4 cases per 100,000.[35] In an 8-year case series from a district hospital population, nearly 10 cases of polyarteritis nodosa were diagnosed for every case of Wegener's granulomatosis.[108] The syndrome has been observed in persons aged 3 months to 75 years, and the peak incidence is in the fourth and fifth decades. There is a slight male predominance in the United States. Wegener's granulomatosis has been observed in whites, blacks, and Hispanics.

Pathogenesis. The cause of Wegener's granulomatosis is unknown. The clinical course of Wegener's granulomatosis, with initial respiratory tract involvement and then later glomerulonephritis, suggests a possible chain of events in which a pathogenic agent gains entry to the respiratory tract and elicits an inflammatory response that later extends to other tissues. Possible immune complex–induced inflam-

mation has been suggested by the findings of glomerular subepithelial deposits adjacent to the basement membrane in some renal biopsies.[109] However, immunohistologic studies reveal the presence of fibrin and, less commonly, immunoglobulins and complement.[23] Circulating immune complexes have been reported infrequently, and cryoglobulins are seldom detected in Wegener's granulomatosis.[110] Elevated serum IgE levels have been found, which may reflect the general elevation of immunoglobulins in this disease.[111]

An alteration of cell-mediated immunity has been suggested by a discrepancy between skin reaction and polymorphonuclear migration inhibition to a number of antigens.[112] The chemotactic response of polymorphonuclear leukocytes from patients with Wegener's granulomatosis has been shown to be decreased.[113] Peripheral blood lymphocytes, monocytes, T lymphocytes, and B lymphocytes appear to be normal in the disease.[114] Genetic susceptibility may be a factor, as indicated by the increased frequency of HLA-DR2[28] and the possible increase in HLA-B8.[115] The beneficial effect of cyclophosphamide in the treatment of Wegener's granulomatosis offers indirect evidence that immunologic factors may be important in its pathogenesis.[116]

Pathology. Wegener's granulomatosis usually starts regionally and may progress to a systemic disease with renal involvement.[117] Necrosis is the first pathologic lesion, and subsequently the characteristic necrotizing granuloma with palisading histiocytes in the periphery develops. The temporal progression of pathologic lesions from micronecrosis to macronecrosis, with granuloma formation and ultimately fibrosis, has been demonstrated on the basis of lung biopsies.[118] The primary necrotizing granulomatous inflammatory process may or may not involve adjacent arteries and veins (Fig. 64–11). Vasculitis, although present in most cases, is not necessary for the diagnosis of Wegener's granulomatosis.[107]

The histopathologic differentiation of Wegener's granulomatosis from those diseases that present with

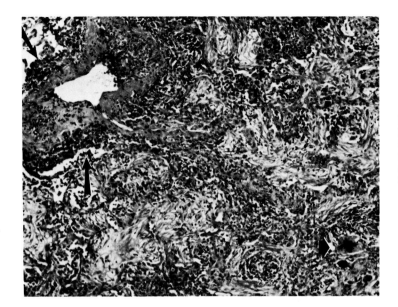

Figure 64–11. Wegener's granulomatosis involving lung. There is necrotizing inflammation of small blood vessel (*long arrow*), with infiltration of vascular wall by mononuclear cells. Granulomatous inflammatory reaction with multinucleated giant cells (*short arrow*) has replaced normal lung tissue.

similar histopathologic findings is important because the management may be different. Infections, especially those with *Mycobacterium, Nocardia,* or fungi, must be ruled out by special stains and appropriate cultures. Vasculitis seen in association with infections is usually not necrotizing. Tuberculous granulomas, rheumatoid nodules, and Churg-Strauss granulomas may have similar histopathologic changes, and the clinical features will influence diagnosis. Lymphomatoid granulomatosis is diagnosed by demonstrating intracellular polyclonal immunoglobulins by immunoperoxidase stains as well as by immunophenotyping with monoclonal antibodies.[119] Lymphomatoid granulomatosis is now considered a lymphoproliferative disease rather than a granulomatous vasculitis.

The most common renal lesion in Wegener's granulomatosis is focal necrotizing glomerulonephritis.[106] However, the spectrum of renal involvement ranges from diffuse proliferative glomerulonephritis and interstitial nephritis to hyalinization of glomeruli. Glomerular crescent formation may be found. Granulomatous inflammation around glomeruli and a necrotizing vasculitis of small renal arteries have been reported, but they are not common.

Granulomatous involvement of the sinuses is common, and it may spread to contiguous structures, such as the orbit.[120] Focal vasculitis of the eye may affect the conjunctiva, sclera, uveal tract, optic nerve, or retinal arteries. Granulomatous or vasculitic involvement may be present in other organs, principally the skin, central nervous system, cranial nerves, peripheral nerves, and heart. The pathologic changes found in skin lesions range from leukocytoclastic vasculitis to necrotizing granulomatous vasculitis.[121] The central nervous system may be involved by contiguous spread of granulomatous involvement of the sinuses, but separate granulomas may be found intracerebrally or in the meninges.[122] Vasa nervorum lesions result in mononeuritis multiplex.[101] Granulomas or vasculitis has been found in the heart in 30

percent of the autopsy cases. The pericardium, myocardium, and coronary arteries may be involved.[106] Granulomatous vasculitis may be rarely found in other sites, including the trachea, larynx, parotid gland, mastoid bone, and temporal bone.

Clinical Features. The earliest complaints are usually referable to the upper respiratory tract, such as chronic sinusitis, chronic rhinitis, nasal ulceration, and serous otitis media. These manifestations may be accompanied by systemic symptoms of fever, weight loss, and anorexia. Suppurative otitis, mastoiditis, a saddle-nose defect, and hearing loss may occur. On examination, ulceration of the nasal mucosa, palatal ulcers, or destructive sinusitis may be found and should suggest the possibility of Wegener's granulomatosis. Sinus roentgenograms may show mucosal thickening of the maxillary sinus and destruction of bony walls. Secondary bacterial infections often develop in the sinuses and are caused by *Staphylococcus aureus.*[123]

The lower respiratory tract is usually affected at some time during the course of the disease, and the initial symptoms may be related to the lungs. Symptoms are cough, hemoptysis, dyspnea, and, less commonly, pleuritic pain and tracheal obstruction. Pulmonary infiltrates are the most common roentgenologic finding. These may be transient or asymptomatic, and they may be discovered incidentally on chest roentgenograms. Cavitation may occur, but secondary infection is not common. Pleural effusion may be found in 20 percent.[124] Pulmonary function tests have revealed obstruction to airway flow in 55 percent of patients with stenosis.[125] The subglottic region is frequently involved and may lead to stenosis and distal atelectasis.[126]

Renal involvement is not usually the initial finding but will eventually become clinically manifest in as many as 85 percent of cases.[123] Manifestations include proteinuria, hematuria, red blood cell casts, and renal insufficiency. Hypertension is not common.

The skin is affected in approximately half the cases. Purpura, the most common dermatologic finding, develops over the lower extremities, but the trunk, upper extremities, and face may be included. Less commonly, the lesions are nodular or ulcerating.

Joint pains occur in as many as 70 percent of the cases. They are usually present early in the course of the disease and resolve without residual effects. Joint swelling is less common. A nondeforming arthritis involving the large lower extremity joints may occur.

The eye is involved in approximately 50 percent of cases. Orbital involvement may result from extension of a purulent sinusitis. This can cause dacryocystitis, proptosis, cavernous sinus thrombosis, or impaired vision. Other ocular manifestations of the vasculitis are conjunctivitis, scleritis, episcleritis, corneoscleral ulcers, uveitis, retinal artery occlusion, and optic neuritis.

About 20 percent of the patients will have nervous system involvement. One half will have central nervous system involvement, including cranial nerves II, V, VII, VIII, IX, and XII. Granulomas extending from the sinuses may affect the pituitary, resulting in diabetes insipidus. Cerebral vasculitis may occur. The other half of the patients will have vasculitis of the peripheral nerves, resulting in the multiple mononeuropathies and a symmetric polyneuropathy.[127]

Clinical manifestations related to granulomatous or vasculitic lesions of the heart are not common. However, arrhythmias and coronary arteritis leading to death have been observed. Also, pericarditis and congestive cardiomyopathy may occur. Granulomas and vasculitis may also be found in other organs, such as the gut, but this is uncommon, and clinical manifestations will reflect the site and extent of involvement.

Based on an analysis of 151 patients, kidney involvement appeared to be the most significant prognostic factor during the first year after diagnosis. Thereafter kidney involvement did not affect the prognosis statistically, and lung involvement was then the most significant prognostic factor.[128]

Laboratory Tests. Normochromic normocytic anemia, moderate leukocytosis without eosinophilia, elevated erythrocyte sedimentation rate, thrombocytosis, and hypergammaglobulinemia are common laboratory abnormalities found in Wegener's granulomatosis.[123] Levels of the C-reactive protein are elevated and can be used to monitor the activity of Wegener's granulomatosis.[129] Levels of all immunoglobulins may be elevated, but the IgA elevation has been stressed. Rheumatoid factor has been detected in more than 50 percent of patients and is noted most often in those with extensive disease. Antinuclear antibodies and cryoglobulins are usually absent. Serum levels of whole complement and of C3 are normal or elevated. Immune complexes are present in about half the active cases, as detected by C1q binding and Raji assay.[123] Urinalysis with proteinuria

and renal sediment abnormalities indicate glomerular involvement.

Anticytoplasmic Antibodies. In 1982 and 1984 Davies and associates[130] and Hall and colleagues[131] independently described the presence of antibodies directed against cytoplasmic components of neutrophils in patients with segmental necrotizing glomerulonephritis and systemic vasculitis. Van der Woude and coworkers[132] reported the presence of these anticytoplasmic antibodies in Wegener's granulomatosis. These antibodies in the serum of patients with Wegener's granulomatosis cause a characteristic cytoplasmic granular staining pattern by immunofluorescence. These antibodies are called antineutrophil cytoplasmic antibodies (ANCAs). Falk and Jennette[133] described antibodies with a perinuclear staining that are frequently seen in patients with glomerulonephritis, various forms of vasculitis, and collagen vascular disease. These antibodies appear to be directed against myeloperoxidase and against elastase. They do not seem to have any disease specificity and are not necessarily related to Wegener's granulomatosis. The term c-ANCA is used for cytoplasmic staining antineutrophil cytoplasmic antibody, and p-ANCA for perinuclear staining antineutrophil cytoplasmic antibody. The c-ANCA is a 29-kilodalton (kD) molecule found in azurophilic granules of human neutrophils. It appears to be a serine protease distinct from elastase and cathepsin G.[134]

It appears that c-ANCA is specific for Wegener's granulomatosis, being found in 90 percent of cases in large series.[135] c-ANCAs have not been detected in various types of collagen vascular disease, including relapsing polychondritis, polyarteritis nodosa, and other granulomatous or infectious diseases. c-ANCAs have been detected in patients with a systemic necrotizing small vessel vasculitis (microscopic PAN).[136] c-ANCAs are also found in cases of isolated rapidly progressive glomerulonephritis. It is possible that the microscopic polyarteritis and rapidly progressive glomerulonephritis represent ends of the spectrum of Wegener's granulomatosis and are part of Wegener's granulomatosis.

Titers of c-ANCA parallel disease activity. However, titers from one patient cannot be compared with those from another patient, and a baseline titer must be established for each patient.[107] The presence of c-ANCAs is not as frequent in the limited Wegener's granulomatosis occurring in about 60 percent of those cases. A negative c-ANCA test does not rule out the diagnosis of Wegener's granulomatosis. The c-ANCA test has provided the clinician with an important diagnostic tool, but it will have to be used with discretion until experience is greater.

Diagnosis. The diagnosis of Wegener's granulomatosis is based on the clinical features and the histopathologic demonstration of necrotizing granulomas with vasculitis (Table 64–6). The diagnosis should be suspected in a patient who has features of a systemic illness and the presence of c-ANCAs. The presence of nasal mucosal ulcerations, proptosis,

Table 64–6. 1990 CRITERIA FOR THE CLASSIFICATION OF WEGENER'S GRANULOMATOSIS (TRADITIONAL FORMAT)*

Criterion	Definition
1. Nasal or oral inflammation	Development of painful or painless oral ulcers or purulent or bloody nasal discharge
2. Abnormal chest radiograph	Chest radiograph showing the presence of nodules, fixed infiltrates, or cavities
3. Urinary sediment	Microhematuria (<5 red blood cells per high-power field) or red cell casts in urine sediment
4. Granulomatous inflammation on biopsy	Histologic changes showing granulomatous inflammation within the wall of an artery or in the perivascular or extravascular area (artery or arteriole)

*For purposes of classification, a patient with vasculitis shall be said to have Wegener's granulomatosis if at least 2 of these 4 criteria are present. The presence of any 2 or more criteria yields a sensitivity of 88.2% and a specificity of 92.0%.

From Leavitt, R. Y., et al.: The American College of Rheumatology 1990 Criteria for the Classification of Wegener's granulomatosis. Arthritis Rheum. 33:1101, 1990; with permission.

lung infiltrates or cavitation, proteinuria, and abnormalities in urinary sediment should further suggest this diagnosis. Anemia, an elevated erythrocyte sedimentation rate, leukocytosis, the presence of rheumatoid factor, and elevated immunoglobulin levels confirm the systemic nature of the patient's illness.

Renal biopsy will rarely be distinctive enough to be definitive. Since most of the patients with Wegener's granulomatosis have upper respiratory tract involvement early in the course of their illness, biopsy of the nasal mucosa or involved sinus tissues offers the best opportunity for securing a histologic diagnosis. A generous portion of tissue must be obtained to allow adequate pathologic examination. Involved lung tissue may be obtained, preferably by open biopsy.

Treatment and Course. Before the 1960s, Wegener's granulomatosis was almost uniformly fatal, and renal failure was the main cause of death.[137] Glucocorticoid therapy resulted in improvement in some cases, but the overall mortality was not altered appreciably.[138] With the use of cytotoxic drugs in the treatment, the course of the disease has been altered favorably. Cyclophosphamide, azathioprine, methotrexate, chlorambucil, and nitrogen mustard have been used.[139] All have been relatively effective, but experience with cyclophosphamide has been the most extensive.[123] It is clear that cyclophosphamide is more effective than azathioprine in inducing a remission. It is used in doses of 2 mg per kg orally. Intermittent high-dose intravenous cyclophosphamide may not offer any advantage in achieving control of disease.[140] Azathioprine may be used in maintenance in those patients who have had an adverse reaction to cyclophosphamide.[123] Some patients with limited Wegener's granulomatosis may be controlled with trimethoprim-sulfamethoxazole alone.[141] In patients who have failed standard treatment, trimethoprim-sulfamethoxazole has been added, with control of disease in about 80 percent of cases. Exacerbations are noted after discontinuation of trimethoprim-sulfamethoxazole; consequently, once this drug is started, it probably should be continued indefinitely as suppressive therapy.

In patients with significant systemic features,

prednisone should be given concomitantly with cyclophosphamide in a dose of 1 mg per kg in divided doses. When the systemic features of disease are controlled, the prednisone can be tapered.

Despite the benefits of treatment with cyclophosphamide and prednisone, there is still significant disease and treatment-related morbidity. Morbidity from irreversible features of disease occurs in more than 80 percent, and side effects of treatment in more than 40 percent. In a recent review in Hoffman et al.[13] 7 percent died of their disease or complications of treatment.[141a]

Response to treatment can be judged by evaluation of the clinical features and the erythrocyte sedimentation rate or the C-reactive protein level. Relapses may occur and are usually successfully managed by increasing the cyclophosphamide and sometimes the prednisone, depending on the severity of the relapse.[123] Infectious complications, such as staphylococcal infections of the sinuses, can simulate a flare-up of Wegener's granulomatosis. Bacterial or viral infections can also exacerbate the inflammatory disease of Wegener's granulomatosis.[142] Maintenance cyclophosphamide should be continued for 1 year after control of symptoms, then gradually tapered.

Patients who have significant renal insufficiency due to Wegener's granulomatosis have a poor outcome, despite the use of cytotoxic agents and prednisone.[143] Those surviving with end-stage renal failure will require hemodialysis. A number of these patients whose disease was otherwise controlled have done well after renal transplantation.[144]

TAKAYASU'S ARTERITIS

The names used for this disease include aortic arch arteritis, aortitis syndrome, pulseless disease, brachiocephalic arteritis, and occlusive thromboarthropathy. Takayasu's arteritis affects large arteries and occurs primarily in children and young women. The aorta and its primary branches are involved most extensively. Varying degrees of narrowing, occlusion, or dilatation develop in the involved segments, leading to a wide range of symptoms.

Epidemiology. The prevalence and incidence are not accurately known. Cases have been described in countries in all parts of the world. The largest number of reports, however, have come from Japan. Nasu found 100 cases in slightly fewer than 300,000 autopsies registered in Japan over a 16-year period (0.03 percent).[145] In one study, the incidence of Takayasu's arteritis in whites was found to be 2.6 cases per million persons per year.[146] Eighty to 90 percent of cases occur in females. In the majority of instances, the onset of the disease is between the ages of 10 and 30 years.[147]

Pathogenesis. The cause remains obscure. Infections with spirochetes, tubercle bacilli, or streptococcal organisms have been suggested as causes, but there is little solid evidence for this. The presence of another connective tissue disease in occasional patients, elevated levels of globulins, and the finding of antiaorta antibodies in the serum of some patients with this condition have suggested an immunologic cause and possibly an autoimmune process. Ueda and coworkers[148] found antiaorta antibodies at a titer of 1:10 or higher in 21 of 34 patients with aortitis but in only 17 of 154 patients with other diseases. Collagenase treatment of aortic tissue that was used as substrate (antigen) resulted in reduced antiaorta antibody titers. HLA studies have detected an increased frequency of HLA-Bw52 in Asians.[149] HLA-Bw52 is in linkage disequilibrium with DR4. In North Americans, there is an increased frequency of MB3 and DR4 in patients with Takayasu's disease.[29] MB3 was present in all ten patients studied. These findings may indicate an inherited susceptibility to Takayasu's arteritis.

Pathology. The disease may be localized to the aortic arch or its branches, the ascending thoracic aorta, or the abdominal aorta, or it may involve the entire aorta.[145, 150] Postmortem examinations on patients who have Takayasu's arteritis have usually shown patchy or continuous involvement of all portions of the aorta, innominate, common carotid, and subclavian arteries. Changes in the subclavian and carotid arteries may be more extensive on the left side than on the right. Other arteries commonly affected include the vertebral, celiac, mesenteric, renal, pulmonary, iliac, and coronary arteries. The inflammatory processes cause thickening of the arterial wall, which is most pronounced in the aortic arch and its branches. Abnormalities of the aortic valve are found in one third of autopsy cases. Aortic valve leaflets may become distorted, with the edges being rolled and contracted. The aortic ring may become dilated and cause aortic insufficiency. Atheromatous changes in the intima are common but are usually mild.[151] Pulmonary artery involvement may also be found by angiography or at postmortem examination in some cases but produces clinical manifestations in only a minority of cases.[152]

Histologically, panarteritis is present in established cases. Early changes are found in the adventitia and outer part of the media. These include granulomatous inflammation with infiltration of lymphocytes, plasma cells, histiocyte cells, multinucleated giant cells, and occasionally polymorphonuclear leukocytes. Lymphocytes collect around the vasa vasorum. As the arteritis continues, the elastic fibers and smooth muscle cells in the media undergo fragmentation and necrosis. Pronounced intimal thickening occurs in areas with inflamed outer layers. The thickened intima and the contraction of the fibrotic media and adventitia cause narrowing or obliteration of the arterial lumen. Thrombosis commonly occurs in stenotic areas. Old areas of obstruction may recanalize. Dissections or aneurysms may form in areas where the arterial wall has been weakened by the inflammatory processes.

Clinical Features. In the early disease (prepulseless phase), systemic symptoms such as fatigue, weight loss, and low-grade fever are common.[153] Arthralgia or mild transient or persistent arthritis has been noted in half the patients.[154] In some cases, skin lesions resembling erythema nodosum are found that, on biopsy, show vasculitis involving small blood vessels.[155] Later (during the pulseless phase), evidence of vascular insufficiency due to large-artery narrowing or obstruction becomes apparent. Important findings on examination, which are present in most patients at some time, are tenderness, diminished pulsations, and bruits over one or more brachial, subclavian, or carotid arteries. The upper extremities become cool. Decreased lower extremity pulsations and femoral or abdominal bruits may also be present. Claudication of the extremities develops in many patients. Occlusions of the vessels may lead to ischemic ulcers on the extremities. Frequently, there is evidence of collateral circulation about the shoulders and elsewhere.

Hypertension is found in half or more of patients and can be caused by narrowing of the thoracic or abdominal aorta, decreased elasticity of the aortic wall, or renal artery involvement.[156] Blood pressure may be difficult to assess because the arteries are narrowed or occluded. It may be measured by using a wide cuff on the legs, by ophthalmodynamometry, or by direct measurements in the ascending aorta. Pulmonary arteritis leads to dyspnea, hemoptysis, and pulmonary hypertension.[157]

Vertigo, syncope, convulsions, dementia, headaches, and reduced visual acuity may occur from decreased cerebral blood flow as a result of obstructed arteries in the neck or because of hypertension. Advance retinopathy with preretinal hemorrhages and arteriovenous anastomoses around the disc occurs in patients with severe narrowing or occlusion of both common carotid and vertebral arteries. Symptoms are accentuated by physical activity. Abdominal pain, diarrhea, and gastrointestinal ischemia and hemorrhage result from mesenteric artery stenosis. Angina pectoris develops from coronary artery ostial narrowing.

Laboratory Tests. In cases of active disease, blood tests reflect the inflammatory processes.[158] In

Table 64–7. 1990 CRITERIA FOR THE CLASSIFICATION OF TAKAYASU ARTERITIS (TRADITIONAL FORMAT)*

Criterion	Definition
Age at disease onset ≤40 years	Development of symptoms or findings related to Takayasu arteritis at age ≤40 years
Claudication of extremities	Development and worsening of fatigue and discomfort in muscles of 1 or more extremities while in use, especially the upper extremities
Decreased brachial artery pulse	Decreased pulsation of 1 or both brachial arteries
BP difference >10 mm Hg	Difference of >10 mm Hg in systolic blood pressure between arms
Bruit over subclavian arteries or abdominal aorta	Bruit audible on auscultation over 1 or both subclavian arteries or abdominal aorta
Arteriogram abnormality	Arteriographic narrowing or occlusion of the entire aorta, its primary branches, or large arteries in the proximal upper or lower extremities, not due to arteriosclerosis, fibromuscular dysplasia, or similar causes; changes usually focal or segmental

*For purposes of classification, a patient with vasculitis shall be said to have Takayasu arteritis if at least 3 of these 6 criteria are present. The presence of any 3 or more criteria yields a sensitivity of 90.5% and a specificity of 97.8%. BP = blood pressure (systolic; difference between arms).

From Arend, W. P., et al.: The American College of Rheumatology 1990 Criteria for the Classification of Takayasu Arteritis. Arthritis Rheum. 33:1129, 1990; with permission.

most, moderate anemia is present, which is usually normochromic but may be hypochromic. The leukocyte count tends to be normal or slightly elevated. Hypoalbuminemia and increased levels of alpha₂ globulin, fibrinogen, and gamma globulin are commonly found. The erythrocyte sedimentation rate is typically high early in the disease, but may be normal after the inflammatory phase.

Diagnosis. Early diagnosis may be difficult, and it is often delayed for a year or more because the symptoms usually are nonspecific in the prepulseless phase of the disease.[154] The diagnosis depends on the recognition of symptoms of vascular ischemia and the finding of bruits or decreased pulses, and it is confirmed by arteriography (Table 64–7). The arteriographic changes are generally most pronounced in the region of the aortic arch and its primary branches, but instances in which changes were con-

fined to the abdominal aorta and its branches have been reported (Fig. 64–12). Typical arteriograms show vascular segments with smooth-walled, tapered, focal, or prolonged narrowing, with other areas of dilatation.

Treatment and Course. Glucocorticoids effectively suppress the systemic symptoms and are helpful in reversing arterial stenoses in the early stage of the disease.[154, 159] Pulses may improve rapidly, and ischemic symptoms such as claudication may be ameliorated. After fibrous tissue has been laid down and after thrombosis has occurred, the response is diminished. An initial daily dose of 45 to 60 mg of prednisone, or the equivalent, may be given. When the symptoms and the erythrocyte sedimentation rate are controlled, the dosage may be gradually reduced until the minimum dose that suppresses the disease is found. Use of a long-term, low-maintenance-dose

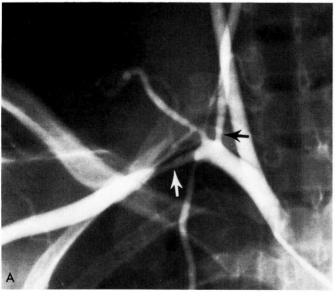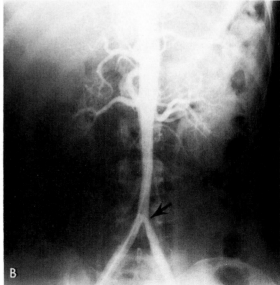

Figure 64–12. Arteries of aortic arch. *A,* Angiogram shows smooth-walled, tapered narrowing of right subclavian artery (*white arrow*). Vertebral and thyrocervical trunk arteries. *B,* Abdominal aorta shows smooth-walled tubular narrowing of middle and lower portions and constriction of left common iliac artery at its origin (*arrow*).

glucocorticoid may prevent progression of the disease. Alternate-day glucocorticoid therapy has not been evaluated. Anticoagulants and vasodilators have been used, but the effects are uncertain. Cytotoxic drugs have been prescribed, but the outcome is similar to the results when glucocorticoids are used alone.[154, 159] The addition of a cytotoxic drug to prednisone is probably necessary only rarely. Salicylates may help control systemic symptoms. Digitalis preparations and antihypertensive drugs may be indicated in certain instances. Arterial patch grafts, angioplasty, or bypass grafts may be considered in late cases when ischemic symptoms are not influenced by therapy with glucocorticoids.[154]

The course of Takayasu's arteritis tends to be prolonged, with possible intermittent exacerbations and an increasingly impaired circulation.[160] After a number of years, the inflammatory component may become less active and the systemic symptoms are replaced by those of vascular ischemia—the pulseless phase of the disease. A few patients have been observed to have spontaneous remissions, but others have been followed in whom there has apparently been continued activity for more than 20 years.[153] Death may occur as a result of congestive heart failure or cerebrovascular ischemia. Rupture of an aneurysm is not common. In one follow-up study of 54 patients, an 83 percent 5-year survival rate was observed.[160] In another study of 32 patients seen at the Mayo Clinic, the 5-year survival was 94 percent.[156] Severe hypertension, functional impairment, and cardiac involvement may indicate a poor prognosis.

KAWASAKI'S DISEASE (MUCOCUTANEOUS LYMPH NODE SYNDROME)

See Chapter 72.

COGAN'S SYNDROME

Cogan's syndrome is a rare disease affecting young people and characterized by the presence of nonsyphilitic interstitial keratitis, autovestibular symptoms, and frequently systemic features.[161] It may be associated with small, medium, and large-artery inflammation. The cause of the disease is unknown. The mean age at onset is 25 years, and the sex incidence is equal. The early eye symptoms include redness and photophobia. Vision may be affected. Ophthalmologic examination reveals interstitial keratitis and occasionally conjunctivitis and uveitis. Vertigo and tinnitus are frequent findings, and loss of hearing usually occurs and may be bilateral. Ataxia and nystagmus may be present. One half of the patients have nonspecific systemic manifestations, including fever, weight loss, and fatigue. One third of the patients have arthralgias and myalgias. Approximately 10 percent of the patients have features of vasculitis, with skin, peripheral nerve, visceral, or kidney involvement. Another 10 percent will develop aortic insufficiency and associated cardiac abnormalities.[162]

The most common laboratory abnormality is an elevated erythrocyte sedimentation rate. Patients may also have leukocytosis, anemia, and thrombocytosis. Audiograms and electronystagmography are usually abnormal and may be helpful in following the course of the disease. Angiographic studies may demonstrate abnormalities, frequently showing large-artery involvement.

Deafness occurs in over half the cases, and blindness may occur in 10 percent. Ten percent of the patients may die as a result of their disease.[163] Topical glucocorticoids are indicated for eye involvement. High doses of oral glucocorticoids are required for control of severe eye involvement, audiovisual symptoms, and systemic features of the disease. Cytotoxic agents may be considered in patients who have evidence of persistent inflammation despite adequate treatment with glucocorticoids. Aortic valve replacement and vascular bypass surgery may be necessary when inflammation is controlled.

BEHÇET'S DISEASE

In 1937, Behçet described a chronic relapsing syndrome of aphthous oral ulceration, genital ulceration, and a uveitis leading to blindness.[164] Additional features include arthritis, dermal infiltrates or vasculitis, meningitis, cerebral or systemic vasculitis, arterial aneurysms, phlebitis, and discrete gut ulcers.[165] The disease is more common and severe in the Mediterranean countries and Japan than in the United States.

Diagnostic Criteria. An international study group has proposed new diagnostic criteria.[166] Recurrent aphthous oral ulcers must exist with two of the following: recurrent genital ulcerations, uveitis or retinal vasculitis, cutaneous pustules or erythema nodosum, or cutaneous pathergy. This set of diagnostic criteria is weighted in the direction of nonspecific mucocutaneous lesions. Since North American patients seldom have cutaneous pathergy, in its place we may substitute any of the following: large-vessel vasculitis, meningoencephalitis, or cerebral vasculitis.[167] Incomplete forms of the syndrome pose problems in diagnosis. The combination of aphthous stomatitis and vulvar ulcerations in girls or young women may be a forme fruste of the disease or may be accompanied, after many years, by a more ominous internal lesion such as cerebral vasculitis. Many years may elapse between the onset of aphthous ulcers and the development of eye or neurologic disease.

Clinical Features. Aphthous oral ulcers (Fig. 64–13; see color section at the front of this volume) are usually the first and most persistent feature. They occur as 2- to 12-mm discrete, painful, round or oval red-rimmed single or multiple ulcers in crops on the

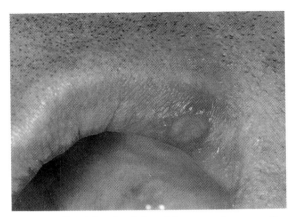

Figure 64–13. Painful oral aphtha of the upper lip; an erythematous border surrounds a necrotic yellow ulcer. (Courtesy of Dr. R. Rogers III.)

mucous membranes of the cheeks, tongue, palate, and pharynx. Lesions heal in 1 to 3 weeks, with little or no scarring. In a typical patient, the ulcers are to be found more than one half of the time.

Recurrent ulcers on the penis, scrotum, vulva, cervix, or vagina resemble the oral lesions and are usually painful. Their recurrence rate is less, typically three or four times per year.

Behçet's original description was of "hypopyon-uveitis."[164] Although this implies an anterior uveitis, it still carries a guarded prognosis for vision. Hypopyon (Fig. 64–14; see color section at the front of this volume) and other severe ocular lesions are less common in North American patients than in eastern Mediterranean patients.[168] Eye involvement may appear several years after the oral lesions begin. Both eyes participate in tandem episodes, but occasionally a previously uninvolved eye can suddenly lose sight many years after its counterpart. Eye inflammation is usually painless and ultimately affects both anterior and posterior chambers of the eye. Ordinarily, anterior uveitis is detected as cells in the anterior chamber by slit-lamp biomicroscopy. An ophthal-

mologic evaluation includes funduscopy, slit-lamp examinations of the anterior and posterior chambers, and indirect ophthalmoscopy.[168] Fluorescence angiograms may show staining of the retina and disc resulting from vascular permeability, implying vasculitis. Some Middle Eastern clinics report visual loss progressing to blindness within 4 to 10 years in a majority of patients.[169]

Erythema nodosum–like lesions, papules, pustules, folliculitis, and ulcers may be seen, and all are not specific. In general, skin findings are mild.

The pathergy response is a nodule or pustule, 3 to 10 mm, appearing 24 to 48 hours after puncture of the forearm skin with a sterile 20 gauge needle. This controversial reaction is seen in 25 to 75 percent of patients with Behçet's disease from the high prevalence countries but in fewer than 25 percent of North American patients.

About 40 percent of patients, if followed prospectively for 1 to 2 years, will be found to have synovitis.[170] The pattern is monoarticular or oligoarticular and involves knees, ankles, wrists, and hands. The synovitis is recurrent and seldom destructive and lasts for a few weeks. During attacks, synovial fluid has white blood cell counts in the range of 5000 to 35,000 cells per mm^3, mostly polymorphonuclear leukocytes.[171] Occasionally, sacroiliitis is evident on radiograph, and then only in HLA-B27–positive patients.

Headache, fever, and stiff neck with cerebrospinal fluid lymphocytosis implies meningitis.[172] Sooner or later focal neurologic deficits develop. The prevalence of neurologic lesions (30 percent) may be higher among North American than among Middle Eastern patients (5 to 10 percent). Magnetic resonance imaging (MRI) reveals a predilection of the disease for the periventricular white matter and brain stem.[173] Accordingly, clinical findings are corticospinal tract disease, cerebellar ataxia, and pseudobulbar palsy.[167] MRI is superior to computed tomography, even with contrast enhancement, in detecting these deep lesions. Arteritis may be demonstrated on cerebral angiography.[174] During active phases, the cerebrospinal fluid shows elevated total protein, elevated IgA and IgG, mononuclear pleocytosis, and an elevated IgM index, implying intrathecal immunoglobulin synthesis.[175] Between episodes, the cerebrospinal fluid is normal.

Venous occlusions affecting the venae cavae and their tributaries as well as extremity veins, superficial or deep, are detected in 7 to 37 percent of patients.[176] Pulmonary embolism is rare. Budd-Chiari syndrome from a hepatic vein occlusion extending from the inferior vena cava can present with ascites or frank liver failure. Dural vein thrombosis causes headache and elevated cerebrospinal fluid pressure and is proved by digital subtraction angiography.[177] Occlusions and aneurysms of large systemic arteries leading to limb ischemia, stroke, and myocardial infarction have been reported. Hemoptysis may occur owing to a pulmonary artery-to-bronchus fistula.

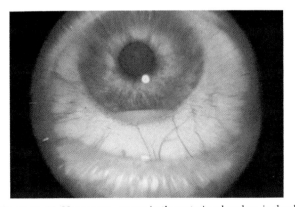

Figure 64–14. Hypopyon, or pus in the anterior chamber, is clearly shown as a yellow segment in front of the iris at 6 o'clock. Previously common in Behçet's disease, anterior uveitis of this severity is now uncommon. (Courtesy of Dr. Dennis Robertson.)

Such potentially fatal lesions can be detected by pulmonary angiogram.

Laboratory Findings. There are no laboratory indices that are diagnostic of Behçet's disease. Circulating immune complexes are found in the serum of more than half the patients and correlate with disease activity. Levels of serum complement are normal but drop during preactive phases. Cryoprecipitates in sera are rare. The level of interferon is higher in Behçet's disease patients than in control subjects. Acute phase reactants, such as erythrocyte sedimentation rate, are not very useful, especially in uveal disease, in which they may be normal. HLA-B51, a subset of HLA-B5, is more common in Behçet's disease patients than in control subjects.

Pathology. In the mouth, perivascular round cell infiltrates in the dermis infiltrate into the epidermis, causing necrosis and slough.[178] Biopsy of some ulcers may reveal a vasculitis, especially in the scrotum or vulva.[179] Enucleated eyes have revealed vasculitic occlusions of retinal veins and arteries. Erythema nodosum lesions display lymphocytes and monocytes and, at times, neutrophilic collections in the dermis and subcutaneous fat (i.e., a panniculitis). In the skin lesions, frank vasculitis may occasionally be present,[180, 181] and C_3 and IgM can be found in dermal vessels. Brain histology reveals vasculitis and perivasculitis of small cerebral arteries and veins. Old lesions seen at autopsy reveal gliosis and demyelination resembling multiple sclerosis. Lesions in the pulmonary arterial system may be a thromboangiitis or panarteritis with aneurysms. There may be lesions in the systemic circulation resembling polyarteritis nodosa as well as occlusive vasculopathy or aneurysms.

Differential Diagnosis. Crohn's disease of the colon can mimic Behçet's disease, even showing discrete colorectal and mucocutaneous ulcers. It differs by having histologic granulomatous enteritis, and central nervous system disease is rare. Mucous membrane pemphigoid and lichen planus are distinguished clinically and by biopsy. The hypereosinophilic syndrome may present with oral and genital ulcers and pronounced eosinophilia. Pseudo-Behçet's syndrome is a form of Munchausen's syndrome in which there is narcotic overuse, factitious skin or mucosal lesions, and multiple operations, but no ocular or central nervous system disease.

Treatment. The response to prednisone is disappointing, since neither ocular nor central nervous system disease is satisfactorily controlled.[167]

Topical applications of triamcinolone in pastes or gels palliate the pain of oral or genital ulcers. Dapsone, in doses of 50 to 100 mg per day, reduces orogenital ulcerations but causes hemolytic anemia. Thalidomide can have a remarkable benefit in mucosal lesions but is not generally available.[182]

Cytotoxic agents, especially the alkylating agents chlorambucil and cyclophosphamide, are the most effective. The disease is usually suppressed and, after chronic treatment, may remit entirely. Chlorambucil,

in a dose of 0.1 mg per kg per day, usually suppresses ocular or central nervous system lesions when used for 1 to 4 years in a dose sufficient to cause lymphopenia.[183] Concurrent prednisone is not needed or, if it is in use for central nervous system disease, can usually be withdrawn. The dose of chlorambucil is lowered as evidence of uveitis or retinal vasculitis recedes, usually manifesting as improved or stable visual acuity. Episodes of meningitis or cerebral vasculitis are also controlled.[172] Bolus therapy with cyclophosphamide or nitrogen mustard can quickly induce remission.[174] Seventy-three percent of forty chlorambucil-treated patients with eye or brain involvement showed inactive disease at 6 years.[183] Two patients acquired carcinomas and one a dysmyelopoietic syndrome. After a year's remission, it is usually possible to stop therapy. Complications include cytopenias, amenorrhea, and, occasionally, infections. Relapses may require reinstitution of therapy. Azathioprine is less effective in suppressing eye disease.[184]

Cyclosporine, beginning in doses of 10 mg per kg per day, was more effective than colchicine in suppressing ocular attacks in a Japanese study.[185] Maintenance treatment with 5.0 mg per kg per day or less is usually effective. These patients must be monitored for renal toxicity.

Surgical resection of perforating bowel lesions, cataracts, and arterial aneurysms may be required and are well tolerated. Anticoagulant therapy is hazardous, as bowel ulcers or pulmonary aneurysms may bleed. The small subset of patients having recurrent deep vein thrombosis are also being selected for immunosuppressive therapy, perhaps in conjunction with short-term heparin.

References

1. Kussmaul, A., and Maier, R.: Ueber eine bisher nicht beschriebene eigenthumliche Arterienerkrankung (Periarteritis nodosa), die mit Morbus Brightii und rapid fortschreitender allgemeiner Muskellahmung einhergeht. Dtsch. Arch. Klin. Med. 1:484, 1866.
2. Zeek, P. M.: Periarteritis nodosa: A critical review. Am. J. Clin. Pathol. 22:777, 1952.
3. Rose, G. A., and Spencer, H.: Polyarteritis nodosa. Q. J. Med. 26:43, 1957.
4. Alarcon-Segovia, D.: The necrotizing vasculitides: A new pathogenetic classification. Med. Clin. North Am. 61:241, 1977.
5. Hunder, G. G., and Lie, J. T.: The vasculitides. Clin. Cardiovasc. Dis. 13:261, 1983.
6. Conn, D. L., Dickson, E. R., and Carpenter, H. A.: The association of Churg-Strauss vasculitis with temporal artery involvement, primary biliary cirrhosis, and polychondritis in a single patient. J. Rheumatol. 9:744, 1982.
7. Fauci, A. S., Haynes, B. F., and Katz, P.: The spectrum of vasculitis: Clinical, pathologic, immunologic, and therapeutic considerations. Ann. Intern. Med. 89:660, 1978.
8. Lightfoot, R. W., Michel, B. A., Bloch, D.A., et al.: The American College of Rheumatology 1990 Criteria for the Classification of Polyarteritis Nodosa. Arthritis Rheum. 33:1088, 1990.
9. Masi, A. T., Hunder, G. G., Lie, J. T., et al.: The American College of Rheumatology 1990 Criteria for the Classification of Churg-Strauss Syndrome (Allergic Granulomatosis and Angiitis). Arthritis Rheum. 33:1094, 1990.
10. Leavitt, R. Y., Fauci, A. S., Bloch, D. A., et al.: The American College of Rheumatology 1990 Criteria for the Classification of Wegener's Granulomatosis. Arthritis Rheum. 33:1101, 1990.
11. Calabrese, L. H., Michel, B. A., Bloch, D. A., et al.: The American

College of Rheumatology 1990 Criteria for the Classification of Hypersensitivity Vasculitis. Arthritis Rheum. 33:1108, 1990.

12. Mills, J. A., Michel, B. A., Bloch, D. A., et al.: The American College of Rheumatology 1990 Criteria for the Classification of Henoch-Schönlein Purpura. Arthritis Rheum. 33:1114, 1990.

13. Hunder, G. G., Bloch, D. A., Michel, B. A., et al.: The American College of Rheumatology 1990 Criteria for the Classification of Giant Cell Arteritis. Arthritis Rheum. 33:1122, 1990.

14. Arend, W. P., Michel, B. A., Bloch, D. A., et al.: The American College of Rheumatology 1990 Criteria for the Classification of Takayasu Arteritis. Arthritis Rheum. 33:1129, 1990.

15. Rich, A. R.: The role of hypersensitivity in periarteritis nodosa: As indicated by seven cases developing during serum sickness and sulfonamide therapy. Bull. Johns Hopkins Hosp. 71:123, 1942.

16. Lawley, T. J., Bielory, L., Gascon, P., et al.: A prospective clinical and immunologic analysis of patients with serum sickness. N. Engl. J. Med. 311:1407, 1988.

17. Gocke, D. J., Hsu, K., Morgan, C., et al.: Association between polyarteritis and Australian antigen. Lancet 2:1149, 1970.

18. Gocke, D. J., Hsu, K., Morgan, C., et al.: Vasculitis in association with Australian antigen. J. Exp. Med. 134(Special Issue):330s, 1971.

19. Conn, D. L.: Polyarteritis. Rheum. Dis. Clin. North Am. 16(2):341, 1990.

20. Sanchez-Guerrero, J., Guiterrez-Urena, S., Vidaller, A., et al.: Vasculitis as a paraneoplastic syndrome. Report of 11 cases and review of the literature. J. Rheumatol. 17:1458, 1990.

21. Gabriel, S. E., Conn., D. L., Philiky, R. L., et al.: Vasculitis in hairy cell leukemia: Review of literature and consideration of possible pathogenic mechanisms. J. Rheumatol. 13:6, 1986.

22. Conn, D. L., McDuffie, F. C., Holley, K. E., et al.: Immunologic mechanisms in systemic vasculitis. Mayo Clin. Proc. 51:511, 1976.

23. Ronco, P., Verroust, P., Mignon, F., Lourilsky, O., et al.: Immunopathological studies of polyarteritis nodosa and Wegener's granulomatosis: A report of 43 patients with 51 renal biopsies. Q. J. Med. 52:212, 1983.

24. Cochrane, C. G., Weigle, W. O., and Dixon, F. J.: The role of polymorphonuclear leukocytes in the initiation and cessation of Arthus vasculitis. J. Exp. Med. 110:481, 1959.

25. Lockwood, C. M., Worlledge, S., Nicholas, A., et al.: Reversal of impaired splenic function in patients with nephritis or vasculitis (or both) by plasma exchange. N. Engl. J. Med. 300:524, 1979.

26. Smiley, J. D., and More, S. E., Jr.: Southwestern Internal Medicine Conference: Immune-complex vasculitis: Role of complement and IgG-Fc receptor functions. Am. J. Med. Sci. 298:267, 1989.

27. Sergent, J. S., Lockshin, M. D., Christian, C. L., et al.: Vasculitis with hepatitis B antigenemia: Long-term observations in nine patients. Medicine (Baltimore) 55:1, 1976.

28. Elkon, K. B., Sutherland, D. C., Rees, A. J., et al.: HLA-A antigens of patients with Wegener's granulomatosis. Tissue Antigens 11:129, 1978.

29. Volkman, D. J., Mann, D. L., and Fauci, A. S.: Association between Takayasu's arteritis and B-cell alloantigen in North Americans. N. Engl. J. Med. 306:464, 1982.

30. Woolf, A. D., Wakerley, G., Wallington, T. B., et al.: Factor VIII–related antigen in the assessment of vasculitis. Ann. Rheum. Dis. 46:441, 1987.

31. Kanaide, H., Takeshita, A., and Nakamura, M.: Etiologic aspects of coagulopathy in Takayasu's aortitis. Am. Heart J. 104:1039, 1982.

32. Burns, J. C., Glode, M. P., Clarke, S. H., et al.: Coagulopathy and platelet activation in Kawasaki syndrome: Identification of patients at the high risk of development of coronary artery aneurysms. J. Pediatr. 105:206, 1984.

33. Jordan, J. M., Allen, N. B., and Pizzo, S. V.: Defective release of tissue plasminogen activator in systemic and cutaneous vasculitis. Am. J. Med. 82:397, 1987.

34. Conn, D. L., McDuffie, F. C., and Dyck, P. J.: Immunopathologic study of sural nerves in rheumatoid arthritis. Arthritis Rheum. 15:135, 1972.

35. Michet, C. J.: Epidemiology of vasculitis. Rheum. Dis. Clin. North Am. 16(2):261, 1990.

36. Moskowitz, R. W., Baggenstoss, A. H., and Slocumb, C. H.: Histopathologic classification of periarteritis nodosa: A study of 56 cases confirmed at necropsy. Proc. Staff Meet. Mayo Clin. 38:345, 1963.

37. Arkin, A.: A clinical and pathological study of periarteritis nodosa: A report of five cases, one histologically healed. Am. J. Pathol. 6:401, 1930.

38. Sack, M., Cassidy, J. T., and Bole, G. G.: Prognostic factors in polyarteritis. J. Rheumatol. 2:411, 1975.

39. Diaz-Perez, J. L., and Winkelmann, R. K.: Cutaneous periarteritis nodosa. Arch. Dermatol. 110:407, 1974.

40. Cohen, R. D., Conn, D. L., and Ilstrup, D. M.: Clinical features, prognosis, and response to treatment in polyarteritis. Mayo Clin. Proc. 55:146, 1980.

41. Lovshin, L. L., and Kernohan, J. W.: Peripheral neuritis in periarteritis nodosa: A clinicopathologic study. Proc. Staff Meet. Mayo Clin. 24:48, 1949.

42. Ford, R. G., and Sieker, R. G.: Central nervous system manifestations of periarteritis nodosa. Neurology 15:114, 1965.

43. Ladefoged, J., Nielsen, B., Raaschou, F., et al.: Acute anuria due to polyarteritis nodosa. Am. J. Med. 46:827, 1969.

44. Wold, L. E., and Baggenstoss, A. H.: Gastrointestinal lesions of periarteritis nodosa. Proc. Staff Meet. Mayo Clin. 24:28, 1949.

45. Holsinger, D. R., Osmundson, P. J., and Edwards, J. E.: The heart in periarteritis nodosa. Circulation 25:610, 1962.

46. Kielar, R. A.: Exudative retinal detachment and scleritis in polyarteritis. Am. J. Ophthalmol. 48:1, 1952.

47. Morgan, C. J., and Harris, E. D., Jr.: Non-giant cell temporal arteritis: Three cases and a review of the literature. Arthritis Rheum. 21:362, 1978.

48. Ettlinger, R. E., Nelson, A. M., Burke, E. D., et al.: Polyarteritis nodosa in childhood. Arthritis Rheum. 22:820, 1979.

49. Duffy, J., Lidsky, M. D., Sharp, J. T., et al.: Polyarthritis, polyarteritis and hepatitis B. Medicine (Baltimore) 55:19, 1976.

50. Gorevic, P. D., Kassab, H. Y. J., Levo, Y., et al.: Mixed cryoglobulinemia: Clinical aspects and long-term follow-up of 40 patients. Am. J. Med. 69:287, 1980.

51. Trepo, C. G., Zuckerman, A. J., Bird, R. C., et al.: The role of circulating hepatitis B antigen/antibody immune complexes in the pathogenesis of vascular and hepatic manifestations in polyarteritis nodosa. J. Clin. Pathol. 27:863, 1974.

52. Luthra, H. S., McDuffie, F. C., Hunder, G. G., et al.: Immune complexes in sera and synovial fluids of patients with rheumatoid arthritis. J. Clin. Invest. 56:458, 1975.

53. Leib, E. S., Hibrawi, H., Chia, D., et al.: Correlation of disease activity in systemic necrotizing vasculitis with immune complexes. J. Rheumatol. 8:258, 1981.

54. Weiss, M. A., and Crissman, J. D.: Segmental necrotizing glomerulonephritis: Diagnostic, prognostic, and therapeutic significance. Am. J. Kidney Dis. 6:199, 1985.

55. Fisher, R. G., Graham, D. Y., Granmayeh, M., et al.: Polyarteritis nodosa and hepatitis-B surface antigen: Role of angiography in diagnosis. Am. J. Roentgenol. 129:77, 1977.

56. Ewald, E. A., Griffin, D., and McCuen, W. J.: Correlation of angiographic abnormalities with disease manifestations and disease severity in polyarteritis nodosa. J. Rheumatol. 14:952, 1987.

57. Travers, R. K., Allison, D. J., Brettle, R. P., et al.: Polyarteritis nodosa: A clinical and angiographic analysis of 17 cases. Semin. Arthritis Rheum. 8:184, 1979.

58. Mokri, B., Stanson, A. W., and Housen, O. W.: Spontaneous dissections of the renal arteries in a patient with previous spontaneous dissections of the internal carotid arteries. Stroke 16:959, 1985.

59. Fauci, A. S., Katz, P., Haynes, B. F., et al.: Cyclophosphamide therapy of severe systemic necrotizing vasculitis. N. Engl. J. Med. 301:235, 1979.

60. Leib, E. S., Restivo, C., and Paulus, H. E.: Immunosuppressive and corticosteroid therapy of polyarteritis nodosa. Am. J. Med. 67:941, 1979.

61. Guillevin, L., Du, L. T. H., Godeau, P., et al.: Clinical findings and prognosis of polyarteritis and Churg-Strauss angiitis: A study in 165 patients. Br. J. Rheumatol. 27:258, 1988.

62. Neild, G. H., and Lee, H. A.: Methylprednisolone pulse therapy in the treatment of polyarteritis nodosa. Postgrad. Med. J. 53:381, 1977.

63. Chalopin, J. M., Rifle, G., Turc, J. M., et al.: Immunological findings during successful treatment of HbsAg-associated polyarteritis nodosa by plasmapheresis alone. Br. Med. J. 280:368, 1980.

64. Baggenstoss, A. H., Shick, R. M., and Polley, H. F.: The effect of cortisone on the lesions of periarteritis nodosa. Am. J. Pathol. 27:537, 1951.

65. Conn, D. L., Tompkins, R. B., and Nichols, W. L.: Glucocorticoids in the management of vasculitis—a double-edged sword? J. Rheumatol. 15:1181, 1988.

66. Scott, D. G. I., Bacon, P. A., and Tribe, C. R.: Systemic rheumatoid vasculitis: A clinical and laboratory study of 50 cases. Medicine 60:288, 1981.

67. Lakhanpal, S., Conn, D. L., and Lie, J. T.: Clinical and prognostic significance of vasculitis as an early manifestation of connective tissue disease syndromes. Ann. Intern. Med. 101:743, 1984.

68. Conn, D. L., and McDuffie, F. C.: Neuropathy: The pathogenesis of rheumatoid neuropathy (Session III). In Organic Manifestations and Complications in Rheumatoid Arthritis (Symposium Hernstein). Stuttgart-New York, F. K. Schattauer Verlag, November 2–5, 1975.

69. Scott, D. G. I., Bacon, P. A., Allen, C., et al.: IgG rheumatoid factor, complement, and immune complexes in rheumatoid synovitis and vasculitis: Comparative and serial studies during cytotoxic therapy. Clin. Exp. Immunol. 43:54, 1981.

70. Kemper, J. W., Baggenstoss, A. H., and Slocumb, C. H.: The relationship of therapy with cortisone to the incidence of vascular lesions in rheumatoid arthritis. Ann. Intern. Med. 46:831, 1957.

71. Vollertsen, R. S., Conn, D. L., Ballard, D. J., et al.: Rheumatoid vasculitis: Survival and associated risk factors. Medicine 65:365, 1986.

72. Sokoloff, L., and Bunim, J. J.: Vascular lesions in rheumatoid arthritis. J. Chronic Dis. 5:668, 1957.
73. Bywaters, E. G. L.: Peripheral vascular obstruction in rheumatoid arthritis and its relationship to other vascular lesions. Ann. Rheum. Dis. 16:84, 1957.
74. Segal, R.: Accelerated nodulosis and vasculitis during methotrexate therapy for rheumatoid arthritis. Arthritis Rheum. 31:1182, 1988.
75. Abel, T., Andrews, B. S., Cunningham, P. H., et al.: Rheumatoid vasculitis: Effect of cyclophosphamide on the clinical course and levels of circulating immune complexes. Ann. Intern. Med. 93:407, 1980.
76. Scott, D. G. I., Bacon, P. A., Bothamley, J. E., et al.: Plasma exchange in rheumatoid vasculitis. J. Rheumatol. 8:433, 1981.
77. Zeek, P. M., Smith, C. C., and Weeter, J. C.: Studies on periarteritis nodosa. III. The differentiation between the vascular lesions of periarteritis nodosa and hypersensitivity. Am. J. Pathol. 24:889, 1948.
78. Gilliam, J. N., and Smiley, J. D.: Cutaneous necrotizing vasculitis and related disorders. Ann. Allergy 37:328, 1976.
79. Green, J. M., Langley, S., Edwards, N. L., et al.: Vasculitis associated with malignancy: Experience with 13 patients and literature review. Medicine 67:220, 1988.
80. Soter, N. A., Mihm, M. C., Gigli, I., et al.: Two distinct cellular patterns in cutaneous necrotizing angiitis. J. Invest. Dermatol. 66:344, 1976.
81. Smaller, B. R., McNutt, S., and Conireras, F.: The natural history of vasculitis: What histopathology tells us about pathogenesis. Arch. Dermatol. 126:84, 1990.
82. Sams, W. M., Jr., Mihm, M. C., Gigli, I., et al.: Leukocytoclastic vasculitis. Arch. Dermatol. 112:219, 1976.
83. Zax, R. H., Hodge, S. J., and Cullen, J. P.: Cutaneous leukocytoclastic angiitis serial histopathologic evaluation demonstrates the dynamic nature of the infiltrate. Arch. Dermatol. 126:69, 1990.
84. Mullick, F. G., McAllister, H. A., Jr., Wagner, B. M., et al.: Drug-related vasculitis: Clinicopathologic correlations in 30 patients. Hum. Pathol. 10:313, 1979.
85. Farley, T. A., Gillespie, S., Rasoulpour, M., et al.: Epidemiology of a cluster of Henoch-Schönlein purpura. Am. J. Dis. Child. 143:798, 1989.
86. Levy, M., Broyer, M., Arsan, A., et al.: Anaphylactoid purpura nephritis in childhood: Natural history and immunopathology. Adv. Nephrol. 6:183, 1976.
87. Agnello, V.: Complement deficiency states. Medicine 57:1, 1978.
88. Cream, J. J., Gumpel, J. M., and Peachey, R. D. G.: Schönlein-Henoch purpura in the adult: A study of 77 adults with anaphylactoid or Schönlein-Henoch purpura. Q. J. Med. 39:461, 1970.
89. Roth, D. A., Wilz, D. R., and Theil, G. B.: Schönlein-Henoch syndrome in adults. Q. J. Med. 55:145, 1985.
90. Allen, D. M., Diamond, L. K., and Howell, D. A.: Anaphylactoid purpura in children (Schönlein-Henoch syndrome): Review with a follow-up of the renal complications. Am. J. Dis. Child. 99:833, 1960.
91. McDuffie, F. C., Sams, W. M., Jr., Maldonado, J. E., et al.: Hypocomplementemia with cutaneous vasculitis and arthritis: Possible immune complex syndrome. Mayo Clin. Proc. 48:340, 1973.
92. Wisnieski, J. J., and Naff, G. B.: Serum IgG antibodies to C1q in hypocomplementemic urticarial vasculitis syndrome. Arthritis Rheum. 32:1119, 1989.
93. Schwartz, H. R., McDuffie, F. C., Black, L. F., et al.: Hypocomplementemic urticarial vasculitis: Association with chronic obstructive pulmonary disease. Mayo Clin. Proc. 57:231, 1982.
94. LoSpalluto, J., Dorward, B., Miller, W., Jr., et al.: Cryoglobulinemia based on interaction between a gamma macroglobulin and 75 gamma globulin. Am. J. Med. 32:142, 1962.
95. Meltzer, M., Franklin, E. C., Elias, K., et al.: Cryoglobulinemia—a clinical and laboratory study. II. Cryoglobulins with rheumatoid factor activity. Am. J. Med. 40:837, 1966.
96. Boom, B. W., Brand, A., Bavinck, J., et al.: Severe leukocytoclastic vasculitis of the skin in a patient with mixed cryoglobulinemia treated with high-dose gammaglobulin intravenously. Arch. Dermatol. 124:1550, 1988.
97. Churg, J., and Strauss, L.: Allergic granulomatosis, allergic angiitis, and periarteritis nodosa. Am. J. Pathol. 27:277, 1951.
98. Chumbley, L. C., Harrison, E. G., Jr., and DeRemee, R. A.: Allergic granulomatosis and angiitis (Churg-Strauss syndrome): Report and analysis of 30 cases. Mayo Clin. Proc. 52:477, 1977.
99. Lanham, J. G., Elkon, K. B., Pusey, C. D., et al.: Systemic vasculitis with asthma and eosinophilia: A clinical approach to the Churg-Strauss syndrome. Medicine 63:65, 1984.
100. Dicken, C. H., and Winkelmann, R. K.: The Churg-Strauss granuloma: Cutaneous, necrotizing, palisading granuloma in vasculitis syndromes. Arch. Pathol. Lab. Med. 102:576, 1978.
101. Dyck, P. J., Conn, D. L., and Okazaki, H.: Necrotizing angiopathic neuropathy: Three-dimensional morphology of fiber degeneration related to sites of occluded vessels. Mayo Clin. Proc. 47:461, 1972.
102. Klinger, H.: Grenzformen der Periarteritis nodosa. Frankfurt, Ztschr. Pathol. 42:455, 1931.
103. Wegener, F.: Uber eine eigenartige rhinogene Granulomatose mit

besonderer Beteiligung des Arteriensystems und der Nieren. Beitr. Pathol. Anat. Allg. Pathol. 102:36, 1939.
104. Godman, G. C., and Churg, J.: Wegener's granulomatosis: Pathology and review of the literature. Arch. Pathol. 58:533, 1954.
105. Carrington, C. B., and Liebow, A. A.: Limited forms of angiitis and granulomatosis of Wegener's type. Am. J. Med. 41:497, 1966.
106. Fauci, A. S., and Wolff, S. M.: Wegener's granulomatosis: Studies in eighteen patients and a review of the literature. Medicine (Baltimore) 52:535, 1973.
107. Specks, U., and DeRemee, R. A.: Granulomatous vasculitis: Wegener's granulomatosis and Churg-Strauss syndrome. Rheum. Dis. Clin. North Am. 16(2):377, 1990.
108. Scott, D. G. I., Bacon, P. A., Elliott, P. J., et al.: Systemic vasculitis in a district general hospital 1972–1980: Clinical and laboratory features, classification, and prognosis of 80 cases. Q. J. Med. 103:292, 1982.
109. Horn, R. G., Fauci, A. S., Rosenthal, A. S., et al.: Renal biopsy pathology in Wegener's granulomatosis. Am. J. Pathol. 74:423, 1974.
110. Howell, S. B., and Epstein, W. V.: Circulating immunoglobulin complexes in Wegener's granulomatosis. Am. J. Med. 60:259, 1976.
111. Conn, D. L., Gleich, G. J., DeRemee, R. A., et al.: Raised serum immunoglobulin E in Wegener's granulomatosis. Ann. Rheum. Dis. 35:17, 1976.
112. Shillitoe, E. J., Lehner, T., Lessof, M. H., et al.: Immunological features of Wegener's granulomatosis. Lancet 1:281, 1974.
113. Niinaka, T., Okochi, T., Watanabe, Y., et al.: Chemotactic defect in Wegener's granulomatosis. J. Med. 8:161, 1977.
114. Dale, D. C., Fauci, A. S., and Wolff, S. M.: The effect of cyclophosphamide on leukocyte kinetics and susceptibility to infection in patients with Wegener's granulomatosis. Arthritis Rheum. 16:657, 1973.
115. Katz, P., Alling, D. W., Haynes, B. F., et al.: Association of Wegener's granulomatosis with HLA-B8. Clin. Immunol. Immunopathol. 14:268, 1979.
116. Wolff, S. M., Fauci, A. S., Horn, R. G., et al.: Wegener's granulomatosis. Ann. Intern. Med. 81:513, 1974.
117. Fienberg, R.: The protracted superficial phenomenon in pathergic (Wegener's) granulomatosis. Hum. Pathol. 12(5):458, 1981.
118. Mark, E. J., Matsubara, O., Tan-Liu, N. S., et al.: The pulmonary biopsy in the early diagnosis of Wegener's (pathergic) granulomatosis: A study based on 35 open lung biopsies. Hum. Pathol. 19:1065, 1988.
119. Jaffe, E. S., Lipford, E. H., Jr., Margolick, J. B., et al.: Lymphomatoid granulomatosis and angiocentric lymphoma: A spectrum of post-thymic T-cell proliferations. Semin. Respir. Med. 10:167, 1989.
120. Haynes, B. F., Fishman, M. L., Fauci, A. S., et al.: The ocular manifestations of Wegener's granulomatosis: Fifteen years experience and review of the literature. Am. J. Med. 63:131, 1977.
121. Hu, C. H., O'Loughlin, S., and Winkelmann, R. K.: Cutaneous manifestations of Wegener's granulomatosis. Arch. Dermatol. 113:175, 1977.
122. Sahn, E. E., and Sahn, S. A.: Wegener's granulomatosis with aphasia. Arch. Intern. Med. 136:87, 1976.
123. Fauci, A. S., Haynes, B. F., Katz, P., et al.: Wegener's granulomatosis: Prospective clinical and therapeutic experience with 85 patients for 21 years. Ann. Intern. Med. 98:76, 1983.
124. Maguire, R., Fauci, A. S., Doppman, J. L., et al.: Unusual radiographic findings in Wegener's granulomatosis. Am. J. Roentgenol. 130:233, 1978.
125. Rosenberg, D. M., Weinberger, S. E., Fulmer, J. D., et al.: Functional correlates of lung involvement in Wegener's granulomatosis. Am. J. Med. 69:387, 1980.
126. Lampman, J. H., Querubin, R., and Kondapalli, P.: Subglottic stenosis in Wegener's granulomatosis. Chest 79:230, 1981.
127. Drachman, D. A.: Neurological complications of Wegener's granulomatosis. Arch. Neurol. 8:45, 1963.
128. DeRemee, R. A., McDonald, T. J., and Weiland, L. H.: Aspekte zur Therapie und Verlaufsbeobachtungen der Wegenerschen Granulomatose. Med. Welt. 38:470, 1987.
129. Hind, C. R. K., Winearls, C. G., Lockwood, C. M., et al.: Objective monitoring of activity in Wegener's granulomatosis by measurement of serum C-reactive protein concentration. Clin. Nephrol. 21:341, 1984.
130. Davies, D. J., Moran, J. E., Niall, J. F., et al.: Segmental necrotizing glomerulonephritis with antineutrophil antibody: Possible arbovirus aetiology? Br. Med. J. 285:606, 1982.
131. Hall, J. B., Wadham, B. M. N., Wood, C. J., et al.: Vasculitis and glomerulonephritis: A subgroup with an antineutrophil cytoplasmic antibody. Aust. N. Z. J. Med. 14:277, 1984.
132. van der Woude, F. J., Labatto, S., Permin, H., et al.: Autoantibodies against neutrophils and monocytes: Tool for diagnosis and marker of disease activity in Wegener's granulomatosis. Lancet 1:425, 1985.
133. Falk, R. L., and Jennette, J. C.: Anti-neutrophil cytoplasmic autoantibodies with specificity for myeloperoxidase in patients with systemic vasculitis and idiopathic necrotizing and crescentic glomerulonephritis. N. Engl. J. Med. 318:1651, 1988.
134. Goldschmeding, R., van der Schoot, C. E., ten Bokkel Huinink, D., et al.: Wegener's granulomatosis autoantibodies identify a novel diiso-

propylfluorophosphate-binding protein in the lysosomes of normal human neutrophils. J. Clin. Invest. 84:1577, 1989.

135. Nolle, B., Specks, U., Ludemann, J., et al.: Anticytoplasmic autoantibodies: Their immunodiagnostic value in Wegener's granulomatosis. Ann. Intern. Med. 11:28, 1989.

136. Savage, C. O. S., Winearls, C. G., Evans, D. J., et al.: Prospective study of radioimmunoassay for antibodies against neutrophil cytoplasm in diagnosis of systemic vasculitis. Lancet 1:1389, 1987.

137. Hollander, D., and Manning, R. T.: The use of aklylating agents in the treatment of Wegener's granulomatosis. Ann. Intern. Med. 67:393, 1967.

138. Raitt, J. W.: Wegener's granulomatosis: Treatment with cytotoxic agents and adrenocorticoids. Ann. Intern. Med. 74:344, 1971.

139. Novack, S. N., and Pearson, C. M.: Cyclophosphamide therapy in Wegener's granulomatosis. N. Engl. J. Med. 284:938, 1971.

140. Hoffman, G. S., Leavitt, R. Y., Fleisher, T. A., et al.: Treatment of Wegener's granulomatosis with intermittent high-dose intravenous cyclophosphamide. Am. J. Med. 89:403, 1990.

141. DeRemee, R. A.: The treatment of Wegener's granulomatosis with trimethoprim/sulfamethoxazole: Illusion or vision? Current controversies in rheumatology. Arthritis Rheum. 31(8):1068, 1988.

141a. Wegener Granulomatosis: An Analysis of 158 Patients.

142. Pinching, A. J., Rees, A. J., Pussell, B. A., et al.: Relapses in Wegener's granulomatosis: The role of infection. Br. Med. J. 281:836, 1980.

143. Pinching, A. J., Lockwood, C. M., Pussell, B. A., et al.: Wegener's granulomatosis: Observations on 18 patients with severe renal disease. Q. J. Med. 52:435, 1983.

144. Kuross, S., Davin, T., and Kjellstrand, C. M.: Wegener's granulomatosis with severe renal failure: Clinical course and results of dialysis and transplantation. Clin. Nephrol. 16:172, 1981.

145. Nasu, T.: Takayasu's truncoarteritis in Japan: A statistical observation of 76 autopsy cases. Pathol. Microbiol. (Basel) 43:140, 1975.

146. Ishikawa, K.: Natural history and classification of occlusive thromboaortopathy (Takayasu's disease). Circulation 57:27, 1978.

147. Lupi-Herrera, E., Sanchez-Torres, G., Marcushamer, J., et al.: Takayasu's arteritis: Clinical study of 107 cases. Am. Heart J. 93:94, 1977.

148. Ueda, H., Saito, Y., Ito, I., Yamaguchi, H., et al.: Further immunological studies of aortitis syndrome. Jpn. Heart J. 12:1, 1971.

149. Isohisa, I., Numano, F., Maezawa, H., et al.: HLA-Bw52 in Takayasu's disease. Tissue Antigens 12:246, 1978.

150. Committee on Study of Arteritis: Clinical and pathological studies of aortitis syndrome. Jpn. Heart J. 9:76, 1968.

151. Cipriano, P. R., Silverman, J. F., Perlroth, M. G., et al.: Coronary arterial narrowing in Takayasu's aortitis. Am. J. Cardiol. 39:744, 1977.

152. Sharma, S., Kamalakar, T., Rajani, M., et al.: The incidence and patterns of pulmonary involvement in Takayasu arteritis. Clin. Radiol. 42:177, 1990.

153. Strachan, R. W.: The natural history of Takayasu's arteriopathy. Q. J. Med. 33:57, 1964.

154. Hall, S., Barr, W., Lie, J. T., et al.: Takayasu arteritis. A study of 32 North American patients. Medicine 64:89, 1985.

155. Perniciaro, C. V., Winkelmann, R. K., and Hunder, G. G.: Cutaneous manifestations of Takayasu's arteritis. A clinicopathologic correlation. J. Am. Acad. Dermatol. 17:998, 1987.

156. Ask-Upmark, E.: On the pathogenesis of the hypertension in Takayasu's syndrome. Acta Med. Scand. 169:467, 1961.

157. Lupi, H. E., Sanchez, T. G., Horwitz, S., et al.: Pulmonary artery involvement in Takayasu's arteritis. Chest 67:69, 1975.

158. Fraga, A., Mintz, G., Valle, L., et al.: Takayasu's arteritis: Frequency of systemic manifestations (study of 22 patients) and favorable response to maintenance steroid therapy with adrenocorticosteroids (12 patients). Arthritis Rheum. 15:617, 1972.

159. Shelhamer, J. H., Volkman, D. J., Parriollo, J. E., et al.: Takayasu's arteritis and its therapy. Ann. Intern. Med. 103:121, 1985.

160. Subramanyan, R., Joy, J., and Bolokrishnan, K. G.: Natural history of aortoarteritis (Takayasu's disease). Circulation 80:429, 1989.

161. Cogan, D. G.: Syndrome of nonsyphilitic interstitial keratitis and vestibuloauditory symptoms. Arch. Ophthalmol. 33:144, 1945.

162. Vollertsen, R. S., McDonald, T. J., Younge, B. R., et al.: Cogan's syndrome: 18 cases and a review of the literature. Mayo Clin. Proc. 61:344, 1986.

163. Haynes, B. F., Kaiser-Kupper, M. I., Mason, P., et al.: Cogan syndrome: Studies in thirteen patients, long-term follow-up and a review of the literature. Medicine 59:426, 1980.

164. Behçet, H.: Uber rezidivierende aphthose, durch ein virus verusachte geschwure am mund. am auge und an den genitalien. Derm. Wschr. 105:1151, 1937.

165. Plotkin, G. R.: Miscellaneous clinical manifestations. In Plotkin, G. R., Calabro, J. J., and O'Duffy, J. D. (eds.): Behçet's Disease: A Contemporary Synopsis. New York, Futura Publishing Company, 1988.

166. International Study Group for Behçet's Disease: Criteria for diagnosis of Behçet's disease. Lancet 335:1078, 1990.

167. O'Duffy, J. D., and Goldstein, N. P.: Neurologic involvement in seven patients with Behçet's disease. Am. J. Med. 61:170, 1976.

168. Colvard, D. M., Robertson, D. M., and O'Duffy, J. D.: The ocular manifestations of Behçet's disease. Arch. Ophthalmol. 95:1813, 1977.

169. BenEzra, D., and Cohen, E.: Treatment and visual prognosis in Behçet's disease. Br. J. Ophthalmol. 70:589, 1986.

170. Yurkadul, S., Yazici, H., Tuzun, Y., et al.: The arthritis of Behçet's disease: A prospective study. Ann. Rheum. Dis. 42:505, 1983.

171. Caporn, N., Higgs, E. R., Dieppe, P. A., et al.: Arthritis in Behçet's syndrome. Br. J. Radiol. 56(662):87, 1983.

172. O'Duffy, J. D., Robertson, D. M., and Goldstein, N. P.: Chlorambucil in the treatment of uveitis and meningoencephalitis of Behçet's disease. Am. J. Med. 76:75, 1984.

173. Willeit, J., Schmutzhard, E., Aichner, F., et al.: CT and MR imaging in neuro-Behçet's disease. J. Comput. Assist. Tomogr. 10(2):313, 1986.

174. Zenlenski, J. D., Capraro, J. A., Holden, D., et al.: Central nervous system vasculitis in Behçet's syndrome: Angiographic improvement after therapy with cytotoxic agents. Arthritis Rheum. 32(2):217, 1989.

175. Hirohata, S., Takeuchi, A., and Miyamoto, T.: Association of cerebrospinal fluid IgM index with central nervous system involvement in Behçet's disease. Arthritis Rheum. 29(6):793, 1986.

176. Wechsler, B., Piette, J. C., Conard, J., et al.: Les thromboses veineuses profondes dans la maladie de Behçet's: 106 localisations sur une serie de 177 malades. Presse Med. 16(14):661, 1987.

177. Harper, C. M., O'Neill, C. P., O'Duffy, J. D., et al.: Intracranial hypertension in Behçet's disease: Demonstration of sinus occlusion with use of digital subtraction angiography. Mayo Clin. Proc. 60(6):419, 1985.

178. Lehner, T.: Progress report: Oral ulceration in Behçet's syndrome. Gut 18:491, 1977.

179. O'Duffy, J. D., Carney, J. A., and Deodhar, S.: Behçet's disease: Report of 10 cases: 3 with manifestations. Ann. Intern. Med. 75:561, 1971.

180. Su, W. P. D., Chun, S. I., Lee, S., et al.: Erythema nodosum–like lesions in Behçet's syndrome. A histopathologic study of 30 cases. In O'Duffy, J. D., and Kokmen, E. (eds.): Behçet's Disease: Basic and Clinical Aspects. Proceedings of the Fifth International Conference on Behçet's Disease. New York, Marcel Dekker, Inc., 1992, pp. 229–240.

181. O'Duffy, J. D.: Vasculitis in Behçet's disease. Rheum. Dis. Clin. North Am. 16:423, 1990.

182. Jorizzo, J. L., Schmalstieg, F. C., Solomon, A. R., et al.: Thalidomide effects in Behçet's syndrome and pustular vasculitis. Arch. Intern. Med. 146:878, 1986.

183. Matteson, E. L., and O'Duffy, J. D.: Treatment of Behçet's disease with chlorambucil. In O'Duffy, J. D., and Kokmen, E. (eds.): Behçet's Disease: Basic and Clinical Aspects. Proceedings of the Fifth International Conference on Behçet's Disease. New York, Marcel Dekker, Inc., 1992, pp. 575–580.

184. Yazici, H., Pazarli, H., Barnes, C. G., et al.: A controlled trial of azathioprine in Behçet's disease. N. Engl. J. Med. 322(5):281, 1990.

185. Masuda, K., Nakajima, A., et al.: Double-masked trial of cyclosporin versus colchicine and long-term open study of cyclosporin in Behçet's Disease. Lancet 1:1093, 1989.

Giant Cell Arteritis and Polymyalgia Rheumatica

INTRODUCTION

A close relationship exists between giant cell arteritis and polymyalgia rheumatica. However, the precise nature of the association is not known. Both conditions affect the same patient population and frequently occur in the same individual. Some investigators have suggested that polymyalgia rheumatica is a manifestation of arteritis, whereas others have taken the view that the two are separate processes frequently occurring together. Because the association between giant cell arteritis and polymyalgia rheumatica has been documented by many authors, these two conditions are discussed together in this chapter.

DEFINITIONS

Giant Cell Arteritis. Giant cell arteritis[1] is also referred to as temporal arteritis,[2] cranial arteritis,[3] and granulomatous arteritis.[4] Nearly all patients are older than 50 years of age when the disease develops. The inflammatory lesions in giant cell arteritis involve the cranial branches of the arteries originating from the arch of the aorta most prominently, but they may be more widespread.

Polymyalgia Rheumatica. Polymyalgia rheumatica, a term suggested by Barber,[5] is a clinical syndrome characterized by aching and morning stiffness in the proximal portions of the extremities and torso. Definitions have commonly included the presence of symptoms in two of the three commonly affected areas (shoulder girdle, hip girdle, and neck) for 1 month or longer, plus evidence of a systemic reaction, such as an erythrocyte sedimentation rate elevation to above 40 or 50 mm in 1 hour by the Westergren method.[6, 7] Some definitions have also included a rapid response to small doses of glucocorticoids, such as 10 mg of prenisone daily.[8, 9] The presence of another specific disease, such as rheumatoid arthritis, chronic infection, polymyositis, and malignancy, excludes the diagnosis of polymyalgia rheumatica.

EPIDEMIOLOGY

Giant cell arteritis appears to be relatively common in Europe and in the United States. Reported annual incidence rates have varied from 0.49 to 23.3 per 100,000 persons aged 50 years and older.[10–18] Among the population of Olmsted County, Minnesota, 94 cases were identified over a 34-year period,[18] these representing an average annual incidence rate of 17.0 cases per 100,000 population aged 50 years and older, and a prevalence of persons with a history of giant cell arteritis of 223 per 100,000 population aged 50 years and older. The incidence increased during the 25 years of the study, from 6.2 per 100,000 population per year from 1950 to 1959, to 24.1 per 100,000 population per year from 1980 to 1985, representing either an increased awareness of this disease in the later years or an increased frequency. The age-specific incidence rate increased from 2.6 per 100,000 in the age group 50 to 59 years to 44.7 per 100,000 in the age group 80 and older. In a Danish county in 1982 an incidence rate of 23.3 per 100,000 persons older than 50 years of age was observed for biopsy-proven arteritis.[14] An increased incidence with age has been noted in the Scandinavian studies, similar to that in Minnesota.[12, 14]

Autopsy studies suggest that giant cell arteritis may be more common than is clinically apparent. Östberg found arteritis in 1.6 percent of 889 postmortem cases in which sections of the temporal artery and two transverse sections of the aorta were made.[19]

Polymyalgia rheumatica, when considered as the primary process, has been less well studied but appears to be more common than giant cell arteritis.[20] In Olmsted County, Minnesota, over a 10-year period from 1970 through 1979, 97 cases were found, providing an average annual incidence rate of 53.7 cases per 100,000 persons aged 50 and older.[21] The prevalence of polymyalgia rheumatica (active plus remitted cases) was approximately 500 per 100,000 persons aged 50 and older.[21]

ETIOLOGY AND PATHOGENESIS

A variety of causes have been suggested for polymyalgia rheumatica and giant cell arteritis, but none has been substantiated. Although the increasing incidence of giant cell arteritis and polymyalgia rheumatica after the age of 50 years implies a relationship to aging, the meaning of this observation is not understood. A number of reports of familial aggregation and an apparent increased frequency of these conditions in northern Europe and in persons in the United States with similar ethnic backgrounds suggest a genetic or hereditary predisposition.[22–24] In several studies of HLA antigens in polymyalgia rheumatica and giant cell arteritis, HLA-DR4 appears to be associated with these conditions more commonly than would be expected by chance alone.[25–27]

Both the humoral and the cellular immune systems have been implicated in the pathogenesis. The granulomatous histopathology of giant cell arteritis has suggested the presence of a cell-mediated immune reaction directed at antigens in or near elastic tissue in the arterial walls.[11, 28, 29] Tests of cellular immunity in patients with giant cell arteritis and polymyalgia rheumatica have shown no consistent abnormality.[30]

Immunoglobulins and complement deposits have been demonstrated intracellularly and adjacent to the internal elastic lamina in some involved temporal arteries.[31, 32] These deposits may represent antibodies to arterial wall antigens or immune complexes deposited from blood. Leukocyte elastase has been noted along the elastic lamina also.[33] However, the specificity of the deposits and correlation with the inflammatory lesions need to be defined further. Reduced peripheral blood cytotoxic/suppressor T cells have been found in similar patients.[34, 35] Interleukin-6 activity has been found to be increased in sera from patients with polymyalgia rheumatica and giant cell arteritis, which declined in most patients after treatment.[36]

Sera from patients with giant cell arteritis, polymyalgia rheumatica, or both have been found to contain increased levels of circulating immune complexes during active disease.[37] Immune complex concentrations showed a positive correlation with the erythrocyte sedimentation rate and gamma globulin levels and dropped to normal levels after treatment or resolution of the inflammatory response.

PATHOLOGY

In giant cell arteritis, inflammation is found most often in vessels that originate from the arch of the aorta, but almost any artery of the body may be affected occasionally as well as some veins.[19, 38] The inflammation tends to affect the arteries in a segmental or patchy fashion, but long portions of arteries may be involved.[39] In patients who died during the active phase of giant cell arteritis, the highest incidence of severe involvement was noted in the superficial temporal arteries, vertebral arteries, and ophthalmic and posterior ciliary arteries.[28] The internal carotid, external carotid, and central retinal arteries were affected somewhat less frequently.[28] In other post-mortem studies lesions were found commonly in the proximal and distal aorta and internal and external carotid, subclavian, brachial, and abdominal arteries.[10, 40] Intracranial arteries are involved infrequently.[28] In some instances, follow-up biopsy or autopsy surveys have shown persistence of mild chronic inflammation even though symptoms had resolved.[41]

In early cases or in regions of arteries with minimal involvement, collections of lymphocytes may be confined to the region of the internal or external elastic lamina or adventitia. Intimal thickening, with prominent cellular infiltration, is usually present. In areas with more marked involvement, all layers are affected (Fig. 65–1). Necrosis of portions of the arterial wall (including the elastic laminae) and granulomas containing multinucleated histiocytic and foreign body giant cells, histiocytes, lymphocytes (which are predominantly T helper cells), and some plasma cells and fibroblasts are found.[42–44] Interdigitating reticulum cells and cells with interleukin-2 receptor expression have been observed.[43] Eosinophils may be seen, but polymorphonuclear leukocytes are rare.[44] Thrombosis may develop at sites of active inflammation; later, these areas may recanalize. The inflammatory process is usually most marked in the inner portion of the media adjacent to the internal elastic lamina. Fragmentation and disintegration of elastic fibers occur, closely associated with an accumulation of giant cells (Fig. 65–2). However, giant cells are not seen in all sections and, therefore, are not required for the diagnosis if other features are compatible. Fibrinoid necrosis seen in necrotizing arteritis is less common.[44] The more sections that are examined in the area of arteritis, the more likely it is that giant cells will be found.[11]

Aside from vasculitis, when present, there has been relatively little found pathologically in polymyalgia rheumatica. Granulomatous myocarditis and hepatitis have been noted.[45–47] Muscle biopsies have been normal or have shown nonspecific type II muscle atrophy.[48] However, a number of reports

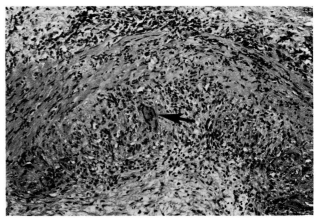

Figure 65–1. Giant cell arteritis. In transverse section of temporal artery, adventitia is at top and intima is at central portion of bottom. Multinucleated giant cell (*arrow*) is present at junction of media and intima. There is extensive disruption of all layers of vessel wall. Hematoxylin of eosin, × 100. (Courtesy of Dr. J. T. Lie.)

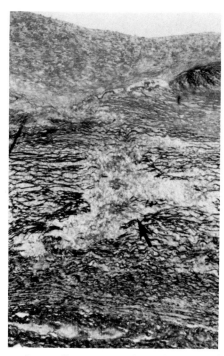

Figure 65–2. Giant cell arteritis involving the proximal aorta in a patient dying of a ruptured ascending aorta. This section of the ascending aorta is distal to the ruptured portion and shows destruction of elastic fibers (*arrow*). Elastic van Gieson stain, × 64. Neighboring sections stained with hematoxylin and eosin showed infiltrations of mononuclear leukocytes in the areas of disrupted fibers.

Table 65–1. INITIAL MANIFESTATION IN 100 PATIENTS WITH GIANT CELL ARTERITIS

Headache	32
Polymyalgia rheumatica	25
Fever	15
Visual symptoms without loss	7
Weakness/malaise/fatigue	5
Tenderness over arteries	3
Myalgias	4
Weight loss/anorexia	2
Jaw claudication	2
Permanent loss of vision	1
Tongue claudication	1
Sore throat	1
Vasculitis on angiogram	1
Stiffness of hands and wrists	1
	Total 100

Data from Calamia, K. T., and Hunder, G. G.: Clin. Rheum. Dis. 6:389, 1980.

are shown in Tables 65–1 and 65–2. Headache is probably the most common symptom and is present in two thirds or more of patients.[55] It usually begins early in the course of the disease and is commonly an initial symptom. The pain is frequently marked, boring, or lancinating in quality and is often localized

Table 65–2. GIANT CELL ARTERITIS: CLINICAL FINDINGS IN 100 PATIENTS

Finding	Number
Sex (female/male)	69/31
Duration of manifestations before diagnosis (months)*	7 (1–48)
Onset (gradual/sudden)	64/36
Weight loss or anorexia	50
Malaise, fatigue, or weakness	40
Fever	42
Polymyalgia rheumatica	39
Other musculoskeletal pains	30
Synovitis	15
Symptoms related to arteries	83
Headache	68
Visual symptoms	
Transient	
Fixed	16
Jaw claudication	14
Swallowing claudication or dysphagia	45
Tongue claudication	8
Limb claudication	6
Signs related to arteries	4
Artery tenderness	66
Decreased temporal artery pulsations	27
Erythematous, nodular, or swollen scalp arteries	46
Large artery bruits	23
Decreased large artery pulses	21
Ophthalmologic	7
Visual loss	20
Ophthalmoscopic	14
Extraocular muscle weakness	18
Raynaud's phenomenon	2
Central nervous system abnormalities	3
Sore throat	15
	9

Data from Calamia, K. T., and Hunder, G. G.: Clin. Rheum. Dis. 6:389, 1080.
*Shown as mean with range in parentheses.

have shown the presence of lymphocytic synovitis in the knees, sternoclavicular joints, and shoulders and evidence of a similar reaction in sacroiliac joints.[49–53] Synovitis (mostly subclinical) has been shown in bone scans demonstrating an increased uptake of technetium pertechnetate in the joints of 24 of 25 patients with polymyalgia rheumatica.[50]

CLINICAL FEATURES

The mean age at onset of giant cell arteritis and polymyalgia rheumatica is approximately 70 years, with a range of about 50 to more than 90 years of age. Younger patients have been reported, but these are atypical. Women are affected about twice as often as men.[54]

The onset may be abrupt or insidious, but in most instances the symptoms have been present for weeks or months before the diagnosis is established. Constitutional symptoms, including fatigue, anorexia, and weight loss, are present in the majority of patients and may be an early or even an initial finding.

Giant Cell Arteritis. The majority of patients with giant cell arteritis have symptoms related to the arteries at some time during the course of the illness. However, the presenting symptoms vary widely. The initial manifestations and clinical findings in 100 patients with giant cell arteritis seen consecutively to the regions along the arteries of the scalp, but it may be less well defined. Headaches may be severe even when the cranial arteries are normal to palpation and may subside even though the disease activity continues.

Scalp tenderness is a common symptom in patients and especially in those with headache. Usually tenderness is localized to the temporal or occipital arteries, but it may be diffuse (Fig. 65–3). Tender spots or nodules may be present for several days over any part of the scalp.

Visual symptoms are common and include diplopia, ptosis, and transient or permanent, partial or complete blindness. Visual loss is generally caused by ischemia of the optic nerve or tracts secondary to arteritis of the branches of the ophthalmic or posterior ciliary arteries and, less commonly, is caused by occlusion of the retinal arterioles.[28, 56] Rarely, arterial lesions cause infarction of the occipital cortex with visual loss. The early funduscopic appearance seen in blindness is ischemic optic neuritis with slight pallor and edema of the optic disc and scattered cotton-wool patches and small hemorrhages (Fig. 65–4). Later, optic atrophy occurs. Blindness may be the initial symptom but tends to follow other symptoms by several weeks or months. Visual impairment may fluctuate initially, but once established, the visual

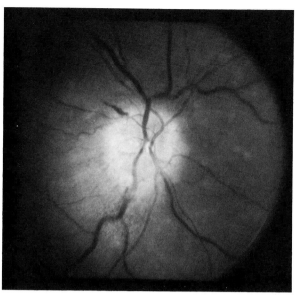

Figure 65–4. Ophthalmoscopic view of the acute phase of ischemic optic neuropathy as seen in patients with giant cell arteritis and loss of vision. The optic disc is pale and swollen, the retinal veins are dilated, and a flame-shaped hemorrhage is visible. (Courtesy of Dr. J. Trautmann.)

deficit is usually permanent. Visual loss may be unilateral or bilateral. If present on one side initially, involvement in the contralateral eye often occurs within 1 or 2 weeks if treatment is not started. Ophthalmoscopic examination in patients without eye involvement is generally normal. In recent reports, the incidence of blindness has been 20 percent or less.[9, 20, 41, 55, 57, 58] Older studies often listed an incidence of 40 to 60 percent of visual loss. The lower incidence of blindness today may reflect earlier recognition (in those patients without eye symptoms) and treatment. In a series of 166 patients, permanent visual loss occurred in 14, and transient visual impairment (amaurosis fugax) in 17. Permanent visual loss was preceded by transient loss in only 2 of 14 patients, and thus amaurosis fugax is not a strong predictor of blindness.[58]

Intermittent claudication may occur in the muscles of mastication (jaw claudication), the extremities, and occasionally the muscles of the tongue or those involved in swallowing. In the jaw muscles, the discomfort is noted especially when chewing meat and may involve the muscles on one side of the mandible more than those on the other. In some instances, however, facial artery involvement results in spasm of the jaw muscles. More marked vascular narrowing may, rarely, lead to gangrene of an extremity, the scalp, or the tongue.

Neurologic problems occur in approximately 30 percent of patients.[58] These are diverse, but most common are neuropathies and transient ischemic attacks or strokes. The former include mononeuropathies and peripheral polyneuropathies and may affect the upper or lower extremities. Presumably they are secondary to involvement of nutrient arte-

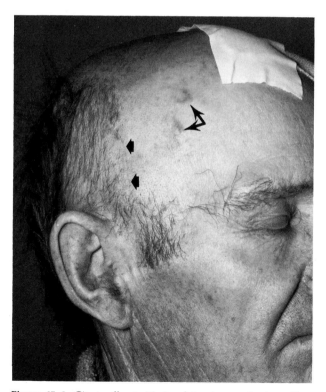

Figure 65–3. Giant cell arteritis involving temporal artery. Short segments of curved artery were erythematous and tender (*long arrows*). Bandage on scalp is over similar artery that was biopsied and showed giant cell arteritis. Previous biopsy of a proximal segment of right temporal artery, which was normal on physical examination, was normal histologically. Faint scar of this biopsy can be seen above and anterior to right ear (*short arrows*).

ries, but little pathologic documentation is available. Hemiparesis or brainstem events are due to narrowing or occlusion of the carotid or vertebrobasilar artery.

Prominent respiratory tract symptoms occur in about 10 percent of patients.[59] These include cough with or without sputum, sore throat, and hoarseness. When these symptoms are severe or an initial manifestation of giant cell arteritis, they may direct the attention of the examining physician away from the underlying arteritis. The vasculitis may induce these symptoms by causing ischemia or hyperirritability of the affected tissues.

Clinical evidence of large artery involvement is present in 10 to 15 percent of cases.[37] The findings are upper extremity claudication; bruits over the carotid, subclavian, axillary, and brachial arteries; absent or decreased pulses in the neck or arms; and Raynaud's phenomenon (Fig. 65–5). In some instances, aortic dissection and rupture occur. Angiographic features that suggest giant cell arteritis are smooth-walled arterial stenoses or occlusions alternating with areas of normal or increased caliber in the absence of irregular plaques and ulcerations, located especially in the carotid, subclavian, axillary, and brachial arteries.[53]

Angina pectoris, congestive heart failure, and myocardial infarction secondary to coronary arteritis have been reported.[60] A low-grade fever is present in as many as half the patients.[20] Approximately 15 percent of patients present with "fever of unknown origin," with a temperature frequently higher than 39°C.[9, 47] Patients may experience shaking chills coincident with fever spikes. The temperature curve does not follow a single or characteristic pattern.

Polymyalgia Rheumatica. As is the case in giant cell arteritis, patients are characteristically in good health before developing polymyalgia rheumatica. Systemic manifestations, such as low-grade fever and weight loss, are present in more than half the patients

and may be the initial symptoms. High, spiking fevers are uncommon in polymyalgia rheumatica in the absence of giant cell arteritis, however.[21] Arthralgias and myalgias may develop abruptly or evolve insidiously over several weeks or months.[6] Malaise, fatigue, and depression, along with aching and stiffness, may be present for months before the diagnosis is made. In the majority of patients, the shoulder girdle is the first to become symptomatic. In the remainder, the hips or neck are involved at the onset. The discomfort may begin in one shoulder or hip but usually becomes bilateral within weeks and may involve most of the proximal limb, axial musculature, and tendinous attachments. Morning stiffness and "gelling" after inactivity are usually prominent. Morning stiffness, characteristic of that in rheumatoid arthritis, is accentuated by minimal movement of the joints of affected regions. If the symptoms are severe, aching is more persistent. Although movement of the joints accentuates the pain, it is often felt in the proximal extremities rather than in the joints.[55] Pain at night is common, and movement during sleep may awaken the patient. Muscular strength is generally unimpaired, although the pain with movement makes interpretation of muscle testing difficult. Pain with movement also makes it difficult for patients to get out of bed or the bathtub. In the later stages of the syndrome, muscle atrophy may develop, and contacture of the shoulder capsule may result in limitation of passive motion as well as active motion.

As noted earlier, the presence of synovitis in polymyalgia rheumatica has been described by many but not all authors and is undoubtedly the cause of many of the findings in this condition.[61] A careful examination may reveal transient synovitis of the knees and sternoclavicular joints. The shoulders and hips are covered by heavy muscles, and minimal effusions of slight synovitis are not palpable on physical examination. Synovitis has been documented by biopsies, synovial analysis, and joint scintiscans.[6, 21, 50, 51, 53]

RELATIONSHIP BETWEEN POLYMYALGIA RHEUMATICA AND GIANT CELL ARTERITIS

It was suggested by Paulley and Hughes[62] that the symptoms of polymyalgia rheumatica might be an expression of an underlying arteritis that was not always clinically evident. Alestig and Barr[63] supported this observation when they found temporal arteritis in patients with polymyalgia rheumatica who had no symptoms or signs of vasculitis. In several reports of giant cell arteritis, polymyalgia rheumatica has been noted in about 40 to 60 percent of patients and was the initial symptom complex in 20 to 40 percent.[54] Conversely, in series of patients with polymyalgia rheumatica, giant cell arteritis has been found in 0 to 80 percent of cases.[54] The cause of this latter variability is uncertain but may be explained in

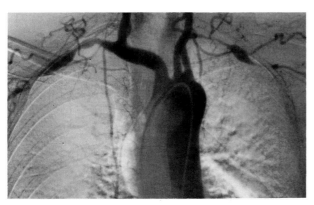

Figure 65–5. Giant cell arteritis of large arteries. Arch aortogram. Both subclavian and axillary arteries are affected. Smooth-walled segmental constrictions alternate with areas of normal caliber or aneurysmal dilation. (From Klein, R. G., et al.: Large artery involvement in giant cell [temporal] arteritis. Ann. Intern. Med. 83:806, 1975. Reprinted by permission of Annals of Internal Medicine.)

part by selection of cases. In some series temporal artery biopsies were done infrequently, or only small artery segments were taken which may not have included an inflamed area. In other studies, biopsies were done when giant cell arteritis was suspected on the basis of symptoms. This inevitably increased the frequency of diagnosis of arteritis. In an epidemiologic study in Olmsted County, Minnesota, in which all diagnosed cases of polymyalgia rheumatic over a 10-year period were studied, 15 percent were considered to have giant cell arteritis.[21] Although the incidence of giant cell arteritis in patients with polymyalgia rheumatica who have no symptoms or signs of arteritis may differ from one population to another, positive temporal artery biopsies will be found in perhaps 10 to 15 percent. Thus, most patients with biopsy-proven giant cell arteritis have symptoms related to artery involvement in addition to musculoskeletal aching.

Polymyalgia rheumatica may begin before, appear simultaneously with, or develop after the symptoms related to the arteries. Mild aching and stiffness may persist for months or years after other findings of giant cell arteritis have remitted. Aside from the symptoms related to arteries themselves, few differences have been noted between patients with polymyalgia rheumatica who have been shown to have giant cell arteritis and those whose temporal artery biopsies are normal.[41]

Although it is tempting to conclude that the musculoskeletal symptoms are related to vasculitis, good evidence for this is lacking. Many patients with giant cell arteritis do not have polymyalgia rheumatica, even when large vessels such as the subclavian, axillary, and brachial arteries are clinically involved. In addition, the finding of joint swelling in some patients argues that polymyalgia rheumatica may be a particular form of proximal synovitis. It has been speculated that a single etiologic factor may educe two pathologic processes, both arteritis and synovitis. The varied clinical and pathologic manifestations that develop (giant cell arteritis, polymyalgia rheumatica, or both) would be the result perhaps of genetic susceptibility or other factors.

LABORATORY STUDIES

Except for the findings on arterial biopsy, laboratory results in polymyalgia rheumatica and giant cell arteritis are similar.[41] A mild to moderate normochromic anemia is usually present in both diseases during their active phases. Leukocyte and differential counts are generally normal. A markedly elevated erythrocyte sedimentation rate is characteristic of both. Levels of over 100 mm in 1 hour (Westergren method) are common, but occasionally untreated biopsy-proven cases of giant cell arteritis or polymyalgia rheumatica may have normal or nearly normal erythrocyte sedimentation rates. Platelet counts are often increased.

Nonspecific changes in plasma proteins are often present and include a decrease in the concentration of albumin and an increase in alpha$_2(\alpha)$-globulins, fibrinogen, and other acute phase reactant proteins. Slight increases in gamma globulins and complement may be present.[64] Tests for antinuclear antibodies and rheumatoid factor are generally negative.

Tests measuring liver function have been found to be mildly abnormal in approximately one third of patients with giant cell arteritis and slightly less in polymyalgia rheumatica.[21, 55] An increased alkaline phosphatase level is the most common abnormality, but increases in aspartate aminotransferese and prolonged prothrombin time may also be found.[65] Liver biopsies are generally normal; granulomatous hepatitis has been observed.[46, 47]

Renal function and urinalysis are usually normal. Red blood cell casts are found in some instances, but their presence does not correlate with clinical large artery involvement.[37]

Levels of serum creatine kinase and other enzymes reflecting muscle damage are normal. Electromyograms have usually been reported to be normal, and muscle biopsy shows normal histology or only the mild atrophy characteristic of disuse.[48]

In the relatively few synovial fluid analyses reported in giant cell arteritis or polymyalgia rheumatica, there has been evidence of mild inflammation, including a poor mucin clot and synovial fluid leukocyte counts varying from 1000 to 20,000 cells per mm^3, with 40 to 50 percent polymorphonuclear leukocytes.[51] Synovial fluid complement levels usually have been normal.[66] In some instances, synovial biopsy has shown lymphocytic synovitis.[49–51]

Factor VIII/von Willebrand's factor levels have been found to be elevated in patients with giant cell arteritis and polymyalgia rheumatica.[67, 68] Values are highest in active giant cell arteritis, but the concentrations do not closely follow changes in the erythrocyte sedimentation rate or other clinical parameters of disease activity. These findings indicate that factor VIII is not simply a measure of inflammation but may be related in some way to the degree of vascular damage.

DIAGNOSIS

The diagnosis of giant cell arteritis should be considered in any patient older than 50 years of age who has a new form of headache, transient or sudden loss of vision, polymyalgia rheumatica, unexplained prolonged fever or anemia, and high erythrocyte sedimentation rate. Because the manifestations may vary in severity or may be transient, patients suspected of having this disease must be questioned carefully about recent as well as current symptoms. The arteries of the head, neck, upper torso, and arms should be examined for tenderness, enlargement, thrombosis, and bruits. Diagnostic artery biopsy is recommended in all patients suspected of having

Table 65–3. 1990 CRITERIA FOR THE CLASSIFICATION OF GIANT CELL (TEMPORAL) ARTERITIS (TRADITIONAL FORMAT)*

Criterion	Definition
1. Age at disease onset ≥50 years	Development of symptoms or findings beginning at age 50 or older
2. New headache	New onset of or new type of localized pain in the head
3. Temporal artery abnormality	Temporal artery tenderness to palpation or decreased pulsation, unrelated to arteriosclerosis of cervical arteries
4. Elevated erythrocyte sedimentation rate	Erythrocyte sedimentation rate ≥50 mm/hour by the Westergren method
5. Abnormal artery biopsy	Biopsy specimen with artery showing vasculitis characterized by a predominance of mononuclear cell infiltration or granulomatous inflammation, usually with multinucleated giant cells

*For purposes of classification, a patient with vasculitis shall be said to have giant cell (temporal) arteritis if at least 3 of these 5 criteria are present. The presence of any 3 or more criteria yields a sensitivity of 93.5% and a specificity of 91.2%.

From Hunder, G. G., et al.: The American College of Rheumatology 1990 Criteria for the Classification of Giant Cell Arteritis. Arthritis Rheum. 33:1125, 1990. Reprinted by permission of Arthritis and Rheumatism.

giant cell arteritis. The temporal artery is biopsied frequently, but a specimen of the occipital or facial artery can also be taken for histologic study. Because the involvement may be focal, a symptomatic or clinically abnormal segment of the artery should be chosen for biopsy (see Fig. 65–3). If the temporal artery is clearly abnormal on physical examination, only a small specimen needs to be removed for histopathologic inspection. But when the extracranial arteries are normal and giant cell arteritis is suspected, it is important to biopsy a segment of a temporal artery of several centimeters and to examine histologic sections at several levels and consider a contralateral biopsy if the first side is normal. Ocular pneumoplethysmography may help in the diagnosis of giant cell arteritis. In one study, patients with a positive temporal artery biopsy had a lower calculated ocular blood flow than that of patients with visual symptoms due to other diseases.[69] An angiographic examination of the aortic arch and its branches should be performed in patients with symptoms or findings of large artery involvement (see Fig. 65–4).[70]

Temporal artery biopsies should be performed in patients with polymyalgia rheumatica who have symptoms or findings suggesting the presence of giant cell arteritis. If clinical evidence for giant cell arteritis is absent, the decision regarding artery biopsy is often more difficult and should be based on the findings in each patient. If symptoms are mild and of recent onset or are stable and of long duration (e.g., a year or longer in duration without current or previous evidence of arteritis), it may be possible to follow the patient closely without biopsy. Blindness is uncommon in such patients. Opinions are divided about the prognostic significance of a negative temporal artery biopsy.[71] In one study, 88 patients with negative temporal artery biopsies were followed up after a mean period of 56 months. The negative biopsy predicted the absence of both clinical giant cell arteritis and the need for glucocorticoid treatment in 78, or about 90 percent.[72]

Generally there is little difficulty in distinguishing giant cell arteritis, polyarteritis, hypersensitivity vasculitis, and Wegener's granulomatosis because of the different distribution of lesions, histopathology, and organ involvement. However, in occasional cases these forms of necrotizing vasculitis appear to involve the temporal artery, and in rare instances there is some overlapping histopathology.[73, 74] Occasionally jaw or arm claudication may be present in patients with primary systemic amyloidosis with vascular involvement.[75]

Giant cell arteritis can be distinguished from isolated angiitis of the central nervous system, Takayasu's arteritis, and other similar arteritides by the age of the patient and the distribution of lesions, even though the histopathologic findings and roentgenologic findings may be indistinguishable at times (see Chapter 64). Recently, criteria for the classification of giant cell arteritis have been formulated. These criteria differentiate this arteritis from other forms of vasculitis and should be used in any study on this disease (Table 65–3).[76]

The diagnosis of polymyalgia rheumatica is clinical and depends on eliciting the symptoms and findings noted earlier. Polymyalgia rheumatica can usually be differentiated from late-onset rheumatoid arthritis by the absence of prominent peripheral joint pain and swelling. However, some patients with findings of polymyalgia rheumatica develop persistent joint swelling, which is consistent with a diagnosis of rheumatoid factor–negative rheumatoid arthritis, and occasionally giant cell arteritis occurs in patients with seropositive rheumatoid arthritis.[77, 78] In patients with polymyositis, the muscular weakness is the predominant factor limiting movement, whereas in patients with polymyalgia rheumatica pain causes limited function. In addition, in polymyositis, levels of muscle enzymes are elevated, and electromyograms are abnormal. Although patients with neoplasms may have generalized musculoskeletal aching, there is no association between polymyalgia rheumatica and malignancy, and a search for an underlying tumor is not necessary unless some clinical evidence for a tumor is present. Some patients with chronic infections, such as bacterial endocarditis, may have findings simulating polymyalgia rheumatica, and blood cultures should be obtained in patients with fever. Patients with functional myalgias usually do not have typical morning stiffness and have laboratory tests that are normal or nearly so.

TREATMENT AND COURSE

Once the diagnosis of giant cell arteritis is established, glucocorticoid treatment should be instituted. In patients strongly suspected of having giant cell arteritis, especially those with impending vascular complications such as visual loss, therapy may be started immediately or after a hemoglobin and erythrocyte sedimentation rate are obtained. Steroid treatment alters the histopathologic picture, but in most instances inflammatory changes are still recognizable for several days after glucocorticoids have been started. If the temporal (or other) artery biopsies show no arteritis, but the clinical suspicion of arteritis is strong as a result of vascular symptoms or findings, a trial of glucocorticoid treatment still may be instituted. An initial amount of 40 to 60 mg of prednisone or equivalent, in divided daily doses, is adequate in nearly all cases. If desired, an initial larger dose or two can be given parenterally. If the patient does not respond promptly, the dose should be increased. Intravenous pulse methylprednisolone can be tried in patients with recent visual loss. The effective starting dose should be continued until all reversible symptoms and findings have gone and laboratory tests have reverted to normal. This usually occurs within 2 to 4 weeks. After that, the dose can be gradually reduced by a maximum of 10 percent of the total daily dose each week or every 2 weeks. The reduction program is gauged by the symptoms and blood tests. The erythrocyte sedimentation rate is generally the most convenient and helpful laboratory test in following patients. The hemoglobin, albumin, and α_2-globulin concentrations may also be used but are somewhat less sensitive indicators of disease activity. Other acute phase reactants have been advocated and can be used to follow the course of the arteritis.[79] At some point in the reduction program, the erythrocyte sedimentation rate may rise above normal once again, and further reductions of prednisone may be temporarily interdicted. Subsequent reductions may have to be smaller and to be made at longer intervals. It is not uncommon to find that it is necessary to continue doses of 15 to 25 mg or more of prednisone daily for several months before making further reductions. Gradual reductions allow the identification of the minimal suppressive dose and also help avoid "exacerbations" resulting from too rapid withdrawal of prednisone. Spontaneous recrudescences occur, however, in an unpredictable fashion. Generally, these occur during the first 2 years of the disease.

Giant cell arteritis runs a self-limited course over several months to several years, commonly 1 or 2 years, and eventually the glucocorticoids can be reduced and discontinued in most patients.[11] A small proportion of patients appear to need low doses of prednisone for several years or more in order to control musculoskeletal symptoms. Alternate-day glucocorticoid therapy is less effective than daily administration and cannot be depended on to control acute symptoms.[55] It may be tried, however, in patients who have developed disturbing side effects from daily treatment. The effects of cytotoxic drugs, dapsone, antimalarials, and penicillamine or other drugs have not been studied in a systematic fashion in this disease but may be considered in cases not responding to glucocorticoids.

In patients with polymyalgia rheumatica without vascular symptoms or signs and especially in those who have temporal artery biopsies that are normal, nonsteroidal drugs may be tried. Salicylates and the nonsteroidal anti-inflammatory drugs adequately control symptoms in some patients with milder symptoms.[21] If the patients do not respond satisfactorily in 2 to 4 weeks, 5 to 15 mg daily doses of prednisone, or equivalent, may be started. These amounts usually result in rapid improvement of the musculoskeletal aching and stiffness but may not suppress an underlying arteritis if it is present. Thus, the patient must be followed carefully even though the aching improves. In patients with polymyalgia rheumatica, the dose should be reduced gradually as soon as symptoms permit. The erythrocyte sedimentation rate generally returns to normal more slowly with small doses of glucocorticoids than that observed with 40 to 60 mg per day. If the laboratory tests become normal while the patient is receiving the smaller doses, the likelihood of an underlying active vasculitis would seem to be much less, and the risk of vascular complications smaller. However, this does not hold in all instances, because active arteritis has been observed even though the sedimentation rate was improved.[80]

References

1. Gilmour, J. R.: Giant-cell arteritis. J. Pathol. Bacteriol. 53:263, 1941.
2. Horton, B. T., Magath, T. B., and Brown, G. E.: An undescribed form of arteritis of the temporal vessels. Proc. Staff Meet. Mayo Clin. 7:700, 1982.
3. Kilbourne, E. D., and Woliff, H. H.: Cranial arteritis: A critical evaluation of the syndrome of "temporal arteritis" with report of a case. Ann. Intern. Med. 24:1, 1946.
4. McMillan, G. C.: Diffuse granulomatous aortitis with giant cells: Associated with partial rupture and dissection of the aorta. Arch. Pathol. 49:63, 1950.
5. Barber, H. S.: Myalgic syndrome with constitutional effects: Polymyalgia rheumatica. Ann. Rheum. Dis. 16:230, 1957.
6. Hunder, G. G., Disney, T. F., and Ward, L. E.: Polymyalgia rheumatica. Mayo Clin. Proc. 44:849, 1969.
7. Healey, L. A., Parker, F., and Wilske, K. R.: Polymyalgia rheumatica and giant cell arteritis. Arthritis Rheum. 14:138, 1971.
8. Dixon, A. St. J., Beardwell, C., Kay, A., Wanka, J., and Wong, Y. T.: Polymyalgia rheumatica and temporal arteritis. Ann. Rheum. Dis. 25:203, 1966.
9. Healey, L. A., and Wilske, K. R.: The Systemic Manifestations of Temporal Arteritis. New York, Grune & Stratton, 1978.
10. Hamrin, B.: Polymyalgia arteritica. Acta Med. Scand. (Suppl.) 533:1, 1972.
11. Huston, K. A., Hunder, G. G., Lie, J. T., Kennedy, R. H., and Elveback, L. R.: Temporal arteritis: A 25-year epidemiologic, clinical and pathologic study. Ann. Intern. Med. 88:162, 1978.
12. Nordborg, E., and Bengtsson, B.-A.: Epidemiology of biopsy-proven giant cell arteritis (GCA). J. Intern. Med. 227:233, 1990.

13. Jonasson, F., Cullen, J. F., and Elton, R. A.: Temporal arteritis: A 14-year epidemiologic, clinical and prognostic study. Scot. Med. J. 24:111, 1979.
14. Boesen, P., and Sorensen, S. F.: Giant cell arteritis, temporal arteritis and polymyalgia rheumatica in a Danish county: a prospective investigation, 1982–1985. Arthritis Rheum. 30:294, 1987.
15. Barrier, J., Pion, P., Massari, R., Peltier, P., Rojouan, J., and Grolleaw, J. W.: Epidemiologic approach to Horton's disease in Department of Loire-Atlantique: 110 cases in 10 years (1970–1979). Rev. Med. Interne 3:13, 1983.
16. Smith, C. A., Fidler, W. J., and Pinals, R. S.: The epidemiology of giant cell arteritis: report of a ten-year study in Shelby County, Tennessee. Arthritis Rheum. 26:1214, 1983.
17. Friedman, G., Friedman, B., and Benbassat, J.: Epidemiology of temporal arteritis in Israel. Isr. J. Med. Sci. 18:241, 1986.
18. Machado, E. B. V., Michet, C. J., Ballard, D. J., Hunder, G. G., Beard, C. M., Chu, C. P., and O'Fallon, W. M.: Trends in incidence and clinical presentation of temporal arteritis in Olmsted County, Minnesota, 1950–1985. Arthritis Rheum. 31:745, 1988.
19. Östberg, G.: On arteritis with special reference to polymyalgia arteritica. Acta Pathol. Microbiol. Scand. (A) Suppl. 237:1, 1973.
20. Calamia, K. T., and Hunder, G. G.: Clinical manifestations of giant cell arteritis. Clin. Rheum. Dis. 6:389, 1980.
21. Chuang, T. Y., Hunder, G. G., Ilstrup, D. M., and Jurland, L. T.: Polymyalgia rheumatica. A 10-year epidemiologic and clinical study. Ann. Intern. Med. 97:672, 1982.
22. Liang, G. C., Simkin, P. A., Hunder, G. G., Wilske, K. R., and Healey, L. A.: Familial aggregation of polymyalgia rheumatica and giant cell arteritis. Arthritis Rheum. 17:19, 1974.
23. Kemp, A.: Monozygotic twins with temporal arteritis and ophthalmic arteritis. Acta Ophthalmol. (Copenh.) 55:183, 1977.
24. Mathewson, J. A., and Hunder, G. G.: Giant cell arteritis in two brothers. J. Rheumatol. 13:190, 1986.
25. Calamia, K. T., Moore, S. B., Elveback, L. R., and Hunder, G. G.: HLA-DR locus antigens in polymyalgia rheumatica and giant cell arteritis. J. Rheumatol. 8:6, 1981.
26. Cid, M. C., Ercilla, G., Vilaseca, J., Sanmarti, R., Villalta, J., Ingelmo, M., and Urbano-Marquez, A.: Polymyalgia rheumatica: A syndrome associated with HLA-DR4 antigen. Arthritis Rheum. 31:678, 1988.
27. Sakkas, L. I., Loqueman, N., Panayi, G. S., Myles, A. B., and Welsh, K. I.: Immunogenetics of polymyalgia rheumatica. Br. J. Rheumatol. 29:331, 1990.
28. Wilkinson, I. M. S., and Russell, R. W. R.: Arteries of the head and neck in giant cell arteritis: A pathological study to show the pattern of arterial involvement. Arch. Neurol. 27:378, 1972.
29. Shiiki, H., Shimokama, T., and Watanabe, T.: Temporal arteritis: cell composition and the possible pathogenetic role of cell-mediated immunity. Hum. Pathol. 20:1057, 1989.
30. Papaioannou, C. C., Hunder, G. G., and McDuffie, F. C.: Cellular immunity in polymyalgia rheumatica and giant cell arteritis: Lack of response to muscle or artery homogenates. Arthritis Rheum. 22:740, 1979.
31. Park, J. R., and Hazleman, B. L.: Immunological and histological study of temporal arteries. Ann. Rheum. Dis. 37:238, 1978.
32. Wells, K. K., Folberg, R., Goeken, J. A., and Kemp, J. D.: Temporal artery biopsies. Correlation of light microscopy and immunofluorescence microscopy. Ophthalmology 96:1058, 1989.
33. Velvart, M., Felder, M., and Fehr, K.: Temporal arteritis in polymyalgia rheumatica: immune complex deposits and the role of leukocyte elastase in pathogeneses. Z. Rheumatol. 42:320, 1983.
34. Dasgupta, B., Duke, O., Timms, A. M., Pitzalis, C., and Panayi, G. S.: Selective depletion and activation of CD8+ lymphocytes from peripheral blood of patients with PMR and giant cell arteritis. Ann. Rheum. Dis. 48:307, 1989.
35. Benlahrache, C., Segond, P., Anquier, L., and Bouvet, J. P.: Decrease of OKT8 positive T cell subset in polymyalgia rheumatica. Lack of correlation with disease activity. Arthritis Rheum. 26:1472, 1983.
36. Dasgupta, B., and Panayi, G. S.: Interleukin-6 in serum of patients with polymyalgia rheumatica and giant cell arteritis. Br. J. Rheumatol. 29:456, 1990.
37. Papaioannou, C. C., Gupta, R. C., Hunder, G. G., and McDuffie, F. C.: Circulating immune complexes in giant cell arteritis polymyalgia rheumatica. Arthritis Rheum. 23:1021, 1980.
38. Klein, R. G., Hunder, G. G., Stanson, A. W., and Sheps, S. G.: Large artery involvement in giant cell (temporal) arteritis. Ann. Intern. Med. 83:806, 1975.
39. Klein, R. G., Campbell, R. J., Hunder, G. G., and Carney, J. A.: Skip lesions in temporal arteritis. Mayo Clin. Proc. 51:504, 1976.
40. Ostberg, G.: Temporal arteritis in a large necropsy series. Ann. Rheum. Dis. 30:224, 1971.
41. Fauchald, P., Rygvold, O., and Oystese, B.: Temporal arteritis and polymyalgia rheumatica: Clinical and biopsy findings. Ann. Intern. Med. 77:845, 1972.
42. Parker, F., Healey, L. A., Wilske, K. R., and Odland, G. F.: Light and electron microscopic studies on human temporal arteries with special reference to alterations related to senescence, atherosclerosis and giant cell arteritis. Am. J. Pathol. 79:57, 1975.
43. Cid, M. C., Campo, E., Ercilla, G., Palacin, A., Vilaseca, J., Villalta, J., and Ingelmo, M.: Immunohistochemical analysis of lymphoid and macrophage cell subsets and the immunological activation markers in temporal arteritis. Arthritis Rheum. 32:884, 1989.
44. Banks, P. M., Cohen, M. D., Ginsburg, W. W., and Hunder, G. G.: Immunohistologic and cytochemical studies of temporal arteritis. Arthritis Rheum. 26:120, 1983.
45. Hamrin, B., Johsson, N., and Hellsten, S.: "Polymyalgia arteritica": Further clinical and histopathological studies with a report of six autopsy cases. Ann. Rheum. Dis. 27:397, 1968.
46. Long, R., and James, O.: Polymyalgia rheumatica and liver disease. Lancet 1:77, 1974.
47. Calamia, K. T., and Hunder, G. G.: Giant cell arteritis (temporal arteritis) presenting as fever of undetermined origin. Arthritis Rheum. 24:1414, 1981.
48. Brooke, M. H., and Kaplan, H.: Muscle pathology in rheumatoid arthritis, polymyalgia rheumatica, and polymyositis: A histochemical study: Arch. Pathol. 94:101, 1972.
49. Henderson, D. R. F., Tribe, C. R., and Dixon, A. St. J.: Synovitis in polymyalgia rheumatica. Rheumatol. Rehabil. 14:244, 1975.
50. O'Duffy, J. D., Hunder, G. G., and Wahner, H. W.: A follow-up study of polymyalgia rheumatica: Evidence of chronic axial synovitis. J. Rheumatol. 7:685, 1980.
51. Healey, L. A.: Long-term follow-up of polymyalgia rheumatica: evidence for synovitis. Semin. Arthritis Rheum. 13:322, 1984.
52. Douglas, W. A., Martin, B. A., and Morris, J. H.: Polymyalgia rheumatica: an arthroscopic study of the shoulder joint. Ann. Rheum. Dis. 42:311, 1983.
53. Chow, C. T., and Schumacher, H. R., Jr.: Clinical and pathologic studies of synovitis in polymyalgia rheumatica. Arthritis Rheum. 27:1107, 1984.
54. Hunder, G. G., and Allen, G. L.: Giant cell arteritis: A review. Bull. Rheum. Dis. 29:980, 1978–79.
55. Hunder, G. G., Sheps, S. G., Allen, G. L., and Joyce, J. W.: Daily and alternate-day corticosteroid regimens in treatment of giant cell arteritis: Comparison in a prospective study. Ann. Intern. Med. 82:613, 1975.
56. Hollenhorst, R. W., Brown, J. R., Wagener, H. P., and Shick, R. M.: Neurologic aspects of temporal arteritis. Neurology 10:490, 1960.
57. Soelberg Sorensen, P., and Lorenzen, I.: Giant-cell arteritis, temporal arteritis and polymyalgia rheumatica: A retrospective study of 63 patients. Acta Med. Scand. 201:207, 1977.
58. Casselli, R. J., Hunder, G. G., and Whisnant, J. P.: Neurologic disease in biopsy-proven giant cell (temporal) arteritis. Neurology 38:352, 1988.
59. Larson, T. S., Hall, S., Hepper, N. G. G., and Hunder G. G.: Respiratory tract symptoms as a clue to giant cell arteritis. Ann. Intern. Med. 101:594, 1984.
60. Lie, J. T., Failoni, D. D., and Davies, D. C., Jr.: Temporal arteritis with giant cell aortitis, coronary arteritis and myocardial infarction. Arch. Pathol. Lab. Med. 110:857, 1986.
61. Kyle, V., Tudor, J., Waight, E. P., Gresham, G. A., and Hazleman, B. L.: Rarity of synovitis in polymyalgia rheumatica. Ann. Rheum. Dis. 49:155, 1990.
62. Paulley, J. W., and Hughes, J. P.: Giant-cell arteritis, or arteritis of the aged. Br. Med. J. 2:1562, 1960.
63. Alestig, K., and Barr, J.: Giant-cell arteritis: A biopsy study of polymyalgia rheumatica, including one case of Takayasu's disease. Lancet 1:228, 1963.
64. Malmvall, B.-E., Bengtsson, B.-A., Kaijser, B., Nilsson, L.-A., and Alestig, K.: Serum levels of immunoglobulin and complement in giant cell arteritis. J.A.M.A. 236:1876, 1976.
65. Dickson, E. R., Maldonado, J. E., Sheps, S. G., and Cain, J. A., Jr.: Systemic giant-cell arteritis with polymyalgia rheumatica: Reversible abnormalities of liver function. J.A.M.A. 224:1496, 1973.
66. Bunch, T. W., Hunder, G. G., McDuffie, F. C., O'Brien, P. C., and Markowitz, H.: Synovial fluid complement determination as a diagnostic aid in inflammatory joint disease. Mayo Clin. Proc. 49:715, 1974.
67. Persellin, S. T., Daniels, T. M., Rings, L. J., Kazmier, F. J., Bowie, E. J. W., and Hunder, G. G.: Factor VIII-von Willebrand factor in giant cell arteritis and polymyalgia rheumatica. Mayo Clin. Proc. 60:457, 1985.
68. Olsson, A., Elling, P., and Elling, H.: Serologic and immunochemical determination of von Willebrand factor antigen in serum and biopsy specimens from patients with arteritis temporalis and polymyalgia rheumatica. Clin. Exp. Rheumatol. 8:55, 1990.
69. Bosley, T. M., Salvino, P. J., Sergott, R. C., Eagle, R. C., Sandy, R., and Gee, W.: Ocular pneumoplethysmography can help in the diagnosis of giant-cell arteritis. Arch. Ophthalmol. 107:379, 1989.
70. Stanson, A. W., Klein, R. G., and Hunder, G. G.: Extracranial angiographic findings in giant cell (temporal) arteritis. Am. J. Roentgenol. 127:957, 1976.
71. Allsop, C. J., and Gallagher, P. J.: Temporal artery biopsy in giant cell arteritis. A reappraisal. Am. J. Surg. Pathol. 5:317, 1981.

72. Hall, S., Persellin, S., Kurland, L., O'Brien, P. O., and Hunder, G. G.: The therapeutic impact of temporal artery biopsy. Lancet 2:1217, 1983.

73. Morgan, G. J., Jr., and Harris, E. D., Jr.: Non–giant cell temporal arteritis: Three cases and a review of the literature. Arthritis Rheum. 21:362, 1978.

74. Papaioannou, C. C., Hunder, G. G., and Lie, J. T.: Vasculitis of the gallbladder in a 70-year-old man with giant cell (temporal) arteritis. J. Rheumatol. 6:71, 1979.

75. Gertz, M. A., Kyle, R. A., Griffing, W. L., and Hunder, G. G.: Jaw claudication in primary systemic amyloidosis. Medicine 65:173, 1986.

76. Hunder G. G., Bloch, D. A., Michel, B. A., Stevens, M. B., Arend, W. P., Calabrese, L. H., Edworthy, S. M., Fauci, A. S., Leavitt, R. Y., Lit, J. T., Lightfoot, R. W., Masi, A. T., McShane, D. J., Mills, J. A., Wallace, S. L., and Zvaifler, N. J.: The American College of Rheumatology 1990 Criteria for the Classification of Giant Cell Arteritis. Arthritis Rheum. 33:1122, 1990.

77. Hall, S., Ginsburg, W. W., Vollertsen, R. S., and Hunder, G. G.: The coexistence of rheumatoid arthritis and giant cell arteritis. J. Rheumatol. 10:995, 1983.

78. Ginsburg, W. W., Cohen, M. D., Hall, S. B., Vollertsen, R. S., and Hunder, G. G.: Seronegative polyarthritis in giant cell arteritis. Arthritis Rheum. 28:1362, 1985.

79. Liozon, E., Venot, J., Liozon, F., Vidal, E., Weinbreck, P., Bordessoule, D., and Loustaud, V.: Proteines de l'inflammation dans la maladie de Horton. Ann. Med. Interne 141:319, 1990.

80. Rynes, R. I., Mika, P., and Bartholomew, L. E.: Development of giant cell (temporal) arteritis in a patient 'adequately' treated for polymyalgia rheumatica. Ann. Rheum. Dis. 36:88, 1977.

Section X

Connective Tissue Diseases Characterized by Fibrosis

Chapter 66

James R. Seibold

Scleroderma

INTRODUCTION

Systemic sclerosis [scleroderma] is a generalized disorder of connective tissue characterized clinically by thickening and fibrosis of the skin (scleroderma) and by distinctive forms of involvement of internal organs, notably the heart, lungs, kidneys, and gastrointestinal tract. The etiology and pathogenesis are unknown. Any unifying hypothesis concerning the pathogenesis must explain the following: (1) the remarkable heterogeneity of patterns of disease extent, progression, and internal organ involvement; (2) the accelerated rate of accumulation of extracellular matrix in both skin and internal organs; (3) the frequent and somewhat characteristic immunologic abnormalities; (4) the variable contributions of acute and chronic inflammatory change; and (5) the ubiquitous and characteristic abnormalities of vascular function and structure.

Systemic sclerosis is often of tragic consequence to the patient. Morbidity and mortality are substantial and are directly related to the extent and severity of visceral involvement. Although supportive care of the individual with systemic sclerosis is available, there are no therapies known to modify the natural course of the disease. This is due in part to the dearth of appropriately designed clinical studies of potentially effective agents.

DEFINITION AND CLASSIFICATION

The term *scleroderma* (Gr. *skleros*, hard, plus *derma*, skin) is a descriptive construct that includes a number of clinical disorders otherwise minimally related or unrelated to systemic sclerosis (Table 66–1). A multicenter study of the American College of Rheumatology (ACR) proposed preliminary criteria for the classification of systemic sclerosis based on

clinical and laboratory assessments of nearly 800 patients with early-diagnosed connective tissue disease, including systemic sclerosis, systemic lupus erythematosus (SLE), inflammatory muscle disease, and isolated Raynaud's phenomenon.[1] Sclerodermatous skin change in any location proximal to the metacarpophalangeal joints was the single major criterion for classification of systemic sclerosis, with sensitivity of 91 percent and specificity greater than 99 percent. The presence of two or more of the following features contributed further as minor criteria: sclerodactyly, digital pitting scars of fingertips or loss of digital finger pad substance, and bibasilar pulmonary fibrosis.[1] It is recognized that many patients with confident diagnoses of systemic sclerosis do not fulfill these criteria.[2] Furthermore, proximal skin thickening is an intrinsic clinical feature of many of the disorders listed in Table 66–1. Thus, while the ACR criteria are useful in assuring uniformity in clinical research, they are without value in clinical differential diagnosis.[3]

Most observers recognize subgroups of clinical and prognostic importance within the diagnosis of systemic sclerosis[4, 5] that are not discriminated by the classification criteria[1] and that are the subject of terminologic controversy.[3] A consensus proposal on nomenclature has been developed to permit separation of systemic sclerosis by clinical features alone with extent of skin involvement serving as a principal guide (Table 66–2).[6] Some think that patients with skin thickening proximal to the fingers yet sparing the trunk (acrosclerosis) represent an intermediate group between those with diffuse cutaneous scleroderma and those with finger involvement only (sclerodactyly).[5] It should be recognized that virtually all the proposed stratifications of systemic sclerosis are somewhat arbitrary and are likely subject to clinical ascertainment bias. The majority of the clinical and

Table 66–1. DIFFERENTIAL DIAGNOSIS OF SCLERODERMA/SYSTEMIC SCLEROSIS

I. Systemic sclerosis (see Table 66–2)
II. Disorders characterized by or associated with skin thickening on the fingers and hands
  Bleomycin-induced scleroderma
  Digital sclerosis of diabetes mellitus
  Chronic reflex sympathetic dystrophy
  Mycosis fungoides
  Vinyl chloride disease
  Amyloidosis
  Acrodermatitis chronica atrophicans
  Adult celiac disease
  Vibration disease
III. Disorders characterized by or associated with generalized skin thickening but typically sparing the fingers and hands
  Scleroderma adultorum of Buschke
  Scleromyxedema
  Eosinophilic fasciitis
  Eosinophilic-myalgia syndrome
  Generalized subcutaneous morphea
  Pentazocine-induced scleroderma
  Human graft-versus-host disease
  Porphyria cutanea tarda
  Amyloidosis
  Human adjuvant disease (silica-induced scleroderma)
IV. Disorders characterized by asymmetric skin change
  Morphea
  Linear scleroderma
  Coup de sabre
V. Disorders characterized by similar internal organ involvement
  Primary pulmonary hypertension
  Primary biliary cirrhosis
  Intestinal pseudo-obstruction
  Collagenous colitis
  Infiltrative cardiomyopathy
  Idiopathic pulmonary fibrosis
VI. Disorders characterized by Raynaud's phenomenon (see Table 66–4)

laboratory information upon which classification is based has been derived from cross-sectional or point prevalence surveys or retrospective study of some specific feature of illness.[3, 6, 7]

INCIDENCE AND EPIDEMIOLOGY

The majority of the available studies suggest an occurrence in between 4 and 12 individuals per million population per year.[8] An analysis of mortality data from England and Wales for the years 1968 to 1985 reveals a small but significant increase in mortality of 3 percent a year over this period.[9] These data suggest an increasing incidence, best explained by improved diagnosis of less severe cases, since advances in supportive therapy would be expected to have lessened disease mortality during this same period. An ongoing study of Raynaud's phenomenon in South Carolina has found evidence of substantial numbers of previously undiagnosed individuals.[10] Data suggest that true prevalence may be more than fourfold higher than previously recognized. These figures suggest that there are 100,000 to 200,000 cases of systemic sclerosis in the United States. It is likely

that many cases are unrecognized or are misdiagnosed as Raynaud's phenomenon only or as having a related connective tissue disease.[10]

Systemic sclerosis is found in all geographic areas and all racial groups, although blacks may be at moderately increased risk.[8, 11] Although all age groups may be affected, disease onset is highest between ages 30 and 50.[8] Systemic sclerosis is three to four times more common in women than in men,[11, 12] with women of childbearing age at peak risk.[11] The majority of cases occur sporadically without reference to season, geography, occupation, and socioeconomic status.[8] There are weak links with exposure to environmental toxins including vinyl chloride,[13] epoxy resins,[14] and trichloroethylene.[15] Silica exposure, either occupational[16, 17] or via silicone implants for augmentative mammoplasty,[18, 19] is associated with an increased incidence of systemic sclerosis. There are rare reports of familial occurrence of systemic sclerosis.[8, 20] Detailed study of HLA phenotypes has failed to reveal consistent associations with either systemic sclerosis or any of its clinical subsets.[21, 22] While first-degree relatives of patients with systemic sclerosis are more likely to have serum antinuclear antibody,[23] there is not an increased familial occurrence of more specific serologic features such as serum anticentromere antibody.[24, 25]

INITIAL PRESENTATIONS

Raynaud's Phenomenon and Systemic Sclerosis

Raynaud's phenomenon is the initial complaint in approximately 70 percent of patients with systemic sclerosis and in virtually all patients destined to evolve into systemic sclerosis with limited scleroderma (formerly CREST syndrome: Calcinosis; Raynaud's phenomenon; Esophageal dysmotility; Scle-

Table 66–2. CLASSIFICATION OF SYSTEMIC SCLEROSIS

1. *With diffuse cutaneous scleroderma:* skin thickening present on the trunk in addition to face, proximal and distal extremities
2. *With limited cutaneous scleroderma:* skin thickening limited to sites distal to the elbow and knee but also involving the face and neck. Synonym: CREST syndrome (C, calcinosis; R, Raynaud's phenomenon; E, esophageal dysmotility; S, sclerodactyly; T, telangiectasias)
3. *Sine scleroderma:* characteristic internal organ manifestations, vascular and serologic abnormalities but without clinically detectable skin change
4. *In overlap:* any of 1–3 (above) occurring concomitantly with diagnosis of systemic lupus erythematosus, inflammatory muscle disease, or rheumatoid arthritis. Synonyms: mixed connective tissue disease, lupoderma, sclerodermatomyositis (see Chapter 63)
5. *Undifferentiated connective tissue disease:* Raynaud's phenomenon with clinical or serologic features of systemic sclerosis (digital ulceration, abnormal nailfold capillary loops, serum anticentromere antibody, finger edema) but without skin thickening and without internal organ abnormalities of systemic sclerosis

rodactyly; *Telangiectasias*) (see Table 66–2).[26] Individuals with diffuse scleroderma are more likely to present with finger and hand swelling, complaints of arthritis, evidence of specific internal organ involvement, or with skin thickening.[26, 27] In diffuse scleroderma, any of these features may occur either contemporaneously or within 1 to 2 years of the development of Raynaud's phenomenon. The small subgroup of patients who never develop Raynaud's phenomenon are more frequently male, are at high risk for developing renal and myocardial involvement, and have poor survival.[27]

The exact incidence of Raynaud's phenomenon is not known. However, it is viewed as an important index characteristic for epidemiologic study of systemic sclerosis.[28] Population surveys have suggested prevalences of 5 to 10 percent in nonsmokers[29, 30] and up to 22 percent in premenopausal females[31] (many of whom had symptoms dating from menarche). Reconciliation of the prevalence of Raynaud's phenomenon with the relative rarity of systemic sclerosis is difficult. The experiences of academic centers are probably subject to referral bias that selects for cases of relative clinical severity thereby skewing case-mix toward secondary forms of this syndrome.

Recent advances in techniques of laboratory diagnosis permit the dismissing of older clinically based studies of the natural history of Raynaud's phenomenon and its potential to evolve to systemic sclerosis.[30] There have been remarkably few patients encountered in any modern study of Raynaud's phenomenon who at initial assessment were free of clinical and laboratory abnormality and at some later time developed features of systemic sclerosis. Support for this view derives from studies of architectural abnormalities of the nailfold capillary bed[32, 33]; serologic abnormalities including antinuclear and anticentromere antibodies[33–35]; physiologic assessments of digital perfusion[36, 37]; and measures of in vivo platelet activation,[38, 39] red cell filterability,[40] and serum endothelial cytotoxic activity.[41] To term patients with systemic sclerosis at the stage of Raynaud's phenomenon only as "transitional" from primary Raynaud's phenomenon describes a biologic and clinical sequence that is virtually never encountered. Classifying such patients as "undifferentiated connective tissue disease" allows for diverse subsequent clinical outcomes including systemic sclerosis[42] (Fig. 66–1).

Edematous Change

An intrinsic feature of undifferentiated connective tissue disease is the painless swelling of the fingers and hands known as early "puffy" or edematous scleroderma. Similar presentations are described in rheumatoid arthritis and systemic lupus erythematosus and as the most typical early sign of overlap syndromes[42] (see Chapter 63). From the clinical standpoint, the longer an individual patient remains at this stage, the more favorable the long-term

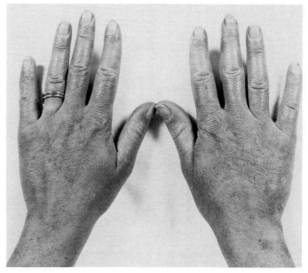

Figure 66–1. The hands of a young woman with undifferentiated connective tissue disease. The fingers are swollen with mild pitting edema, and there is digital tip cyanosis. The skin is not yet thickened.

prognosis. Symptoms of morning stiffness and arthralgia are typical and median nerve compression a frequent occurrence. Pitting edema of the fingers and dorsa of the hands is easily elicited on physical examination. The edema is also typically present in unexpected locations such as the upper arms, face, and trunk even in patients with clear diagnoses of limited scleroderma. Clinical observations do not confirm differences in extent and severity of skin edema related to either duration or classification of disease.

The edema is due in part to deposition of hydrophilic glycosaminoglycan in the dermis[43] but may also reflect local inflammation, hydrostatic effects, and microvascular disruption.[44] It is not known what causes the edema to regress, in fact there are some data to suggest that it does not. In one study, 180 uniform and trimmed punch biopsies from the forearms of patients with systemic sclerosis were weighed fresh and again after desiccation. The percentage contribution to weight of tissue water was remarkably consistent (about 70 percent) in all patients irrespective of their clinical classification, duration of disease, or degree of clinical skin thickness and edema at the site of biopsy.[45] Similar observations were noted by Rodnan in studies of skin core biopsy weights.[46] It is possible that the edema does not resolve but the clinical ability to detect such changes becomes more limited as the dermis becomes more fibrosed.

SKIN INVOLVEMENT

Clinical Findings

The skin thickening of systemic sclerosis begins on the fingers and hands in nearly all cases. The skin

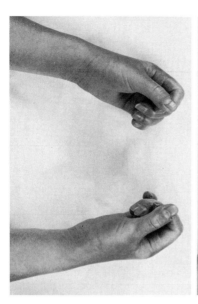
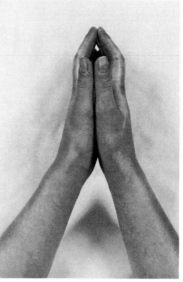

Figure 66–2. The hands of a young woman with several months of rapidly progressive scleroderma. The skin is taut and indurated, and there is limitation of both fist closure and finger extension.

initially appears shiny and taut and may be erythematous at early stages (Fig. 66–2). Superficial landmarks such as transverse digital skin creases are obscured and hair growth is sparse. The skin of the face and neck is usually involved next and associated with an immobile and pinched facies (Fig. 66–3). The lips become thin and pursed and radial furrowing may develop about the mouth (Fig. 66–4). Skin tightening and thickening may limit the oral aperture, impairing effective dental hygiene. The skin change may stay restricted to fingers, hands, and face and may remain relatively mild. Extension to the forearms is followed by spontaneous arrest of

progression (limited scleroderma) or by rapid centripetal spread to the upper arms, shoulders, anterior chest, back, abdomen, and legs (diffuse scleroderma). Impressive areas of hyper- and hypopigmentation may develop (Fig. 66–5), or there may be generalized deepening of skin tone.

In diffuse scleroderma, the pace of extension of skin change is somewhat variable, ranging from development of total body skin thickening within a few months to more insidious progression over several years. Some data suggest that untreated diffuse scleroderma is uniphasic, with peaking of skin involvement in both extent and severity within 3 years of disease onset[47, 48] (Fig. 66–6). In contrast, patients with limited scleroderma inexorably worsen with

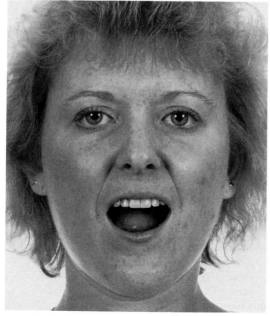

Figure 66–3. The face of a young woman with several months of rapidly progressive scleroderma. The facial skin is taut, with an immobile facies and limitation of the oral aperture.

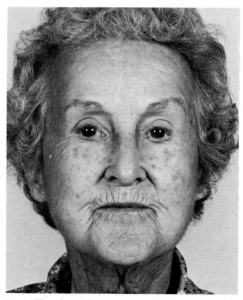

Figure 66–4. The face of a woman with long-standing diffuse scleroderma exhibiting multiple telangiectasias and exaggerated radial furrowing about the lips.

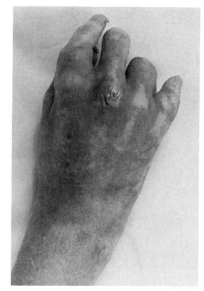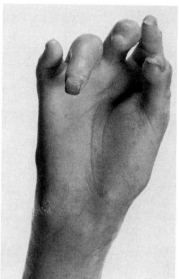

Figure 66–5. Advanced changes of scleroderma in the hand of a woman with long-standing disease. The skin is taut and thickened with irregular pigmentary change and palmar telangiectasias. Ulcerations are present over bony prominences, and the fingers reveal extensive trophic abnormalities.

time without periods of spontaneous improvement or arrest. However, these patients may enjoy so slow a rate of progression of skin change as to be clinically unchanged from year to year.

At very late stages of disease, atrophy develops, leading to fragility and laxity of the superficial dermis although tethering to deeper tissues may still be appreciated. The clinical observation of improving skin change in late diffuse scleroderma[47, 48] may reflect this atrophic phase. This renders interpretation of clinical trials difficult.

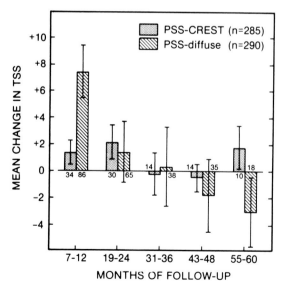

Figure 66–6. The natural history of scleroderma skin involvement as assessed by the total skin score (TSS) in a large number of patients followed for periods as long as 5 years. Individuals with diffuse scleroderma worsen in extent and severity for the first 2 to 3 years of disease but thereafter improve spontaneously. Limited scleroderma (CREST syndrome) is typified by slow but continual worsening. (From Medsger, T. A.: Progressive systemic sclerosis. Clin. Rheum. Dis. 9:655, 1983; used by permission.)

Assessment and Classification

The diagnosis of systemic sclerosis is usually clinically obvious once skin thickening has developed, and skin biopsies are rarely necessary. However, virtually all of the proposed classification schemes[3-6] are based on clinical determinations of the extent of sclerodermatous skin change (see Table 66–2). As discussed in detail in subsequent sections, there are important relations between classification and prognosis. A useful aphorism is that the relative risk of accruing new internal organ involvement closely parallels the pace, progression, and extent of skin involvement. Since internal organ involvement is the principal determinant of morbidity and mortality, the clinical ability to accurately recognize the extent of and serial changes in skin involvement is paramount.

A variety of methods for monitoring skin change in systemic sclerosis have been proposed including roentgenography, biopsy, and clinical palpation. The Rodnan total skin score[48] employs a qualitative rating scale (0—normal skin, 1—mild, 2—moderate, 3—severe, and 4—extreme skin thickening) of findings on clinical palpation of multiple body areas and thus permits a semiquantitative tool for clinical research as well as a measure of clinical progress in the individual patient (Fig. 66–7). Other proposed systems estimate both skin thickening and tethering.[49] Skin thickness ratings of experienced clinical investigators by clinical palpation correlate closely with skin core biopsy weights as well as total hydroxyproline content.[46] The total skin score and more simplified versions (fewer body areas and 0 to 3 rating scales: normal, mild, moderate, and severe thickening) are increasingly used in clinical research reports. There are, however, few data validating reproducibility or measuring interobserver variability. The author, as coordinator of several multicenter trials, has

TOTAL SKIN SCORE BY PALPATION

Right		Left
0 1 2 ③ 4	Fingers	0 1 2 ③ 4
0 1 2 ③ 4	Hands	0 1 2 ③ 4
0 1 ② 3 4	Forearms	0 1 ② 3 4
0 1 ② 3 4	Arms	0 1 ② 3 4
0 ① 2 3 4	Shoulders	0 ① 2 3 4
0 ① 2 3 4	Neck	
0 1 ② 3 4	Face	
0 1 ② 3 4	Chest	
0 ① 2 3 4	Breasts	0 ① 2 3 4
0 ① 2 3 4	Abdomen	
0 ① 2 3 4	Upper Back	
⓪ 1 2 3 4	Lower Back	
⓪ 1 2 3 4	Thighs	⓪ 1 2 3 4
⓪ 1 2 3 4	Legs	⓪ 1 2 3 4
0 ① 2 3 4	Feet	0 ① 2 3 4
0 1 ② 3 4	Toes	0 1 ② 3 4

TOTAL 3̲7̲

Figure 66–7. An example of the total skin score technique (Rodnan) of assessing scleroderma skin thickening by clinical palpation. The presence of skin change on the trunk permits classification of the condition of this patient as systemic sclerosis with diffuse scleroderma. Serial examinations are used to follow the clinical course and to assess the response to therapy.

been impressed by the relative inability of experienced examiners to discriminate thickness from tethering or to recognize skin edema in typical diffuse scleroderma.

Histopathologic Findings

The tightening and thickening of the skin in systemic sclerosis are due to the accumulation of excess collagen and other extracellular matrix constituents including glycosaminoglycan and fibronectin. Skin biopsies from early stages of illness disclose an increase in compact hyalinized collagen fibers in the lower dermis and upper subcutaneum in association with perivascular and interstitial lymphocyte and histiocyte infiltrates[46, 50–52] (Fig. 66–8). Direct skin immunofluorescence is lacking[52] and electron microscopy reveals an increase in fine collagen fibrils of diameter 10 to 20 nm and ground substance.[50, 53] At later stages, atrophic change is noted, including thinning of the epidermis with loss of rete pegs and of dermal appendages.[46, 50]

Abnormalities of Extracellular Matrix

Collagen accumulation by cultured fibroblasts derived from the skin of patients with systemic sclerosis is increased.[54–56] The relative proportion of the two major skin procollagens, types I and III, is that of normal skin,[56] which with some forms of keloid separates systemic sclerosis as unique among fibrosing disorders (see Chapter 20). There is some evidence of disproportionately increased synthesis of type V (basement membrane) collagen[57] as well as of fibronectin[58] and glycosaminoglycan.[43, 59] The collagen is biochemically normal. Preliminary and somewhat limited studies with cDNA probes for pro-alpha 1(I), alpha 2(I), and alpha 1(IV) collagens have failed to reveal disease-associated genomic polymorphism[60] or differences in comparison of limited and generalized patients.[61] The increased synthesis of types I and III collagen is associated with a coordinate increase in mRNA levels.[62–64]

Collagen degradation in systemic sclerosis is normal.[55] Activity of intracellular enzymes responsible for post-translational modification of collagen, prolyl hydroxylase, and lysyl hydroxylase is increased[65] and the response of scleroderma fibroblasts

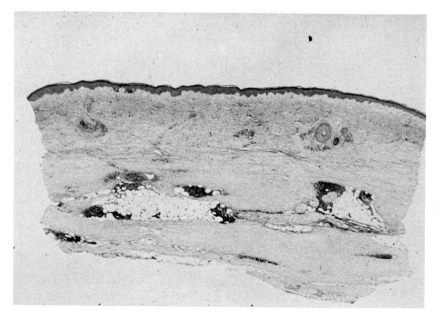

Figure 66–8. Photomicrograph of a punch skin biopsy obtained from a patient with early diffuse scleroderma. The epidermis is thinned and shows loss of appendages. The lower dermis and subcutis are markedly thickened from an increase in compact hyalinized collagen. Lymphocyte infiltrates (typically T-helper phenotype) are readily apparent in the lower dermis and at the dermal-subcuticular interface.

to feedback regulation by the aminopropeptide of collagen is normal.[66]

The data all support the hypothesis that the matrix accumulation of systemic sclerosis is secondary to some as yet unidentified signal operative at the transcriptional level. Theoretically, this may be viewed as either an across the board "activation" of the fibroblast or alternatively as the result of a preferential selection of fibroblasts of high matrix-producing capacity.[67, 68]

Influences on Matrix Metabolism

To assume that the fibrosis of systemic sclerosis is a secondary event casts focus on potential primary signals of connective tissue activation (Table 66–3). A diverse array of cytokines and growth factors are capable of inducing or modulating the scleroderma fibroblast phenotype (enhanced proliferation and synthetic function)[69] (see Chapter 20). For example, serum from patients with systemic sclerosis increases collagen accumulation by and proliferation of fibroblasts from both systemic sclerosis and normals.[70, 71]

Mast cell infiltration[72, 73] and degranulation[72] have been demonstrated in scleroderma skin preceding clinically apparent fibrosis. Similar findings are noted in murine models of scleroderma including the tight skin (Tsk) mouse[74] and chronic graft-versus-host disease[75] as well as in a variety of other fibrosing conditions.[76] Mast cell release of histamine may stimulate fibroblast proliferation,[77] and, indeed, patients with systemic sclerosis have increased plasma levels of histamine.[78]

Mast cell or monocyte release of tumor necrosis factor might be implicated.[79] Tumor necrosis factor-alpha (TNF-α) and lymphotoxin (TNF-β) are mitogenic for fibroblasts, inhibitory to endothelium, and pleotropic for matrix synthesis[69] and may represent the prime mitogenic signal released by monocytes.[80] Their effects are augmented by interferon-gamma (IFN-γ). Rosenbloom et al. have demonstrated that recombinant IFN-γ causes potent inhibition of fibroblast collagen production and an associated coordinate decrease in types I and III procollagen mRNA levels in studies of systemic sclerosis.[64] This effect is noted at very low concentrations of IFN-γ[64] and has been shown to persist through serial passages of cultured scleroderma fibroblasts.[81]

Antigen- and mitogen-stimulated T lymphocytes release factors that are both chemotactic for fibroblasts[82] and stimulatory to both fibroblast proliferation and collagen accumulation.[83] Soluble mediators derived from concanavalin A–incubated normal human mononuclear cells have been shown to induce systemic sclerosis–like fibroblast growth and glycosaminoglycan synthesis.[84] Phytohemagglutinin-stimulated monocytes from systemic sclerosis enhance collagen accumulation.[85]

Platelet-derived growth factors have been implicated,[69] perhaps most importantly, transforming growth factor-beta (TGF-β). TGF-β stimulates fibroblast proliferation and matrix synthesis[63] in part by stimulation of autocrine release of platelet-derived growth factor and in part by being inhibitory to endothelium.[86] TGF-β, when injected subcutaneously, causes intense mononuclear cell infiltrate, neoangiogenesis, and fibrosis.[87] Continued investigation of these various influences on connective tissue metabolism in systemic sclerosis may lead to effective approaches to therapeutic manipulation.[69, 69a]

Table 66–3. IMPLICATED GROWTH FACTOR AND CYTOKINE EFFECTS IN SYSTEMIC SCLEROSIS

Receptor-Ligand System	Likely Cell of Origin
Fibroblast Proliferation and Collagen Accumulation	
Histamine	Mast cell
Tumor necrosis factor	Mast cell
	Monocytes
	Lymphocytes
Transforming growth factor-β	Platelet
	Monocyte
Platelet-derived growth factor	Platelet
Basic fibroblast growth factor	Monocyte
	Lymphocyte
Interleukin-1 β	Monocyte
Interleukin-4	Lymphocyte
Interleukin-2	Lymphocyte
	Monocyte
Endothelial Injury and Growth Suppression	
Tumor necrosis factor	Monocyte
	Lymphocyte
Transforming growth factor-β	Platelet
Interleukin-2	Lymphocyte
	Monocyte
Basic fibroblast growth factor	Monocyte
	Lymphocyte

VASCULAR AND MICROVASCULAR ABNORMALITIES

A vascular hypothesis for the pathogenesis of systemic sclerosis is supported by a variety of clinical and laboratory observations. Characteristic structural alterations of the small artery and microvasculature are present at the earliest recognizable stages of illness, and clinical manifestations reflecting the vascular derangement dominate aspects of the disease course in all forms of the disorder.

Raynaud's Phenomenon

As discussed before, Raynaud's phenomenon is the most typical presenting manifestation of systemic sclerosis. The digital arteries of patients with systemic sclerosis exhibit marked intimal hyperplasia consisting predominantly of collagen and to a lesser degree of ground substance[26] (Fig. 66–9). Medial changes are relatively inconspicuous but adventitial fibrosis is seen in 40 percent of cases.[26] Severe narrowing (> 75 percent) of the arterial lumen results, which may

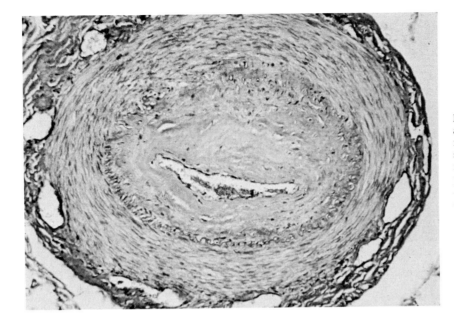

Figure 66–9. Photomicrograph of a digital artery in cross-section obtained at post mortem from a patient with long-standing systemic sclerosis. The intima shows dramatic collagenous hyperplasia, with a 90 percent reduction of the arterial lumen. Medial changes are inconspicuous, but the adventitia is mildly fibrosed.

in itself be of sufficient severity to account for Raynaud's phenomenon. Normal vasoconstrictor response to cold or emotional stimuli, superimposed on the anatomic obstruction, could cause complete or near complete occlusion of the arterial lumen.[26] Similar histopathologic changes are evident in the small arteries and arterioles of affected internal organs[88, 89] (Fig. 66–10). Certain important clinical syndromes such as scleroderma renal crisis[90] and pulmonary hypertension[91] are due principally to the presence of this fibrotic arteriosclerotic lesion.

Mechanisms of Raynaud's Phenomenon

Perfusion to the skin is ordinarily 10- to 20-fold that required for nutrition and oxygenation. Altera-

tions in skin blood flow are thus a principal mechanism of body thermoregulation. Peripheral vasoconstriction in response to cold is physiologic, and vasoconstriction sufficient to produce digital pallor or cyanosis may occur in normals, given a prolonged or severe enough cold exposure. Individuals with Raynaud's phenomenon, irrespective of etiology, have undue intolerance to environmental cold. No single pathophysiologic mechanism adequately explains cold-induced vasospasm in all forms of the syndrome, and, in fact, there is no single form of Raynaud's phenomenon for which the pathophysiology is entirely understood.[92] Sufficient information is available to classify Raynaud's phenomenon according to reasonable estimations regarding the predominant pathophysiologic abnormality[93, 94] (Table 66–4).

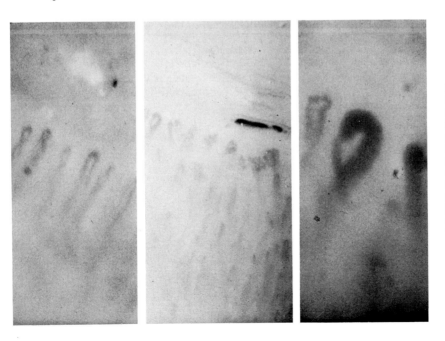

Figure 66–10. Nailfold capillary loop photography. On the left are the delicate and symmetric hairpin loops of normal nailfold circulation. The center photograph reveals tortuosity and redundancy of multiple capillary loops and might be encountered in systemic sclerosis as well as other connective tissue disorders. The right photograph reveals change and disease-specific changes of systemic sclerosis including a paucity of capillary loops and a single loop with gross dilatation of both the venular and the arteriolar limbs. (Courtesy of Dr. M. F. R. Martin.)

Table 66–4. MECHANISTIC CLASSIFICATION OF RAYNAUD'S PHENOMENON

I. **Vasospastic**
   Primary Raynaud's phenomenon (Raynaud's disease)
   Drug induced
      Ergot
      Methysergide
      β-Adrenergic blockers
   Pheochromocytoma
   Carcinoid syndrome
   Primary with other vasospastic syndromes (migraine,
      variant angina)

II. **Structural**
   Large and medium arteries
      Thoracic outlet syndrome
      Crutch pressure
      Brachiocephalic trunk disease (Takayasu's disease,
         atherosclerosis)
   Small arteries and arterioles
      Vibration disease
      Arteriosclerosis and thromboangiitis obliterans
      Cold injury (frostbite, pernio)
      Polyvinyl chloride disease
      Chemotherapy (bleomycin, vinblastine)
      Connective tissue disease
         Systemic sclerosis
         Systemic lupus erythematosus
         Inflammatory myopathy (dermatomyositis >>
            polymyositis)
         Overlap syndromes

III. **Hemorrheologic**
   Cryoglobulinemia
   Cryofibrinogenemia
   Paraproteinemia and hyperviscosity syndromes
   Cold agglutinin disease
   Polycythemia (essential thrombocythemia, polycythemia
      vera)

Although structural features perforce dominate consideration of the mechanism of Raynaud's phenomenon in systemic sclerosis, other factors are doubtless participatory. Platelet activation in vivo[38, 39] is associated with the local release of substances that exert powerful local effects on vascular smooth muscle tone. Potentially important are unstable products of arachidonic acid metabolism, such as thromboxane A_2, and stable constituents of the platelet dense granule, principally serotonin. Whereas unaggregated platelets do not cause contraction of human digital artery muscle strips, addition of platelets following induced aggregation causes brisk contraction of these preparations.[95] Of likely relevance is the observation that cooling to 24°C augments platelet-induced vasoconstrictive response.[96]

The status of the endothelium is felt to have important influences on arterial smooth muscle response to serotonin and thromboxane. Endothelial release of prostacyclin and endothelial monoamine oxidase activity in the catabolism of serotonin represent the opposing vasodilatory influences.[97] Ketanserin, an experimental S_2-serotonergic antagonist, improves digital artery perfusion across a broad range of temperatures in both short-term oral and intravenous usage in patients with systemic sclerosis,[98] suggesting a continual level of in vivo seroto-

nergic tone. The antiplatelet effects of calcium channel blockers such as nifedipine may be partially responsible for their favorable effects in treatment of Raynaud's phenomenon complicating systemic sclerosis.[99] Iloprost, an experimental stable prostacyclin, improves cold tolerance, lessens Raynaud's phenomenon, and facilitates healing of ischemic digital ulcers in patients with systemic sclerosis.[100, 101] Individuals with primary Raynaud's phenomenon do not have evidence of in vivo platelet activation,[38, 102] nor is such detectable in the venous effluent of cold-exposed extremities.[103] However, both ketanserin[104] and dazoxiben,[105] a thromboxane synthetase inhibitor, are associated with improved recovery from Raynaud's phenomenon episodes. Their lack of efficacy in attenuation of the initial cold-induced vasoconstriction implies that platelet activation is intermittent in primary Raynaud's phenomenon.

Adrenergic influences in the Raynaud's phenomenon of systemic sclerosis are felt to be minor.[92] The responsiveness to catecholamines of arterial smooth muscle obtained from patients with systemic sclerosis is reduced at lower temperatures,[106] and peripheral vasoconstrictor responses to reflex increases in sympathetic tone are either normal or reduced.[107] There is histopathologic evidence of destructive change in the peripheral sympathetic ganglia[108] and physiologic evidence of reduced electrical resistance of skin[109] in systemic sclerosis.

Hemorrheologic abnormalities including mild thrombocytosis and diminished red blood cell filterability[40] and increased plasma viscosity,[110] which correlates with plasma levels of fibrinogen, are present in systemic sclerosis and are thought to influence perfusion of the microvasculature (radius 2–10 nm).

Internal Organ Raynaud's Phenomenon

Fibrotic arteriosclerosis changes of the small artery and arteriole are present in the internal organs of patients with systemic sclerosis[88, 89] and have clinical and functional significance. This has long been suspected from clinical observation such as the increased incidence of scleroderma renal crisis during cold weather months[111] and is now supported by a variety of modern clinical physiologic investigations (Table 66–5).

Myocardial involvement from systemic sclerosis has been particularly well studied in this regard. Intermittent ischemia is suggested by histopathologic study revealing myocardial contraction band necrosis.[112] Recent clinical physiologic studies have supported this notion, including demonstrations of a high prevalence of both fixed and reversible thallium perfusion abnormalities in individuals with diffuse scleroderma[113] and a comparable prevalence of fixed perfusion defects in patients with limited skin involvement.[114] Thallium perfusion abnormalities have been demonstrated to improve in response to nifedipine[115] as have myocardial perfusion and met-

Table 66-5. EVIDENCE OF REVERSIBLE COLD-INDUCED PERFUSION CHANGES IN THE INTERNAL ORGANS IN SYSTEMIC SCLEROSIS

Myocardial
Fixed and reversible thallium perfusion defects in diffuse scleroderma
Fixed thallium perfusion defects in limited scleroderma (CREST syndrome)
Reversible thallium perfusion defects with nifedipine and dipyridamole
Transient regional wall motion abnormalities by echocardiography
Transient left ventricular dysfunction by gated ventriculoscintigraphy

Pulmonary
Transient perfusion changes by [81]M krypton scanning
Attenuated rise in diffusing capacity during cold challenge
Transient elevation in pulmonary artery pressure

Renal
Transient elevation of plasma renin activity
Transient reduction in renal cortical perfusion by xenon washout

abolic function assayed by positron emission tomography.[116] Transient regional wall motion abnormalities have been demonstrated to occur during cold challenge by both echocardiographic[117] and scintigraphic[118] techniques, suggesting a Raynaud-like reactivity of the coronary microvasculature.

It is perhaps not technically correct to term these transient changes in visceral perfusion as Raynaud's phenomenon, since the phases of cyanosis and of reactive erythema have not been successfully demonstrated. The increase in pulmonary diffusing capacity seen in normals during cold exposure is lacking in patients with systemic sclerosis.[119] However, similar findings are noted with assumption of recumbent posture (another maneuver that increases central venous volume and elevation of diffusing capacity).[120] This suggests an inability of a fibrosed pulmonary vasculature to accommodate increased venous return rather than cold-induced vasospasm. However, other sensitive techniques such as [81]M krypton lung scanning have demonstrated transient cold-induced perfusion decreases in around one half of patients.[121]

Microvascular Abnormalities

Concomitant with and possibly antedating the arteriolar abnormalities are characteristic architectural abnormalities of the microvasculature (see Fig. 66-10),[32-34] which are easily appreciated by widefield microscopy of the nailfold capillary bed.[126] The changes of systemic sclerosis include enlargement and tortuosity of individual capillary loops interspersed with areas of capillary loop dropout.[126] The mechanism of the capillary loop injury remains unresolved. Tissue pressure in the proximal digit is known to exceed that of the capillary bed; thus it is possible that hydrostatic effects contribute to capillary "varicosity."[44]

Ultrastructural study has demonstrated loss of endothelium and associated basement membrane thickening and reduplication in systemic sclerosis.[89, 127] The finding of increased plasma von Willebrand factor activity, factor VIII/von Willebrand factor antigen,[128] tissue plasminogen activator,[129] and endothelin-1[130] in patients with systemic sclerosis suggests that in vivo endothelial cell injury is ongoing. The factor or factors responsible for initiation and perpetuation of endothelial injury are unknown. Circulating immune complexes are present in many patients[131] but immunohistologic evidence for tissue deposition is largely lacking. Sparse deposits of antibody have been noted in areas of serum protein exudate in biopsies of the nailfold capillary bed.[132]

A serum factor specifically cytotoxic to endothelial cells in culture has been described in patients with systemic sclerosis.[41] The biologic activity of this factor is abolished by preincubation with a variety of protease inhibitors.[132] However, other laboratories have found this activity in only 7 to 40 percent of patients with systemic sclerosis[134, 135] and have called into question its specificity both for endothelium[134, 135] and for systemic sclerosis.[135] These disparate results are difficult to reconcile, since each of these studies employed similar techniques of endothelial culture derived from the same source of human umbilical vein. One study of rapidly progressive diffuse scleroderma, in which serum was found to support endothelial growth, noted that products of platelet aggregation suppressed endothelial growth and suggested that this suppression was due to release of transforming growth factor-β.[136]

The initial lesion of vascular injury, by whatever mechanism, can be seen as perpetuating a variety of local tissue responses, important among which are platelet activation and the attendant release of platelet-derived growth factors[86, 87] and vasoconstrictive substances. Exposure of subendothelial matrix constituents may induce an "amplification loop" of immunologically mediated vascular injury including the development of circulating antibodies to type IV collagen[137] and antibody-dependent endothelial injury.[138] T lymphocytes from patients with systemic sclerosis both proliferate[139] and express interleukin-2 receptor (CD 25 positivity)[140] on exposure to subendothelial laminin.

IMMUNOLOGIC FEATURES

As is discussed in detail in Chapter 63, systemic sclerosis is known to occur in overlap with other connective tissue disorders, most commonly systemic lupus erythematosus and polymyositis but also rheumatoid arthritis, Sjögren's syndrome, and organ-specific autoimmune disorders such as Hashimoto's thyroiditis and primary biliary cirrhosis. More frequently, patients with systemic sclerosis will present with clinical features and laboratory abnormalities reminiscent of a specific concomitant disorder but insufficient to sustain a second diagnosis.

Serologic Abnormalities—Nonspecific

Antinuclear antibodies are present in the sera of over 90 percent of patients with systemic sclerosis,[141] and most typically include patterns of homogeneous, speckled, and nucleolar immunofluorescent staining when sought on fixed tissue substrates. With few exceptions, these antinuclear antibodies are not complement-fixing[141] and persist following antigen denaturation with ribonuclease and deoxyribonuclease.[141] Similarly, by direct testing, antibody to native DNA is either lacking[142] or present in extremely low titer. As a rule, patients with systemic sclerosis lack anti-Sm antibody[143] and only about 20 percent have antibody directed against nuclear ribonucleoprotein (anti-nRNP).[144] There are no consistent clinical associations of any of these serologic features. Around 30 percent of patients have serum rheumatoid factor, and serum cryoglobulins are detectable in low concentration in as many as 50 percent.[110] While there is a single case report of circulating anticoagulant in systemic sclerosis,[145] anticardiolipin antibodies are either lacking (IgG) or present in low titer (IgM).[146]

Serum immune complexes have been found in systemic sclerosis in studies employing a variety of measurement techniques.[131] While their significance remains speculative, the presence of immune complexes has been correlated with cardiopulmonary involvement,[121, 131] overall severity of disease, and other evidence of serologic abnormality.[131, 147] Additional laboratory features include polyclonal hypergammaglobulinemia and other evidence of acute phase response.

Anticentromere Antibodies

Utilizing tissue culture substrates for indirect immunofluorescent study, most notably the human laryngeal carcinoma cell line HEp-2, anticentromere antibodies give rise to coarse, speckled patterns on interphase nuclei and appear as centromeric clustering on metaphase nuclei. The original reports suggested that between 50 and 96 percent of patients with limited systemic sclerosis had detectable serum anticentromere antibody.[34, 148, 149] In contrast, anticentromere antibody is found in fewer than 10 percent of individuals with diffuse scleroderma and is infrequent in other non–systemic sclerosis connective tissue diseases. Inasmuch as its presence parallels limited systemic sclerosis, serum anticentromere antibody confers a favorable prognosis[149, 150] and is a useful tool in the assessment and classification of patients with early systemic sclerosis. In comparisons of patients with clinical diagnoses of limited scleroderma, those with serum anticentromere antibody were more likely to have telangiectasias and calcinosis and less likely to have restrictive lung disease than those lacking anticentromere antibody.[151] Retrospective analysis of banked sera suggests that anticentromere titers do not change with time or disease course.[152] The presence of serum anticentromere antibody is of great value in the recognition of limited scleroderma at the stage of Raynaud's phenomenon only.[34, 35, 38, 153] The origin and biologic role of anticentromere antibody remain unclear.

Anti-DNA-Topoisomerase I (Scl-70)

Between 20 and 40 percent of patients classified as having systemic sclerosis have serum antibody reactive with an extractable nuclear antigen of 70 kD termed Scl-70.[154, 155] The antigen has been definitely characterized as DNA-topoisomerase I, an intracellular enzyme involved in the initial uncoiling of supercoiled DNA prior to transcription and present at both centromeric and other intracellular locations.[156] Anti-topoisomerase I antibodies inhibit function of the enzyme.[157] There are data to suggest that Scl-70 is a fragment of protease degradation of a 96-kD topoisomerase[158] and similarly of an 86-kD antigen,[159] both of which have kinetochore localization and DNA-topoisomerase function.

Antigenicity to DNA-topoisomerase I has been isolated to an 11-amino acid sequence that contains 6 sequential amino acids of identity with a sequence present in the group-specific p30^{gag} of mammalian retrovirus.[160] Serum antibody to retroviral p24^{gag} is present in 25 percent of patients with diffuse scleroderma but is unrelated to the presence of anti-DNA-topoisomerase I.[161] Others have identified at least two independent antigenic epitopes of DNA-topoisomerase I unrelated to the region of retroviral homology.[162] It remains possible that antibody elicited by previous or persistent retrovirus cross-reacts with intracellular topoisomerase. A retroviral etiology of disease would be consistent with the sporadic occurrence, variable latency, and broad spectrum of disease expression that typify systemic sclerosis.

Abnormalities of Cellular Immunity

Lymphocyte infiltration of the lower dermis occurs early in systemic sclerosis (see Fig. 66–8) and consists largely of T lymphocytes typically expressing surface markers of T helper phenotype.[51, 52, 163] Mononuclear cell infiltration has been correlated with the severity of local skin thickening[163] and is most frequent at early stages of disease. Since a variety of studies have suggested that lymphokines and monokines may stimulate collagen accumulation by fibroblasts,[82–85] it is likely that these infiltrating cells are important participants in the evolution of disease.

While total peripheral lymphocyte counts are typically normal or slightly reduced in untreated systemic sclerosis, analysis of T lymphocyte subpopulations has noted a relative increased proportion of CD4+ (T helper) cells due mainly to an absolute reduction in CD8+ (T suppressor) cells.[140, 164–166] Within the CD4+ subpopulation, the percentage of CD4/4B4+ cells (inducers of help) is lowered, whereas the CD4/2H4+ cells (inducers of suppression) are increased.[140] Soluble plasma levels of the CD8 molecule are elevated, suggesting increased turnover or activation of the CD8+ population.[140]

Serum or plasma levels of soluble interleukin-2 receptors are increased in patients with systemic sclerosis[167–169] and correlate with disease severity, progression, and mortality.[167, 168] The proportion of T lymphocytes expressing interleukin-2 receptors (CD25+) is slightly increased in systemic sclerosis.[140] Exposure to mitogen (phytohemagglutinin and conconavalin A) stimulates CD25+ expression comparable to that of lymphocytes from normal controls.[140] Laminin, a putative autoantigen in systemic sclerosis,[139] induces CD25 expression without enhancing lymphocyte proliferation or release of soluble interleukin-2 receptors.[140]

In vitro abnormalities include diminished lymphocyte response to phytohemagglutinin,[140, 170] which is improved after removal of adherent monocytes[170] and reductions in both antibody-dependent and phytohemagglutinin-induced lymphocyte cytotoxicity in individuals with extensive visceral involvement.[171]

Interleukin-1 production by peripheral blood mononuclear cells is diminished in systemic sclerosis.[172, 173] Elevated levels of serum interleukin-2, by both immunoreactive and biologic assay, have been reported and are correlated with extent of skin involvement and disease activity.[174] Others have found less consistent[168] or absent[167] elevations of this cytokine. Ongoing studies are finding inconsistent elevations of interleukin-4, interleukin-6, and tumor necrosis factor.[69a]

There is thus ample evidence of T lymphocyte activation and turnover from early stages of systemic sclerosis. Whether or not this is attributable to a specific cytokine effect or to an as yet unidentified cytokine inhibitor is unclear. Although the macrophage-activating effects of IFN-γ were just discussed, additional information links platelet-derived autocoids including serotonin via the S_2-serotonergic receptor to macrophage activation in scleroderma[175–177] or via the effects of transforming growth factor-β.[87] Clinically, patients with systemic sclerosis are not prone to opportunistic or even an increased incidence of infection, and cutaneous delayed hypersensitivity is normal.

A THEORY OF PATHOGENESIS

Experimental Models

Convincing animal models of systemic sclerosis have been lacking. The tight skin mouse (Tsk) develops thickened and adherent skin due to collagen and glycosaminoglycan accumulation in the dermis.[178, 179] Dermal fibroblasts derived from the Tsk mouse produce increased amounts of types I and III collagen in association with mast cell and lymphocyte tissue infiltration,[74, 180] and disodium cromoglycate therapy attenuates the dermis fibrosis of the Tsk mouse.[74] Similar evidence of mast cell infiltration and

of in vivo degranulation is noted in chronic graft-versus-host disease in BALB/c mice,[75] another animal model characterized by dermal fibrosis in the setting of mononuclear cell infiltrate.[181] The predictability of these models of dermal fibrosis is seen as providing a mechanism for the screening of potential therapies of systemic sclerosis.

The "scleroderma chicken" describes an inherited fibrotic disorder of White Leghorn chickens characterized by dermal and esophageal fibrosis and diffuse occlusive change of small and medium-sized arteries.[182] While the blood vessel changes are largely medial as opposed to the intimal disruption of human systemic sclerosis, arthritis, peripheral vascular insufficiency (digital and comb necrosis), and extensive visceral involvement, in the presence of diverse autoantibody formation and evidence of T cell infiltration in affected tissues,[182, 183] offer many parallels with human disease.

Human Models

Augmentation mammoplasty, with silicone-gel envelope implants in the United States and with direct injection of silica-related polymers and paraffin in Japan, is associated with the development of scleroderma-like skin changes both locally, and on occasion, with more extensive skin involvement.[18, 19, 184] Human adjuvant disease is the termed employed to describe those individuals who progress to a systemic connective tissue disorder.[184] This includes evolution of typical systemic sclerosis occurring years after surgery.[18, 19] Electron microscopy of affected tissue has confirmed "leakage" of silica.[18] Although definitive epidemiologic study is lacking, there are sufficient cases being identified to make silica-induced systemic sclerosis a likely route of pathogenesis. It is unclear whether such patients benefit from removal of their prostheses.

Human graft-versus-host disease, while uncommon, is associated with scleroderma-like skin thickening, sicca syndrome, and interstitial lung disease.[185]

Pathogenic Interrelationships

In general, hypotheses with regard to the pathogenesis of systemic sclerosis can be segregated by their emphasis on vascular, immunologic, or collagen abnormalities. As discussed before, virtually all of the available evidence suggests that accumulation of collagen and other matrix constituents is a secondary process. The principal research questions revolve around the determination of which of the various cytokine/growth factors have biologic relevance in systemic sclerosis and by what mechanism they operate. It is fair to emphasize that the dermal fibrosis from which the disorder is named is the least consistent clinical feature of disease. Scleroderma skin change is limited in around one half of patients to the fingers, hands, and face and in the case of systemic sclerosis sine scleroderma and undifferentiated connective tissue disease either absent or trivial. Furthermore, fibrotic change of visceral tissues is inconsistent and difficult in many cases to differentiate from vascular and inflammatory change as to its contribution to organ dysfunction. Lastly, there is evidence that even in diffuse scleroderma, progressive fibrosis of skin is typical only of early stages of disease.

As an intellectual strategy in a disease as complex as systemic sclerosis, it would seem appropriate to address the abnormalities present at the first recognizable stages of illness, which typically directs attention to the clinical presentation of Raynaud's phenomenon. However, modern investigations of such patients have revealed that immunologic features,[34, 35] abnormalities of microvascular architecture and endothelial integrity,[32, 33, 38, 39, 41] and abnormalities of arteriolar structure and function[36, 37] are well established at this earliest stage of disease. The issues of pathogenesis become paradigms of "the chicken or the egg" and would include the inability to elucidate whether or not platelet activation in systemic sclerosis is a primary event or is secondary to vascular injury of alternative mechanisms and the inability to recognize whether the specific immunologic features are fundamental to pathogenesis or epiphenomena of chronic tissue injury. There is no known "prescleroderma" clinical syndrome, and the absence of convincing kindreds of scleroderma has made investigation of potential host factors difficult. If there is a principal exogenous agent that triggers the disease in the susceptible individual, the absence of geographic and seasonal clusters of case outbreaks has rendered its identification problematic.

Figure 66–11 is one attempt to link the various descriptive abnormalities of systemic sclerosis. While there is reason or evidence to implicate each and all of these various possibilities in the development and expression of disease, their relative importance remains entirely speculative.

CLINICAL FEATURES

The individual with systemic sclerosis is confronted with a wide array of symptoms and difficulties ranging from complaints attributable to specific internal organ involvement to the protean manifestations of chronic, catabolic illness. Fever, even low grade, is uncommon in systemic sclerosis and should prompt a search for alternate etiology. Malaise and fatigue are virtually universal complaints as is weight loss even in the absence of gastrointestinal involvement. Many patients suffer waxing and waning of systemic symptoms in a pattern reminiscent of systemic lupus erythematosus and rheumatoid arthritis. Reactive depression is common, and diminished self-esteem and concern over cosmetic features of scleroderma can dominate the patient's sense of well-being. Systemic sclerosis is uncommon enough that many patients have neither met another with the illness nor heard of the disease until diagnosed. The burden on the psyche is made greater by the lack of understanding of cause and by the absence of consistently effective treatments.

Musculoskeletal Features

Generalized arthralgia and morning stiffness are typical symptoms of systemic sclerosis and may be confused with early rheumatoid arthritis. Clinically appreciable joint inflammation is uncommon, although erosive arthropathy has been demonstrated to occur in some series in as many as 29 percent of patients.[186, 187] Inexorable loss of hand function is the rule as skin thickening worsens and the underlying joints become tethered and restricted in motion.

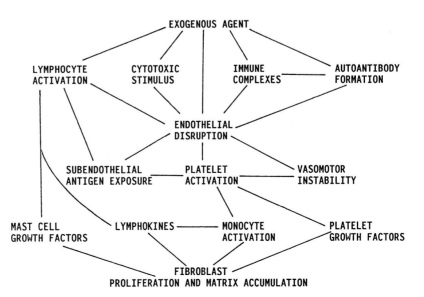

Figure 66–11. Potential pathogenic interrelationships in systemic sclerosis.

Inflammatory and fibrinous involvement of tendon sheaths may mimic arthritis. Leathery tendon friction rubs are appreciated by palpation during active or passive motion of involved areas and on rare occasions are audible. While most typically present over the wrists, ankles, and knees, occurrence of tendon friction rubs in the subscapular bursae may mimic the auscultatory findings of pleural friction rubs, and deep involvement surrounding the hip girdle may cause anterior thigh pain on weight bearing and suggest possible aseptic necrosis of the hip.

Insidious muscle weakness, both proximal and distal, occurs in many patients with systemic sclerosis secondary to disuse atrophy. There is also ample evidence of a primary myopathy characterized by mild proximal muscle weakness and mild elevations of serum muscle enzymes including aldolase and creatine phosphokinase[188, 189] in many patients. Electromyographic abnormalities are typical and include increased polyphasic potentials of normal and decreased amplitude and duration but without the insertional irritability and fibrillation that are hallmarks of polymyositis/dermatomyositis.[189, 190] Muscle biopsy reveals interstitial fibrosis and fiber atrophy with less conspicuous evidence of inflammatory cell infiltration and muscle fiber degeneration.[189, 190] An indolent clinical course characterized by waxing and waning of symptoms and laboratory features, generally unresponsive to glucocorticoid therapy, serves further to differentiate the simple myopathy of systemic sclerosis from inflammatory myositis occurring in overlap syndromes.

Although seldom a source of clinical complaint, osteopenia is common in systemic sclerosis and is related to impaired intestinal absorptive function, disuse, and diminished perfusion. Resorption and dissolution of the digital tufts (acro-osteolysis) (Fig. 66–12) occur in long-standing disease and are best explained by chronic digital ischemia. Resorption of

the mandibular condyles and thickening of the periodontal membrane have been reported.[191]

Subcutaneous calcinosis occurs in around 40 percent of patients with long-standing limited scleroderma and less frequently in diffuse disease. The most characteristic locations include the fingers (see Fig. 66–12), preolecranon area, olecranon and prepatellar bursae, and the anterior compartment of the lower extremity. Widespread involvement of tendon sheaths may occur as well as involvement of bizarre and strategically troublesome locations such as the ischial tuberosities, lateral malleoli, and at the thoracic outlet. These deposits are intermittently inflamed and a source of discomfort and spontaneous extrusion through the skin with complicating superinfection a frequent problem. Protein rich in γ-carboxyglutamic acid is increased locally[192] in the calcinosis both of dermatomyositis and of systemic sclerosis.

Gastrointestinal Involvement

Involvement of the gastrointestinal tract is the third most common manifestation of systemic sclerosis following only scleroderma skin change and Raynaud's phenomenon. Particularly with reference to esophageal dysmotility, there is no significant difference in prevalence or severity between individuals with generalized and limited scleroderma, and esophageal involvement is a principal feature of systemic sclerosis sine scleroderma.

Impaired function of the lower esophageal sphincter is associated with symptoms of intermittent heartburn, typically described as retrosternal burning pain but with frequent radiation cephalad and associated sour or bitter regurgitation. Disordered peristalsis of the lower two thirds of the esophagus presents as dysphagia and odynophagia for solid foods. Patients frequently complain of a "sticking" sensation of extraordinary reproducibility in location and severity. The lower esophageal dysmotility also serves to exacerbate the symptoms of reflux by allowing pooling of acid in the esophagus.[193]

Histopathologic study at late stages of illness has emphasized smooth muscle atrophy with fibrous replacement of the muscularis, fibrosis of the submucosa and lamina propria, and varying degrees of mucosal thinning and erosion.[88] Motility studies of early esophageal involvement have suggested that disordered cholinergic neural function is present in the nutritive vasculature,[194] and capillary alterations of endothelial swelling and basement membrane lamination are typical.[195] It seems likely that impaired perfusion and microvascular disruption contribute to the pathogenesis, first as disordered myoelectrical function and later as influences on muscle atrophy and fibrosis.

Esophageal function may be assessed by a variety of techniques including manometrics,[194] thin-barium recumbent cine-esophagraphy (Fig. 66–13),

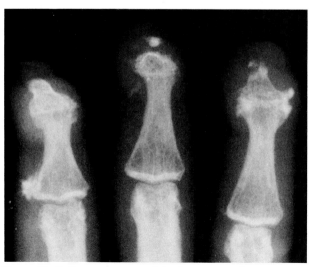

Figure 66–12. Roentgenogram of the fingers, revealing resorption and dissolution of the phalangeal tufts and multiple areas of punctate subcutaneous calcinosis.

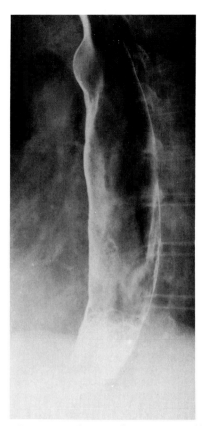

Figure 66–13. Barium esophagram demonstrating dilatation and aperistalsis of the distal esophagus and a patulous lower esophageal sphincter.

radionuclide transit studies,[196, 197] and esophagoscopy.[193] The abnormalities of esophageal function are not unique to systemic sclerosis.[198] It is also clear that there are patients within the spectrum of idiopathic intestinal hypomotility syndromes who share immunologic features of systemic sclerosis such as serum antinuclear antibody but in whom confident diagnosis cannot be sustained.

Complications of chronic esophageal reflux include erosive esophagitis with bleeding, Barrett's esophagus, and lower esophageal stricture,[193] which when present further contributes to solid food dysphagia. The presence of lower esophageal dysmotility is the principal influence on the development of erosive esophagitis, which may be present in surprising degree even in the asymptomatic patient.[193] Upper esophageal dysmotility and impaired deglutition occur rarely. Aspiration is often clinically unrecognized but should be suspected if patients present with productive cough or pulmonary infiltrates.

Involvement of the stomach occurs in systemic sclerosis and presents clinically as ease of satiety and on occasion as either functional gastric outlet obstruction or acute gastric dilatation. Telangiectases of the gastrointestinal tract may rarely be the cause of both upper and lower intestinal bleeding.

Small bowel involvement is one of the most vexing complications of systemic sclerosis and is more likely encountered in patients with long-standing limited scleroderma. Symptoms include intermittent bloating with abdominal cramps, intermittent or chronic diarrhea, and presentations suggestive of intestinal obstruction. Malabsorption occurs in a minority of patients and is most readily detected as impaired D-xylose absorption or as increased quantitative fecal fat elimination. The basic mechanism of small bowel dysfunction is similar to that of the esophagus where fibrosis and smooth muscle atrophy are noted in either a patchy or diffuse distribution.[194] Bacterial overgrowth in areas of intestinal stasis occurs frequently and is often responsive to empirical courses of broad-spectrum oral antibiotics such as tetracycline, vancomycin, or metronidazole.[199] Jejunal cultures and the bile acid breath test are useful in diagnosis.[200] Pneumatosis intestinalis cystoides may occur and is an ominous clinical sign. Volvulus and perforation are reported complications.

Colon involvement is present in the majority of patients with systemic sclerosis but is infrequently a prominent cause of clinical symptoms. Constipation, obstipation, and pseudo-obstruction may occur and are related to abnormal colonic motility.[201] Wide-mouthed diverticula along the antimesenteric border of the colon occur but are seldom the site of bleeding or of diverticular abscess. Rectal prolapse and fecal incontinence reflect scleroderma involvement of the anal sphincter.

Primary biliary cirrhosis is well described as occurring in overlap with systemic sclerosis, principally in individuals with long-standing limited disease.[202] In one series, 17 percent of patients classified as "primary" biliary cirrhosis had clinical evidence of systemic sclerosis,[203] and anticentromere antibody was detected in 10 of 110 consecutive patients, all of whom had clinical features of systemic sclerosis.[204] The antimitochondrial antibodies of systemic sclerosis most typically react with a DNAse sensitive antigen rather than the mitochondrial ATPase typical of primary biliary cirrhosis.[205] Hepatic and biliary tract fibrosis are distinctly uncommon.

Pulmonary Manifestations

As the ability to manage other complications of systemic sclerosis has improved, pulmonary involvement has emerged as the leading cause of mortality and a principal source of morbidity. No organ illustrates the diversity of pathologic processes operative in scleroderma as well as the lung, where any combination of vascular obliteration, fibrosis, and inflammation may be present. Clinical onset is frequently insidious, perhaps because of the relative physical inactivity of many patients with systemic sclerosis. Progressive dyspnea on exertion, limited effort tolerance, and nonproductive cough are typical, whereas chest pain, pleuritic symptoms, and increased sputum are less likely. Physical findings include fine early inspiratory crackling rales in the

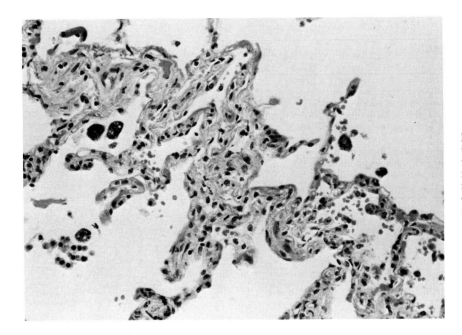

Figure 66–14. Photomicrograph of lung tissue obtained post mortem from a patient with interstitial pulmonary involvement from systemic sclerosis. There is interstitial thickening and fibrosis and continuing evidence of interstitial inflammation.

case of interstitial fibrotic disease or may instead reflect signs of pulmonary hypertension including an audibly increased and palpable pulmonic component of the second heart sound, right ventricular gallops, murmurs of pulmonic and tricuspid insufficiency, jugular venous distention, hepatojugular reflux, and pedal edema.[91, 206]

As a general rule, patients with diffuse scleroderma are at risk for progressive interstitial fibrotic lung disease. Histologic changes of diffuse fibrosis and variable degrees of inflammatory infiltrate are seen of alveoli, interstitium, and the peribronchiolar tissues[207] (Fig. 66–14). Individuals with limited systemic sclerosis may also develop interstitial disease but are also at risk for progressive pulmonary hyper-

tension in the absence of interstitial change, a complication most typical of long-standing disease.[91] Autopsy studies have defined the presence of intimal proliferation and medial myxomatous change in the small to medium-sized pulmonary arteries in 29 to 47 percent of patients[88, 207] (Fig. 66–15). In a prospective clinical study of 49 patients with systemic sclerosis, pulmonary arterial hypertension was detected by right heart catheterization in 33 percent of all patients and five of ten with limited scleroderma.[208]

Chest radiography reveals increased interstitial markings most prominently at the bases but is a relatively insensitive screening test. High-resolution computerized tomography is more sensitive. Pulmonary function testing remains the mainstay of

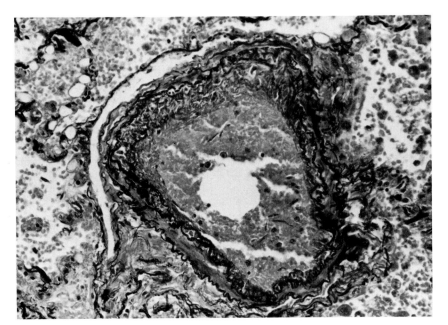

Figure 66–15. Intimal proliferation with reduplication of the internal elastic lamella and medial myxomatous change are seen in this photomicrograph of a pulmonary arteriole obtained at post mortem from a patient with long-standing limited scleroderma and severe pulmonary hypertension. The surrounding interstitium is thickened and reveals a mild inflammatory infiltrate, emphasizing the heterogeneity of pathologic processes operative in scleroderma lung (Verhoeff–van Gieson stain for elastin).

clinical diagnosis and serial assessment. Evidence of restriction including reduced vital capacity, diminished compliance, and increased ratios of forced expiratory volume to vital capacity is typical.[209, 210] Reduction of diffusing capacity is the most likely abnormality and if isolated or disproportionately decreased should suggest pulmonary vascular involvement.[91, 210] Most of the studies to date have suggested that pulmonary involvement, once established, is continually progressive and that prevalence increases in parallel with duration of systemic sclerosis.[209] Occasional patients improve their measures of either volume or diffusing capacity,[209] although variability in testing or difficulties in performance of pulmonary function testing such as diminished oral aperture might be contributory. Isolated reduction in diffusing capacity confers a poor prognosis.[211] Obstructive disease is usually attributed to cigarette smoking. Complications typical of interstitial lung disease such as spontaneous pneumothorax secondary to cicatricial emphysema occur only rarely.

Gallium lung scanning has been advocated in the assessment of the inflammatory component[212] but is generally less sensitive than in idiopathic interstitial fibrosis. Bronchoalveolar lavage reveals elevated proportions of neutrophils, lymphocytes, and occasionally eosinophils in the majority of patients[213–215] as well as selectively increased concentrations of immune complexes[213] and fibronectin.[216] It is unclear based on current data if the presence of inflammation should guide subsequent therapy.

Myocardial Involvement

Pathologic series have noted patchy myocardial fibrosis in as many as 81 percent of patients with systemic sclerosis.[88] These studies, as do large retrospective clinical analyses,[217] suggest that myocardial involvement is a principal determinant of survival in systemic sclerosis.

As discussed earlier (see Table 66–5), the fibrosis seems inseparable from and may be due to intermittent microvascular ischemia of the myocardium, perhaps mediated by myocardial mast cell infiltrates.[218] Physical findings are nonspecific and include ventricular gallops, sinus tachycardia, signs of congestive heart failure, and occasional pericardial friction rubs. Echocardiography reveals evidence of pericardial thickening or fluid in about one half of patients, but clinical presentations of pericarditis and of tamponade are infrequent.[219]

Resting electrocardiographic abnormalities including atrial and ventricular arrhythmias and conduction disturbances are encountered in nearly 50 percent of patients.[220] Ambulatory electrocardiographic features include a high prevalence of both supraventricular and ventricular tachyarrhythmias[221] with the latter being strongly associated with both overall mortality and the syndrome of sudden death.[221] Of the plethora of available techniques of cardiovascular assessment, Holter monitor studies are sensitive and yield information of potential therapeutic benefit.[222] Patients with limited systemic sclerosis are at only slightly decreased risk of myocardial involvement.[114, 222] Discrimination of the relative roles of heart and lung involvement in the clinical complaints of the individual patient is often difficult.[222]

Renal Involvement

The sudden onset of accelerated to malignant hypertension, rapidly progressive renal insufficiency, hyper-reninemia, and evidence of microangiopathic hemolysis describe the syndrome of "scleroderma renal crisis."[90, 111, 125] The clinical setting is usually in an individual with diffuse scleroderma who is relatively early in disease and at a stage of rapid progression of skin involvement.[223] Onset is most typically in cold weather months,[90, 223] although exceptions to all these statements are frequent. The predominance of cases in early diffuse scleroderma contributes substantially to the shortened survival of this classification of disease.[217]

Histopathologic study reveals the typical intimal proliferative lesion of systemic sclerosis (Fig. 66–16) with accompanying evidence of fibrinoid necrosis of the media,[88, 90, 111] the latter a nonspecific finding of malignant hypertension. Changes are most conspicuous in the interlobular and arcuate arteries and are in anatomic relation to areas of renal cortical necrosis. Sparse deposits of complement and immunoglobulin are noted in vessel walls but vasculitis is uncommon.[224]

Patients at risk for development of scleroderma renal disease cannot be identified by elevations of plasma renin activity,[223] and pathologic evidence of renal vascular disease is present in many patients without clinical renal disease.[88] Transient elevations of plasma renin activity[125] and diminished cortical perfusion[90, 125] may be evoked with cold challenge but do not reliably identify impending renal disease. Nonetheless, markedly elevated plasma renin activity is encountered in virtually all patients at the onset of hypertension.[223] Functional vasospasm superimposed on the intimal proliferative lesion is hypothesized to result in sufficient renal cortical hypoperfusion to trigger the release of renin.[225, 226] Ultimately, the vasoconstrictive effects of angiotensin II perpetuate the renal cortical ischemia, and the accelerated hypertension contributes the element of injury to the media, resulting in a fixed and irreversible deprivation of cortical blood flow and necrosis. Diffuse extrarenal vascular injury occurs as well with intimal disruption, fibrin deposition, and microangiopathic hemolysis. Although renal Raynaud's phenomenon is doubtless participatory in many cases, other factors may evoke scleroderma renal crisis including sudden depletion of intravascular fluid. Normotensive renal failure related to arteriolar thrombosis is associated with previous glucocorticoid therapy.[227]

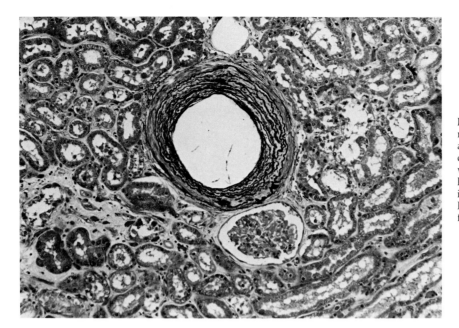

Figure 66–16. Photomicrograph of a small renal artery obtained from a patient with a successfully aborted scleroderma renal crisis. The intimal proliferative changes with reduplication of the internal elastic lamella are characteristic and highly reminiscent of the digital artery changes of Figure 66–9 (Verhoeff–van Gieson stain for elastin).

Profound drops in hemoglobin may occur as well as thrombocytopenia. Peripheral blood smears demonstrating fragmented red cells are often key to early diagnosis. Serum fibrinogen levels are usually normal although frequently decreased from previous values, and fibrin degradation products may be detected. Urinary sediment typically reveals modest protein and red cells but casts and nephrosis are unusual. Progression to anuric renal failure is the expected outcome if diagnosis is not promptly established and hypertension controlled.

Endocrine Features

Histologic evidence of thyroid gland fibrosis was found in 14 percent of a series of autopsied cases of scleroderma.[228] Evidence of hypothyroidism, frequently occult, is noted in as many as one fourth of patients and is best detected by abnormal responses to thyrotropin releasing hormone.[229] Serum antithyroid antibodies, lymphocytic infiltration of the gland, and clinical presentations of acute autoimmune thyroiditis are uncommon. Impotence is described as an early feature of scleroderma[230] and is felt to represent an abnormality of penile vascular function.[231]

Exocrine Features

Sicca syndrome occurs in 20 to 30 percent of patients with systemic sclerosis. Fibrosis in the absence of mononuclear cell infiltration is noted on minor salivary gland biopsy.[232] Antibodies to the Sjögren's syndrome precipitins (SS-A and SS-B) occur in approximately one half of patients.[233] Clinical presentations include dry eyes and dry mouth but salivary gland enlargement is uncommon.[233] Dry mouth coupled with the mechanical problems of limited oral aperture and impaired hand function serves to make adequate dental hygiene a formidable task.[234] Pancreatic insufficiency has been reported but pathologic evidence of pancreatic fibrosis is lacking.

Pregnancy

There is little known concerning the effects of scleroderma on pregnancy and vice versa. Irregular menses and amenorrhea occur in severely ill patients, and women with scleroderma frequently have difficulty with conception. Intrauterine growth retardation and low birth weights have been reported.[235] In general, pregnancy does not worsen the scleroderma,[235] although the course of pregnancy is typified by worsened symptoms of reflux esophagitis and by exacerbation of cardiopulmonary compromise.

Neurologic Manifestations

Systemic sclerosis spares the central nervous system. However, entrapment neuropathies including carpal tunnel syndrome, meralgia paresthetica, trigeminal neuropathy, and facial nerve palsies[236] are well known. Subclinical autonomic dysfunction has been demonstrated,[237] and physiologic study has suggested that gastrointestinal cholinergic and peripheral adrenergic nervous function are impaired.

Scleroderma and Malignancy

The coincidence of malignancy and scleroderma has been described[238] including the occurrence of lung carcinoma superimposed on long-standing interstitial pulmonary disease.[239] In one series, the relative risk of lung cancer in systemic sclerosis was 16.5.[239] In contrast, a detailed epidemiologic comparison including over 1000 patient years of experience found 14 malignancies, mainly pulmonary, versus an expected 7 to 8 and a relative risk of 1.81.[240] While there was no increase in breast carcinoma, a biologic relationship was suggested by its occurrence in close temporal relationship to the onset of scleroderma.[240] Esophageal carcinoma is so rare that regular surveillance is not felt to be cost-effective.[241]

THERAPY FOR SYSTEMIC SCLEROSIS

The Impact of Classification

Individuals at early stages of diffuse scleroderma are most likely to manifest increasing extent and severity of scleroderma skin thickening and are at the highest risk of developing new internal organ involvement.[47, 48, 223] At later stages of diffuse disease, slowly improving skin change is typical.[47, 48] Spontaneous regression to clinical features of limited disease occurs but complete remission is exceedingly rare.[242] In later disease, the risk of developing new visceral involvement is much reduced although still present, and it should be emphasized that spontaneous improvement in established internal organ dysfunction is most uncommon.

Limited scleroderma is typified by insidious progression of skin involvement, often so slow as to be unrecognizably changed from year to year. Internal organ involvement including heart and lung is known to occur with frequencies close to that of diffuse disease, but onset of involvement is typically delayed for years. Other than the association of renal disease with diffuse scleroderma and of pulmonary hypertension with limited scleroderma, there is little difference between these subgroups at very late stages of disease. Patients with chronic diffuse and limited scleroderma, matched for sex, age, and disease duration, are found to differ only in terms of frequency of skeletal muscle involvement and, by definition, extent of scleroderma.[243]

Although vast gaps remain in our understanding of the natural history of systemic sclerosis, it would seem apparent that the syndrome is clinically divergent at early stages and clinically convergent late in the disease course. Assuming that truly remittive or effective drug therapy were available, the goals of treatment in any given subgroup would be somewhat different (Table 66–6). An agent of potential effectiveness in the prevention of new skin involvement would be most appropriately employed and most easily assessed in patients with early diffuse disease, but improvement from baseline might not be detected for 1 to 3 years. However, benefit over placebo in attenuating new skin involvement would be more easily demonstrated. It should also be emphasized

Table 66–6. IMPACT OF CLASSIFICATION AND NATURAL HISTORY OF SYSTEMIC SCLEROSIS ON CHOICE OF THERAPY

Clinical Subgroup	Goal and Relevance of Therapy (Duration of Therapy Required)			
	Sclerodermatous Skin Change		Internal Organ Involvement	
	PREVENT NEW INVOLVEMENT	IMPROVE EXISTING DISEASE	PREVENT NEW INVOLVEMENT	IMPROVE EXISTING DISEASE
Early, diffuse	+ + + + (1–3 y)	+ + (1–3 y)	+ + + + (1–3 y)	+ (1–3 y)
Early, limited	NA	NA	+ (>3 y)	+ (1–3 y)
Late, diffuse	+ (1–3 y)	+ + + (1–3 y)	+ + (>3 y)	+ + + (1–3 y)
Late, limited	NA	+ (1–3 y)	+ (>3 y)	+ + (1–3 y)

NA, not applicable.

that the clinical progression of skin involvement in early diffuse disease is somewhat variable. Many patients can have prolonged periods of months or more in which skin thickening appears unchanged. Others can seem to improve rapidly, although this probably represents waxing and waning of skin edema rather than changes in dermal collagen accumulation. In later years of diffuse disease, placebo-treated patients would be predicted to somewhat improve in extent and severity of skin involvement. Agents chosen to affect skin involvement would not be applicable to patients with limited scleroderma.

Parallel arguments apply to consideration of therapeutic agents for visceral involvement. Study of therapies directed toward pre-existing internal organ dysfunction would again need to consider the slowness of tissue remodeling. Irrespective of which element of pathogenesis were approached and with which modality, including antifibrotic agents, immunomodulators, or therapies directed against vascular features of systemic sclerosis, clinical benefit would be difficult to prove.

Therapeutic studies of systemic sclerosis can be easily criticized for lack of controls matched for duration, severity, and classification of disease; inappropriate choices of study duration; unclear therapeutic end points; and lack of standardization of measures of outcome. The paradox of adequately designed therapeutic studies of systemic sclerosis is that any trial of less than 1 year's duration is likely to risk false negative outcome, whereas any trial of longer than 3 years risks false positive results.

Disease-Modifying Therapies

There are NO drug therapies of proven value in the management of systemic sclerosis. Controlled and prospective clinical trials have been performed but with disappointing, uniformly negative results. A variety of trials of one or more agents have claimed to demonstrate clinical benefit but have been, by and large, of inadequate design.[243a]

Glucocorticoids have no efficacy in slowing the progress of systemic sclerosis. Their usefulness is limited to management of inflammatory myositis occurring in overlap with systemic sclerosis, and potentially in inflammatory stages of interstitial lung disease.[215] Short courses of low-dose glucocorticoid have palliative benefit in the arthralgias and myalgias of early edematous scleroderma and in management of painful tendinous involvement. High-dose glucocorticoid ($\geq$30 mg prednisone per day) is linked etiologically to the syndrome of normotensive renal failure[227] and other vaso-occlusive complications of disease.

Immunosuppressive agents have been relatively well studied. A 3-year controlled trial of chlorambucil, which incorporated detailed laboratory assessments of internal organ involvement, found no benefit of drug over placebo.[244] Azathioprine employed for periods up to 23 months was similarly ineffective.[245] A 6-month study of 5-fluorouracil failed to demonstrate clinically important change.[246] Pilot studies of cyclosporin A suggested usefulness for skin involvement but have ceased because of unacceptable renal toxicity. In view of the prominent abnormalities of cellular and humoral immune dysfunction present at early stages of systemic sclerosis, immunosuppressive therapy would seem a rational approach to management but one that is not supported by the trial results to date.

Apheresis has been claimed to be effective in systemic sclerosis. A preliminary report of a blinded and controlled trial of lymphoplasmapheresis in patients with early disease suggested improvement in skin involvement as well as in global assessments by patient, physician, and physical therapist.[247] Clinical improvement was also reported in 14 of 15 patients receiving prednisone, cyclophosphamide, and plasmapheresis in an uncontrolled trial,[248] whereas no benefit was demonstrated in an open experience with plasmapheresis as the sole therapy.[249] Apheresis is complicated by problems of venous access and expense. Lack of homogeneity of treated subjects and the use of concomitant immunosuppressives render problematic the interpretation of its purported benefit. Further study is warranted.

Ketotifen, an antihistamine claimed to also inhibit mast cell degranulation, produced no benefit in skin involvement, pulmonary function, or other clinical parameters in a 6-month controlled trial.[250] Recombinant IFN-γ was the subject of an as yet unreported open trial in early diffuse disease. Although a minority of patients seemed to improve, clinical effect was quite inconsistent. Photophoresis employs extracorporeal ultraviolet A irradiation to activate 8-methoxypsoralen[251] and is an approved therapy for cutaneous T cell lymphoma. A short-term comparison with D-penicillamine treatment suggested minor benefits including improved sense of well-being in photophoresed subjects but inconsistent and poorly quantified effects on skin.[251a]

Some well-designed and well-performed studies have been directed at the vascular aspects of systemic sclerosis including the chronic in vivo platelet activation. Vasodilators, including captopril,[252] α-methyldopa with propranolol,[253] an as yet unreported long-term trial of the S_2-serotonergic antagonist ketanserin,[98] and a controlled study of aspirin with dipyridamole,[254] were found to have no clinical or laboratory benefit.

A variety of therapies of less apparent rationale have been attempted including dimethylsulfoxide, colchicine, N-acetylcysteine, anabolic steroids, griseofulvin, and potassium aminobenzoate.[255]

The most commonly employed agent in systemic sclerosis is D-penicillamine. In a large and detailed retrospective analysis, D-penicillamine, given at high dosage and for prolonged periods, was reported to improve skin involvement and to be associated with a lesser incidence of new visceral involvement, notably renal, and improved survival in comparison with a matched group of patients receiving other therapies.[48, 48a] Theoretically, D-penicillamine, by virtue of its interference with the intermolecular cross-linking of collagen and possibly due to immunomodulatory effects, might be predicted to benefit scleroderma. Indeed, there are now two retrospective experiences suggesting modest efficacy in established interstitial lung disease.[256, 257] Adverse effects occur in around 30 percent of patients,[258] and there is no evidence that D-penicillamine therapy improves vascular and immunologic features of systemic sclerosis. Controlled and prospective study is needed. At present, D-penicillamine must be accorded cautious optimism. Such therapy is best reserved for individuals with early diffuse scleroderma in whom internal organ involvement is minimal; its clinical rationale in limited scleroderma and in long-standing established diffuse disease remains unclear.

Although there are obvious benefits to controlled and prospective trials in systemic sclerosis, the reader should be aware that such trials are expensive, particularly if they incorporate laboratory measures of internal organ status, and the number of patients required is substantial. The relative rarity of systemic sclerosis has accorded this disorder low priority in privately sponsored therapeutic research.

Supportive Measures

A lot of supportive therapy is available for the individual patient with systemic sclerosis. Proper clinical management mandates an awareness of the multiplicity of symptoms and the palliative potential of the modern therapeutic armamentarium. All patients benefit from education about their condition. Although the clinician may feel somewhat frustrated by the lack of disease-modifying therapeutic options, attentive and individualized monitoring can help many patients to lead full and productive lives.

Management of Raynaud's phenomenon should focus both on reduction of frequency and severity of episodes of cold-induced vasospasm and on prevention of digital tip ischemic ulcerations. All patients benefit from cessation of smoking and commonsense advice regarding lifestyle. Dress can be important and, in addition to mittens and warm footwear, should include hats and layered clothing on the trunk to minimize the contribution of reflex responses to central body cold stimuli. Choice of drug therapy is a complicated issue in systemic sclerosis, and response is dominated by the degree of fixed obstructive change in the digital vasculature. Calcium channel blockers including nifedipine,[99, 259] diltiazem,[260] verapamil,[260] and nicardipine[261] are subjectively effective in many patients, although physiologic benefit is less consistently demonstrable. The availability of sustained-release preparations of both nifedipine and diltiazem has increased their usefulness by permitting higher dosage with improved tolerance. These agents cause vascular smooth muscle relaxation by interference with trans-sarcolemmal influx of calcium through membrane channels termed *slow-channels*[262] and likely function as antivasoconstrictors rather than as vasodilators. Their clinical use is somewhat limited by their potential to interfere with esophageal motility, and they may, in some patients, actually worsen peripheral vascular resistance by increasing perfusion of the fixed distal vasculature. Prazosin, an orally active selective antagonist of α_1-adrenoceptors, is effective occasionally.[263] Other therapies including sympatholytics, biofeedback, and Pavlovian conditioning are more useful in primary Raynaud's phenomenon.[93, 94] An occasional patient may benefit from sympathectomy and can be chosen by monitoring short-term response to sympathetic ganglion instillation of bupivacaine.

Digital ischemic ulcerations (Fig. 66–17) require attention to the role of superinfection and consideration of the possible contribution of underlying calcinosis. In addition to agents for peripheral vasodilatation, aspirin and dipyridamole are theoretically helpful although of dubious clinical efficacy,[254] and pentoxifylline may be added for enhancement of microvascular perfusion.[264] The S_2-serotonergic receptor antagonist ketanserin is unavailable in the United States.[98] Iloprost, an intravenously administered stable prostacyclin analogue, remains investigational but appears efficacious for both control of Raynaud's phenomenon and healing of digital tip ulcerations.[100, 265, 266] The ischemically compromised digit is an indication for angiography, which permits localization of the site of vascular occlusion, recognition of emboli, and assessment of the component of reversible vasoconstriction.

Nonsteroidal anti-inflammatory agents are generally useful in the management of arthralgias and myalgia although occasional patients require low doses of oral glucocorticoids. While few patients maintain normal hand function, the early institution of a vigorous and sustained physical therapy program can attenuate the effects of the inexorably progressive tethering and atrophy responsible for loss of function.

Skin care is important and should include moisturizing agents and prompt treatment of infected ulcerations. There are no current effective therapies for subcutaneous calcinosis.

Symptoms of reflux esophagitis are typical of systemic sclerosis, but they are generally amenable to therapy. Patients should be encouraged to avoid large meals and tight clothing to minimize increased gastric pressure. Reflux can be minimized by avoidance of postprandial recumbency and by elevation of the head of the bed. Histamine-2 receptor blockade with cimetidine, ranitidine, famotidine, or nizatidine supplemented with antacid is generally useful as is mucosal protection, with sucralfate[267] administered postprandially. Omeprazole, an inhibitor of gastric acid secretion due to inhibition of the $H+/K+/ATPase$ proton pump of the parietal cell, is remarkably effective in palliation of pyrosis but is

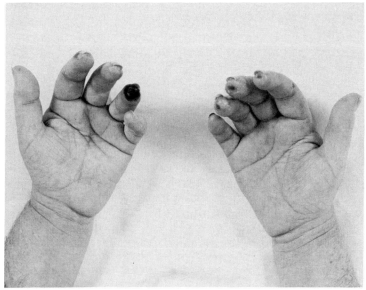

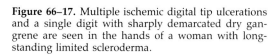
Figure 66–17. Multiple ischemic digital tip ulcerations and a single digit with sharply demarcated dry gangrene are seen in the hands of a woman with longstanding limited scleroderma.

limited by expense and a theoretical potential for gastric carcinogenesis with unduly prolonged therapy.[268] Dysphagia can be minimized by careful mastication of small quantities of food. Occasional patients benefit clinically from the esophageal motility–enhancing effects of metoclopramide.[269] Refractory dysphagia should suggest lower esophageal stricture and the need for mechanical dilatation. Symptoms of small bowel involvement may respond to broad-spectrum antibiotics and occasionally to dietary lactose restriction. Constipation is best managed with agents that soften and increase the bulk of stool.

Although myocardial perfusion abnormalities have been demonstrated to improve in response to nifedipine and dipyridamole, evidence of clinical efficacy is lacking.[115] Symptomatic pericarditis responds to both nonsteroidal anti-inflammatory agents and glucocorticoids. While cardiac arrhythmias are felt to have important prognostic value, studies demonstrating enhanced survival by treatment of these arrhythmias are lacking.

Pulmonary involvement is at the present time not consistently amenable to therapy. Theoretically, a patient in whom there was evidence of pulmonary interstitial inflammation might be treated with glucocorticoids and immunosuppressives in the hope of arresting development of interstitial fibrosis. Clinical trials demonstrating the usefulness of this approach, including use of methotrexate, cyclophosphamide, cyclosporine, and azathioprine, remain to be reported. Interstitial fibrosis has been treated with D-penicillamine,[256, 257] although substantial questions concerning its efficacy remain unanswered.[270]

Pulmonary hypertension has emerged as a principal cause of morbidity and mortality in late systemic sclerosis. Vasodilator therapy is generally without clinical benefit and may on occasion lead to paradoxical worsening of pulmonary artery pressure and pulmonary vascular resistance.[206, 271–273] Supplemental oxygen and careful attention to fluid balance are the mainstays of symptomatic management.

The key to management of scleroderma renal involvement is prompt recognition of the diagnosis and aggressive treatment of the accompanying accelerated hypertension. Patients at high risk, namely early generalized scleroderma, should be taught ambulatory self-monitoring of blood pressure. While pulmonary hypertension was previously refractory to all but the most desperate therapies such as bilateral nephrectomy, a variety of modern and effective antihypertensive agents have revolutionized clinical management. Angiotensin converting enzyme inhibitors such as captopril and enalapril are mechanistically suited to the hyper-reninemic hypertension of scleroderma renal crisis and are the treatment of choice.[110, 226, 252, 274] Successful control of hypertension and arrest of progressive renal insufficiency have also been reported with minoxidil, α-methyldopa, and other agents. If blood pressure is controlled before serum creatinine rises to 4.0 mg per dl, arrest of renal insufficiency and occasional improvement of renal function result.[275] Peritoneal

dialysis is the modality of choice for management of uremia and facilitates the option for renal transplantation. While there are reports of regression of scleroderma skin thickening following successful medical management of scleroderma renal crisis,[275] this is uncommon[252] and probably due in part to the spontaneous improvement typical of later stages of diffuse scleroderma.

LOCALIZED SCLERODERMA

Localized scleroderma is the term employed to describe a variety of conditions of clinical and histopathologic similarity to the skin manifestations of systemic sclerosis but in which the characteristic internal organ and vascular features are lacking.[276]

Linear Scleroderma

Linear scleroderma is an uncommon disorder of unknown etiology characterized by a band of sclerotic induration and hyperpigmentation occurring on a single extremity or on the face. Although onset may occur at any age, linear scleroderma is most typically encountered in children and young adults. Women are affected approximately three times as often as men, and the condition is uncommon in blacks.

Onset is heralded by a frequently asymptomatic band of erythema followed by rapid evolution of induration and thickening of skin with tethering to deeper tissues. The original lesion will frequently extend insidiously to involve the entire length of the affected extremity, and satellite lesions of morphea (see later) are common. Irregular atrophy of underlying subcutaneous fat is typical and extension to underlying muscle and bone (melorheostosis) may occur. In the adult, the principal functional impact is contracture of underlying joints. Involvement of the face (coup de sabre) in children (Fig. 66–18) is associated with asymmetric growth and progressive facial disfigurement. Linear scleroderma of an extremity in childhood leads to substantial muscle atrophy and progressive leg length discrepancy (Fig. 66–19).

Peripheral blood eosinophilia and polyclonal hypergammaglobulinemia are present in many patients at clinically active stages of disease,[277] as are antinuclear and anti–single-stranded DNA antibodies. Biopsy of affected skin reveals lower dermal and subcutaneous fibrosis and infiltration with lymphocytes and plasma cells and is essentially indistinguishable from the changes of systemic sclerosis. Augmented accumulation of collagen and glycosaminoglycan is noted in studies of cultured dermal fibroblasts derived from patients with linear scleroderma.[278]

The typical patient has active disease for 2 to 3 years. Involutional atrophic change dominates the later stages of disease.[277, 279] Physical therapy of affected joint groups is useful. D-Penicillamine, topical and systemic glucocorticoids, and hydroxychloroquine have been advocated but convincing evidence of their effectiveness is lacking.

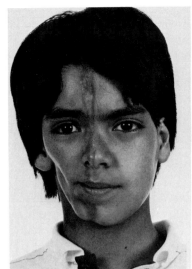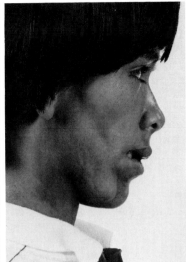

Figure 66–18. Linear scleroderma of the face (coup de sabre) in a 13-year-old boy with 8 years of disease. Atrophy of the subcutaneum and of the mandible is apparent as well as an isolated depression of bone over the forehead. Progressive facial distortion has occurred with ongoing asymmetric growth. Reconstructive surgery is planned for early adulthood.

Morphea

The morphea variety of localized scleroderma may occur at any site and at any age and is characterized by either small discrete spots (guttate morphea) or by larger patches (morphea en plaque) (Fig. 66–20) of sclerodermatous skin induration. Slowly expanding "target" lesions with an erythematous or violaceous border and with central hypopigmentation, tethering, and thickening may occur in many locations either simultaneously or as evolving contin-

ually over several months or years. Involutional atrophy with persistent pigmentary change, spontaneous improvement, and even total clinical resolution of morphea are typical after periods of several months to several years.[276, 279] The clinical consequences of morphea are principally cosmetic although contracture of underlying joint groups may occur. Biopsies at early stages of illness reveal inflammatory infiltrate, felt by some observers to be more intense than that of systemic sclerosis, and fibrosis with the changes principally noted in the lower dermis and upper subcutaneum.

On occasion, morphea can present in an exten-

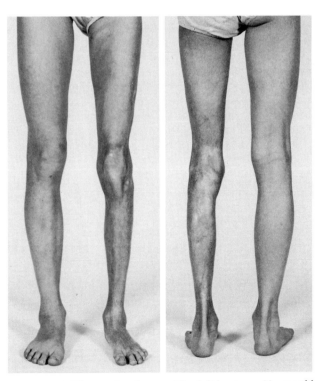

Figure 66–19. Linear scleroderma of the left leg in an 11-year-old girl. Diffuse muscle atrophy is apparent. As this patient enters puberty, progressive leg length discrepancy is expected.

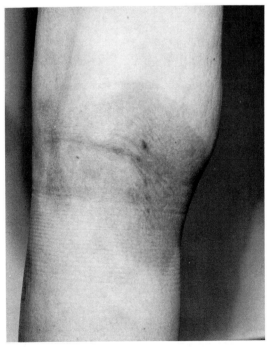

Figure 66–20. Morphea en plaque is seen in the popliteal fossa of this 55-year-old woman. Present for 4 years, the recent course has been marked by progressive softening of this and other lesions.

sively generalized distribution and with protean manifestations of catabolic illness including fatigue, weight loss, and inanition. Generalized subcutaneous morphea describes a rare entity in which inflammation and fibrosis are centered in the subcutaneous tissue with apparent extension to the lower dermis and occasionally to the subtending fascia.[280] In one well-described series of 16 patients, many had features suggestive of systemic sclerosis including interstitial pulmonary disease, esophageal dysmotility, joint complaints, and serum antinuclear antibodies.[280]

Relationship to Systemic Sclerosis

Individuals with otherwise typical systemic sclerosis may on occasion manifest morphea and linear scleroderma–like skin changes[281] as may rare patients with systemic lupus erythematosus and overlap syndromes. As a general rule, the converse occurs so rarely as to confirm a lack of association. The similarities of localized scleroderma to systemic sclerosis are limited to the histopathologic features, the serologic abnormalities, and the shared prevalence in young women.

Scleredema/Scleromyxedema

Scleredema (scleredema adultorum of Buschke) and scleromyxedema (papular mucinosis, lichen myxedematosus) are clinically similar but distinct connective tissue disorders characterized by widespread induration and thickening of the skin resulting from accumulation of collagen and proteoglycan in the dermis. The skin involvement on the face and neck, which progresses acrally, and the sparing of the fingers and hands, as well as the absence of Raynaud's phenomenon and of visceral involvement, permit clinical differentiation from systemic sclerosis. Histopathologically, both scleredema and scleromyxedema show minimal epidermal changes, whereas the dermis is markedly thickened with variable degrees of proteoglycan, hyaluronic acid, and collagen deposits.[282, 283]

The etiology and pathogenesis of both diseases are obscure. Around one half of adult scleredema patients have diabetes mellitus, and both conditions are associated with underlying plasma cell dyscrasia including multiple myeloma.[282, 284] Sera from patients with scleromyxedema have been shown to stimulate DNA synthesis and cell proliferation of normal human skin fibroblasts in culture,[285] and sera from patients with scleredema stimulate collagen and proteoglycan accumulation by autologous and homologous dermal fibroblasts lines.[284] Serologic, internal organ, and vascular features of systemic sclerosis are conspicuously absent and there are no known effective therapies.

Eosinophilic Fasciitis

Eosinophilic fasciitis is a scleroderma-like disorder characterized by inflammation and thickening of the deep fascia. Since the original description by Shulman in 1975, several hundred cases have been reported,[286–288] and the clinical description is still evolving. Extension to subjacent skeletal muscle may occur and extension to overlying subcutaneum and lower dermis is common. Onset frequently follows periods of undue physical exertion and trauma, particularly in males, and the condition has been reported to occur in children and the elderly although it is most frequent in young adults. The rapid onset of pain and swelling of the extremities is soon followed by progressive induration of the skin and subcutaneous tissues of the forearms, legs, and, on occasion, the hands, feet, and trunk. In many cases, exaggerated deep grooving or "furrowing" of the subcutis surrounding superficial veins is noted (Fig. 66–21) and may be enhanced by antidependent posture. The overlying skin is typically shiny and erythematous with a coarse orange-peel appearance. Carpal tunnel syndrome is frequent and contractures

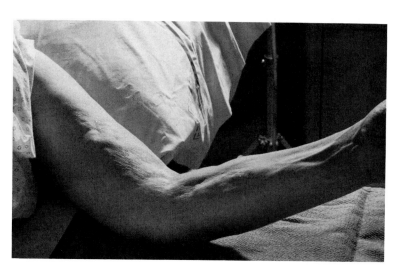

Figure 66–21. The arm of a 59-year-old woman with 4 months of eosinophilic fasciitis. The superficial skin is not thickened but is irregularly tethered to deeper tissues, which have a woody induration. There is a coarse orange-peel appearance and patchy erythema. The exaggerated furrow over the course of superficial veins in the volar forearm is pathognomonic of idiopathic eosinophilic fasciitis and of the fasciitis secondary to the eosinophilia-myalgia syndrome.

of underlying joints develop early in the course of illness.[288]

Raynaud's phenomenon and internal organ features of systemic sclerosis are absent although peripheral vascular entrapment syndromes may occur. There have been several cases reported of accompanying hematologic disorders including aplastic anemia and myeloproliferative syndromes.[289, 290]

Laboratory abnormalities at early stages of illness include peripheral eosinophilia, elevated erythrocyte sedimentation rates, polyclonal hypergammaglobulinemia, and elevated levels of circulating immune complexes.

Diagnosis is best established by a full-thickness (skin to skeletal muscle) wedge biopsy. Early in the course of the illness, the deep fascia and subcutis are edematous and infiltrated with lymphocytes, plasma cells, histiocytes, eosinophils,[291] and mast cells.[292] As the disease progresses, these structures, and often the dermis as well, become thickened and fibrotic (Fig. 66–22).

Glucocorticoids in small doses (prednisone, 10 to 20 mg per day) are useful in the palliation of limb discomfort and readily suppress the peripheral and tissue eosinophilia. Glucocorticoids have not been demonstrated to hasten the resolution of fibrosis nor to modify the long-term course of the disease. Their usage is reserved for individuals with early disease and actively inflamed biopsy lesions and as adjuncts in the management of carpal tunnel syndrome and flexion contracture. Nonsteroidal anti-inflammatory agents are useful for symptomatic relief as well. There is anecdotal evidence of the usefulness of hydroxychloroquine, methotrexate, and D-penicillamine.

The natural history of eosinophilic fasciitis remains to be resolved. Many patients improve spontaneously or while on glucocorticoids over periods of 2 to 5 years, although histopathologic evidence of fascial fibrosis may persist.[293] Other patients experience a course of recurrent relapse and remission and a minority have protracted clinical activity. Later disease can be dominated by painful symmetric joint complaints.

Eosinophilia-Myalgia Syndrome

An epidemic of now more than 1500 cases of abrupt onset of myalgia, fatigue, and peripheral eosinophilia was identified in 1989 and rapidly linked to the use of L-tryptophan dietary supplement for insomnia, premenstrual symptoms, and depression.[294] This syndrome is discussed extensively in Chapter 68.

Other Syndromes

An epidemic of acute pneumonitis followed by a chronic stage of scleroderma-like skin thickening, neuromyopathy, and sicca syndrome affected thousands of individuals in Spain in 1981.[295] A tainted rapeseed oil was implicated epidemiologically although the precise chemical offending substance was not identified and the mechanism of the toxic oil syndrome remains unknown.[296] Scleroderma-like illnesses have been reported in vinyl chloride workers[13] and following trichlorethylene exposure.[15] Intramuscular pentazocine is associated with a local inflammatory fibrosing tissue reaction, which on occasion may become more generalized,[297] and bleomycin therapy may induce scleroderma-like fibrosis of skin and lungs.[298]

The syndromes of localized scleroderma should be considered if not accompanied by Raynaud's phenomenon or if the distribution of skin involvement is atypical for systemic sclerosis. Dermal fibrosis, frequently linked to inflammatory processes of diverse etiology, suggests common pathogenic influences in the spectrum of the scleroderma disorders.

This chapter is dedicated to the memory of Dr. Gerald P. Rodnan. The assistance of Deborah A. McCloskey, Nurse Coordinator, Scleroderma Program, and of the staff and faculty of the Robert Wood Johnson Medical School Clinical Research Center is gratefully appreciated.

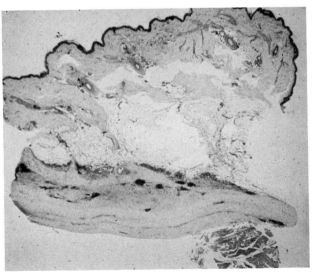

Figure 66–22. Photomicrograph of a full-thickness biopsy from the forearm of a patient with eosinophilic fasciitis. The epidermis and upper dermis are unremarkable. The fascia is several-fold thickened with dense fibrosis and persistent inflammatory infiltrate. Inflammation and patchy fibrosis extend into the subcutaneous fat and to the lower dermis. Although eosinophils were readily apparent on higher magnification in this case, they are inconsistently demonstrated and are easily suppressed by glucocorticoid.

References

1. Subcommittee for Scleroderma Criteria of the American Rheumatism Association Diagnostic and Therapeutic Criteria Committee: Preliminary criteria for the classification of systemic sclerosis (scleroderma). Arthritis Rheum. 23:581, 1980.

2. Medsger, T. A.: Comment on scleroderma criteria cooperative study. *In* Black, C. M., and Myers, A. R. (eds.): Systemic Sclerosis (Scleroderma). 1st ed. New York, Gower Med., 1985.
3. Masi, A. T.: Classification of systemic sclerosis (scleroderma). *In* Black, C. M., and Myers, A. R. (eds.): Systemic Sclerosis (Scleroderma). 1st ed. New York, Gower Med., 1985.
4. Rodnan, G. P., Jablonska, S., and Medsger, T. A.: Classification and nomenclature of progressive systemic sclerosis (scleroderma). Clin. Rheum. Dis. 5:5, 1979.
5. Barnett, A. F.: Scleroderma (progressive systemic sclerosis): Progress and course based on a personal series of 118 cases. Med. J. Aust. 2:129, 1978.
6. LeRoy, E. C., Black, C., Fleischmajer, R., et al.: Scleroderma (systemic sclerosis): Classification, subsets and pathogenesis. J. Rheumatol. 15:202, 1988.
7. Giordano, M., Valentini, G., Migliaresi, S., et al.: Different antibody patterns and different prognoses in patients with scleroderma with various extents of skin sclerosis. J. Rheumatol. 13:911, 1986.
8. Medsger, T. A.: Epidemiology of progressive systemic sclerosis. *In* Black, C. M., and Myers, A. R. (eds.): Systemic Sclerosis (Scleroderma). 1st ed. New York, Gower Med., 1985.
9. Silman, A. J.: Mortality from scleroderma in England and Wales 1968–1985. Ann. Rheum. Dis. 50:95, 1991.
10. Maricq, H. R., Weinrich, M. C., Keil, J. E., et al.: Prevalence of scleroderma spectrum disorders in the general population of South Carolina. Arthritis Rheum. 32:998, 1989.
11. Medsger, T. A., and Masi, A. T.: Epidemiology of systemic sclerosis (scleroderma). Ann. Intern. Med. 74:714, 1971.
12. Medsger, T. A., and Masi, A. T.: The epidemiology of systemic sclerosis (scleroderma) among male U.S. veterans. J. Chronic Dis. 31:73, 1978.
13. Lilis, R., Anderson, H., Nicholason, W. J., et al.: The prevalence of disease among vinyl chloride and polyvinyl chloride workers. Ann. N.Y. Acad. Sci. 246:22, 1975.
14. Yamakage, A., Ishikawa, H., Saito, Y., et al.: Occupational scleroderma-like disorder in men engaged in the polymerization of epoxy resins. Dermatologia 161:33, 1980.
15. Sparrow, G. P.: A connective tissue disorder similar to vinyl chloride disease in a patient exposed to perchloroethylene. Clin. Exp. Dermatol. 2:17, 1977.
16. Erasmus, L. D.: Scleroderma in gold-miners on the Witwatersrand with particular reference to pulmonary manifestations. S. Afr. J. Lab. Clin. Med. 3:209, 1957.
17. Rodnan, G. P., Benedek, T. G., Medsger, T. A., et al.: The association of progressive systemic sclerosis (scleroderma) with coal miners' pneumoconiosis and other forms of silicosis. Ann. Intern. Med. 66:323, 1967.
18. Varga, J., Schumacher, H. R., and Jimenez, S. A.: Systemic sclerosis after augmentation mammoplasty with silicone implants. Ann. Intern. Med. 111:377, 1989.
19. Spiera, H.: Scleroderma after silicone augmentation mammoplasty. J.A.M.A. 260:236, 1988.
20. Gray, R. G., and Altman, R. D.: Progressive systemic sclerosis in a family. Case report of a mother and son and review of the literature. Arthritis Rheum. 20:35, 1977.
21. Whiteside, T. L., Medsger, T. A., and Rodnan, G. P.: Studies of the HLA antigens in progressive systemic sclerosis. *In* Black, C. M., and Myers, A. R. (eds.): Systemic Sclerosis (Scleroderma). 1st ed. New York, Gower Med., 1985.
22. Lynch, C. J., Singh, G., Whiteside, T. L., et al.: Histocompatibility antigens in progressive systemic sclerosis (scleroderma). J. Clin. Immunol. 2:314, 1982.
23. Rothfield, N. F., and Rodnan, G. P.: Serum antinuclear antibodies in progressive systemic sclerosis (scleroderma). Arthritis Rheum. 11:607, 1968.
24. Terregino, C. A., Udasin, I. G., and Seibold, J. R.: Family members of CREST patients lack serum anticentromere antibody. J. Rheumatol. 12:635, 1985.
25. Maddison, P. J., Skinner, R. P., Pereira, R. S., et al.: Antinuclear antibodies in the relatives and spouses of patients with systemic sclerosis. Ann. Rheum. Dis. 45:793, 1986.
26. Rodnan, G. P., Myerowitz, R. L., and Justh, G. O.: Morphologic changes in the digital arteries of patients with progressive systemic sclerosis (scleroderma) and Raynaud phenomenon. Medicine 59:393, 1980.
27. Young, E. A., Steen, V. D., and Medsger, T. A.: Systemic sclerosis without Raynaud's phenomenon. Arthritis Rheum. 29(Suppl. 4):S51, 1986 (abstract).
28. Stallones, R. A.: The epidemiology of systemic sclerosis. *In* Lawrence, R. C., and Shulman, L. E. (eds.): Epidemiology of the Rheumatic Diseases. 1st ed. New York, Gower Med., 1984.
29. Heslop, J., Coggon, D., and Acheson, E. D.: The prevalence of intermittent digital ischaemia (Raynaud's phenomenon) in a general practice. J. R. Coll. Gen. Pract. 33:85, 1983.
30. Gifford, R. W., and Hines, E. A.: Raynaud's disease among women and girls. Circulation 16:1012, 1957.
31. Olsen, N., and Nielson, S. L.: Prevalence of primary Raynaud phenomenon in young females. Scand. J. Clin. Lab. Invest. 37:761, 1978.
32. Maricq, H. R., Spencer-Green, G., and LeRoy, E. C.: Skin capillary abnormalities as indicators of organ involvement in scleroderma (systemic sclerosis), Raynaud's syndrome and dermatomyositis. Am. J. Med. 61:862, 1976.
33. Harper, F. E., Maricq, H. R., Turner, R. E., et al.: A prospective study of Raynaud phenomenon and early connective tissue disease. A five-year report. Am. J. Med. 72:883, 1982.
34. Kallenberg, C. G. M., Pastoor, G. W., Wouda, A. A., et al.: Antinuclear antibodies in patients with Raynaud's phenomenon: Clinical significance of anticentromere antibodies. Ann. Rheum. Dis. 41:382, 1982.
35. Gerbracht, D. D., Steen, V. D., Ziegler, G. L., et al.: Evolution of primary Raynaud's phenomenon (Raynaud's disease) to connective tissue disease. Arthritis Rheum. 28:87, 1985.
36. Maricq, H. R., Downey, J. A., and LeRoy, E. C.: Standstill of nailfold capillary blood flow during cooling in scleroderma and Raynaud's syndrome. Blood Vessels 13:338, 1976.
37. Engelhart, M., and Seibold, J. R.: The effect of local temperature versus sympathetic tone on digital perfusion in Raynaud's phenomenon. Angiology 41:715, 1990.
38. Seibold, J. R., and Harris, J. N.: Plasma beta-thromboglobulin in the differential diagnosis of Raynaud's phenomenon. J. Rheumatol. 12:99, 1985.
39. Kahaleh, M. B., Osborn, I., and LeRoy, E. C.: Elevated levels of circulating platelet aggregates and beta-thromboglobulin in scleroderma. Ann. Intern. Med. 96:610, 1982.
40. Rustin, M.H.A., Kovacs, I. B., Sowemimo-Coker, S. O., et al.: Differences in red cell behaviour between patients with Raynaud's phenomenon and systemic sclerosis and patients with Raynaud's disease. Br. J. Dermatol. 113:265, 1985.
41. Kahaleh, M. B., Sherer, G. K., and LeRoy, E. C.: Endothelial injury in scleroderma. J. Exp. Med. 149:1326, 1979.
42. LeRoy, E. C., Maricq, H. R., and Kahaleh, M. B.: Undifferentiated connective tissue syndromes. Arthritis Rheum. 23:341, 1980.
43. Buckingham, R. B., Prince, R. K., and Rodnan, G. P.: Progressive systemic sclerosis (PSS, scleroderma) dermal fibroblasts synthesize increased amounts of glycosaminoglycans. J. Lab. Clin. Med. 101:659, 1983.
44. Engelhart, M., and Seibold, J. R.: Cyanosis and Raynaud's phenomenon: The relation to underlying disease and venous abnormalities. Angiology 41:432, 1990.
45. Seibold, J. R., Harris, J. N., D'Angelo, W. A., et al.: Skin thickness and skin edema in systemic sclerosis. Arthritis Rheum. 29(Suppl. 1):S3, 1986 (abstract).
46. Rodnan, G. P., Lipinski, E., and Luksick, J.: Skin thickness and collagen content in progressive systemic sclerosis and localized scleroderma. Arthritis Rheum. 22:130, 1979.
47. Medsger, T. A.: Progressive systemic sclerosis. Clin. Rheum. Dis. 9:655, 1983.
48. Steen, V. D., Medsger, T. A., and Rodnan, G. P.: D-Penicillamine therapy in progressive systemic sclerosis (scleroderma). A retrospective analysis. Ann. Intern. Med. 97:652, 1982.
48a. Jimenez, S. A., and Sigal, S. H.: A 15-year prospective study of treatment of rapidly progressive systemic sclerosis with D-penicillamine. J. Rheumatol. 18:1496, 1991.
49. Clements, P. J., Lachenbruch, P. A., Ng, S. C., et al.: Skin score. A semiquantitative measure of cutaneous involvement that improves prediction of prognosis in systemic sclerosis. Arthritis Rheum. 33:1256, 1990.
50. Fleischmajer, R., Damiano, V., and Nedwich, A.: Alteration of subcutaneous tissue in systemic scleroderma. Arch. Dermatol. 105:59, 1972.
51. Fleischmajer, R., Perlish, J. S., and Reeves, I.R.T.: Cellular infiltrates in scleroderma skin. Arthritis Rheum. 20:975, 1977.
52. Haynes, D. C., and Gershwin, M. E.: The immunopathology of progressive systemic sclerosis (PSS). Semin. Arthritis Rheum. 11:331, 1982.
53. Fleischmajer, R., and Prunieras, M.: II. Electron microscopy of collagen, cells, and the subcutaneous tissue. Arch. Dermatol. 106:515, 1972.
54. Buckingham, R. B., Prince, R. K., Rodnan, G. P., et al.: Increased collagen accumulation in dermal fibroblast cultures from patients with progressive systemic sclerosis (scleroderma). J. Lab. Clin. Med. 92:5, 1978.
55. Uitto, J., Bauer, E. A., and Eisen, A. Z.: Scleroderma. Increased biosynthesis of triple-helical Type I and Type III procollagens associated with unaltered expression of collagenase by skin fibroblasts in culture. J. Clin. Invest. 64:921, 1979.
56. Jimenez, S. A., Yankowski, R. I., and Frontino, P. M.: Biosynthetic heterogeneity of sclerodermatous skin in organ cultures. J. Mol. Med. 2:423, 1977.
57. Gay, R. E., Buckingham, R. B., Prince, R. K., et al.: Collagen types

synthesized in dermal fibroblast cultures from patients with early progressive systemic sclerosis. Arthritis Rheum. 23:190, 1980.

58. Fleischmajer, R., Perlish, J. S., Kreig, T., et al.: Variability in collagen and fibronectin synthesis by scleroderma fibroblasts in primary culture. J. Invest. Dermatol. 76:400, 1981.

59. Bashey, R. I., Perlish, J. S., Nochumson, S., et al.: Connective tissue synthesis by cultured scleroderma fibroblasts. II. Incorporation of 3H glucosamine and synthesis of glycosaminoglycans. Arthritis Rheum. 20:879, 1977.

60. Uitto, J., Murray, L. W., Blumberg, B., et al.: Biochemistry of collagen in diseases. Ann. Intern. Med. 105:740, 1986.

61. Mitrane, M. P., Boyd, C. D., Prockop, D. J., et al.: Systemic sclerosis (SS) lacks genomic polymorphism for Type IV collagen. Arthritis Rheum. 29(Suppl. 4):S55, 1986 (abstract).

62. Jimenez, S. A., Feldman, G., Bashey, R. I., et al.: Co-ordinate increase in the expression of Type I and Type III collagen genes in progressive systemic sclerosis. Biochem. J. 237:837, 1986.

63. Varga, J., Rosenbloom, J., and Jimenez, S. A.: Transforming growth factor-beta (TGF-beta) causes a persistent increase in steady-state amounts of type I and type III collagen and fibronectin mRNAs in normal human dermal fibroblasts. Biochem. J. 247:597, 1987.

64. Rosenbloom, J., Feldman, G., Freundlich, B., et al.: Inhibition of excessive scleroderma fibroblast collagen production by recombinant gamma-interferon. Arthritis Rheum. 29:851, 1986.

65. Peltonen, L., Palotie, A., Myllyla, R., et al.: Collagen biosynthesis in systemic scleroderma: Regulation of posttranslational modifications and synthesis of procollagen in cultured fibroblasts. J. Invest. Dermatol. 84:14, 1985.

66. Krieg, T., Horlein, D., Wiestner, M., et al.: Aminoterminal extension peptides from type I procollagen normalize excessive collagen synthesis of scleroderma fibroblasts. Arch. Dermatol. Res. 263:171, 1978.

67. Botstein, G. R., Sherer, G. K., and LeRoy, E. C.: Fibroblast selection in scleroderma. An alternative model of fibrosis. Arthritis Rheum. 25:189, 1982.

68. Goldring, S. R., Stephenson, M. L., Downie, E., et al.: Heterogeneity in hormone responses and patterns of collagen synthesis in cloned dermal fibroblasts. J. Clin. Invest. 85:798, 1990.

69. LeRoy, E. C., Smith, E. A., Kahaleh, M. B., et al.: A strategy for determining the pathogenesis of systemic sclerosis. Is transforming growth factor beta the answer? Arthritis Rheum. 32:817, 1989.

69a. Needleman, B. W., Wigley, F. M., and Stair, R. W.: Interleukin-1, interleukin-2, interleukin-4, interleukin-6, tumor necrosis factor, and interferon-α levels in sera from patients with scleroderma. Arthritis Rheum. 35:67, 1992.

70. Potter, S. R., Bienenstock, J., Goldstein, S., et al.: Fibroblast growth factors in scleroderma. J. Rheumatol. 12:1129, 1985.

71. Keyser, A. J., Nimni, M. E., and Cooper, S. M.: Scleroderma serum stimulates collagen synthesis in normal human dermal fibroblasts. In Black, C. M., and Myers, A. R. (eds.): Systemic Sclerosis (Scleroderma). 1st ed. New York, Gower Med., 1985.

72. Seibold, J. R., Giorno, R. C., and Claman, H. N.: Dermal mast cell degranulation in systemic sclerosis. Arthritis Rheum. 33:1702, 1990.

73. Hawkins, R. A., Claman, H. N., Clark, R.A.F., et al.: Increased dermal mast cell populations in progressive systemic sclerosis: A link in chronic fibrosis? Ann. Intern. Med. 102:182, 1985.

74. Walker, M., Harley, R., Maize, J., et al.: Mast cells and their degranulation in the Tsk mouse model of scleroderma. Proc. Soc. Exp. Biol. Med. 180:323, 1985.

75. Lee Choi, K., Giorno, R., and Claman, H. N.: Cutaneous mast cell depletion and recovery in murine graft-vs-host disease. J. Immunol. 138:4093, 1987.

76. Claman, H. N.: On scleroderma: Mast cells, endothelial cells and fibroblasts. J.A.M.A. 262:1206, 1989.

77. Hamatochi, A., Fujiwara, K., and Ueki, H.: Effects of histamine on collagen synthesis by cultured fibroblasts derived from guinea pig skin. Arch. Dermatol. Res. 277:60, 1985.

78. Falanga, V., Soter, N. A., Altman, R., et al.: Elevated plasma histamine levels in systemic sclerosis (scleroderma). Arch. Dermatol. 126:336, 1990.

79. Okuno, T., and Takagaki, Y.: Natural cytotoxic cell-specific factor produced by IL-3–dependent basophilic/mast cells: Relationship to TNF. J. Immunol. 141:3061, 1988.

80. Austgulen, R., Espevik, T., and Nissen-Meyer, J.: Fibroblast growth-stimulatory activity released from human monocytes. Scand. J. Immunol. 26:621, 1987.

81. Duncan, M. R., and Berman, B.: Persistence of a reduced-collagen-producing phenotype in cultured scleroderma fibroblasts after short-term exposure to interferons. J. Clin. Invest. 79:1318, 1987.

82. Postlethwaite, A. E., Snyderman, R., and Kang, A. H.: The chemotactic attraction of human fibroblasts to a lymphocyte-derived factor. J. Exp. Med. 144:1188, 1976.

83. Wahl, S. M., Wahl, L. M., and McCarthy, J. B.: Lymphocyte-mediated activation of fibroblast proliferation and collagen production. J. Immunol. 121:942, 1978.

84. Worrall, J. G., Whiteside, T. L., Prince, R. K., et al.: Persistence of scleroderma-like phenotype in normal fibroblasts after prolonged exposure to soluble mediators from mononuclear cells. Arthritis Rheum. 29:54, 1986.

85. Perlish, J. S., and Fleischmajer, R.: Effect of mitogen-stimulated scleroderma mononuclear cells on collagen synthesis by normal fibroblasts. In Black, C. M., and Myers, A. R. (eds.): Systemic Sclerosis (Scleroderma). 1st ed. New York, Gower Med., 1985.

86. Takehara, K., LeRoy, E. C., and Grotendorst, G. R.: TGF-beta inhibition of endothelial cell proliferation: Alteration of EGF binding and EGF-induced growth regulatory (competence) gene expression. Cell 49:415, 1987.

87. Roberts, A. B., Sporn, M. B., Assoian, R. K., et al.: Transforming growth factor type B: Rapid induction of fibrosis and angiogenesis in vivo and stimulation of collagen formation in vitro. Proc. Natl. Acad. Sci. U.S.A. 83:4167, 1986.

88. D'Angelo, W. A., Fries, J. F., Masi, A. T., et al.: Pathologic observations in systemic sclerosis (scleroderma). A study of fifty-eight autopsy cases and fifty-eight matched controls. Am. J. Med. 46:428, 1969.

89. Norton, W. L., and Nardo, J. M.: Vascular disease in progressive systemic sclerosis (scleroderma). Ann. Intern. Med. 73:317, 1970.

90. Cannon, P. J., Hassar, M., Cararella, W. J., et al.: The relationship of hypertension and renal failure in scleroderma (progressive systemic sclerosis) to structural and functional abnormalities of the renal cortical circulation. Medicine (Baltimore) 53:1, 1974.

91. Salerni, R., Rodnan, G. P., Leon, D. F., et al.: Pulmonary hypertension in the CREST syndrome variant of progressive systemic sclerosis (scleroderma). Ann. Intern. Med. 86:394, 1977.

92. Seibold, J. R.: Serotonin and Raynaud's phenomenon. In Vanhoutte, P. M. (ed.): Serotonin and the Cardiovascular System. 1st ed. New York, Raven Press, 1985.

93. Spencer-Green, G.: Raynaud phenomenon. Bull. Rheum. Dis. 33:1, 1983.

94. Blunt, R. J., and Porter, J. M.: Raynaud syndrome. Semin. Arthritis Rheum. 10:282, 1981.

95. Moulds, R. F. W., Iwanov, V., and Medcalf, R. L.: The effects of platelet-derived contractile agents on human digital arteries. Clin. Sci. 66:443, 1984.

96. Lindblad, L. E., Shepherd, J. T., and Vanhoutte, P. M.: Cooling augments platelet-induced contraction of peripheral arteries of the dog. Proc. Soc. Exp. Biol. Med. 176:119, 1984.

97. Shepherd, J. T., and Vanhoutte, P. M.: Spasm of the coronary arteries: Causes and consequences (the scientist's viewpoint). Mayo Clin. Proc. 60:33, 1985.

98. Seibold, J. R., and Jageneau, A. H. M.: Treatment of Raynaud's phenomenon with ketanserin, a selective antagonist of the serotonin₂(5-HT₂) receptor. Arthritis Rheum. 27:139, 1984.

99. Malamet, R., Wise, R. A., Ettinger, W. H., et al.: Nifedipine in the treatment of Raynaud's phenomenon. Evidence for inhibition of platelet activation. Am. J. Med. 78:602, 1985.

100. Wigley, F. M., Seibold, J. R., Wise, R. A., et al.: Intravenous iloprost treatment of Raynaud's phenomenon and ischemic ulcers secondary to systemic sclerosis. J. Rheumatol. (in press).

101. Rademaker, M., Cooke, E. D., Almond, N. E., et al.: Comparison of intravenous infusions of iloprost and oral nifedipine in treatment of Raynaud's phenomenon in patients with systemic sclerosis: A double-blind randomized study. Br. Med. J. 298:561, 1989.

102. Kallenberg, C. G. M., Vellenga, E., Wouda, A. A., et al.: Platelet activation, fibrinolytic activity and circulating immune complexes in Raynaud's phenomenon. J. Rheumatol. 9:878, 1982.

103. Hutton, R. A., Mikhailidis, D. P., Bernstein, R. M., et al.: Assessment of platelet function in patients with Raynaud's syndrome. J. Clin. Pathol. 37:182, 1984.

104. Seibold, J. R., and Terregino, C. A.: Selective antagonism of S₂-serotonergic receptors relieves but does not prevent cold induced vasoconstriction in primary Raynaud's phenomenon. J. Rheumatol. 13:337, 1986.

105. Tindall, H., Tooke, J. E., Menys, V. C., et al.: Effect of dazoxiben, a thromboxane synthetase inhibitor, on skin-blood flow following cold challenge in patients with Raynaud's phenomenon. Eur. J. Clin. Invest. 15:20, 1985.

106. Winkelmann, R. K., Goldyne, M. E., and Linscheid, R. L.: Influence of cold on catecholamine response of vascular smooth muscle strips from resistance vessels of scleroderma skin. Angiology 28:330, 1977.

107. Jamieson, G. G., Ludbrook, J., and Wilson, A.: Cold hypersensitivity in Raynaud's phenomenon. Circulation 44:254, 1971.

108. Pawloski, A.: The nerve network of the skin in diffuse scleroderma and clinically similar conditions. Arch. Dermatol. 83:868, 1963.

109. Fries, J. F.: Physiologic studies in systemic sclerosis (scleroderma). Arch. Intern. Med. 123:22, 1969.

110. Blunt, R., George, A., Hurlow, R., et al.: Hyperviscosity and thrombotic changes in idiopathic and secondary Raynaud's phenomenon. Br. J. Haematol. 45:651, 1980.

111. Traub, Y. M., Shapiro, A. P., Rodnan, G. P., et al.: Hypertension and

renal failure (scleroderma renal crisis) in progressive systemic sclerosis. Review of a 25-year experience with 68 cases. Medicine (Baltimore) 62:335, 1983.

112. Bulkley, B. H., Ridolfi, R. L., Salyer, W. R., et al.: Myocardial lesions of progressive systemic sclerosis. A cause of cardiac dysfunction. Circulation 53:483, 1976.

113. Follansbee, W. P., Curtiss, E. I., Medsger, T. A., et al.: Physiologic abnormalities of cardiac function in progressive systemic sclerosis with diffuse scleroderma. N. Engl. J. Med. 310:142, 1984.

114. Follansbee, W. P., Curtiss, E. I., Medsger, T. A., et al.: Myocardial function and perfusion in the CREST syndrome variant of progressive systemic sclerosis. Exercise radionuclide evaluation and comparison with diffuse scleroderma. Am. J. Med. 77:489, 1984.

115. Kahan, A., Devaux, J. Y., Amor, B., et al.: Nifedipine and thallium-201 myocardial perfusion in progressive systemic sclerosis. N. Engl. J. Med. 314:1397, 1986.

116. Duboc, D., Kahan, A., Maziere, B., et al.: The effect of nifedipine on myocardial perfusion and metabolism in systemic sclerosis. A positron emission tomographic study. Arthritis Rheum. 34:198, 1991.

117. Alexander, E. L., Firestein, G. S., Weiss, J. L., et al.: Reversible cold-induced abnormalities in myocardial perfusion and function in systemic sclerosis. Ann. Intern. Med. 105:661, 1986.

118. Ellis, W. W., Baer, A. N., Robertson, R. M., et al.: Left ventricular dysfunction induced by cold exposure in patients with systemic sclerosis. Am. J. Med. 80:385, 1986.

119. Wise, R. A., Wigley, F., Newball, H. H., et al.: The effect of cold exposure on diffusing capacity in patients with Raynaud's phenomenon. Chest 81:695, 1982.

120. Ettinger, W. H., Wise, R. A., Stevens, M. B., et al.: Absence of positional change in pulmonary diffusing capacity in systemic sclerosis. Am. J. Med. 75:305, 1983.

121. Furst, D. E., Davis, J. A., Clements, P. J., et al.: Abnormalities of pulmonary vascular dynamics and inflammation in early progressive systemic sclerosis. Arthritis Rheum. 24:1403, 1981.

122. Siegel, R. J., O'Connor, B., Mena, I., et al.: Left ventricular dysfunction at rest and during Raynaud's phenomenon in patients with scleroderma. Am. Heart J. 108:1469, 1984.

123. Ohar, J. M., Robichaud, A. M., Fowler, A. A., et al.: Increased pulmonary artery pressure in association with Raynaud's phenomenon. Am. J. Med. 81:361, 1986.

124. Fahey, P. J., Utell, M. J., Condemi, J. J., et al.: Raynaud's phenomenon of the lung. Am. J. Med. 76:263, 1984.

125. Kovalchik, M. T., Guggenheim, S. J., Silverman, M. H., et al.: The kidney in progressive systemic sclerosis. A prospective study. Ann. Intern. Med. 89:881, 1978.

126. Maricq, H. R.: Widefield capillary microscopy. Technique and rating scale for abnormalities seen in scleroderma and related disorders. Arthritis Rheum. 24:1159, 1981.

127. Fleischmajer, R., Perlish, J., Shaw, K. V., et al.: Skin capillary changes in early systemic scleroderma. Electron microscopy and "in vitro" autoradiography with tritiated thymidine. Arch. Dermatol. 112:1553, 1976.

128. Kahaleh, M. B., Osborn, I., and LeRoy, E. C.: Increased Factor VIII/von Willebrand factor antigen and von Willebrand factor activity in scleroderma and in Raynaud's phenomenon. Ann. Intern. Med. 94:482, 1981.

129. Godin-Ostro, E., Mitrane, M., Heller, I., et al.: Plasma plasminogen activator in systemic sclerosis. Arthritis Rheum. 28(Suppl. 4):S80, 1985 (abstract).

130. Yamane, K., Kashiwagi, H., Suzuki, N., et al.: Elevated plasma levels of endothelin-1 in systemic sclerosis. Arthritis Rheum. 34:243, 1991.

131. Seibold, J. R., Medsger, T. A., Winkelstein, A., et al.: Immune complexes in progressive systemic sclerosis (scleroderma). Arthritis Rheum. 25:1167, 1982.

132. Thompson, R. P., Harper, F. E., Maize, J. C., et al.: Nailfold biopsy in scleroderma and related disorders. Correlation of histologic, capillaroscopic, and clinical data. Arthritis Rheum. 27:97, 1984.

133. Kahaleh, M. B., and LeRoy, E. C.: Endothelial injury in scleroderma. A protease mechanism. J. Lab. Clin. Med. 101:553, 1983.

134. Shanahan, W. R., and Korn, J. H.: Cytotoxic activity of sera from scleroderma and other connective tissue diseases. Lack of cellular and disease specificity. Arthritis Rheum. 25:1391, 1982.

135. Cohen, S., Johnson, A. R., and Hurd, E.: Cytotoxicity of sera from patients with scleroderma. Effects on human endothelial cells and fibroblasts in culture. Arthritis Rheum. 26:170, 1983.

136. Johnson, T. B., Wong, H., Harris, J. N., et al.: Platelet-derived suppression of endothelial growth in systemic sclerosis. Arthritis Rheum. 31(Suppl. 4):S113, 1988.

137. Mackel, A. M., DeLustro, F., Harper, F. E., et al.: Antibodies to collagen in scleroderma. Arthritis Rheum. 25:522, 1982.

138. Penning, C. A., Cunningham, J., French, M.A.H., et al.: Antibody-dependent cellular cytotoxicity of human vascular endothelium in systemic sclerosis. Clin. Exp. Immunol. 58:548, 1984.

139. Huffstutter, J. E., DeLustro, F. A., and LeRoy, E. C.: Cellular immunity to collagen and laminin in scleroderma. Arthritis Rheum. 28:775, 1985.

140. Degiannis, D., Seibold, J. R., Czarnecki, M., et al.: Soluble and cellular markers of immune activation in patients with systemic sclerosis. Clin. Immunol. Immunopathol. 56:259, 1990.

141. Tan, E. M., and Rodnan, G. P.: Profile of antinuclear antibodies in progressive systemic sclerosis (PSS). Arthritis Rheum. 18:430, 1975.

142. Notman, D. D., Kurata, N., and Tan, E. M.: Profiles of anti-nuclear antibodies in systemic rheumatic diseases. Ann. Intern. Med. 83:464, 1975.

143. Munves, E. F., and Schur, P. H.: Antibodies to Sm and RNP. Prognosticators of disease involvement. Arthritis Rheum. 26:848, 1983.

144. Ginsburg, W. W., Conn, D. L., Bunch, T. W., et al.: Comparison of clinical and serologic markers in systemic lupus erythematosus and overlap syndrome. A review of 247 patients. J. Rheumatol. 10:235, 1983.

145. Albert, J., Ekoe, J-M., Cunningham, M., et al.: Circulating anticoagulant in CREST syndrome. Br. J. Dermatol. 23:20, 1984.

146. Seibold, J. R., Knight, P. J., and Peter, J. B.: Anticardiolipin antibodies in systemic sclerosis. Arthritis Rheum. 29:1052, 1986.

147. Chen, Z., Virella, G., Tung, H. E., et al.: Immune complexes and antinuclear, antinucleolar, and anticentromere antibodies in scleroderma. J. Am. Acad. Dermatol. 11:461, 1984.

148. Moroi, Y., Peebles, C., Fritzler, M. J., et al.: Autoantibody to centromere (kinetochore) in scleroderma sera. Proc. Natl. Acad. Sci. U.S.A. 77:1627, 1980.

149. Fritzler, M. J., Kinsella, T. D., and Garbutt, E.: The CREST syndrome: A distinct serologic entity with anticentromere antibodies. Am. J. Med. 69:520, 1980.

150. McCarty, G. A., Rice, J. R., Bembe, M. L., et al.: Anticentromere antibody. Clinical correlations and association with favorable prognosis in patients with scleroderma variants. Arthritis Rheum. 26:1, 1983.

151. Steen, V. D., Ziegler, G. L., Rodnan, G. P., et al.: Clinical and laboratory associations of anticentromere antibody in patients with progressive systemic sclerosis. Arthritis Rheum. 27:125, 1984.

152. Tramposch, H. D., Smith, C. D., Senecal, J.-L., et al.: A long-term longitudinal study of anticentromere antibodies. Arthritis Rheum. 27:121, 1984.

153. Weiner, E. S., Hildebrandt, S., Senecal, J.-L., et al.: Prognostic significance of anticentromere antibodies and anti-topoisomerase I antibodies in Raynaud's disease. Arthritis Rheum. 34:68, 1991.

154. Tan, E. M., Rodnan, G. P., Garcia, I., et al.: Diversity of antinuclear antibodies in progressive systemic sclerosis. Anti-centromere antibody and its relationship to CREST syndrome. Arthritis Rheum. 23:617, 1980.

155. Jarzabek-Chorzelska, M., Blaszczyk, M., Jablonska, S., et al.: Scl-70 antibody—a specific marker of systemic sclerosis. Br. J. Dermatol. 115:393, 1986.

156. Maul, G. G., French, B. T., van Venrooij, W. J., et al.: Topoisomerase I identified by scleroderma 70 antisera: Enrichment of topoisomerase I at the centromere in mouse mitotic cells before anaphase. Proc. Natl. Acad. Sci. U.S.A. 83:5145, 1986.

157. Samuels, D. S., Tojo, T., Homma, M., et al.: Inhibition of topoisomerase I by antibodies in sera from scleroderma patients. FEBS Lett. 209:231, 1986.

158. Guldner, H.-H., Szostecki, C., Vosberg, H.-P., et al.: Scl-70 autoantibodies from scleroderma patients recognize a 95 kDa protein identified as DNA topoisomerase I. Chromosoma 94:132, 1986.

159. van Venrooij, W. J., Stapel, S. O., Houben, H., et al.: Scl-86, a marker antigen for diffuse scleroderma. J. Clin. Invest. 75:1053, 1985.

160. Maul, G. G., Jimenez, S. A., Riggs, E., et al.: Determination of an epitope of the diffuse systemic sclerosis marker antigen DNA topoisomerase-I: Sequence similarity with retroviral p30 gag protein suggests a possible cause for autoimmunity in systemic sclerosis. Proc. Natl. Acad. Sci. U.S.A. 86:8492, 1989.

161. Dang, H., Garry, R. F., Seibold, J. R., et al.: Serum antibody to retroviral GAG proteins in systemic sclerosis. Arthritis Rheum. 34:1336, 1991.

162. D'Arpa, P., White-Cooper, H., Cleveland, D. W., et al.: Use of molecular cloning methods to map the distribution of epitopes on topoisomerase I (Scl-70) recognized by sera of scleroderma patients. Arthritis Rheum. 33:1501, 1990.

163. Roumm, A. D., Whiteside, T. L., Medsger, T. A., et al.: Lymphocytes in the skin of patients with progressive systemic sclerosis. Quantification, subtyping, and clinical correlations. Arthritis Rheum. 27:645, 1984.

164. Inoshita, T., Whiteside, T. L., Rodnan, G. P., et al.: Abnormalities of T lymphocyte subsets in patients with progressive systemic sclerosis (PSS, scleroderma). J. Lab. Clin. Med. 97:264, 1981.

165. Whiteside, T. L., Kumagai, Y., Roumm, A. D., et al.: Suppressor cell function and T lymphocyte subpopulations in peripheral blood of patients with progressive systemic sclerosis. Arthritis Rheum. 26:841, 1983.

166. Keystone, E. C., Lau, C., Gladman, C. C., et al.: Immunoregulatory T cell subpopulations in patients with scleroderma using monoclonal antibodies. Clin. Exp. Immunol. 48:443, 1982.

167. Degiannis, D., Seibold, J. R., Czarnecki, M., et al.: Soluble interleukin-

2 receptors in patients with systemic sclerosis. Clinical and laboratory correlations. Arthritis Rheum. 33:375, 1990.

168. Clements, P. J., Peter, J. B., Agopian, M. S., et al.: Elevated serum levels of soluble interleukin 2 receptor, interleukin 2 and neopterin in diffuse and limited scleroderma: Effect of chlorambucil. J. Rheumatol. 17:908, 1990.

169. Engel, E. E., Charley, M. R., Steen, V. D., et al.: Soluble interleukin 2 receptors in systemic sclerosis (scleroderma). Arthritis Rheum. 32(Suppl. 4):R39, 1989 (abstract).

170. Lockshin, M. D., Markenson, J. A., Fuzesi, L., et al.: Monocyte-induced inhibition of lymphocyte response to phytohaemagglutinin in progressive systemic sclerosis. Ann. Rheum. Dis. 42:40, 1983.

171. Wright, C., Hughes, P., Rowell, N. R., et al.: Antibody-dependent and phytohaemagglutinin-induced lymphocyte cytotoxicity in systemic sclerosis. Clin. Exp. Immunol. 36:175, 1979.

172. Sandborg, C. I., Berman, M. A., Andrews, B. S., et al.: Interleukin-1 production by mononuclear cells from patients with scleroderma. Clin. Exp. Immunol. 60:294, 1985.

173. Whicher, J. T., Gilbert, A. M., Westacott, C., et al.: Defective production of leucocytic endogenous mediator (interleukin-1) by peripheral blood leucocytes of patients with systemic sclerosis, systemic lupus erythematosus, rheumatoid arthritis and mixed connective tissue disease. Clin. Exp. Immunol. 65:80, 1986.

174. Kahaleh, M. B., and LeRoy, E. C.: Interleukin-2 in scleroderma: Correlation of serum level with extent of skin involvement and disease duration. Ann. Intern. Med. 110:446, 1989.

175. Sternberg, E. M., Trial, J., and Parker, C. W.: Effect of serotonin on murine macrophages: Suppression of Ia expression by serotonin and its reversal by 5-HT2 serotonergic receptor antagonists. J. Immunol. 137:1986, 1986.

176. Sternberg, E. M., Van Woert, M. H., Young, S. N., et al.: Development of a scleroderma-like illness during therapy with L-5-hydroxytryptophan and carbidopa. N. Engl. J. Med. 303:782, 1980.

177. Sternberg, E. M.: Pathogenesis of scleroderma: The interrelationship of the immune and vascular hypotheses. Surv. Immunol. Res. 4:69, 1985.

178. Green, M. C., Sweet, H. O., and Bunker, L. E.: Tight skin, a new mutation of the mouse causing excessive growth of connective tissue and skeleton. Am. J. Pathol. 82:493, 1976.

179. Menton, D. N., and Hess, R. A.: The ultrastructure of collagen in the dermis of tight skin (Tsk) mutant mice. J. Invest. Dermatol. 74:139, 1980.

180. Jimenez, S. A., Williams, C. J., and Myers, J. C.: Increased collagen biosynthesis and increased expression of Type I and Type III procollagen genes in tight skin (Tsk) mouse fibroblasts. J. Biol. Chem. 261:657, 1986.

181. Jaffee, B. D., and Claman, H. N.: Chronic graft-vs-host disease as a model for scleroderma. I. Description of model systems. Cell. Immunol. 77:1, 1983.

182. van de Water, J., and Gershwin, M. E.: Avian scleroderma. An inherited fibrotic disease of white leghorn chickens resembling progressive systemic sclerosis. Am. J. Pathol. 120:478, 1985.

183. van de Water, J., Haapanen, L., Boyd, R., et al.: Identification of T cells in early dermal lymphocytic infiltrates in avian scleroderma. Arthritis Rheum. 32:1031, 1989.

184. Kumagai, Y., Shiokawa, Y., Medsger, T. A., and Rodnan, G. P.: Clinical spectrum of connective tissue disease after cosmetic surgery. Observations on eighteen patients and a review of the Japanese literature. Arthritis Rheum. 27:1, 1984.

185. Furst, D. E., Clements, P. J., Graze, P., et al.: A syndrome resembling progressive systemic sclerosis after bone marrow transplantation. A model for scleroderma? Arthritis Rheum. 22:904, 1979.

186. Rabinowitz, F., Twersky, J., and Guttadauria, M.: Similar bone manifestations of scleroderma and rheumatoid arthritis. Am. J. Roentgenol. 121:35, 1974.

187. Blocka, K. L. N., Bassett, L. W., Furst, D. E., et al.: The arthropathy of advanced progressive systemic sclerosis: A radiographic survey. Arthritis Rheum. 24:874, 1981.

188. Medsger, T. A., Rodnan, G. P., Moossy, J., et al.: Skeletal muscle involvement in progressive systemic sclerosis (scleroderma). Arthritis Rheum. 11:554, 1968.

189. Clements, P. J., Furst, D. E., Campion, D. S., et al.: Muscle disease in progressive systemic sclerosis. Diagnostic and therapeutic considerations. Arthritis Rheum. 21:62, 1978.

190. Medsger, T. A.: Progressive systemic sclerosis: Skeletal muscle involvement. Clin. Rheum. Dis. 5:103, 1979.

191. Osial, T. A., Avakian, A., Sassouni, V., et al.: Resorption of the mandibular condyles and coronoid processes in progressive systemic sclerosis (scleroderma). Arthritis Rheum. 24:729, 1981.

192. Lian, J. B., Pachman, L. M., Gundberg, C. M., et al.: Gamma-carboxyglutamate excretion and calcinosis in juvenile dermatomyositis. Arthritis Rheum. 25:1094, 1982.

193. Zamost, B. J., Hirschberg, J., Ippoliti, A. F., et al.: Esophagitis in scleroderma. Prevalence and risk factors. Gastroenterology 92:421, 1987.

194. Cohen, S., Laufer, I., Snape, W. J., et al.: The gastrointestinal manifestations of scleroderma: Pathogenesis and management. Gastroenterology 79:155, 1980.

195. Russell, M. L., Friesen, D., Henderson, R. D., et al.: Ultrastructure of the esophagus in scleroderma. Arthritis Rheum. 25:1117, 1982.

196. Davidson, A., Russell, C., and Littlejohn, G. O.: Assessment of esophageal abnormalities in progressive systemic sclerosis using radionuclide transit. J. Rheumatol. 12:472, 1985.

197. Carette, S., Lacourciere, Y., Lavoie, S., et al.: Radionuclide esophageal transit in progressive systemic sclerosis. J. Rheumatol. 12:478, 1985.

198. Schneider, H. A., Yonker, R. A., Longley, S., et al.: Scleroderma esophagus: A nonspecific entity. Ann. Intern. Med. 100:848, 1984.

199. Salen, G., Goldstein, F., and Wirts, C. W.: Malabsorption in scleroderma: Relation to bacterial flora and treatment with antibiotics. Ann. Intern. Med. 64:834, 1966.

200. Isaacs, P. E. T., and Kim, Y. S.: The contaminated small bowel syndrome. Am. J. Med. 67:1049, 1979.

201. Battle, W. M., Snape, W. J., Wright, S., et al.: Abnormal colonic motility in progressive systemic sclerosis. Ann. Intern. Med. 94:749, 1981.

202. Miller, F., Lane, B., and D'Angelo, W. A.: Primary biliary cirrhosis and scleroderma. The possibility of a common pathogenetic mechanism. Arch. Pathol. Lab. Med. 103:505, 1979.

203. Clarke, A. K., Galbraith, R. M., Hamilton, E. B. D., et al.: Rheumatic disorders in primary biliary cirrhosis. Ann. Rheum. Dis. 37:42, 1978.

204. Bernstein, R. M., Callender, M. E., Neuberger, J. M., et al.: Anticentromere antibody in primary biliary cirrhosis. Ann. Rheum. Dis. 41:612, 1982.

205. Gupta, R. C., Seibold, J. R., Krishnan, M. R., et al.: Precipitating autoantibodies to mitochondrial proteins in progressive systemic sclerosis. Clin. Exp. Immunol. 58:68, 1984.

206. Seibold, J. R., Molony, R. R., Turkevich, D., et al.: Acute hemodynamic effects of ketanserin in pulmonary hypertension secondary to systemic sclerosis. J. Rheumatol. 14:519, 1987.

207. Young, R. H., and Mark, G. J.: Pulmonary vascular changes in scleroderma. Am. J. Med. 64:998, 1978.

208. Ungerer, R. G., Tashkin, D. P., Furst, D., et al.: Prevalence and clinical correlates of pulmonary arterial hypertension in progressive systemic sclerosis. Am. J. Med. 75:65, 1983.

209. Greenwald, G. I., Tashkin, D. P., Gong, H., et al.: Longitudinal changes in lung function and respiratory symptoms in progressive systemic sclerosis. Prospective study. Am. J. Med. 83:83, 1987.

210. Owens, G. R., Fino, G. J., Herbert, D. L., et al.: Pulmonary function in progressive systemic sclerosis: Comparison of CREST syndrome variant with diffuse scleroderma. Chest 84:546, 1983.

211. Stupi, A. M., Steen, V. D., Owens, G. R., et al.: Pulmonary hypertension in the CREST syndrome variant of systemic sclerosis. Arthritis Rheum. 29:515, 1986.

212. Baron, M., Feiglin, D., Hyland, R., et al.: 67Gallium lung scans in progressive systemic sclerosis. Arthritis Rheum. 26:969, 1983.

213. Silver, R. M., Metcalf, J. F., and LeRoy, E. C.: Interstitial lung disease in scleroderma. Immune complexes in sera and bronchoalveolar lavage fluid. Arthritis Rheum. 29:525, 1986.

214. Rossi, G. A., Bitterman, P. B., Rennard, S. I., et al.: Evidence for chronic inflammation as a component of the interstitial lung disease associated with progressive systemic sclerosis. Am. Rev. Respir. Dis. 130:650, 1985.

215. Konig, G., Luderschmidt, C., Hammer, C., et al.: Lung involvement in scleroderma. Chest 85:318, 1984.

216. Kinsella, M. B., Smith, E. A., Miller, K. S., et al.: Spontaneous production of fibronectin by alveolar macrophages in patients with scleroderma. Arthritis Rheum. 32:577, 1989.

217. Medsger, T. A., Masi, A. T., Rodnan, G. P., et al.: Survival with systemic sclerosis (scleroderma). A life-table analysis of clinical and demographic factors in 309 patients. Ann. Intern. Med. 75:369, 1971.

218. Lichtbroun, A. S., Sandhaus, L. M., Giorno, R. C., et al.: Myocardial mast cells in systemic sclerosis: A report of three fatal cases. Am. J. Med. 89:372, 1990.

219. McWhorter, J. E., and LeRoy, E. C.: Pericardial disease in scleroderma (systemic sclerosis). Am. J. Med. 57:566, 1974.

220. Follansbee, W. P., Curtiss, E. I., Rahko, P. S., et al.: The electrocardiogram in systemic sclerosis (scleroderma). Study of 102 consecutive cases with functional correlations and review of the literature. Am. J. Med. 79:183, 1985.

221. Kostis, J. B., Seibold, J. R., Turkevich, D., et al.: Prognostic importance of cardiac arrhythmias in systemic sclerosis. Am. J. Med. 84:1007, 1988.

222. Follansbee, W. P.: The cardiovascular manifestations of systemic sclerosis (scleroderma). Curr. Probl. Cardiol. 11(5):242, 1986.

223. Steen, V. D., Medsger, T. A., Osial, T. A., et al.: Factors predicting development of renal involvement in progressive systemic sclerosis. Am. J. Med. 76:779, 1984.

224. Lapenas, D., Rodnan, G. P., and Cavallo, T.: Immunopathology of the renal vascular lesion of progressive systemic sclerosis (scleroderma). Am. J. Pathol. 91:243, 1978.

225. Cannon, P. J.: Medical management of renal scleroderma. N. Engl. J. Med. 299:886, 1978.
226. Whitman, H. H., Case, D. B., Laragh, J. H., et al.: Variable response to oral angiotensin-converting-enzyme blockade in hypertensive scleroderma patients. Arthritis Rheum. 25:241, 1982.
227. Helfrich, D. J., Banner, B., Steen, V. D., et al.: Normotensive renal failure in systemic sclerosis. Arthritis Rheum. 32:1128, 1989.
228. Gordon, M. B., Klein, I., Dekker, A., et al.: Thyroid disease in progressive systemic sclerosis: Increased frequency of glandular fibrosis and hypothyroidism. Ann. Intern. Med. 95:431, 1981.
229. Kahl, L. E., Medsger, T. A., Klein, I., et al.: Prospective evaluation of thyroid function in patients with progressive systemic sclerosis (PSS). Arthritis Rheum. 26(Suppl. 4):S62, 1983 (abstract).
230. Lally, E. V., and Jimenez, S. A.: Impotence in progressive systemic sclerosis. Ann. Intern. Med. 95:150, 1981.
231. Nowlin, N. S., Brick, J. E., Weaver, D. J., et al.: Impotence in scleroderma. Ann. Intern. Med. 104:794, 1986.
232. Cipoletti, J. F., Buckingham, R. B., Barnes, E. L., et al.: Sjögren's syndrome in progressive systemic sclerosis. Ann. Intern. Med. 87:535, 1977.
233. Osial, T. A., Whiteside, T. L., Buckingham, R. B., et al.: Clinical and serologic study of Sjögren's syndrome in patients with progressive systemic sclerosis. Arthritis Rheum. 26:500, 1983.
234. Naylor, W. P.: Oral management of the scleroderma patient. J. Am. Dent. Assoc. 105:814, 1982.
235. Steen, V. D., Conte, C., Day, N., et al.: Pregnancy in women with systemic sclerosis. Arthritis Rheum. 32:151, 1989.
236. Teasdall, R. D., Frayha, R. A., and Shulman, L. E.: Cranial nerve involvement in systemic sclerosis (scleroderma): A report of 10 cases. Medicine (Baltimore) 59:149, 1980.
237. Sonnex, C., Paice, E., and White, A. G.: Autonomic neuropathy in systemic sclerosis: A case report and evaluation of six patients. Ann. Rheum. Dis. 45:957, 1986.
238. Talbott, J. H., and Barrocas, M.: Progressive systemic sclerosis (PSS) and malignancy, pulmonary and non-pulmonary. Medicine (Baltimore) 58:182, 1979.
239. Peters-Golden, M., Wise, R. A., Hochberg, M., et al.: Incidence of lung cancer in systemic sclerosis. J. Rheumatol. 12:1136, 1985.
240. Roumm, A. D., and Medsger, T. A.: Cancer and systemic sclerosis. An epidemiologic study. Arthritis Rheum. 28:1336, 1985.
241. Segel, M. C., Campbell, W. L., Medsger, T. A., et al.: Systemic sclerosis (scleroderma) and esophageal adenocarcinoma: Is increased patient screening necessary? Gastroenterology 89:485, 1985.
242. Black, C., Dieppe, P., Huskisson, T., et al.: Regressive systemic sclerosis. Ann. Rheum. Dis. 45:384, 1986.
243. Furst, D. E., Clements, P. J., Saab, M., et al.: Clinical and serological comparison of 17 chronic progressive systemic sclerosis (PSS) and 17 CREST syndrome patients matched for sex, age, and disease duration. Ann. Rheum. Dis. 43:794, 1984.
243a. Siebold, J. R., Furst, D. E., and Clements, P. J.: Why everything (or nothing) seems to work in the treatment of scleroderma. J. Rheumatol. 19:673, 1992.
244. Furst, D. E., Clements, P. J., Hillis, S., et al.: Immunosuppression with chlorambucil, versus placebo, for scleroderma: Results of a three-year, parallel, randomized, double-blind study. Arthritis Rheum. 32:584, 1989.
245. Jansen, G. T., Barraza, D. F., Ballard, J. L., et al.: Generalized scleroderma—treatment with an immunosuppressive agent. Arch. Dermatol. 97:690, 1968.
246. Casas, J. A., Saway, P. A., Villarreal, I., et al.: 5-Fluorouracil in the treatment of scleroderma: A randomised, double-blind, placebo-controlled international collaborative study. Ann. Rheum. Dis. 49:926, 1990.
247. Weiner, S. R., Kono, D. H., Osterman, H. A., et al.: Preliminary report on a controlled trial of apheresis in the treatment of scleroderma. Arthritis Rheum. 30(Suppl. 4):S27, 1987 (abstract).
248. Dau, P. C., Kahaleh, M. B., and Sagebiel, R. W.: Plasmapheresis and immunosuppressive drug therapy in scleroderma. Arthritis Rheum. 24:1128, 1981.
249. Guillevin, L., Leon, A., Levy, Y., et al.: Treatment of progressive systemic sclerosis with plasma exchange. Seven cases. Int. J. Artif. Organs 6:315, 1983.
250. Gruber, B. L., and Kaufman, L. D.: A double-blind randomized controlled trial of ketotifen versus placebo in early diffuse scleroderma. Arthritis Rheum. 34:362, 1991.
251. Rook, A. H., Freundlich, B., Nahass, G. T., et al.: Treatment of autoimmune disease with extracorporeal photochemotherapy: Progressive systemic sclerosis. Yale J. Biol. Med. 62:639, 1989.
251a. Rook, A. H., Freundlich, B., Jegasothy, B. V., et al: Treatment of systemic sclerosis with extracorporeal photochemotherapy: results of a multicenter trial. Arch. Dermatol. 128:1517, 1992.
252. Beckett, V. L., Donadio, J. V., Brennan, L. A., et al.: Use of captopril as early therapy for renal scleroderma: A prospective study. Mayo Clin. Proc. 60:763, 1985.
253. Fries, J. F., Wasner, C., Brown, J., et al.: A controlled trial of antihypertensive therapy in systemic sclerosis (scleroderma). Ann. Rheum. Dis. 43:407, 1984.
254. Beckett, V. L., Conn, D. L., Fuster, V., et al.: Trial of platelet-inhibiting drugs in scleroderma. Double-blind study with dipyridamole and aspirin. Arthritis Rheum. 27:1137, 1984.
255. D'Angelo, W. A.: Progressive systemic sclerosis: Management. Part I: Introduction and general commentary. Clin. Rheum. Dis. 5:263, 1979.
256. Steen, V. D., Owens, G. R., Redmond, C., et al.: The effect of D-penicillamine on pulmonary findings in systemic sclerosis. Arthritis Rheum. 28:882, 1985.
257. De Clerck, L. S., Dequeker, J., Francx, L., et al.: D-Penicillamine therapy and interstitial lung disease in scleroderma. A long-term follow-up study. Arthritis Rheum. 30:643, 1987.
258. Steen, V. D., Blair, S., and Medsger, T. A.: The toxicity of D-penicillamine in systemic sclerosis. Ann. Intern. Med. 104:699, 1986.
259. Rodeheffer, R. J., Rommer, J. A., Wigley, F. M., et al.: Controlled double-blind trial of nifedipine in the treatment of Raynaud's phenomenon. N. Engl. J. Med. 308:880, 1983.
260. Smith, C. R., and Rodeheffer, R. J.: Treatment of Raynaud's phenomenon with calcium channel blockers. Am. J. Med. 78(Suppl. 2B):39, 1985.
261. Rupp, P. A. F., Mellinger, S., Kohler, J., et al.: Nicardipine for the treatment of Raynaud's phenomena: A double-blind cross-over trial of a new calcium entry blocker. J. Rheumatol. 14:745, 1987.
262. Snyder, S. H., and Reynolds, I. J.: Calcium-antagonist drugs. Receptor interactions that clarify therapeutic effects. N. Engl. J. Med. 313:995, 1985.
263. Russell, I. J., and Lessard, J. A.: Prazosin treatment of Raynaud's phenomenon: A double-blind single cross-over study. J. Rheumatol. 12:94, 1985.
264. Seibold, J. R., O'Byrne, M., and Harris, J. N.: Open trial of pentoxifylline in prophylaxis of digital ulceration in systemic sclerosis. Arthritis Rheum. 30(Suppl. 4):S120, 1987 (abstract).
265. Yardumian, D. A., Isenberg, D. A., Rustin, M., et al.: Successful treatment of Raynaud's phenomenon with Iloprost, a chemically stable prostacyclin analogue. Br. J. Rheumatol. 27:220, 1988.
266. McHugh, N. J., Csuka, M., Watson, H., et al.: Infusion of Iloprost, a prostacyclin analogue for treatment of Raynaud's phenomenon in systemic sclerosis. Ann. Rheum. Dis. 47:43, 1988.
267. Castell, D. O.: Medical therapy for reflux esophagitis: 1986 and beyond. Ann. Intern. Med. 104:112, 1986.
268. Adams, M. H., Ostrosky, J. D., and Kirkwood, C. F.: Therapeutic evaluation of omeprazole. Clin. Pharm. 7:725, 1988.
269. Ramirez-Mata, M., Ibanez, G., and Alarcon-Segovia, D.: Stimulatory effect of metoclopramide on the esophagus and lower esophageal sphincter of patients with PSS. Arthritis Rheum. 20:30, 1977.
270. Medsger, T. A.: D-Penicillamine treatment of lung involvement in patients with systemic sclerosis (scleroderma). Arthritis Rheum. 30:833, 1987.
271. Sfikakis, P. P., Kyriakidis, M. K., Vergos, C. G., et al.: Cardiopulmonary hemodynamics in systemic sclerosis and response to nifedipine and captopril. Am. J. Med. 90:541, 1991.
272. Thurm, C. A., Wigley, F. M., Dole, W. P., et al.: Failure of vasodilator infusion to alter pulmonary diffusing capacity in systemic sclerosis. Am. J. Med. 90:547, 1991.
273. Packer, M.: Vasodilator therapy for primary pulmonary hypertension: Limitations and hazards. Ann. Intern. Med. 103:258, 1985.
274. Lopez-Ovejero, J. A., Saal, S. D., D'Angelo, W. A., et al.: Reversal of vascular and renal crisis of scleroderma by oral angiotensin-converting-enzyme blockade. N. Engl. J. Med. 300:1417, 1979.
275. D'Angelo, W. A.: Long-term survival of scleroderma renal crisis and malignant hypertension with captopril. In Black, C. M., and Myers, A. R. (eds.): Systemic Sclerosis (Scleroderma). 1st ed. New York, Gower Med., 1985.
276. Rodnan, G. P.: When is scleroderma not scleroderma? The differential diagnosis of progressive systemic sclerosis. Bull. Rheum. Dis. 31:7, 1981.
277. Falanga, V., Medsger, T. A., Reichlin, M., et al.: Linear scleroderma. Clinical spectrum, prognosis, and laboratory abnormalities. Ann. Intern. Med. 104:849, 1986.
278. Buckingham, R. B., Prince, R. K., Rodnan, G. P., et al.: Collagen accumulation by dermal fibroblast cultures of patients with linear localized scleroderma. J. Rheumatol. 7:130, 1980.
279. Christianson, H. B., Dorsey, C. S., O'Leary, P. A., et al.: Localized scleroderma. A clinical study of two hundred thirty-five cases. Arch. Dermatol. 74:629, 1956.
280. Person, J. R., and Su, W. P. D.: Subcutaneous morphea: A clinical study of sixteen cases. Br. J. Dermatol. 100:371, 1979.
281. Dubois, E. L., Chandor, S., Friou, G. J., et al.: Progressive systemic sclerosis (PSS) and localized scleroderma (morphea) with positive LE test and unusual systemic manifestations compatible with systemic lupus erythematosus (SLE): Presentation of 14 cases including one set of identical twins, one with scleroderma and the other SLE. Review of the literature. Medicine (Baltimore) 50:199, 1971.

282. Venencie, P. Y., Powell, F. C., Su, W. P. D., et al.: Scleredema: A review of thirty-three cases. J. Am. Acad. Dermatol. 11:128, 1984.

283. Feldman, P., Shapiro, L., Pick, A. I., et al.: Scleromyxedema. Arch. Dermatol. 99:51, 1969.

284. Ohta, A., Uitto, J., Oikarinen, A. I., et al.: Paraproteinemia in patients with scleredema. Clinical findings and serum effects on skin fibroblasts in vitro. J. Am. Acad. Dermatol. 16:96, 1987.

285. Harper, R. A., and Rispler, J.: Lichen myxedematosus serum stimulates human skin fibroblast proliferation. Science 199:545, 1978.

286. Shulman, L. E.: Diffuse fasciitis with eosinophilia: A new syndrome? Trans. Assoc. Am. Physicians 88:70, 1975.

287. Moore, T. L., and Zuckner, J.: Eosinophilic fasciitis. Semin. Arthritis Rheum. 9:228, 1980.

288. Michet, C. J., Doyle, J. A., and Ginsburg, W. W.: Eosinophilic fasciitis. Report of 15 cases. Mayo Clin. Proc. 56:27, 1981.

289. Hoffman, R., Dainiak, N., Sibrack, L., et al.: Antibody-mediated aplastic anemia and diffuse fasciitis. N. Engl. J. Med. 300:718, 1979.

290. Littlejohn, G. O., and Keystone, E. C.: Eosinophilic fasciitis and aplastic anemia. J. Rheumatol. 7:730, 1980.

291. Barnes, L., Rodnan, G. P., Medsger, T. A., et al.: Eosinophilic fasciitis. A pathologic study of twenty cases. Am. J. Pathol. 96:493, 1979.

292. Gabrielli, A., De Nictolis, M., Campanati, G., et al.: Eosinophilic fasciitis: A mast cell disorder? Clin. Exp. Rheumatol. 1:75, 1983.

293. Moutsopoulos, H. M., Webber, B. L., Pavlidis, N. A., et al.: Diffuse fasciitis with eosinophilia. A clinicopathologic study. Am. J. Med. 68:710, 1980.

294. Martin, R. W., Duffy, J., Engel, A. G., et al.: The clinical spectrum of the eosinophilia-myalgia syndrome associated with L-tryptophan ingestion. Clinical features in 20 patients and aspects of pathophysiology. Ann. Intern. Med. 113:124, 1990.

295. Tabuenca, J. M.: Toxic-allergic syndrome caused by ingestion of rapeseed oil denatured with aniline. Lancet 2:567, 1981.

296. Mateo, I. M., Fernandez-Dapica, M. P., Izquierdo, M., et al.: Toxic epidemic syndrome: Musculoskeletal manifestations. J. Rheumatol. 11:333, 1984.

297. Palestine, R. F., Millens, J. L., and Sligel, G. T.: Skin manifestations of pentazocine abuse. J. Am. Acad. Dermatol. 2:47, 1980.

298. Finch, W. R., Rodnan, G. P., Buckingham, R. B., et al.: Bleomycin-induced scleroderma. J. Rheumatol. 7:651, 1980.

Chapter 67

Localized Fibrotic Disorders

Carlo L. Mainardi

Fibrotic disorders affecting vital organs are among the most common conditions with which clinicians are faced, and rheumatologists are familiar with organ fibrosis because it is a major component of progressive systemic sclerosis (PSS) and is often an accompaniment of other systemic rheumatic diseases (e.g., rheumatoid lung). Despite the frequent occurrence of diseases such as hepatic cirrhosis and the various fibrotic lung diseases, medical management of these disorders is inadequate, and our understanding of their pathogenesis is fragmentary. Rheumatologists are familiar with the sense of frustration associated with treating patients with PSS, but localized fibrotic disorders are equally as difficult to treat successfully. In addition to PSS, there are several other sclerosing disorders that are of interest to the practice of rheumatology because of the involvement of the musculoskeletal system (Dupuytren's contracture) or because of the expression of abnormal antibodies suggesting a relationship to immune complex disease (e.g., idiopathic pulmonary fibrosis).

In this chapter, selected clinical conditions characterized by localized sclerosis are briefly reviewed. Morphea and its variants are covered along with scleroderma in Chapter 66. These represent a spectrum of conditions ranging from indolent, mild disorders such as keloids or Dupuytren's contracture to life-threatening, subacute diseases such as idiopathic pulmonary fibrosis and retroperitoneal fibrosis. In fact, the severity of any of these disorders is related to the specific organ involvement and the time required for progression to an end-stage lesion.

FIBROTIC PULMONARY DISEASE

Of the clinical conditions discussed in this chapter, the entity of interstitial pulmonary fibrosis is the most important to the rheumatologist. This general category encompasses a large group of interstitial pulmonary diseases that share the feature of resulting in fibrotic lung disease. In some of these conditions, the etiologic agent is apparent (silicosis), and in others, the pulmonary disease is only a single manifestation of a systemic disease (rheumatoid arthritis, sarcoidosis), and a large group of these patients have idiopathic pulmonary fibrosis (IPF). Regardless of the

cause or associated disease, these conditions are to be considered serious and life-threatening.

The rheumatologist encounters fibrotic pulmonary disease in three distinct settings: (1) patients with IPF are often referred to the rheumatologist, (2) patients with a systemic rheumatic disorder may develop pulmonary fibrosis as a manifestation of the primary disorder, and (3) pulmonary fibrosis is an uncommon untoward effect of certain antirheumatic and cytotoxic drugs.

Idiopathic Pulmonary Fibrosis

This is a systemic disease of middle-aged men and women characterized by interstitial pulmonary inflammation and subsequent fibrosis. There have been several terms used to identify this condition. In honor of the investigators who first described the condition, it is often referred to as the Hamman-Rich syndrome. The disorder originally described by these investigators was a rapidly progressive illness,[1] and the term IPF includes those patients as well as those with less fulminant disease.[2]

The disease presents subjectively with breathlessness and a nonproductive cough. These symptoms are often accompanied by systemic complaints such as weight loss, fever, malaise, and arthralgias. With the exception of digital clubbing, the physical findings are limited to the chest. Diffuse rales and rhonchi are heard in the early stages, and as the disease progresses, dry, crackling rales are classically heard. In these later stages, signs of pulmonary hypertension (augmented P2) and right-sided heart failure are observed. The disease characteristically progresses to respiratory failure, but other causes of death include congestive heart failure, lung cancer, infection, and pulmonary embolism.[3]

Laboratory evaluation reveals an elevated erythrocyte sedimentation rate (ESR) in almost all patients. In addition, serum immunoglobulins are often elevated, and cryoglobulins are sometimes positive. Of particular interest to the rheumatologist is the significant incidence of positive antinuclear antibodies in IPF.[4] Circulating immune complexes have been found.[5] These clinical observations have led many to believe that IPF is an immune-mediated disease. Therefore, these patients are often referred to the rheumatologist to rule out a connective tissue disease.

Physiologically, these patients have normal indicators of airways resistance but have a depressed total lung volume and diffusion capacity. Resting hypoxia with mild hypocapnia and an exercise-induced impairment of gas exchange are the rule in IPF, but these physiologic studies do not necessarily correlate well with the histologic features of increased cellularity and fibrosis.[6, 7] Early in the disease the chest roentgenogram may have a diffuse, hazy, ground-glass appearance or may have a reticulonodular pattern. In the later stages, the classic "honeycomb lung" fibrotic appearance is observed. Pulmonary fibrosis can be assessed by computed tomography (CT) scanning, particularly high-resolution CT.[8] Characteristic findings include subpleural reticular opacities, and the distribution of fibrosis is peripheral. Cystic airspaces (honeycomb cysts) are frequently found.

Lung biopsy has been the mainstay of diagnosis in IPF. This can be obtained by an open technique or through bronchoscopy, although the former technique is preferable owing to the larger sample obtained. Histologic examination of lung invariably reveals thickening of the alveolar septa with fibrosis. In addition, alveolitis, manifest by infiltration of the interstitium with inflammatory cells with or without desquamation, occurs in a somewhat patchy manner.[2, 7] In later stages, the inflammatory component becomes less prominent, and fibrosis prevails.

Analysis of the fluid obtained by bronchoalveolar lavage (BAL) has become a standard procedure in the evaluation of patients with pulmonary fibrosis. The analysis of the cells in BAL fluid can be compared with synovial fluid analysis in rheumatoid arthritis. Although the cells in the fluid are not necessarily representative of the cells in the interalveolar tissue, the procedure has some diagnostic and prognostic value. The cellularity of this fluid is increased during the inflammatory phase of this disease, and patients with IPF (as well as connective tissue disease–associated pulmonary fibrosis) have been reported to exhibit a relative increase in neutrophils, whereas patients with sarcoidosis and hypersensitivity pneumonitis have a relative increase in lymphocytes.[9, 10] Subsequent studies have shown that BAL fluid lymphocytosis correlated with moderate to severe septal inflammation with little honeycombing and predicted a response to glucocorticoids. On the other hand, neutrophilia or eosinophilia predicted a poor response to steroids.[11, 12] A favorable clinical response to therapy is associated with a normalization of the BAL fluid cellularity and differential count.[13] Gallium scanning is of some value in the initial evaluation because most of the isotope will concentrate in inflamed tissue. Its correlation with disease activity and response to therapy, however, is suboptimal, and the procedure is generally considered to be of limited value in the follow-up of these patients.

Therapy of IPF includes the early institution of glucocorticoids. Only about half the patients experience a satisfactory response. Attempts have been made to correlate certain clinical parameters with a favorable response to steroids.[14] It seems logical that the fibrotic component is irreversible and that the effect of therapy is directed at the inflammatory component.[4] This concept is supported somewhat in that patients tend to respond more frequently if therapy is initiated early in the disease, and patients with a significant amount of fibrosis are much less likely to respond. Many patients fail to respond despite early therapy, however, and the reasons for this are not exactly clear. In one study, an increase in lymphocytes in the BAL fluid was associated with a favorable response, whereas an increase in neutrophils or eosinophils was associated with an unfavorable response.[15] The use of cytotoxic agents is controversial, but it is relatively common practice to use these agents in steroid failures.[16] Because improvement of certain hepatic fibroses has been reported with colchicine therapy (see later), this agent is currently under investigation for the treatment of pulmonary fibrosis.

Pulmonary Fibrosis as a Manifestation of Systemic Connective Tissue Diseases

This is the most common setting in which the rheumatologist will encounter interstitial lung disease. It can be a manifestation of rheumatoid arthritis,[17, 18] systemic lupus erythematosus,[19, 20] PSS,[21, 22] or dermatopolymyositis.[23, 24] Most investigators agree that the interstitial pulmonary disease associated with these systemic disorders is virtually indistinguishable from IPF because the clinical and pathologic pictures are very similar. As with IPF, BAL fluid analysis has been reported to be of value in the early diagnosis of rheumatoid lung.[25] The therapeutic approach is the same as for IPF, although the patients with an underlying connective tissue disease are less likely to respond to glucocorticoids. Agents such as D-penicillamine and methotrexate[26, 27] have been used in these conditions, although these agents have been reported to cause interstitial lung disease.[28, 29] This association, along with the immunologic abnormalities reported in some patients with IPF, suggests an overlap between these diseases.

Drug-Induced Pulmonary Fibrosis and the Rheumatologist

The spectrum of drugs reported to induce interstitial pulmonary fibrosis is vast and beyond the scope of this chapter. Certain of these drugs, however, are commonly used by rheumatologists and include gold, D-penicillamine, methotrexate, chlorambucil, and cyclophosphamide.[28–31] Generally speaking, the clinical pattern is similar to that described previously. This usually presents a perplexing problem to the clinician in that it is sometimes uncertain whether the pulmonary condition is due to the underlying disease or to the therapeutic agent. The withdrawal of a potentially offending agent, however, is always warranted considering the lack of specific therapy for the lung disease.

FIBROTIC LIVER DISEASE

The liver is the parenchymal organ most commonly diseased in a fibrotic state. The obvious reason for this is the prevalence of alcoholic liver disease in our society. This entity is not discussed in this chapter. There are, however, certain chronic disorders of the liver that ultimately lead to fibrosis and are of interest to rheumatologists. These include diseases such as chronic active hepatitis, primary biliary cirrhosis, and sclerosing cholangitis, which have features common to certain connective tissue diseases.[32]

Chronic Active Liver Disease

This term includes a spectrum of disorders characterized by chronic inflammation of the liver, which is followed by a fibrotic response. Most of the cases that fall into this category are related to viral hepatitis (both hepatitis B and hepatitis C). These patients do not generally present to a rheumatologist. A small group of patients with chronic active liver disease (CALD), however, have a disease characterized by chronic hepatitis, immunologic abnormalities, and extrahepatic manifestations.[33] This subgroup was once called *lupoid hepatitis*, but this term has fallen into disfavor[34] and has been replaced by the terms *autoimmune chronic hepatitis* or *chronic active hepatitis of unknown etiology*. These patients are mostly young and middle-aged women who present with signs and symptoms of acute hepatitis. Extrahepatic manifestations are not infrequent, and arthritis/arthralgias occur in as many as 25 percent of these patients. Other manifestations include skin rash, pleuropericarditis, fever, chronic diarrhea, and interstitial pulmonary disease.

Laboratory evaluation suggests an immune-mediated disease. Lupus erythematosus cells are positive in 10 to 20 percent (hence the term *lupoid hepatitis*), and a diffuse elevation of immunoglobulins is found in most of the patients. In addition, autoantibodies including antinuclear antibodies and anti–smooth muscle antibodies are present in a majority of patients. Thus, the overlap with systemic lupus erythematosus is significant, and the distinction may not be clear. The major distinguishing characteristic is the prominence of liver involvement. If left untreated, these patients progress to fibrotic liver disease, but the response to glucocorticoids is more favorable in this group when compared with other subgroups of CALD.[35]

Primary Biliary Cirrhosis

Primary biliary cirrhosis (PBC) is a progressive hepatic disease in which symptoms and signs of cholestasis result from an inflammatory and fibrotic reaction of the intrahepatic bile ducts.[36] The overwhelming majority of the patients are female (90 percent), and most are middle-aged. The most common presenting symptom is pruritus owing to cholestasis. The serum cholesterol is elevated, which leads to the formation of xanthomata. The disease progresses to cirrhosis, resulting in jaundice, portal hypertension, and hepatic failure.

There is an abundance of circumstantial evidence pointing toward immune mechanisms in the pathogenesis. Serum immunoglobulins (especially IgM) are elevated, and the hallmark of diagnosis is the presence of antimitochondrial antibody in the serum. Circulating immune complexes have been found, and other abnormal antibodies are often present (including antinuclear antibodies, rheumatoid factor, and anti–smooth muscle antibody). Of these autoantibodies, the antimitochondrial antibody has been a useful clinical test in establishing the diagnosis of PBC. The autoantigens responsible reactive with antimitochondrial antibodies have been characterized. These antigens are enzymes of the 2-oxo-acid dehydrogenase family, with the major reactive antigen being the E2 subunit of pyruvate dehydrogenase.[38] More circumstantial evidence is provided by the association with certain immunologic and connective tissue diseases.[36] Sjögren's syndrome has been reported with incidences ranging from 5 to 100 percent (see Chapter 55), and it is probable that more than half these patients have Sjögren's syndrome. In addition, a significant number of patients with PBC have either rheumatoid arthritis, PSS, or CREST* syndrome.[36, 37, 39, 40]

Of further interest to the rheumatologist is the frequent occurrence of metabolic bone disease. This is generally manifest as bone pain, and it has been reported that 20 percent of patients will experience vertebral collapse. Osteomalacia occurs owing to insufficient absorption of the fat-soluble vitamin D; in addition, cholestasis leads to insufficient bile salts in the intestine and results in excessive intestinal fat, which complexes with calcium preventing its absorption. The relative vitamin D deficiency is presumably due to impaired absorption (secondary to insufficient intestinal bile salts) and impaired hepatic conversion to 25-hydroxy-vitamin D.[41, 42]

Treatment is mostly supportive with dietary supplementation of medium-chain triglycerides and vitamin D and calcium. The pruritus is controlled with cholestyramine or ursodeoxycholate. This latter compound may be of general benefit to the disease process, and biochemical improvement may be

---

*Calcinosis, Raynaud's phenomenon, esophageal hypomotility, sclerodactyly, and telangiectasia.

seen.[37, 43] Other therapies are of marginal benefit and include steroids, immunosuppressives, and D-penicillamine.[37, 44] There has been recent interest in the use of colchicine for PBC as well as other forms of hepatic fibrosis. Trials have reported mixed results, with no reports of dramatic improvement of the majority of patients. The value of colchicine in these disorders remains to be determined.[45, 46]

Sclerosing Cholangitis

This is an unusual disorder in which chronic inflammation and subsequent fibrosis occur in the extrahepatic biliary tree. More than half the cases are associated with inflammatory bowel disease (usually ulcerative proctocolitis), and there is some association with retroperitoneal fibrosis. Serum immunoglobulins (IgM) are often elevated suggesting an immunologic role. The disease is progressive and leads to biliary cirrhosis. There is no known effective medical therapy, although liver transplantation has been successful.[47-49]

DUPUYTREN'S CONTRACTURE

This is an extremely common condition with which rheumatologists are familiar. It is characterized by a nodular thickening of the palmar fascia and an associated contraction of fourth and fifth digits. It is associated with alcoholic liver disease and epilepsy and is often familial. Its association with other localized fibroses (plantar fasciitis and Peyronie's disease) has led to the concept of a *Dupuytren's diathesis*.[50]

Pathologically, there is a thickening of the palmar fascia resulting in a shortened fascia without an apparent inflammatory reaction. The thickening takes the form of a firm fibrous band or of a nodular, fusiform area.[51-52] This tissue has been the subject of microscopic and biochemical analysis. The total collagen content is increased, and about 25 percent of the collagen is type III, which is not normally present in fascia. In addition, the content of hydroxylysine is elevated as are reducible cross-links. These observations indicate a clear-cut abnormality of the collagen present in the abnormal fascia. Of further interest is the presence of myofibroblasts (contractile smooth muscle–like cells) in these nodules. It has been hypothesized that the contraction of the fascia is related to the presence of these contractile cells. These cells may be responsible for the increase in type III collagen.[53-56]

KELOIDS

Keloids are hypertrophic scars that are seen frequently in black patients. Keloid formation can be considered to be wound healing in which the control mechanisms are abnormal. The dermis is hypercellular, and the collagen content is increased.[57] The rate of collagen synthesis by keloid tissue is increased,[58] and this is also true with keloid fibroblasts.[59, 60] Keloid fibroblasts exhibit abnormal growth characteristics in that they have a reduced requirement for growth factors.[61] The regulation of collagen synthesis is also abnormal in these cells in that they exhibit a reduced sensitivity to the inhibitory effect of glucocorticoids.[62]

The management of keloids is difficult and frustrating owing to the tendency for recurrence. Therefore, a varied spectrum of treatment modalities has been reported, including excision, radiotherapy, systemic chemotherapy, and intralesional steroids.[63] Although most would agree that the most logical approach is excision of the growth with measures to prevent recurrence, there is no universally accepted treatment modality.

RETROPERITONEAL FIBROSIS

Retroperitoneal fibrosis (RPF) is a disorder in which the retroperitoneal fat is the site of a subacute and chronic inflammatory reaction and is subsequently replaced by dense fibrotic tissue. The presentation is that of flank and abdominal pain. Systemic symptoms are common and include malaise, weight loss, and fever. As the disease progresses, the result of compression of retroperitoneal structures becomes clinically apparent and includes anuria and azotemia, Leriche's syndrome, constipation, and hypertension from obstruction of the renal artery. Laboratory abnormalities include a mild anemia, elevation of the ESR, hypoalbuminemia, and hyperglobulinemia. The diagnosis is made by the demonstration of a soft tissue retroperitoneal mass, which is usually periaortic by CT. Although the "mass" is fibrotic tissue, it displaces normal structures including ureters. Classic intravenous pyelography findings include narrowing of the ureters at the L-4–L-5 level, medial displacement of the ureters, and dilatation of the calyceal system.

The natural course of the disease is variable, and spontaneous remission is not uncommon. The major therapeutic modality is surgery with release of the ureters from the fibrotic mass. Surgery is often indicated for pathologic confirmation of the diagnosis. Glucocorticoid therapy is of benefit in these patients, usually in conjunction with surgical release of the ureters.[64-66]

The relationship between RPF and periaortitis is unclear. In some cases of abdominal aortic aneurysm, periaortic inflammation and fibrosis occur. This combination has been referred to as perianeurysmal fibrosis or inflammatory abdominal aortic aneurysm.[67] In RPF, the fibrosis is typically periaortic, but aneurysm is not typically present. It has been suggested that RPF is a periaortic inflammatory reaction as a manifestation of an immune response to a lipid/protein antigen leaking through the aorta from atheromatous plaques.[68] This hypothesis remains to be proved but would not explain the cases of RPF that are associated with drugs (ergot alkaloids, bromocriptine) rather than with atherosclerosis.

OTHER LOCALIZED FIBROSES

Carcinoid tumors are associated with localized fibrosis, and the pathogenesis is believed to be related to the release of vasoactive substances from the tumors. The most familiar of these is the association of endocardial fibrosis with metastatic carcinoids. Right-sided valvular involvement occurs with liver metastases, and left-sided cardiac involvement is associated with lung metastases.[69] RPF has been associated with carcinoid tumors.[70] A promising approach to the carcinoid syndrome is the use of octreotide (SMS 201–995), a long-acting somatostatin analogue.[71]

Peyronie's disease is a fibrotic disorder involving the shaft of the penis that results in pain and discomfort with difficulty in sexual function. It tends to occur in conjunction with other localized fibroses (Dupuytren's contracture)[72, 73] and has been associated with β-adrenergic blocking agents.[74, 75] Intralesional injection of clostridial collagenase has been reported to be of benefit to patients with this disorder.[76]

Pseudotumor of the orbit is a rare fibrotic disorder in which orbital inflammation and fibrosis result in a protrusion of the eye.[77] This disorder has also been reported to occur in association with other localized fibroses as well as with polyarteritis nodosa.[78, 79]

Riedel's struma is a condition in which fibrotic tissue replaces normal thyroid gland and extends beyond the thyroid to involve other structures in the neck.[80] Like some of the diseases already mentioned, Riedel's struma occurs in association with other fibroses, including RPF, sclerosing cholangitis, and pseudotumor of the orbit.[81–83]

References

1. Hamman, L., and Rich, A. R.: Acute diffuse interstitial fibrosis of the lungs. Bull. Johns Hopkins Hosp. 74:177, 1944.
2. Crystal, R. G., Fulmer, J. D., Roberts, W. C., Moss, M. L., Line, B. R., and Reynolds, H. Y.: Idiopathic pulmonary fibrosis. Clinical, histologic, radiographic, physiologic, scintigraphic, cytologic, and biochemical aspects. Ann. Intern. Med. 85:769, 1976.
3. Panos, R. J., Mortenson, R. L., Niccoli, S. A., and King, T. E.: Clinical deterioration in patients with idiopathic pulmonary fibrosis: Causes and assessment. Am. J. Med. 88:396, 1990.
4. Nagaya, H., and Seiker, H. O.: Pathogenic mechanisms of interstitial pulmonary fibrosis in patients with serum antinuclear factor. A histologic and clinical correlation. Am. J. Med. 52:51, 1972.
5. Dreisin, R. B., Schwartz, M. I., Theophilopoulos, A. N., and Stanford, R. E.: Circulating immune complexes in idiopathic interstitial pneumonias. N. Engl. J. Med. 298:353, 1978.
6. Fulmer, J. D., Roberts, W. C., von Gal, E. R., and Crystal, R. G.: Morphologic-physiologic correlates of the severity of fibrosis and degree of cellularity in idiopathic pulmonary fibrosis. J. Clin. Invest. 63:665, 1979.
7. Crystal, R. G., Gadek, J. E., Ferrans, V. J., Fulmer, J. D., Line, B. R.,
and Hunninghake, G. W.: Interstitial lung disease: Current concepts of pathogenesis, staging, and therapy. Am. J. Med. 70:542, 1981.
8. Muller, N. L., and Miller, R. R.: Computed tomography of chronic diffuse infiltrative lung disease. Part 1. Am. Rev. Resp. Dis. 142:1206, 1990.
9. Reynolds, H. Y., Fulmer, J. D., Kazmierowski, J. A., Roberts, W. C., Frank, M. M., and Crystal, R. G.: Analysis of cellular and protein content of broncho-alveolar lavage fluid from patients with idiopathic pulmonary fibrosis and chronic hypersensitivity pneumonitis. J. Clin. Invest. 59:165, 1977.
10. Weinberger, S. E., Kelman, J. A., Elson, N. A., Young, R. C., Reynolds, H. Y., Fulmer, J. D., and Crystal, R. G.: Bronchoalveolar lavage in interstitial lung disease. Ann. Intern. Med. 89:459, 1978.
11. Watters, L. C., Schwarz, M. I., Cherniack, R. M., et al.: Idiopathic pulmonary fibrosis: Pretreatment bronchoalveolar lavage cellular constituents and their relationships with lung histopathology and clinical response to therapy. Am. Rev. Resp. Dis. 135:696, 1987.
12. Haslam, P. L., Turton, C. W. G., Lokoszek, A., et al.: Bronchoalveolar lavage fluid cell counts in cryptogenic fibrosing alveolitis and their relation to therapy. Thorax 35:328, 1980.
13. Turner-Warwick, M., and Haslam, P. L.: The value of serial bronchoalveolar lavages in assessing the clinical progress of patients with cryptogenic fibrosing alveolitis. Am. Rev. Resp. Dis. 135:26, 1987.
14. Turner-Warwick, M., Burrows, B., and Johnson, A.: Cryptogenic fibrosing alveolitis: Response to corticosteroid therapy and its effect on survival. Thorax 35:593, 1980.
15. Rudd, R. M., Halsam, P. L., and Turner-Warwick, M.: Cryptogenic fibrosing alveolitis. Relationships of pulmonary physiology and bronchoalveolar lavage to response to treatment and prognosis. Am. Rev. Resp. Dis. 124:1, 1981.
16. Winterbauer, R. H., Hammar, S. P., Hallman, K. O., Hays, J. E., Pardee, N. E., Morgan, E. H., Allen, J., Moores, K. D., Bush, W., and Walker, J.: Diffuse interstitial pneumonitis. Clinicopathologic correlations in 20 patients treated with prednisone and azathioprine. Am. J. Med. 65:661, 1978.
17. Popper, M. S., Bogdonoff, M. L., and Hughes, R. L.: Interstitial rheumatoid lung disease. A reassessment and review of the literature. Chest 62:243, 1972.
18. Gordon, D. A., Stein, J. L., and Broder, I.: The extra-articular manifestations of rheumatoid arthritis. A systemic analysis of 127 cases. Am. J. Med. 54:445, 1973.
19. Gross, M., Esterly, J. R., and Earle, R. H.: Pulmonary alterations in systemic lupus erythematosus. Am. Rev. Resp. Dis. 105:572, 1972.
20. Eisenberg, H., Dubois, E. L., Sherwin, R. P., and Balchum, O. J.: Diffuse interstitial lung disease in systemic lupus erythematosus. Ann. Intern. Med. 79:37, 1973.
21. Spain, D. M., and Thomas, A. G.: The pulmonary manifestations of scleroderma. An anatomic-physiologic correlation. Ann. Intern. Med. 32:152, 1950.
22. Wilson, R. J., Rodnan, G. P., and Robin, E. D.: An early pulmonary physiologic abnormality in progressive systemic sclerosis (diffuse scleroderma). Am. J. Med. 36:361, 1964.
23. Songcharoen, S., Raju, S. F., and Pennebaker, J. B.: Interstitial lung disease in polymyositis and dermatomyositis. J. Rheumatol. 7:353, 1980.
24. Salmeron, G., Greenberg, S. D., and Lidsky, M. D.: Polymyositis and diffuse interstitial lung disease. A review of the pulmonary histopathologic findings. Arch. Intern. Med. 141:1005, 1981.
25. Tishler, M., Grief, J., Firemen, E., Yaron, M., and Topilsky, M.: Bronchoalveolar lavage—a sensitive tool for early diagnosis of pulmonary involvement in rheumatoid arthritis. J. Rheumatol. 13:547, 1986.
26. Goodman, M., and Turner-Warwick, M.: Pilot study of penicillamine therapy in corticosteroid failure patients with widespread pulmonary fibrosis. Chest 74:338, 1978.
27. Scott, G. I., and Bacon, P. A.: Response to methotrexate in fibrosing alveolitis associated with connective tissue disease. Thorax 35:725, 1980.
28. Turner-Warwick, M.: Adverse reactions affecting the lung: possible association with D-penicillamine. J. Rheumatol. 8(Suppl. 7):166, 1981.
29. Weiss, R. B., and Muggia, F. M.: Cytotoxic drug-induced pulmonary disease: Update 1980. Am. J. Med. 68:259, 1980.
30. Podell, J. E., Klinenberg, J. R., Kramer, L. S., and Brown, H. V.: Pulmonary toxicity with gold therapy. Arthritis Rheum. 23:347, 1980.
31. Godard, Ph., Marty, J. P., and Michel, P. B.: Interstitial pneumonia and chlorambucil. Chest 76:471, 1979.
32. Golding, P. L., Smith, M., and Williams, R.: Multisystem involvement in chronic liver disease. Studies on the incidence and pathogenesis. Am. J. Med. 55:772, 1973.
33. Boyer, J. L., and Miller, D. J.: Chronic hepatitis. In Schiff, L., and Schiff, E. R. (eds.): Diseases of the Liver. 5th ed. Philadelphia, J. B. Lippincott Co., 1982, p. 771.
34. Soloway, R. D., Summerskill, W. H. J., Baggenstoss, A. H., and Schoenfeld, L. J.: "Lupoid hepatitis," a non-entity in the spectrum of chronic active liver disease. Gastroenterology 63:458, 1972.
35. Reynolds, T. B.: Chronic hepatitis: Current dilemmas. Am. J. Med. 69:485, 1980.

36. Christensen, E., Crowe, J., Doniach, D., Popper, H., Ranek, L., Rodes, J., Tygstrup, N., and Williams, R.: Clinical pattern and course of disease in primary biliary cirrhosis based on an analysis of 236 patients. Gastroenterology 78:236, 1980.

37. Triger, D. R.: Update on primary biliary cirrhosis. Dig. Dis. 8:61, 1990.

38. Gershwin, M. E., and Mackay, I. R.: Primary biliary cirrhosis: Paradigm or paradox for autoimmunity. Gastroenterology 100:822, 1991.

39. MacGregor, G. A.: Primary biliary cirrhosis is a dry gland syndrome. Lancet 2:535, 1980.

40. Crowe, J. P., Christensen, E., Butler, J., Wheeler, P., Doniach, D., Keenan, J., and Williams, R.: Primary biliary cirrhosis: The prevalence of hypothyroidism and its relationship to thyroid autoantibodies and sicca syndrome. Gastroenterology 78:1437, 1980.

41. Long, R. C., Wills, M. R., Skinner, R. K., and Sherlock, S.: Serum 1-25-hydroxy-vitamin D in untreated parenchymal and cholestatic liver disease. Lancet 2:650, 1976.

42. Long, R. G.: Hepatic osteodystrophy: outlook good but some problems unsolved. Gastroenterology 78:644, 1980.

43. Poupon, P., Chretien, Y., Poupon, R. E., et al.: Is ursodeoxycholic acid an effective treatment for primary biliary cirrhosis? Lancet 1:834, 1987.

44. Crowe, J., Christensen, E., Smith, M., Cochrane, M., Ranek, L., Watkinson, G., Doniach, D., Popper, H., Tygstrup, N., and Williams, R.: Azathioprine in primary biliary cirrhosis: Preliminary report of an international trial. Gastroenterology 78:1005, 1980.

45. Kaplan, M. M., Alling, D. W., Zimmerman, H. J., Wolfe, H. J., Sepersky, R. A., Hirsch, G. S., Elta, G. H., Glick, K. A., and Eagen, K. A.: A prospective trial of colchicine for primary biliary cirrhosis. N. Engl. J. Med. 315:1448, 1986.

46. Kershenobich, D., Vargas, F., Garcia-Tsao, G., Perez-Tamayo, R., Gent, M., and Rojkind, M.: Colchicine in the treatment of cirrhosis of the liver. N. Engl. J. Med. 318:1709, 1988.

47. Chapman, R. W. G., Arborgh, B. A. M., Rhodes, J. M., Summerfield, J. A., Dick, R., Scheuer, P. J., and Sherlock, S.: Primary sclerosing cholangitis: A review of its clinical features, cholangiography, and hepatic histology. Gut 21:870, 1980.

48. Lindor, K. D., Wiesner, R. H., MacCarty, R. L., Ludwig, J., and LaRusso, N. F.: Advances in primary sclerosing cholangitis. Am. J. Med. 89:73, 1990.

49. Marsh, J. W., Jr., Iwatsuki, S., Makowka, L., et al.: Orthotopic liver transplantation for primary sclerosing cholangitis. Ann. Surg. 207:21, 1988.

50. Wheeler, E. S., and Meals, R. A.: Dupuytren's diathesis: A broad spectrum disease. Plast. Reconstr. Surg. 68:781, 1981.

51. Gelberman, R. H., Amiel, D., Rudolph, R. M., and Vance, R. M.: Dupuytren's contracture. An electron microscopic, biochemical, and clinical correlative study. J. Bone Joint Surg. 62-A:425, 1980.

52. Vande Berg, J. S., Rudolph, R., Gelberman, R., and Woodward, M. R.: Ultrastructural relationship of skin to nodule and cord in Dupuytren's contracture. Plast. Reconstr. Surg. 69:835, 1982.

53. Hanyu, T., Tajima, T., Takagi, T., Sasaki, S., Fujimoto, D., Isemura, M., and Yosizawa, Z.: Biochemical studies on the collagen of the palmar aponeurosis affected with Dupuytren's disease. Tokohu J. Exp. Med. 142:437, 1984.

54. Iwasaki, H., Mueller, H., Stutte, H. J., and Breenscheidt, U.: Palmer fibromatosis (Dupuytren's contracture): Ultrastructural and enzyme histochemical studies in 43 cases. Virchows Arch. (A) 405:41, 1984.

55. Brickley-Parsons, D., Climcher, M. J., Smith, R., Albin, R., and Adams, J. P.: Biochemical changes in the collagen of the palmar fascia in patients with Dupuytren's disease. J. Bone Joint Surg. 63-A:787, 1981.

56. Bailey, A. J., Sims, T. J., Gabbiani, G., Bazin, S., and LeLouis, M.: Collagen of Dupuytren's disease. Clin. Sci. 53:499, 1977.

57. Peacock, E. E., Jr., Madden, J. W., and Trier, W. C.: Biologic basis for treatment of keloids and hypertrophic scars. South. Med. J. 63:755, 1970.

58. Cohen, I. K., Keiser, H. R., and Sjoerdsma, A.: Collagen synthesis in human keloid and hypertrophic scar. Surg. Forum 22:488, 1971.

59. Abergel, R. P., Pizzurro, D., Meeker, C. A., Lask, G., Matsuoka, L. Y., Minor, R. R., Chu, M. L., and Uitto, J.: Biochemical composition of the connective tissue in keloids and analysis of collagen metabolism in keloid fibroblast cultures. J. Invest. Dermatol. 84:384, 1985.

60. Diegelmann, R. F., Cohen, I. K., and McCoy, B. J.: Growth kinetics and collagen synthesis of normal skin, normal scar, and keloid fibroblasts in vitro. J. Cell. Physiol. 98:341, 1979.

61. Russell, S. B., Russell, J. D., and Trupin, J. S.: Alteration of amino acid transport by hydrocortisone. Different effects in human fibroblasts derived from normal skin and keloid. J. Biol. Chem. 257:9525, 1982.

62. Russell, S. B., Trupin, K. N., Rodriguez-Eaton, S., and Russell, J. D.: Reduced growth factor requirement of keloid-derived fibroblasts may account for tumour growth. Proc. Nat. Acad. Sci. U.S.A. 85:587, 1988.

63. Datubo-Brown, D. D.: Keloids: A review of the literature. Br. J. Plast. Surg. 43:70, 1990.

64. Lepor, H., and Walsh, P. C.: Idiopathic retroperitoneal fibrosis. J. Urol. 122:1, 1979.

65. Larrieu, A. J., Weiner, I., Abston, S., and Warren, M. M.: Retroperitoneal fibrosis. Surg. Gynecol. Obstet. 150:699, 1980.

66. Higgins, P. M., and Aberm, G. M.: Idiopathic retroperitoneal fibrosis— an update. Dig. Dis. 8:206, 1990.

67. Brooks, A. P.: Computed tomography of idiopathic retroperitoneal fibrosis ("periaortitis"): Variants, variations, patterns, and pitfalls. Clin. Radiol. 42:75, 1990.

68. Bullock, N.: Idiopathic retroperitoneal fibrosis. Br. Med. J. 297:240, 1988.

69. Sjoerdsma, A., and Roberts, W. C.: The cardiac disease associated with the carcinoid syndrome (carcinoid heart disease). Am. J. Med. 36:5, 1964.

70. Morin, L. J., and Zuerner, R. T.: Retroperitoneal fibrosis and carcinoid tumor. J.A.M.A. 216:1647, 1971.

71. Wynick, D., and Bloom, S. R.: The use of the long acting somatostatin analog, octreotide, in the treatment of gut neuroendocrine tumors. J. Clin. Endocrinol. Metab. 73:1, 1991.

72. Smith, B. H.: Peyronie's disease. Am. J. Clin. Pathol. 45:670, 1966.

73. Dupuytren's contracture, fibroma plantae, periarthrosis humeri, induration penis plastica, and epilepsy, with attempt at pathogenetic valuation. Acta Psychiat. Neurol. Scand. 16:465, 1941.

74. Yudkin, J. S.: Peyronie's disease in association with metoprolol. Lancet 2:1355, 1977.

75. Wallis, A. A., Bell, R., and Sutherland, P. W.: Propranolol and Peyronie's disease. Lancet 2:980, 1977.

76. Gelbard, M. K., Lindner, A., and Kaufman, J. J.: The use of collagenase in the treatment of Peyronie's disease. J. Urol. 134:208, 1985.

77. Jackson, H.: Pseudotumor of the orbit. Br. J. Ophthalmol. 42:212, 1958.

78. Arnott, E. J., and Greaves, D. P.: Orbital involvement in Riedel's thyroiditis. Br. J. Ophthalmol. 49:1, 1965.

79. Walton, E. W.: Pseudotumor of the orbit and polyarteritis nodosa. J. Clin. Pathol. 12:419, 1959.

80. Woolner, L. B., McConahey, W. M., and Beahrs, O. H.: Invasive fibrous thyroiditis (Riedel's struma). J. Clin. Endocrinol. 17:201, 1957.

81. Turner-Warwick, M., Nabarro, J. D. N., and Domiach, D.: Riedel's thyroiditis and retroperitoneal fibrosis. Proc. R. Soc. Med. 59:596, 1966.

82. Bartholomew, L. G., Cain, J. C., Woolner, L. B., Utz, D. C., and Ferris, D. O.: Sclerosing cholangitis. Its possible association with Riedel's struma and fibrous retroperitonitis—report of two cases. N. Engl. J. Med. 269:8, 1963.

83. deLange, W. E., Freling, N. J., Molenaar, W. M., and Doorenbos, H.: Invasive fibrous thyroiditis, Riedel's struma: A manifestation of multifocal fibrosclerosis? A case report with review of the literature. Q. Med. J. 72:709, 1989.

Chapter 68

Eosinophilia-Myalgia Syndrome

Bruce Freundlich

The eosinophilia-myalgia syndrome (EMS) was first recognized as an entity in October 1989, when three patients who had ingested L-tryptophan and developed severe myalgias with a peripheral blood eosinophilia were reported to the New Mexico State Health Department and the Centers for Disease Control (CDC).[1] Additional cases were rapidly identified, and two case-control studies established a strong connection between the syndrome and L-tryptophan usage.[2]

In addition to myalgias, patients also frequently exhibited rashes, transient dyspnea, extremity edema, and cutaneous thickening.[3] Subsequent reports of neuropathies, myopathies, cardiopulmonary involvement, and gastrointestinal involvement made it clear that EMS was a multisystem process.[4] By August 1990, 1536 cases had been reported to the CDC.[5] Only a handful of further new cases were reported as late as January 1991. The mean age of patients with EMS has been 49 years, with 73 percent being between 35 and 64.[4] Eighty-four percent of cases were women, and 97 percent were white.[4]

The CDC established case surveillance definition criteria, which are delineated in Table 68–1.[6] The consumption of L-tryptophan was not a part of the case definition, although 97 percent of patients meeting the criteria did consume this product.[4] The criteria, although important as an investigational tool, excluded a potentially large group of patients with myalgias that were not incapacitating or who did not have an eosinophil count assessed near the onset of their symptoms, when it was more likely to have been elevated. Therefore, the surveillance criteria have undoubtedly led to an underestimation of the true prevalence of this syndrome.[6a]

L-Tryptophan is an essential amino acid that is abundant in the average diet in the United States. Patients with EMS had consumed an average of approximately 2 g of supplemental daily L-tryptophan (range, 10 mg to 15 g).[4] Since 1974, L-tryptophan has been available as a single over-the-counter food supplement, sold mostly in health food stores. It is estimated that millions of U. S. citizens have consumed this product, most frequently to treat insomnia based on the rationale that serotonin, a major L-tryptophan metabolite, may be important in sleep induction.[8] Patients who developed EMS were also taking L-tryptophan for depression, premenstrual syndrome, bulimia, arthritis, anxiety, behavioral disorders, headaches, tinnitus, smoking cessation, and substance abuse. The use of L-tryptophan appeared to have increased almost threefold from 1986 to mid-1988 in one metropolitan survey.[7] This increase was inconsonant, however, with the clustered temporal presentation of EMS that occurred during the summer and autumn of 1989.[4] It was therefore unlikely that this was a pre-existing rare syndrome that increased in incidence owing to a higher rate of consumption.

CLINICAL FINDINGS

EMS can roughly be divided into two stages. Once patients discontinued L-tryptophan, the mean latency to onset of symptoms was 84 days (range, 1 to 2858).[4] Initially almost all patients complained of the abrupt onset of myalgias and were found to have an elevated peripheral eosinophil count. Other early findings included rashes, fever, peripheral and periorbital edema, weight change, a nonproductive cough with dyspnea, and arthralgias. Within weeks to a few months, with the notable exception of myalgias, the majority of these symptoms and findings cleared. Subsequent problems have included cutaneous thickening and various degrees of myopathy and neuropathy. Table 68–2 is a listing of the more common signs, symptoms, and laboratory findings of patients with EMS.

NEUROMUSCULAR FINDINGS

Myalgias have been the predominant symptom of EMS. They have been rapid in onset, severe, incapacitating, and persistent. Several weeks into the

Table 68–1. THE CDC CASE SURVEILLANCE DEFINITION CRITERIA FOR THE EOSINOPHILIA-MYALGIA SYNDROME

Peripheral eosinophil count $\geq$ 1000 cells/mm^3
Severe myalgias that interfere with daily activities
Exclusion of infectious, neoplastic, or other illnesses that might account for the above two findings

Table 68–2. CLINICAL SIGNS, SYMPTOMS, AND LABORATORY FINDINGS OF EOSINOPHILIA-MYALGIA SYNDROME

Clinical Finding	% Patients	Laboratory Finding	% Patients
Arthralgia	73	Leukocytosis	85
Rash	60	Aldolase increase	46
Peripheral edema	59	Creatine kinase increase	10
Cough or dyspnea	59	Sedimentation rate increase	33
Fever	36		
Thickened skin	32	Liver function abnormality	43
Periorbital edema	28	Chest roentgenogram	
Alopecia	28	Infiltrates	17
Neuropathy	27	Pleural effusions	12
Hepatomegaly	5		

Adapted from Swygart, L. A., Maes, E. F., Sewell, L. E., Miller, L., Falk, H., and Kilbourne, E. M.: J.A.M.A. 264:1698–1703, 1990.

syndrome, muscle spasms also commonly appear. These spasms frequently affect the calves and abdominal muscles. The upper limbs, hands, jaw, neck, ocular muscles, and tongue may also be involved. Movement and change in position may bring the spasms on, leaving some patients almost completely immobilized. The specific location of myalgias and spasms has limited ambulation, utensil use, ability to write or read, mastication, and speech in selected patients. Symmetric lower limb weakness has not been uncommon and may be due to myopathy or neuropathy but may on occasion be more apparent than real owing to effort-associated pain. Serum aldolase levels are reported to be elevated in half of tested patients;[4] however, creatinine kinase levels are only infrequently high and in fact are commonly below normal values.[9, 10] This does not appear to be due to an inhibitor in the serum, although plasma has not been studied.[9] Electrophysiologic studies have demonstrated various combinations of myopathic and neuropathic patterns.[11–13]

Muscle histology from EMS patients has revealed mononuclear cell infiltrates in the endomysium and perimysium.[1, 10, 12] These infiltrates are frequently perivascular with only occasional eosinophils (Fig. 68–1). Thickened vessel walls and swollen endothelial cells have been found; however, fibrinoid necrosis of vessel walls, thrombosis, and obvious vasculitis have been mostly absent.[12, 14] About one third of the infiltrating cells have been acid phosphatase–positive macrophages.[12] In some cases, vessel necrosis could be demonstrated on an ultrastructural level.[14] However, in only a few cases were myofibril destruction and fiber necrosis present.[12, 13] Type II fiber atrophy and denervation atrophy were not uncommon.[12]

Neuropathies have been reported in more than one quarter of patients.[4] Patients may complain of a burning sensation, paresthesias, hypesthesias, or weakness in the absence of myopathy. Nerve conduction studies confirmed by biopsy have demonstrated combinations of demyelinization and axonal degeneration.[13] Biopsies of affected nerves show epineural, perineural, and perivascular cellular infiltrates (Fig. 68–2). The neuropathies have been mostly sensorimotor or sensory predominant,[12, 15] although ascending motor paralysis has been described.[16, 17] Bell's palsy has been rarely noted, whereas other cranial neuropathies have been absent. There are two reports of patients who had encephalopathy.[10, 12] One had electroencephalographic findings of bilateral slowing without focal abnormalities.[12] Cerebrospinal fluid was normal, but magnetic resonance imaging (MRI) showed areas of increased signal intensity in the white matter. Patients not infrequently complain of memory loss and a diminished ability to concentrate. Chronic pain may play a role in this process, but this has not been formally analyzed.

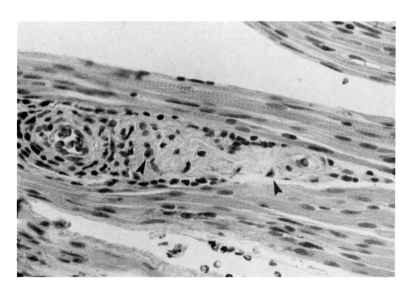

Figure 68–1. Perimyositis is characteristic of muscle histopathology in EMS. Two eosinophils are present (*arrows*). (Courtesy of Victoria Werth, M.D., University of Pennsylvania.)

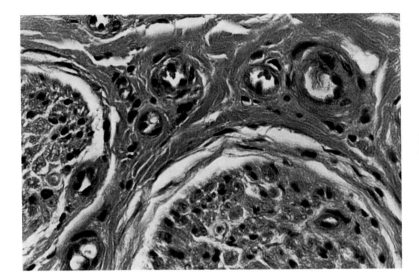

Figure 68–2. Epineural and perivascular infiltrates from a sural nerve biopsy of a patient with EMS.

CUTANEOUS FINDINGS

Cutaneous nonpitting edema in the arms and legs found in up to 60 percent of cases has been the most recognized cutaneous finding in EMS patients.[4] This occurred particularly early during the disease course and appears to have been frequently due to fascial inflammation. The edema, especially in the upper extremities, may improve with prednisone; however, some edematous areas progressively harden with a peau d'orange appearance characteristic of eosinophilic fasciitis.

Other early cutaneous manifestations of EMS have included urticaria, macule-papules, small purplish brown patches, mucinous papules, dermatographism, serpiginous lesions, subcutaneous nodules, and morphea-like lesions.[10, 16, 18] Alopecia occurred in up to 28 percent of the CDC-reported cases.[4] Diffuse erythema and cutaneous mottling particularly over the extremities may occur.[16] Pruritus was prominent in some series.[10]

The fasciitis itself by clinical and histologic criteria appears indistinguishable from eosinophilic fasciitis.[12, 19, 20] Mononuclear cell infiltrates that may include eosinophils and commonly have a perivascular component are found in the fascia, subcutaneous fat, and lower dermis (Fig. 68–3). The general infiltrate pattern differs from scleroderma, in which mononuclear cells are predominantly found in the dermis. Increased cutaneous collagen synthesis of EMS patients has been observed,[23] but collagen content of the dermis with rare exception appears substantially less than in scleroderma. Clinically, the skin may feel woody, with a peau d'orange appearance as in eosinophilic fasciitis, which is likely to be due to the inflammatory infiltrates and fibrosis in the subcutaneous fibrous bands that run perpendicular to the skin surface. There may be a "groove sign" with prominent tethering of surface veins in the upper medial part of the arm. In recent years, many patients who had been diagnosed as having eosinophilic fasciitis in retrospective analysis had consumed

L-tryptophan.[19] In one study, eight of eight patients who had been given a diagnosis of eosinophilic fasciitis between 1988 and 1990 were discovered to have ingested L-tryptophan, whereas only one of 40 patients with systemic sclerosis and zero of three with morphea had taken this product.[19] L-Tryptophan consumption has not, however, been a universal phenomenon in patients with a diagnosis of eosinophilic fasciitis, particularly when the diagnosis was established before 1988.[21] Since the summer of

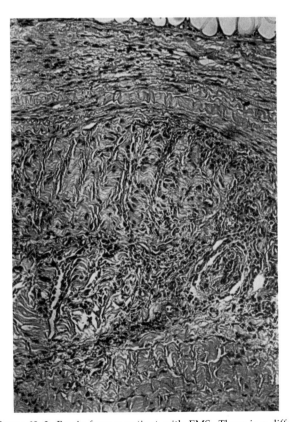

Figure 68–3. Fascia from a patient with EMS. There is a diffuse and perivascular mononuclear cell infiltrate with scattered eosinophils.

1990, almost no further new cases of L-tryptophan–associated eosinophilic fasciitis have been diagnosed; however, at the University of Pennsylvania, two patients with a recent onset of eosinophilic fasciitis were seen with no history of L-tryptophan consumption. One presented after unusual physical exertion, a feature previously described in eosinophilic fasciitis and unusual in cases of L-tryptophan–induced eosinophilic fasciitis.

The non–L-tryptophan–associated eosinophilic fasciitis cases appear to have fewer systemic complaints and less internal organ involvement.[22] The characteristic severe myalgias and cramps of EMS are not a feature among the non–L-tryptophan eosinophilic fasciitis patients. Severe cytopenias and aplastic anemia, uncommon but potentially lethal complications of the non–L-tryptophan eosinophilic fasciitis, have been described in two L-tryptophan–associated cases (Hertzman, P.: Personal communication, 1991).

CARDIOPULMONARY FINDINGS

Complaints of a nonproductive cough and dyspnea have been common,[4] particularly in the first weeks of illness. These symptoms have been occasionally associated with transient pulmonary infiltrates similar to Löffler's syndrome. Eosinophils, neutrophils, and mast cells have been seen by biopsy or during bronchoalveolar lavage.[24, 25] One case of pulmonary vasculitis was described.[26]

Abnormal pulmonary function tests showing restrictive or obstructive patterns have been noted.[9, 15] Interpretation of these tests may be complicated by poor effort owing to pain and muscle spasm. Decreased carbon monoxide diffusing capacity was noted in more than half of patients in one series.[9] Diffuse or bibasilar interstitial infiltrates have been reported in several series.[16, 24, 25] A minority of patients tested had gallium scans demonstrating increased lung parenchymal uptake.[9, 12] Several cases of pleural effusions have been documented.[9, 15, 16, 24, 26] These were mostly bilateral, transient, and mild. In two cases,[12, 16] pleurocentesis revealed an exudative effusion with few eosinophils.

There have been at least seven reports of mostly mild pulmonary hypertension.[9, 10, 12, 21, 24] One had associated myocarditis, pericarditis, and a negative pulmonary angiogram ruling out pulmonary emboli.[12] This patient had an endomyocardial biopsy, which revealed a mononuclear cell infiltrate with myocyte necrosis. Although the heart itself appears to be relatively spared in this disease, several cases were reported with right-sided heart enlargement by chest radiograph or right-sided strain by electrocardiogram.[1, 9, 10, 12, 21, 27a]

GASTROINTESTINAL FINDINGS

There have been several reports of dysphagia and dyspepsia; however, this does not appear to be as prominent a manifestation as in patients with scleroderma. There may be abnormal peristaltic motion by upper gastrointestinal series,[9, 25] but unlike scleroderma, this is not confined to the lower esophagus. Diarrhea that may be watery or bloody has been noted infrequently.[1, 9, 10, 25] Biopsies of the small intestine in some of these cases have revealed inflammatory infiltrates with eosinophils.[1, 25]

Eosinophilic infiltrates have also been found in the stomach[1] and liver.[1, 9] Liver enzymes were elevated in 43 percent of cases, but frank liver disease has been rare.[4] One patient had an obstructive biliary lesion owing to a fibrotic mass infiltrated with eosinophils blocking the common bile duct and extending into the liver.[12]

MISCELLANEOUS FINDINGS

Hypothyroidism has been described in several patients.[9, 19] A few cases of carpal tunnel syndrome associated with EMS were reported.[9, 26] One patient each had a vaginal ulceration and an ovarian biopsy with an eosinophilic infiltrate.[1] Eosinophils were also found on biopsy of a urinary bladder.[12] Hepatomegaly, splenomegaly, and lymphadenopathy are all rare in this syndrome.

LABORATORY FINDINGS

The most characteristic laboratory abnormalities in this entity are high peripheral blood eosinophil and white blood cell counts. Eosinophil counts were as high as 36×10^9 cells per liter (mean, 6.3×10^9).[4] Eosinophilia with leukocytosis was generally manifest during the first few weeks of the syndrome or until the L-tryptophan was discontinued. Patients have been seen with many of the symptoms of EMS in whom an eosinophil count was not obtained when these symptoms began, and the follow-up count months after having discontinued L-tryptophan was normal. Eosinophilia was quite sensitive to glucocorticoids and generally did not recur after several weeks. Mild immunoglobulin E (IgE) elevations were noted in 17 percent of patients,[4] but polyclonal gammopathies were generally not seen.

Antinuclear antibodies were frequently positive.[9, 12, 16, 19] The speckled pattern, although not exclusively seen, was most common. Other autoantibodies such as anti-dsDNA, RNP, Smith, SSA, and SSB were absent, and complement values were not decreased. Two patients with positive antimitochondrial antibodies were reported.[9, 27]

In patients complaining of weakness, creatinine kinase levels were usually normal or low with elevated aldolase.[4] Erythrocyte sedimentation rates were abnormal in one third of cases[4] but were only rarely above 50 mm Hg. More than 200 patients tested negative for *Trichinella* serology,[4] and in many patients ova and parasites were excluded.

DIFFERENTIAL DIAGNOSIS

An important consideration in the differential diagnosis of EMS is the exclusion of alternative explanations for myalgias, eosinophilia, and cutaneous thickening. The full-blown triad of prior L-tryptophan consumption, elevated peripheral eosinophil counts, and severe myalgias is relatively unique. Polymyositis uncommonly causes significant myalgias, but neither polymyositis nor polymyalgia rheumatica is associated with eosinophilia. Trichinosis, which can present with myalgias, fever, weakness, periorbital edema, and eosinophilia, is rare in the United States. Serum creatinine phosphokinase levels are frequently elevated, and serologic tests are available.

Eosinophilia from allergic reactions or neoplasms is not generally associated with myalgias. Patients with Churg-Strauss syndrome and variations of polyarteritis nodosa with eosinophilia may have myalgias, but the former follows a history of asthma, and a necrotizing medium-vessel vasculitis on tissue biopsy is characteristic of these entities.

EMS patients not infrequently have thickened skin, which may be mistaken for systemic sclerosis. Raynaud's phenomenon and severe hand involvement, which are the rule in the latter disease, are usually not present in EMS. Also dysphagia with abnormal manometry of the lower two thirds of the esophagus, telangiectasias, and calcinosis are frequent findings in systemic sclerosis. Systemic sclerosis may rarely have high eosinophil counts, but this is much more common in eosinophilic fasciitis.[28]

The hypereosinophilic syndrome (HES) has been associated with fevers, pulmonary infiltrates, neuropathies, and cutaneous eruptions[29, 30]; however, these similarities are probably superficial. The pulmonary infiltrates, which are associated with a chronic cough, and the fevers in HES tend to occur at times of worsening disease rather than early in the disease course. HES patients with neurologic involvement often have diffuse central nervous system dysfunction. Maculopapular rashes rather than fasciitis are common. An eosinophilic polymyositis has rarely been described with HES.[31]

Various rare forms of eosinophilia with myositis or perimyositis have been documented.[31-34] One patient with this latter entity was later discovered to have ingested L-tryptophan.[1, 35]

PATHOGENESIS

There have been basically two nonmutually exclusive theories to explain the pathogenesis of this apparently new entity. The simplest involves a product contaminant, whereas an alternative hypothesis evokes an aberration of tryptophan metabolism in susceptible individuals. Although a contaminant has been implicated, the contribution of an aberrant metabolic pathway has not been ruled out as a pathogenic element. Only a small percentage of people who consumed L-tryptophan developed EMS, and only a few predisposing factors have been elucidated.

In a Minneapolis-based survey, the prevalence of tryptophan use among females at least 15 years of age was 8.6 per 1000 in 1988 and 19.1 per 1000 in 1989.[7] The use in 1988 was approximately three times that during the years 1980 to 1984. Also, the prevalence of L-tryptophan use in females in 1988 and 1989 was roughly four times that found in males. All the patients identified from Minneapolis had dated the onset of their symptoms between September, 1988, and November, 1989. A similar type of survey conducted in Oregon[36] demonstrated that over 92 percent of EMS patients developed their first symptoms after July 1, 1989. Only 26 cases, or less than 2 percent of the total cases reported to the CDC, have been reported to have experienced EMS symptoms before 1988.[4] Further, combining data from the Minneapolis and Oregon surveys, 74 of 76 (97 percent) EMS patients in whom it could be ascertained had consumed L-tryptophan manufactured by a single company. This was compared with 29 of 76 (38 percent) control subjects who had consumed L-tryptophan without developing EMS. The temporal clustering of cases and the implication of one specific L-tryptophan manufacturer, Showa Denko (Japan), make it highly probable that a contaminant was involved in the etiology of EMS.

Samples of L-tryptophan belonging to patients who developed EMS have been studied. One particular contaminant identified as a discrete absorbance peak, called *peak E* or *peak 97*, by high-performance liquid chromatography[7] was associated with clinical EMS cases. Spectral and chemical studies have demonstrated that the implicated peak contained 1,1'-ethylidenebis [tryptophan], a novel amino acid.[38] The chemical structure can be seen in Figure 68–4. A total of 32 other peaks of non–L-tryptophan trace chemicals were also found in contaminated lots.[7] These lots, however, contained 99.6 percent pure L-tryptophan that conformed with the standards of the United States Pharmacopeia.[7] The etiologic agent therefore appears to have had a high biologic activity. The appearance of the contaminated lots has been related to changes of the L-tryptophan manufacturing process at Showa Denko that predated the epidemic. Epidemiologically, the most important changes have been traced to the use of a smaller quantity of powdered carbon during a purification step and the introduction of a new strain of *Bacillus amyloliquefaciens*, the bacterium used in the fermentation process to manufacture L-tryptophan.[7]

Contaminated lots or purified L-tryptophan was fed in a blinded fashion to Lewis rats, a rodent known to be susceptible to various inflammatory diseases. Animals that had consumed the implicated but not the purified L-tryptophan developed histologic evidence of fasciitis and perimyositis[38] mimicking two of the more characteristic features of EMS in humans. Mononuclear cell infiltrates were found encircling blood vessels similar to the human pa-

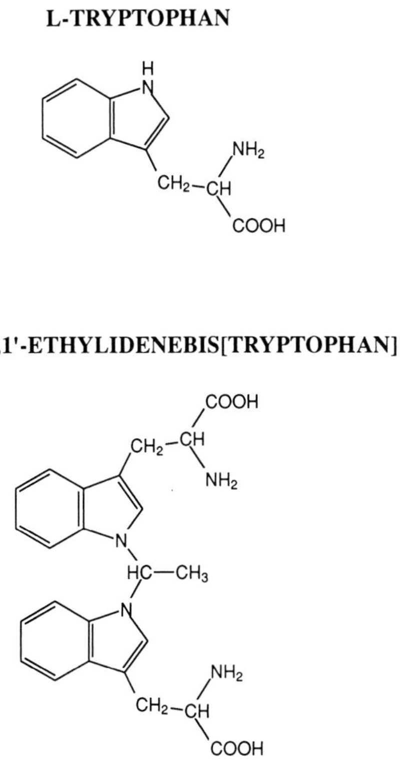

L-TRYPTOPHAN

1,1'-ETHYLIDENEBIS[TRYPTOPHAN]

Figure 68–4. Chemical structure of L-tryptophan and the implicated contaminant from "peak E" or "peak 97."

thology. Different from human EMS, however, peripheral blood and tissue eosinophilia were not observed in the diseased animals. This study raises questions about the role of eosinophils in human EMS.

Although hypereosinophilia is a part of the case definition of EMS, this tends to be transient, occurring early in the disease process. Eosinophils, although occasionally present in tissue from EMS specimens, have frequently been absent. Eosinophils may still exert an indirect adverse influence through the release of toxic cationic proteins. The eosinophil products, major basic protein and eosinophil-derived neurotoxin, were shown to be elevated in the sera and urine of EMS patients compared with control subjects.[12] Major basic protein deposits were also demonstrated by immunofluorescence in affected organs, even occasionally in the absence of cellular infiltrates, indicating that these products could have a distant effect or that the eosinophils disintegrated after degranulation.[12] These products have also been found in patients with other disorders with eosinophilia such as in allergic reactions with dissimilar manifestations to EMS.[1]

The eosinophils present in EMS patients have been found to have abnormal sedimentation properties (hypodense).[39] Further, eosinophils from normal controls when incubated with sera from EMS patients developed hypodense phenotypes.[39] This effect could be blocked by neutralizing antibodies to interleukin-5 (IL-5) but not to other eosinophilopoietic substances such as interleukin-3 (IL-3) or

granulocyte/macrophage colony-stimulating factor (GM-CSF). These hypodense eosinophils had a prolonged viability and an enhanced biologic response to ligand activation. Preliminary results suggest that IL-3, IL-5, and GM-CSF levels are not elevated in sera from EMS patients.[40]

Little is known about the phenotype of other hematopoietic cells involved in EMS. In the few cases in which peripheral blood lymphocytes have been studied, phenotype does not appear to be substantially altered.[25] Macrophages may account for up to 30 percent of mononuclear cells found in tissue infiltrates.[12] HLA typing has not yet been performed on a large sample of patients.

The function of the tryptophan metabolic pathway in the pathogenesis of EMS remains an as yet unanswered question. This pathway is shown in Figure 68–5. There are two major branches that lead toward 5-hydroxytryptamine (serotonin) and kynurenine and its by-products. Vitamin B_6 is involved in both arms of the pathway. There are several lines of data that suggest a potential role for this pathway in sclerosing diseases such as scleroderma and eosinophilic fasciitis. Patients with carcinoid syndrome in whom there is an excess of circulating serotonin may have fibrotic skin changes.[41, 42] Also, animals that have been injected subcutaneously with serotonin develop cutaneous fibrosis.[43] Finally, methysergide, a serotonin analogue, may lead to internal organ fibrosis.[44]

In 1980, Sternberg et al.[45] reported a patient that developed a syndrome that appeared to be identical to EMS with skin thickening and eosinophilia in a 70-year-old man who had been taking L-5-hydroxytryptophan and carbidopa for intention myoclonus. A high plasma kynurenine level was found, which lingered on discontinuation of these medications. Other patients without skin thickening had normal plasma levels. A skin biopsy of the patient revealed dermal perivascular infiltrates and increased collagen deposition. A full-thickness biopsy was not performed, so the presence of fasciitis cannot be determined. Because of the dermal sclerosis, however, the authors were prompted to study tryptophan metabolites in a group of scleroderma patients. It was determined that half the scleroderma patients had an elevated plasma kynurenine. A more recent study involving EMS patients found significantly higher plasma kynurenine and quinolinic acid levels in EMS patients with active disease compared with patients in whom eosinophilia had resolved and healthy control subjects.[15] It is therefore possible that the kynurenine branch of the tryptophan pathway and in particular the neurotoxic substance quinolinic acid[46] may have been involved in the pathogenesis of EMS.

A final possible clue into the pathogenesis of EMS may relate to the toxic oil syndrome (TOS), another epidemic that occurred in the early 1980s in Spain claiming almost 20,000 victims.[47] The TOS was characterized by early fever and pneumonitis followed rapidly by eosinophilia, gastrointestinal findings, and later fibrosing cutaneous lesions and severe

1156　Connective Tissue Diseases Characterized by Fibrosis • 68

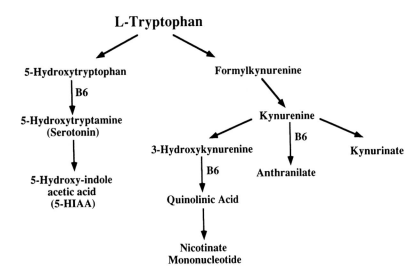

Figure 68–5. Catabolic pathways of L-tryptophan.

neuromuscular problems including incapacitating myalgias. There is a striking resemblance of TOS, which has been linked to a contaminated cooking oil, to EMS.[22] One conjecture has been that anilid impurities found in the Spanish cooking oil were responsible for the TOS,[48] although it does not appear that these products were present in L-tryptophan.

TREATMENT AND PROGNOSIS

Although it is still premature to delineate clearly the prognosis of patients with EMS, several observations may be posited. Prognosis as yet seems better for the majority of patients who have not developed severe disease and have stopped taking L-tryptophan. In these patients, pains and muscle spasms may persist and remain an annoyance for years, occasionally affecting functional abilities, but generally more serious organ involvement does not develop after the patient abstains from taking L-tryptophan for several months. In contrast, patients with extensive fasciitis, neurologic involvement, and other internal organ involvement tend to have a worse prognosis. These patients may be plagued with relentless incapacitating muscle spasms and pain. They may become and remain nonambulatory, spending the majority of their time confined to a bed owing to a combination of motor deficit and pain. To date, there have been 29 reported deaths caused by EMS, and complications associated with an ascending motor neuropathy have been shown to be a common cause of death (CDC: Personal communication, 1991). Of concern is a group of TOS patients who have had late hepatic and right-sided cardiopulmonary complications.[49, 50] Although EMS cardiopulmonary disease has also been right-sided, it is not clear whether late cases will also evolve.

The response to glucocorticoids has not been uniformly positive.[12, 16, 19] The eosinophilia responds rapidly, and most but not all patients have some improvement of myalgias, early edema, and possibly the cutaneous thickening. High doses of glucocorticoids seem to be more effective initially. Patients, however, who have not responded after 4 to 6 weeks of this treatment will probably not benefit from continued glucocorticoid therapy. Patients who remain seriously ill do not appear to benefit from long-term glucocorticoids even if there was some initial response.[51] Other treatments that have been tried anecdotally have included methotrexate, vitamin B6, cyclosporine, cyclophosphamide, and plasmapheresis.[52] Isotretinoin, which can block collagen synthesis in vitro, may be of some benefit for the cutaneous thickening and flexion contractures.[19]

The myalgias and muscle spasms have been extremely resistant to therapeutic interventions. Quinine sulfate, tricyclic antidepressants, methocarbamol, cyclobenzaprine, dantrolene, baclofen, and benzodiazepines including clonazepam may have a limited effectiveness in specific patients. Narcotics are occasionally necessary for analgesia.

References

1. Hertzman, P. A., Blevins, W. L., Mayer, J., Greenfield, B., Ting, M., and Gleich, G.: Association of the eosinophilia-myalgia syndrome with the ingestion of L-tryptophan. N. Engl. J. Med. 13:864, 1990.
2. Eosinophilia-myalgia syndrome and L-tryptophan–containing products—New Mexico, Minnesota, Oregon and New York, 1989. M. M. W. R. 38:785, 1989.
3. Eosinophilia-myalgia syndrome. New Mexico. M. M. W. R. 38:765, 1989.
4. Swygert, L. A., Maes, E. F., Sewell, L. E., Miller, L., Falk, H., and Kilbourne, E. M.: Eosinophilia-myalgia syndrome: Results of national surveillance. J.A.M.A. 264:1698, 1990.
5. Update eosinophilia-myalgia syndrome associated with ingestion of L-tryptophan—United States, through August 24, 1990. M. M. W. R. 39:587, 1990.
6. Kilbourne, E. M., Swygert, L. A., Philen, R. M., Sun, R. K., Auerbach, S. B., Miller, L., Nelson, D. E., and Falk, H.: Interim guidance on the eosinophilia-myalgia syndrome. Ann. Intern. Med. 112:85, 1990.
6a. Kamb, M. L., Murphy, J. J., Jones, J. L., Caston, J. C., Nederlof, K., Horney, L. F., Swaggert, L. A., Folk, H., and Kilbourne, E. M.: Eosinophilia-myalgia syndrome in L-tryptophan–exposed patients. J.A.M.A. 267:77, 1992.
7. Belongia, E. A., Hedberg, C. W., Gleich, G. J., White, K. E., Mayeno, A., N., Loegering, D. A., Dunette, S. L., Pirie, P. L., MacDonald, K. L., and Osterholm, M. T.: An investigation of the cause of eosinophilia-myalgia syndrome associated with tryptophan use. N. Engl. J. Med. 323:357, 1990.

8. Schneider-Helmert, D., and Spinweber, C. L.: Evaluation of L-tryptophan for treatment of insomnia: A review. Psychopharmacology 89:1, 1986.
9. Varga, J., Heimen-Patterson, T. D., Emery, D. L., Griffin, R., Lally, E. V., Uitto, J. J., and Jimenez, S. A.: Clinical spectrum of the systemic manifestations of the eosinophilia-myalgia syndrome. Semin. Arthritis Rheum. 19:313, 1990.
10. Glickstein, S. L., Gertner, E., Smith, S. A., Roelofs, R. I., Hathaway, D. E., Schlesinger, P. A., and Schned, E. S.: Eosinophilia-myalgia syndrome associated with L-tryptophan use. J. Rheumatol. 17:1534, 1990.
11. Smith, B. E., and Dyck, P. J.: Peripheral neuropathy in the eosinophilia-myalgia syndrome associated with L-tryptophan ingestion. Neurology 40:1035, 1990.
12. Martin, R. W., Duffy, J., Engel, A. G., Lie, J. T., Bowles, C. A., Moyer, T. P., and Gleich, G. J.: The clinical spectrum of the eosinophilia-myalgia syndrome associated with L-tryptophan ingestion. Ann. Intern. Med. 113:124, 1990.
13. Chartash, E. K., Given, W. P., Vishnubhakat, S. M., Susin, M., Coffey, E. J., Jr., Farmer, P. M., Albanese, J. M., Kaplan, M. H., and Furie, R. A.: L-Tryptophan–induced eosinophilia-myalgia syndrome. J. Rheumatol. 17:1527, 1990.
14. Smith, S. A., Roelofs, R. I., and Gertner, E.: Microangiopathy in the eosinophilia-myalgia syndrome. J. Rheumatol. 17:1544, 1990.
15. Silver, R. M., Heyes, M. P., Maize, J. C., Quearry, B., Voinnet-Fuasset, M., and Sternberg, E. M.: Scleroderma, fasciitis with eosinophilia associated with the ingestion of tryptophan. N. Engl. J. Med. 322:874, 1990.
16. Kaufman, L. D., Seidman, R. J., and Gruber, B. L.: L-Tryptophan–associated eosinophilia perimyositis, neuritis and fasciitis. Medicine 69:187, 1990.
17. Heiman-Patterson, T. D., Bird, S. J., Parry, G. J., Varga, J., Shy, M. E., Culligan, N. W., Edelsohn, L., Tatarisin, G. T., Heyes, M. P., Garcia, C. A., and Tahmoush, A. J.: Peripheral neuropathy associated with eosinophilia-myalgia syndrome. Ann. Neurol. 28:522, 1990.
18. Clauw, D. J., Nashel, D. J., Umhau, A., and Katz, P.: Tryptophan-associated eosinophilia connective tissue disease. A new clinical entity? J.A.M.A. 263:1502, 1990.
19. Freundlich, B., Werth, V. P., Rook, A. H., O'Connor, C. R., Schumacher, H. R., Leyden, J. J., and Stolley, P. D.: L-Tryptophan ingestion associated with eosinophilic fasciitis but not progressive systemic sclerosis. Ann. Intern. Med. 112:758, 1990.
20. Jaffe, I., Kopelman, R., Baird, R., Grossman, M., and Hays, A.: Eosinophilic fasciitis associated with the eosinophilic-myalgia syndrome. Am. J. Med. 68:542, 1990.
21. Medsger, T. A.: Tryptophan-induced eosinophilia-myalgia syndrome. N. Engl. J. Med. 322:926, 1990.
22. Shulman, L. E.: The eosinophilia-myalgia syndrome associated with ingestion of L-tryptophan. Arthritis Rheum. 33:913, 1990.
23. Varga, J., Petonen, J., Uitto, J., and Jimenez, S. A.: Development of diffuse fasciitis with eosinophilia during L-tryptophan treatment: Demonstration of elevated type I collagen gene expression in affected tissues. Ann. Intern. Med. 112:344, 1990.
24. Tazelaar, H. D., Meges, J. L., Drage, C. W., King, T. F., Aguayo, S., and Colby, T. V.: Pulmonary disease associated with L-tryptophan–induced eosinophilia-myalgia syndrome. Chest 97:1232, 1990.
25. Strongwater, S. L., Woda, B. A., Hood, R. A., Rybak, E., Sargent, J., DeGirolami, U., Smith, T. W., Varnis, C., Allen, S., Murphy, K., Malhotra, R., and Romain, P. L.: Eosinophilia-myalgia syndrome associated with L-tryptophan ingestion. Arch. Intern. Med. 150:2178, 1990.
26. Travis, W. D., Kalafer, M. E., Robin, H. S., and Luibel, F. J.: Hypersensitivity pneumonitis and pulmonary vasculitis with eosinophilia in a patient taking an L-tryptophan preparation. Ann. Intern. Med. 112:301, 1990.
26a. Bulpitt, K. J., Verity, M. A., Clements, P. J., and Paulus, H. E.: Association of L-tryptophan and an illness resembling eosinophilic fasciitis. Arthritis Rheum. 33:918, 1990.
27. Roubenoff, R., Cote, T., Watson, R., Levin, M. L., and Hochberg, M. C.: Eosinophilia-myalgia syndrome due to L-tryptophan ingestion. Arthritis Rheum. 33:930, 1990.
27a. James, T. N., Kamb, M. L., Sandberg, G. A., Silver, R. M., and Kilbourne, E. M.: Postmortem studies of the heart in three fatal cases of the eosinophilia-myalgia syndrome. Ann. Intern. Med. 115:102, 1991.
28. Falanga, V., and Medsger, T. A.: Frequency, levels and significance of

29. Chusid, M. J., Dale, D. C., West, B. C., and Wolff, S. M.: The hypereosinophilia syndrome. Medicine 85:1, 1975.
30. Fauci, A. S., Harley, J. B., Roberts, W. C., Ferrons, V. J., Gralnick, H. R., and Björnson, B. H.: The idiopathic hypereosinophilia syndrome. Ann. Intern. Med. 97:78, 1982.
31. Layzer, R. B., Shearn, M. A., and Satya-Murti, S.: Eosinophilia polymyositis. Ann. Neurol. 1:65, 1977.
32. Sladek, G. D., Vasey, F. B., Sieger, B., Behnke, D. A., Germain, B. F., and Espinoza, L. R.: Relapsing eosinophilic myositis. J. Rheumatol. 10:467, 1983.
33. Symmons, W. A., Beresford, C. H., and Burton, D.: Cyclic eosinophilic myositis and hyperimmunoglobulin-E. Ann. Intern. Med. 104:26, 1986.
34. Serratrice, G., Pellissier, J. F., Cros, D., Gastaut, J. L., and Brindisi, G.: Relapsing eosinophilic perimyositis. J. Rheumatol. 7:199, 1980.
35. Lakhanpal, S., Duffy, J., and Engel, A. G.: Eosinophilia associated with perimyositis and pneumonitis. Mayo Clin. Proc. 63:37, 1988.
36. Slutsker, L., Hoesly, F. C., Miller, L., Williams, P., Watson, J. C., and Fleming, D. W.: Eosinophilia-myalgia syndrome associated with exposure to tryptophan from a single manufacturer. J.A.M.A. 264:213, 1990.
37. Mayeno, A. N., Lin, F., Foote, C. S., Loegering, D. A., Ames, M. M., Craig, W. H., and Gleich, G. J.: Characterization of "Peak E," a novel amino acid associated with eosinophilia-myalgia syndrome. Science 250:1707, 1990.
38. Crofford, L. J., Rader, J. I., Dalakas, M. C., Hill, R. H., Page, S. W., Needham, L. L., Brady, L. S., Heyes, M. P., Wilder, R. L., Gold, P. W., Illa, I., Smith, C., and Sternberg, E.: L-Tryptophan implicated in human eosinophilia-myalgia syndrome causes fasciitis and perimyositis in the Lewis rat. J. Clin. Invest. 86:1757, 1990.
39. Owen, W. F., Jr., Petersen, J., Sheff, D. M., Folkerth, R. D., Anderson, R. J., Corson, J. M., Sheffer, A. L., and Austen, K. F.: Hypodense eosinophils and interleukin-5 activity in the blood of patients with the eosinophilia-myalgia syndrome. Proc. Natl. Acad. Sci. 87:8647, 1990.
40. Bowles, C., Duffy, J., Martin, R., Engel, A., Lie, J., Abrams, A., and Gleich, G.: Eosinophilia-myalgia syndrome associated with L-tryptophan ingestion. Arthritis Rheum. 33:S18, 1990.
41. Zarafonetis, D. L., Lorber, S. H., and Hanson, S. M.: Association of functioning carcinoid syndrome and scleroderma. Am. J. Med. Sci. 236:1, 1958.
42. Fries, J. F., Lindgren, J. A., and Bull, J. M.: Scleroderma-like lesions and the carcinoid syndrome. Arch. Intern. Med. 131:550, 1973.
43. Macdonald, R. A., Robbins, S. L., and Mallory, G. K.: Dermal fibrosis following subcutaneous injection of serotonin creatinine sulphate. Proc. Soc. Exp. Biol. Med. 97:334, 1958.
44. Graham, J. R.: Cardiac and pulmonary fibrosis during methysergide therapy for headache. Am. J. Med. Sci. 254:1, 1967.
45. Sternberg, E. M., Van Woert, M. H., Young, S. N., Magnussen, J., Baker, Q., Gauthier, S., and Osterland, C. K.: Development of a scleroderma-like illness during therapy with L-5-hydroxytryptophan and carbidopa. N. Engl. J. Med. 303:782, 1980.
46. Houpt, J. B.: Tryptophan. New questions for an old amino acid. J. Rheumatol. 17:1431, 1990.
47. Kilbourne, E. M., Rigau-Perez, J. G., Heath, C. W., Jr., Zack, M. M., Falk, H., Martin-Marcos, M., and DeCarlos, A.: Clinical epidemiology of toxic oil syndrome: manifestations of a new illness. N. Engl. J. Med. 309:1408, 1983.
48. Kilbourne, E. M., Bernert, J. T., Jr., Posada, de la Paz, M., Hill, R. H., Jr., Borda, I. A., Kilbourne, B. W., Zack, M. M., and the Toxico-Epidemiologic Study Group: Chemical correlates of pathogenicity of oils related to the toxic oil syndrome in Spain. Am. J. Epidemiol. 127:1210, 1988.
49. Solis-Herruzo, J. A., Vidal, J. V., Colina, F., Castellano, G., Munoz-Yague, M. T., and Morillas, J. D.: Clinico-biochemical evolution and late hepatic lesions in the toxic oil syndrome. Gastroenterology 93:558, 1987.
50. Gomez-Sanchez, M. A., Mestre de Juan, M. J., Gomez-Pajuelo, C., Lopez, J. I., Diaz de Atauri, M. J., and Martinez-Tello, F. J.: Pulmonary hypertension due to toxic oil syndrome. Chest 95:325, 1989.
51. Culpepper, R. C., Williams, R. G., Mease, P. J., Koepsell, T. D., and Kobayashi, J. M.: The natural history of the eosinophilia-myalgia syndrome. Ann. Intern. Med. 115:437, 1991.
52. Martinez-Osuna, P., Wallach, P. M., Seleznick, M. J., Levin, R. W., Silveira, L. H., Jara, L. J., and Espinoza, L. R.: Treatment of the eosinophilia-myalgia syndrome. Semin. Arthritis Rheum. 21:110, 1991.

Section XI
Inflammatory Diseases of Muscle

Chapter 69

Robert L. Wortmann

Inflammatory Diseases of Muscle

INTRODUCTION

The inflammatory diseases of muscle are a heterogeneous group of conditions characterized by proximal muscle weakness and nonsuppurative inflammation of skeletal muscle. Traditionally, the terms polymyositis and polymyositis-dermatomyositis syndrome (or complex) have been used to represent a variety of diagnoses including adult and childhood forms of polymyositis and dermatomyositis, myositis associated with other defined collagen vascular diseases, myositis associated with malignancy, inclusion body myositis, and other rare conditions. These groupings reflect a lack of understanding of the precise nature and causes of these diseases. Because of this limited understanding, it is perhaps more appropriate to use the term *idiopathic inflammatory myopathy* to represent the entire group and reserve the terms *polymyositis* and *dermatomyositis* for more specific conditions or subsets of patients. This allows differentiation from the inflammatory myopathies related to known infectious or toxic causes (Table 69–1).

STRUCTURE AND FUNCTION OF SKELETAL MUSCLE

To understand the changes that occur in inflammatory diseases of muscle or other myopathic conditions, it is useful to understand the normal anatomy, physiology, and biochemistry of this tissue. Skeletal muscle is composed of motor units that consist of a lower motor neuron, which originates in a spinal cord anterior horn cell; a neuromuscular junction; and the muscle cells or fibers innervated by the motor neuron. Muscle fibers are anatomically grouped in fascicles, with different fibers within a fascicle innervated by different motor neurons. Muscle fibers contain contractile proteins termed myofilaments (Fig. 69–1). The structural anatomy of muscle and biochemical events during contraction are described in Chapter 5.

Contraction and relaxation are active processes and require the activities of three adenosine triphosphatase (ATPase) proteins: a sodium-potassium ATPase, which maintains normal membrane polarity; a magnesium-dependent ATPase, which provides for actin myosin cross-linking; and a calcium-dependent ATPase, which pumps calcium from the sarcoplasm into the sarcoplasmic reticulum. Consequently, normal muscle function requires adequate levels of the various electrolytes and ATP.

Normally, skeletal muscle uses fatty acids and carbohydrates as substrates to provide ATP. Each substrate is processed by different pathways, with the importance of a particular pathway varying with the activity state and nutritional status of the individual. These pathways work in concert to maintain intracellular ATP concentrations at constant levels

Table 69–1. CLASSIFICATION OF INFLAMMATORY DISEASES OF MUSCLE

I. Idiopathic Inflammatory Myopathies
   Polymyositis
   Dermatomyositis
   Juvenile (childhood) dermatomyositis
   Myositis associated with collagen vascular disease
   Myositis associated with malignancy
   Inclusion body myositis
   Myositis associated with eosinophilia
   Myositis ossificans
   Localized or focal myositis
   Giant cell myositis
II. Myopathies Caused by Infection
III. Myopathies Caused by Drugs and Toxins

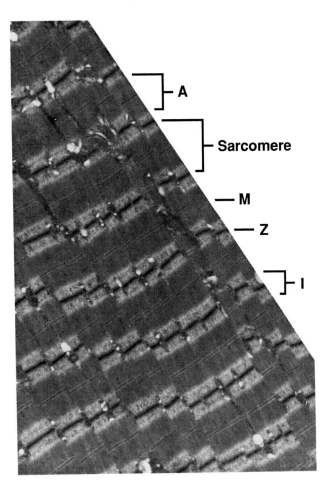

Figure 69–1. Ultrastructure of skeletal muscle seen by electron microscopy. The zones of lines and bands and cross-striated appearance of skeletal muscle are the result of the organization and varying refractile indices of myofilaments. The functional contractile unit of a muscle fiber is called the sarcomere and is defined as the area between two Z lines. The M line, the midpoint of the sarcomere, is produced by bulges in the thick filaments (myosin). A bands are composed of the thick filaments. The I bands are the areas occupied by the thin filaments (troponin, tropomyosin, and actin), not overlapped by thick filaments. With contraction the I bands shorten as the Z lines move toward the M lines.

under most conditions and to restore them to those levels if vigorous activity or hypoxia has caused ATP concentrations to fall.

Creatine phosphokinase (CK) activity plays a pivotal role in maintaining intracellular ATP concentrations. CK catalyzes the reversible transphosphorylation of creatine and adenine nucleotides and functions to buffer changes in cytosolic ATP concentration (Fig. 69–2). At rest, creatine phosphate acts as a reservoir of high-energy phosphates. With muscle

activity and ATP degradation, CK catalyzes the transfer of those phosphates to rapidly restore ATP levels to normal. The enzyme, along with its products, creatine and creatine phosphate, also serves as a shuttle mechanism for energy transport between mitochondria (where ATP is generated by oxidative metabolism) and the myofibrils (where ATP is consumed in the processes of muscle contraction and relaxation).[1]

Free fatty acids provide the major source of ATP

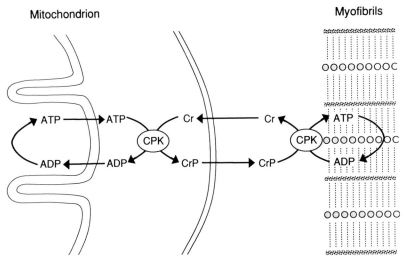

Figure 69–2. Skeletal muscle cells (muscle fibers) maintain constant levels of ATP despite large variations in production and degradation through the activity of CK. At rest, when ATP is generated in excess of demand, high-energy phosphate is transferred to creatine, forming creatine phosphate. When energy is consumed, the reaction runs in reverse, rapidly restoring ATP levels to normal. The enzyme also acts to shuttle adenine nucleotides between the mitochondria and the cytosol. CK = creatine phosphokinase; ATP = adenosine triphosphate; ADP = adenine diphosphate; Cr = creatine; Cr-P = creatine phosphate.

during fasting intervals, at rest, and with muscular activities of low intensity and long duration. To be processed for energy, the free fatty acid must enter the mitochondria, where large quantities of ATP are generated by oxidative metabolism (Fig. 69–3). To enter mitochondria, long-chain fatty acids must be combined with the carrier molecule carnitine. The combination of the long-chain fatty acid to carnitine and its release into the mitochondrial matrix are catalyzed by two enzymes found in the mitochondrial inner membrane, carnitine palmitoyltransferase (CPT) I and CPT II, respectively. Once in the mitochondria, two carbon fragments of acetylcoenzyme A (acetylCoA) are split off by the process of beta (β)-oxidation and metabolized sequentially by the tricar-

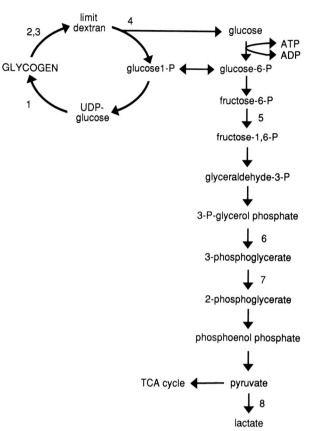

Figure 69–4. Pathway of glycogen synthesis and breakdown (glycogenolysis) and glycolysis. Under aerobic conditions, glucose is metabolized to pyruvate, which enters the tricarboxylic acid (TCA) cycle. This metabolic route generates 38 molecules of ATP per molecule of glucose. Under anaerobic conditions, pyruvate is converted to lactate, netting 2 molecules of ATP per molecule of glucose. Nine inborn errors of glycogen biochemistry that affect skeletal muscle function have been described. These include deficiencies of (1) brancher enzyme, (2) phosphorylase b kinase, (3) myophosphorylase, (4) debrancher enzyme, (5) phosphofructokinase, (6) phosphoglycerate kinase, (7) phosphoglycerate mutase, (8) lactate dehydrogenase, and acid maltase (not shown). Acid maltase catalyzes the release of glucose from maltase, oligosaccharides, and glycogen in lysosomes. Its role in cytosolic metabolism is unknown.

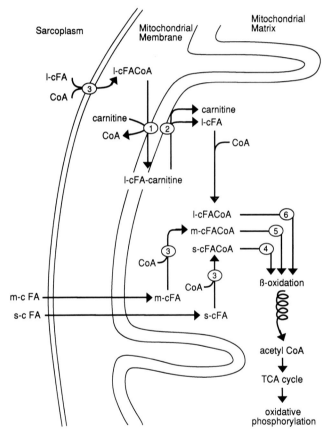

Figure 69–3. Free fatty acids must enter mitochondria to be metabolized for energy. Long-chain fatty acids, such as palmitate, combine with the carrier-molecule carnitine for transport across the mitochondrial inner membrane. The binding and release from carnitine are catalyzed by two enzymes located in the inner mitochondrial membrane, carnitine palmitoyltransferase (CPT) I and CPT II. Short- and medium-chain fatty acids enter mitochondria without a carrier. Once inside a mitochondrion, fatty acids are converted to their respective CoA esters and sequentially shortened by the process of β-oxidation, releasing acetylCoA. The initial step of β-oxidation is catalyzed by a flavin-containing acylCoA-dehydrogenase specific for fatty acid CoA esters of specific lengths. l-cFA = long-chain fatty acid (more than 12 carbons); m-cFA = medium-chain fatty acid (6 to 12 carbons); s-cFA = short-chain fatty acid (4 to 6 carbons); 1 = CPT I; 2 = CPT II; 3 = acylCoA synthetase; 4 = short-chain acylCoA dehydrogenase; 5 = medium-chain acylCoA dehydrogenase; 6 = long-chain acylCoA dehydrogenase.

boxylic acid cycle and oxidative phosphorylation. By this metabolic route, one molecule of palmitate results in the net gain of 131 molecules of ATP.

Glycogen, the major storage form of carbohydrate in the body, is the primary source of ATP generation when physical activity is intense or when anaerobic conditions exist.[2] Under such conditions, glycogen is mobilized to form glucose-6-phosphate by the process of glycogenolysis (Fig. 69–4). The process is initiated by the activity of myophosphorylase. Glucose-6-phosphate is metabolized through the glycolytic pathway. Under aerobic conditions, this pathway produces pyruvate, which can enter the tricarboxylic acid cycle. Under anaerobic conditions, pyruvate is converted to lactate. The aerobic metabolism of one molecule of glucose nets 38 molecules of ATP, whereas the anaerobic processing results in the generation of only two molecules of ATP.

The purine nucleotide cycle is another important regulatory pathway used to maintain adequate ATP levels[3] (Fig. 69–5). This cycle comes into play when ATP concentrations fall. Generally under those conditions, glycolysis becomes the major route for ATP regeneration.[4] The first step of the purine nucleotide cycle is catalyzed by myoadenylate deaminase activity, which converts adenosine-5'-monophosphate (AMP) to inosine-5'-monophosphate (IMP) with the release of ammonia. Both IMP and ammonia stimulate glycolytic activity. As ATP concentrations fall, IMP concentrations rise stoichiometrically until muscle activity decreases and recovery can occur. During recovery, oxidative pathways function and AMP is regenerated from IMP by a two-step process with the liberation of fumarate. Fumarate is converted to malate, which enters mitochondria and participates as an intermediate in the tricarboxylic acid cycle. The higher concentrations of malate thus act to "drive" the cycle, causing efficient regeneration of ATP by oxidative phosphorylation.[5]

Muscle fibers are heterogenous with respect to how they metabolize ATP and respond to stimuli. A variety of fiber-type classifications have emerged, based on different biochemical and physiologic properties.[6–8] For most purposes, fibers are divided among three types (Table 69–2). Type 1 fibers, also called slow-twitch oxidative (SO) fibers, respond to electrical stimulation more slowly with a moderate contractile intensity and are fatigue resistant with repeated stimulation. Lipid content, myoglobin concentrations, and oxidative enzyme activities are higher. In contrast, type 2b fibers, known as fast-twitch glycolytic (FG) fibers, respond more rapidly with greater force of contraction but fatigue rapidly. Glycogen content and the activities of glycolytic enzymes and myoadenylate deaminase are higher in these fibers. Type 2a fibers, termed fast-twitch oxidative glycolytic (FOG), have properties that range in between those of the other two. A type 2c fiber is included in some classification schemes. These fibers are believed to

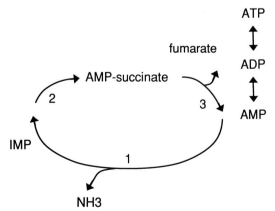

Figure 69–5. The purine nucleotide cycle is composed of a sequence of reactions that has a significant role in skeletal muscle metabolism when ATP levels decrease. It is composed of the activities of (1) myoadenylate deaminase, (2) AMP-succinate synthetase, and (3) AMP-succinate lyase.

Table 69–2. CHARACTERISTICS OF SKELETAL MUSCLE FIBER TYPES

	Fiber Type Nomenclature		
	1 SO RED	*2a* FOG RED	*2b* FG WHITE
Physiologic			
Twitch speed	Slow	Fast	Fast
Susceptibility to fatigue	Resistant	Resistant	Susceptible
Histochemical			
ATPase, pH 9.4	1+	3+	3+
ATPase, pH 4.6	3+	0	3+
ATPase, pH 4.4	3+	0	0
NADH-tetrazolium reductase	3+	2+	1+
Succinic dehydrogenase	3+	2+	1+
Myophosphorylase	1+	3+	3+
Myoadenylate deaminase	1+	2+	3+
PAS (glycogen)	1+	3+	2+
Oil red O (lipid)	3+	2+	1+

FG, fast-twitch glycolytic; FOG, fast-twitch oxidative glycolytic; SO, slow-twitch oxidative.

represent undifferentiated cells. The individual fiber characteristics are originally determined during development and are maintained through interaction with the motor neuron through which the fiber is innervated. Fiber type specificity and distribution can be altered by reinnervation with a different type of motor neuron, physical training, or disease processes.[9, 10]

CLASSIFICATIONS OF INFLAMMATORY DISEASES OF MUSCLE

Although polymyositis and dermatomyositis were recognized as clinical entities over 100 years ago, it was not until 1975 that generally accepted criteria for the diagnosis of these conditions were proposed by Bohan and Peter (Table 69–3).[11] Their work allowed, for the first time, a more systematic approach to the study of the inflammatory myopathies. In general, according to these criteria, patients with polymyositis manifest (1) proximal muscle weakness, (2) elevated serum levels of enzymes derived from skeletal muscle, (3) myopathic changes demonstrated by electromyography, and (4) muscle biopsy evidence of inflammation. The addition of a skin rash (criterion 5) affords the diagnosis of dermatomyositis. Patients are assigned to other categories, based on their age and the coexistence of another disease. Bohan and Peter divided the idiopathic inflammatory myopathies among five groups: (1) primary idiopathic polymyositis; (2) primary idiopathic dermatomyositis; (3) dermatomyositis or polymyositis associated with neoplasia; (4) childhood dermatomyositis (or polymyositis) associated with vasculitis; and (5) polymyositis or dermatomyositis with associated collagen vascular disease. Subsequently additional classification schemes have been proposed by Walton and Adams,[12] the Research

Table 69–3. CRITERIA TO DEFINE POLYMYOSITIS-DERMATOMYOSITIS PROPOSED BY BOHAN AND PETER

1. Symmetric weakness of limb-girdle muscles and anterior neck flexors, progressing over weeks to months, with or without dysphagia or respiratory muscle involvement.
2. Skeletal muscle histology showing evidence of necrosis of type 1 and 2 muscle fibers, phagocytosis, regeneration with basophilia, large sarcolemmal nuclei and prominent nucleoli, atrophy in a perifascicular distribution, variation in fiber size, and an inflammatory exudate.
3. Elevation of serum skeletal muscle enzymes (CK, aldolase, SGOT, SGPT, and LDH).
4. Electromyographic triad of short, small, polyphasic motor units; fibrillations, positive waves, and insertional irritability; and bizarre high-frequency discharges.
5. Dermatologic features including a lilac (heliotrope) discoloration of the eyelids with periorbital edema; a scaly, erythematous dermatitis over the dorsa of the hands, especially over the metacarpophalangeal and proximal interphalangeal joints (Gottron's sign), and involvement of the knees, elbows, medial malleoli, face, neck, and upper torso.

LDH, lactate dehydrogenase; SGOT, serum glutamic-oxaloacetic transaminase; SGPT, serum glutamic-pyruvic transaminase.
From Bohan, A., and Peter, J. B.: Polymyositis and dermatomyositis (first of two parts). N. Engl. J. Med. 292:344, 1975. Reprinted by permission of The New England Journal of Medicine.

Group on Neuromuscular Diseases of the World Federation of Neurology,[13] DeVere and Bradley,[14] and Banker and Engel.[15] However, none of these have been universally accepted. Most studies have continued to use the criteria and classification scheme proposed by Bohan and Peter for defining patients to be included. Recently, the group of inclusion body myositis (IBM) emerged from studies of patients who fulfilled criteria for polymyositis but were generally resistant to therapy. Criteria for the diagnosis of inclusion body myositis have been proposed and employed for investigation of this diagnostic group (Table 69–4).[16] The application of criteria for the diagnosis of polymyositis, dermatomyositis, and inclusion body myositis has proved quite useful, but these criteria have not been validated in a fashion similar to those proposed by the American College of Rheumatology for the diagnosis of rheumatoid arthritis or systemic lupus erythematosus.

EPIDEMIOLOGY

The idiopathic inflammatory myopathies are relatively rare diseases. Accurate estimates of their occurrence are difficult to obtain because the diseases are uncommon and lack universally accepted specific diagnostic criteria. Furthermore, these conditions are treated by physicians in several different specialties and may be managed on an outpatient basis. Estimates of incidence range from 0.5 to 8.4 cases per million.[17, 18] The incidence appears to be increasing, although this may simply reflect increased awareness and more accurate diagnosis.

Racial differences are apparent. In adults the lowest rates are reported in the Japanese, and the highest in blacks in the United States. The incidence for childhood dermatomyositis is significantly higher for Asians and Africans than for Europeans and Americans, and the incidence among blacks in the United States is twice that among whites.[19] Overall, the age at onset for the idiopathic inflammatory myopathies has a bimodal distribution, with peaks between ages 10 and 15 years in children and between 45 and 54 years in adults. However, the mean ages for specific groups differ. The age at onset for myositis associated with another collagen vascular disease is similar to that for the associated condition. Both myositis associated with malignancy and inclusion body myositis are more common after age 50. Women are affected more frequently than men by a two-to-one ratio, with the exception of inclusion body myositis, in which the ratio is reversed. Female predominance is especially great between ages 15 and 44, in myositis associated with other collagen vascular diseases and in blacks.

GENETIC MARKERS

Familial cases of idiopathic inflammatory myopathies are reported in monozygotic twins, siblings, parent-child pairs, and first-degree relatives of patients. These familial occurrences indicate an immunogenetic relationship in some cases. Although no direct relationships have been established between an inflammatory myopathy and a specific genetic marker, several observations support the premise that different pathogenetic mechanisms are involved in different diagnostic groups. The strongest associations exist for HLA-B8 and HLA-DR3 phenotypes

Table 69–4. DIAGNOSTIC CRITERIA PROPOSED FOR INCLUSION BODY MYOSITIS (IBM)

Pathologic Criteria
Electron Microscopy
1. Microtubular filaments in the inclusions
Light Microscopy
1. Lined vacuoles
2. Intranuclear and/or intracytoplasmic inclusions
Clinical Criteria
1. Proximal muscle weakness (insidious onset)
2. Distal muscle weakness
3. Electromyographic evidence of a generalized myopathy (inflammatory myopathy)
4. Elevation of muscle enzyme levels (creatine phosphokinase and/or aldolase)
5. Failure of muscle weakness to improve on a high-dose corticosteroid regimen (at least 40–60 mg/day for 3–4 months)

Definite IBM = pathologic electron microscopy criterion 1 and clinical criterion 1 plus one other clinical criterion. Probable IBM = pathologic light microscopy criterion 1 and clinical criterion 1 plus 3 other clinical criteria. Possible IBM = pathologic light microscopy criterion 2 plus any 3 clinical criteria.
From Calabrese, L. H., Mitsumoto, H., and Chous, S. M.: Inclusion body myositis presenting as treatment-resistant polymyositis. Arthritis Rheum. 30:397, 1987; used by permission.

in both children and adults with polymyositis and dermatomyositis.[19, 20] In one study, white patients had a 48 percent prevalence of HLA-DR3 with a 96 percent linkage to B8, whereas black patients had no increase in HLA-DR3 but a 50 percent linkage to B8. The frequency of HLA-B8 and HLA-DR3 is especially high in the subset of white patients with anti-Jo-1 antibodies.[21] All patients with anti-Jo-1 antibodies carry HLA-DRw52. Others have shown a greater frequency of HLA-B14 in whites and HLA-B7 and HLA-DRw6 in blacks with polymyositis, but not with dermatomyositis. Inclusion body myositis is more likely associated with the HLA-DR1 as well as DR3 phenotype.[22]

CLINICAL FEATURES

The dominant clinical feature of the idiopathic inflammatory myopathies is symmetric proximal muscle weakness.[14, 22–24] Although strength may be essentially normal at the time of presentation, virtually all patients will develop significant muscle weakness during the course of their illness. The weakness can be accompanied by myalgias, tenderness, and, eventually, atrophy and fibrosis. Laboratory investigation reveals elevated serum enzyme levels of skeletal muscle origin, electromyography demonstrates changes consistent with inflammation, and histology of skeletal muscle shows changes characteristic of inflammation. These manifestations can occur in a variety of combinations or patterns. No single feature is specific or diagnostic. Thus, the presence of any one feature should suggest the diagnosis of inflammatory myopathy, but the diagnosis is made by ruling out other causes for the abnormalities observed.

Polymyositis in the Adult

Typically adult-onset polymyositis begins insidiously over 3 to 6 months with no identifiable precipitating event. Only very rarely is the onset abrupt and associated with clinically evident rhabdomyolysis and myoglobinuria.[25] The weakness initially affects the muscles of the shoulder and pelvic girdles, with the latter slightly more common. Distal weakness is uncommon initially but can develop over time in severe cases. Weakness of neck muscles, particularly the flexors, occurs in about half the patients. Ocular muscles are virtually never involved. Facial and bulbar muscle weakness is rare, but dysphagia may develop secondary to esophageal dysfunction or cricopharyngeal obstruction. Pharyngeal muscle weakness may cause dysphonia and difficulty in swallowing. In severe cases, attempts to swallow fluids may result in liquid coming out the nose or in aspiration.

Polymyositis is a systemic disease and patients may develop morning stiffness, fatigue, anorexia, weight loss, and fever. Arthralgias are not uncommon, but frank synovitis is less usual. Raynaud's phenomenon is sometimes present. Muscle pain and tenderness are present in about half of patients. Periorbital edema may occur. The neurologic portion of the physical examination is normal except for motor function.

Pulmonary manifestations may occur at any time during the course of the disease.[26] "Velcro"-like crackles may be heard on chest auscultation, and changes indicative of interstitial fibrosis may be seen on chest radiograph. Interstitial pneumonitis may cause dyspnea, a nonproductive cough, and hypoxemia. Aspiration pneumonia may complicate the disease course in patients with esophageal dysmotility, swallowing difficulties, or dysphonia. Cardiac involvement is usually absent or is restricted to electrocardiographic abnormalities. However, heart block, supraventricular arrhythmia, or cardiomyopathy may develop, causing syncope, palpitations, or congestive heart failure.[27]

The CK level is elevated in almost every patient with polymyositis at some time during the course of the disease. Normal levels of CK may be found in patients who present very early in the course of their disease, in advanced cases with significant muscle atrophy late in the course, or as a result of circulating inhibitors of CK activity that may be present during active disease and can lower serum levels to within the normal range.[28] However, in most patients, elevation of the serum CK level is a helpful indicator of the severity of muscle damage. Although the range of CK elevations observed is great, levels peak at ten times normal in the average case. Levels of other muscle enzymes (aldolase, serum glutamic-oxaloacetic transaminase [SGOT], serum glutamic-pyruvic transaminase [SGPT], and lactate dehydrogenase [LDH]) are also found to be elevated in most cases, if the appropriate enzymes are measured repeatedly throughout the course of the disease. The erythrocyte sedimentation rate is normal in half the patients with polymyositis but is elevated above 50 mm per hour (Westergren's method) in only 20 percent of patients.

Electromyographic evaluation of patients with polymyositis classically reveals the triad of (1) increased insertional activity, fibrillations, and sharp positive waves; (2) spontaneous, bizarre high-frequency discharges; and (3) polyphasic motor unit potentials of low amplitude and short duration. In larger series, the complete triad is found in approximately 40 percent of patients. In contrast, 10 percent of patients may have completely normal studies.[23] Electromyographic abnormalities are limited to the paraspinal muscles in a small number of patients, even in the presence of widespread weakness.[29]

Although the histopathology of polymyositis is well described, no specific change is pathognomonic.[12, 30, 31] Wide variations in pathologic change can be observed within the tissue of an individual patient as well as from individual to individual (Fig. 69–6). In the typical case, muscle fibers are found to be in varying stages of necrosis and regeneration. The inflammatory cell infiltrate is predominantly fo-

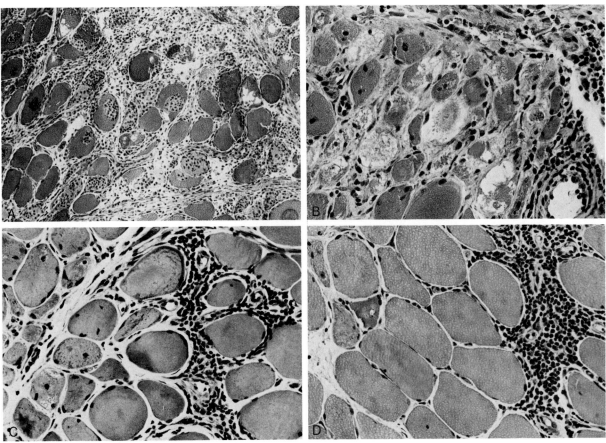

Figure 69–6. Pathologic changes in idiopathic inflammatory myopathies. Classic changes in polymyositis show fiber necrosis and regeneration with endomysial mononuclear cell infiltration. Typical infiltrates in dermatomyositis are perimysial. It is not uncommon to find elements of each on an individual biopsy. *A,* Extensive endomysial infiltration of inflammatory cells, with fiber invasion and necrosis. *B,* Necrotic fibers, regenerating fibers, and perivascular mononuclear cell infiltration. *C,* Variation in fiber size with endomysial infiltration. *D,* Primarily perimysial inflammatory infiltrate. (Courtesy of A. R. Sulaiman.)

cal and endomysial, although perivascular accumulations may also occur. In some cases, T lymphocytes, especially T8+ cytotoxic cells, accompanied by a smaller number of macrophages are found surrounding and invading initially non-necrotic fibers.[32] In other cases, degeneration is seen in the absence of inflammatory cells in the immediate area. Using hematoxylin and eosin staining, regenerating cells are identified by basophilic staining, large centrally located nuclei, and prominent nucleoli. Intact fibers may vary in size. Destroyed fibers are replaced by fibrous connective tissue and fat. However, in some cases, no fiber necrosis is observed, and the only recognized change is type 2 fiber atrophy (Fig. 69–7).

Dermatomyositis in the Adult

The clinical features of dermatomyositis include all those described for polymyositis plus cutaneous manifestations. Rash is often the presenting complaint and may antedate the onset of myopathic symptoms by more than a year. The skin involvement varies widely from patient to patient. In some, the severity of the rash and muscle weakness coincide. In other patients, the activity of the skin disease and muscle weakness have no relationship. The rash may change from one type to another during the course of the disease.

A variety of skin changes can be observed. More characteristic cutaneous changes include heliotrope (lilac) discoloration of the eyelids; erythematous rash over the face, neck, and upper torso; and Gottron's sign, pink to violaceous scaling areas typically found over the knuckles, elbows, and knees. Periungual erythema is common. Linear erythematous discolorations may develop around nailbeds. These subsequently can develop scaling, become pigmented or depigmented, and eventually result in areas of brawny induration. Darkened, or dirty-appearing, horizontal lines may be noted across the lateral and palmar aspects of the fingers. These changes are termed "machinist hands" because of the similarity to changes often noted in people who do manual labor.[33] Raynaud's phenomenon is more common in dermatomyositis and is often associated with nailfold capillary changes similar to those observed in patients with scleroderma or lupus erythematosus and Raynaud's phenomenon.[34] Cutaneous vasculitis may occur, with livedo reticularis, digital infarcts, or palpable, white-centered petechiae.

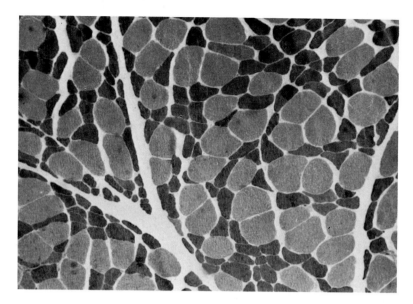

Figure 69–7. Histochemical staining of muscle for ATPase activity, pH 9.4 allows differentiation between type 2 fibers (darker) and type 1 fibers (lighter). Type 2 fiber atrophy, shown here, is a nonspecific change that may occur in inflammatory muscle disease, steroid myopathy, cachectic states, upper motor neuron deficit, peripheral nerve disease, myasthenia gravis, and hyperparathyroidism. (Courtesy of A. R. Sulaiman.)

The muscle biopsy histopathology of adult dermatomyositis may be identical to that of polymyositis. However, fiber invasion by T lymphocytes is rare, and a perivascular distribution of inflammatory cells, composed of higher percentages of B lymphocytes and T4+ helper lymphocytes, is the rule.[35] Occasional biopsies reveal perifascicular atrophy (Fig. 69–8). Skin histopathology varies according to the stage of the disease and the type of lesion. Epidermal thickening; prominent dermal blood vessels; infiltration of lymphocytes, plasma cells, and histiocytes; and edema of the superficial layers of the dermis are seen in the earlier erythematous edematous regions. Epidermal thinning, inflammatory cell infiltrates in the dermis, and increased connective tissue are seen in thickened, pigmented areas.

Juvenile (Childhood) Dermatomyositis

The usual inflammatory myopathic process observed in children has a highly characteristic pattern, although a disease similar to adult polymyositis is occasionally encountered in that age group.[19, 36, 37] The general features of juvenile dermatomyositis include rash and weakness. This process differs from that of the adult form in many patients, however, because of the coexistence of vasculitis, ectopic calcification, and lipodystrophy. Classically, the child develops cutaneous manifestations followed by muscle weakness. The rash is typically erythematous and is found on the malar region as well as the extensor surfaces of the elbows, knuckles, and knees. These lesions often are scaling and may become pigmented

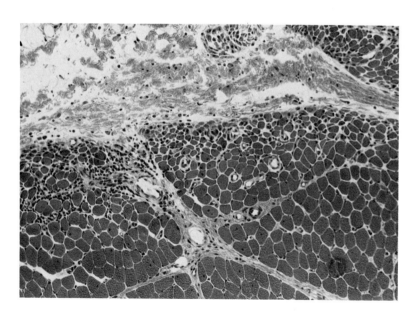

Figure 69–8. Hematoxylin and eosin stain of skeletal muscle revealing perifascicular atrophy. This change is characteristic of juvenile dermatomyositis but may also be seen in adults with dermatomyositis and other inflammatory myopathies. (Courtesy of A. R. Sulaiman.)

and depigmented. The weakness, myalgias, and stiffness are most severe in the proximal muscles and neck flexors but may be generalized. Involved muscles are tender and swollen to palpation.

In juvenile dermatomyositis the skin lesions and weakness are almost always coincidental, but the severity and progression of each can vary greatly from case to case. In some, remission is complete with little or no therapy. In severe cases accompanied by vasculitis, progression may be devastating in spite of therapy. Weakness can become profound and affect the patient's ability to chew, phonate, swallow, and breathe. Occasionally, respiratory failure results. Gastrointestinal ulcerations resulting from vasculitis may cause hemorrhage or perforation of a viscus. Ectopic calcifications may occur in the subcutaneous tissues or in the muscles. Subcutaneous calcifications can develop in association with vasculitis in some patients or independently in others. The calcifications may be accompanied by ulceration of the overlying skin, may affect posture and mobility, and may become a major cause of morbidity over time. Additional disability may result from flexion contractures, a common consequence of chronic weakness.

The histologic changes in muscle of patients with juvenile dermatomyositis are essentially the same as those for the adult form, although perifascicular atrophy (see Fig. 69–8) is much more prevalent.[38] Prominent changes are often observed in the intramuscular arteries and veins. These include endothelial hyperplasia and deposition of IgG, IgM, and complement (C3) within the vessel wall. Blood vessel changes are not limited to skeletal muscle. Perivascular collections of inflammatory cells, intimal hyperplasia, and fibrin thrombi lead to arteritis, phlebitis, and, subsequently, infarction in skin, intestines, nerves, and fat.

Myositis and Other Collagen Vascular Diseases

Muscle weakness is a frequent finding in patients with collagen vascular diseases (Table 69–5). In some cases, the weakness may result from the systemic effects of cytokines (i.e., interleukin-1, interleukin-6, tumor necrosis factors) or side effects of therapies (i.e., glucocorticosteriods, D-penicillamine, hydroxychloroquine). However, in some patients, the proximal muscle weakness and other myopathic manifestations are indistinguishable from those of typical polymyositis, including high CK levels and typical electromyographic changes. On the other hand, weakness may be accompanied by normal enzyme levels and an absence of abnormalities on electromyographic examination.

The features of idiopathic inflammatory myopathy (see Table 69–1) may dominate the clinical picture in some patients with scleroderma, systemic lupus erythematosus, rheumatoid arthritis, mixed connective tissue disease, and Sjögren's syndrome. This

Table 69–5. COLLAGEN VASCULAR DISEASES THAT MAY BE ASSOCIATED WITH INFLAMMATORY MYOPATHY

Allergic granulomatosis
Giant cell arteritis
Hypersensitivity vasculitis
Mixed connective tissue disease
Polyarteritis nodosum
Polymyalgia rheumatica
Rheumatoid arthritis
Scleroderma
Sjögren's syndrome
Systemic lupus erythematosus
Wegener's granulomatosis

picture is rarer in the vasculitic syndromes, raising the question of whether the concurrence is anything more than coincidental. In vasculitic syndromes, muscle weakness is more commonly related to arteritis and nerve involvement than to nonsuppurative inflammatory changes of muscles.

The histology of muscle in patients with myositis secondary to another diffuse connective tissue disease may be identical to that for patients with polymyositis. In some patients, however, differences more representative of the associated condition are recognized. The myositis of scleroderma is characterized by fiber size variation, occasional necrosis of single muscle fibers, increased amounts of connective tissue in the endomysial and perimysial regions, and mononuclear cell infiltration around perimysial blood vessels.[39] The histologic changes in systemic lupus are similar to those in adult dermatomyositis. Florid inflammatory change is rare in rheumatoid arthritis and less common in Sjögren's syndrome. More commonly, the findings consist of type 2 fiber atrophy, nonspecific degenerative changes of muscle fibers, or essentially normal architecture associated with the presence of an occasional lymphocyte.[40] Arteritis can be seen in muscle in severe cases of rheumatoid vasculitis. The muscle pathology in patients with mixed connective tissue disease can be identical to changes seen in dermatomyositis or scleroderma.

Myositis and Malignancy

The first association of myositis and malignancy was reported in 1935.[39] Observations that followed promoted the concept that patients with polymyositis and dermatomyositis had an increased risk of malignancy. This issue has been reinvestigated many times since Bohan and Peter published their criteria. In spite of this, questions still remain concerning the frequency of malignancy in patients with myositis and whether the risk is higher for those with dermatomyositis.[42, 43]

In studies reported after 1976, the frequency of malignancy associated with myositis is about 20 percent (with a range from 6 to 60 percent). Although this seems quite high, it is no different from the frequency of malignancy for the general population when appropriate control groups are analyzed.[44] Some studies show that malignancy is more commonly associated with dermatomyositis than with polymyositis, but others demonstrate no difference between the two subsets. Malignancy can develop before, at the same time as, or after the diagnosis of myositis. Occasionally both conditions seem to follow a parallel course, but more commonly the two seem to have only a temporal relationship, having developed within 1 year of each other. CK levels are elevated in most but not all cases of myositis with malignancy. Finding normal CK levels on repeated testing in patients with other features of myositis indicates an increased likelihood of malignancy.

Some evidence supports the premise that myositis and malignancy are associated more commonly in the elderly. However, the two conditions are also well reported to coexist in adults younger than 40 years of age. Earlier studies indicated that ovarian and gastric cancers were the most common. It now appears that the sites or types of malignancy that occur in patients with myositis are those expected for the age group and sex of the individual. Malignancy is not generally associated with childhood inflammatory myopathies, but it can occur with those conditions.[45] (See Chapter 94.)

Inclusion Body Myositis

Inclusion body myositis is the most recently identified subset of inflammatory myopathies.[46] Criteria have been proposed for making the diagnosis (see Table 69–4).[16] Recent reports indicate that this diagnosis makes up 15 to 28 percent of all inflammatory myopathies.[47] The actual incidence of inclusion body myositis is unknown because it is a rare disease and many physicians are unaware of this diagnosis. In addition, the clinical presentation may be identical to that of polymyositis, and special handling (histochemical examination of frozen sections) of biopsy specimens or electron microscopy is necessary to see the characteristic pathology.

Although a small number of cases of inclusion body myositis have been diagnosed in patients younger than 40 years and rarely in childhood,[48] this disease affects primarily older individuals. The onset of symptoms is typically insidious, and progression is slow. Symptoms may have been present for 5 or 6 years prior to a diagnosis. The clinical picture in some patients differs from that of typical polymyositis in that it may include focal, distal, or asymmetric weakness. Myalgia and muscle tenderness are rare. Dysphagia, noted in about 20 percent of cases, tends to be a late occurrence but occasionally is a significant presenting symptom. Facial weakness is rare, and no cases with ptosis or ophthalmoplegia have been reported. The cardiovascular features are similar to those observed in polymyositis.

As the muscle weakness becomes severe, it is accompanied by atrophy and diminished deep tendon reflexes. In some patients, the disease continues a slow, steady progression. In others, it seems to plateau, leaving the individual with fixed weakness and atrophy of the involved musculature.[49] Present therapies seem to have limited or no effect in the majority of individuals with inclusion body myositis. No clear relationship exists between inclusion body myositis and malignancy, but the diagnosis has been observed to be associated with interstitial pneumonitis, scleroderma, systemic lupus erythematosus, dermatomyositis, Sjögren's syndrome, immune thrombocytopenia, sarcoidosis, psoriasis, and diabetes. The frequency of these associations is quite low, and their significance is uncertain.

Serum CK levels are only slightly elevated in most cases of inclusion body myositis and are normal in 25 percent. No correlation exists between the level of CK and the acuteness or severity of the disease. Elevated erythrocyte sedimentation rates or positive tests for antinuclear antibodies are present in fewer than 20 percent of patients. Most patients have myopathic changes on electromyograms, with approximately half the patients having electromyographic features consistent with neurogenic or mixed neurogenic and myopathic changes.[50] In some cases, the changes are believed to be very characteristic of the disease process, but in other cases they are similar to changes observed in the chronic stages of other inflammatory myopathies.

The diagnosis is defined primarily by pathology. Histologic changes include necrosis and inflammation consistent with polymyositis, although perivascular exudates are rare and "ragged-red" fibers and angulated atrophic fibers may be seen. The characteristic change is the presence of intracellular lined vacuoles (Fig. 69–9). On paraffin sections, the vacuoles appear lined with eosinophilic material, but on frozen preparations they appear lined with basophilic granules. Lined vacuoles are not specific for inclusion body myositis. Similar vacuoles have been described in oculopharyngeal muscular dystrophy and distal myopathy (conditions that, arguably, could be considered variants of the same disease). Vacuolar changes are also prominent features in muscle from patients with a wide variety of myopathies (Table 69–6).

Electron microscopy reveals either intracytoplasmic or intranuclear tubular or filamentous inclusions (Fig. 69–10). These structures are straight, rigid-appearing with periodic transverse and longitudinal striations and resemble paramyxovirus nucleocapsid. Myelin figures, which are also called myeloid bodies or membranous whorls, are common in inclusion body myositis but are also seen in chloroquine myopathy, colchicine myopathy, adult-onset acid maltase deficiency, and, occasionally, myotonic and limb-girdle dystrophies.

Myositis and Eosinophils

Eosinophilic myositis is a rare disorder characterized by the subacute onset of proximal weakness,

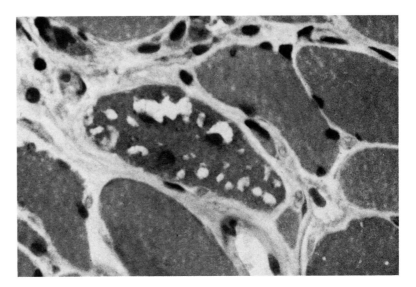

Figure 69–9. Hematoxylin and eosin–stained section of muscle from a patient with inclusion body myositis showing degenerating fibers with "lined vacuoles," atrophic and angulated fibers, increased endomysium, and scattered mononuclear cells. (From Cohen, M. R., Sulaiman, A. R., et al.: Clinical heterogeneity and treatment response in inclusion body myositis. Arthritis Rheum. 32:734, 1989; used by permission.)

myalgias, elevated serum levels of muscle enzymes, myopathic electromyographic findings, and an eosinophilic inflammatory infiltrate in skeletal muscle. In some patients, eosinophilic myositis is a focal disorder, but in others, it is associated with a predominant overlying eosinophilic fasciitis (Schulman's disease).[52] It may also represent one manifestation of a generalized hypereosinophilic syndrome.[53]

The term eosinophilia-myalgia syndrome is used for a neuromuscular condition caused by ingestion of L-tryptophan that was contaminated during production.[54–56] This syndrome reached epidemic status during the autumn of 1989, but reports of new cases disappeared by January 1990 after L-tryptophan was removed from sale and the toxicity resulting from its use was publicized. The syndrome typically began with the subacute onset of myalgias and subjective weakness that progressed to become incapacitating in many patients. Over half the patients also developed fatigue, rash, peripheral edema, and neurologic problems, including agitation, memory loss, profound paresthesias, distal motor weakness, demyelinating changes, or ascending neuropathy. One third experienced arthralgias, alopecia, fever, weight loss, and pulmonary problems, which included dyspnea on exertion, interstitial infiltrates, and decreased diffusing capacity. These symptoms developed in the presence of profound peripheral blood hypereosinophilia (more than 1000 eosinophils per mm^3). Serum aldolase levels were elevated in two thirds of patients, but CK levels were virtually always normal (a curious and unexplained phenomenon). Biopsies of muscle revealed inflammatory infiltrates containing eosinophils in the perimysium and fascia and

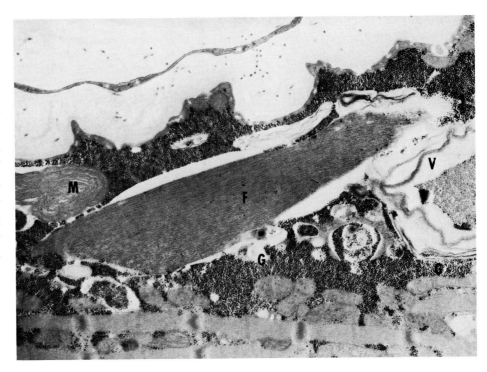

Figure 69–10. Electron micrograph of muscle tissue from a patient with inclusion body myositis. Seen are a cytoplasmic inclusion (F) beneath the sarcolemma, a myelin figure (M), a vacuole (V), and pools of cytoplasmic glycogen (G). (From Cohen, M. R., Sulaiman, A. R., et al.: Clinical heterogeneity and treatment response in inclusion body myositis. Arthritis Rheum. 32:734, 1989; used by permission.)

Table 69–6. MYOPATHIES ASSOCIATED WITH VACUOLES

Inflammatory	Adult dermatomyositis
	Inclusion body myositis
Dystrophic	Duchenne's muscular dystrophy (acute lesions)
	Oculopharyngeal muscular dystrophy
Toxic	Alcohol
	Chloroquine
	Colchicine
	Zidovudine (AZT)
Metabolic	Acid maltase deficiency
	Other glycogen storage disease
	Carnitine deficiency
Infectious	Echovirus
Miscellaneous	Distal myopathy
	Lafora's disease
	Periodic paralysis

microangiopathic changes. Perimysial fibrosis and perifascicular atrophy were also seen, usually in more advanced stages. Discontinuation of the L-tryptophan led to resolution of symptoms in some patients, and glucocorticoid therapy was helpful in others. However, some patients continue to have persistent myalgias and paresthesia, and others have died primarily from progressive pulmonary complications.

Myositis Ossificans

Myositis ossificans can be divided into two types, localized and widespread. Localized myositis ossificans invariably follows trauma, although the trauma may have seemed trivial or even may have been forgotten. Initially, a warm, tender swelling of a doughy consistency is noted in the muscle. If the swelling is close to a joint, the picture may simulate an acute monoarticular arthritis.[57] Soon thereafter,

the area takes on the consistency of a mass and becomes firm and hard. At about 1 month, calcifications are seen on radiographs or with computed tomography (CT) scanning. Surgical excision is often necessary and leads to a good outcome.[58] Histologically lesions have three zones. A highly cellular core containing fibroblasts, pleomorphic histiocytes, and rare giant cells is surrounded by a zone of compact layers of connective tissue running parallel to each other, with areas of well-formed bone at the periphery (Fig. 69–11).

The widespread, progressive form is termed myositis ossificans progressiva and is inherited in the autosomal dominant pattern.[59] Warm, tender swelling in many muscles is typically first noted during childhood. The lesions gradually shrink, become hard, and may disappear only to recur, especially in the muscles of the spine, abdominal wall, chest, and extremities.[60] Most patients also have some congenital skeletal defects, including microdactyly of the great toe and thumb, exostosis, and absence of the two upper incisors as well as hypogenitalism, absence of the ear lobules, and deafness. Treatment with ethane-1-hydroxy-1,1-diphosphonate (EHDP) has been effective in halting the progression of the disease in some patients.[61]

Localized or Focal Myositis

Histologic changes identical to those observed in polymyositis occasionally are present in biopsies of focal nodules from patients with only one muscle or one extremity involved. Occasionally, this disorder remains focal and confined to one limb for several years.[62] In other cases, this condition represents an unusual presentation of polymyositis and progresses to a more typical distribution after a few days or weeks.[63] These lesions must be differentiated from a skeletal muscle tumor.

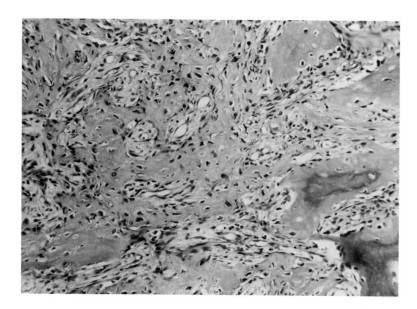

Figure 69–11. Hematoxylin and eosin–stained section of muscle from localized area of myositis ossificans. (From Siegert, J. J., and Wortmann, R. L.: Myositis ossificans simulating acute monoarticular arthritis. J. Rheumatol. 13:652, 1986; used by permission.)

Giant Cell Myositis

Multinucleated giant cells may occur in skeletal muscle in a variety of conditions, including foreign body reactions, tuberculosis, sarcoidosis,[64] or the syndrome of giant cell (granulomatous) myositis, giant cell myocarditis, and myasthenia gravis with or without thymoma.[65] Regenerating muscle cells are multinucleate and may closely resemble giant cells. Therefore, the histopathology and overall clinical status of the patient should be reviewed carefully whenever giant cells are found in skeletal muscle.

PATHOGENESIS

The idiopathic inflammatory myopathies are believed to be immune-mediated processes that are triggered by environmental factors in genetically susceptible individuals. This hypothesis is based on the specifics of the inflammatory changes in muscle, immunogenetic observations, animal models, prevalence and type of circulating autoantibodies, association with other autoimmune and connective tissue diseases, and response to immunosuppressive therapy.

The pathologic changes in muscle provide the strongest evidence that these diseases have an immune-mediated pathogenesis. The changes in polymyositis and inclusion body myositis appear to result from cell-mediated, antigen-specific cytotoxicity.[66, 67] Non-necrotic muscle fibers are seen surrounded by and invaded by CD8+ mononuclear cells, with cytotoxic cells outnumbering suppressor cells by a ratio of 3 to 1 in the CD8+ population.[32] B cells and natural killer cells do not appear to play a significant role in polymyositis or inclusion body myositis. The fibers invaded by T cells show increased major histocompatibility complex class I expression, a necessary condition for T cell–mediated cytotoxicity.[68] Using electron microscopy, the CD8+ cells are found to adhere to the fibers, sending spider-like projections through a seemingly intact membrane, indicating that these cells are attached to specific antigens on the sarcolemma. Other T cell–activating antigens are also present, including interleukin-2 receptors, Ta-1 (an activation marker also associated with anamestic responses), and TLiSA-1 (a late marker associated with cytotoxic T cell differentiation).[69, 70] Together, these findings imply that the pathology of polymyositis and inclusion body myositis involves recognition of an antigen on the surface of muscle fibers by antigen-specific T cells.

In contrast, humoral immune mechanisms appear to play a greater role in dermatomyositis.[32, 66] Invasion of non-necrotic fibers is quite universal, and the cellular infiltrates are predominantly perivascular in location. B cells outnumber T cells. Among T lymphocytes, CD4+ cells are common, whereas CD8+ cells and activated T cells are rare. In the circulation, DR+ cells and B cells (CD20+ cells) are

increased, whereas T cells (CD3+ cells) are decreased.[70] The vasculopathy that is so prominent in juvenile dermatomyositis and occasionally present in the adult form of the disease also appears to be immune mediated through humoral mechanisms. Immunoglobulins and complement components including the C5-9 membrane attack complex are also deposited in the capillaries and small arterioles in this disease, but not in polymyositis.[71]

Two observations have provided strong support for the hypothesis that the idiopathic inflammatory myopathies are disorders of autoimmunity. First is the recognized association with other autoimmune diseases, including the collagen vascular diseases (see Table 69–5), Hashimoto's thyroiditis, Graves' disease, myasthenia gravis, type 1 diabetes mellitus, primary biliary cirrhosis, dermatitis herpetiformis, and primary vitiligo. Second is the high prevalence of circulating autoantibodies.[72] Many individuals with polymyositis and dermatomyositis have antibodies that appear to be unique to these diseases. These are termed myositis-associated antibodies and are directed at cytoplasmic antigens related to transfer RNA (tRNA) and protein synthesis (Table 69–7). The most commonly recognized myositis-associated antibody is directed at histidyl-tRNA synthetase and is termed anti-Jo-1.[73] Other autoantibodies are directed at the aminoacyl-tRNA synthetases for threonine (anti-PL-7),[74] alanine (anti-PL-12),[75] isoleucine (anti-OJ), and glycine (anti-EJ).[76] These antibodies do not cross-react with each other, and only one is found in an individual patient. These antibodies have a property characteristic of autoantibodies; that is, they inhibit the function of the respective antigen by interaction with the active site.

The presence of a particular myositis-associated autoantibody indicates a particular clinical subset. Most individuals with anti-Jo-1 are younger adults and have polymyositis. More than 60 percent have interstitial lung disease, arthritis, and Raynaud's phenomenon. Onset is usually sudden and occurs in the first half of the year. This is in contrast with children with juvenile dermatomyositis and adults

Table 69–7. MYOSITIS-ASSOCIATED AUTOANTIBODIES

Antibody	Antigen
anti-Jo-1	Histidyl-tRNA synthetase
anti-PL-7	Threonyl-tRNA synthetase
anti-PL-12	Alanyl-tRNA synthetase and alanyl-tRNA
anti-OJ	Isoleucyl-tRNA synthetase
anti-EJ	Glycyl-tRNA synthetase
anti-SRP	Signal recognition particle
anti-KJ	Translocation factor
anti-Fer	Elongation factor 1-alpha
anti-Mas	Small RNA
anti-Mi-2	220-kD nuclear protein complex
anti-56-kD	Ribonucleoprotein component

From Targoff, I. N., and Reichlein, M.: Humoral immunity in polymyositis and dermatomyositis. Mt. Sinai J. Med. (N.Y.) 55:487, 1988; used by permission.

with polymyositis and anti-SRP antibodies who do not have lung disease or arthritis and whose onset of disease is in the latter half of the year.[77]

Viruses have been strongly implicated as the pathogens of the idiopathic inflammatory myopathies. Certainly the seasonal variation of onset of different subsets is indirect evidence that infectious agents may play a role.[78] Interestingly, certain picornaviruses can serve as a substrate for aminoacyl-tRNA synthetase activity and be charged with the respective amino acid. Furthermore, some homology exists among amino acid sequences near the active site of *Escherichia coli* histidyl-tRNA synthetase (Jo-1), muscle proteins, and a capsid protein of encephalomyocarditis virus, a picornavirus that induces a model of myositis in mice.[79] Although no homology exists between human and *E. coli* histidyl-tRNA synthetase, antibodies initially directed against a virus or a virus-enzyme complex could react with homologous areas of host proteins, resulting in autoantibody production by the process of molecular mimicry.

Although evidence exists suggesting that viruses could cause autoantibody production, more compelling evidence supports the hypothesis that the idiopathic inflammatory myopathies are actually caused by viruses. Clearly, some viruses such as coxsackievirus A9, which has been cultured from muscle, can cause myositis.[80] Elevated titers to coxsackievirus have been found in children with juvenile dermatomyositis compared with matched control subjects.[81] Mumps virus antigen has been identified in inclusions in muscle from patients with inclusion body myositis, using an immunoperoxidase staining technique.[82] Recent studies using techniques of molecular biology have identified enteroviral genomes in muscle from some patients with polymyositis and dermatomyositis, but not in control subjects.[83, 84] The most striking evidence of a viral cause for the idiopathic inflammatory myopathies is found in animal models in which chronic myositis develops following infection with a picornavirus and persists long after virus can no longer be detected in the tissue. The best described model is produced by injecting coxsackievirus B1 into neonatal Swiss mice. Virus cannot be cultured after 2 weeks, although changes characteristic of juvenile dermatomyositis persist for up to 70 days. Nude and athymic Swiss mice are able to clear the virus without sequelae, indicating the importance of T cells in the pathogenesis of this disorder.[86] In contrast, injection of adult BALB/c mice with encephalomyocarditis virus-221A produces a virus-dose–dependent model of polymyositis. Mice with different H2 (immunoresponse) haplotypes show different susceptibilities to the virus. The viral genome has been shown to persist in skeletal muscle 3 to 4 weeks after inoculation using in situ hybridization; however, muscle inflammation can persist beyond that point.[87]

The importance of genetic factors is further evident in studies of class II immunohistocompatibility antigens in humans. Individuals with HLA-DR3 are at an increased risk to develop inflammatory muscle disease, including polymyositis and juvenile dermatomyositis.[19, 20] All patients with anti-Jo-1 antibodies have the HLA antigen DR52, with white patients also having a high prevalence of HLA-DR3 and DR6.[88] Patients with anti-SRP antibodies carry HLA-DR5, and those with anti-Mi2 express DR7 and DRw53. HLA-DR1 is increased threefold in patients with inclusion body myositis compared with control subjects.[22]

It is therefore likely that the inflammatory myopathies are the result of and are perpetuated by an immune response mounted against an environmental factor (probably viral) in genetically predisposed individuals. The muscle weakness that occurs in an inflammatory myopathy may result directly from the loss of muscle fibers destroyed by that immune response and subsequent fibrosis. On the other hand, additional mechanisms must come into play, at least in part, because weakness occurs in some individuals with muscle histology showing no inflammatory cells or evidence of fiber necrosis. These observations suggest that abnormalities of the contractile process or membrane defects may underlie the symptoms of muscle weakness. Both muscle contraction and maintenance of membrane integrity are energy (ATP)-dependent processes. It is possible, therefore, that disordered energy metabolism in skeletal muscle fibers is responsible for at least some of the muscle weakness in the idiopathic inflammatory myopathies.

The hypothesis that inflammatory myopathies are associated with altered muscle cell energetics is supported by studies of animal and human disease. Alterations in glucose utilization have been demonstrated in myositic muscle from coxsackievirus B1–infected Swiss mice and littermate controls studied 30 days after inoculation. When incubated with equal amounts of glucose, the myositis muscle produces twofold greater carbon dioxide and fivefold greater lactate than does control muscle. The carbon dioxide that is generated is produced by pentose phosphatase shunt activity, a pathway normally not active in normal skeletal muscle.[89] Enzyme analyses reveal that the myositic muscle has 50 percent greater activity of glucose-6-phosphate dehydrogenase and 6-phosphogluconate dehydrogenase, similar activities of carnitine palmitoyltransferase, and 50 percent less activity of myophosphorylase and myoadenylate deaminase.[90] A high percentage of adults with polymyositis have an acquired deficiency of myoadenylate deaminase activity. The deficiency is attributable to reduced transcript availability and correlates with the severity of myositis.[91] Furthermore, studies using magnetic resonance spectroscopy, a noninvasive method of measuring high-energy phosphate compounds in tissue, have shown that patients with polymyositis deplete ATP pools more rapidly and take longer to restore baseline levels than do healthy control subjects.[92] These studies indicate that metabolic abnormalities of skeletal muscle may cause weakness, but more information is needed to determine the relationship of these phenomena to the immune response.

DIFFERENTIAL DIAGNOSIS

Although the idiopathic inflammatory myopathies are relatively rare diseases, the list of diseases that cause myopathic symptoms for which patients seek medical attention is long (Table 69–8). Myopathic symptoms include fixed muscle weakness, or the inability to perform specific tasks, such as climbing stairs or raising one's hands above the head; early or premature fatigue; and cramping or myalgia after muscular activity. The symptoms of myopathic diseases can range from chronic and mild to acute and fulminant. Some symptoms allow individuals to live comfortably, provided that they sufficiently limit their physical activity; others are severe and are associated with profound disability or rhabdomyolysis, myoglobinuria, and renal failure.

Neurologic Diseases

Neurologic diseases (Table 69–9) generally can be differentiated from polymyositis because of the occurrence of asymmetric weakness, distal extremity involvement, altered sensorium, or abnormal cranial nerve function. Generally, myopathies cause only proximal and symmetric weakness. Exceptions include some cases of mitochondrial myopathies, which may have ocular problems, and some cases of inclusion body myosis, which may have some "neuropathic" features.

Table 69–8. CATEGORIES OF DISEASES AND DISORDERS THAT CAN CAUSE MYOPATHIC SYMPTOMS

Collagen vascular diseases
Neuropathic diseases
  Muscular dystrophies
  Denervating conditions
  Neuromuscular junction disorders
  Proximal neuropathies
  Myotonic diseases
Neoplasia
Drug-related conditions
Infections
  Metabolic
    Primary
      Storage diseases and inborn errors of metabolism
      Mitochondrial myopathies
    Secondary
      Nutritional-toxic
      Endocrine disorders
Rhabdomyolysis
Miscellaneous causes
  Sarcoidosis
  Fibromyalgia
  Psychosomatic

Table 69–9. NEUROLOGIC DISEASES MOST OFTEN CONFUSED WITH INFLAMMATORY MUSCLE DISEASE

Muscular Dystrophies
  Duchenne's muscular dystrophy
  Becker's muscular dystrophy
  Facioscapulohumeral muscular dystrophy
  Limb-girdle muscular dystrophy
Denervating Conditions
  Spinal muscular atrophies
  Amyotrophic lateral sclerosis
Neuromuscular Junction Disorders
  Myasthenia gravis
  Eaton-Lambert syndrome
Proximal Neuropathies
  Diabetic amyotrophy
  Diabetic plexopathy
  Guillain-Barré syndrome
  Acute intermittent porphyria

The muscular dystrophies often have a positive family history. Limb-girdle muscular dystrophy is perhaps most readily confused with adult polymyositis.[93] The inheritance is autosomal recessive. Upper and lower extremity proximal muscle weakness begins in the second to fourth decades and is eventually accompanied by muscle wasting. Typically, the shoulder and pelvic girdle musculature is involved, but significant variation from this pattern can occur. These muscles are also most commonly affected in Duchenne's muscular dystrophy and Becker's muscular dystrophy. Each of these is passed by X-linked inheritance. The onset of Duchenne's muscular dystrophy is usually by age 5 years. In addition to muscle weakness and wasting, individuals develop winging of the scapulae, a hyperlordotic gait, and pseudohypertrophy of the calf muscles. Patients usually cannot walk after age 11 years and die of respiratory failure by age 20 years. Becker's muscular dystrophy is similar but generally milder, with patients able to walk beyond age 16 years. Facioscapulohumeral muscular dystrophy is an autosomal dominant disorder with a better prognosis. Weakness characteristically develops in the orbicularis oculi, orbicularis oris, periscapular, biceps, brachioradialis, triceps, hip flexor, and anterior tibial muscles.

The spinal muscle atrophies are generally autosomal recessive disorders that cause degeneration of the spinal anterior horn cells.[94] Onset may occur at any age. The distribution of muscles involved is dependent on the specific cord segments affected, and, accordingly, the weakness tends to be localized rather than diffuse. Amyotrophic lateral sclerosis is associated with lower motor neuron denervation, upper motor neuron signs, and bulbar or pseudobulbar palsy.[95]

Although proximal muscle weakness, especially of the upper extremities, may be the dominant clinical feature of myasthenia gravis, extraocular and bulbar muscle involvement as well as the marked fatigability helps differentiate it from polymyositis. Eaton-Lambert syndrome also causes proximal muscle weakness. Although Eaton-Lambert syndrome is usually associated with neoplastic disease, it can occur in the absence of cancer, especially when it develops before age 40 years.[96]

Conditions considered under the classification of proximal neuropathies can cause myopathic symptoms and are occasionally confused with polymyositis. These include diabetic amyotrophy and plexopathy, Guillain-Barré syndrome, and acute intermittent porphyria.

Neoplasia

Cancer must be considered in the evaluation of patients with myopathic symptoms. The association between myositis and malignancy has been discussed earlier. The weakness and fatigue that develop in the progress of a neoplastic disease may result from the systemic effects of cytokines released by the tumor cells or by virtue of the immune response to the malignancy. In addition, prominent neuromuscular changes can develop as features of paraneoplastic syndromes.[97] Eaton-Lambert syndrome is an example of the latter.[98] These individuals have excessive fatigability on exertion and weakness that may be profound and exclusively proximal in distribution. Patients report that their strength is reduced at rest but may increase at the first of repetitive movements, only to decrease with continued exercise. Electromyographic studies readily differentiate this diagnosis from myasthenia gravis and polymyositis. The proximal myopathy that develops in patients with carcinoid syndrome is probably the result of compounds produced by the cancer cells.

Drug-Related Conditions

A long list of drugs can cause myopathic changes.[99] Examples include drugs commonly used in a rheumatology practice (Table 69–10). Glucocor-

Table 69–10. DRUGS THAT CAN CAUSE MYOPATHIC SYMPTOMS OR SYNDROMES*

Alcohol	Hydroxychloroquine
Bezafibrate	Ipecac
D, L-Carnitine	Levodopa
L-Carnitine	Lovastatin
Chloroquine	D-Penicillamine
Cimetidine	Phenytoin
Clofibrate	Procainamide
Cocaine	Rifampin
Colchicine	Sulfonamides
Danazol	L-Tryptophan
Gemfibrozil	Valproic acid
Glucocorticoids	Vincristine
Heroin	Zidovudine (AZT)
Hydralazine	

*Additional causes include any drug or hormone that can raise or lower serum concentrations of sodium, potassium, calcium, phosphorus, or magnesium.

ticoid use causes proximal muscle weakness and wasting.[100, 101] Electromyographic changes are minimal and, if present, nonspecific. Biopsy of muscle shows only type 2 fiber atrophy. This condition may be difficult to diagnosis, since it may develop in patients being treated for inflammatory muscle disease. Colchicine, chloroquine, and hydroxychloroquine can cause an axonal neuromyopathy.[102, 103] This toxicity is invariably associated with high CK levels. Withdrawal of the drug should rapidly lead to clinical improvement and normalization of the CK level. Some patients receiving D-penicillamine develop autoimmune syndromes, including polymyositis and myasthenia gravis.[104]

The exact mechanism by which many drugs cause myopathy is uncertain. Some, such as penicillamine, hydralazine, and procainamide, are immune mediated. Some, such as alcohol, may have direct toxic effects.[105] Still others may cause metabolic or electrolyte abnormalities. For example, clofibrate, lovastatin, and gemfibrozil probably alter muscle fiber energetics[106]; thiazide diuretics induce hypokalemia, which can cause weakness, myalgias, and cramps.

Infections

Numerous infections can cause a myopathy (Table 69–11), and many may be confused with polymyositis. For example, patients, especially children, with influenza A and B viral infections can experience severe myalgias associated with very high (up to 15 times normal) CK levels and nonspecific myopathic changes, including fiber necrosis and inflammatory cell infiltration on muscle biopsy.[107] A subacute myositis has also been described following rubella infection and after immunization with live attenuated rubella virus.[108] The diagnosis of a viral myositis should be based on virus culture from throat, rectum, urine, or skeletal muscle or positive serologic testing.

Acquired immunodeficiency syndrome (AIDS) represents a very complicated situation.[109] Weakness is a common finding in patients suffering from AIDS. The possible causes include the generalized debilitated, cachectic state; central or peripheral nervous system disease; polymyositis emerging as a consequence of the altered immune function; infections with the human immunodeficiency virus (HIV), cytomegalovirus, *Mycobacterium avium-intracellulare*, *Cryptococcus*, or *Toxoplasma*; and the toxic effects of zidovudine (AZT) therapy. Biopsies of muscle from patients with AIDS and the AIDS-related complex (ARC) who have not received AZT therapy are abnormal in 70 to 96 percent of cases.[110, 111] Among the changes noted are "moth-eaten" fibers (76 percent), type 2 fiber atrophy (58 percent), endomysial and/or perimysial and/or perivascular mononuclear cell infiltrates (36 percent), and vasculitis with perifascicular atrophy (4 percent).[112]

Bacterial causes of myositis are important to recognize because the diagnosis will allow effective

Table 69–11. INFECTIOUS CAUSES OF MYOSITIS

Viral
Adenovirus
Coxsackievirus
Cytomegalovirus
Echovirus A9
Epstein-Barr virus
Hepatitis B virus
Human immunodeficiency virus (HIV)
Influenza A and B viruses
Mumps virus
Parainfluenza virus 4b
Rubella virus
Varicella-zoster virus

Bacterial
Borrelia burgdorferi (Lyme spirochete)
Clostridium welchii
Mycobacterium
    Leprosy
    Tuberculosis
Mycoplasma pneumoniae
Rickettsia
Staphylococcus
Streptococcus

Fungal
Cryptococcus

Parasitic
Cysticercus
Sarcocystis
Schistosoma
Toxoplasma
Trichinella
Trypanosoma

treatment with the appropriate antibiotics. Pyomyositis is a rare focal suppurative process usually encountered in the tropics.[113] Typically, abscesses, most often caused by streptococcal infection, are found in one or more proximal muscles, usually in the lower extremities. Among the parasites that cause myositis, *Toxoplasma* is the most common in the United States. Toxoplasmosis can cause an acute or subacute picture resembling polymyositis.[114] Toxoplasmosis is diagnosed by finding raised serum titers of antibodies or, rarely, by identifying the organism in muscle tissue. The observation of raised complement-fixing antibodies to *Toxoplasma* in a fair percentage of patients believed to have idiopathic polymyositis and dermatomyositis has suggested a possible causal relationship for this parasite.[115] Ultrasound evaluation and gallium scans may be useful in localizing areas of infection. Culture of muscle tissue is usually necessary to diagnose a bacterial, fungal, or parasitic infection.

Metabolic Myopathies

The term *metabolic myopathy* represents a heterogenous group of conditions (Table 69–12) that have in common abnormalities in muscle energy metabolism that result in skeletal muscle dysfunction. Some metabolic myopathies should be considered primary and are associated with known or postulated bio-

chemical defects that affect the ability of the muscle fibers to maintain adequate levels of ATP. These may be grouped into abnormalities of glycogen, lipid, purine, and mitochondrial biochemistry. Other metabolic myopathies may be considered secondary and attributed to various endocrine or electrolyte abnormalities.

Primary Metabolic Myopathies

Disorders of Glycogen Metabolism

Myophosphorylase deficiency, or McArdle's disease, was the first described, in 1951.[116] Today, a total of nine diseases have been identified that have in common an underlying defect in glycogen synthesis, glycogenolysis, or glycolysis (see Fig. 69–4). They are often referred to as the glycogen storage diseases because each defect results in the abnormal deposition and accumulation of glycogen in skeletal muscle.

The classic clinical manifestation of a glycogen storage disease is exercise intolerance, which may be attributed to pain, fatigue, stiffness, weakness, or intense cramping.[117] Most afflicted persons are well at rest and can function without difficulty at low levels of activity and during periods when lipids provide the major source of muscle energy. Symptoms develop following activities of high intensity and short duration or of less intensive effort for longer intervals, times when the majority of energy for muscular work is derived from carbohydrate. Some patients experience a "second wind" phenomenon. Although they must stop an activity because of exercise-induced symptoms, they are often able to resume the exercise after a brief rest.[118] Most patients

Table 69–12. METABOLIC MYOPATHIES

Primary	Secondary
Disordered Glycogen Metabolism	*Endocrine*
Myophosphorylase deficiency (McArdle's disease)	Acromegaly
Phosphorylase b kinase deficiency	Hypothyroidism
Phosphofructokinase deficiency	Hyperthyroidism
Debrancher enzyme deficiency	Hyperparathyroidism
Brancher enzyme deficiency	Cushing's disease
Phosphoglycerate kinase deficiency	Addison's disease
Phosphoglycerate mutase deficiency	Hyperaldosteronism
Lactate dehydrogenase deficiency	Carcinoid syndrome
Acid maltase deficiency	*Metabolic-Nutritional*
Disordered Lipid Metabolism	Uremia
Carnitine deficiency	Hepatic failure
Inherited	Malabsorption
Acquired	Periodic paralysis
Carnitine palmitoyltransferase deficiency	Vitamin D deficiency
Fatty acid acylCoA dehydrogenase deficiency	Vitamin E deficiency
Myoadenylate Deaminase Deficiency	*Electrolyte Disorders*
Mitochondrial Myopathies	Hypernatremia
	Hyponatremia
	Hyperkalemia
	Hypokalemia
	Hypercalcemia
	Hypocalcemia
	Hypophosphatemia
	Hypomagnesemia

develop some symptoms during childhood, but significant problems such as severe cramping or exercise-induced rhabdomyolysis and myoglobinuria with renal failure do not develop until the teenage years.[119] A subset of patients, however, complain only of easy fatigability, while others develop the gradual onset of proximal muscle weakness.[120] The latter presentation, which often occurs in adulthood (the oldest patient reported was diagnosed at age 78), may be difficult to differentiate from polymyositis.[121, 122]

Confusion of glycogen storage disease with inflammatory muscle disease results because serum CK levels are commonly elevated and electromyograms show increased insertional irritability, increased numbers of polyphasic motor unit potentials, fibrillations, and positive waves, all of which are nonspecific abnormalities that can also be seen in inflammatory myopathies. On muscle biopsy, fiber necrosis and phagocytosis may be noted.[123]

The diagnosis of *glycogen storage diseases* may be suggested by finding the classic changes of glycogen deposition on muscle biopsy. The finding of excessive glycogen deposition is not specific and can be seen in inclusion body myositis, mitochondrial myopathies, and other diseases. However, these changes may be missed in patients with a glycogen storage disease in the presence of significant rhabdomyolysis. In other cases, the changes may be inapparent using only light microscopy and may require electron microscopy to be appreciated. The forearm ischemic exercise test is a useful method of screening for a glycogen storage disease.[124, 125] Individuals with any glycogen storage disease (including McArdle's syndrome but excluding acid maltase deficiency) will fail to generate lactate during ischemic exercise. The putative diagnosis should always be confirmed by specific enzyme analysis of muscle tissue whenever it is suspected, either by histology or ischemic exercise testing.

Inherited *deficiency of acid maltase* presents in infantile, childhood, and adult forms.[126] The last typically manifests as proximal muscle weakness beginning after age 20 and may be misdiagnosed as polymyositis or limb-girdle muscular dystrophy.[127] Diaphragmatic involvement and respiratory failure may develop in one third of patients.[128] Acid maltase activity is localized to lysosomes and does not affect cytosolic glycogen metabolism. Therefore, a deficiency will not affect the results of ischemic exercise testing. The diagnosis of adult acid maltase deficiency should usually be suspected because of the characteristic electromyographic changes of intense electrical irritability and myotonic discharges in the absence of clinical myotonia.[126]

Disorders of Lipid Metabolism

The recognized disorders of lipid metabolism that cause myopathic problems are due to abnormalities in the transport and processing of fatty acids for energy. Carnitine palmitoyltransferase (CPT) activities are necessary for the transport of long-chain fatty acids into mitochondria (see Fig. 69-3). CPT deficiency is an autosomal recessive disorder that invariably causes attacks of severe malagia and myoglobinuria.[129] These are typically associated with vigorous physical activity but may occur with fasting, infection, or cold exposure. Initiation of ibuprofen therapy has been implicated in one case.[130] Serum CK levels, electromyograms, and muscle histology are normal except during episodes of rhabdomyolysis. The diagnosis is made by assaying muscle tissue for enzyme activity, which reveals a partial deficiency.

Carnitine is an essential intermediate that acts as a carrier of long-chain fatty acids into mitochondria, where they can undergo β-oxidation (see Fig. 69-3). Carnitine deficiency causes abnormal lipid deposition in skeletal muscle and can result from inherited or acquired causes.[131] Primary carnitine deficiencies can be divided into "systemic" and "muscle" types. Symptoms of "systemic carnitine deficiency" develop early in life, with episodes of coma and hypoketotic hypoglycemia similar to Reye's syndrome.[132] This may be associated with deficiency of short-, medium-, or long-chain acylCoA dehydrogenase activities or a defect in cellular uptake of carnitine. Those with "muscle carnitine deficiency" present in later childhood or during the early adult years with chronic muscle weakness.[131] The process affects mainly proximal muscles but may also involve facial and pharyngeal musculature. Acquired carnitine deficiencies have been reported during pregnancy and with renal failure requiring long-term hemodialysis, end-stage cirrhosis, myxedema, adrenal insufficiency, and valproic acid therapy. Myopathic symptoms have developed in individuals who have used D,L-carnitine (but not L-carnitine) as a fitness training supplement.[133]

Carnitine deficiency may be confused with polymyositis because serum CK levels are elevated in more than half the cases and electromyography often reveals polyphasic motor unit potentials of small amplitude and short duration. The diagnosis should be considered when abnormal deposits of lipid are identified by histochemical analysis of muscle tissue. Only 50 percent of patients with carnitine deficiency will respond to dietary supplementation with L-carnitine. Treatment with dietary manipulation, prednisone, or propranolol has provided success in a few patients refractory to L-carnitine treatment.[131, 134, 135]

Deficiencies of the three fatty acid acylCoA dehydrogenase activities have been reported in a 38-year-old male who presented with only a 2-year history of proximal muscle weakness and neck pain.[136] Evaluation revealed high CK levels, myopathic changes on electromyography, and abnormal lipid acceleration in muscle tissue. Riboflavin therapy resulted in normalization of muscle histology and improved strength. Riboflavin therapy was considered because the acylCoA dehydrogenases are flavin-containing proteins.

Myoadenylate Deaminase Deficiency

Myoadenylate deaminase deficiency is the most commonly recognized metabolic myopathy, being found in 2 percent of muscle biopsy specimens in large series of patients. This deficiency is known to exist in primary and secondary forms.[137] The primary form is inherited in an autosomal recessive pattern. Patients report symptoms of exercise intolerance with postexercise cramping and myalgia. When rested, patients are asymptomatic, and the symptoms are only mildly restrictive at first. With time, however, symptoms are brought on by less and less activity and persist longer and longer after completion of exercise, causing significant disability. Symptoms are a consequence of the defect in the purine nucleotide cycle (see Fig. 69–5). A deficiency in myoadenylate deaminase activity impedes the cell's ability to restore ATP levels to normal after they are depleted in the usual, efficient manner.[138]

The secondary forms appear to be acquired in the course of a variety of neuromuscular diseases, including Duchenne's, Becker's, and limb-girdle dystrophies; the spinal muscular atrophies; diabetes mellitus; periodic paralysis; and several collagen vascular diseases, including polymyositis, dermatomyositis, scleroderma, and systemic lupus erythematosus. In fact, 15 percent of all secondary cases have been observed in patients with polymyositis.[139] The reduced myoadenylate deaminase activity in these neuromuscular conditions could simply reflect a general deterioration of muscle fibers caused by the basic disease. However, the reductions of other enzyme activities such as CK and myokinase in the same tissues are not as severe, indicating a more selective effect on myoadenylate deaminase activity.[91]

Patients with primary myoadenylate deaminase deficiency will most often have normal serum CK levels, normal electromyograms, and normal muscle histology. The forearm ischemic exercise test is, however, abnormal.[125] Myoadenylate deaminase–deficient persons can release lactate into the circulation after ischemic exercise but fail to generate ammonia. The deficiency state should always be confirmed by histochemical staining or assay for the enzyme activity in skeletal muscle.

Mitochondrial Myopathies

The term *mitochondrial myopathy* represents a clinically heterogenous group of disorders that have in common morphologic abnormalities in the number, size, or structure of mitochondria. The metabolic abnormalities described in these conditions are numerous and can be attributed to defects in nutrient transport, pyruvate and acetylCoA processing, β-oxidation, the respiratory (electron transport) chain, or energy conservation. It appears that the mitochondrial myopathies are inherited through maternal transmission and are caused by defects in mitochondrial DNA.[140] The clinical spectrum of these conditions is quite diverse and includes progressive muscular weakness, external ophthalmoplegia with or without proximal myopathy, progressive exercise intolerance, and multisystem disease. More than 25 specific enzyme abnormalities have been described, of which at least six may present with exercise intolerance or progressive muscle weakness in adults.[141] In addition, mitochondrial myopathy may develop in patients who have received long-term zidovudine (AZT) therapy.[112]

Secondary Metabolic Myopathies

A host of endocrine and metabolic disorders may lead to myopathic symptoms (see Table 69–12). Both hypothyroidism and hyperthyroidism can produce proximal muscle weakness and elevated serum CK values.[142, 143] Hyperparathyroidism may cause proximal weakness, high CK levels, and myopathic electromyographic changes.[144] The basis for the weakness in these disorders is related, in part, to hormonal or toxic effects on muscle contractility. Electrolyte disorders must also play a crucial role. In fact, virtually any disturbance of electrolyte concentrations or ionization may result in myopathic symptoms[145] (Table 69–13).

Rhabdomyolysis

Rhabdomyolysis is not a disease, rather it is the common result of any cause of extensive muscle necrosis. Although rhabdomyolysis is most commonly associated with severe muscle injury, it may be caused by a variety of conditions[146, 147] (Table 69–14). The clinical result of rhabdomyolysis is intense myalgia associated with muscle tenderness and swelling. Serum CK values may reach levels 2000 times normal. If the cause or offending agent is corrected or removed, the muscle can heal remarkably quickly, with few or no residua. Permanent weakness and atrophy are rare unless significant infarction has occurred or the rhabdomyolysis has developed in relation to myositis or another myopathy.

Potential complications of massive muscle necrosis include hypocalcemia, hyperuricemia, myoglobinuria, and hyperkalemia. Hypocalcemia results from the sequestration of calcium by necrotic muscle, perhaps because the solubility product for calcium

Table 69–13. MYOPATHIC SYMPTOMS RESULTING FROM ELECTROLYTE ABNORMALITIES

Ion	Abnormalities	Weakness	Myalgia	Cramps
Calcium	Hypercalcemia	+	+	−
	Hypocalcemia	+ +	−	+
Magnesium	Hypomagnesemia	+	+	+
Phosphorus	Hypophosphatemia	+ +	+	−
Potassium	Hyperkalemia	+	−	−
	Hypokalemia	+ +	+	+
Sodium	Hypernatremia	+	+	+
	Hyponatremia	+	−	+

Table 69–14. CAUSES OF RHABDOMYOLYSIS

Trauma
Crush injury (with or without coma)
Excessive exercise (marathon running, military training)
Electrical shock (lightning, high-voltage injury, electroshock therapy)
Muscle activity (status epilepticus, delirium tremens)
High temperature (malignant hyperthermia, heatstroke, malignant neuroleptic syndrome, infection)
Ischemic injury (thromboembolism, sickle cell trait)
Drugs and Toxins
Recreational (alcohol, barbiturates, heroin, cocaine)
Lipid-lowering (clofibrate, bezafibrate, gemfibrozil, lovastatin)
Venoms (rattlesnake, sea snake, hornet)
Infections
Viral (influenza virus, coxsackievirus, herpesvirus, echovirus)
Bacterial (*Staphylococcus, Salmonella typhi* [typhoid], *Legionella, Clostridium*)
Metabolic Causes
Genetic (glycogen storage diseases, CPT deficiency)
Electrolyte imbalance (hypocalcemia, hypernatremia, hypophosphatemia, hyperosmolar nonketotic states, acidosis)
Collagen Vascular Causes
Polymyositis and dermatomyositis
Unknown Causes

phosphate is exceeded locally. The risk of hypocalcemia decreases within the first days after the onset. Serum urate concentrations increase as a result of the degradation of purine compounds released from the damaged muscle plus a block in uric acid excretion due to a concomitant acidosis or renal failure.

The most threatening complication of rhabdomyolysis is acute tubular necrosis. The risk of renal failure increases directly with the height of the serum CK, potassium, and phosphorus levels; inversely with serum albumin levels; and in the presence of dehydration or sepsis as the underlying cause.[148] The renal disorder is characterized by oliguria, myoglobin-positive urine containing pigmented granular casts, and a high serum creatinine level. Acute uric acid nephropathy may also complicate the picture. Treatment is essentially supportive. When myoglobinuria is identified, a diuresis should be established in hopes of preventing renal failure. Most nephrologists also recommend alkalinization of the urine, but this has not been proved to alter outcomes unless uric acid nephropathy is a component. The patient should be monitored for hyperkalemia, potentially the most life-threatening complication of the sequence.

TESTING FOR MUSCLE DISEASE

Physical Examination

The findings on physical examination of patients with an inflammatory disease of skeletal muscle are typical of those for most myopathic processes. Abnormalities are generally limited to the motor component of the examination, with weakness in a proximal and symmetric distribution. An objective determination of strength proves very useful in assessing the severity of disease as well as the effectiveness of therapy. Perhaps the most frequently used system for assessing individual muscle groups is that of the Medical Research Council, which grades strength on a scale of 0 (no contraction) to 5 (normal power resistance) (Table 69–15). A useful method for following the progress of the disease is the timed-stands test.[149] This test involves counting the time needed to stand ten times from a chair. The time required to perform this activity is quite reproducible in normal individuals but does increase with age (Fig. 69–12).

Laboratory Testing

Chemistries

Elevation of serum enzymes derived from skeletal muscle including CK, aldolase, SGOT, SGPT, and LDH helps confirm the presence of a myopathic process. High levels of these enzymes are found in the inflammatory diseases of muscle but are not specific for those diagnoses.

CK is a dimer and exists in the serum in three isoforms: MM, MB, and BB. The MM form predominates in skeletal and cardiac muscle. MB is found primarily in cardiac muscle, composing about 25 percent of the total CK activity in that tissue. MB is a very minor component in skeletal muscle but is present in that tissue in greater amounts in embryonal and regenerating fibers.[150] BB is the major isoenzyme in brain and smooth muscle. It is important to determine the tissue source of the CK whenever elevated levels are encountered.

The amount of CK in the serum is the result of that released from tissues less that which is removed from the circulation. Most elevated serum CK levels result from muscle necrosis or leaking membranes. Inflammatory or hypoxic injury, blunt trauma, and sharp trauma (intramuscular injections, electromyographic needle insertion, muscle biopsy) are well-recognized causes of high CK levels.[151] Both isometric and aerobic exercise can also produce elevated CK levels, especially in poorly conditioned individuals.[152, 153] Furthermore, morphine, benzodiazepam, and barbiturate use may elevate the serum CK levels by retarding the elimination of the enzyme from the circulation.[154]

Table 69–15. SYSTEM FOR OBJECTIVE (SEMIQUANTITATIVE) GRADING OF MUSCLE STRENGTH

5	Normal power resistance
4	Power decreased, but muscle contraction possible against resistance
3	Muscle contraction against gravity only
2	Muscle contraction possible only when gravity is eliminated
1	Contraction without motion
0	No contraction

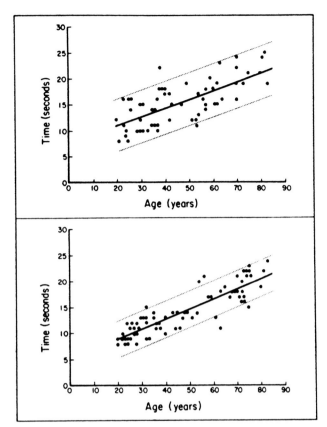

Figure 69–12. Timed-stands test as a function of age in 62 normal women *(top)* and in 77 normal men *(bottom)*. The mean and limits of normal (90 percent prediction region) are shown. (From Csuka, M., and McCarty, D. J.: A simple method for measurement of lower extremity muscle strength. Am. J. Med. 78:77, 1985; used by permission.)

Occasionally, elevated CK levels are observed in asymptomatic individuals. Racial differences in normal CK levels must be considered in this context. Healthy asymptomatic black males have higher total CK levels than those of whites or Hispanics, with the majority of values judged to be abnormal using the usual laboratory values.[155] Men generally have higher values than do women. Many of these asymptomatic elevations can be accounted for by exercise, medications, or hemolysis.[156] Some indicate a carrier state for Duchenne's muscular dystrophy, and others are signs of early or mild myopathies.[157] Some of these asymptomatic elevations, however, remain idiopathic.

Serum aldolase, SGOT, SGPT, and LDH levels are also useful in identifying muscle disease. Levels of all or only one of these may be elevated at different times. Elevations of LDH levels tend to occur later and remain increased longer than do elevations of CK. In most cases, extensive skeletal muscle injury or necrosis is associated with a shift of LDH isoforms in serum to LDH-1 and LDH-2. However, LDH isoenzyme determination is of limited value because of the heterogeneity of skeletal muscle in this regard. For example, the gluteus medius and soleus are richer in LDH-1 and LDH-2, whereas the triceps brachii and gastrocnemius contain higher percentages of LDH-4 and LDH-5.[158]

Myoglobin, the oxygen-binding heme protein, is released from injured skeletal and cardiac muscles and, subsequently, cleared in the urine. The serum myoglobin concentration is a sensitive indicator of muscle fiber integrity. Hypermyoglobinemia can result from any factor or disease that would raise serum CK levels. In some patients, however, serum myoglobin concentrations correlate better with the clinical course than do serum enzyme levels.[159] Myoglobin concentrations may rise rapidly in myositis. The rise in myoglobin may occur prior to elevations of CK levels and may even precede recognized clinical symptoms. Highly sensitive radioimmunoassays are available for quantitation of myoglobin. Myoglobin may be detected in serum even when it goes undetected in urine.[160] Myoglobinuria may occur in the absence of visible pigmenturia. The finding of positive tests for hemoglobin in urine in the absence of red blood cells is indirect evidence of myoglobinuria; the presence of myoglobinuria indicates the potential for acute renal failure.

The average adult man excretes 60 to 100 mg of creatine in the urine per 24 hours. Women excrete approximately twice those amounts. Increased excretion can occur with any cause of muscle atrophy. Muscle atrophy or necrosis also causes increased excretion of the substituted amino acid 3-methylhistidine.[161]

Autoantibodies

Circulating autoantibodies can be detected in the sera in a large number of patients with inflammatory myopathies. Antinuclear antibody (ANA) testing may be positive at low titers in a small percentage of patients with polymyositis, 60 percent of children with childhood dermatomyositis, and the majority of patients with an associated collagen vascular disease. In the latter cases, patients may also have autoantibodies more specific for those diseases (see Chapters 55, 60, 63, 64 and 66): anti-SM, anti-RNP, anti-Ro/La, and anti-Ku antibodies in systemic lupus erythematosus; anti-Ro/La antibodies in Sjögren's syndrome; anti-RNP in mixed connective tissue disease; anti-Scl-70, anti-PM-Scl, anti-Ku, anti-U_2 RNP, and anti-centromere antibodies in scleroderma and CREST (calcinosis, Raynaud's phenomenon, esophageal dysmotility, sclerodactyly, and telangiectasia); and anticytoplasmic antibodies (ANCAs) in Wegener's granulomatosis.

In addition, some patients with polymyositis or dermatomyositis have autoantibodies that are found almost exclusively in those conditions (see Table 69–7).[72] These antibodies tend to be present in genetically restricted groups of patients and may indicate specific patterns of disease. Anti-Mi-2 antibodies are found in 2 to 20 percent of patients with adult-onset dermatomyositis. Anti-Jo-1 antibodies are present in the sera in as many as 50 percent of patients with polymyositis and as many as 15 percent of patients with dermatomyositis.[73] The anti-Jo-1 antibody is a marker for patients whose myositis develops at a younger age, has an acute onset often in the first half of the calendar year, and is associated with interstitial lung disease, arthritis, and Raynaud's phenomenon.[22] This is in contrast with antibodies against SRPs (signal recognition particles), which identify patients with acute onset of severe myositis with a high incidence of dysphagia and an onset in the fall of the year, but little interstitial lung disease and arthritis.[77]

SRPs are proteins of the ribonuclear protein complex that mediate the translocation of nascent polypeptides across the endoplasmic reticulum. The antigen Jo-1 has been identified as histidyl-tRNA synthetase. Antibodies to at least four other amino-tRNA synthetases have been identified in patients with inflammatory muscle disease and interstitial lung disease. These include antibodies directed at threonyl-tRNA synthetase (anti-PL7),[74] alanyl-tRNA synthetase as well as alanyl tRNA (anti-PL12),[75] iso-leucyl-tRNA synthetase (anti-OJ), and glycyl-tRNA synthetase (anti-EJ).[76]

Electromyography

Electromyography is a valuable technique for determining the classification, distribution, and severity of diseases affecting skeletal muscle[162-164] (see Chapter 5). Although the changes identified are not specific, this technique should allow differentiation between myopathic and neuropathic conditions and, in the latter, localize the site of the abnormality to the central nervous system, spinal cord anterior horn cell, peripheral nerves, or neuromuscular junction. In addition, knowledge of the distribution and severity of abnormalities can guide selection of the most appropriate site to biopsy. Both spontaneous and voluntary activity can be affected by temperature, caffeine, and epinephrine as well as the age of the patient.[165, 166]

Normal muscle is electrically silent at rest, with spontaneous activity noted only when the needle electrode passes through the muscle, mechanically stimulating or damaging the fibers. This activity is termed insertional activity and is characterized by a burst of spikes of varying amplitudes.[167] Insertional activity may be increased with conditions causing irritability of fiber membranes or may be decreased if muscle fibers have been replaced by fat or fibrous tissue.

After insertional activity subsides, no potentials are generated in normal muscle unless the electrode is moved or the muscle is contracted. Abnormal spontaneous activity, however, may occur in a variety of disease states. Of the different forms of abnormal spontaneous activity, fibrillation potentials have the most diagnostic importance. These are generated by fibers that have lost their innervation.[168] Most commonly fibrillation potentials are the result of loss of or damage to some part of a lower motor

neuron; however, diseases of the neuromuscular junction and primary myopathies associated with fiber membrane damage will also produce them. The term *positive waves* is used for fibrillation potentials with a characteristic form that are produced by fibers that have been damaged and have lost innervation. Myotonic discharges are another form of spontaneous activity.[169] These differ from fibrillation in the rate and pattern of firing and are attributed to alterations in ion channels within the muscle fiber membrane. Myotonic discharges are not specific for any single disease or even for myopathic conditions.[170] A third form of spontaneous activity is termed "complex repetitive discharges." Also known as "bizarre high-frequency discharges" or "bizarre repetitive potentials," these forms generally, but not invariably, indicate muscle disease and are more commonly observed in chronic disorders.[171]

Additional information is provided from examination of potentials evoked by electrical stimulation or those generated by a voluntary muscle contraction. Both methods cause the fibers within a motor unit to fire in a synchronous fashion, producing motor unit potentials (MUPs). The size and shape of an MUP depend on the number, density, size, conduction velocity, and synchrony of firing of muscle fibers within the recording area as well as any intervening inactive fat or connective tissue.[172] Normal MUPs are triphasic, ranging from 100 µV to 5 mV in amplitude and from 3 to 15 msec in duration. In general, the amplitude reflects the potentials close to the electrode. During voluntary muscle contraction, the number of units activated will increase with the force of contraction. The activation of additional motor units is termed *recruitment*.[173]

Diseases can affect both the appearance of individual MUPs and recruitment. Typically in diseases of muscle, MUPs have reduced amplitude and shortened duration.[174] Although this pattern is often referred to as "myopathic," these changes are not specific and can also be seen in neuropathic conditions such as anterior horn cell disease, diseases of peripheral nerves, and disturbances of neuromuscular transmission. An MUP is termed *polyphasic* if it contains more than four phases, or baseline crossings. Polyphasic MUPs occur when fibers within the unit fire asynchronously. This may result from degeneration and regeneration of fibers (as occurs in many myopathies), segmental fiber destruction, or longitudinal fiber splitting. Myopathies commonly cause altered recruitment, as do other causes that reduce the number of motor units.

Patterns of Myopathic Disorders

The characteristic findings in myopathic disorders include individual MUPs of decreased duration and smaller amplitude, increased numbers of polyphasic potentials, full recruitment pattern generated with full effort despite clinical weakness, and decreased amplitude and increased density of the complex interference pattern. Inflammatory myopathies cause changes that tend to be scattered in distribution and variable in character, but most marked in the proximal muscles and paraspinal muscles. Earlier in the disease, low-amplitude MUPs of short duration and spontaneous fibrillation potentials are observed. The spontaneous fibrillations often fire at a slower rate than those seen in neuropathic disorders. Over time, MUPs tend to become more polyphasic, and more positive waves are present within the fibrillation potentials.[176]

The prominent spontaneous activity, which may also include scattered myotonic discharges and complex repetitive discharges, is characteristic of most inflammatory myopathies and distinguishes them from other myopathies. However, similar patterns of abnormalities can be seen with myasthenia gravis, glycogen storage diseases, carnitine deficiency, congenital myopthies, botulism, Duchenne's muscular dystrophy, hyperkalemic periodic paralysis, rhabdomyolysis, and trauma.

The electromyographic patterns change as the disease progresses and the myositic process becomes chronic.[177] MUPs of longer duration and higher than normal amplitude appear as regenerated fibers are reinnervated. Recruitment is reduced in proportion to the number of motor units damaged or replaced. Insertional activity is diminished with increased fibrosis. Thus, it may be difficult to distinguish chronic myositis from chronic neurogenic atrophy.

The electromyographic features of primary metabolic myopathies are quite variable. Many patients may, in fact, have relatively normal studies. Myophosphorylase deficiency and carnitine deficiency may have so-called "myopathic" MUPs and some fibrillations, occasionally limited to the paraspinal muscles. The electromyographic features of acid maltase deficiency are, in contrast, pronounced, with prominent polyphasic MUPs in proximal muscles and striking fibrillation potentials, myotonic discharges, and complex repetitive discharges.[126]

Disorders of Neuromuscular Transmission

The findings in diseases that disturb neuromuscular transmission are among the most characteristic of electromyographic abnormalities. In myasthenia gravis, a standard electromyographic study may reveal small, short MUPs and fibrillations. The classic finding, however, is a decremental response to repetitive stimulation.[178] Evoked potentials are initially normal but slowly and progressively decrease with successive stimuli. In contrast, repetitive stimulation of motor units in patients with Eaton-Lambert syndrome results in minimal responses initially followed by progressive increases in amplitude.[179]

Neuropathic Disorders

Neuropathic disorders are characterized by denervation and reinnervation. These processes result in spontaneous activity, including fibrillation potential and positive waves; polyphasic MUPs that are of large amplitude and long duration, particularly in areas of denervation; and an incomplete interference pattern. Biphasic MUPs of large amplitude and small duration are produced by denervated motor units, whereas polyphasic MUPs of long duration result from asynchronous firing of scattered reinnervated fibers. The fallout of motor units in neuropathic conditions results in an incomplete interference pattern with full effort contraction.

Muscle Biopsy and Histology

This information is invaluable in assessing myopathic conditions and is essential for establishing the diagnosis of an inflammatory myopathy.[180] Unfortunately, only in the case of an enzyme deficiency state can the examination of muscle tissue provide a specific diagnosis. Too often the changes observed are simply too nonspecific. One should not expect the pathologist to solve difficult clinical problems; rather, the biopsy should be performed with specific questions in mind.

Four types of evaluation can be performed on skeletal muscle: histology, histochemistry, electron microscopy, and assays of enzyme activities or other constituents.[181] The technique for the biopsy depends on which tests are to be done. If only histology is required, a percutaneous needle biopsy may prove satisfactory.[182] On the other hand, if all four evaluations are desired, an open technique is preferred. In the end, the method selected should be agreed on prospectively by the physician ordering the test, the individual who will perform the biopsy, and the pathologist.

The site of the biopsy should be selected carefully. A proximal muscle is preferred for the evaluation of myopathic problems. Ideally the area selected should be actively involved with the process, but the most severely involved area should be avoided. Severely damaged muscle is often too necrotic or scarred for meaningful interpretation. An electromyogram is usually helpful in localizing the site for biopsy. However, EMG needles can traumatize the muscle. Since the distribution of most myopathies is symmetric, it is best to perform the electromyography on one side of the body and take the biopsy from the identified site on the opposite side. Magnetic resonance imaging (MRI) is a noninvasive technique that may also be used to identify the optimal site for biopsy.[183] Technetium-99m pyrophosphate scanning has also been used to define areas of abnormality, but the experience with this technique is quite limited.

Infiltration of the muscle with a local anesthetic must also be avoided. Tissue for histology is fixed in formalin and embedded in paraffin for sectioning. Specimens for histochemical analysis are rapidly frozen in liquid nitrogen and sectioned in a cryostat. Hematoxylin and eosin (H&E) and modified Gomori's trichrome stains are used for most histology. A wide variety of stains are used for histochemistry.

These include *ATPase,* which stains the enzyme of the myofibrils; *NADH* and *succinic dehydrogenases,* both oxidative enzymes in the mitochondria; *myophosphorylase,* which catalyzes the initiation of glycogenolysis; *myoadenylate deaminase,* the first enzyme in the purine nucleotide cycle; *acid phosphatase* and nonspecific esterase, which stain for lysosomes and macrophages; periodic acid–Schiff (PAS) stains for *glycogen;* and oil red O for *lipid.* Staining for ATPase and enzymes of other metabolic systems is useful in determining fiber type, size, and distribution (see Table 69–2).

This combination of histologic and histochemical analysis is generally useful in differentiating myopathic from neuropathic processes. Each process is associated with characteristic, but not necessarily specific, changes. Myopathic changes include rounding and increased random variation of fiber size, internal nuclei, fibrosis, and fatty replacement. Myopathic processes may also cause necrosis associated with phagocytosis. Inflammatory myopathies are associated with fiber atrophy, degeneration, and regeneration plus inflammatory cell infiltrates in both endomysial and perimysial locations. Fiber necrosis, phagocytosis, and regeneration are also typically seen in Duchenne's muscular dystrophy.

Neuropathic conditions that cause denervation, such as disorders of the spinal cord and peripheral nerves, produce small, atrophic angular fibers. Target fibers can also result from denervation. Target fibers are seen using the ATPase stain and are generally type 1 cells. Each fiber has a central clear area surrounded by a zone of increased intensity of staining, with normal staining at the periphery. Reinnervation causes fiber type grouping; that is, aggregation of fibers all of the same type.[184]

Histochemistry is also useful in identifying other neuromuscular diseases. Applying Gomori's trichrome stain to frozen sections identifies nemaline rod and some mitochrondrial myopathies. The "ragged-red" fiber, characteristic of mitochondrial myopathies, is evident with the trichrome stain. Central core disease is apparent when the central portion of each fiber does not stain for mitochondrial enzymes. Abnormal accumulation of glycogen or lipid suggests either a glycogen storage disease or a lipid storage disease, respectively. Enzyme deficiency states may be identified with appropriate histochemical stains but are best diagnosed by subjecting the tissue protein to assays for the specific enzyme activity.[185] Ultrastructural analysis will show characteristic changes in cases of inclusion body myositis, increased numbers or altered morphology of mitochondria in mitochondrial myopathies, and abnormal glycogen or lipid deposition.

Forearm Ischemic Exercise Testing

During vigorous ischemic exercise, skeletal muscle functions anaerobically, generating lactate and ammonia. Lactate is the product of the glycolytic metabolism of glycogen and glucose. Ammonia is generated through the conversion of AMP to IMP by the activity of myoadenylate deaminase. The forearm ischemic exercise test takes advantage of this physiology and has been standardized for use in screening for various metabolic myopathies, including the recognized glycogen storage diseases (except acid maltase deficiency) and myoadenylate deaminase deficiency.[125]

The forearm ischemic exercise test is performed after drawing a venous blood sample for lactate and ammonia, preferably from the nondominant arm at rest and without the use of a tourniquet. Next, a sphygmomanometer is placed around the upper arm of the dominant side and inflated to 20 to 30 mm Hg above systolic pressure. The patient then vigorously exercises that extremity by repeatedly squeezing a ball or grip strength testing device (1 grip every 2 seconds). The exercise is continued, and the cuff inflated, for a total of 2 minutes (many normal people can exercise only for 90 seconds under these conditions if they give maximal effort). This may cause some discomfort, which is immediately relieved when the cuff is deflated. Blood samples for levels of lactate and ammonia are then drawn from the dominant arm at various time points after the cuff is deflated. Most research studies have drawn samples at intervals over 10 minutes. One sample obtained 2 minutes after the tourniquet is removed has proved useful in clinical practice. The normal response to forearm ischemic exercise is at least a three-fold rise over baseline for each metabolite. In individuals with a glycogen storage disease, the ammonia level increases normally, but lactate levels remain at baseline.[116] On the other hand, in myoadenylate deaminase deficiency, lactate levels increase but ammonia levels do not.[137] The forearm ischemic exercise test is an effective screening test, provided that the patient exercises vigorously. A submaximal exercise effort, whether due to pain, weakness, or malingering, can cause a false-positive result.[125] Therefore, failure to generate lactate or ammonia after ischemic exercise does not ensure the diagnosis of the particular enzyme deficiency. Any abnormal result should be confirmed with the appropriate enzyme analysis.

TREATMENT OF IDIOPATHIC INFLAMMATORY MYOPATHIES

To date, only one blinded, controlled therapeutic trial for the treatment of polymyositis has been published.[186] Consequently, the treatment of the inflammatory myopathies is largely empirical.[22, 187, 188] Before initiating treatment with any medication it is important to ensure an accurate diagnosis. Since there is no specific diagnostic test for the idiopathic inflammatory myopathies, these diagnoses must be arrived at by excluding other possible causes. Unfortunately, it is difficult to determine the actual effects of therapy in some patients, because some fail to respond to any treatment and others have only partial resolution of their weakness. It is therefore essential to evaluate the patient's clinical status as objectively as possible. Pretreatment testing of the strength of individual muscle groups and a timed-stands test provide valuable information. These baseline measures can be compared with those obtained after therapy is initiated. Blood pressure, chest examination, chest radiograph, and pulmonary function studies are indicated. Fluoroscopic swallowing studies with contrast material may be important if the patient has difficulty in swallowing, dysphagia, or dysphonia. Precautions that could prevent aspiration must be emphasized for patients at risk. Such precautions include education about swallowing, elevating the head of the bed on blocks, and the use of antacids or H2 blockers to neutralize gastric secretions.

Muscle enzymes including the CK, aldolase, SGOT, SGPT, and LDH should be measured, although only the most abnormal value(s) needs to be tested routinely. In addition, blood cell counts, electrolytes, creatinine, glucose, and other values that might be affected by therapy should be quantitated at baseline. The recognized association between the inflammatory myopathies and malignancy has led some physicians to perform extensive evaluations for an occult neoplasm whenever they encounter a patient with myositis. This, however, is not warranted unless some indication is provided by the history, physical examination, or routine testing.[189]

A physical therapist can prove invaluable in the treatment of the patient with myositis (see Chapter 102). Not only are they well-trained and experienced in muscle group strength testing, but also they can instruct and assist the patient in an exercise program. Exercise programs that take into account the amount of inflammatory activity are important for a good outcome. Bed rest is important, and active range of motion is to be avoided during intervals of severe inflammation. Passive motion is encouraged during these intervals in an effort to maintain range of motion and prevent contractures. A soft cervical collar may greatly benefit patients with weakness of the neck flexor muscles. Only with improvement does the program move on to active-assisted exercises and then active exercises.

Glucocorticoids are the standard first-line medication for patients with idiopathic inflammatory myopathy. Initially prednisone is given in a single dose of 1 to 2 mg per kg (with a usual arbitrary maximum of 100 mg) per day. In very severe cases some would divide the daily dose or substitute daily doses of intravenous methylprednisolone.[190] Once instituted, daily high-dose prednisone is continued until strength improves. Clinical improvement may be noted in the first weeks or gradually over 3 to 6 months. This variability is related, at least in part, to the timing of the treatment, because the earlier in the course of the illness the prednisone is given, the faster and more effectively it works.

Regular evaluations of muscle strength and serum enzymes should be performed during treatment. Ideally, the initial steroid dosage is maintained until strength and CK values have returned to normal and have remained normal for 4 to 8 weeks. Although CK levels are a useful monitor, muscle strength is more important.[191] Objective testing of strength is necessary to make certain that the patients' reported improvement is not simply due to a euphoric or "energizing" side effect of the steroids. Lowered CK values can be observed despite no improvement in strength because of circulating inhibitors present in active disease[28] or as a nonspecific consequence of the effect of the glucocorticoids. On the other hand, CK values may remain high after complete normalization of muscle strength, presumedly because the disease process has resulted in "leaky" cell membranes.

Once remission is apparent, the prednisone dosage can be tapered gradually by reducing the daily dose by about 10 mg per month. As the taper continues, therapy may be changed to an alternate-day schedule.[192] Although alternate-day steroid therapy will cause fewer side effects, if initiated too soon it may well be accompanied by a flare of the disease. To control a flare encountered at any point during a taper will probably require that the dosage be returned to the level that initially brought about the remission.

During the course of treatment, some patients who have had a partial, if not a gratifying, response to glucocorticoid therapy again develop weakness. One is then faced with the dilemma of whether the decline in muscle strength is caused by a flare of the inflammatory disease process or by steroid myopathy.[100, 101] Unfortunately, no specific test will provide the answer. Even a muscle biopsy is of little value. An active inflammatory change can be observed even when steroid myopathy is contributing to the weakness. A provocative challenge with higher doses of glucocorticoids or rapidly tapering the dose is the only way of determining the cause of the clinical decline.

Exactly how many patients will benefit or will be cured by glucocorticoid therapy is not certain. As many as 90 percent of patients will improve at least partially with glucocorticoid therapy, with 50 to 75 percent of those achieving a complete remission.[193] If, however, a patient fails to respond to glucocorticoid therapy after 6 weeks or if a patient has had some improvement but the level of strength has reached a plateau, serious consideration should be given to adding another agent.

The choice of additional therapy is between the immunosuppressive agents azathioprine and methotrexate. The usual dose of azathioprine is 2 to 3 mg per kg (with the usual maximum of 150 mg per day in a single oral dose). Azathioprine is the only drug tested in a blinded, controlled trial.[186] Patients with polymyositis and dermatomyositis whose disease had reached a plateau while receiving prednisone alone were randomized to a group to continue with prednisone alone or to a group to receive prednisone plus azathioprine. Although no difference in the groups was noted at 3 months, the group receiving azathioprine was significantly improved at 1 and 3 years.[194] Beneficial results have also been reported with methotrexate.[195] This agent is usually given on a weekly schedule at doses ranging between 5 and 15 mg orally or 15 and 50 mg intravenously. Measurements of serum SGOT and SGPT levels and pulmonary functions must be performed before initiating methotrexate therapy in order to minimize confusion between changes in these parameters caused by the basic disease and the potential hepatic and pulmonary toxicities of the medication.

Other immunosuppressive agents have been used in steroid-resistant patients. Hydroxychloroquine can be used to treat the cutaneous lesions of dermatomyositis, even in patients with an associated malignancy.[196] However, this drug has no recognized effect on the myositis. Cyclophosphamide given intravenously with concomitant oral prednisone appears to be effective in childhood disease and in some adults, although it has not proved effective in small numbers of patients with long-standing myositis, interstitial pneumonitis, or inclusion body myositis.[197, 198] Anecdotal reports suggest that 6-mercaptopurine and chlorambucil may be helpful. Recently low-dose cyclosporine therapy (2.5 to 7.5 mg per kg of body weight daily) has been observed to be very helpful and safe in children with active juvenile dermatomyositis who were unresponsive to other treatments, and in some adults.[199, 200] Additional treatments that have been employed include plasmapheresis,[201, 201a] lymphapheresis,[202] total-body or total nodal irradiation,[203] and intravenous gamma globulin.[204, 204a] Clinical trials of plasmapheresis have been difficult to evaluate because of concomitant use of immunosuppressive agents. Controlled trials involving larger numbers of patients are definitely needed to prove a benefit for any of these therapies.

The general approach to the therapy outlined previously can be applied to all the idiopathic inflammatory myopathies. However, special consideration should be given to the subset of patients with inclusion body myositis. Since this subset has generally been identified as refractory to therapy, some have suggested that treatment is futile. Indeed, steroid therapy has provided only mild, transient benefit to most patients with inclusion body myositis. However, a small number of patients have had excellent responses.[51] Therefore, it is worth a therapeutic trial for a limited time for patients with inclusion body myositis. Initially, prednisone is used as a single agent. If no benefit is found in 6 weeks, a second immunosuppressive drug should be added. If no benefit is witnessed after 6 more weeks, another agent can be substituted. If that trial fails, then treatment with immunosuppressive agents should be abandoned to avoid toxicity. In contrast, patients with an elevated CK level and an associated collagen vascular disease may have an extremely rapid response to glucocorticoid therapy. This, however, is not always the case.

The prognosis for patients with idiopathic inflammatory myopathies has improved with the availability of immunosuppressive therapy, although some argue about the amount of that improvement.[205] Studies for adults indicate a 5-year survival of 60 percent in the preglucocorticoid era,[206] 68 percent between 1947 and 1968,[207] and 80 percent in more recent reports.[208] The reasons for the improved survival are not certain but may be related to earlier and more accurate diagnosis, improved treatments for associated problems such as infection, and the earlier use of immunosuppressive agents. In general, children have a better prognosis than that of adults. Ninety percent of children with juvenile dermatomyositis who live 10 years lead normal lives. Mortality in children is attributable most often to myocarditis, perforation of a viscus, or infection. Whites have a better prognosis than do blacks. Regardless of age or race, the longer the duration of disease and the more severe the weakness at the time when therapy is initiated, the worse the morbidity and mortality. Pharyngeal muscle weakness, aspiration, and interstitial pulmonary fibrosis bode a poor diagnosis.[209] Patients with myositis and malignancy fare the worst. The actual prognosis for patients with inclusion body myositis is unknown, because of the recent discovery of the disease and the small number of patients identified. Generally, the course is slow and prolonged. Whereas the weakness becomes fixed in some, in others it continues with a relentless progression leading to severe incapacitation and death.

References

1. Erickson-Viitanen, S., Geiger, P., Yang, W. C. T., and Bessman, S. P.: The creatine–creatine phosphate shuttle for energy transport-compartmentation of creatine phosphokinase in muscle. Adv. Exp. Med. Biol. 151:115, 1982.
2. Essen, B., and Henriksson, J.: Glycogen content of individual muscle fibers in man. Acta Physiol. Scand. 90:645, 1974.
3. Goodman, M. N., and Lowenstein, J. M.: The purine nucleotide cycle. Studies of ammonia production by skeletal muscle in situ and in perfused preparations. J. Biol. Chem. 252:5054, 1977.
4. Aragon, J. J., Tornheim, K., and Lowenstein, J. M.: On a possible role of IMP in the regulation of phosphorylase activity in skeletal muscle. FEBS Lett. 117(Suppl.): K56, 1980.
5. Aragon, J. J., and Lowenstein, J. M.: The purine nucleotide cycle. Comparisons of the levels of citric acid intermediates with the operation of the purine nucleotide cycle in rat skeletal muscle during exercise and recovery from exercise. Eur. J. Biochem. 110:371, 1980.
6. Engel, W. K.: Fiber-type nomenclature of human skeletal muscle for histochemical purposes. Neurology 24:344, 1974.
7. Romanul, F. C. A.: Enzymes in muscle. 1. Histochemical studies of enzymes in individual muscle fibers. Arch. Neurol. 11:355, 1964.
8. Tunell, G. L., and Hart, M. N.: Simultaneous determination of skeletal muscle fiber types I, IIA, and IIB by histochemistry. Arch. Neurol. 34:171, 1977.
9. Pette, D., and Staron, R. S.: Molecular basis of the phenotypic characteristics of mammalian muscle fibers. Ciba Found. Symp. 138:22, 1988.
10. Brown, J. M. C., Henriksson, J., and Salmons, S.: Restoration of fast muscle characteristics following cessation of chronic stimulation: physiological, histochemical and metabolic changes during slow-to-fast transformation. Proc. R. Soc. Lond. (Biol.) 235:321, 1989.
11. Bohan, A., and Peter, J. B.: Polymyositis and dermatomyositis (first of two parts). N. Engl. J. Med. 292:344, 1975.
12. Walton, J. N., and Adams, R. D.: Polymyositis. Baltimore, Williams & Wilkins, 1958.
13. Research Group on Neuromuscular Diseases of the World Federation of Neurology: Classification of the neuromuscular disorders. J. Neurol. Sci. 6:165, 1968.
14. DeVere, R., and Bradley, W. G.: Polymyositis: its presentations, morbidity and mortality. Brain 98:637, 1975.

15. Banker, B. Q., and Engel, A. G.: The polymyositis and dermatomyositis syndromes. In Engel, A. G., and Banker, B. Q. (eds.): Myology. Vol 2. New York, McGraw-Hill, 1986.
16. Calabrese, L. H., Mitsumoto, H., and Chou, S. M.: Inclusion body myositis presenting as treatment-resistant polymyositis. Arthritis Rheum. 30:397, 1987.
17. Hochberg, M. C.: Epidemiology of polymyositis/dermatomyositis. Mt. Sinai J. Med. 55:447, 1988.
18. Cronin M. E., and Plotz, P. H.: Idiopathic inflammatory myopathies. Rheum. Dis. Clin. North Am. 16:655, 1990.
19. Pachman, L. M.: Juvenile dermatomyositis. Mt. Sinai J. Med. 55:465, 1988.
20. Walker, G. L., Mastaglia, F. L., and Roberts, D. F.: A search for genetic influence in idiopathic inflammatory myopathy. Acta Neurol. Scand. 66:432, 1982.
21. Arnett, F. C., Hirsch, T. J., Bias, W. B., et al.: The Jo-1 antibody system in myositis: Relationships to clinical features and HLA. J. Rheumatol. 8:925, 1981.
22. Plotz, P. H., Dalakas, M., Leff, R. L., Love, L. A., Miller, F. W., and Cronin, M. E.: Current concepts in the idiopathic inflammatory myopathies: polymyositis, dermatomyositis, and related disorders. Ann. Intern. Med. 111(2): 143, 1989.
23. Bohan, A., Peter, J. B., Bowman, B. S., and Pearson, C. M.: A computer-assisted analysis of 153 patients with polymyositis and dermatomyositis. Medicine 56:255, 1977.
24. Strongwater, S. L.: Overview and clinical manifestations of inflammatory myositis: polymyositis and dermatomyositis. Mt. Sinai J. Med. 55:435, 1988.
25. Misra, A., Singh, R. R., Kapoor, S. K., Kumar, A., and Malaviya, A. N.: A fatal case of acute polymyositis with persistent myoglobinuria and progressive renal failure. J. Assoc. Physicians India 36(2):153, 1988.
26. Tazelaar, H. D., Viggiano, R. W., Pickersgill, J., and Colby, T. V.: Interstitial lung disease in polymyositis and dermatomyositis. Clinical features and prognosis as correlated with histologic findings. Am. Rev. Respir. Dis. 14:272, 1990.
27. Agrawal, C. S., Behari, M., Shrivastava, S., et al.: The heart in polymyositis-dermatomyositis. J. Neurol. 236(4):249, 1989.
28. Kagen, L. J., and Aram, S.: Creatine kinase activity inhibitor in sera from patients with muscle disease. Arthritis Rheum. 30:213, 1987.
29. Szmidt-Salkowska, E., Rowinska-Marcinska, K., and Lovelace, R. E.: EMG dynamics in polymyositis and dermatomyositis in adults. Electromyogr. Clin. Neurophysiol. 29:399, 1989.
30. Ringel, S. P., Carry, M. R., Aguilera, A. J., and Starcevich, J. M.: Quantitative histopathology of the inflammatory myopathies. Arch. Neurol. 43:1004, 1986.
31. Carpenter, S.: Resin histology and electron microscopy in inflammatory myopathies. In Dalakas, M. C. (eds.): Polymyositis and Dermatomyositis. Boston, Butterworths, 1988, pp. 195–215.
32. Arahata, K., and Engel, A. G.: Monoclonal antibody analysis of mononuclear cells in myopathies. V: Identification and quantitation of T8+ cytotoxic and T8+ suppressor cells. Ann. Neurol. 23:493, 1988.
33. Stahl, N. I., Klippel, J. H., and Decker, J. L.: A cutaneous lesion associated with myositis. Ann. Intern. Med. 91:577, 1979.
34. Ganczarczyk, M. L., Lee, P., and Armstrong, S. K.: Nailfold capillary microscopy in polymyositis and dermatomyositis. Arhthritis Rheum. 31:116, 1988.
35. Engel, A. G., and Arahata, K.: Mononuclear cells in myopathies: quantitation of functionally distinct subsets, recognition of antigen-specific cell-mediated cytotoxicity in some diseases, and implications for the pathogenesis of the different inflammatory myopathies. Hum. Pathol. 17:704, 1986.
36. Roberts, L. J., and Fink, C. W.: Childhood polymyositis/dermatomyositis. Clin. Dermatol. 6:36, 1988.
37. Gamstorp, I.: Dermatomyositis and polymyositis in childhood. Brain Dev. 12:345, 1990.
38. Arahata, K., and Engel, A. G.: Monoclonal antibody analysis of mononuclear cells in myopathies. I. Quantitation of subsets according to diagnosis and sites of accumulation and demonstration and counts of muscle fibers invaded by T cells. Ann. Neurol. 16:193, 1984.
39. Ringel, R. A., Brick, J. E., Brick, J. F., et al.: Muscle involvement in the scleroderma syndromes. Arch. Intern. Med. 150:2550, 1990.
40. Brooke, M. H., and Kaplan, H.: Muscle pathology in rheumatoid arthritis, polymyalgia rheumatica and polymyositis. A histochemical study. Arch. Pathol. 94:101, 1972.
41. Bezecny, R.: Dermatomyositis. Arch. Dermatol. Syphilol. 171:242, 1935.
42. Masi, A. T., and Hochberg, M. C.: Temporal association of polymyositis-dermatomyositis with malignancy: methodologic and clinical considerations. Mt. Sinai J. Med. 55:471, 1988.
43. Callen, J. P.: Myositis and malignancy. Curr. Opin. Rheumatol. 1:468, 1989.
44. Lakhanpal, S., Bunch, T. W., Ilstrup, D. M., and Melton, L. J.: Polymyositis-dermatomyositis and malignant lesions: does an association exist? Mayo Clin. Proc. 61:645, 1986.
45. Deroo, H., DeBersaques, J., and Naeyaert, J. M.: Paraneoplastic dermatomyositis in an adolescent. Dermatologica 174:392, 1988.
46. Chou, S. M.: Myxovirus-like structures in a case of human chronic polymyositis. Science 158:1453, 1967.
47. Kula, R. W., Sawchak, J. A., and Sher, J. H.: Inclusion body myositis. Curr. Opin. Rheumatol. 1:460, 1989.
48. Riggs, J. E., Schochet, S. S., Jr., Gutmann, L., and Lerfald, S. C.: Childhood onset inclusion body myositis mimicking limb-girdle muscular dystrophy. J. Child. Neurol. 4:283, 1989.
49. Lotz, B. P., Engel, A. G., Nishino, H., et al.: Inclusion body myositis. Observations in 40 patients. Brain 112:727, 1989.
50. Dumitru, D., and Newell-Eggert, M.: Inclusion myositis. An electrophysiologic study. Am. J. Phys. Med. Rehabil. 69:2, 1990.
51. Cohen, M. R., Sulaiman, A. R., Garancis, J. C., and Wortmann, R. L.: Clinical heterogeneity and treatment response in inclusion body myositis. Arthritis Rheum. 32:734, 1989.
52. Serratrice, G., Pellissier, J. F., Roux, H., and Quilichini, P.: Fasciitis, perimyositis, myositis, polymyositis, and eosinophilia. Muscle Nerve 13:385, 1990.
53. Peison, B., Benisch, B., Lim, M., and Chin, J. C.: Idiopathic hypereosinophilic syndrome with polymyositis. South Med. J. 81:403, 1988.
54. Kaufman, L. D., Seidman, R. J., and Ruber, B. L.: L-Tryptophan–associated eosinophilic perimyositis, neuritis, and fasciitis. Medicine 69:187, 1990.
55. Martin, R. W., Duffy, J., Engel, A. G., et al.: The clinical spectrum of the eosinophilic-myalgia syndrome associated with L-tryptophan ingestion. Ann. Intern. Med. 113:124, 1990.
56. Belongia, E. A., Hedberg, C. W., Gleich, G. J., et al.: An investigation of the cause of the eosinophilia-myalgia syndrome associated with tryptophan use. N. Engl. J. Med. 323:357, 1990.
57. Siegert, J. J., and Wortmann, R. L.: Myositis ossificans simulating acute monoarticular arthritis. J. Rheumatol. 13:652, 1986.
58. Lagier, R., and Cox, J. N.: Pseudomalignant myositis ossificans: a pathologic study of eight cases. Hum. Pathol. 6:653, 1975.
59. Illingworth, R. S.: Myositis ossificans progressiva (Munchmeyer's disease). Brief review with report of two cases treated with corticosteroids and observed for 16 years. Arch. Dis. Child. 46:264, 1971.
60. Coakley, J. H., Smith, P. E., Jackson, M. J., et al.: Myositis ossificans non-progressiva–reversible muscle calcification in polymyositis. Br. J. Rheumatol. 28:443, 1989.
61. Russell, G. G., Smith, R., Bishop, M. C., et al.: Treatment of myositis ossificans progressiva with a diphosphonate. Lancet 1:10, 1972.
62. Noda, S., Umezaki, H., Itoh, H., et al.: Chronic focal polymyositis (letter). J. Neurol. Neurosurg. Psychiatry 51(5):728, 1988.
63. Brown, P., Doyle, D. V., and Evans, M. D.: Localized nodular myositis as the first manifestation of polymyositis. Br. J. Rheumatol. 28:84, 1989.
64. Silverstein, A., and Siltzbach, L. E.: Muscle involvement in sarcoidosis. Asymptomatic myositis and myopathy. Arch. Neurol. 21:235, 1969.
65. Kattah, J. C., Zimmerman, L. E., Kolsky, M. P., et al.: Bilateral orbital involvement in fatal giant cell polymyositis. Ophthalmology 97:520, 1990.
66. Arahata, K., and Engel, A. G.: Monoclonal antibody analysis of mononuclear cells in myopathies. IV. Cell-mediated cytotoxicity and muscle fiber necrosis. Ann. Neurol. 23:168, 1988.
67. Botet, J. C., Grau, J. M., Casademont, J., et al.: Characterization of mononuclear exudates in idiopathic inflammatory myopathies. Virchows Arch. [A] 412:371, 1988.
68. Emslie-Smith, A. M., Arahata, K., and Engel, A.: Major histocompatibility complex class I antigen expression, immunolocalization of interferon subtypes, and T-cell–mediated cytotoxicity in myopathies. Hum. Pathol. 20:224, 1989.
69. Wolf, R. E., and Baethge, B. A.: Interleukin-1 alpha, interleukin-2, and soluble interleukin-2 receptors in polymyositis. Arthritis Rheum. 33:1007, 1990.
70. Miller, F. W., Love, L. A., Barbieri, S. A., et al.: Lymphocyte activation markers in idiopathic myositis: changes with disease activity and differences among clinical and autoantibody subgroups. Clin. Exp. Immunol. 81:373, 1990.
71. Kissel, J. T., Mendell, J. R., and Rammohan, K. W.: Microvascular deposition of complement membrane attack complex in dermatomyositis. N. Engl. J. Med. 314:329, 1986.
72. Targoff, I. N., and Reichlin, M.: Humoral immunity in polymyositis and dermatomyositis. Mt. Sinai J. Med. 55:487, 1988.
73. Goldstein, R., Duvic, M., Targoff, I. N., et al.: HLA-D region genes associated with autoantibody responses to histidyl-transfer RNA synthetase (Jo-1) and other translation-related factors in myositis. Arthritis Rheum. 33:1240, 1990.
74. Targoff, I. N., Arnett, F. C., and Reichlin, M.: Antibody to threonyl-transfer RNA synthetase in myositis sera. Arthritis Rheum. 31:515, 1988.
75. Targoff, I. N., and Arnett, F. C.: Clinical manifestations in patients with antibody to PL-12 antigen (alanyl-tRNA synthetase). Am. J. Med. 88:241, 1990.
76. Targoff, I. N.: Autoantibodies to aminoacyl-transfer RNA synthetases

for isoleucine and glycine. Two additional synthetases are antigenic in myositis. J. Immunol. 144:1737, 1990.

77. Targoff, I. N., Johnson, A. E., and Miller F. W.: Antibody to signal recognition particle in polymyositis. Arthritis Rheum. 33:1361, 1990.

78. Manta, P., Kalfakis, N., and Vassilopoulos, D.: Evidence for seasonal variation in polymyositis. Neuroepidemiology 8:262, 1989.

79. Walker, E. J., and Jeffrey, P. D.: Sequence homology between encephalomyocarditis virus protein VPI and histidyl-tRNA synthetase. Med. Hypotheses 25:21, 1988.

80. Crennan, J. M., Van Scoy, R. E., McKenna, C. H., and Smith, T. F.: Echovirus polymyositis in patients with hypogammaglobulinemia. Failure of high-dose intravenous gammaglobulin therapy and review of the literature. Am. J. Med. 81:35, 1986.

81. Christensen, M. L., Pachman, L. M., Schneiderman, R., et al.: Prevalence of coxsackie B virus antibodies in patients with juvenile dermatomyositis. Arthritis Rheum. 29:1365, 1986.

82. Chou, S. M.: Inclusion body myositis: a chronic persistent mumps myositis? Hum. Pathol. 17:765, 1986.

83. Bowles, N. E., Sewry, C. A., Dubowitz, V., and Archard, L. C.: Dermatomyositis, polymyositis, and coxsackie-B virus infection. Lancet 1:1004, 1987.

84. Yousef, G. E., Isenberg, D. A., and Mowbray, J. F.: Detection of enterovirus specific RNA sequences in muscle biopsy specimens from patients with adult onset myositis. Ann. Rheum. Dis. 49:310, 1990.

85. Ytterberg, S. R., Mahowald, M. L., and Messner, R. P.: Coxsackievirus B1–induced polymyositis. Lack of disease expression in nu/nu mice. J. Clin. Invest. 80:499, 1987.

86. Ytterberg, S. R., Mahowald, M. L., and Messner, R. P.: T cells are required for induction of murine polymyositis by coxsackievirus B1. J. Rheumatol. 15:475, 1988.

87. Cronin, M. E., Love, L. A., Miller, F. W., et al.: The natural history of encephalomyocarditis virus–induced myositis and myocarditis in mice. Viral persistence demonstrated by in situ hybridization. J. Exp. Med. 168:1639, 1988.

88. Goldstein, R., Duvic, M., Targoff, I. N., et al.: Serologic and restriction enzyme studies of HLA-D region genes in myositis. Arthritis Rheum. 31:533, 1988.

89. Chowdhury, S., Ytterberg, S. R., and Wortmann, R. L.: Alteration in intermediary metabolism in murine polymyositis. Arthritis Rheum. 32:R30, 1989.

90. Chowdhury, S. A., Ytterbertg, S. R., and Wortmann R. L.: Abnormal energy metabolism in murine polymyositis. Arthritis Rheum. 32:S125, 1989.

91. Sabina, R. L., Sulaiman, A. R., and Wortmann, R. L.: Reduced transcript availability and myoadenylate deaminase (MAD) activity in polymyositis. Implications for acquired MAD deficiency. Arthritis Rheum. 33:S70, 1990.

92. Park, J. H., Vansant, J. P., Kumar, N. G., et al.: Dermatomyositis: correlative MR imaging and P-31 MR spectroscopy for quantitative characterization of inflammatory disease. Radiology 177:473, 1990.

93. Bradley, W. G.: The limb-girdle syndromes. In Vinken, P. J., and Bruyn, G. W. (eds.): Handbook of Clinical Neurology. Vol. 40. Amsterdam, Elsevier/North-Holland, 1979.

94. Tandan, R., and Bradley, W. G.: ALS and other motor neuron diseases. In Asbury, A. K., McKhann, G. M., and Macdonald, W. I. (eds.): Diseases of the Nervous System. Vol. 2. Philadelphia, W. B. Saunders Co., 1986.

95. Tandan, R., and Bradley, W. G.: Amyotrophic lateral sclerosis. Part 1: Clinical features, pathology and ethical issues in management. Ann. Neurol. 18:271, 1985.

96. Engel, A.: Acquired autoimmune myasthenia gravis. In Engel, A. G., and Banker, B. Q. (eds.): Myology. 1st ed. New York, McGraw-Hill Book Co., 1986.

97. Dropcho, E. J.: Autoimmune aspects of neurologic paraneoplastic syndromes. Clin. Aspects Autoimmunity 4:8, 1989.

98. O'Neill, J. H., Murrary, N. M., and Newsom-Davis, J.: The Eaton-Lambert myasthenic syndrome: a review of 50 cases. Brain 111:577, 1988.

99. Zuckner, J.: Drug-induced myopathies. Semin. Arthritis Rheum. 19:259, 1990.

100. Afifi, A. K., Bergman, R. A., and Harvey, J. C.: Steroid myopathy. Clinical, histologic, and cytologic observations. Johns Hopkins Med. J. 123:158, 1968.

101. Askari, A., Vignos, P. J., and Moskowitz, R. W.: Steroid myopathy in connective tissue disease. Am. J. Med. 61:485, 1976.

102. Kuncl, R. W., Duncan, G., Watson, D., et al.: Colchicine and neuropathy. N. Engl. J. Med. 316:1562, 1987.

103. Estes, M. L., Ewing-Wilson, D., Chou, S. M., et al.: Chloroquine neuromyotoxicity. Clinical and pathologic perspective. Am. J. Med. 82:447, 1987.

104. Halla, J. T., Fallahi, S., and Koopman, W. J.: Penicillamine-induced myositis. Observations and unique features in two patients and review of the literature. Am. J. Med. 77:719, 1984.

105. Urbano-Marquez, A., Estruch, R., Navarro-Lopez, F., et al.: The effects

106. Pierce, L. R., Wysowski, D. K., and Gross, T. P.: Myopathy and rhabdomyolysis associated with lovastatin-gemfibrozil combination therapy. J.A.M.A. 264:71, 1990.

107. McKinlay, I. A., and Mitchell, I.: Transient acute myositis in childhood. Arch. Dis. Child. 51:135, 1976.

108. Hanissian, A. S., Martinez, A. J., Jabbour, J. T., and Duenas, D. A.: Vasculitis and myositis secondary to rubella vaccination. Arch. Neurol. 28:202, 1973.

109. Nordstrom, D. M., Petropolis, A. A., Giorno, R., et al.: Inflammatory myopathy and acquired immunodeficiency syndrome. Arthritis Rheum. 32:475, 1989.

110. Wrzolek, M. A., Sher, J. H., Kozlowski, P. B., and Chandrakant, R.: Skeletal muscle pathology in AIDS: an autopsy study. Muscle Nerve 13:508, 1990.

111. Gabbai, A. A., Schmidt, B., Castelo, A., et al.: Muscle biopsy in ARC: analysis of 50 patients. Muscle Nerve 13:541, 1990.

112. Dalakas, M. C., Illa, I., Pezeshkpour, G. H., et al.: Mitochondrial myopathy caused by long-term zidovudine therapy. N. Engl. J. Med. 332:1098, 1990.

113. Altrocchi, P. H.: Spontaneous bacterial myositis. J.A.M.A. 217:819, 1971.

114. Samuels, B. S., and Rietschal, R. L.: Polymyositis and toxoplasmosis. J.A.M.A. 235:60, 1976.

115. Kagen, L. T., Kimball, A. C., and Christian, C. L.: Serologic evidence of toxoplasmosis among patients with polymyositis. Am. J. Med. 56:186, 1974.

116. McArdle, B.: Myopathy due to a defect in muscle glycogen breakdown. Clin. Sci. 24:13, 1951.

117. DiMauro, S., and Bresolin, N.: Phosphorylase deficiency. In Engel, A. G., and Banker, B. Q. (eds.): Myology. 1st ed. New York, McGraw-Hill Book Co., 1986.

118. Pernow, B. B., Havel, R. J., and Jennings, D. B.: The second-wind phenomenon in McArdle's syndrome. Acta Med. Scand. 472 (Suppl.):294, 1967.

119. Kleinman, D. S., and Kunze, H. E.: McArdle's disease and acute renal failure. Nephron 48:255, 1988.

120. Mastaglia, G. C., McCollum, J. P. K., Larson, P. F., and Hudgson, P.: Steroid myopathy complicating McArdle's disease. J. Neurol. Neurosurg. Psychiatry 33:111, 1970.

121. Pourmand, R., Sander, D. B., and Corwin, H. M.: Late-onset McArdle's disease with unusual electromyographic findings. Arch. Neurol. 40:374, 1983.

122. Damon, M. J., Serenella, S., DiMauro, S., and Vora, S.: Late-onset muscle phosphofructokinase deficiency. Neurology 38:956, 1988.

123. Higgs, J. B., Blaivas, M., and Albers, J. W.: McArdle's disease presenting as treatment-resistant polymyositis. J. Rheumatol. 16:1588, 1989.

124. Munsat, T. L.: A standardized forearm ischemic exercise test. Neurology 20:1171, 1970.

125. Valen, P. A., Nakayama, D., Veum, J. A., et al.: Myoadenylate deaminase deficiency and forearm ischemic exercise testing. Arthritis Rheum. 30:661, 1987.

126. Engel, A. G., Gomez, M. R., Seybold, M. E., and Lambert, E. H.: The spectrum and diagnosis of acid maltase deficiency. Neurology 23:95, 1973.

127. Engel, A. G.: Acid maltase deficiency in adults: studies in four cases of a syndrome which may mimic muscular dystrophy or other myopathies. Brain 93:599, 1970.

128. Keunen, R. W., Lambregts, P. C., Op de Coul, A. A., and Joosten, E. M.: Respiratory failure as initial symptom of acid maltase deficiency. J. Neurol. Neurosurg. Psychiatry 47:549, 1984.

129. DiMauro, S., and Papadimitrion, A.: Carnitine palmitoyltransferase deficiency. In Engel, A. G., and Banker, B. Q. (eds.): Myology. 1st ed. New York, McGraw-Hill Book Co., 1986.

130. Ross, N. S., and Hoppel, C. L.: Partial muscle carnitine palmitoyltransferase-A deficiency. Rhabdomyolysis associated with transiently decreased muscle carnitine content after ibuprofen therapy. J.A.M.A. 257:60, 1987.

131. Engel, A. G.: Carnitine deficiency syndromes and lipd storage myopathies. In Engel, A. G., and Banker, B. Q. (eds.): Myology. 1st ed. New York, McGraw-Hill Book Co., 1986.

132. Strumpf, D. A., Parker, W. D., and Angelini, C.: Carnitine deficiency, organic acidemias, and Reye's syndrome. Neurology 35:1041, 1985.

133. Keith, R. E.: Symptoms of carnitine-like deficiency in a trained runner taking DL-carnitine supplements. J.A.M.A. 255:1137, 1986.

134. VanDyke, D. H., Griggs, K. R. C., Markesbery, W., and DiMauro, S.: Hereditary carnitine deficiency of muscle. Neurology 25:154, 1975.

135. Issacs, H., Heffron, J. J. A., Badenhorst, M., et al.: Weakness associated with the pathological presence of lipid in skeletal muscle: a detailed study of a patient with carnitine deficiency. J. Neurol. Neurosurg. Psychiatry 39:1114, 1976.

136. Turnbull, D. M., Shepherd, I. M., Ashworth, B., et al.: Lipid storage

myopathy associated with low acyl-CoA dehydrogenase activities. Brain 111:815, 1988.

137. Fishbein, W. N.: Myoadenylate deaminase deficiency: Inherited and acquired forms. Biochem. Med. 33:158, 1985.

138. Sabina, R. L., Swain, J. L., Olanow, C. W., et al.: Myoadenylate deaminase deficiency. Functional and metabolic abnormalities associated with disruption of the purine nucleotide cycle. J. Clin. Invest. 73:720, 1984.

139. Shergy, W. J., and Caldwell, D. S.: Polymyositis after propylthiouracil treatment for hyperthyroidism. Ann. Rheum. Dis. 47:340, 1988.

140. Harding, A. E., Petty, R. K. H., and Morgan-Hughes, J. A.: Mitochondrial myopathy: a genetic study of 71 cases. J. Med. Genet. 25:528, 1988.

141. Morgan-Hughes, J. A.: The mitochondrial myopathies. In Engel, A. G., and Banker, B. Q. (eds.): Myology. 1st ed. New York, McGraw-Hill Book Co., 1986.

142. Salvarani, C., Marcello, N., Macchioni, P., et al.: Hypothyroidism simulating polymyositis. Report of two cases. Scand. J. Rheumatol. 17:147, 1988.

143. Shergy, W. J., and Caldwell, D. S.: Polymyositis after propylthiouracil treatment for hyperthyroidism. Ann. Rheum. Dis. 47:340, 1988.

144. Joborn, C., Rastad, J., Stalberg, E., et al.: Muscle function in patients with primary hyperparathyroidism. Muscle Nerve 12:87, 1989.

145. Knochel, J. P.: Neuromuscular manifestations of electrolyte disorders. Am. J. Med. 72:521, 1982.

146. Gabow, P. A., Kaehny, W. D., and Kelleher, S. P.: The spectrum of rhabdomyolysis. Medicine 61:141, 1982.

147. Rowland, L. P.: Myoglobinuria. Can. J. Neurol. Sci. 11:1, 1984.

148. Ward, M. M.: Factors predictive of acute renal failure in rhabdomyolysis. Arch. Intern. Med. 148:1553, 1988.

149. Csuka, M., and McCarty, D. J.: A simple method for measurement of lower extremity muscle strength. Am. J. Med. 78:77, 1985.

150. Larca, L. J., Coppola, J. T., and Honig, S.: Creatine kinase MB isoenzyme in dermatomyositis: a noncardiac source. Ann. Intern. Med. 94:341, 1981.

151. Elin, R. J., Foidart, M., Adornato, B. T., et al.: Quantification of acute phase reactants after muscle biopsy. J. Lab. Clin. Med. 100:566, 1982.

152. Clarkson, P. M., Apple, F. S., Byrnes, W. C., et al.: Creatine kinase isoforms following isometric exercise. Muscle Nerve 10:41, 1987.

153. Nicholson, G. A., Morgan, G. J., Meerkin, M., et al.: The effect of aerobic exercise on serum creatine kinase activities. Muscle Nerve 9:820, 1986.

154. Roberts, R., and Sobel, B. E.: Effect of selected drugs and myocardial infarction on the disappearance of creatine kinase from the circulation in conscious dogs. Cardiovasc. Res. 11:103, 1977.

155. Black, H. R., Quallich, H., and Gareleck, C. B.: Racial differences in serum creatine kinase levels. Am. J. Med. 81:479, 1986.

156. Bais, R., and Edwards, J. B.: Increased creatine kinase activities associated with hemolysis. Pathology 12:203, 1980.

157. Joy, J. L., and Oh, S. J.: Asymptomatic hyper-CK-emia: An electrophysiologic and histopathologic study. Muscle Nerve 12:206, 1989.

158. Takasu, T., and Hughes, B. P.: Lactate dehydrogenase isozyme patterns in human skeletal muscle. J. Neurol. Neurosurg. Psychiatry 32:175, 1969.

159. Nishikai, M., and Reichlin, M.: Radioimmunoassay of serum myoglobin in polymyositis and other conditions. Arthritis Rheum. 20:1514, 1977.

160. Kagen, L. J., and Furevich, R.: "Myoglobinolytic" activity of human skeletal muscle and other tissues. Proc. Soc. Exp. Biol. Med. 130:923, 1969.

161. Long, C. L., Dillard, D. R., Bodzin, J. H., et al.: Validity of 3-methylhistidine excretion as an indicator of skeletal muscle protein breakdown in humans. Metabolism 37:844, 1988.

162. Kimura, J.: Electrodiagnosis in Diseases of Nerve and Muscle: Principles and Practice. 1st ed. Philadelphia, F. A. Davis, 1983.

163. Daube, J. R.: Electrodiagnostics of muscle disorders. In Engel, A. G., and Banker, B. Q. (eds.): Myology. 1st ed. New York, McGraw-Hill Book Co., 1986.

164. Bradley, W. G., and Fries, T. J.: Neuromuscular testing. In Kelley, W. N., Harris, E. D., Jr., Ruddy, S., and Sledge, C. B. (eds.): Textbook of Rheumatology. 3rd ed. Philadelphia, W. B. Saunders, 1989.

165. Buchthal, F., Pinelli, P., and Kosenfalck, P.: Action potential parameters in normal human muscle and their physiological determinants. Acta Physiol. Scand. 32:219, 1954.

166. Bolton, C. F., Sawa, G. M., and Carter, K.: The effects of temperature on human compound action potentials. J. Neurol. Neurosurg. Psychiatry 44:407, 1981.

167. Meadows, J. C.: Observations on the responses of muscle to mechanical and electrical stimuli. J. Neurol. Neurosurg. Psychiatry 34:57, 1971.

168. Thesleff, S.: Fibrillation in denervated mammalian skeletal muscle. In Culp, W. J., and Ochoa, J. (eds.): Abnormal Nerves and Muscles as Impulse Generators. New York, Oxford University Press, 1982.

169. Bryant, S. H.: Abnormal repetitive impulse production in myotonic muscle. In Culp, W. J., and Ochoa, J. (eds.): Abnormal Nerves and Muscles as Impulse Generators. New York, Oxford University Press, 1982.

170. Brumlik, J., Dreschsler, B., and Vannin, T. M.: The myotonic discharge in various neurological syndromes: a neurophysiological analysis. Electromyography 10:369, 1970.

171. Eisen, A. A., and Karpati, G.: Spontaneous electrical activity in muscle: description of two patients with motor neurone disease. J. Neurol. Sci. 12:121, 1971.

172. Gath, I., and Stalberg, E.: On the volume conduction in human skeletal muscle: in situ measurements. Electroencephalogr. Clin. Neurophysiol. 43:106, 1977.

173. Milner-Brown, H. S., and Stein, R. B.: The relation between the surface electromyogram and muscular force. J. Physiol. (Lond.) 246:549, 1975.

174. Gath, I., Sjaastad, O., and Loken, A. C.: Myopathic electromyographic changes correlated with histopathology in Wohlfart-Kugelberg-Welander disease. Neurology (Minneap.) 19:344, 1969.

175. Lindstrom, L., and Petersen, I.: Power spectra of myoelectric signals: motor unit activity and muscle fatigue. In Stalberg, E., and Young, R. R. (eds.): Clinical Neurophysiology. London, Butterworths, 1981.

176. Streib, E. W., Wilbourn, A. J., and Mitsumoto, H.: Spontaneous electrical muscle fiber activity in polymyositis and dermatomyositis. Muscle Nerve 2:14, 1979.

177. Mechler, F.: Changing electromyographic findings during the chronic course of polymyositis. J. Neurol. Sci. 23:237, 1974.

178. Ozdemir, C., and Young, R. R.: The results to be expected from electrical testing in the diagnosis of myasthenia gravis. Ann. N.Y. Acad. Sci. 274:203, 1976.

179. Lambert, E. H., Rooke, E. D., Eaton, L. M., and Hodgson, C. H.: Myasthenic syndrome occasionally associated with bronchial neoplasm: Neurophysiologic studies. In Viets, H. (ed.): Second International Symposium on Myasthenia Gravis. Springfield, IL, Charles C Thomas, 1961.

180. Pamphlett, R.: Muscle biopsy. In Mastaglia, F. L. (ed.): Inflammatory Diseases of Muscle. 1st ed. Oxford, Blackwell Scientific Publications, 1988.

181. Dubowitz, V.: Muscle Biopsy, A Modern Approach. London, Balliere Tindall, 1985.

182. Edwards, R., Young, A., and Wiles, M.: Needle biopsy of skeletal muscle in the diagnosis of myopathy and the clinical study of muscle function and repair. N. Engl. J. Med. 302:261, 1980.

183. Murphy, W. A., Totty, W. G., and Carrol, J. E.: MRI of normal and pathologic skeletal muscle. Radiology 162:251, 1987.

184. Fewings, J. D., Harris, J. B., Johnson, M. A., and Bradley, W. G.: Progressive denervation of skeletal muscle induced by spinal irradiation in rats. Brain 100:157, 1977.

185. Mitsumoto, H.: McArdle's disease: phosphorylase activity in regenerating muscle fibers. Neurology 29:258, 1979.

186. Bunch, T. W., Worthington, J. W., Combs, J. J., et al.: Azathioprine with prednisone for polymyositis. A controlled, clinical trial. Ann. Intern. Med. 92:365, 1980.

187. Dalakas, M.: Treatment of polymyositis and dermatomyositis. Curr. Opin. Rheumatol. 1:443, 1989.

188. Bunch, T. W.: The therapy of polymyositis. Mt. Sinai J. Med. 55:483, 1988.

189. Cox, N. H., Langtry, J. A. A., Lawrence, C. M., and Ive, F. A.: Dermatomyositis and malignancy: an audit of the value of extensive investigations. Br. J. Dermatol. 121:47, 1989.

190. Yanagisawa, T., Sueishi, M., Nawata, Y., et al.: Methylprednisolone pulse therapy in dermatomyositis. Dermatologica 167:47, 1983.

191. Oddis, C. V., and Medsger, T. A., Jr.: Relationship between serum creatine kinase level and corticosteroid therapy in polymyositis-dermatomyositis. J. Rheumatol. 15:807, 1988.

192. Uchino, M., Araki, S., Yoshida, O., et al.: High single-dose, alternate-day corticosteroid regimens in treatment of polymyositis. J. Neurol. 232:175, 1985.

193. Henriksson, K. G., and Sandstedt, P.: Polymyositis—treatment and prognosis. A study of 107 patients. Acta Neurol. Scand. 65:280, 1982.

194. Bunch, T. W.: Prednisone and azathioprine for polymyositis: long-term follow-up. Arthritis Rheum. 24:45, 1981.

195. Metzger, A. L., Bohan, A., Goldberg, L. S., et al.: Polymyositis and dermatomyositis: combined methotrexate and corticosteroid therapy. Ann. Intern. Med. 81:182, 1974.

196. Woo, T. Y., Callen, J. P., Voorhees, J. J., et al.: Cutaneous lesions of dermatomyositis are improved by hydroxychloroquine. J. Am. Acad. Dermatol. 10:592, 1984.

197. al-Janadi, M., Smith, C. D., and Karsh, J.: Cyclophosphamide treatment of interstitial pulmonary fibrosis in polymyositis/dermatomyositis. J. Rheumatol. 16:1592, 1989.

198. Bombardieri, S., Hughes, G. R., Neri, R., et al.: Cyclophosphamide in severe polymyositis (letter). Lancet 1:1138, 1989.

199. Heckmatt, J., Hasson, N., Saunders, C., et al.: Cyclosporine in juvenile dermatomyositis. Lancet 1:1063, 1988.

200. Jongen, P. J., Joosten, E. M., Berden, J. H., and Ter-Laak, H. J.:

Cyclosporine therapy in chronic slowly progressive polymyositis—preliminary report of clinical results in three patients. Transplant. Proc. 20(Suppl. 4):335, 1988.

201. Clarke, C. R., Dyall-Smith, D. J., Mackay, I. R., et al.: Plasma exchange in dermatomyositis/polymyositis: beneficial effects in three cases. J. Clin. Lab. Immunol. 27:149, 1988.

201a. Miller, F. W., Leitman, S. F., Cronin, M. E., et al.: Controlled trial of plasma exchange and leukapheresis in polymyositis and dermatomyositis. N. Engl. J. Med. 326:1380, 1992.

202. Howard, J. F., Jr.: Therapeutic apheresis and polymyositis. J. Clin. Apheresis 5:61, 1990.

203. Kelly, J. J., Mudoc-Jones, H., Adelman, L. S., et al.: Response to total body irradiation in dermatomyositis. Muscle Nerve 11:120, 1988.

204. Cherin, P., Herson, S., Wechsler, B., et al.: Intravenous immunoglobulin for polymyositis and dermatomyositis (letter). Lancet 336(8707):116, 1990.

204a. Cherin, P., Herson, S., Wechsler, B., et al.: Efficacy of intravenous gammaglobulin therapy in chronic refractory polymyositis and dermatomyositis: an open study with 20 adult patients. Am. J. Med. 91:162, 1991.

205. Tuffanelli, D. L., and Lavoie, P. E.: Prognosis and therapy of polymyositis/dermatomyositis. Clin. Dermatol. 6:93, 1988.

206. O'Leary, P. A., and Waisman, M.: Dermatomyositis. Arch. Dermatol. 41:1001, 1940.

207. Medsger, T. A., Robinson, H., and Masi, A. T.: Factors affecting survivorship in polymyositis. A life-table study of 124 patients. Arthritis Rheum. 15:168, 1986.

208. Hochberg, M. C., Feldman, D., and Stevens, M. B.: Adult onset polymyositis/dermatomyositis: an analysis of clinical and laboratory features and survival in 76 patients with a review of the literature. Semin. Arthritis Rheum. 15:168, 1986.

209. Arsura, E. L., and Greenberg, A. S.: Adverse impact of interstitial pulmonary fibrosis on prognosis in polymyositis and dermatomyositis. Semin. Arthritis Rheum. 18:29, 1988.

Rheumatic Diseases of Childhood

Chapter 70

James T. Cassidy

Juvenile Rheumatoid Arthritis

Juvenile rheumatoid arthritis (JRA) is the most frequent major connective tissue disease in children.[1] It is one of the more common chronic illnesses of childhood and is a major cause of functional disability and of eye disease leading to blindness.

JRA differs in many respects from rheumatoid arthritis (RA) in adults. Oligoarthritis is common, and systemic onset is seen more frequently. Large joints such as the knees, wrists, and ankles are more prominently involved than small joints, and there are less frequent complaints of joint pain. Subcutaneous nodules and rheumatoid factor (RF) seropositivity are unusual, but antinuclear antibody (ANA) seropositivity is a hallmark of this disease. Inflammation and ankylosis of the posterior apophyseal joints of the upper cervical spine are particularly characteristic along with atlantoaxial subluxation, but neurologic sequelae are rare.

Management of the disease in the child is affected to a large extent by recognition of the importance of fostering normal growth patterns, both physical and psychologic. A satisfactory recovery for properly managed children is approximately 85 percent.

EPIDEMIOLOGY

JRA is not a rare disease. The incidence rate is approximately equal to those for juvenile diabetes mellitus and all forms of childhood cancer. In a study in Michigan, the minimal estimate of the incidence of the disease was 0.01 percent of children at risk per year.[2] Laaksonen[3] in Finland reported a similar experience of approximately 0.008 percent of children under age 15 affected per year. Studies in 1986 from Finland estimated that the incidence of JRA was 18.2 cases per 100,000 children[4] and from Sweden in 1983 12 per 100,000.[5] A report from Rochester, Minnesota, estimated that the incidence of JRA was 13.9 per 100,000 children with confidence limits of 9.9 to 18.8.[6]

Although JRA rarely occurs in siblings, unfolding data on human leukocyte antigen (HLA) segregation underscore a hereditary basis to the immunopathogenesis of the disease. As an illustration, in children with early-onset oligoarthritis, there is a striking increase in the frequency of HLA-A2; HLA-DR5, -w6, -w8, and -w52; HLA-DQw1; and HLA-DPw2.1.[7-9] In children with seropositive polyarticular disease, HLA-DR4, HLA-Dw4 and w14 are increased,[10-13] and in seronegative arthritis, HLA-DRw8.1, HLA-DQw4, and HLA-DP3 are increased.[14]

Earlier studies of Ansell et al.[15] reported that female relatives of children with JRA had a 13-fold increased frequency of seronegative erosive polyarthritis. In identical twins, a 44 per cent concordance rate has been reported and a 4 percent rate in dizygotic twins. Similar patterns of onset and course of JRA have been found in families.[16]

By definition, JRA begins before the age of 16 years.[17] Even though onset before 6 months is unusual, the age of onset is characteristically young, 1 to 3 years, but with a substantial number of cases beginning throughout childhood (Fig. 70–1).[2] Systemic onset may be an exception, with no increased frequency at any particular age. Girls account for the majority of patients in the early peak of the distribution curve and are affected overall at least twice

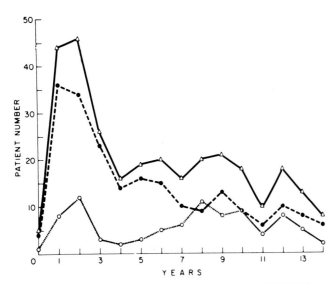

Figure 70–1. Age at onset (0 to 14 years) for a group of 300 children with JRA (△—△), and for girls (●---●) and boys (○······○) separately. For the total group, a single large peak at 1 to 2 years is observed. Age at onset for boys, however, shows a bimodal distribution, with the first peak at 2 years and the second at 8 years. Age at onset for girls does not clearly show a second peak. No definite accentuation in frequency of onset was seen in either sex at 10 to 14 years.

as often as boys except again for systemic onset, in which the sex ratio is equal.

ETIOLOGY AND PATHOGENESIS

The etiology and pathogenesis of JRA are unclear in spite of numerous investigations.[18] JRA may represent not a single disease but a syndrome of diverse etiologies. Abnormal immunoregulation, cytokine production, immunogenetic predisposition, and latent viral infection may all play a role. Viral antibody titers may be increased in some children with JRA.[19] Many viral diseases such as rubella and parvovirus have arthritis associated with their course. Persistent rubella virus infection in the synovia of children with JRA has been implicated as a potential cause of this disease.[20] A role for overt or subtle immunodeficiency in the causation of arthritis in children is underlined by the frequent occurrence of chronic arthritis in children with selective immunoglobulin A (IgA) deficiency,[21] agammaglobulinemia or hypogammaglobulinemia,[22] and heterozygous C2 complement-component deficiency.[18] Antibodies and cellular immune reactivity to types I and II collagens have been demonstrated in children with JRA.

It has been noted in several studies that serum antibodies from children with JRA react with T cells of the suppressor-inducer type and that such cells are absent in children with active disease. Morimoto et al.[23] reported that these antibodies specifically reacted with the CD4 cell subset and to a lesser extent with the CD8 suppressor population. Barron

et al.,[24] while confirming the validity of these studies, also found anti–T cell antibodies in children with systemic lupus erythematosus (SLE).

CLINICAL MANIFESTATIONS

Constitutional Signs and Symptoms

Morning stiffness, gelling following inactivity or in the evening, and night pain are probably encountered as often in JRA as in adult disease; however, children may not directly communicate these symptoms, and their presence will be suspected only by careful observation of the child or questioning of the parent. The child's more obvious presentation may be one of increased irritability, assumption of a posture of guarding the joints, or refusal to walk. Fatigue and low-grade fever are common at onset of disease. Anorexia, weight loss, and failure to grow are seen in many children. Extreme degrees of inanition and muscle atrophy are sometimes encountered. Psychologic regression to a more infantile pattern of behavior is often encountered in children who are experiencing moderate to severe disease.

Types of Onset

The diagnosis of JRA has been materially aided by recognition of three distinct types of onset of disease (Table 70–1). These are defined by a constellation of clinical signs and symptoms during the first 6 months of illness.[17]

Polyarthritis

JRA begins in five or more joints in slightly less than half of the children. The onset may be acute but is often insidious, with gradual development of progressive joint involvement. The arthritis is often of an indolent nature and generally involves the large joints, knees, wrists, elbows, and ankles and may include the small joints of the hands or feet either early or late in the course. The pattern of joint involvement is most often symmetric but may be asymmetric or affect only one side of the body. The joints are swollen from periarticular soft tissue edema and synovial effusions. They are warm but are not usually erythematous. Often the child does not complain of pain[25, 26]; however, the joints may be tender or painful on motion.

Palpable synovial cysts are an unusual complication of JRA. These cysts, when they occur in the popliteal space, may dissect into the calf of the leg (Baker cyst). Much less frequently, they develop in the antecubital area or anterior to the shoulder. Ultrasonography may aid in their correct diagnosis. These cysts are not confined to polyarticular disease

Table 70–1. TYPES OF ONSET OF JUVENILE RHEUMATOID ARTHRITIS

	Polyarthritis	Oligoarthritis	Systemic Disease
Relative frequency	40%	50%	10%
Number of joints involved	≥ 5	≤ 4	Variable
Sex ratio (F:M)	3:1	5:1	1:1
Extra-articular involvement	Moderate	Not present	Prominent
Chronic uveitis	5%	20%	Rare
Seropositivity			
Rheumatoid factors	15%*	Rare	Rare
Antinuclear antibodies	40%	85%†	10%
Clinical course	Systemic disease generally mild; articular involvement often unremitting	Systemic disease absent; major cause of morbidity is uveitis	Systemic disease often self-limited; arthritis chronic and destructive in half
Prognosis	Moderately good	Excellent	Moderate

*RF seropositivity forms a risk group in children with polyarthritis of older age at onset.
†ANA seropositivity forms a risk group for chronic uveitis in children with oligoarthritis of young age at onset.

but are also seen in systemic onset and occasionally in oligoarthritis.

The pattern of small joint involvement of the hands is not remarkably different from that observed in adults. The terminal interphalangeal joints are affected, however, in approximately 10 to 45 percent of children. Radial deviation at the metacarpophalangeal joints is more frequent than ulnar drift with ulnar rotation and subluxation of the carpus (Fig. 70–2). The wrist is the most commonly involved joint of the upper extremity.

Arthritis of the apophyseal joints of the spine is

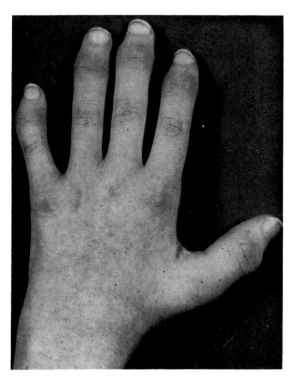

Figure 70–2. Hand of a 7-year-old girl with marked inflammatory involvement of the interphalangeal joint of the thumb and the terminal interphalangeal joints of the fingers. Arthritis began as systemic disease at 5½ years of age with fever, maculopapular rash, hepatosplenomegaly, and arthritis of the hands, feet, and left knee.

common. Involvement of the cervical spine occurs in half of the children with polyarthritis. The neck is usually painful and stiff; an alarmingly rapid loss of extension and rotation may follow. Occasionally torticollis is encountered. Involvement of the thoracolumbar apophyseal joints is seldom recognized clinically; however, scoliosis is increased in children with JRA.

Temporomandibular joint involvement, often asymmetric, is relatively common in children with polyarthritis and leads to limitation of bite and micrognathia. Ankylosis is uncommon. Of the remaining joints of the chest wall, the sternoclavicular joints are often affected and the acromioclavicular and manubriosternal less often so. Although involvement of the vocal cords by rheumatoid nodules can occur and cause hoarseness, cricoarytenoid arthritis is rare in JRA.

Systemic manifestations in polyarthritis are usually not as acute or persistent as in children with systemic onset of JRA. Low-grade fever and slight to moderate hepatosplenomegaly and lymphadenopathy may be present. Clinically evident pericarditis is infrequent, and chronic uveitis occurs in only 5 percent.

Oligoarthritis

The onset of JRA in half of the children involves four or fewer joints, particularly the knees and ankles of the lower extremities, in a low-grade inflammatory process. In one third to one half of these children, this onset type begins in only a single joint.[27] Monarthritis may occur in any joint, but the knee is affected in 75 percent (Figs. 70–3 and 70–4). Hip involvement at onset is unusual. There is probably little value in distinguishing a monarticular from a pauciarticular onset because both pursue the same general course. The hips are usually spared at least initially in this pattern of disease. Extra-articular manifestations, save for chronic uveitis, are quite unusual.

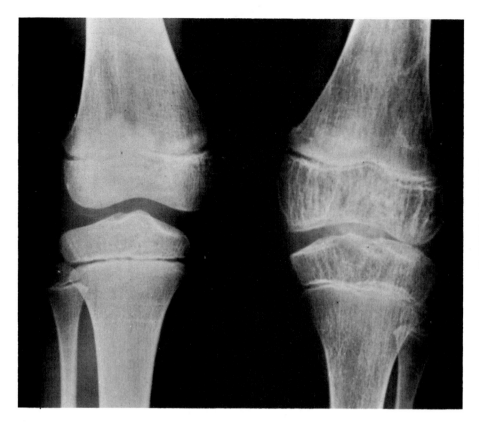

Figure 70–3. Radiographs of the knees of a boy with monarthritis of the left knee. There is marked osteoporosis on the left with coarsening of the trabeculae and enlargement of the epiphyses. The joint space is narrowed laterally, and there is lengthening of the left leg with a moderate valgus deformity. Erosions are not present.

Systemic Onset

Some children have severe constitutional and systemic involvement at onset of disease that may precede development of overt arthritis. These pa-

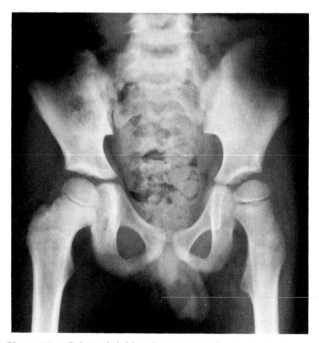

Figure 70–4. Pelvis of child in Figure 70–3. Coxa valga is present on the left and moderate stunting of growth of the ischium secondary to arthritis of the left knee. The hip was not involved in the inflammatory process; however, its deformity accounts in part for the ipsilateral leg length discrepancy.

tients make up 10 percent of the children with JRA. Arthritis may appear concurrent with the onset of systemic signs or many weeks to months later. The longest interval between the onset of systemic disease and objective signs of arthritis is seldom greater than 3 years. The systemic pattern of disease generally establishes its identity at onset and does not later intervene during the course of the other two types of JRA.

A hallmark of systemic onset is the high-spiking fever, which in combination with the rheumatoid rash is virtually diagnostic of the disease.[28] Daily (quotidian) or twice-daily temperature elevations rise to 39°C or higher with a rapid return to the baseline (Fig. 70–5). JRA is one of the few diseases in which the temperature actually becomes subnormal at this point. This intermittent pattern is highly suggestive of the diagnosis of JRA. The fever may occur at any time of the day but is characteristically seen in the late afternoon, evening, or early morning hours. The temperature may be subnormal in the morning. Chills are frequent, but rigor is unusual. The children are quite often strikingly ill while febrile and surprisingly well the rest of the day.

This intermittent fever is usually accompanied by a rheumatoid rash (Fig. 70–6).[29] This rash consists of discrete, 2- to 5-mm erythematous morbilliform macules and is most commonly seen on the trunk, on the proximal extremities, and over pressure areas. It may occur on the face, palms and soles, and axillae. A signal characteristic is its evanescent nature: Lesions are of short duration in any specific location, and the rash tends to be migratory. Each macule may be surrounded by a zone of pallor, and the larger

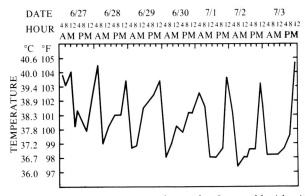

DATE   6/27   6/28   6/29   6/30   7/1   7/2   7/3

Figure 70–5. High, intermittent fever of a 3-year-old girl with systemic onset of JRA. The majority of the febrile spikes occurred in the late evening to early morning hours and were accompanied by a rheumatoid rash.

lesions show central clearing. The rash may resemble urticaria but is seldom pruritic. Although seen regularly in children with systemic disease, the rheumatoid rash also occurs occasionally in patients with

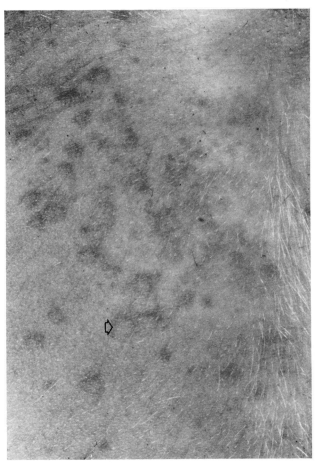

Figure 70–6. Rheumatoid rash of the patient in Figure 70–8. This was a faintly erythematous (salmon-colored), macular rash that was most prominent over the back but involved the extremities and face as well. The individual lesions were transient, appeared in crops, and generally conformed to a linear distribution. Some of the lesions had central clearing (*arrow*).

polyarthritis but is rarely observed in oligoarthritis. Because of the transient nature of the rash and its usual occurrence late in the day during febrile episodes, it is frequently missed by physicians caring for a child with "fever of unknown origin." The individual lesions may be induced, however, by rubbing or scratching the skin, the Koebner phenomenon, or isomorphic response. A hot bath or psychologic stress may also precipitate it.

Systemic onset of JRA is also accompanied by prominent visceral involvement such as hepatosplenomegaly and pericarditis or other evidence of serositis. Hepatosplenomegaly and lymphadenopathy of varying degree occur in most children with active systemic disease and can be striking in their development. A true hepatitis, not related to salicylate therapy, may occur; however, even massive hepatomegaly is usually associated with only a mild derangement of liver function. Hepatic disease is most common at or near the onset of JRA and regresses with time. Progressive liver disease is not seen. Occasionally a fatty liver develops with glucocorticoid administration. Enlargement of the spleen, which occurs in a quarter of the children, is generally most prominent the first year of disease. The degree of splenomegaly may be extreme but is not usually associated in children with the hematologic abnormalities of Felty syndrome. Lymphadenopathy, particularly in the cervical, axillary, and epitrochlear areas, may be marked and is usually symmetric. A similar pattern of systemic onset with spiking fevers, rash, and arthritis is seen occasionally in the older age groups, the so-called adult-onset Still's disease.[30, 31]

Extra-articular Manifestations of Disease

Pericarditis, often subclinical, is especially common in children with systemic onset of disease.[32, 33] It is unusual for pericarditis to precede the development of arthritis, but it may occur at any time during the course of JRA, usually accompanied by a systemic exacerbation. Its occurrence is not influenced by the sex or age of the child. Each episode generally persists for a week to 4 months; however, pericarditis may be recurrent in the face of poorly controlled disease. Echocardiography has been the most useful aid to diagnosis. Pericardial effusion does not usually progress to tamponade and rarely results in chronic constrictive pericarditis.

Myocarditis is much less common but may also lead to cardiac enlargement and failure. Valvular lesions, although rare, have been reported.[34] Systolic murmurs are generally functional; however, rheumatoid nodules have been described on the valve leaflets and visceral pericardium.

Other rare extra-articular manifestations of JRA include diffuse interstitial pulmonary fibrosis[35] and central nervous system disease. Rarely, a child will have idiopathic pulmonary hemosiderosis as the first manifestation of the disease. Pulmonary rheumatoid nodules have not been noted. Although the occurrence of central nervous system involvement has been described in children with JRA, this complication is more likely related to the presence of other contributory factors such as salicylate toxicity, viral infection, fever, embolism, or other systemic disease.

A renal glomerulitis as evidenced by intermittent hematuria is apparently part of the clinical course of JRA in some children and can present real problems of differential diagnosis relative to analgesic administration or gold therapy.[36, 37] Other children may develop renal papillary necrosis.[38, 39]

Tenosynovitis and myositis are manifestations of active disease. Inflammation of the tendon sheaths develops principally over the dorsa of the wrists and around the ankles. Loss of extension of the fingers can result from a stenosing synovitis of the flexor tendon sheaths. Unusual presentations may occur such as a stenosing tenosynovitis of the superior oblique muscle (Brown's syndrome). Atrophy of muscles around involved joints is characteristic of established disease.

Subcutaneous rheumatoid nodules are not as common as in adults (5 to 10 percent versus 35 percent).[40] They are associated with RF seropositivity in more than three fourths of the patients and are typically seen in children with polyarthritis. Benign rheumatoid nodules occur in a rare child without arthritis; a few of these patients later develop JRA. At least some of these reports may represent subcutaneous granuloma annulare. Rheumatoid polyarteritis has been described in a few instances, usually in the older child with RF seropositivity.

Chronic Uveitis

One of the most devastating complications of JRA is a chronic nongranulomatous uveitis, which can lead to blindness.[41, 42] Uveitis is especially likely to occur *in girls of early age of onset of oligoarthritis who have ANA seropositivity.*[41] Because the onset of chronic uveitis is usually insidious and asymptomatic, routine ophthalmologic examination must be performed at the time of diagnosis in every child with JRA and should be repeated at frequent intervals during the first years of the disease. Fewer than 2 percent of patients have a symptomatic onset of uveitis with redness, pain, or decreased visual acuity.

Approximately two thirds of children with uveitis have bilateral disease. If the initial involvement is unilateral, the second eye will usually be affected within a year. The earliest manifestations of inflammation are an increased number of cells in the anterior chamber of the eye, a proteinaceous flare on slit-lamp examination, or a punctate keratic precipitate on the posterior surface of the cornea. Inflammation that is inadequately controlled results in posterior synechiae, which produce an irregular or poorly reactive pupil (Fig. 70–7). Band keratopathy

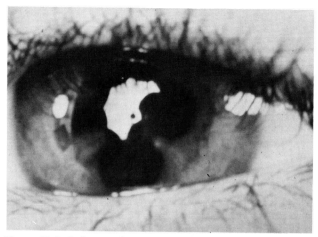

Figure 70–7. Left eye of a 7-year-old boy showing an irregular pupil that resulted from adhesions of the iris to the anterior surface of the lens (posterior synechiae). Onset of polyarthritis was at 9 months of age. Chronic uveitis was first detected at 2½ years in the right eye and 5 years later in the left eye. The patient subsequently had cataract extractions and developed glaucoma. Eyesight remains precariously at approximately 20/200. His arthritis has progressed to severe disease with marked muscular atrophy. Antinuclear antibody tests have been persistently negative.

occurs as a late degenerative lesion. It is not as common now as formerly, perhaps because of earlier diagnosis and better treatment of the initial ocular lesions. Complicated cataracts, secondary glaucoma, and phthisis bulbi are still encountered, however, in certain children with chronic uveitis in spite of vigorous long-term treatment of the disease.[43]

Growth Retardation

Disturbances of growth are characteristic and predictable features of JRA.[27, 44] During periods of active disease, linear growth is usually retarded. Full stature will seldom be attained if chronic rheumatic activity persists for many years. There is often delayed development of secondary sexual characteristics. Growth hormone secretion may be impaired or absent.[45]

Growth retardation may also occur in selective areas, such as in the jaw (Fig. 70–8). Micrognathia is caused by failure of normal development of one or both of the temporomandibular growth centers or results from contiguous involvement of the cervical spine.[46] The most extreme degrees of micrognathia are due to disease of long duration that had its onset before the fourth birthday.

Secondary growth deformities are frequent in children with limited joint disease involving the knee and result in unequal leg lengths.[27, 46, 47] The involved leg usually grows longer. Early during active disease, development of the ossification centers or epiphyses is accelerated, and later stunting, dwarfing, and premature fusion of the involved bones may result. Brachydactyly of the digits develops from premature closure of the epiphyseal growth plates.

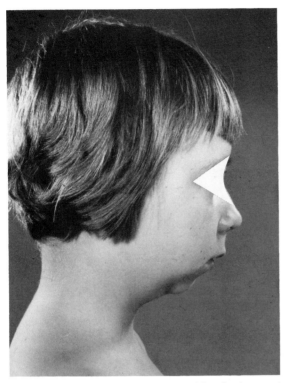

Figure 70–8. Micrognathia in an 11-year-old girl whose polyarthritis began at 18 months of age. There was no restriction of motion of the temporomandibular joints. Extension, rotation, and lateral binding of the cervical spine were absent, and flexion was limited to 10 degrees.

PATHOLOGY

JRA is characterized by many of the same histologic findings that have been identified in adult RA. There is villous hypertrophy of the synovium and hyperplasia of the synovial lining layer. The subsynovial tissues are edematous and hyperemic, and there is often prominent vascular endothelial hyperplasia and infiltration of lymphocytes and plasma cells. Electron microscopy has confirmed the similarity of the juvenile and adult synovial response to inflammation.[48] Pannus formation may result, and the articular cartilage and later contiguous bone become progressively eroded and destroyed. These events usually take place much later in the course of JRA than in adult disease. The synovial histopathology in oligoarthritis is not distinguishable from that seen in polyarthritis.[27] Rheumatoid nodules and necrotizing vasculitis have not been observed in synovial biopsy specimens from children.

Rheumatoid nodules in children probably do not differ in major pathologic characteristics from the nodules of adults, especially in seropositive patients.[40] When seen in the seronegative child, they may resemble more closely the nodules of rheumatic fever. The serosal lining surfaces of the major cavities (pleura, pericardium, and peritoneum) may develop a nonspecific fibrous serositis that is characterized by pain, exudation, and effusions. Nonspecific follicular

hyperplasia results in enlargement of lymph nodes that rarely simulates the picture of lymphoma. Hepatic histology usually shows a nonspecific periportal collection of inflammatory cells and hyperplasia of Kupffer cells.[49]

The rash of JRA is one of the most characteristic clinical features of the disease. Histologically there is a slight infiltration of round cells surrounding capillaries and venules in the subdermal tissues.[29] Neutrophilic perivasculitis may accompany the more flagrant lesions.

LABORATORY EXAMINATION

Many children with polyarthritis or systemic disease develop a normocytic, hypochromic anemia during periods of activity of disease. This may be moderately severe, in the range of 7 to 10 g per dl. Hypoplastic crisis or a hemophagocytic syndrome may rarely occur. Leukocytosis is common with active disease, especially in children with systemic onset. White blood cell counts of 30,000 to 50,000 per mm^3 are not uncommon; polymorphonuclear neutrophils (PMNs) predominate. Thrombocytosis routinely accompanies active disease and may also occur as a prelude to an exacerbation. Oligoarthritis is seldom associated with an anemia or leukocytosis.

The erythrocyte sedimentation rate (ESR) is a useful measure of the acute-phase reaction for following a child with active disease and is occasionally helpful in monitoring therapeutic efficacy. Determination of the C-reactive protein (CRP) is also a reasonably reliable indicator of the inflammatory response. Neither is a totally valid guide to activity of the arthritis, nor can the ESR or CRP be substituted for good clinical judgment. Increases in the serum concentrations of the immunoglobulins are also correlated in general with activity of the disease. Extreme degrees of hypergammaglobulinemia occur in the sickest children and return toward normal with improvement of the disease. Serum complement components are usually elevated in children with JRA. Serum AA (amyloid-like) protein is increased in concentration in children with JRA as a nonspecific indicator of inflammation. Soluble immune complexes can be detected in the sera of certain children with JRA, particularly those with systemic onset of disease.[50]

The latex fixation test or sensitized sheep cell agglutination for RFs is positive in children less frequently than in adults.[51, 52] Fewer than 4 percent of children with JRA are seropositive at onset of the disease. RFs tend to be present in the child of late age of onset or in the older child, in one with subcutaneous rheumatoid nodules or articular erosions, or in those in a poorer functional class.

Children who are strongly seropositive for RFs may represent a subset of disease different from that of the larger group of seronegative children. Although the frequency of classic RF seropositivity may

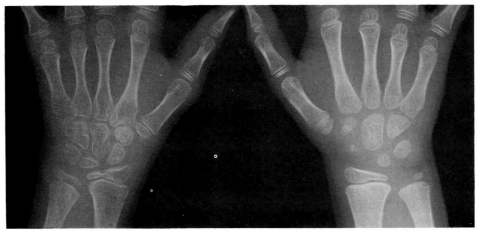

Figure 70–9. Accelerated maturation of the left carpus in a 9-year-old girl with arthritis for 7 years. Marked osteoporosis and atrophy of soft tissue is present. The individual carpal bones on the left are smaller, and eventual mature growth is already stunted.

not increase with continuing active disease of long duration, the frequency of RFs rises progressively as the age of onset or duration of disease of the cohort group under study increases. These findings, although not unequivocal, tend to suggest that seropositivity may be a result rather than a determinative event in children with JRA who go on to unremitting, disabling disease in the early adult years.

Hidden 19S IgM RFs have been described by Moore et al.,[53] using acid elution-gel filtration, in sera of children with JRA. These hidden RFs are found with all types of onset of disease (not just polyarticular) and correlated best with activity of the articular disease.

Tests for ANAs are positive in approximately 40 percent of children with JRA.[54, 55] These antibodies are heterogeneous and directed at a variety of nuclear antigens including histones.[56] The pattern of fluorescent staining on mouse liver substrate or HEp-2 cells is usually homogeneous or speckled, and the standardized serum dilution titer is generally low to moderate (≤1:256). The frequency of ANAs increases in girls of younger age of disease onset and decreases in older boys and in children with systemic disease and reach their highest prevalence in children who have oligoarthritis and uveitis (65 to 85 percent).[41, 54, 55] Thus, ANAs are of critical importance in the initial diagnostic program of a child suspected of having JRA and in selecting for closer observation children at risk for developing chronic uveitis. They are not frequently found in other childhood illnesses except for diseases such as SLE and scleroderma. Anti–double-stranded DNA antibody assays are normal in children with classic JRA.[57] The finding of an elevated DNA-binding activity would usually indicate supervention of active immune-complex disease of the lupus type.[58]

Immunogenetic typing has added an important dimension to the laboratory assessment of rheumatic disease in selected children, as the presence of HLA-B27 is characteristic of the spondyloarthropathies.[59]

As already stated, studies have shown an impressive association of subtypes of JRA with HLA antigens in the DR, DQ, and DP loci.[7-14]

Synovial fluid examination in JRA is usually typical of group II or inflammatory fluid. The white blood cell count does not always correlate, however, with the degree of clinical activity. Low counts have been observed in fluids from joints clinically involved by active inflammatory disease. Conversely, counts in the range of infectious arthritis, e.g., 100,000 cells per mm^3, have been recorded in patients with otherwise classic JRA. As in adult RA, levels of glucose may be low in the synovial fluid. Complement levels are not as characteristically or uniformly depressed as in adult disease.[60]

Urinalysis is usually normal in children with JRA except for the proteinuria associated with fever. Persistent proteinuria is often the first indication of amyloidosis in reports from Europe.[36] Intermittent hematuria may occur and be evidence of a mild glomerulitis associated with JRA, of drug toxicity (interstitial nephritis or renal papillary necrosis),[37-39] or of the development of another disease such as SLE.[58]

RADIOLOGIC EXAMINATION

Early radiographic changes consist of soft tissue swelling, juxta-articular osteoporosis, and periosteal new bone formation.[46, 61] Premature epiphyseal closure may lead to stunting of bone growth, especially in the phalanges. Conversely, there may be accelerated epiphyseal development stimulated by the local inflammatory changes (Fig. 70–9). Marked bony overgrowth owing to enlargement of the epiphyses may occur at the interphalangeal joints. Widening of the phalanges from periosteal new bone apposition is another characteristic feature in children with JRA. Marginal erosions and narrowing of the cartilaginous space may occur in disease of long duration. These

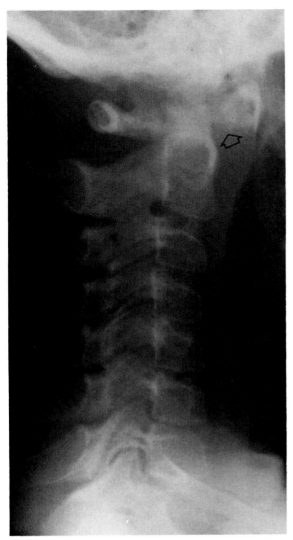

Figure 70–10. Radiograph of the cervical spine of a young girl with polyarthritis. There is an atlantoaxial subluxation (*arrow*) and fusion of the C2-C3 apophyseal joint. Three years later subluxation developed at the C3-C4 vertebral interspace.

changes are not observed early in the course of JRA, e.g., generally not before 2 years of active disease even in the child with polyarthritis. Indeed, in some children with oligoarthritis, erosions have not occurred even after one or two decades of joint disease.

Fusion of the upper cervical apophyseal joints is the most characteristic change in the cervical spine (Fig. 70–10).[46, 62] Atlantoaxial subluxation is a potential complication of this involvement. The upper limit of the atlanto-odontoid space in children is 4 mm measured on a lateral film in flexion. The odontoid is often eroded and can impinge onto the upper cervical cord or migrate superiorly (Fig. 70–11). Vertebral bodies at areas of fusion fail to grow normally and are smaller than contiguous vertebrae or have an altered ratio of height to width. The intervertebral spaces at these levels are also narrowed, and calcification of the discs is occasionally seen. Apophyseal joint disease also occurs in the thoracic and lumbar

spines but is less often recognized. Sacroiliac arthritis in children with JRA is not characterized by the degree of change, particularly reactive sclerosis, that is seen in juvenile ankylosing spondylitis. Late fusion occurs, however, particularly in children with severe polyarticular disease who have been bedridden.

Fractures related to generalized osteoporosis are all too frequent in young children, particularly if they have had severe disease, immobilization, or glucocorticoid therapy. The supracondylar area of the femur is a characteristic site of fracture, often following manipulation for contracture of the knee. Recurrent vertebral compression fractures are a potential complication in children who have been treated with glucocorticoids.

There is considerable clinical interest in the role of other objective techniques to document the presence of inflammation or destruction in joints.[63] Radionucleid bone scanning, thermography, ultrasonography, computed tomography (CT), and magnetic resonance imaging (MRI) have been studied to delineate their precise roles in the diagnosis or follow-up of JRA and in determining the extent of soft tissue or bone involvement.

DIAGNOSIS

Classification Criteria

Criteria for the classification of JRA have been revised (Table 70–2).[17] Arthritis in one or more joints

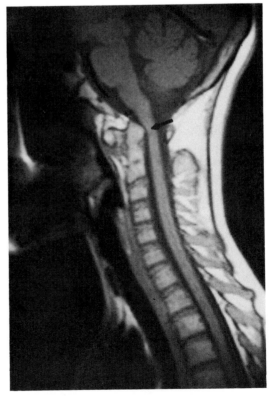

Figure 70–11. Magnetic resonance image of the cervical spine in a 10-year-old girl with severe polyarticular JRA and an atlantoaxial subluxation of 11 mm. The arrow points to the odontoid, which has not encroached on the upper cervical cord.

Table 70–2. DIAGNOSTIC CRITERIA FOR
THE CLASSIFICATION OF JUVENILE
RHEUMATOID ARTHRITIS

Age at onset less than 16 years
Arthritis in one or more joints defined as swelling or effusion,
    or the presence of two or more of the following signs:
    limitation of range of motion, tenderness or pain on motion,
    and increased heat
Duration of disease of ≥ 6 weeks
Type of onset of disease during the first 6 months classified as
    Polyarthritis—5 joints or more
    Oligoarthritis—4 joints or fewer
    Systemic disease with arthritis and intermittent fever
Exclusion of other forms of juvenile arthritis

Modified from Cassidy, J. T., Levinson, J. E., Bass, J. G., et al.: A study of classification criteria for a diagnosis of juvenile rheumatoid arthritis. Arthritis Rheum. 29:274, 1986.

for 6 weeks may be sufficient for diagnosis. Arthritis present for 3 months provides even more assurance that JRA is the correct diagnosis. Objective arthritis must be distinguished from arthralgia or pain in the joints.

There is no world-wide agreement on the use of diagnostic terms for JRA or on criteria for classification.[64] The criteria that have been presented for JRA are the only ones subjected in recent years to extensive review and testing by a subcommittee of the American College of Rheumatology. The term *juvenile arthritis* is most appropriately used when referring to all of the rheumatic diseases of childhood associated with arthritis.

Exclusions for Diagnosis of Juvenile Rheumatoid Arthritis

JRA is often a diagnosis of exclusion. Because many of the more common types of juvenile arthritis may be confused with JRA, serious consideration must be given at onset of the disease to the other rheumatic and connective-tissue diseases, especially rheumatic fever, SLE, and spondyloarthropathy. Particular attention must also be accorded the possibility of infectious arthritis, serum sickness, Henoch-Schönlein purpura, the inflammatory enteropathies such as ulcerative colitis and regional enteritis, and hematologic diseases, especially leukemia, sickle cell anemia, and hemophilia.

A number of clinical observations are helpful in the differential diagnosis of JRA.[65, 66] The child with oligoarthritis has involvement of one to four joints, generally including the knees. In this type of onset, the joint is swollen with effusion, but is generally not very painful, tender, or red. It is often slightly warm. Such a child is not systemically ill. If a child with limited joint disease has an acutely painful and erythematous joint or systemic signs of illness, one should suspect a septic process or another disease such as acute rheumatic fever. Synovial fluid aspiration is almost always indicated in such a patient to exclude pyogenic synovitis.

Lyme disease has presented diagnostic difficulties in children with arthritis in the endemic geographic areas such as the Northeast and upper Midwest.[67] It most often has onset in the summer months, and the characteristic rash, erythema chronicum migrans, occurs in half of the children coincident with the tick bite. Arthritis is delayed until 1 to 2 months after onset and is often a monarthritis or oligoarthritis. It is recurrent and episodic in two thirds of the children. Occasionally polyarthritis occurs; 10 percent of children develop a chronic arthritis with erosions.

Internal derangements of the knee are not common in children. Episodic arthritis, especially of the knee, however, is unusually frequent in hypermobile children.[68] Tumors that present as monarticular disease such as pigmented villonodular synovitis are rare. The finding of chronic nongranulomatous uveitis in a child with oligoarthritis almost always indicates that the diagnosis is JRA. Other causes of uveitis must be considered, however, such as sarcoidosis or psoriatic arthritis.[69] Needle biopsy of the synovial membrane is occasionally useful in monarthritis to exclude other diagnoses such as specific granuloma or tumor. A nonreactive tuberculin skin test in a child virtually eliminates tuberculosis as a consideration. Other types of infection may cause a monarthritis, particularly gonorrhea, and trauma may do so transiently.

Certain malignancies enter into the differential diagnosis of JRA. Among the more prominent considerations are neuroblastoma, histiocytosis X, and leukemia, particularly in systemic-onset disease. Acute leukemia in childhood may present as arthritis because of the presence of red marrow in the metaphyseal portions of the bones and infiltration of malignant cells into the periosteum and joint capsule. The presence of bone pain on weight bearing may be a clue to its presence. This pain in leukemia is often out of proportion to the observed swelling. Sickle cell anemia, because of involvement of the periosteum and microinfarcts of bones, can give rise to periarthritis or dactylitis that mimics a true arthritis. The hand-foot syndrome is an example of this hemoglobinopathy in early infancy.

Arthritis involving either the peripheral joints or the spine is seen in 5 to 15 percent of children with regional enteritis or ulcerative colitis.[70] Although Whipple's disease has been described in children, it is rare. Reiter's syndrome and psoriatic arthritis are common in some geographic areas.[59]

Onset of hip disease in the very young child may represent a septic process or congenital dislocation of the hip. In the somewhat older child, aseptic necrosis of the femoral head (Legg-Calvé-Perthes disease) is another diagnostic consideration. In the adolescent child, particularly if an obese boy, a slipped capital femoral epiphysis may initially mimic JRA. Transient synovitis of the hip is a self-limited condition of uncertain origin. Results of laboratory and radiologic studies are normal. Osgood-Schlatter disease of the tibial tubercle can usually be easily distinguished from involvement of the knee in JRA.

Although the child with systemic onset of JRA has many of the manifestations of an acute infectious process, finding the rheumatoid rash or typical polyarthritis points to a diagnosis of JRA. The fever in these children is of the septic type; a sustained fever readily responsive to salicylate therapy would be more characteristic of acute rheumatic fever. Likewise, although many children with systemic onset of disease have pericarditis and effusion, these are isolated cardiac findings: A pericardial effusion in conjunction with evidence of endocarditis such as a diastolic murmur would point away from JRA and toward a disease such as rheumatic fever or bacterial endocarditis. The onset of acute rheumatic fever in developed countries of the world is usually between the ages of 5 and 15 years. Although its diagnosis may be difficult, arthritis in this disease is characteristically acute, painful, asymmetric, and migratory and involves the peripheral joints without sequelae.[71] The total duration of a single attack is usually less than 6 weeks and seldom as long as 3 months. The antistreptolysin O (ASO) titer is chronically elevated in one third of the children with JRA and should not be taken as an indication of recent streptococcal infection without a documented rise or fall in the titer.

There are three diseases that present long-term, more difficult problems in the diagnosis of JRA. These conditions are SLE, juvenile ankylosing spondylitis (JAS), and the arthritis of immunodeficiency.

The child with SLE can have an arthritis that mimics that seen in JRA, and the correct diagnosis may not be evident until one of the more characteristic clinical findings of lupus occurs later in the course of the disease. This arthritis is often nondeforming and nonerosive but not always so. Serologic tests may confirm the presence of lupus and should always be performed when a diagnostic question arises.[57] Ragsdale and associates[58] have presented the course of 10 children who developed SLE after an initial diagnosis of JRA. In all cases, serum anti-DNA antibodies were present before the development of clinical symptoms characteristic of SLE.

The child with JAS will usually have arthritis of the lower extremities accompanied by enthesitis, rather than lumbar pain or stiffness.[72] Pain in the groin or buttock may be an early sign. Two thirds of these individuals are boys. Remittent oligoarthritis is most frequent, and involvement of the wrists or joints of the hands is rare. Other helpful diagnostic points are onset of disease after the age of 7 to 9 years, infrequent cervical spine involvement, seronegativity for RFs or ANAs, and a family history of similar disease. Approximately 92 percent of these children will be positive for the lymphocyte surface antigen HLA-B27.[59] A firm diagnosis of JAS depends on demonstration of the characteristic radiologic features in the sacroiliac joints. These changes are often present at onset of the disease if technically adequate,

angulated views of the sacroiliac joints are obtained[46]; however, a definite diagnosis may be delayed by months to years in unusual cases.

Children with immunologic deficiencies, particularly selective IgA deficiency,[21] common variable immunodeficiency and X-linked agammaglobulinemia,[22] and heterozygous C2 complement component deficiency,[18] may have an arthritis that mimics JRA. Indeed, one hesitates at this time to separate all of these children from the larger group with JRA because it is not known on an etiologic basis what JRA entails. It is mandatory in any child with chronic arthritis who has other features of unexpected autoimmunity or infection (i.e., sinopulmonary disease) to obtain studies for humoral immunologic deficiency, particularly quantitation of the serum immunoglobulins, and to determine the hemolytic complement titer.

TREATMENT

Conservative management of JRA attempts to control the clinical manifestations of the disease and to prevent deformity. It almost always involves a coordinated, multidisciplinary team approach: pediatric rheumatologist, social worker, physical therapist, occupational therapist, nurse, and orthopedic surgeon. Because JRA is characterized by chronic inflammation of the joints and varying systemic manifestations, treatment in most children is prolonged over many years. This long duration of therapy must be accepted ultimately by the child and family and judged safe by the physician. Although prognosis is excellent in a majority of the children, it is not possible at onset to predict with certainty who will recover and who will have unremitting disease. Therefore, treatment must be vigorous in all cases and aimed at suppression of articular inflammation, prevention of secondary deformities, and control of systemic disease.

The philosophy of management of children with JRA is to begin with the simplest, safest, and most conservative measures. If this treatment proves inadequate, the physician should choose other therapeutic modalities in an orderly fashion (Table 70–3).[1, 73] In children, potentially toxic regimens such as immunosuppressive drugs should be employed only in life-threatening disease with full explanation of the risk-to-benefit ratio and only in approved experimental protocols.

Nonsteroidal Anti-inflammatory Drugs

Aspirin is the single most useful nonsteroidal anti-inflammatory drug (NSAID) in the treatment of JRA and has analgesic, anti-inflammatory, and antipyretic actions. It is relatively inexpensive and has a proved record of long-term safety. Treatment with aspirin is started at 75 to 90 mg per kg per day

Table 70–3. MANAGEMENT OF JUVENILE
RHEUMATOID ARTHRITIS

Stage I
  Basic program
    Nonsteroidal anti-inflammatory drug
    Local and general rest
    Physical and occupational therapy
    Education of patient and family
    Involvement of school and community agencies

Stage II
  Hydroxychloroquine
  Gold salts
  Penicillamine
  Sulfasalazine

Stage III
  Hospitalization
  Intra-articular steroids
  Systemic glucocorticoid drugs

Stage IV
  Methotrexate

Stage V
  Preventive surgery
  Reconstructive surgery
  Experimental therapy

depending on the child's age and weight. Higher doses are tolerated best in younger children weighing less than 25 kg. It should be given four times a day with meals and at bedtime with milk to minimize gastrointestinal irritation. Awakening the child at night to administer aspirin is not necessary because the serum half-life of salicylate is prolonged (>16 hours) once therapeutic levels have been achieved. Salicylate blood levels are occasionally useful as a guide to correct dosage or when signs of toxicity such as tinnitus or inattention develop. The appropriate serum level is 20 to 25 mg per dl measured 2 hours after the morning dose. It may be difficult to reach therapeutic levels in children with systemic disease, but increasing the daily amount of aspirin beyond 100 mg per kg usually results in toxicity. If higher doses are required initially for control, they should be gradually reduced to maintenance levels on subsidence of the systemic manifestations. The febrile pattern will usually respond to adequate salicylate dosage in 1 to 4 weeks.

Magnesium or choline salts of salicylate may be useful in certain children who have experienced gastrointestinal irritation from the use of aspirin alone. Buffered preparations of aspirin or enteric-coated tablets are preferred by some families.

Studies have indicated that children who chew aspirin develop gingival inflammation and erosions of the biting surfaces of the teeth. Children must be taught to swallow the pills, or if they cannot, a liquid preparation may be temporarily indicated. The teeth may be coated by a dentist to protect against the effects of aspirin.

Some children develop hepatitis related to salicylate therapy, although clinical manifestations of liver disease appear to be uncommon. Biopsies have

shown a mild periportal round cell infiltration and scattered single cell necrosis. This type of hepatitis occurs most frequently when the serum salicylate concentration is in the toxic range (>25 mg per dl), although the transaminase enzymes (aspartate transaminase [AST] and alanine transaminase [ALT]) may be intermittently increased in as many as 50 percent of the children on therapeutic levels of aspirin.[74, 75] Transient elevation of these enzymes in a child who is otherwise not showing signs of toxicity is not an indication for stopping the drug. If levels of the enzymes remain elevated or are high, for example, AST level five times normal, aspirin should be temporarily stopped or the dosage reduced by at least 20 percent until they return to normal.

Epidemiologic studies have demonstrated a potential association between the administration of salicylates and the development of Reye's syndrome.[76] Salicylates and other NSAIDs should be stopped in any sick child who is vomiting or who potentially has influenza or varicella. NSAIDs should be discontinued in children directly exposed to these viral diseases for the duration of the incubation period. All children with JRA should be vaccinated for influenza as an added precaution (there is not uniform agreement on this recommendation) and for varicella when that vaccine is released for general use.

A few children with JRA may develop signs of analgesic nephropathy when seemingly taking only aspirin. These are often children who are severely disabled, confined to wheelchairs or dependent on adults for their needs, and undoubtedly chronically dehydrated.[38, 39] Many reports have emphasized adverse effects of the other NSAIDs on renal function. These drugs appear to have little influence on glomerular filtration and renal blood flow in normal adults but may suppress both in patients with compromised renal function or occasionally in otherwise normal children. This toxicity results in signs of fluid and sodium retention, congestive heart failure, and azotemia. Caution should be exercised in the chronic use of acetaminophen as an analgesic in children on an NSAID. Its safety from the viewpoint of interstitial nephritis has been questioned because it is the active metabolite of phenacetin.[77]

If a child does not respond to aspirin after a maximum 3-month trial or the response is inadequate, a limited number of other NSAIDs can be considered.[78, 79] Most of the newer NSAIDs have not been approved for use in children in the United States by the Food and Drug Administration. Among approved agents, tolmetin, 25 mg per kg per day (4 times a day); naproxen, 15 mg per kg per day (2 times a day); and ibuprofen, 35 mg per kg per day (4 times a day), have been used extensively. The latter two medications are also available as suspensions for younger children who have difficulty swallowing tablets.

Satisfactory treatment of the arthritis will be achieved in 50 to 70 percent of children with NSAIDs alone. Such therapy is generally continued for 2 years after all manifestations of activity have been suppressed to avoid stopping anti-inflammatory therapy with short, self-limited remissions.

Advanced Drug Therapy

When children do not respond to an initial trial of NSAIDs alone or respond inadequately, a limited number of other medications can be added to the antirheumatic program.[80, 81] Agents that should be considered are hydroxychloroquine, gold, sulfasalazine, and D-penicillamine.

Antimalarial Drugs

Hydroxychloroquine is a useful adjunctive agent for treatment of the older child with JRA.[82] The initial dose is 5 to 7 mg per kg per day (≤600 mg), and the total period of initial treatment should not be prolonged beyond 2 years if at all possible. An ophthalmologic examination must be performed before institution of therapy and every 4 months thereafter. Children younger than 4 to 7 years of age often have enough difficulty on color vision testing that use of hydroxychloroquine cannot be justified. Although it would be unusual for retinal toxicity to occur with the above-recommended dose, the drug should be discontinued at any suspicion of retinopathy because its effects are cumulative. Corneal deposition may occur and is an indication for lowering the dose.

Intramuscular Gold

Intramuscular gold is an effective treatment of children with JRA.[80, 83] Preparations that are available are gold sodium thiomalate and aurothioglucose. Gold therapy is indicated in children whose polyarthritis has been unresponsive to a conservative program of management. It may be used in conjunction with an NSAID and hydroxychloroquine. Before beginning therapy, the child's hematologic, renal, and hepatic function must be normal. A test dose of 5 mg of one of the organic gold compounds should be given initially. Weekly injections are gradually increased thereafter until a dose of approximately 0.75 to 1 mg per kg per week is reached (≤50 mg). This program is continued for 20 weeks to a total dose of approximately 15 mg per kg (≤1000 mg). If satisfactory improvement or remission has been achieved, maintenance therapy is instituted every 2 weeks for 3 months and then every 3 weeks for 3 months. At that juncture, if objective signs of improvement continue, the child is placed on gold injections every 4 weeks, periodically adjusted on the basis of growth and increased body weight.

A complete blood count and urinalysis must be obtained before each administration of the drug, and assessment of the child for any toxicity, especially stomatitis, dermatitis, bone marrow suppression, hematuria, or proteinuria, should be done. Assessment

of renal and hepatic function (biochemistry panel) is performed approximately every 6 weeks. A decrease in the white blood cell count to fewer than 4500 per mm³; a fall in the absolute neutrophil count by 50 percent; the development of eosinophilia, proteinuria, or hematuria; or clinical signs of gold toxicity are indications for at least a temporary interruption of therapy. Absolute contraindications to reinstitution of gold therapy are severe leukopenia, neutropenia, proteinuria, or exfoliative dermatitis.

Children with systemic onset may be at greater risk for reactions from any of the antirheumatic drugs, especially gold, with neutropenia and diffuse intravascular coagulation (DIC) as predominant reported toxicities.[84]

Oral Gold

Triethylphosphine gold, auranofin, has been introduced into the treatment of JRA.[85, 86] Dosage is 0.15 mg per kg per day (≤9 mg). In pediatric studies, auranofin appeared to be well tolerated but not necessarily more effective than an NSAID. It was associated with loose stools in approximately 10 percent of children, a side effect that can often be controlled by decreasing the dose. Toxicity is otherwise similar to that of injectable gold. Initial evaluation before starting auranofin therapy is the same as with the other gold compounds; thereafter, a complete blood count and urinalysis are performed every 2 weeks and a biochemistry panel every 6 weeks.

Sulfasalazine

Although there are few published studies on the use of sulfasalazine in JRA, it appears to be effective, relatively safe, and with a clinical response evaluable at approximately 6 to 8 weeks.[87] Toxicities include gastrointestinal irritation; oral ulcerations; dermatitis, including the Stevens-Johnson syndrome; and bone marrow suppression. Sulfasalazine should not be used in infants or children with known hypersensitivity to sulfa or salicylate, impaired renal or hepatic function, or with specific contraindications such as porphyria or glucose-6-phosphate dehydrogenase deficiency.

The maintenance dose for children is 40 to 60 mg per kg per day in three to four divided doses taken with food or milk. This dosage is reached by gradual increments from once-a-day administration to multiple doses with meals over a period of 4 to 6 weeks. The enteric-coated 500-mg tablets are preferred in the older child; a suspension is available for use in younger children. After the initial treatment period, the maintenance dose should be gradually reduced to approximately 25 mg per kg per day as long as improvement is sustained. Baseline evaluation should be as with gold salts. Clinical assessment of the patient along with a complete blood count, urine, and biochemical studies should be done approximately every month.

D-Penicillamine

The indications for the use of D-penicillamine are the same as those for gold; these two agents are not combined therapeutically.[73, 80, 82] The maintenance dose is 10 mg per kg per day (≤750 mg per day) taken early in the morning on an empty stomach. This dose is achieved after three increments of 8 to 12 weeks duration, for example, 3 mg per kg initial dose. A complete blood count and urinalysis are done once a week and a biochemistry panel every 6 weeks. Important side effects of D-penicillamine are drug-induced lupus, dermatitis, thrombocytopenia, and proteinuria. Toxicity is not necessarily dose related. Children who developed toxicity while receiving gold therapy are more likely to develop toxicity to D-penicillamine, often similar to that which occurred with the gold salt. A large multicenter study has been reported on the use of D-penicillamine or hydroxychloroquine in the treatment of severe JRA during a 12-month therapeutic trial.[82] In the presence of an NSAID, neither drug was shown to be superior to placebo.

Glucocorticoids

The glucocorticoid drugs are useful in the treatment of JRA resistant to more conservative forms of therapy. They are often combined with an NSAID and another antirheumatic drug. They may be given orally in severe disease or in combination with ophthalmic steroid for the treatment of chronic uveitis. Intra-articular steroid is limited to use in one or two joints that continue to be actively involved in a child who has otherwise responded satisfactorily to conservative therapy.

Although glucocorticoids are among the most potent anti-inflammatory drugs available for the treatment of arthritis, the benefits of prolonged systemic use need to be weighed carefully because steroids result in superimposition of Cushing's syndrome and growth suppression, osteopenia and fractures, and increased susceptibility to infection. Reasonable caloric restrictions are necessary in most children, antacids are given for symptoms of dyspepsia, and the child may need moderate restriction of sodium intake and attention to early symptoms of hypokalemia or hyperglycemia.

Prednisone is the glucocorticoid usually chosen for use orally. For uncontrolled systemic disease with marked disability, it may be given as a single morning dose of 0.1 to 1 mg per kg per day (≤40 mg) or in divided doses for more severe disease. After satisfactory control is reached or it is obvious that adequate control is not going to be achieved, the drug should be gradually decreased and eventually discontinued. *Steroid pseudorheumatism* may make even slow withdrawal of the drug difficult.

There are no studies that indicate that glucocorticoid therapy, even in high dosage, limits the duration of the disease, prevents extra-articular complications, or alters the eventual prognosis. It is important that both the child, if possible, and the parents understand that total control of the signs and symptoms of JRA may not be possible and that it will be necessary to accept some degree of activity of the disease in exchange for less glucocorticoid toxicity. Although use of steroids to suppress joint inflammation alone is to be avoided, low-dose, alternate-day prednisone may be useful in some children with severe, relatively unresponsive polyarthritis.

Growth retardation is the most significant untoward effect of steroid toxicity in children. A dose of 5 mg per day is usually inhibitory; as little as 3 mg in the child under 25 kg of body weight may be suppressive. JRA in itself retards normal development and growth. A child may regain loss in height with time, be it the result of either disease or therapy, but this does not happen often if a significant deficit has occurred or is not complete in terms of resumption of growth in the previous isodevelopmental channel. Recombinant growth hormone therapy may or may not be effective for these patients.

Increased glucocorticoid dosage is necessary for stress in any child who has been on the drug and who has a serious infection or traumatic injury or who is about to undergo a surgical procedure. The requirement of increased amounts of glucocorticoid during acute stress should be noted to the parents, and in addition, each child should wear a Med-Alert necklace or bracelet indicating that he or she is receiving a glucocorticoid medication. As an additional precaution, children on glucocorticoid drugs should not receive live virus vaccines (OPV, MMR).

To minimize the daily steroid requirement or avoid it altogether, intravenous steroid-pulse therapy has been introduced into the treatment of the more severe manifestations of JRA. The rationale for this approach is to achieve an immediate anti-inflammatory effect and minimize toxicity related to long-term continuous therapy. Methylprednisolone is the drug of choice in a dose of 10 to 30 mg per kg per pulse administered in a variety of protocols. These have consisted of a single intravenous pulse to three pulses administered on alternate days. Intravenous steroid-pulse therapy can cause serious and fatal complications involving electrolyte and fluid imbalance and cardiac arrhythmia. The child needs continuous monitoring during the pulse and for a number of hours thereafter.

The treatment of chronic uveitis with glucocorticoids should be supervised by an experienced ophthalmologist. Initial therapy consists of steroid eye drops and mydriasis. A short-acting mydriatic drug is preferred once a day in the evening, so pupillary dilatation does not interfere with school. It is often advisable to use supplemental oral prednisone in low dosage (2 to 4 mg once a day). A significant proportion of children may actually require larger amounts to control their disease. Even ophthalmic steroid administration may result in the development of Cushing's syndrome.

Although the slit-lamp examination may return to normal soon after treatment is initiated, it is inadvisable to stop glucocorticoids completely at that time because of the frequent reappearance of signs of inflammation. Uveitis generally remains active for many years after onset and requires long-term surveillance by an experienced ophthalmologist. The improved prognosis for sight in recent years may be the result of earlier detection of chronic uveitis and its prompt treatment or may relate to the diagnosis of relatively benign forms of the disease.[88] Management of glaucoma remains unsatisfactory, but results of lensectomy-vitrectomy for complicated cataract are good.[43]

Prednisolone tertiary butylacetate and triamcinolone acetonide, 5 to 40 mg, are intra-articular preparations that may be used in one or two joints that do not respond satisfactorily to a conservative program or as a short-term aid to physical therapy.[89] Intra-articular injections should not be given more than a limited number of times, e.g., three times in a single joint during a 3-month period of time.

Immunosuppressive Agents

Immunosuppressive and cytotoxic agents should be used only in approved experimental protocols and for life-threatening illness or unremitting progression of arthritis and disability. The drugs most commonly employed are azathioprine, cyclophosphamide, chlorambucil, and methotrexate. Leukopenia or bone marrow suppression may result from any of these agents. The development of malignancy and mutagenic effects is the most critical long-term consideration. Sterility and amenorrhea have been associated with most of the immunosuppressive agents, particularly those of the alkylating variety. A unique indication for the use of immunosuppressive therapy in children with JRA may be the development of amyloidosis.[90] The benefit of cytotoxic agents in the treatment of intractable uveitis is outweighed by the risk of serious side effects.[43]

Methotrexate

Methotrexate has been introduced into the treatment of children with severe polyarticular disease who have failed to respond to adequate and often prolonged courses of other medications including the slow-acting antirheumatic drugs.[91] The advantages of methotrexate are its efficacy at relatively low doses and its apparent lack of oncogenicity or production of sterility. Potential systemic toxicity includes bone marrow suppression, gastrointestinal ulceration, diarrhea, headache, acute interstitial pneumonitis, alopecia, dermatitis, and hepatic cirrhosis. Cirrhosis of the liver is not an expected toxicity in children on weekly therapy; certain risks should be avoided, however, such as malnutrition, viral hepatitis, diabetes mellitus, obesity, or alcoholism.

Baseline studies before therapy is started include a complete blood count, urinalysis, monitoring for renal and hepatic function and serum albumin levels, ophthalmologic examination, pulmonary function testing, and a chest roentgenogram. The drug is given as a single weekly dose on an empty stomach with clear liquids 60 minutes before breakfast. The liquid injectable preparation (25 mg per ml) can be used orally in children to give the correct amount. A starting dose of 10 mg per M^2 per week is chosen with adjustment on the basis of 1-hour and 24-hour blood levels obtained at 1 month and periodically thereafter.[92] Additional monitoring during the course of the treatment includes a complete blood count and urinalysis every 2 weeks and serum transaminase assays every month. Some NSAIDs may interfere with the protein binding and excretion of methotrexate, and their dosage should be kept constant during treatment.

Experimental Therapies

Intravenous human immune globulin has been investigated as adjunctive therapy for polyarticular and systemic onset JRA.[93] Protocols have varied: Monthly infusions of intravenous immunoglobulin in a range of 1 g per kg per day for 2 consecutive days have been recommended. Other experimental approaches have included cyclosporin A[94] and plasmapheresis.

Physical and Occupational Therapy

Maintenance of function and prevention of deformity by exercises and splinting cannot be overemphasized and are vitally important in the total management of the child with JRA.[95, 96] This is particularly true for children who are initially confined to bed or a wheelchair because of the activity of their disease or pain. During periods of acute inflammation of the joints, the physical therapist might best use range of motion exercises after a warm whirlpool bath. Heat aids in the relief of joint pain and stiffness and prepares a child for the exercise program. Atrophy of the extensor muscles and later of the flexors begins early in disease, and a program should be instituted as soon as possible to strengthen these muscle groups. As weight bearing is sometimes difficult because of pain or contractures, passive and then active motion of selected joints must be begun early.

A balanced program of increased rest at night or during the day after school is advisable in many children. A child will usually best determine his or her own level of activity; only rarely does encouragement beyond present capabilities or undue restriction of daily activity profit the child. Normal play should be encouraged, and the only activities that are potentially undesirable are those that place unacceptable levels of stress on weight-bearing joints that are inflamed, such as basketball and certain forms of gymnastics. Tricycle riding and swimming are almost always helpful and avoid putting weight on involved joints.

Cock-up splints for the wrists and night splints for the elbows or knees are used to prevent malpositioning or as aids in the long-term correction of deformity. Leg length discrepancy should be minimized by a heel or sole lift for the shorter extremity. If the hips are involved, a prone lining board will help prevent hip flexion contractures. For severe contractures of a knee, elbow, or wrist, serial casting with active exercises every 2 to 4 days each time the cast is removed may be tried; forced extension should be avoided. Maintenance of reduced contractures often requires gentle stretching and the use of resting splints. Malpositioning of the cervical spine may be minimized by the use of a soft collar and a desk with a tilt top on which the child can do homework. If atlantoaxial subluxation is present, a firm collar should be worn while riding in an automobile.

Orthopedic Surgery

Synovectomy does not affect the long-term course of JRA but may be useful in carefully selected children for relief of mechanical impairment of joint motion related to synovial hypertrophy, joint pain, or decreased range of motion.[97, 98] Open arthrotomy should be avoided if at all possible because remobilization of a postsurgical joint in a child is often difficult. Arthroscopy offers an attractive alternative.[99] Tenosynovectomy may be indicated to decrease the risk of tendon rupture over the dorsum of the wrist or for adhesive tenosynovitis and trigger finger. A well thought out plan of reconstructive surgery can be of critical importance in children who enter the late teenage years or adulthood with marked disability. Total joint replacement, particularly of the hip, is usually undertaken only after bone growth has ceased (e.g., 18 years of age). Children with micrognathia may eventually benefit cosmetically from orthodontic management.

Education and Counseling of Family and Patient

Because the prognosis for JRA is excellent, it is vitally important that parents and child, if possible, understand the disease and share in its management.[100–103] A considerable amount of time and effort must be expended in explaining to them the nature of JRA, reasonable expectations during the period of initial therapy, and the course of the disease. This counseling should be initiated by the pediatric rheumatologist and reinforced by the nurse and social worker. These educational efforts must be an ongoing process; it is often useful to ask a parent to write down problems and questions and bring the list to the next appointment. More than half the families of children with JRA display psychiatrically important disruption (divorce, separation, death, or adoption) and often severe emotional disturbances. A priority in the management of the child with JRA is to foster the formation of normal psychologic and social development.[104, 105] Attendance at school is strongly encouraged; only rarely is home instruction indicated.

Nutrition

The child's nutrition is an important aspect of the long-term management of JRA. Vitamin supplementation is often indicated. Increasing attention needs to focus on the development of osteoporosis during periods of active disease and approaches to its prevention and management.[106–108]

COURSE OF DISEASE AND PROGNOSIS

Functional Disability

In general, 70 to 90 percent of children with JRA make a satisfactory recovery from their disease without serious disability.[109] A small percentage of children have a recurrence of arthritis as adults. Soon after onset, the course of JRA is especially unpredictable. The type of onset to some extent is associated with the future unfolding of the clinical disease (Table 70–4).[110–112] After the pattern of the disease is well established, the course tends to be repetitive and somewhat more predictable.

The functional result in children with unremitting polyarthritis is least favorable. The child who has oligoarthritis does best from the standpoint of joint disease but worst from the risk of uveitis. Children with systemic onset are the most prone to develop life-threatening and sometimes fatal complications.[1] Regardless of the type of onset or pattern of disease, 83 percent of children in the 15-year follow-up series at Taplow were able to work or function normally.[109] Laaksonen[3] reported that complete resolution of disease was present in 30 percent of patients at reassessment (which averaged 16 years from onset of disease); there was slight disability in 40 percent and incapacitation in 30 percent. Complete recovery was most common when duration of disease was 7 years or less (51 percent) and least when it was 16 years or longer (10 percent).

Approximately 10 percent of children with JRA enter adulthood with significant functional disability. The child most at risk is the one with polyarthritis of late age of onset, early involvement of the small joints of the hands or feet, rapid appearance of erosions, unremitting inflammatory activity, prominent systemic manifestations, RF seropositivity, and subcutaneous nodules.[52] Although the small joints may be involved in any of the various types of onset

Table 70-4. ONSET TYPES AND COURSE SUBTYPES OF JUVENILE RHEUMATOID ARTHRITIS

Onset Type (Number)	Course Subtype (Number)	Profile	Outcome
Polyarthritis (78)	RF seropositive (16)	Female	Poor
		Older age	
		Hand/wrist	
		Erosions	
		Nodules	
		Unremitting	
	ANA seropositive (38)	Female	Good
		Young age	
	Seronegative (24)	Variable	Good
Oligoarthritis (121)	ANA seropositive (66)	Female	Excellent (except eyes)
		Young age	
		Chronic uveitis	
	RF seropositive (8)	Polyarthritis	Poor
		Erosions	
		Unremitting	
	HLA-B27 positive (12)	Male	Good
		Older age	
	Seronegative (35)	Variable	Excellent
Systemic disease (51)	Oligoarthritis (30)	Variable	Good
	Polyarthritis (21)	Erosions	Poor

Modified from Cassidy, J. T., Levinson, J. E., Brewer, E. J., Jr: The development of classification criteria for children with juvenile rheumatoid arthritis. Bull. Rheum. Dis. 38:1, 1989.

of disease, widespread symmetric involvement of the metacarpophalangeal and proximal interphalangeal joints of the hands, the so-called adult pattern of RA, is characteristically associated with a poorer prognostic outlook than disease that confines itself to large joints. Hip disease is a major cause of disability in JRA and is justifiably interpreted as a relatively poor prognostic sign when it occurs (Fig. 70-12).[113]

The course of children with oligoarthritis may become monarticular or be confined to the joints of initial involvement in over one third of the children.[27] Another one third with onset of disease in a single joint will have involvement of one or two additional joints. The remaining children will progress after 6 months to an articular pattern similar to that described for polyarthritis. Children with established oligoarthritis, however, do not later develop acute manifestations of disease typical of the systemic onset type. Because of the limited nature of the joint involvement in this pattern of the disease, serious functional disability is uncommon, and these children have a generally excellent prognostic outlook if they do not develop uveitis. Osteoarthritis may occur later in the course of the disease after clinical remission of active inflammation, particularly in the weight-bearing joints of the knees or ankles.

The acute manifestations of the systemic onset type of JRA are variable in duration, lasting from weeks to months or even years, and tend to recur during the initial years of the disease, usually in association with exacerbations of the child's arthritis. About half the children with systemic onset will eventually recover completely, especially if only a limited number of joints are involved. The other half continue to show progressive arthritis and moderate to severe disability. Systemic symptoms alone are not a cause of permanent disability and seldom persist longer than 5 years.

Death

Death occurred historically in 2 to 7 percent of children with JRA but is the unfortunate outcome in less than 1 percent of children in North America at the present time. The major causes of death in 46 children followed at Taplow were renal failure, in half of the cases associated with amyloidosis, and infections.[114] Excess mortality was identified at the 15-year evaluation in girls who had developed disease early in life. The majority of the deaths associated with JRA in the United States occur in children with systemic onset of disease. Errors of steroid management are a particular risk in this group.

Children with cervical spine disease present special problems with intubation before general anesthesia. In the presence of atlantoaxial subluxation, instability, or odontoid erosion or loosening, forced extension of the neck (from intubation or an automobile accident) has resulted in respiratory arrest and death in a few patients.

Although the development of amyloidosis is rare in North America, in certain areas of the world it occurs in approximately 7 percent of patients with JRA, often heralded by proteinuria and the nephrotic syndrome, diarrhea, or unexplained anemia.[90, 114, 115] It usually develops in the more severely affected children with disease activity of long duration. It is rarely encountered as early as 1 year after onset and has been observed as late as 23 years. Amyloidosis has followed all types of onset of disease and has

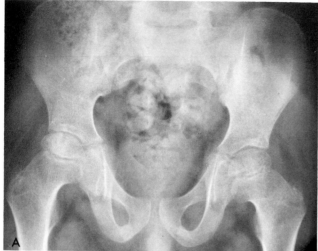
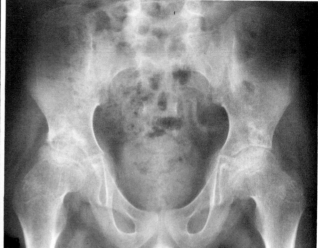
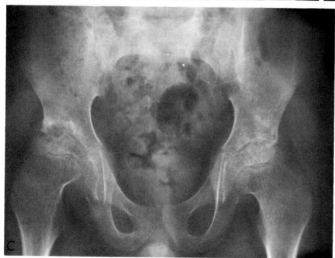

Figure 70–12. *A,* Pelvis at age 5 years in a boy with severe systemic disease and polyarthritis. There is bilateral hip disease, narrowing of the joint spaces, and remodeling of the femoral head. *B,* Two years later, destructive hip disease has progressed, and there is more marked involvement of the acetabular bone with sclerosis and multiple cystic lucencies, also seen now along the margins of the femoral heads. *C,* One year after *B,* generalized osteopenia is marked, coxa valga on the right is more extreme, and there is beginning subluxation of the right femoral head. Clinically this child had severe pain in the hips with weight bearing and virtually no rotation. Flexion contractures of approximately 35 degrees were present bilaterally.

been nearly always fatal in spite of the use of chlorambucil. The mean duration of life after diagnosis has been 8 years. A diagnosis of amyloidosis may be confirmed by rectal biopsy.

Blindness

The prognosis for sight in children with chronic uveitis is probably improving because of earlier detection and better management; however, blindness occurred previously in approximately 50 to 70 percent of children with this complication.[116, 117] Kanski's review[43] of the Taplow experience indicated that visual prognosis was good in 25 percent and fair in 50 percent. The remaining 25 percent developed visual impairment from cataract or glaucoma.

Perspective

A child's potential for growth is an important factor working in favor of the pediatric rheumatologist and the therapeutic program. To a large extent,

it is this endowment for future physical and psychologic development that enables so much to be accomplished in the majority of children with JRA.

References

1. Cassidy, J. T., and Petty, R. E.: Textbook of Pediatric Rheumatology. 2nd ed. New York, Churchill Livingstone, 1990.
2. Sullivan, D. B., Cassidy, J. T., and Petty, R. E.: Pathogenic implications of age of onset in juvenile rheumatoid arthritis. Arthritis Rheum. 18:251, 1975.
3. Laaksonen, A. -L.: A prognostic study of juvenile rheumatoid arthritis. Analysis of 544 cases. Acta Paediatr. Scand. (Suppl.) 166:1, 1966.
4. Kunnmo, I., Kallio, P., and Pelkonen, P.: Incidence of arthritis in urban Finnish children. Arthritis Rheum. 29:1232, 1986.
5. Gare, A., Fasth, A., and Anderson, J.: Incidence and prevalence of juvenile chronic arthritis: A population survey. Ann. Rheum. Dis. 45:277, 1987.
6. Towner, S. R., Michet, C. J., Jr., O'Fallon, W. M., et al.: The epidemiology of juvenile arthritis in Rochester, Minnesota. Arthritis Rheum. 26:1208, 1983.
7. Oen, K., Petty, R. E., and Schroeder, M. -L.: An association between HLA-A2 and juvenile rheumatoid arthritis in girls. J. Rheumatol. 9:916, 1982.
8. Giannini, E. H., Malagon, C. N., Van Kerckhove, C., et al.: Longitudinal analysis of HLA-associated risks for iridocyclitis in juvenile rheumatoid arthritis. J. Rheumatol. 18:9, 1991.
9. Malagon, C., Van Kerckhove, C., Giannini, E. H., et al.: The iridocyclitis of early-onset pauciarticular juvenile rheumatoid arthritis: out-

come in immunogenetically characterized patients. J. Rheumatol. 19:160, 1992.

10. Sher, M. R., Schultz, J. S., Ragsdale, C. G., et al.: HLA-DR and MT associations with the clinical and serologic manifestations of pauciarticular onset juvenile rheumatoid arthritis. J. Rheumatol. 12:114, 1985.

11. Hoffman, R. W., Shaw, S., Francis, L. C., et al.: HLA-DP antigens in patients with pauciarticular juvenile rheumatoid arthritis. Arthritis Rheum. 29:1057, 1986.

12. Nepom, B. S., Nepom, G. T., Mickelson, E., et al.: Specific HLA-DR4 associated histocompatibility molecules characterize patients with seropositive juvenile rheumatoid arthritis. J. Clin. Invest. 74:287, 1984.

13. Vehe, R. K., Begovich, A. B., and Nepom, B. S.: HLA susceptibility genes in rheumatoid factor positive juvenile rheumatoid arthritis. J. Rheumatol. 17(Suppl. 26):11, 1990.

14. Fernandez-Vina, M. A., Fink, C. W., and Stastny, P.: HLA antigens in juvenile arthritis: Pauciarticular and polyarticular juvenile arthritis are immunogenetically distinct. Arthritis Rheum. 33:1787, 1990.

15. Ansell, B. M., Bywaters, E. G., and Lawrence, J. S.: Familial aggregation and twin studies in Still's disease. Juvenile chronic polyarthritis. Rheumatology 2:37, 1969.

16. Rosenberg, A. M., and Petty, R. E.: Similar patterns of juvenile rheumatoid arthritis within families. Arthritis Rheum. 23:951, 1980.

17. Cassidy, J. T., Levinson, J. E., Bass, J. C., et al.: A study of classification criteria for a diagnosis of juvenile rheumatoid arthritis. Arthritis Rheum. 29:274, 1986.

18. Lang, B. A., and Shore, A.: A review of current concepts on the pathogenesis of juvenile rheumatoid arthritis. J. Rheumatol. 17(Suppl. 21):1, 1990.

19. Cassidy, J. T., Shillis, J. L., Brandon, F. B., et al.: Viral antibody titers to rubella and rubeola in juvenile rheumatoid arthritis. Pediatrics 54:239, 1974.

20. Chantler, J. K., Tingle, A. J., Petty, R. E.: Persistent rubella virus infection associated with chronic arthritis in children. N. Engl. J. Med. 313:1117, 1985.

21. Cassidy, J. T., Petty, R. E., and Sullivan, D. B.: Occurrence of selective IgA deficiency in children with juvenile rheumatoid arthritis. Arthritis Rheum. 20:181, 1977.

22. Petty, R. E., Cassidy, J. T., and Tubergen, D. G.: Association of arthritis with hypogammaglobulinemia. Arthritis Rheum. 20:441, 1977.

23. Morimoto, C., Reinherz, E. L., Borel, Y., et al.: Autoantibody to an immunoregulatory inducer population in patients with juvenile rheumatoid arthritis. J. Clin. Invest. 67:753, 1981.

24. Barron, K. S., Lewis, D. E., Brewer, E. J., et al.: Cytotoxic anti–T cell antibodies in children with juvenile rheumatoid arthritis. Arthritis Rheum. 27:1272, 1984.

25. Laaksonen, A. -L., and Laine, V.: A comparative study of joint pain in adult and juvenile rheumatoid arthritis. Ann. Rheum. Dis. 20:386, 1961.

26. Sherry, D. D., Bohnsack, J., Salmonson, K., et al.: Painless juvenile rheumatoid arthritis. J. Pediatr. 116:921, 1990.

27. Cassidy, J. T., Brody, G. L., and Martel, W.: Monarticular juvenile rheumatoid arthritis. J. Pediatr. 70:867, 1967.

28. McMinn, F. J., and Bywaters, E. G. L.: Differences between the fever of Still's disease and that of rheumatic fever. Ann. Rheum. Dis. 18:293, 1959.

29. Isdale, I. C., and Bywaters, E. G. L.: The rash of rheumatoid arthritis and Still's disease. Quart. J. Med. 25:377, 1956.

30. Reginato, A. J., Schumacher, H. R., Jr., Baker, D. G., et al.: Adult-onset Still's disease: Experience in 23 patients and literature review with emphasis on organ failure. Semin. Arthritis Rheum. 17:39, 1987.

31. Ohta, A., Yamaguchi, M., Tsunematsu, T., et al.: Adult Still's disease: A multicenter survey of Japanese patients. J. Rheumatol. 17:1058, 1990.

32. Sury, B., and Vesterdal, J.: Extra-articular lesions in juvenile rheumatoid arthritis. A survey based upon a study of 151 cases. Acta Rheumatol. Scand. 14:309, 1968.

33. Svantesson, H., Bjorkhem, G., and Elbough, R.: Cardiac involvement in juvenile rheumatoid arthritis. A follow-up study. Acta Paediatr. Scand. 72:345, 1983.

34. Delgado, E. A., Petty, R. E., Malleson, P. N., et al.: Aortic valve insufficiency and coronary artery narrowing in a child with polyarticular juvenile rheumatoid arthritis. J. Rheumatol. 15:144, 1988.

35. Athreya, B., Doughty, R. A., Bookspan, M., et al.: Pulmonary manifestations of juvenile rheumatoid arthritis: A report of eight cases and review. Clin. Chest Med. 1:361, 1980.

36. Anttila, R.: Renal involvement in juvenile rheumatoid arthritis. A clinical and histopathological study. Acta Paediatr. Scand. (Suppl.) 277:3, 1972.

37. Malleson, P. N., Lockitch, G., Mackinnon, M., et al.: Renal disease in chronic arthritis of childhood: A study of urinary N-acetyl-β-glucosaminidase and β₂-microglobulin excretion. Arthritis Rheum. 33:1560, 1990.

38. Wortmann, D. W., Kelsch, R. C., Kuhns, L., et al.: Renal papillary necrosis in juvenile rheumatoid arthritis. J. Pediatr. 97:37, 1980.

39. Allen, R. C., Petty, R. E., Lirenman, D. S., et al.: Renal papillary necrosis in children with chronic arthritis. J. Pediatr. 140:16, 1986.

40. Bywaters, E. G. L., Glynn, L. E., and Zeldis, A.: Subcutaneous nodules of Still's disease. Ann. Rheum. Dis. 17:278, 1958.

41. Cassidy, J. T., Sullivan, D. B., and Petty, R. E.: Clinical patterns of chronic iridocyclitis in children with juvenile rheumatoid arthritis. Arthritis Rheum. 20:224, 1977.

42. Chylack, L. T., Jr.: The ocular manifestations of juvenile rheumatoid arthritis. Arthritis Rheum. 20:217, 1977.

43. Kanski, J. J.: Juvenile arthritis and uveitis. Surv. Ophthalmol. 34:253, 1990.

44. Ansell, B. M., and Bywaters, E. G. L.: Growth in Still's disease. Ann. Rheum. Dis. 15:295, 1956.

45. Butenandt, O.: Rheumatoid arthritis and growth retardation in children: Treatment with human growth hormone. Eur. J. Pediatr. 130:15, 1979.

46. Martel, W., Holt, J. F., and Cassidy, J. T.: Roentgenologic manifestations of juvenile rheumatoid arthritis. Am. J. Roentgenol. Radium Ther. Nucl. Med. 88:400, 1962.

47. Vostrejs, M., and Hollister, J. R.: Muscle atrophy and leg length discrepancies in pauciarticular juvenile rheumatoid arthritis. Am. J. Dis. Child. 142:343, 1988.

48. Wynne-Roberts, C. R., Anderson, C., Turano, A. M., et al.: Light-and electron-microscopic findings of juvenile rheumatoid arthritis synovium. Comparison with normal juvenile synovium. Semin. Arthritis Rheum. 7:287, 1978.

49. Schaller, J., Beckwith, B., Wedgwood, R. J.: Hepatic involvement in juvenile rheumatoid arthritis. J. Pediatr. 77:203, 1970.

50. Scott, J. P., Gerber, P., Maryjowski, M. C., et al.: Evidence for intravascular coagulation in systemic onset, but not polyarticular, juvenile rheumatoid arthritis. Arthritis Rheum. 28:256, 1985.

51. Petty, R. E., Cassidy, J. T., and Sullivan, D. B.: Serologic studies in juvenile rheumatoid arthritis. A review. Arthritis Rheum. 20:260, 1977.

52. Cassidy, J. T., and Valkenburg, H. A.: A five-year prospective study of rheumatoid factor tests in juvenile rheumatoid arthritis. Arthritis Rheum. 10:83, 1967.

53. Moore, T., Osborn, T. G., and Dorner, R. W.: 19S IgM rheumatoid factor–7S IgG rheumatoid factor immune complexes in sera of patients with juvenile rheumatoid arthritis. Pediatr. Res. 20:977, 1986.

54. Petty, R. E., Cassidy, J. T., and Sullivan, D. B.: Clinical correlates of antinuclear antibodies in juvenile rheumatoid arthritis. J. Pediatr. 83:386, 1973.

55. Schaller, J. G., Johnson, G. D., Holborow, E. J., et al.: The association of antinuclear antibodies with the chronic iridocyclitis of juvenile rheumatoid arthritis (Still's disease). Arthritis Rheum. 17:409, 1974.

56. Rosenberg, A. M.: The clinical associations of antinuclear antibodies in juvenile rheumatoid arthritis. Clin. Immunol. Immunopath. 49:19, 1988.

57. Cassidy, J. T., Walker, S. E., Soderstrom, S. J., et al.: Diagnostic significance of antibody to native deoxyribonucleic acid in children with juvenile rheumatoid arthritis and connective tissue diseases. J. Pediatr. 93:416, 1978.

58. Ragsdale, C. G., Petty, R. E., Cassidy, J. T., et al.: The clinical progression of apparent juvenile rheumatoid arthritis to systemic lupus erythematosus. J. Rheumatol. 7:50, 1980.

59. Petty, R. E.: HLA-B27 and rheumatic diseases of childhood. J. Rheumatol. 17(Suppl. 26):7, 1990.

60. Rynes, R. I., Ruddy, S., Spragg, J., et al.: Intraarticular activation of the complement system in patients with juvenile rheumatoid arthritis. Arthritis Rheum. 19:161, 1976.

61. Cassidy, J. T., and Martel, W.: Juvenile rheumatoid arthritis: Clinicoradiologic correlations. Arthritis Rheum. 20:207, 1977.

62. Hensinger, R. N., DeVito, P. D., and Ragsdale, C. G.: Changes in the cervical spine in juvenile rheumatoid arthritis. J. Bone Joint Surg. 68:189, 1986.

63. Poznanski, A. K., Conway, J. J., Shkolnik, A., et al.: Radiological approaches in the evaluation of joint disease in children. Rheum. Dis. Clin. North Am. 13:57, 1987.

64. Kvien, T. K., Høyeraal, H. M., and Kåss, E.: Diagnostic criteria for rheumatoid arthritis in children. Scand. J. Rheumatol. 11:187, 1982.

65. Brewer, E. J., Jr.: Pitfalls in the diagnosis of juvenile rheumatoid arthritis. Pediatr. Clin. North Am. 33:1015, 1986.

66. Cassidy, J. T.: Miscellaneous conditions associated with arthritis in children. Pediatr. Clin. North Am. 33:1015, 1986.

67. Williams, C. L., Strobino, B., Lee, A., et al.: Lyme disease in childhood: Clinical and epidemiologic features of ninety cases. Pediatr. Infect. Dis. J. 9:10, 1990.

68. Gedalia, A., Person, D. A., Brewer, E. J., Jr., et al.: Hypermobility of the joints in juvenile episodic arthritis/arthralgia. J. Pediatr. 107:873, 1985.

69. Shore, A., and Ansell, B. M.: Juvenile psoriatic arthritis—an analysis of 60 cases. J. Pediatr. 100:529, 1982.

70. Lindsley, C. B., and Schaller, J. G.: Arthritis associated with inflammatory bowel disease in children. J. Pediatr. 84:16, 1974.

71. Kaplan, E. L.: Rheumatic fever. Curr. Opin. Rheumatol. 2:836, 1990.

72. Ladd, J. R., Cassidy, J. T., and Martel, W.: Juvenile ankylosing spondylitis. Arthritis Rheum. 14:579, 1971.

73. Kvien, T. K.: Drug Management of Patients with Juvenile Rheumatoid Arthritis. Oslo Sanitetsforening Rheumatism Hospital, Oslo, Norway, 1986.

74. Athreya, B. H., Moser, G., Cecil, H. S., et al.: Aspirin-induced hepatotoxicity in juvenile rheumatoid arthritis. A prospective study. Arthritis Rheum. 18:347, 1975.

75. Bernstein, B. H., Singsen, B. H., King, K. K., et al.: Aspirin-induced hepatotoxicity and its effect on juvenile rheumatoid arthritis. Am. J. Dis. Child. 131:659, 1977.

76. Rennebohm, R. M., Heubi, J. E., Daugherty, C. C., et al.: Reye's syndrome in children receiving salicylate therapy for connective tissue disease. J. Pediatr. 107:877, 1985.

77. Sandler, D. P., Smith, J. C., Weinberg, C. R., et al.: Analgesic use and chronic renal disease. N. Engl. J. Med. 320:1238, 1989.

78. Lovell, D. J., Giannini, E. H., and Brewer, E. J., Jr.: Time course of response to nonsteroidal antiinflammatory drugs in juvenile rheumatoid arthritis. Arthritis Rheum. 27:1433, 1984.

79. Giannini, E. H., Brewer, E. J., Miller, M. L., et al.: Ibuprofen suspension in the treatment of juvenile rheumatoid arthritis. J. Pediatr. 117:645, 1990.

80. Manners, P. J., and Ansell, B. M.: Slow-acting antirheumatic drug use in systemic onset juvenile chronic arthritis. Pediatrics 77:99, 1986.

81. Grondin, C., Malleson, P., and Petty, R. E.: Slow-acting antirheumatic drugs in chronic arthritis of childhood. Semin. Arthritis Rheum. 18:38, 1988.

82. Brewer, E. J., Giannini, E. H., Kuzmina, H., et al.: Penicillamine and hydroxychloroquine in the treatment of severe juvenile rheumatoid arthritis: Results of the U.S.A.–U.S.S.R., double-blind, placebo-controlled trial. N. Engl. J. Med. 314:1269, 1986.

83. Kvien, T. K., Høyeraal, H. M., and Sandstad, B.: Gold sodium thiomalate and D-penicillamine. A controlled, comparative study in patients with pauciarticular and polyarticular juvenile rheumatoid arthritis. Scand. J. Rheumatol. 14:346, 1985.

84. Hadchouel, M., Prieur, A. -M., and Griscelli, C.: Acute hemorrhagic, hepatic, and neurologic manifestations in juvenile rheumatoid arthritis: Possible relationship to drugs or infection. J. Pediatr. 106:561, 1985.

85. Giannini, E. H., Brewer, E. J., Jr., Kuzmina, N., et al.: Auranofin in the treatment of juvenile rheumatoid arthritis: Results of the U.S.A.–U.S.S.R. double-blind, placebo-controlled trial. Arthritis Rheum. 33:466, 1989.

86. Giannini, E. H., Barron, K. S., Spencer, C. H., et al.: Auranofin therapy for juvenile rheumatoid arthritis: results of the five-year open-label extension trial. J. Rheumatol. 18:1240, 1991.

87. Ozdogan, H., Turunc, M., Deringol, B., et al.: Sulphasalazine in the treatment of juvenile rheumatoid arthritis: A preliminary open trial. J. Rheumatol. 13:124, 1986.

88. Wolf, M. D., Lichter, P. R., and Ragsdale, C. G.: Prognostic factors in the uveitis of juvenile rheumatoid arthritis. Ophthalmology 94:1242, 1987.

89. Allen, R. C., Gross, K. R., Laxer, R. M., et al.: Intraarticular triamcinolone hexacetonide in the management of chronic arthritis in children. Arthritis Rheum. 29:997, 1986.

90. Ansell, B. M., Eghtedari, A., and Bywaters, E. G. L.: Chlorambucil in the management of juvenile chronic arthritis complicated by amyloidosis. Ann. Rheum. Dis. 30:331, 1971.

91. Giannini, E. H., Brewer, E. J., Kuzmina, N., et al.: Low-dose methotrexate in resistant juvenile rheumatoid arthritis. Results of the U.S.A.-U.S.S.R. double-blind placebo-controlled trial. N. Engl. J. Med. 326:1043, 1992.

92. Wallace, C. A., Bleyer, W. A., Sherry, D., et al.: Toxicity and serum levels of methotrexate in children with juvenile rheumatoid arthritis. Arthritis Rheum. 32:677, 1989.

93. Silverman, E. D., Laxer, R. M., Greenwald, M., et al.: Intravenous gamma globulin therapy in systemic juvenile rheumatoid arthritis. Arthritis Rheum. 33:1015, 1990.

94. Ostensen, M., Høyeraal, H. M., and Kass, E.: Tolerance of cyclosporin A in children with refractory juvenile rheumatoid arthritis. J. Rheumatol. 15:10, 1988.

95. Emery, H. M., and Kucinski, J.: Management of Juvenile Rheumatoid Arthritis. A Handbook for Occupational and Physical Therapists. Chicago, IL, LaRabida Children's Hospital and Research Center, 1987.

96. Schull, S. A., Dow, M. B., and Athreya, B. H.: Physical and occupational therapy for children with rheumatic diseases. Pediatr. Clin. North Am. 33:1053, 1986.

97. Arden, G. P., and Ansell, B. M. (eds.): Surgical Management of Juvenile Chronic Polyarthritis. London, Academic Press, 1978.

98. Kvien, T. K., Pahle, J. A., Høyeraal, H. M., et al.: Comparison of synovectomy and no synovectomy in patients with juvenile rheumatoid arthritis. A 24-month controlled study. Scand. J. Rheumatol. 16:81, 1987.

99. Rydholm, U.: Arthroscopy of the knee in juvenile chronic arthritis. Scand. J. Rheumatol. 15:109, 1986.

100. Hobbs, N., and Perrin, J. M. (eds.): Issues in the Care of Children with Chronic Illness. A Source Book on Problems, Services, and Policies. San Francisco, Jossey-Bass, Inc., 1985.

101. Hobbs, N., Perrin, J. M., and Ireys, H. T.: Chronically Ill Children and Their Families. Problems, Prospects, and Proposals From the Vanderbilt Study. San Francisco, Jossey-Bass, Inc., 1985.

102. Rapoff, M. A., Lindsley, C. B., and Christophersen, E. R.: Parent perception of problems experienced by their children in complying with treatments for juvenile rheumatoid arthritis. Arch. Phys. Med. Rehabil. 66:427, 1985.

103. Atreya, B. H., and McCormick, M. C.: Impact of chronic illness on families. Rheum. Dis. Clin. North Am. 13:123, 1987.

104. Henoch, M. J., Batson, J. W., and Baum, J.: Psychosocial factors in juvenile rheumatoid arthritis. Arthritis Rheum. 21:229, 1978.

105. Ungerer, J. A., Horgan, B., Chaitwo, J., et al.: Psychosocial functioning in children and young adults with juvenile arthritis. Pediatrics 81:195, 1988.

106. Hopp, R., Degan, J., Gallagher, J. C., et al.: Estimation of total body calcium and bone density in children with juvenile rheumatoid arthritis. Clin. Res. 37:964A, 1989.

107. Bianchi, M. L., Baldare, M., Caraceni, M. P., et al.: Bone metabolism in juvenile rheumatoid arthritis. Bone Miner. 9:153, 1990.

108. Reed, A., Haugen, M., Packman, L. M., et al.: Abnormalities in serum osteocalcin values in children with chronic rheumatic diseases. J. Pediatr. 116:574, 1990.

109. Ansell, B. M., and Wood, P. H. N.: Prognosis in juvenile chronic polyarthritis. Clin. Rheum. Dis. 2:397, 1976.

110. Allen, R. C., and Ansell, B. M.: Juvenile chronic arthritis—clinical sub-groups with particular relationship to adult patterns of disease. Postgrad. Med. J. 62:821, 1986.

111. Prieur, A. M., Ansell, B. M., Bardfeld, R., et al.: Is onset type evaluated during the first 3 months of disease satisfactory for defining the sub-groups of juvenile chronic arthritis? A EULAR Cooperative Study (1983–1986). Clin. Exp. Rheumatol. 8:321, 1990.

112. Cassidy, J. T., Levinson, J. E., and Brewer, E. J., Jr.: The development of classification criteria for children with juvenile rheumatoid arthritis. Bull. Rheumat. Dis. 38:1, 1989.

113. Blane, C. E., Ragsdale, C. G., and Hensinger, R. N.: Late effects of JRA on the hip. J. Pediatr. Orthop. 7:677, 1987.

114. Bywaters, E. G. L.: Deaths in juvenile chronic polyarthritis. Arthritis Rheum. 20:256, 1977.

115. Smith, M. E., Ansell, B. M., and Bywaters, E. G. L.: Mortality and prognosis related to the amyloidosis of Still's disease. Ann. Rheum. Dis. 27:137, 1968.

116. Smiley, W. K.: The eye in juvenile rheumatoid arthritis. Trans. Ophthalmol. Soc. U.K. 94:817, 1974.

117. Rosenberg, A. M.: Uveitis associated with juvenile rheumatoid arthritis. Semin. Arthritis Rheum. 16:158, 1987.

Rheumatic Fever

DEFINITION

Rheumatic fever is an inflammatory disease that occurs as a delayed sequela to pharyngeal infection with group A streptococci. It involves the heart, joints, central nervous system, skin, and subcutaneous tissues. In the acute form its common clinical manifestations are migratory polyarthritis, fever, carditis, and, less frequently, Sydenham's chorea, subcutaneous nodules, and erythema marginatum. No single symptom, sign, or laboratory test result is pathognomonic of rheumatic fever, although several combinations of them are diagnostic. Although involvement of the joints justifies grouping this syndrome with the rheumatic diseases, its importance relates to involvement of the heart, which can be fatal during the acute stage of the disease or can lead to rheumatic heart disease, a chronic condition due to scarring and deformity of the heart valves.

ETIOLOGY AND PATHOGENESIS

The evidence that has established the group A streptococcus as the etiologic agent of rheumatic fever is all indirect because group A streptococci are not recoverable from the lesions and no satisfactory experimental model of the disease has been demonstrated. Nonetheless, the evidence is overwhelming and can be summarized briefly according to four main lines of observation.

Clinical Evidence

It has been recognized for more than a hundred years that acute rheumatic fever (ARF) is often preceded by acute pharyngitis. The inconsistency of this relationship, however, has been noted repeatedly.[1] At least one third of patients with ARF deny antecedent sore throat. At the onset of the rheumatic attack cultures of the throat are usually negative and cultures of the blood are virtually always sterile. Rheumatic recurrences are even more difficult to relate to an antecedent sore throat because subclinical streptococcal infection so often reactivates the disease. On clinical grounds alone, therefore, the group A streptococcus is difficult to establish as the only etiologic agent.

Epidemiologic Evidence

Factors such as latitude, altitude, crowding, dampness, socioeconomic status, and age all affect the incidence of rheumatic fever because they are related to the incidence and severity of streptococcal pharyngitis in general. Careful military epidemiologic studies over a period of 20 years show a clear sequential relationship of outbreaks of streptococcal pharyngitis to rheumatic fever. Despite epidemics caused by a variety of other respiratory pathogens, ARF is absent in the same population when streptococcal infection is controlled by chemotherapy.[2] Military recruits are healthy, young adults, physically highly trained, optimally nourished, and socially and ethnically heterogeneous—yet rheumatic fever occurred more frequently in those with previous histories of ARF.[3]

Immunologic Evidence

Initial (primary) or recurrent (secondary) rheumatic fever does not occur without a streptococcal antibody response.[4] Furthermore, the magnitude of the antibody response is strongly correlated with the attack rate of rheumatic fever following streptococcal pharyngitis.[5] This is true for both primary and secondary attacks.[6]

Prophylactic Evidence

The most convincing evidence of all is the complete prevention of rheumatic recurrences by continuous chemoprophylaxis against streptococcal infection in rheumatic subjects and the prevention of initial attacks by prompt and effective penicillin therapy of streptococcal sore throat.[7, 8]

PATHOGENESIS

Despite the clear implication of the group A streptococcus as the causative agent of rheumatic fever, the pathogenesis of the disease remains an enigma. Four requirements for the pathogenesis seem firmly established: (1) the presence of the group A streptococcus, (2) location of the infection in the throat, (3) persistence of the organism in the pharynx for a sufficient period of time, and (4) a streptococcal antibody response indicative of actual recent infection.

Site of Infection

Lymphatic connections between the pharynx and the heart are suspected of playing a role in the pathogenesis of ARF. Streptococcal infections at other sites, such as in skin, wound infections, puerperal sepsis, or pneumonia, have not been associated with rheumatic fever.

Strain of Group A Streptococcus

The severity of streptococcal sore throat bears a general relationship to the attack rate of rheumatic fever,[9] and this observation is reflected in the correlation of attack rate with the magnitude of the antibody response.[5] Moreover, strains of only a relatively limited number of streptococcal M serotypes (e.g., types 3, 5, 14, 18, 19, and 24) have been strongly epidemiologically associated with epidemics of rheumatic fever.[10] When freshly isolated, such strains are often heavily encapsulated as well as rich in M protein.[7] On the other hand, certain M protein serotypes (e.g., types 2, 4, and 12) and those associated with skin infections have not been shown to produce ARF.[11–13] Furthermore, nephritogenic group A streptococci rarely if ever have been shown to cause rheumatic fever in well-defined epidemics of nephritis.[14] Strains of the streptococcal serotypes most strongly associated with ARF have been isolated with decreased frequency in the United States during the past two decades,[15, 16] during which the incidence of rheumatic fever has declined precipitously,[17] only to reappear in the mid-1980s in association with outbreaks of ARF.

These observations provide strong evidence that individual strains of group A streptococci vary in their ability to elicit ARF, as they do glomerulonephritis. This concept has been advanced by several investigators for many years, and further evidence for its validity has been presented elsewhere.[7, 10, 12, 13, 18–20] Whether rheumatogenic strains are simply those of unusual virulence, owing to their encapsulation and high content of M protein, or whether a qualitative difference in the antigens they possess is a key factor, remains conjectural.

Several recent findings raise the possibility of a role for M protein in the pathogenesis of ARF. These include the existence of shared epitopes between M proteins of rheumatogenic group A streptococcal serotypes and human heart,[21–23] the recognition of distinct structural differences between M proteins of rheumatogenic and nonrheumatogenic types,[24, 25] and the finding that M protein functions as a superantigen,[26] capable of strongly activating a broad range of T lymphocytes.

The role of the hyaluronate capsule of the streptococcus as a virulence factor, and possibly in the pathogenesis of the disease, has been repeatedly noted.[7, 18] The recent outbreaks of rheumatic fever in the United States are significant in this regard, because of their association with mucoid (highly encapsulated) strains of M3 and M18.[27–29] Such strains were frequently encountered during the notorious military recruit camp epidemics in the United States during and after World War II.

Immunologic Theories

Bacterial allergy or autoimmunity is the most popular pathogenetic theory of rheumatic fever, although none of the streptococcal antibodies described to date, including those reactive with the heart, has been shown to be cytotoxic. However, rheumatic fever patients are, in general, the population that is most intensively hyperimmune to all antigenic streptococcal products that have been tested. Moreover, circulating immune complexes in patients with ARF have been found to contain streptococcal antigens.[30, 31]

Autoimmunity. A comprehensive discussion of the possible relation of autoimmunity to the pathogenesis of rheumatic fever is beyond the scope of this chapter and has been reviewed elsewhere.[32] Some of the most relevant aspects of autoimmunity to group A streptococcal infection are considered below.

Cross-Reactions Between Streptococci and Human Heart and Other Organs. In the early 1960s, Kaplan and associates demonstrated that rabbit antisera against certain group A streptococci react with human heart preparations in the immunofluorescent test.[33, 34] In the years since, additional immunologic cross-reactions have been described between streptococci and human tissues. The purification of the streptococcal M proteins and the identification of M protein peptides, which cross-react with cardiac myosin and sarcolemma and which are contained in some "rheumatogenic" M protein serotypes,[21–23] may now permit more incisive immunologic research concerning the pathogenetic significance, if any, of this autoimmune phenomenon. The concept of autoimmunity in ARF has been extended to Sydenham's chorea by studies demonstrating antibody to caudate and subthalamic nuclei in sera from patients with this rheumatic manifestation.[35] This antibody could be absorbed with group A streptococcal membranes, which also cross-react with the sarcolemmal membranes of the heart.

Group A carbohydrate antibodies that cross-react with the glycoprotein of the human heart persist longer after rheumatic fever in patients with rheumatic heart disease than in those rheumatic fever patients who escape heart damage.[36] Moreover, in subsequent studies, it was found that the level of group A antibodies decreased after valvectomy but not after valvotomy, suggesting that the group A antibody persists in patients with rheumatic heart disease because of self-reimmunization with valvular components.[37]

Although purified hyaluronate extracted from encapsulated group A streptococci was previously considered to be nonantigenic in animals and humans, more recent studies have demonstrated antigenicity when more sensitive methods, such as the enzyme-linked immunosorbent assay (ELISA), were employed. Moreover, the immune responses were shown by monoclonal antibody techniques to be specific for epitopes of hyaluronate itself and not due to contaminants, as previously suspected.[38, 39] Hyaluronate is a widely distributed component of the ground substance of the heart's connective tissues and therefore the mucoid (heavily encapsulated) strains of M protein–rich streptococci associated with epidemic rheumatic fever make the possibility of autoimmunity to hyaluronate or M protein component peptides a reasonable possibility.

Host Factors

Rheumatic fever is a ubiquitous malady that exhibits no obvious racial or ethnic predilection. Nevertheless, there is strong circumstantial evidence to suggest a genetic predisposition to the development of this disease. It is believed to be immunologically mediated and tends to cluster in family groups. Although the concordance rate for rheumatic fever among monozygotic twins is relatively low (18.7 percent), it is sevenfold higher than that in dizygotic twins.[40] Moreover, even in severe epidemics of acute pharyngitis caused by highly virulent and rheumatogenic streptococci, only a small proportion of infected individuals develop rheumatic fever.

Studies of the distribution of class I HLA antigens in patients with rheumatic fever and control subjects have been inconclusive. A statistically significant association has been reported, however, between certain class II HLA antigens (DR4 in whites,[41, 42] and DR2 in blacks[41]) and rheumatic fever. Moreover, certain alloantigens are expressed in a significantly higher frequency on B cells of rheumatic fever and rheumatic heart disease patients and their family members than on B cells of patients with poststreptococcal nephritis and their family members or normal controls.[43, 44] The extent to which expression of this phenotype is inherited or acquired remains to be determined.

Immune Response of Rheumatic Fever Patients

Virtually every immune response, humoral and cellular, to all streptococcal antigens that have been studied shows a statistically significant increase in rheumatic subjects compared with nonrheumatics recovering from streptococcal pharyngitis. Rheumatic

fever patients respond normally to other antigens, such as diphtheria toxoids. The increased immune response may represent a greater magnitude, antigenically, of streptococcal infection in the rheumatic patient or, alternatively, more frequent or severe previous infections. The genetic control of immune responses, however, and their strong association with certain HLA haplotypes in other rheumatic diseases make the issue of genetic predisposition still quite viable especially with regard to certain complications such as mitral stenosis and chorea.

EPIDEMIOLOGY

Global Epidemiology of Rheumatic Fever

ARF continues to occur with great frequency in many of the developing countries of the world (e.g., the Indian subcontinent, the Muslim countries of the Middle East, and Africa), and in those areas rheumatic heart disease remains the leading cause of cardiovascular morbidity and mortality in the 5–24-year age-group.[45, 46] In contrast, the incidence of the disease has declined dramatically in North America, western Europe, and Japan.[47] In the United States, the disease became exceedingly rare among middle-class populations and tended to persist primarily among disadvantaged black and Hispanic residents of the inner cities.[17, 48–50] The reasons for the decline are most likely multifactorial, including improvements in social conditions and improved access to health care. Although the advent of effective antimicrobial therapy for the prevention of rheumatic fever has been beneficial, the decline actually began long before the antimicrobial era.[51] The profound decline in ARF incidence occurred in the absence of any evidence of a decline in the incidence of streptococcal pharyngitis.

Resurgence of Rheumatic Fever in the United States

Quite unexpectedly, a series of outbreaks of ARF occurred in the United States in the mid-1980s. The largest outbreak occurred in Salt Lake City, Utah, in 1985,[27] and by the end of 1989 approximately 200 cases had occurred.[52] Smaller outbreaks were reported from Columbus[28] and Akron, Ohio,[53] Pittsburgh, Pennsylvania,[54] New York, New York,[55] Nashville[56] and Memphis,[57] Tennessee, Kansas City, Missouri,[58] Dallas, Texas,[59] and Morgantown, West Virginia.[60] As surprising as the resurgence of ARF was the fact that a number of the outbreaks involved white children of middle-class suburban families (Salt Lake City, Columbus, Akron, and Pittsburgh) who would presumably have had ready access to health care. Moreover, two outbreaks of ARF occurred among military recruits undergoing basic training (Fig. 71–1).[29, 61] Such outbreaks, which had been

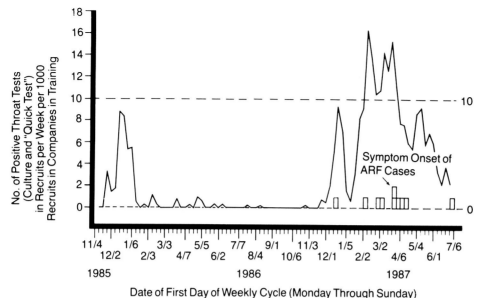

Figure 71–1. Incidence of group A streptococcal pharyngitis among recruits at the Naval Training Center, San Diego, CA. Dashed line indicates the epidemic threshold defined by the Armed Forces Epidemiologic Board. Squares represent cases of acute rheumatic fever. (From Wallace, M. R., et al. The return of acute rheumatic fever in young adults. J.A.M.A. Nov. 10, 1989, 262:2557, with permission.)

commonplace during and immediately after World War II, had not been seen for some two decades. Group A streptococci recovered from ARF patients, their families, and community and training camp surveys were generally highly mucoid and belonged to well-known rheumatogenic serotypes (e.g., 3, 18), which had rarely been recovered from patients with streptococcal pharyngitis in recent years.

At approximately the same time that the resurgence of ARF in the United States became evident, cases of invasive, life-threatening streptococcal infections began to be reported in the United States,[62–65] the United Kingdom,[66, 67] Scandinavia,[68] and elsewhere in Europe. These included streptococcal bacteremias and a syndrome characterized by localized or generalized rash, hypotension, and multiorgan failure. The latter syndrome occurs primarily in adults, is frequently secondary to cutaneous or soft-tissue infection, is often due to streptococci of M-type 1 as well as strains producing pyrogenic exotoxin A, and has been referred to as the "toxic strep syndrome."[62–65] The resurgence of ARF, the appearance of life-threatening streptococcal infections, and the isolation of group A streptococci that exhibit certain biologic characteristics known to be associated with severe forms of illness suggest that the recent changes in streptococcal epidemiology reflect basic changes in the virulence of prevalent streptococcal strains.

Attack Rate of Rheumatic Fever

Among military populations, patients who were ill with exudative streptococcal pharyngitis caused by several common and virulent pharyngeal strains of rheumatogenic group A streptococci developed rheumatic fever at a remarkably predictable rate of approximately 3 percent regardless of their age, race,

or ethnic group and regardless of the season or year in which the study was made.[69] The major variables that seemed related to this attack rate were the magnitude of the immune response and the duration of carriage of the organism.[5, 70]

Rheumatic fever occurs less frequently following the endemic, sporadic form of streptococcal disease seen in civilian practice. In studies of Chicago school children, the absence of rheumatic fever was noteworthy in some 300 patients who had nonexudative sore throat, a positive throat culture for group A streptococci, and a significant increase in antistreptolysin O (ASO) titer.[7, 71, 72] In contrast to the military studies, few of the streptococcal strains prevalent among the Chicago children belonged to the virulent M-serotypes now recognized to be highly rheumatogenic.

Host Factors and the Course of Rheumatic Fever

Rheumatic fever is to be found in every race and ethnic group exposed to rheumatogenic streptococcal disease, and there is no convincing evidence of a particular predilection among any of these groups. The effect of other host variables such as sex on the frequency of certain complications of rheumatic fever suggests that host factors undoubtedly play some part. The incidence of chorea is equal among prepubescent boys and girls, but this manifestation is absent in the sexually mature male and exaggerated during pregnancy. Other examples of sex predilection are the increased frequency of tight mitral stenosis in the female and aortic stenosis in the male.

After rheumatic fever is acquired, its reactivation following streptococcal infection is many times greater in rheumatic subjects than the attack rate in the general population. The recurrence rate per infection (R/I) may be as high as 50 percent during the first year and decreases sharply until 4 to 5 years after the attack when it levels off at approximately 10 percent.[73] Thereafter, it does not seem to decrease any further.[74]

PATHOLOGIC CHANGES

General Pathologic Findings

The earliest structural change of rheumatic inflammation is found in the collagen of the connective tissues of the heart, and is called fibrinoid degeneration. "Mucoid edema," a basophilic-staining swelling of the ground substance, is observed most prominently in the dense collagen of the valves and endocardium. The collagen fibers themselves in these mucoid areas become swollen and eosinophilic, forming a meshwork of rigid, waxlike fibers. These changes in the myocardium are followed within a couple of weeks by the development of the most characteristic lesion of rheumatic fever, the Aschoff nodule.

Aschoff nodules are virtually pathognomonic of rheumatic fever. Some believe that Aschoff lesions derive from injured muscle cells,[75, 76] but most pathologists believe the epithelioid cells and so-called Anitschkow myocytes are actually derived from cells of the histiocyte and macrophage lineage.[77–80] Whatever the origin of the Aschoff nodule, its functional role in rheumatic carditis is also controversial. Acute rheumatic myocarditis is associated with a toxic effect on the myocardium that is not always reflected in the morbid anatomy of the disease. The persistence of Aschoff nodules for many years after a rheumatic attack has been recognized by all pathologists. Biopsies of the left atrial appendage obtained during mitral valve surgery have shown persistence of these lesions in patients who no longer have clinical or laboratory evidence of rheumatic activity. The persistence of Aschoff nodules seems to be correlated, however, with the tendency in the host to develop progressive fibrosis and stenosis of the mitral valve.[81]

Pathologic Changes of the Heart

Rheumatic carditis is characteristically a pancarditis; all layers of the heart are involved. On gross inspection, fresh exudative pericardial lesions, dilation of the myocardium, and verrucous valvular lesions are almost always evident. Pericarditis involves both layers of the pericardium, which are thickened and covered by a fibrinous exudate. Serosanguineous fluid often fills the pericardial sac. Microscopically, mucoid edema and fibrinoid changes present in other layers of the heart are also found in the pericardium. With healing, fibrosis and adhesions occur, but constrictive pericarditis is not a complication of rheumatic pericarditis.

Myocarditis is characterized by the focal cellular lesions described before, but in addition to Aschoff bodies, a diffuse cellular infiltrate is present in interstitial tissues, consisting of lymphocytes, polymorphonuclear neutrophils (PMNs), histiocytes, and eosinophils. The greatest damage to myocardial fibers occurs in the vicinity of Aschoff nodules and around blood vessels, leading to myocytolysis, loss of striation, fatty degeneration, and vacuolation of muscle fibers. Despite the great frequency of delayed atrioventricular conduction in acute rheumatic fever, involvement of the bundle of His by visible anatomic changes is rare.

Endocarditis is characterized by verrucous lesions at the free borders of the valve cusps. They are amorphous masses of eosinophilic material staining as fibrin. At the base and edges of the valve, the cells line up in palisades at right angles to the base. During healing, granulation tissue develops and vascularization and progressive fibrosis take place. The annulus is involved as well as the cusps. The chordae tendineae are also frequently affected and thickened and shortened. Subendocardial scarring also occurs with the formation of characteristic broad bands of eosinophilic granular or hyaline material, which often heals as a thickened, scarred, and even calcified layer.

Rheumatic Valvular Deformities

The lesions of the mitral, aortic, and tricuspid valves are described elsewhere[7] and will not be detailed here. It should be noted, however, that some of the progressive changes and continued fibrosis of the heart valves seem to be unrelated to the original rheumatic process or to rheumatic recurrences alone. Rapid platelet destruction and turnover[82] and progressive thrombosis and fibrosis can occur along with calcification in deformed and scarred heart valves (Fig. 71–2).

Extracardiac Lesions

The characteristic pathologic changes in the *arthritis* of rheumatic fever are swelling and edema of the articular and periarticular structures with serous effusion into the joint space but without erosion of the joint surface and without pannus formation. The synovial membrane is reddened, thickened, and covered by a fibrinous exudate. Microscopically, the picture is one of acute exudative inflammation with focal and diffuse cellular infiltrates of PMNs and lymphocytes. Later, focal fibrinoid lesions and histiocytic granulomas may appear, but fibrosis is absent.

Subcutaneous nodules are composed of a central zone of fibrinoid necrosis surrounded by histiocytes and fibroblasts. Lymphocytes and PMNs collect around small blood vessels and present an appearance resembling the histology of Aschoff bodies. These lesions heal rapidly, leaving no apparent scars.

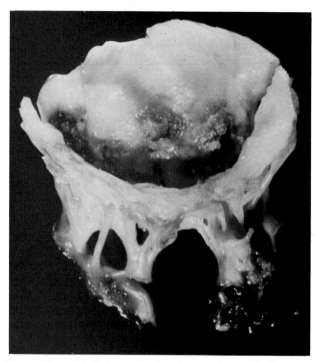

Figure 71–2. Calcified mitral valve from patient with rheumatic heart disease. (Courtesy of A. Morales, M.D.)

The pathology of *chorea* has caused considerable confusion for several reasons. Few patients die of "pure" chorea, whereas those who die of severe carditis may have central nervous system lesions without chorea. No single site is consistently involved; Aschoff nodules are not found in the brain. It has not been possible to correlate clinical findings with pathologic changes.[83]

CLINICAL MANIFESTATIONS

Antecedent Streptococcal Infection

One third or more of patients do not remember having any upper respiratory illness in the month preceding the onset of a first attack of rheumatic fever. Rheumatic recurrences may be preceded by asymptomatic streptococcal infections in more than 50 percent of instances. Streptococcal pharyngitis may be strongly immunogenic when caused by virulent rheumatogenic strains without always producing severe symptoms. Furthermore, when streptococcal pharyngitis causes symptoms, they may last for only a few days even in the absence of specific therapy and may not be remembered.

Latent Period

Between the onset of symptoms of pharyngitis and the onset of rheumatic fever there is always a time lag or latent period, which is, on the average,

approximately 19 days. It is rarely less than 1 week or longer than 5 weeks. The latent period does not shorten with recurrent rheumatic attacks. During the latent period there is neither clinical nor laboratory evidence of active inflammation.

Major Manifestations of an Acute Rheumatic Attack

Certain manifestations that follow streptococcal infections with a frequency far exceeding chance may occur simultaneously, in rapid succession, or singly. These major manifestations consist of arthritis, carditis, chorea, subcutaneous nodules, and erythema marginatum. The term *major* refers to their importance as diagnostic criteria rather than to their importance in the severity of the process, its activity, or prognosis.

Arthritis. The arthritis of rheumatic fever usually involves the large joints, particularly the knees, ankles, elbows, and wrists. The hips are less commonly involved, and the spine is only rarely affected. The smaller joints of the fingers and toes are also less commonly inflamed. Almost any joint, however, may be affected. In the classic attack, several joints are involved in quick succession and each for a brief period of time, resulting in the typical picture of migratory polyarthritis accompanied by signs and symptoms of an acute febrile illness.

Each joint remains inflamed for usually no more than a week before it begins to subside, and the inflammation usually abates spontaneously in 2 or 3 weeks. The course of the entire bout of polyarthritis is usually severe for a week in approximately two thirds of patients and for an additional week or two in the remainder, but by the end of 4 weeks it subsides with only rare exceptions. Flare-ups may occur, however, in a small percentage of patients treated with antirheumatic therapy for 4 to 6 weeks but rarely after a second 6-week course of antirheumatic treatment.

Rheumatic fever never causes permanent joint deformities, with the rare exception of the so-called Jaccoud type of deformity of the metacarpophalangeal joints.[84, 85] This condition is a "postrheumatic" periarticular fibrosis and not a synovitis. Because it occurs so rarely, its relationship to rheumatic fever is not clear, but it usually occurs in patients with severe rheumatic heart disease and is not associated with other evidence of active rheumatic fever.

The time of onset of rheumatic polyarthritis is sharply defined in relation to the antecedent streptococcal infection. Acute polyarthritis virtually never occurs more that 35 days from the onset of the antecedent streptococcal infection. For that reason, it is almost always associated with a rising or peak titer of streptococcal antibodies, an association useful in identifying an isolated bout of polyarthritis as rheumatic or, more accurately, of excluding rheumatic fever as a cause for a given bout of polyarthritis when streptococcal antibodies are not increased.

Arthritis occurs in approximately three fourths of patients during the acute stage of rheumatic fever. Joint involvement becomes more common with increasing age of the patient. When arthritis is the only major manifestation of rheumatic fever, the diagnosis is most difficult, and arthritis should be carefully distinguished from arthralgia, a less specific symptom and one more difficult to assess when objective signs are lacking. To be acceptable as a criterion for the diagnosis of rheumatic fever, the polyarthritis should involve two or more joints, should be associated with at least two minor manifestations such as fever and increase in the erythrocyte sedimentation rate (ESR), and should be associated with high titers of ASO or some other streptococcal antibody (Table 71–1). The prognostic significance of more atypical forms of poststreptococcal arthritis, unaccompanied by other manifestations of ARF, remains a matter of debate.[86–88]

Carditis. In its most severe form, carditis causes death from acute cardiac failure. More commonly, however, it is less intense, and its predominant effect is scarring of the heart valves. In contrast to the seriousness of its prognosis, rheumatic carditis often causes no symptoms of its own. It is usually diagnosed in the course of examination of a patient with arthritis or chorea, which directs the physician's attention to the heart, where the murmurs of rheumatic carditis are detected. If other symptoms of rheumatic fever are absent or if the carditis is not severe enough to cause heart failure, the pain of pericarditis, or prolonged or severe fever, carditis is frequently undetected. Patients with undiagnosed carditis may later be found to have rheumatic heart

Table 71–1. JONES CRITERIA (REVISED) FOR GUIDANCE IN THE DIAGNOSIS OF RHEUMATIC FEVER*

Major Manifestations	Minor Manifestations
Carditis	Clinical
Polyarthritis	Previous rheumatic fever or
Chorea	rheumatic heart disease
Erythema marginatum	Arthralgia
Subcutaneous nodules	Fever
	Laboratory
	Acute phase reactants
	Erythrocyte sedimentation rate
	C-reactive protein
	Leukocytosis
	Prolonged P-R interval

Supporting Evidence of Streptococcal Infection
Increased titer of antistreptococcal antibodies (ASO or others)
Positive throat culture for group A streptococcus
Recent scarlet fever

*The presence of two major criteria, or of one major and two minor criteria, indicates a high probability of acute rheumatic fever, if supported by evidence of preceding group A streptococcal infection.
From "Jones Criteria (revised) for Guidance in the Diagnosis of Rheumatic Fever." Circulation 69(1):204A, 1984. Reproduced with permission. Copyright American Heart Association.

disease, and they often recall no history of a previous rheumatic attack.

The incidence of carditis in initial rheumatic attacks varies from 40 to 90 percent in different reports. The source and selection of clinical material greatly influence the statistics.

The major criteria for the clinical diagnosis of carditis are (1) an organic heart murmur not previously present, (2) an enlarged heart, (3) congestive heart failure, and (4) pericardial friction rubs or signs of effusion. In a patient with active rheumatic fever, any one of the criteria that is unequivocal justifies the diagnosis of carditis. New murmurs indicative of rheumatic carditis include those of mitral regurgitation or aortic insufficiency, as well as a mitral diastolic flow murmur (Carey-Coombs murmur). One of these murmurs is nearly always audible in the patient with acute carditis except in the presence of very low cardiac output, extreme tachycardia, loud pericardial rub, or large pericardial effusion. For further details regarding the clinical findings of rheumatic carditis, the reader is referred to the classic monograph by Stollerman.[7]

Subcutaneous Nodules. Subcutaneous nodules are a major manifestation of rheumatic fever. They are not pathognomonic because they also occur in rheumatoid arthritis (RA) and in systemic lupus erythematosus (SLE). They are associated most often with severe carditis and rarely appear as an isolated manifestation of rheumatic fever. The nodules are round, firm, painless, freely movable subcutaneous lesions varying in size from 0.5 to 2.0 cm. They are located over bony prominences and over tendons, particularly the extensor tendons of the hands and feet. They occur in crops varying in number from one to a few dozen. One should look for them over the scalp, especially the occiput, over the vertebral spines, and over the elbows, wrists, knees, ankles, and Achilles tendons. Nodules are evanescent, disappearing often in a matter of days but usually lasting a week or two. They tend to be much smaller, more discrete, and less persistent than rheumatoid nodules.

Erythema Marginatum. The rash of erythema marginatum is a less common feature of rheumatic fever than the other manifestations, but it is so characteristic as to have major diagnostic significance. It is quite useful in diagnosis when the other manifestations are equivocal. Like chorea, it may persist long after other clinical signs of active inflammation have abated. Erythema marginatum is not pathognomonic of rheumatic fever, because it has been reported in sepsis, drug reactions, and glomerulonephritis, and in patients in whom no etiologic factor can be identified. Erythema marginatum appears as a bright pink ring spreading serpiginously through the skin. It is nonpruritic, nonpainful, and neither indurated nor raised; it blanches completely on pressure. It is evanescent, changing before one's eyes. It may first appear as a pink spot, but the center then fades and the periphery forms an irregular but sharp outer line. The individual lesions appear on the trunk and the proximal parts of the extremities but not on the face. They rarely extend more peripherally than the elbows and knees.

Sydenham's Chorea (Chorea Minor, St. Vitus's Dance). Chorea is a neurologic disorder characterized by involuntary, purposeless, rapid movements, muscular weakness, and emotional lability. It may be associated with other rheumatic manifestations but may also appear as the sole expression of the disease—so-called pure chorea. Its sex distribution is different from that of the other manifestations in that it is present after puberty exclusively in females, and its incidence declines rapidly after adolescence. It is seen occasionally in adult women but virtually never in sexually fully developed men.

The movements of chorea are abrupt and erratic and not rhythmic or repetitive like those of athetosis. Even in the most violent attacks, all choreiform movements disappear during sleep. They are less violent with rest and sedation. The involuntary movements affect all muscles, but those in the hands, face, and feet are most apparent. The patient cannot sustain a tetanic muscular contraction for long.

Chorea may last from a week to more than 2 years but it usually runs its course in 8 to 15 weeks. It is never seen simultaneously with arthritis but often coexists with carditis. When chorea appears alone, the other minor clinical and laboratory signs of acute rheumatic fever may be absent. The ESR and the C-reactive protein (CRP) may be normal. Even more confusing, in such cases streptococcal antibody titers may not be increased. These observations are explained by the long latent period (as long as 1 to 6 months) between the antecedent streptococcal infection and the onset of chorea.[89, 90]

Minor Manifestations of a Rheumatic Attack

Fever. Temperature is increased in almost all rheumatic attacks and ranges from 38.4° to 40°C. Usually fever decreases in approximately a week without antipyretic treatment and becomes low grade for another week or two. It rarely lasts for more than 3 to 4 weeks.

Abdominal Pain. The abdominal pain of rheumatic fever resembles that of other conditions associated with acute microvascular mesenteric inflammation such as sepsis, endotoxin or anaphylactic shock, transfusion reactions, anaphylactoid purpura, or sickle cell crises. It usually occurs at or near the onset of the rheumatic attack so that other manifestations may not yet be present to clarify the diagnosis.

Epistaxis. Epistaxis in the past occurred most prominently and severely in patients with severe and protracted rheumatic carditis. In some studies in the 1930s its frequency was reported as high as 48 percent, but it declined to as low as 4 to 9 percent in

the late 1950s and perhaps occurs even less frequently now. Although epistaxis has been correlated in the past with the severity of rheumatic inflammation, it is difficult to assess retrospectively the possible thrombasthenic effect of large doses of salicylates administered for prolonged periods of protracted attacks.

Rheumatic Pneumonia. Rheumatic pneumonia may appear in the lung in the course of severe rheumatic carditis.[91] As noted earlier, this inflammatory process is very difficult to distinguish from pulmonary edema or the alveolitis associated with respiratory distress syndromes due to a variety of pathophysiologic states.

LABORATORY FINDINGS

The diagnosis of rheumatic fever cannot be established by laboratory tests, but these may be helpful in two ways: demonstrating that antecedent streptococcal infection has occurred and documenting the presence or persistence of an inflammatory process. The course of carditis should be followed by serial chest radiographs, and the electrocardiogram may reflect the toxic effect of the rheumatic process on the conduction system.[92] A variety of laboratory tests may be required to exclude the large list of conditions from which rheumatic fever must be differentiated.

Evidence of Antecedent Streptococcal Infection

Throat cultures are usually negative by the time rheumatic fever appears. When they are positive for group A streptococci, their interpretation may be difficult because the organism isolated may, indeed, represent convalescent carriage of the inciting rheumatogenic strain but could also be the result of an intercurrent infection with a different strain. Streptococcal antibodies are more useful because (1) they reach a peak titer at about the time of onset of rheumatic fever, (2) they indicate true infection rather than transient carriage, and (3) by performing several tests for different antibodies, any significant recent streptococcal infection can be detected.

The specific antibody tests that have been used to diagnose streptococcal infections most frequently are those directed against extracellular products found in the supernatant broth of streptococcal cultures. They include ASO, anti-DNAase B, antihyaluronidase, anti-NADase (anti-DPNase), and antistreptokinase. The ASO test has been the most widely used and is generally available in hospitals in the United States.

ASO titers vary with age, season, geography, and other factors that affect the frequency and intensity of streptococcal disease. They reach peak levels in the young, school-aged population. Titers of 200 to 300 Todd units per ml are common, therefore, in healthy children of elementary school age who live in crowded cities of the temperate zone of the United States. Following streptococcal sore throat, the antibody response peaks at about 4 to 5 weeks, which is usually during the second or third week of rheumatic fever (depending on how early it is detected). Thereafter, antibody titers fall off rapidly in the next several months, and after 6 months they decline more slowly. Evidence of increased streptococcal antibodies should be present therefore in all patients at the onset of the rheumatic attack unless the onset is ill defined. One exception is "pure" chorea. Because the latent period between the antecedent streptococcal infection and onset of Sydenham's chorea may be as long as several months, streptococcal antibody titers may have declined to an equivocal or normal range by the time chorea appears.

Anti-DNAase B is the most widely used ancillary test, with antihyaluronidase a useful third assay. A product has been marketed that is a concentrate of extracellular streptococcal antigens (Streptozyme). Sheep cells sensitized with this concentrate will agglutinate in the presence of streptococcal antibodies providing a simple, rapid, and sensitive measure of the streptococcal immune response.[93] The antigens involved are poorly characterized and standardized, however. Because of reports of significant variability in the potency of various lots of reagents, this test is not recommended for routine use.[94]

Streptococcal antibodies, when present in high titer, support but do not prove the diagnosis of acute rheumatic fever. One should not diagnose the disease on the basis of increased titers of streptococcal antibodies alone. Streptococcal antibodies are not a measure of rheumatic activity. In the absence of intercurrent streptococcal infection, titers decline during the rheumatic attack despite the persistence or severity of rheumatic activity.

Acute Phase Reactants

The two tests that have gained widest use are the CRP and ESR determinations because both are almost invariably abnormal during the active rheumatic process if it is not suppressed by antirheumatic drugs. "Pure" chorea and persistent erythema marginatum are exceptions. CRP and ESR are not of great value when rheumatic manifestations are obvious clinically. During treatment, however, they are quite useful, especially CRP, to measure the effectiveness of the suppression of the inflammatory process. Particularly when treatment has been discontinued or is being tapered off, the CRP is efficient in monitoring "rebounds" of rheumatic inflammation, which indicate that the rheumatic process in still active. When CRP and ESR remain normal a few weeks after antirheumatic treatment has been terminated, the attack may be considered ended unless chorea appears. Even then, however, there will be no exacerbation of the systemic inflammatory component of the attack, and chorea will be an isolated manifestation.

Anemia

The anemia of rheumatic fever is the normochromic normocytic anemia of chronic infection or inflammation. It is of mild to moderate degree and is corrected partially or completely by suppression of inflammation, particularly with glucocorticoids. Anemia is a useful index of the severity and chronicity of rheumatic fever.

Electrocardiography

The electrocardiogram (ECG) has no characteristic pattern in rheumatic fever, and the diagnosis of carditis should never be made on the basis of ECG changes alone. Neither the course of the acute rheumatic attack nor the subsequent development of valvular or myocardial damage can be predicted from ECG changes. Patients with abnormal ECG changes but without the criteria described earlier for carditis recover completely without stigmata of rheumatic heart disease.[92]

Echocardiography

The utility of echocardiography in the study of primary attacks of rheumatic fever is now being assessed. Ultrasound should greatly improve the detection of pericardial effusions in acute rheumatic carditis. In the Utah epidemic,[27] carditis was confirmed by auscultation in 72 percent of patients with ARF. Doppler ultrasound examination revealed inaudible valvular regurgitation in an additional 19 percent of patients. The prognostic significance of such echocardiographic findings in regard to the subsequent development of rheumatic heart disease, however, remains to be determined.

DIAGNOSIS

Manifestations of rheumatic fever that are not clearly expressed pose a dilemma because of the importance of identifying a first rheumatic attack clearly to establish the need for prophylaxis of recurrences. Some of the isolated manifestations, particularly polyarthritis, may be difficult or impossible to distinguish from those of other diseases, especially at their onset. The *Jones criteria* for the diagnosis of rheumatic fever[95] have been widely utilized as a scheme to avoid the overdiagnosis of the disease, because of the significant implications of such a diagnosis for future management of the patient. The revised criteria (see Table 71–1) emphasize the importance of establishing the presence of antecedent streptococcal infection by demonstration of increased titers of streptococcal antibodies. If supported by such evidence, two major, or one major and two minor, manifestations constitute a high probability of the diagnosis of rheumatic fever. The diagnosis can usually be made with confidence, however, when "pure" chorea is the sole manifestation because of the rarity with which this syndrome is due to any other cause and the fact that streptococcal antibody titers may be unimpressive.

The polyarthritis of rheumatic fever, when it appears as the sole major manifestation of the disease, constitutes the greatest problem, because of the frequency with which polyarthritis may be due to other causes. The exclusion of bacteremia by appropriate blood cultures before antibiotic therapy is initiated is essential. Because gonococcal polyarthritis cannot be unequivocally excluded by cultures of the joints or blood in the majority of cases, a trial of antigonococcal therapy should be used when the epidemiologic and clinical picture is compatible with disseminated gonococcal infection. Subacute bacterial endocarditis must always be considered whenever a patient with rheumatic heart disease develops polyarthritis and unexplained fever. Certain viral infections, such as rubella, or the persistent viremias causing immune complex disease, such as type B hepatitis, are often problems in a young patient who may coincidentally also have increased titers of streptococcal antibodies. The serum sickness–like syndromes, especially penicillin allergy following treatment of streptococcal pharyngitis, cause diagnostic confusion. It is well to bear in mind that rheumatic fever does not cause urticaria, angioneurotic edema, or with extremely rare exceptions,[96] clinically overt glomerulonephritis, and that serum complement levels are increased rather than decreased in rheumatic fever. Although collagen vascular disease is a frequent differential diagnostic consideration, antinuclear and other autoantibodies do not appear in the course of rheumatic fever, no matter how persistent the disease.

With regard to carditis, when functional or organic murmurs are typical, there is little problem for the experienced physician in distinguishing between them. At times, however, a nondescript murmur, especially in the obese or heavy-chested individual, may defy sharp distinctions, and repeated examinations and other studies may be necessary. Such murmurs are classified as "doubtful" or "questionable" when no other decision can be made. Myocarditis in its severe and chronic form due to other diseases may be impossible to distinguish from chronic rheumatic carditis if the heart is dilated and mitral regurgitation is prominent. This situation is encountered when rheumatic fever patients have heart failure with no associated extracardiac manifestations to provide clues. In rheumatic carditis, as the patient recovers cardiac compensation, the valvular lesions usually persist and the murmurs may become louder, whereas the reverse is true in viral and other forms of acute and subcutaneous myocarditis.

COURSE, PROGNOSIS, AND NATURAL HISTORY

The clinical course of rheumatic fever is quite variable, but in general there is a characteristic sequence of the major manifestations and a predictable duration. Most attacks begin with fever and joint symptoms. Carditis, if it is going to occur, does so early in the attack—within the first few weeks. The latent period between streptococcal infection and the onset of rheumatic fever is shortest in arthritis and erythema marginatum and longest in chorea, with carditis and subcutaneous nodules in between. The average duration of a rheumatic attack is less than 3 months. When severe carditis is present, clinical rheumatic activity may continue for 6 months or more. Less than 5 percent of attacks persist for more than 6 months, however. Such cases are classified as "chronic rheumatic fever."

The age of onset and severity of carditis influence its chronicity. Children younger than 3 years of age who develop rheumatic fever have the highest incidence of carditis (more than 90 percent). The incidence of carditis declines to approximately one third in the 14- to 17-year age group. When carditis is mild, it usually disappears rapidly. Severe carditis prolongs the attack, causes persistent cardiac enlargement and persistent valvular disease, and may produce protracted or permanent heart failure. Antirheumatic therapy "masks" rheumatic inflammation but tends to prolong rather than terminate the attack. The majority of prolonged attacks occur in patients who have had one or more previous attacks, particularly those with carditis, and the incidence of chronic rheumatic fever increases with the number of recurrences. When antirheumatic therapy is withdrawn and no "rebound" of inflammation is noted for 8 weeks or more, the attack is over and will not be reactivated without a new streptococcal infection.[97]

Prognosis

Rheumatic fever does not recur when streptococcal disease is prevented. Prognosis is therefore excellent for the rheumatic subject who escapes carditis during the initial attack.[98, 99] Prognosis is poorer for those with severe carditis in the initial attack. The presence of heart failure is followed by complete healing in 30 percent at 5 years and 40 percent at 10 years (Fig. 71–3).[99]

Recurrences of Rheumatic Fever

In epidemics of pharyngitis caused by rheumatogenic streptococci, first attacks of rheumatic fever

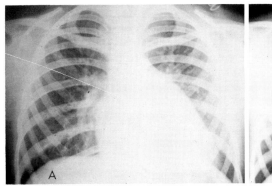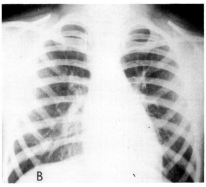

Figure 71–3. Healing of acute rheumatic carditis. *A,* Greatly enlarged heart and congestive heart failure. *B,* Same patient approximately 6 months later when the attack had subsided. (From Stollerman, G. H.: Rheumatic Fever and Streptococcal Infection. New York, Grune & Stratton, 1975, p. 153, with permission.)

following untreated infection[5] occur with a frequency of approximately 1 to 3 percent. The ARF attack rate following endemically occurring streptococcal pharyngitis in civilian populations may be 1 percent or less. In contrast, the rate of reactivation of rheumatic fever by streptococcal pharyngitis in patients who have had rheumatic fever previously may exceed 50 percent.[73] Recurrence rates decline with the time elapsed from the last attack. The presence or absence of rheumatic heart disease is a second major factor that influences the risk of rheumatic recurrences. The third important factor influencing the ARF recurrence rate is the severity of the streptococcal infection as reflected in the magnitude of the streptococcal immune response. Rheumatic recurrences, therefore, are most likely to occur within the first several years after the rheumatic attack in those with rheumatic heart disease who are exposed to virulent streptococcal pharyngitis.[73]

The natural history of rheumatic fever after an initial rheumatic attack has abated is now fairly predictable, and a period of convalescence enables assessment of the degree of healing of carditis. If cardiac healing is complete, prevention of recurrences should guarantee freedom from rheumatic heart disease. Persistent mild mitral regurgitation, although usually quite compatible with normal longevity if recurrences and infective endocarditis are prevented, must be observed continuously because of the small but significant group of patients, predominantly women, in whom mitral stenosis evolves despite careful, continuous antistreptococcal prophylaxis.[99]

TREATMENT AND MANAGEMENT

General

The manifestations and severity of the rheumatic attack will determine to a large extent the management of a given patient. In general, however, rheumatic fever is unpredictable at the onset of the attack, and patients should be put to bed for the duration of the acute, febrile phase of the illness until clinical and laboratory evidence of inflammation abates.

The administration of anti-inflammatory medi-

cines should be withheld until the disease process is clearly expressed to establish the diagnosis and avoid confusion. Furthermore, in isolated polyarthritis a trial of antimicrobial therapy may be essential to eliminate the diagnosis of septic arthritis, especially of disseminated gonococcal disease in adolescents and young adults. If pain must be controlled, codeine or meperidine is effective and will not mask inflammation.

When the diagnosis is established, treatment is started with the completion of a course of penicillin adequate to eradicate pharyngeal carriage of group A streptococci. Massive penicillin therapy will not alter the course of the disease or the frequency or severity of cardiac involvement.[100] The usual penicillin regimen recommended for the optimal treatment of streptococcal pharyngitis will suffice (see later).

Antirheumatic Therapy

The selection of an antirheumatic agent is not critical to the outcome of most attacks of rheumatic fever. Several controlled studies have failed to show a superiority of glucocorticoids over salicylates with regard to alteration of the course of the attack or prevention of cardiac stigmata.[98, 99, 101] These studies have been critically reviewed in detail.[7, 102] Glucocorticoids and salicylates can be regarded as useful symptomatic and supportive therapeutic agents, but they are not curative and may actually prolong the course of the attack. Nonetheless, they control the toxic manifestations of the disease, contribute to the comfort of the patient, and combat constitutional symptoms. Glucocorticoids are more potent than salicylates in suppressing acute exudative inflammation, and some patients in whom salicylates fail to control the disease respond quickly to relatively large doses of glucocorticoids. The effect of such doses on the course of chronic rheumatic carditis is disappointing, however, and their use in early cases of acute carditis has not been proved to decrease residual heart disease. Prolonged use of large doses of glucocorticoids beyond the period of time required to control the acute manifestations is not justified.

Patients with mild arthritis or arthralgias and no carditis may be treated with analgesics only, such as codeine, as needed. This choice has two advantages: (1) the diagnosis may be established with greater certainty by a more characteristic arthritis when symptoms and signs are borderline, and (2) the course of the attack will not be prolonged by "rebounds." Most patients, however, who have frank arthritis and no evidence of carditis may be given salicylates initially as a therapeutic trial for the diagnosis of rheumatic polyarthritis because of the consistency (but not specificity) of the response to them in patients with this manifestation. Patients with mild carditis are usually given glucocorticoids but without conviction that they are superior to salicylates. Patients with severe carditis are usually treated promptly with glucocorticoids, particularly if heart failure is evident, and with the precaution of adequate doses of diuretics and restriction of salt intake to combat sodium retention.

Approximately 75 to 80 percent of attacks of ARF subside within 6 weeks; 90 percent are over in 12 weeks; and 5 percent persist for 6 months or more. In mild attacks, therefore, one may plan a 4-week course of treatment and taper off the dose of antirheumatic drugs during the ensuing 2 weeks. For detailed discussion of treatment of ARF, the reader is referred elsewhere.[7, 102, 103]

PREVENTION OF RHEUMATIC FEVER

Secondary prophylaxis is the term used to describe protection against rheumatic recurrences by continuous antistreptococcal prophylaxis. Limiting prophylaxis of recurrences to the treatment of overt streptococcal infections in rheumatic subjects is hazardous, as many such infections that reactivate rheumatic fever are subclinical. Furthermore, it is a difficult task to abort a recurrence by administering penicillin after a streptococcal sore throat is already symptomatic.

The most effective form of continuous prophylaxis is a single injection of 1.2 million units of benzathine penicillin G every 4 weeks (Table 71–2).[94] Using this form of prophylaxis, an attack rate of less than one recurrence per 250 patient-years was documented in the extensive studies by the Irvington House group.[104, 105] This method circumvents the vagaries of gastrointestinal absorption of penicillin, does not require daily fidelity to an oral regimen, and facilitates closer surveillance of the patient by the managing physician. Although the reaction rate is somewhat higher for all injectable forms of penicillin compared with oral penicillin, reactions are rare after the first months of continuous prophylaxis. In patients who are at highest risk for developing recurrences, especially those with rheumatic heart disease, with recent rheumatic fever, and in a challenging environment for streptococcal exposure, benzathine penicillin G is undoubtedly the preferred form of prophylaxis. In fact, in certain developing countries, in which the incidence of ARF and the

Table 71–2. SECONDARY PREVENTION OF RHEUMATIC FEVER (PREVENTION OF RECURRENT ATTACKS)*

Agent	Dose and Frequency	Route
Benzathine penicillin G	1,200,000 units every 4 weeks	Intramuscular
	OR	
Sulfadiazine	0.5 g once daily for patients <60 lb	Oral
	1.0 g once daily for patients ≥60 lb	Oral
	OR	
Penicillin V	250 mg twice daily	Oral
For individuals allergic to penicillin and sulfadiazine:		
Erythromycin stearate	250 mg twice daily	Oral

*Author's recommendations, which vary slightly from those of the American Heart Association. Modified from Dajani, A. S., Bisno, A. L., et al.: Prevention of rheumatic fever. A statement for health professionals by the Committee on Rheumatic Fever, Endocarditis, and Kawasaki Disease of the Council on Cardiovascular Disease in the Young, American Heart Association. Circulation 78:1082, 1988. Reproduced with permission. Copyright American Heart Association.

risk of recurrence are particularly high, administration of benzathine penicillin G every 3 weeks rather than every 4 weeks has been advocated for secondary prevention of rheumatic fever.[106, 107] This is not required in the United States. In affluent societies and in countries in which rheumatic fever has become rare,[17] it is unlikely that intramuscular prophylaxis will be preferred by the average managing physician except when the major risk factors of recurrences coexist: severity of rheumatic heart disease, recent previous attack, and exposure to streptococcal pharyngitis in locales where rheumatic fever still occurs.

Oral prophylaxis is less reliable than repository penicillin prophylaxis. Daily doses of either sulfadiazine or penicillin V should be employed if the requirement for prophylaxis is less stringent or the intramuscular form is not acceptable or feasible. For the rare patient who is sensitive to both penicillin and sulfonamides, erythromycin may be substituted (see Table 71–2).

It has been difficult to make a single arbitrary recommendation concerning the duration for which continuous prophylaxis must be maintained in all rheumatic subjects because of the large number of variables that influence the attack rate of recurrences following streptococcal infections. Exceptions to maintaining prophylaxis should be made in adults only, and then after assessing carefully the risk of exposure to streptococcal infection in communities in which rheumatic fever still persists. Patients with significant rheumatic heart disease, a history of repeated recurrences, or a recent attack at any age require most careful consideration before discontinuing prophylaxis, a decision that is still to be regarded as a calculated risk.

Primary prophylaxis is the term applied to the prevention of first rheumatic attacks by prompt treatment of the antecedent streptococcal infection. In

Table 71–3. PRIMARY PREVENTION OF RHEUMATIC FEVER (TREATMENT OF STREPTOCOCCAL TONSILLOPHARYNGITIS)

Agent	Dose	Mode	Duration
Benzathine penicillin G	600,000 units for patients <60 lb 1,200,000 units for patients >60 lb OR	Intramuscular	Once
Penicillin V (phenoxymethyl penicillin)	250 mg 3 times daily	Oral	10 days
For individuals allergic to penicillin:			
Erythromycin estolate	20–40 mg/kg/day 2–4 times daily (maximum 1 g/day)	Oral	10 days
ethylsuccinate	40 mg/kg/day 2–4 times daily (maximum 1 g/day)	Oral	10 days

The following agents are acceptable but usually not recommended: amoxicillin, dicloxacillin, oral cephalosporins, and clindamycin. The following are not acceptable: sulfonamides, trimethoprim, tetracyclines, and chloramphenicol.

Recommendations of the American Heart Association.

From Dajani, A. S., Bisno, A. L., et al.: Prevention of rheumatic fever. A statement for health professionals by the Committee on Rheumatic Fever, Endocarditis, and Kawasaki Disease of the Council on Cardiovascular Disease in the Young, American Heart Association. Circulation 78:1082, 1988, reproduced with permission. Copyright American Heart Association.

classic studies in military populations, penicillin therapy of streptococcal pharyngitis causing high attack rates of rheumatic fever reduced the rate from 3 to 0.3 percent.[8] It has been more difficult to apply primary prevention to civilian populations, particularly children with sporadic or endemic streptococcal pharyngitis. Such infections are difficult to differentiate clinically from viral pharyngitis. In patients, particularly children or adolescents, in whom an alternative diagnosis (e.g., influenza, common cold) is not apparent, a throat culture is indicated to detect the presence of beta hemolytic streptococci. A positive culture does not reliably discriminate between acutely infected patients and asymptomatic streptococcal carriers with superimposed viral pharyngitis. It does, however, identify those patients in whom therapy is indicated. Moreover, the majority of persons with acute pharyngitis will have a negative throat culture, a finding that obviates the necessity for antimicrobial therapy. A number of commercial kits are now on the market that allow identification of group A streptococcal antigen from a throat swab. Unlike the throat culture, which requires overnight incubation, these kits provide an answer within a matter of minutes. Most of the licensed kits are quite specific, and a positive test obviates the need for a throat culture. The kits are somewhat less sensitive than the culture, however, and the American Heart Association recommends confirming a negative antigen test with a throat culture.[94]

Effective therapy, that is, treatment adequate to prevent rheumatic fever, requires eradication of the infecting organisms rather than clinical improvement alone. To accomplish this end, penicillin must be at effective levels for 10 days.[108] Many patients fail to extend oral therapy for 10 days because symptoms abate within a day or two. A single injection of benzathine penicillin G intramuscularly is highly effective and obviates the problem of compliance. The recommended dose is 600,000 units in children weighing less than 27 kg (60 lb) and 1.2 million units in those who are heavier (Table 71–3). Intramuscular benzathine penicillin G is no longer used extensively in populations in which rheumatic fever has virtually disappeared. It is still the treatment of choice, however, for those populations in which the disease is still a serious problem. If given orally, penicillin V is recommended in doses of 250 mg units three times daily. For those sensitive to penicillin, erythromycin may be substituted. Dosages of erythromycin vary with the preparation chosen (see Table 71–3). Sulfonamides, although effective in prevention of streptococcal infections, are not indicated for treatment of an established streptococcal sore throat because they do not eradicate carriage and do not prevent initial rheumatic attacks.

Mass penicillin prophylaxis is effective in populations in which streptococcal pharyngitis is epidemic. Mass administration of 1.2 million units of benzathine penicillin G intramuscularly to all members of the affected population has been extremely effective in military training camps.[2]

It may be possible to induce protective antibodies with small doses of purified streptococcal M protein. The M proteins of several serotypes have been purified to molecular homogeneity and are antigenic in laboratory animals and in humans.[109, 110] Their potential for the preparation of streptococcal vaccines has been emphasized.[111]

References

1. Zagala, J. G., and Feinstein, A. R.: The preceding illness of acute rheumatic fever. J.A.M.A. 179:863, 1962.
2. Frank, P. F., Stollerman, G. H., and Miller, L. F.: Protection of a military population from rheumatic fever. J.A.M.A. 193:755, 1965.
3. Rammelkamp, C. H.: Epidemiology of streptococcal infections. Harvey Lect. 51:113, 1955.
4. Stollerman, G. H.: The epidemiology of primary and secondary rheumatic fever. In Uhr, J. W. (ed.): The Streptococcus, Rheumatic Fever and Glomerulonephritis. Baltimore, Williams & Wilkins, 1964, p. 311.
5. Stetson, C. A.: The relation of antibody response to rheumatic fever. In McCarty, M. (ed.): Streptococcal Infections. New York, Columbia University Press, 1954, p. 208.
6. Taranta, A.: Rheumatic fever in children and adolescents. IV. Relation of the rheumatic fever recurrence rate per streptococcal infection to the titers of streptococcal antibodies. Ann. Intern. Med. 50(Suppl. 5):47, 1964.
7. Stollerman, G. H.: Rheumatic Fever and Streptococcal Infection. New York, Grune & Stratton, 1975.
8. Wannamaker, L. W., Rammelkamp, C. H., Jr., Denny, F. W., Brink, W. R., Houser, H. B., and Hahn, E. O.: Prophylaxis of acute rheumatic fever by treatment of preceding streptococcal infection with various amounts of depot penicillin. Am. J. Med. 10:673, 1951.
9. Spagnuolo, M., Pasternak, B., and Taranta, A.: Risk of rheumatic fever recurrences after streptococcal infections. N. Engl. J. Med. 285:641, 1971.
10. Bisno, A. L.: The concept of rheumatogenic and non-rheumatogenic group A streptococci. In Read, S. E., and Zabriskie, J. B. (eds.):

Streptococcal Diseases and the Immune Response. New York, Academic Press, 1980, p. 789.

11. Wannamaker, L. W.: Medical progress. Differences between streptococcal infections of the throat and of the skin. N. Engl. J. Med. 282:23, 78, 1970.
12. Stollerman, G. H.: Nephritogenic and rheumatogenic group A streptococci. J. Infect. Dis. 120:258, 1969.
13. Bisno, A. L., Pearce, I. A., Wall, H. P., Moody, M. D., and Stollerman, G. H.: Contrasting epidemiology of acute rheumatic fever and acute glumerulonephritis. Nature of the antecedent streptococcal infection. N. Engl. J. Med. 283:561, 1970.
14. Potter, E. V., Svartman, M., Poon-King, T., and Earle, D. P.: The families of patients with acute rheumatic fever or glomerulonephritis in Trinidad. Am. J. Epidemiol. 106:130, 1977.
15. Kaplan, E. L., Top, F. H., Jr., Dudding, B. A., and Wannamaker, L. W.: Diagnosis of streptococcal pharyngitis: Differentiation of active infection from the carrier state in the symptomatic child. J. Infect. Dis. 123:490, 1971.
16. Schwartz, B., Facklam, R. R., and Breiman, R. F.: Changing epidemiology of group A streptococcal infection in the USA. Lancet 336:1167, 1990.
17. Land, M. A., and Bisno, A. L.: Acute rheumatic fever—a vanishing disease in suburbia. J.A.M.A. 249(7):895, 1983.
18. Stollerman, G. H.: The relative rheumatogenicity of strains of group A streptococci. Mod. Concepts Cardiovasc. Dis. 44:35, 1975.
19. Bisno, A. L., Pearce, I. A., and Stollerman, G. H.: Streptococcal infections that fail to cause recurrences of rheumatic fever. J. Infect. Dis. 136:278, 1977.
20. Bisno, A. L.: Group A streptococcal infections and acute rheumatic fever. N. Engl. J. Med. 325(11):783, 1991.
21. Dale, J. B., and Beachey, E. H.: Protective antigenic determinant of streptococcal M protein shared with sarcolemmal membrane protein of human heart. J. Exp. Med. 156:1165, 1982.
22. Dale, J. B., and Beachey, E. H.: Epitopes of streptococcal M proteins shared with cardiac myosin. J. Exp. Med. 162:583, 1985.
23. Dale, J. B., and Beachey, E. H.: Multiple heart cross-reactive epitopes of streptococcal M proteins. J. Exp. Med. 161:113, 1985.
24. Khandke, K. M., Fairwell, T., and Manjula, B. N.: Difference in the structural features of streptococcal M-proteins from nephritogenic and rheumatogenic serotypes. J. Exp. Med. 166:151, 1987.
25. Bessen, D., Jones, K. F., and Fischetti, V. A.: Evidence for two distinct classes of streptococcal M protein and their relationship to rheumatic fever. J. Exp. Med. 169:269, 1989.
26. Tomai, M., Kotb, M., Majumdar, G., and Beachey, E. H.: Superantigenicity of streptococcal M protein. J. Exp. Med. 172:359, 1990.
27. Veasy, L. G., Wiedmeier, S. E., Orsmond, G. S., Ruttenberg, H. D., Boucek, M. M., Roth, S. J., Tait, V. F., Thompson, J. A., Daly, J. A., Kaplan, E. L., and Hill, H. R.: Resurgence of acute rheumatic fever in the intermountain area of the United States. N. Engl. J. Med. 316:421, 1987.
28. Hosier, D. M., Craenen, J. M., Teske, D. W., and Wheller, J. J.: Resurgence of acute rheumatic fever. Am. J. Dis. Child. 141:730, 1987.
29. Centers for Disease Control: Acute rheumatic fever among Army trainees—Fort Leonard Wood, Missouri, 1987–1988. MMWR 37:519, 1988.
30. Friedman, J., van de Rinj, I., Ohkuni, H., Fischetti, V. A., and Zabriskie, J. B.: Immunological studies of post-streptococcal sequelae: Evidence for presence of streptococcal antigens in circulating immune complexes. J. Clin. Invest. 74:1027, 1984.
31. Gupta, R. C., Badhwar, A. K., Bisno, A. L., and Berrios, X.: Detection of C-reactive protein, streptolysin O, and antistreptolysin O antibodies in immune complexes isolated from the sera of patients with acute rheumatic fever. J. Immunol. 137:2173, 1986.
32. Stollerman, G. H.: Autoimmunity and rheumatic fever. In Cohen, I. R. (ed.): Perspectives on Autoimmunity. Boca Raton, FL, CRC Press, 1987.
33. Kaplan, M. H.: Immunologic relation of streptococcal and tissue antigens. I. Properties of an antigen in certain strains of group A streptococci exhibiting an immunologic cross reaction with human heart tissue. J. Immunol. 90:595, 1963.
34. Kaplan, M. H., and Suchy, M. L.: Immunologic relation of streptococcal and tissue antigens II. Cross reactions of antisera to mammalian heart tissue with a cell wall constituent of certain strains of group A streptococci. J. Exp. Med. 119:643, 1964.
35. Husby, G., van de Rijn, I., Zabriskie, J. B., Abdin, Z. H., and Williams, R. C., Jr.: Antibodies reacting with cytoplasm of subthalamic and caudate nuclei neurons in chorea and rheumatic fever. J. Exp. Med. 144:1094, 1976.
36. Dudding, B. A., and Ayoub, E. M.: Persistence of streptococcal group A antibody in patients with rheumatic valvular disease. J. Exp. Med. 128:1081, 1968.
37. Ayoub, E. M., Taranta, A., and Bartley, T. D.: Effect of valvular surgery on antibody to the group A streptococcal carbohydrate. Circulation 50:144, 1974.

38. Fillit, H. M., McCarty, M., and Blake, M.: Induction of antibodies to hyaluronic acid by immunization of rabbits with encapsulated streptococci. J. Exp. Med. 164:762, 1986.
39. Fillit, H. M., Blake, M., MacDonald, C., and McCarty, M.: Immunogenicity of liposome-bound hyaluronate in mice. J. Exp. Med. 168:971, 1988.
40. Taranta, A., Torosdag, S., Metrakos, J., Jegier, W., and Uchida, I.: Rheumatic fever in monozygotic and dizygotic twins. Circulation 20:778, 1959.
41. Ayoub, E. M., Barrett, D. J., Maclaren, N. K., and Krischer, J. P.: Association of class II human histocompatibility leukocyte antigens with rheumatic fever. J. Clin. Invest. 77:2019, 1986.
42. Anastasiou-Nana, M. I., Anderson, J. L., Carlquist, J. F., and Nanas, J. N.: HLA-DR typing and lymphocyte subset evaluation in rheumatic heart disease: A search for immune response factors. Am. Heart J. 112:992, 1986.
43. Khanna, A. K., Buskirk, D. R., Williams, R. C., Jr., Gibofsky, A., Crow, M. K., Menon, A., Fotino, M., Reid, H. M., Poon-King, T., Rubinstein, P., and Zabriskie, J. B.: Presence of a non-HLA B cell antigen in rheumatic fever patients and their families as defined by a monoclonal antibody. J. Clin. Invest. 83:1710, 1989.
44. Regelmann, W. E., Talbot, R., Cairns, L., Martin, D., Miller, L. C., Zabriskie, J. B., Braun, D., and Gray, E. D.: Distribution of cells bearing "rheumatic" antigens in peripheral blood of patients with rheumatic fever/rheumatic heart disease. J. Rheumatol. 16:931, 1989.
45. Agarwal, B. L.: Rheumatic heart disease unabated in developing countries. Lancet 2:910, 1981.
46. Markowitz, M.: The decline of rheumatic fever: Role of medical intervention. Lewis W. Wannamaker Memorial Lecture. J. Pediatr. 106:545, 1985.
47. Stollerman, G. H.: Global changes in group A streptococcal diseases and strategies for their prevention. Adv. Intern. Med. 27:373, 1982.
48. Brownell, K. D., and Bailen-Rose, F.: Acute rheumatic fever in children: Incidence in a borough of New York City. J.A.M.A. 224:1593, 1973.
49. Gordis, L., Lilienfeld, A., and Rodriguez, R.: Studies in the epidemiology and preventability of rheumatic fever-1. Demographic factors and the incidence of acute attacks. J. Chronic Dis. 21:645, 1969.
50. Quinn, R. W., and Federspiel, C. F.: The incidence of rheumatic fever in metropolitan Nashville, 1963–1969. Am. J. Epidemiol. 99(4):273, 1974.
51. Gordis, L.: The virtual disappearance of rheumatic fever in the United States: Lessons in the rise and fall of disease. Circulation 72:1155, 1985.
52. Veasy, L. G., and Hill, H. R.: Clinical features of acute rheumatic fever recrudescence in the inter-mountain area of the United States. In Proceedings of the XI Lancefield Symposium on Streptococci and Streptococcal Diseases. Siena, Italy, 1990, p. L6.
53. Congeni, B., Rizzo, C., Congeni, J., and Sreenivasan, V. V.: Outbreak of acute rheumatic fever in Northeast Ohio. J. Pediatr. 111:176, 1987.
54. Wald, E. R., Dashefsky, B., Feidt, C., Chiponis, D., and Byers, C.: Acute rheumatic fever in Western Pennsylvania and the Tristate area. Pediatrics 80:371, 1987.
55. Griffiths, S. P., and Gersony, W. M.: Acute rheumatic fever in New York City (1969 to 1988): A comparative study of two decades. J. Pediatr. 116:882, 1990.
56. Westlake, R. M., Graham, T. P., and Edwards, K. M.: An outbreak of acute rheumatic fever in Tennessee. Pediatr. Infect. Dis. J. 9:97, 1990.
57. Leggiadro, R. J., Birnbaum, S. E., Chase, N. A., and Myers, L. K.: A resurgence of acute rheumatic fever in a mid-south children's hospital. South. Med. J. 83:1418, 1990.
58. Jackson, M. A., Sotiropoulos, S. V., Christensen, B., Diehl, A. M., and Kaplan, E. L.: Mucoid group A streptococcal disease in Kansas City, MO. Pediatr. Res. 23:372A (Abst 1024), 1988.
59. Burns, D. L., and Ginsburg, C. M.: Recrudescence of acute rheumatic fever in Dallas, Texas. Pediatr. Res. 21:256A (Abst 496), 1987.
60. Mason, T., Fisher, M., and Kujala, G.: Acute rheumatic fever in West Virginia: Not just a disease of children. Arch. Intern. Med. 151:133, 1991.
61. Wallace, M. R., Garst, P. D., Papadimos, T. J., and Oldfield, E. C. III.: The return of acute rheumatic fever in young adults. J.A.M.A. 262:2557, 1989.
62. Stevens, D. L., Tanner, M. H., Winship, J., Swarts, R., Ries, K. M., Shlievert, P. M., and Kaplan, E. L.: Severe group A streptococcal infections associated with a toxic shock-like syndrome and scarlet fever toxin A. N. Engl. J. Med. 321:1, 1989.
63. Cone, L. A., Woodard, D. R., Schlievert, P. M., and Tomory, G. S.: Clinical and bacteriologic observations of a toxic shock-like syndrome due to Streptococcus pyogenes. N. Engl. J. Med. 317:146, 1987.
64. Bartter, T., Dascal, A., Carroll, K., and Curley, F. J.: "Toxic strep syndrome." A manifestation of group A streptococcal infection. Arch. Intern. Med. 148:1421, 1988.
65. Stollerman, G. H.: Changing group A streptococci—the reappearance of streptococcal "toxic shock." Arch. Intern. Med. 148:1268, 1988.

66. Francis, J., and Warren, R. E.: *Streptococcus pyogenes* bacteremia in Cambridge—a review of 67 episodes. Q. J. Med. 68:603, 1988.
67. Gaworzewska, E., and Colman, G.: Changes in the pattern of infection caused by *Streptococcus pyogenes*. Epidemiol. Infect. 100:257, 1988.
68. Martin, P. R., and Hiby, E. A.: Streptococcal serogroup A epidemic in Norway 1987–1988. Scand. J. Infect. Dis. 22:421, 1990.
69. Rammelkamp, C. H., Denny, F. W., and Wannamaker, L. W.: Studies on the epidemiology of rheumatic fever in the armed services. *In* Thomas, L. (ed.): Rheumatic Fever. Minneapolis, University of Minnesota Press, 1952, p. 72.
70. Rammelkamp, C. H., Jr.: The Lewis A. Connor Memorial Lecture. Rheumatic heart disease—a challenge. Circulation 17:842, 1958.
71. Siegel, A. C., Johnson, E. E., and Stollerman, G. H.: Controlled studies of streptococcal pharyngitis in a pediatric population. I. Factors related to the attack rate of rheumatic fever. N. Engl. J. Med. 265:559, 1961.
72. Stollerman, G. H., Siegel, A. C., and Johnson, E. E.: Variable epidemiology of streptococcal disease and the changing pattern of rheumatic fever. Mod. Concepts Cardiovasc. Dis. 34:35, 1965.
73. Taranta, A., Kleinberg, E., Feinstein, A. R., Wood, H. F., Tursky, E., and Simpson, R.: Rheumatic fever in children and adolescents. A long-term epidemiologic study of subsequent prophylaxis, streptococcal infections, and clinical sequelae. V. Relation of the rheumatic fever recurrence rate per streptococcal infection to pre-existing clinical features of the patients. Ann. Intern. Med. 60(Suppl. 5):58, 1964.
74. Johnson, E. E., Stollerman, G. H., and Grossman, B. J.: Rheumatic recurrences in patients not receiving continuous prophylaxis. J.A.M.A. 190:407, 1964.
75. Murphy, G. E.: Nature of rheumatic heart disease with special reference to myocardial disease and heart failure. Medicine 39:289, 1960.
76. Becker, C. G., and Murphy, G. E.: On the pathology of rheumatic heart disease. *In* Read, S. E., and Zabriskie, J. B. (eds.): Streptococcal Diseases and the Immune Response. New York, Academic Press, 1980, p. 23.
77. Husby, G. H., Arora, R., Williams, R. C., Kwaw, B. A., Haber, E., and Butler, C.: Immunofluorescent studies of florid rheumatic Aschoff lesions. Arthritis Rheum. 29:207, 1986.
78. Pienaar, J. G., and Price, H. M.: Ultrastructure and origin of the Antischkow cell. Am. J. Pathol. 51:1063, 1977.
79. Love, G. L., and Restrepo, C.: Aschoff bodies of rheumatic carditis are granulomatous lesions of histiocytic origin. Mod. Pathol. 1:256, 1988.
80. Chopra, P.: Origin of Aschoff nodule: An ultrastructural, light microscopic and histochemical evaluation. Jpn. Heart J. 26:227, 1985.
81. Virmani, R., and Roberts, W. C.: Aschoff bodies in operatively excised atrial appendages and in papillary muscles. Frequency and clinical significance. Circulation 55:559, 1977.
82. Steele, P. P., Weily, H. S., Davies, H., and Genton, E.: Platelet survival in patients with rheumatic heart disease. N. Engl. J. Med. 290:537, 1974.
83. Buchanan, D. N.: Pathologic changes in chorea. Am. J. Dis. Child. 62:443, 1941.
84. Zvaifler, N. J.: Chronic postrheumatic-fever (Jaccoud's) arthritis. N. Engl. J. Med. 267:10, 1962.
85. Meyers, O. L., and Chalmers, I. M.: Jaccoud's arthropathy. Report of seven cases. S. Afr. Med. J. 51:753, 1977.
86. Herold, B. C., and Shulman, S. T.: Poststreptococcal arthritis. Pediatr. Infect. Dis. J. 7:681, 1988.
87. de Cunto, C. L., Giannini, E. H., Fink, C. W., Brewer, E. J., and Person, D. A.: Prognosis of children with poststreptococcal reactive arthritis. Pediatr. Infect. Dis. J. 7:683, 1988.
88. Arnold, M. H., and Tyndall, A.: Poststreptococcal reactive arthritis. Ann. Rheum. Dis. 48:686, 1989.
89. Taranta, A., and Stollerman, G. H.: The relationship of Sydenham's chorea to infection with group A streptococci. Am. J. Med. 20:170, 1956.
90. Berrios, X., Quesney, F., Morales, A., Blazquez, J., and Bisno, A. L.: Are all recurrences of "pure" Sydenham's chorea true recurrences of acute rheumatic fever? J. Pediatr. 107:867, 1985.
91. Raz, I., Fisher, J., Israeli, A., Gottehrer, N., Chisin, R., and Kleinman, Y.: An unusual case of rheumatic pneumonia. Arch. Intern. Med. 145:1130, 1985.
92. Reddy, D. V., Chun, L. T., and Yamamoto, L. G.: Acute rheumatic fever with advanced degree/AV block. Clin. Pediatr. 28:326, 1989.
93. Bisno, A. L., and Ofek, I.: Serologic diagnosis of streptococcal infection. Comparison of a rapid hemagglutination technique with conventional antibody tests. Am. J. Dis. Child. 127:676, 1974.
94. Dajani, A. S., Bisno, A. L., Chung, K. J., Durack, D. T., Gerber, M. A., Kaplan, E. L., Millard, H. D., Randolph, M. F., Shulman, S. T., and Watanakunakorn, C.: Prevention of rheumatic fever. A statement for health professionals by the Committee on Rheumatic Fever, Endocarditis, and Kawasaki Disease of the Council on Cardiovascular Disease in the Young, American Heart Association. Circulation 78:1082, 1988.
95. Jones criteria (revised) for guidance in the diagnosis of rheumatic fever. Circulation 69:204A, 1984.
96. Bisno, A. L.: Coexistence of acute rheumatic fever and acute glomerulonephritis. Arthritis Rheum. 32:230, 1989.
97. Stollerman, G. H., Lewis, A. J., Schultz, I., and Taranta, A.: Relationship of immune response to group A streptococci to the course of acute, chronic and recurrent rheumatic fever. Am. J. Med. 20:163, 1956.
98. United Kingdom and United States Joint Report on Rheumatic Heart Disease.: The natural history of rheumatic fever and rheumatic heart disease. Five-year report of a cooperative clinical trial of ACTH, cortisone and aspirin. Circulation 22:503, 1960.
99. United Kingdom and United States Joint Report on Rheumatic Heart Disease.: The natural history of rheumatic fever and rheumatic heart disease: Ten-year report of a cooperative clinical trial of ACTH, cortisone and aspirin. Circulation 194:1284, 1965.
100. Vaisman, S., Guash, J., Vignau, A., Correa, E., Schuster, A., Mortimer, E. A., Jr., and Rammelkamp, C. H., Jr.: The failure of penicillin to alter acute rheumatic vasculitis. J.A.M.A. 194:1284, 1965.
101. Combined Rheumatic Fever Study Group, 1965: A comparison of the short-term, intensive prednisone and acetylsalicylic acid therapy in the treatment of acute rheumatic fever. N. Engl. J. Med. 272:63, 1965.
102. Markowitz, M., and Gordis, L.: Rheumatic Fever. Philadelphia, W. B. Saunders Company, 1972.
103. Bisno, A. L.: Nonsuppurative sequelae of group A streptococcal infection. *In* Kass, E. H., and Platt, R. (eds.): Current Therapy in Infectious Diseases—2. Philadelphia, B. C. Decker, Inc., 1986, p. 341.
104. Stollerman, G. H., Rusoff, J. H., and Hirschfeld, I.: Prophylaxis against group A streptococci in rheumatic fever. The use of single monthly injections of benzathine penicillin G. N. Engl. J. Med. 252:787, 1955.
105. Albam, B., Epstein, J. A., Feinstein, A. R., Gavrin, J. B., Jonas, S., Kleinberg, E., and Wood, H. F.: Rheumatic fever in children and adolescents. A long-term epidemiologic study of subsequent prophylaxis, streptococcal infections, and clinical sequelae. Ann. Intern. Med. 60(Suppl. 5):No. 2, Part II, 1964.
106. Lue, H. C., Wu, M., Hsieh, K., Lin, G. J., Hsieh, R. P., and Chiou, J. F.: Rheumatic fever recurrences: Controlled study of 3-week versus 4-week benzathine penicillin prevention programs. J. Pediatr. 108:299, 1986.
107. Padmavati, S., Gupta, V., Prakash, K., and Sharma, K. B.: Penicillin for rheumatic fever prophylaxis: 3-weekly or 4-weekly schedule? J. Assoc. Physicians India 35:753, 1987.
108. Schwartz, R. H., Wientzen, R. L., Jr., Pedreira, F., Feroli, E. J., Mella, G. W., and Guandolo, V. L.: Penicillin V for group A streptococcal pharyngotonsillitis: A randomized trial of seven days' versus ten days' therapy. J.A.M.A. 246:1790, 1981.
109. Beachey, E. H., Stollerman, G. H., Johnson, R. H., Ofek, I., and Bisno, A. L.: Human immune response to immunization with a structurally defined polypeptide fragment of streptococcal M protein. J. Exp. Med. 150:862, 1979.
110. Hasty, D. L., Beachey, E. H., Simpson, W. A., and Dale, J. B.: Hybridoma antibodies against protective and nonprotective antigenic determinants of a structurally defined polypeptide fragment of streptococcal M protein. J. Exp. Med. 155:1010, 1982.
111. Beachey, E. H., Gras-Masse, H., Tarter, A., Jolivet, M., Audibert, F., Chedid, L., and Seyer, J. M.: Opsonic antibodies evoked by hybrid peptide copies of types 5 and 24 streptococcal M proteins synthesized in tandem. J. Exp. Med. 163:1451, 1986.

Systemic Lupus Erythematosus, Juvenile Dermatomyositis, Scleroderma, and Vasculitis

Four of the other major connective tissue diseases of children are discussed in this chapter. Clinical data already covered in the chapter on juvenile rheumatoid arthritis (JRA) are not repeated, especially those relevant to treatment and drug dosages. Likewise, an attempt has been made to limit discussion to aspects of these diseases important or unique to children and avoid repetition of data already presented elsewhere in this text. Studies on the incidence and prevalence of these diseases are not as complete as for JRA. Intraclinic frequency, however, is available from four pediatric rheumatology services in North America (Table 72–1) that reflects reasonably accurate estimates of the relative prevalence of these disorders.[1, 2]

SYSTEMIC LUPUS ERYTHEMATOSUS

Systemic lupus erythematosus (SLE) is a multisystem disorder characterized by widespread inflammatory involvement of the connective tissues and immune-complex vasculitis. It is a prototype of autoimmune diseases in humans that results from altered immunologic reactivity and a genetic predisposition to the disease.

Epidemiology

The incidence of SLE in children has been estimated at 0.6 cases per 100,000.[3–5] Asians, Polynesians, North American Indians, and blacks are more at risk than whites.

Onset of SLE is unusual in a child younger than 4 years of age and becomes increasingly more common after the age of 9 and during the teenage years.[1] The female to male ratio in children is approximately 4.3:1; in the younger age group, relatively more boys are affected.[6, 7]

Another connective tissue disease occurs in approximately one out of every ten families with SLE. SLE has been described in identical twins with a concordance rate of 24 percent.[8] It is also associated with sporadic or familial immunodeficiency such as selective immunoglobulin A (IgA) deficiency[9] and inherited disorders of complement components such as heterozygous C2 deficiency.[10] Human leukocyte

Table 72–1. FREQUENCIES OF THE MAJOR PEDIATRIC CONNECTIVE TISSUE DISEASES (%)

	Michigan (1961–1979)	Southern California (1952–1977)	British Columbia (1979–1987)	Saskatchewan (1981–1989)
Number	*587*	*1460*	*396*	*204*
Juvenile rheumatoid arthritis	79	83	76.5	76.5
Systemic lupus erythematosus	10.6	8.5	7.6	5.4
Juvenile dermatomyositis	6.3	4	2.3	2.6
Scleroderma	3.2	3.5	2.3	3.4†
Vasculitis	1*	1*	11.9	12

*Does not include Kawasaki disease.
†Localized scleroderma only.

antigen (HLA)-A1, HLA-B8, HLA-DR2/DR3, and HLA-C4A null form an extended haplotype associated with SLE. HLA-DQw1 or w2 are also increased in frequency in this disease.

Etiology and Pathogenesis

A number of factors have been implicated in the pathogenesis of SLE.[11] The F1 hybrid of the New Zealand Black and White mice has a disease as similar to SLE as one is likely to find in an experimental animal. Outbred dogs also develop an SLE-like disease and, identical to their mouse counterparts, have circulating antibodies to native DNA and immune-complex deposition in tissues.

The basic pathogenesis of SLE appears to be variable immunologic abnormalities of homeostatic control affecting reactivity to nuclear and cytoplasmic antigens that may be antigen driven.[12] Environmental triggers such as sun exposure, a drug reaction, or a slow virus infection may precipitate the onset. Antibodies found in children with SLE include those that are tissue specific as well as ones related to nuclear antigens. These antibodies result in manifestations of the disease such as acute hemolytic anemia, leukopenia, thrombocytopenia, and thrombosis and in antigen-antibody complex deposition resulting in widespread vasculitis and lupus nephritis.

Clinical Manifestations

SLE is an extremely variable disease and may present with any degree of severity from acute, rapidly fatal illness to insidious, chronic disability with repeated exacerbations.[13–15] In more than 80 percent of children, SLE is correctly diagnosed within the first half year after onset, but diagnosis may be delayed by 4 to 5 years.[1]

Constitutional symptoms such as fever, malaise, and weight loss are common. Table 72–2 lists the clinical manifestations of SLE in children. Enormous variability exists in presenting signs and symptoms and in eventual organ involvement. The disease with each exacerbation tends to mimic previous acute episodes and in this manner often establishes within the first 2 years a pattern of involvement. Serious renal disease, if it is going to develop, usually declares itself during this same time period. The only major exception to the predictability of SLE is in the occurrence of central nervous system illness, which may intervene at any time.[16]

Mucocutaneous involvement is common and extremely varied in character and distribution. A malar erythematous rash in a butterfly distribution is characteristic of acute disease.

Arthralgia and arthritis affect the majority of children. Arthritis commonly involves the hands, wrists, elbows, shoulders, knees, and ankles. Characteristics of this arthritis are its transient character

Table 72–2. CLINICAL MANIFESTATIONS OF SYSTEMIC LUPUS ERYTHEMATOSUS IN CHILDHOOD

Skin (75%)
    Malar erythema (55%)
    Alopecia (20%)
    Photosensitivity (15%)
    Raynaud's phenomenon (25%)
Kidneys (85–100%)
    Hypertension (30%)
    Renal failure (10%)
Musculoskeletal system
    Arthritis (75%)
    Myositis (20%)
Cardiopulmonary system
    Pericarditis (45%)
    Pleuritis (35%)
    Pulmonary hemorrhage (5%)
Gastrointestinal tract
    Oral or nasopharyngeal ulcerations (15%)
    Mesenteric thrombosis (10%)
    Sterile peritonitis (5%)
Hepatosplenomegaly (45%)
Nervous system
    Central (30%)
    Peripheral (30%)

and the fact that it may be migratory. Pain may be more severe than is warranted by objective inflammatory findings. The arthritis of SLE is almost never destructive nor does it often result in permanent deformity. SLE may evolve, however, from JRA.[17]

Raynaud's phenomenon is frequent and often present at onset. Digital vasculitic ulceration occurs in a few children. Ischemic necrosis of bone, particularly of the femoral heads and tibial plateaus, is common, especially after treatment with glucocorticoids.

Pericarditis is the most common manifestation of cardiac disease. The child may develop congestive heart failure, arrhythmia, or cardiomegaly. Valvular insufficiency may occur, and Libman-Sacks verrucous endocarditis is particularly characteristic. Pleuritis is also common and may involve the diaphragmatic pleura accompanied by basilar pneumonitis. Pulmonary hemorrhage is rare.[18]

Many gastrointestinal complications of SLE are encountered. Mesenteric thrombosis and acute pancreatitis are often life-threatening events. Hepatomegaly and splenomegaly are common.

The two systems whose involvement correlates most closely with survivorship are the nervous system and the kidneys. Diseases of the central and peripheral nervous systems are common causes of morbidity in children. Severe recurrent headaches, focal or generalized seizures, chorea closely resembling that seen in rheumatic fever, and psychiatric manifestations of disordered personality to frank psychosis all occur. A labile, inappropriate affect is particularly common in the older child and adolescent. Intracranial hemorrhage and thrombosis may result from hypertension,[19] thrombocytopenia, or a circulating anticoagulant.[20] Pseudotumor cerebri may be a complication of SLE or of glucocorticoid therapy.

Systemic polyneuropathy, Guillain-Barré syndrome, transverse myelopathy, or involvement of the cranial nerves have all been reported. The so-called cytoid body of retinal vasculitis is often associated with lupus crisis or central nervous system vasculitis.

Lupus nephritis to some degree is present in virtually all children with SLE. Even severe nephritis may not be reflected in changes in the creatinine clearance, proteinuria, or an abnormal urinary sediment.[21] Evidence of immune-complex disease, however, such as increased circulating anti-native DNA antibodies or hypocomplementemia, correlate with active nephritis in most patients.

Laboratory Examination

The acute-phase reactants are generally increased in active systemic disease. Thrombocytopenia and acute hemolytic anemia may be present. Coombs' antibodies are often demonstrated in these children. Other causes of anemia besides systemic disease include polymenorrhagia, septicemia, and gastrointestinal bleeding. SLE may present as thrombocytopenic purpura. Persistent leukopenia is particularly characteristic. The majority of children are leukopenic at onset, with neutrophils predominating in the peripheral count. Often leukocytosis does not develop to an appropriate degree even with septicemia.

Antinuclear antibodies (ANAs) are a hallmark of the immunologic abnormalities of SLE, and as stated earlier, anti-native DNA antibodies are central to evaluating the degree of activity of the immune-complex disease.[22] ANAs are present in the vast majority of children with SLE (more than 95 percent). They generally occur in high titer in a homogeneous or peripheral pattern. The peripheral nuclear pattern is virtually diagnostic of the presence of anti-native DNA antibodies. Although historically important, the LE-cell test is seldom performed at this time. LE-cell phenomena are still present in the majority of children at onset of the disease and during acute exacerbations.

A minority of children with an SLE-like disease, often with prominent discoid lesions (subacute cutaneous lupus), have negative ANA serology by the usual laboratory techniques (rodent tissues); instead they have specific ANAs present, anti-Ro (SS-A) antibodies.[23] These antibodies are also associated with neonatal lupus.

Rheumatoid factors (RFs) are often present in high titer in children with SLE. Other children develop antitissue antibodies such as antithyroglobulin. Cold agglutinins and cryoglobulins may also be present and result in peripheral anoxic phenomena and gangrene. Circulating anticoagulant antibodies (antiphospholipid antibodies) that cross-react with cardiolipin of the Venereal Disease Research Laboratory (VDRL) test for syphilis occur in children with SLE.[20]

A young person with a biologic false-positive test for syphilis is at risk for the development of SLE.

Both the classic and the alternative complement pathways are activated in children with the immune-complex vasculitis of SLE.[24] A depressed whole hemolytic complement (CH50) determination reflects the status of the total complement cascade; a low concentration of C4 is usually a reliable indicator of active disease; the C3 concentration appears to be abnormally low less frequently. Dyslipoproteinemia is characteristic of active disease and is also a consequence of glucocorticoid therapy.[25]

Pathology

The basic inflammatory lesion of SLE is an immune-complex vasculitis with fibrinoid necrosis, inflammatory cell infiltrates, and sclerosis of collagen. Vascular deposition of immune complexes affects both arterioles and venules and is widespread throughout the parenchymal organs and in the supporting tissues underlying the dermis and the mucosal and serosal surfaces. Abnormal tubuloreticular (myxovirus-like) structures occur within endothelial cells and in circulating lymphocytes. Although originally interpreted as adding support to an etiologic role of viruses, these structures probably reflect degenerative or regenerative alterations in the cytoplasmic constituents of the endothelial cells.

In the kidney, immune complexes are deposited first in the mesangial areas and then in subendothelial spaces beneath the glomerular basement membrane.[26] Diffuse proliferative glomerulonephritis is regarded as a more severe form of focal proliferative nephritis, and progression from one to the other has been demonstrated in sequential biopsies. On the other hand, membranous disease may be immunologically a different entity. In this disorder, immune complexes form along the epithelial side of the glomerular basement membrane when circulating antibody forms complexes in situ with antigens that are fixed to that surface. Circulating DNA has been shown to have affinity for basement membrane.

Diagnosis

SLE is an episodic disease that is associated with persistent ANA seropositivity. The 11 criteria that have been developed by the American College of Rheumatology for the classification of SLE are generally applicable to children.[27] In adults, the presence of four of these criteria has a sensitivity of 90 percent and a specificity of 98 percent.

Renal biopsy is warranted in the majority of children with SLE to establish the classification of type, activity, and chronicity of the disease, unless there is no clinical or serologic evidence of significant involvement of the kidneys.[28] Occasionally a skin biopsy is also useful diagnostically in difficult cases.

Soluble immune complexes (IgG, C3) are deposited in the vascular endothelium and along the dermal-epidermal junction, the so-called lupus-band test, in both involved and uninvolved skin.

A number of other diseases should be considered in the differential diagnosis. Among these are JRA, acute poststreptococcal glomerulonephritis, hemolytic anemia, leukemia, allergic or contact dermatitis, idiopathic seizure disorder, mononucleosis, rheumatic fever, and septicemia. Chronic active hepatitis is associated as an overlap syndrome with SLE.

Primary Sjögren's syndrome is a multisystem disorder that may be misdiagnosed as SLE, in particular because of the presence of high titers of multiple autoimmune antibodies (Ro/La).[29] It is insidious in onset in many cases and often slowly progressive. Sjögren's syndrome is rare in children and may present as recurrent parotid and lacrimal swelling, dry mouth, and persistent conjunctivitis.

Treatment

In general, expert long-term supportive care of the child with SLE should include adequate nutrition, attention to fluid and electrolyte balance (sodium, potassium), prompt treatment of infections, and control of hypertension if present. Unnecessary restraints on a child's general level of activity and psychosocial peer group interactions are undesirable.

Because SLE is an extremely serious disease, most children with this disorder benefit from contact with the same medical team over the course of their illness. This team needs to emphasize to these children and their families the current treatment program and prophylactic measures of avoiding unnecessary drug exposure, transfusions, or excessive sunlight. Appropriate clothing and sunscreens are prescribed. Prompt attention to any fever or potential infection is mandatory. Pneumonitis, septicemia, and pyelonephritis are particular concerns.

Nonsteroidal anti-inflammatory drugs such as aspirin are helpful in treating minor manifestations of SLE such as arthralgia and myalgia. Hydroxychloroquine is used as an adjunctive medication in the treatment of SLE to control dermatitis or to moderate glucocorticoid dosage.[30] Glucocorticoid drugs are, however, the mainstay of the basic regimen for children with this disease. A negative result on testing with purified protein derivative (PPD) for tuberculosis should be verified before a child is started on glucocorticoids. Prednisone is often the preferred analogue. As low a dose as possible should be used to achieve the objectives of the treatment program. Initial therapy usually requires a split dosage regimen. Low-dose therapy, defined as 0.5 mg per kg per day, is used to treat persistent fever, dermatitis, arthritis, or serositis. These manifestations are often suppressed promptly. Weeks are usually required to control anemia, to suppress anti-DNA antibodies, or to return hypocomplementemia

toward normal. Relatively low-dose glucocorticoid programs are often sufficient to control the clinical disease in children with mesangial or focal glomerulonephritis.

High-dose prednisone therapy, defined as 1 to 2 mg per kg per day in divided doses, is employed for lupus crisis, central nervous system disease, acute hemolytic anemia, or the more severe forms of nephritis. Hypertension, azotemia, and pre-existing psychosis are relative contraindications to prolonged high-dosage regimens. Although a controversial area, the precise glucocorticoid program and consideration of immunosuppressive drugs are often predicated on the degree and type of involvement of the kidneys.

Treatment of the child with active SLE is monitored by the clinical course and physical examination and by periodic assessment of anti-DNA antibodies and serum complement levels. Exacerbation of the disease during a steroid taper may be signaled by a deterioration of the serologic indices.

Intravenous-pulse therapy with methylprednisolone may be used in an acute exacerbation along with other experimental therapies such as plasmapheresis.[31] Immunosuppressive agents are unfortunately necessary in some children in addition to glucocorticoids. Although azathioprine has been employed extensively, data suggest that intravenous cyclophosphamide pulse therapy is preferable (500 to 750 mg per M^2 every 4 weeks), especially in patients with severe nephritis.[32] Dialysis and kidney transplantation have been successfully used in end-stage renal disease.

Course of Disease and Prognosis

SLE is characterized by repeated exacerbations and remissions; active disease is often prolonged over many years. Although the course of the disease and its severity are highly variable, prognosis has improved dramatically during the past 25 years.[33-35] There has been especially a marked reduction in deaths within the first year of disease. Therefore, a guardedly optimistic attitude toward these children is justified. It is currently estimated that 85 percent of children will survive for 10 years.[36] It is generally stated that serious renal lesions are more common in children with SLE than in adults, prognosis for renal disease is more guarded, and the correct approach to long-term therapy is based on a careful evaluation of the renal status. Life table analysis in a study from Minnesota also indicated that survivorship in 21 children with diffuse proliferative glomerulonephritis was 80 percent at 10 years; however, end-stage renal failure or death had occurred in approximately 35 percent of the total series.

Prognosis for a specific child with SLE is unpredictable, and generalizations about outcome are especially unreliable during the first 1 to 2 years. Later a more realistic estimate can be discussed with the family based on the degree of systemic activity and its response to therapy and the severity of nephritis, immune-complex vasculitis, and parenchymal organ involvement. Outcome is poorest in diffuse proliferative nephritis or with development of the organic brain syndrome, and best in minimal or controlled systemic disease and mesangial nephritis and in patients who have had a prompt response to steroid therapy. Morbidity is often underestimated.[37]

Although nephritis and central nervous system disease have been leading causes of death,[38] infection has replaced them in some series as the most common event leading to death. Functional asplenia may contribute to this problem by predisposing the child to increased risk of septicemia.[39] Malignant hypertension, gastrointestinal bleeding or perforation, acute pancreatitis, and pulmonary hemorrhage are also prominent in the fatalities that have been reported. Accelerated atherosclerosis of the coronary arteries is a late cause of death.

Drug-Induced Systemic Lupus Erythematosus

A few children have acute SLE precipitated by a drug reaction. Among the medications that are often implicated are hydralazine, isoniazid, penicillin, and the sulfonamides. In children, as might be expected, anticonvulsant drugs have been common precipitating events.[40] Among these are phenylhydantoin, mephenytoin, trimethadione, and ethosuximide.

Most of the drugs are associated with a self-limited illness that clears on withdrawal of the offending agent. The most frequent clinical manifestations in drug-induced SLE are fever, dermatitis, and pleuropericardial disease. Antibodies to double-stranded DNA are usually not present, the serum complement concentration remains normal, and central nervous system disease and nephritis are uncommon. ANA reactivity specific for the DNA-histone antigens is particularly characteristic. Although the precise pathogenic mechanisms have not been elucidated in drug-induced SLE, some of these medications such as hydralazine may sensitize cutaneous DNA to degradation by ultraviolet light.

Lupus Phenomena in the Newborn Period

Children of mothers who have active SLE may develop lupus-like syndromes in the neonatal period related to transplacental passage of specific maternal IgG ANAs.[41, 42] It is convenient to separate these disorders into two types: a transient syndrome and complete congenital heart block.

Infants with the transient neonatal lupus syndrome (NLS) demonstrate high-titered ANAs, LE-cell phenomena, and depressed complement levels. This disorder results from the placental transport of maternal anti-Ro/La antibodies. In the majority of babies, there is no associated clinical disease, and

the serologic abnormalities abate within the first few months of life with metabolic decay of maternal immunoglobulin. In some infants, malar erythema develops along with discoid or annular lesions either immediately after birth or within the first 2 months of life (Fig. 72–1). Thrombocytopenia may be present along with mild hemolytic anemia or leukopenia. SLE may develop in young adults who had had transient manifestations of neonatal lupus.[43]

Usually this form of NLS requires no specific treatment. Occasionally glucocorticoids are indicated for severe dermatologic disease or gastrointestinal bleeding. Not all of the rashes completely disappear, and areas of pigmentation or hypopigmentation may remain.

Complete congenital heart block (CCHB) alone or associated with other cardiac defects such as widespread inflammation of the myocardium, endocardial cushion defects, and endomyocardial fibroelastosis has been described as a distinct and permanent neonatal lupus syndrome.[44] Approximately one third of the affected babies are born of mothers who have SLE or who develop SLE. The primary immunologic characteristic is ANA with anti-Ro (SS-A) antibody directed against a small cytoplasmic RNA-protein complex.[45] This antibody, and in most cases antibody to the La (SS-B) ribonucleoprotein complex, has been found in virtually every child and mother who have been studied with this syndrome. The predominant anti-Ro specificity is to the 52 kD

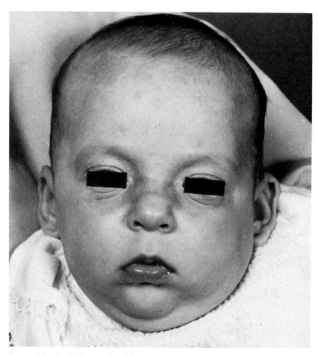

Figure 72–1. A 4-month-old white girl with the erythematous rash of neonatal lupus across the bridge of the nose, the lower eyelids, and the superior forehead. This baby was born at 33 weeks with complete congenital heart block. The electrocardiogram showed a normal QRS interval, and she did not require a cardiac pacemaker. Her mother had high titers of anti-Ro antibody.

peptide.[46] Anti-Ro antibody binds to fetal cardiac epitopes and results in heart block, which occurs after maturation of the fetal heart at 16 weeks of age. The atrioventricular node is absent and replaced by fibrous tissue and areas of calcification. More than 90 percent of affected mothers are HLA-DR3 positive.

CCHB can be recognized in utero by fetal echocardiography. The correct approach to the obstetric problem of CCHB is unclear but includes the use of glucocorticoids and potentially plasmapheresis.[47] Extreme bradycardia in utero results in fetal hydrops. Surviving infants eventually need cardiac pacing.

JUVENILE DERMATOMYOSITIS

Juvenile dermatomyositis (JDM) is a multisystem disease characterized by nonsuppurative inflammation of striated muscle, skin, and gastrointestinal tract.[1, 48, 49] The disease is typified early in its course by an immune-complex vasculitis of varying severity and late by the development of calcinosis.

Epidemiology

JDM, a relatively uncommon rheumatic disease of children, constitutes approximately 5 percent of the new diagnoses in a pediatric rheumatology clinic each year.[1] At all ages, the disease is slightly more frequent in girls than boys with a sex ratio of approximately 1.6:1. Age of onset is especially common from the fourth to the tenth year of childhood. A precise incidence rate has not been verified but is probably in the range of 0.3 to 0.4 cases per 100,000.

JDM has been reported in patients with selective IgA deficiency[9] and C2-complement component deficiency.[10] There may be an immunogenetic predisposition to the development of JDM: HLA-B8 and DR3 are increased in frequency in this disorder.[50]

Etiology and Pathogenesis

Although the etiology of JDM remains unknown, data indicate that it is autoimmune in pathogenesis and represents primary aberrations in the control of cell-mediated immunity.[51] Immune-complex vasculitis may be an important initiating or perpetuating event.[52] Immunoglobulins and complement are deposited in the walls of small blood vessels in the skeletal muscle.[53]

JDM is rarely associated with malignancy in contrast to dermatomyositis in adults except for a few reports in conjunction with leukemia. The disease has also followed infections, vaccination, hypersensitivity reactions to drugs, and sunburn. A number of studies have indicated that coxsackie B virus or toxoplasmosis may play a role in pathogenesis.[54] Acute transient inflammatory myositis has been reported after certain viral infections in otherwise normal children, e.g., influenza A and B.[55] A usually fatal myositis has been described in a few children with agammaglobulinemia in association with echovirus infection.

Clinical Manifestations

JDM usually presents with proximal muscle weakness, dermatitis, fever, and constitutional symptoms.[56] Table 72–3 lists the most important clinical manifestations. The majority of affected children have fatigue, malaise, weight loss, and anorexia. The muscle groups that are affected initially are the proximal limb-girdle muscles of the lower extremities followed by the shoulder girdle and proximal arm muscles. Weakness of the anterior neck flexors and back leads to an inability to hold the head upright or maintain a sitting posture. Facial and extraocular muscles are less commonly involved. Later in the disease or in children with an especially acute onset, the distal muscles of the extremities may be affected. Rarely there may be generalized acute inflammation of the entire striated musculature, a type of disease that may be more common in infants.

Fever may be the event that prompts referral to a physician. A child, however, may also complain of muscle pain, tenderness, or stiffness and stop walking or be unable to dress or climb stairs. There is usually a pronounced inability to get up off the floor (Gowers' sign) or out of bed. Although muscle weakness may be impressive, the deep tendon reflexes are well preserved.

Affected muscles are occasionally edematous and indurated. Ten percent of children with JDM develop pharyngeal, hypopharyngeal, or palatal muscle weakness. Dysphonia results along with dys-

Table 72–3. CLINICAL MANIFESTATIONS OF JUVENILE DERMATOMYOSITIS

Musculoskeletal system (100%)
   Proximal pelvic girdle (95%)
   Proximal shoulder girdle (75%)
   Neck flexors (60%)
   Pharyngeal muscles (30%)
   Distal muscles of the extremities (30%)
   Facial and extraocular muscles (5%)
   Arthritis (30%)
Skin (85–100%)
   Heliotrope rash of eyelids and periorbital edema (30%)
   Malar rash (40%)
   Periungual and articular rash (Gottron's papules) (80%)
   Photosensitivity (30%)
   Ulcerations (25%)
   Raynaud's phenomenon (15%)
   Calcinosis (40%)
Gastrointestinal tract (50%)
   Pharyngitis (40%)
   Dysphagia (15%)
   Hemorrhage (5%)
Pulmonary tract (80%)
   Restrictive disease (80%)
   Fibrosis (<1%)

phagia, which may also be related to esophageal hypomotility. These children are at particular risk for aspiration. Palatal speech and nasal regurgitation of liquids are early warning signs of impending respiratory compromise. Profound involvement of the thoracic and respiratory muscles is seen in a few children and leads to acute respiratory insufficiency, aspiration, or death.

The majority of children have the classic rash. Occasionally this rash may be the first sign of the disease. Cutaneous involvement is of variable severity and is distinctive over the malar areas, upper eyelids, and dorsal surfaces of the knuckles (Fig. 72–2), elbows, and knees. The basic cutaneous lesion is angiitis. At onset there is often indurative edema of the skin and subcutaneous tissues with periorbital edema. Later there is epidermal thinning and atrophy of the accessory structures with loss of hair and telangiectases. Vasculitic ulcers at the corners of the eyes, around the axillae, and in stretch marks may become a serious problem. Although a few cases of JDM in children have presented with calcinosis, this development is more characteristic of the healing phase of the disease.

Nail fold capillary loop abnormalities are present in half of the children with JDM as additional evidence of an early vascular abnormality.[57] These changes can be identified though the +40 lens of an ophthalmoscope or a microscope. The nail folds show

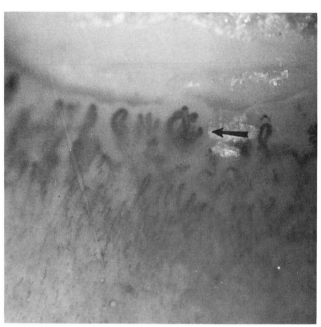

Figure 72–3. Abnormal nail fold capillary pattern, 100 × magnification. The vessels are thickened and tortuous and show a peripheral bushy pattern of arborization (*arrow*). The clear areas between the capillaries represent dropout areas. (Courtesy of Dr. Jay Kenik.)

simultaneous dilation of isolated loops, drop-out of surrounding vessels, and an arborized cluster of capillary loops that are distinctive for JDM (Fig. 72–3).

Laboratory Examinations

Nonspecific tests of inflammation such as the erythrocyte sedimentation rate and C-reactive protein tend to correlate with the degree of clinical disease. Leukocytosis and anemia are uncommon at onset except in the child with associated gastrointestinal bleeding. Although the frequency of RFs and ANAs is variable, specific antibodies such as to the PM-1 antigens have been described in a minority of children.[58] Half of the affected children have circulating immune complexes.

The serum concentrations of the muscle enzymes (creatine kinase, aldolase, aspartate transaminase, and alanine transaminase) are elevated in active disease. The extent of the increase is variable but may range from 20 to 40 times normal for the creatine kinase or aspartate transaminase.

A number of children at onset of disease have repeated episodes of microscopic hematuria that probably represent mild renal glomerulitis. Progression to renal insufficiency has not been described.

Pathology

The characteristic histopathology of JDM involves the striated muscles, skin, and gastrointestinal

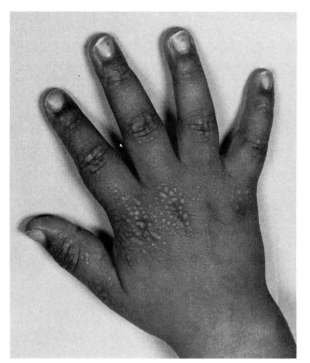

Figure 72–2. Gottron's papules in a 4-year-old black girl with JDM who had this skin rash since the age of 18 months. There is a remarkable development of raised hypopigmented papules on an erythematous base over the dorsum of the hand with accentuation over the metacarpophalangeal, proximal interphalangeal, and distal interphalangeal joints.

tract. The initial lesion is an acute patchy inflammatory round-cell infiltration (Fig. 72–4). Concomitant degeneration and regeneration of muscle fibers follow and result in a moderate variation in fiber size. All fiber types are involved. Areas of focal necrosis are replaced during the healing phase by an interstitial proliferation of connective tissue and fat.

An immune-complex necrotizing vasculitis occurs in arterioles, capillaries, and venules and may lead to infarction, ulceration, and hemorrhage, especially in the gastrointestinal tract.[59] In early studies, vasculitis was cited as an important prognostic factor in the survival of children with JDM.[60] More recently, additional distinctive features of a noninflammatory vasculopathy identified on electron microscopy have been related to a poorer outcome.[61, 62] Zonal loss of the capillary bed, areas of focal infarction of muscle, lymphocytic non-necrotizing vasculitis, and a noninflammatory endarteropathy have been associated with progressive infarction of muscles and gastrointestinal tract and cutaneous ulcerations.[62, 63] IgG is not deposited in these vascular lesions; diffuse linear and occasionally granular deposits of IgM, C3d, and fibrin are present in the areas of noninflammatory vasculopathy. Thus, capillary endothelial damage may play a central role in the pathogenesis of JDM. Electron microscopic examination of muscle biopsy specimens from children has also revealed abnormal tubuloreticular structures within the endothelial cells that are similar to the myxovirus-like particles found in renal biopsy specimens of patients with SLE.

Except for isolated vasculitis, smooth muscle is not affected. The heart is generally not involved in the primary pathologic process. A few children with cardiac disease have been described with focal myocardial fibrosis and contraction-band necrosis. The

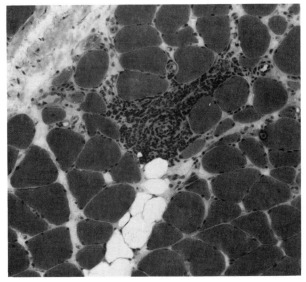

Figure 72–4. Muscle biopsy specimen (H & E, 100 ×). In the center is a perivascular mononuclear cell inflammatory infiltrate with arterial thickening and prominent endothelial cells. (Courtesy of Dr. George McClellan.)

detection of MB bands on the isozyme pattern of serum creatine kinase in children with JDM is usually evidence of regeneration of the striated muscle and not of cardiac damage.

Diagnosis

The acute onset of proximal muscle weakness accompanied by characteristic dermatitis is pathognomonic of JDM.[64] The one fourth of children who do not have the classic rash almost invariably have an atypical rash that is still suggestive of this diagnosis. Polymyositis, that is, inflammatory myositis without dermatitis, is a rare presentation in children.[65]

The three most important diagnostic findings are elevated serum muscle enzymes in 98 percent of the children, abnormal electromyographic changes in 96 percent, and specific histopathologic abnormalities in the muscle biopsy in 79 percent. Sequential determinations of the serum muscle enzymes are important for diagnosis and in monitoring effective therapy. Electromyography (EMG) is useful in confirming the diagnosis of JDM and in aiding in the selection of the best site for performing a muscle biopsy. The notable EMG changes are those of myopathy and denervation. An EMG should be performed on one side of the body only so the biopsy can be done on the opposite extremity without any confusion over inflammation created by the needle insertions. Atrophy, fatty infiltration, and signal abnormalities indicative of active disease can also be demonstrated by magnetic resonance imaging (MRI).

A muscle biopsy is generally indicated in initial evaluation of a child to be certain of the diagnosis, assess prognosis, and provide support for instituting long-term glucocorticoid therapy or immunosuppressive drugs. The muscle to be biopsied should be clinically involved as demonstrated by muscle testing or EMG but not atrophied. The best sites are generally a deltoid or quadriceps. This biopsy should be generous and is usually performed by the open technique.

The differential diagnosis of JDM includes the other connective tissue diseases that present as multisystem illnesses. There is seldom any confusion with the acute systemic onset of JRA or with SLE. Mild forms of JDM presenting predominantly as arthritis may, however, be confused with either of these two diseases. An occasional child may develop an overlap syndrome with specific features of the different connective tissue diseases.[66] Eosinophilic fasciitis[67, 68] and mixed connective tissue disease[69–71] are distinctive syndromes within this category. Scleroderma poses unique diagnostic problems in that approximately 25 percent of children with this disorder have a primary myositis not unlike that seen in dermatomyositis. Although early cutaneous abnormalities of scleroderma and JDM are quite different, during the courses of these diseases the skin changes tend to merge in character.

In the child with muscular dystrophy, there should be a selective pattern of muscle weakness, insidious onset of progressive or remitting illness, and a positive family history. Dermatitis is absent. The serum creatine kinase is elevated in the first-degree relatives of children with muscular dystrophy, especially in the mothers of children with X-linked disease. Myoadenylate deaminase deficiency may be a primary or associated defect.[72] The other congenital myopathies, myotonias, and hypotonic syndromes and the metabolic and endocrine myopathies must also be considered. Paroxysmal myoglobulinuria and thyrotoxic myopathy may occasionally be encountered. Myasthenia gravis is rare in children.

Rhabdomyolysis may follow an acute infection, trauma, or extreme muscular exertion. The onset is abrupt and characterized by profound weakness, myoglobinuria, and occasionally oliguria and renal failure. Trichinosis and toxoplasmosis cause myositis of varying severity, and severe pustular acne may occasionally be associated with inflammatory disease of muscle. Influenza B, coxsackie B virus infection, poliomyelitis, and Guillain-Barré syndrome are other diagnostic possibilities.

Treatment

Introduction of glucocorticoid drugs into the management of JDM has dramatically improved the prognostic outlook for children.[56, 73] General supportive care and a coordinated team approach are important, including individualized bed rest and positioning along with physical therapy to minimize contractures.

For treatment of acute disease, it is generally necessary to use 2 mg per kg per day of prednisone in four divided doses for at least the first month; then, if indicated by clinical response and a fall in the serum muscle enzyme concentrations, a lower dose in the range of 1 mg per kg per day is prescribed. Thereafter daily steroid is slowly tapered in amount and frequency of administration by monitoring improvement in the clinical status of the child, the degree of muscle weakness, and level of the serum muscle enzymes. Satisfactory control is not achieved until serum muscle enzymes have returned to normal or nearly normal levels and remain there during tapering of the steroids and an increase in the level of physical activity of the child. Because long-term steroid administration is not without significant toxicity in growing children, the aim of management is to lower the steroid dose as much as possible concomitant with continued improvement in the disease. Alternate-day steroid therapy may be useful late in the recovery phase. Addition of hydroxychloroquine aids in controlling the dermatitis and appears to be steroid-sparing.[74]

Many approaches to the therapy of calcinosis

have been tried, including colchicine, probenecid, aluminum salts, warfarin, and the diphosphonates. In general, none of these has met with uniform success except for surgical excision of calcific tumors in areas of ulceration or pressure.

Acute complications of the disease such as cutaneous ulcerations or a course that fails to respond to steroid management may be indications for the use of immunosuppressive agents. Methotrexate has achieved a degree of success in the treatment of adults and has been used in resistant children. Intravenous cyclophosphamide[62] and steroid-pulse therapy[75] have also been recommended. Initial reports of the use of cyclosporin A have been published.[76]

Course of Disease and Prognosis

The course of JDM in most children can be divided into four clinical phases (Table 72–4).[77] Approximately 80 percent of children pursue a uniphasic course that lasts approximately 2 years.[56] Durations of disease as short as 8 months have been reported. The remaining 20 percent of the children continue to have acute exacerbations and remissions; a few eventually develop a disease that is more typical of systemic vasculitis. A small number of children late in the course may assume more of the characteristics of scleroderma with profound sclerodactyly and cutaneous atrophy. Other children even years after onset have persistent elevations of the serum muscle enzymes (especially the creatine kinase) and characteristic histopathologic features of the disease if a muscle biopsy is performed.[78]

The course of dermatitis may not follow that of myositis. Many clinicians are convinced that children who have a generalized rash and develop cutaneous ulcerations have the poorest prognosis.[1, 56] The characteristic nail fold loop abnormalities along with the noninflammatory vasculopathy correlate prognostically with more severe disease.[57]

During the healing phase of JDM, deposits of calcium salts (hydroxyapatite or fluorapatite) may develop in the skin and subcutaneous tissues, about the joints, and within the interfascial planes of the muscles in approximately half of the children.[79] Subsequently calcification may be slowly resorbed spontaneously (Figs. 72–5 and 72–6).

In spite of the aforementioned, the average child with JDM pursues a progressively improving course

Table 72–4. CLINICAL PHASES OF JUVENILE DERMATOMYOSITIS

Prodromal period with nonspecific symptoms (weeks to months)
Progressive muscle weakness and dermatitis (days to weeks)
Persistent myositis and dermatitis (up to 2 years)
Recovery with residual muscle atrophy and contractures with or without calcinosis

Modified from Hanson, V.: Dermatomyositis, scleroderma, and polyarteritis nodosa. Clin. Rheum. Dis. 2:445, 1976.

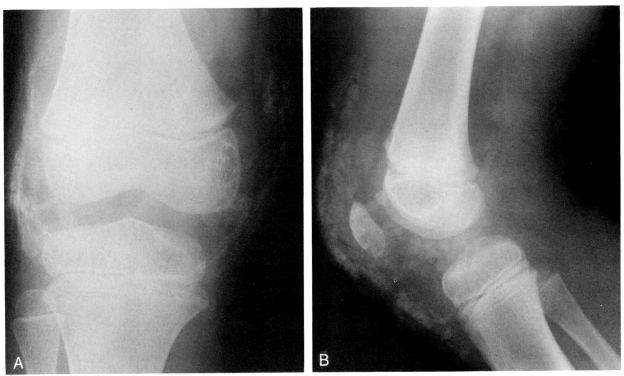

Figure 72–5. There are massive deposits of calcium salts in the subcutaneum and fascia about the right knee in this 11-year-old boy. Calcinosis followed by 3 years the acute phase of JDM. Anteroposterior (*A*) and lateral (*B*) views.

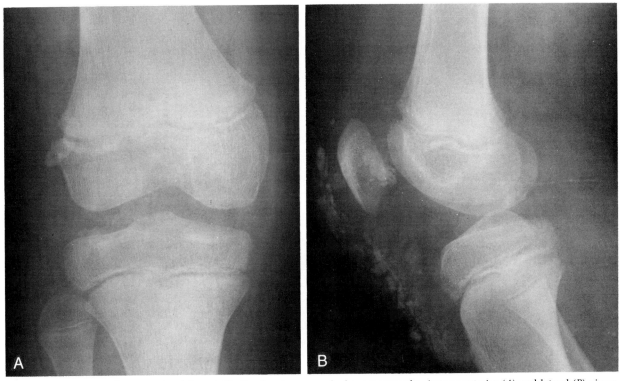

Figure 72–6. Two years later, much of the calcification has been resorbed spontaneously. Anteroposterior (*A*) and lateral (*B*) views.

to functional recovery (Table 72–5).[73, 80, 81] During the convalescent phase, the physical therapy program should focus on normalizing function as nearly as possible and minimizing development of contractures secondary to muscle weakness or atrophy. Muscle strengthening should be added to the exercise program only when clinical evidence of acute inflammation has subsided.

In the preglucocorticoid era, JDM was associated with a mortality rate that approached 50 percent.[82] Surviving children often had devastating residual problems of contractures, muscle atrophy, and widespread calcinosis. At the present time, JDM is rarely fatal, and long-term survival approaches 90 percent. In addition, functional outcome has been greatly improved. The majority of children should be able to function independently as adults, although some will have residual atrophy of skin or muscle groups. Difficulties during pregnancy have been described in women who have had JDM.[83]

The greatest risk of death is within the first 2 years after onset of disease. The basic nature of the inflammatory disease, its early response to treatment, whether vasculitis is present, or progressive involvement of other organ systems, such as the gastrointestinal or pulmonary tracts, are major factors that influence outcome. Acute gastrointestinal complications are seen in a minority of children and may not be well controlled by steroid therapy alone. They have been a leading cause of death. Respiratory insufficiency leading to hypoxia with or without aspiration is also a serious, often preterminal event. Functional outcome appears best in children who have been seen early and treated vigorously.

SCLERODERMA

The sclerodermas are connective tissue diseases of unknown etiology whose development in a child is often unrecognized at first because each is so rare.[84–86] Systemic or generalized scleroderma is seen in children as well as the more common localized diseases of morphea and linear scleroderma. In the former, there is often a diagnostic delay of up to 5 years because of the subtle, insidious nature of the onset.

Systemic Disease

Systemic disease is divided into classic scleroderma and the CREST (calcinosis, Raynaud's phe-

Table 72–5. OUTCOME FOR CHILDREN WITH JUVENILE DERMATOMYOSITIS

Complete functional recovery	70%
Minimal disease (atrophy or contractures)	20%
Calcinosis	40%
Significant disability or dependence	5%
Death	5%

nomenon, esophageal abnormalities, sclerodactyly, and telangiectases) syndrome and the overlap syndromes with SLE and JDM. Some authors also include other distinctive disorders such as mixed connective tissue disease and eosinophilic fasciitis in this category.

Epidemiology

Girls are affected more frequently than boys (3:1) except in the youngest age group.[1] There is no peak age of onset during childhood or racial predilection.[87] In comparison to the other major connective tissue diseases, scleroderma accounts for 3 percent of diagnoses in a pediatric rheumatology clinic.[1, 85]

Etiology and Pathogenesis

Angiitis may be the basic initial lesion in scleroderma. The skin and gastrointestinal tract are involved early along with the lungs, heart, and kidneys. A number of disorders have been described that mimic or duplicate abnormalities found in scleroderma and may provide a clue to its pathogenesis. Scleroderma-like changes are seen in children with diabetes mellitus, phenylketonuria, and progeria. Scleroderma-like disease has also followed exposure to vinyl chloride, bleomycin, pentazocine, and prosthetic implants. It has occurred in an epidemic in Spain relating to a toxic oil syndrome (rapeseed oil). It occurs as a component of graft-versus-host disease in bone marrow transplantation patients.[88]

Clinical Manifestations

Clinical manifestations of scleroderma are summarized in Table 72–6. The onset is often characterized by the appearance of Raynaud's phenomenon; tightening, thinning, and atrophy of the skin of the hands and face; or the appearance of cutaneous telangiectases.[85] Classic two to three color change Raynaud's phenomenon occurs in most children and may antedate the onset of cutaneous abnormalities. It is characterized by obstructive digital arterial disease and sympathetic hyperactivity. It is often progressive, and digital gangrene may supervene with small atrophic pits on the fingertips.

Skin tightening is virtually universal and tends to become more generalized with time. Hypopigmentation and hyperpigmentation are characteristic along with subcutaneous calcification and deposition of calcium salts around joints (Fig. 72–7). Erythema and ulcerations may develop over the elbows, knees, and malleoli. Cutaneous evidence of vasculitis is also evident in the early appearance of telangiectases about the face, upper trunk, and hands.

Characteristic abnormalities of the nail fold capillaries have been identified in children with scleroderma.[89] These changes are virtually universal at onset and characteristic of the diagnosis. There is a reduction in the number of vessels and a marked

Table 72–6. CLINICAL MANIFESTATIONS OF SCLERODERMA IN CHILDHOOD

Skin (100%)
   Raynaud's phenomenon (75%)
   Ulcerations (30%)
   Subcutaneous calcification (20%)
   Telangiectases (30%)
   Pigmentary changes (20%)
Gastrointestinal tract
   Dysphagia (20%)
   Abnormal esophageal motility (75%)
   Colonic sacculations (20%)
   Duodenal dilatation (5%)
Pulmonary tract
   Dyspnea (20%)
   Abnormal diffusion (75%)
   Abnormal vital capacity (70%)
Musculoskeletal system
   Joint contractures (75%)
   Resorption of digital tufts (60%)
   Muscle weakness and pain (25%)
Heart
   Electrocardiographic abnormalities (30%)
   Cardiomegaly (15%)
   Congestive failure (15%)

tortuosity and puddling of the remaining capillaries. Scattered white fibrotic areas are prominent.

Many children have arthralgias and contractures about joints, and a few present with objective arthritis. Others develop crepitant tenosynovitis. Dyspnea on exertion may be related to skin tightness, muscle weakness, or pulmonary disease. Myocarditis and cardiomyopathy also lead to dyspnea, arrhythmia, and signs of heart failure. Muscle pain and tenderness are present in approximately 20 percent of patients. Elevation of the serum muscle enzymes tends to be mild to moderate and not as striking as in JDM.

Although widespread gastrointestinal involvement occurs in the majority of children, symptomatic disease is often confined to the esophagus with complaints of dysphagia or reflux esophagitis. Esophageal ulceration and constriction may develop. Malabsorption may become severe and lead to a fatal outcome.

Laboratory Examinations

Routine laboratory studies are usually normal. ANAs, however, are found in the majority of children and on the HEp-2 cell substrate are often characterized by high-titered speckled patterns. Distinct antigenic specificity may be present: anticentromere in the CREST syndrome,[90] anti–Scl-70 (topoisomerase 1), or antinucleolar antibodies.

Pulmonary diffusion and spirometry are sensitive measures of involvement of the respiratory tract. These studies document a decrease in the timed vital capacity and forced expiratory flow, an early decrease in diffusion, and an increase in functional residual volume. These findings are present in most children at onset of the disease and often progressive.

Plethysmography is abnormal in children with Raynaud's phenomenon and documents the obstructive nature of the vascular disease and involvement of the sympathetic nervous system. Arteriography should not be performed as a diagnostic measure because it may precipitate an acute exacerbation of digital anoxia.

Radiologic Examination

Even in early disease, upper gastrointestinal films often reveal disordered motility of the distal esophagus. Esophageal motility studies by manometry are, however, a more sensitive indicator of peristaltic and functional abnormalities. Dilation of the second portion of the duodenum and pseudo-sacculations of the colon may also be present.

Acro-osteolysis of the digital tufts may be present on radiographs of the hands (Fig. 72–8). In most of these cases, this resorption is accompanied by focal areas of soft tissue calcification.

Pathology

In systemic or generalized scleroderma, there is thinning of the epidermis, loss of the rete pegs, and atrophy of the dermal appendages. In the deeper layers, there is homogenization of the collagen fibers with loss of structural detail, an increased density and thickness of collagen deposition, and a predom-

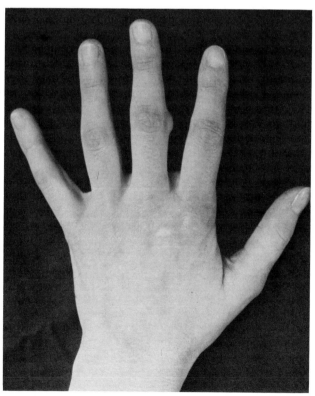

Figure 72–7. Subcutaneous nodule of calcification in a teenaged girl with acrosclerosis.

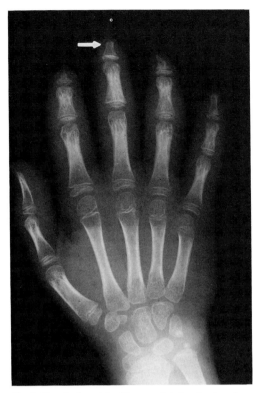

Figure 72–8. Hand of a girl with complaints of scleroderma for 2 years showing acro-osteolysis. The arrow points to early resorption of the tuft of a distal phalanx.

overlap syndromes who have the immune complex characteristics of SLE: Antibodies to native DNA and to the Sm nuclear antigen are present in this latter group.

MCTD was reported at first as a disease of favorable prognosis and an excellent initial response to relatively low-dose glucocorticoid therapy.[69] Progression into a more scleroderma-like disease has occurred, however, with sclerodactyly and gastrointestinal involvement or an SLE-like disease. Nephritis may be more frequent in children than in adults and more severe. Children may have less pulmonary disease (hypertension) and more hematologic complications than adults.

Eosinophilic Fasciitis. This disorder has been exceptionally rare in children, and only approximately 13 cases have been described.[67, 68] These children present with marked induration of the cutaneous and subcutaneous tissues of the upper or lower extremities and occasionally the trunk or face. Onset of the disease may have been preceded by unusual physical exertion. Raynaud's phenomenon, nail fold capillary abnormalities, and visceral disease are absent.

The diagnosis of eosinophilic fasciitis is confirmed by a full-thickness biopsy of skin, fascia, and muscle. Inflammation is present in all layers, but the most characteristic feature is thickened fascia with

inance of embryonal fibers. Perivascular infiltrates of mononuclear cells are often present, which have been shown in some studies to be predominantly T lymphocytes. The arterioles undergo eventual hyalinization and fibrosis (Fig. 72–9).

Diagnosis

The early clinical picture of scleroderma is usually classic but often quite subtle. Diagnostic criteria are the same as for adults.[91] Differential diagnoses should include JDM, SLE, and less frequently JRA. Patients with the CREST syndrome have predominant calcinosis, Raynaud's phenomenon, esophageal abnormalities, sclerodactyly, and telangiectases. Other overlap syndromes, mixed connective tissue disease, and eosinophilic fasciitis should also be considered.

Mixed Connective Tissue Disease. Mixed connective tissue disease (MCTD) has been described in approximately 90 children who presented with arthritis, myositis, and cutaneous disease characteristic of scleroderma, SLE, or JDM.[69–71] These findings are associated with very high titers of ANAs, often in a speckled pattern, to an extractable nuclear antigen (ENA) and ribonucleoprotein (RNP). Epitope specificity is to the U_1RNP 70 kD peptide, along with the A and C peptides. Prominent HLA associations in these patients are to DR4, 2, and w53. Other ANAs characteristically delineate the subset of children with

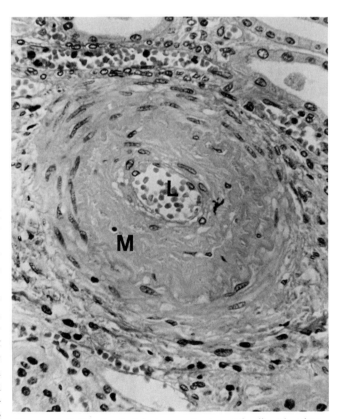

Figure 72–9. Renal arteriole in a patient acutely ill with scleroderma and a hypertensive crisis. There is virtual obliteration of the vessel lumen (L) by intimal proliferation and medial mucoid hyperplasia (M).

round cell infiltration of histiocytes and often eosinophils and a prominent perivascular infiltrate of lymphocytes and plasma cells. IgG, IgM, and C3 may be deposited in areas of inflammation. Associated laboratory findings include a remarkable peripheral eosinophilia of 40 to 60 percent and hypergammaglobulinemia in approximately half of the children.

This disorder as originally reported was self-limited with spontaneous resolution after months to years. There was often marked relief with the administration of small amounts of the glucocorticoid drugs. Occasionally, however, a more severe form of the disease evolved with hematologic abnormalities. These complications may be more common in the childhood type of onset.

Treatment

No uniformly effective therapy is available for scleroderma.[1] Nonsteroidal anti-inflammatory drugs may relieve some of the musculoskeletal symptoms of this disease. Penicillamine or colchicine may be useful in management of the cutaneous manifestations if prescribed early. Captopril is effective in treatment of hypertension and may have some effect on the skin and subcutaneous tissues. Often children who present with gastrointestinal problems require special therapeutic intervention for esophageal stricture or obstruction, reflux esophagitis, or malabsorption.

Glucocorticoid drugs are probably contraindicated in the majority of children. They may exacerbate small blood vessel disease and renal involvement with hypertension. Renal failure and acute hypertensive encephalopathy may supervene as a potentially fatal outcome in a few children. At least in the adult literature, this event seems more likely to occur early in the course of the disease. It merits emergency lowering of the blood pressure to normal and expert intensive care.

Raynaud's phenomenon is best treated with alpha-blocking agents such as phenoxybenzamine or prazocin or the calcium-channel blockers such as nifedipine. Some investigators recommend early treatment of the angiitis of scleroderma by these drugs. Plasmapheresis has been used in severe systemic disease and biofeedback for less threatening vasospasm. Children with prominent Raynaud's phenomenon must also learn to dress appropriate to the season and avoid cold liquids and objects that can exacerbate not only peripheral anoxia, but also vascular spasm within viscera. Vigorous physical therapy is important in the majority of these patients to prevent or minimize joint contractures.

Course of Disease and Prognosis

The prognosis of generalized scleroderma is poor in children as well as in adults.[85, 92] Death is often related to cardiopulmonary failure or gastrointestinal complications including severe inanition.[1] Cardiac arrhythmias may develop during the course of the disease, and congestive heart failure is often a terminal event. The frequency of a fatal outcome has not been determined in any large series of children because of the rarity of this disease. It is not judged to be any more favorable, however, than in adults, in whom prognosis for life at 7 years was only 35 percent.[92] A child, however, may live decades after onset; therefore, an optimistic but realistic attitude should be taken in discussions with the parents. Patients with the CREST syndrome were originally thought to have a more favorable prognosis; evidence for this judgment is not present in studies of children, albeit this diagnosis is very rare in that age group.

Localized Scleroderma

In morphea and linear scleroderma, fibrosis of the connective tissues is limited to the dermis, subdermis, and superficial striated muscles.[86, 93] The localized sclerodermas are about twice as common as systemic disease. Linear scleroderma is approximately twice as frequent as morphea in children.

Morphea can be subdivided into single or multiple plaques, smaller lesions in a more general distribution (guttate morphea), or generalized, coalescent, cutaneous involvement. In early disease, acute inflammatory erythema and edema are present in one or more circumscribed lesions followed later by hypopigmentation and induration surrounded by hyperpigmentation (Fig. 72–10). These lesions are located anywhere on the trunk or extremities. The child may complain of paresthesia or pain over the lesions. The patches may coalesce or enlarge centrifugally and involve larger areas of the body.

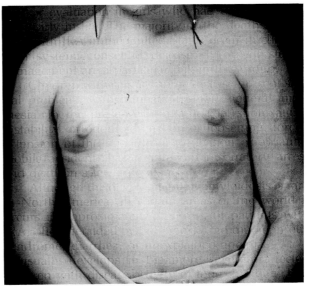

Figure 72–10. Typical morphea with central hypopigmentation and an active border on the left thorax of this young girl. Another extensive lesion is present on the outer left arm.

Linear scleroderma is characterized by the presence of one or more areas of linear involvement of the skin of the head, trunk, or extremities.[86] Underlying bone is often affected in this disorder, with resultant growth abnormalities, deformity, or contractures of joints. Because lesions of the face or scalp may have the appearance of scars from dueling, the term *en coup de sabre* has been used.

Linear scleroderma develops primarily in the first two decades of life. It often affects only one side of the body producing hemiatrophy of the involved areas. Indeed it is this lack of normal development that causes the most severe disabilities from this disease, e.g., hemifacial atrophy or failure of an extremity to grow in proportion to its opposite member (Fig. 72–11).

Laboratory abnormalities are few indeed in localized scleroderma with the exception of ANAs in approximately one half of the children. Antibodies to centromere or Scl-70 characteristic of systemic disease are generally not present in the localized forms.

Localized scleroderma may regress spontaneously without treatment, or fibrosis of the involved skin and subcutaneous tissues may progress and produce hide-binding and marked contractures of an extremity. Active disease may undergo exacerbations and remissions for many months to 2 to 3 years.

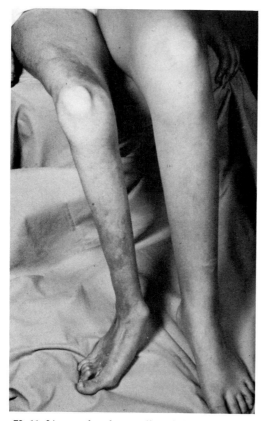

Figure 72–11. Linear scleroderma affected the right leg of this 14-year-old girl beginning at the age of 6 years. There is severe atrophy and shortening of the extremity.

Prognosis is generally excellent in the absence of systemic involvement. Occasionally visceral disease or a seizure disorder develops late in the course of localized scleroderma. A few children may evolve into an overlap syndrome with another connective tissue disease such as SLE. Penicillamine may be effective if used early in the more generalized form of morphea.[94] Morphea may also regress with age. Although linear lesions may also improve with age, significant abnormalities of local growth unfortunately persist.

VASCULITIS

Inflammatory vasculitis is a prominent component of virtually all of the systemic connective tissue diseases. Several attempts have been made to classify the various forms of idiopathic vasculitis, and that proposed by Zeek in 1953 and later modified has been adopted for this review.[95] This classification is based on the size of the vessel involved, the location of visceral involvement, and whether the predominant histopathology is necrosis of vessel wall or a granulomatous response.

All forms of vasculitis except for Henoch-Schönlein purpura and Kawasaki's disease are rare in children. Hypersensitivity angiitis was previously more commonly encountered than at the present time as a reaction to sulfa drugs and penicillin. A major study of classification criteria for the vasculitic diseases has been reported by a Committee of the American College of Rheumatology.[96]

Necrotizing Vasculitis of Medium-Sized and Small Arteries

In these diseases, the medium-sized muscular arteries are involved, and the predominant histologic change is fibrinoid necrosis of the entire thickness of the vessel wall. The lesions tend to be segmental with a predilection for the bifurcations of the vessels. Biopsy specimens usually show vasculitis in all stages of development from acute to chronic.

Polyarteritis Nodosa

The classic form of polyarteritis nodosa (PAN) was initially described more than 100 years ago, and reports of small numbers of cases have periodically appeared in the pediatric literature.[97–99] The course and progression of this disease are highly variable, and multisystem involvement leads to confusion with a broad spectrum of other diseases. Early diagnosis and correct classification are often difficult.

Clinical Manifestations. The onset of PAN is frequently insidious, and constitutional symptoms of fever and weight loss may be the presenting complaints. No single pattern of clinical presentation is characteristic; however, renal, gastrointestinal, and

Table 72–7. CLINICAL MANIFESTATIONS OF POLYARTERITIS NODOSA IN CHILDHOOD

Hypertension	80%
Skin	70%
Gastrointestinal tract	70%
Musculoskeletal system	65%
Nervous system	40%
Central nervous system	30%
Peripheral neuropathy	20%
Kidneys	25%
Heart	45%
Myocardial infarction	20%
Pulmonary tract	15%

cardiac disease are often prominent along with involvement of both the central and peripheral nervous systems (Table 72–7). Cutaneous lesions are frequent, but arthritis is unusual. Dermatitis includes a broad spectrum of lesions of purpura, peripheral gangrene, and nodular vasculitis (Fig. 72–12). The initial diagnosis may be renovascular hypertension or a surgical abdomen. Severe sensorimotor peripheral neuropathy that is symmetric is frequently observed, so-called mononeuritis multiplex.

Laboratory Studies. The degree and extent of multisystem involvement are often reflected in anemia, leukocytosis, marked elevation of the erythrocyte sedimentation rate, urinary sediment changes, and abnormalities in the serum immunoglobulin concentrations. Classic RFs and ANAs are unusual. A few children will be positive for hepatitis B–associated antigens, e.g., fewer than 5 percent. Diagnosis is invariably dependent on biopsy of an involved, accessible site (skin, muscle, nerve) or an angiogram that demonstrates aneurysms in the celiac or renal vasculature.[1]

Treatment. Glucocorticoid therapy is the mainstay of the management of children with PAN.[1] Suppressive amounts of prednisone are indicated in the range of 1 to 2 mg per kg per day in divided dosage. The aggressiveness of the therapeutic program needs to be modified depending on the extent of cardiac or renal involvement or the presence of hypertension.

A child may not respond adequately to the use of oral prednisone alone or to intravenous steroid-pulse therapy. Extensive systemic involvement, particularly of the abdominal vasculature with aneurysms and thrombosis, is generally accepted as an indication for the use of cyclophosphamide in conjunction with glucocorticoids. Although most reports have been based on the use of daily oral cyclophosphamide, intravenous-pulse therapy may be preferable in this type of disease.

Course of Disease and Prognosis. PAN pursues a chronic relapsing course over many years, with eventual remission possible in some children. Death most commonly occurs secondary to renal failure, myocardial infarction, or hypertensive encephalopathy. It is difficult to estimate the long-term prognosis for this syndrome because of past confusion in published series that has resulted from a failure to distinguish among the several forms of polyarteritis when reporting therapeutic results.

Previously a number of very young infants with a febrile illness that lasted for a few weeks to months were described with a syndrome referred to as *infantile polyarteritis nodosa*. Dermatitis, conjunctivitis, and evidence of involvement of internal organs, usually the heart and kidneys, were often present. Many of these children died suddenly from acute myocardial infarction. The disease was more common in boys and was often misdiagnosed initially as a viral infection. The course was generally brief, and often the correct diagnosis was made only at necropsy. It is now thought that infantile PAN probably represented undiagnosed Kawasaki's disease.

Kawasaki's Disease

An acute febrile illness associated with systemic vasculitis primarily affecting infants and young children was first noted by Kawasaki in 1961 in Japan.[100] The first descriptions in the English literature appeared in the 1970s under the designation *mucocutaneous lymph node syndrome*.[101, 102]

Epidemiology. Kawasaki's disease (KD) may occur sporadically or in mini-epidemics in any one geographic location.[102, 103] Within the United States, most patients present in the fall and spring. The mean age of onset is young, approximately 1½ years, and the male to female ratio is 1.5:1. The disease is distinctly more common in children of Japanese descent: In the United States, the risk factor for KD for

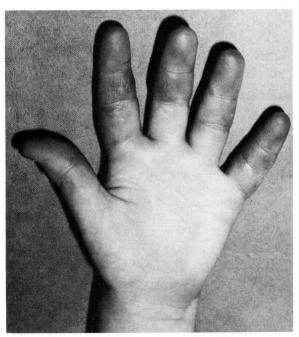

Figure 72–12. Marked digital cyanosis and swelling were present in this young boy with PAN. The digital anoxia was accompanied by chronic pain that was exacerbated during acute vasospastic episodes.

Table 72–8. CRITERIA FOR DIAGNOSIS OF
KAWASAKI DISEASE*

Fever lasting 5 days or more (100%)
Bilateral conjunctivitis (85%)
Changes of lips and oral cavity (90%)
   Dry, red, fissured lips
   Strawberry tongue
   Diffuse erythema of mucous membranes
Changes of peripheral extremities (70%)
   Erythema of palms and soles
   Indurative edema of hands and feet
   Desquamation from digital tips
Polymorphous rash (primarily on trunk) (80%)
Acute nonpurulent swelling of cervical lymph node to >1.5 cm
   in diameter (70%)

*Five criteria are required for diagnosis. One of the signs listed under changes of lips and oral cavity and changes of peripheral extremities is sufficient to establish these criteria.

Modified from the Japan Mucocutaneous Lymph Node Syndrome Research Committee, 1984. Sekiguchi, M., Takao, A., Endo, M., et al: On the mucocutaneous lymph nodes syndrome or Kawasaki disease. In Yu, P. N., Goodwin, J. F. (eds.): Progress in Cardiology 13. Philadelphia, Lea & Febiger, 1985, p. 97.

those of Japanese ancestry is 17 times that of white children. The disease is not only more common in the male of very young age, but risk factors for the single most important complication of KD, coronary aneurysms, are also associated with a young age of onset and maleness.[104] The disease rarely occurs beyond the age of 11 years. The occurrence of KD in adults has been questioned: Those cases that have been reported may represent this disease or another similar disorder such as toxic shock syndrome or severe scarlet fever.

Etiology and Pathogenesis. Observations concerning the onset and epidemiology of KD suggest an infectious vector that is currently unidentified; however, secondary cases in a home are unusual.[105] Many etiologies have been suggested but none proved. Numerous immunologic abnormalities have been studied.[106] There is no simple relationship to antigens of the major histocompatibility complex in North American white children. A similar disease can be induced in mice by intraperitoneal injection of *Lactobacillus casei.*[107]

Clinical Manifestations. Clinical criteria were established by the Japanese in 1974 to aid in the diagnosis of KD. The revised criteria are listed in Table 72–8.

Fever is universal at onset. The fever is usually sustained and remittent. Temperatures to 40°C are common; even higher temperatures may occur. The febrile phase lasts from 5 to 25 days, with a mean of approximately 10 days. The young child may present with a febrile seizure, although other causes for central nervous system involvement must be carefully excluded. Extreme irritability is common.

Mucocutaneous changes are prominent in KD. Nonsuppurative conjunctival injection is usually bilateral and may persist for several weeks. Erythema of the lips with cracking, peeling, and bleeding is present in the majority of children. Pharyngeal erythema and a strawberry tongue (white changing to red) often accompany these changes and are similar to those observed in scarlet fever.

Edema and erythema of the hands, fingers, feet, and toes occur within a few days after onset. These changes are often painful, and the child may refuse to walk. During recovery, characteristic desquamation of the skin of the extremities occurs, with peeling beginning underneath the nails. This change can be extensive (Fig. 72–13) and is most commonly seen during the third week after onset and persists for 1 to 2 weeks. Desquamation and indurative edema can occur elsewhere including the perineal area. Late in the disease, Beau's lines of the fingernails can be identified.

A polymorphous rash develops in most children. Vesiculation does not occur. The rash accompanies the fever throughout the entire acute phase of the disease and then gradually fades. These cutaneous changes represent a small blood vessel vasculitis and perivasculitis of the dermis and subcutaneous tissues.

Although lymphadenopathy occurs in approximately half of the children reported from the United

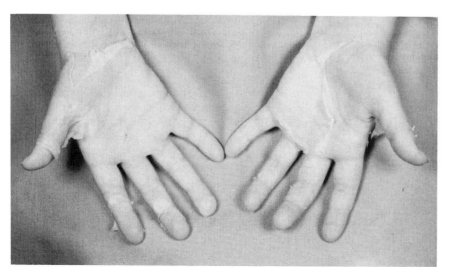

Figure 72–13. Marked desquamation of the skin of the hands during the late subacute phase of KD. Although this change is often striking, it is not accompanied by pain.

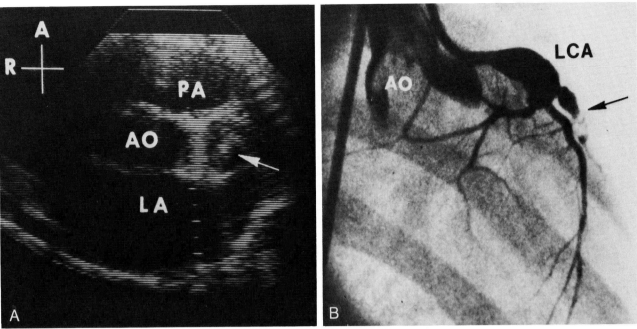

Figure 72–14. *A,* Echocardiographic demonstration of an aneurysm of the left coronary artery *(arrow). B,* Angiography of this giant aneurysm in a young boy with KD *(arrow).*

States, it is often not prominent. Involvement of the cervical nodes is most common and may be unilateral. A sentinel cervical node of 1 to 2 cm is the most suggestive physical finding. Lymphadenopathy disappears rapidly toward the end of the febrile period.

There are many other ancillary features of KD. In fact, involvement of almost any system can occur. Relatively common at presentation and during the initial course are pneumonitis, tympanitis, meningitis, photophobia and uveitis; diarrhea, meatitis, and sterile pyuria; and arthritis or arthralgia.

Relatively uncommon clinical findings are pleural effusions, abdominal colic, hydrops of the gallbladder, jaundice, tonsillar exudate, or an unusual character to the rash such as vesicles, petechiae, or pruritus. The kidneys are not involved in KD.

The most serious manifestations of KD are myocarditis and coronary vasculitis.[104, 108] It is assumed that a panmyocarditis occurs during the acute febrile phase of the disease. A variable number of children progress to develop coronary vasculitis with necrosis of vessel wall, aneurysm formation, or thrombosis. Aneurysms of the coronary arteries are often present at onset of the disease or appear as early as the second week of the illness. These aneurysms reach their peak development during the subacute period, are usually multiple, and are found in approximately 20 percent of children in the United States. In children with the risk factors for coronary aneurysms (male, age of onset less than 18 months, Japanese ancestry, and an acute toxic febrile course with early clinical myocarditis), these aneurysms are increased in frequency to more than 50 percent.[104] Aneurysms also occur in arteries other than the coronaries including the brachial, subclavian, and axillary.

Radiologic Examination. Echocardiography is the most sensitive technique for delineating the proximal coronary aneurysms (Fig. 72–14). It should be performed immediately on suspecting the diagnosis of KD in a febrile child. Angiography in selected cases may demonstrate lesions of the proximal or peripheral cardiac vessels including narrowing or infarction.

Treatment. The current approach to treatment of KD is divided into two parts: the administration of salicylate first in anti-inflammatory doses and then as an antiplatelet agent, and the use of intravenous immunoglobulin therapy.[1] High-dose salicylate therapy, e.g., 100 mg per kg per day in divided doses, is instituted during the acute phase of the illness. Larger doses than the above-mentioned may be required because of poor absorption of salicylate in children with KD. With onset of the subacute period, resolution of the fever, and the appearance of thrombocytosis, antiplatelet doses of salicylate are employed, e.g., 5 mg per kg per day of acetylsalicylic acid. This dose is continued once a day for months or even years in children at risk to have had coronary artery involvement.

High-dose intravenous immunoglobulin therapy of 400 mg per kg per day for 4 days has been employed in controlled studies and demonstrated to be efficacious in children with KD.[109] In general, this type of therapy may be most effective if started within the initial 10 days of the illness. Children often have a dramatic response to institution of intravenous immunoglobulin in terms of fever, constitutional symptoms, and general well-being. In addition, intravenous immunoglobulin reduces the frequency, size, or severity of the coronary aneurysms or improves the outcome in comparison to control groups. Such therapy is expensive, however, and additional investigations need to be performed to select those children who are most likely to respond to its use. Current studies recommend single infusions of 2000 mg per kg of immunoglobulin as a more efficient approach to treatment.[110] Glucocorticoid drugs are contraindicated in KD because of early studies in Japan showing an increase in coronary aneurysms in children treated with glucocorticoids compared with those receiving no therapy or treated with salicylate alone.

In the presence of developing, progressive, or unstable cardiac disease, close observation of the child in the hospital with cardiac monitoring is extremely important. Only by detecting the initial signs of cardiac decompensation or arrhythmia can appropriate emergency measures be taken to save the life of a severely affected child. A child who develops an infarction may be a candidate for coronary bypass surgery.

Course of Disease and Prognosis. The disease course, although monocyclic, is divided into three phases that aid in diagnosis and approach to treatment (Table 72–9).[1, 102] The acute febrile onset of the disease has already been described. The subacute period begins with return of the temperature to normal and elevation of the platelet count. It ends with a return of that count to normal. The convalescent phase follows.

Although survivorship has greatly improved among children with Kawasaki's disease,[111] almost all of the early deaths and most of the long-term disability are related to involvement of the heart. Myocardial infarction had been described historically in approximately 2.5 percent of reported cases. This event occurs most commonly in the subacute phase of the disease. The child may die from infarction, coronary thrombosis, or rupture of an aneurysm. Giant aneurysms (greater than 8 mm) are an especially serious prognostic development. The extreme thrombocytosis that is observed (greater than 550,000 to 1,000,000 per mm^3) may contribute to thrombus formation on a damaged vascular endothelium.

Late death may occur related to coronary occlusive disease, rupture of an aneurysm several years after onset, or small blood vessel disease and premature atherosclerosis. Children who have survived an initial severe coronary insult may develop extensive scar formation, arterial calcification, multiple areas of stenosis, or recanalization. Progressive myo-

cardial dysfunction may occur secondary to these changes.

A careful history for previous KD is indicated in all older children or young adolescents presenting for presport physical examinations. If a history is obtained of a febrile illness accompanied by features suggestive of KD, whether a diagnosis of KD was made or not, that examination must include specific measures of cardiac function that otherwise would not be performed (stress testing and echocardiography).

Necrotizing Vasculitis of Small Vessels

Necrotizing vasculitis affecting the smaller blood vessels including the postcapillary venules is referred to as leukocytoclastic vasculitis.[95] The necrotic vessel wall is infiltrated with polymorphonuclear leukocytes, and nuclear debris is scattered around the lesions. This form of vasculitis may be encountered as a sequela to drug hypersensitivity or in cases of infectious endocarditis or hematologic malignancy.

An isolated *cutaneous vasculitis* is occasionally seen in a child who presents with palpable purpura, painful nodules, or ridges that develop along the course of involved vessels without systemic or constitutional symptoms. The clinical course is variable and is characterized by remissions and recurrences, often over many years. Although each exacerbation may respond to glucocorticoids or occasionally even to aspirin, this disease is frequently of such long duration that it is difficult to treat the growing child with prednisone during the entire course. Alternate-day dosage may offer a more acceptable approach to the therapy of such children.

Hypocomplementemic urticarial vasculitis has also been described in children. Girls apparently are more at risk. The eruption affects principally the face, upper extremities, and trunk. The urticarial lesions last for 1 to 2 days with each exacerbation and then fade without scarring. Systemic features may accompany the cutaneous disease. The degree of hypocomplementemia parallels the severity of the illness. Some of these children warrant treatment with glucocorticoid drugs.

Cryoglobulinemia, either essential or secondary to another disease, causes an immune-complex vasculitis that can mimic other forms of vasculitis. Depending on the disease and the nature of the involvement, therapy consists of specific treatment of the underlying problem, the use of prednisone or immunosuppressive agents, or plasmapheresis.

Hypersensitivity Angiitis

In hypersensitivity angiitis, the smaller blood vessels are typically involved, including arterioles, capillaries, and venules.[1, 96] Cutaneous disease is common and consists of painful, palpable purpura or hemorrhagic infarcts. The inflammatory lesions

Table 72–9. CLINICAL PHASES OF KAWASAKI'S DISEASE

Acute febrile period of approximately 1 to 1½ weeks
Subacute phase of approximately 2 to 4 weeks characterized by thrombocytosis
Convalescent period lasting months to years during which coronary artery disease may first be noted

are at a similar stage of development in all involved vessels in the biopsy specimen, and the cellular infiltrate often contains many eosinophils. Immune complexes can be demonstrated in the circulation of many of these children and by fluorescent histopathology at the site of inflammatory changes along with polymorphonuclear leukocytes, karyorrhexis, and fibrinoid necrosis. The postcapillary venules are often the most characteristically involved.

This disease was previously more common than at present, related to the therapeutic use of heterologous antisera and the introduction of the sulfa drugs and penicillin. In addition to these medications, iodides, antithyroid agents, and indeed many other drugs have been implicated in reported cases.

Hypersensitivity angiitis is characterized by a variable course whose outcome is often determined by the presence or severity of the cardiac, pulmonary, or renal abnormalities. Prednisone is usually effective in suppressing this disorder and in preventing severe complications or death. Often the disease runs its course over approximately a 6-week period of time.

Henoch-Schönlein Purpura

Henoch-Schönlein purpura (HSP) is a form of vasculitis involving the small blood vessels that occurs rather commonly in children and young adults.[112] Diagnosis is based on the triad of arthritis, abdominal pain, and hematuria in the presence of nonthrombocytopenic purpura. The classic purpuric skin rash is generally thought to be essential for diagnosis (Fig. 72–15).

Epidemiology. HSP most commonly occurs in children after an upper respiratory tract infection or

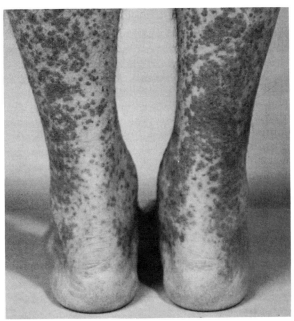

Figure 72–15. A profuse petechial and papular rash over the lower extremities of this teenage boy are typical of Henoch-Schönlein purpura.

other illness, often in the spring of the year.[113, 114] In some cases, streptococcal disease has been identified, and other reports have been related to vaccination, varicella, hepatitis B infection, insect bites, dietary allergens, carcinoma, or mycoplasmal disease.

Occasionally a familial occurrence is noted, but no definite HLA association has been demonstrated. HSP also occurs in children with heterozygous C2 complement-component deficiency.[11]

Clinical Manifestations. The clinical manifestations of HSP are directly dependent on the extent of the underlying vasculitis. The skin, gastrointestinal tract, joints, and kidneys are the primary organs affected. The central nervous system may be involved, and isolated central nervous system vasculitis has been described in a few cases.

The onset of the disease is often acute with sequential manifestations appearing over a few days to weeks. Purpura is the first sign in more than half of the children. The buttocks and lower extremities are most often affected. The trunk is usually spared. The lesions often appear in crops; some may develop central hemorrhage or ulceration, and others mimic urticaria. Individual purpuric lesions may coalesce to form larger areas of involvement interspersed with petechiae.

Subcutaneous edema is observed in one fourth of the children. It is nonpitting and commonly involves the dorsa of the hands and feet and less commonly the scalp, forehead, periorbital areas, perineum, and scrotum. Extensive edema is most common in the child under the age of 2 years.

More than 85 percent of affected children have gastrointestinal symptoms. These include colicky abdominal pain, melena, ileus, vomiting, and hematemesis. Extensive submucosal and mucosal edema, hemorrhage, perforation, or intussusception occur in less than 5 percent of children. These complications are more common in the child older than 4 years.

Arthritis is a prominent finding in approximately three fourths of the children with HSP. Although usually painful at onset, it may be less dramatic and is usually not migratory. It may be symmetric or asymmetric and involves predominantly the larger joints. The knees and ankles are most commonly affected, but wrists, elbows, and fingers may also be involved. The examination is characterized by prominent periarticular swelling and tenderness, usually without erythema or warmth. Joint effusions per se are unusual. The arthritis is transient and often resolves within a few days. It leads to no residual damage.

Evidence of glomerulitis occurs in approximately half of the children: 5 percent progressed to end-stage renal disease in early reports.[114]

Laboratory Studies. A moderate leukocytosis occurs along with normochromic anemia, which may be related to gastrointestinal blood loss. The platelet count and coagulation studies are normal. Hemolytic and C3 complement levels are normal, but the concentration of properdin and factor B may be decreased in one half of the children during the acute illness. Serum IgA and IgM concentrations are elevated in half of the patients. Split fibrin products are increased in the circulation and urine as evidence of involvement of the fibrinolytic system.

Pathology. There is a leukocytoclastic vasculitis with deposition of IgA and C3 in the lesions in all affected organs, with the skin, synovium, gastrointestinal tract, and glomeruli being most commonly involved.[115] A kidney biopsy is generally not indicated except to clarify the extent and nature of the renal disease in children who are severely affected. The degree of renal involvement may vary from mild inflammation to extensive crescentic disease. Fibrin is deposited within the lesions of the disease. Mesangial involvement is prominent at onset and is similar to that seen in Berger's nephropathy.

Diagnosis. It has been traditional to conclude that purpura is necessary for a diagnosis of HSP along with a normal platelet count; however, there are undoubtedly children who either do not develop purpura or do not have it at onset of the disease. A skin biopsy may be done for diagnosis in difficult cases.[115] It will demonstrate a leukocytoclastic vasculitis characterized by deposition of IgA and C3. HSP must be carefully differentiated from a wide variety of other illnesses, including acute poststreptococcal glomerulonephritis, rheumatic fever, SLE, septicemia, and disseminated intravascular coagulation. Other causes of an acute surgical abdomen or gastrointestinal bleeding must be considered along with intussusception or pancreatitis.

Treatment. General measures of support are critically important in the seriously ill child with HSP. In general, glucocorticoids have demonstrated usefulness only in gastrointestinal vasculitis and hemorrhage or in severe symptomatic disease. The response to the use of these drugs in such cases may be dramatic. Generally prednisone, in the range of 1 to 2 mg per kg per day in divided doses, is used for at least a week followed by a gradual reduction depending on response to therapy and the extent of the bleeding. It is not thought that prednisone otherwise modifies the disease, shortens its course, or has any direct effect on the frequency or severity of renal involvement. Clinical studies, however, have not thoroughly evaluated the efficacy of glucocorticoids administered early to children with nephritis. In the face of progressive renal disease, consideration should be given to their use and to cytotoxic agents. Antiplatelet drugs should also be considered in these cases.

Renal transplantation has been successfully performed in children with renal failure related to HSP. Unfortunately, nephritis has recurred in the allografts of some of these patients.[1]

Course of Disease and Prognosis. Most cases of HSP are self-limited and consist of a single episode of the disease. Although approximately one third of young children have a second or third exacerbation, an increasing percentage of older children will develop recurrences.

The majority of children run a course of approximately 4 weeks. The younger the child, the shorter the course and the fewer recurrences that may be expected. The majority of exacerbations occur within the initial 6-week period. Generally the disease is over by 3 months. An unusual child may experience recurrences for as long as 2 years after onset.

Prognosis is generally excellent and is dependent on the extent of the involvement and the age of the child, being better in the younger child. Morbidity and mortality are often related to involvement of the gastrointestinal tract or kidneys.[116, 117]

Allergic Granulomatosis

Allergic granulomatosis is a systemic vasculitis that occurs predominantly in young males on a background of chronic asthma and peripheral eosinophilia.[1, 96] Other manifestations of this syndrome are similar to those seen in PAN, especially in the gastrointestinal tract, central nervous system, and musculoskeletal system. Renal disease is, however, less frequent. Pulmonary disease is often the single most important manifestation with prominent radiologic changes. The histopathologic pattern is that of a necrotizing vasculitis with an eosinophilic infiltrate and extravascular necrotizing granulomata. Glucocorticoid drugs are the main approach to treatment. Prognosis is variable; death often involves cardiopulmonary failure.

Giant Cell Arteritis

Giant cell arteritis in adults is discussed in Chapter 65. Although this disease is rare in children, it has been reported.[118]

Takayasu's arteritis is a giant cell arteritis that is predominantly seen in children, especially teenaged girls, and involves the aorta, its major branches, and the pulmonary arteries. Stenosis, occlusion, dilation (Fig. 72–16), and aneurysms occur.[119–121] The disease has often been referred to as "pulseless disease" because of the obliteration of the radial pulses, or "reverse coarctation."

Granulomatous Arteritis

Wegener's granulomatosis is a classic but rare example of granulomatous arteritis in children.[122, 123] The disease has been described as early as 3 months of age. It is characterized by a necrotizing granulomatous angiitis with involvement of the sinopulmonary tract (sinuses, nasal passages, and lungs) and kidneys. In unusual cases, granulomata are also found in the skin, heart, central nervous system, gastrointestinal tract, and synovia.

Constitutional symptoms are almost always prominent. Unexplained pain, rhinorrhea, mucosal ulceration, or bleeding from the upper respiratory

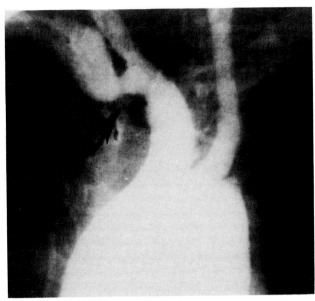

Figure 72–16. Aortic angiogram showing tortuosity and dilation of the right carotid vessels in a young girl with Takayasu's disease.

tract is characteristic. Destruction of nasal cartilage may result in a saddle nose. Hemoptysis and pleuritic pain are frequent. The pulmonary disease may progress to hemorrhage, obstruction, atelectasis, or repeated episodes of infection. Chest films demonstrate multiform pulmonary infiltrates.

More than 80 percent of the patients have renal disease, although hypertension may be less common than in other types of nephritis. The renal disease may become rapidly progressive.

The differential diagnosis in a child with suspected Wegener's granulomatosis includes other types of vasculitis, sarcoidosis, berylliosis, Löffler's syndrome, tuberculosis, syphilis, or lymphoma. Disseminated fungal disease is particularly important as a diagnostic consideration along with *Malleomyces* if the child is from a farm. Goodpasture's syndrome, lymphomatoid granulomatosis, and other rare forms of granulomatous arteritis are sometimes confused with Wegener's granulomatosis.

Biopsy of an affected organ is essential to an early diagnosis. Generally this involves the nasal mucosa or an open lung biopsy. Necrotizing granulomata with leukocytic, lymphocytic, and giant cell infiltration are seen. Overt vasculitis may not be evident.

In most cases, death from renal or pulmonary complications occurs in a matter of months, but long-term survivorship in the absence of specific therapy may be possible. Glucocorticoid treatment may be effective early in the disease, but reports confirm that immunosuppressive drugs, especially cyclophosphamide, are essential in the long-term management of these patients.[123, 124]

References

1. Cassidy, J. T., and Petty, R. E.: Textbook of Pediatric Rheumatology. New York, Churchill Livingstone, 1990.
2. Rosenberg, A. M.: Analysis of a pediatric rheumatology clinic population. J. Rheumatol. 17:827, 1990.
3. Nobrega, F. T., Ferguson, R. H., Kurland, L. T., et al.: Lupus erythematosus in Rochester, Minnesota 1950–65: A preliminary study. In Bennett, P. H., and Wood, P. H. N. (eds.): Population Studies of the Rheumatic Diseases. International Congress Series, No. 148. Amsterdam, Excerpta Medica Foundation, 1968.
4. Siegel, M., and Lee, M. L.: The epidemiology of systemic lupus erythematosus. Semin. Arthritis Rheum. 3:1, 1973.
5. Fessel, W. J.: Epidemiology of systemic lupus erythematosus. Rheum. Dis. Clin. North Am. 14:15, 1988.
6. Lehman, T. J. A., Reichlin, M., Santner, T. J., et al.: Maternal antibodies to Ro (SS-A) are associated with both early onset of disease and male sex among children with systemic lupus erythematosus. Arthritis Rheum. 32:1414, 1989.
7. Lahita, R. G., Chiorazzi, N., Gibofsky, A., et al.: Familial systemic lupus erythematosus in males. Arthritis Rheum. 26:39, 1983.
8. Deapen, D., Escalante, A., Weinrib, L., et al.: A revised estimate of twin concordance in systemic lupus erythematosus. Arthritis Rheum. 35:311, 1992.
9. Petty, R. E., Palmer, N. R., Cassidy, J. T., et al.: The association of autoimmune diseases and anti-IgA antibodies in patients with selective IgA deficiency. Clin. Exp. Immunol. 37:83, 1979.
10. Atkinson, J. P.: Complement deficiency. Predisposing factor to autoimmune syndromes. Am. J. Med. 85(Suppl. 6A):45, 1988.
11. Kaufman, D. B., Laxer, R. M., Silverman, E. D., et al.: Systemic lupus erythematosus in childhood and adolescence—the problem, epidemiology, incidence, susceptibility, genetics, and prognosis. Curr. Probl. Pediatr. 16:545, 1986.
12. Miller, M. L., Magilavy, D. B., and Warren, R. W.: The immunologic basis of lupus. Pediatr. Clin. North Am. 33:1191, 1986.
13. Meislin, A. G., and Rothfield, N. F.: Systemic lupus erythematosus in childhood. Analysis of 42 cases with comparative data on 200 adult cases followed concurrently. Pediatrics 42:37, 1968.
14. Ansell, B. M.: Perspectives in pediatric systemic lupus erythematosus. J. Rheumatol. 13:177, 1987.
15. King, K. K., Kornreich, H. K., Bernstein, B. H., et al.: The clinical spectrum of systemic lupus erythematosus in childhood. Arthritis Rheum. 20:287, 1977.
16. Yancey, C. L., Doughty, R. A., and Athreya, B. H.: Central nervous system involvement in childhood systemic lupus erythematosus. Arthritis Rheum. 24:1389, 1981.
17. Ragsdale, C. G., Petty, R. E., Cassidy, J. T., et al.: The clinical progression of apparent juvenile rheumatoid arthritis to systemic lupus erythematosus. J. Rheumatol. 7:50, 1980.
18. Delgado, E. A., Malleson, P. N., Pirie, G. E., et al.: The pulmonary manifestations of childhood onset systemic lupus erythematosus. Semin. Arthritis Rheum. 19:285, 1990.
19. Ostrov, B. E., Min, W., Eichenfield, A. H., et al.: Hypertension in children with systemic lupus erythematosus. Semin. Arthritis Rheum. 19:90, 1989.
20. Appan, S., Boey, M. L., and Lim, K. W.: Multiple thromboses in systemic lupus erythematosus. Arch. Dis. Child. 62:739, 1987.
21. Weis, L. S., Pachman, L. M., Potter, E. V., et al.: Occult lupus nephropathy: A correlated light, electron and immunofluorescent microscopic study. Histopathology 1:401, 1977.
22. Tan, E. M.: Antinuclear antibodies: Diagnostic markers and clues to the basis of systemic autoimmunity. Pediatr. Infect. Dis. 7:53, 1988.
23. Gillespie, J. P., Lindsley, C. B., Linshaw, M. A., et al.: Childhood systemic erythematosus with negative antinuclear antibody test. J. Pediatr. 98:578, 1981.
24. Ting, C. K., and Hsieh, K. H.: A long-term immunological study of childhood-onset systemic lupus erythematosus. Ann. Rheum. Dis. 51:45, 1992.
25. Ilowhite, N. T., Samuel, P., Ginzler, E., et al.: Dyslipoproteinemia in pediatric systemic lupus erythematosus. Arthritis Rheum. 31:859, 1988.
26. Churg, J.: Renal Disease. Classification and Atlas of Glomerular Diseases. New York, Igaku-Shoin, 1982.
27. Tan, E. M., Cohen, A. S., Fries, J. F., et al.: The 1982 revised criteria for the classification of systemic lupus erythematosus. Arthritis Rheum. 25:1271, 1982.
28. Malleson, P. N.: The role of the renal biopsy in childhood onset systemic lupus erythematosus: A viewpoint. Clin. Exp. Rheumatol. 7:563, 1989.
29. Krause, A., and Alarcon-Segovia, D.: Primary juvenile Sjögren's syndrome. J. Rheumatol. 15:803, 1988.
30. The Canadian Hydroxychloroquine Study Group: A randomized study of the effect of withdrawing hydroxychloroquine sulfate in systemic lupus erythematosus. N. Engl. J. Med. 324:150, 1991.
31. Barron, K. S., Person, D. A., Brewer, E. J., Jr., et al.: Pulse methylprednisolone therapy in diffuse proliferative lupus nephritis. J. Pediatr. 101:137, 1982.
32. Lehman, T. J. A., Sherry, D. D., Wagner-Weiner, L., et al.: Intermittent intravenous cyclophosphamide therapy for lupus nephritis. J. Pediatr. 114:1055, 1989.

33. Walravens, P. A., and Chase, H. P.: The prognosis of childhood systemic lupus erythematosus. Am. J. Dis. Child. 130:929, 1976.
34. Abeles, M., Urman, J. D., Weinstein, A., et al.: SLE in the younger patient: Survival studies. J. Rheumatol. 7:515, 1980.
35. Glidden, R. S., Mantzouranis, E. C., and Borel, Y.: Systemic lupus erythematosus in childhood: Clinical manifestations and improved survival in fifty-five patients. Clin. Immunol. Immunopathol. 29:196, 1983.
36. Platt, J. L., Burke, B. A., Fish, A. J., et al.: Systemic lupus erythematosus in the first two decades of life. Am. J. Kidney Dis. 2:212, 1982.
37. Lacks, S., and White, P.: Morbidity associated with childhood systemic lupus erythematosus. J. Rheumatol. 17:941, 1990.
38. Cassidy, J. T., Sullivan, D. B., Petty, R. E., et al.: Lupus nephritis and encephalopathy. Prognosis in 58 children. Arthritis Rheum. 20:315, 1977.
39. Malleson, P., Petty, R. E., Nadel, H., et al.: Functional asplenia in childhood onset systemic lupus erythematosus. J. Rheumatol. 15:1648, 1988.
40. Singsen, B. H., Fishman, L., and Hanson, V.: Antinuclear antibodies and lupus-like syndromes in children receiving anticonvulsants. Pediatrics 57:529, 1976.
41. Ramsey-Goldman, R., Hom, D., Deng, J. S., et al.: Anti-SS-A antibodies and fetal outcome in maternal systemic lupus erythematosus. Arthritis Rheum. 29:1269, 1986.
42. Gross, K. R., Petty, R. E., Lum, V. L., et al.: Maternal autoantibodies and fetal disease. Clin. Exp. Rheumatol. 7:651, 1989.
43. Fox, R. J., Jr., McCuistion, C. H., and Schoch, E. P., Jr.: Systemic lupus erythematosus. Association with previous neonatal lupus erythematosus. Arch. Dermatol. 115:340, 1979.
44. Buyon, J., Roubey, R., Swersky, S., et al.: Complete congenital heart block: Risk of occurrence and therapeutic approach to prevention. J. Rheumatol. 15:1104, 1988.
45. Taylor, P. V., Taylor, K. F., Norman, A., et al.: Prevalence of maternal Ro(SSA) and La(SSB) autoantibodies in relation to congenital heart block. Br. J. Rheumatol. 27:128, 1988.
46. Buyon, J. P., Ben-Chetrit, E., Karp, S., et al.: Acquired congenital heart block. Pattern of maternal antibody response to biochemically defined antigens of the SSA/Ro-SSB/La system in neonatal lupus. J. Clin. Invest. 84:627, 1989.
47. Singsen, B. H., Akhter, J. E., Weinstein, M. M., et al.: Congenital complete heart block and SSA antibodies: Obstetric implications. Am. J. Obstet. Gynecol. 512:655, 1985.
48. Malleson, P. N.: Controversies in juvenile dermatomyositis. J. Rheumatol. 17(Suppl. 23):1, 1990.
49. Ansell, B. M.: Juvenile dermatomyositis. J. Rheumatol. 19(Suppl. 33):60, 1992.
50. Friedman, J. M., Pachman, L. M., Maryjowski, M. L., et al.: Immunogenetic studies of juvenile dermatomyositis: HLA-DR antigen frequencies. Arthritis Rheum. 26:214, 1983.
51. Cambridge, G., Faith, A., Saunders, C, et al.: A comparative study of in vitro proliferative responses to mitogens and immunoglobulin production in patients with inflammatory muscle disease. Clin. Exp. Rheumatol. 7:27, 1989.
52. Spencer, C. H., Jordan, S. C., and Hanson, V.: Circulating immune complexes in juvenile dermatomyositis. Arthritis Rheum. 23:750, 1980.
53. Whitaker, J. N., and Engel, W. K.: Vascular deposits of immunoglobulin and complement in idiopathic inflammatory myopathy. N. Engl. J. Med. 286:333, 1972.
54. Christensen, M. L., Pachman, L. M., Schneiderman, R., et al.: Prevalence of Coxsackie B virus antibodies in patients with juvenile dermatomyositis. Arthritis Rheum. 29:1365, 1986.
55. Dietzman, D. E., Schaller, J. G., Ray, C. G., et al.: Acute myositis associated with influenza B infection. Pediatrics 57:255, 1976.
56. Sullivan, D. B., Cassidy, J. T., and Petty, R. E.: Dermatomyositis in the pediatric patient. Arthritis Rheum. 20:327, 1977.
57. Spencer-Green, G., Crowe, W. E., and Levinson, J. E.: Nailfold capillary abnormalities and clinical outcome in childhood dermatomyositis. Arthritis Rheum. 25:954, 1982.
58. Pachman, L. M., Friedman, J. M., Maryjowski-Sweeney, M. L., et al.: Immunogenetic studies of juvenile dermatomyositis. III. Study of antibody to organ-specific and nuclear antigens. Arthritis Rheum. 28:151, 1985.
59. Bowyer, S. L., Clark, R. A., Ragsdale, C. G., et al.: Juvenile dermatomyositis: Histological findings and pathogenic hypothesis for the associated skin changes. J. Rheumatol. 13:753, 1986.
60. Banker, B. Q., and Victor, M.: Dermatomyositis (systemic angiopathy) of childhood. Medicine 45:261, 1966.
61. Banker, B. Q.: Dermatomyositis of childhood. Ultrastructural alternations of muscle and intramuscular blood vessels. J. Neuropathol. Exp. Neurol. 34:46, 1975.
62. Crowe, W. E., Bove, K. E., Levinson, J. E., et al.: Clinical and pathogenetic implications of histopathology in childhood polydermatomyositis. Arthritis Rheum. 25:126, 1982.
63. Silver, R. M., and Maricq, H. R.: Childhood dermatomyositis: Serial microvascular studies. Pediatrics 83:278, 1989.

64. Bohan, A., and Peter, J. B.: Polymyositis and dermatomyositis. N. Engl. J. Med. 292:344, 1975.
65. Hanissian, A. S., Masi, A. T., Pitner, S. E., et al.: Polymyositis and dermatomyositis in children: An epidemiologic and clinical comparative analysis. J. Rheumatol. 9:390, 1982.
66. Allen, R. C., St-Cyr, C., Maddison, P. J., et al.: Overlap connective tissue syndromes. Arch. Dis. Child. 61:284, 1986.
67. Sills, E. M.: Diffuse fasciitis with eosinophilia in childhood. Johns Hopkins Med. J. 151:203, 1982.
68. Patrone, N. A., and Kredich, D. W.: Eosinophilic fasciitis in a child. Am. J. Dis. Child. 138:363, 1984.
69. Sharp, G. G., Irvin, W. S., Tan, E. M., et al.: Mixed connective tissue disease—an apparently distinct rheumatic syndrome associated with a specific antibody to an extractable nuclear antigen (ENA). Am. J. Med. 52:148, 1972.
70. Singsen, B. H., Bernstein, B. H., Kornreich, H. K., et al.: Mixed connective tissue disease in childhood. J. Pediatr. 90:893, 1977.
71. Peskett, S. A., Ansell, B. M., Fizzman, P., et al.: Mixed connective tissue disease in children. Rheumatol. Rehab. 17:245, 1978.
72. Sabina, R. L., Swain, J. L., and Holmes, E. W.: Myoadenylate deaminase deficiency. In Scriver, C. R., Beaudet, A. L., Sly, W. S., et al. (eds.): The Metabolic Basis of Inherited Disease. 6th ed. New York, McGraw-Hill, 1989, p. 1077.
73. Sullivan, D. B., Cassidy, J. T., and Petty, R. E.: Prognosis in childhood dermatomyositis. J. Pediatr. 80:555, 1972.
74. Olson, N. Y., and Lindsley, C. B.: Adjunctive use of hydroxychloroquine in childhood dermatomyositis. J. Rheumatol. 16:1545, 1989.
75. Laxer, R. M., Stein, L. D., and Petty, R. E.: Intravenous pulse methylprednisolone treatment of juvenile dermatomyositis. Arthritis Rheum. 30:328, 1987.
76. Heckmatt, J., Saunders, C., Thompson, N., et al.: Cyclosporine in juvenile dermatomyositis. Lancet 1:1063, 1989.
77. Spencer, C. H., Hanson, V., Singsen, B. H., et al.: Course of treated juvenile dermatomyositis. J. Pediatr. 105:399, 1984.
78. Miller, J. J., III, and Koehler, J. P.: Persistance of activity in dermatomyositis of childhood. Arthritis Rheum. 20:332, 1977.
79. Bowyer, S. L., Blane, C. E., Sullivan, D. B., et al.: Childhood dermatomyositis: Factors predicting functional outcome and development of dystrophic calcification. J. Pediatr. 103:882, 1983.
80. Miller, L. C., Michael, A. F., and Kim, Y.: Childhood dermatomyositis. Clinical course and long-term follow-up. Clin. Pediatr. 26:561, 1987.
81. Taieb, A., Guichard, C., Salamon, R., et al.: Prognosis in juvenile dermatopolymyositis: A cooperative retrospective study of 70 cases. Pediatr. Dermatol. 2:275, 1985.
82. Wedgwood, R. J. P., Cook, C. D., and Cohen, J.: Dermatomyositis: Report of 26 cases in children with a discussion of endocrine therapy in 13. Pediatrics 12:447, 1953.
83. Gutierrez, G., Dagnino, R., and Mintz, G.: Polymyositis/dermatomyositis and pregnancy. Arthritis Rheum. 27:291, 1984.
84. Ansell, B. M., Nasseh, G. A., and Bywaters, E. G. L.: Scleroderma in childhood. Ann. Rheum. Dis. 35:198, 1976.
85. Cassidy, J. T., Sullivan, D. B., Dabich, L., et al.: Scleroderma in children. Arthritis Rheum. 20:351, 1977.
86. Kornreich, H., Koster King, K., Bernstein, N., et al.: Scleroderma in childhood. Arthritis Rheum. 20:343, 1977.
87. Medsger, T. A., and Masi, A. T.: Epidemiology of systemic sclerosis (scleroderma). Ann. Intern. Med. 74:714, 1971.
88. Chosidow, O., Bagot, M., Vernant, J. P., et al.: Sclerodermatous chronic graft-versus-host disease. Analysis of seven cases. J. Am. Acad. Dermatol. 26:49, 1992.
89. Spencer-Green, G., Schlesinger, M., Bove, K. E., et al.: Nailfold capillary abnormalities in childhood rheumatic diseases. J. Pediatr. 102:341, 1983.
90. Fritzler, M. J., Kinsella, T. D., and Garbutt, E.: The CREST syndrome: A distinct serologic entity with anticentromere antibodies. Am. J. Med. 69:520, 1980.
91. Masi, A. T., Rodnan, G. P., Medsger, T. A., et al.: Preliminary criteria for the classification of systemic sclerosis (scleroderma). Arthritis Rheum. 23:581, 1980.
92. Medsger, T. A., Masi, A. T., Rodnan, B. P., et al.: Survival with systemic sclerosis (scleroderma): A life-table analysis of clinical and demographic factors in 358 male U.S. veteran patients. J. Chronic Dis. 26:647, 1973.
93. Jablonska, S., and Rodnan, G. P.: Localized forms of scleroderma. Clin. Rheum. Dis. 5:215, 1979.
94. Moynahan, E. J.: Penicillamine in the treatment of morphoea and keloid in children. Postgrad. Med. J. 50(Suppl. 2):39, 1974.
95. Zeek, P. M.: Periarteritis nodosa and other forms of necrotizing angiitis. N. Engl. J. Med. 248:764, 1953.
96. Hunder, G. G., Arend, W. P., Block, D. A., et al.: The American College of Rheumatology 1990 criteria for the classification of vasculitis: Introduction. Arthritis Rheum. 33:1065, 1990.
97. Reimold, E. W., Weinberg, A. G., Fink, C. W., and Battles, N. D.: Polyarteritis in children. Am. J. Dis. Child. 130:534, 1976.

98. Magilavy, D. B., Petty, R. E., Cassidy, J. T., et al.: A syndrome of childhood polyarteritis. J. Pediatr. 91:25, 1977.
99. Ettlinger, R. E., Nelson, A. M., Burke, E. C., et al.: Polyarteritis nodosa in childhood. A clinical pathologic study. Arthritis Rheum. 22:820, 1979.
100. Kawasaki, T.: Acute febrile mucocutaneous syndrome with lymphoid involvement with specific desquamation of the fingers and toes. Japan J. Allergy 16:178, 1967.
101. Melish, M. E., Hicks, R. M., and Larson, E. J.: Mucocutaneous lymph node syndrome in the United States. Am. J. Dis. Child. 130:599, 1976.
102. Wortman, D. W., and Nelson, A. M.: Kawasaki syndrome. Rheum. Dis. Clin. North Am. 16:363, 1990.
103. Cook, D. H., Antia, A., Attie, F., et al.: Results from an international survey of Kawasaki disease in 1979–82. Can. J. Cardiol. 5:389, 1989.
104. Nakano, H., Ueda, K., Saito, A., et al.: Scoring method for identifying patients with Kawasaki disease at high risk of coronary artery aneurysms. Am. J. Cardiol. 158:739, 1986.
105. Melish, M. E., and Hicks, R. V.: Kawasaki syndrome: Clinical features, pathophysiology, etiology and therapy. J. Rheumatol. 17(Suppl. 24):2, 1990.
106. Leung, D. Y. M.: Immunologic aspects of Kawasaki syndrome. J. Rheumatol. 17(Suppl. 24):15, 1990.
107. Lehman, T. J. A., Walker, S. M., Mahnovski, V., et al.: Coronary arteritis in mice following the systemic injection of group B *Lactobacillus casei* cell walls in aqueous suspension. Arthritis Rheum. 28:652, 1985.
108. Rose, V.: Kawasaki syndrome—cardiovascular manifestations. J. Rheumatol. 17(Suppl. 24):11, 1990.
109. Newburger, J. W., Takahashi, M., Burns, J. C., et al.: The treatment of Kawasaki syndrome with intravenous gammaglobulin. N. Engl. J. Med. 315:341, 1986.
110. Newburger, J. W., Takahashi, M., Beiser, A. S., et al.: A single intravenous infusion of gamma globulin as compared with four infusions in the treatment of acute Kawasaki syndrome. N. Engl. J. Med. 324:1633, 1991.
111. Nakamura, Y., Yanagawa, H., and Kawasaki, T.: Mortality among children with Kawasaki disease in Japan. N. Engl. J. Med. 326:1246, 1992.
112. Emery, H., Larter, W., Schaller, J. G.: Henoch-Schönlein vasculitis. Arthritis Rheum. 20:385, 1977.
113. Farley, T. A., Gillespie, S., Rasoulopour, M., et al.: Epidemiology of a cluster of Henoch-Schönlein purpura. Am. J. Dis. Child. 143:798, 1989.
114. Levy, M., Broyer, M., Assan, A., et al.: Anaphylactoid purpura nephritis in childhood: Natural history and immunopathology. Adv. Nephrol. 6:183, 1976.
115. Giangiacomo, J., and Tsai, C. C.: Dermal and glomerular deposition of IgA in anaphylactoid purpura. Am. J. Dis. Child. 131:981, 1977.
116. Allen, D. M., Diamond, L. K., and Howell, D. A.: Anaphylactoid purpura in children (Henoch-Schönlein syndrome): Review with a follow-up of the renal complications. Am. J. Dis. Child. 99:833, 1960.
117. Counahan, R., Winterborn, M. H., White, R. H. R., et al.: Prognosis of Henoch-Schönlein nephritis in children. Br. Med. J. 2:11, 1977.
118. Lie, J. T., Gordon, L. P., and Titus, J. L.: Juvenile temporal arteritis: Biopsy study of four cases. J.A.M.A. 234:496, 1975.
119. Hall, S., Barr, W., Lie, J. T., et al.: Takayasu arteritis. A study of 32 North American patients. Medicine 64:89, 1985.
120. Gronemeyer, P. S., and DeMello, D. E.: Takayasu's disease with aneurysm of right common iliac artery and iliocaval fistula in a young infant: Case report and review of the literature. Pediatrics 69:626, 1982.
121. Hall, S., and Nelson, A. M.: Takayasu's arteritis and juvenile rheumatoid arthritis. J. Rheumatol. 13:431, 1986.
122. Isaeva, L. A., Fedorova, A. N., Lysinka, G. A., et al.: Wegener's granulomatosis in children. Pediatriia 51:67, 1972.
123. Hall, S. L., Miller, L. C., Duggan, E., et al.: Wegener granulomatosis in pediatric patients. J. Pediatr. 106:739, 1985.
124. Moorthy, A. V., Chesney, R. W., Segar, W. E., et al.: Wegener granulomatosis in childhood: Prolonged survival following cytotoxic therapy. J. Pediatr. 91:616, 1977.
125. Fauci, A., Haynes, B., Katz, P., et al.: Wegener's granulomatosis: Prospective clinical and therapeutic experience with 85 patients for 21 years. Ann. Intern. Med. 98:76, 1983.

Section XIII

Syndromes of Impaired Immune Function

Chapter 73

Silviu Itescu
Robert J. Winchester

Rheumatologic Manifestations of HIV Infection

The principal feature of infection with the human immunodeficiency virus type 1 (HIV-1) is a progressive deterioration of the immune system primarily resulting from failure in the function of T cells of the CD4 lineage. This results in the appearance of diverse opportunistic infections, including those involving the musculoskeletal system. As might be anticipated, antecedent classic autoimmune illnesses, such as rheumatoid arthritis and systemic lupus erythematosus, are rarely found among HIV-infected individuals and when seen are reported to improve with progression of HIV infection,[1-3] emphasizing the probable importance of CD4 T cells in their immunopathogenesis. In contrast, certain other rheumatic diseases such as Reiter's syndrome, which are also considered to have an autoimmune basis, are found, frequently in more severe forms, among HIV-infected individuals, emphasizing their distinct mechanisms of immunologic drive independent from the CD4 lineage. Moreover, the occurrence of certain novel disorders emphasizes the broad spectrum of host-virus relationships that can occur in HIV infection. The rheumatologic diseases that occur in individuals infected with HIV can be placed in three categories, as follows:

1. Those arising as a direct consequence of a deficient helper arm of the immune response associated with CD4 T cell depletion; these include infectious arthritis and osteomyelitis caused by conventional and opportunistic pathogens.
2. Disorders considered to have an immunopathogenesis yet occurring with the same or enhanced intensity in individuals with selective depletion of CD4 lineage T cells; Reiter's disease, psoriatic arthritis, and various undifferentiated spondyloarthropathy syndromes are the principal examples of this category.
3. Diseases apparently occurring as a direct result of the host response to HIV infection; these include polymyositis; various vasculitides; diffuse infiltrative lymphocytosis syndrome (DILS), which superficially resembles Sjögren's disease; and syndromes associated with the production of autoantibodies.

IMMUNOLOGIC CONSEQUENCES OF HIV INFECTION

T Cell Defects

In addition to the characteristic progressive depletion of CD4-positive T cells, HIV-infected individuals develop a qualitative helper cell defect, evident as a deficient T cell proliferative response first to recall soluble antigens and then to T cell mitogens.[4] These abnormalities are accompanied by diminished production of and response to interleukin-2 (IL-2).[5, 6] These defects, which frequently precede the decline in CD4 cell numbers, lead to increased susceptibility to conventional and opportunistic infections and are most simply demonstrated clinically by cutaneous anergy to routine recall test antigens.

While CD4-positive cells are the primary targets

1249

of HIV infection, most patients develop an increase in the numbers of CD8-positive T cells early in the course of disease.[7] Functional studies in HIV-positive individuals have frequently demonstrated circulating HIV-specific MHC class I–restricted as well as class I–unrestricted CD8 cytotoxic cells,[8,9] which are particularly prominent early in the course of HIV infection and tend to diminish with disease progression. The biologic significance of these cellular host immune responses remains to be determined. As the stage of infection progresses, the CD8 T cell numbers return to normal levels or decline to levels below normal, in parallel with progressive diminution in CD4 T cells. Because of the role of CD4 T cells in inducing CD8 T cell maturation, the progressive loss of CD4-derived inductive signals, particularly IL-2, leads to a functional deficiency of CD8 cell cytotoxicity against opportunistic pathogens, such as cytomegalovirus (CMV).

The Paradox of B Cell Hyporesponsiveness and Polyclonal Activation

Involvement of the humoral (B cell) arm of the immune system is reflected by the presence of polyclonal hypergammaglobulinemia, circulating immune complexes, increased spontaneous B cell proliferation, and B cell lymphomas.[10] These features occur despite an inability to mount antigen-specific B cell responses,[11] and poor B cell responsiveness to T cell factors involved in proliferation and differentiation.[12] Peripheral blood B cells from HIV-infected individuals are polyclonally activated and spontaneously secrete high levels of immunoglobulins.[11] This may be the result of coinfection with known polyclonal B cell–activating viruses, such as Epstein-Barr virus (EBV) or CMV,[12] or the direct consequence of effects on B cells by HIV-encoded proteins,[13] or of B cell stimulation of IL-6, which is induced in monocytes by HIV infection.[14] In addition, rare circulating B cells are CD4 positive, and such cells have been shown to be capable of direct infection with HIV.[15]

Despite the B cell hyper-reactivity in HIV infection, the well-characterized autoantibodies associated with classic rheumatic syndromes are not commonly observed. Circulating immune complexes, measured by the C1q binding assay, are elevated in HIV-infected individuals at all stages of disease, reflecting, at least in part, viral-antiviral complexes. However, C3 and C4 levels are not significantly decreased,[16] and evidence of immune complex disease is not common. Rheumatoid factors are rarely detected.[10,17] Low titers of antinuclear antibodies are seen in a few patients, without being associated with analogous clinical syndromes in HIV-negative individuals.[17,18] One exception is the presence of antinuclear antibodies with a speckled pattern in a minority of patients with DILS. These individuals also demonstrate antibodies to components of SSA/Ro and SSB/La, in contrast with the majority of individuals with DILS,

who do not exhibit autoantibodies.[19] High titers of IgG anticardiolipin antibodies occur in 20 to 30 percent of HIV-infected individuals.[20] While apparently not associated with the development of thrombotic events, these antibodies have been reported to be associated with thrombocytopenia.[21] Autoantibodies against circulating lymphocytes have been reported in HIV-positive individuals at all stages of infection.[22,23] These may be lymphocytotoxic, recognizing an extracellular domain of the CD4 molecule that is distinct from the HIV-1 gp120-binding region,[24] or may be directed against the gp41 component of the HIV-1 envelope.[25] In addition to these reactivities, antibodies directed to autologous red blood cell or neutrophil antigens have been reported; however, the specificity and functional significance of such autoantibodies are not clear.[10]

IMMUNOLOGIC HOST RESPONSE AND DIAGNOSIS

Following infection with HIV-1, specific antibodies develop that are directed against the major structural products of the viral genes *gag* (p55, p24, p18), *pol* (p68, p53, p34), and *env* (gp160, gp120, gp41). The presence of these antibodies is detected by an enzyme-linked immunosorbent assay (ELISA) screen. Because this assay is limited by a relatively high frequency of false-positive results among low-risk populations, the immunoblot (Western blot) technique is used to confirm positive results. IgM antibodies against *gag* or *env* proteins usually appear within 2 weeks of the acute clinical illness associated with primary HIV infection and, by 3 months,[26] are replaced by IgG antibodies. The development of antibodies is, however, sometimes delayed for several months or more after initial infection. Antibodies to p24 are the first to appear, followed by antibodies to gp41, gp120, and gp160.[26]

Several techniques are available for the direct detection of the virus, including p24 antigen capture assays, HIV culture, and viral DNA amplification using the polymerase chain reaction (PCR). Free p24 antigenemia can usually be detected shortly after infection, becomes undetectable concomitantly with seroconversion, and becomes detectable again years later as a prelude to, or associated with, clinical symptoms of progressive infection.[27] In vitro culture of viral isolates demonstrates preferential tropism for either lymphocytes or monocytes-macrophages.[28] Among strains that are lymphotropic in vitro, there is a correlation between the ease of isolation of viral strains growing rapidly in culture and the in vivo presence of both antigenemia[28] and high viral RNA loads within host peripheral blood mononuclear cells.[29] In addition, PCR analysis has clearly demonstrated that the primary reservoir for HIV-1 is the CD4 T cell, and that whereas only 1 in 1000 to 1 in 10,000 CD4-positive cells contain viral DNA in asymptomatic HIV-infected individuals, the number of infected cells progressively increases to more than 1 in 100 CD4 T cells among those with acquired immunodeficiency syndrome (AIDS).[30, 31]

Factors Predicting Progression to AIDS

The rate of progression to AIDS increases with the duration of HIV infection, from 1 to 2 percent per year in the early years following HIV infection to as high as 10 percent per year in those infected for longer periods.[32, 33] The median duration from infection to the development of AIDS is 7 to 10 years.[34, 35] Laboratory parameters that have become most established as predictive of progression from asymptomatic status to AIDS are declining numbers of CD4 lymphocytes,[27, 36, 37] persistent p24 antigenemia,[27, 38, 39] and elevated serum β_2-microglobulin levels.[36, 40] In addition, increased rates of progression of AIDS have been reported in HIV-infected individuals with HLA-B35[41, 42] and the HLA-A1,B8,DR3 haplotype,[43, 44] suggesting the importance of host immunogenetics in influencing the response to HIV infection.

DISORDERS OCCURRING AS A DIRECT RESULT OF CD4 HELPER T CELL DYSFUNCTION

Musculoskeletal Infections, Including Septic Arthritis, Osteomyelitis, and Pyomyositis

The profound cell-mediated and humoral immunodeficiency associated with HIV-1 infection predisposes individuals to a variety of infectious complications. In addition, the various high-risk behavior patterns or underlying conditions associated with HIV infection may themselves independently predispose to infection with particular pathogens. Among HIV-infected intravenous drug users, *Staphylococcus aureus* infection accounts for more than 70 percent of cases of nongonococcal septic arthritis.[45] Pyogenic sacroiliitis occurs predominantly among intravenous drug users and is usually caused by infection with *S. aureus* or gram-negative organisms, including *Fusobacterium* and *Pseudomonas aeruginosa*.[46] There appears to be an increased incidence of septic arthritis among HIV-infected hemophiliacs compared with those uninfected,[47] with the predominant cultured organisms being *S. aureus* and *Streptococcus pneumoniae*. Staphylococcal infections causing septic bursitis,[48, 49] juxta-articular osteomyelitis,[50] extensive periarticular soft tissue involvement, and pyomyositis[51] have been encountered in patients with acquired immunodeficiency syndrome (AIDS). Organisms reported to have caused osteomyelitis in HIV-infected individuals include *Candida albicans*,[52] *Mycobacterium kansasii*,[53] and *Nocardia asteroides*.[54] Opportunistic infections of various joints, including knee, wrist, metacarpophalangeal, and interphalangeal, have

been reported. Organisms cultured have included *Sporothrix schenckii*,[55] *Cryptococcus neoformans*,[56] *Histoplasma capsulatum*,[57] and *Mycobacterium avium–intracellulare* species.[58] Other unusual pathogens cultured from septic joints include *Salmonella* species and *Campylobacter fetus*.[59]

Clinical Features and Differential Diagnosis

Staphylococcal or streptococcal septic arthritis usually presents as an acutely swollen, painful, erythematous process in one or several joints, accompanied by systemic symptoms of bacteremia. Gram's stain and culture of synovial fluid specimens are diagnostic and are frequently accompanied by positive blood cultures. The pronounced pain, exquisite localized tenderness, asymmetry, and lack of involvement of other joints help differentiate pyogenic sacroiliitis from inflammatory sacroiliitis associated with the spondyloarthropathies. Scintigraphy demonstrating unilateral involvement is more suggestive of infection, especially when found in the absence of enthesopathy and other arthritis; however, diagnostic aspiration may be required. Staphylococcal juxta-articular osteomyelitis involving the olecranon process[50] or distal clavicle[60] may present with subacute or chronic joint pain and swelling. Extensive periarticular infections, usually by *S. aureus*, can simulate dactylitis or arthritis. Acute onset of unilateral thigh pain associated with soft tissue swelling, erythema, and woody induration of the distal thigh is characteristic of pyomyositis.[45, 51, 61] In the majority of cases, the cause is a single staphylococcal abscess; however, multiple collections may occur within the quadriceps muscle. Diagnosis is facilitated by imaging techniques, including ultrasound, computed tomographic (CT), and magnetic resonance imaging (MRI) scans.

Septic arthritis caused by opportunistic organisms tends to be a more indolent and subtle process, often with minimal inflammation. In these patients, the underlying disorder may be suggested by the presence of associated extra-articular manifestations, such as necrotic, crusted skin lesions in sporotrichosis.[55] Synovial fluid aspirate often reveals low numbers of leukocytes with a relative increase in the proportion of monocytes. In addition to culture, fungal infections may be diagnosed by the demonstration of synovial fluid hyphae or positive India ink stains and molecular biologic methods.

Treatment

These individuals are in an advanced stage of HIV infection and require a comprehensive immunologic staging evaluation and most probably zidovudine therapy. Septic arthritis or bursitis is treated with broad-spectrum coverage until culture results are available. Although streptococcal and staphylococcal joint infections in HIV-positive individuals often respond as well to conventional antibiotic treatment as infections in HIV-negative intravenous drug users,[45] septic bursitis is difficult to eradicate and requires prolonged therapy.[49] Opportunistic infections are treated with appropriate antibiotic therapy, including intravenous amphotericin B for fungal infections. Surgical drainage is required for appropriate treatment of osteomyelitis and pyomyositis in HIV infection in addition to antibiotics. Osteomyelitis may require permanent antimicrobial maintenance. The duration of therapy must be given individual consideration in light of an assessment of the integrity of the residual immune function and with the knowledge that most infections in HIV-positive individuals require prolonged therapy and sometimes chronic suppressive therapy.

IMMUNE-MEDIATED ARTHRITIS OCCURRING WITH THE SAME OR INCREASED INTENSITY AND FREQUENCY IN INDIVIDUALS WITH SELECTIVE DEPLETION OF CD4 LINEAGE T CELLS

Reiter's Disease, Reactive Arthritis, and Undifferentiated Spondyloarthropathy Syndromes

Infection with HIV has served to blur further the distinctions between the various seronegative spondyloarthropathies. Although HIV-infected patients presenting with classic Reiter's syndrome are at one end of the spectrum and those with classic psoriasis and psoriatic arthritis are at the other, many develop features of an undifferentiated spondyloarthropathy with or without cutaneous manifestations. For these patients, established criteria for Reiter's syndrome or psoriatic arthritis are not proving adequate for classification. Moreover, in the setting of HIV infection, a subset of individuals with Reiter's syndrome have a more distinctively fulminant and extensive disorder simulating psoriatic arthritis with disproportionately severe enthesopathy, upper limb joint manifestations, and cutaneous involvement, which often becomes indistinguishable from pustular psoriasis.

Epidemiology

It appears that both forms of Reiter's syndrome, the sexually transmitted venereal or endemic form preceded and apparently initiated by urethritis and the epidemic or postdysenteric form following infection of the gastrointestinal tract, are seen in association with HIV infection. The frequency with which Reiter's syndrome and the related spondyloarthropathies occur in HIV-positive individuals is presently the subject of inquiry. Prevalence rates of Reiter's syndrome and related spondylopathic disorders among HIV-infected individuals ranging up to nearly 5 percent have been reported when ascertainment was performed by rheumatologists.[62, 63] In these studies, a variety of undifferentiated spondyloarthropa-

thy syndromes were observed that do not fulfill criteria for "complete" Reiter's syndrome. In contrast, the prevalence rates of Reiter's syndrome were found to be similar in both HIV-negative and HIV-positive homosexuals in two large cohort studies, although elevated in both groups to three to five per 1000,[64, 65] a 100-fold higher rate than in nonhomosexual populations. This reflects higher rates of sexually transmitted diseases among homosexuals. Discrepancies in prevalence rates among the studies could reflect methodologic differences such as ascertainment by the use of questionnaires versus detailed rheumatologic examinations, differences in diagnostic criteria employed, and variation in clinical stage of HIV infection. The central point among HIV-positive persons remains that, in contrast to the diminished frequency of rheumatoid arthritis, that of Reiter's syndrome is undiminished if not increased.

Clinical Features

The predominant finding in HIV-infected individuals with Reiter's syndrome is often relatively severe arthritis and enthesopathy, frequently accompanied by skin and nail disease. The course of the arthritis in HIV-associated Reiter's syndrome can take two general forms: an accumulative pattern evolving to full intensity over several weeks to months, or more commonly a milder intermittent pattern with recrudescences and remissions. The accumulative form is often associated with widespread polyarticular but asymmetric arthritis and is characterized by synovial thickening, erosions, and juxta-articular osteoporosis. The degree of upper extremity involvement and the accumulative pattern suggest features seen in psoriatic arthritis. The intermittent form usually has oligoarticular knee or ankle joint involvement and more closely resembles the clinical evolution of Reiter's syndrome in HIV-negative individuals.

The foot and ankle are the most commonly involved sites. Severe enthesopathy of the Achilles tendon, plantar fascia, and anterior or posterior tibial tendons may cause some patients to exhibit a characteristic broad-based "AIDS" gait, walking with the feet in inversion and extension in an attempt to diminish pain by distributing weight on the lateral margins. New bone formation at the insertion of the Achilles tendon or plantar fascia may often be seen radiographically as typical fluffy periostitis. Multidigit dactylitis frequently occurs and in combination with plantar fasciitis and extensor tenosynovitis, may simulate cellulitis or pedal edema (Fig. 73–1). Although synovitis of the knee is prominent, hip disease and shoulder-girdle involvement are uncommon. The prevalence of axial involvement appears to be significantly less common than in the HIV-negative forms of the disease, with sacroiliitis only occasionally being seen and spinal ankylosis very rarely. Synovitis at the elbow and wrist may result in early flexion contractures and fusion, whereas asymmetric distal interphalangeal (DIP) joint involve-

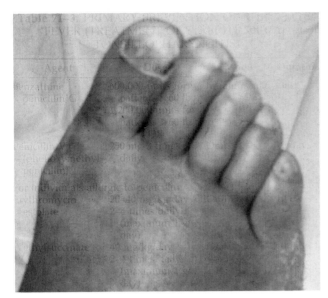

Figure 73–1. Multidigit dactylitis and extensor tenosynovitis in an HIV-infected individual simulating cellulitis or pedal edema.

ment may cause progressive hand deformities (Fig. 73–2).

The cutaneous manifestations of HIV-associated Reiter's syndrome vary considerably from individual to individual but are often very conspicuous and sustained, in contrast to HIV-negative Reiter's syndrome. The most prominent is keratoderma blennorrhagicum, a papulosquamous and pustular eruption that usually occurs on the palms and soles. In some instances (Fig. 73–3), the sole is involved with a uniform dyskeratosis. The rash may progressively spread over the body in a pattern indistinguishable from pustular psoriasis except that there is a greater tendency for involvement of the groin and intertriginous regions (inverse or sebopsoriasis). A progressive intensification of changes in the distal digits

is often prominent. Acrokeratosis is common, often associated with erythema and periungual pseudo-paronychia formation. Severe alterations in the nails of the hands and feet often accompanies DIP involvement and is manifested clinically as onychodystrophy with or without subungual hyperkeratoses and yellow discoloration of the nails (see Fig. 73–2). Milder degrees of onychodystrophy are present without DIP joint involvement. Conjunctivitis and iritis appear to be much less prominent than in HIV-negative Reiter's syndrome.

Pathogenesis

The frequency of HLA-B27 in HIV-positive white individuals with Reiter's syndrome approaches 80 percent,[59, 63, 66] the same frequency observed in conventional Reiter's syndrome.[67] More than 30 percent of cases are preceded by gastrointestinal infection with *Shigella flexneri*, *Salmonella* species, *Yersinia enterocolitica* and *Y. pseudotuberculosis*, and *Campylobacter jejuni*.[59, 66] Temporal associations of Reiter's syndrome with infection by other organisms, including *Giardia lamblia* and atypical *Mycobacteria*, have also been observed but are of unknown significance.[59] High titers of antichlamydial antibodies have been reported in 33 percent of HIV-positive individuals not necessarily afflicted with Reiter's syndrome, compared with 1.7 percent in normal subjects.[68] Of interest, we have observed that circulating antibodies against the recombinant chlamydial 57 kd heat shock protein are found in one third of HIV-positive individuals with Reiter's syndrome.

Progressive CD4 cell depletion in HIV infection may be a permissive factor for greater severity and possibly increased prevalence of Reiter's syndrome by allowing the establishment of persistent infection with, or greater invasiveness of, gut microorganisms such as *C. jejuni*,[69] or by diminishing help for B cell–

Figure 73–2. Extensive psoriasiform skin involvement of the hand, with onychodystrophy, subungual hyperkeratosis, fusiform swelling, and flexion contracture of the digits in an HIV-positive patient with Reiter's syndrome.

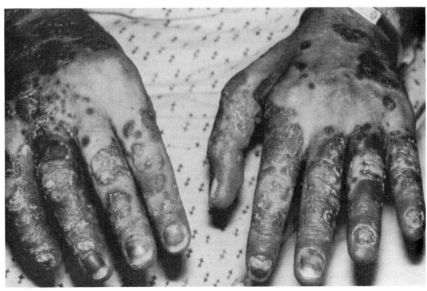

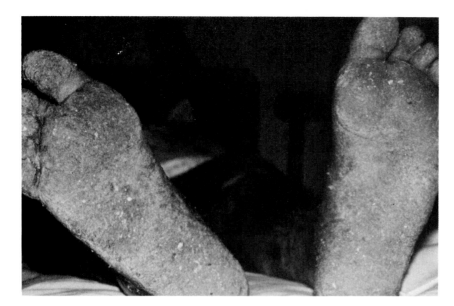

Figure 73–3. Severe keratoderma blennorrhagicum on the soles of an HIV-infected individual with lower limb arthritis and extensive psoriasiform skin lesions.

dependent bacterial clearance mechanisms, which have been shown to be important in attenuating experimental chlamydial arthritis.[70] In addition to quantitative CD4 cell depletion, infection with HIV also leads to qualitative defects reflected by diminished interleukin-2 (IL-2) production following antigenic challenge.[5] Such defects have been observed in HLA-B27 positive individuals developing Reiter's syndrome after a *Salmonella* epidemic,[71] and may contribute to selective microbial persistence and the development of Reiter's syndrome in HIV-infected individuals.

The occurrence of Reiter's syndrome in the setting of HIV-induced immunosuppression and CD4 T cell depletion suggests that the critical cells involved in disease pathogenesis may be residual components of the immune system such as CD8 T lymphocytes or cells of the monocyte lineage. Immunopathologic studies of synovium from HIV-infected patients with Reiter's syndrome demonstrate a lymphocytic infiltrate that is predominantly CD8 positive.[72] HIV has been cultured from synovial fluid,[73] abundant p24 antigen can be demonstrated in synovial tissue,[66, 72] and HIV DNA has been detected in synovial dendritic cells,[74] suggesting that the cellular infiltrate may at least in part be reactive to retroviral peptides. As the natural ligand for the CD8 structure on the surface of cytotoxic/suppressor cells is an MHC class I molecule such as HLA-B27, we have postulated that in Reiter's syndrome, cells of the CD8 lineage may be critically involved in an immune recognition event interacting with a particular antigen presented by HLA-B27 molecules on the surface of cells of the monocyte/macrophage lineage.[75, 76]

Immunophenotypic studies in patients with HIV-associated Reiter's syndrome demonstrate a higher proportion of circulating activated CD4 positive cells, expressing MHC class II molecules and IL-2 receptors, than in other HIV-infected individuals.[77]

Parallel transactivation of HIV in this inflammatory milieu[78] may act to increase HIV replication within these activated monocytes and T cells and lead to more rapid progression to AIDS. In support of this possibility is the fact that the appearance of Reiter's syndrome is an unfavorable prognostic sign, with many patients developing their first opportunistic infection within several months after the initial manifestations of Reiter's syndrome.[62]

Treatment

The management of Reiter's syndrome and undifferentiated spondyloarthropathies in HIV-infected individuals poses a difficult challenge (Fig 73–4). Joint erosions, ankylosis, and osteolysis together with chronic or recurrent enthesopathy can rapidly lead to fibrosis, deformity, and functional disability. These are frequently compounded by generalized weakness, resulting from progressive muscle loss, and cachexia. Physical and rehabilitative therapy to maintain joint range of motion, prevent contractures, and strengthen muscle function is a central component in the comprehensive care of these patients. Optimal management involves a team-oriented approach including rheumatologists, physical and occupational therapists, and mental health care experts for management of the reactive depression that frequently accompanies the severe physical disability.

Although mild cases may respond to conventional nonsteroidal anti-inflammatory agents, severe manifestations of the spondyloarthropathy syndromes in HIV infection are more effectively treated with phenylbutazone, given in 100 mg doses twice to three times daily. Monitoring of hematologic parameters is recommended during this therapy, although no untoward cytopenias have been observed. Sulfasalazine, at doses of 0.5 to 1.5 g twice daily, may be administered together with phenylbutazone

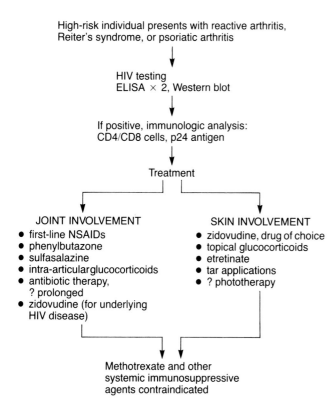

High-risk individual presents with reactive arthritis,
Reiter's syndrome, or psoriatic arthritis

↓

HIV testing
ELISA × 2, Western blot

↓

If positive, immunologic analysis:
CD4/CD8 cells, p24 antigen

↓

Treatment

JOINT INVOLVEMENT
- first-line NSAIDs
- phenylbutazone
- sulfasalazine
- intra-articular glucocorticoids
- antibiotic therapy,
  ? prolonged
- zidovudine (for underlying
  HIV disease)

SKIN INVOLVEMENT
- zidovudine, drug of choice
- topical glucocorticoids
- etretinate
- tar applications
- ? phototherapy

Methotrexate and other
systemic immunosuppressive
agents contraindicated

Figure 73–4. Management of spondyloarthropathy syndromes in HIV infection.

in severe cases. Although controlled studies have not been performed, at least one third of patients respond to this slow-acting drug. Maintenance sulfasalazine therapy is continued, while phenylbutazone is gradually withdrawn. Intra-articular glucocorticoid injection may sometimes be beneficial and has not been associated with deleterious effects, in contrast to systemic glucocorticoids, which may cause extensive candidiasis and opportunistic infections in these patients.[59, 79] Injections through skin lesions should be avoided. Methotrexate and other immunosuppressive agents, although clearly effective, are contraindicated in the treatment of these disorders in HIV infection because they have been associated with the development of opportunistic infections and Kaposi's sarcoma.[59] Prolonged and aggressive antibiotic therapy may in theory be of benefit in diminishing microbial persistence.

Although zidovudine has no documented beneficial effect on the arthritic symptoms per se, therapy with this agent should be considered in all patients with Reiter's syndrome, whether presenting at advanced stages of immunosuppression or as the initial manifestation of HIV infection, to prevent the enhanced HIV replication that may secondarily occur as a result of CD4 cell activation. Serial assessment of HIV antigenemia and T cell phenotyping for activation markers should be a guide to therapy. Zidovudine-induced myopathy may become a confounding variable in the rehabilitative management of the generalized weakness, muscle loss, and disability

associated with Reiter's syndrome and related disorders, as discussed subsequently.

Psoriasis and Psoriatic Arthritis

Epidemiology

Psoriasiform lesions, with or without arthritis, may be the first clinical manifestations of HIV infection. Alternatively in individuals with pre-existent psoriasis, infection with HIV may significantly exacerbate the psoriatic condition, including the joint manifestations. In general, psoriasiform lesions in HIV infection are of greater severity than in HIV-negative individuals and sometimes distinctive in distribution.[79] There is some divergence in studies on the prevalence of the psoriasiform disorders. Certain groups have found an increased prevalence of both psoriasiform lesions and musculoskeletal involvement plus psoriasiform skin lesions in HIV infection.[62, 63, 80, 81] These studies have suggested that the prevalence of arthritis that resembles psoriatic arthritis in HIV infection is 1 to 3 percent, compared with 0.05 to 0.14 percent in HIV-negative individuals and of psoriasiform lesions is 3 to 6 percent compared with 1 to 3 percent in the negative population. Other studies have found similar prevalence rates of psoriasiform lesions but lower rates of arthritis approximating those in the general population.[79, 82] Possible explanations for these discrepancies may be differences in categorization of patients between centers, ethnic differences, variable use of diagnostic procedures such as confirmatory skin biopsies, and the high frequency of undifferentiated spondyloarthropathy syndromes in HIV infection that do not fully meet criteria for either psoriatic arthritis or Reiter's syndrome.

Clinical Features

There is a striking temporal relationship between the onset or exacerbation of psoriasis, with or without arthritis, and the development of severe immune deficiency and opportunistic infections.[79] The cutaneous psoriasiform manifestations include lesions of psoriasis vulgaris, guttate psoriasis, keratoderma or pustular psoriasis, sebopsoriasis of the groin and axilla, and erythroderma. Among the spectrum of psoriasiform skin diseases in HIV patients, atypical features are present that are not seen in classic psoriasis, suggesting the existence of distinct disease mechanisms.[85] The spondyloarthropathy-like peripheral musculoskeletal involvement is equivalent to that described earlier in the section on Reiter's disease and oligoarthritis syndromes but also includes individuals with preponderant DIP joint disease including pencil-in-cup deformities. Enthesopathy and dactylitis, especially of the foot, are particularly prominent. Onychodystrophy is a common presenting symptom and is highly correlated with arthritis, especially in DIP joints of the hands or feet. A significant number of patients with psoriatic skin manifestations or onychodystrophy have only limited musculoskeletal findings such as dactylitis or enthesopathy and do not meet the criteria for psoriatic arthritis.[62, 63, 84]

Pathogenesis

Although psoriasis vulgaris and psoriatic arthritis in the general population are associated with increased frequencies of HLA class I alleles Cw6, B13, B17, and B38,[85, 86] no HLA associations have been detected with these disorders in HIV-infected individuals in two independent studies,[62, 79] suggesting differences in underlying pathogenesis and further arguing against a necessity for these conditions to occur at similar frequencies. In contrast, the presence of pustular psoriasis and the arthritis that may accompany it is associated with an increased frequency of HLA-B27 in both HIV-negative and HIV-positive individuals.[62, 86] It is this subgroup that most resembles Reiter's syndrome.

Infectious agents thought to trigger psoriasis in the general population include streptococci in guttate psoriasis[87] and staphylococci in pustular psoriasis.[88] Both organisms have also been implicated in psoriatic arthropathy.[89, 90] In HIV infection, the presence of psoriasis or psoriatic arthritis has been reported to be exacerbated by staphylococcal infections in almost 50 percent of individuals.[79] In addition, infusion of glucan, a component of staphylococcal and streptococcal cell walls, into patients with AIDS-related complex (ARC) or AIDS resulted in epidermal proliferation resembling keratoderma and pustular psoriasis.[91]

Biopsy of involved tissue in HIV-associated psoriasis is superficially similar to that in the idiopathic variety, demonstrating epidermal proliferation, dermal inflammatory cell infiltrate, tortuous dermal capillaries, and decreased numbers of epidermal Langerhans's cells. Similar blood vessel changes, inflammatory cell infiltrate, and proliferative tissue are also present in psoriatic synovium.[92] The depletion of epidermal Langerhans's cells, which are CD4 positive and readily infected by HIV in vivo,[93, 94] may be a permissive factor for the development of psoriatic lesions. In addition, products of the HIV proviral DNA may directly cause epidermal proliferation.[95] In this regard, mice transgenic for the HIV tat gene preferentially express the tat protein in the skin and develop epidermal hyperkeratosis and acanthosis.[96]

Treatment

The psoriatic skin and nail disease in HIV-infected individuals is difficult to manage and is refractory to conventional therapy.[79, 82] Although methotrexate and other immunosuppressive agents are contraindicated, etretinate and local applications of tar and glucocorticoids may be of some benefit. Phototherapy may be helpful but has been associated with the appearance or exacerbation of Kaposi's sarcoma.[79] Zidovudine has been reported to improve skin disease.[82, 97] Nonsteroidal anti-inflammatory agents may be of use in the treatment of psoriatic arthritis. As with Reiter's syndrome, phenylbutazone, given in 100 mg doses two to three times a day, is often efficacious. Zidovudine should be added, although less dramatic effects have been reported with respect to the treatment of arthritis.

DISORDERS OCCURRING AS A DIRECT RESULT OF THE HOST RESPONSE TO HIV INFECTION

Diffuse Infiltrative Lymphocytosis Syndrome: A Sjögren's Syndrome–Like Disease

The concept of a syndrome of keratoconjunctivitis sicca, xerostomia, and polyarthritis, originally described by Sjögren, has expanded over the past decade. The sicca syndrome has been recognized as a consequence of chronic graft-versus-host disease following bone marrow transplantation,[98] in individuals infected with human T-cell lymphotropic virus type 1 (HTLV-1),[99] and most recently in HIV infection.[100, 101] The sicca syndrome occurring in HIV infection, which has been designated *diffuse infiltrative lymphocytosis syndrome*, differs from classic Sjögren's syndrome in a number of important clinical, immunologic, and immunogenetic features (Table 73–1) and appears to reflect a specific host immune response to HIV.

Epidemiology

At presentation to a physician, most patients meet criteria for ARC, or stage 3B,[102] with fevers, lymphadenopathy, and weight loss. In a New York City series of adults with DILS, 77 percent are males, presumably reflecting the male bias among all HIV-positive individuals, and 53 percent are black. Of special interest, DILS is encountered in a bimodal age distribution, being seen in children up to age 14, frequently as the first manifestation of perinatally acquired HIV infection, and in adults ranging in age from 22 to 62 years. Risk factors for HIV infection are equally distributed between homosexuality and intravenous drug use, with heterosexual transmission accounting for 20 percent of cases.

Clinical Features

Bilateral parotid gland enlargement is present in more than 90 percent of patients, being massive in two thirds. Enlarged submandibular glands may be observed. Xerostomia occurs in 85 percent, whereas xerophthalmia and keratoconjunctivitis sicca, diagnosed by Schirmer's test or rose bengal staining of

Table 73–1. CONTRASTING FEATURES BETWEEN SJÖGREN'S SYNDROME AND DIFFUSE INFILTRATIVE LYMPHOCYTOSIS SYNDROME IN HIV INFECTION

	Sjögren's Syndrome	DILS
Glandular Manifestations	Moderate parotid enlargement Frequent xerostomia, frequent xerophthalmia	Massive parotid enlargement Frequent xerostomia, occasional xerophthalmia
Extraglandular Manifestations	Infrequent May have pulmonary, gastrointestinal, renal, and neurologic involvement	Prominent Pulmonary, gastrointestinal, renal, and neurologic involvement
Infiltrative Lymphocytic Phenotype	CD4	CD8
Autoantibodies	High frequency Rheumatoid factor ANA Anti-Ro/SS-A Anti-La/SS-B	Low frequency Rheumatoid factor ANA Anti-Ro/SS-A Anti-La/SS-B
HLA Association	B8 DR2, DR3 DR4 (rheumatoid arthritis)	DR5, DR6 (blacks) DR6 (whites)

DILS, Diffuse infiltrative lymphocytosis syndrome.

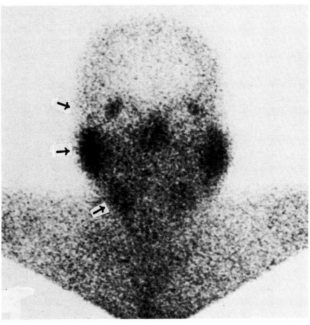

Figure 73–5. Gallium scan demonstrating increased uptake bilaterally in the lacrimal, parotid, and submandibular glands (*arrows*) in an HIV-infected individual with diffuse infiltrative lymphocytosis syndrome.

the cornea, occur less frequently, in 40 percent. Sicca symptoms are much less evident in children with DILS. Patients commonly complain of pain or discomfort in the enlarged salivary glands. The decreased glandular secretions and associated lymphoid tissue enlargement predisposes to recurrent sinus and middle ear infections, the latter of which may cause conduction deafness. Gallium scanning demonstrates bilateral isotope uptake in the parotid, submandibular, and lacrimal glands (Fig. 73–5). CT scans and MRI techniques show massive symmetric and often cystic enlargement of major salivary glands (Fig. 73–6). Definitive diagnosis rests on microscopic examination of minor salivary gland tissues, which by conventional histologic studies demonstrates focal lymphocytic infiltration indistinguishable from that of classic Sjögren's syndrome. There is a spectrum from complete preservation of glandular architecture to varying degrees of atrophic duct epithelium, canal dilatation, and interstitial fibrosis.

Extraglandular involvement is particularly prominent. The development and extent of glandular and visceral lymphocytic infiltration in DILS is loosely correlated with the absolute numbers of circulating CD8 T cells, suggesting that lymphocytic infiltration is a direct consequence of the expanded population of circulating CD8 cells in these patients. Pulmonary involvement as a result of lymphocytic interstitial pneumonitis (LIP), which occurs in more than 50 percent of patients, appears to be the most serious

complication of DILS and may be the initial manifestation of the syndrome. Affected patients may progress to frank respiratory insufficiency and end-stage lung disease. Chest radiograph reveals bilateral interstitial infiltrates, and gallium scanning often shows diffuse uptake throughout the lung fields. Diagnosis requires histologic confirmation, and pulmonary infections, particularly *Pneumocystis carinii* or *Mycobac-*

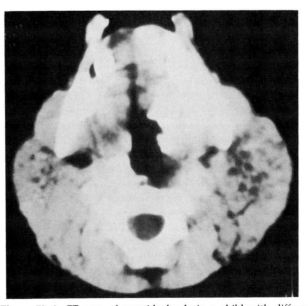

Figure 73–6. CT scan of parotid glands in a child with diffuse infiltrative lymphocytosis syndrome, demonstrating bilateral glandular enlargement with cystic changes. (Courtesy of Dr. P. Winchester.)

terium tuberculosis, must be excluded. Superimposed bacterial pneumonias can complicate LIP. Gastrointestinal manifestations include lymphocytic hepatitis, causing hepatomegaly and moderate elevations in transaminases and alkaline phosphatase, and gastric lymphocytic infiltration, causing disorders in food intake resembling a linitis plastica. Lymphocytic interstitial nephritis, without glomerular involvement, may cause aseptic progressive renal insufficiency and a type IV renal tubular acidosis. Neurologic involvement may cause lymphocytic meningitis, unilateral or bilateral VII cranial nerve palsy, and symmetric sensorimotor neuropathies. Other manifestations have included lymphocytic mastitis, uveitis, and lymphocytic thymoma.

HIV-infected individuals with DILS have a relatively low rate of progression to frank immune deficiency.[103] Opportunistic infections and disseminated fungal or viral infections are rarely seen, and few constitutional manifestations of HIV infection occur. Patients with DILS, however, appear to be at a considerably increased risk of developing high-grade B cell salivary gland lymphomas. This complication should be suspected when there is a sudden, generalized increase in the size of the parotid glands or when there is marked asymmetry. Circulating cryoglobulins or monoclonal light chains may appear with lymphomatous transformation.[104]

Pathogenesis

DILS is characterized by circulating CD8 lymphocytosis, marked reversal of the CD4/CD8T cell ratio, and predominant infiltration of salivary gland and visceral organs by CD8 T cells. Immunophenotypic analysis demonstrates that the expanded circulating and infiltrative lymphocyte population in DILS preferentially expresses the CD8+ CD29+ phenotype, characteristic of memory, effector cells.[103] These lymphocytes also express the beta$_2$ integrin molecule CD11a/CD18(LFA-1), associated with adhesion properties and cytotoxicity.[105, 106] The infiltrating lymphocytes are oligoclonal[107] and in contrast to those in the periphery, express major histocompatibility complex (MHC) class II molecules, suggesting antigen-driven activation. Whether these cells actually recognize HIV-derived peptides remains to be determined; however, the striking diminution in salivary gland size seen in some patients after treatment with zidovudine and ability to culture virus from salivary tissue[108] suggest a direct causal role for HIV infection. Predisposition to DILS is associated in blacks with HLA-DR5[101] and DRw6. DNA sequence analysis demonstrates preferential association with the DRB1.1102 subtype of HLA-DR5,[109] which is extremely rare in whites.[110, 111] This presumably accounts for the lack of association with HLA-DR5 in whites with DILS and the increased frequency of the DRB1.1301 subtype of HLA-DRw6, which shares critical beta$_1$ chain diversity regions with DRB1.1102. In contrast, there is a significantly decreased fre-

quency, in both blacks and whites with DILS, of the MHC class I allele HLA-B35, a specificity that is conversely positively associated with accelerated progression to AIDS.[41, 42] Rheumatoid factors are found in only 17 percent of individuals with DILS and antinuclear antibodies with speckled pattern in 13 percent, all at titers less than 1:640. Antibodies against SSA/Ro and SSB/La, determined by enzyme-linked immunosorbent assay (ELISA) using bovine and rabbit substrates as antigen sources,[112] are present in only 8 percent of patients.

Diagnosis

HIV infection should be considered in all high-risk individuals presenting with the sicca syndrome or in those with atypical features, such as pediatric onset, male gender, prominent extraglandular manifestations, low or absent titers of autoantibodies, and reversed circulating CD4/CD8T cell ratio. Tentative criteria that we employ for the diagnosis of DILS are (1) HIV-seropositivity documented by ELISA and Western blot analysis; (2) the presence of bilateral salivary gland enlargement or xerostomia persisting for more than 6 months; and (3) histologic confirmation of salivary or lacrimal gland lymphocytic infiltration, in the absence of granulomatous or neoplastic involvement. Typically two or more foci of at least 50 lymphocytes per 4 mm^2 of minor salivary gland tissue are seen, or grade 4 according to the criteria of Chisholm and Mason.[113]

Treatment

Figure 73–7 shows a management plan for DILS. Recurrent sinus and middle ear infections, after culture sensitivity results, are generally successfully treated with brief courses of appropriate antibiotic therapy. Therapy with zidovudine has often but not uniformly resulted in diminution of salivary gland enlargement and improvement in the associated facial pain and discomfort. Discontinuation of zidovudine may result in re-enlargement of parotid glands. Immunosuppressive therapy is reserved for progressive visceral lymphocytic infiltration. After tissue confirmation of lymphocytic interstitial pneumonitis, either by transbronchial or open lung biopsy, gallium scanning and pulmonary function studies are performed to assess the degree of pulmonary involvement. Lymphocytic infiltration of other tissues is documented by appropriate biopsy. Symptomatic and progressive visceral involvement is treated with 40 to 60 mg of prednisone daily, or other immunosuppressive agents such as chlorambucil, for 8 to 12 weeks. Before commencing this therapy, the degree of circulating HIV antigen load is assessed usually by evaluating for the presence of p24 antigenemia. Circulating p24 antigen is uncommon in DILS but if elevated would constitute a relative contraindication to immunosuppressive therapy.

Circulating T cell subsets are monitored regu-

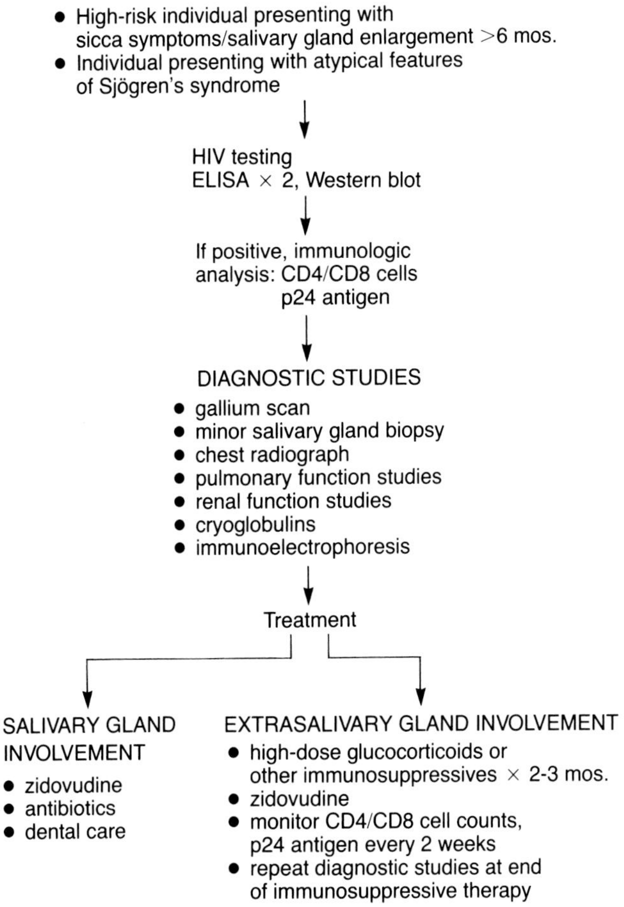

- High-risk individual presenting with sicca symptoms/salivary gland enlargement >6 mos.
- Individual presenting with atypical features of Sjögren's syndrome

↓

HIV testing
ELISA × 2, Western blot

↓

If positive, immunologic
analysis: CD4/CD8 cells
p24 antigen

↓

DIAGNOSTIC STUDIES

- gallium scan
- minor salivary gland biopsy
- chest radiograph
- pulmonary function studies
- renal function studies
- cryoglobulins
- immunoelectrophoresis

↓

Treatment

SALIVARY GLAND INVOLVEMENT

- zidovudine
- antibiotics
- dental care

EXTRASALIVARY GLAND INVOLVEMENT

- high-dose glucocorticoids or other immunosuppressives × 2-3 mos.
- zidovudine
- monitor CD4/CD8 cell counts, p24 antigen every 2 weeks
- repeat diagnostic studies at end of immunosuppressive therapy

Figure 73–7. Management of diffuse infiltrative lymphocytosis syndrome.

larly. Patients responding to the above-mentioned regimen have demonstrated progressive diminution in CD8 cell numbers and either no change or a concomitant increase in CD4 cells. Parameters of viral replication should be measured throughout therapy, such as p24 antigen assays and HIV reverse transcriptase levels, by cocultivation techniques. Evidence of enhanced viral replication ascertained by these methods in patients being treated with prednisone would be an indication for discontinuation of therapy. Complications of long-term glucocorticoid therapy are similar to those in other rheumatic diseases. Oral candidiasis may become troublesome and require antifungal troches or ketoconazole. Opportunistic infections related to immunosuppressive therapy have to date not been observed; however, the underlying lung damage caused by LIP does leave patients more susceptible to superimposed bacterial pneumonias. Treatment of salivary gland lymphomas must be aggressive, as these are high-grade tumors and are associated with poor outcome.

Myopathy

Clinical Features

HIV-infected individuals may develop a myopathy as a result of polymyositis-like inflammatory

muscle disease, zidovudine therapy, or opportunistic infections (e.g., toxoplasmosis).[114, 115–120] Most patients with HIV-associated polymyositis present with an insidious onset of proximal muscle weakness and atrophy as well as muscle pain and tenderness. Systemic features such as fever and weight loss may be present, and typical skin lesions of dermatomyositis may be seen, such as heliotropic discoloration, periungual erythema, and erythematous plaques over the wrists and knuckles. In approximately 50 percent of patients with myopathy, the myopathy is the initial manifestation of HIV infection, whereas in the remainder, myopathy develops after the occurrence of opportunistic infections. Differential diagnosis includes vasculitic syndromes, which are usually associated with neuropathies and systemic organ involvement, and pyomyositis, which is usually a discrete unilateral process. Most patients with either HIV-1–associated inflammatory myopathy or zidovudine-induced myopathy have elevations of muscle enzymes as well as similar abnormalities on electromyography (EMG). In one study, 16 percent of all HIV-infected individuals taking zidovudine for more than 6 months developed abnormally elevated muscle enzymes, although only a few became symptomatic.[115]

Diagnosis and Pathogenesis

Muscle biopsy is the procedure of choice for determining the cause of HIV-associated myopathy. In HIV-infected individuals with polymyositis, classic myopathic changes are seen, including variation in fiber size, vacuolar change, and fiber destruction. In addition, type II atrophy and nemaline rod myopathy have been described.[116, 120, 121] Most prominent, however, is the inflammatory perivascular and interstitial mononuclear cell infiltrate.[116, 117] The infiltration consists predominantly of CD8-positive lymphocytes, although CD4 positive T cells and macrophages are also present.[122] HIV antigens have been demonstrated by immunofluorescence techniques in both muscle tissue and infiltrating mononuclear cells[117, 122]; however, HIV-1 has not been cultured from muscle fibers in patients with polymyositis. The possible role of coinfection with HTLV-1, which is tropic for myocytes[122a] and may be associated clinically with a myositis,[123] remains to be determined. In contrast, muscle biopsy in zidovudine-associated myopathy demonstrates similar myopathic changes but much less of an inflammatory infiltrate.[115, 124] In addition, ragged red fibers suggestive of abnormal mitochondria are consistently observed. Electron microscopic studies confirm mitochondrial damage, with wide size variation, swelling, degeneration, and laminar bodies present in these organelles.[115, 124] These mitochondrial abnormalities may be a result of inhibition by zidovudine of gamma-DNA polymerase,[125] an enzyme required for mitochondrial DNA replication.[126]

Treatment

Therapy of zidovudine-induced myopathy requires discontinuation of the drug. In most cases, clinical improvement and decrease in creatine kinase values occur within 1 to 2 weeks. Careful reinstitution of lower dose zidovudine may then be attempted. If no improvement occurs after zidovudine withdrawal or if the affected individual was not taking the drug, muscle biopsy should be performed. Significant inflammatory infiltrates without evidence of mitochondrial changes or opportunistic pathogens indicate an immune-mediated myositis, which usually responds to glucocorticoid therapy. Although these individuals appear to tolerate 40 to 60 mg of prednisone daily, the fact that many patients with polymyositis are at advanced stages of HIV disease as well as reports of Kaposi's sarcoma developing after treatment with prednisone and methotrexate[122] emphasize the need to taper steroids to the lowest dose effective in symptomatic control and to remain vigilant for possible infectious or malignant complications. Zidovudine therapy should be initiated or continued in polymyositis because it appears to be of benefit in the diminution of myopathic symptoms.[124, 127]

Vasculitis

Epidemiology

A number of vasculitic syndromes have been reported in HIV-infected individuals.[128] Whether some or all of these are causally related to infection with HIV is not clear. Such determinations are complicated by (1) the relative infrequency of these reports; (2) the similarity in clinical manifestations between vasculitides and specific neurologic, renal, pulmonary, or cardiac manifestations of HIV infection; and (3) the high frequency of coexistent infections such as Epstein-Barr virus, cytomegalovirus, and hepatitis B, all of which have been causally related to various vasculitic syndromes.[129]

Clinical Features

The reported vasculitic syndromes in HIV infection range from involvement of small vessels in the hypersensitivity vasculitis group[130–132] to lesions of medium-sized vessels in the polyarteritis nodosa (PAN) group,[133–135] systemic granulomatous processes,[137] and primary angiitis of the central nervous system.[138, 139] Hypersensitivity vasculitis has been reported to occur either limited to the skin, presenting as palpable purpura, or in association with gut and renal involvement as part of Henoch-Schönlein purpura.[139] PAN-like forms of arteritides primarily involve muscles and nerves and cause symmetric sensorimotor neuropathies, mononeuritis multiplex, muscle pain, and digital ischemia.[128] Skin, gastrointestinal, and renal involvement are less common. EMG studies help differentiate this condition from

myopathy, demonstrating an axonal loss pattern. Churg-Strauss syndrome, characterized by purpuric skin lesions, bronchospasm, and eosinophilia, has been reported.[140] Other granulomatous processes, including lymphomatoid granulomatosis, have been reported in HIV-infected individuals, presenting chiefly with pulmonary and central nervous system disease.[136] Primary angiitis of the central nervous system may present either as a progressive loss of neurologic function or as a rapidly fulminant encephalitic illness. Diagnosis is made by angiography or tissue biopsy. Positive HIV serology or cultures in these cases may not be present in the periphery and may be limited to the cerebrospinal fluid.[138]

Pathogenesis

Biopsy of involved skin in hypersensitivity angiitis demonstrates typical small vessel leukocytoclastic vasculitis with immunoglobulin deposition within dermal capillaries. PAN-like disorders are associated with necrotizing vasculitic lesions in medium-sized vessels within muscle or epineurium. HIV p24 antigen has been reported within the vascular lesions,[141] suggesting a possible direct viral role in disease pathogenesis. In addition, p24 antigen has been detected within vascular endothelial cells in the midst of granulomatous inflammation associated with lymphomatoid granulomatosis or with primary central nervous system angiitis.[128, 136] The latter is further characterized by multinucleated giant cells within the internal elastic lamina on the surface of the cortex, brainstem, and associated leptomeninges. These findings may also be found in central nervous system angiitis associated with herpes zoster infection.[142]

Treatment

Life-threatening vasculitic complications involving the lungs, kidneys, or central nervous system require treatment with glucocorticoids or other immunosuppressive agents. Additional treatment required may include antiretroviral agents and prophylactic therapy for herpes zoster and *P. carinii* pneumonia.

References

1. Bijlsma, J. W., Derksen, R. W., Huber-Bruning, O., and Borleffs, J. C.: Does AIDS 'cure' rheumatoid arthritis? [letter]. Ann. Rheum. Dis. 47(4):350, 1988.
2. Amor, B.: Rheumatoid arthritis and AIDS. J. Rheumatol. 16:845, 1989.
3. Calabrese, L. H., Wilke, W. S., Perkins, A. D., et al.: Rheumatoid arthritis complicated by infection with the human immunodeficiency virus and the development of Sjogren's syndrome. Arthritis Rheum. 32:1453, 1989.
4. Fahey, J. L.: Immunologic aspects of human immunodeficiency virus infection and AIDS. Clin. Asp. Autoimm. 1:12, 1986.
5. Antonen, J., and Krohn, K.: Interleukin-2 production in HTLV III/LAV infection. Evidence of defective antigen-induced, but normal mitogen-induced, IL-2 production. Clin. Exp. Immunol. 65:489, 1986.
6. Prince, H. E., and John, J. K.: Abnormalities of interleukin-2 receptor expression associated with decreased antigen-induced lymphocyte

proliferation in patients with AIDS and related disorders. Clin. Exp. Immunol. 67:236, 1987.

7. Zolla-Pazner, S., Des Jarlais, D. C., Friedman, S. R., et al.: Nonrandom development of immunologic abnormalities after infection with human immunodeficiency virus: implications for immunologic classification of the disease. Proc. Natl. Acad. Sci. U.S.A. 84:5404, 1987.

8. Walker, B. D., Chakrabarti, S., Moss, B., Paradis, T. J., Flynn, T., Durno, A. G., et al.: HIV-specific cytotoxic T lymphocytes in seropositive individuals. Nature 328:345, 1987.

9. Riviere, Y., Tanneau-Salvadori, F., Regnault, A., et al.: HIV-specific cytotoxic responses of seropositive individuals: distinct type of effector cells mediate killing of targets expressing gag and env proteins. J. Virol. 63:2270, 1989.

10. Solinger, A. M., and Hess, E. V.: Induction of autoantibodies by HIV infection and their significance. Rheum. Dis. Clin. North Am. 17(1):157, 1991.

11. Lane, H. C., Masur, H., Edgar, L. C., et al.: Abnormalities of B cell activation and immunoregulation in patients with the acquired immunodeficiency syndrome. N. Engl. J. Med. 309:453, 1983.

12. Lane, H. C., and Fauci, A. S.: Immunologic abnormalities in the acquired immune deficiency syndrome. Annu. Rev. Immunol. 3:477, 1985.

13. Pahwa, S., Pahwa, R., Saxinger, C., et al.: Influence of the human T-lymphotropic virus/lymphadenopathy-associated virus and functions of human lymphocytes: Evidence of immunosuppressive effects and polyclonal B-cell activation by banded viral and lymphocyte preparations. Proc. Natl. Acad. Sci. U.S.A. 82:8198, 1985.

14. Nakajima, K., Martinez-Maza, O., Hirano, T., et al.: Induction of IL-6 (B cell stimulatory factor 2/IFN-β2) production by HIV. J. Immunol. 142:531, 1989.

15. Levy, J. A., Shimabukuro, J., McHugh, T., et al.: AIDS-associated retrovirus (ARV) can productively infect other cells besides human T helper cells. Virology 147:441, 1985.

16. Mayer-Sinta, R., Keil, L. B., and De Bari, V. A.: Autoantibodies and circulating immune complexes in subjects infected with human immunodeficiency virus. Med. Microbiol. Immunol. (Berlin) 177:189, 1988.

17. Solinger, A. M., Adams, L. E., Friedman-Kien, A. E., et al.: Acquired immune deficiency syndrome (AIDS) and autoimmunity—mutually exclusive entities? J. Clin. Immunol. 8:32, 1988.

18. Rynes, R. I.: HIV and rheumatologic autoimmune phenomena: imitator or illuminator. Clin. Exp. Rheumatol. 8:103, 1990.

19. Buyon, J. P., Itescu, S., Slade, S. G., and Winchester, R.: Antibodies to components of SSA/Ro-SSB/La in patients with diffuse infiltrative lymphocytosis syndrome (DILS) (abstr.). Arthritis Rheum. 33:533, 1990.

20. Bernard, C., Exquis, B., Reber, A., et al.: Determination of anticardiolipin and other antibodies in HIV-1–infected patients. J. AIDS 3:536, 1990.

21. Canoso, R. T., Zon, L. I., and Groopman, J. E.: Anticardiolipin antibodies associated with HTLV-III infection. Br. J. Haematol. 65:495, 1987.

22. Williams, R. C., Masur, H., and Spera, T. J.: Lymphocyte-reactive antibodies in acquired immunodeficiency syndrome. J. Clin. Immunol. 4:118, 1984.

23. Dorsett, B. H., Cronin, W., and Joachim, H. L.: Presence and prognostic significance of antilymphocyte antibodies in symptomatic and asymptomatic human immunodeficiency virus infection. Arch. Intern. Med. 150:1025, 1990.

24. Kowalski, M., Ardman, B., Basiripour, L., et al.: Antibodies to CD4 in individuals infected with human immunodeficiency virus type 1. Proc. Natl. Acad. Sci. U.S.A. 86:3346, 1989.

25. Golding, H., Robey, F. A., Gates, F. T., et al.: Identification of homologous regions in HIV-Igp41 and MHC class II beta 1 domain. I. Monoclonal antibodies against the gp41-derived peptide and patients' sera react with native HLA class II antigens, suggesting a role for autoimmunity in the pathogenesis of AIDS. J. Exp. Med. 167:914, 1988.

26. Tindall, B., Imre, A., Donovan, B., Penny, R., and Cooper, D. A.: Primary HIV infection: clinical, immunologic and serologic aspects. In Sande, M. A., and Volberding, P. A. (eds.): The Medical Management of AIDS. Philadelphia, W. B. Saunders Company, 1990, pp. 68–84.

27. De Wolf, F., Lange, J. M. A., Houweling, J. T. M., et al.: Numbers of CD4+ cells and the levels of core antigens of and antibodies to the human immunodeficiency virus as predictors of AIDS among seropositive homosexual men. J. Infect. Dis. 158:615, 1988.

28. Fenyo, E. M., Albert, J., and Asjo, B.: Replicative capacity, cytopathic effect and cell tropism of HIV. AIDS 3:S5, 1989.

29. Asjo, B., Morfeldt-Manson, L., Albert, J., et al.: Replicative capacity of human immunodeficiency virus from patients with varying severity of HIV infection. Lancet 2:660, 1986.

30. Schnittman, S. M., Psallidopoulos, M. C., Lane, H. C., et al.: The reservoir for HIV-1 in human peripheral blood is a T-cell that maintains expression of CD4. Science 245:305, 1989.

31. Schnittman, S. M., Greenhouse, J. J., Psallidopoulos, M. C., Baseler, M., Salzman, N. P., Fauci, A. S., and Lane, H. C.: Increasing viral burden in CD4+ T cells from patients with human immunodeficiency virus (HIV) infection reflects rapidly progressive immunosuppression and clinical disease. Ann. Intern. Med. 113:438, 1990.

32. Jaffee, H. W., Darrow, W. W., Echenberd, D. F., et al.: AIDS in a cohort of homosexual men. Ann. Intern. Med. 103:210, 1985.

33. Goedert, J. J., Biggar, R. J., Weiss, S. H., Eyster, M. E., Melbye, M., Wilson, S., Ginzburg, H. M., Grossman, R. J., DiGioia, R. A., Sanchez, W. C., et al.: Three-year incidence of AIDS in five cohorts of HTLV-III–infected risk group members. Science 231:992, 1986.

34. Lui, K.-J., Darrow, W. W., and Rutherford, G. W., III: A model-based estimate of the mean incubation period for AIDS in homosexual men. Science 240:1333, 1988.

35. Bacchetti, P., and Moss, A. R.: Incubation time of AIDS in San Francisco. Nature 338:251, 1989.

36. Moss, A. R., Bacchetti, P., Osmond, D., Krampf, W., Chaisson, R. E., Stites, D., Wilber, J., Allain, J. P., and Carlson, J.: Seropositivity for HIV and the development of AIDS or AIDS-related conditions: three-year follow-up of the San Francisco General Hospital cohort. Br. Med. J. 296:745, 1988.

37. Goedert, J. J., Biggar, R. J., Melbye, M., et al.: Effect of T4 count and cofactors on the incidence of AIDS in homosexual men infected with human immunodeficiency virus. J.A.M.A. 257:331, 1987.

38. Pedersen, C., Moller-Nielsen, C., Vestergaard, B. F., Gerstoft, J., Krogsgaard, K., and Nielsen, J. O.: Temporal relation of antigenaemia and loss of antibodies to core antigens to development of clinical disease in HIV infection. Br. Med. J. 295:567, 1987.

39. Allain, J.-P., Laurian, Y., Paul, D., et al.: Long-term evaluation of HIV antigen and antibodies to p24 and gp41 in patients with hemophilia. N. Engl. J. Med. 317:1141, 1987.

40. Jacobson, M. A., Abrams, D. I., Volberding, P. A., et al.: Serum β2-microglobulin decreases in patients with AIDS or ARC treated with azidothymidine. J. Infect. Dis. 159:1029, 1989.

41. Scorza Smeraldi, R., Fabio G., Lazzarin, A., Eisera, N. B., Moroni, M., and Zanussi, C.: HLA-associated susceptibility to acquired immunodeficiency syndrome in Italian patients with human-immunodeficiency-virus infection. Lancet 2:1187, 1986.

42. Itescu, S., Mathur-Wagh, U., Skovron, M. L., Brancato, L. J., Marmor, M., Zeleniuch-Jacquotte, A., Winchester, R.: HLA-B35 is associated with accelerated progression to AIDS. J. AIDS 5:37, 1992.

43. Steel, C. M., Ludlam, C. A., Beatson, D., et al.: HLA-haplotype A1 B8 DR3 as a risk factor for HIV-related disease. Lancet 1:1185, 1988.

44. Kaslow, R. A., Duquesnoy, R., VanRaden, M., et al.: A1, Cw7, B8, DR3 HLA antigen combination associated with rapid decline of T-helper lymphocytes in HIV-1 infection. Lancet 335:927, 1990.

45. Goldenberg, D. L.: Septic arthritis and other infections of rheumatologic significance. Rheum. Dis. Clin. North Am. 17(1):149, 1991.

46. Guyot, D. R., Manoli, II, A., and Kling, G. A.: Pyogenic sacroiliitis in IV drug abusers. A. J. R. 149:1209, 1987.

47. Pappo, A. S., Buchanan, G. R., and Johnson, A.: Septic arthritis in children with hemophilia. Am. J. Dis. Child. 143:1226, 1989.

48. Buskila, D., and Tenenbaum, J.: Septic bursitis in human immunodeficiency virus infection. J. Rheumatol. 16:1374, 1989.

49. Jacobson, M. A., Geller, H., and Chambers, H.: Staphylococcus aureus bacteremia and recurrent staphylococcal infection in patients with acquired immunodeficiency syndrome and AIDS-related complex. Am. J. Med. 85:172, 1988.

50. Goh, B. T., Jawad, A. S., Chapman, D., et al.: Osteomyelitis presenting as a swollen elbow in a patient with the acquired immune deficiency syndrome. Ann. Rheum. Dis. 47:695, 1988.

51. Gaut, P., Wong, P. K., and Meyer, R. D.: Pyomyositis in a patient with the acquired immunodeficiency syndrome. Arch. Intern. Med. 148:1608, 1988.

52. Boix, V., Tovar, J., and Martin-Hidalgo, A.: Candida spondylodiscitis, chronic illness due to heroin analgesia in an HIV positive person. J. Rheumatol. 17:563, 1990.

53. Crawford, E. J. P., and Baird, P. R. E.: An orthopedic presentation of AIDS: Brief report. J. Bone Joint Surg. 69B:672, 1987.

54. Masters, D. L., and Lentino, J. R.: Cervical osteomyelitis related to Nocardia asteroides. J. Infect. Dis. 149:824, 1984.

55. Lipstein-Kresch, E., Isenberg, H. D., Singer, C., Cooke, O., and Greenwald, R. A.: Disseminated Sporothrix schenkii infection with arthritis in a patient with acquired immunodeficiency syndrome. J. Rheumatol. 12:805, 1985.

56. Ricciardi, D. D., Sepkowitz, D. V., Berkowitz, L. B., Bienenstock, H., and Maslow, M.: Cryptococcal arthritis in AIDS patients. J. Rheumatol. 13:455, 1986.

57. Calabrese, L. H.: The rheumatic manifestations of infection with the human immunodeficiency virus. Semin. Arthritis Rheum. 18:225, 1989.

58. Blumenthal, D. R., Zucker, J. R., and Hawkins, C. C.: Mycobacterium avium complex–induced septic arthritis and osteomyelitis in a patient with the acquired immunodeficiency syndrome. Arthritis Rheum. 33:757, 1990.

59. Winchester, R., Bernstein, D. H., Fischer, H. D., Enlow, R., and Solomon, G.: The co-occurrence of Reiter's syndrome and acquired immunodeficiency. Ann. Intern. Med. 106:19, 1987.
60. Zimmermann, B., Erickson, A. D., and Mikolich, D. J.: Septic acromioclavicular arthritis and osteomyelitis in a patient with acquired immunodeficiency syndrome. Arthritis Rheum. 32:1175, 1989.
61. Watts, R. A., Hoffbrand, B. I., Paton, D. F., et al.: Pyomyositis associated with human immunodeficiency virus infection. Br. Med. J. 294:1524, 1987.
62. Winchester, R., Brancato, L., Itescu, S., Skovron, M. L., and Solomon, G.: Implications from the occurrence of Reiter's syndrome and related disorders in association with advanced HIV infection. Scand. J. Rheumatol. 74:89, 1988.
63. Berman, A., Espinoza, L. R., Aguillar, J. L., Rolando, T., Vasey, F. B., Germain, B. F., and Lockey, R. F.: Rheumatic manifestations of human immunodeficiency virus infection. Am. J. Med. 85:59, 1988.
64. Clark, M., Kinsolving, M, and Chernoff, D.: The prevalence of arthritis in two HIV-infected cohorts (Abstract). Arthritis Rheum. 32 (Suppl.):585, 1989.
65. Hochberg, M. C., Fox, R., Nelson, K. E., and Saah, A.: HIV infection is not associated with Reiter's syndrome: Data from the Johns Hopkins Multicenter AIDS cohort study. AIDS 4:1149, 1990.
66. Forster, S. M., Seifert, M. H., Keat, A. C., Rowe, I. F., Thomas, B. J., Taylor-Robinson, D., Pinching, A. J., and Harris, J. R.: Inflammatory joint disease and human immunodeficiency virus infection (Abstract). Br. Med. J. 296:1625, 1988.
67. Tiwari, J. L., and Terasaki, P. I.: HLA and Disease Associations. New York, Springer Verlag, 1985.
68. Gutierrez, F., Espinoza, L. R., et al.: Serologic evidence for chlamydia infection in human immunodeficiency virus–infected patients (Abstract). Revista Mexicana de Rheumatologica 5(Suppl.):62, 1990.
69. Perlman, D. M., Ampel, N. M., Schifman, R. B., Cohn, D. L., Patton, C. M., Aguirre, M. L., Wang, W-L. L., and Blaser, M. J.: Persistent Campylobacter jejuni infections in patients infected with human immunodeficiency virus (HIV). Ann. Intern. Med. 108:540, 1988.
70. Rank, R. G., Ramsey, K. H., and Hough, A. J.: Antibody-mediated modulation of arthritis induced by Chlamydia. Am. J. Pathol. 132(2):372, 1988.
71. Inman, R. D., Chiu, B., Johnson, M. E., Vas, S., and Falk, J.: HLA class I-related impairment in IL-2 production and lymphocyte response to microbial antigens in reactive arthritis. J. Immunol. 142:4256, 1989.
72. Espinoza, L., Aguilar, J., Espinoza, C., Berman, A., Gutierrez, F., Vasey, F., and Germain, B.: HIV-associated arthropathy: HIV antigen demonstration in the synovial membrane. J. Rheumatol. In press, 1990.
73. Withington, R. H., Cornes, P., Harris, J. R. W., et al.: Isolation of HIV from synovial fluid of a patient with reactive arthritis. Br. Med. J. 294:484, 1987.
74. Hughes, R. A., Macatonia, S. E., Rowe, I. F., et al.: The detection of HIV DNA in dendritic cells from the joints of patients with aseptic arthritis. Br. J. Rheumatol. 29:166, 1990.
75. Meiser, S. C., Schlossman, S. F., and Reinhertz, E. L.: Clonal analysis of human cytotoxic T lymphocytes: T4+ and T8+ effector cells recognize products of different major histocompatibility complex regions. Proc. Natl. Acad. Sci. U.S.A. 79:4395, 1982.
76. Swain, S. L.: T cell subsets and the recognition of MHC class. Immunol. Rev. 74:129, 1983.
77. Itescu, S., Dalton, J., Brancato, L. B., Skovron, M. L., Solomon, G., and Winchester, R.: Increased circulating gamma-delta cells in HIV infection and in Reiter's syndrome (Abstract). Clin. Res. 38:230A, 1990.
78. Siekevitz, M., Josephs, S. F., Dukovich, M., Peffer, N., Wong-Staal, F., and Green, W. C.: Activation of the HIV-1 LTR by the T-cell mitogens and the trans-activator protein of HTLV-1. Science 238:1575, 1987.
79. Duvic, M., Johnson, T. M., Rapini, R. P., Freeze, T., Brewton, G., and Rios, A.: Acquired immunodeficiency syndrome associated psoriasis and Reiter's syndrome. Arch. Dermatol. 123:1622, 1987.
80. Calabrese, L. H., Kelly, D. M., Myers, A., O'Connell, M., and Easley, K.: Rheumatic symptoms and human immunodeficiency virus infection: The influence of clinical and laboratory variables in a longitudinal cohort study. Arthritis Rheum. 34:257, 1991.
81. Solinger, A. M., and Hess, E. V.: HIV and arthritis. Arthritis Rheum. 17:562, 1990.
82. Kaplan, M. H., Sadick, N. S., Weider, J., and et al.: Anti-psoriatic effects of zidovudine in HIV-associated psoriasis. J. Am. Acad. Dermatol. 20:76, 1989.
83. Kaplan, M. H., Sadick, N., McNutt, S., Meltzer, M., Sarngadharan, M. G., and Pahwa, S.: Dermatologic findings and manifestations of acquired immunodeficiency syndrome (AIDS). J. Am. Acad. Dermatol. 16:485, 1987.
84. Espinoza, L. R., Berman, A., Vasey, F. B., Cahalin, C., Nelson, R., and Germain, B. F.: Psoriatic arthritis and acquired immunodeficiency syndrome. Arthritis Rheum. 31(8):1034, 1988.
85. White, S. H., Newcomer, V. D., Mickey, M. R., et al.: Disturbance of HL-A antigen frequency in psoriasis. N. Engl. J. Med. 287:740, 1972.

86. Arnett, F. C.: Psoriatic arthritis: Relationship to other spondyloarthropathies. In Gerber, L. H., and Espinoza, L. R. (eds): Psoriatic Arthritis. Orlando, Grune & Stratton, 1985, p. 95.
87. Whyte, H. J., and Baughman, R. D.: Acute guttate psoriasis and streptococcal infection. Arch. Dermatol. 89:350, 1964.
88. McFayden, T., and Lyell, A.: Coagulase positive staphylococci in pustular psoriasis: Evidence for bacteremia and good response to treatment. In Farber, E., and Cox, A. (eds.): International symposium on psoriasis. Stanford, CA, Stanford University Press, 1971, p. 79.
89. Mustakellio, K. K., and Lassus, A.: Staphylococcal alpha-antitoxin in psoriatic arthropathy. Br. J. Dermatol. 76:544, 1964.
90. Vasey, F. B., et al.: Possible involvement of group A streptococci in the pathogenesis of psoriatic arthritis. J. Rheumatol. 9:719, 1982.
91. Duvic, M., Reisman, M., Finley, V. et al.: Glucan-induced keratoderma in AIDS. Arch. Dermatol. 123:751, 1987.
92. Espinoza, L. R., et al.: Vascular changes in psoriatic synovium. Arthritis Rheum. 25:677, 1982.
93. Grelen, V., Schnitt, D., Degritter-Dambuyant, C., Nicholas, J. F., and Thivolet, J.: AIDS and Langerhans cells: CD1, CD4 and HLA class II antigen expression. J. Invest. Dermatol. 89:324A, 1987.
94. Belsito, D. V., Sanchez, M. R., Baer, R. L., Valentine, F., and Thorbecke, G. J.: Reduced Langerhans cell IA antigen and ATPase activity in patients with AIDS. N. Engl. J. Med. 310:1279, 1984.
95. Ensoli, B., Barillari, G., Salahuddin, G. Z., Gallo, J. R. C., and Wong-Staal, F.: Tat protein of HIV-1 stimulates growth of cells derived from Kaposi's sarcoma lesions of AIDS patients. Nature 345:84, 1990.
96. Vogel, J., Henrichs, S. H., Reynolds, R. K., et al.: The HIV tat gene induces dermal lesions resembling Kaposi's sarcoma in transgenic mice. Nature 335:606, 1988.
97. Ruzicka, T., Froschl, M., Hohenleutner, V., et al.: Treatment of HIV-induced retinoid-resistant psoriasis with zidovudine. Lancet 2:1469, 1987.
98. Fox, R. I., Robinson, C. A., Curd, J. G., Kozin, F., and Howell, F. V.: Sjogren's syndrome: Criteria for classification. Arthritis Rheum. 29:577, 1986.
99. Vernant, J. C., Buisson, G., Magdeleine, J., De Thore, J., Jouannelle, A., Neisson-Vernant, C., and Monplaisir, N.: T-lymphocyte alveolitis, tropical spastic paresis, and Sjogren syndrome [letter]. Lancet 1(8578):177, 1988.
100. Couderc, L. J., D'Agay, M. F., Danon, F., Harzic, M., Brocheriou, C., and Clauvel, J. P.: Sicca complex and infection with human immunodeficiency virus. Arch. Intern. Med. 147:898, 1987.
101. Itescu, S., Brancato, L. J., and Winchester, R.: A sicca syndrome in HIV infection: Association with HLA-DR5 and CD8 lymphocytosis. Lancet (2):466, 1989.
102. Haverkos, H. W., Gotlieb, M. S., Killen, J. Y., et al.: Classification of HTLV-III/LAV-related diseases. J. Infect. Dis. 152:1095, 1985.
103. Itescu, S., Brancato, L. J., Buxbaum, J., Gregersen, P. K., Rizk, C. C., Croxson, S., Solomon, G., and Winchester, R.: A diffuse infiltrative CD8 lymphocytosis syndrome in human immunodeficiency virus (HIV) infection: A host immune response associated with HLA-DR5. Ann. Intern. Med. 112:3, 1990.
104. Itescu, S.: Diffuse infiltrative lymphocytosis syndrome in human immunodeficiency virus infection—a Sjogren's-like disease. Rheum. Dis. Clin. North Am. 17:99, 1991.
105. Springer, T. A., Dustin, M. L., Kishimoto, T. K., and Marlin, S. D.: The lymphocyte function-associated LFA-1, CD2, and LFA-3 molecules: Cell adhesion receptors of the immune system. Annu. Rev. Immunol. 5:223, 1987.
106. Martz, E.: LFA-1 and other accessory molecules functioning in adhesions of T and B lymphocytes. Hum. Immunol. 18:3, 1986.
107. Dwyer, E., Itescu, S., and Winchester, R.: Selective αβ T cell receptor usage in diffuse infiltrative lymphocytosis syndrome. (Abstract) Clin. Res. 39(2):255A, 1991.
108. Lecatsas, A., Houff, S., Macher, A., et al.: Retrovirus-like particles in salivary glands, prostate and testes of AIDS patients. Proc. Soc. Exp. Biol. Med. 178:653, 1985.
109. Itescu, S., Brancato, L. J., Dwyer, E., Gregersen, P. K., and Winchester, R.: Susceptibility to HIV-associated Sjogren's syndrome requires interaction of MHC class I and II gene products (Abstract). Arthritis Rheum. 33:9(Suppl.):S79, 1990.
110. Johnson, A. H., Rosen-Bronson, S., and Hurley, C. K.: Heterogeneity of the HLA-D region in American Blacks. Transplant. Proc. 21:3872, 1989.
111. Fernandez-Vina, M., Shumway, J. W., and Stastny, P.: DNA typing for class II HLA antigens with allele-specific or group specific amplification. II. Typing for alleles of the DRw52-associated group. Hum. Immunol. 28:51, 1990.
112. Buyon, J. P., Ben-Chetrit, E., Karp, S., Roubey, R. A. S., Pompeo, L., Reeves, W. H., Tan, E. M., and Winchester, R.: Acquired congenital heart block. J. Clin. Invest. 84:627, 1989.
113. Chisholm, D. M., and Mason, D. K.: Labial salivary gland biopsy in Sjogren's disease. J. Clin. Pathol. 21:656, 1968.
114. Snider, W. D., Simpson, D. M., Nielsen, S., Gold, J. W., Metroka, C.

E., and Posner, J. B.: Neurological complications of acquired immunodeficiency virus: Analysis of 50 patients. Ann. Neurol. 14:403, 1983.
115. Till, M., and MacDonell, K. B.: Myopathy with HIV-1 infection: HIV-1 or zidovudine? Ann. Intern. Med. 113:492, 1990.
116. Simpson, D. M., and Bender, A. N.: Human immunodeficiency virus–associated myopathy: Analysis of 11 patients. Ann. Neurol. 24:79, 1988.
117. Dalakas, M. C., Pezeshkpour, G. H., Gravell, M., and Sever, J. L.: Polymyositis associated with AIDS retrovirus. J.A.M.A. 256:2381, 1986.
118. Dalakas, M. C., and Pezeshkpour, G. H.: Neuromuscular diseases associated with human immunodeficiency virus infection. Ann. Neurol. 23(Suppl.):S38, 1988.
119. Baguley, E., Wolfe, C., and Hughes, G. R.: Dermatomyositis in HIV infection. Br. J. Rheumatol. 27:493, 1988.
120. Panegyres, P. K., Tan, N., Kakulas, B. A., Armstrong, J. A., and Hollingsworth, P.: Necrotising myopathy and zidovudine. Lancet 1:1050, 1988.
121. Dalakas, M. C., Pezeshkpour, G. H., and Flaherty, M.: Progressive nemaline (rod) myopathy associated with HIV infection. N. Engl. J. Med. 317:1602, 1987.
122. Espinoza, L. R., Aguilar, J. L., Espinoza, C. G., Gresh, J., Jara, J., Silveira, L. H., Martinez-Osuna, P., and Seleznick, M.: Characteristics and pathogenesis of myositis in human immunodeficiency virus infection—distinction from azidothymidine-induced myopathy. Rheum. Dis. Clin. North Am. 17(1):117, 1991.
122a. Wiley, C. A., Nerenberg, M., Cros, D., and Soto-Aguilar, M. C.: HTLV-I polymyositis in a patient also infected with the human immunodeficiency virus. N. Engl. J. Med. 320:992, 1989.
123. Mora, C. A., Garruto, R. M., Brown, P., et al.: Seroprevalence of antibodies to HTLV-1 in patients with chronic neurological disorders other than tropical spastic paraparesis. Ann. Neurol. 23(Suppl.):S192, 1988.
124. Dalakas, M. C., Illa, I., Pezeshkpour, G. H., et al.: Mitochondrial myopathy caused by long-term zidovudine therapy. N. Engl. J. Med. 322:1098, 1990.
125. Mitsuya, H., and Broder, S.: Inhibition of the in vitro infectivity and cytopathic effect of human T-lymphotrophic virus type III/lymphadenopathy-associated virus (HTLV-III/LAV) by 2′,3′-dideoxynucleosides. Proc. Natl. Acad. Sci. U.S.A. 83:1911, 1986.
126. Zimmerman, W., Cher, S. M., Bolden, A., and Weissbach, A.: Mitochondrial DNA replication does not involve DNA polymerase-alpha. J. Biol. Chem. 255:11847, 1980.
127. Simpson, D. M.: Myopathy associated with human immunodeficiency virus (HIV) but not with zidovudine. Ann. Intern. Med. 109:842, 1988.
128. Calabrese, L. H.: Vasculitis and infection with the human immunodeficiency virus. Rheum. Dis. Clin. North Am. 17(1):131, 1991.

129. Sergent, J.: Vasculitis associated with viral infection. Clin. Rheum. Dis. 6:339, 1980.
130. Chren, M. M., Silverman, R. A., Sorsensen, R. U., et al.: Leukocytoclastic vasculitis in a patient infected with human immunodeficiency virus. J. Am. Acad. Dermatol. 21:1161a, 1989.
131. Farthing, C. F., Staughton, R. C. D., and Rowland Payne, C. M. E.: Skin disease in homosexual patients with acquired immune deficiency syndrome (AIDS) and lesser forms of human T cell leukaemia virus (HTLV-III) disease. Clin. Exp. Dermatol. 10:3, 1985.
132. Potashner, W., Buskila, D., Patterson, B., Karasik, A., and Keystone, E. C.: Leukocytoclastic vasculitis in association with human immunodeficiency virus infection [Letter]. J. Rheumatol. 17(8):1104, 1990.
133. Gherardi, R., Lebargy, F., Gaulard, P., et al.: Necrotizing vasculitis and HIV replication in peripheral nerves (Letter). N. Engl. J. Med. 31:685, 1989.
134. Said, G., Lacroix-Ciaudo, C., Fugimura, H., et al.: The peripheral neuropathy of necrotizing arteritis: A clinicopathological study. Ann. Neurol. 23:461, 1988.
135. Valeriano, J., Lolita, B., and Kerry, L. D.: HIV-associated polyarteritis nodosa (PAN) diagnosed by rectal biopsy; a case report (Abstract). Arthritis Rheum. 32(Suppl.):S44, 1989.
136. Anders, K. H., Latta, H., Chang, B. S., et al.: Lymphoid granulomatosis and malignant lymphoma of the central nervous system in acquired immunodeficiency syndrome. Hum. Pathol. 20:326, 1989.
137. Scaravalli, F., Daniel, S. E., Harcourt-Webster, N., et al.: Chronic basal meningitis and vasculitis in acquired immunodeficiency syndrome. Arch. Pathol. Lab. Med. 113:192, 1989.
138. Yanker, B. A., Skolnik, P. R., Shoukimas, G. M., et al.: Cerebral granulomatous angiitis associated with isolation of human T-lymphotrophic virus III from the central nervous system. Ann. Neurol. 20:362, 1986.
139. Thompson, I., Cooper, D., Savdie, E., et al.: Henoch-Schoenlein purpura and IgA glomerulonephritis associated with HIV infection (Abstract). Abstracts of the V International Conference on AIDS: The scientific and social challenge. Quebec MBP278, 1989.
140. Cooper, L. M., and Patterson, J. A. K.: Allergic granulomatosis and angiitis of Churg-Strauss: Case report in a patient with antibodies to human immunodeficiency virus and hepatitis B virus. Int. J. Dermatol. 28:597, 1989.
141. Bardin, T., Kuntz, D., Gavdoven, C., et al.: Necrotizing vasculitis in human immunodeficiency virus (HIV) infection (Abstract). Arthritis Rheum. 30:S105, 1987.
142. Eidelberg, D., Sotrel, A., Horoupian, D. S., et al.: Thrombotic cerebral vasculopathy associated with herpes zoster. Ann. Neurol. 19:7, 1986.

Specific Immunodeficiency Diseases, Excluding AIDS

INTRODUCTION

Since the first example of a human host deficit was described four decades ago,[1] nearly 50 genetically determined immunodeficiency syndromes have been reported in the world's literature.[2] These defects involve one or more components of the immune system, including T, B, and NK lymphocytes; phagocytic cells; and complement proteins. This chapter covers only those non–acquired immunodeficiency syndrome (AIDS) immunodeficiency disorders known to involve lymphocytes. Complement deficiency states are reviewed in Chapter 75, phagocytic cell defects are discussed in Chapter 11, and AIDS is discussed comprehensively in Chapter 73.

Immunodeficiency diseases are characterized by undue susceptibility to infection. Identification of pathogens by culture is of crucial importance in assessment of such defects because knowledge of the causative infectious agents and the body sites affected can provide important clues as to the most likely host deficit. It is important to keep in mind that patients with antibody, phagocytic cell, or complement deficiencies have problems with recurrent infections with high-grade encapsulated bacterial pathogens. Thus, the patient with repeated viral infections is not as likely to have disorders of these components. In contrast, patients with deficiencies in T cell function usually manifest opportunistic infections with viral and fungal agents and often have persistent or intractable diarrhea. They begin to fail to thrive shortly after these problems develop. Infants with AIDS may present in a similar manner but have generalized lymphadenopathy, or hepatosplenomegaly, or both, which are unusual in genetic defects of immunity.

Paradoxically, many immunodeficiency syndromes are also characterized by excessive production of immunoglobulin E (IgE) antibodies[3] or of autoantibodies.[4] Because of the availability of effective means of controlling bacterial infections, often allergic or autoimmune diseases are significant causes of morbidity among this patient population. Finally, there is an increased incidence of malignancy in patients with immunodeficiency diseases.[5] Whether the latter is due to increased susceptibility to infection with agents predisposing to malignancy or to defective tumor immunosurveillance is unknown.

With the exception of selective IgA deficiency, genetically determined immunodeficiency is rare.[2] B cell defects far outnumber those affecting T cells, phagocytic cells, or complement proteins. Although general population statistics are not available in the United States, it has been estimated that agammaglobulinemia occurs with a frequency of one in 50,000 and severe combined immunodeficiency with a frequency of one in 100,000 to one in 500,000 live births. Selective absence of serum and secretory IgA is the most common defect, with reported incidences ranging from one in 333 to one in 700.[6, 7] Primary immunodeficiency is seen more often in infants and children (60 per cent) than in adults (40 per cent). During childhood, there is a 5:1 male to female sex predominance for these disorders. This later reverses so there is a slight predominance (1:1.4) in females in adulthood.

EVALUATION OF PATIENT WITH RECURRENT INFECTION

Despite an exponential rise in the number of patients with human immunodeficiency virus (HIV) infections over the past decade, the number of individuals suspected of having either acquired or genetically determined immunodeficiency will far exceed the true incidence of these diseases. For this reason, it is essential that the clinical and laboratory tests selected for immunologic assessment be broadly informative, reliable, and cost-effective. Most of these disorders can be ruled out at little cost to the patient if the proper choice of screening tests is made (Table 74–1). The complete blood count and sedimentation rate are among the most cost-effective screening tests. If the sedimentation rate is normal, chronic bacterial infection is unlikely. If the absolute neutrophil count is normal, congenital and acquired neutropenias and severe chemotactic defects are eliminated. If the absolute lymphocyte count is normal, the patient is not likely to have a severe T cell defect. It is important to remember, however, that infant lymphocyte counts are normally very high. For example, at 9 months of age—an age when infants affected with severe T cell immunodeficiency are likely to present—the lower limit of normal is 4500

Table 74–1. INITIAL EVALUATION OF PATIENT WITH SUSPECTED IMMUNODEFICIENCY

Suspected Deficiency	Tests
All immunodeficiency	Complete and differential blood counts, platelet count, examination of red cells for Howell-Jolly bodies, erythrocyte sedimentation rate
Antibody deficiency	Immunoglobulin quantification (particularly IgA), isoagglutinin titers (anti-A, anti-B), diphtheria and tetanus antibody titers, pneumococcal antibody titers, *Haemophilus influenzae* antibody titers. If titers abnormal, repeat after immunizations
T cell deficiency	Absolute lymphocyte count, intradermal skin test to *Candida albicans* 1:1000 or 1:100
Phagocytic cell deficiency	Absolute neutrophil count, nitroblue tetrazolium test
Complement deficiency	CH50

lymphocytes per mm³.[8, 9] Examination of red cells for Howell-Jolly bodies will help exclude congenital asplenia. If the platelet count is normal, Wiskott-Aldrich syndrome is excluded.

Beyond this, it is well to keep in mind that tests that measure immune function are far more informative and cost-effective than those measuring milligrams of immunoglobulins or characterizing and enumerating lymphocyte subpopulations with monoclonal antibodies. Taking the B cell system first, a simple screening test is to determine the presence and titer of antibodies to type A and B red blood cells, i.e., isohemagglutinins (see Table 74–1). As assayed in most blood banks, this test measures predominantly IgM antibodies. Because most infants, children, and adults have received DPT immunizations, measurement of antibodies to diphtheria or tetanus toxoids before and 2 weeks after a pediatric or an adult D-T booster is helpful in assessing the capacity to form IgG antibodies to protein antigens. To evaluate the ability to respond to polysaccharide antigens, antipneumococcal antibodies can be measured before and 3 weeks after immunization with Pneumovax, and baseline anti–*Haemophilus influenzae* titers can be obtained. As a rule, patients with B cell defects for which intravenous immunoglobulin (IVIG) replacement therapy is indicated do not have either IgM or IgG antibodies in their sera.[10] The finding of normal IgM and IgG antibodies, however, does not exclude selective IgA deficiency, transient hypogammaglobulinemia of infancy, or protein-losing states. Those patients usually make both IgM and IgG antibodies normally; thus, IVIG therapy is not indicated in those conditions.[10, 11] IgA deficiency would be missed on serum electrophoresis because that test does not quantify individual immunoglobulin isotypes. Immunoelectrophoresis is also not quantitative and, for that reason, not useful in evaluating immunocompetence. IgA deficiency, how-

ever, can be excluded by measuring serum IgA. This is one of the most cost-effective immunologic tests; if the IgA concentration is normal, this also rules out all of the permanent types of agammaglobulinemia, since IgA is usually very low or absent in those conditions as well. If IgA is low, IgG and IgM should also be quantified. It is extremely important to remember, however, that serum concentrations of IgG and IgA in infants and children are both normally lower than in adults until 6 to 7 years of age. Therefore, any values obtained (other than extremely low ones) that are below published normal ranges should be investigated further in a laboratory that has its own age-appropriate normal values before beginning IVIG therapy. Very high serum concentrations of one or more immunoglobulin classes suggest HIV infection or chronic granulomatous disease.

The most cost-effective test for assessing T cell function is the *Candida* skin test (see Table 74–1). Adults and children older than 6 years should be tested intradermally with 0.1 ml of a 1:1000 dilution of a known potent *Candida albicans* extract. If the test is negative at 24, 48, and 72 hours, a 1:100 dilution should be tested. This dilution is, in fact, a useful starting one for infants and young children. Seventy-five per cent of normal infants react to the 1:100 strength of *Candida* by 9 months of age. If the test is positive, as defined by erythema and induration of 10 mm or more at 48 hours, virtually all primary T cell defects are excluded, and this will obviate the need for more expensive in vitro tests.

Killing defects of phagocytic cells, which should be suspected if the patient has problems with recurrent staphylococcal, gram-negative bacterial, or fungal infections, can be screened for by a nitroblue tetrazolium dye test (see Table 74–1). Complement defects can be screened for most cost effectively by a CH50 assay, which measures the intactness of the entire complement pathway. This test is a time-dependent and temperature-dependent bioassay, however; thus, the specimen should be delivered to the laboratory immediately or the serum frozen immediately and shipped on dry ice to ensure that the result is not artifactually low.

If these screening tests are abnormal or even if they are normal and clinical features of the patient still strongly suggest a host defect, the patient should be evaluated at a center where more definitive immunologic studies can be done before any type of immunologic treatment is begun. Some "abnormalities" may be laboratory artifacts, and conversely, what may appear to be a straightforward diagnosis may prove to be a more complex underlying problem.

Patients found to have abnormalities on any of the screening tests should be characterized as fully as possible. B cells, T cells, T cell subpopulations, NK cells, and monocytes can be enumerated by reacting them with monoclonal antibodies to unique cell surface antigens and analyzing them on a fluorescence-activated cell sorter. This type of test is particularly useful in screening for leukocyte adhesion deficiency (LAD).

There is currently a tendency among many primary care physicians to measure IgG subclasses as part of the routine evaluation of the patient with recurrent infections. Patients who are deficient in IgG2 are often unable to make antibodies to polysaccharide antigens; however, this can be true even when the IgG2 concentration is normal. Conversely, patients who are receiving steroid therapy often have low IgG concentrations but make antibodies normally. Thus, antibody measurements are far more cost-effective than IgG subclass determinations. The capacity of blood B lymphocytes to differentiate into plasma cells that synthesize and secrete immunoglobulin can be assessed in in vitro cultures to which pokeweed mitogen is added as a differentiating agent. If all of these tests prove to be normal and the immunoglobulins are still low, trace label studies of serum proteins should be carried out to make certain that the immunoglobulins are not being lost, such as in the nephrotic syndrome, protein-losing enteropathy, or intestinal lymphangiectasia. Measurement of IgA in secretions can prove useful in excluding the extremely rare situation in which serum IgA is normal and secretory IgA is missing owing to a lack of secretory piece.

For the T cell system, the capacity of blood T cells to proliferate in response to the mitogens, phytohemagglutinin, and concanavalin A or in mixed lymphocyte culture is a useful indicator of their functional capacities. Other functional assays detect the generation of cytotoxic T cells and NK cells and the production of cytokines (i.e., interleukin-2 [IL-2], interferon-gamma [IFN-γ]) by T lymphocytes and monocytes or their responses to them.

GENETICS OF IMMUNODEFICIENCY DISORDERS

Considerable information has accrued about inheritance patterns, clinical features, and cellular abnormalities in each of the conditions to be discussed, and the primary biologic errors have been identified in a growing number. Examples of the latter include an adhesion protein deficiency, now known to be due to genetic abnormalities in a 95 kD beta (β) chain (CD18, encoded by a gene on chromosome 21q22.3) common to three different leukocyte surface glycoprotein heterodimers,[13] and combined immunodeficiencies owing to abnormalities of purine salvage pathway enzymes, either adenosine deaminase (ADA) (encoded by a gene on chromosome 20q13-ter)[14] or purine nucleoside phosphorylase (PNP) (encoded by a gene on chromosome 14q13.1)[15] (Table 74–2).

The faulty genes in many other immunodeficiencies are known to be on the X chromosome.[16, 17] They have been localized to specific sites in the case of X-linked agammaglobulinemia,[18] X-linked severe combined immunodeficiency,[19] the Wiskott-Aldrich syndrome,[20] X-linked lymphoproliferative disease,[22] properdin deficiency,[16] and X-linked chronic granu-

Table 74–2. PROBABLE CHROMOSOMAL MAP LOCATIONS FOR FAULTY GENES IN PRIMARY IMMUNODEFICIENCY DISEASES INVOLVING LYMPHOCYTES

Chromosome	Disease
2p11	Kappa chain deficiency
6p21.3	(?)Common variable immunodeficiency and selective IgA deficiency
11q22.3	Ataxia telangiectasia
14q13.1	Purine nucleoside phosphorylase deficiency*
14q32.3	Immunoglobulin heavy chain deletion
20q13-ter	Adenosine deaminase deficiency*
21q22.3	Leukocyte adhesion deficiency (CD11:CD18 deficiency)*
Xp11–11.3	Wiskott-Aldrich syndrome
Xq13–21.1	Severe combined immunodeficiency
Xq21.3–22	X-linked immunodeficiency
Xq24–27	Immunodeficiency with hyper IgM
Xq24–26	X-linked lymphoproliferative syndrome

*Gene cloned and sequenced, gene product known.

lomatous disease (CGD) but only in the last-mentioned case has the abnormal gene been identified.[16] Lethal immunodeficiency can also be due to broad deficiencies of human leukocyte antigen (HLA) class I and II antigens, and these have been shown to be due to different mutations in transacting factors governing the surface expression of these molecules.[22–24] Because trace amounts of immunoglobulins of all five isotypes can usually be found in the serum of most agammaglobulinemics, it is unlikely that most immunoglobulin deficiency states are attributable to deletions of immunoglobulin genes. Exceptions include rare patients with deletions of genes encoding the kappa (κ) light chain or the heavy chains of immunoglobulin G or A subclasses (Table 74–3).[25]

GENETICALLY DETERMINED IMMUNODEFICIENCY SYNDROMES INVOLVING LYMPHOCYTES

Various attempts have been made by World Health Organization (WHO) committees over the past 22 years to classify the known primary immunodeficiency disorders involving lymphocytes as well as the other components of the immune system.[2] Tables 74–3 and 74–4 list the current state of knowledge about 20 of the more well-known primary immunodeficiency syndromes involving lymphocytes, giving the most prominent functional deficits and the presumed cellular or molecular level of the defects. The descriptions of specific diseases do not include all of the currently recognized immunodeficiency states; the ones selected were chosen because of new information about them, their frequency, recent recognition, or relevance to rheumatologic diseases.

Table 74–3. ANTIBODY DEFICIENCY DISORDERS

Disorder	Functional Deficiencies	Presumed Cellular Level of Defect
X-linked agammaglobulinemia	Antibody	Pre-B cell
Common variable immunodeficiency ("acquired" hypogamma-globulinemia)	Antibody	B lymphocyte
IgG subclass deficiencies; kappa chain deficiency	Antibody	B lymphocyte; immunoglobulin heavy or light chain gene deletions
Selective IgA deficiency	IgA antibody	IgA B lymphocyte
Secretory component deficiency	Secretory IgA	Mucosal epithelium
Selective IgM deficiency	IgM antibody	T helper cells
Immunodeficiency with elevated IgM	IgG and IgA antibodies	B lymphocytes; "switch" T cells
Transient hypogammaglobulinemia of infancy	None; immunoglobulins low but antibodies present	Unknown
Antibody deficiency with near-normal immunoglobulins	Antibody	Unknown; ?B cell
X-linked lymphoproliferative disease	Anti-EBNA antibody	B cell; ?also T cell

EBNA, Epstein-Barr nuclear antigen.

ANTIBODY DEFICIENCY DISORDERS

Antibody deficiency may occur clinically either as a congenital or as an "acquired" abnormality, although in both situations it appears to be genetically determined. There may be deficiencies in all immunoglobulin classes (agammaglobulinemia or hypogammaglobulinemia) or in one or more but not all isotypes (selective immunoglobulin deficiencies) (see Table 74–3). In addition, antibody deficiency may occur in the presence of normal or near-normal concentrations of serum immunoglobulins or immunoglobulin subclasses. Most patients with these disorders are recognized because they have recurrent infections with high-grade bacterial pathogens, but some with selective IgA deficiency or infants with transient hypogammaglobulinemia may have few or no infections.

X-Linked (Bruton's) Agammaglobulinemia

This was the first recognized immunodeficiency disorder, discovered by Colonel Ogden Bruton in 1952.[1]

Clinical Features. Most boys afflicted with this malady remain well during the first 6 to 9 months of life, presumably by virtue of maternally transmitted IgG antibodies. Thereafter, they repeatedly acquire infections with extracellular pyogenic organisms such as pneumococci, streptococci, and *Haemophilus* unless given prophylactic antibiotics or gamma globulin therapy. Infections with other organisms such as meningococci, staphylococci, *Pseudomonas*, and various *Mycoplasma* species[26] occur less frequently.[27] These include not only mucous membrane infections (sinusitis, pneumonia, otitis, and conjunctivitis), but also life-threatening systemic infections (septic arthritis, meningitis, and septicemia).[27] Despite these

Table 74–4. CELLULAR AND COMBINED IMMUNODEFICIENCY DISORDERS

Disorder	Functional Deficiencies	Presumed Cellular Level of Defect
DiGeorge's syndrome	T cellular, some antibody	Dysmorphogenesis of third and fourth branchial pouches
Nezelof's syndrome (including PNP deficiency)	T cellular, some antibody	Unknown, ?thymus, ?T cell, metabolic defects
Severe combined immunodeficiency syndromes (autosomal recessive, ADA deficiency, X-linked recessive, defective expression of HLA antigens, reticular dysgenesis)	Antibody and T cellular, phagocytic in reticular dysgenesis	Unknown, metabolic defect(s), ?T cell, ?stem cell, ?thymus, regulatory gene defects
Wiskott-Aldrich syndrome	Antibody, T cellular	Unknown, ?CD43 expression
Ataxia telangiectasia	Antibody, T cellular	B lymphocyte, helper T lymphocyte
Cartilage-hair hypoplasia	T cellular	G1 cycle of many cells
Immunodeficiency with thymoma	Antibody, some T cellular	B lymphocyte, excessive T suppressor cells
Hyperimmunoglobulinemia E	Specific immune responses, excessive IgE	Unknown, ?deficiency of CD43RO+ TH1 memory cells
Leukocyte adhesion deficiency (CD11/18 deficiency)	Cytotoxic lymphocytes, phagocytic cells	95 Kd molecular weight beta chain (CD18) of LFA-1, CR3 and p150,95
Lymphocyte activation defects	T cellular, some antibody	Decreased CD3/Ti expression, defective signal transduction, defective IL-2 and other cytokine production

PNP, Purine nucleoside phosphorylase; ADA, adenosine deaminase; HLA, human leukocyte antigen.

chronic or recurrent infections, patients with this disorder usually grow normally unless they develop bronchiectasis or persistent enterovirus infections.[28, 29] Chronic fungal infections are not usually present, and *Pneumocystis carinii* pneumonia rarely occurs unless there is an associated neutropenia. Viral infections are also usually handled normally, with the notable exceptions of the hepatitis viruses and the enteroviruses.[28, 29] Several examples of meningoencephalitis or paralysis after live poliovirus (an enterovirus) vaccine administration have occurred as a result of failure of immune elimination of the vaccine virus by secretory IgA antibodies, subsequent viremia, then central nervous system infection because of a lack of circulating IgG antibody. In addition, chronic, progressive, eventually fatal central nervous system infections with various echoviruses and coxsackie viruses have occurred in more than 40 such patients.[29] Of interest is the fact that several of these patients have presented with a dermatomyositis-like picture before neurologic abnormalities were apparent, raising the possibility of a viral cause for many of the collagen-like diseases described in these patients[28, 29] (Fig. 74–1). These observations suggest a primary role for antibody, particularly secretory IgA, in host defense against this group of viruses, since normal T cell function has been present in all X-linked agammaglobulinemics with persistent enterovirus infections reported thus far.

Other associated conditions frequently seen in X-linked agammaglobulinemia are rheumatoid arthritis[27, 30] and lymphoreticular malignancy.[5, 27] The arthritis, which may occur in as many as 20 per cent of cases,[27] may be due to acute pyogenic bacterial infections or to viral or *Mycoplasma* infections, or the cause may be unknown. The arthritis usually involves only one or a few joints and characteristically involves large joints. Septic arthritis is rare after IVIG replacement therapy is initiated. Infections with *Ureaplasma urealyticum*[26] and viral agents such as echoviruses, coxsackie viruses and adenovirus, however, have been identified from joint fluid cultures of patients on replacement therapy.[27] There is generally no radiographic evidence of joint destruction, and biopsies revealed a mononuclear round cell infiltrate but no pannus or abnormalities of cartilage.[27] There is no increased incidence of arthritis in first-degree relatives of such patients, suggesting that the arthritis is unrelated genetically to rheumatoid arthritis or Still's disease.[30]

Immunologic Defects. The diagnosis of X-linked agammaglobulinemia is suspected if serum concentrations of IgG, IgA, and IgM are far below the 95 per cent confidence limits for appropriate age-matched and race-matched controls (i.e., usually <100 mg per dl total immunoglobulin). Tests for natural antibodies to blood group substances, for antibodies to antigens given during standard courses of immunization (e.g., diphtheria, tetanus, *H. influenzae*, and pneumococcal) and for antibodies to bacteriophage ØX174, are useful in distinguishing this disorder from transient hypogammaglobulinemia of infancy. Polymorphonuclear functions are usually normal if heat-stable opsonins (e.g., IgG antibodies) are provided, but some patients with this condition have had transient, persistent, or cyclic neutropenia.

The number of T cells is usually increased, and the percentages of T cell subsets have been found to be normal in most of these patients. By contrast, blood lymphocytes bearing surface immunoglobulin, "Ia-like" antigens, or the Epstein-Barr virus (EBV) receptor or reacting with monoclonal antibodies specific for B cell antigens are absent or present in very low number.[31] Nevertheless, pre-B cells can be found in the bone marrow in low number. Hypoplasia of adenoids, tonsils, and peripheral lymph nodes is the rule. Germinal centers are not found in these tissues, and plasma cells are rarely found. Mixed lymphocyte responsiveness, cell-mediated lympholysis, and lymphocyte proliferative responses to antigens and mitogens are normal. Cell-mediated immune responses can be detected in vivo, and the capacity to reject allografts is intact. Natural killer cell function is normal. The thymus is morphologically normal. Hassall's corpuscles are present, and lymphoid cells are abundant in thymus-dependent areas of peripheral lymphoid tissues.

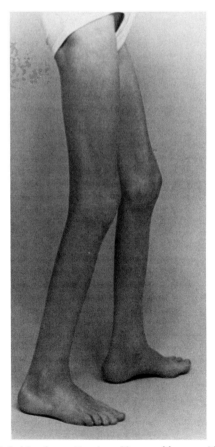

Figure 74–1. Muscle wasting in a 20-year-old man with X-linked agammaglobulinemia who developed a dermatomyositis-like clinical picture. Blood and spinal fluid cultures grew an echovirus.

Pathogenesis. The fundamental defect remains unknown, but it affects very early B lineage cells.[17] Studies suggest that there is a maturation block in the transition between terminal deoxynucleotidyl transferase positive, $c\mu^-$ pre-pre-B cells and $c\mu^+$ pre-B cells.[32] The abnormal gene in X-linked agammaglobulinemia was mapped to a region on the proximal part of the long arm of the X chromosome.[18] This was accomplished by restriction fragment length polymorphism (RFLP) studies, using DNA probes for the loci DXS17 and DXS3 that mapped the abnormal gene to the q21.3-q22 region.[16, 17] Carriers can be detected by the finding of nonrandom X-chromosome inactivation in B cells in RFLP studies of hamster-human B cell hybrids[33] or differences in methylation patterns.[16]

Treatment and Prognosis. Except in those unfortunate patients who develop polio, persistent enterovirus infection, rheumatoid arthritis, or lymphoreticular malignancy (an incidence as high as 6 per cent has been reported), the overall prognosis is reasonably good if IgG replacement therapy is instituted early. Systemic infection can be prevented by administration of intravenous immune serum globulin (IVIG) at a dose of 400 mg per kg every 3 to 4 weeks.[10, 11] Such preparations are known to be free of hepatitis viruses and the AIDS viruses. Many patients go on to develop crippling sinopulmonary disease despite IVIG therapy, since no effective means exists for replacing secretory IgA at the mucosal surface. Chronic antibiotic therapy is usually necessary in addition for the management of such patients.

Common Variable Immunodeficiency

Clinical Features. Common variable immunodeficiency (CVID), also known as *"acquired" hypogammaglobulinemia* or *idiopathic late-onset immunoglobulin deficiency*, may appear similar clinically in many respects to X-linked agammaglobulinemia.[2, 34] The kinds of infections experienced and bacterial etiologic agents involved are generally the same for the two defects. Fortunately, however, for unknown reasons echovirus meningoencephalitis is rare in patients with CVID.[29] The principal differences are the generally later age of onset, the somewhat less severe infections, an almost equal sex distribution, a tendency to autoantibody formation, normal-sized or enlarged tonsils and lymph nodes, and splenomegaly in approximately 25 per cent.

CVID has been variably associated with a sprue-like syndrome, nodular follicular lymphoid hyperplasia of the intestine, thymoma, alopecia areata (Fig. 74–2), hemolytic anemia, gastric atrophy, achlorhydria, and pernicious anemia. In addition, such patients have frequent thyroid abnormalities, vitiligo, keratoconjunctivitis sicca, and arthritis. The arthritis in such patients is usually mild to moderate in severity and symmetric, affecting both large and small joints (Fig. 74–3).[35] It is usually nonerosive,

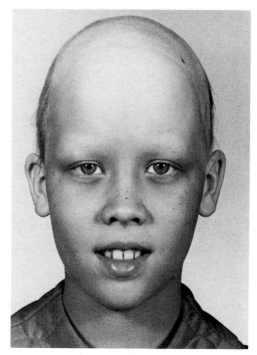

Figure 74–2. Alopecia areata totalis in a girl with common variable immunodeficiency who also had an autoimmune Coombs's-positive hemolytic anemia.

and subcutaneous nodules do not occur. Synovial biopsies have revealed capillary proliferation, but an absence of lining cell hyperplasia and only variable infiltration by chronic inflammatory cells.[35] Finally, there are now several cases of lupus erythematosus converting to CVID.[36] Frequent complications include giardiasis (seen far more often here than in X-linked agammaglobulinemia), bronchiectasis, gastric carcinoma, lymphoreticular malignancy, and cholelithiasis. Lymphoid interstitial pneumonia; pseudolymphoma; amyloidosis; and noncaseating granulomata of the lungs, spleen, skin, and liver have also been seen. There is a 438-fold increase in lymphomas in affected women in the fifth and sixth decades.[37]

Immunologic Defects. The serum immunoglobulin and antibody deficiencies in CVID may be as

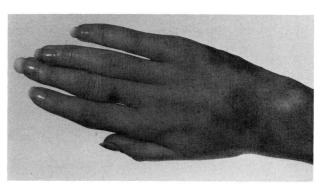

Figure 74–3. Arthritis in a girl with common variable immunodeficiency and a macular skin lesion with a lymphocyte infiltrate.

profound as in the X-linked disorder. Despite normal numbers of circulating immunoglobulin-bearing B lymphocytes and the presence of lymphoid cortical follicles, blood lymphocytes from CVID patients do not differentiate into immunoglobulin-producing cells when stimulated with pokeweed mitogen in vitro, even when co-cultured with normal T cells.[34, 38] T cells and subsets are usually present in normal percentages, although T cell function may be depressed in some patients.[35]

Pathogenesis. In most patients, the defect appears to be intrinsic to the B cell, resulting in abnormal terminal differentiation.[34, 38] Because this disorder occurs in first-degree relatives of patients with selective IgA deficiency (A Def) and some patients with A Def later become panhypogammaglobulinemic, it is possible that these diseases have a common genetic basis. The high incidences of abnormal immunoglobulin concentrations, autoantibodies, autoimmune disease, and malignancy in families of both types of patients also suggest a shared hereditary influence.[4] This concept is supported by the finding of rare alleles or deletions of class III major histocompatibility complex (MHC) genes in individuals with either A Def[4, 39] or CVID,[39, 40] suggesting that the susceptibility gene(s) are in this region on chromosome 6.

Treatment. The treatment of patients with CVID is essentially the same as for X-linked agammaglobulinemia.[10, 11]

IgG Subclass Deficiency

A number of patients have been reported to have deficiencies of one or more subclasses of IgG, despite normal total IgG serum concentrations.[41] Most of those with absent or very low concentrations of IgG2 have been patients with selective IgA deficiency (see later).[42] It is difficult to know the biologic significance of the multiple moderate deficiencies of IgG subclasses that have been reported, particularly when completely asymptomatic individuals have been described who totally lacked IgG1, IgG2, IgG4, and IgA1 owing to gene deletion.[25] The more relevant question to ask is "what is the capacity of the patient to make specific antibodies to protein and polysaccharide antigens?" because profound deficiencies of antipolysaccharide antibodies have been noted even in the presence of normal concentrations of IgG2.[43] IVIG should not be given to IgG subclass deficient patients unless they are shown to have a deficiency of antibodies to a broad array of antigens.[10, 11]

Selective IgA Deficiency

An isolated absence or near-absence (i.e., <10 mg per dl) of serum and secretory IgA is thought to be the most common well-defined immunodeficiency disorder, a frequency of one in 333 being reported among some blood donors.[6, 7]

Clinical Features. Although this disorder has been observed in apparently healthy individuals,[6] it is commonly associated with ill health. As would be expected when there is a deficiency of the major immunoglobulin of external secretions, infections occur predominantly in the respiratory, gastrointestinal, and urogenital tracts.[7] Bacterial agents responsible are essentially the same as in other types of antibody deficiency syndromes. There is no clear evidence that patients with this disorder have an undue susceptibility to viral agents. Similar to CVID, there is a frequent association of A Def with collagen vascular and autoimmune diseases.[4] These include (among others) systemic lupus erythematosus, rheumatoid arthritis, ankylosing spondylitis, dermatomyositis, pernicious anemia, thyroiditis, diabetes mellitus, Addison's disease, Sjögren's syndrome, chronic active hepatitis, idiopathic thrombocytopenic purpura, Coombs'-positive hemolytic anemia, pulmonary hemosiderosis, regional enteritis, and ulcerative colitis. A sprue-like syndrome has occurred in adults with A Def; the latter may or may not respond to a gluten-free diet. In further similarity to patients with CVID, there is an increased incidence of malignancy.[5]

Immunologic Defects. Serum concentrations of other immunoglobulins are usually normal in patients with selective IgA deficiency, although IgG2 subclass deficiency has been reported,[42] and IgM (usually elevated) may be monomeric. Children with IgA deficiency vaccinated with killed poliovirus intranasally produced local IgM and IgG antibodies. Several of them later contracted rubella, and IgM and IgG antirubella antibodies were found in their secretions during convalescence. Of possible etiologic and great clinical significance is the presence of antibodies to IgA in the sera of as high as 44 per cent of patients with selective IgA deficiency.[6] IgG anti-IgA antibodies can fix complement and remove IgA from the circulation four to 20 times faster than the normal catabolic rate for IgA. A number of IgA-deficient patients have had severe or fatal anaphylactic reactions after intravenous administration of blood products containing IgA, and anti-IgA antibodies (particularly IgE anti-IgA antibodies[44]) have been implicated. For this reason, only five times–washed (in 200 ml volumes) normal donor erythrocytes or blood products from other IgA-absent individuals should be administered to these patients. Patients with A Def also frequently have IgG antibodies against cow milk and ruminant serum proteins. These antiruminant antibodies often falsely detect "IgA" in immunoassays that employ goat (but not rabbit) antisera.[7] A high incidence of autoantibodies has also been noted.[45]

Pathogenesis. The basic defect leading to selective IgA deficiency is unknown. In ten of 11 IgA-deficient individuals studied, more than 80 per cent of the IgA-bearing B cells also coexpressed surface IgM and IgD (similar to cord blood B cells), as compared with less than 10 per cent triple isotype-bearing IgA B cells in healthy persons, suggesting an IgA isotype-specific B cell maturation arrest.[46] In others, treatment with dilantin, sulfasalazine,[47] D-penicillamine, or gold has been suspected as being the cause. The occurrence of IgA deficiency in both males and females and in families is consistent with autosomal inheritance; in some families, this appears to be dominant with variable expressivity. As already noted, this defect occurs in pedigrees with CVID patients, and molecular genetic studies suggest that the susceptibility genes for these two defects may reside in the MHC class III region on chromosome 6.[4, 39, 40, 48]

Treatment and Prognosis. Currently there is no treatment for A Def beyond the vigorous treatment of specific infections with appropriate antimicrobial agents. IVIG (which is greater than 99 per cent IgG) is not indicated because most A Def patients make IgG antibodies normally.[10] Moreover, many IVIG preparations contain sufficient IgA to cause anaphylactic reactions.[10, 44] Even if serum IgA could be replaced (a dangerous thing to attempt), it could not be transported into the external secretions because the latter is an active process involving only locally and endogenously produced IgA. In some A Def patients, the defect may spontaneously disappear with time,[49] whereas in others it may evolve into CVID.

Secretory Component Deficiency

A patient with chronic intestinal candidiasis and diarrhea was found to lack IgA in his external secretions, despite having a normal serum IgA concentration.[50] This was ultimately traced to a lack of secretory piece, which prevented the normal secretion of locally produced IgA onto his mucous membrane surfaces.

Selective IgM Deficiency

There are very few well-documented cases of selective IgM deficiency (<10 mg per dl IgM).[2] Septicemia due to meningococci and other gram-negative organisms, pneumococcal meningitis, tuberculosis, recurrent staphylococcal pyoderma, periorbital cellulitis, bronchiectasis, recurrent otitis, and other respiratory infections have been reported in this disorder. In vivo production of IgM antibodies is markedly impaired. There is no specific treatment for this disorder; early and vigorous treatment with antibiotics is recommended to avoid fatal septicemia.

Immunodeficiency with Elevated IgM

Clinical Features. Patients with immunodeficiency with elevated IgM (Hyper M) may become symptomatic during the first or second year of life with recurrent pyogenic infections, including otitis media, sinusitis, pneumonia, and tonsillitis.[2] In contrast to patients with X-linked agammaglobulinemia, however, the frequent presence of lymphoid hyperplasia in patients with Hyper M is often misleading.

Coexistent neutropenia is considered a possible explanation for the occurrence of *Pneumocystis carinii* pneumonia and extensive verruca vulgaris lesions in some such patients.

Immunologic Defects. Hyper M is characterized by very low serum IgG and IgA but either a normal or more frequently a markedly elevated concentration of polyclonal IgM. Some of these patients have low molecular weight IgM molecules that give falsely high IgM values in radial immunodiffusion assays. High titers of IgM antibodies to blood group substances and to *Salmonella* O antigen have been found in some patients, but very low titers or no IgM antibody has been noted in others. Even more than with some of the other antibody-deficiency syndromes, there is an increased frequency of autoimmune disorders in the Hyper IgM syndrome.[2] Hemolytic anemia and thrombocytopenia have been seen in several patients, and transient, persistent, or cyclic neutropenia is a common feature. Thymic-dependent lymphoid tissues and T cell functions are usually normal, but several have had partial T cell deficiencies.

Pathogenesis. Normal or only slightly reduced numbers of IgM or IgD B lymphocytes have been found in the blood of these patients. Cultured B cell lines from such patients, however, have shown the capacity to synthesize only IgM and a defect of switch recombination.[51] B cells from a few such patients have shown the capacity to synthesize IgM, IgA, and IgG when co-cultured with a "switch" T cell line, suggesting that in those patients the defect lay in T lineage cells.[52] A sex-linked mode of inheritance has been noted in some pedigrees. The abnormal gene in the X-linked type has been localized to Xq24-Xq27.[16, 17] Several examples in females suggest that this phenotype has more than one genetic cause.

Treatment. Because these patients have an inability to make IgG antibodies, the treatment for this condition is the same as for agammaglobulinemia, i.e., monthly IVIG infusions.[10, 11]

Transient Hypogammaglobulinemia of Infancy

Unlike patients with X-linked agammaglobulinemia or CVID, patients with transient hypogammaglobulinemia of infancy (THI) can synthesize antibodies to human type A and B erythrocytes and to diphtheria and tetanus toxoids, usually by 6 to 11 months of age, and well before immunoglobulin concentrations become normal.[53] Lymphocyte studies in vitro show no abnormalities in the percentages of cells in the different subpopulations or in their responses to mitogens. THI has been found in pedigrees of patients with other immune defects, including CVID and severe combined immunodeficiency disorders (SCID). The finding of only 11 cases of THI among more than 10,000 patients whose sera were sent to the author for immunoglobulin studies over a 12-year period suggests that this is not a common entity.[53]

IVIG therapy is not indicated in this condition.[10, 11] In addition to the known risk of inducing anti-allotype antibodies, passively administered IgG antibodies could suppress endogenous antibody formation to infectious agents in the same manner that RhoGAM suppresses anti-D antibodies in Rh-negative mothers delivering Rh-positive infants. IVIG may also suppress immune responses by Fc-receptor interaction and by the induction of anti-idiotypic antibodies.

Antibody Deficiency with Near-Normal Immunoglobulins

Only scattered reports have appeared in the literature describing patients with apparently normal T cell function and normal or near-normal immunoglobulin concentrations but with deficient antibody responses.[43, 54] Such individuals have recurrent pyogenic infections similar to those with agammaglobulinemia. Indeed, with time, serum immunoglobulin concentrations may decline to levels seen in CVID patients. This has led to speculation that this condition may be an early stage of CVID. Blood group antibody titers are frequently absent; diphtheria, tetanus, H. influenzae, and pneumococcal antibody titers are significantly lower than normal; and primary immune responses to bacteriophage ØX174 are far below the normal range. Because these patients do not have the ability to produce antibodies normally, they are candidates for monthly IVIG infusions.[10, 11]

X-Linked Lymphoproliferative Disease

X-linked lymphoproliferative disease, also referred to as Duncan's disease (after the original kindred in which it was described), is a recessive trait characterized by an inadequate immune response to infection with EBV.[21] The defective gene has been localized to the Xq26-q27 region near DXS42 and DXS37.[21] Affected individuals are apparently healthy until they experience infectious mononucleosis.[21] The mean age of presentation is less than 5 years. The most common form of presentation (75 per cent) is severe fatal (80 per cent) mononucleosis, primarily owing to extensive liver necrosis caused by polyclonally activated alloreactive cytotoxic T cells that recognize EBV-infected autologous B cells.[21] Most patients surviving the primary infection developed global cellular immune defects involving T, B, and NK cells; lymphomas; or hypogammaglobulinemia. There is a marked impairment in production of antibodies to the EBV nuclear antigen (EBNA), whereas titers of antibodies to the viral capsid antigen have ranged from zero to markedly elevated. Antibody-dependent cell-mediated cytotoxicity (ADCC) against EBV-infected cells has been low in many, and natural killer (NK) function is also depressed. There is also a deficiency in long-lived T cell immunity to EBV. Studies of T lymphocyte subpopulations with monoclonal antibodies have frequently revealed elevated percentages of CD8+ cells. Immunoglobulin synthesis in response to pokeweed mitogen stimulation in vitro is markedly depressed. Thus, both EBV-specific and nonspecific immunologic abnormalities occur in these patients.

Cellular and Combined Immunodeficiency Disorders

In general, patients with partial or absolute defects in T cell function have infections or other clinical problems for which there is no effective treatment or which are of a more severe nature than those with antibody deficiency disorders (see Table 74–4). It is also rare that such individuals survive beyond infancy or childhood.

Thymic Hypoplasia (DiGeorge's Syndrome)

Thymic hypoplasia results from dysmorphogenesis of the third and fourth pharyngeal pouches during early embryogenesis, leading to hypoplasia or aplasia of the thymus and parathyroid glands.[2] Other structures forming at the same age are also frequently affected, resulting in anomalies of the great vessels (right-sided aortic arch), esophageal atresia, bifid uvula, congenital heart disease (atrial and ventricular septal defects), a short philtrum of the upper lip, hypertelorism, an antimongoloid slant to the eyes, mandibular hypoplasia, and low-set, often notched ears (Fig. 74–4). The diagnosis is usually first suggested by the presence of hypocalcemic seizures during the neonatal period. Since the original description of the syndrome, it has become apparent that a variable degree of hypoplasia is more frequent than total aplasia of the thymus and parathyroid glands. Some children have little trouble with life-threatening infections and grow normally; such patients are often referred to as having partial DiGeorge's syndrome. Those with complete DiGeorge's syndrome may resemble patients with SCID in their susceptibility to infections with opportunistic pathogens (i.e., fungi, viruses, and P. carinii) and to graft-versus-host disease (GVHD) from nonirradiated blood transfusions.

Immunologic Defects

Concentrations of serum immunoglobulins are usually near normal for age, but IgA may be diminished in some, and IgE may be elevated. T cell numbers are decreased; as a result, there is a relative increase in the percentage of B cells. Monoclonal antibody analyses have demonstrated that, despite decreased numbers of CD3+ T cells, there are usually normal proportions of CD4 and CD8+ cells. Responses of blood lymphocytes following mitogen stimulation, like the intradermal delayed hypersensitivity response, have been absent, reduced, or normal, depending on the degree of thymic defi-

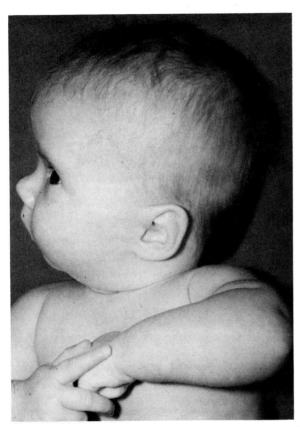

Figure 74–4. An infant with DiGeorge's syndrome illustrating the hypertelorism, mandibular hypoplasia, and low-set ears resulting from the dysembryogenesis of the upper pharyngeal pouches.

ciency. Thymic tissue, when found, does contain Hassall's corpuscles and a normal density of thymocytes; corticomedullary distinction is present. Lymphoid follicles are usually present, but lymph node paracortical areas and thymus-dependent regions of the spleen show variable degrees of depletion.

Pathogenesis. DiGeorge's syndrome has occurred in both males and females, and chromosomal abnormalities (monosomy 22q11 and 10p13) have been noted in approximately 10 to 15 per cent. It has been hypothesized that deletion of contiguous genes on chromosome 22 results in DiGeorge's syndrome and that the critical region may be in proximity to the BCRL2 locus.[55] Familial occurrence is rare but has been reported. Because the characteristic facies and conotruncal heart lesions seen in DiGeorge patients have also been noted in the fetal alcohol syndrome, it has been proposed that the DiGeorge anomaly may be a polytypic field defect of diverse etiology involving cephalic neural crest cells.

Treatment. Because of variability in the severity of the immunodeficiency, it is difficult to evaluate claimed benefits of fetal thymus transplantation. Three patients have experienced immunologic reconstitution following unfractionated HLA-identical bone marrow transplantation.[56]

Cellular Immunodeficiency with Immunoglobulins (Nezelof's Syndrome)

Clinical Features. Patients with Nezelof's syndrome present during infancy with recurrent or chronic pulmonary infections, failure to thrive, oral or cutaneous candidiasis, chronic diarrhea, recurrent skin infections, gram-negative sepsis, urinary tract infections, or severe varicella.[2] Other findings include neutropenia and eosinophilia.

Immunologic Defects. Serum immunoglobulins may be normal or elevated for all classes, but selective IgA deficiency, marked elevation of IgE, and elevated IgD levels have been found in some cases. Although antibody-forming capacity has been impaired in a majority, it has not been absent and has been apparently normal in roughly one third of the reported cases. Moreover, plasma cells are usually abundant in the lamina propria and lymph nodes.

Studies of cellular immune function have shown delayed cutaneous anergy to ubiquitous antigens in all such patients; lymphopenia; and extremely low but not absent lymphocyte proliferative responses to mitogens, antigens, and allogeneic cells in vitro. Nezelof's syndrome is the primary immunodeficiency disorder most likely to be confused with AIDS in the pediatric age group. Nezelof patients, however, have profound deficiencies of CD3+ T cells but usually normal proportions of CD4 and CD8 positive cells, in contrast to patients with AIDS, who characteristically have a selective deficiency of CD4+ cells. Peripheral lymphoid tissues demonstrate paracortical lymphocyte depletion. The thymuses are very small and have a paucity of thymocytes and usually no Hassall's corpuscles; however, again in contrast to AIDS, thymic epithelium is intact.

Pathogenesis and Treatment. An autosomal recessive pattern of inheritance is often seen. Although patients with this disorder have been successfully reconstituted by matched sibling bone marrow transplants, most other forms of therapy have been unsuccessful. Despite the profound cellular immunodeficiency, however, Nezelof patients usually survive longer than do infants with severe combined immunodeficiency.

Nezelof's Syndrome with Purine Nucleoside Phosphorylase Deficiency. Thirty-three patients with Nezelof's syndrome have been found to have purine nucleoside phosphorylase (PNP) (encoded by a gene on chromosome 14q13.1) deficiency.[15] In contrast to patients with adenosine deaminase (ADA) deficiency (see later),[14] serum and urinary uric acid are markedly deficient, and no characteristic physical or skeletal abnormalities have been noted. Deaths have occurred from generalized vaccinia, varicella, lymphosarcoma, and GVHD mediated by allogeneic T cells in nonirradiated blood or bone marrow. Two thirds of patients have neurologic abnormalities ranging from spasticity to mental retardation. One third of patients develop autoimmune diseases, the most common of which is autoimmune hemolytic anemia. Idiopathic thrombocytopenic purpura and systemic lupus erythematosus have also been reported. Unlike most Nezelof patients, the thymuses of PNP-deficient patients have had occasional Hassall's corpuscles at postmortem examination, reminiscent of some patients with ADA deficiency. Analyses of lymphocyte subpopulations with monoclonal antibodies have demonstrated a marked deficiency of T cells and T cell subsets but increased numbers of cells with NK phenotype and function. Prenatal diagnosis is possible. Attempts to correct the immunologic and enzymatic deficiencies of PNP-deficient patients by enzyme replacement or deoxycytidine therapy have not been successful. Bone marrow transplantation is the treatment of choice but has thus far been successful in only a few such patients. Gene therapy may be available in the future.

Severe Combined Immunodeficiency Disorders

The syndromes of SCID are characterized by (1) absence of all adaptive immune function from birth and (2) great cellular, molecular, and genetic diversity.[2, 14, 57, 58, 58a] Patients with this group of disorders have the most severe of all of the recognized immunodeficiencies. Unless immunologic reconstitution can be achieved through immunocompetent tissue transplants or enzyme replacement therapy or gnotobiotic isolation can be carried out, death usually occurs before the patient's first birthday and almost invariably before the second.

Autosomal Recessive Severe Combined Immunodeficiency Disease

This was the first described of the SCID syndromes, reported initially by Swiss workers in 1958. Affected infants present within the first few months of life with frequent episodes of diarrhea, pneumonia, otitis, sepsis, and cutaneous infections. Growth may appear normal initially, but extreme wasting usually develops after infections and diarrhea begin. Persistent infections with opportunistic organisms such as *C. albicans, P. carinii,* varicella, measles, parainfluenzae 3, cytomegalovirus, EBV, and bacillus Calmette-Guérin lead to death. These infants also lack the ability to reject foreign tissue and are therefore at risk for GVHD. GVHD reactions can result from maternal immunocompetent cells crossing the placenta or from the administration of nonirradiated blood products or allogeneic bone marrow containing T lymphocytes.

Infants with SCID have profound lymphopenia (Fig. 74–5);[9] an absence of lymphocyte proliferative responses to mitogens, antigens, and allogeneic cells in vitro; and delayed cutaneous anergy.[2, 57, 58a] Serum immunoglobulin concentrations are diminished to absent, and no antibody formation occurs following immunization. Analyses of lymphocyte populations and subpopulations have demonstrated marked heterogeneity among SCID patients, even among those

with similar inheritance patterns[57, 58, 58a] or with ADA deficiency.[14] Despite the uniformly profound lack of T or B cell function, many patients have elevated percentages of B cells.[57, 58, 58a] Monoclonal antibody studies have generally shown extremely low percentages of T cells and subsets. There is no increase in circulating lymphocytes bearing CD1, an antigen present on immature cortical thymocytes. Thus, the few T lymphocytes present appear to have acquired surface markers characteristic of mature T cells. All or most of the circulating lymphocytes in some SCID infants are large granular lymphocytes with NK cell phenotype and function,[59] whereas NK cells and function are totally lacking in other SCID patients. Typically, SCID patients have very small thymuses (less than 1 g), which usually fail to descend from the neck, contain few thymocytes, and lack corticomedullary distinction and Hassall's corpuscles. It should be noted that despite the profound thymocyte depletion in SCID patients, thymic epithelium appears histologically normal, in contrast to the situation in AIDS, in which there is marked epithelial atrophy. Both the follicular and the paracortical areas of the peripheral lymph nodes are depleted of lymphocytes in SCID patients; tonsils, adenoids, and Peyer's patches are absent or extremely underdeveloped.

Replacement therapy with IVIG fails to halt the progressively downhill course of SCID.[10, 11] Conversely, transplantation of bone marrow cells from

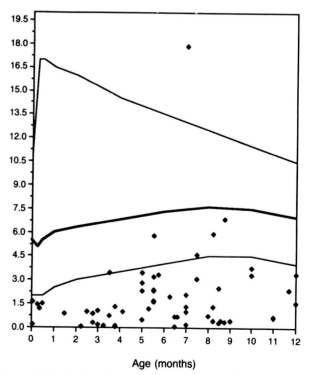

Figure 74–5. Absolute lymphocyte counts in 59 infants with severe combined immunodeficiency disorder (SCID). The light lines indicate the normal 95 per cent confidence limits, and the heavy line indicates the normal mean. (Normative data are from Altman.[9])

HLA identical or haploidentical donors has resulted in correction of the immunologic defect in a number of these patients, with more than 200 known long-term survivors.[60, 61, 61a]

Autosomal Recessive Severe Combined Immunodeficiency Disease with Adenosine Deaminase Deficiency. An absence of the enzyme ADA (encoded by a gene mapped to chromosome 20q.13-ter) has been observed in approximately 40 per cent of patients with autosomal recessively inherited SCID.[14] Marked accumulations of adenosine, 2'-deoxyadenosine and 2'-O-methyladenosine directly or indirectly lead to lymphocyte toxicity, which causes the immunodeficiency. Adenosine and deoxyadenosine are apparent suicide inactivators of the enzyme, S-adenosylhomocysteine (SAH) hydrolase, resulting in the accumulation of SAH. SAH is a potent inhibitor of virtually all cellular methylation reactions. Such patients usually have more profound lymphopenia than other SCID infants and rarely have elevated percentages of B cells.[57] In further contrast to infants with other types of SCID, a few ADA-deficient patients have been found to have rare Hassall's corpuscles in their thymuses and changes suggestive of early differentiation.

Other distinguishing features of ADA-deficient SCID have included the presence of rib cage abnormalities similar to a rachitic rosary and multiple skeletal abnormalities of chondro-osseous dysplasia on radiographic examination; these occur predominantly at the costochondral junctions, at the apophyses of the iliac bones, and in the vertebral bodies. As with other types, ADA-deficient SCID can be cured by HLA-identical or haploidentical T cell–depleted bone marrow transplantation, which remains the treatment of choice.[57, 61a] Enzyme replacement therapy with polyethylene glycol–modified bovine ADA (PEG-ADA) administered subcutaneously once weekly has resulted in both clinical and immunologic improvement in more than 15 ADA-deficient patients.[62] This therapy should not be initiated, however, if bone marrow transplantation is contemplated because it will confer graft-rejection capability. ADA-deficient SCID became the first genetic defect in which gene therapy was attempted. That particular effort, however, is not likely to be successful because mature T cells rather than stem cells were transfected with a vector carrying the normal ADA gene.

X-Linked Recessive Severe Combined Immunodeficiency Diseases

This is thought to be the most common form of SCID in the United States.[58] The abnormal gene has been mapped by RFLP analysis to the Xq13–21.1 region.[19] Carriers can be detected by demonstration of the presence of nonrandom X-chromosome inactivation in T lymphocytes.[58] Clinically, immunologically, and histopathologically, patients with the X-linked form usually appear similar to those with the autosomal recessive form except that they generally tend to have higher percentages of B cells.[58] Results of X-chromosome inactivation and functional[63] studies, however, suggest that the genetic defect affects their B lineage cells as well as those of T lineage.

Defective Expression of Major Histocompatibility Complex Antigens

There are two main forms: (1) class I MHC antigen deficiency (bare lymphocyte syndrome) and (2) class I MHC antigen deficiency plus absence of class II MHC antigens.[22] These conditions are inherited in an autosomal recessive pattern. The defect is *not* linked to genes encoding MHC antigens on chromosome 6 (6p21.3). In some patients lacking class II MHC antigens, the defect appears to be due to a defective X-box binding protein that binds to the HLA-DR promoter.[22–24] Sera from affected infants contain normal quantities of class I MHC antigens and beta$_2$-microglobulin. Patients (usually of North African descent) present with persistent diarrhea in early infancy and have oral candidiasis, bacterial pneumonia, *Pneumocystis* infection, septicemia, and undue susceptibility to enteroviruses, herpes, and other viral agents. Those with both class I and II antigen deficiencies also have malabsorption. There is variable hypogammaglobulinemia, with decreased serum IgM and IgA and poor to absent antibody production. B cell percentages are usually normal, but plasma cells are absent in tissues. Lymphopenia is only moderate; T cell functions are decreased in vivo and in vitro but are not absent. The thymus and other lymphoid organs are severely hypoplastic. Most affected patients die in the first 3 years of life. The associated defects of both B and T cell immunity and of HLA expression emphasize the important biologic role for HLA determinants in effective immune cell cooperation.

Severe Combined Immunodeficiency with Leukopenia (Reticular Dysgenesis)

In 1959, identical twin male infants were described who exhibited a total lack of both lymphocytes and granulocytes in their peripheral blood and bone marrow. Seven of the eight infants thus far reported with this defect died between 3 and 119 days of age from overwhelming infections; the eighth underwent complete immunologic reconstitution from a bone marrow transplant.[2] Mature normal-appearing granulocytes (although markedly reduced in number) were noted in three patients and a normal percentage of E rosetting T cells in the cord blood of a fourth patient, arguing against a total failure of stem cell differentiation in this defect. Despite the normal percentage of T cells in the latter patient's cord blood, however, the cells failed to give an in vitro proliferative response to mitogens. The thymus glands have all weighed less than 1 g, no Hassall's corpuscles have been present, and few or no thymocytes have been seen. An autosomal-recessive mode of inheritance seems most likely.

Partial Combined Immunodeficiency Disorders

Immunodeficiency with Thrombocytopenia and Eczema (Wiskott-Aldrich Syndrome)

Wiskott-Aldrich syndrome is an X-linked recessive syndrome that is characterized clinically by the triad of eczema, thrombocytopenic purpura with normal-appearing megakaryocytes but small defective platelets and undue susceptibility to infection.[2, 3] The abnormal gene responsible for this defect was shown by de Saint Basile et al.[20] to be closely linked to the novel hypervariable locus DXS255 on the proximal arm of the X chromosome between DXS7 (Xp11.3) and DXS14 (Xp11). Carriers can be detected by nonrandom X-chromosome inactivation in several hematopoietic cell lineages.[64] Often there is prolonged bleeding from the circumcision site or bloody diarrhea during infancy. The thrombocytopenia appears to be caused by an intrinsic platelet abnormality; survival times of homologous but not autologous ^{51}Cr-labeled platelets have been normal in these patients.

Atopic dermatitis and recurrent infections also usually develop during the first year of life. In younger patients, infections are commonly those produced by pneumococci and other bacteria having polysaccharide capsules, resulting in episodes of otitis media, pneumonia, meningitis, and sepsis. Later, infections with agents such as P. carinii and the herpesviruses become more frequent. Survival beyond the teens is rare; infections and bleeding are major causes of death, but there is also a 12 per cent incidence of fatal malignancy in this condition.

Patients with this defect uniformly have an impaired humoral immune response to polysaccharide antigens, as evidenced by absent or markedly diminished isohemagglutinins and poor or absent antibody responses after immunization with polysaccharide antigens.[2] Antibody titers to proteins also fall with time, and anamnestic responses are often poor or absent. Studies of immunoglobulin metabolism have shown an accelerated rate of synthesis as well as hypercatabolism of albumin, IgG, IgA, and IgM, resulting in highly variable concentrations of different immunoglobulins, even within the same patient. The predominant pattern is a low serum IgM, elevated IgA and IgE, and a normal or slightly low IgG concentration. Lymphocyte responses to mitogens are moderately depressed, and cutaneous anergy is a frequent finding. Analyses of blood lymphocytes have shown moderately reduced percentages of T cells reacting with monoclonal antibodies to CD3, CD4, and CD8. In addition, there is defective expression of the sialoglycoprotein, CD43, on all circulating leukocytes and platelets of Wiskott-Aldrich patients, owing to instability of this molecule on the cell surfaces.[3] Sialophorin is encoded by a gene on the short arm of chromosome 16, whereas the susceptibility gene for this immunodeficiency disease is on the short arm of the X chromosome. The interrelationship of the two genes or their products (if any) in causing this disorder is unknown.

Several patients who required splenectomy for uncontrollable bleeding had impressive rises in their platelet counts and have done well clinically while on long-term antibiotic and antibody replacement therapy with IVIG. A number of patients with this disorder have had complete corrections of both the platelet and the immunologic abnormalities by HLA-identical sibling bone marrow transplants after being conditioned with irradiation or busulfan and cyclophosphamide.[60] Success has been minimal with T cell–depleted haploidentical stem cell transplants in this condition, primarily because of the requirement for pretransplant immunosuppression to permit engraftment, the long time course to immunoreconstitution when T cells are depleted, and the high mortality from pre-existing opportunistic infections in that setting.

Ataxia Telangiectasia

Ataxia telangiectasia is a complex syndrome with neurologic, immunologic, endocrinologic, hepatic, and cutaneous abnormalities. Inheritance follows an autosomal recessive pattern.[2, 65] The abnormal gene has been mapped to the long arm of chromosome 11 (11q22–23).[65, 66] The most prominent clinical features are progressive cerebellar ataxia, oculocutaneous telangiectasias, chronic sinopulmonary disease, a high incidence of malignancy, and variable humoral and cellular immunodeficiency. Ataxia typically becomes evident soon after the child begins to walk and progresses until he or she is confined to a wheelchair, usually by the age of 10 to 12 years. The telangiectasias develop between 3 and 6 years of age. Recurrent, usually bacterial, sinopulmonary infections occur in roughly 80 per cent of these patients, but common viral exanthems and smallpox vaccination have not usually resulted in untoward sequelae. Fatal varicella, however, occurred in one of the author's patients.

Cells from patients as well as those of heterozygous carriers have increased sensitivity to ionizing radiation, defective DNA repair, and frequent chromosomal abnormalities.[65, 66] The sites of chromosomal breakage involve chromosomes 7 and 14 in more than 50 per cent of cases. The breakpoints involve the genes that code for the T cell receptor and immunoglobulin heavy chains, most likely accounting for the combined T and B cell abnormalities seen. Inversion of chromosome 7-inv (7) (p14q35) is the most frequent rearrangement seen, although others involve chromosome 14 and the X chromosome. These rearrangements may be clonal and may either be stable or undergo malignant transformation. The malignancies reported in this condition have usually been of the lymphoreticular type, but adenocarcinoma and other forms have also been seen; there is also an increased incidence of malignancy in unaffected relatives. The most frequent humoral immunologic abnormality is the selective absence of IgA, found in from 50 to 80 per cent of these patients; hypercatabolism of IgA is also known to occur.[65] IgE concentrations are usually low, and the IgM may be of the low molecular weight variety. IgG2 or total IgG may be decreased. Specific antibody titers may be decreased or normal. In vivo there is impaired (but not absent) cell-mediated immunity, as evidenced by delayed cutaneous anergy and prolonged allograft survival. In vitro tests of lymphocyte function have generally shown moderately depressed proliferative responses to T and B cell mitogens. There are moderately reduced percentages of CD3+ and CD4+ T cells, with normal or increased percentages of CD8+ T cells and elevated numbers of gamma/delta T cell receptor-positive cells.[67] Studies of immunoglobulin synthesis have shown both helper T cell and intrinsic B cell defects. The thymus is hypoplastic, exhibits poor organization, and is lacking in Hassall's corpuscles. No satisfactory treatment has been found.[65]

Cartilage-Hair Hypoplasia

In 1965, an unusual form of short-limbed dwarfism with frequent and severe infections was reported among the Pennsylvania Amish; non-Amish cases have since been described.[2, 68] Features include short and pudgy hands; redundant skin; hyperextensible joints of hands and feet but an inability to extend the elbows completely; and fine, sparse light hair and eyebrows. Radiographically, the bones show scalloping and sclerotic or cystic changes in the metaphyses and flaring of the costochondral junctions of the ribs. Severe and often fatal varicella infections, progressive vaccinia, and vaccine-associated poliomyelitis have been observed.

The severity of the immunodeficiency varies; in one series, 11 of 77 patients died before age 20, but two were still alive at age 76. Three patterns of immune dysfunction have emerged: defective antibody mediated immunity, defective cellular immunity (most common form), and severe combined immunodeficiency. In vitro studies have shown decreased numbers of T cells and defective T cell proliferation owing to an intrinsic defect related to the G1 phase, resulting in a longer cell cycle for individual cells.[68] This abnormality also occurs in fibroblasts from these patients. NK cells, however, are increased in number and function. Cartilage-hair hypoplasia appears to be inherited as an autosomal recessive condition with variable penetrance. Bone marrow transplantation has resulted in immunologic reconstitution in some cartilage-hair hypoplasia patients with the SCID phenotype.

Immunodeficiency with Thymoma

Patients with immunodeficiency with thymoma are adults who almost simultaneously develop recurrent infections, panhypogammaglobulinemia, deficits in cell-mediated immunity, and benign thymoma.[2] They may also have eosinophilia or eosinopenia, aregenerative or hemolytic anemia, agranulocytosis, thrombocytopenia, or pancytopenia. Antibody formation is poor, and progressive lymphopenia develops, although percentages of Ig-bearing B lymphocytes are usually normal. Several patients with this disorder have been shown to have excessive suppressor T cell activity. The thymomas are predominantly of the spindle cell variety, although other types of benign and malignant thymic tumors have also been seen.

Hyperimmunoglobulinemia E Syndrome

The hyperimmunoglobulinemia E (hyper IgE) syndrome is a relatively rare primary immunodeficiency syndrome characterized by recurrent severe staphylococcal abscesses and markedly elevated levels of serum IgE.[69] The disorder was first reported by the author and her coworkers in two young boys in 1972; since then she has evaluated a total of 30 patients with the condition, and many other examples have been reported. These patients all have histories of staphylococcal abscesses involving the skin, lungs, joints, and other sites from infancy; persistent pneumatoceles develop as a result of their recurrent pneumonias. The pruritic dermatitis that occurs is not typical atopic eczema, and it does not always persist; respiratory allergic symptoms are usually absent.

Laboratory features include exceptionally high serum IgE; elevated serum IgD; usually normal concentrations of IgG, IgA, and IgM; pronounced blood and sputum eosinophilia; abnormally low anamnestic antibody responses to booster immunizations; and poor antibody-mediated and cell-mediated responses to neoantigens. In vitro studies have shown normal percentages of CD2+, CD3+, CD4+, and CD8+ lymphocytes, and there is no increase in the percentage of IgE-bearing B lymphocytes. Most have normal lymphocyte proliferative responses to mitogens but very low or absent responses to antigens or allogeneic cells from family members. Possibly related to this is the observation by the author of a decreased percentage of T cells with the memory (CD45RO) phenotype in the blood of these patients. Blood, sputum, and histologic sections of lymph nodes, spleen, and lung cysts show striking eosinophilia. Hassall's corpuscles and normal thymic architecture were observed at postmortem examination of one patient.

Phagocytic cell ingestion, metabolism, killing, and total hemolytic complement activity have been normal in all patients. Variable defects of mononuclear or polymorphonuclear chemotaxis have been present in some but not all patients and hence are not the basic problem in these patients.[69]

The fact that both men and women have been affected, as have members of succeeding generations, suggests an autosomal dominant form of inheritance with incomplete penetrance. The most effective management for this condition consists of long-term therapy with a penicillinase-resistant penicillin, with the addition of other antibiotics or antifungal agents as required for specific infections, and appropriate thoracic surgery for superinfected pneumatoceles or those persisting beyond 6 months.

Leukocyte Adhesion Deficiency (CD11/CD18 Deficiency)

This condition is due to mutations in the gene on chromosome 21q22.3 encoding the 95 kd molecular weight β subunit (CD18) shared by three adhesive heterodimers: LFA-1 on B, T, and NK lymphocytes; complement receptor type 3 (CR3) on neutrophils, monocytes, macrophages, eosinophils, and NK cells; and p150,95 (another complement receptor).[16, 73] The alpha chains of these three molecules (encoded by genes on chromosome 16) are not expressed because of the abnormal β chain. Those so affected have histories of delayed separation of the umbilical cord, omphalitis, gingivitis, recurrent skin infections, repeated otitis media, pneumonia, peritonitis, perianal abscesses, and impaired wound healing. Severe, widespread, and life-threatening bacterial and fungal infections account for the high mortality. They do not have increased susceptibility to viral infections or malignancy. All cytotoxic lymphocyte functions are markedly impaired because of a lack of the adhesion protein LFA-1; deficiency of LFA-1 also interferes with immune cell interaction and immune recognition. CR3 binds fixed iC3b fragments of C3 and β-glucans; its absence causes abnormal phagocytic cell adherence and chemotaxis and a reduced respiratory burst with phagocytosis. Blood neutrophil counts are usually significantly elevated even when no infection is present. Deficiencies of these glycoproteins can be screened for by cytofluorography of blood leukocytes with any of the following monoclonal antibodies: anti-Mac-1, OKM1, Leu 15, or anti-Mol, which react with the α chain of CR3, or with anti-Leu-M5, specific for the α chain of p150,95. This disease can be corrected by bone marrow transplantation.[60] Since the CD18 gene has been cloned and sequenced, this disorder is also considered a leading candidate for gene therapy.

T Cell Activation Defects

These conditions are characterized by the presence of T cells that appear phenotypically normal by many criteria but that fail to proliferate or produce cytokines in response to stimulation with mitogens, antigens, or other signals delivered to the T cell antigen receptor (TCR). A number of these have

been characterized at the molecular level, including patients who had (1) defective surface expression of the CD3/TCR complex, owing to failure of the CD3 zeta chain to associate with the rest of the components of CD3;[71] (2) defective signal transduction from the TCR to intracellular metabolic pathways;[72, 73] or (3) pretranslational defects in IL-2 (T cell growth factor) or other cytokine production.[74] These patients have clinical problems similar to those of other T cell–deficient individuals, although somewhat less severe than in SCID patients.

Seventy per cent of the circulating CD3+ T cells of a patient whose sibling had died with thymic dysplasia were found to bear disulfide-bonded gamma/delta TCRs.[75] She was lymphopenic, and her T cells exhibited a progressive decline in mitogen responsiveness over 5 years. A thymic biopsy revealed only a single Hassall's corpuscle and a deficiency of both medullary epithelium and thymocytes. Despite these abnormalities, her clinical history was unremarkable.

INTRAUTERINE DIAGNOSIS AND CARRIER DETECTION

Intrauterine diagnoses of ADA[14] and PNP[15] deficiencies can be made by enzyme analyses on amnion cells (fresh or cultured) obtained before 20 weeks gestation and of several X-linked defects by RFLP studies of the X chromosome in amnion cells from male infants whose mothers have been identified as carriers and who are heterozygous for informative DNA polymorphisms.[76] Diagnosis of enzyme-normal SCID or other severe T cell deficiencies, MHC class I or II antigen deficiencies, CGD or Wiskott-Aldrich syndrome (by platelet size) can be made by appropriate tests of phenotype or function on small samples of blood obtained by fetoscopy at 18 to 22 weeks of gestation. In the case of those disorders for which the defective gene has been cloned and cDNA probes are available (CGD, ADA, PNP, and LAD), the diagnosis can be made by deletional or RFLP analyses of chorionic villus samples obtained during the first trimester.

Carriers of ADA and PNP deficiency can be detected by quantitative enzyme analyses of blood samples. Carriers of X-linked agammaglobulinemia,[33] X-linked SCID,[58] or the Wiskott-Aldrich syndrome[64] can be identified by one of two techniques designed to detect nonrandom X chromosome inactivation in one or more blood cell lineages.[16] One method employs somatic cell hybrids that selectively retain the active X chromosome, and the other depends on methylation differences between the active and inactive X chromosomes. Either method can be used successfully even when only one member of a family (or no previous members) has been affected, since neither of these methods depends on linkage analysis.[16, 58]

TREATMENT

The principal modes of therapy for the primary immunodeficiency disorders include protective isolation, use of antibiotics for the eradication or prevention of bacterial and fungal infections, and attempted replacement of missing humoral or cellular immunologic functions. The complexities of both the immunodeficiency diseases and their treatment emphasize the need for all such patients to be evaluated in centers where detailed studies of immune function can be conducted before therapy is selected or begun.

Antibody Deficiency Disorders

Judicious use of antibiotics and regular administration of antibodies are the only treatments that have proved effective for this group of disorders. Patients with agammaglobulinemia, X-linked immunodeficiency with hyper IgM, antibody deficiency with near-normal immunoglobulins, Wiskott-Aldrich syndrome, and all forms of SCID are candidates for immunoglobulin replacement therapy.[10, 11] The most common form of replacement therapy currently is with immune serum globulin (ISG) modified for safe intravenous use (IVIG). All seven IVIG preparations in the United States approved by the Food and Drug Administration consist primarily of IgG antibodies, with small amounts of antibodies of the other classes.[10] Experience suggests that 400 mg per kg per month of IVIG permits achievement of trough IgG levels close to the normal range. HIV is inactivated by the ethanol used in preparation of ISG and IVIG; such preparations are also free of hepatitis antigen. Systemic reactions to IVIG may occur, but rarely are these true anaphylactic reactions. Anaphylactic reactions caused by IgE antibodies (in the patient) to IgA (in the IVIG preparation) may, however, occur in patients with common variable immunodeficiency who have absent serum IgA.[44] All newly diagnosed patients with the latter defect should be screened for anti-IgA antibodies through the American Red Cross before undergoing IVIG therapy. If such antibodies are detected, IVIG therapy may still be possible by use of IVIG containing almost no IgA (Gammagard, Baxter-Hyland, or a similar preparation from the American Red Cross).[10]

Immunoglobulin replacement therapy is contraindicated in patients with selective absence of serum and secretory IgA, owing to the high frequency of anti-IgA antibodies[6, 44] and because these patients usually have normal quantities of IgG antibodies.[10, 11] IVIG should also not be given to infants with transient hypogammaglobulinemia of infancy because it could suppress their innate capacity to form antibodies. There is no indication for the use of gammaglobulin therapy in patients with IgG subclass deficiencies unless they have been shown to have a broad defect in antibody-forming capacity,

and it is futile to give it to patients with low IgG owing to protein-losing states.[10]

Cellular Immunodeficiency

The only adequate therapy for patients with severe forms of cellular immunodeficiency is immunologic reconstitution by means of an immunocompetent tissue transplant.[57, 60, 61, 61a] Bone marrow cells that are MHC compatible or haploidentical with the recipient are the treatment of choice. There is no convincing evidence that thymic transplants cause

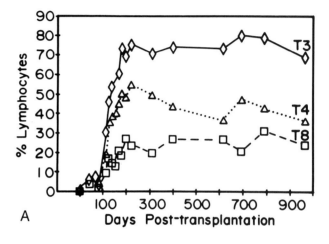

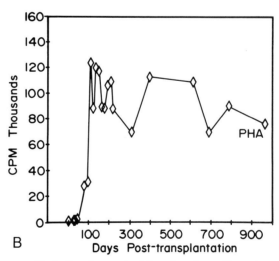

Figure 74–6. Development of lymphocytes with mature T cell phenotypes (top) and function (bottom) in a male infant with severe combined immune deficiency after a maternal bone marrow stem cell transplant. All cells dividing in response to phytohemagglutinin had a female karyotype. The 90- to 100-day lag before the maternal stem cells have been matured completely by the infant's thymus is reminiscent of the time it takes for mature T cells to appear in the human embryo. (From Buckley, R. H.: Normal and abnormal development of the immune system. *In* Joklik, W. K., et al. [eds.]: Zinsser Microbiology. 19th ed. East Norwalk, CT, Appleton & Lange, 1988, p. 226, used by permission.)

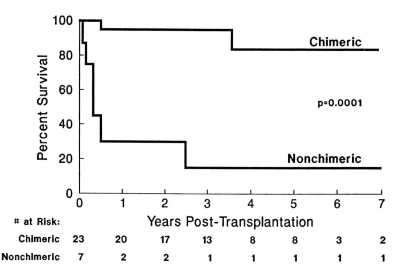

Figure 74–7. Kaplan-Meier estimates of probability of survival in severe combined immunodeficiency disorder (SCID) patients transplanted with T cell–depleted haploidentical marrow, with and without chimerism. Once chimerism is achieved, survival matches that of recipients of unfractionated HLA-identical marrow.

# at Risk:	0	1	2	3	4	5	6	7
Chimeric	23	20	17	13	8	8	3	2
Nonchimeric	7	2	2	1	1	1	1	1

immunologic reconstitution in DiGeorge's syndrome, whereas unfractionated HLA-identical bone marrow transplantation has been effective in all three DiGeorge patients in whom this was attempted.[56] The major risk to the recipient from transplants of bone marrow or fetal tissues is that of GVHD. The development of techniques to deplete all post-thymic T cells from donor marrow has, however, permitted the safe and successful use of haploidentical (half-matched) bone marrow cells for the correction of SCID (Fig. 74–6).[57, 60, 61, 61a] These techniques have employed (1) initial incubation with soybean lectin followed by two rosette-depletion steps with sheep erythrocytes (the most successful approach) or (2) incubation with monoclonal antibodies to T cells plus complement. Both methods enrich the final cell suspension for stem cells. To date, more than 150 infants with SCID who lacked an HLA-identical donor have been treated with T cell–depleted haploidentical pa-

rental bone marrow, with usually little or no GVHD; approximately 60 per cent survive with successful immune reconstitution (Fig. 74–7). Patients with less severe forms of cellular immunodeficiency reject such grafts unless they are treated with immunosuppressive agents before transplantation, and even then there has been a high incidence of resistance to engraftment of T cell–depleted, half-matched marrow cells.[60, 61, 61a] Several patients with Wiskott-Aldrich syndrome and other forms of partial cellular immunodeficiency have been treated successfully with (usually HLA-identical) bone marrow transplants after immunosuppression. Cytokine therapy has been considered as a potential approach to the treatment of patients who for various reasons have not been candidates for bone marrow transplantation. Limited clinical trials with recombinant IL-2 (or T cell growth factor) therapy have shown beneficial effects in some patients with T cell activation defects

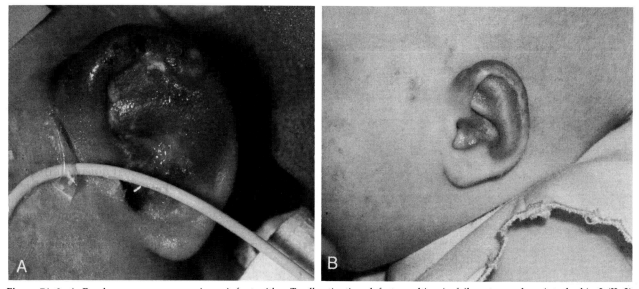

Figure 74–8. A, Pyoderma gangrenosum in an infant with a T cell activation defect resulting in failure to produce interleukin-2 (IL-2). B, After 2 weeks of therapy with recombinant IL-2.

(Fig. 74–8).[77] Finally, it is entirely possible that a number of genetic defects, including ADA and PNP deficiencies, LAD, and CGD, will be correctable in the future by gene therapy.

References

1. Bruton, O. C.: Agammaglobulinemia. Pediatr. 9:722, 1952.
2. Primary immunodeficiency diseases—report of a WHO sponsored meeting. Immunodef. Rev. 1:173, 1989.
3. Remold-O'Donnell, E., and Rosen, F. S.: Sialophorin (CD43) and the Wiskott-Aldrich syndrome. Immunodef. Rev. 2:151, 1990.
4. French, M. A., and Dawkins, R. L.: Central MHC genes, IgA deficiency and autoimmune diseases. Immunol. Today 11:271, 1990.
5. Penn, I.: Lymphoproliferative diseases in disorders of the immune system. Cancer Detect. Prev. 14:415, 1990.
6. Clark, J. A., Callicoat, P. A., and Brenner, N. A.: Selective IgA deficiency in blood donors. Am. J. Clin. Pathol. 80:210, 1983.
7. Buckley, R. H.: Clinical and immunologic features of selective IgA deficiency. In Bergsma, D., Good, R. A., Finstad, J., and Paul, N. W. (eds.): Immunodeficiency in Man and Animals. Stamford, CT, Sinauer Associates, 1975.
8. Altman, P. L.: Blood leukocyte values: Man. In Dittmer, D. S. (ed.): Blood and Other Body Fluids. Washington, D. C., Federation of American Societies for Experimental Biology, 1961.
9. Gossage, D. L., and Buckley, R. H.: Prevalence of lymphocytopenia in severe combined immunodeficiency. N. Engl. J. Med. 323:1422, 1990.
10. Buckley, R. H., and Schiff, R. I.: The use of intravenous immunoglobulin in immunodeficiency diseases. N. Engl. J. Med. 325:110, 1991.
11. Eibl, M. M., and Wedgwood, R. J.: Intravenous immunoglobulin: A review. Immunodef. Rev. 1(Suppl.):1, 1989.
12. Buckley, R. H.: Abnormal development of the immune system. In Joklik, W. K., et al. (eds.): Zinsser Microbiology. 20th ed. East Norwalk, CT, Appleton & Lange, 1992, p. 327.
13. Fischer, A., Lisowska-Grospierre, B., Anderson, D. C., and Springer, T. A.: Leukocyte adhesion deficiency: Molecular basis and functional consequences. Immunodef. Rev. 1:39, 1988.
14. Hirschhorn, R.: Adenosine deaminase deficiency. Immunodef. Rev. 2:175, 1990.
15. Markert, M. L.: Purine nucleoside phosphorylase deficiency. Immunodef. Rev. 3:45, 1991.
16. Winkelstein, J. A., and Fearon, E.: Carrier detection of the X-linked primary immunodeficiency diseases using X-chromosome inactivation analysis. J. Allerg. Clin. Immunol. 85:1090, 1990.
17. Schwaber, J., and Rosen, F. S.: X chromosome linked immunodeficiency. Immunodef. Rev. 2:233, 1990.
18. Kwan, S. P., Kunkel, L., and Bruns, G.: Mapping of the X-linked agammaglobulinemia locus by use of restriction fragment-length polymorphism. J. Clin. Invest. 77:649, 1986.
19. deSaint Basile, G., Arveiler, B., and Oberle, I.: Close linkage of the locus for X chromosome-linked severe combined immunodeficiency to polymorphic DNA markers in Xq11-q13. Proc. Natl. Acad. Sci. U.S.A. 84:7576, 1987.
20. de Saint Basile, G., Fraser, N. J., Craig, I. W., et al.: Close linkage of hypervariable marker DXS255 to disease locus of Wiskott-Aldrich syndrome. Lancet 2:1319, 1989.
21. Sullivan, J. L., and Woda, B. A.: X-linked lymphoproliferative syndrome. Immunodef. Rev. 1:325, 1989.
22. Griscelli, C., Lisowska-Grospierre, B., and Mach, B.: Combined immunodeficiency with defective expression in MHC class II genes. Immunodef. Rev. 1:135, 1989.
23. Hume, C. R., and Lee, J. S.: Congenital immunodeficiencies associated with absence of HLA Class II antigens on lymphocytes result from distinct mutation in transacting factors. Hum. Immunol. 26:288, 1989.
24. Reith, W., Satola, S., and Herrero Sanchez, C.: Congenital immunodeficiency with a regulatory defect in MHC Class II gene expression lacks a specific HLA-Dr promoter binding protein, RF-X. Cell 53:897, 1988.
25. Lefranc, M. P., Hammarstrom, L., Smith, C. I. E., and Lefranc, G.: Gene deletions in the human immunoglobulin heavy chain constant region locus: Molecular and immunological analysis. Immunol. Rev. 2:265, 1991.
26. Mohiuddin, A. A., Corren, J., Harbeck, R. J., Teague, J. L., Volz, M., and Gelfand, E. W.: Ureaplasma urealyticum chronic osteomyelitis in a patient with hypogammaglobulinemia. J. Allergy Clin. Immunol. 87:104, 1991.
27. Lederman, H. M., and Winkelstein, J. A.: X-linked agammaglobulinemia: An analysis of 96 patients. Medicine 64:145, 1985.
28. Wilfert, C. M., Buckley, R. H., Mohanakumar, T., et al.: Persistent and fatal central nervous system Echovirus infections in patients with agammaglobulinemia. N. Engl. J. Med. 296:1485, 1977.
29. McKinney, R. E., Katz, S. L., and Wilfert, C. M.: Chronic enteroviral meningoenceophalitis in agammaglobulinemic patients. Rev. Infect. Dis. 9:334, 1987.
30. Working Party on Hypogammaglobulinemia: Hypogammaglobulinemia in the United Kingdom. Medical Research Council Special Report Series 310:1, 1971.
31. Leickly, F. E., and Buckley, R. H.: Variability in B cell maturation and differentiation in X-linked agammaglobulinemia. Clin. Exp. Immunol. 65:90, 1986.
32. Campana, D., Farrant, J., Inamdar, N., Webster, A. D. B., and Janossy, G.: Phenotypic features and proliferative activity of B cell progenitors in X-linked agammaglobulinemia. J. Immunol. 145:1675, 1990.
33. Conley, M. E., Brown, P., Pickard, A. R., et al.: Expression of the gene defect in X-linked agammaglobulinemia. N. Engl. J. Med. 315:5648, 1986.
34. Cunningham-Rundles, C.: Clinical and immunologic analyses of 103 patients with common variable immunodeficiency. J. Clin. Immunol. 9:22, 1989.
35. Webster, A. D., Loewi, G., Dourmashkin, R. D., Golding, D. N., Ward, D. J., and Asherson, G. L.: Polyarthritis in adults with hypogammaglobulinaemia and its rapid response to immunoglobulin treatment. Br. Med. J. 1:1314, 1976.
36. Baum, C. G., Chiorazzi, N., Frankel, S., and Shepherd, G. M.: Conversion of systemic lupus erythematosus to common variable hypogammaglobulinemia. Am. J. Med. 87:449, 1989.
37. Cunningham-Rundles, C., Siegal, F. P., Cunningham-Rundles, S., and Lieberman, P.: Incidence of cancer in 98 patients with common varied immunodeficiency. J. Clin. Immunol. 7:294, 1987.
38. Spickett, G. P., Webster, A. D. B., and Farrant, J.: Cellular abnormalities in common variable immunodeficiency. Immunodef. Rev. 2:199, 1990.
39. Schaffer, F. M., Palermos, J., Zhu, Z. B., Barger, B. D., Cooper, M. D., and Volanakis, J. E.: Individuals with IgA deficiency and common variable immunodeficiency share complex polymorphisms of major histocompatibility complex class III genes. Proc. Natl. Acad. Sci. U.S.A. 86:8015, 1989.
40. Howe, H. S., So, A. K. L., Farrant, J., and Webster, A. D. B.: Common variable immunodeficiency is associated with polymorphic markers in the human major histocompatibility complex. Clin. Exp. Immunol. 84:387, 1991.
41. Preud'Homme, J. L., and Hanson, L. A.: IgG subclass deficiency. Immunodef. Rev. 2:129, 1990.
42. Oxelius, V. A., Laurell, A. B., and Lindquist, B.: IgG subclasses in selective IgA deficiency. N. Engl. J. Med. 304:1476, 1981.
43. Ambrosino, D. M., Umetsu, D. T., Siber, G. R., et al.: Selective defect in the antibody response to Haemophilus influenzae type b in children with recurrent infections and normal IgG subclass levels. J. Allergy Clin. Immunol. 81:1175, 1988.
44. Burks, A. W., Sampson, H. A., and Buckley, R. H.: Anaphylactic reactions after gamma globulin administration in patients with hypogammaglobulinemia. N. Engl. J. Med. 314:560, 1986.
45. Goshen, E., Livne, A., Krupp, M., et al.: Antinuclear and related autoantibodies in sera of healthy subjects with IgA deficiency. J. Autoimmun. 2:51, 1989.
46. Conley, M. E., and Cooper, M. D.: Immature IgA B cells in IgA deficient patients. N. Engl. J. Med. 305:495, 1981.
47. Leickly, F. E., and Buckley, R. H.: Development of IgA and IgG2 subclass deficiency after sulfasalazine therapy. J. Pediatr. 108:481, 1986.
48. Cobain, T. J., Stuckey, M. S., McCluskey, J., et al.: The coexistence of IgA deficiency and 21-hydroxylase deficiency marked by specific MHC supratypes. Ann. N. Y. Acad. Sci. 458:76, 1985.
49. Plebani, A., Monafo, V., Ugazio, A. G., and Burgio, G. R.: Clinical heterogeneity and reversibility of selective immunoglobulin A deficiency in 80 children. Lancet 1:829, 1986.
50. Strober, W., Krakauer, R., Klaeveman, H. L., Reynolds, H. Y., and Nelson, D. L.: Secretory component deficiency. N. Engl. J. Med. 294:351, 1976.
51. Akahori, Y., Kurosawa, Y., Kamachi, Y., Torii, S., and Matsuoka, H.: Presence of immunoglobulin (Ig) M and IgG double isotype-bearing cells and defect of switch recombination in hyper IgM immunodeficiency. J. Clin. Invest. 85:1722, 1990.
52. Mayer, L., Swan, S. P., and Thompson, C.: Evidence for a defect in "switch" T cells in patients with immunodeficiency and hyperimmunoglobulinemia M. N. Engl. J. Med. 314:409, 1986.
53. Tiller, T. L., and Buckley, R. H.: Transient hypogammaglobulinemia of infancy: Review of the literature, clinical and immunologic features of 11 new cases, and long-term follow-up. J. Pediatr. 92:347, 1978.
54. Knutsen, A. P., Merten, D. F., and Buckley, R. H.: Colonic nodular lymphoid hyperplasia in a child with antibody deficiency and near normal immunoglobulins. J. Pediatr. 98:420, 1981.
55. Fibison, W. J., Budarf, M., McDermid, H., Greenberg, F., and Emanuel, B. S.: Molecular studies of DiGeorge syndrome. Am. J. Hum. Genet. 46:888, 1990.

56. Goldsobel, A. B., Haas, A., and Stiehm, E. R.: Bone marrow transplantation in DiGeorge syndrome. J. Pediatr. 111:40, 1987.
57. Buckley, R. H., Schiff, S. E., Sampson, H. A., et al.: Development of immunity in human severe primary T cell deficiency following haploidentical bone marrow stem cell transplantation. J. Immunol. 136:2398, 1986.
58. Conley, M. E., Buckley, R. H., Hong, R., et al.: X-linked severe combined immunodeficiency. Diagnosis in males with sporadic severe combined immunodeficiency and clarification of clinical findings. J. Clin. Invest. 85:1548, 1990.
58a. Fischer, A.: Severe combined immunodeficiencies. Immunodef. Rev. 3:83, 1992.
59. Sindel, L. J., Buckley, R. H., Schiff, S. E., et al.: Severe combined immunodeficiency with natural killer cell predominance: Abrogation of graft-versus-host disease and immunologic reconstitution with HLA-identical bone marrow cells. J. Allergy Clin. Immunol. 73:829, 1984.
60. Buckley, R. H.: Bone marrow transplantation in treatment of severe primary T cell immunodeficiency: Recent advances. Pediatr. Ann. 16:412, 1987.
61. O'Reilly, R. J., Keever, C. A., Small, T. N., and Brochstein, J.: The use of HLA-non-identical T cell depleted marrow transplants for correction of severe combined immunodeficiency disease. Immunodef. Rev. 1:273, 1989.
61a. Fischer, A., Landais, P., Friedrich, W., et al.: European experience of bone marrow transplantation for severe combined immunodeficiency. Lancet 336:850, 1990.
62. Hershfield, M. S., Buckley, R. H., Greenberg, M. L., et al.: Treatment of adenosine deaminase deficiency with polyethylene glycol-modified adenosine deaminase (PEG-ADA). N. Engl. J. Med. 316:589, 1987.
63. Gougeon, M. L., Drean, G., LeDeist, F., et al.: Human severe combined immunodeficiency disease. Phenotypic and functional characteristics of peripheral B lymphocytes. J. Immunol. 145:2873, 1990.
64. Greer, W. L., Kwong, P. C., Peacocke, M., Ip, P., Rubin, L. A., and Siminovitch, K. A.: X-chromosome inactivation in the Wiskott-Aldrich syndrome: A marker for detection of the carrier state and identification of cell lineages expressing the gene defect. Genomics 4:60, 1989.
65. Gatti, R. A., Boder, E., Vinters, H. V., Sparkes, R. S., Norman, A.,

and Lange, K.: Ataxia-telangiectasia: An interdisciplinary approach to pathogenesis. Medicine 70:99, 1991.
66. Swift, M.: Genetic aspects of ataxia telangiectasia. Immunodef. Rev. 2:67, 1990.
67. Carbonari, M., Cherchi, M., Paganelli, R., et al.: Relative increase of T cells expressing the gamma/delta rather than the alpha/beta receptor in ataxia telangiectasia. N. Engl. J. Med. 322:73, 1990.
68. Polmar, S. H., and Pierce, G. F.: Cartilage hair hypoplasia: Immunological aspects and their clinical implications. Clin. Immunol. Immunopathol. 40:87, 1986.
69. Buckley, R. H., and Sampson, H. A.: The hyperimmunoglobulinemia E syndrome. In Franklin, E. C. (ed.): Clinical Immunology Update. New York, Elsevier North-Holland, 1981.
70. Todd, R. F., and Freyer, D. R.: The CD11/CD18 leukocyte glycoprotein deficiency. Hematol. Oncol. Clin. North Am. 2:13, 1988.
71. Alarcon, B., Regueiro, J. R., Arnaiz-Villena, A., and Terhorst, C.: Familial defect in the surface expression of the T cell receptor CD3 complex. N. Engl. J. Med. 319:1203, 1988.
72. Chatila, T., Wong, R., Young, M., Miller, R., Terhorst, C., and Geha, R. S.: An immunodeficiency characterized by defective signal transduction in T lymphocytes. N. Engl. J. Med. 320:696, 1989.
73. Rijkers, G. T., Scharenberg, J. G. M., VanDongen, J. J. M., Neijens, H. J., and Zegers, B. J. M.: Abnormal signal transduction in a patient with severe combined immunodeficiency disease. Pediatr. Res. 29:306, 1991.
74. Weinberg, K., and Parkman, R.: Severe combined immunodeficiency due to a specific defect in the production of interleukin-2. N. Engl. J. Med. 322:1718, 1990.
75. Geisler, C., Pallesen, G., and Platz, P.: Novel primary thymic defect with T lymphocytes expressing gamma/delta T cell receptor. J. Clin. Pathol. 43:705, 1989.
76. Puck, J. M., Krauss, C., Puck, S. M., Buckley, R. H., and Conley, M. E.: Prenatal exclusion of X chromosome linked severe combined immunodeficiency using maternal nonrandom T cell X inactivtion and linkage analysis. N. Engl. J. Med. 321:1063, 1990.
77. Pahwa, R., Chatila, T., Pahwa, S., et al.: Recombinant interleukin 2 therapy in severe combined immunodeficiency disease. Proc. Natl. Acad. Sci. U.S.A. 86:5069, 1989.

Complement Deficiencies and Rheumatic Diseases

INTRODUCTION

Homozygous or, in the case of C4, heterozygous deficiency of classic pathway complement components, e.g., C1, C4, or C2, is associated with an increased frequency of diseases caused by immune complexes such as systemic lupus erythematosus (SLE).[1,2] Homozygous deficiency of components that form the membrane attack complex, e.g., C5, C6, C7, or C8, predisposes to recurrent *Neisseria* infections,[3] including recurrent gonococcal arthritis. For both of these reasons, knowledge of complement genetics and deficiencies is clinically important.[4] Information about the basic functions of the complement system is contained in Chapter 10.

COMPLEMENT GENETICS

All of the genes for the complement proteins have been cloned and many have been localized to particular chromosomes. Two important linkage groups are known: (1) those located in the major histocompatibility region on the sixth chromosome, including C2, factor B, and C4 (MHC group);[5,6] and (2) the group located on the first chromosome, including C4 binding protein (C4BP), factor I, decay accelerating factor (DAF), and other regulators of complement activation (the RCA group)[7,8]

Complement Genes in the MHC

On the short arm of the sixth human chromosome, about 700 Kb downstream from the HLA-A, B, and C loci that code for the class I histocompatibility antigens, is a stretch of approximately 100 Kb containing the genes for the class III products of the MHC, including C2, factor B (Bf), and the two genes for C4, (C4A and C4B) (Fig. 75–1). These four genes are not only closely linked, they are also functionally related, being involved in the formation of C3 convertases.[9] Two genes related to the 21-beta (β) hydroxylase enzymes of steroid metabolism, 21A and 21B, are in tandem with the C4A and C4B genes. Factors B and C2 exhibit extensive sequence homology as well as the functional homology of providing the enzymatically active site for the alternative and classic pathway convertases, respectively. The C2 gene probably arose by tandem gene duplication from factor B (Bf), which occupies a more primitive place in phylogeny. Both are polymorphic, with more than ten electrophoretic variants known for Bf and at least five isoelectric variants for C2.[10] Gene duplication presumably also accounts for the two C4 genes (C4A and C4B), which differ slightly in amino acid sequence and very much in activity.[11,12] Products of

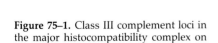
Supported by NIH Grant Numbers AR07079–15, AI28532–03, and AI 13049–15.

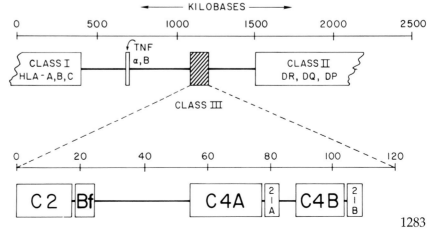

Figure 75–1. Class III complement loci in the major histocompatibility complex on chromosome 6.

the C4A gene tend to combine covalently in amide linkages with free amino groups, and are hemolytically less active on a weight basis than C4B gene products, which preferentially link via ester linkages to hydroxyl residues.[12] The human erythrocyte blood grouping "antigens," Chido and Rodgers, are actually fragments of C4B and C4A, respectively, which are deposited on erythrocytes when the complement system is activated as blood clots.[13]

Certain combinations of alleles within the MHC occur with much greater frequency than would be predicted from chance recombination among an outbred population.[14] Such "supratypes" tend to appear as chunks or blocks of DNA even among unrelated individuals.[15] One such example is the combination HLA-B8 C4AQ0 C4B1 BfS C2C DR3, which contains the "Q0" allele coding for nonsynthesis of C4A;[16] another is HLA-B18 C4A4 C4B2 BfS C2Q0 DR2, coding for nonsynthesis of C2.[17] Both of these are associated with increased susceptibility to autoimmune disorders such as SLE or type I diabetes, yet they remain as stable allelic combinations within the population.

Regulators of Complement Activation

The genes for six proteins that control the activity of C3 convertases are located in a region spanning 1000 to 1500 Kb in the q32 band of the first human chromosome.[7, 8, 18] These include the C4b/C3b receptor (CR1), the C3d receptor (CR2), decay accelerating factor (DAF), C4 binding protein (C4BP), factor H (H), and membrane cofactor protein (MCP). All members of this group share homologous short consensus repeats (SCRs) of 60 amino acids, characterized by a framework of four very highly conserved cysteines. Although many of the members of the RCA group share the function of binding to C3, the SCRs are not directly homologous with this function. They are also found in other complement proteins, including C2 and factor B (three each) and C1r and C1s (two each) as well as in a protein of unknown function (beta (β)-2 glycoprotein I), the interleukin-2 receptor (CD25), the leukocyte common antigen (CD45), and factor XIII of the clotting system.[19]

SPECIFIC DEFICIENCY STATES FOUND WITH RHEUMATIC DISEASES

Detection of Deficiency States

With the exception of C4, which is controlled by two genes, and properdin, which is X-linked, deficiencies of complement proteins are inherited codominantly as "null alleles," with a single null gene coding for approximately half-normal levels, and two null alleles coding for complete deficiency.[20] For the classic activation pathway (C1, C4, C2) or the terminal sequence (C5-C9), the total hemolytic comple-

ment performed with sheep erythrocytes coated with rabbit antibody is a reliable screen for homozygous deficiency. For the alternative pathway, lysis of rabbit erythrocytes in the absence of exogenous antibody is the screening test of choice. Homozygous deficiency states of all nine of the classic components, three of the four plasma control proteins, and two of the three alternative pathway factors have been described. Because of the wide range of normal for most complement proteins, detection of the heterozygous deficiency state requires family studies. This is particularly true for C4, in which inheritance of null alleles at either the C4A or the C4B locus is possible.

C1q Deficiency

Following an initial report of selective deficiency of the C1q subcomponent of C1 in a young Turkish male with skin disease and nephritis, complete absence of this protein was demonstrated in the sera of three siblings who also had renal and cutaneous lesions.[21] Renal biopsies showed mesangioproliferative glomerulonephritis with deposits of IgM and C3. The skin disease had both clinical and pathologic features of congenital poikiloderma (Rothmund-Thomson syndrome). In a third kindred, one child had a severe lupus-like syndrome, while the other was normal; a dysfunctional C1q molecule, which was antigenically deficient and devoid of activity, was found.[22]

C1r Deficiency

The first patient to be described with C1r deficiency was a female with chronic glomerulonephritis that progressed to end-stage renal disease and required transplantation.[23] The second kindred had for its propositus a 16-year-old Puerto Rican boy with a lupus-like syndrome, including fever, malar rash, arthralgias, and subacute focal membranous glomerulonephritis. Although immunoglobulins and C3 were demonstrated by immunofluorescence as deposited along the glomerular basement membrane, studies of biopsies of the skin lesions, which were typical of discoid lupus erythematosus, failed to reveal the deposits of immunoglobulin and C3 usually observed in such lesions. Serology for antinuclear antibodies and LE cells was negative.[24] The 24-year-old sister of the proband had arthralgias and skin ulcers and was said to have had a malar rash. Her skin biopsy was also negative for deposits of immunoglobulins and C3. Two other siblings had died in infancy of gastroenteritis of unknown cause; a third had died at age 12 of lupus erythematosus. Affected individuals have no detectable total hemolytic complement activity or immunochemical C1r. Levels of C1s are approximately 40 percent of normal, but all other components, including C1q, are normal or elevated. Family studies have identified heterozygotes with 60 to 90 percent of normal mean C1r levels, indicating an autosomal recessive mode of inheritance.

C1s Deficiency

A six-year-old girl with cutaneous manifestations of SLE was the first reported case of C1s deficiency.[25] Tests for antinuclear antibody and for deposits of immunoglobulin in the skin were both positive. Subsequenty a second kindred containing two individuals with C1s deficiency and a lupus-like disease manifested by polyarthritis, alopecia, discoid lupus, Raynaud's phenomenon, and a positive antinuclear antibody test has been reported.[26] Another sibling with the same syndrome had normal complement levels; two others with C1s deficiency were well.

C1 Inhibitor Deficiency

Inherited absence or reduced levels of this important control protein are regularly associated with the clinical syndrome of hereditary angioedema manifested by recurrent swellings of the subepithelial areas of the skin and upper respiratory and gastrointestinal tracts.[27] Patients with C1 inhibitor deficiency have continuous activation of their classic pathway, which results in depressed plasma levels of C4 and C2. They also have an increased frequency of systemic or discoid lupus. In one kindred, a mother with SLE and C1 inhibitor deficiency gave birth to identical twin boys who had discoid lupus.[28] Although measurements of antinuclear antibody were not available for the mother's serum, she did have a false positive VDRL and a negative LE cell test. The twins both had weakly positive antinuclear antibody tests with antibodies to single- but not double-stranded DNA. Measurements of metabolism indicated the profoundly depressed plasma levels and increased fractional catabolic rates for this component usually found in C1 inhibitor deficiency. Another set of twins has one member with symptoms of hereditary angioedema since the age of 6 years who developed classic SLE with positive antinuclear antibodies and antibodies to double-stranded DNA at the age of 14.[29] Her C4 levels before the onset of SLE were less than 4 percent of normal. The twin without symptoms of hereditary angioedema did not develop SLE; her C4 levels ranged between 10 and 15 percent of normal. Three other unrelated patients with C1 inhibitor deficiency and lupus-like disease, manifested predominantly as rash, have been reported.[30] Among 220 patients with C1 inhibitor deficiency, the occurrence of lupus erythematosus–like disease was approximately 2 percent, a figure considerably in excess of the usual estimates of the frequency of this disease (0.1 to 0.01 percent).[30]

C4 Polymorphisms and Deficiency

The possibility of inheriting null (Q0) alleles at either or both of the C4 loci complicates the inheritance of deficiency of this component.[31] Plasma levels roughly correspond to the number of expressed C4 genes. Individuals homozygous for null alleles at both loci (C4AQO, BQO/C4AQO, BQO) are rare, but single null alleles account for 12 percent of C4A types and 14 percent of C4B types among whites.[32] An increased frequency of C4AQO has been found in myasthenia gravis, in type I diabetes mellitus,[33] and most frequently in association with SLE.[16, 34–36] More than half of whites with SLE have one C4AQ0 allele, and 10 to 15 percent are homozygous C4A deficient.[37] As noted before, the C4AQ0 gene is usually found as part of a "supratype" containing HLA-B8 and DR3.

Homozygous C4 deficiency was first described in an 18-year-old girl with cutaneous and renal involvement typical of SLE.[38] Serologic tests for antinuclear antibodies and DNA binding were negative, and immunofluorescent studies of skin did not demonstrate binding of immunoglobulins or complement components. The patient's mother had approximately half-normal levels of C4. A second kindred had for its propositus a five-year-old boy with rash, fever, arthralgias, and hepatosplenomegaly who subsequently developed diffuse proliferative glomerulonephritis. Antinuclear antibodies were present and DNA binding was increased with the onset of the glomerulonephritis.[39] Subsequent reports have included patients with SLE and renal involvement, lupus-like disease, Henoch-Schönlein purpura, Sjögren's syndrome, and SLE with pulmonary infection.

C2 Deficiency

C2 deficiency is by far the most frequent of the complement component deficiencies.[40] It is inherited as an autosomal codominant, heterozygotes having levels between 30 and 70 percent of the normal mean. The gene frequency appears to be approximately 1 percent. Although the probands of the first two kindreds with C2 deficiency appeared to be normal,[41] those of the subsequently reported kindreds have had diseases such as SLE, discoid lupus erythematosus, polymyositis, glomerulonephritis, Henoch-Schönlein purpura, Hodgkin's disease, or vasculitis. In one tabulation, 14 of 38 homozygous C2-deficient individuals had either systemic or discoid lupus erythematosus.[40] The female:male ratio for such individuals was consistent with the predominance of females generally seen in these diseases. Although a few patients with florid lupus including fulminant renal disease, have been described, the features of the disease are somewhat atypical in most patients with C2 deficiency. Five of eight patients with SLE had weak or absent antibodies to native double-stranded DNA. Five of seven tested had no immunoglobulins or complement deposited in the skin, and the remaining two had only IgG present. The frequency of discoid lupus is also quite high. Although skin involvement may be the typical erythematous raised scaly rash, subacute cutaneous lupus is more common. Immunofluorescent studies of skin lesions often do not demonstrate the presence of immunoglobulin or complement along the epidermal-dermal junction that is typical of the usual form of this disease. These patients also have a high frequency of antibodies to the Ro or SS-A antigen. C2 was the first of the complement component deficiencies to be linked to the MHC[42] and typically occurs in linkage disequilibrium with the genes for HLA-A10, B18, C4A4, C4B2, and DR2.

C3 Deficiency

Homozygous deficiency of C3 is usually associated with profound defects in host defenses, consistent with the pivotal role of this component in both the classic and the alternative activation pathways.[43] Recurrent infections with both pyogenic gram-positive and gram-negative bacteria result in severe furunculosis, pneumonia, meningitis, and septic arthritis.[44] Syndromes resembling SLE have also been observed, however.[45] Vasculitis with circulating immune complexes has been found in a Dutch family with complete C3 deficiency,[45] as well as in familial partial deficiency.[46] A 34-month-old male with fever, skin rash, and arthralgias had homozygous C3 deficiency and improved dramatically following transfusion therapy.[47]

Other Deficiencies

Although more frequently associated with recurrent *Neisseria* infections, complete deficiency of C5 has been found in a patient with SLE manifested by Raynaud's phenomenon, arthritis, hemolytic anemia, and membranous glomerulonephritis.[48] Antinuclear antibodies and anti-DNA were present as well as typical immunofluorescent deposits on skin biopsy. A ten-year-old half-sister also had 1 to 2 percent of normal C5 levels and recurrent pyogenic infections, including two episodes of pneumonia. One of two propositi of C7-deficient kindreds has been found to have severe Raynaud's phenomenon and sclerodactyly.[49] Both SLE and rheumatoid arthritis have also been described in homozygous C7-deficient individuals;[50, 51] in the patient with rheumatoid arthritis, platelet aggregation induced by thrombin was found to be impaired. Absence of C8 has been found in a patient with SLE manifested by membranous glomerulonephritis, photosensitivity, and a positive LE cell test.[52]

Significance of Association Between Complement Deficiencies and Rheumatic Diseases

Although the list of deficiency states with diseases compiled in Table 75–1 is long, some of the associations may be artifacts of sampling—"ascertainment bias"—reflecting the fact that patients with rheumatic disease or nephritis tend to have their complement levels determined more frequently than normal individuals. Even if there were no true association with rheumatic diseases, deficiency states would be found more frequently among such patients simply because their levels are more frequently measured. One example of such an artifact is the finding that the probands of the first two kindreds with C2 deficiency were both immunologists, another group that has its complement levels measured more frequently than normal because of proximity and availability to the measuring laboratory. Only prospective determinations of the occurrence of complement deficiency and rheumatic disease in a randomly sampled population would serve to establish such an association beyond all doubt; because of the low frequency of both of these events, a very large sample size is required. No inherited complete deficiencies of early-acting complement proteins were found in a study of 146,000 healthy Japanese blood donors in Osaka, establishing the rarity of such deficiencies.[53] In a case-control study, the prevalence of C2 deficiency in a group of patients with rheumatic diseases was compared with that of a group of control blood donors.[54] The increase in C2 deficiency in patients with SLE or juvenile rheumatoid arthritis was highly significant. Both of these studies support the conclusion that the association between C2 deficiency and rheumatic diseases has not occurred by chance alone. Given the small numbers of cases and the absence of reliable estimates of gene frequencies for deficiencies of the other complement proteins, the significance of their association with rheumatic diseases is

Table 75–1. RHEUMATIC DISEASES ASSOCIATED WITH COMPLEMENT DEFICIENCIES

Protein	Disease
C1q	Glomerulonephritis and poikiloderma congenita
C1r	Glomerulonephritis, lupus-like syndrome
C1s	Lupus-like syndrome
C1INH	Discoid lupus, SLE, lupus-like syndrome
C4	SLE, Sjögren's syndrome
C2	SLE, discoid lupus, polymyositis, Henoch-Schönlein purpura, Hodgkin's disease, vasculitis, glomerulonephritis, common variable hypogammaglobulinemia
C3	Vasculitis, lupus-like syndrome, glomerulonephritis
C5	SLE, *Neisseria* infection
C6	*Neisseria* infection
C7	SLE, rheumatoid arthritis, Raynaud's phenomenon and sclerodactyly, vasculitis, *Neisseria* infection
C8	SLE, *Neisseria* infection

less certain. One tabulation indicated that 7 percent of patients with deficiencies of the late-acting (C5-C9) components had SLE or a related illness.[50]

Mechanism for Increased Frequency of Rheumatic Diseases

Since the genes for C4, C2, and factor B are located in the major histocompatibility complex, the same region that contains immune response genes, the association of complement deficiency and rheumatic diseases may reflect inheritance of an altered immune response. This seems unlikely because (1) deficiency states with increased susceptibility include several components that are not linked to the MHC, including the deficiencies of C4 and C2 that are secondary to C1 inhibitor deficiency and (2) the range of diseases is such that a single etiologic agent is probably not responsible for all of them. Since virtually all the diseases described have in common the finding of circulating immune complexes, impairment of the clearance or processing of such complexes by the reticuloendothelial system may be involved. In patients with hereditary angioedema who have low levels of C4 and no detectable C2, the survival of IgM-coated erythrocytes is grossly prolonged, essentially equivalent to that of erythrocytes that have not been exposed to antibody.[55] The clearance is normalized by prior treatment of the IgM-coated erythrocytes with a source of normal serum, and is correlated with the deposition of C3b on the cell membranes. Patients with SLE also have defective clearance of antibody-coated erythrocytes, although this phenomenon seems more likely to be a result than a cause of their disease.[56]

The most likely explanation for the predispositon of complement deficiencies to immune complex diseases involves the function of complement in preventing the precipitation of immune complexes[57] or in solubilizing those that have already precipitated.[58] The former depends chiefly on the classic pathway and the latter on the alternative. Both involve the covalent binding of C3b to the immune complex and the intercalation of C3b into the antigen-antibody lattice.[59] Sera from individuals deficient in the early-reacting components, in whom the overall prevalence of SLE was 41 percent, were ineffective in solubilizing immune complexes, whereas those with C5, C6, C7, or C8 deficiency, in whom the prevalence of SLE is much lower, were normally active in this regard.[50] The failure of patients' sera to prevent the precipitation of immune complexes is not always correlated with hypocomplementemia, however, and other factors may be involved.[60, 61] The strong association of heterozygous C4A deficiency with SLE may reflect the relative potency of this subtype of C4 in promoting binding to complement receptors, rather than an effect on immune precipitation.[62]

RECURRENT NEISSERIA INFECTIONS IN DEFICIENCY OF MEMBRANE ATTACK COMPONENTS

Although not usually considered a "rheumatic" disease, recurrent or disseminated gonococcal infection is frequently encountered by the practicing rheumatologist. Although the capacity of serum to kill gram-negative bacteria in vitro had been known since the beginning of the century, only during the mid 1970s was the clinical correlate of this identified, namely, increased Neisseria infections in individuals deficient in constituents of the membrane attack complex (C5-C9). The first such instance occurred in an 18-year-old female with chills, polyarthralgia, painful fingertip lesions, and a history of gonococcal arthritis some 13 months earlier; C6 deficiency was found.[63] The first patient with C8 deficiency also had recurrent gonococcal infections.[64] Both the C6- and the C8-deficient serum had no bactericidal activity against Neisseria gonorrhoeae, but addition of the appropriate purified component restored this activity to normal. Patients with C5 deficiency or C7 deficiency have also been described with disseminated Neisseria infections. Among 24 cases of homozygous deficiency of C6, C7, or C8, 13 had at least one episode and usually two or more episodes of Neisseria meningitidis or Neisseria gonorrhoeae bacteremia, or both.[3] Even among sporadic cases of meningococcal disease, 3 of 20 patients had deficiencies of either C6 or C8, and 3 others had depletion of multiple complement proteins associated with underlying SLE.[65] Recurrent Neisseria infections have also been observed with factor D deficiency,[66] and fulminant meningococcal infection is commonly associated with properdin deficiency.[67, 68]

The striking association of these deficiencies with recurrent infections, specifically Neisseria infections, has two implications. First, formation of the membrane attack complex and subsequent bacterial lysis has a central and probably critical role in host defense against serum-sensitive Neisseria organisms, particularly in preventing dissemination. Second, and most important for the rheumatologist, any patient with recurrent gonococcal infections should be screened for a deficiency of the late complement components by measurement of total hemolytic complement (CH50). Measurements most commonly available in clinical pathology laboratories, namely, immunodiffusion tests for C3 and C4, will not detect deficiencies of the late-reacting components important in defense against Neisseria. While most complement-deficient individuals with Neisseria infections have responded promptly to appropriate antibiotic therapy, transfusions with fresh plasma might prove life-saving when response to the more common therapeutic modalities remains unsatisfactory.

SUMMARY AND CONCLUSIONS

Deficiencies of individual complement proteins may be accompanied by SLE or related syndromes.

Most commonly, deficiencies of the classic activation pathway are involved, including those that are secondary to C1 inhibitor deficiency. In the case of C2, the evidence is strong that this association occurs more frequently than would be expected by chance. Often the clinical picture differs from classic SLE. There is an increased frequency of skin involvement, a decreased frequency of renal disease, low or absent levels of antibody to native DNA, and infrequent deposits of immunoglobulins and complement in the skin. The mechanism for the association may involve the effects of C3 and C4 on the precipitation or solubilization of the immune complexes, or on their processing through cell surface complement receptors. Disseminated or recurrent *Neisseria* infections are common in patients lacking the constituents of the terminal membrane attack complex.

References

1. Agnello, V., deBracco, M. M. E., and Kunkel, H. G.: Hereditary C2 deficiency with some manifestations of systemic lupus erythematosus. J. Immunol. 108:837, 1972.
2. Ruddy, S.: Complement, rheumatic diseases and the major histocompatibility complex. Clin. Rheum. Dis. 3:215, 1977.
3. Petersen, B. H., Lee, T. J., Snyderman, R., and Brooks, G. F.: *Neisseria meningitidis* and *Neisseria gonorrhoeae* bacteremia associated with C6, C7, or C8 deficiency. Ann. Intern. Med. 90:917, 1979.
4. Morgan, B. P., and Walport, M.: Complement deficiency and disease. Immunol. Today 12:301, 1991.
5. Carroll, M. C., Campbell, R. D., Bentley, D. R., and Porter, R. R.: A molecular map of the human major histocompatibility complex class III region linking complement genes C4, C2 and factor B. Nature 307:237, 1984.
6. Perlmutter, D. H., and Colten, H. R.: Molecular basis of complement deficiencies. Immunodefic. Rev. 1:105, 1989.
7. Holers, V. M., Cole, J. L., Lublin, D. M., Seya, T., and Atkinson, J.: Human C3b- and C4b-regulatory proteins: A new multi-gene family. Immunol. Today 6:188, 1985.
8. Carroll, M. C., Alicot, E. M., Katzman, P. J., Klickstein, L. B., Smith, J. A., and Fearon, D. T.: Organization of the genes encoding complement receptors type 1 and 2, decay-accelerating factor, and C4-binding protein in the RCA locus on human chromosome 1. J. Exp. Med. 167:1271, 1988.
9. Campbell, R. D., Carroll, M. C., and Porter, R. R.: The molecular genetics of components of complement. Adv. Immunol. 38:203, 1986.
10. Colten, H. R., Borsos, T., and Rapp, H. J.: Isoelectric focusing of human and guinea-pig C2: Polymorphism of guinea-pig C2. Immunology 18:467, 1970.
11. Rosenfeld, S. I., Ruddy, S., and Austen, K. F.: Structural polymorphism of the fourth component of human complement. J. Clin. Invest. 48:2283, 1969.
12. Law, S. K., Dodds, A. W., and Porter, R. R.: A comparison of the properties of two classes, C4A and C4B, of the human complement component C4. EMBO J. 3:1819, 1984.
13. O'Neill, G. J., Yang, S. Y., Berger, R., Tegoli, J., and Dupont, B.: Chido and Rodgers blood groups are distinct antigenic components of complement C4. Fed. Proc. 37:1269, 1978 (abstract).
14. Alper, C. A., Awdeh, Z. L., and Yunis, E. J.: Complotypes, extended haplotypes, male segregation distortion, and disease markers. Hum. Immunol. 15:366, 1986.
15. Awdeh, Z. L., Raum, D., Yunis, E. J., and Alper, C. A.: Extended HLA/complement allele haplotypes: Evidence for a T/t like complex in man. Proc. Natl. Acad. Sci. U.S.A. 80:259, 1983.
16. Reveille, J. D., Arnett, F. C., Wilson, R. W., Bias, W. B., and Mclean, R. H.: Null alleles of the fourth component of complement and HLA haplotypes in familial systemic lupus erythematosus. Immunogenetics 21:299, 1985.
17. Hauptmann, G., Tongio, M. M., Goetz, J., et al.: Association of the C2-deficiency gene (C2*Q0) with the C4A*4, C4B*2 genes. J. Immunol. 9:127, 1982.
18. Weis, J. H., Morton, C. C., Bruns, G. A., et al.: A complement receptor locus: Genes encoding C3b/C4b receptor and C3d/Epstein-Barr virus receptor map to 1q32. J. Immunol. 138:312, 1987.
19. Reid, K. B., Bentley, D. R., Campbell, R. D., et al.: Complement system

proteins which interact with C3b or C4b. A superfamily of structurally related proteins. Immunol. Today 7:230, 1986.
20. Colten, H. R., and Dowton, S. B.: Regulation of complement gene expression. Biochem. Soc. Symp. 51:37, 1986.
21. Mampaso, F., Ecija, J., Fogue, L., Moneo, I., Gallego, N., and Leyva-Cobian, F.: Familial C1q deficiency in 3 siblings with glomerulonephritis and Rothmund-Thomson syndrome. Nephron 28:179, 1981.
22. Chapuis, R. M., Hauptmann, G., Grosshans, E., and Isliker, H.: Structural and functional studies in C1q deficiency. J. Immunol. 129:1509, 1982.
23. Pickering, R. J., Naff, G. B., Stroud, R. M., Good, R. A., and Gewurz, H.: Deficiency of C1r in human serum effects on the structure and function of macromolecular C1. J. Exp. Med. 131:803, 1970.
24. Moncada, B., Day, N. K., Good, R. A., and Windhorst, D. B.: Lupus erythematosus-like syndrome associated with a familial defect of the first component of complement. N. Engl. J. Med. 286:689, 1972.
25. Pondman, K. W., Stoop, J. W., Cormane, R. H., and Hannema, A. J.: Abnormal C1 in a patient with systemic lupus erythematosus. J. Immunol. 101:811, 1968 (abstract).
26. Chase, P. H., Barone, R., Blum, L., and Wallace, S. L.: "Lupus-like" syndrome associated with deficiency of C1s: Family studies. Ann. R. Coll. Phys. Surg. 9:93, 1976.
27. Donaldson, V. H., and Evans, R. R.: A biochemical abnormality in hereditary angioneurotic edema. Absence of serum inhibitor of C'1-esterase. Am. J. Med. 35:37, 1963.
28. Kohler, P. F., Percy, J., Campion, W. M., and Smyth, C. J.: Hereditary angioedema and "familial" lupus erythematosus in identical twin boys. Am. J. Med. 56:406, 1974 (abstract).
29. Rosenfeld, G. B., Partridge, R. E. H., Bartholomew, W. R., Murphey, W. H., and Singleton, C. M.: Hereditary angioedema and "familial" lupus erythematosus in identical twin boys. J. Allergy Clin. Immunol. 53:68, 1974.
30. Donaldson, V. H., Hess, E. V., and McAdams, A. J.: Lupus erythematosus-like disease in three unrelated women with hereditary angioneurotic edema. Ann. Intern. Med. 86:312, 1977.
31. Awdeh, Z. L., and Ochs, H. D.: Genetic analysis of C4 deficiency. J. Clin. Invest. 67:260, 1981.
32. Schendel, D. J., O'Neill, G. J., and Wank, R.: MHC-linked class III genes. Analysis of C4 gene frequencies, complotypes and associations with distinct HLA haplotypes in German Caucasians. Immunogenetics 20:23, 1984.
33. McCluskey, J., McCann, V. J., Kay, P. H., et al.: HLA and complement allotypes in type 1 (insulin dependent) diabetes. Diabetologia 24:162, 1983.
34. Fielder, A. H., Walport, M. J., Batchelor, J. R., et al.: Family study of the major histocompatibility complex in patients with systemic lupus erythematosus: Importance of null alleles of C4A and C4B in determining disease susceptibility. Br. Med. J. 286:425, 1983.
35. Goldstein, R., Arnett, F. C., Mclean, R. H., Bias, W. B., and Duvic, M.: Molecular heterogeneity of complement component C4-null and 21-hydroxylase genes in systemic lupus erythematosus. Arthritis Rheum. 31:736, 1988.
36. Kumar, A., Kumar, P., and Schur, P. H.: DR3 and nonDR3 associated complement component C4A deficiency in systemic lupus erythematosus. Clin. Immunol. Immunopathol. 60:55, 1991.
37. Arnett, F. C., Bias, W. B., Mclean, R. H., et al.: Connective tissue disease in southeast Georgia. A community based study of immunogenetic markers and autoantibodies. J. Rheumatol. 17:1029, 1990.
38. Hauptmann, G., Grosshans, E., and Heid, E.: Lupus erythemateux aigus et deficits hereditaires en complement. A propos d'un cas par deficit complet en C4. Ann. Dermatol. Syphiligraphie 101:479, 1974.
39. Ochs, H. D., Rosenfeld, S. I., Thomas, E. D., et al.: Linkage between the gene (or genes) controlling synthesis of the fourth component of complement and the major histocompatibility complex. N. Engl. J. Med. 296:470, 1977.
40. Agnello, V.: Complement deficiency states. Medicine 57:1, 1978.
41. Klemperer, M. R., Austen, K. F., and Rosen, F. S.: Hereditary deficiency of the second component of complement (C'2) in man: Further observations on a second kindred. J. Immunol. 98:72, 1967.
42. Fu, S. M., Kunkel, H. G., Brusman, H. P., Allen, F. H., Jr., and Fotino, M.: Evidence for linkage between HL-A histocompatibility genes and those involved in the synthesis of the second component of complement. J. Exp. Med. 140:1108, 1974.
43. Day, N. K.: Component deficiencies. 4. The third component. Prog. Allergy 39:267, 1986.
44. Sano, Y., Nishimukai, H., Kitamura, J., et al.: Hereditary deficiency of the third component of complement in a patient with repeated infections. Clin. Immunol. Immunopathol. 8:543, 1978.
45. Toord, J. J., Daha, M., Kuis, W., et al.: Hereditary deficiency of the third component of complement in two sisters with systemic lupus erythematosus-like symptoms. Arthritis Rheum. 24:1255, 1981.
46. Mclean, R. H., Weinstein, A., Chapitis, J., Lowenstein, M., and Rothfield, N. F.: Familial partial deficiency of the third component of complement (C3) and the hypocomplementemic cutaneous vasculitis syndrome. Am. J. Med. 68:549, 1980.

47. Osofsky, S. G., Thompson, B. H., Lint, T. F., and Gewurz, H.: Hereditary deficiency of the third component of complement in a child with fever, skin rash and arthralgias, and response to whole blood transfusion. J. Pediatr. 90:180, 1977.

48. Rosenfeld, S. I., Kelly, M. E., and Leddy, J. P.: Hereditary deficiency of the fifth component of complement in man. I. Clinical, immuno-chemical, and family studies. J. Clin. Invest. 57:1626, 1976.

49. Boyer, J. T., Gall, E. P., Norman, M. E., Nilsson, U. R., and Zimmerman, T. S.: Hereditary deficiency of the seventh component of complement. J. Clin. Invest. 56:905, 1975.

50. Zeitz, H. J., Miller, G. W., Lint, T. F., Ali, M. A., and Gewurz, H.: Deficiency of C7 with systemic lupus erythematosus: Solubilization of immune complexes in complement deficiency sera. Arthritis Rheum. 24:87, 1981.

51. Alcalay, M., Bontous, D., Wautier, J. I., Vilde, J. M., Vial, M. C., and Peltier, A. P.: Deficit hereditaire en 7e composant du complement avec trouble de l'aggregation plaquettaire, associe a une polyarthrite rhumatoide. Une observation. Nouv. Presse Med. 9:2147, 1980.

52. Jasin, H. E.: Absence of the eighth component of complement in association with systemic lupus erythematosus-like disease. J. Clin. Invest. 60:709, 1977.

53. Inai, S., Akagaki, Y., Moriyama, T., et al.: Inherited deficiencies of the late-acting complement components other than C9 found among healthy blood donors. Int. Arch. Allergy Appl. Immunol. 90:274, 1989.

54. Glass, D., Raum, D., Gibson, D. J., Stillman, J., and Schur, P. H.: Inherited deficiency of the second component of complement. Rheumatic disease associations. J. Clin. Invest. 58:853, 1976.

55. Atkinson, J., and Frank, M. M.: Studies on the in vivo effects of antibody: Interaction of IgM antibody and complement in the immune clearance and destruction of erythrocytes in man. J. Clin. Invest. 54:339, 1974.

56. Frank, M. M., Hamburger, M. I., Lawley, T. J., Kimberley, R. P., and Plotz, P. H.: Defective reticuloendothelial system Fc receptor function in systemic lupus erythematosus. N. Engl. J. Med. 300:518, 1979.

57. Schifferli, J. A., Woo P., and Peters, D. K.: Complement-mediated inhibition of immune precipitation. I. Role of the classical and alternative pathways. Clin. Exp. Immunol. 47:555, 1982.

58. Miller, G. W., and Nussenzweig, V.: A new complement function: Solubilization of antigen antibody aggregates. Proc. Natl. Acad. Sci. U.S.A. 72:418, 1975.

59. Whaley, K., and Ahmed, A. E.: Control of immune complexes by the classical pathway. Behring Inst. Mitt. 111, 1989.

60. Naama, J. K., Mitchell, W. S., Zoma, A., Veitch, J., and Whaley, K.: Complement-mediated inhibition of immune precipitation in patients with immune complex diseases. Clin. Exp. Immunol. 51:292, 1983.

61. Ahmed, A. E., Veitch, J., and Whaley, K.: Mechanism of action of an inhibitor of complement-mediated prevention of immune precipitation. Immunology 70:139, 1990.

62. Gatenby, P. A., Barbosa, J. E., and Lachmann, P. J.: Differences between C4A and C4B in the handling of immune complexes: The enhancement of CR1 binding is more important than the inhibition of immunoprecipitation. Clin. Exp. Immunol. 79:158, 1990.

63. Leddy, J. P., Frank, M. M., Gaither, T. A., Baum, J., and Klemperer, M. R.: Hereditary deficiency of the sixth component of complement in man. I. Immunochemical, biologic and family studies. J. Clin. Invest. 53:544, 1974.

64. Petersen, B. H., Graham, J. A., and Brooks, G. F.: Human deficiency of the eighth component of complement: The requirement of C8 for serum *Neisseria gonorrhoeae* bactericidal activity. J. Clin. Invest. 57:283, 1976.

65. Ellison, R. T., Kohler, P. F., Curd, J. G., Judson, F. N., and Reller, L. B.: Prevalence of congenital or acquired complement deficiency in patients with sporadic meningococcal disease. N. Engl. J. Med. 308:913, 1983.

66. Hiemstra, P. S., Langeler, E., Compier, B., et al.: Complete and partial deficiencies of complement factor D in a Dutch family. J. Clin. Invest. 84:1957, 1989.

67. Nielsen, H. E., Koch, C., Magnussen, P., and Lind, I.: Complement deficiencies in selected groups of patients with meningococcal disease. Scand. J. Infect. Dis. 21:389, 1989.

68. Gelfand, E. W., Rao, C. P., Minta, J. O., Ham, T., Purkall, D., and Ruddy, S.: Inherited deficiency of properdin and C2 in a patient with recurrent bacteremia. Am. J. Med. 82:671, 1987.

Section XIV
Crystal-Associated Synovitis

Chapter 76

William N. Kelley
H. Ralph Schumacher, Jr.

Gout

INTRODUCTION

"Gout is a term representing a heterogeneous group of diseases found exclusively in man, which in their full development can be manifest by (a) an increase in the serum urate concentration; (b) recurrent attacks of a characteristic type of acute arthritis, in which crystals of monosodium urate monohydrate are demonstrable in leukocytes of synovial fluid; (c) aggregated deposits of sodium urate monohydrate (tophi) occurring chiefly in and around the joints of the extremities and sometimes leading to severe crippling and deformity; (d) renal disease involving glomerular, tubular, and interstitial tissues and blood vessels; and (e) uric acid urolithiasis. These manifestations can occur in different combinations."[1]

Gout has been called the "king of diseases" and the "disease of kings." Several excellent narrative and pictorial histories of gout have appeared.[2-11] The major events in the history of gout are summarized in Table 76-1.

EPIDEMIOLOGY

A true serum urate value above 7.0 mg per dl is abnormal: In physiochemical terms, it represents supersaturation; in epidemiologic terms, it carries an increased risk of gout or renal stones. This value corresponds to a concentration of 7.5 to 8.0 mg per dl as determined by chemical methods and automatic analyzers.

A variety of factors appear to be associated with higher mean serum urate concentration. Studies of several indigenous Pacific peoples have disclosed populations with mean serum urate levels significantly higher than those in white populations.[1] Serum urate values show positive correlations with weight and with surface area in peoples of widely differing races and cultures throughout the world,[12] although specific exceptions do exist. For example,

in epidemiologic studies, body bulk (as estimated by body weight, surface area, or ponderal index) has proved to be one of the most important predictors of hyperuricemia.[13] There may also be an association of higher serum urate values with greater intelligence, drive, achievement, leadership, range of activities, or education.[1] In commenting on these associations, Acheson and Chan[13] have expressed the situation well by stating, "The associates of a high uric acid are the associates of plenty."

The serum urate concentration varies with the age and sex of the patient.[14] Children of both sexes normally have a serum urate concentration in the range of 3 to 4 mg per dl. At puberty, males exhibit a further elevation in the serum urate concentration of 1 to 2 mg per dl, which is generally sustained throughout life, whereas females exhibit little if any change in the serum urate concentration at this time; at menopause, however, the serum urate concentration rises and begins to approach the value for adult males.

Large population studies have confirmed the influence of age and sex on urate concentration with a normal distribution for serum urate levels for both males and females.[15-17] Mean urate levels of adult male volunteers in a longitudinal study of human aging rose steadily during a 17-year period.[18]

The mechanism of the lower serum urate levels in females as compared with males is related to a higher fractional excretion of urate secondary to lower tubular urate postsecretory reabsorption.[19] Although changes in plasma 17-beta-estradiol did not modify this,[19] increases in testosterone to estradiol ratios are associated with hyperuricemia.[20]

In adults, serum urate levels correlate strongly with serum creatinine, body weight, height, age, urea nitrogen, blood pressure, and alcohol intake.[21-23]

The incidence of gout in populations varies from 0.20 to 0.35 per 1000, with an overall prevalence of 2 to 2.6 per 1000.[16, 23-24] The prevalence seems to increase substantially with age and increasing serum

Table 76–1. MAJOR EVENTS IN THE HISTORY OF GOUT

Date	Event	Author(s)	Reference
5th century B.C.	Aphorisms on gout	Hippocrates	11
1st century A.D.	Familial nature	Seneca	661
3rd century	Tophi described	Galen	662
13th century	The term gout originated	de Vielehardouin	2
1679	Crystals in gouty tophi	van Leeuwenhoek	663
1776	Uric acid in stones	Scheele	253
1797	Urate in tophi	Wollaston	254
1814	Specificity of colchicine in acute gout	Want	664
1848	Hyperuricemia in gout	Garrod	255
1899	Urate crystals cause gouty arthritis	Freudweiler	517
1950	Introduction of effective uricosuric agents	Talbott	165
1963	Introduction of allopurinol	Gutman and Yu	666
1967	First specific enzyme defect described in patients with gout	Rundles et al. Kelley et al.	667 444

urate concentration.[22, 23] For example, the prevalence was 15 per 1000 in males in the 35 to 44 age range.[22] The annual incidence rate of gout is 4.9 percent for urate levels greater than 9 mg per dl, 0.5 percent for 7.0 to 8.9 mg per dl, and 0.1 percent for values less than 7.0 mg per dl.[25] For serum urate values greater than 9 mg per dl, the cumulative incidence of gout reaches 22 percent after 5 years.[25] In a study of male physicians, the cumulative incidence of gout was 8.6 percent over a median of 19.5 years of follow-up. The health impact of gout was shown by major limitations of activity in 9.2 percent of all men with gout.[26]

CLINICAL FEATURES

In the full development of its natural history, gout passes through four stages: asymptomatic hyperuricemia, acute gouty arthritis, intercritical gout, and chronic tophaceous gout.

Asymptomatic Hyperuricemia

Asymptomatic hyperuricemia is the situation in which the serum urate level is raised, but gout as manifested by arthritic symptoms, tophi, or uric acid stones has not yet appeared. In male subjects at risk for the classic form of primary gout, this stage begins at puberty, whereas in females at risk, hyperuricemia is usually delayed until menopause. By contrast, in patients with hyperuricemia secondary to a specific enzyme deficiency, this trait is present from birth.

Asymptomatic hyperuricemia usually lasts throughout the lifetime of the individual, with no recognizable consequences. The tendency toward acute gout increases with the height of the serum urate concentration value. The risk of nephrolithiasis increases with the height of the serum urate value and with the magnitude of the daily uric acid excretion.[1] The approach to the patient with asymptomatic hyperuricemia is discussed in Chapter 31.

The phase of asymptomatic hyperuricemia ends with the first attack of gouty arthritis or of urolithiasis. In most instances, gouty arthritis comes first and usually after at least 20 to 30 years of sustained hyperuricemia. Between 10 and 40 percent of gouty subjects, however, will have had one or more attacks of renal colic before the first articular event, sometimes more than a decade earlier. A diagnosis of gout should be reserved for the disease marked by urate crystal deposition and not used to describe the patient with hyperuricemia or renal stones.

Acute Gouty Arthritis

The basic pattern of clinical gout is one of acute attacks of exquisitely painful arthritis, at first usually monoarticular and associated with few constitutional symptoms, later often polyarticular and febrile, lasting a variable but limited time and separated by intervals of complete freedom from all symptoms. Attacks recur at shorter intervals and eventually resolve incompletely, leaving chronic arthritis that progresses slowly to a crippling disease on which acute exacerbations are superimposed with decreasing frequency and severity. The peak age at onset of acute gouty arthritis is between the fourth and sixth decades[27–30] in various studies. There is a marked predominance for males, with a peak age at onset at 50 years.[31] Onset before the age of 30 should raise the question of an unusual form of gout, perhaps related to a specific enzymatic defect that leads to marked overproduction of purines or rarely to an unusual form of parenchymal renal disease.

In about 85 to 90 percent of first attacks, a single joint is involved. In at least one half of initial acute attacks, the first metatarsophalangeal joint is the site of the paroxysm (podagra). In Scudamore's[32] series of 516 cases collected in 1817, 60 percent of initial attacks involved the great toe of one foot only. Both great toes were involved simultaneously in 5 percent of subjects in the first attack. The percentage of patients in whom the initial attack is polyarticular varies from 3 to 14 percent.

Ninety percent of gouty patients experience acute attacks in the great toe at some time during the course of the disease. Next in order of frequency as sites of initial involvement are the insteps, ankles, heels, knees, wrists, fingers, and elbows. Acute gout is predominantly a disease of the lower extremity, but any joint of any extremity may be involved. Acute attacks may affect the shoulders, hips, or spine and sacroiliac, sternoclavicular, and temporomandibular joints, but attacks at such sites are very rare. The more distal the site of involvement, the more typical is the character of the attack. Acute gouty bursitis occurs and mainly involves the prepatellar or olecranon bursa.[33]

Some patients report numerous short trivial episodes of "ankle sprains," or sore heels, or twinges of pain in the great toe before the first dramatic gouty attack, sometimes going back over several years. The patient may "walk these off" in a few hours. In most patients, however, the initial visitation of the gout occurs with explosive suddenness during apparent excellent health. Commonly the first attack begins at night. In some patients, symptoms are first detected when the foot is placed on the floor after awakening. In others, the pain awakens the victim. Within a few hours, the affected joint becomes hot, dusky red, and extremely tender. Initially, the joint is only slightly swollen, but signs of inflammation may progress to resemble a bacterial cellulitis. Occasionally, lymphangitis may be evident. Systemic signs of inflammation may include leukocytosis, fever, and elevation of the erythrocyte sedimentation rate. Radiographs generally show only soft tissue swelling during uncomplicated early episodes, but radiographs can be helpful in searching for clues to other causes of podagra or other acute arthritis. Not all podagra in hyperuricemic patients is due to gout.[34]

It is difficult to improve on Sydenham's[35] classic description of the acute attack:

The victim goes to bed and sleeps in good health. About two o'clock in the morning he is awakened by a severe pain in the great toe; more rarely in the heel, ankle or instep. This pain is like that of a dislocation, and yet the parts feel as if cold water were poured over them. Then follow chills and shivers and a little fever. The pain, which was at first moderate, becomes more intense. With its intensity the chills and shivers increase. After a time this comes to its full height, accommodating itself to the bones and ligaments of the tarsus and metatarsus. Now it is a violent stretching and tearing of the ligaments—now it is a gnawing pain and now a pressure and tightening. So exquisite and lively meanwhile is the feeling of the part affected, that it cannot bear the weight of bedclothes nor the jar of a person walking in the room. The night is passed in torture, sleeplessness, turning of the part affected, and perpetual change of posture; the tossing about of the body being as incessant as the pain of the tortured joint, and being worse as the fit comes on. Hence the vain effort by change of posture, both in the body and the limb affected, to obtain an abatement of the pain.

The course of untreated acute gout is highly variable. Mild attacks may subside in several hours or persist for only a day or two and never reach the intensity described by Sydenham. Severe attacks may last days to weeks. The skin over the joint may desquamate as the attack subsides. On recovery, the patient will re-enter an asymptomatic phase termed the intercritical period. Resolution is usually complete, and the patient is once again perfectly well. There are a number of less common presentations of acute gout. Although classically occurring as a mono-articular arthritis, polyarticular gout occurs and may be clinically confusing, especially since some patients are normouricemic on presentation.[36–38] These patients usually have a history of acute gout and involvement of joints in the lower extremities.

Urate deposition and subsequent gout appear to occur more often in previously damaged joints. Hence the occurrence of gout in the Heberden's nodes of older women has been appropriately emphasized.[39–41] The simultaneous presence of both gout and septic arthritis can be confusing clinically, with the former masking the latter.[42–44]

Drugs may precipitate acute gout by either increasing or decreasing serum urate levels acutely. The occurrence of gout following the initiation of antihyperuricemic therapy is well established. Drug-induced gout secondary to increased serum urate levels occurs in association with diuretic therapy, intravenous heparin, and cyclosporin.[45–49] Diuretic therapy in the elderly appears to be a particularly important precipitating factor for gouty arthritis.[45–49]

Provocative factors may include trauma, alcohol ingestion, surgery, dietary excess, hemorrhage, venisection, foreign protein therapy, infections, and radiographic therapy.

Although the diagnosis of acute gouty arthritis can be strongly suggested by the typical picture described here, the definitive diagnosis is best established by aspiration of the joint for identification of classic intracellular needle-shaped or rod-shaped, bi-refringent crystals showing negative elongation with compensated polarized light.[50] Caution must be exercised, however, when relying on crystal identification because every study that has examined quality control has shown discrepancies in identification of crystals.[51–54] A variety of lipid and other crystals have been described that can mimic monosodium urate and are especially common after delay in examination of joint fluid.[55, 56] Preliminary criteria have been described for clinical diagnosis of gout[57] that can help support a clinical impression. A clinical diagnosis has been said to be supported by a dramatic response to colchicine. Diseases other than gout reported to improve on this regimen are serum sickness,[58] pseudogout,[59] hydroxyapatite calcific tendinitis,[60] sarcoid arthritis,[61] erythema nodosum,[62] rheumatoid arthritis,[63] and familial Mediterranean fever.[64] Only rarely will the response in any of these diseases meet the criteria set forth by Wallace and associates[65] for an acceptable response in gout.

Intercritical Gout

The intervals between gouty attacks are called intercritical periods. Some patients never have a second attack. In others, the next attack occurs after an intercritical period of 5 to 10 years. In most patients, a second attack occurs within 6 months to 2 years. In Gutman's[66] series, 62 percent had recurrences within the first year, 16 percent in 1 to 2 years, 11 percent in 2 to 5 years, and 4 percent in 5 to 10 years; 7 percent had no recurrence in 10 or more years. The frequency of the gouty attacks usually increases with time in the untreated patients. Later attacks are often polyarticular, more severe, longer, and perhaps febrile. Roentgenographic changes may develop, and the attacks may abate more gradually than before, but the joints may nevertheless recover complete symptomless function. Eventually the patient may enter a phase of chronic polyarticular gout with no pain-free intercritical periods. At this stage, gout may be easily confused with rheumatoid or degenerative arthritis.

The course described here is the usual one. If the patient is seen late in the disease, a clear and detailed description of the initial attacks and of the completely asymptomatic intervals between attacks of sudden onset and rapid offset can usually be obtained and is exceedingly valuable in pointing toward the correct diagnosis. Not all patients, however, will have followed this course. Rarely the disease may run a fulminant febrile course. In addition, a percentage of patients progress directly from the initial acute attack into a subchronic and then chronic illness, with no remissions and early development of tophi and incapacity.

The diagnosis of gout in a hyperuricemic patient with a history of acute attacks of monarthritis may be difficult or inconclusive during the intercritical phase. Aspiration of an asymptomatic joint, however, may be a useful adjunct in the diagnosis of gout if urate crystals are demonstrated.[67, 68] Joint fluid obtained from gouty patients during the intercritical phase revealed monosodium urate crystals in 12.5 to 58 percent of knees and 52 percent of metatarsophalangeal joints.[69–71] Such crystals in asymptomatic joints were often associated with mild synovial fluid leukocytosis, suggesting the potential for contribution to joint damage even in the interim between attacks.[72, 73] Postmortem detection of intracellular crystals in 4 to 18 percent of synovial fluids obtained from first metatarsophalangeal joints has been reported even though there was no significant association with antecedent recognized gouty arthritis.[74, 75]

Chronic Tophaceous Gout

The duration of time from the initial attack to the beginning of chronic symptoms or visible tophaceous involvement was highly variable in untreated patients, in the experience of Hench[76] ranging from 3 to 42 years, with an average of 11.6 years. Ten years after the first acute attack, about half were still nontophaceous, and most of the remainder still had only minimal deposits. Thereafter the proportion of

nontophaceous patients slowly declined to 28 percent after 20 years. The percentage of patients with severe crippling disease reached appreciable proportions (24 percent) some 20 years after the initial attack.

The principal determinant of the rate of urate deposition in and about the joints is the serum urate level. In Gutman's[77] series, the mean serum urate concentration was 9.1 mg per dl (uricase method) in 722 nontophaceous patients, 10 to 11 mg per dl in 456 patients with minimal to moderate tophaceous deposits, and greater than 11 mg per dl in 111 patients with extensive tophaceous involvement. The rate of formation of tophaceous deposits in primary gout thus correlates with both the degree and duration of hyperuricemia. The rate of formation of tophi is also correlated with the severity of renal disease, which in turn is related to the duration of hyperuricemia as well as being a factor in determining its degree.[78] The ability to control hyperuricemia has been associated with a striking reduction in the frequency with which tophi develop in the gouty population. The decreasing incidence of tophi in patients with gout is shown in Table 76–2.

Although there has been a declining incidence of tophaceous gout to as low as 3 percent,[79] in one study 35 percent of gouty male veterans were noted to have tophi on physical examination.[80] This group was characterized by an early age of onset (40.5 years), long duration of disease (18.7 years), four attacks per year, mean serum urate value of 9.2 mg per dl, and a high frequency (71 percent) of polyarticular episodes. Although tophi generally develop with longstanding gout, rarely tophi may develop without preceding acute gouty arthritis.[81] Elderly patients with impaired renal function receiving anti-inflammatory and urate-retaining drugs may be at high risk for developing tophi without preceding gouty arthritis.

Tophaceous gout is a consequence of the progressive inability to dispose of urate as rapidly as it is produced. The urate pool expands and crystalline deposits of urate appear in cartilage, synovial membranes, tendons, soft tissues, and elsewhere. Occasionally, palpable tophi may be present at the time of the initial acute attack. This is unusual in primary gout but was recorded by Yu[82] in nearly 0.5 percent

Table 76–2. CHANGING TREND IN THE INCIDENCE OF TOPHI IN PRIMARY GOUT

Years	Patients (No.)	Tophi No.	Tophi %
1948–1953	165	88	53
1954–1958	369	154	42
1959–1963	522	172	33
1964–1968	355	112	32
1969–1973	289	49	17
Total	1700	575	—

From Yu, T., and Yu, T.-F.: Milestones in the treatment of gout. Am. J. Med. 56:676, 1974. Reproduced by permission of the American Journal of Medicine.

of subjects with gout secondary to myeloproliferative disease and may also occur in juvenile gout, for example, complicating glycogen storage disease[83] or the Lesch-Nyhan syndrome.[84]

A classic location of tophi is the helix or less commonly, the antihelix of the ear (Fig. 76–1), but this is no longer the most common site. Tophaceous deposits may produce irregular asymmetric, moderately discrete tumescences of fingers (Fig. 76–2), hands, knees, or feet, requiring larger gloves or shoes. The classic gouty shoe is one with a window cut to accommodate an irregularly prominent joint, usually the first metatarsophalangeal. Tophi commonly form lumps along the ulnar surface of the forearm, or saccular distentions of olecranon bursae (Fig. 76–3), or fusiform or lumpy enlargements of the Achilles tendon (Fig. 76–4). Occasionally they develop subcutaneously along the tibial surface.

As tophi and renal disease advance, acute attacks recur less frequently and are milder. Dialysis therapy further reduces the frequency of acute attacks.[85]

The process of tophaceous deposition advances insidiously, and although the tophi themselves are relatively painless, there is often progressive stiffness and persistent aching of affected joints. Eventually extensive destruction of joints and large subcutaneous tophi may lead to grotesque deformities, particularly of hands and feet, and to progressive crippling. The tense, shiny thin skin overlying the tophus may ulcerate and extrude white chalky or pasty material composed of myriads of fine needle-like crystals. Bony ankylosis may rarely occur.[86]

Tophi may produce a marked limitation of joint movement by the direct involvement of the joint structure or of tendons serving the joint. Any joint may be involved, although those of the lower extremity are chiefly affected. Spinal joints do not escape urate deposition,[87] but acute gouty spondylitis is unusual. Symptoms related to spinal cord compression by tophi have been rarely observed.[88, 89] Tophi may also occur in myocardium, valves,[90, 91] cardiac conduction system, and various parts of the eye[92, 93]

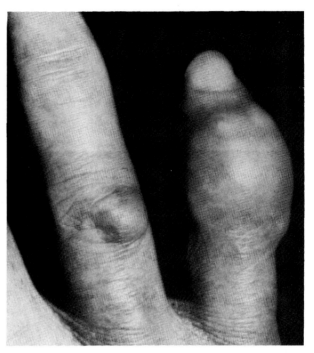

Figure 76–2. Tophus of fifth digit, with smaller tophus over fourth proximal interphalangeal joint.

as well as the larynx. Before the advent of antihyperuricemic agents, 50 to 70 percent of gouty patients developed visible tophi, permanent joint changes, or chronicity of symptoms.[94, 95] Typical radiologic changes, particularly erosions (sharply marginated lucent pockets), occur with the development of tophi.[96-98] These may be difficult to distinguish from rheumatoid erosions. A thin overhanging edge favors a gouty etiology. Tophi can calcify. See Chapter 37 for further discussion.

Associated Conditions

Obesity. The association of gout with obesity and overeating has been recognized for hundreds of years.[6, 99, 100] In 6000 subjects in Tecumseh, Michigan, hyperuricemia was found in only 3.4 percent of those with a relative weight at or below the twentieth percentile, in 5.7 percent of those between the twenty-first and seventy-ninth percentile, and in 11.4 percent of those at or above the eightieth percentile.[101] Other population studies have also demonstrated a positive correlation between serum urate and weight or body surface area.[17, 102, 103, 104]

As expected from the data cited here, obesity is also common in subjects selected because of hyperuricemia or gout. Gouty patients show body weights above ideal values for age and height in a large percentage of subjects. Emmerson and Knowles[105] noted that subjects with primary gout were an average of 17.8 percent overweight (compared with patients with lead gout who were an average of 1.3

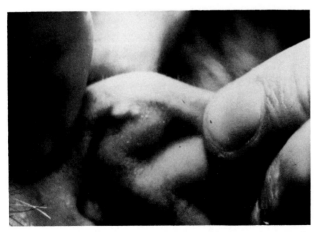

Figure 76–1. Tophus of the helix of the ear adjacent to the auricular tubercle.

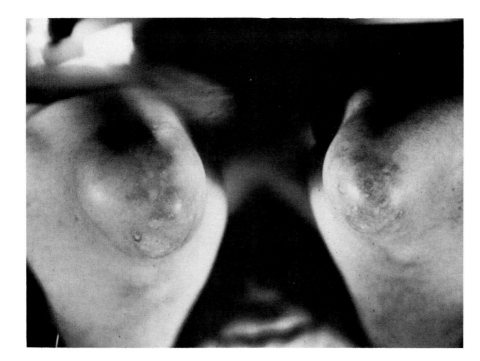

Figure 76–3. Saccular tophaceous enlargements of olecranon bursae, with small cutaneous deposits of overlying skin.

percent overweight). Brochner-Mortensen[106] found that 78 percent of his gouty subjects were more than 10 percent overweight and 57 percent more than 30 percent overweight. Grahame and Scott[29] noted that 48 percent of 355 patients with gout were more than 15 percent overweight. Obesity seems to be a common factor relating diabetes,[107–109] hyperlipidemia,[110] hypertension,[111] and atherosclerosis.[101]

Diabetes Mellitus. Hyperuricemia has been reported in 2 to 50 percent of patients with diabetes, whereas gouty arthritis has been reported in from less than 0.1 percent to 9.0 percent of diabetic subjects.[112] Abnormal glucose tolerance tests have been noted in 7 to 74 percent of patients with gout,[113–115] depending, in part, on the criteria used. When overt clinical diabetes is present in such patients, it tends to be mild. Engelhardt and Wagner[107] called attention to obesity as an integral part of a triad with gout and diabetes; others have since noted this association.[107–109] Thus, obesity may predispose to both hyperuricemia and hyperglycemia.

Despite these observations, epidemiologic stud-

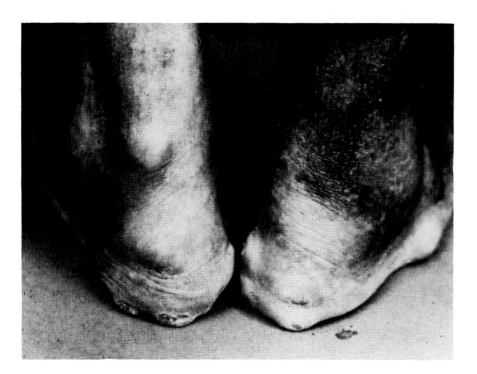

Figure 76–4. Tophi of Achilles tendons and their insertions in a black patient with gout.

ies have not demonstrated any relation between gout and diabetes or between serum urate and blood glucose concentrations.[9, 112, 116] In such studies, the mean serum urate concentration is actually lower in patients with overt diabetes. This has been attributed to the apparent uricosuric effect of high blood glucose levels.[117, 118]

Hyperlipidemia. Hypertriglyceridemia has been reported in 75 to 84 percent of patients with gout[99, 115, 119] and hyperuricemia in up to 82 percent of patients with hypertriglyceridemia. A rank order correlation of serum urate and serum triglyceride values has been described but also disclaimed.[110] The gouty patients who drank alcohol excessively had a mean serum triglyceride level that was higher than that of their obesity-matched controls and that of nondrinking gouty patients. It appears that diet and possibly defective clearance of triglyceride may be the etiologic factors associated with elevated triglycerides and lipoprotein concentrations in gouty individuals.[120–126] Although individual gouty subjects are frequently hypercholesterolemic,[127, 128] many studies have failed to show a correlation between serum urate and cholesterol values.[99, 105, 110, 129, 130]

Hypertension. Hyperuricemia has been reported in 22 to 38 percent of untreated hypertensives.[131–133] This is significantly greater than the prevalence of hyperuricemia expected in an unselected population. When therapy and renal disease are not excluded, the prevalence increases to 47 to 67 percent.[131–135] The overall prevalence of gout in hypertension has been variously reported as 2 to 12 percent.[132, 134] In the population study of 6000 residents of Tecumseh, Michigan, Myers et al.[101] found no correlation between serum urate concentrations adjusted for age, sex, relative body weight, and levels of blood pressure.

Hypertension is present in one fourth to one half of patients with classic gout.[136, 137] The incidence of both moderate and severe hypertension was unrelated to duration of gout, but that of moderate hypertension rose with increasing age of onset.

The serum urate concentration correlates inversely with renal blood flow and urate clearance and directly with renal vascular and total resistance.[135, 138–140] Therefore, the association between hypertension and hyperuricemia may be related to reduction of renal blood flow in the former condition. Further, it has been proposed that an elevation of the serum urate concentration may be an indicator of renal vascular involvement in essential hypertension. Weight changes may be important modifiers of hypertension and hyperuricemia. Loss of weight may improve both variables.[141, 142]

Atherosclerosis. In 1951, Gertler et al.[143] noted a statistically significant excess of hyperuricemia in a group of young patients with coronary heart disease. Several other reports have noted the association of hyperuricemia with the manifestations of atherosclerosis,[144–146] and hyperuricemia has been proposed as a risk factor for coronary heart disease.[147] In the Tecumseh study,[101, 148] there was no clear association between levels of blood pressure, blood sugar, or serum cholesterol and serum urate concentrations when adjustments were made for effects of age, sex, and relative weight. When these variables were taken into account, the figures showed that the serum urate levels of persons with coronary heart disease were not significantly different from the mean of the population. Myers et al.[101] concluded that an elevated serum urate concentration value could not be taken as an attribute associated with coronary heart disease.

In a retrospective study on the cause of death in patients with gout treated with antihyperuricemic drugs,[149] however, cerebrovascular disease and cardiovascular disease accounted for more than 50 percent of the mortality. The majority of these patients had either hypertension or hyperlipidemia. It seems likely that in patients with hyperuricemia, clinical correlates such as hypertension, diabetes mellitus, hyperlipidemia, and obesity[1, 150–153] may all contribute to the observed association between elevated serum urate concentration and arteriosclerosis. Many other studies suggest that hyperuricemia is a risk factor for cardiovascular mortality.[154–157] In multivariate analysis, however, serum urate levels do not add independently to the prediction of coronary heart disease.[157, 158] Platelet aggregation and adhesion are not enhanced by hyperuricemia, removing this potential mechanism associating hyperuricemia and vascular disease.[158, 159]

Ethanol. Alcohol consumption has long been associated with hyperuricemia and, in susceptible persons, the precipitation of acute gouty arthritis. Although studies indicated that a decrease in the renal excretion of uric acid could account for ethanol-induced hyperuricemia,[160–163] an increase in uric acid production now seems to be a more important factor. Ethanol increases uric acid production by accelerating the turnover of adenosine triphosphate (ATP).[164, 165] Beer may have more potent effects on uric acid production as a result of its guanosine content.[166]

Acute Illness. Studies of acutely ill patients in intensive care units indicate that markedly elevated serum urate levels in the range of 20 mg per dl are associated with a poor prognosis[167] and hypotensive events.[168] This may be related to two factors. First, ischemic tissue may foster the degradation of ATP to purine end products, thus enhancing the synthesis of uric acid. The finding of elevated plasma ATP degradation products associated with hyperuricemia in adult respiratory distress syndrome supports this possibility.[169] Second, the conversion of hypoxanthine to uric acid by xanthine oxidase during ischemia produces oxidant radicals.[170] The latter are themselves associated with tissue injury. It is possible that inhibition of xanthine oxidase with allopurinol may be a useful therapy in this setting.

The substantial antioxidant properties of uric acid have been the subject of speculation[171–174]; it is possible that these properties may counteract the potent oxidant properties of xanthine oxidase during uric acid synthesis.

Pregnancy. Maternal serum urate levels normally decrease during pregnancy until the twenty-fourth week and then increase until 12 weeks after delivery.[175-177] An increase in the serum urate level occurs in pre-eclampsia and toxemia of pregnancy[175-183] owing to decrease in the renal clearance of urate. Perinatal mortality is markedly increased when maternal plasma urate levels are raised, generally in association with early-onset pre-eclampsia.[181, 182] The highest mortality is seen with serum urate levels in excess of 6.0 mg per dl and diastolic blood pressure in excess of 110 mm Hg.[181]

Labor itself is associated with an increasing serum urate level.[184] The mechanism may be related to decreased renal clearance of urate, since there is an associated increase in plasma urea levels. The serum urate level remains elevated for 1 to 2 days postpartum.[185] Increased production of urate may occur as well, although direct evidence for this is lacking.

Negative Disease Associations. A negative association appears to exist between gout and rheumatoid arthritis.[186-189] The basis for the decreased concurrence of these disorders, however, is unclear. There may be difficulty in distinguishing acute gout from a flare of rheumatoid arthritis; the low synovial fluid complement in rheumatoid arthritis may inhibit the expression of clinical gout; and treatment with full doses of aspirin is often used, which would delay or prevent the onset of gout owing to the uricosuric effect of high doses of aspirin. Patients with rheumatoid arthritis and persistent hyperuricemia above 7.5 mg per dl have been said to have minimally active disease.[190] Hyperuricemia inhibits mononuclear cell activation to produce rheumatoid factor, suggesting one possible mechanism.[191] In addition, if the interaction of crystal-bound IgG with Fc receptors is important in the pathogenesis of gout, this may be blocked by rheumatoid factor.[192] Systemic lupus and gout coexist infrequently[193-195] because they in part tend to affect different populations.

Parenchymal Renal Disease

After gouty arthritis, renal disease appears to be the most frequent complication of hyperuricemia. Several types of renal disease have been associated with hyperuricemia. The first type, urate nephropathy, is attributed to the deposition of monosodium urate crystals in the renal interstitial tissue and is thought to be associated with chronic hyperuricemia. In contrast, uric acid nephropathy is related to the formation of uric acid crystals in the collecting tubules, pelvis, or ureter, with subsequent impairment of urine flow. This disorder is caused by elevated concentrations of uric acid in the urine and can appear as either acute uric acid nephropathy or uric acid calculi. In addition, calcium oxalate nephrolithi-

asis occurs more commonly in patients with hyperuricemia or gout than in normouricemic subjects. Other renal disease associations have been observed in gout caused by uncertain mechanisms.

Urate Nephropathy

Although urate nephropathy appears to exist as a distinct entity, it is not believed to be an important contributor to declining renal function in the majority of gouty patients.[8, 13, 150, 196-199] The deposition of urate crystals in the interstitium of the medulla and pyramids with a surrounding giant cell reaction is a distinctive histologic finding characteristic of gouty kidney (Fig. 76–5).[200] Twenty to 40 percent of patients with gout have albuminuria, which is usually mild and often intermittent.[201] Although up to one third of patients with gout appear to have hypertension, a number of abnormalities in renal function are observed in gouty patients, such as a reduced glomerular filtration rate, proteinuria, and a reduced renal concentrating ability, even when hypertensive patients are eliminated from the study population.[193, 194]

Renal failure has accounted for 10 percent of deaths of gouty patients.[202] Although it is clear that renal disease is associated with gout, it has not been evident to what extent this is related to hyperuricemia per se or to the deposition of monosodium urate in the renal tissue. Indeed, it appears at this time that moderate hyperuricemia per se has little, if any, harmful effect on renal function. Other factors, such as coexistent hypertension, chronic lead exposure, ischemic heart disease, and primary pre-existent renal insufficiency, may be more important than urate in the pathogenesis of the lesion previously considered to be "urate" nephropathy.[194-196]

Administration of nonsteroidal anti-inflammatory drugs in gouty arthritis may lead to deterioration of renal function and exacerbate existing renal disease. Although increasing age does lead to deterioration of renal function in both gouty and control populations,[196, 197] the aging phenomenon appears to be accentuated in the gouty patients,[196] especially in the presence of hypertension, ischemic heart disease, or pre-existent renal disease.[197] On the other hand, extreme hyperuricemia, in excess of 13 mg per dl in males or 10.0 mg per dl in females, may be implicated in the etiology of renal damage.[150] These extremes of hyperuricemia may exist in the presence of inherited enzyme deficiencies, leading to urate overproduction and blood dyscrasias with oliguria and urolithiasis.[197]

The gouty kidney, as described by Garrod,[203] may be rare at the present time. However, two studies have reported a substantial incidence of urate deposition not associated with clinical gout.[204, 205] In one study, 17 of 62 patients dying of renal insufficiency had renal medullary tophi, which were attributed to the hyperuricemia of chronic renal insufficiency; however, only four of these patients had attacks of articular gout. In another study, medullary

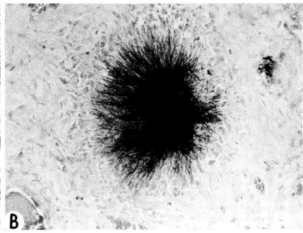

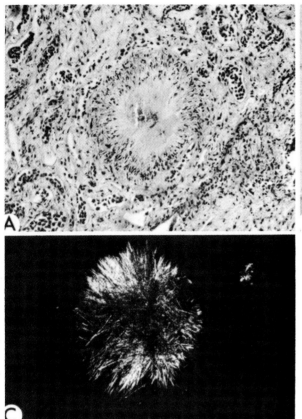

Figure 76–5. *A,* Urate deposit in the medulla of the kidney as seen in alcohol-fixed section stained with hematoxylin and eosin (×250). *B,* Adjacent section of deposit shown in *A,* stained with methenamine silver (×250). *C,* Adjacent section of deposit shown in *A* as seen with polarized light (×250).

microtophi were found in 8 percent of unselected autopsies. Although these deposits were most frequently associated with a history of gout or the presence of pre-existing nongouty renal disease, in 26 percent of patients there was no clear cause. Each of these studies suggests that, in some instances, urate deposition in the renal medulla may be a consequence rather than a direct cause of renal failure. In addition, factors other than hyperuricemia that are unclear at present contribute to urate deposition in the kidney.

Uric Acid Nephropathy

Acute Uric Acid Nephropathy. Acute renal failure can result from the precipitation of uric acid crystals in the collecting ducts and ureters.[206, 207] This complication most commonly occurs in patients with leukemias and lymphomas as a result of rapid malignant cell turnover, often during chemotherapy.[207–210] This syndrome, the *acute tumor lysis syndrome,* has been more clearly defined as hyperuricemia, lactic acidosis, hyperkalemia, hyperphosphatemia, and hypocalcemia; it is described in aggressive, rapidly proliferating tumors, including lymphoproliferative disorders and metastatic medulloblastoma.[208–211] The large amount of nucleic acid and nucleotides liberated with massive cytolysis is converted rapidly to uric acid. Marked hyperphosphatemia also contributes to the toxicity of this syndrome.[210] Renal failure may also result acutely or chronically from uric acid over-

production secondary to an enzyme deficiency such as hypoxanthine-guanine phosphoribosyltransferase deficiency.[211]

The pathogenesis of acute renal failure in uric acid nephropathy is related to the precipitation of uric acid in the distal tubules and in collecting ducts,[207, 215] which are the sites of maximal acidification and concentration of the urine. Typically, there is marked hyperuricemia, with a mean serum urate level of 20 mg per dl (range, 12 to 36 mg per dl).[208] Oliguria or even anuria as well as azotemia may occur. There may be gravel or sand noted in the urine. The ratio of urinary uric acid to creatinine in these patients typically exceeds 1.0, whereas in patients with most other causes of acute renal failure, it is 0.4 ± 0.3.[216]

Renal Calculi. Uric acid calculi, which account for approximately 10 percent of all stones in patients in the United States, range from as low as 5 percent in some countries to 40 percent in countries such as Israel and Australia.[217, 220] Renal stones occur in 10 to 25 percent of patients with primary gout, a prevalence more than 1000 times greater than that in the general population.[221] The likelihood of stones in a given patient with gout increases with the serum urate concentration and with urinary uric acid excretion.[221, 222] It reaches 50 percent with a serum urate value of 13 mg per dl or above or with urinary uric acid excretion rates in excess of 1100 mg per dl. The yearly risk for the development of urolithiasis in established gouty arthritis is about 1 percent; in asymptomatic hyperuricemia, it is about 0.27 percent.[150]

Although renal calculi are uncommon in gout secondary to lead nephropathy, the incidence of renal calculi in other patients with secondary gout may be as high as 42 percent, particularly after vigorous cytolytic therapy. The high incidence of uric acid calculi in secondary gout is related to higher serum urate levels and urinary uric acid excretion in this group.[223] Uric acid stones are also reported to occur in patients with no history of gouty arthritis, but only approximately 20 percent of this group are hyperuricemic. This may be related to a lower fasting urine pH in some patients with uric acid calculi.[223] However, a report of uric acid as a major constituent in a stone obtained from a patient with no apparent abnormalities of uric acid metabolism should suggest the possibility that the constituent is actually 2,8-dihydroxyadenine and that the patient has adenine phosphoribosyltransferase deficiency.[224, 225]

Other stone disease is associated with hyperuricemia and gout. Gouty subjects also have an increased incidence of stones that contain calcium. In addition, studies have demonstrated that about 30 percent of patients with recurrent calcium stone disease either may have an elevated urinary uric acid excretion rate or are hyperuricemic. Patients with recurrent calcium oxalate stones consume greater quantities of dietary purines than do normal subjects, tend to excrete larger quantities of uric acid even with purine restriction, and have a higher renal clearance of uric acid. Evidence that uric acid is associated etiologically with recurrent calcium oxalate calculi is the reduction of the stone frequency with allopurinol therapy.[226–228]

There is an association between cystinuria and gout.[223, 229] As many as 50 percent of cystinuric patients are hyperuricemic, and a similar percentage have mixed stones of cystine and uric acid.[223] Xanthine and oxipurinol calculi have been reported in patients with Lesch-Nyhan syndrome on allopurinol therapy.[227]

Other Nephropathy in Gout

Familial Urate Nephropathy. Several families have been reported in which there is (1) a high incidence of hyperuricemia with gout beginning at an unusually young age; (2) involvement of females or involvement of both sexes with hypertension; (3) progressive renal disease leading to death before the age of 40; (4) no evidence for any metabolic abnormality that increases uric acid production; and (5) frequently an autosomal dominant mode of inheritance.[231–236] These patients are unusual for several reasons. Although hyperuricemia and gout may be familial and may be associated with progressive renal disease, it is unusual for renal disease to be the cause of early death in primary gout. Usually these patients with familial urate nephropathy do not exhibit other

features suggestive of hereditary renal disease.[237, 238] Specific diagnosis may be relevant, since stabilization of renal function has occurred in some patients following allopurinol therapy.[231]

Hyperuricemia has been associated with other familial nephropathies, such as medullary cystic disease[231] and focal tubulointerstitial disease.[239] It is possible that the primary interstitial nephropathy leads to a relatively selective defect in uric acid secretion, causing hyperuricemia. The possibility that renal disease is the primary event in other families as well cannot be overlooked.

Polycystic Kidney Disease. About one third of patients with polycystic kidney disease are reported to have gout.[240, 241] The hyperuricemia and gouty arthritis appear to precede the development of renal failure.[240–242] Although the basis for this association remains unclear, altered renal handling of uric acid may be an early manifestation of the underlying renal lesion.

Lead Intoxication. Hyperuricemia and gout are well-recognized complications of chronic lead intoxication. Although a renal defect appears to be present, it has not been well defined. Campbell et al.[199] have reported that patients with primary gout have elevated blood lead levels when compared with age-matched and sex-matched controls despite the absence of a history of overt lead exposure. This suggests that occult chronic lead intoxication may play an etiologic role in some cases of primary gout. In addition, there is evidence that patients with gout who have renal impairment, as compared with gouty patients with normal renal function, have an increased quantity of mobilizable lead. This observation suggests an important potential role for lead in the pathogenesis of gouty nephropathy.[198] On the other hand, in a study of patients with a history of moonshine ingestion, no correlation was found between extent of depression in clearance of uric acid or creatinine and amount of lead excretion following ethylenediaminetetra-acetic acid (EDTA) infusion.[240]

Studies of lead intoxication indicate that there is considerable variation in the occurrence of gout. In one study, in excess of 50 percent of patients with a diagnosis of plumbism had gout, and gout secondary to lead accumulation constituted 36 percent of all gouty patients.[244] In another setting, only 6 percent of lead-intoxicated adults had documented gout, whereas 20 percent complained of arthralgias.[245] The presence of gout in chronic renal failure is a useful marker to suggest chronic lead poisoning.[246–250]

Factors other than renal alterations may account for the relatively frequent occurrence of gout in lead intoxication. The addition of lead to a urate solution induces nucleation of lead urate at lower concentrations than is required for the nucleation of monosodium urate.[251] In addition, lead urate crystals can serve as nucleation sites for monosodium urate. In contrast, the inhibition of guanine aminohydrolase by lead[252] is difficult to relate to the etiology of gout in lead intoxication.

PURINE METABOLISM

Recognition of the role of purines in human disease began with the observation that uric acid, a purine base, was a component of some renal calculi,[253] and in its ionized form, monosodium urate, was (1) a major constituent of tophi,[254] (2) elevated in the serum of gouty patients,[255] and (3) present, in its crystalline form, in synovial fluid during the acute attack of gouty arthritis. The biochemistry of purine compounds and the biosynthesis of the purine ring have been extensively investigated and reviewed.[1]

Biochemistry of Purine Compounds

The parent compound, the purine base, is composed of a six-membered pyrimidine ring fused to the five-membered imidazole ring. The origins of individual atoms of the purine ring are shown in Figure 76–6.

The most important purine bases are adenine, guanine, hypoxanthine, xanthine, and uric acid. The purines all show lactam-lactim isomerism and may be written in either form, as shown for uric acid in Figure 76–7.

Purine nucleosides are composed of a purine base plus a pentose joined to the base by a β-*N*-glycosyl bond between carbon atom 1 of the pentose and nitrogen atom 9 of the purine base. There are two series of nucleosides: the ribonucleosides, which contain D-ribose as the sugar component, and the deoxyribonucleosides, which contain 2-deoxy-D-ribose (Fig. 76–8).

Purine nucleotides and deoxynucleotides consist of a nucleoside or deoxynucleoside with a phosphate group in ester linkage with carbon 5 of the pentose (Fig. 76–9). The nucleosides and deoxynucleosides may exist as 5′-monophosphates, 5′-diphosphates, and 5′-triphosphates (Fig. 76–10). The phosphoric acid residues of these compounds are designated by the symbols α, β, and γ. These compounds serve (1) as building blocks for RNA and DNA; (2) as precursors of the cyclic nucleotides, adenosine 3′,5′-cyclic phosphate, and guanosine 3′,5′-cyclic phosphate; (3) as a source of chemical energy; and (4) as precursors of various purine cofactors and coenzymes such as nicotinamide adenine dinucleotide (NAD).

Formation of Uric Acid. The free purine bases that result from nucleoside cleavage are adenine, guanine, hypoxanthine, and xanthine. Because purine nucleoside phosphorylase acts most readily on inosine and guanosine,[256] the major bases generated are very likely hypoxanthine and guanine. Guanine

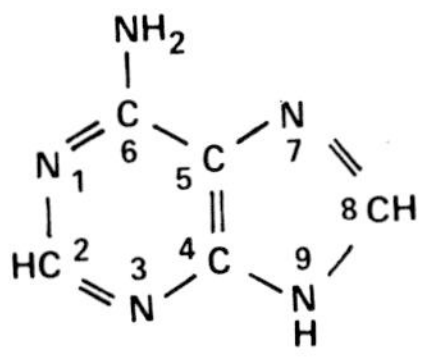
Adenine

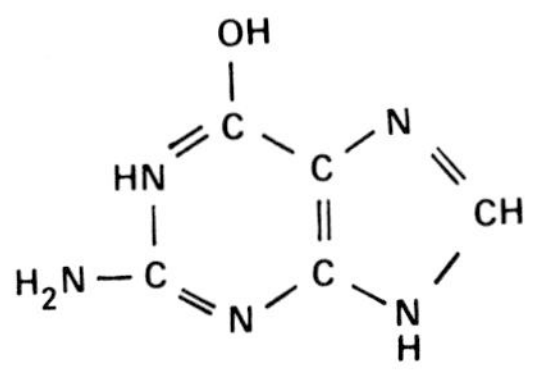
Guanine

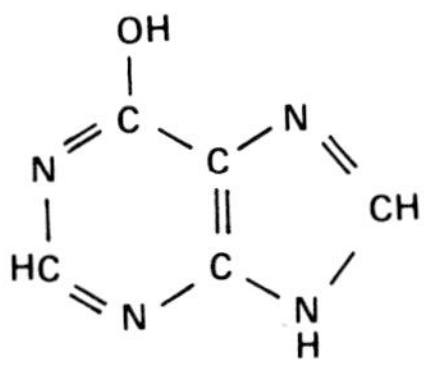
Hypoxanthine

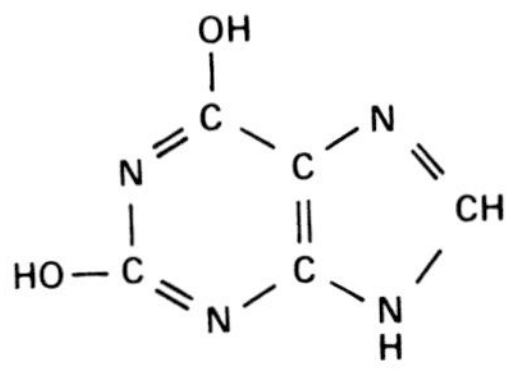
Xanthine

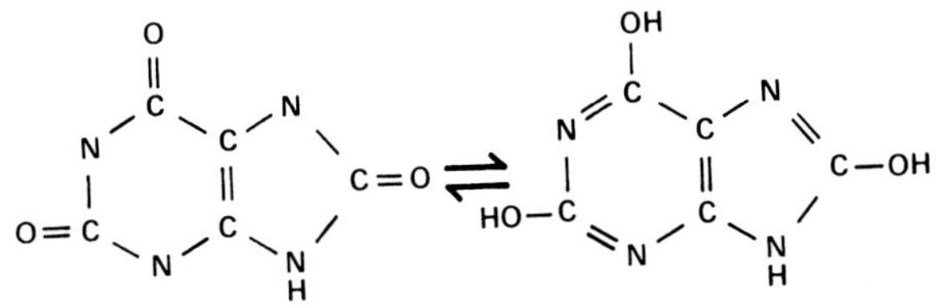
(Lactam) (Lactim)

Uric acid

Figure 76–7. Structure of uric acid. All purine bases may exist in the lactam form in a reversible manner as shown for uric acid.

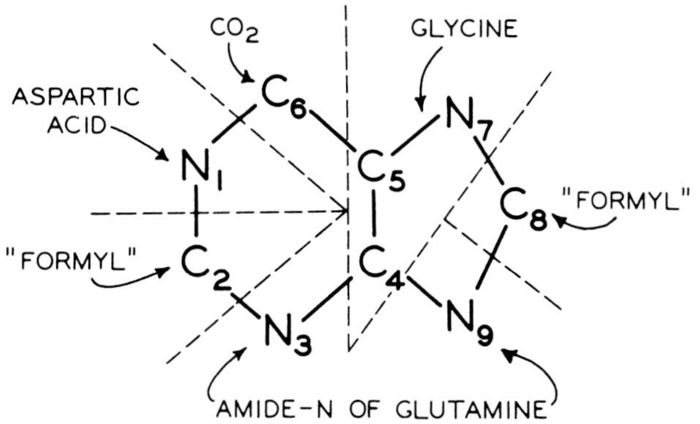

Figure 76–6. Origins of atoms of the purine ring.

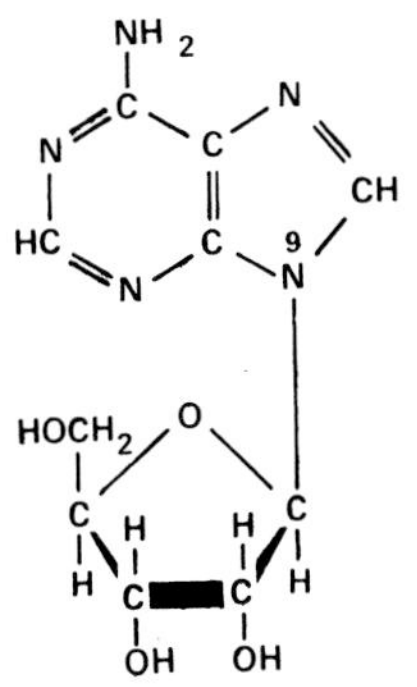
Adenosine

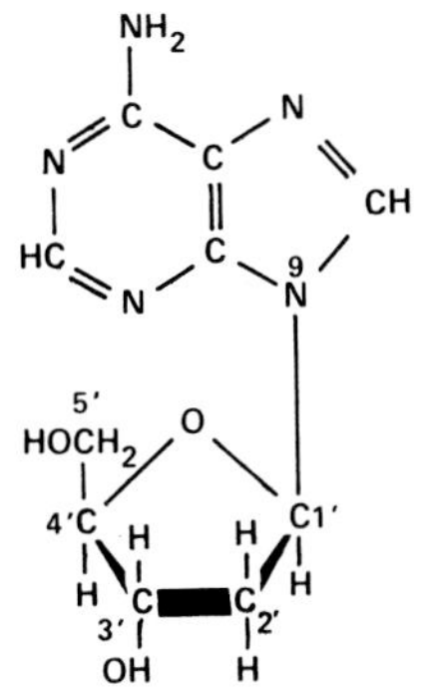
2′ – Deoxyadenosine

Figure 76–8. Structures of adenosine and 2′-deoxyadenosine as examples of nucleosides and 2′-deoxynucleosides, respectively.

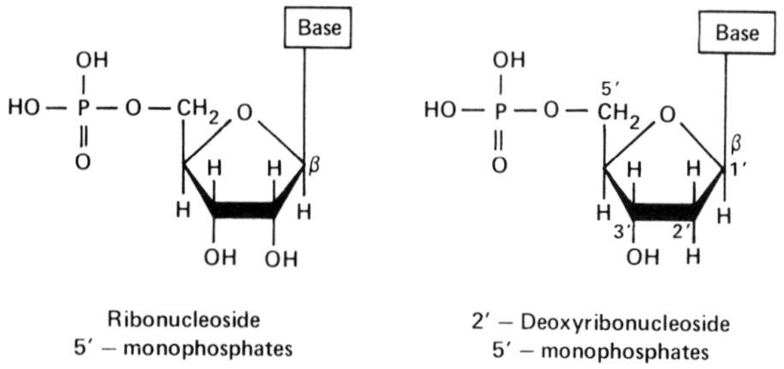

OH
|
HO — P — O — CH₂ O   Base
‖
O   H   H   β

H   H

OH   OH

Ribonucleoside
5′ — monophosphates

OH
|
HO — P — O — CH₂ O   Base
‖   5′
O   H   H   β   1′

H   H
3′   2′
OH   H

2′ — Deoxyribonucleoside
5′ — monophosphates

Figure 76–9. General structures of nucleoside and deoxynucleoside 5′-monophosphates.

is deaminated to xanthine by guanase (Fig. 76–11). Hypoxanthine is oxidized to xanthine by xanthine oxidase and then further oxidized to uric acid by the same enzyme (Reaction 8, Fig. 76–11).[254] Thus, although adenine, hypoxanthine, and guanine arise exclusively by cleavage of the corresponding nucleoside, xanthine potentially has three direct precursors: xanthosine (or deoxyxanthosine), hypoxanthine, and guanine. Xanthine oxidase is a flavoprotein containing both iron and molybdenum that oxidizes a wide variety of purines and pteridines.[258, 259] A soluble form of the enzyme having dehydrogenase activity (xanthine dehydrogenase of D-form[260]) has been isolated from a variety of sources.[260–263] The D-form is converted to the oxidase form by the oxidation of thiol groups in the protein, especially in the presence of high concentrations of oxygen.[264–267] It is the D-form of xanthine oxidase that is responsible for the formation of uric acid as the final metabolic product in human purine metabolism. This enzyme converts hypoxanthine to xanthine and xanthine to uric acid (Reaction 8, Fig. 76–11):

$$\text{Hypoxanthine} + H_2O + 2O_2 \rightarrow$$
$$\text{Xanthine} + 2O^{2-} + 2H^+$$

$$\text{Hypoxanthine} + H_2O + O_2 \rightarrow \text{Xanthine} + H_2O_2$$

$$\text{Xanthine} + H_2O + 2O_2 \rightarrow \text{Uric acid} +$$
$$2O^{2-} + 2H^+$$

or

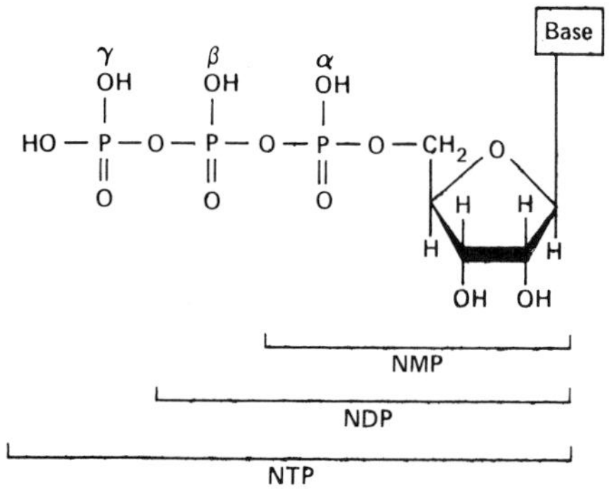

γ   β   α
OH   OH   OH   Base
| | |
HO — P — O — P — O — P — O — CH₂ O
‖   ‖   ‖
O   O   O   H   H

H   H

OH   OH

NMP

NDP

NTP

Figure 76–10. Comparison of the structures of nucleoside, monophosphates, diphosphates, and triphosphates.

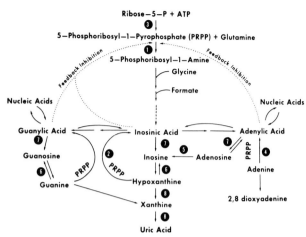

Figure 76–11. Outline of purine metabolism. (1) Amidophosphoribosyltransferase; (2) hypoxanthine-guanine phosphoribosyltransferase; (3) PRPP synthetase; (4) adenine phosphoribosyltransferase; (5) adenosine deaminase; (6) purine nucleoside phosphorylase; (7) 5′-nucleotidase; (8) xanthine oxidase. (From Seegmiller, J. E., et al.: Enzyme defect associated with a sex-linked human neurological disorder and excessive purine synthesis. Science 155:1682, 1967. Copyright 1967 by the AAAS.)

$$\text{Xanthine} + H_2O + O_2 \rightarrow \text{Uric acid} + H_2O_2$$

Superoxide anion or hydrogen peroxide is thus generated.[170] Hydrogen peroxide may then be converted to free hydroxyl radicals:

$$Fe^{2+} + H_2O_2 \rightarrow Fe^{3+} + OH^- + OH^{\cdot}$$

These compounds, O^{2-}, H_2O_2, OH^-, and $OH^{\cdot}$ are important mediators of inflammation and tissue destruction. Xanthine oxidase may have a significant pathophysiologic role in states of ischemia or tissue injury that lead to accelerated adenine nucleotide breakdown.[264]

In humans, xanthine oxidase is found in high activity only in liver and small intestinal mucosa.[267, 268] Trace amounts of activity are found in other tissues, but none is detectable in leukocytes, erythrocytes, or fibroblasts in tissue culture.[268] The enzyme protein is detected by sensitive immunohistochemical techniques in endothelial cells, where xanthine oxidase has been postulated to have a role in defense against injury and microbial invasion.[269] These same studies localize xanthine oxidase activity to hepatic sinusoidal lining cells in the liver, accounting for the abundance of enzyme activity in this organ.[269] Because of this restricted distribution of xanthine oxidase, uric acid synthesis appears largely to be a hepatic process in humans. Presumably, purine degradation products of other tissues are transported to the liver for further oxidation. Plasma contains small quantities of xanthine and hypoxanthine, together amounting to about 0.1 to 0.3 mg per dl,[270, 271] but no other uric acid precursors have been detected in normal plasma in significant quantity, with the possible exception of inosine-5′-monophosphate (IMP) following anoxic muscle injury.[272]

Regulation of Purine Metabolism

Nucleotide Synthesis de Novo. Data obtained in bacterial,[273] avian,[274, 275] and mammalian[276–279] systems indicate that adenylic acid (AMP) and guanylic acid (GMP) inhibit amidophosphoribosyltransferase (Reaction 1, Fig. 76–11), the initial and rate-limiting step of de novo purine biosynthesis, by interacting at separate sites on the enzyme termed the 6-amino and 6-hydroxy sites. Inhibition of the human enzyme by purine nucleotides is competitive with respect to PP-ribose-P, and the kinetics of the reaction shift from a hyperbolic to a sigmoidal function when PP-ribose-P is the variable substrate. Adenylic acid and guanylic acid are also inhibitors of formylglycinamide ribonucleotide (FGAR) amidotransferase, although the importance of this feedback site to the control of the rate of purine synthesis de novo is not established.[277]

A regulatory role of PP-ribose-P was suggested by several observations in human cell culture as well as in humans in vivo.[281–284] Under normal conditions, depletion of PP-ribose-P in vitro and in vivo decreases the rate of purine biosynthesis de novo.[281–284] Elevation of PP-ribose-P by several different mechanisms is associated with an increased rate of purine biosynthesis de novo.[282, 285, 286] In addition, when PP-ribose-P concentrations are initially elevated and then reduced to levels that are still supranormal, there is no inhibitory effect on purine biosynthesis de novo.[281] Finally, the normal intracellular concentration of PP-ribose-P is considerably less than the Michaelis constant established for amidophosphoribosyltransferase in lower organisms[273, 287–289] or in mammalian cells.

The mechanism by which PP-ribose-P and purine ribonucleotides interact to regulate the activity of amidophosphoribosyltransferase was provided by direct study of the enzyme from a human source, and, in subsequent studies, from Chinese hamster fibroblasts and mouse liver.[290, 291] Two forms of human amidophosphoribosyltransferase are apparent following gel filtration; the small form has a molecular weight of about 133,000, and the large form has a molecular weight of about 270,000.[279] The larger species appears to be catalytically inactive, whereas the smaller species appears to be catalytically active. Purine ribonucleotides shift the active smaller species to the inactive larger molecular species: PP-ribose-P converts the large inactive species back to the small active species (Fig. 76–12). Direct in vivo confirmation of this model has now been obtained in mouse liver.[291]

Regulation of Purine Ribonucleotide Interconversions. The first branch point in the pathway leading to the synthesis de novo of adenylic acid and guanylic acid occurs with the synthesis of inosinic acid (see Fig. 76–11). In bacterial systems, each nucleotide appears to regulate its own de novo formation by inhibiting the appropriate nucleotide interconversion; guanylic acid inhibits inosinic acid

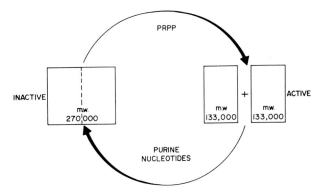

Figure 76–12. Model of interconversion of small (active) and large (inactive) forms of amidophosphoribosyltransferase. (From Kelley, W. N., et al.: Current concepts on the regulation of purine biosynthesis de novo in man. Arthritis Rheum. 18:673, 1975.)

dehydrogenase that catalyzes the formation of xanthylic acid (XMP) from inosinic acid,[292] and adenylic acid inhibits the formation of adenylosuccinic acid (AMP-S) from inosinic acid that is catalyzed by adenylosuccinic acid synthetase. An analysis, however, of the regulation of adenylosuccinic acid synthetase and inosinic acid dehydrogenase[293] from a human source suggests that the utilization of inosinic acid by each of the alternative pathways may be governed by the intracellular concentration of guanylic acid triphosphate (GTP). GTP is a substrate of adenylosuccinate synthetase with a K_m ranging from 31 to 72 μM and an inhibitor of inosinic acid dehydrogenase.[293] Although those observations cannot be applied directly to the setting in vivo, they suggest that as inosinic acid is formed, it is used for the synthesis of XMP, guanylic acid, guanylic acid diphosphate (GDP), and GTP. As GTP reaches a critical concentration in the cell, probably in the micromolar range, it may then increase the activity of AMP-S synthetase, allowing inosinic acid to be effectively used in the synthesis of adenylic acid. As GTP reaches an even higher level, not only can it promote the flux of inosinic acid in the direction of adenylic acid, but also it can then function as a direct inhibitor of the conversion of inosinic acid to XMP and thus guanylic acid. Indirect evidence in support of this mode of regulation derives from studies with cultured murine lymphoma cells partially deficient in adenylosuccinic acid synthetase. AMP synthesis is maintained at the expense of elevated GTP and IMP.[294]

Ribonucleotide Cleavage. In circumstances in which accelerated purine biosynthesis de novo results in production of a surfeit of inosinic acid, there is a rapid conversion of the excess ribonucleotide to uric acid. The controls that lead to this result, rather than to continual expansion of pools of adenyl and guanyl nucleotides, are not well characterized but may depend on tight regulation of nucleotide biosynthetic pathways plus improved competition of 5'-nucleotidase for inosinic acid as its concentration is raised.

Ribonucleotide Degradation. In vivo and in vitro evidence indicates that nucleotide breakdown is regulated in a complex manner.[295-297] When cultured ascites tumor cells are incubated with 2-deoxyglucose or glucose, these compounds are rapidly phosphorylated by ATP.[297] The abrupt decrease of ATP from its rapid utilization results in elevations of AMP and IMP. These nucleotides are dephosphorylated to purine nucleosides by 5'-nucleotidases and are subsequently catabolized or reused.

Regulation of nucleotide degradation is critically controlled by AMP deaminase and 5'-nucleotidases. AMP deaminase is an allosteric enzyme that is activated by ATP and adenosine diphosphate (ADP) and inhibited by GTP and Pi.[1] Release of inhibition of AMP deaminase results in accelerated production of uric acid. Regulation at the level of dephosphorylation is complex and is the focus of intensive investigation. At least three soluble 5'-nucleotidase activities have been described.[298-301] One form has a micromolar K_m for both AMP and IMP and is inhibited by nucleotides.[298, 300] A second form, isolated from a wide variety of sources, hydrolyzes IMP and GMP preferentially but with millimolar K_m values for these substrates.[302-306] This "high K_m" form is activated by ATP and ADP and inhibited by Pi. Finally, nonspecific phosphatases cleave AMP and have millimolar K_m values. This activity is inhibited by Pi.

Although the interactions of these enzymatic activities are incompletely understood at present, their catalytic and regulatory properties indicate that both nucleotides themselves, especially ATP and ADP, as well as Pi are key modulators of nucleotide catabolism. Intracellular ATP and ADP levels activate AMP deaminase and the "high K_m" nucleotidase, whereas they inhibit "low K_m" nucleotidase.[298, 299, 307] In addition, the relative levels of these nucleotides determine the rates of AMP formation by adenylate kinase. Adenylate kinase reversibly catalyzes the conversion of ATP and AMP to ADP. The direction and rate of this reaction are influenced by the relative concentrations of AMP, ADP, and ATP. GTP activates "high K_m" nucleotidase but inhibits AMP deaminase and "low K_m" nucleotidase activity.[299, 308]

Inorganic phosphate levels are also critical. Pi (1 to 5 mM) inhibits AMP deaminase, "high K_m" 5'-nucleotidase, and nonspecific phosphatases but not "low K_m" nucleotidases. Examination of ATP degradation in cellular systems employing different substrates such as deoxyglucose, rotenone, or dinitrophenol reveals marked differences in degradative patterns.[309, 310] The latter two compounds cause increased Pi levels, and ATP degrades through adenosine. The use of 2-deoxyglucose decreases Pi levels and causes degradation by AMP deaminase.

A comparison of the K_m values of cytoplasmic 5'-nucleotidases with reactions of inosinic acid leading to synthesis of adenylic acid or guanylic acid suggests that increasing concentrations of inosinic acid will saturate adenylosuccinic acid synthetase and inosinic acid dehydrogenase first and then activate the 5'-nucleotidases reaction. The latter will lead to

hydrolysis of inosinic acid to inosine, which can then be cleaved by phosphorolysis to form hypoxanthine, followed by oxidation to xanthine and uric acid. Adenylic acid and guanylic acid may be relatively protected from this fate by their higher K_m values and slower rates of hydrolysis in the 5'-nucleotidase reaction and by their conversions to triphosphates, which are poor 5'-nucleotidase substrates.[1, 305, 311]

The purine phosphoribosyltransferases are inhibited by the nucleoside monophosphate products of each reaction. Whether such product inhibition is of any physiologic significance in the control of these pathways remains uncertain.

ORIGIN OF URIC ACID IN HUMANS

Exogenous Contribution. Unless an individual is in a total fast or ingesting a highly artificial purine-free diet, there is a significant exogenous contribution to the body load and urinary excretion of uric acid. The magnitude of this contribution depends on both the amount and the type of purine in the diet, but it is often considerable. For example, when Griebsch and Zollner[312] placed healthy young males on an isocaloric purine-free formula diet, serum urate values declined in 10 days from about 4.9 mg per dl to 3.1 ± 0.4 mg per dl, and urinary excretion of uric acid declined from 500 to 600 mg per day to 336 ± 39 mg per day. Roughly 50 percent of the RNA purines and 25 percent of DNA purines are absorbed and excreted in the urine as uric acid.[313] The difference between amounts of purine administered and excreted may be due to partial hydrolysis, incomplete absorption, enteric decomposition, suppression of purine synthesis de novo, or a combination of some or all of these factors.[312]

Endogenous Formation of Uric Acid. Urinary uric acid excretion declines to constant low values after 5 to 7 days of dietary purine elimination or severe restriction. Mean values then range from 336 ± 39 to 426 ± 81 mg per 24 hours. These values reflect the continued synthesis and turnover of endogenous purines. The urinary uric acid excretion, however, accounts for only a part of the daily disposition of uric acid. Thus, the true rate of endogenous purine turnover cannot be accurately determined by measurement of urinary uric acid excretion but requires the use of isotope dilution techniques in subjects in whom the exogenous contribution has been reduced to a minimum by severe dietary purine restriction.

EXTRARENAL DISPOSITION OF URIC ACID

Urinary recoveries of intravenously administered uric acid are incomplete in normal subjects. Recoveries of infused ^{15}N-uric acid or 2-^{14}C-uric acid ranging from 55 to 95 percent have been reported.[314-317] The average of 14 studies with ^{15}N-uric acid was 75.6

percent. These studies suggested extrarenal disposal of 25 to 50 percent of infused uric acid.

Studies of the turnover of uric acid in normal humans have uniformly shown that the quantity of uric acid turning over each day exceeds the quantity appearing in urine. Surplus amounts have ranged from 100 to 365 mg per day.[318, 320] Thus, these studies also indicate that a significant quantity of uric acid is disposed of by routes other than the kidney. In fact, in comparative studies the fraction of the turnover appearing in urine is essentially the same as the fraction of injected isotopic uric acid recovered in urine.[321-323]

Sorensen[319] estimated that 100 mg or more of uric acid enters the alimentary tract in saliva, gastric juice, and bile. An equal quantity may enter in pancreatic and intestinal juices. These quantities of uric acid are larger than once thought[324, 325] and are sufficient to account for the degradation of one third of the uric acid normally turned over each day.

The total amount of uricolysis that can be attributed to human tissues is unknown but has been estimated to be less than 2 percent of the turnover of the uric acid pool.[326] Thus, for all practical purposes, extrarenal disposal of uric acid is synonymous with intestinal uricolysis.

RENAL HANDLING OF URIC ACID IN NORMAL HUMANS

Several investigators have proposed a four-component model for renal handling of uric acid. This consists of glomerular filtration, early proximal tubular reabsorption, tubular secretion, and finally postsecretory tubular reabsorption.

Within the vertebrate phylum, there is an impressive variety of patterns for the renal disposition of uric acid. In some animals, net secretion of urate is the rule—e.g., birds,[327] reptiles,[328, 329] guinea pigs,[330] Dalmation coach hounds,[331] and certain species of monkeys.[332] In others, net reabsorption is the rule—e.g., rats,[333, 334] non-Dalmatian dogs,[333] cats,[330] several species of New World monkeys,[332] the great apes,[332] and humans.[335] In many of these species, there is evidence for bidirectional transport. In some species in which net secretion occurs, clearance ratios (i.e., C_{urate}/C_{inulin}) fall below 1.0 in the presence of inhibitors of urate secretion.[327, 336, 337] In almost all animals exhibiting net reabsorption, there is evidence that secretion of urate also occurs but is normally masked by extensive reabsorption.[334-342]

The species most nearly comparable to humans in the renal handling of urate is the chimpanzee, and next the *Cebus* monkey. The ratio, C_{urate}/GFR, is about 0.07 to 0.11 in these species,[338, 339, 346] as in humans. Both species respond appropriately to substances that are uricosuric in humans.[346-349] The discussion to follow emphasizes studies performed in humans or in these lower primates.

Glomerular Filtration of Uric Acid. Glomerular ultrafiltration of uric acid was first conclusively demonstrated by micropuncture studies of Bowman's space in the snake and frog, in which urate concentrations in the glomerular fluid were the same as in plasma.[350] Although comparable studies have not been performed with a mammalian glomerulus, micropuncture of the earliest portion of the proximal tubule of the rat also discloses urate concentrations of tubular fluid equal to those of plasma.[340] It is reasonable to assume that ultrafiltration of uric acid also occurs in humans.

Whether all urate in plasma is freely filterable at the glomerulus is uncertain. Although some urate may be bound to plasma protein, this fraction is currently thought to be small, perhaps less than 5 percent. If the fraction is larger, as some studies suggest, binding could result in the incomplete filtration of urate at the glomerulus.

Reabsorption of Uric Acid. Comparisons of renal clearance of uric acid with those of inulin or creatinine disclose a mean ratio of about 0.07 to 0.10 in normal human subjects. If complete glomerular ultrafiltration of plasma urate is assumed, such clearance ratios indicate tubular reabsorption of at least 90 to 93 percent of filtered urate.

Almost all studies of uric acid reabsorption indicate that the process takes place in the proximal tubule. Most localizations have been made with the stop-flow technique in lower animals. Results of free-flow micropuncture studies in *Cebus albifrons* are essentially in accord with results of stop-flow experiments in specifying that most urate reabsorption occurs in the proximal tubule.[351] Distal tubular fluid, however, contains a greater fraction of filtered urate than does final urine. This finding, confirmed in additional animals,[352] may signify reabsorption of a small fraction of filtered or secreted urate in collecting ducts. Thus, although net urate reabsorption occurs largely in proximal tubules in all animals in which the process has been localized (with the exception of the rat, in which it may take place in the loop of Henle), the possibility exists of reabsorption in more distal segments, at least in certain animals.

Available evidence suggests that urate reabsorption occurs by a mechanism of *active transport*. In lower animals, ouabain and metabolic poisons inhibit urate reabsorption.[345, 353] In rats, the net urate reabsorption in the proximal tubule is an active transport process, although passive movement of urate into and out of the proximal tubule has been demonstrated.[354] This active transport mechanism has been shown to have saturable kinetics, indicating that urate reabsorption in the rat proximal tubule is probably carrier mediated.[355] By way of contrast, urate reabsorption in the rabbit proximal tubule has been shown to consist of both passive and facilitated mechanisms. In these studies, it appeared that the net absorptive flux in the rabbit proximal tubule was passive.[356] In nonhuman primates and in humans, the concentration of uric acid in urine may approach one tenth the concentration in plasma during diuresis and inhibition of urate secretion with pyrazinoate.[357] In free-flowing micropuncture samples in the chimpanzee and monkey, the concentrations of urate average 0.6 of the concentrations in plasma and in individual samples may be as low as 0.2. Thus, urate reabsorption may occur against a concentration gradient. According to Weiner and Fanelli[352] the transepithelial potential difference in the proximal tubule is too small to account for this phenomenon by passive forces.

There is a close link between reabsorption of sodium and reabsorption of a number of other components of the glomerular filtrate such as glucose,[358] phosphate,[359] calcium,[360] and bicarbonate,[361] and also uric acid.[360, 362, 363] In conditions associated with an increase in proximal reabsorption of sodium, the clearance of uric acid is reduced (Table 76–3); in conditions leading to decreased proximal reabsorption of sodium, the clearance of uric acid is increased (Table 76–4). In addition, sodium reabsorption per nephron is decreased[364] and uric acid excretion per nephron is increased[365] in chronic renal failure in humans.

The responses of proximal sodium reabsorption to changes in extracellular fluid volume or filtration fraction have been attributed to changes of hydrostatic and effective oncotic pressure ("physical factors") in the peritubular capillaries.[366] Tubular reabsorption of many solutes in addition to sodium is affected.[360] Uric acid is among the solutes that respond to changes in "physical factors."[363]

The pH of the fluid in the proximal tubule is approximately the same as that of plasma.[367] Since the pK_{a1} of uric acid is 5.75, over 98 percent of this compound will be in the form of the monovalent urate ion in the proximal tubule. Excretion of uric acid is largely independent of changes in pH of urine,[368] but acidification is a distal tubular function and would not be expected to affect proximal processes. In highly acidified distal tubular fluid, uric acid will be minimally ionized. One might anticipate that uric acid would then undergo reabsorption by nonionic diffusion. If so, the contribution to urate reabsorption is too small to be readily detected, for unlike other weak organic acids, the overall process of uric acid reabsorption does not follow principles of nonionic diffusion.[352]

Secretion of Uric Acid. The first evidence for uric acid secretion in humans was published in 1950, when Praetorius and Kirk[369] reported the case of a young man with a plasma urate concentration of less than 0.6 mg per dl and a urate/inulin clearance ratio of 1.46. Subsequently, Gutman et al.[341] achieved urate/inulin clearance ratios as high as 1.23 in normal subjects following urate loading, mannitol diuresis, and large doses of probenecid. Each of these studies indicated net tubular secretion of urate in humans under these special conditions. The biphasic effects of salicylate on uric acid excretion were interpreted as representing inhibition of urate secretion with urate retention at low salicylate doses plus inhibition of urate reabsorption with urate diuresis at higher salicylate doses.[370] Diamond et al.[371] have suggested that this apparent paradoxical effect of salicylate on uric acid excretion is due to inhibition of reabsorption by salicylate itself with inhibition of secretion owing to a metabolite, salicylurate. Regardless of the mechanism, bidirectional transport of uric acid is apparent.

The site within the nephron of humans where uric acid secretion occurs is not definitely established. In the only study of this process in humans, the proximal nephron transported uric acid from plasma to tubular fluid but the distal nephron was unable to do so.[372]

In animals in which net secretion occurs, urate moves into the proximal lumen against an electrical potential difference. Thus, the process qualifies as an active transport mechanism. In animals in which net movement of urate is reabsorptive, secretory flux of urate normally proceeds in the direction of a favorable concentration gradient. The process, however, can be inhibited by certain chemicals[344, 345, 373, 374] and possesses specificity; it cannot therefore represent simple diffusion. Weiner and Fanelli[352] have evidence that the mechanism is capable of transport against a gradient and is therefore active. In the chimpanzee,[375] the mercurial diuretic mersalyl is sufficiently uricosuric to unmask net secretion of urate.

Table 76–3. CONDITIONS ASSOCIATED WITH HYPERURICEMIA OR REDUCED RENAL URIC ACID CLEARANCE

Condition	Δ Serum Urate	Δ Uric Acid Clearance	Δ Extracellular Fluid Volume	Δ Filtration Fraction	Predicted Δ Proximal Tubular Sodium Reabsorption*
Salt restriction	↑	↓	↓	–	↑
Diuretic therapy without salt replacement	↑	↓	↓	–	↑
Diabetes insipidus	↑	↓	↓	↑	↑
Hypertension	↑	↓	–	↑	↑
Angiotensin infusion (without increased lactate or ketones)	–	↓	–	↑	↑
Norepinephrine (without increased lactate or ketones)	–	↓	–	↑	↑

*Proximal tubular sodium reabsorption was not evaluated directly in the reported studies; the changes listed represent a prediction from the observed changes in extracellular fluid volume and filtration fraction.

From Holmes, E. W., et al.: The kidney and uric acid excretion in man. Kidney Int. 2:115, 1972. Reproduced with permission.

Table 76–4. CONDITIONS ASSOCIATED WITH REDUCTION IN SERUM URATE LEVELS

Condition	Δ Serum Urate	Δ Uric Acid Clearance	Δ Extracellular Fluid Volume	Δ Filtration Fraction	Predicted Δ Proximal Tubular Sodium Reabsorption
Salt	↓	↑	↑	–	↓
Diuretic therapy with salt replacement	↓	↑	↑	–	↓
Inappropriate secretion of ADH	↓	↑	↑	–	↓
Pregnancy (early)	↓	↑	↑	–	↓

From Holmes, E. W., et al.: The kidney and uric acid excretion in man. Kidney Int. 2:115, 1972. Reproduced with permission.

These results suggest a model involving two oppositely oriented active transport systems in the proximal tubule.

Although a number of authors have expressed the view that urate is secreted by the same mechanism responsible for the secretion of other organic anions, e.g., p-aminohippurate (PAH),[344, 376] there is reason to consider an alternative hypothesis: that urate and PAH are secreted by different transport systems. Two types of observation support this concept. In the reptile, transport of PAH and urate is not strictly coextensive along the nephron. In the chimpanzee[357, 358] and humans,[377] pyrazinoate reduces urate excretion to very low levels at concentrations that do not influence clearance or T_m of PAH.

A number of organic acids inhibit uric acid excretion in animals and humans. These include lactate,[163, 378] β-hydroxybutyrate,[379] acetoacetate,[379] and branched-chain keto acids.[380] These effects have been interpreted as representing inhibition of tubular secretion of urate,[370, 381] for which there is evidence in micropuncture studies.[382]

Postsecretory Reabsorption. In patients with Wilson's disease[383] or Hodgkin's disease[384] and hypouricemia associated with raised renal urate clearance values, pyrazinamide suppresses the hyperuricosuria. In both chimpanzees[339] and humans,[385, 386] the uricosuric response to probenecid is virtually abolished by pretreatment with pyrazinamide or pyrazinoate. Finally, the uricosuric responses to intravenous chlorothiazide[386] or volume expansion with hypertonic sodium chloride[387] are substantially diminished by pretreatment with pyrazinamide.

In 1973, Steele and Boner,[385] Steele,[388] and Diamond and Paolino[389] proposed a model to account for these observations, in which extensive postsecretory reabsorption of urate was postulated. In this model, the effects of pyrazinamide are explained in terms of reduced secretory delivery to the late reabsorptive sites. The location of the postsecretory reabsorptive process could be coextensive with the secretory mechanism, or separate and distal to it, or both. Fanelli and Weiner have attempted to demonstrate that the observations on which this model is based are consistent with coextensive secretion and reabsorption.[390] The latter possibilities are supported in some animals by evidence for urate reabsorption beyond the proximal tubule, as cited earlier. A pa-

tient with renal urate wasting, presumably on the basis of a defect in postsecretory reabsorption, has now been described.[391] Additionally, in two kindreds with familial hyperuricemia owing to diminished renal clearance of urate, it was proposed that the defect was due to increased postsecretory reabsorption.[235, 392] Thus, postsecretory reabsorption may be more important than previously recognized.

Additional Factors Controlling Renal Clearance of Uric Acid in Normal Subjects

Urine Flow. In 1940, Brochner-Mortensen[392] observed that uric acid excretion and clearance were increased at high rates of urine flow in humans. He reported an augmentation limit of 2 ml per minute, above which further increases of rates of urine flow did not affect uric acid clearance. Others have reported that uric acid excretion in dogs is also dependent on the rate of urine flow.[337, 343]

Diamond et al.[393] found that uric acid excretion increased from 290 to 410 μg per minute as urine flow increased from 2.7 to 6.4 ml per minute in response to oral and intravenous fluid loading in humans. The effects of flow may be difficult to distinguish from those of osmotic diuresis.[100] Nevertheless, both the basal uric acid excretion and the increment accompanying diuresis were greatly reduced by pyrazinamide. Diamond and Meisel[394] suggest that the uricosuria of water diuresis can be attributed to diminished postsecretory reabsorption of urate, perhaps in the collecting duct.

Estrogens. The serum urate concentration is relatively low in children, increases in males and to a lesser extent also in females at puberty, and in females increases again at the menopause. Changes in renal urate clearance are at least partly responsible. Wolfson et al.[395] and Scott and Pollard[396] observed that the mean clearance of uric acid was 2.3 and 1.2 ml per minute higher in females than in males. Nicholls et al.[397] found that exogenous estrogens produced a significant increase in mean C_{urate} values from 6.3 to 9.1 ml per minute in 22 transsexual males.

Surgery. Snaith and Scott[398] observed an increase in the excretion of uric acid and in the urinary uric acid to creatinine ratio in 10 patients undergoing abdominal surgery. Little or no change in serum urate concentration occurred. Factors such as anesthetics, increased endogenous steroids, intravenous fluids, intestinal manipulation, and vagotomy were suggested as possibly affecting urate clearance. The only patient not exhibiting a postoperative increase in uric acid excretion was one of two who did not have a vagotomy.

Autonomic Nervous System. In 1937, Grabfield[399] noted that the uricosuric effect of cincophen depended on an intact renal nerve supply in the dog. Denervation increased the renal clearance of uric acid to values attained with cincophen in the intact dog. Cincophen had no additional uricosuric effect in the denervated dog. The effects of cincophen were blocked by ergotamine but not by atropine. Excretion of allantoin, which is cleared by glomerular filtration without subsequent tubular reabsorption, was unchanged by denervation.

Postlethwaite et al.[400] noted that several anticholinergic agents increased renal clearance of uric acid in some subjects. One interpretation is that the parasympathetic nervous system plays a role in controlling the renal excretion of uric acid, perhaps through an effect on peritubular blood flow.

Physical Properties of Uric Acid

Ionization and Salt Formation. The weakly acidic nature of uric acid is due to ionization of hydrogen atoms at position 9 (pK_a = 5.75) and position 3 (pK_a = 10.3).[401] The hydrogen atoms at positions 1 and 7 do not ionize significantly. The ionized forms of uric acid readily form salts such as monosodium and disodium or potassium urates. In extracellular fluids in which sodium is the principal cation, about 98 percent of uric acid is in the form of the monosodium salt at pH 7.4. When the solubility limits of body fluids are exceeded, the crystals that occur in the synovial fluid or the tophi of gouty patients are composed of monosodium urate monohydrate.

Solubility in Water. Monosodium urate is soluble in water to the extent of 120 mg per dl, compared with the much more limited solubility of uric acid in water of only 6.5 mg per dl.[401] The solubility product of monosodium urate is 4.9×10^{-5}. Based on this value, aqueous solutions having the sodium content of serum, 0.13 M, are saturated with urate at 6.4 mg per dl at 37°C.[401] Allen et al.[402] and Loeb[403] have found that urate solubility in solutions of 140 mEq per liter sodium content is markedly temperature dependent, with a twofold drop in solubility between 37°C and 25°C (Table 76–5). Wilcox et al.[404] have carefully reinvestigated the solubility of uric acid and monosodium urate and have found that both are dependent on pH; with increasing pH, uric acid is more soluble, whereas monosodium urate is less so. The solubility of monosodium urate is dependent on sodium concentration and ionic strength as well. No stoichiometric relationship between urate and sodium (or potassium) exists. Binding of monovalent

Table 76–5. SOLUBILITY OF URATE ION (U⁻) AS A FUNCTION OF TEMPERATURE IN THE PRESENCE OF 140 mM Na⁺

Temperature (°C)	Maximal Equilibrium Concentration of U⁻ in the Presence of 140 mM Na⁺ (mg/dl)
37	6.8
35	6.0
30	4.5
25	3.3
20	2.5
15	1.8
10	1.2

From Allen, D. J., Milosovich, G., and Mattocks, A. M.: Inhibition of monosodium urate crystal growth.: Arthritis Rheum. 8:1123, 1965. Reproduced by permission.

cations is a complex function of crystal shape, ion concentration, time, pH, and ion competition.[405]

Solubility in Plasma. The solubility of urate in plasma is somewhat greater than the saturation value in aqueous solutions of 0.13 M sodium. Actual determinations of solubility of monosodium urate in human plasma (or serum) indicate that saturation occurs at concentrations of about 7 mg per dl.[406, 407] Considerably higher concentrations of monosodium urate in plasma can be achieved in supersaturated solutions. Concentrations approaching 400 mg per dl can be obtained by dissolving free uric acid in serum at 38°C.[406] These solutions are unstable, and monosodium urate readily precipitates out. At somewhat lower concentrations of 100 to 200 mg per dl, the solution may remain in a stable supersaturated state for longer periods of time, and no crystallization may occur for 24 hours or more, or until a seed crystal of monosodium urate is added. Stable supersaturated solutions of monosodium urate ranging up to 40 to 90 mg per dl have been observed in patients with leukemia or lymphoma following aggressive therapy with cytotoxic drugs in the absence of allopurinol therapy.[208, 408] The factors responsible for enhanced urate solubility in such patients are not clear and may include both the natural tendency for urate to form stable supersaturated solutions and an increase in plasma of substances capable of solubilizing urate.[409] Even at these remarkable plasma concentrations, however, all urate is digestible by uricase.[408]

The physicochemical state of urate in plasma has been a controversial subject for decades. Some early investigators claimed substantial binding of urate to nondiffusible elements of plasma,[410] whereas others concluded that all urate was in true solution because it was readily ultrafilterable[411] and dialyzable.[412] Even studies of urate localization following filter paper electrophoresis of serum yielded conflicting data in different laboratories.[413] In one laboratory, a careful study of urate binding[414] disclosed no more than 4 to 5 percent of urate bound to plasma protein, a figure agreeing with results of earlier studies in vitro using equilibrium dialysis[412] as well as with studies in vivo.[415] These studies confirm that the binding of uric acid to plasma proteins at 37°C is small and probably of little physiologic significance.

Solubility in Urine. As the urine is acidified along the renal tubule, a portion of urinary urate is converted to uric acid. The solubility of uric acid in aqueous solutions is substantially less than that of urate. At pH 5, urine is saturated with uric acid at 15 mg per dl, whereas at pH 7, urine will accommodate 158 to 200 mg per dl in solution.[401, 407] The limited solubility of uric acid in urine of pH 5 is of particular significance in patients with gout, many of whom display a tendency toward excretion of unusually acidic urine.

At any pH value, human urine will dissolve more urate than can be carried in water. The solubilizing effects of urine have been attributed to urea,[416] proteins, and a mucopolysaccharide that resembles the Tamm-Horsfall mucopolysaccharide.[417, 418] It was initially anticipated that habitual uric acid stone formers would show deficits of this mucopolysaccharide, but this could not be demonstrated.[418]

Crystalline Forms. Monosodium urate occurs as a monohydrate and forms crystals in tissue and joint fluids that are needle-shaped or rod-shaped as described earlier.

Free uric acid crystallizes from pure solutions in an orthorhombic system, forming rhombic plates. Crystals formed in urine incorporate pigments and exist in a variety of crystalline forms. Tissue deposits are composed of monosodium urate monohydrate

and urinary stones largely of uric acid.[419, 420] Both urate and uric acid crystals are birefringent with strong negative elongation when viewed under compensated polarized light. These features permit ready identification of urate crystals in synovial fluid, leukocytes, or tissue deposits and thus constitute an important diagnostic aid.[420, 421]

CLASSIFICATION AND PATHOGENESIS OF HYPERURICEMIA AND GOUT

The biochemical hallmark and prerequisite of gout is hyperuricemia. The concentration of uric acid in body fluids is determined by the balance between rates of production and elimination of urate. The development of hyperuricemia may be due to an excessive rate of uric acid production, a decrease in the renal excretion of uric acid, or a combination of both events.[422, 423]

Hyperuricemia and gout may be classified as primary, secondary, or idiopathic (Table 76–6). Primary hyperuricemia or gout refers to those cases that appear to be innate, that are neither secondary to another acquired disorder nor a subordinate manifestation of an inborn error that leads initially to a major disease unlike gout. Although some cases of primary gout will have a genetic basis, others do not. Secondary hyperuricemia or gout refers to those cases that develop in the course of another disease or as a consequence of drugs. Finally, idiopathic hyperuricemia or gout represents those cases in

Table 76–6. CLASSIFICATION OF HYPERURICEMIA AND GOUT

Type	Metabolic Disturbance	Inheritance
Primary		
Molecular defects undefined		
Underexcretion (90% of primary gout)	Not established	Polygenic
Overproduction (10% of primary gout)	Not established	Polygenic
Associated with specific enzyme defects		
PP-ribose-P synthetase variants; increased activity	Overproduction of PP-ribose-P and of uric acid	X-linked
Hypoxanthine-guanine phosphoribosyltransferase deficiency, partial	Overproduction of uric acid; increased purine biosynthesis de novo driven by surplus PP-ribose-P; Kelley-Seegmiller syndrome	X-linked
Secondary		
Associated with increased purine biosynthesis de novo		
Hypoxanthine-guanine phosphoribosyltransferase deficiency, "virtually complete"	Overproduction of uric acid; increased purine biosynthesis de novo driven by surplus PP-ribose-P; Lesch-Nyhan syndrome	X-linked
Glucose-6-phosphatase deficiency or absence	Overproduction plus underexcretion of uric acid; glycogen storage disease, type I (von Gierke)	Autosomal recessive
Associated with increased ATP degradation		
Associated with increased nucleic acid turnover	Overproduction of uric acid	Most not familial
Associated with decreased renal excretion of uric acid	Decreased filtration of uric acid; inhibited tubular secretion of uric acid; or enhanced tubular reabsorption of uric acid	Some autosomal dominant; some not familial; most unknown
Idiopathic		Unknown

which a more precise classification cannot be assigned. Further subdivisions within each major category are based on the identification of overproduction or underexcretion or both as responsible for the hyperuricemia.

Primary Gout

Renal Handling of Uric Acid in Primary Gout.
Over a century ago, Garrod proposed that diminished excretion of uric acid by the kidneys was one of the possible causes of hyperuricemia. A careful comparison of uric acid clearances and excretion rates over wide but comparable ranges of filtered loads of urate indicates that most gouty subjects have a lower C_{urate}/C_{inulin} ratio than nongouty subjects.[78, 424-429] This ratio increases in gouty subjects as in normal controls when the plasma urate level is raised by feeding of RNA or by infusion of lithium urate, but higher plasma urate values are required in gouty subjects to achieve a given clearance ratio.[428, 429] When the data from these studies are plotted as rates of uric acid excretion at various serum urate levels, the curve of excretion rates has the same form in gouty subjects as in nongouty controls, and the capacity of the excretory mechanism for uric acid is not reduced in gout (Fig. 76–13). The excretion curve, however, is shifted such that gouty subjects require serum urate values 2 or 3 mg per dl higher than those of controls to achieve equivalent uric acid excretion rates. Perhaps 75 to 90 percent of patients with primary gout exhibit the renal defect as defined by this abnormal substrate-velocity curve. Patients with gout caused by one of the specific enzymatic defects usually exhibit a normal uric acid/inulin (or creatinine) clearance ratio.[423]

Theoretically, the shift in the substrate-velocity curve in gouty subjects could be due to (1) reduced filtration of uric acid, (2) enhanced reabsorption, or (3) decreased secretion. Attempts to localize the site of the defect of uric acid transport in the nephron have been thwarted by the limitations of available techniques. At present, there are no unequivocal data to establish any one of these three mechanisms.

Glomerular Filtration. Enhanced binding of urate to proteins in gouty subjects could result in precisely the abnormal substrate-velocity curve described. Although such an abnormality has been proposed in the hyperuricemic Maori,[430] it has yet to be confirmed. Reduced urate binding to proteins has also been described in some gouty subjects by two different groups of investigators.[409, 431]

Tubular Reabsorption. Increased reabsorption of uric acid as a cause of the altered substrate-velocity curve has not received serious consideration in the past. Since reabsorption of secreted urate occurs, the extent of reabsorption in the nephron may be well in excess of 100 percent of the filtered urate. Thus, increased reabsorption could be an important factor in the pathogenesis of hyperuricemia.

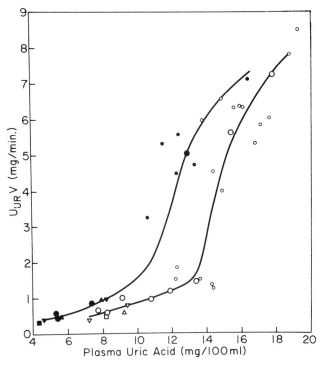

Figure 76–13. Rate of uric acid excretion at various plasma urate levels in nongouty (solid symbols) and gouty (open symbols) subjects. Large symbols represent mean values; small symbols represent individual data of a few mean values selected to illustrate the degree of scatter within groups. Studies were conducted under basal conditions, after RNA feeding, and after infusions of lithium urate. ▲, △, Nugent and Tyler[422]; ▼, ▽, Seegmiller et al.[423]; ●, ○, Yu et al.[424]; ■, □, Latham and Rodnan.[425] (From Wyngaarden, J. B.: Gout. Adv. Metabol. Dis. 2:2, 1965. Reproduced by permission of Academic Press.)

Tubular Secretion. Rieselbach et al.[432] have postulated diminished renal urate secretion *per nephron* as a basis for hyperuricemia in some patients with primary gout without demonstrable overproduction of uric acid. The evidence for this was based on the pyrazinamide suppression test, the reliability of which has now been questioned. According to the current interpretation of the test by Steele,[388] the data presented in support of decreased secretion in these patients would now be reinterpreted as enhanced reabsorption distal to the urate secretory site. Nevertheless, decreased secretion could lead to the abnormal substrate-velocity curve and should be considered further. If one assumes that benzbromarone selectively inhibits tubular reabsorption of secreted urate,[433, 434] maximum uricosuria induced by this drug could be equated with the minimal secretory rate. Using this measure, gouty patients with normal production hyperuricemia had a significantly lower secretory rate in comparison with patients with an overproduction of uric acid.[433-435]

Overproduction of Uric Acid in Primary Gout.
Determination of the 24-hour urinary uric acid excretion is essential in defining the role of uric acid overproduction as a cause of hyperuricemia. Before and during the collection period, the patient should

not be taking medications that alter the metabolism or excretion of uric acid. For adults on a purine-free diet, up to 600 mg per day is considered within the normal range, with a mean value of about 425 mg per day or 5.6 mg per kg per 24 hours.[423, 436] Under usual circumstances, however, it is not practical to place patients on a purine-free diet for 3 to 5 days before the collection of a 24-hour urine sample. With patients on a regular purine diet, a value in excess of 1000 mg per day is clearly abnormal, whereas 800 to 1000 mg per day is considered a borderline value.

It has been suggested that an overproduction of uric acid can be assessed simply by determining the ratio of uric acid to creatinine in the urine or the ratio of the uric acid clearance to the creatinine clearance.[437] Comparison of these two ratios with the 24-hour urinary uric acid excretion, however, reveals a poor correlation between the urinary uric acid excretion in 24 hours in most patients and these ratios.[438] This is largely because of a striking diurnal variation in the excretion of uric acid. Only specific enzymatic deficiencies or rapid cell lysis in treatment of leukemia or lymphoma lead to such a substantial increase in uric acid production that the ratio of uric acid to creatinine in the urine is consistently greater than 0.75. It is necessary, therefore, in most gouty patients to measure the 24-hour uric acid excretion before proper classification of the patient is possible. Attempts to correlate de novo purine synthesis in circulating lymphocytes with clinical assessment of uric acid production status also have been unsuccessful.[439] Therefore, the measurement of purine synthesis in vitro will not predict urate overproduction.

Patients classified as exhibiting an overproduction of uric acid probably represent 10 percent or less of the gouty population. In these patients with primary gout caused by an overproduction of uric acid, there is an acceleration in the rate of purine biosynthesis de novo. Three specific defects that appear to be important as a cause of uric acid overproduction include hypoxanthine-guanine phosphoribosyltransferase deficiency, phosphoribosylpyrophosphate (PRPP) synthetase overactivity, and glucose-6-phosphatase deficiency; these are discussed subsequently. Hers and Van Den Berghe[440] have proposed that abnormalities of AMP deaminase could lead to accelerated nucleotide degradation, increased production of uric acid, and gout. In addition, a deficiency in adenylosuccinate synthetase in cultured cells leads to overexcretion of purine metabolites and increased de novo purine synthesis.[294] These observations predict that a similar deficiency in humans could lead to increased synthesis of uric acid.

Hypoxanthine-Guanine Phosphoribosyltransferase Deficiency. In 1967, Seegmiller, Rosenbloom, and Kelley described a virtually complete deficiency of an enzyme of purine metabolism, hypoxanthine-guanine phosphoribosyltransferase (HPRT) (Fig. 76–14), in erythrocyte lysates from three children and in cultured skin fibroblasts from a fourth patient with the Lesch-Nyhan syndrome,[441] a disorder characterized by choreoathetosis, striking growth and mental retardation, spasticity, self-mutilation, and marked hyperuricemia, with excessive uric acid production and uric acid crystalluria (see Fig. 76–15).[442] The enzyme defect was subsequently confirmed in other tissues as well as in cultured skin fibroblasts and erythrocytes from many similarly affected subjects.[443] Adolescent and adult patients were then described with a "partial" rather than a "complete" deficiency of HPRT.[444] These patients presented with uric acid calculi or gouty arthritis and did not have the devastating neurologic and behavioral features characteristic of children with the complete enzyme defect.[321] This has been referred to as the Kelley-Seegmiller syndrome.

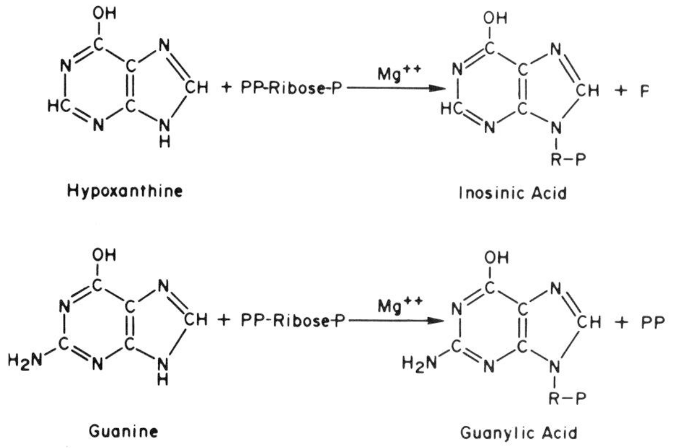

Partial HPRT deficiency is considered to be a form of primary hyperuricemia, since the major clinical manifestations are a direct result of the hyperuricemia and hyperuricaciduria. Patients with the Lesch-Nyhan syndrome and a virtually complete deficiency of HPRT are considered to have secondary hyperuricemia because their major clinical manifestations are unrelated to hyperuricemia per se.

Clinical Features. Patients with a partial deficiency of HPRT typically exhibit a markedly increased production of uric acid, and accordingly, the daily urinary excretion of uric acid is high when expressed on the basis of body weight. Values range from 10 to 36 mg per kg per day in patients with a "partial" deficiency of HPRT.[321] The upper limits of normal in children and adults are 18 and 10 mg per kg per day.[445]

Because of the increased quantity of uric acid in the urine, most patients experience uric acid crystalluria at some time. Some patients develop symptomatic uric acid nephrolithiasis, which may lead eventually to obstructive uropathy with severe and unrelenting azotemia. The older the patient before institution of proper therapy, the more likely that uric acid concretions will develop. Nineteen of the initial 28 patients described with partial HPRT deficiency had a history of uric acid calculi. In at least nine, this was the initial symptom prompting the

Figure 76–14. Reactions catalyzed by hypoxanthine-guanine phosphoribosyltransferase.

patient to seek medical care.[321] The hyperuricaciduria may also lead to pitressin-resistant polyuria.[446]

The serum urate concentration may range from 7 to as high as 18 mg per dl in the absence of renal insufficiency. In an occasional patient, particularly before puberty, a random value will fall within the normal range.[447–449] The serum urate concentration may provide an initial clue to the diagnosis; however, it is not an infallible screening test because of its variability, especially in the younger patients. A history of gouty arthritis was present in 20 of the initial 23 patients with the partial defect who were older than 13 before effective antihyperuricemic therapy was instituted.[321] Over half of this latter group had developed tophi. The likelihood that gouty arthritis or tophi will develop reflects the duration and severity of hyperuricemia prior to antihyperuricemic therapy.

Six of the initial 28 patients with a partial deficiency of HPRT had evidence of neurologic dysfunction.[321, 450–452] In four of these, the neurologic features suggested a forme fruste relationship to the devastating neurologic disease found in patients with the Lesch-Nyhan syndrome. Two siblings had a spinocerebellar syndrome characterized by nystagmus, hyperreflexia, and an inability to perform heel-to-toe walking. Another patient had a delayed onset of speech as a child and a lifelong history of spasticity. A fourth patient had a long history of a seizure disorder. Three of these four patients were mildly retarded, with IQ values ranging from 67 to 75 by formal testing. Most patients with partial HPRT deficiency, however, are normal neurologically.

A number of investigators have confirmed the presence of macrocytic erythrocytes in the peripheral blood and megaloblastic changes in the bone marrow in patients with partial HPRT deficiency.[453–455] Such changes may be present even in the absence of overt anemia. The cause of the megaloblastic changes remains unclear.

Biochemical Features—Nature of the Enzyme Defect. The level of HPRT activity in erythrocytes and cultured B lymphoblasts derived from patients with the partial enzyme defect is the same within a family but often differs between families, with values ranging from 0.01 to nearly 70 percent of normal (Table 76–7).[321, 450–452] Direct evidence for heterogeneous mutations responsible for HPRT deficiency was first provided by detailed studies of highly purified enzyme from five unrelated patients.[456–460] Data acquired by a variety of techniques—including cloning, polymerase chain reaction (PCR) amplification, and direct sequencing of mutant genes—have defined at least 50 different mutations. Among these, major and minor deletions and rearrangements as well as base substitutions are represented (Table 76–8).[458, 459, 461–471] Additional independent mutations continue to be described.[462]

The excessive production of uric acid characteristic of partial HPRT deficiency results from an ac-

Table 76–7. BIOCHEMICAL AND GENETIC CHARACTERISTICS OF HPRT DEFICIENCY

Patients	Specific Activity (% Control)	Immunoreactive Protein (% Control)	Electrophoretic Properties	Kinetic Properties	mRNA
Lesch-Nyhan					
1. D.A., E.C., H.D. D.M., B.S.	<0.7	<0.6	N.D.*	N.M.†	+
2. HPRT$_{Midland}$	<0.7	<0.6	N.D.	N.M.	+
3. HPRT$_{Flint}$	<0.7	<0.6	N.D.	N.M.	+
4. GM1899	<0.7	1.3	N.D.	N.M.	+
5. GM6804	<0.7	<0.6	N.D.	N.M.	Variant‡
6. McA	<0.7	<0.6	N.D.	N.M.	−§
7. W.E., GM2292	<0.7	<0.6	N.D.	N.M.	−
8. HPRT$_{Yale}$	<0.7	92	Cathodal	N.M.	+
9. HPRT$_{Kinston}$	<0.7	72	Cathodal	↑ Km Hx + PRPP	+
10. HPRT$_{New Haven}$	<0.7	50	Anodal	N.M.	+
Gout					
11. R.T., J.M.	<0.7 to 1.4	0.8–3	N.D.	N.M.	+
12. B.D.	<0.7	2	N.D.	N.M.	−
13. HPRT$_{Ann Arbor}$	10	11	Neutral	↑ Km Hx + PRPP	+
14. HPRT$_{Ashville}$	<0.7	4	Cathodal	↑ Km Hx + PRPP	+
15. HPRT$_{Toronto}$	33	52	Anodal	Normal	+
16. HPRT$_{Munich}$	3	79	Cathodal	↑ Km Hx and ↓ Vmax	+
17. HPRT$_{London}$, D.B.	59–69	35–52	Neutral and ↓ apparent size	↑ Km Hx	+

*N.D., not determined owing to limited residual enzyme protein.
†N.M., not measured because of limited catalytic activity of residual enzyme.
‡This mRNA is slightly larger than normal. Southern analysis indicates internal duplication of exons 2 and 3.
§The entire structural gene is deleted.
Adapted from Wilson, J. M., et al.: A molecular survey of hypoxanthine-guanine phosphoribosyltransferase deficiency in man. J. Clin. Invest. 77:188, 1986.

Table 76–8. MUTATIONS IN THE HUMAN HPRT GENE ASSOCIATED WITH THE LESCH-NYHAN SYNDROME OR GOUT

Variant	Mutation	Predicted Amino Acid Change	Reference
Point Mutations			
1151	$G_3{\to}A$	$Met_1{\to}Ile$	461
Gravesend	$G_{20}{\to}A$	$Gly_7{\to}Asp$	462
Mashad	$A_{59}{\to}T$	$Asp_{20}{\to}Val$	462
Detroit	$T_{122}{\to}C$	$Leu_{41}{\to}Pro$	463
Heapy	$T_{125}{\to}C$	$Ile_{42}{\to}Thr$	462
1265	$C_{149}{\to}T$	$Ala_{50}{\to}Val$	461
754-4	$C_{151}{\to}T$	$Arg_{51}{\to}Stop$	461
Shefford	$C_{151}{\to}T$	$Arg_{51}{\to}Stop$	462
Banbury	$G_{152}{\to}C$	$Arg_{51}{\to}Pro$	462
Toronto	N.D.[a]	$Arg_{51}{\to}Gly$	464
955-2, 1510, New Haven	$G_{209}{\to}A$	$Gly_{70}{\to}Glu$	461–463
Yale	$G_{212}{\to}C$	$Gly_{71}{\to}Arg$	465
Flint	$T_{222}{\to}C$	$Phe_{74}{\to}Leu$	466
1522	$C_{222}{\to}A$	$Phe_{74}{\to}Leu$	461
Arlington	$A_{239}{\to}T$	$Asp_{80}{\to}Val$	463
Munich	N.D.[a]	$Ser_{104}{\to}Arg$	467
London	$C_{329}{\to}T$	$Ser_{110}{\to}Leu$	458
Midland	$T_{389}{\to}A$	$Val_{130}{\to}Asp$	468
375	$T_{389}{\to}A$	$Val_{130}{\to}Asp$	461
Runcorn	$T_{395}{\to}C$	$Ile_{132}{\to}Thr$	462
Ann Arbor	$T_{396}{\to}G$	$Ile_{132}{\to}Met$	469
Milwaukee	$G_{481}{\to}T$	$Ala_{161}{\to}Ser$	463
Farnham	$C_{486}{\to}G$	$Ser_{162}{\to}Arg$	462
1321 & North Mymms	$C_{508}{\to}T$	$Arg_{170}{\to}Stop$	461, 462
Marlow	$C_{527}{\to}T$	$Pro_{176}{\to}Leu$	462
1734	$T_{548}{\to}C$	$Ile_{183}{\to}Thr$	461
Kinston	N.D.[a]	$Asp_{194}{\to}Asn$	459
New Britain	$T_{595}{\to}G$	$Phe_{199}{\to}Val$	463
Ashville	$A_{602}{\to}G$	$Asp_{201}{\to}Gly$	468
779	$A_{611}{\to}G$	$His_{204}{\to}Arg$	461
Reading	$G_{617}{\to}A$	$Cys_{206}{\to}Tyr$	462
Deletions			
1423	$ATT_{80{\to}82}$[b]	ΔTyr_{28}	461
1052	Exon 4	Premature termination	461
1757 & 1758[c]	Exon 4	Premature termination	461
Bamber Ridge	Exon 4	Premature termination	462
Coulsdon	Exon 7	Premature termination	462
DAG25	Exon 7	Premature termination	462
DAG33	Exon 7	Premature termination	462
Connersville	Exon 8	Premature termination	463
Cheltenham	$GT_{288{\to}289}$	Premature termination	462
Michigan	$GTT_{535{\to}537}$	Premature termination	463
Brierley Hill	$GT_{617{\to}618}$[d]	Premature termination	462
Evansville	Deletion$_{643{\to}663}$	Premature termination	463
Insertions			
Chicago	T_{56}[e]	Premature termination	463
1650	$G_{206-211}$[f]	Premature termination	461
Codicote	T_{298}[g]	Premature termination	462
1656	$T_{435-437}$[h]	Premature termination	461
1266	$GT_{511-517}$[i]	Premature termination	461

[a]N.D. not determined. The amino acid substitutions in these variants were determined by amino acid sequencing. Amino acid substitutions were deduced from nucleotide substitutions in the others.
[b]The exact position of this deletion could be 80–82 or 81–83.
[c]Cell lines 1757 and 1758 are derived from siblings.
[d]Ambiguous; may occur at either 617–618 or 619–620.
[e]The nucleotide insertion could occur at nucleotide position 56, 57, or 58.
[f]The exact position is unclear; insertion could be at any site from 206 to 211.
[g]Actual nucleotide position ambiguous. A track of deoxythymidines occurs at 294 to 298.
[h]The exact position is unclear; insertion could be at any site from 435 to 437.
[i]The exact position is unclear; insertion could be at 511 to 512, 514 to 515, or 516 to 517.

celerated rate of purine biosynthesis de novo. There are at least three possible mechanisms by which a deficiency of HPRT could result in excessive purine synthesis. First, the deficiency could lead to enhanced purine synthesis by virtue of decreased concentrations of either IMP or GMP, since these nucleotides are normally important inhibitors of de novo purine biosynthesis.[277, 279] Attempts to measure intracellular levels of IMP and GMP in these cells have been of only limited value, partly because of the very low intracellular concentration of these compounds under normal conditions.[473, 474] Second, the increased concentration of PP-ribose-P characteristic of HPRT deficiency could increase de novo purine biosynthesis by providing more substrate for the enzyme that catalyzes the presumed limiting step of this pathway, amidophosphoribosyltransferase. The altered concentration of PP-ribose-P appears to be the more important factor responsible for the accelerated rate of purine biosynthesis de novo occurring with HPRT deficiency. Third, a decreased reutilization of hypoxanthine occurs in HPRT deficiency,[305] where the loss of enzyme activity leaves hypoxanthine only one pathway of metabolism, i.e., oxidation to uric acid. The loss of hypoxanthine reutilization leads to decreased consumption of phosphoribosylpyrophosphate and increased intracellular concentrations of this compound.

Genetic Features. The familial nature of partial HPRT deficiency was recognized in the original report of this syndrome.[444] Major clinical manifestations occur in affected males, with evidence of transmission through carrier females. The X-linked nature of the inheritance has been confirmed by many different techniques.

Several observations indicate that heterozygotes for a deficiency of HPRT exhibit subtle biochemical abnormalities in vivo, even though they are generally asymptomatic clinically. An elevated serum urate concentration has been noted in a number of such patients, and at least four have had recurrent monoarticular arthritis thought clinically to represent gout. In addition, several obligate heterozygotes have excreted greater than normal quantities of uric acid in their urine.[475, 476] Finally, studies on the incorporation of ^{14}C-glycine into urinary uric acid in heterozygous individuals have demonstrated a moderate increase in the rate of purine synthesis de novo.[477, 478] Based on the data cited here, some cases of gout in the female occurring after menopause may be related to heterozygosity for HPRT deficiency.

Increased PRPP Synthetase Activity. Sperling et al.[479] demonstrated a markedly accelerated rate of PP-ribose-P synthesis in two gouty brothers with flamboyant overproduction of urate and showed[480] that this was a consequence of altered kinetic properties of PP-ribose-P synthetase (Fig. 76–15). Subsequently, at least 20 additional families have been discovered in which excessive rates of PP-ribose-P synthesis can be attributed to abnormalities of this enzyme. At least five distinct molecular alterations

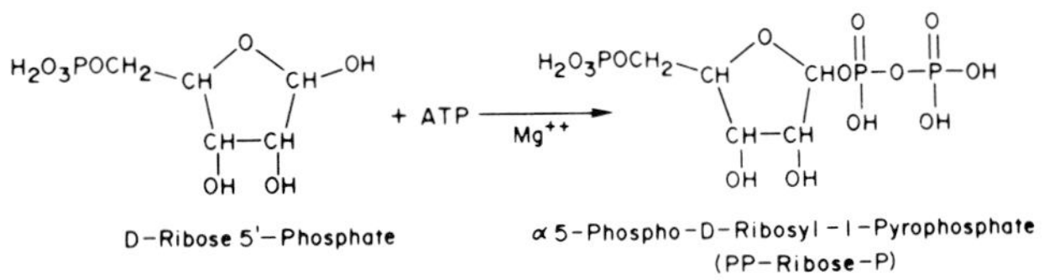

Figure 76–15. Reaction catalyzed by PP-ribose-P synthetase.

have been noted among these families.[481–486] Affected male subjects had clinical gout. Age of onset of gout has ranged from 21 to 39 years. Three of the patients had a history of renal calculi, with onset as early as age 18 in one. None of the patients had tophi. Hyperuricemia ranged from 9.6 to 13.6 mg per dl, and urinary uric acid excretion values ranged from 950 to 2400 mg per day.

The enzyme is now known to be coded by DNA in the X chromosome,[487] and thus males are affected through asymptomatic carrier females. Studies suggest mosaicism in female family members and X-linked dominant transmission of this trait.[488]

Although the biochemical cause of the increased PRPP synthetase activity is different in each family, the net result of all three types of defects is an excessive rate of generation of PP-ribose-P. There is little question now that increased PP-ribose-P synthetase activity represents a specific genetic subtype of gout. This class of defects is probably rare. Several hundred additional gouty overproducers have been screened for abnormal PP-ribose-P synthetase activity in several laboratories in the United States, Europe, Japan, and Israel, with discovery of only a few other possible examples.

Secondary Gout

Renal Handling of Uric Acid in Secondary Gout. Numerous secondary causes of hyperuricemia and gout can be attributed to a decrease in the renal excretion of uric acid. A reduction in the glomerular filtration rate leads to a decrease in the filtered load of uric acid and thus to hyperuricemia; patients with renal disease will be hyperuricemic on this basis. Other factors, such as decreased secretion of uric acid, have been postulated in patients with some types of renal disease, e.g., polycystic kidney disease and lead nephropathy. Gout is a rare complication of the secondary hyperuricemia resulting from renal insufficiency.

Diuretic therapy currently represents one of the most important causes of secondary hyperuricemia in humans. Diuretic-induced volume depletion leads to enhanced tubular reabsorption of uric acid as well as a decreased filtered load of uric acid. Decreased secretion of uric acid has also been postulated as a possible mechanism in diuretic-induced hyperuricemia. A number of other drugs lead to hyperuricemia by a renal mechanism, although the nature of the abnormality remains less clear; these agents include low-dose aspirin, pyrazinamide, nicotinic acid, ethambutol, ethanol, and cyclosporine.[489]

Decreased renal excretion of uric acid is thought to be an important mechanism for the hyperuricemia associated with several disease states. Volume depletion may be an important factor in patients with hyperuricemia associated with adrenal insufficiency and nephrogenic diabetes insipidus. An accumulation of organic acids on any basis is thought to competitively inhibit uric acid secretion and thus lead to hyperuricemia on that basis. This is the case in patients with starvation, alcoholic ketosis, diabetic ketoacidosis, maple syrup urine disease, and lactic acidosis of any cause, e.g., hypoxemia, respiratory insufficiency, chronic beryllium disease, and acute alcohol intoxication. The renal basis of the hyperuricemia in conditions such as chronic lead intoxication, hyperparathyroidism, hypoparathyroidism, pseudohypoparathyroidism, and hypothyroidism remains unclear.

Overproduction of Uric Acid in Secondary Gout. There are many causes of secondary hyperuricemia associated with an increased production of uric acid. In some, the increased excretion of uric acid is related, as it is in primary gout, to an accelerated rate of purine biosynthesis de novo. Patients with glucose-6-phosphatase deficiency (von Gierke's glycogen storage disease) uniformly exhibit an increased production of uric acid as well as an accelerated rate of purine biosynthesis de novo. A major cause of increased uric acid synthesis results from an accelerated breakdown of ATP. This occurs during hypoglycemia-induced glycogen degradation with the subsequent elevated concentrations of phosphorylated sugars in the liver in glucose-6-phosphatase deficiency.[311, 490, 491] Indeed, the acceleration of purine synthesis de novo observed in this disorder is secondary to a primary depletion of the adenine nucleotide pool. Patients with the Lesch-Nyhan syndrome, which is due to a virtually complete deficiency of HPRT, also uniformly exhibit a profound overproduction of uric acid and an accelerated rate of purine biosynthesis de novo (Fig. 76–16). In these patients, as in those with gout caused by a partial deficiency of HPRT, the basic mechanism is thought to be related to a decreased consumption of PRPP and perhaps to decreased reutilization of hypoxanthine.

In the majority of patients with secondary hyperuricemia caused by an overproduction of uric acid, the predominant abnormality appears to be an increased turnover of nucleic acids. A number of diseases, including the myeloproliferative and lymphoproliferative disorders, multiple myeloma, secondary polycythemia, pernicious anemia, certain hemoglobinopathies, thalassemia, other hemolytic anemias, infectious mononucleosis, and some carcinomas, may be associated with increased marrow activity or increased cell turnover at other sites and an associated increased turnover of nucleic acids. The increased turnover in nucleic acids leads in turn to hyperuricemia, hyperuricaciduria, and a compensatory increase in the rate of purine biosynthesis de novo.

An important cause for overproduction of uric acid in secondary hyperuricemia appears to be related to the acceleration of ATP degradation to uric acid. Hyperuricemia observed in acutely ill patients may be related to the accelerated degradation of ATP.[167–170, 311] Patients with myocardial infarction, acute smoke inhalation, respiratory failure, and status epilepticus appear to fall into this category. Strenuous exercise leads to the excessive degradation of muscle ATP to uric acid.[492] This can lead to increased serum urate levels, which can be substantial with extreme exercise, as seen in status epilepticus.[493, 494] Myogenic hyperuricemia has been reported in patients with three glycogen storage diseases with muscle involvement either in the basal state or following exercise.[494–504] This abnormality has been observed in debranching enzyme deficiency (type III), myophosphorylase deficiency (type V), and muscle phosphofructokinase deficiency (type VII). The mechanism for this disorder is related to excessive ATP degradation in muscle tissue during exercise secondary to decreased formation of carbohydrate substrates necessary for ATP synthesis (Fig. 76–17).

Normal and ischemic exercise cause increased formation of ATP degradation products, including inosine, hypoxanthine, and xanthine, as compared with the resting subject;[495, 496, 501, 502] the degradation of these compounds to uric acid may lead to hyperuricemia. Excessive formation of ATP degradation products following ischemic exercise also occurs in carnitine palmitoyl transferase deficiency and myoadenylate deaminase deficiency and could potentially cause hyperuricemia.[506, 507]

As described earlier, hyperuricemia occurs in glucose-6-phosphatase deficiency (glycogen storage disease, type I). In this disorder, hypoglycemia can stimulate uric acid synthesis. Glucagon contributes to this response by activating ATP degradation to uric acid.[311, 490, 491] Excessive alcohol consumption, although associated with hyperlacticacidemia, also appears to be associated with increased synthesis of uric acid owing to accelerated degradation of ATP.[166, 167]

GENETICS OF GOUT

Gout has been recognized as a familial disorder since antiquity. Garrod[508] found the ancestral trait to be almost 80 percent among his patients and commented that "breed is stronger than pasture." A familial incidence of gout of 50 to 80 percent has been reported by English observers,[509] but these contrast with figures as low as 11 percent in Denmark.[28] In the United States, the familial incidence has generally ranged from 6 to 18 percent,[510, 511] but figures up to 75 percent[512] have been obtained after persistent questioning. In two large series from clinics with a special interest in gout, one English[29] and

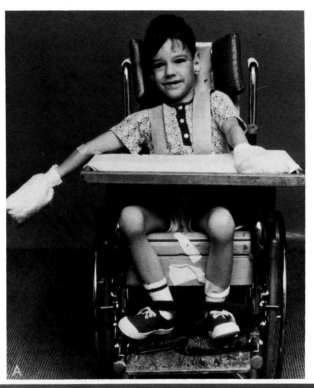

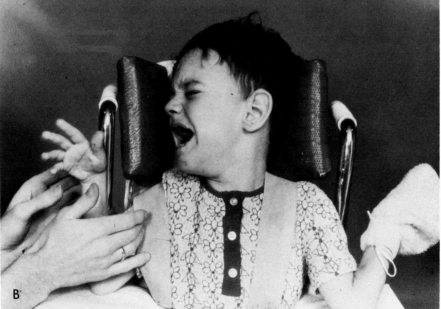

Figure 76–16. *A,* Patient H. D. *B,* Note agitated appearance and the attempt by the patient to bite his fingers after the wrapping is removed from his hands.

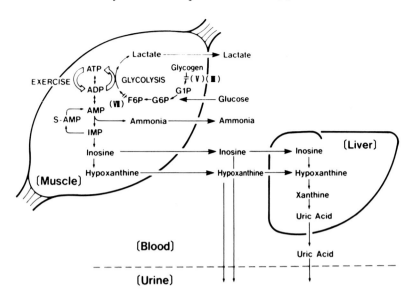

Figure 76–17. Mechanism of myogenic hyperuricemia in glycogen storage diseases. In the three glycogen storage diseases associated with metabolic myopathy, there is impairment of the metabolic pathways providing substrate necessary for adenosine triphosphate (ATP) synthesis. Thus, when ATP is consumed by muscle contraction, accelerated degradation of ATP may occur. (Adapted from information appearing in Mineo, I., et al.: Myogenic hyperuricemia. A common pathophysiologic feature of glycogenosis types III, V, and VII. N. Engl. J. Med. 317:75, 1987. Used by permission.)

one American,[513] about 40 percent of the gouty subjects gave a positive family history of gout. These wide discrepancies may be attributed in part to variations of diligence in pursuing genealogic data. Population studies of families suggested the highest correlations between the mothers' serum urate and their children's, mainly their sons'.[23]

When all available data are considered, they suggest that serum uric acid concentrations are controlled by multiple genes.[514] The probability of isolating an apparently dominant genetic factor increases when the basis of selection is racial, when the group is an isolate, or when the study concerns several generations of families in which gout occurs. Evidence for polygenic control will be more prominent when the population is heterogeneous or when only sibs of gouty subjects are studied.

The modes of inheritance of known rare subtypes of primary gout were described earlier. These include X-linked inheritance of both HPRT deficiency and PRPP synthetase overactivity and autosomal inheritance of glucose-6-phosphatase deficiency and some types of gout associated with a renal defect and a high incidence of renal disease.

ACUTE GOUTY ARTHRITIS

Role of the Urate Crystal in the Acute Attack

Garrod[515] proposed in 1859 that the acute gouty paroxysm was triggered by precipitation of sodium urate crystals in the joint or neighboring tissues: "The deposited urate of soda may be looked upon as the cause, and not the effect, of the gouty inflammation." In 1899, Freudweiler[516] reproduced acute gouty attacks by injection of microcrystals of sodium urate and also of other crystals such as those of hypoxanthine or xanthine.[517] Subcutaneous injection of urate crystals was followed by evolution of a

histologically characteristic tophus.[518] Freudweiler also proposed a central role for the urate crystal in the genesis of the acute gouty attack. In 1961, a study of joint fluid by McCarty and Hollander[50] led to a renewed interest in crystals of sodium urate in gouty effusions[519] and particularly in the diagnostic value of large numbers of negatively birefringent crystals within synovial fluid leukocytes during the acute attack as demonstrated with the use of polarized light.[520, 521] Urate crystals are virtually constant in acute gouty arthritis.[421, 522] At the height of the response, the majority of the crystals are intracellular, although the extracellular proportion increases as inflammation subsides. Urate crystals may also rarely occur in synovial fluid in a spherulite form.[523] The large "beach ball"–like structures are negatively birefringent and are digestible with the addition of uricase to the slide. Since the simultaneous occurrence of gout and infection in the same joint has been observed,[524, 525] the identification of urate crystals does not rule out a concomitant septic arthritis. The importance and use of urate crystals in the diagnosis of gouty arthritis is reviewed in Chapter 40.

In 1962, Faires and McCarty[526] and Seegmiller et al.[527–529] rediscovered the capacity of microcrystals of sodium urate to evoke an inflammatory response in skin, subcutaneous tissues, and joints of animals and humans. In both normouricemic and gouty humans, the inflammatory response strikingly resembles the acute gouty attack. It may be successfully treated with[530] or prevented by[531] colchicine. The response is not limited to crystals of sodium urate but may also be evoked by calcium oxalate,[526] calcium pyrophosphate dihydrate,[532] sodium orotate,[527] and certain steroids,[526] but not by diamond dust.[533]

Synovial Membrane Tophi in Acute Gout. Agudelo and Schumacher[534] have observed urate crystals and microtophi in the synovial membrane 2 days after the onset of the first attack of acute gout. This finding as well as others suggests that acute gout may be superimposed on a joint in which urate deposition and low-grade chronic inflammation may have developed silently at an earlier time. The crystals of the synovium are often in a superficial location near the joint space. Thus, it seems possible that crystals could flake off the synovial membrane and enter the joint space, there to trigger an inflammatory attack when engulfed by polymorphonuclear or synovial cells in the synovial fluid.

Mechanism of Crystal Formation. The factors leading to precipitation of monosodium urate crystals in tissue and the mechanisms by which these crystals induce inflammation are complex and poorly understood. The mystery of crystal deposition in some tissues and not others is not yet satisfactorily explained, but some interesting clues are emerging from studies of the chemistry of cartilage. A relationship between the process by which the acute attack is triggered and that by which visible urate deposits form is not yet established, but both processes involve crystal formation, and it is reasonable to surmise that a pathogenetic connection exists. This link too may reside in the behavior of certain cartilage constituents.

Supersaturation of serum or synovial fluid with monosodium urate is a necessary but not sufficient precondition for the development of acute gouty arthritis. To be sure, there is a correlation between the degree of hyperuricemia and the prevalence of gouty arthritis,[535] but it is also true that most hyperuricemic subjects never develop gout, and that those who do are often hyperuricemic for years before an attack supervenes. In addition, subjects with a history of gout may develop acute gouty arthritis at a time when their serum urate concentration is well below saturation. Perhaps the best example of this phenomenon is the occurrence of acute gouty arthritis in the patient recently started on antihyperuricemic therapy.

In subjects with gouty synovitis, the concentration of urate in the synovial fluid is usually similar to its concentration in serum.[536, 537] Urate has less of a tendency to precipitate in plasma than in synovial fluid, since plasma is a significantly better solvent for monosodium urate than synovial fluid.[538] Thus, an important question is what makes monosodium urate crystals form in some subjects but not in others despite a similarity in serum urate concentrations. Specific factors in gouty synovial fluid or tissue may enhance urate crystallization. Addition of synovial fluids from gout patients to a supersaturated solution of sodium urate under physiologic conditions greatly enhanced urate nucleation, whereas fluids from degenerative joint disease patients moderately enhanced nucleation, and fluids from rheumatoid patients had only a slight effect.[539] Gamma globulin and insoluble type I collagen have been shown to promote urate formation in vitro.[540] Additional factors may regulate the deposition of urate in human tissues. These include lower intra-articular tempera-

ture, the presence of proteoglycans, changes in pH, reduced binding of urate to plasma protein, trauma, aging, and dysequilibrium, which can result from extracellular fluid reabsorption from a joint space at a faster rate than urate.[403, 414, 415, 528, 529, 541–553]

Mediation of the Inflammatory Response. An important role for the complement system[554–556] in this process has been suggested by the monosodium urate–mediated, C-reactive protein–dependent, or IgG-dependent complement depletion of plasma and activation of the classic and alternative complement pathways.[557–559] In excess of 30 crystal-associated polypeptides have been identified, including C1q, C1r, C1s, fibronectin, fibrinogen, IgG, lysosomal enzymes, and apolipoproteins.[557, 560–572] Crystal-bound apolipoprotein B is an inhibitor of synovitis by blocking phagocytosis, superoxide generation, and cytolysis associated with neutrophils.[551, 552] These properties of lipoproteins may be related to inhibition of physical association of crystals with cell membranes. The latter may explain why crystals may be present in asymptomatic joints (see later).

The multiplicity of factors identified in the acute inflammation associated with monosodium urate crystals makes it difficult to identify those that are critical from those that may be playing a facilitating role. Other factors may be involved in mediating the chronic inflammation and joint destruction that occur in gout. The release of latent collagenase and prostaglandin E_2 (PGE_2) from cultured synovial fibroblasts may have a role in the latter process.[563] Synovial lining cells may also produce a chemotactic factor.[564]

Role of the Leukocyte

The acute inflammatory response to urate crystals depends on the presence of polymorphonuclear leukocytes. In dogs rendered leukopenic with vancomycin[565] or with antipolymorphonuclear leukocyte serum,[566] urate crystals fail to induce an inflammatory response; responsiveness is restored by cross circulation with replacement of leukocytes[565] or when time for recovery is allowed.[566] The neutrophil remains the central focus for crystal-induced synovitis, although a role has been proposed for platelet mediators as well. The neutrophil is attracted by crystal-induced chemotactic factor,[567–572] which is degraded after binding to its specific receptor.[573] There appears to be no correlation between crystal sizes, shapes, or numbers and the intensity of inflammation.[574] Protein-coated crystals of sodium urate are taken up within the phagosomes of polymorphs and merge with lysosomes. The interaction between the crystals and the lysosomal membrane involves binding and then membranolysis. The crystal surface and membrane interaction may be electrostatic in nature,[575–577] since monosodium urate crystals have a high negative surface potential. Crystals stimulate oxygen radical formation by neutrophils,[559, 560, 578, 579] and hence the release of lysosomal mediators as well as the release of superoxide anion contributes to the local inflammation. The stimulation of oxygen radical formation is inhibited by supernatants of polymorphonuclear leukocytes exposed to monosodium urate crystals.[579] Since polymorphonuclear leukocyte lysis occurs during crystal-induced synovitis, this provides possible explanation for the self-limitation of acute gouty attacks.

Other mediators released from polymorphonuclear leukocytes appear to have importance in the urate-induced inflammation. These include leukotriene B_4, kinins, latent collagenase, kallikrein, PGE_2, and 6-keto-PGF_1-alpha and interleukin-1.[580–584] The further metabolism and deactivation of leukotriene B_4, an important local mediator of inflammation, is partly inhibited by monosodium urate crystals, thus potentiating its activity.[576] Clearly, Hageman factor XII is not essential for the development of crystal-induced synovitis because gout may occur even when there is a deficiency of this factor.[585] The interaction of urate crystals with mononuclear phagocytes stimulates the production of interleukin-1, the peptide mediator of fever and other features of inflammation.[584] The dissemination of this hormone-like substance may account for the systemic effects of acute gouty arthritis, including fever, peripheral neutrophilia, acute phase reactants, and polyarticular inflammation. A number of mediators of inflammation in addition to interleukin-1, including tumor necrosis factor (TNFα) and interleukin-6, are released by monocytes and synovial phagocytic cells exposed to monosodium urate crystals and can be identified in gouty joint fluid.[586, 587] Possibly most interesting is that interleukin-8, a potent neutrophil chemotactic factor, is also released.[588] This could be one important factor involved in the attraction of neutrophils into the joint space to initiate acute arthritis in gout.

Unexplained Features

Self-Limited Nature of the Attack. Although it is not known why acute gouty arthritis is self-limited, several contributing factors may be postulated: (1) The increased heat of inflammation may increase urate solubility, diminishing the tendency toward new crystal formation and favoring dissolution of existing crystals. (2) The increased blood flow may help transport urate away from the joint and lessen the tendency toward formation of local regions of supersaturation. (3) Some of the ingested urate crystals may be destroyed by the myeloperoxidase of the leukocytes, thus diminishing the load of crystals released by ruptured cells and capable of perpetuating the inflammatory response. (4) Adrenal cortical hormones secreted as a part of the alarm reaction of acute attack may suppress the inflammatory process. (5) Superoxide anion generated during crystal-leukocyte interaction during acute gout may alter crystal properties and the proteins bound to the crystals.[589] (6) Proteins exuding into the joint or materials re-leased from lysis of leukocytes may displace IgG from the surface of the crystals and thus decrease their phlogistic properties.[590, 591]

Crystals Present with Minimal Inflammation. The work of McCarty[520] and others[421, 524] has shown that urate crystals are a virtually constant finding in the synovial fluid during an acute attack, and a great deal of work has been directed toward the mechanism or mechanisms by which urate crystals may trigger the attack. Urate crystals, however, are also often found in the joints of patients with chronic gout at times when there is only indolent soreness of low intensity. Also, as mentioned earlier, urate crystals may be present in the synovium of joints during the quiescent phase between acute attacks. Clearly, more than the presence of crystals is involved in the pathogenesis of the gouty paroxysm.

TREATMENT OF GOUT

The therapeutic aims in gout are (1) to terminate the acute attack as promptly and gently as possible; (2) to prevent recurrences of acute gouty arthritis; (3) to prevent or reverse complications of the disease resulting from deposition of sodium urate or uric acid crystals in joints, kidneys, or other sites; and (4) to prevent or reverse associated features of the illness that are also deleterious, such as obesity, hypertriglyceridemia, or hypertension.

In considering these aims, an important distinction must be made between the means employed in the management of the acute inflammatory manifestations on the one hand and the control of hyperuricemia (and hyperuricaciduria) on the other. With one possible exception, those agents that are so highly effective in the treatment of acute gout are of no value in the control of hyperuricemia. Conversely, those drugs useful in the control of hyperuricemia are of no immediate or direct value in the treatment of the acute gouty attack.

Asymptomatic Hyperuricemia

There are relatively few indications for institution of drug therapy in patients with asymptomatic hyperuricemia, for the incidence of gout is low. Because advice on the indications for drug therapy of asymptomatic hyperuricemia is so often solicited, this is reviewed in Chapter 35.

Acute Gouty Arthritis

The affected joint should be placed at rest and suitable therapy instituted as soon as possible. The pharmacology of agents of value in the treatment of acute gout has been considered in Chapter 46. The acute gouty attack may be effectively terminated by any of several drugs. For practical purposes, the choice in most situations is among colchicine, indomethacin, the other newer nonsteroidal anti-inflammatory drugs (NSAIDs), and rarely phenylbutazone or its analogue oxyphenbutazone.

Drugs that affect the serum urate concentration should not be changed, i.e., started or stopped, during an acute attack. Just as sudden fluctuations in serum urate levels may tend to precipitate an acute attack, an inflammatory reaction already in progress may be made substantially worse by a major change in the urate concentration. Antihyperuricemic drug therapy should not be instituted until an attack has resolved. Antihyperuricemic drugs already in place should not be stopped unless the drug has just been started and has itself possibly contributed to the attack.

If an appropriately treated attack has not begun to resolve within 48 hours, one should consider the possibility that another disease, such as infection, may be contributing to the inflammatory process. If no other disease can be incriminated, one should then consider changing the medication. For example, in protracted attacks, phenylbutazone will sometimes succeed where colchicine has failed. If after several days the attack is still disabling and inflammation does not abate, intra-articular glucocorticoids may be indicated.

Colchicine

Oral Administration. Colchicine may be administered orally in a dose of 0.5 or 0.6 mg (1 tablet) at hourly intervals until the joint symptoms ease; until the patient develops nausea, vomiting, or diarrhea; or until he or she has taken a maximum of 12 doses (6 mg). In most patients, the side effects precede or coincide with improvement in joint symptoms. If the attack is treated within the first few hours, a favorable response can be predicted over 90 percent of the time, often without the need for the maximum dose.[65] If treatment is delayed beyond 12 hours, only 75 percent of the patients with acute gouty arthritis treated in this manner will respond within 12 to 48 hours.[65] The major disadvantage of the oral colchicine regimen is that 50[591] to 80 percent[592] of patients treated in the usual manner develop increased peristalsis, cramping abdominal pain, diarrhea, nausea, or vomiting before relief from gout occurs or coincident with relief. The drug must be stopped promptly and symptomatic treatment given as needed for the gastrointestinal side effects. One may use oral colchicine when the diagnosis of gout is uncertain and the patient's response might be of diagnostic help. In the uncomplicated gouty patient with an established diagnosis, we use indomethacin or another NSAID as noted subsequently.

Intravenous Administration. Colchicine has been used intravenously since at least 1951.[592, 596] When used properly, the drug abolishes the acute attack without the high incidence of gastrointestinal side effects observed with oral administration.

An initial dose of 2 mg is followed, if relief is not obtained, by an additional 1 mg every 6 to 12 hours to a maximum dose of 4 mg during the treatment period. The colchicine should be diluted with 20 ml of normal saline before administration and given slowly into an established venous access to minimize sclerosis of the vein. In addition, oral colchicine should be discontinued, and no additional colchicine should be given for at least 7 days because of the slow excretion of this drug.

The use of intravenous colchicine is associated with some risk.[595] The most common complication is local extravasation during or immediately after injection. This can lead to inflammation and necrosis that may be painful. The presence of small veins that are difficult to inject represents a relative contraindication to intravenous use of this drug. Because one loses gastrointestinal symptoms as an indicator of toxicity, bone marrow suppression may be the first complication. The drug should not be used in patients who are neutropenic. In addition, the total dose should be reduced if the patient has been receiving oral colchicine chronically or if he or she has significant liver or renal disease. Intravenous colchicine should not be given if there is combined renal and liver disease, creatinine clearance less than 10 ml per minute, or extrahepatic biliary obstruction. Although serious toxicity has been rare, it has occurred when these factors have not been considered.

Although colchicine remains efficacious, the reports of severe bone marrow toxicity and death[592–599] and myopathy and neuropathy[600] indicate that the drug should be used with caution, if at all, to treat acute gouty arthritis.

Nonsteroidal Anti-inflammatory Drugs. Indomethacin was first shown to be effective in the treatment of acute gouty arthritis in 1963.[601–603] This response has subsequently been confirmed by many investigators. The drug may be effective in doses as low as 25 mg given four times a day. We recommend an initial dose of 50 to 75 mg followed by 50 mg every 6 hours, with a maximum dose of 200 mg in the first 24 hours. In most instances, substantial relief will have occurred within this time. To prevent relapse, it is reasonable to continue this dose for an additional 24 hours, then taper to 50 mg every 8 hours for 24 hours, and then 25 mg every 8 hours for 24 hours.

Cuq[604] treated 20 patients with acute gouty arthritis with naproxen and recorded a response in 75 percent. Sturge et al.[605] found that naproxen, 750 mg as the initial dose, followed by 250 mg three times per day, was as effective in the treatment of acute gouty arthritis as phenylbutazone, 200 mg four times per day.

Several studies document the effectiveness of fenoprofen in the treatment of acute gouty arthritis.[606] Wanasukapunt and colleagues[607] treated 27 patients with gouty arthritis with fenoprofen, 800 mg every 6 hours, until improvement occurred followed by taper of the drug. Nineteen patients had a good response within 48 hours.

Ten patients with acute gouty arthritis were treated with ibuprofen, 800 mg every 8 hours orally.[608] With resolution, the dose was reduced to 400 mg every 6 hours for an additional 24 to 72 hours. All ten patients showed complete resolution within 72 hours.

In comparative studies, the efficacy of sulindac, 400 mg daily, was found to be similar to that of phenylbutazone, 600 mg daily.[605]

The administration of piroxicam, 40 mg per day for 5 days, is an effective therapy in acute gout.[609, 610] The dose of 40 mg per day was more effective than 20 mg per day in that a higher percentage of patients received faster and complete relief within 5 days (53 versus 28 percent).[611] Substantial improvement was seen by 24 hours, and most patients were improved or free of symptoms by 5 days.

Ketoprofen (100 mg three times a day) was found to be as effective as indomethacin (50 mg three times a day). Toxicity, however, was common in this study as in many others. Thirty-one of 59 patients experienced side effects, and three in each group withdrew from the study.[612] NSAID toxicity is even more likely in patients with antecedent gastrointestinal or renal disease, who are usually excluded from clinical trials.

Contraindications or causes of concern for the use of NSAIDs include active peptic ulcer disease, regional enteritis, ulcerative colitis, severe infection, and mental disease. Inflammatory bowel disease is considered a relative contraindication because of reports[613, 614] of bowel perforation occurring after indomethacin use in this setting. NSAIDs also should be used with caution in patients with impaired renal function or coronary artery disease. Although they may often cause only a transient rise of blood urea nitrogen and creatinine, severe azotemia may result in patients with diminished glomerular filtration rate from congestive heart failure.[615] Acute renal failure has occasionally been observed in patients with normal renal function.[616] Indomethacin decreases coronary blood flow and increases coronary vascular resistance in patients with coronary artery disease.[617] These properties are probably related to inhibition of prostaglandin synthesis; these side effects may occur with other nonsteroidal drugs.[615, 618]

Glucocorticoids

Systemic adrenocorticosteroids are frequently used in practice for acute polyarticular gout when there are contraindications to NSAIDS or colchicine.[619, 620] Effective doses have varied between 20 and 50 mg prednisone per day; optimal steroid regimens have not been systematically studied. Rebound attacks may occur as steroids are withdrawn unless other prophylactic measures can be used.

Intra-articular glucocorticoids are useful in the treatment of acute gout limited to a single joint or bursa. Triamcinolone hexacetonide injected intra-articularly into the involved joint is useful in treating acute gout limited to a single joint or bursa; relief

from pain is usually prompt and complete within 12 hours.[621] When this local measure was accompanied by administration of colchicine, no recurrence was noted.

The time of initiation of therapy may be as important as the choice of drug. With any of these agents, the sooner the drug is started, the more likely the patient is to have a rapid and complete response. If the patient cannot take medications by mouth or has active peptic ulcer disease, intravenous colchicine can be given. For most patients in whom the diagnosis is secure, the acute attack should be treated with indomethacin or another NSAID.

Patients with established gout should have their preferred anti-inflammatory agent immediately available to them, and they should be instructed to start taking the drug at the first "twinge" of an acute attack. The attack may often be aborted with less than a full therapeutic dose of the drug. Some patients can terminate an incipient acute attack with a single dose of 50 to 100 mg of indomethacin.

The anti-inflammatory agents are reviewed extensively in Chapters 41 and 43.

Prophylaxis

The practice of giving small daily doses of colchicine as prophylaxis against acute attacks of gout was introduced by Cohen in 1936[622] and advocated by Talbott and Coombs in 1938.[623] In 1952, Gutman and Yu[102] reported that 18 of 31 patients who ingested colchicine daily for 18 months or more experienced a conspicuous reduction in the frequency of acute attacks. This program enabled restoration of full employment for 13 patients who had been virtually incapacitated because of frequent episodes of gout.

Gutman[624] reported observations in 260 patients who were given 0.5 to 2 mg of colchicine a day (in 66 percent the dose was 1.0 mg) over a mean period of 6.4 years. Colchicine alone was given in 117 patients; the remainder received uricosuric agents in addition. In 74 percent, there was complete or virtually complete cessation of attacks; in 20 percent, the response was satisfactory; and in 6 percent, the regimen was a failure. In patients who received both uricosuric drugs and colchicine, discontinuance of colchicine alone was sometimes followed by recurrence of attacks, whereas this did not happen in patients in whom the uricosuric drug alone was stopped. The effectiveness of prophylactic colchicine has been confirmed by Paulus et al.[625] However, even relatively low maintenance doses of colchicine such as 0.6 mg twice a day given to patients with chronic renal insufficiency can produce neuromyopathy, so that patients must be monitored during chronic use.[600]

In the patient unable to tolerate even one colchicine tablet per day, indomethacin has been used prophylactically at a dose of 25 mg two times per day with some subjective success.

A program of maintenance colchicine or indomethacin may make the difference between frequent incapacitation and uninterrupted daily activities. If for a period of a year the serum urate value has been maintained well within the normal range and there have been no acute attacks or tophi, maintenance colchicine may be discontinued. Here, again, it is advisable to warn the patient that this alteration in the therapeutic program may be followed by an exacerbation of acute gouty arthritis.

Control of Hyperuricemia and Monosodium Urate Deposition

Based on our current concepts, the first episode of acute gouty arthritis represents the initial clinical evidence of urate deposition in most patients. Control of hyperuricemia with antihyperuricemic agents can prevent and, in fact, reverse urate deposition. A spectrum of opinion exists as to when in the course of gout antihyperuricemic therapy should be started, and how important maintenance of normal serum urate levels may prove to be in the absence of renewed symptoms. Some physicians regard the first gouty attack as already a late event in a disorder marked by years of antecedent silent deposition of microcrystalline deposits of urate in cartilage and other connective tissue. There is some morphologic evidence for this.[534]

Many physicians take the position that since tophi and symptomatic chronic gouty arthritis develop only in a minority of cases of gout—ordinarily very slowly after many years of recurrent acute attacks—unnecessary or premature medication can be avoided, without demonstrable penalty, by withholding antihyperuricemic drugs until there is an indication that recurrent attacks cannot be prevented by a prophylactic program alone or that tophaceous deposits are indeed forming.[626] For example, some patients never have a second attack even in the absence of therapy. The probability of such a course is greatest in patients with only minimally elevated serum urate values and with normal 24-hour urinary uric acid values. In the Framingham population study,[535] intervals between attacks were longer early in the course of the disease and in subjects with serum urate values under 8 mg per dl as compared with those with higher values. In the experience of Yu and Gutman,[627] only 62 percent of patients experienced a second attack of acute gout within 1 year and 78 percent within 2 years. Seven percent had no further attacks for 10 years or more even without antihyperuricemic drugs or maintenance colchicine therapy.

Antihyperuricemic drugs provide a definitive method for controlling hyperuricemia. Although it is important to treat and prevent acute attacks of gouty arthritis with anti-inflammatory agents, it is the long-term control of hyperuricemia that ultimately modifies the manifestations of the gouty diathesis. In general, the aim of antihyperuricemic therapy is to reduce the serum urate concentration to below the concentration at which monosodium urate saturates extracellular fluid (6.4 mg per dl). When this is achieved, urate deposits will resolve (Fig. 76–18). Reduction to these levels may be achieved pharmacologically at present by the use of uricosuric agents or allopurinol. Antihyperuricemic drugs generally do not have anti-inflammatory properties (the exception is aspirin in high doses). Uricosuric agents reduce the serum urate concentration by enhancing the renal excretion of uric acid. Although a large number of drugs exhibit this property, the most effective agents available in the United States today are probenecid and sulfinpyrazone. These two drugs are effective in lowering the serum urate in 75 to 80 percent of patients with hyperuricemia and gout. The prototypic drug available to decrease uric acid synthesis is allopurinol. Allopurinol inhibits xanthine oxidase, the enzyme that catalyzes the oxidation of hypoxanthine to xanthine and xanthine to uric acid. These agents are discussed extensively in Chapter 50.

The choice of an antihyperuricemic drug should have a rational basis because the treatment of hyperuricemia in gout is ordinarily carried on indefinitely. In those patients with gout who excrete less than 700 mg of uric acid per day and have normal renal function, a reduction in serum urate concentration can be achieved equally well with allopurinol or a uricosuric drug such as probenecid or sulfinpyrazone. Each of these agents may prevent the deterioration of renal function in patients with primary gout.[628-635] There is no clear-cut evidence that uricosuric drugs are superior to the inhibitors of xanthine oxidase or vice versa in preventing renal damage from hyperuricemia in subjects with a normal excre-

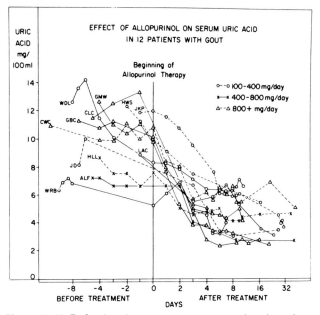

Figure 76–18. Reductions in serum urate concentrations in patients receiving allopurinol. (From Wyngaarden, J. B., and Kelley, W. N.: Gout and Hyperuricemia. New York, Grune & Stratton, 1976.)

tion of uric acid and no history of renal calculi. All other things being equal, a uricosuric drug might be tried first because these agents are not known to influence purine or pyrimidine metabolism as allopurinol does.[636, 637] In general, the candidate for uricosuric agents at present is the gouty patient under 60 years of age with normal renal function (creatinine clearance greater than 80 ml per minute), uric acid excretion of less than 700 mg per 24 hours on a general diet, and no history of renal calculi. There is very little to lead one to choose either probenecid or sulfinpyrazone over the other, although an advantage of the latter is its added antiplatelet effect. There are certain situations in which an inhibitor of xanthine oxidase is clearly the drug of choice in the gouty patient (Table 76–9). Gouty individuals with a history of renal calculi of any type should be treated with an inhibitor of xanthine oxidase. Likewise, patients with tophi generally should receive allopurinol to decrease the load of uric acid that must be handled by the kidney. Patients with gout and mild renal insufficiency can be tried on either type of agent, but uricosuric drugs would not be expected to work when the glomerular filtration rate is less than 30 ml per minute.[638] Allopurinol doses must be decreased in the presence of reduced glomerular filtration. A final indication for allopurinol is the failure of uricosuric drugs to produce a serum urate of less than 7.0 mg per dl or patient intolerance of the uricosuric agent. Occasionally, allopurinol and a uricosuric drug may be used in combination when the patient has tophaceous gout and it is not possible to reduce the serum urate below 7.0 mg per dl with allopurinol alone.

Another indication for allopurinol therapy in the gouty patient relates to the level of uric acid excretion. The incidence of renal calculi is greater than 34 percent in patients with primary gout who excrete more than 700 mg per day of uric acid.[222] Likewise, it is the magnitude of uric acid excreted per day that correlates best with the development of acute uric acid nephropathy.[207] Therefore, these individuals run a risk of developing renal disease. They are also at greater risk for developing uric acid stones or acute uric acid nephropathy on initiation of uricosuric therapy. The logical choice of therapy in these patients is, therefore, an agent, such as allopurinol,

Table 76–9. INDICATIONS FOR ALLOPURINOL

Hyperuricemia Associated with Increased Uric Acid Production
Urinary uric acid excretion of 1000 mg or more in 24 hours
Hyperuricemia associated with HPRT deficiency or PP-ribose-P synthetase overactivity
Uric acid nephropathy
Nephrolithiasis
Prophylaxis before cytolytic therapy
Intolerance or Reduced Efficacy of Uricosuric Agents
Gout with renal insufficiency (GFR <60 ml per minute)
Allergy to uricosurics

that decreases uric acid synthesis. For the same reason, patients with certain neoplastic diseases that are associated with hyperuricemia caused by increased nucleotide catabolism with increased uric acid synthesis may be treated with allopurinol. The effectiveness of allopurinol as an antihyperuricemic agent is illustrated in Figure 76–18. There is evidence to suggest that allopurinol is overprescribed.[639]

Management of Acute Uric Acid Nephropathy

Acute uric acid nephropathy may be effectively prevented in patients at high risk by alkalinizing the urine above pH 6.5, maintaining high urine flow, and prophylactically administering allopurinol.[640] These measures decrease the uric acid concentration and increase uric acid solubility.

More detailed studies of the acute tumor lysis syndrome indicate that despite allopurinol therapy, urinary uric acid may still increase and urinary excretion of xanthine can increase to concentrations capable of precipitating xanthine nephropathy.[641] Alternative approaches using increased destruction of uric acid may be indicated. The administration of urate oxidase appears promising in prophylaxis against renal damage.[642, 643] Polyethylene glycol modified uricase may be particularly useful because it has a prolonged half-life and appears to be nonantigenic.[644]

If the patient develops acute renal failure, the rapid application of preventive measures may reverse the problem. If this fails, the only effective therapy is hemodialysis, which is 10 to 20 times more effective than peritoneal dialysis in clearing uric acid, since uric acid crosses the peritoneum relatively poorly.

Management of Nephrolithiasis

In potential formers of stones of any type, the first rule is to maintain a large urinary volume by the liberal ingestion of fluids, about 2 or 3 liters per day. This is particularly important in those hyperuricemic subjects whose daily urinary uric excretion is excessive; these patients constitute about 20 to 25 percent of the total. In gouty subjects with persistently acid urine, regular use of suitable alkalinizing agents may be attempted to adjust urine pH up to 6.0 to 6.5, which will shift uric acid to its more soluble urate form.

The treatment of choice in nephrolithiasis of gout is allopurinol, which lowers both serum and urinary uric acid values. Allopurinol has greatly ameliorated the uric acid stone problem in gout. There is also evidence that its use reduces the rate of recurrence of calcium stones in hyperuricemic or hyperuricaciduric subjects.[226–228, 645] However, it does not seem effective in patients with calcium stones in the absence of hyperuricemia or hyperuricaciduria.[646]

Ancillary Factors

In addition to anti-inflammatory agents, colchicine prophylaxis, and antihyperuricemic therapy, other factors may be decisive in determining whether recurrent attacks, chronic arthritis, stone, or nephropathy will develop.

Role of Diet

Weight Reduction. Many gouty patients are overweight, and restoration of ideal weight through regulated caloric restriction is to be advocated strongly. Crash weight-reduction programs are to be avoided because these may precipitate attacks of gout. Some gouty subjects respond to gradual weight loss with a reduction in serum urate concentration and urinary uric acid excretion;[647, 648] others do not.[649]

Alcohol Ingestion. Many gouty patients consume liberal amounts of alcohol. Acute excesses may lead to exacerbations of hyperuricemia, in large part secondary to the temporary hyperlactacidemia found during inebriation. Chronic ingestion of alcohol may stimulate increased purine production, resulting in increased hyperuricemia and hyperuricaciduria.[164, 650] The added purine load resulting from regular ingestion of beer may also be detrimental. The gouty patient should be instructed in the deleterious effects of too liberal use of alcoholic beverages.

Avoidance of Acute Attack. Some gouty subjects are susceptible to acute attacks following use of alcoholic beverages, especially heavy wines and champagnes, or of rich foods, notably those high in purines, proteins, or fats. Others describe idiosyncratic responses, such as acute gout following eating of asparagus, but such relationships are rare and questionable. In gouty subjects, the dietary indiscretions of holidays, feast days, and weddings are especially prone to end in gouty arthritis. A diet designed to avoid indiscretions known to be associated with the precipitation of an acute gouty attack in a particular individual may be helpful.

Reduction in Body Load of Purines. In the pursuit of this objective by dietary means, one may limit the ingestion of preformed purines that add to the burden of the uric acid pool and urinary disposal as well as the ingestion of dietary constituents that promote endogenous production of purines. The introduction of potent uricosuric agents in the management of gout led to a general loss of attention to the purine content of the diet on the part of both physician and patient. Although the use of rigid purine restriction is indeed superseded by the use of uricosuric agents and allopurinol, the neglect of dietary factors in gout has been a disservice to some patients. It is still prudent to avoid excessive intake of purines in the average gouty patient. A diet restricted in purine content will reduce the urinary excretion of uric acid by 200 by 400 mg per day and lower the mean serum urate value about 1 mg per dl.[102] In some patients, the reduction is even greater.[431] For example, increased serum urate levels, hyperuricosuria, dysuria, and uric acid crystalluria have been associated with the substantial purine content in high-dose pancreatic extract therapy in cystic fibrosis.[651, 652] Under these specific conditions, reduction of pancreatic enzyme therapy dose decreases serum urate levels and urinary uric acid. Severe dietary purine restriction is not often necessary, unless renal function is very poor and the control of hyperuricemia with drugs is unsatisfactory. The purine content of certain foods is summarized in Table 76–10. Unfortunately, the low purine diet may be atherogenic in this setting. In addition, a diet with a high fructose content may increase the levels of both uric acid and triglycerides.[125, 653–657]

In both normal and gouty humans, the rate of endogenous purine production is somewhat greater on a high protein than on a more moderate protein diet.[658] It may be desirable to limit the intake of nitrogenous precursors of uric acid by restriction of dietary proteins to levels of 70 or 80 g per day. The benefits of dietary protein restriction, however, are small compared with those of purine restriction. Excessive loads of dietary fructose may result in sudden acceleration of adenyl nucleotide catabolism and accelerated rates of uric acid synthesis[655, 659] and should also be avoided.

Control of Hypertriglyceridemia. Seventy-five percent or more of patients with primary gout have hypertriglyceridemia, which may or may not be related to alcohol ingestion. The initial step in management of hypertriglyceridemia is reduction to ideal weight. If triglycerides are still over 300 mg per dl after 6 weeks of appropriate dietary regulation and weight reduction, clofibrate (2 g per day) may be tried. In unresponsive patients, nicotinic acid (1.5 to 3.0 g per day), less pleasant to take, will usually lower triglycerides, although if caloric restriction and weight maintenance do not return the triglycerides to completely normal values, drugs rarely will, and control, not "cure," becomes the highest expectation.[660] The hyperuricemic effect of nicotinic acid should not prevent its use in the patient with gout so long as antihyperuricemic therapy is modified accordingly.

Management of Hypertension. About one third of gouty subjects are hypertensive. The complications of hypertension are potentially more serious than those of hyperuricemia, and one should not hesitate to use whatever drugs are necessary to control the hypertension. Angiotensin converting enzyme inhibitors and calcium channel blockers are effective and probably the safest agents in the treatment of hypertension in patients with concomitant gout.

Many hypertensive gouty patients require a thiazide diuretic. If needed to control hypertension, one should not hesitate to use one and to adjust the antigout program. The combined control of hypertension and hyperuricemia (and hyperlipidemia if present) should give the patient the best possible

Table 76–10. PURINE CONTENT OF CERTAIN FOODS*

List 1. Foods that contain very large amounts (150–1000 mg) of purine bodies in 100 g

Heart, sheep	174	Meat extracts	236–356	Smelts	168
Herring	172	Mussels	154	Sweetbreads	426
Herring roe	484	Sardines	234	Yeast	570–990

List 2. Foods that contain a large amount (75–150 mg) of purine bodies in 100 g: anchovies, bacon, codfish, goose, grouse, haddock, liver, kidneys, mackerel, mutton leg, partridge, pheasant, pigeon, salmon, scallops, trout, turkey, veal, venison

List 3. Foods that contain a moderate amount (up to 75 mg) of purine bodies in 100 g: asparagus, bass, beef, bouillon, brains, chicken, crab, duck, eel, halibut, ham, kidney beans, lentils, lima beans, liverwurst, lobster, mushrooms, mutton chop, navy beans, oysters, peas, plaice, pork, rabbit, roe, shrimp, spinach, tongue, tripe

List 4. Foods that contain an insignificant amount of purine or no purine:

1. Beverages
    Carbonated
    Chocolate
    Cocoa
    Coffee
    Fruit juices
    Postum
    Tea
2. Butter†
3. Breads and breadstuffs (refined and whole grain)
4. Caviar
5. Cereals (refined and whole grain)
6. Miscellaneous cereal products
    Arrowroot
    Hominy
    Macaroni
    Noodles
    Sago
    Spaghetti
7. Cheese of all kinds†
8. Eggs
9. Fats of all kinds (but eat in moderation)†
10. Fruits of all kinds
11. Gelatin
12. Milk
    Buttermilk
    Condensed milk
    Malted milk
13. Nuts of all kinds
    Peanut butter
14. Pies (except mincemeat)†
15. Sugar and sweets
16. Vegetables (except those in List 3)
17. Vegetables and cream soups (to be made with allowed vegetables and without meat stock)
18. Vitamin concentrates
    Cod liver oil
    Halibut oil

*To calculate the purine or "purine bodies" in a given food, the purine nitrogen is multiplied by 3: for example, 200 mg of purine nitrogen equals 600 mg of purine bodies.

†These foods are high in fats.

Source: Hench, P. S.: In Cecil, R. L., and Loeb, R. F. (eds.): Textbook of Medicine. 9th ed. From Bridges, M. A.: Food and Beverage Analyses. 3rd ed. Philadelphia, Lea & Febiger, 1950, pp. 188–192; and Dirr, K., and Decker, P.: Biochem. Z. 316:239, 1944. Reprinted with permission.

outlook with respect to avoidance of gouty attacks, preservation of renal function, and maintenance of cardiovascular and cerebrovascular status.

References

1. Wyngaarden, J. D., and Kelley, W. N.: Gout and Hyperuricemia. New York, Grune & Stratton, 1976.
2. Copeman, W. S. C.: A Short History of the Gout. Berkeley, University of California Press, 1964.
3. Neuwirth, E.: Milestones in the diagnosis and treatment of gout. Arch. Intern. Med. 72:377, 1943.
4. Schnitker, M. A.: A history of the treatment of gout. Bull. Inst. Hist. Med. 4:89, 1936.
5. Talbott, J. H.: Gout. 3rd ed. New York, Grune & Stratton, 1967, p. 5.
6. Rodnan, G. P.: A gallery of gout. Being a miscellany of prints and caricatures from the 16th century to the present day. Arthritis Rheum. 4:27, 1961.
7. Rodnan, G. P., and Benedek, T. G.: Cotton Mather and the gout. Arthritis Rheum. 6:789, 1963.
8. Rodnan, G. P., and Benedek, T. G.: Ancient therapeutic arts in the gout. Arthritis Rheum. 6:317, 1963.
9. Bywaters, E. G. L.: Gout in the time and person of George IV: A case history. Ann. Rheum. Dis. 21:325, 1962.
10. Strauss, M. B.: Familiar Medical Quotations. Boston, Little, Brown & Company, 1968, p. 186.
11. Hippocrates: The Genuine Works of Hippocrates, Vols. I and II. Translated from the Greek with a preliminary discourse and annotations by Francis Adams. New York, Wood, 1886.
12. Evans, J. G., Prior, I. A. M., and Harvey, J. P. B.: Relation of serum uric acid to body bulk, haemoglobin and alcohol intake in two South Pacific Polynesian populations. Ann. Rheum. Dis. 27:319, 1968.
13. Acheson, R. M., and Chan, Y. K.: The prediction of serum uric acid on haemoglobin and other factors in the general population. Lancet 2:777, 1966.
14. Mikkelsen, W. M., Dodge, H. J., and Valkenburg, H.: The distribution of serum uric acid values in a population unselected as to gout or hyperuricemia: Tecumseh, Michigan, 1959–1960. Am. J. Med. 39:242, 1965.
15. Harlan, W. R., Cornoni-Huntley, J., and Leaverton, P. E.: Physiologic determinants of serum urate levels in adolescence. Pediatrics 63:569, 1979.
16. Akzuki, S.: A population study of hyperuricaemia and gout in Japan: Analysis of sex, age and occupational differences in thirty-four thousand people living in Nagano Prefecture. Ryumachi 22:201, 1982.
17. Harlan, W. R., Hull, A. L., Schmouder, R. P., Thompson, F. E., Larkin, F. A., and Landis, J. R., Jr.: Dietary intake and cardiovascular risk factors, part II. Serum urate, serum cholesterol, and correlates. In Vital and Health Statistics, United States, 1971–75. Series 11, No. 227. DHHS Pub. No. (PHS) 83–1677. Washington, D.C., Public Health Service, March 1983.
18. Glynn, R. J., Campion, E. W., and Silbert J. E.: Trends in serum uric acid levels 1961–1980. Arthritis Rheum. 26:87, 1983.
19. Anton, F. M., Garcia-Puig, J., Ramos, T., Gonzalez, P., and Ordas, J.: Sex differences in uric acid metabolism in adults: Evidence for a lack of influence of estradiol-17 beta (E₂) on the renal handling of urate. Metabolism 35:343, 1986.
20. Marinello, E., Giuseppe, R.-S., and Marcolongo, R.: Plasma follicle-stimulating hormone, luteinizing hormone, and sex hormones in patients with gout. Arthritis Rheum. 28:127, 1985.
21. Kuntz, D., Chretien, J. M., Ryckewaert, A., et al.: Distribution and correlations of serum uric acid in two French adult populations. Semin. Hop. Paris 55:241, 1979.
22. Zalokar, J., Lellouch, J., and Claude, J. R.: Serum urate and gout in 4663 young male workers. Semin. Hop. Paris 57:664, 1981.
23. Nishioka, K., and Mikanagi, K.: Hereditary and environmental factors influencing on the serum uric acid throughout ten years population study in Japan. Adv. Exp. Med. Biol. 122A:155, 1980.
24. Currie, W. J. C.: Prevalence and incidence of the diagnosis of gout in Great Britain. Ann. Rheum. Dis. 38:101, 1979.
25. Campion, E. W., Glynn, R. J., and deLabry, L. O.: Asymptomatic hyperuricemia: The risks and consequences. Am. J. Med. 82:421, 1987.
26. Roubenoff, R.: Gout and hyperuricemia. Rheum. Dis. North Am. 16:539, 1990.

27. Delbarre, F., Braun, S., and St. George-Bhaumet, F.: La goutte feminine (analyse de quarante observations). Semin. Hop. Paris 43:623, 1967.
28. Arnold, W. J., and Grobner, W.: Clinical manifestations of hyperuricemia. Clin. Rheum. Dis. 3:51, 1977.
29. Grahame, R., and Scott, J. T.: Clinical survey of 354 patients with gout. Ann. Rheum. Dis. 29:461, 1970.
30. Harth, M., and Robinson, C. E. G.: Gouty arthritis in a D. V. A. hospital. A retrospective study. Med. Serv. J. Can. 18:671, 1962.
31. Nishioka, N., and Mikanagi, K.: Clinical features of 4,000 gouty subjects in Japan. Adv. Exp. Med. Biol. 122A:47, 1980.
32. Scudamore, C.: A Treatise on the Nature and Cure of Gout and Rheumatism, Including General Considerations on Morbid States of the Digestive Organs: Some Remarks on Regimen, and Practical Observations on Gravel. 2nd ed. London, Longman, 1817.
33. Canoso, J. J., and Yood, R. A.: Acute gouty bursitis: report of 15 cases. Ann. Rheum. Dis. 38:326, 1979.
34. Bonal J., and Schumacher, H. R.: Podagra is more than gout. Bull. Rheum. Dis. 34:1, 1984.
35. Sydenham, T.: The Works of Thomas Sydenham, translated from the Latin by R. G. Lathan, Vol. II. London, New Sydenham Society, 1850, p. 124.
36. Hadler, N. M., Franck, W. A., Bress, N. M., et al.: Acute polyarticular gout. Am. J. Med. 56:715, 1974.
37. Raddatz, D. A., Mahowald, M. L., and Bilka, P. J.: Acute polyarticular gout. Ann. Rheum. Dis. 42:117, 1983.
38. Mody, G. M., and Naidoo, P. D.: Gout in South African blacks. Ann. Rheum. Dis. 43:394, 1984.
39. Simkin, P. A., Campbell, P. M., and Larson, E. B.: Gout in Heberden's nodes. Arthritis Rheum. 26:94, 1983.
40. Parhami, N., Greenstein, N., and Juozevicius, J. L.: Erosive osteoarthritis and gout: Gout in 36 joints. J. Rheumatol. 11:469, 1986.
41. Lally, E. V., Zimmerman, B., Ho, G., and Kaplan, S. R.: Urate-mediated inflammation in nodal osteoarthritis: Clinical and roentgenographic correlations. Arthritis Rheum. 32:86, 1989.
42. Baer, P. A., Tennenbaum, J., Fam, A. G., and Little, H.: Coexistent septic and crystal arthritis. Report of four cases and literature review. J. Rheumatol. 13:604, 1986.
43. Boulware, D. W., Lopez, M., and Gum, O. B.: Tuberculous podagra (Letter). J. Rheumatol. 12:1022, 1985.
44. O'Connell, P. G., Milburn, B. M., and Nashel, D. J.: Coexistent gout and septic arthritis: A report of two cases and literature review. Clin. Exp. Rheumatol. 3:265, 1985.
45. Wordsworth, B. P., and Mowat, A. G.: Rapid development of gouty tophi after diuretic therapy. J. Rheumatol. 12:376, 1985.
46. Khalifa, P., Sereni, D., Boissonnas, A., Bremer, G., and Laroche, C.: Attacks of gout and thromboembolic disease: Role of heparin therapy. Ann. Intern. Med. 136:582, 1985.
47. Tiller, D. J., Hall, B. M., Horvath, J. S., Buggin, G. G., and Thompson, J. F.: Gout and hyperuricaemia in patients on cyclosporin and diuretics (Letter). Lancet 1:453, 1985.
48. Schousboe, J. T., Davey, K., Gilchrist, N. L., and Sainsbury, R.: Chronic polyarticular gout in the elderly: A report of six cases. Age Ageing 15:8, 1986.
49. Myers, O. L., and Monteagudo, F. S. E.: Gout in females: An analysis of 92 patients. Clin. Exp. Rheumatol. 3:105, 1985.
50. McCarty, D. J., Jr., and Hollander, J. L.: Identification of urate crystals in gouty synovial fluid. Ann. Intern. Med. 54:452, 1961.
51. Schumacher, H. R., Sieck, M., and Clayburne, G.: Development and evaluation of a method for preservation of synovial fluid wet preparations for quality control testing of crystal identification. J. Rheumatol. 17:1369, 1990.
52. Schumacher, H. R., Sieck, M. S., Rothfuss, S., et al.: Reproducibility of synovial fluid analysis. Arthritis Rheum. 29:770, 1987.
53. Hasselbacher, P.: Variation in synovial fluid analysis by hospital laboratories. Arthritis Rheum. 30:637, 1987.
54. Gordon, C., Swan, A., and Dieppe, P.: Detection of crystals in synovial fluids by light microscopy: Sensitivity and reliability. Ann. Rheum. Dis. 48:737, 1989.
55. Schumacher, H. R., and Reginato, A. J.: Atlas of Synovial Fluid Analysis and Crystal Identification. Philadelphia, Lea & Febiger, 1991.
56. Kerolous, G., Clayburne, G., and Schumacher, H. R.: Is it mandatory to examine synovial fluids promptly after arthrocentesis? Arthritis Rheum. 32:271, 1989.
57. Wallace, S. L., and Singer, J. Z.: Review: Systemic toxicity associated with the intravenous administration of colchicine guidelines for use. J. Rheumatol. 15:495, 1988.
58. Mugler, A., Wackenheim, A., and Grappe, J.: Nouvelle observations de maladies allergiques traitees par la colchicine par boie intraveineuse. Bull. Mem. Soc. Med. Hop. Paris 67:821, 1951.
59. McCarty, D. J., Jr.: Crystal-induced inflammation; syndromes of gout and pseudogout. Geriatrics 18:467, 1963.
60. Thompson, G. R., Ting, M. Y., Riggs, G. A., et al.: Calcific tendinitis and soft-tissue calcification resembling gout. J.A.M.A. 203:464, 1968.
61. Kaplan, H.: Further experience with colchicine in the treatment of sarcoid arthritis. N. Engl. J. Med. 268:761, 1963.
62. Blomgren, S. E.: Conditions associated with erythema nodosum. N.Y. State J. Med. 72:2302, 1972.
63. Zuckner, J.: Colchicine therapeutic trial responses in rheumatoid arthritis (abstr.) Arthritis Rheum. 5:329, 1962.
64. Goldfinger, S. E.: Colchicine for familial Mediterranean fever. N. Engl. J. Med. 287:1302, 1972.
65. Wallace, S. L., Bernstein, D., and Diamond, H.: Diagnostic value of the colchicine therapeutic trial. J.A.M.A. 199:525, 1967.
66. Gutman, A. B.: Gout. In Beeson, P. B., and McDermott, W. (eds.): Textbook of Medicine. 12th ed. Philadelphia, W. B. Saunders Company, 1958, p. 595.
67. Weinberger, A., and Schumacher, H. R.: Urate crystals in asymptomatic metatarsophalangeal joints. Ann. Intern. Med. 91:56, 1979.
68. Roualt, T., Caldwell, D. S., and Holmes, E. W.: Aspiration of the asymptomatic metatarsophalangeal joint in gout patients and hyperuricemic controls. Arthritis Rheum. 25:209, 1982.
69. Gordon, T. P., Bertouch, J. V., Walsh, B. R., and Brooks, P. M.: Monosodium urate crystals in asymptomatic knee joints. J. Rheumatol. 9:967, 1982.
70. Kennedy, T. D., Higgens, C. S., Woodrow, D. F., and Scott, J. T.: Crystal deposition in the knee and great toe joints of asymptomatic gout patients. J. Soc. Med. 77:747, 1984.
71. Bomalaski, J. S., Lluberas, G., and Schumacher, H. R., Jr.: Monosodium urate crystals in the knee joints of patients with asymptomatic nontophaceous gout. Arthritis Rheum. 29:1480, 1986.
72. Pascual, E.: Persistence of monosodium urate crystals and low grade inflammation in the synovial fluid of patients with untreated gout. Arthritis Rheum. 34:141, 1991.
73. Louthrenoo, W., Sieck, M., Clayburne, G., et al.: Supravital staining of cells in non-inflammatory synovial fluids. Analysis of the effects of crystals on cell populations. J. Rheumatol. 18:409, 1991.
74. Wall, B., Agudelo, C. A., Tesser, J. R. P., Mountz, J., Holt, D., and Turner, R. A.: An autopsy study of the prevalence of monosodium urate and calcium pyrophosphate dihydrate crystal deposition in first metatarsophalangeal joints. Arthritis Rheum. 26:1522, 1983.
75. Moens, C., Moens, D., and Moens, P. H.: Prevalence of monosodium urate and calcium pyrophosphate dihydrate crystals in postmortem knee synovial fluid. Arthritis Rheum. 28:1319, 1985.
76. Hench, P. S.: The diagnosis of gout and gouty arthritis. J. Lab. Clin. Med. 220:48, 1936.
77. Gutman, A. B.: The past four decades of progress in the knowledge of gout, with an assessment of the present status. Arthritis Rheum. 16:431, 1973.
78. Gutman, A. B., and Yu, T.-F.: Renal function in gout with a commentary on the renal regulation of urate excretion and the role of the kidney in the pathogenesis of gout. Am. J. Med. 23:600, 1957.
79. O'Duffy, J. D., Hunder, G. G., and Kelly, P. J.: Decreasing prevalence of tophaceous gout. Mayo Clin. Proc. 50:227, 1975.
80. Nakayama, D. A., Barthelemy, C., Carrera, G., Lightfoot, R. W., Jr., and Wortmann, R. L.: Tophaceous gout: A clinical and radiographic assessment. Arthritis Rheum. 27:468, 1984.
81. Hollingworth, P., Scott, J. T., and Burry, H. C.: Nonarticular gout: Hyperuricemia and tophus formation without gouty arthritis. Arthritis Rheum. 26:98, 1983.
82. Yu, T.-F.: Secondary gout associated with myeloproliferative diseases. Arthritis Rheum. 8:765, 1965.
83. Symythe, C. M., and Cutchin, J. H.: Primary juvenile gout. Am. J. Med. 32:799, 1962.
84. Wood, M. H., Fox, R. M., Vincent, L., et al.: The Lesch-Nyhan syndrome: Report of three cases. Aust. N.Z. J. Med. 1:57, 1972.
85. Chou, C. T., Wasserstein, A., Schumacher, H. R., et al.: Musculoskeletal manifestations in hemodialysis patients. J. Rheumatol. 12:1149, 1985.
86. Good, A. E., and Rapp, R.: Bony ankylosis: A rare manifestation of gout. J. Rheumatol. 5:335, 1978.
87. Varga, J., Giampaolo, C., and Goldenberg, D. L.: Tophaceous gout of the spine in a patient with no peripheral tophi: Case report and review of the literature. Arthritis Rheum. 18:1312, 1985.
88. Sequeira, W., Bouffard, A., Salgia, K., et al.: Quadriparesis in tophaceous gout. Arthritis Rheum. 24:1428, 1981.
89. Magid, S. K., Gray, G. E., and Anand, A.: Spinal cord compression by tophi in a patient with chronic polyarthritis: Case report and literature review. Arthritis Rheum. 24:1431, 1981.
90. Scalapino, J. N., Edwards, W. D., Steckelberg, J. M., Wooten, R. S., Callahan, J. A., and Ginsburg, W. W.: Mitral stenosis associated with valvular tophi. Mayo Clin. Proc. 59:509, 1984.
91. Gawoski, J. M., Balogh, K., and Landis, W. J.: Aortic valvular tophus: Identification by x-ray diffraction of urate and calcium phosphates. J. Clin. Pathol. 38:873, 1985.
92. Martinez-Cordero, E., Barriera-Maercado, E., and Katona, G.: Eye tophi deposition in gout (Letter). J. Rheumatol. 11:471, 1986.

93. Ferry, A. P., Safir, A., and Melikian, H. E.: Ocular abnormalities in patients with gout. Ann. Ophthalmol. 17:632, 1985.
94. Bauer, W., and Klemperer, F.: Gout. In Duncan, G. G. (ed.): Diseases of Metabolism. 2nd ed. Philadelphia, W. B. Saunders Company, 1947, p. 6121.
95. Bartels, E. C., and Matossian, G. S.: Gout: Six year follow-up on probenecid (Benemid) therapy. Arthritis Rheum. 2:193, 1959.
96. Bloch, C., Hermann, G., and Yu, T.-F.: A radiologic reevaluation of gout: A study of 2,000 patients. Am. J. Radiol. 134:781, 1980.
97. Resnick, D., and Broderick, T. W.: Intraosseous calcifications in tophaceous gout. Am. J. Radiol. 17:1157, 1981.
98. Stockman, A., Darlington, L. G., and Scott, J. T.: Frequency of chondrocalcinosis of the knees and avascular necrosis of the femoral heads in gout: A controlled study. Ann. Rheum. Dis. 39:7, 1980.
99. Benedek, T. G.: Correlations of serum uric acid and lipid concentrations in normal, gouty, and atherosclerotic men. Ann. Intern. Med. 66:851, 1967.
100. Acheson, R. M., and Florey, C. du V.: Body-weight, ABO blood groups, and altitude of domicile as determinants of serum-uric-acid in military recruits in four countries. Lancet 2:391, 1969.
101. Myers, A., Epstein, F. H., Dodge, H. J., et al.: The relationship of serum uric acid to risk factors in coronary heart disease. Am. J. Med. 45:520, 1968.
102. Gutman, A. B., and Yu, T.-F.: Gout, a derangement of purine metabolism. Adv. Intern. Med. 5:227, 1952.
103. O'Brien, W. M., Burch, T. A., and Bunim, J. J.: Genetics of hyperuricemia in Blackfeet and Pima Indians. Ann. Rheum. Dis. 25:117, 1966.
104. Brauer, G. W., and Prior, I. A. M.: A prospective study of gout in New Zealand Maoris. Ann. Rheum. Dis. 37:466, 1978.
105. Emmerson, B. T., and Knowles, B. R.: Triglyceride concentrations in primary gout of chronic lead nephropathy. Metabolism 20:721, 1971.
106. Brochner-Mortensen, K.: 100 gouty patients. Acta Med. Scand. 106:81, 1941.
107. Engelhardt, H. T., and Wagner, E. L.: Gout, diabetes mellitus and obesity, a poorly recognized syndrome. South. Med. J. 43:51, 1950.
108. Prior, I. A. M., Rose, B. S., Harvey, H. P. B., et al.: Hyperuricaemia, gout, and diabetic abnormality in Polynesian people. Lancet 1:333, 1966.
109. Healey, L. A., and Hall, A. P.: The epidemiology of hyperuricemia. Bull. Rheum. Dis. 20:600, 1970.
110. Gibson, T., and Grahame, R.: Gout and hyperlipidaemia. Ann. Rheum. Dis. 33:298, 1974.
111. Kahn, H. A., Medalie, J. H., Newfeld, H. N., et al.: The incidence of hypertension and associated factors: The Israel ischemic heart disease study. Am. Heart J. 84:171, 1972.
112. Mikkelsen, W. M.: The possible association of hyperuricemia and/or gout with diabetes mellitus. Arthritis Rheum. 8:853, 1965.
113. Denis, G., and Launay, M. P.: Carbohydrate intolerance in gout. Metabolism 18:770, 1969.
114. Bernheim, C., Ott, H., Zahnd, G., et al.: Goutte et diabete. 1. La goutte et ses relations avec le diabete. Schweiz. Med. Wochenschr. 98:33, 1968.
115. Berkowitz, D.: Gout, hyperlipidemia and diabetes interrelationships. J.A.M.A. 197:77, 1966.
116. Herman, J. B., Mount, F. W., Medalie, J. H., et al.: Diabetes prevalence and serum uric acid: Observations among 10,000 men in a survey of ischemic heart disease in Israel. Diabetes 16:858, 1967.
117. Herman, J. B., and Keynan, A.: Hyperglycemia and uric acid. Isr. J. Med. Sci. 5:1048, 1969.
118. Skeith, M. D., Healey, L. A., and Cutler, R. E.: Urate excretion during mannitol and glucose diuresis. J. Lab. Clin. Med. 70:213, 1967.
119. Barlow, K. A.: Hyperlipidemia in primary gout. Metabolism 17:289, 1968.
120. Naito, H. K., and Mackenzie, A. H.: Secondary hypertriglyceridemia and hyperlipoproteinemia in patients with primary asymptomatic gout. Clin. Chem. 25:371, 1979.
121. Jiao, S., Kameda, K., Matsuzawa, Y., and Tarui, S.: Hyperlipoproteinaemia in primary gout: Hyperlipoproteinaemic phenotype and influence of alcohol intake and obesity in Japan. Ann. Rheum. Dis. 45:308, 1986.
122. Laskarzewski, P. M., Khoury, P., Morrison, J. A., Kelly, K., and Glueck, C. J.: Familial hyper- and hypouricemias in random and hyperlipidemic recall cohorts. Metabolism 32:230, 1983.
123. MacFarlane, D. G., Midwinter, C. A., Dieppe, P. A., Bolton, C. H., and Hartog, M.: Demonstration of an abnormality of C apoprotein of very low density lipoprotein in patients with gout. Ann. Rheum. Dis. 44:390, 1985.
124. Ferns, G. A., Lanham, J., Stocks, J., Ritchie, C., Katz, J., and Galton, D. J.: The measurement of high density lipoprotein subfractions in patients with primary gout using a simple precipitation method. Ann. Clin. Biochem. 22:526, 1985.
125. Fox, I. H., John, D., Debruyne, S., Dwosh, I., and Marliss, E. B.: Hyperuricemia and hypertriglyceridemia: Metabolic basis for the association. Metabolism 34:741, 1985.

126. Ferns, G. A., Lanham, J., and Galton, D. J.: The association between primary gout and hypertriglyceridemia may be due to genetic linkage. Monogr. Atheroscler. 13:121, 1985.
127. Harris-Jones, J. N.: Hyperuricemia and essential hypercholesterolemia. Lancet 1:857, 1957.
128. Salvini, L., and Verdi, G.: Statistical study on correlation between blood level of cholesterol beta/alpha lipoprotein ratio and uric acid of normal and arteriosclerotic subjects. Gerontologia 3:327, 1959.
129. Jensen, J., Blankenhorn, D. H., and Dornerup, V.: Blood-uric acid levels in familial hypercholesterolemia. Lancet 1:298, 1966.
130. Strejcek, J., and Kucerova, L.: Idiopathic hyperlipidemia and gout. Acta Rheumatol. Scand. 14:95, 1968.
131. Cannon, P. J., Stason, W. B., Demartini, F. E., et al.: Hyperuricemia in primary and renal hypertension. N. Engl. J. Med. 275:457, 1966.
132. Breckenridge, A.: Hypertension and hyperuricemia. Lancet 1:15, 1966.
133. Garrick, R., Bauer, G. E., Ewan, C. E., et al.: Serum uric acid in normal and hypertensive Australian subjects: From a continuing epidemiological survey on hypertension commenced in 1955. Aust. N.Z. J. Med. 2:351, 1972.
134. Dollery, C. T., Duncan, H., and Schumer, B.: Hyperuricemia related to treatment of hypertension. Br. Med. J. 2:832, 1960.
135. Simon, N. M., Smucker, J. E., O'Conor, J., Jr., et al.: Differential uric acid excretion in essential and renal hypertension. Circulation 39:121, 1969.
136. Kuzell, W. C., Schaffarzick, R. W., Naugler, W. E., et al.: Some observations on 520 gouty patients. J. Chronic Dis. 2:645, 1955.
137. Barlow, K. A., and Beilin, L. J.: Renal disease in primary gout. Q. J. Med. 37:79, 1968.
138. Messerli, F. H., Frohlich, E. D., Dreslinski, G. R., et al.: Serum uric acid in essential hypertension: An indicator of renal vascular involvement. Ann. Intern. Med. 93:817, 1980.
139. Prebis, J. W., Gruskin, A. B., Polinsky, M. S., et al.: Uric acid in childhood essential hypertension. J. Pediatr. 98:702, 1981.
140. Saito, I., Saruta, T., Kondo, K., et al.: Serum uric acid and the reninangiotensin system in hypertension. J. Am. Geriatr. Soc. 26:241, 1978.
141. Heyden, S., Borhani, N. O., Tyroler, H. A., Schneider, K. A., Langford, H. G., Hames, C. G., Hutchinson, R., and Oberman, A.: The relationship of weight change to changes in blood pressure, serum uric acid, cholesterol and glucose in the treatment of hypertension. J. Chronic. Dis. 38:281, 1985.
142. The Hypertension Detection and Follow-up Program Cooperative Research Group: Mortality findings for stepped-care and referred-care participants in the hypertension detection and follow-up program, stratified by other risk factors. Prev. Med. 14:312, 1985.
143. Gertler, M. M., Gam, S. M., and Levine, S. A.: Serum uric acid in relation to age and physique in health and in coronary artery disease. Ann. Intern. Med. 34:1421, 1951.
144. Upmark-Ask, E., and Adner, L.: Coronary infarction and gout. Acta Med. Scand. 139:1, 1950.
145. Kramer, D. W., Perlistein, P. K., and DeMedeiros, A.: Metabolic influences in vascular disorders with particular reference to cholesterol determinations in comparison with uric acid levels. Angiology 9:162, 1958.
146. Hansen, O. E.: Hyperuricemia, gout and atherosclerosis. Am. Heart J. 72:570, 1966.
147. Kohn, P. M., and Prozan, G. B.: Hyperuricemia—relationship to hypercholesterolemia and acute myocardial infarction. J.A.M.A. 17:1909, 1959.
148. Editorial: Serum uric acid and coronary heart disease. Lancet 1:358, 1969.
149. Nishioka, K., and Miknangi, K.: A retrospective study on the cause of death, in Japan, of patients with gout. Ryumachi 21(Suppl.):29, 1981.
150. Fessel, W. J.: Renal outcomes of gout and hyperuricemia. Am. J. Med. 67:74, 1979.
151. Johnson, M. W., and Mitch, W. E.: The risks of asymptomatic hyperuricemia and the use of uricosuric diuretics. Drugs 21:220, 1981.
152. Tweddale, M. G., and Fodor, J. G.: Elevated serum uric acid: A cardiovascular risk factor. Nephron 23:3, 1979.
153. Fessel, W. J.: High uric acid as an indicator of cardiovascular disease, independence from obesity. Am. J. Med. 68:401, 1980.
154. Reunanen, A., Takkunen, H., Knekt, P., and Aromaa, A.: Hyperuricemia as a risk factor for cardiovascular mortality. Acta Med. Scand. 668:49, 1982.
155. Peterson, B., and Trell, E.: Raised serum urate concentration as risk factor for premature mortality in middle aged men: Relation to death from cancer. Br. Med. J. 287:7, 1983.
156. Beard, J. T.: Serum uric acid and coronary heart disease. Am. Heart J. 106:397, 1983.
157. Brand, F. N., McGee, D. L., Kannel, W., Stokes, J., III, and Castelli, W. P.: Original contributions: Hyperuricemia as a risk factor of coronary heart disease: The Framingham Study. Am. J. Epidemiol. 121:11, 1985.

158. MacFarlane, D. G., Slade, R., Hopes, P. A., and Hartog, M.: A study of platelet aggregation and adhesion in gout. Clin. Exp. Rheumatol. 1:63, 1983.
159. Ciompi, M. L., Decaterina, R., Bertolucci, D., Bernini, W., Michelassi, C., and Labbate, A.: Uric acid levels and platelet function in humans. An in-vivo ex-vivo study. Clin. Exp. Rheumatol. 1:143, 1983.
160. Lieber, C. S., and Davidson, C. S.: Some metabolic effects of ethanol accumulation. Am. J. Med. 33:319, 1962.
161. Lieber, C. S., Jones, D. P., Losowsky, M. S., and Davidson, C. S.: Interrelation of uric acid and ethanol metabolism in man. J. Clin. Invest. 41:1863, 1962.
162. Beck, L. H.: Clinical disorders of uric acid metabolism. Med. Clin. North Am. 65:401, 1981.
163. Yu, T.-F., Sirota, J. H., Berger, L., Halpern, M., and Gutman, A. B.: Effect of sodium lactate infusion on urate clearance in man. Proc. Soc. Exp. Biol. Med. 96:809, 1957.
164. Faller, J., and Fox, I. H.: Ethanol-induced hyperuricemia: Evidence for increased urate production by activation of adenine nucleotide turnover. N. Engl. J. Med. 307:1598, 1982.
165. Puig, J. G., and Fox, I. H.: Ethanol induced activation of adenine nucleotide turnover. Evidence for a role of acetate. J. Clin. Invest. 74:936, 1984.
166. Gibson, T., Rodgers, A. V., Simmonds, H. A., and Toseland, P.: Beer drinking and its effect on uric acid. Br. J. Rheumatol. 23:203, 1984.
167. Woolliscroft, J. O., Colfer, H., and Fox, I. H.: Hyperuricemia in acute illness: A poor prognostic sign. Am. J. Med. 72:58, 1982.
168. Woolliscroft, J. O., and Fox, I. H.: Increased body fluid purines during hypotensive events: Evidence for ATP degradation. Am. J. Med. 81:472, 1986.
169. Grum, C. M., Simon, R. H., Dantzker, D. R., and Fox, I. H.: Biochemical indicators of cellular hypoxia in critically ill patients. Evidence for ATP degradation. Chest 88:763, 1985.
170. McCord, J.: Oxygen-derived free radicals in postischemic tissue injury. N. Engl. J. Med. 312:159, 1985.
171. Ames, B. N., Cathcart, R., Schwiers, E., and Hochstein, P.: Uric acid provides an antioxidant defense in humans against oxidant- and radical-caused aging and cancer: A hypothesis. Proc. Natl. Acad. Sci. U.S.A. 78:6858, 1981.
172. Smith, R. C., and Lawing, L.: Antioxidant activity of uric acid and 3-N-ribosyluric acid with unsaturated fatty acids and erythrocyte membranes. Arch. Biochem. Biophys. 223:166, 1983.
173. Kittridge, K. J., and Willson, R. L.: Uric acid substantially enhances the free radical-induced inactivation of alcohol dehydrogenase. Fed. Eur. Biochem. Soc. 170:162, 1984.
174. Meadows, J., Smith, R. C., and Reeves, J.: Uric acid protects membranes and linolenic acid from ozone-induced oxidation. Biochem. Biophys. Res. Commun. 137:536, 1986.
175. Boyle, J. A., Campbell, S., Duncan, A. M., Greig, W. R., and Buchanan, W. W.: Serum uric acid levels in normal pregnancy with observations on the renal excretion of urate in pregnancy. J. Clin. Pathol. 19:501, 1966.
176. Hill, L. M.: Subject review. Metabolism of uric acid in normal and toxemic pregnancy. Mayo Clin. Proc. 53:743, 1978.
177. Lind, T., Godfrey, K. A., and Otun, H.: Changes in serum uric acid concentrations during normal pregnancy. Br. J. Obstet. Gynaecol. 91:128, 1984.
178. Schaffer, N. K., Dill, L. V., and Cadden, J. F.: Uric acid clearance in normal pregnancy and pre-eclampsia. J. Clin. Invest. 22:201, 1943.
179. Seitzchik, J.: Observations on the renal tubular reabsorption of uric acid. Am. J. Obstet. Gynecol. 65:981, 1953.
180. Carswell, W., and Semple, P. F.: The effect of frusemide on uric acid levels in maternal blood, fetal blood and amniotic fluid. J. Obstet. Gynecol. 81:472, 1974.
181. Redman, C. W. G., Beilin, L. J., Bonnar, J., and Wilkinson, R. H.: Plasma-urate measurements in predicting fetal death in hypertensive pregnancy. Lancet 1:1370, 1976.
182. Haeckel, R., Riedel, H., and Buttner, J.: Estimation of decision criteria for the uric acid concentration for the early diagnosis of gestosis. J. Clin. Chem. Clin. Biochem. 19:173, 1981.
183. Liedholm, H., Montan, S., and Aberg, A.: Risk grouping of 113 patients with hypertensive disorders during pregnancy, with respect to serum urate, proteinuria and time of onset of hypertension. Acta Obstet. Gynecol. Scand. (Suppl.) 118:43, 1984.
184. Crawford, M. D.: The effect of labour on plasma uric acid and urea. J. Obstet. Gynecol. 46:540, 1939.
185. Hamilton, W. F. D., Robertson, G. S., and Campbell, D.: Changes in serum uric acid concentrations after caesarean section using methoxyflurane. Br. J. Anaesth. 47:508, 1975.
186. Jessee, E. F., Toone, E., Owen, D. S., et al.: Coexistent rheumatoid arthritis and chronic tophaceous gout. Arthritis Rheum. 23:244, 1980.
187. Atdjian, M., and Fernandez-Madris, F.: Coexistence of chronic tophaceous gout and rheumatoid arthritis. J. Rheumatol. 8:989, 1981.
188. Rizzoli, A. J., Trujeque, L., and Bankhurst, A. D.: The coexistence of gout and rheumatoid arthritis: Case reports and a review of the literature. J. Rheumatol. 7:316, 1980.

189. Wallace, D. J., Klineberg, J. R., Morhaim, D., et al.: Coexistent gout and rheumatoid arthritis. Arthritis Rheum. 22:81, 1979.
190. Agudelo, C. A., Turner, R. A., Panetti, M., and Pisko, E.: Does hyperuricemia protect from rheumatoid inflammation? A clinical study. Arthritis Rheum. 27:443, 1984.
191. Gordon, T. P., Ahern, M. J., Reid, C., and Roberts-Thomson, P. J.: Studies on the interaction of rheumatoid factor with monosodium urate crystals and case report of coexistent tophaceous gout and rheumatoid arthritis. Ann. Rheum. Dis. 44:384, 1985.
192. Turner, R. A., Pisko, E. J., Agudelo, C., Counts, G. B., Foster, S. L., and Treadway, W. J.: Uric acid effects on in vitro models of rheumatoid inflammatory and autoimmune processes. Ann. Rheum. Dis. 42:338, 1983.
193. Lally, E. V., Parker, V. S., and Kaplan, S. R.: Acute gouty arthritis and systemic lupus erythematosus. J. Rheumatol. 9:308, 1982.
194. Moidel, R. A., and Good, A. E.: Coexistent gout and systemic lupus erythematosus. Arthritis Rheum. 24:969, 1981.
195. Wall, B. A., Agudelo, C. A., Weinblatt, M. E., et al.: Acute gout and systemic lupus erythematosus: Report of 2 cases and literature review. J. Rheumatol. 9:305, 1982.
196. Gibson, T., Highton, J., Potter, C., et al.: Renal impairment and gout. Ann. Rheum. Dis. 39:417, 1980.
197. Yu, T.-F., and Berger, L.: Renal function in gout: Its association with hypertensive vascular disease and intrinsic renal disease. Am. J. Med. 72:95, 1982.
198. Batuman, V., Maesaka, J. K., Haddad, B., et al.: The role of lead in gout nephropathy. N. Engl. J. Med. 304:520, 1981.
199. Campbell, B. C., Moore, M. R., Goldberg, A., et al.: Subclinical lead exposure: A possible cause of gout. Br. Med. J. 2:1403, 1978.
200. Sokoloff, L.: The pathology of gout. Metabolism 6:230, 1957.
201. Talbott, J. H., and Terplan, K. L.: The kidney in gout. Medicine 39:405, 1960.
202. Yu, T.-F., and Berger, L.: Renal disease in primary gout. Semin. Arthritis Rheum. 3:293, 1975.
203. Garrod, A. B.: A Treatise on Gout and Rheumatic Gout. 3rd ed. London, Longman, Green and Co., 1876.
204. Verger, D., Leroux-Robert, G. P., and Richet, G.: Depots d'urate intrarenaux chez les insuffisants renaux chroniques hyperuricemiques. Urol. Nephrol. 73:314, 1967.
205. Linnane, J. W., Burry, A. F., and Emmerson, B. T.: Urate deposits in the renal medulla: Prevalence and associations. Nephron 29:216, 1981.
206. Frei, E., Bentzel, C. J., Rieselbach, R. E., and Block, R. B.: Renal complications of neoplastic disease. J. Chronic Dis. 16:757, 1963.
207. Rieselbach, R. E., Bentzel, C. J., Cotlove, E., et al.: Uric acid excretion and renal function in the acute hyperuricemia of leukemia. Am. J. Med. 37:872, 1964.
208. Kjellstrand, C. M., Campbell, D. C., von Hartitzsch, B., et al.: Hyperuricemic acute renal failure. Arch. Intern. Med. 133:349, 1974.
209. Lilje, E.: Hyperurikaemi og akut nyriensuffciens. Ugeskr. Laeger. 132:12, 1970.
210. Cohen, L. F., Balow, J. E., Poplack, D. G., et al.: Acute tumor lysis syndrome: A review of 37 patients with Burkitt's lymphoma. Am. J. Med. 68:486, 1980.
211. Tomlinson, G. C., and Solberg, L. A., Jr.: Acute tumor lysis syndrome with metastatic medulloblastoma. A case report. Cancer 53:1783, 1984.
212. Boccia, R. V., Longo, D. L., Lieber, M. L., Jaffe, E. S., and Fisher, R. I.: Multiple recurrences of acute tumor lysis syndrome in an indolent non-Hodgkin's lymphoma. Cancer 56:2295, 1985.
213. Andreoli, S. P., Clark, J. H., McGuire, W. A., and Bergstein, J. M.: Purine excretion during turnover lysis in children with acute lymphocytic leukemia receiving allopurinol: Relationship to acute renal failure. J. Pediatr. 109:292, 1986.
214. Batch, J. A., Riek, R. P., Gordon, R. B., Burke, J. R., and Emmerson, B. T.: Renal failure in infancy due to over-production of urate. J. Med. 14:852, 1984.
215. Stavric, B., Johnson, W. J., and Grice, H. C.: Uric acid nephropathy: An experimental model. Proc. Soc. Exp. Biol. Med. 130:512, 1969.
216. Kelton, J., Kelley, W. N., and Holmes, E. W.: A rapid method for the diagnosis of acute uric acid nepropathy. Arch. Intern. Med. 138:612, 1978.
217. Atsmon, A., DeVries, A., and Frank, M.: Uric Acid Lithiasis. Amsterdam, Elsevier, 1963.
218. Hughes, J., Coppridge, W. M., Roberts, L. C., et al.: Oxalate urinary tract stones. J.A.M.A. 172:774, 1960.
219. Nicholas, H. O.: Urinary calculi. II. Further observations on calculi from patients in the southeast Texas area. Clin. Chem. 7:175, 1961.
220. Leonard, R. H.: Quantitative composition of kidney stones. Clin. Chem. 7:546, 1961.
221. Gutman, A. B., and Yu, T.-F.: Uric acid nephrolithiasis. Am. J. Med. 45:756, 1968.
222. Yu, T.-F., and Gutman, A. B.: Uric acid nephrolithiasis in gout. Predisposing factors. Ann. Intern. Med. 67:1133, 1967.
223. Yu, T.-F.: Review article. Urolithiasis in hyperuricemia and gout. J. Urol. 126:424, 1981.
224. Cartier, M. B., and Hamet, M.: Une nouvelle maladie metabolique: Le

deficit complet en adeninephosphoribosyltransferase avec lithiase de 2,8-dihydroxyadenine. C.R. Acad. Sci. Paris 270:883, 1974.

225. Simmonds, H. A., and Van Acker, K. J.: Adenine phosphoribosyltransferase deficiency: 2,8-dihydroxyadenine lithiasis. In Stanbury, J. B., Wyngaarden, J. B., Fredrickson, D. S., Goldstein, J. L., and Brown, M. S. (eds.): The Metabolic Basis of Inherited Disease. New York, McGraw-Hill Book Company, 1983.

226. Maschio, G., Tessitore, N., Dangelo, A., Fabris, A., Pagano, F., Tasca, A., Graziani, G., Aroldi, A., Surian, M., Colussi, G., Mandressi, A., Trinchieri, A., Rocco, F., Ponticelli, C., and Minetti, L.: Prevention of calcium nephrolithiasis with low dose thiazide, amiloride and allopurinol. Am. J. Med. 71:623, 1981.

227. Pak, C., Peters, P., Hurt, G., Kadesky, M., Fine, M., Reisman, D., Splann, F., Caramela, C., Feeman, A., Britton, F., Sakhaee, K., and Breslau, N. A.: Is selective therapy of recurrent nephrolithiasis possible? Am. J. Med. 71:615, 1981.

228. Ettinger, B., Tang, A., Citron, J. T., Livermore, B., and Williams, T.: Randomized trial of allopurinol in the prevention of calcium oxalate calculi. N. Engl. J. Med. 27:1386, 1986.

229. Smith, A., and Wilcken, B.: Homozygous cystinuria in New South Wales. A study of 110 individuals with cystinuria ascertained by methods other than neonatal screening. Med. J. Aust. 141:500, 1984.

230. Brock, W. A., Golden, J., and Kaplan, G. W.: Xanthine calculi in the Lesch-Nyhan syndrome. J. Urol. 130:157, 1983.

231. Thompson, G. R., Weiss, J. J., Goldman, R. T., et al.: Familial occurrence of hyperuricemia, gout and medullary cystic disease. Arch. Intern. Med. 138:1614, 1978.

232. Massari, P. W., Hsu, C. H., Barnes, R. V., et al.: Familial hyperuricemia and renal disease. Arch. Intern. Med. 140:680, 1980.

233. Simmonds, H. A., Cameron, J. S., Potter, C. V., et al.: Renal failure in young subjects with familial gout. Adv. Exp. Med. Biol. 122A:15, 1980.

234. Simmonds, H. A., Warren, D. J., Cameron, J. S., et al.: Familial gout and renal failure in young women. Clin. Nephrol. 14:176, 1980.

235. Stapleton, F. B., Nyhan, W. L., Borden, M., et al.: Renal pathogenesis of familial hyperuricemia: Studies in two kindreds. Pediatr. Res. 15:1447, 1981.

236. MacDermot, K. D., Allsop, J., and Watts, R. W.: The rate of purine synthesis de novo in blood mononuclear cells in vitro from patients with familial hyperuricaemic nephropathy. Clin. Sci. 67:249, 1984.

237. Whalen, R. E., and McIntosh, H. D.: The spectrum of hereditary renal diseases. Am. J. Med. 33:282, 1962.

238. Perkoff, G. R.: The hereditary renal diseases. N. Engl. J. Med. 277:79, 1967.

239. Leumann, E. P., and Wegmann, W.: Familial nephropathy with hyperuricemia and gout. Nephron 34:51, 1983.

240. Rivera, J. V., Martinex-Maldonado, M. M., Ramirez de Arellano, G. A., and Ehrlich L.: Association of hyperuricemia and polycystic kidney disease. Bol. Asoc. Med. PR 57:251, 1965.

241. Newcombe, D. S.: Gouty arthritis and polycystic kidney disease. Ann. Intern. Med. 79:605, 1973.

242. Rivera, J. V.: Gout and polycystic disease of kidney. Ann. Intern. Med. 80:427, 1974.

243. Reynolds, P. P., Knapp, M. J., Baraf, H. S. B., and Holmes, E. W.: Moonshine and lead: Relationship to the pathogenesis of hyperuricemia in gout. Arthritis Rheum. 26:1057, 1983.

244. Halla, J. T., and Ball, G. V.: Saturnine gout: A review of 42 patients. Semin. Arthritis Rheum. 11:307, 1982.

245. Cullen, M. R., Robins, J. M., and Eskenazi, B.: Adult inorganic lead intoxication: Presentation of 31 new cases and a review of recent advances in the literature. Medicine 62:221, 1983.

246. Batuman, V., Landy, E., Maesaka, J. K., and Wedeen, R. P.: Contribution of lead to hypertension with renal impairment. N. Engl. J. Med. 309:17, 1983.

247. Wright, L. F., Saylor, R. P., and Cecere, F. A.: Occult lead intoxication in patients with gout and kidney disease. J. Rheumatol. 11:517, 1984.

248. Craswell, P. W., Price, J., Boyle, P. D., Heazlewood, V. J., Baddeley, H., Lloyd, H. M., Thomas, B. J., and Thomas, B. W.: Chronic renal failure with gout: A marker of chronic lead poisoning. Kidney Int. 26:319, 1984.

249. Behringer, D., Craswell, P., Mohl, C., Stoeppler, M., and Ritz, E.: Urinary lead excretion in uremic patients. Nephron 42:323, 1986.

250. Colleoni, N., and Damico, G.: Chronic lead accumulation as a possible cause of renal failure in gouty patients. Nephron 44:32, 1986.

251. Tak, H. K., Wilcox, W. R., and Cooper, S. M.: The effect of lead upon urate nucleation. Arthritis Rheum. 224:1291, 1981.

252. Farkas, W. R., Stanowitz, T., and Schneider, M.: Saturnine gout: Lead induced formation of guanine crystals. Science 99:786, 1978.

253. Scheele, K. W.: Examen chemicum calculi urinarii. Opuscula 2:73, 1776.

254. Wollaston, W. H.: On gouty and urinary concretions. Philos. Trans. R. Soc. Lond. 87:386, 1848.

255. Garrod, A. B.: Observations on certain pathological conditions of the blood and urine in gout, rheumatism and Bright's disease. Trans. M-Chir. Soc. Edinb. 31:83, 1848.

256. Friedkin, N., and Kalckar, H.: Nucleoside phosphorylases. In Boyer, P. D., Lardy, H., and Myrback, K. (eds.): The Enzymes, Vol. 5. New York, Academic Press, 1961, p. 237.

257. Bergmann, F., and Dikstein, S.: Studies on uric acid and related compounds. III. Observations on the specificity of mammalian xanthine oxidase. J. Biol. Chem. 223:765, 1956.

258. Bray, R. C.: Molybdenum iron-sulfur flavin hydrolases and related enzymes. In Boyer, R. D. (ed.): The Enzymes, Vol. 12. 3rd ed. New York, Academic Press, 1975, p. 229.

259. Waud, W. R., and Rajagopalan, K. V.: The mechanism of conversion of rat liver xanthine dehydrogenase from an NAD^+-dependent form (type D) to an O_2-dependent form (type O). Arch. Biochem. Biophys. 172:265, 1976.

260. Della Corte, E., and Stirpe, F.: The regulation of rat liver xanthine oxidase. Involvement of thiol groups in the conversion of the enzyme activity from dehydrogenase (type D) into oxidase (type O) and purification of the enzyme. Biochem. J. 126:739, 1972.

261. Roussos, G. G.: Xanthine oxidase from bovine small intestine. Methods Enzymol. 12:5, 1967.

262. Bruder, G., Heid, H., Jafrasch, E.-D., Keenan, T. W., and Mather, I. H.: Characteristics of membrane-bound and soluble forms of xanthine oxidase from milk and endothelial cells of capillaries. Biochim. Biophys. Acta 701:357, 1982.

263. Nakamura, M., Kurebayashi, H., and Yamazaki, I.: One-electron and two-electron reductions of acceptors by xanthine oxidase and xanthine dehydrogenase. J. Biochem. 83:9, 1978.

264. Kaminski, Z. W., and Jezewska, M. M.: Involvement of a single thiol group in the conversion of the NAD^+-dependent activity of rat liver xanthine oxidoreductase to the O_2-dependent activity. Biochem. J. 207:341, 1982.

265. Battelli, M. G.: Enzymic conversion of rat liver xanthine oxidase from dehydrogenase (D-form) to oxidase (O-form). FEBS Lett. 113:47, 1980.

266. Lynch, R. E., and Fridovich, I.: Effects of superoxide on the erythrocyte membrane. J. Chem. 253:1838, 1982.

267. Engleman, K., Watts, R. W. E., Klinenberg, J. R., et al.: Clinical physiological and biochemical studies of a patient with xanthinuria and pheochromocytoma. Am. J. Med. 37:839, 1964.

268. Watts, R. W. E., Watts, J. E. M., and Seegmiller, J. E.: Xanthine oxidase activity in human tissues and its inhibition by allopurinol (4-hydropyrazolo [3,4-d] pyrimidine). J. Lab. Clin. Med. 66:688, 1965.

269. Jarasch, E.-D., Burder, G., and Heid, H. W.: Significance of xanthine oxidase in capillary endothelial cells. Acta Physiol. Scand. (Suppl.) 548:39, 1986.

270. Segal, S., and Wyngaarden, J. B.: Plasma glutamine and oxypurine content in patients with gout. Proc. Soc. Exp. Biol. Med. 88:342, 1955.

271. Jorgensen, S., and Poulsen, H. E.: Enzymatic determination of hypoxanthine and xanthine in human plasma and urine. Acta Pharmacol. 11:223, 1955.

272. Hoffman, G. T., Rottino, A., and Albaum, H. G.: Levels of nucleotide in the blood during shock. Science 114:188, 1951.

273. Nierlich, D. P., and Magasanik, B.: Regulation of purine ribonucleotide synthesis by end product inhibition: The effect of adenine and guanine ribonucleotides on the 5'-phos-phoribosylpyrophosphate amidotransferase of Aerobacter aerogenes. J. Biol. Chem. 239:2570, 1964.

274. Wyngaarden, J. B., and Ashton, D. M.: The regulation of activity of phosphoribosylpyrophosphate amidotransferase by purine ribonucleotides: A potential feedback control of purine biosynthesis. J. Biol. Chem. 234:1492, 1959.

275. Caskey, C. T., Ashton, D. M., and Wyngaarden, J. B.: The enzymology of feedback inhibition of glutamine phosphoribosylpyrophosphate amidotransferase by purine ribonucleotides. J. Biol. Chem. 239:2570, 1964.

276. Henderson, J. F.: Feedback inhibition of purine biosynthesis in ascites tumor cells. J. Biol. Chem. 237:2631, 1962.

277. Holmes, E. W., McDonald, J. A., McCord, M. M., Wyngaarden, J. B., and Kelley, W. N.: Human glutamine phosphoribosylpyrophosphate amidotransferase: Kinetic and regulatory properties. J. Biol. Chem. 248:144, 1973.

278. Wood, A. W., and Seegmiller, J. E.: Properties of 5-phosphoribosyl-1-pyrophosphate amidotransferase from human lymphoblasts. J. Biol. Chem. 248:138, 1973.

279. Holmes, E. W., Wyngaarden, J. B., and Kelley, W. N.: Human glutamine phosphoribosylpyrophosphate amidotransferase: Two molecular forms interconvertible by purine ribonucleotide and phosphoribosylpyrophosphate. J. Biol. Chem. 248:6035, 1973.

280. Howard, W. J., and Appel, S. I.: Control of purine biosynthesis: FGAR amidotransferase (abstr.). Clin. Res. 16:344, 1968.

281. Kelley, W. N., Fox, I. H., and Wyngaarden, J. B.: Regulation of purine biosynthesis in cultured human cells. I. Effects of orotic acid. Biochim. Biophys. Acta 215:512, 1970.

282. Kelley, W. N., Fox, I. H., and Wyngaarden, J. B.: Essential role of phosphoribosylpyrophosphate (PRPP) in regulation of purine biosynthesis in cultured human fibroblasts. Clin. Res. 18:457, 1970.

283. Fox, I. H., and Kelley, W. N.: Phosphoribosylpyrophosphate in man: Biochemical and clinical significance. Ann. Intern. Med. 74:424, 1971.

284. Kelley, W. N., Greene, M. I., Fox, I. H., Rosenbloom, F. M., Levy, R. H., and Seegmiller, J. E.: Effects of orotic acid on purine and lipoprotein metabolism in man. Metabolism 19:1025, 1970.

285. Henderson, J. F., and Khoo, M. K. Y.: Synthesis of 5-phosphoribosyl-1-pyrophosphate from glucose in Ehrlich ascites tumor cells in vitro. J. Biol. Chem. 240:2349, 1965.

286. Lindsay, R. H., Cash, A. G., and Hill, J. B.: TSH stimulation of orotic acid conversion of pyrimidine nucleotides and RNA in bovine thyroid. Endocrinology 84:534, 1969.

287. Rottman, R., and Guarino, A. J.: The inhibition of phosphoribosylpyrophosphate amidotransferase activity by cordecepin monophosphate. Biochim. Biophys. Acta 89:465, 1964.

288. Nagy, M.: Regulation of biosynthesis of purine nucleotides in Schizosaccharomyces pombe. I. Properties of the phosphoribosylpyrophosphate glutamine amidotransferase of the wild strain and of a mutant desensitized towards feedback modifiers. Biochim. Biophys. Acta 198:471, 1970.

289. Rowe, P. B., Coleman, M. D., and Wyngaarden, J. B.: Glutamine phosphoribosylpyrophosphate amidotransferase: Catalytic and conformational heterogeneity of the pigeon liver enzyme. Biochemistry 9:1498, 1970.

290. King, G., Meade, J. C., Borinous, C. G., and Holmes, E. W.: Demonstration of ammonia utilization for purine biosynthesis by the intact cell and characterization of the enzymatic activity catalyzing this reaction. Metabolism 28:348, 1979.

291. Itakura, M., Sabina, R., Heald, P., and Holmes, E. W.: Basis for the control of purine biosynthesis by purine ribonucleotides. J. Clin. Invest. 67:994, 1981.

292. Magasanik, B., and Karibian, D.: Purine nucleotide cycles and their metabolic role. J. Biol. Chem. 235:2672, 1960.

293. Holmes, E. W., Pehlke, D. M., and Kelley, W. N.: The role of human inosinic acid dehydrogenase in the control of purine biosynthesis de novo. Biochim. Biophys. Acta 364:209, 1974.

294. Ullman, B., Wormstead, M. A., Cohen, M. B., and Martin, D. W.: Purine oversecretion in cultured murine lymphoma cells deficient in adenylosuccinate synthetase: Genetic model for hyperuricemia and gout. Proc. Natl. Acad. Sci. U.S.A. 79:2673, 1982.

295. Hers, H.-G.: The mechanism of adenosine triphosphate depletion in the liver after a fructose load. A kinetic study of liver adenylate deaminase. Biochem. J. 162:601, 1977.

296. Zoref, E., DeVries, A., and Sperling, O.: Kinetic aspects of purine metabolism in cultured fibroblasts. A comparative study of cells from patients overproducing purines due to HGPRT deficiency and PRPP synthetase superactivity. Monogr. Hum. Genet. 10:96, 1978.

297. Lomax, C. A., Bagnara, A. S., and Henderson, J. F.: Studies of the regulation of purine nucleotide catabolism. Can. J. Biochem. 53:231, 1975.

298. Madrid-Marina, V., and Fox, I. H.: Human placental cytoplasmic 5'-nucleotidase. Kinetic properties and inhibition. J. Biol. Chem. 261:444, 1986.

299. Kaminska-Berry, J., Madrid-Marina, V., and Fox, I. H.: Purification and properties of human placental cytoplasmic 5'-nucleotide. J. Biol. Chem. 261:449, 1986.

300. Naito, Y., and Tsushima, K.: Cytosol 5'-nucleotidase from chicken liver. Purification and some properties. Biochim. Biophys. Acta 438: 159, 1976.

301. Fritzson, P.: Nucleotidase activities in the soluble fraction of rat liver homogenate. Partial purification and properties of a 5'-nucleotidase with pH optimum 6.3. Biochim. Biophys. Acta 178:534, 1969.

302. Fritzson, P.: Regulation of nucleotidase activities in animal tissues. Adv. Enz. Reg. 16:43, 1978.

303. Carson, D. A., Kaye, J., and Wasson, D. B.: The potential importance of soluble deoxynucleotidase activity in mediating deoxyadenosine toxicity in human lymphoblasts. J. Immunol 126:348, 1981.

304. Carson, D. A., and Wasson, W. B.: Characterization of an adenosine 5'-triphosphate- and deoxyadenosine 5'-triphosphate-activated nucleotidase from human malignant lymphocytes. Cancer Res. 42:4321, 1982.

305. Bagnara, A. S., and Hershfield, M. S.: Mechanism of deoxyadenosine-induced catabolism of adenine ribonucleotides in adenosine deaminase-inhibited human T lymphoblastoid cells. Proc. Natl. Acad. Sci. U.S.A. 79:2673, 1982.

306. Fox, I. H., and Marchant, P. J.: Purine catabolism in man: Inhibition of 5'-phosphomonesterase activities from placental microsomes. Can. J. Biochem. 54:1055, 1976.

307. Barankiewicz, J., Battell, M. L., and Henderson, J. F.: Role of orthophosphate concentration in the regulation of ribose phosphate synthesis and purine metabolism in Ehrlich ascites tumor cells. Can. J. Biochem. 55:834, 1977.

308. Lomax, C. A., and Henderson, J. F.: Adenosine formation and metabolism during adenosine triphosphate catabolism in Ehrlich ascites tumor cells. Cancer Res. 33:2825, 1973.

309. Barankiewicz, J., and Cohen, A.: Nucleotide catabolism and nucleoside cycles in human thymocytes. Role of orthophosphate. Biochem. J. 219:197, 1984.

310. Matsumoto, S. S., Raivio, K., and Seegmiller, J. E.: Adenine nucleotide degradation during energy depletion in human lymphoblasts. Adenosine accumulation and adenylate energy charge correlation. J. Biol. Chem. 254:8956, 1979.

311. Fox, I. H.: Metabolic basis for disorders of purine nucleotide degradation. Metabolism 30:616, 1981.

312. Griebsch, A., and Zollner, N.: Effect of ribonucleotides given orally on uric acid production in man. In Sperling, O., de Vries, A., and Wyngaarden, J. B. (eds.): Purine Metabolism in Man, Vol. 41B. New York, Plenum Press, 1974, p. 443.

313. Zollner, N.: Influence of various purines on uric acid metabolism. Bibl. "Nutr. Diet" No. 19. Basel, Karger, 1973, pp. 34–43.

314. Buzard, J., Bishop, C., and Talbott, J. H.: Recovery in humans of intravenously injected isotopic uric acid. J. Biol. Chem. 196:179, 1952.

315. Wyngaarden, J. B.: The effect of phenylbutazone on uric acid metabolism in two normal subjects. J. Clin. Invest. 34:256, 1955.

316. Sorensen, L. B.: The elimination of uric acid in man studies by means of C^{14}-labeled uric acid. Scand. J. Clin. Lab. Invest. 12 (Suppl. 54):1, 1960.

317. Spilman, E. L.: Uric acid synthesis in the nongouty and gouty human (abstr.). Fed. Proc. 13:302, 1954.

318. Benedict, J. D., Forsham, P. H., and Stetten, DeW., Jr.: The metabolism of uric acid in the normal and gouty human studied with the aid of isotopic uric acid. J. Biol. Chem. 18:183, 1949.

319. Sorensen, L. B.: Degradation of uric acid in man. Metabolism 8:687, 1959.

320. Scott, J. T., Holloway, V. P., Glass, H. I., et al.: Studies of uric acid pool size and turnover rate. Ann. Rheum. Dis. 28:366, 1969.

321. Kelley, W. N., Greene, M. L., Rosenbloom, F. M., et al.: Hypoxanthine-guanine phosphoribosyltransferase deficiency in gout. Ann. Intern. Med. 70:155, 1969.

322. Seegmiller, J. C., Grayzel, A. I., Laster, L., et al.: Uric acid production in gout. J. Clin. Invest. 40:1304, 1961.

323. Kelley, W. N., Rosenbloom, F. M., Seegmiller, J. E., et al.: Excessive production of uric acid in type I glycogen storage disease. J. Pediatr. 72:488, 1968.

324. Lucke, H.: Das Harnsaureproblem und seine klinische Bedeutung. Ergeb. Inn. Med. Kinderheilk. 44:499, 1932.

325. Kurti, L.: Untersuchungen uber den Harnsauerstoffwechsel bei Nierenkranken. Z. Klin. Med. 122:585, 1932.

326. Wyngaarden, J. B.: Gout. In Stanbury, J. B., Wyngaarden, J. B., and Fredrickson, D. S. (eds.): The Metabolic Basis of Inherited Disease. New York, McGraw-Hill Book Company, 1960, p. 728.

327. Shannon, J. A.: The excretion of uric acid by the chicken. J. Cell. Comp. Physiol. 11:135, 1938.

328. Dantzler, W. H.: Comparison of renal tubular transport of urate and PAH in water snakes. Evidence for differences in mechanisms and sites of transport. Comp. Biochem. Physiol. 34:609, 1970.

329. Dantzler, W. H.: Characteristics of urate transport by isolated perfused snake proximal renal tubules. Am. J. Physiol. 224:445, 1973.

330. Mudge, G. H., McAlary, B., and Berndt, W. O.: Renal transport of uric acid in the guinea pig. Am. J. Physiol. 214:875, 1969.

331. Kessler, R. H., Hierholzer, K., and Gurd, R. S.: Localization of urate transport in the nephron of mongrel and Dalmation dog kidney. Am. J. Physiol. 197:601, 1959.

332. Fanelli, G. M., Bohn, D., and Russo, H. F.: Renal clearance of uric acid in nonhuman primates. Comp. Biochem. Physiol. 33:459, 1970.

333. Boudry, J. F.: Mecanismes de l'excretion d'acide urique chez le rat. Pfluegers Arch. Ges. Physiol. 328:265, 1971.

334. Boudry, J. F.: Effet d'inhibiteurs des transports transtubulaires sur l'excretion renale d'acide urique chez le rat. Pfluegers Arch. Ges. Physiol. 328:279, 1971.

335. Berliner, R. W., Hilton, J. G., Yu, T.-F., et al.: The renal mechanism for urate excretion in man. J. Clin. Invest. 29:296, 1950.

336. Berger, L., Yu, T.-F., and Gutman, A. B.: Effects of drugs that alter uric acid excretion in man on uric acid clearance in the chicken. Am. J. Physiol. 198:575, 1960.

337. Yu, T.-F., Berger, L., Kupfer, S., et al.: Tubular secretion of urate in the dog. Am. J. Physiol. 199:1199, 1960.

338. Fanelli, G. M., Jr., Bohn, D., and Stafford, S.: Functional characteristics of renal urate transport in the Cebus monkey. Am. J. Physiol. 218:627, 1970.

339. Fanelli, G. M., Jr., Bohn, D. L., and Reilly, S. S.: Renal urate transport in the chimpanzee. Am. J. Physiol. 220:613, 1971.

340. Greger, R., Lang, F., and Deetjen, P.: Handling of uric acid by the rat kidney. I. Microanalysis of uric acid in proximal tubular fluid. Eur. J. Physiol. 324:279, 1971.

341. Gutman, A. B., Yu, T.-F., and Berger, L.: Tubular secretion of urate in man. J. Clin. Invest. 39:1778, 1959.

342. Lathem, W., Davis, B. B., and Rodnan, G. P.: Renal tubular secretion of uric acid in the mongrel dog. Am. J. Physiol. 199:9, 1960.

343. Mudge, G. H., Cucchi, J., Platts, M., et al.: Renal excretion of uric acid in the dog. Am. J. Physiol. 215:404, 1968.

344. Nolan, R. P., and Foulkes, E. C.: Studies on renal urate secretion in the dog. J. Pharmacol. Exp. Ther. 179:429, 1971.
345. Zins, G. R., and Weiner, I. M.: Bidirectional urate transport limited to the proximal tubule in dogs. Am. J. Physiol. 215:411, 1968.
346. Blanchard, K. C., Marooske, D., May, D. G., et al.: Uricosuric potency of 2-substituted analogs of probenecid. J. Pharmacol. Exp. Ther. 180:397, 1972.
347. Fanelli, G. M., Jr., Bohn, D. L., and Reilly, S. S.: Renal effects of uricosuric agents in the Cebus monkey. J. Pharmacol. Exp. Ther. 175:259, 1970.
348. Fanelli, G. M., Jr., Bohn, D. L., and Reilly, S. S.: Renal effects of uricosuric agents in the chimpanzee. J. Pharmacol. Exp. Ther. 177:591, 1971.
349. Fanelli, G. M., Jr., Bohn, D. L., Reilly, S. S., et al.: Renal excretion and uricosuric properties of halofenate, a hypolipidemic uricosuric agent, in the chimpanzee. J. Pharmacol. Exp. Ther. 180:377, 1972.
350. Bordley, J., III, and Richards, A. N.: Quantitative studies of the composition of glomerular urine. VIII. The concentration of uric acid in glomerular urine of snakes and frogs, determined by an ultramicro adaption of Folin's method. J. Biol. Chem. 101:193, 1933.
351. Roch-Ramel, F., and Weiner, I. M.: Excretion of urate by the kidneys of Cebus monkeys: A micropuncture study. Am. J. Physiol. 224:1369, 1973.
352. Weiner, I. M., and Fanelli, G. M., Jr.: Renal urate excretion in animal models. Nephron 14:33, 1975.
353. Berndt, W. O., and Beechwood, E. C.: Influence of inorganic electrolytes and ouabain on uric acid transport. Am. J. Physiol. 208:642, 1965.
354. Weinman, E. J., Senekjian, H. O., Sansom, S. C., et al.: Evidence for active and passive urate transport in the rat proximal tubule. Am. J. Physiol. 240:F90, 1981.
355. Sansom, S. C., Senekjian, H. O., Knight, T. F., et al.: Determination of the apparent transport constants for urate absorption in the rat proximal tubule. Am. J. Physiol. 240:F406, 1981.
356. Senekjian, H. O., Knight, T. F., and Weinman, E. J.: Urate transport by the isolated perfused S2 segment of the rabbit. Am. J. Physiol. 240:F530, 1981.
357. Fanelli, G. M., Jr., and Weiner, I. M.: Pyrazinoate excretion in the chimpanzee. Relation to urate disposition and the actions of uricosuric drugs. J. Clin. Invest. 52:1946, 1973.
358. Robson, A. M., Srivastave, P. L., and Bricker, N. S.: The influence of saline loading on renal glucose reabsorption in the rat. J. Clin. Invest. 47:329, 1968.
359. Bricker, N. S.: On the pathogenesis of the uremic state: The "trade-off hypothesis." N. Engl. J. Med. 286:1093, 1972.
360. Cannon, P. J., Svahn, D. S., and DeMartini, F. E.: The influence of hypertonic saline infusion upon the fractional reabsorption of urate and other ions in normal and hypertensive man. Circulation 41:97, 1970.
361. Kurtzman, N. A.: Regulation of renal bicarbonate reabsorption by extracellular volume. J. Clin. Invest. 49:586, 1970.
362. Holmes, E. W., Kelley, W. N., and Wyngaarden, J. B.: The kidney and uric acid excretion in man. Kidney Int. 2:115, 1972.
363. Weinman, E. J., Eknoyan, G., and Suki, W. N.: The influence of the extracellular fluid volume on the tubular reabsorption of uric acid. J. Clin. Invest. 55:283, 1975.
364. Kahn, T., Mohammed, G., and Stein, R. M.: Alterations in renal tubular sodium and water reabsorption in chronic renal disease in man. Kidney Int. 2:164, 1972.
365. Steele, T. H., and Rieselbach, R. E.: The contributions of residual nephrons within the chronically diseased kidney to rate homeostasis in man. Am. J. Med. 43:876, 1967.
366. Martino, J. A., and Earley, L. E.: Demonstration of a role of physical factors as determinants of the natriuretic response to volume expansion. J. Clin. Invest. 56:1963, 1967.
367. Malnic, G., Aires, M. M., and Giebisch, G.: Micropuncture study of renal tubular hydrogen ion transport in the rat. Am. J. Physiol. 222:147, 1972.
368. Weiner, I. M., and Mudge, F. H.: Renal tubular mechanisms for excretion of organic acids and bases. Am. J. Med. 36:743, 1964.
369. Praetorius, D., and Kirk, J. E.: Hypouricemia: With evidence for tubular elimination of uric acid. J. Lab. Clin. Med. 35:865, 1950.
370. Yu, T.-F., and Gutman, A. B.: Study of the paradoxical effects of salicylate in low, intermediate and high dosage on the renal mechanisms for excretion of urate in man. J. Clin. Invest. 38:1298, 1959.
371. Diamond, H. S., Sterba, G., Jayadeven, K., and Meisel, A. D.: On the mechanism of the paradoxical effect of salicylate on urate excretion. In Ropade, A., Watts, R. W. E., and DeBruyn, C. H. M. (eds.): Third International Symposium on Purine Metabolism in Man. New York, Plenum Publishing Co., 1980, pp. 221–225.
372. Podevin, R., Ardaillou, R., Paillar, F., et al.: Etude chez l'homme de la cinetique d'apparition dans l'urine de l'acide urique-2¹⁴C. Nephron 5:134, 1968.
373. Nechay, B. R., and Nechay, L.: Effects of probenecid, sodium lactate,

374. Moller, J. V.: The tubular site of urate transport in the rabbit kidney and the effect of probenecid on urate secretion. Acta Pharmacol. Toxicol. 23:329, 1965.
375. Fanelli, G. M., Jr., Bohn, D. L., Reilly, S. S., et al.: Effects of mercurial diuretics on renal transport of urate in the chimpanzee. Am. J. Physiol. 224:985, 1973.
376. Moller, J. V.: The relation between secretion of urate and p-aminohippurate in the rabbit kidney. J. Physiol. 192:505, 1967.
377. Boner, G., and Steele, T. H.: Relationship of urate and p-aminohippurate secretion in man. Am. J. Physiol. 225:100, 1967.
378. Reem, G. H., and Vanamee, P.: Effect of sodium lactate on urate clearance in the Dalmatian and mongrel dog. Am. J. Physiol. 207:113, 1964.
379. Goldfinger, S., Klinenberg, J. R., and Seegmiller, J. E.: Renal retention of uric acid induced by infusion of betahydroxybutyrate and acetoacetate. N. Engl. J. Med. 272:351, 1965.
380. Schulman, J. F., Lustberg, T. J., Kennedy, J. L., et al.: A new variant of maple syrup urine disease (branched chain ketoaciduria). Clinical and biochemical evaluation. Am. J. Med. 49:118, 1970.
381. Gutman, A. B., and Yu, T.-F.: Renal mechanisms for regulation of uric acid excretion with special reference to normal and gouty man. Semin. Arthritis Rheum. 2:1, 1972.
382. Greger, R., Lang, R., and Deetjen, P.: Handling of uric acid by the rat kidney. II. Microperfusion studies on bidirectional transport of uric acid in the proximal tubule. Eur. J. Physiol. 335:257, 1972.
383. Wilson, D. M., and Goldstein, N. P.: Renal urate excretion in patients with Wilson's disease. Kidney Int. 4:331, 1973.
384. Bennet, J. S., Bond, J., Singer, I., et al.: Hypouricemia in Hodgkin's disease. Ann. Intern. Med. 76:751, 1972.
385. Steele, T. H., and Boner, G.: Origins of the uricosuric response. J. Clin. Invest. 52:1368, 1973.
386. Gutman, W. B., and Yu, T.-F.: A three-component system for regulation of renal excretion of urate in man. Trans. Assoc. Am. Physicians 74:353, 1961.
387. Manuel, M. A., and Steele, T. H.: Pyrazinamide suppression of the uricosuric response to sodium chloride infusion. J. Lab. Clin. Med. 83:417, 1974.
388. Steele, T. H.: Urate secretion in man: The pyrazinamide suppression test. Ann. Intern. Med. 79:734, 1973.
389. Diamond, H. S., and Paolino, J. S.: Evidence for a postsecretory reabsorptive site for uric acid in man. J. Clin. Invest. 52:1491, 1973.
390. Fanelli, G. M., Jr., and Weiner, I. M.: Urate excretion: Drug interactions. J. Pharmacol. Exp. Ther. 210:186, 1979.
391. Tofuku, Y., Mitsuhiko, K., and Takeda, R.: Hypouricemia due to renal urate wasting. Nephron 30:39, 1982.
392. Brochner-Mortensen, K.: The uric acid content in blood and urine in health and disease. Medicine 19:161, 1940.
393. Diamond, H. S., Lazarus, R., Kaplan, E., et al.: Effect of urine flow rate on uric acid excretion in man. Arthritis Rheum. 15:338, 1972.
394. Diamond, H. S., and Meisel, A. D.: Collecting duct urate reabsorption in man. Program abstracts, 39th Annual Meeting of American Rheumatism Association, Section of Arthritis Foundation, New Orleans, June 4–6, 1977.
395. Wolfson, W. Q., Hunt, H. D., Levine, R., et al.: The transport and excretion of uric acid in man; sex difference and urate metabolism with note on clinical and laboratory findings in gouty women. J. Clin. Endocrinol. Metab. 9:749, 1949.
396. Scott, J. T., and Pollard, A. D.: Uric acid excretion in the relatives of patients with gout. Ann. Rheum. Dis. 29:397, 1970.
397. Nicholls, A., Snaith, M. L., and Scott, J. T.: Effect of oestrogen therapy on plasma and urinary levels of uric acid. Br. Med. J. 1:449, 1973.
398. Snaith, M. L., and Scott, J. T.: Uric acid excretion and surgery. Ann. Rheum. Dis. 31:162, 1972.
399. Grabfield, B. P.: A pharmacologic study of the mechanism of gout. Ann. Intern. Med. 11:651, 1937.
400. Postlethwaite, A. E., Ramsdell, C. M., and Kelley, W. N.: Uricosuric effect of an anticholinergic agent in hyperuricemic subjects. Arch. Intern. Med. 134:270, 1974.
401. Peters, J. P., and Van Slyke, K. K.: Quantitative Clinical Chemistry, Vol. 1. 2nd ed. Baltimore, Williams & Wilkins, 1946, p. 937.
402. Allen, D. J., Milosovich, G., and Mattocks, A. M.: Inhibition of monosodium urate crystal growth. Arthritis Rheum. 8:1123, 1965.
403. Loeb, J. N.: The influence of temperature on the solubility of monosodium urate. Arthritis Rheum. 15:189, 1972.
404. Wilcox, W. R., Khalaf, A., Weinberger, A., et al.: The solubility of uric acid and monosodium urate. Med. Biol. Eng. 10:522, 1972.
405. McNabb, R. A., and McNabb, F. M. A.: Physiological chemistry of uric acid: solubility, colloid, and ion-binding properties. Comp. Biochem. Physiol. 67A:27, 1980.
406. Seegmiller, J. E.: The acute attack of gouty arthritis. Arthritis Rheum. 8:714, 1965.

2,4-dinitrophenol, and pyrazinamide on renal secretion of uric acid in chickens. J. Pharmacol. Exp. Ther. 126:291, 1959.

407. Klinenberg, J. R., Goldfinger, S. E., and Seegmiller, J. E.: The effectiveness of a xanthine oxidase inhibitor on the treatment of gout. Ann. Intern. Med. 62:639, 1965.
408. Gold, G. L., and Fritz, R. D.: Hyperuricemia associated with the treatment of acute leukemia. Ann. Intern. Med. 47:428, 1957.
409. Alvsaker, J. O.: Uric acid in human plasma. V. Isolation and identification of plasma proteins interacting with urate. Scand. J. Clin. Lab. Invest. 18:228, 1966.
410. Adlersberg, D., Brishman, E., and Sobotka, H.: Uric acid partition in gout and hepatic disease. Arch. Intern. Med. 70:101, 1942.
411. Yu, T.-F., and Gutman, A. B.: Ultrafilterability of plasma urate in man. Proc. Soc. Exp. Biol. Med. 84:21, 1953.
412. Wyngaarden, J. B.: Uric Acid. *In* Persol, G. M. (ed.): The Cyclopedia of Medicine, Surgery Specialties. Philadelphia, F. A. Davis Company, 1955, p. 341.
413. Morris, J. E.: The transport of uric acid in serum. Am. J. Med. Sci. 235:43, 1958.
414. Kovarsky, J., Holmes, E., and Kelley, W. N.: Absence of significant urate binding to human serum proteins. J. Lab. Clin. Med. 93:85, 1979.
415. Postlethwaite, A. E., Gutman, R. A., and Kelley, W. N.: Salicylate-mediated increase in urate removal during hemodialysis: Evidence of urate binding to protein in vivo. Metabolism 23:771, 1974.
416. Medes, G.: Solubility of calcium oxalate and uric acid in solutions of urea. Proc. Soc. Exp. Biol. Med. 30:281, 1932.
417. Atsmon, A., DeVries, A., and Kedem, O.: Uric Acid Lithiasis. Amsterdam, Elsevier, 1963, p. 63.
418. Sperling, O., DeVries, A., and Kedem, O.: Studies on the etiology of uric acid lithiasis. IV. Urinary non-dialyzable substances in idiopathic uric acid lithiasis. J. Urol. 94:286, 1965.
419. Prien, E. L., and Prien, E. L., Jr.: Composition and structure of urinary stone. Am. J. Med. 45:654, 1968.
420. Howell, R. R., Eanes, E. D., and Seegmiller, J. E.: X-ray diffraction studies on the tophaceous deposits in gout. Arthritis Rheum. 6:97, 1963.
421. Zwaifler, N. J., and Pekin, T. J.: Significance of urate crystals in synovial fluids. Ann. Intern. Med. 111:99, 1963.
422. Nugent, C. A., and Tyler, F. H.: The renal excretion of uric acid in patients with gout and in nongouty subjects. J. Clin. Invest. 38:1890, 1959.
423. Seegmiller, J. E., Grayzel, A. I., Howell, R. R., et al.: The renal excretion of uric acid in gout. J. Clin. Invest. 41:1094, 1962.
424. Yu, T.-F., Berger, L., and Gutman, A. B.: Renal function in gout. II. Effect of uric acid loading on renal excretion of uric acid. Am. J. Med. 33:829, 1962.
425. Lathem, W., and Rodnan, G. P.: Impairment of uric acid excretion in gout. J. Clin. Invest. 41:1955, 1962.
426. Houpt, J. B., and Ogryzlo, M. A.: Persistence of impaired uric acid excretion in gout during reduced synthesis with allopurinol (abstr.). Arthritis Rheum. 7:316.
427. Snaith, M. L., and Scott, J. T.: Uric acid clearance in patients with gout and normal subjects. Ann. Rheum. Dis. 30:285, 1971.
428. Wyngaarden, J. B.: Gout. Adv. Metabol. Dis. 2:2, 1965.
429. Nugent, C. A., MacDiarmid, W. D., and Tyler, F. H.: Renal excretion of urate in patients with gout. Arch. Intern. Med. 113:115, 1964.
430. Campion, D. S., Olsen, R. W., Caughey, D., et al.: Does increased free serum urate concentration cause gout? (abstr.). Clin. Res. 23:109A, 1974.
431. Klinenberg, J. R., and Kippen, I.: The binding of urate to plasma proteins determined by means of equilibrium dialysis. J. Lab. Clin. Med. 75:503, 1970.
432. Rieselbach, R. E., Sorensen, L. B., Shelp, W. D., et al.: Diminished renal urate secretion per nephron on a basis for primary gout. Ann. Intern. Med. 73:359, 1970.
433. Levinson, D. J., and Sorensen, L. B.: Renal handling of uric acid in normal and gouty subject: Evidence for a 4-component system. Ann. Rheum. Dis. 39:173, 1980.
434. Levinson, D. J., Decker, D. E., and Sorensen, L. B.: Renal handling of uric acid in man. Ann. Clin. Lab. Sci. 12:73, 1982.
435. Puig, J. G., Anton, F. M., Jimenez, M. L., and Gutierrez, P. C.: Renal handling of uric acid in gout: Impaired tubular transport of urate not dependent on serum urate levels. Metabolism 35:1147, 1986.
436. Kavalich, A. G., Moran, E., and Coe, F. L.: Dietary purine consumption by hyperuricosuric calcium oxalate stone formers and normal subjects. J. Chronic Dis. 29:745, 1976.
437. Simkin, P. A., Hoover, P. L., Paxson, C. S., et al.: Uric acid excretion: Quantitative assessment from spot, midmorning serum and urine samples. Ann. Intern. Med. 91:44, 1979.
438. Wortmann, R. L., and Fox, I. H.: Limited value of uric acid to creatinine ratios in estimating uric acid excretion. Ann. Intern. Med. 93:822, 1980.
439. Gordon, R. B., Counsilman, A. C., Cross, S. M. C., and Emmerson, B. T.: Purine synthesis de novo in lymphocytes from patients with gout. Clin. Sci. 63:429, 1982.
440. Hers, H.-G., and Van Den Berghe, G.: Enzyme defect in primary gout. Lancet 1:585, 1979.
441. Seegmiller, J. E., Rosenbloom, R. M., and Kelley, W. N.: An enzyme defect associated with a sex-linked human neurological disorder and excessive purine synthesis. Science 155:1682, 1967.
442. Lesch, M., and Nyhan, W. L.: A familial disorder of uric acid metabolism and central nervous system function. Am. J. Med. 36:561, 1964.
443. Kelley, W. N.: Hypoxanthine-guanine phosphoribosyltransferase deficiency in the Lesch-Nyhan syndrome and gout. Fed. Proc. 27:1060, 1968.
444. Kelley, W. N., Rosenbloom, E. M., Henderson, J. F., et al.: A specific enzyme defect in gout associated with overproduction of uric acid. Proc. Natl. Acad. Sci. USA 57:1735, 1967.
445. Michener, W. M.: Hyperuricemia and mental retardation with athetosis and self-mutilation. Am. J. Dis. Child. 133:195, 1967.
446. Marie, J., Royer, P., and Rappaport, R.: Hyperuricemie cogenitale avec troubles neurologiques, renaux et sanguins. Arch. Fr. Pediatr. 23:970, 1966.
447. van Bogaert, L., Damme, J. V., and Verschueren, M.: Sur un syndrome professif d'hypertonie extrapyramidale avec osteoarthropathies goutteuses chez deux freres. Rev. Neurol. 114:15, 1966.
448. Riley, J. D.: Gout and cerebral palsy in a three-year-old boy. Arch. Dis. Child. 35:293, 1960.
449. Berman, P. H., Balis, M. E., and Dancis, J.: Congenital hyperuricemia: An inborn error of purine metabolism associated with psychomotor retardation athetosis, and self-mutilation. Arch. Neurol. 20:44, 1969.
450. Kogut, M. D., Donnell, G. N., Nyhan, W. L., et al.: Disorder of purine metabolism due to partial deficiency of hypoxanthine-guanine phosphoribosyltransferase: A study of a family. Am. J. Med. 48:148, 1970.
451. Sperling, O., Frank, M., Ophir, R., et al.: Partial deficiency of hypoxanthine-guanine phosphoribosyltransferase associated with gout and uric acid lithiasis. Eur. J. Clin. Biol. Res. 15:942, 1970.
452. Delbarre, F., Cartier, P., Auscher, C., et al.: Gouttes enzymopathiques dyspurinies par deficit en hypoxanthineguanine phosphoribosyl-transferase. Frequence et caracteres cliniques de l'anenzymose. Presse Med. 78:729, 1970.
453. Marie, J., Royer, P., and Rappaport, R.: Hyperuricemie congenitale avec troubles neurologiques, renaux et sanguins. Arch. Fr. Pediatr. 25:501, 1967.
454. Manzke, H.: Hyperuricamie mit cerebralparese Syndrome eines hereditaren Purinstoffwechselleidens. Helv. Paediat. Acta 22:258, 1967.
455. van der Zee, S. P. M., Schretien, E. D. A. M., and Monnens, L. A. H.: Megaloblastic anemia in the Lesch-Nyhan syndrome (letter). Lancet 1:1427, 1968.
456. Wilson, J. M., Baugher, B. W., Landa, L., et al.: Human hypoxanthine-guanine phosphoribosyltransferase: Purification and characterization of mutant forms of the enzyme. J. Biol. Chem. 256:10306, 1981.
457. Wilson, J. M., Baugher, B. W., Mattes, P. M., et al.: Human hypoxanthine-guanine phosphoribosyltransferase: Demonstration of structural variants in lymphoblastoid cells derived from patients with a deficiency of the enzyme. J. Clin. Invest. 69:706, 1982.
458. Wilson, J. M., Tarr, G. E., and Kelley, W. N.: Human hypoxanthine-guanine phosphoribosyltransferase: A single amino acid substitution in a mutant form of the enzyme isolated from a patient with gout. Proc. Natl. Acad. Sci. U.S.A. 80:870, 1983.
459. Wilson, J. M., and Kelley, W. N.: The molecular basis of hypoxanthine-guanine phosphoribosyltransferase deficiency in a patient with the Lesch-Nyhan syndrome. J. Clin. Invest. 71:1331, 1983.
460. Wilson, J. M., Young, A. B., and Kelley, W. N.: Hypoxanthine-guanine phosphoribosyltransferase deficiency: The molecular basis of the clinical syndrome. N. Engl. J. Med. 309:900, 1983.
461. Tarle, S. A., Davidson, B. L., Wu, V. C., Zidar, F. J., Seegmiller, J. E., Kelley, W. N., and Palella, T. D.: Determination of the mutations responsible for the Lesch-Nyhan syndrome in seventeen subjects. Genomics 10:499, 1991.
462. Davidson, B. L., Tare, S. A., Van Antwerp, M., et al.: Identification of 17 independent mutations responsible for human hypoxanthine-guanine phosphoribosyl transferase (HPRT) deficiency. Am. J. Hum. Genet. 48:951, 1991.
463. Davidson, B. L., Tarle, S. A., Palella, T. D., and Kelley, W. N.: The molecular basis of HPRT deficiency in ten subjects determined by direct sequencing of amplified transcripts. J. Clin. Invest. 84:342, 1989.
464. Wilson, J. M., Kobayashi, R., Fox, I. H., and Kelley, W. N.: Human hypoxanthine phosphoribosyltransferase. Molecular abnormality in a mutant form of the enzyme ($HPRT_{Toronto}$). J. Biol. Chem. 258:6458, 1983.
465. Fujimori, S., Davidson, B. L., Kelley, W. N., and Palella, T. D.: Identification of a single nucleotide change in the hypoxanthine-guanine phosphoribosyltransferase gene ($HPRT_{Yale}$) responsible for Lesch-Nyhan syndrome. J. Clin. Invest. In press.
466. Davidson, B. L., Pashmforoush, M., Kelley, W. N., and Palella, T. D.: Genetic basis of hypoxanthine guanine phosphoribosyltransferase deficiency in a patient with the Lesch-Nyhan syndrome ($HPRT_{Flint}$). Gene. 63:331, 1988.

467. Wilson, J. M., and Kelley, W. N.: Human hypoxanthine-guanine phosphoribosyltransferase: Structural alteration in a dysfunctional enzyme variant (HPRT_Munich) isolated from a patient with gout. J. Biol. Chem. 259:27, 1984.
468. Davidson, B. L., Palella, T. D., and Kelley, W. N.: Personal communication, 1988.
469. Fujimori, S., Hidaka, Y., Davidson, B. L., Palella, T. D., and Kelley, W. N.: Identification of a single nucleotide change in a mutant HPRT gene (HPRT_Ann Arbor). Hum. Genet. In press.
470. Brennard, J., Chinault, A. C., Konecki, D. S., et al.: Cloned cDNA sequences of the hypoxanthine-guanine phosphoribosyltransferase gene from a mouse neuroblastoma cell line found to have amplified genomic sequences. Proc. Natl. Acad. Sci. U.S.A. 79:1950, 1982.
470a. Jolly, D., Esty, A. C., Bernard, H. U., and Friedmann, T.: Isolation of a genomic clone partially encoding human hypoxanthine phosphoribosyltransferase. Proc. Natl. Acad. Sci. U.S.A. 79:5038, 1982.
471. Wilson, J. M., Stout, J. T., Palella, T. D., Davidson, B. L., Kelley, W. N., and Casky, C. T.: A molecular survey of hypoxanthine-guanine phosphoribosyltransferase deficiency in man. J. Clin. Invest. 77:188, 1986.
471a. Yang, T. P., Patel, P. I., Chinault, A. C., Stout, J. T., Jackson, L. G., Hildebrand, B. M., and Caskey, C. T.: Molecular evidence for new mutation at the HPRT locus in Lesch-Nyhan patients. Nature 310:412, 1984.
472. Gibbs, R. A., and Caskey, C. T.: Identification and localization of mutations at the Lesch-Nyhan locus by ribonuclease A cleavage. Science 236:303, 1987.
473. Rosenbloom, F. M., Henderson, J. F., Caldwell, I. C., et al.: Biochemical bases of accelerated purine biosynthesis de novo in human fibroblasts lacking hypoxanthine-guanine phosphoribosyltransferase. J. Biol. Chem. 243:1166, 1968.
474. Nuki, G., Lever, J., and Seegmiller, J. E.: Biochemical characteristics of 8-azaguanine resistant human lymphoblast mutants selected in vitro. In Sperling, O., DeVries, A., and Wyngaarden, J. B. (eds.): Purine Metabolism in Man. New York, Plenum Press, 1974, p. 255.
475. Hoefnagel, D., Andrew, E. D., Mireault, N. G., et al.: Hereditary choreoathetosis, self-mutilation, and hyperuricemia in young males. N. Engl. J. Med. 273:130, 1965.
476. Shapiro, S. L., Sheppard, G. L., Jr., Dreifuss, F. E., et al.: X-linked recessive inheritance of a syndrome of mental retardation with hyperuricemia. Proc. Soc. Exp. Biol. Med. 122:609, 1966.
477. Emmerson, B. T., and Wyngaarden, J. B.: Purine metabolism in heterozygous carriers of hypoxanthine-guanine phosphoribosyltransferase deficiency. Science 166:1533, 1969.
478. Emmerson, B. T.: Urate metabolism in heterozygotes for HGPRTase deficiency. In Sperling, O., DeVries, A., and Wyngaarden, J. B. (eds.): Purine Metabolism in Man. New York, Plenum Press, 1974, p. 287.
479. Sperling, O., Eilam, G., Persky-Brosh, S., et al.: Accelerated erythrocyte 5'-phosphoribosyl-1-pyrophosphate synthesis. A familial abnormality associated with excessive uric acid production and gout. Biochem. Med. 6:310, 1972.
480. Sperling, O., Persky-Brosh, S., Boer, P., et al.: Human erythrocyte phosphoribosylpyrophosphate synthetase mutationally altered in regulatory properties. Biochem. Med. 7:389, 1973.
481. Becker, M. A., Meyer, L. J., Wood, A. W., et al.: Purine overproduction in man associated with increased phosphoribosylpyrophosphate synthetase activity. Science 179:1123, 1973.
482. Becker, M. A., Meyer, L. J., and Seegmiller, J. E.: Gout with purine overproduction due to increased phosphoribosylpyrophosphate synthetase activity. Am. J. Med. 55:232, 1973.
483. Becker, M. A., Kostel, P. J., Meyer, L. J., et al.: Human phosphoribosylpyrophosphate synthetase: Increased enzyme-specific activity in a family with gout and excessive purine synthesis. Proc. Natl. Acad. Sci. U.S.A. 70:2749, 1973.
484. Becker, M. A., Meyer, L. J., Dostel, P. J., et al.: Increased 5-phosphoribosyl-1-pyrophosphate (PRPP) synthetase activity and gout. Diversity of structural alterations the enzyme (abstr.). J. Clin. Invest. 53:4a, 1974.
485. Akaoka, I., Fujimori, S., Kamatani, N., et al.: A gouty family with increased phosphoribosylpyrophosphate synthetase activity: Case reports, familial studies, and kinetic studies of the abnormal enzyme. J. Rheumatol. 8:563, 1981.
486. Becker, M. A., Losman, M. J., Itkin, P., et al.: Gout with superactive phosphoribosylpyrophosphate synthetase due to increased enzyme catalytic rate. J. Lab. Clin. Med. 99:495, 1982.
487. Yen, R. C. K., Adams, W. B., Lazar, C., and Becker, M. A.: Evidence for x-linkage of human phosphoribosylpyrophosphate synthetase. Proc. Natl. Acad. Sci. U.S.A. 75:482, 1978.
488. Takeuchi, F., Hanaoka, F., Yano, E., et al.: The mode of genetic transmission of a gouty family with increased phosphoribosylpyrophosphate synthetase activity. Hum. Genet. 58:322, 1981.
489. Lin, H. Y., Rocher, L. L., McQuillan, M. A., et al.: Cyclosporine-induced hyperuricemia and gout. N. Engl. J. Med. 321:287, 1989.
490. Greene, H. L., Wilson, F. A., Heffernan, P., Terry, A. B., Moran, J.

R., Slonim, A. E., Claus, T. M., and Burr, I. M.: ATP depletion, a possible role in the pathogenesis of hyperuricemia in glycogen storage disease type I. J. Clin. Invest. 62:321, 1978.
491. Cohen, J. L., Vinik, A., Faller, J., and Fox, I. H.: Hyperuricemia in glycogen storage disease type I: Contributions by hypoglycemia and hyperglucagonemia to increased urate production. J. Clin. Invest. 75:251, 1985.
492. Sutton, J., Toews, C. J., Ward, G. R., and Fox, I. H.: Purine metabolism during strenuous muscular exercise in man. Metabolism 29:254, 1980.
493. Knochel, J. P., Dotin, L. N., and Hamburger, R. J.: Heat stress, exercise and muscle injury: Effects on urate metabolism and renal function. Ann. Intern. Med. 81:321, 1974.
494. Warren, D. J., Leitch, A. G., and Leggett, R. J. E.: Hyperuricaemic acute renal failure after epileptic seizures. Lancet 2:385, 1975.
495. Agamanolis, D., Askari, A. D., Di Mauro, S., et al.: Muscle phosphofructokinase deficiency. Two cases with unusual polysaccharide accumulation and immunologically active enzyme protein. Muscle Nerve 3:346, 1980.
496. Hays, A. P., Hallett, M., Delfs, J., Morris, B. M., Sotrel, A., and Shevchunk, M. M.: Muscle phosphofructokinase deficiency. Abnormal polysaccharide in a case of late-onset myopathy. Neurology 31:1077, 1981.
497. Zanella, A., Mariani, M., Meola, G., Fagnani, G., and Sirchia, G.: Phosphofructokinase (PFK) deficiency due to a catalytically inactive mutant M-type subunit. Am. J. Hematol. 12:215, 1982.
498. Vora, S., Davidson, M., Seaman, C., et al.: Heterogeneity of the molecular lesions in inherited phosphofructokinase deficiency. J. Clin. Invest. 72:1995, 1983.
499. Mineo, I., Kono, N., Shimizu, T., et al.: Excess purine degradation in exercising muscles of patients with glycogen storage disease types V and VII. J. Clin. Invest. 76:556, 1985.
500. Kono, N., Mineo, I., Shimizu, T., Hara, N., Yamada, Y., and Nonaka, K.: Increased plasma uric acid after exercise in muscle phosphofructokinase deficiency. Neurology 36:106, 1986.
501. Fogelfeld, L., Sarova-Pinhas, I., and Meytes, D.: Glycogen storage disease type VII myopathy (Tarui) associated with hemolysis and gout. J. Neurol. 232(Suppl.):186, 1985.
502. Brunberg, J. B., McCormick, W. F., and Schochet, S. S.: Type III glycogenosis. An adult with diffuse weakness and muscle wasting. Arch. Neurol. 25:171, 1971.
503. Murase, T., Ikeda, H., Muro, T., Nakao, K., and Sugita, H.: Myopathy associated with type III glycogenosis. J. Neurol. Sci. 20:287, 1973.
504. Mineo, I., Kono, N., Hara, N., et al.: Myogenic hyperuricemia: A common pathophysiologic feature of glycogenosis types III, V, and VIII. N. Engl. J. Med. 317:75, 1987.
505. Brooke, M. H., Patterson, V. H., and Kaiser, K. K.: Hypoxanthine and McArdle disease. A clue to metabolic stress in the working forearm. Muscle Nerve 6:204, 1983.
506. Bertorini, T. E., Shively, V., Taylor, B., Palmieri, G. M. A., and Fox, I. H.: ATP degradation products after ischemic exercise: hereditary lack of phosphorylase or carnitine palmitoyltransferase. Neurology 35:1355, 1985.
507. Sabina, R. L., Swain, J. L., Olanow, C. W., Bradley, W. G., Fishbein, W. N., Di Mauro, S., and Holmes, E. W.: Myoadenylate deaminase deficiency. Functional and metabolic abnormalities associated with disruption of the purine nucleotide cycle. J. Clin. Invest. 73:720, 1984.
508. Garrod, A. B.: A Treatise on Gout and Rheumatic Gout (Rheumatic Arthritis). 3rd ed. London, Longman, Green and Company, 1876, p. 584.
509. Cohen, H.: Gout. In Dopeman, W. S. C. (ed.): Textbook of the Rheumatic Diseases. Edinburgh, Churchill Livingstone, 1955, p. 361.
510. Neel, J. V.: The clinical detection of the genetic carriers of inherited disease. Medicine 26:115, 1947.
511. Rosenberg, E. F.: Gout and male hermaphroditism: Report of a case. Ann. Rheum. Dis. 2:175, 1941.
512. Talbott, J. G.: Gout. J. Chronic Dis. 1:338, 1955.
513. Yu, T.-F.: Milestones in the treatment of gout. Am. J. Med. 56:676, 1974.
514. Morton, N. E.: Genetics of hyperuricemia in families with gout. Am. J. Med. Genet. 4:103, 1979.
515. Garrod, A. B.: The Nature and Treatment of Gout and Rheumatic Gout. London, Walton & Maberly, 1859.
516. Freudweiler, M.: Experimentelle Untersuchungen uber das Wesen der Gichtknoten. Dtsch. Arch. Klin. Med. 63:266, 1899.
517. Freudweiler, M.: Experimentelle Untersuchungen uber die Entstehung der Gichtknoten. Dtsch. Arch. Klin. Med. 69:155, 1909. (English translation: Experimental investigations into the origin of gouty tophi. Arthritis Rheum. 1:270, 1965.)
518. His, W. J.: Schicksal und Wirkungend des sauren harnsauren Natrons in Bauch und Gelenkohle des Kaninchens. Dtsch. Arch. Klin. Med. 67:81, 1900.
519. Roberts, W.: The Croonian Lectures. On the chemistry and therapeutics of uric acid gravel and gout. Br. Med. J. 2:61, 1892.

520. McCarty, D. J., Jr.: Phagocytosis of urate crystals in gouty synovial fluid. Am. J. Med. Sci. 243:288, 1962.
521. Phelps, P., Steele, A. D., and McCarty, J. D., Jr.: Compensated polarized light microscopy. J.A.M.A. 203:508, 1968.
522. Seegmiller, J. E., Laster, L., and Howell, R. R.: Biochemistry of uric acid and its relation to gout. N. Engl. J. Med. 268:712, 1963.
523. Flechtner, J. J., and Simkin, P. A.: Urate spherulites in gouty synovia. J.A.M.A. 245:1533, 1981.
524. Hamilton, M. E., Parris, T. M., Gibson, R. S., et al.: Simultaneous gout and pyarthrosis. Arch. Intern. Med. 140:917, 1980.
525. Itzkowitch, D. F., Famaey, J.-P., and Appelboom, T.: Crystal arthropathy as a complication of septic arthritis. J. Rheumatol. 8:3, 1981.
526. Faires, J. S., and McCarty, D. J., Jr.: Acute synovitis in normal joints of man and dog produced by injections of microcrystalline sodium urate, calcium oxalate and corticosteroid esters (abstr.). Arthritis Rheum. 5:295, 1962.
527. Malawista, S. E., Howell, R. R., and Seegmiller, J. E.: Factors modifying the inflammatory response to injected microcrystalline sodium urate (abstr.). Arthritis Rheum. 5:307, 1962.
528. Seegmiller, J. E., and Howell, R. R.: The old and new concepts of acute gouty arthritis. Arthritis Rheum. 5:616, 1962.
529. Seegmiller, J. E., Howell, R. R., and Malawista, S. E.: Inflammatory reaction to sodium urate: Its possible relationship to genesis of acute gouty arthritis. J.A.M.A. 180:469, 1962.
530. Seegmiller, J. E., Howell, R. R., and Malawista, S. E.: A mechanism of action of colchicine in acute gouty arthritis (abstr.). J. Clin. Invest. 41:1399, 1962.
531. Malawista, S. E., and Seegmiller, J. E.: The effect of pretreatment with colchicine on the inflammatory response to injected microcrystalline monosodium urate: A model for gouty inflammation. Ann. Intern. Med. 62:648, 1965.
532. McCarty, D. J., and Gatter, R. A.: Pseudogout syndrome. Bull. Rheum. Dis. 14:331, 1964.
533. Tse, R., and Phelps, P.: Polymorphonuclear leukocyte motility in vitro: V. Release of chemotactic activity following phagocytosis of calcium pyrophosphate crystals, diamond dust and urate crystals. J. Lab. Clin. Med. 76:403, 1970.
534. Agudelo, C. A., and Schumacher, H. R.: The synovitis of acute gouty arthritis: A light and electron microscopic study. Hum. Pathol. 4:265, 1973.
535. Hail, A. P., Barry, P. E., Dawber, T. R., et al.: Epidemiology of gout and hyperuricemia: A long-term population study. Am. J. Med. 42:27, 1967.
536. Ropes, M. W., and Bauer, W.: Synovial Fluid Changes in Joint Disease. Cambridge, Harvard University Press, 1953, p. 150.
537. Seegmiller, J. E.: Serum uric acid. In Cohen, A. S., (ed.): Laboratory Diagnostic Procedures in the Rheumatic Diseases. 2nd ed. Boston, Little Brown & Company, 1974, p. 216.
538. Dorner, R. W., Weiss, T. E., Baldassare, A. R., et al.: Plasma and synovial fluid as solvents for monosodium urate. Ann. Rheum. Dis. 40:70, 1981.
539. Tak, H.-K., Cooper, S. M., and Wilcox, W. R.: Studies on the nucleation of monosodium urate at 37°C. Arthritis Rheum. 23:574, 1980.
540. McGill, N. W., and Dieppe, P. A.: The role of serum and synovial fluid components in the promotion of urate crystal formation. J. Rheumatol. 18:1042, 1991.
541. Katz, W. A., and Schubert, M.: The interaction of monosodium urate with connective tissue components. J. Clin. Invest. 49:1783, 1970.
542. Brugsch, T., and Citron, J.: Uber die Absorption der Harnsaure Durch Knorpel. Z. Exp. Pathol. Ther. 5:401, 1908.
543. Dainty, J., and House, C. R.: "Unstirred layers" in frog skin. J. Physiol. 182:66, 1966.
544. Katz, W. A., and Ehrlich, G. E.: The solubility of monosodium urate in serum and connective tissue fractions. Arthritis Rheum. 11:492, 1968.
545. Perricone, E., and Brandt, K. D.: Enhancement of urate solubility by connective tissue. I. Effect of proteoglycan aggregates and buffer cation. Arthritis Rheum. 21:453, 1978.
546. Perricone, E., and Brandt, K. D.: Enhancement of urate solubility by connective tissue. II. Inhibition of sodium urate crystallization by cation exchange. Ann. Rheum. Dis. 38:467, 1979.
547. Roch-Ramel, F., Dieze-Chomety, F., Rougemont, D., et al.: Renal excretion of uric acid in the rat: A micro-puncture and microperfusion study. Am. J. Physiol. 230:768, 1976.
548. Horvath, S. M., and Hollander, J. L.: Intra-articular temperature as a measure of joint reaction. J. Clin. Invest. 28:469, 1949.
549. Hollander, J. L., Stoner, E. K., Brown, E. M., Jr., et al.: Joint temperature measurements in the evaluation of antiarthritic agents. J. Clin. Invest. 30:701, 1951.
550. Hollander, J. L., and Horvath, S. M.: The influence of physical therapy procedures on intra-articular temperature of normal and arthritic subjects. Am. J. Med. Sci. 218:543, 1949.
551. Simkin, P. A.: Concentration of urate by differential diffusion: A hypothesis for initial urate deposition. In Sperling, O., DeVries, A., and Wyngaarden, J. B. (eds.): Purine Metabolism in Man. New York, Plenum Press, 1974, p. 547.
552. Howell, D. S.: Preliminary observations on local pH in gout tophi and synovial fluid. Arthritis Rheum. 8:736, 1965.
553. Spilberg, I., Tanphaichitr, D., and Kantor, O.: Synovial fluid pH in acute gouty arthritis (letter). Arthritis Rheum. 20:142, 1977.
554. Naff, G. B., and Byers, P. H.: Complement as a mediator of inflammation in acute gouty arthritis. I. Studies on the reaction between human serum complement and sodium urate crystals. J. Lab. Clin. Med. 81:747, 1973.
555. Hasselbacher, P.: C3 activation by monosodium urate monohydrate and other crystalline material. Arthritis Rheum. 22:571, 1979.
556. Giclas, P. C., Ginsberg, M. H., and Cooper, N. R.: Immunoglobulin G independent activation of the classical complement pathway by monosodium urate crystals. J. Clin. Invest. 63:759, 1979.
557. Terkeltaub, R., Tenner, A. J., Kozin, F., and Ginsberg, M. H.: Plasma protein binding by monosodium urate crystals. Arthritis Rheum. 26:775, 1983.
558. Fields, T. R., Abramson, S. B., Weissmann, G., Kaplan, A. P., and Ghebrehiwet, B.: Activation of the alternative pathway of complement by monosodium urate crystals. Clin. Immunol. Immunopathol. 26:249, 1983.
559. Russell, I. J., Papaioannou, C., McDuffie, F. C., MacIntyre, S., and Kushner, I.: Effect of IgG and C-reactive protein on complement depletion by monosodium urate crystals. J. Rheumatol. 10:425, 1983.
560. Cherian, P. V., and Schumacher, H. R., Jr.: Immunochemical and ultrastructural characterization of serum proteins associated with monosodium urate crystals (MSU) in synovial fluid cells from patients with gout. Ultrastruct. Pathol. 10:209, 1986.
561. Terkeltaub, R., Curtiss, L. K., Tenner, A. J., and Ginsberg, M. H.: Lipoproteins containing apoprotein B are a major regulator of neutrophil responses to monosodium urate crystals. J. Clin. Invest. 73:1719, 1984.
562. Terkeltaub, R., Smeltzer, D., Curtiss, L. K., and Ginsberg, M. H.: Low density lipoprotein inhibits the physical interaction of phlogistic crystals and inflammatory cells. Arthritis Rheum. 29:363, 1986.
563. Hasselbacher, P.: Stimulation of synovial fibroblasts by calcium oxalate and monosodium urate monohydrate: A mechanism of connective tissue degradation in oxalosis and gout. J. Lab. Clin. Med. 100:977, 1982.
564. Phelps, P., Andrews, R., and Rosenbloom, J.: Demonstration of chemotactic factor in human gout: Further characterization of occurrence and structure. J. Rheumatol. 8:889, 1981.
565. Phelps, P., and McCarty, D. J., Jr.: Crystal induced inflammation in canine joints. II. Importance of polymorphonuclear leukocytes. J. Exp. Med. 124:115, 1966.
566. Chang, Y.-H., and Gialla, E. J.: Suppression of urate crystal-induced canine joint inflammation by heterologous antipolymorphonuclear leukocyte serum. Arthritis Rheum. 11:145, 1968.
567. Phelps, P.: Polymorphonuclear leukocyte motility in vitro. III. Possible release of a chemotactic substance after phagocytosis of urate crystals by polymorphonuclear leukocytes. Arthritis Rheum. 12:197, 1969.
568. Phelps, P.: Appearance of chemotactic activity following intraarticular injection of monosodium urate crystals. Effect of colchicine. J. Lab. Clin. Med. 76:622, 1970.
569. Spilberg, I., Mandell, B., and Wochner, R. D.: Studies on crystal induced chemotactic factor. I. Role of protein synthesis and neutral protease activity. J. Lab. Clin. Med. 83:56, 1974.
570. Phelps, D.: Polymorphonuclear leukocyte motility in vitro. IV. Colchicine inhibition of chemotactic activity formation after phagocytosis of urate crystals. Arthritis Rheum. 13:1, 1970.
571. Spilberg, I., Gallacher, A., Mehta, J. M., and Mandell, B.: Urate crystal-induced chemotactic factor. Isolation and partial characterization. J. Clin. Invest. 58:815, 1976.
572. Spilberg, I., and Mehta, J.: Demonstration of a specific neutrophil receptor for a cell-derived chemotactic factor. J. Clin. Invest. 63:85, 1979.
573. Spilberg, I., and Mehta, J.: Binding characteristics of radioiodinated crystal-induced chemotactic factor to human neutrophils. J. Lab. Clin. Med. 104:939, 1984.
574. Antommattei, O., Schumacher, H. R., Reginato, A. J., and Clayburne, G.: Prospective study of morphology and phagocytosis of synovial fluid monosodium urate crystals in gouty arthritis. J. Rheumatol. 11:741, 1984.
575. Burt, H. M., Kalkman, P. H., and Mauldin, D.: Membranolytic effects of crystalline monosodium urate monohydrate. J. Rheumatol. 10:440, 1983.
576. Herring, F. G., Lam, E. W. N., and Burt, H. M.: A spin label study of the membranolytic effects of crystalline monosodium urate monohydrate. J. Rheumatol. 13:623, 1986.
577. Burt, H. M., Evans, E., Lam, E. W. N., Gehrs, P. F., and Herring, F. G.: Membranolytic effects of monosodium urate monohydrate: Influence of grinding. J. Rheumatol. 13:778, 1986.

578. Higson, F. K., and Jones, O. T. G.: Oxygen radical production by horse and pig neutrophils induced by a range of crystals. J. Rheumatol. 11:735, 1984.

579. Rosen, M. S., Baker, D. G., Schumacher, H. R., Jr., and Cherian, P. V.: Products of polymorphonuclear cell injury inhibit IgG enhancement of monosodium urate–induced superoxide production. Arthritis Rheum. 29:1473, 1986.

580. Rae, S. A., Davidson, E. M., and Smith, M. J. H.: Leukotriene B4, an inflammatory mediator in gout. Lancet 2:1122, 1982.

581. Damas, J., Remacle-Volon, G., and Adam, A.: Inflammation in the rat paw due to urate crystals. Involvement of the kinin system. Arch. Pharmacol. 325:76, 1984.

582. Wigley, F. M., Fine, I. T., and Newcombe, D. S.: The role of the human synovial fibroblast in monosodium urate crystal–induced synovitis. J. Rheumatol. 10:602, 1983.

583. Duff, G. W., Atkins, E., and Malawista, S. E.: The fever of gout: Urate crystals activate endogenous pyrogen production from human and rabbit mononuclear phagocytes. Trans. Assoc. Am. Phys. 96:234, 1983.

584. Malawista, S. E., Duff, G. W., Atkins, E., Cheung, H. S., and McCarty, D. J.: Crystal-induced endogenous pyrogen production. A further look at gouty inflammation. Arthritis Rheum. 28:1039, 1985.

585. Londino, A. V., Jr., and Luparello, F. J.: Factor XII deficiency in a man with gout and angioimmunoblastic lymphadenopathy. Arch. Intern. Med. 144:1497, 1984.

586. Digiovine, F. S., Malawista, S. F., Thornton, E., et al.: Urate crystals stimulate production of tumor necrosis factor-alpha from human blood monocytes and synovial cells. Cytokine messenger RNA and protein kinetics and cellular distribution. J. Clin. Invest. 87:1375, 1991.

587. Guerne, P. A., Terkeltaub, R., Zuraw B., et al.: Inflammatory microcrystal stimulate interleukin-6 production and secretion by human monocytes and synoviocytes. Arthritis Rheum. 32:1443, 1989.

588. Terkeltaub, R., Zachariae, C., Santoro, D. et al.: Monocyte-derived neutrophil chromatic factor/interleukin-8 is a potential mediator of crystal-induced inflammation. Arthritis Rheum. 34:894, 1991.

589. Marcolongo, R., Calabria, A. A., Lallumera, M., Gerli, R., Allessandrini, C., and Cavallo, G.: The "switch-off" mechanism of spontaneous resolution of acute gout attacks. J. Rheumatol. 15:101, 1988.

590. Rosen, M. S., Baker, D., and Schumacher, H. R.: Products of polymorphonuclear cell injury inhibit IqG enhancement of monosodium urate induced superoxide production. Arthritis Rheum. 29:1480, 1986.

591. Ortiz-Bravo, E., Clayburne, G., and Sieck, M.: Immunolabelling of proteins coating monosodium urate crystal in sequential samples from acute gouty arthritis and MSU induced inflammation in the rat subcutaneous air pouch (abstr.). Arthritis Rheum. 33(Suppl.):555, 1990.

592. Boardman, P. L., and Hart, F. D.: Indomethacin in the treatment of acute gout. Practitioner 194:560, 1965.

593. Davis, J. S., Jr.: Guest editorial. V. Med. Mon. 78:335, 1951.

594. Davis, J. S., Jr., and Bartfield, H.: The effect of intravenous colchicine on acute gout. Am. J. Med. 16:218, 1954.

595. Wallace, S. L., Robinson, H., Masi, A. T., et al.: Preliminary criteria for the classification of the acute arthritis of primary gout. Arthritis Rheum. 20:895, 1977.

596. Freeman, D. L.: Frequent doses of intravenous colchicine can be lethal. N. Engl. J. Med. 309:310, 1983.

597. Stanley, M. W., Taurog, J. D., and Snover, D. C.: Fatal colchicine toxicity: Report of a case. Clin. Exp. Rheumatol. 2:167, 1984.

598. Ferrannini, E., and Pentimone, F.: Marrow aplasia following colchicine treatment for gouty arthritis. Clin. Exp. Rheumatol. 2:173, 1984.

599. Neuss, M. N., McCallum, R. M., Brenckman, W. D., and Silberman, H. R.: Long-term colchicine administration leading to colchicine toxicity and death. Arthritis Rheum. 29:448, 1986.

600. Kunck, R. W., Duncan, G., Watson, D., Alderson, K., Rogawski, M. A., and Peper, M.: Colchicine myopathy and neuropathy. N. Engl. J. Med. 316:1562, 1987.

601. Smyth, C. J., Velayos, E. E., and Amoroso, C.: A method for measuring swelling of hands and feet. II. Influence of a new anti-inflammatory drug, indomethacin, in acute gout. Acta Rheumatol. Scand. 9:306, 1963.

602. Hart, F. D., and Boardman, P. L.: Indomethacin: A new non-steroid anti-inflammatory agent. Br. Med. J. 2:965, 1963.

603. Norcross, B. M.: Treatment of connective tissue disease with a new non-steroidal compound (indomethacin) (abstr.). Arthritis Rheum. 6:290, 1963.

604. Cuq, P.: Experience française du traitement de la crise de goutte aigue par le naproxen-C 1674. Scand. J. Rheumatol. (Suppl.) 2:64, 1973.

605. Sturge, R. A., Scott, J. T., Hamilton, E. B. D., et al.: Multicentre trial of naproxen and phenylbutazone in acute gout. Ann. Rheum. Dis. 36:80, 1977.

606. Wallace, S. L.: Colchicine and new anti-inflammatory drugs for the treatment of acute gout. Arthritis Rheum. (Suppl.) 18:847, 1975.

607. Wanasukapunt, S., Lertratanakul, Y., and Rubinstein, H. M.: Effect of fenoprofen calcium on acute gouty arthritis. Arthritis Rheum. 19:933, 1976.

608. Schweitz, M. D., Nashel, D. J., and Alepa, F. P.: Ibuprofen in the treatment of acute gouty arthritis. J.A.M.A. 239:34, 1978.

609. Brogden, R. N., Heel, R. C., Speight, T. M., and Avery, G. S.: Sulindac: Review of its pharmacologic properties and therapeutic efficacy. Drugs 16:97, 1978.

610. Widmark, P. H.: Piroxicam: Its safety and efficacy in the treatment of acute gout. Am. J. Med. 72:63, 1982.

611. Bluestone, R. H.: Safety and efficacy of piroxicam in the treatment of gout. Am. J. Med. 72:66, 1982.

612. Altman, R. D., Honig, S., Levin, J. M., and Lightfoot, R. W.: Ketoprofen versus indomethacin in patients with acute gouty arthritis: A multicenter, double-blind comparative study. J. Rheumatol. 18:1422, 1988.

613. Shack, M. E.: Drug-induced ulceration and perforation of the small bowel. Ariz. Med. 23:517, 1966.

614. O'Brian, W. M.: Indomethacin: A survey of clinical trials. Clin. Pharmacol. Ther. 9:94, 1968.

615. Simon, L. S., and Mills, J. A.: Medical intelligence: Nonsteroidal antiinflammatory drugs. N. Engl. J. Med. 302:1179, 1980.

616. Gary, N. E., Dodelson, R., and Eisinger, R. P.: Indomethacin-associated acute renal failure. Am. J. Med. 69:135, 1980.

617. Friedman, P. L., Brown, E. J., Gunther, S., et al.: Coronary vasoconstrictor effect of indomethacin in patients with coronary-artery disease. N. Engl. J. Med. 305:1171, 1981.

618. Kimberly, R. P., Bowden, R. E., Keiser, H. R., et al.: Reduction of renal function by newer nonsteroidal anti-inflammatory drugs. Am. J. Med. 64:804, 1978.

619. Groff, G. D., Franck, W. A., and Raddatz, D. A.: Systemic steroid therapy for acute gout: A clinical trial and review of the literature. Semin. Arthritis Rheum. 19:329, 1990.

620. Axelrod, D., and Preston, S.: Comparison of parenteral adrenocorticotropic hormone with oral indomethacin in the treatment of acute gout. Arthritis Rheum. 31:803, 1988.

621. Hollander, J. L.: Intra-articular hydrocortisone in arthritis and allied conditions. J. Bone Joint Surg. 35A:983, 1953.

622. Cohen, A.: Gout. Am. J. Med. Sci. 192:448, 1936.

623. Talbott, J. H., and Coombs, F. S.: Metabolic studies on patients with gout. J.A.M.A. 110:1977, 1938.

624. Gutman, A. B.: Treatment of primary gout: The present status. Arthritis Rheum. 8:911, 1965.

625. Paulus, H. E., Schlosstein, L. H., Godfrey, R. G., et al.: Prophylactic colchicine therapy of intercritical gout. A placebo-controlled study of probenecid-treated patients. Arthritis Rheum. 17:609, 1974.

626. Gutman, A. B.: Medical management of gout. Postgrad. Med. 51:61, 1972.

627. Yu, T.-F., and Gutman, A. B.: Efficacy of colchicine prophylaxis. Prevention of recurrent gouty arthritis over a mean period of five years in 208 gouty subjects. Ann. Intern. Med. 55:179, 1961.

628. Rundles, R. W., Metz, E. N., and Siberman, H. R.: Allopurinol in the treatment of gout. Ann. Intern. Med. 64:220, 1966.

629. Robinson, W. D.: The present status of colchicine and uricosuric agents in the management of gout. J.A.M.A. 173:1076, 1960.

630. Emmerson, B. T.: The use of the xanthine oxidase inhibitor, allopurinol, in the control of hyperuricemia, gout and uric acid calculi. Aust. Ann. Med. 16:205, 1967.

631. Levin, N. W., and Abrahams, O. L.: Allopurinol in patients with impaired renal function. Ann. Rheum. Dis. 25:681, 1966.

632. Ogryzlo, M. A., Urowitz, M., Weber, H. M., and Haupt, J. B.: Effects of allopurinol on gouty and nongouty uric acid nephropathy. Ann. Rheum. Dis. 25:673, 1966.

633. Stoberg, K.-H.: Allopurinol therapy of gout with renal complications. Ann. Rheum. Dis. 25:688, 1966.

634. Rundles, R. W.: Allopurinol in gouty nephropathy and renal dialysis. Ann. Rheum. Dis. 25:694, 1966.

635. Wilson, J. D., Simmonds, H. A., and North, J. D. K.: Allopurinol in the treatment of uremic patients with gout. Ann. Rheum. Dis. 26:136, 1967.

636. Fox, R. M., Royse-Smith, D., and O'Sullivan, W. J.: Oroditinuria induced by allopurinol. Science 168:861, 1970.

637. Kelley, W. N., and Beardmore, T. D.: Allopurinol: Alteration in pyrimidine metabolism in man. Science 169:388, 1970.

638. Gutman, A. B., and Yu, T.-F.: Protracted uricosuric therapy in tophaceous gout. Lancet 2:1258, 1957.

639. Zell, S. C., and Carmichael, J. M.: Evaluation of allopurinol use in patient with gout. Am. J. Hosp. Pharm. 46:1813, 1989.

640. Fox, I. H., and Kelley, W. N.: Management of gout. J.A.M.A. 242:361, 1979.

641. Hande, K. R., Hixson, C. V., and Chabner, B. A.: Postchemotherapy purine excretion in lymphoma patients receiving allopurinol. Cancer Res. 41:2273, 1981.

642. Davis, S., and Park, Y. K.: Hypouricaemic effect of polyethyleneglycol modified urate oxidase. Lancet 1:281, 1981.

643. Masera, G., Jankovic, M., Zurlo, M. G., Lacasciulli, A., Rossi, M. R.,

Uderzo, C., and Reccjoa, M.: Urate-oxidase prophylaxis of uric acid-induced renal damage in childhood leukemia. J. Pediatr. 100:152, 1982.

644. Chua, C. C., Greenberg, M. L., Viau, A. T., et al.: Use of polymethylene glycol-modified uricase to treat hyperuricemia in a patient with non-Hodgkins lymphoma. Ann. Intern. Med. 1096:114, 1988.

645. Coe, F. L., and Kavalach, A. K.: Hypercalcemia and hyperuricosuria in patients with calcium nephrolithiasis. N. Engl. J. Med. 291:1344, 1974.

646. Sanchez-Bayle, M., Garcia-Vao, C., Ramo-Mancheno, C., and Vazquez-Martul, M.: Hyperuricemia and increase in postsecretory reabsorption of uric acid. Nephron 43:151, 1986.

647. Emmerson, B. T.: Alteration of urate metabolism by weight reduction. Aust. N.Z. J. Med. 3:410, 1973.

648. Heyden, S.: Risikofaktoren fur das Herz. Ergebnisse und Konsequenzen der post-Framingham-Studien. Boehringer Manheim GmbH, 1974, p. 53.

649. Nicholls, A., and Scott, J. T.: Effect of weight-loss on plasma and urinary levels of uric acid and acute attacks of gout. Lancet 2:1223, 1972.

650. MacLachlan, M. J., and Rodnan, G. P.: Effect of food, fast and alcohol on serum uric acid and acute attacks of gout. Am. J. Med. 42:38, 1967.

651. Stapleton, F. B., Kennedy, J., Nousia-Arvanitakis, S., and Linshaw, M. A.: Hyperuricosuria due to high-dose pancreatic extract therapy in cystic fibrosis. N. Engl. J. Med. 295:246, 1976.

652. Sack, J., Blau, H., Goldfarb, D., Ben-Zaray, S., and Katznelson, D.: Hyperuricosuria in cystic fibrosis patients treated with pancreatic enzyme supplements. A study of 16 patients in Israel. Isr. J. Med. Sci. 16:417, 1980.

653. Fox, I. H., and Kelley, W. N.: Studies on the mechanism of fructose-induced hyperuricemia in man. Metabolism 21:713, 1972.

654. Narins, R. G., Weisberg, J. S., and Meyers, A. R.: Effects of carbohydrate on uric acid metabolism. Metabolism 23:455, 1974.

655. Perheentupa, J., and Raivio, K.: Fructose-induced hyperuricemia. Lancet 2:528, 1967.

656. Bode, J. C., Zelder, O., Rumpelt, H. J., et al.: Depletion of liver adenosine phosphates and metabolic effects of intravenous infusion of fructose or sorbital in man and in the rat. Eur. J. Clin. Invest. 3:436, 1973.

657. Emmerson, B. T.: Effect of oral fructose on urate production. Ann. Rheum. Dis. 33:276, 1974.

658. Bien, E. J., Yu, T.-F., Benedict, J. D., et al.: The relation of dietary nitrogen consumption to the rate of uric acid synthesis in normal and gouty man. J. Clin. Invest. 32:778, 1953.

659. Maenpaa, P. H., Raivio, K. E., and Kekomaki, M. P.: Liver adenine nucleotides: Fructose-induced depletion and its effect on protein syntheses. Science 161:1253, 1968.

660. Fredrickson, D. S., and Levy, R. I.: Familial hyperlipoproteinemia. In Stanbury, J. B., Wyngaarden, J. B., and Fredrickson, D. S. (eds.): The Metabolic Basis of Inherited Disease. 3rd ed. New York, McGraw-Hill Book Company, 1972, p. 545.

661. Garrison, F. H.: An Introduction to the History of Medicine: With Medical Chronology, Suggestions for Study and Bibliographic Data. 4th ed. Philadelphia, W. B. Saunders Co., 1929.

662. Galen, C.: Opera Omina, ed. by Kuhn. Leipzig, 1821–1883.

663. McCarty, D. J.: A historical note: Leeuwenhoek's description of crystals from a gouty typhus. Arthritis Rheum. 13:414, 1970.

664. Want, J.: The use of Colchicum autumnale in rheumatism. Med. Physiol. J. Lond. 32:312, 1814.

665. Talbott, J. H., Bishop, C., Norcross, B. M., et al.: The clinical and metabolic effects of Benemid in patients with gout. Trans. Assoc. Am. Physicians 64:372, 1951.

666. Gutman, A. B., and Yu, T.-F.: Benemid (P-(di-n-propylsulfamyl)-benzoic acid) as uricosuric agent in chronic gouty arthritis. Trans. Assoc. Am. Physicians 64:279, 1951.

667. Rundles, R. W., Wyngaarden, J. B., Hitchings, G. H., et al.: Effects of a xanthine oxidase inhibitor on thiopurine metabolism, hyperuricemia and gout. Trans. Assoc. Am. Physicians 76:126, 1963.

Diseases Associated with the Deposition of Calcium Pyrophosphate or Hydroxyapatite

INTRODUCTION

McCarty and Hollander in 1961 reported finding nonurate crystals in the affected joints of two patients with presumed gout.[1] Six additional cases of arthritis with similar nonurate crystals in synovial fluid were noted soon after.[2] Roentgenographic examination of the joints of these patients was characterized by abnormal calcifications in or around numerous joints; calcification of articular hyaline cartilage and fibrocartilage was particularly distinctive. These findings were similar to those described by Zitnan and Sitaj,[3] who presented detailed clinical features of 27 patients with articular chondrocalcinosis; 21 of the patients were members of five different families, suggesting that the disease was hereditary in nature. Although there appeared to be some differences in the findings described by these two groups of investigators, it became apparent that they represented a similar disease state. These seminal observations led to a broad expansion of knowledge of a group of primary and secondary articular disorders due to calcium crystal deposition.

CALCIUM PYROPHOSPHATE CRYSTAL DEPOSITION DISEASE

McCarty, Kohn, and Faires[2] coined the term "pseudogout syndrome" to describe their series of patients who demonstrated acute attacks of monarthritis similar to those seen in gout, in association with radiologic deposition of calcium in hyaline cartilage and fibrocartilage, and crystals of calcium pyrophosphate dihydrate (CPPD) in synovial fluid. The observation that subacute and chronic arthritis was also seen in patients afflicted with this disorder led to new, more accurate terminology. McCarty designated the total disease state associated with calcium pyrophosphate dihydrate crystal deposition as calcium pyrophosphate deposition disease (CPDD); this term accented the basic characteristics of the disorder rather than its symptomatology.[4] The term "chondrocalcinosis" is still widely used, although it lacks the specificity of nomenclature defined on the basis of crystal type.

Epidemiology

As with all diseases, prevalence statistics will differ depending on case-finding techniques, whether clinical, radiologic, or pathologic. This is particularly true in CPDD, since many cases are asymptomatic (lanthanic), may be symptomatic but without radiologic evidence of articular cartilage calcification, or may demonstrate evidence of calcification only with sensitive radiologic techniques.[5] Nevertheless, observations over the past 25 years support inclusion of CPDD as one of the more common connective tissue disorders.[6, 7] Studies at the Mayo Clinic in which the prevalence of gout and pseudogout was compared noted a prevalence ratio of 1.5 to 2.2 per 1000 and 0.9 per 1000, respectively.[8] No specific sexual or ethnic preponderance has yet been defined.

In a prevalence study, 100 consecutive patients admitted to an acute-care geriatric unit were examined for clinical and radiographic evidence of osteoarthritis and articular chondrocalcinosis; 34 patients had evidence of the latter.[7] Prevalence increased from 15 percent in patients aged 65 to 74 years, to 44 percent in patients older than 84 years. Commonly involved joints were the knee (25 percent), symphysis pubis (15 percent), and wrist (19 percent). These findings are similar to observations of others, who noted a frequency of CPDD of 10 to 15 percent at ages 65 to 75 years, rising to 30 to 60 percent in those older than age 85.[7, 9]

Classification Criteria

Cases of chondrocalcinosis can be classified as sporadic (idiopathic), hereditary, or secondary (due to underlying disorders) (Table 77-1).

Sporadic (idiopathic) cases are identified as patients who demonstrate neither clinical evidence of associated underlying disorders leading to calcium pyrophosphate deposition nor evidence of familial disease occurrence. It is likely that a number of sporadic cases will bear reclassification as improved diagnostic studies and more accurate understanding of basic disease pathophysiologic mechanisms are developed.

Support for a hereditary familial form of chondrocalcinosis was provided in the detailed review by Zitnan and Sitaj,[3] in which 21 of 27 patients studied were members of five different families; the precise type of hereditary transmission could not be determined. Subsequently, a series of well-defined hereditary forms of CPDD has been documented in a number of countries.[10–22a] Although the mode of inheritance appears to be autosomal dominant with variable penetrance in almost all the series, differences in decade at onset, ratio of male to female involvement, and severity of arthritis suggest differences in genetic defects. Several studies suggested that the hereditary and sporadic types of chondrocalcinosis were indistinguishable with respect to clinical and radiologic appearances.[18, 20, 21] In only one family series has an HLA association been documented, an association of chondrocalcinosis with the haplotype HLA-A2,W5.[10, 17] It is likely that the relative rarity of familial forms of the disease relates to difficulties in detection. In particular, prevalence studies are made difficult by the increasing mobility of the population and by late onset of disease expression, which limits examination required of the several generations at risk. Similarly, lack of a definable defect limits definition of asymptomatic "carrier" members of involved families.

Associated Diseases

A number of secondary associations have been reported in patients with CPDD (see Table 77–1). The high prevalence of CPDD coupled with the common occurrence of some of the putative associated entities, such as diabetes mellitus and hyperuricemia, makes it difficult to ascertain whether a true cause and effect relationship exists or whether the observed "association" is coincidental. A more convincing association can be made with certain rare conditions such as hypophosphatasia[23] and Bartter's syndrome,[24] since CPDD is less likely to cluster as a coincidental finding in the presence of such rare disorders.

The best substantiated associations of CPDD with underlying metabolic disorders are those occurring with hyperparathyroidism,[25–28] hemochromatosis,[29, 30] hypophosphatasia,[23] and hypomagnesemia.[24, 31, 32] Additional conditions or diseases with which variable associations have been described include osteoarthritis,[7, 33, 34] aging,[5, 7, 9, 34] hypermobility syndrome,[35] hypothyroidism,[36–38] and amyloidosis.[39] Even more

Table 77–1. CLASSIFICATION AND POSSIBLE DISEASE ASSOCIATIONS OF CPDD

Sporadic (Idiopathic)
Hereditary
Secondary
Association Strong
  Hyperparathyroidism
  Hemochromatosis
  Hypomagnesemia
  Aging
Association Likely
  Osteoarthritis
  Amyloid disease
  Bartter's syndrome
  Hypermobility syndrome
  Hypocalciuric hypercalcemia
Association Weak
  Hypothyroidism
  Ochronosis
  Paget's disease
  Wilson's disease
  Acromegaly
  Diabetes mellitus
  Gout

tentative associations are the occurrence of CPDD and Wilson's disease,[40] ochronosis,[41] Paget's disease, hyperuricemia, and diabetes mellitus.

An association of CPDD with hemochromatosis is well documented.[29, 30, 42] In these patients, chondrocalcinosis is associated with the classic features of hemochromatosis arthropathy, characterized by subchondral cystic changes and sclerosis and loss of articular cartilage. Cartilage calcifications are similar in distribution to those seen in other sporadic forms of chondrocalcinosis; in particular, fibrocartilage and hyaline articular cartilage involvement of the knees, wrists, and hips is common. Calcification is frequently observed in the symphysis pubis and in the intervertebral discs of the lumbar spine.

The pathophysiologic mechanism by which chondrocalcinosis develops in association with hemochromatosis is uncertain. A relationship to iron is suggested by observations of CPDD in patients with transfusion hemochromatosis[43] and hereditary spherocytosis. In addition, it has been demonstrated that ferrous ions inhibit some inorganic pyrophosphatases[44] and may permit precipitation of insoluble pyrophosphate crystals.

Conversely, recent studies reported that ferrous (Fe^{2+}) ions at biologic concentrations may function as an inhibitor of CPPD formation, and that therapeutic depletion of Fe^{2+} ions may thereby facilitate CPPD crystal deposition in articular tissues.[45] Alternatively, it has been postulated that iron leads directly to cartilage degeneration, with deposition of calcium pyrophosphate crystals being a secondary response.

CPDD is a common finding in patients with hyperparathyroidism; an incidence as high as 40 percent has been reported.[25–28] Conversely, patients with hyperparathyroidism constitute up to 15 percent of individuals with CPDD. Several factors appear to influence the development of chondrocalcinosis in these patients. Although it is likely that persistently elevated levels of serum calcium play a role, observations suggest that hypercalcemia alone is not a sufficient stimulus for CPPD crystal deposition.[27] In both hyperparathyroid and normal control groups, the incidence of chondrocalcinosis rose steadily with age.[25, 27] It was postulated that chondrocalcinosis seen in patients with hyperparathyroidism is the result of both sustained hypercalcemia and age-related changes in articular cartilage that make it more prone to calcification. It is of interest that parathyroidectomy is generally not followed by resolution of pre-existing cartilage calcification.[25]

Studies relating parathyroid hormone levels to CPPD deposition show conflicting results.[46, 47] Although initial studies demonstrated elevated parathyroid hormone levels in patients with CPDD,[47] other investigators found no significant differences in mean laboratory test values for serum calcium, phosphorus, alkaline phosphatase, and parathormone levels[46] between CPDD patients and controls.

Parathyroidectomy is often followed by acute episodes of pseudogout; such attacks frequently coincide with the nadir of postoperative hypocalcemia.[28] It was suggested that rapid calcium shifts are associated with shedding of calcium pyrophosphate crystals into synovial fluid and subsequent induction of acute synovitis.

Although an association between chondrocalcinosis and osteoarthritis exists,[7, 33, 34] it has yet to be determined whether this association is causal or coincidental. In patients in whom crystal deposition appears to antedate osteoarthritis, such crystal deposition may alter calcium matrix, predisposing it to degenerative change. Conversely, osteoarthritis may appear first, leading to a milieu of cartilage changes that favor precipitation and deposition of crystals. Finally, since chondrocalcinosis and osteoarthritis are diseases seen more commonly in the elderly, some component of the associated incidence may be coincidental.

A destructive arthropathy in patients with articular chondrocalcinosis[48] is seen more frequently when generalized osteoarthritis and chondrocalcinosis coexist. It is of interest that, in contrast to idiopathic osteoarthritis, involvement of non-weight-bearing joints such as the elbows and wrists is seen in addition to involvement of weight-bearing joints. Halverson and McCarty analyzed synovial and knee radiographs from 59 patients with symptomatic osteoarthritis.[49] Patients with basic calcium phosphate (BCP) and CPPD crystals had more widespread joint degeneration than did those with no crystals or those with CPPD crystals alone. Knee joint compartment narrowing and osteophytes in all three compartments were correlated with BCP crystals; CPPD crystals correlated with patient age. Accordingly, some of the observations relating osteoarthritis to CPPD crystals may reflect previously undetected correlations with basic calcium phosphate crystal deposition.

As noted earlier, a number of studies have confirmed the increased incidence of chondrocalcinosis with aging, dramatic increases occurring in decades over age 60 years.[5, 7, 9] Although studies demonstrated that chondrocalcinosis is significantly associated with osteoarthritis after controlling for age, findings also suggested that chondrocalcinosis and osteoarthritis increase independently with age.[34]

Osteoarthritis and chondrocalcinosis have been described in relation to generalized joint hypermobility.[35] This association may represent a systemic defect of connective tissue that predisposes to both hypermobility and chondrocalcinosis; alternatively, local mechanical factors related to laxity may result in chondrocalcinosis.

Chondrocalcinosis has been observed in association with other metabolic diseases.[36–39] A causal relationship appears reasonable based on the relative infrequency of the metabolic disorders in which CPPD crystal deposition has been described. The fact that pseudogout is associated with a number of these different metabolic disorders suggests that deposition of calcium pyrophosphate represents the end result of a variety of metabolic disturbances.

Hypophosphatasia, a metabolic disorder associated with CPDD, is characterized by subnormal circulating alkaline phosphatase activity, increased urinary excretion of inorganic pyrophosphate, and defective bone mineralization.[23] Plasma pyrophosphate levels are elevated in these patients; however, the lack of an increased frequency of CPDD in other disorders associated with high plasma pyrophosphate, such as renal failure,[50] suggests that plasma pyrophosphate does not provide the complete explanation for crystal deposition in these patients. The arthropathy seen in patients with hypophosphatasia resembles not only that seen in primary CPDD but also that seen in hemochromatosis.[24] In a recent study of crystal deposition associated with hypophosphatasia, polyarticular chondrocalcinosis due to CPPD deposition was associated with spinal hyperostosis and with a paradoxical occurrence of calcific periarthritis due to apatite.[23]

Chondrocalcinosis is associated with hypomagnesemia.[31, 32] Calcification may be due to the dependence of pyrophosphatase enzyme activity on the presence of magnesium ions, a direct relationship between calcium pyrophosphate solubility and concentration of magnesium, and an influence of magnesium on the type of crystals formed by calcium and pyrophosphate in aqueous solution. Hypomagnesemia may play a role in the development of CPPD crystal deposition in patients with Bartter's syndrome.[24]

CPDD has been described in patients with hypocalciuric hypercalcemia.[51]

An association between CPPD deposition and hypothyroidism has been suggested, with some studies showing a higher than expected incidence of CPPD deposition in the presence of this metabolic disorder.[36, 37] In more recent studies, hypothyroid patients had no greater prevalence of chondrocalcinosis compared with euthyroid subjects matched for age and sex.[38] It should be noted that hypothyroidism is frequently associated with musculoskeletal complaints, and patients with this disorder may be overly represented in a rheumatology clinic. In addition, both hypothyroidism and CPDD increase with age, increasing the potential for coincidental occurrence.

An association was reported between chondrocalcinosis and senile amyloid disease.[39] Enhancement of glycosaminoglycan synthesis and pyrophosphate release in response to amyloid fibrils,[52] and subsequent binding of pyrophosphate and amyloid,[53] may represent the mechanism linking the two disorders.

Clinical Features

The identification of CPDD by McCarty and colleagues[2] evolved from the observation that acute attacks of monoarthritis appeared to be due to CPPD rather than urate crystals. Accordingly, in early descriptions of this disorder, acute attacks of arthritis were deemed classic, characteristic components of the disorder, and the term "pseudogout" was used in its definition. It soon became apparent on the basis of additional observations, and has been confirmed now in extensive clinical studies, that CPDD is a great "simulator," mimicking a number of forms of connective tissue disease.[54-56] Acute, subacute, and chronic arthralgias and arthritis have been described; in many patients, acute and chronic symptoms overlap at various phases of disease expression. McCarty has classified CPDD into six clinical patterns.[54] Type A pattern, pseudogout, is marked by acute or subacute arthritis attacks that last from 1 or 2 days to several weeks. The knees are the most frequently involved joints; podagra involving the great toe has been noted only infrequently.[55] Other joints commonly affected include the wrists, elbows, shoulders, and ankles. Acute attacks may be monoarticular or polyarticular; not infrequently, acute involvement of one joint is followed by migratory involvement of additional joints. In some patients, low-grade, relatively brief attacks of mild severity simulate "petit" attacks described in true gout.

Acute inflammation may be associated with systemic reactions with moderately high fever;[57] in older patients, a confusional state may be observed. As in true gout, acute attacks of pseudogout may be precipitated by stress situations, such as surgery or acute vascular accidents, or after marked diuresis as in treatment of congestive heart failure.[8] Precipitation of acute attacks following such illnesses may be related to a fall in serum and synovial fluid ionized calcium, which results in dissolution of crystals from their cartilaginous matrix.[8] Support exists for both "crystal shedding"[54] and acute intra-articular crystallization as a cause of acute attacks.

Type B presentation, pseudorheumatoid arthritis, is characterized by a subacute or chronic synovitis of large joints, particularly the knees, wrists (Fig. 77–1), or elbows. Morning stiffness may be observed. Polyarticular involvement is usually less widespread than in rheumatoid arthritis, and involvement of small joints of the hands and feet is uncommon. This form of CPDD may be difficult to differentiate from rheumatoid arthritis with coexistent pyrophosphate deposition.[58] It is of interest that articular chondrocalcinosis was observed less frequently in a group of patients with seropositive rheumatoid arthritis as compared with a control group of age- and sex-matched patients with low back pain or extra-articular rheumatism.[59] Articular chondrocalcinosis occurred in the older patients with rheumatoid arthritis and was observed in those with the shortest duration of the disease.

Types C and D patterns, pseudo-osteoarthritis, are associated with low-grade chronic symptoms in multiple joints, with evidence of degenerative joint disease. In patients with type C disease, low-grade arthralgias and degenerative changes are associated with superimposed acute attacks; type D patients have chronic symptoms alone, without acute episodes. One should consider this form of CPDD in patients who have generalized joint complaints "more severe than one would expect for osteoarthritis, but less severe than anticipated for chronic rheumatoid arthritis."

Type E patients (lanthanic form) represent the most common form of CPDD. In such patients, calcium deposition is noted as a coincidental observation on roentgenograms involving asymptomatic joints in known CPDD patients or in patients in whom roentgenographic studies are performed for other illnesses.

Type F, a pseudoneurotrophic arthritis, was originally reported by Jacobelli et al.[60] In this series, neuropathic arthritis of the knees was described in patients with concomitant pyrophosphate deposition and late syphilis. The authors suggested that neurotrophic joints developed as a synergistic response in tabetic patients with underlying CPPD crystal deposition. Subsequently, severely destructive disease similar to changes described in characteristic Charcot joints has been described in CPDD, even in the absence of neurologic deficits or syphilis.[9, 48]

Although not a disease pattern in the same sense as those previously described, arthropathy with a pattern resembling that of CPDD has been described in patients receiving long-term renal dialysis.[61, 62] Twenty-three of 28 patients receiving dialysis had arthritic complaints, and 14 had an arthropathy; in six of the latter, the arthropathy had a pattern resembling CPDD. Factors that appeared to predispose to metabolic arthropathy were elevated ferritin levels; a history of hyperparathyroidism; elevated serum levels of parathormone; hyperphosphatemia; hypercalcemia; HLA haplotypes A3, B7, or B14; and hyperaluminemia. The arthropathy appeared to represent a composite of etiologic factors including CPPD crystals, hydroxyapatite, other calcium-containing sub-

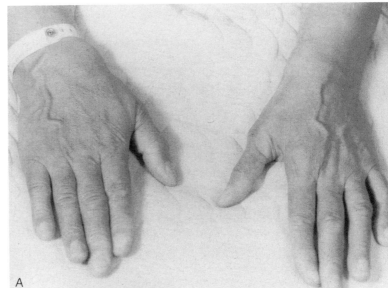

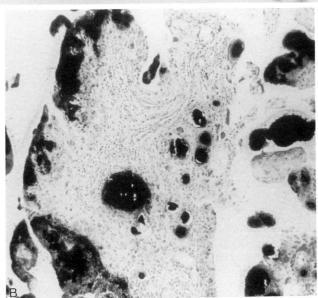

Figure 77–1. *A,* Pseudorheumatoid form of CPDD involving both wrists. Swelling is visible; wrist limitation was present bilaterally. *B,* Synovial biopsy, left wrist. Calcific deposits are diffusely distributed throughout areas of synovial inflammation (von Kossa × 80). (From Moskowitz, R. W., et al.: Chronic synovitis as a manifestation of calcium crystal deposition disease. Arthritis Rheum. 14:114, 1971. Used by permission.)

stances in joints, or a number of dialysis-induced metabolic abnormalities.

Laboratory Findings

In the sporadic or familial forms of the disease, routine blood chemistries and urine determinations are normal. At the time of initial diagnosis, screening studies to exclude underlying metabolic disorders should be performed. Serum calcium, phosphorus, alkaline phosphatase, iron, iron-binding capacity/saturation, and magnesium determinations are helpful in excluding hyperparathyroidism, hemochromatosis, hypophosphatasia, and hypomagnesemia. Other studies to be considered include blood glucose and serum uric acid levels. Given that the associations of pyrophosphate arthropathy and dia-

betes mellitus and gout are less well defined, these studies are optional at present.

Diagnostic confirmation of CPDD is based on synovial fluid analysis, with demonstration of characteristic CPPD crystals, and on characteristic cartilaginous calcifications on roentgenographic study.

Synovial fluid findings vary, depending on the degree of inflammatory response. In acute attacks, the fluid appears grossly cloudy to turbid, and viscosity is diminished. The total leukocyte count may approach that seen in acute septic arthritis; more commonly, however, it is fewer than 50,000 cells per mm^3; polymorphonuclear cells are increased. Synovial fluid sugar may be less than half a simultaneously determined fasting blood specimen.

Analysis of synovial fluid for crystals is of obvious import. Findings on ordinary light microscopy are helpful,[63] but more specific identification is made

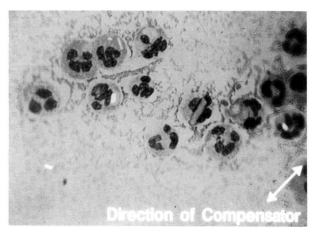

Figure 77–2. Calcium pyrophosphate crystals in synovial fluid; crystals are intra- and extracellular. The blue color of crystals lying parallel to the axis of the line of slow vibration (*arrow*), and yellow at right angles to the axis, is consistent with positive birefringence. (Courtesy of Syntex Inc., and Jeanne Riddle, Ph.D.)

possible by subsequent use of a first-order red plate compensator in a polarizing microscopy system. Studies should be performed soon after joint aspiration, if possible. The importance of prompt examination of synovial fluid samples was demonstrated in a study in which synovial fluids were kept at room temperature or at refrigerator temperature and reexamined serially at periods of up to 6 hours, 3 days, 3 weeks, and 2 months.[64] Studies revealed that leukocyte counts tended to decrease within a few hours. CPPD crystals became much less abundant after even 1 day; monosodium urate crystals tended to remain detectable throughout the 8 weeks of the study, but they became smaller, less birefringent, and less numerous with time. Clumps of apatite-like crystals persisted for several months. New, artifactual crystals developed with time. If crystals are not observed and a diagnosis of CPDD is strongly considered, it is well to follow up "negative studies" with examination of synovial fluid after mild centrifugation so as to concentrate cells and debris in which crystals may be more readily demonstrated.

Calcium pyrophosphate dihydrate crystals are linear or rhomboid (Fig. 77–2). Although the linear form of these crystals may resemble monosodium urate, calcium pyrophosphate rods tend to have blunt ends; monosodium urate crystals are characteristically sharply pointed (Table 77–2). A presumptive diagnosis of pyrophosphate-induced acute synovitis can usually be made on screening light microscopy, based on crystal morphology. The ability to utilize the ordinary light microscope as an appropriate tool for provisional detection and identification of crystals in synovial fluid was formally evaluated in comparison with polarized light microscopy.[63] High sensitivity and specificity of crystal identification was noted utilizing the morphologic characteristics described earlier; namely, fluids containing only acicular crystals were likely to contain monosodium urate, whereas synovial fluids with parallelepiped and rhomboidal as well as acicular structures were most likely to contain CPPD crystals. More definitive identification of the crystals as CPPD, however, requires use of a polarizing system, as noted. CPPD crystals are generally nonbirefringent or weakly positively birefringent; that is, they appear blue when lying parallel to the axis of the line of slow vibration of the first-order red compensator, and yellow at right angles (see Fig. 77–2). Absolute identification of crystals, which requires a more specialized technique such as x-ray or electron diffraction, is generally not needed for practical clinical diagnostic purposes.

CPPD crystals must be differentiated from other crystals found in pathologic states, such as cholesterol crystals seen in chronic effusions and xanthine crystals seen in xanthinuria. Like urate crystals, the latter are strongly birefringent. In addition, crystals introduced iatrogenically into the fluid during collection need to be considered. Such crystals include calcium oxalate or lithium heparin[65] used as anticoagulants, steroid crystals following recent joint injection, and crystals of talc in starch dusting powders used on sterile rubber gloves at the time of joint fluid aspiration.

Calcium oxalate crystals have also been demonstrated in patients undergoing hemodialysis for chronic renal failure.[66] Dicalcium phosphate dihydrate, a brightly positively birefringent crystal, occurs at times, usually in association with CPPD crystal deposition.[67] Several reports have described lipid liquid crystal spherulites that appear as Maltese crosses in joint fluids.[68] A possible phlogistic action of these crystals has been suggested.

Calcium stains, such as alizarin red, allow visualization of calcium-containing crystals in synovial fluid (Fig. 77–3).[69, 69a] This stain should be used only as a screening test, however, since it is not totally specific for calcium-containing crystals.

Roentgenographic Features

The diagnostic accuracy with which joint chondrocalcinosis can be identified depends on the skeletal roentgenographic technique utilized.[70–72] Although high-resolution techniques using industrial films or magnification will more accurately delineate

Table 77–2. DIFFERENTIATION OF CALCIUM PYROPHOSPHATE DIHYDRATE (CPPD) AND MONOSODIUM URATE (MSU) CRYSTALS

	CPPD Crystals	MSU Crystals
Shape	Linear or rhomboid	Linear, needle-shaped
Crystal ends	Blunt	Sharp
Birefringence (direction)	Weak or absent (positive)	Strong (negative)

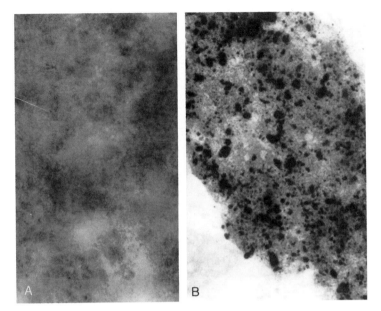

Figure 77–3. Synovial fluid smears to which alizarin red solution has been added as a stain for crystals containing calcium. *A*, Normal synovial fluid lacking calcium crystals. *B*, Positive crystal staining for calcium is seen in fluid obtained from a patient with CPDD. (Courtesy of Dr. R. Schumacher.)

chondrocalcinosis, they are generally not required for routine clinical studies.

Characteristic radiologic features of chondrocalcinosis include linear and punctate calcification of fibrocartilage and hyaline cartilage of involved joints (Figs. 77–4 to 77–6). Fibrocartilages that are most frequently and extensively calcified include the knee menisci (see Fig. 77–4), triangular fibrocartilage of the wrist (see Fig. 77–5), and pubic symphysis; the glenoid and acetabular labra and intervertebral discs are less often affected. Hyaline cartilage calcification differs from that seen in fibrocartilage; it is more linear and finer and parallels subchondral bone (see Fig. 77–6). Capsular calcification is not uncommon and may be seen in smaller joints, such as the metacarpophalangeal and metatarsophalangeal articulations, as well as in larger joints, including the knees, shoulders, and hips. Periarticular soft tissue calcifications are occasionally observed in tendinous structures, such as the Achilles tendon at the heel, the quadriceps, and supraspinatus. The synovial lining of joints may calcify at times. Roentgenograms to include both knees, pelvis, and both wrists will effectively screen for the presence of chondrocalcinosis in the majority of patients with CPDD (Table 77–3).

In addition to cartilage calcification, CPDD patients frequently exhibit characteristic arthropathic

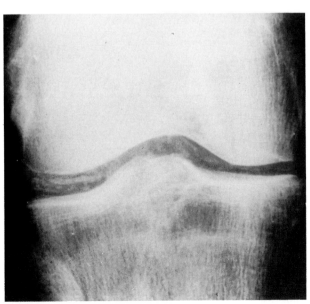

Figure 77–4. Punctate calcification of fibrocartilage in knee meniscus of a patient with CPDD.

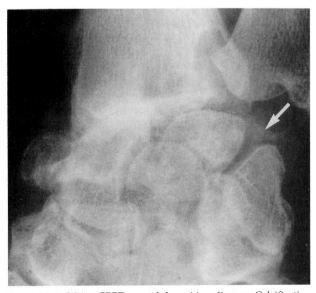

Figure 77–5. Wrist, CPPD crystal deposition disease. Calcification of the triangular fibrocartilage is noted (*arrow*). In addition, pyrophosphate arthropathy characterized by narrowing of the radionavicular joint, subchondral sclerosis, and cysts in the distal radius and carpal bones is readily seen.

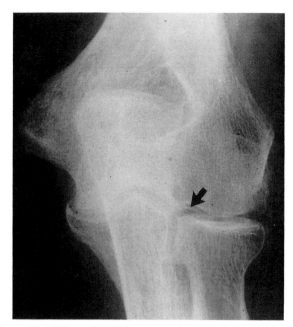

Figure 77–6. Elbow, CPDD. Linear calcification of hyaline cartilage is seen at the radiohumeral articulation (*arrow*).

changes, which include joint space narrowing, eburnation, and subchondral cyst formation. Resnick and Utsinger[73] have described a characteristic wrist arthropathy in patients with pseudogout (see Fig. 77–5). Changes include narrowing of the radionavicular joint space; subchondral sclerosis; multiple subchondral lucencies or cysts, especially of the navicular or lunate bones; and chondrocalcinosis of the triangular fibrocartilage; the distal radioulnar and first carpometacarpal joints are not involved, however. These changes are so characteristic that, in their presence, a diagnosis of CPDD should be considered even in the absence of demonstrable calcific deposits.

Patellofemoral compartmental disease characterized by joint space narrowing, osteophyte formation, and a "wrap-around" appearance of the patella on the femur may be observed (Fig. 77–7). Similar patellofemoral changes are seen in patients with hyperparathyroidism or renal osteodystrophy, with or without crystal deposition.

As noted earlier, osteoarthritic degenerative

Table 77–3. CPDD—JOINTS RECOMMENDED FOR SCREENING ROENTGENOGRAPHIC STUDIES TO SHOW STRUCTURES INVOLVED BY CHARACTERISTIC LESIONS

Knees—*to show*
Meniscal and hyaline articular cartilage calcification
AP Pelvis—*to show*
Acetabular labra, and hip hyaline articular cartilage calcification
Symphysis pubis fibrocartilaginous disc calcification
Lower lumbar spine disc calcification
Wrists—*to show*
Triangular fibrocartilage calcification
Characteristic arthropathy

changes are not uncommon as a corollary finding in the joints of patients with CPDD. In some patients, rapidly progressive destructive changes may ensue; bony collapse and fragmentation of subchondral bone resemble Charcot joints.[74] These destructive changes may develop in otherwise uncomplicated CPPD deposition disease or in association with neurologic deficits.[75]

Although symptoms and roentgenographic evidence of joint cartilage calcification frequently correlate, joint calcification often occurs without symptoms.[55] Conversely, symptoms may be present in the absence of demonstrable calcium on routine radiologic examination. In such cases, a diagnosis of pseudogout depends on finding calcium pyrophosphate crystals in synovial fluid or in synovial tissue at biopsy.

McCarty has suggested that cases of CPPD crystal deposition disease be identified as possible, probable, or definite, depending on the presence or absence of certain required clinical, roentgenographic, or crystal criteria (Table 77–4).[76] For example, chemical, electron, or x-ray diffraction identification of crystals as CPPD represents a definite diagnosis. Identification of crystals consistent with CPPD in synovial fluid requires associated roentgenographic demonstration of calcifications for a diagnosis of definite disease. Synovial fluid crystal identification or roentgenographic calcification of cartilage alone represents a probable diagnosis. In most pa-

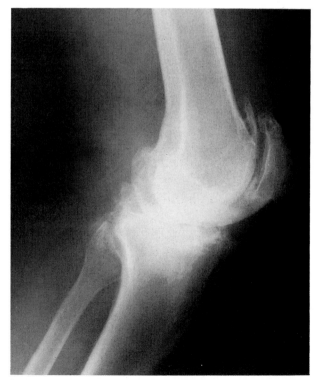

Figure 77–7. Patellofemoral compartmental disease is prominent in this patient with CPDD. In addition to joint space narrowing and osteophyte formation, the "wraparound" appearance of the patella on the femur suggests the diagnosis.

Table 77-4. CPDD—DIAGNOSTIC CRITERIA

Criteria
I. Definitive identification of CPPD crystals, e.g., chemical analysis, x-ray or electron diffraction studies
II. (a) Synovial fluid crystals consistent with CPDD in morphology/birefringence
    (b) Typical calcifications on roentgenogram
III. (a) Acute arthritis attacks, especially knees, wrists
    (b) Subacute or chronic arthritis, with or without acute episodes

Categories
A. Definite—criterion I, or II(a) *plus* (b)
B. Probable—criterion II(a) *or* (b)
C. Possible—criterion III in any combination

Modified from Ryan, L. M., and McCarty, D. J.: *In* McCarty, D. J. (ed.): Arthritis and Allied Conditions. 10th ed. Philadelphia, Lea & Febiger, 1985, p. 1522. Reproduced with permission.

tients the relationship of CPPD crystal deposition and the symptoms can usually be made by careful assessment of roentgenographic, synovial fluid, and clinical findings.

Unusual (Atypical, Variant) Clinical Presentations

In addition to the more common presentations of CPDD described previously, calcium pyrophosphate deposition may be associated with somewhat more unusual clinical patterns. While it is apparent that acute attacks of pseudogout may resemble septic arthritis,[57, 77] it is important to note that septic arthritis and acute pyrophosphate-induced arthritis may co-exist.[78] In certain patients this may result from the fact that joints already altered by pyrophosphate crystals may serve as a locus of increased susceptibility to deposition of bacterial organisms. Conversely, patients with acute septic arthritis may develop an acute crystal-induced synovitis when hydrolytic enzymes released during the course of joint infection digest cartilage matrix, releasing "innocent bystander" deposits of CPPD. The term "enzymatic strip-mining" has been used to describe this mechanism of crystal release.[78] This same mechanism of "enzymatic strip-mining" is postulated to occur when pseudogout occurs in patients with joint diseases other than septic arthritis.

Tophaceous deposition of calcium pyrophosphate leads to acute, subacute, and chronic soft tissue inflammatory responses. Such deposits have been described in a number of areas, including the extremities and spinal and paraspinal structures, and in and around peripheral nerves.[79-86] Particularly striking are large calcific tumors composed of CPPD crystals leading to pseudotumor formation in and around the temporomandibular joint[83]; parotid tumors may be simulated. Although rare, this pathologic entity becomes a diagnostic consideration in patients with a preauricular mass.

Subacute attacks of inflammation due to tophaceous deposits of calcium pyrophosphate involving

the fingers have been described.[79, 84] Radiographs reveal fluffy calcification overlying the area of inflammation. As in patients with parotid area disease, tophaceous pseudogout appears to be a local rather than a generalized process.

CPPD deposition disease is a differential diagnostic consideration in patients with acute olecranon bursitis[81] and needs to be excluded from similar clinical presentations observed in patients with acute septic or gouty arthritis.

Various roentgenographic and clinical findings related to the spine have been described in patients with CPDD.[82, 85, 86] Changes included calcifications of the intervertebral discs, diffuse idiopathic skeletal hyperostosis (DISH), and cervical myelopathy secondary to involvement of the ligamentum flavum with CPPD crystals.[86] Although myelopathic symptoms may be related to hypertrophy of the ligamentum flavum alone, a contributing role for CPPD crystal deposition in augmentation of observed symptoms was considered likely.

A case of progressive foramen magnum syndrome due to deposits of CPPD was described[86]; symptoms responded to transoral decompression of the cervicomedullary junction.

Calcium pyrophosphate dihydrate deposits were noted in lumbar disc fibrocartilage in four patients undergoing surgery for spinal cord or nerve root compression.[87, 88] Patients had had prior surgery at the same or adjacent vertebral level; it was suggested that surgical trauma to fibrocartilaginous disc remnants stimulated pyrophosphate production and deposition. The suggestion that CPPD deposition may be promoted in the presence of altered or damaged cartilage is supported by a study that noted an increased frequency of localized chondrocalcinosis in knees following meniscectomy.[89] Chondrocalcinosis was detected roentgenographically in 20 percent of operated knees and in 4 percent of unoperated knees.

Pathology and Pathogenesis

Mechanisms of Crystal Deposition

Pathologic deposits of CPPD crystals generally parallel those seen roentgenographically.[6] In particular, crystal deposits are heaviest in fibrocartilaginous structures, such as menisci (Figs. 77-4 and 77-8), triangular cartilages of the wrists, acetabular and glenoid labra, and symphysis pubis. Calcification may involve other joint structures, however, including articular hyaline cartilage, synovium (see Fig. 77-1B), joint capsules, and intra-articular ligamentous and tendinous structures. Intra- and extra-articular deposits of pyrophosphate appear grossly as white chalky structures similar to those seen in urate gout (Fig. 77-9). Alterations in cartilage matrix seen in association with CPPD deposition include variable losses of metachromatic stain, chondrocyte "clon-

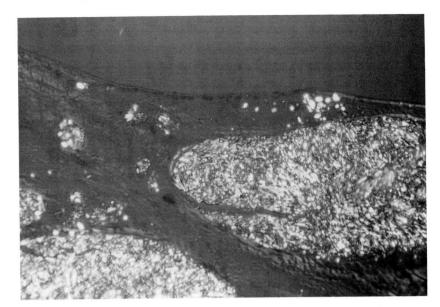

Figure 77–8. Meniscal deposition of calcium pyrophosphate dihydrate crystals is readily observed by utilizing polarized light. (Courtesy of Dr. R. Schumacher.)

ing," and collagen fibril fragmentation. These changes are nonspecific and may be related to osteoarthritic changes associated with pyrophosphate deposition. It is as yet uncertain whether such changes precede, follow, or are coincidental to crystal deposition.

Conceptual mechanisms to be considered in the pathogenesis of sporadic or familial CPDD include primary abnormalities of the cartilage matrix with secondary calcification, or biochemical abnormalities that lead to elevated serum and synovial fluid levels of calcium or inorganic pyrophosphate (PPi). Morphologic alterations in articular cartilage from areas without calcification in CPDD patients, and abnormalities in glycosaminoglycan deposition not due to osteoarthritis or aging,[90] supported primary changes in cartilage matrix in the pathogenesis of CPPD deposition.

In studies of CPPD crystal deposition using an in vitro model system of native collagen gels, chondroitin sulfate was shown to inhibit formation of CPPD; chondroitin sulfate was a more impotent inhibitor of CPPD crystal formation than was keratan sulfate.[91] The increase in keratan sulfate:chondroitin sulfate ratio that occurs in human hyaline articular cartilage with aging might thus conceivably facilitate the deposition of CPPD crystals.

Dieppe et al.[74] proposed an "amplification loop" hypothesis, whereby joint damage plays a primary role in predisposing cartilage to CPPD crystal deposition. This hypothesis is based on demonstration of a pre-existing condition known to damage joints in 70 percent of patients with CPDD.[74] Shedding of secondarily deposited crystals into the synovial space then leads to activation of inflammatory mediators that contribute to further joint destruction. This augmented joint damage sets up an amplification loop with further circular predisposition to crystal deposition.[9]

In other studies, increased intracellular levels of pyrophosphate (PPi) were demonstrated in skin fibroblasts and lymphoblasts from affected members of a large kindred with familial CPDD.[92] Ryan and colleagues[93] demonstrated elevated levels of PPi from skin fibroblasts derived from patients with sporadic as well as familial forms of CPDD; however, nucleoside triphosphate pyrophosphohydrolase (NTPPPH) activity was elevated only in the sporadic form.

Investigations detailing alterations in enzyme activity important in pyrophosphate production have provided new directions in understanding the underlying pathophysiology of pyrophosphate deposition. Studies have demonstrated augmented generation of pyrophosphate by extracts of cartilages from

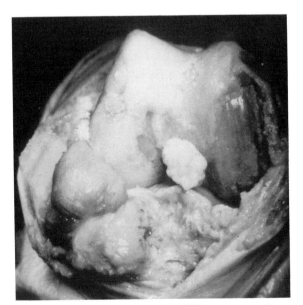

Figure 77–9. Knee from patient with CPDD at autopsy. Deposits of calcium pyrophosphate dihydrate appear grossly as white chalky structures, similar to those seen in urate gout. (Courtesy of Dr. R. Schumacher.)

patients with CPDD compared with osteoarthritic or normal cartilages; high levels of 5' nucleotidase (5'NTase) activity were also noted.[94] The authors postulated that the pathway by which adenosine triphosphate is hydrolyzed to adenosine monophosphate (AMP) and PPi by ATP pyrophosphohydrolase plays a major role in the pathogenesis of CPPD deposition. Further investigations[95-98] have provided evidence identifying NTPPPH as an ectoenzyme capable of acting on extracellular substrate. The external location of this enzyme, shown to be elevated in synovial fluids and cartilage extracts of some patients with CPDD, is consistent with the hypothesis that PPi generation occurs at the perilacunar site where crystals form. Further studies have shown ATP levels to be elevated in the synovial fluid of patients with CPDD; lesser elevations occurred in osteoarthritic synovial fluid as compared with normal synovial fluid.[99, 99a] ATP, a naturally occurring extracellular substrate for the ectoenzyme NTPPPH, was present in a variety of pathologic synovial fluids, with highest levels noted in CPDD.

Based on these studies, which have demonstrated elevated levels of NTPPPH and 5'NTase and diminished levels of pyrophosphatase activity in cartilages of patients with CPDD, a schema for pyrophosphate deposition has been suggested (Fig. 77–10). Increased adenosine triphosphate pyrophosphohydrolase activity could generate increased amounts of pyrophosphate; adenosine triphosphate degradation would be enhanced by removal of adenosine monophosphate by 5'NTase, and removal of pyrophosphate would be diminished in the presence of low pyrophosphatase activity. These alterations in enzyme activity would explain increased pyrophosphate accumulation.

Of interest in regard to the above hypothesis are studies that assessed the influence of alterations in ambient pH, various hormones, serum, and serum factors on inorganic pyrophosphate elaboration in in vitro studies of cartilage and chondrocytes.[100, 101] Al-terations in ambient pH, thyroid-stimulating hormone, and parathyroid hormone did not affect pyrophosphate accumulation.[100] Exposing cartilage to 10 percent fetal bovine serum significantly enhanced the egress of pyrophosphate from the tissue[100]; similarly, exposure of the culture system to human serum, and to an acid-ethanol extract of human platelets resulted in increased pyrophosphate production.[101] The platelet factor responsible for stimulation of pyrophosphate by cartilage was not mitogenic for chondrocytes, nor was it platelet-derived growth factor (PDGF).[102] Increased pyrophosphate production in response to serum and platelet factors occurred without increases in NTPPPH activity in the tissue; this suggests that increased NTPPPH activity may not be a necessary condition for CPDD in vivo.[101, 102]

Transforming growth factor-β alone and in synergy with epidermal growth factor was also shown to stimulate pyrophosphate elaboration by cartilage explants.[103] As with other serum and platelet factors, NTPPPH activity in cartilage did not increase significantly, suggesting stimulation of cartilage pyrophosphate production through another pathway.[103]

Dissociation of sulfate incorporation and pyrophosphate secretion indicates that it is not likely that glycosaminoglycan sulfation is the source of pyrophosphate emanating from chondrocytes in formation of crystals in the extracellular matrix.[104]

As is the case in hyperuricemia and gout, it is likely that multiple mechanisms are responsible in different forms of CPDD.

The availability of an animal model of CPDD would facilitate studies of the pathophysiology of this disorder. CPDD, described in rhesus monkeys (Macaca mulatta), was characterized by focal radiodensities in lumbar intervertebral discs, menisci, and articular cartilage.[105, 106] Crystal deposits were identified as CPPD. The presence of CPDD and osteoarthritis that resembled spontaneous human disease with respect to age, sex, joint histology, and cartilage

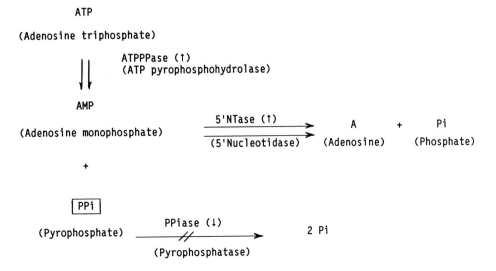

Figure 77–10. Schema of enzyme alterations leading to pyrophosphate deposition. Pyrophosphate (PPi) concentration increases as a result of increased formation and decreased breakdown.

composition may provide the opportunity for more detailed studies of both CPDD and osteoarthritis.

Mechanisms of Crystal-Induced Inflammation

Activation of inflammatory mediators by CPPD crystals is similar in many respects to those mechanisms described for acute gouty arthritis.[107–110] Phagocytosis of calcium pyrophosphate crystals by polymorphonuclear cells has been regularly noted, particularly in patients with acute crystal-induced attacks (see Fig. 77–2). Polymorphonuclear cells exposed in vitro to calcium pyrophosphate crystals do not, however, show the extensive cell death of, or as rapid phagocytosis of crystals as, that seen in similar experiments with MSU crystals.[109] Small-sized fractions of monosodium urate monohydrate and CPPD crystals give neutrophil cytolysis values of higher percentages than those of large-sized crystals.[111] High density lipoprotein (HDL) and low density lipoprotein (LDL) bound in significant amounts to both CPPD and MSU and strongly inhibited neutrophil cytolysis; HDL and LDL bound to urate and CPPD crystals may play important roles in the regulation of crystal-induced inflammation.

Crystal phagocytosis by polymorphonuclear leukocytes is, in turn, accompanied by release of prostaglandins, leukotrienes, reactive oxygen species, and lysosomal enzymes as general responses.

Monosodium urate and CPPD crystals and, to a lesser extent, hydroxyapatite crystals increased interleukin-6 (IL-6) production by synoviocytes and monocytes in vitro.[112] High levels of IL-6 were found in synovial fluid from patients with gout and pseudogout. IL-6 production in synoviocytes and monocytes may be an important mediator of inflammatory responses in acute gout and pseudogout.

In vitro studies have shown that incubation of CPPD or MSU crystals with neutrophils leads to the generation of an apparently identical chemotactic glycopeptide.[110] This factor, injected intra-articularly into rabbit joints, mimics inflammatory attacks of acute gout or pseudogout; colchicine at therapeutic concentrations suppresses production of the factor.[113]

The mechanism by which CPPD crystals gain access to the joint space needs further validation. One hypothesis suggests that calcium pyrophosphate crystallizes within synovial fluid, related to elevated synovial fluid levels of inorganic pyrophosphate.[114] Alternatively, crystals seen in synovial fluid may emanate from preformed deposits in cartilage via crystal shedding or enzymatic "strip-mining" of crystal deposits.[115] Crystal shedding may be triggered by any factor that enhances CPPD crystal solubility, such as the fall in ionized calcium that occurs after surgical procedures, especially after parathyroidectomy.[28] A fall in total and ionized plasma and synovial fluid calcium levels would enhance CPPD crystal solubility and lead to a loosening of crystals from their cartilaginous matrix.

Crystal-induced inflammation occurring as a concomitant process in patients with other forms of joint inflammation, such as septic, gouty, or rheumatoid arthritis, may result from enzymatic digestion of cartilage, with subsequent loosening of crystal deposits.[78] Once inflammation begins, secondary joint fluid pH changes and enzymatic digestion of the matrix perpetuate the process. Thus, crystal release may be the result as well as the cause of inflammation.

It appears that eventual dissolution of CPPD crystals occurs within fixed synovial cells after endocytosis,[116, 117] based on rapid disappearance of crystals from the joint space with concentration in the synovium, localization of crystals within synovial cells, and a relative insolubility of crystals in body fluids.

Management

At present, no available therapy has been shown to consistently remove pyrophosphate deposits already present or to retard further crystal deposition. Even treatment of underlying metabolic defects, such as hemochromatosis[42] or hyperparathyroidism,[25] does not affect established pyrophosphate deposition. Accordingly, therapy is symptomatic, being directed at treatment and prevention of acute attacks and management of subacute and chronic symptoms (Table 77–5). Acute attacks respond to aspiration alone with removal of inflammogenic crystals, mediators, and leukocytes; response is hastened by the addition of intra-articular injection of glucocorticoids.

Although relief of acute attacks with oral colchicine may at times be satisfactory, responses are generally inconsistent.[55] Intravenous colchicine, on the other hand, is more uniformly successful.[118] The use of intravenous colchicine for acute attacks is, however, rarely indicated, given a uniformly successful response to various of the nonaspirin nonsteroidal anti-inflammatory drugs (NSAIDs), used in full dose.

Colchicine in doses of 0.6 mg b.i.d. has been shown to be effective in the prevention of recurrent acute pseudogout attacks.[119, 120] Although not formally studied, it is likely that low doses of NSAIDs

Table 77–5. CPDD—MANAGEMENT

Acute Attacks
  Joint fluid aspiration
  Intra-articular glucocorticoids
  Nonaspirin NSAIDs (full dose)
  Colchicine, intravenous route
Prophylaxis of Acute Attacks
  Colchicine 0.6 mg b.i.d. daily
  Nonaspirin NSAIDs (low dose daily)
Subacute/Chronic Symptoms
  Salicylates
  NSAIDs
  Analgesics (e.g., acetaminophen, propoxyphene)
  Physical therapy

daily would have a similar prophylactic effect. Fortunately, most patients with CPDD have acute episodes of arthritis at widely spaced intervals and can be managed by treatment of acute attacks as they occur, without the need to utilize prophylactic therapy.

Subacute and chronic symptoms are treated in the same fashion as management of osteoarthritis. In particular, use of salicylates or NSAIDs on a continuing basis provides symptomatic relief. Avoidance of overuse of the affected joint, in addition to appropriate exercises, is indicated, particularly when osteoarthritic changes are associated.

BASIC CALCIUM PHOSPHATE (CALCIUM APATITE) CRYSTAL DEPOSITION DISEASES

Acute, subacute, and chronic musculoskeletal symptoms, such as bursitis and tendinitis, are well known to occur in response to calcium apatite deposition (Table 77–6).[121] Similar acute episodes of periarthritis, tendinitis, or bursitis related to calcific deposits at joints other than the shoulder have now been well described (Fig. 77–11). In these studies, recurrent painful periarticular inflammation was associated with roentgenographically demonstrable periarticular calcifications at multiple sites near articulations.[122, 123] Common areas of involvement included the shoulder, greater trochanter of the hip, lateral epicondyle of the elbow, tendons about the wrist, and tendon attachments at the medial and lateral aspects of the knee. Material aspirated from the involved site often had a milky or cheesy consistency. Microscopic study revealed typical globular bodies with a "shiny coin" appearance, which probably represent clusters of apatite crystals. Disappearance of the calcific deposits noted on roentgenographic study was not uncommon over a period of weeks or months following an acute inflammatory episode.

A second form of apatite crystal–induced inflammation has been observed in patients undergoing hemodialysis for chronic renal failure.[124] Inflammation appeared to be related to calcific deposits of apatite crystals found in and around involved joints.

Table 77–6. BCP (APATITE) CRYSTAL DEPOSITION DISEASE STATES

Calcific bursitis or tendinitis
Calcific periarthritis—soft tissue deposition
   Primary
      Unifocal
      Multifocal
   Secondary
      Chronic renal failure
      Progressive systemic sclerosis, dermatomyositis
   Familial
Intra-articular
   Acute arthritis
   Chronic erosive disease

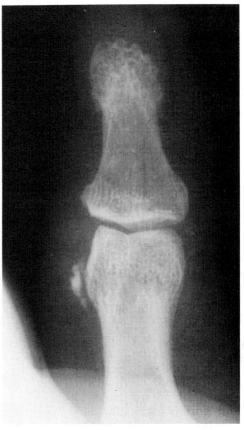

Figure 77–11. Apatite deposition in para-articular soft tissue of the finger in this patient led to an acute inflammatory reaction suggesting septic arthritis.

Studies suggest that calcification in these patients is related to elevated serum phosphorus concentration. Increased frequency and efficiency of dialysis to maintain normal serum phosphate levels, coupled with regular use of aluminum hydroxide to bind phosphate in the gastrointestinal tract, has led to prevention and control of these crystal-related symptoms.

Interstitial calcinosis with deposition of variably sized deposits of calcium apatite in soft tissues is well known to occur in patients with certain connective tissue diseases, such as scleroderma and dermatomyositis. In contrast with calcifications observed in patients undergoing renal dialysis in whom calcium deposition is metastatic secondary to raised calcium or phosphate concentrations, ectopic calcification seen in patients with scleroderma and dermatomyositis is dystrophic in character, secondary to local tissue damage. Drainage of calcific material coupled with moderate to marked inflammatory responses not infrequently leads to a misdiagnosis of septic cellulitis.

Idiopathic familial chondrocalcinosis due to apatite crystal deposition has been described.[125] Clinical features of the disease included morning stiffness, pain and limitation of motion of the dorsolumbar spine, and arthritis of peripheral joints. Radiographic studies revealed multiple intervertebral disc calcifications, located mainly at the area of the nucleus pulposus. Periarticular calcific deposits were also observed in and around small joints of the hands.

In contrast with reports of periarticular inflammatory responses secondary to apatite deposition, an association of intra-articular apatite crystals and joint disease has been described.[126-130] In 1976, Dieppe and coworkers[126] reported seven patients with osteoarthritis in whom synovial fluid studies revealed crystals morphologically similar to those of pure crystalline calcium hydroxyapatite; inflammatory responses were induced when apatite crystals were injected into rat intrapleural space and into skin. Similar observations were reported by Schumacher and colleagues,[127] who identified needle-shaped crystals in synovial fluid by transmission electron microscopy in a variety of joint diseases. Seven of 11 patients studied had acute undiagnosed arthritis, or inflammatory exacerbations of osteoarthritis. The joints involved included the knee, small joints of the hands, and wrists.

Erosive arthritis also occurs in association with apatite crystal deposition. McCarty and colleagues gave the term "Milwaukee shoulder" to a rapidly progressive, destructive arthritis, seen predominantly in older women and characterized by recurrent large shoulder effusions and decreased mobility or stability (Fig. 77–12).[129, 131] Roentgenographic evidence of a complete tear of the fibrous rotator cuff was common. Additional roentgenographic findings included degenerative changes of the humeral head or glenoid of the scapula, degenerative changes of the acromoclavicular joint, and calcification of the tendinous rotator cuff. Multiple filling defects on arthrography were seen at times, consistent with osteochondromatosis.

Synovial fluids from patients with this disorder contained few leukocytes, and were often blood-tinged.[131] Basic calcium phosphate crystals, that is, carbonate-substituted hydroxyapatite, octacalcium phosphate, and, occasionally, tricalcium phosphate, were identified; particulate collagens were also noted in nearly all fluids. Synovial fluid collagenase activity was detectable in some, but not all, patients. Knee joints were involved with a similar process in about 50 percent of patients. In contrast with primary osteoarthritis in which the medial tibial femoral compartment is most frequently involved, lateral tibial femoral compartment involvement was common in BCP disease. Factors that appeared to predispose to this syndrome included associated deposition of CPPD crystals, direct injury or chronic overuse of joints, and neurologic disorders. In addition to involvement of shoulders and knees, erosive destructive arthritis related to BCP crystal deposition disease has been described in other joints, including hips, elbows, ankles, and interphalangeal joints of the hands.[49]

The role of apatite in the etiopathogenesis of these lesions is still somewhat contested. McCarty and colleagues suggest that BCP crystals, phagocytosed by synovial macrophage-like cells, activate collagenase and neutral protease.[129, 130] Active enzymes then lead to joint destruction, "enzymatic strip-mining," and release of additional crystals and particulate collagen into the joint space, thereby augmenting the destructive response. Following endocytosis by synovial lining cells, BCP crystals stimulate increased synthesis and secretion of proteases, collagenase, and prostaglandin E_2.[129, 130] In addition, BCP crystals are potent mitogens, possibly contributing to the synovial proliferation seen in this disorder.[132] BCP crystals appear to stimulate mitogenesis and collagenase production by different mechanisms.[133] Blocking crystal dissolution inhibited the mitogenic effect of BCP crystals but did not inhibit collagenase synthesis. Dieppe and colleagues caution that joint apatite deposition may be a secondary event in damaged cartilage or, at times, may be coincidental.[134]

Several similarities between synovial fluid findings in CPDD and BCP have been demonstrated.[135] In particular, synovial fluid inorganic pyrophosphate concentration was found to be elevated in arthropathies associated with BCP crystals as well as in CPPD disease. In addition, synovial fluid NTPPPH activity was elevated and appeared to correlate with the severity of joint degeneration.

Laboratory Findings

Alterations in calcium and phosphorus metabolism are generally not observed in patients with BCP disease, other than in those with underlying associated diseases, such as uremic syndrome, who are

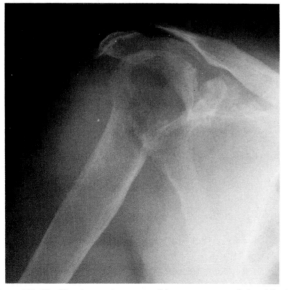

Figure 77–12. Classic roentgenographic appearance of shoulder in patient with "Milwaukee shoulder syndrome." Destructive arthritis is characterized by bony erosions, cyst formation, and loss of joint space, noted particularly at the inferior aspect of the joint.

undergoing dialysis therapy. Synovial fluid crystals may be sparse or may be sufficiently profuse to make the fluid grossly milky. Synovial fluid leukocyte counts and polymorphonuclear predominance may be marked; counts generally tend to be lower, however, with more monocytes than those seen in acute gout and CPDD.[129, 136]

Specific identification of BCP crystals in synovial fluid by light microscopy is difficult, owing to their small size (less than 1 μm in length). Certain light microscopic findings may, however, suggest the diagnosis (Table 77–7). Shiny nonbirefringent irregular cytoplasmic inclusions that may result from clumps of crystals have been described.[123] When seen extracellularly, they take on the appearance of "shiny coins" (Fig. 77–13). Similarly, purplish cytoplasmic inclusions seen on Wright-stained smears suggest the diagnosis. Clumps of crystals stain strongly with alizarin red[69] or von Kossa stain. Alizarin red solution mixed with synovial fluid will stain calcium-containing materials (see Fig. 77–3); this technique has been suggested as a screening study.[69] Various forms of calcium crystals, such as CPPD, calcium apatite, and calcium oxalate, as well as phosphate-containing crystals, are not differentiated. Further lack of specificity is seen in the positive staining of some synovial fluids from patients with osteoarthritis, renal-failure dialysis, rheumatoid arthritis, and gout, although calcium crystal deposition associated with these other disorders cannot be excluded. Specific identification of BCP crystals requires use of techniques such as electron probe or transmission electron microscopy.

Roentgenographic Features

Roentgenographic findings in patients with BCP disease are variable. In patients with periarticular calcific deposition, calcium deposits are readily visible contiguous to involved joints. In patients with intra-articular BCP-related disease, articular hyaline cartilage or meniscal calcifications seen with CPDD are not observed unless CPPD crystal deposition is associated. Roentgenograms may show absence of calcification despite demonstration of apatite on intra-articular study. Erosive destructive arthritis and changes of osteoarthritis are not infrequent.

Management

Patients with acute arthritis or periarthritis secondary to calcium apatite deposition respond to

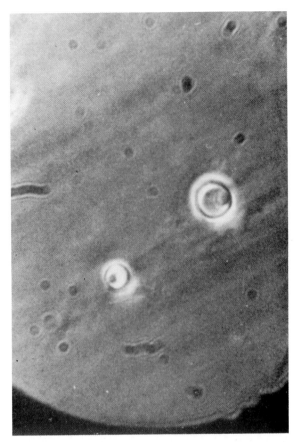

Figure 77–13. "Shiny coins" seen on light microscopic examination of a patient with apatite deposition disease and associated synovitis. These structures probably result from clumping of crystals in an extracellular location. (From McCarty, D. J., and Gatter, R. A.: Recurrent acute inflammation associated with focal apatite crystal deposition. Arthritis Rheum. 9:808, 1966. Used by permission.)

NSAIDs used in full dosages as recommended for acute gouty attacks. In addition, colchicine utilized in full oral or intravenous doses is frequently salutary. As in other forms of crystal deposition disease, intra-articular glucocorticoid injection following aspiration of the inflammatory effusion has a high rate of success.

In patients with chronic forms of the disease, daily administration of NSAIDs in lower doses is helpful. As in all forms of subacute and chronic arthritis, appropriate attention to physical therapy programs, including heat and exercise, is important in maintaining joint range of motion and providing further symptomatic relief. Large periarticular deposits of crystals may occasionally require surgical excision if more conservative approaches are not efficacious; the need for this is rare. Efforts directed toward removing calcium deposits themselves, such as the use of disodium etidronate, have not been uniformly successful.[137]

Table 77–7. SYNOVIAL FLUID LIGHT MICROSCOPIC FINDINGS IN BCP DEPOSITION DISEASE

Morphologically discrete crystals absent
Nonbirefringent cytoplasmic inclusions
Extracellular "shiny coins"
Positive von Kossa or alizarin red staining

References

1. McCarty, D. J., and Hollander, J. L.: Identification of urate crystals in gouty synovial fluid. Ann. Intern. Med. 54:452, 1961.

2. McCarty, D. J., Kohn, N. N., and Faires, J. S.: The significance of calcium phosphate crystals in the synovial fluid of arthritis patients: the "pseudogout syndrome." I. Clinical aspects. Ann. Intern. Med. 56:711, 1962.

3. Zitnan, D., and Sitaj, S.: Chondrocalcinosis articularis. Ann. Rheum. Dis. 22:142, 1963.

4. McCarty, D. J.: Calcium pyrophosphate dihydrate deposition disease— 1975. Arthritis Rheum. 19:275, 1976.

5. Ellman, M. H., and Levin, B.: Chondrocalcinosis in elderly persons. Arthritis Rheum. 18:43, 1975.

6. McCarty, D. J., Hogan, J. M., Gatter, R. A., et al.: Studies on pathological calcifications in human cartilage. I. Prevalence and types of crystal deposits in the menisci of two hundred fifteen cadavera. J. Bone Joint Surg. 48A:308, 1966.

7. Wilkins, E., Dieppe, P., Maddison, P., and Evison, G.: Osteoarthritis and articular chondrocalcinosis in the elderly. Ann. Rheum. Dis. 42:280, 1983.

8. O'Duffy, J. D.: Clinical studies of acute pseudogout attacks. Comments on prevalence, predispositions, and treatment. Arthritis Rheum. 19(Suppl.):349, 1976.

9. Doherty, M., and Dieppe, P.: Crystal deposition disease in the elderly. Clin. Rheum. Dis. 12:97, 1986.

10. Nyulassy, S., Stefanovic, J., Sitaj, S., and Zitnan, D.: HLA system in articular chondrocalcinosis. Arthritis Rheum. 19(Suppl.):391, 1976.

11. Reginato, A. J., Hollander, J. L., Martinez, V., et al.: Familial chondrocalcinosis in the Chiloe Islands, Chile. Ann. Rheum. Dis. 34:260, 1975.

12. Reginato, A. J., Schiapachasse, V., Zmijewski, C. M., Schumacher, H. R., Fuentes, C., and Galdamez, M.: HLA antigens in chondrocalcinosis and ankylosing chondrocalcinosis. Arthritis Rheum. 22:928, 1979.

13. Gaucher, A., Faure, G., Netter, P., Pourel, J., Raffoux, C., Streiff, F., Tongio, M-M., and Mayer, S.: Hereditary diffuse articular chondrocalcinosis. Scand. J. Rheumatol. 6:217, 1977.

14. Gaudreau, A., Camerlain, M., Piborot, M. L., Beauregard, G., Lebiun, A., and Petitclere, C.: Familial articular chondrocalcinosis in Quebec. Arthritis Rheum. 24:611, 1981.

15. Bjelle, A., Nordström, S., and Hagstam, A.: Hereditary pyrophosphate arthropathy (familial articular chondrocalcinosis) in Sweden. Clin. Genet. 21:174, 1982.

16. Richardson, B. C., Chafetz, N. I., Ferrell, L. D., Zulman, J. I., and Genant, H. K.: Hereditary chondrocalcinosis in a Mexican-American family. Arthritis Rheum. 26:1387, 1983.

17. Nunez-Roldan, A., Sanchez-Burson, J., Prieto, J., and Pujol, E.: Familial chondrocalcinosis and HLA system. Arthritis Rheum. 24:1590, 1981.

18. Fernandez Dapica, M. P., and Gomez-Reino, J. J.: Familial chondrocalcinosis in the Spanish population. J. Rheumatol. 13:631, 1986.

19. Rodriguez-Valverde, V., Zuniga, M., Casanueva, B., Sanchez, S., and Merino, J.: Hereditary articular chondrocalcinosis. Clinical and genetic features in 13 pedigrees. Am. J. Med. 84:101, 1988.

20. Riestra, J. L., Sanchez, A., Rodriguez-Valverde, V., Alonso, J. L., de la Hera, M., and Merino, J.: Radiographic features of hereditary articular chondrocalcinosis. A comparative study with the sporadic type. Clin. Exp. Rheumatol. 6:369, 1988.

21. Balsa, A., Martin-Mola, E., Gonzalez, T., Cruz, A., Ojeda, S., and Gijon-Banos, J.: Familial articular chondrocalcinosis in Spain. Ann. Rheum. Dis. 49:531, 1990.

22. Eshel, G., Gulik, A., Halperin, N., Avrahami, E., Schumacher, H. R., McCarty, D. J., and Caspi, D.: Hereditary chondrocalcinosis in an Ashkenazi Jewish family. Ann. Rheum. Dis. 49:528, 1990.

22a. Doherty, M., Hamilton, E., Henderson, J., Mista, H., and Dixey, J.: Familial chondrocalcinosis due to calcium pyrophosphate dihydrate crystal deposition in English families. Br. J. Rheumatol. 30:10, 1991.

23. Chuck, A. J., Pattrick, M. G., Hamilton, E., Wilson, R., and Doherty, M.: Crystal deposition in hypophosphatasia: a reappraisal. Ann. Rheum. Dis. 48:571, 1989.

24. Salvarani, C., Rossi, F., Macchioni, P. L., Baricchi, R., Capozzoli, N., Castellani, S., Ghirelli, L., Veneziani, M., Scarti, L., and Portioli, I.: Bartter's syndrome and chondrocalcinosis: a possible role for hypomagnesemia in the deposition of calcium pyrophosphate dihydrate (CPPD) crystals. Clin. Exp. Rheumatol. 7:415, 1989.

25. Pritchard, M. H., and Jessop, J. D.: Chondrocalcinosis in primary hyperparathyroidism—influence of age, metabolic bone disease, and parathyroidectomy. Ann. Rheum. Dis. 36:146, 1977.

26. Rynes, R. I., and Merzig, E. G.: Calcium pyrophosphate crystal deposition disease and hyperparathyroidism: a controlled, prospective study. J. Rheumatol. 5:460, 1978.

27. McGill, P. E., Grange, A. T., and Royston, S. M.: Chondrocalcinosis in primary hyperparathyroidism—influence of parathyroid activity and age. Scand. J. Rheumatol. 13:56, 1984.

28. Geelhoed, G. W., and Kelly, T. R.: Pseudogout as a clue and complication in primary hyperparathyroidism. Surgery 106:1036, 1989.

29. Dymock, I. W., Hamilton, E. B., Laws, J. W., et al.: Arthropathy of hemochromatosis. Ann. Rheum. Dis. 29:469, 1970.

30. Huaux, J. P., Geubel, A., Koch, M. C., Malghem, J., Maldague, B., Devogelaer, J. P., and Nagant de Deuxchaisnesm, C.: The arthritis of hemochromatosis. A Review of 25 cases with special reference to chondrocalcinosis, and a comparison with patients with primary hyperparathyroidism and controls. Clin. Rheumatol. 5:317, 1986.

31. Milazzo, S. C., Ahern, M. J., Cleland, L. G., and Henderson, D. R. F.: Calcium pyrophosphate dihydrate deposition disease and familial hypomagnesemia. J. Rheumatol. 8:767, 1981.

32. Resnick, D., and Rausch, J. M.: Hypomagnesemia with chondrocalcinosis. J. Assoc. Can. Radiol. 35:214, 1984.

33. Hernborg, J., Linden, B., and Nilsson, B. O.: Chondrocalcinosis: a secondary finding in osteoarthritis of the knee. Geriatrics 32:123, 1977.

34. Felson, D. T., Anderson, J. J., Naimark, A., Kannel, W., and Meenan, R. F.: The prevalence of chondrocalcinosis in the elderly and its association with knee osteoarthritis: The Framingham study. J. Rheumatol. 16:1241, 1989.

35. Bird, H. A., Tribe, C. R., and Bacon, P. A.: Joint hypermobility leading to osteoarthritis and chondrocalcinosis. Ann. Rheum. Dis. 37:203, 1978.

36. Dorwart, B. B., and Schumacher, H. R.: Joint effusions, chondrocalcinosis, and other rheumatic manifestations in hypothyroidism. Am. J. Med. 59:780, 1975.

37. Alexander, G. M., Dieppe, P. A., Doherty, M., and Scott, D. G.: Pyrophosphate arthropathy: a study of metabolic associations and laboratory parameters. Ann. Rheum. Dis. 41:377, 1982.

38. Komatireddy, G. R., Ellman, M. H., and Brown, N. L.: Lack of association between hypothyroidism and chondrocalcinosis. J. Rheumatol. 16:807, 1989.

39. Ryan, L. M., Liang, G., and Kozin, F.: Amyloid arthropathy: possible association with chondrocalcinosis. J. Rheumatol. 9:273, 1982.

40. Feller, E. R., and Schumacher, H. R.: Osteoarticular changes in Wilson's disease. Arthritis Rheum. 15:259, 1972.

41. Reginato, A. J., Schumacher, H. R., and Martinez, V. A.: Ochronotic arthropathy with calcium pyrophosphate crystal deposition. Arthritis Rheum. 16:705, 1973.

42. Hamilton, E. B. D., Bomford, A. B., Laws, J. W., and Williams, R.: The natural history of arthritis in idiopathic haemochromatosis: progression of the clinical and radiological features over ten years. Q. J. Med. 199:321, 1981.

43. Wardle, E. N., and Patton, J. E.: Bone and joint changes in hemochromatosis. Ann. Rheum. Dis. 28:15, 1969.

44. McCarty, D. J., and Pepe, P. F.: Erythrocyte neutral inorganic pyrophosphate in pseudogout. J. Lab. Clin. Med. 79:277, 1972.

45. Cheng, P. T., and Pritzker, K. P.: Ferrous [Fe^{++}] but not ferric [Fe] ions inhibit de novo formation of calcium pyrophosphate dihydrate crystals: possible relationships to chondrocalcinosis and hemochromatosis. J. Rheumatol. 15:321, 1988.

46. Ellman, M. H., Brown, N. L., and Porat, A. P.: Laboratory investigations in pseudogout patients and controls. J. Rheumatol. 7:77, 1980.

47. Phelps, P., and Hawker, C. D.: Serum parathyroid hormone levels in patients with calcium pyrophosphate crystal deposition disease (chondrocalcinosis, pseudogout). Arthritis Rheum. 16:590, 1973.

48. Richards, A. J., and Hamilton, E. B. D.: Destructive arthropathy in chondrocalcinosis articularis. Ann. Rheum. Dis. 33:196, 1974.

49. Halverson, P. B., and McCarty, D. J.: Patterns of radiographic abnormalities associated with basic calcium phosphate and calcium pyrophosphate dihydrate crystal deposition in the knee. Ann. Rheum. Dis. 45:603, 1986.

50. Russell, R. G. G.: Metabolism of inorganic pyrophosphate (PPi). Arthritis Rheum. 19(Suppl.):465, 1976.

51. Marx, S. J., Attie, M. F., Levine, M. A., et al.: The hypocalciuric or benign variant of familial hypercalcemia: clinical and biochemical features in fifteen kindreds. Medicine 60:397, 1981.

52. Palmoski, M., and Brandt, K.: Stimulation of glycosaminoglycan biosynthesis by amyloid fibrils. Biochem. J. 148:145, 1975.

53. Kula, R., Engel, W., and Line, B.: Scanning for soft tissue amyloid. Lancet 1:92, 1977.

54. McCarty, D.: Crystals, joints and consternation. Ann. Rheum. Dis. 42:243, 1983.

55. Moskowitz, R. W., and Katz, D.: Chondrocalcinosis and chondrocalsynovitis (pseudogout syndrome)—analysis of twenty-four cases. Am. J. Med. 43:322, 1967.

56. Doherty, M.: Pyrophosphate arthropathy—recent clinical advances. Ann. Rheum. Dis. 42(Suppl.):38, 1983.

57. Rahman, M. U., Shenberger, K. N., and Schumacher, H. R., Jr.: Initially unrecognized calcium pyrophosphate dihydrate deposition disease as a cause of fever. Am. J. Med. 89:115, 1990.

58. Moskowitz, R. W., and Katz, D.: Chondrocalcinosis coincidental to other rheumatic disease. Arch. Intern. Med. 115:680, 1965.

59. Brasseur, J. P., Huaux, J. P., Devogelaer, J. P., and De Deuxchaisnes, C. N.: Articular chondrocalcinosis in seropositive rheumatoid arthritis. Comparison with a control group. J. Rheumatol. 14:40, 1987.

60. Jacobelli, S. G., McCarty, D. J., Silcox, D. C., et al.: Calcium pyrophosphate dihydrate crystal deposition in neuropathic joints: four cases of polyarticular involvement. Ann. Intern. Med. 79:340, 1973.

61. Menerey, K., Braunstein, E., Brown, M., Swartz, R., Brown, C., and Fox, I. H.: Musculoskeletal symptoms related to arthropathy in patients receiving dialysis. J. Rheumatol. 15:1848, 1988.
62. Braunstein, E. M., Menerey, K., Martel, W., Swartz, R., and Fox, I. H.: Radiologic features of a pyrophosphate-like arthropathy associated with long-term dialysis. Skeletal Radiol. 16:437, 1987.
63. Pascual, E., Tovar, J., and Teresa Ruiz, M.: The ordinary light microscope: an appropriate tool for provisional detection and identification of crystals in synovial fluid. Ann. Rheum. Dis. 48:983, 1989.
64. Kerolus, G., Clayburne, G., and Schumacher, H. R.: Is it mandatory to examine synovial fluids promptly after arthrocentesis? Arthritis Rheum. 32:271, 1989.
65. Tanphaiachit, R. K., Spilberg, I., and Hahn, B. H.: Lithium heparin crystals simulating CPPD crystals. Arthritis Rheum. 19:966, 1976.
66. Reginato, A. J., Ferreiro Seoane, J. L., Barbaza Alvarez, C., Mitja Piferrer, J., Vidal Meijon, L., Pascual Turon, R., Vasconez, F., Rivera, E. R., Clayburne, G., and Rothfuss, S.: Arthropathy and cutaneous calcinosis in hemodialysis oxalosis. Arthritis Rheum. 29:1387, 1986.
67. Moskowitz, R. W., Harris, B. K., Schwartz, A., et al.: Chronic synovitis as a manifestation of calcium crystal deposition disease. Arthritis Rheum. 14:109, 1971.
68. Choi, S. J., Schumacher, H. R., Jr., Clayburne, G., Rothfuss, M. S., and Sieck, M.: Liposome-induced synovitis in rabbits. Arthritis Rheum. 29:889, 1986.
69. Paul, H., Reginato, A. J., and Schumacher, H. R.: Alizarin red S staining as a screening test to detect calcium compounds in synovial fluid. Arthritis Rheum. 26:191, 1983.
69a. Hamilton, E., Patrick, M., Hobby, J., Derrick, G., and Doherty, M.: Synovial fluid calcium pyrophosphate crystal and alizarin red positivity: analysis of 3000 samples. Br. J. Rheumatol. 29:101, 1990.
70. Parlee, D. E., Freundlich, I. M., and McCarty, D. J., Jr.: Comparative study of roentgenographic techniques for detection of calcium pyrophosphate dihydrate deposits (pseudogout) in human cartilage. Am. J. Roentgenol. Radium Ther. Nucl. Med. 99:688, 1967.
71. Genant, H. K., Doi, K., and Mall, J. C.: Optical versus radiographic magnification for fine-detail skeletal radiography. Invest. Radiol. 10:169, 1975.
72. Doi, K., Genant, H. K., and Rossmann, K.: Effect of film graininess and geometric unsharpness of image quality in fine-detail skeletal radiography. Invest. Radiol. 10:35, 1975.
73. Resnick, D., and Utsinger, P. D.: The wrist arthropathy of "pseudogout" occurring with and without chondrocalcinosis. Radiology 113:633, 1974.
74. Dieppe, P. A., Alexander, G. J. M., Jones, H. E., Doherty, M., Scott, D. G. I., Manhire, A., and Watt, I.: Pyrophosphate arthropathy: a clinical and radiological study of 105 cases. Ann. Rheum. Dis. 41:371, 1982.
75. Martel, W., Champion, C. K., Thompson, G. R., et al.: A roentgenologically distinctive arthropathy in some patients with pseudogout syndrome. Am. J. Roentgenol. 109:587, 1970.
76. Ryan, L., and McCarty, D. J.: Calcium pyrophosphate crystal deposition disease; pseudogout; articular chondrocalcinosis. In McCarty, D. J. (ed.): Arthritis and Allied Conditions. 10th ed. Philadelphia, Lea & Febiger, 1985, p. 1522.
77. Jobanputra, P., and Gibson, T.: Diagnosis of pseudogout and septic arthritis. Br. J. Rheumatol. 26:379, 1987.
78. Lurie, D. P., and Musil, G.: Staphylococcal septic arthritis presenting as acute flare of pseudogout: clinical, pathological and arthroscopic findings with a review of the literature. J. Rheumatol. 10:503, 1983.
79. Schumacher, H. R., Bonner, H., Thompson, J. J., Kester, W. L., and Benner, J. J.: Tumor-like soft tissue swelling of the distal phalanx due to calcium pyrophosphate dihydrate crystal deposition. Arthritis Rheum. 27:1428, 1984.
80. Goodwin, D. R. A., and Arbel, R.: Pseudogout of the wrist presenting as acute median nerve compression. J. Hand Surg. 10B:261, 1985.
81. Gerster, J.-C., Lagier, R., and Boivin, G.: Olecranon bursitis related to calcium pyrophosphate dihydrate crystal deposition disease. Arthritis Rheum. 25:989, 1982.
82. Richards, A. J., and Hamilton, E. B. D.: Spinal changes in idiopathic chondrocalcinosis articularis. Rheumatol. Rehabil. 15:138, 1976.
83. Hutton, C. W., Doherty, M., and Dieppe, P. A.: Acute pseudogout of the temporomandibular joint: a report of three cases and review of the literature. Br. J. Rheumatol 26:51, 1987.
84. el-Khoury, G. Y., Foucar, E., Blair, W. F., Strottmann, M. P., Malvitz, T. A., and Smoker, W. R.: Case report 364: Massive calcium pyrophosphate dihydrate crystal deposition disorder (MCPDD) involving thumb. Skeletal Radiol. 15:313, 1986.
85. Bergausen, E. J., Balogh, K., Landis, W. J., Lee, D. D., and Wright, A. M.: Cervical myelopathy attributable to pseudogout. Case report with radiologic, histologic, and crystallographic observations. Clin. Orthop. 214:217, 1987.
86. Ciricillo, S. F., and Weinstein, P. R.: Foramen magnum syndrome from pseudogout of the atlanto-occipital ligament. Case report. J. Neurosurg. 71:141, 1989.

87. Ellman, M. H., Vazquez, L. T., Brown, N. L., and Mandel, N.: Calcium pyrophosphate dihydrate deposition in lumbar disc fibrocartilage. J. Rheumatol. 8:955, 1981.
88. Andres, T. L., and Trainer, T. D.: Intervertebral chondrocalcinosis—a coincidental finding possibly related to previous surgery. Arch. Pathol. Lab. Med. 104:269, 1980.
89. Doherty, M., Watt, I., and Dieppe, P. A.: Localised chondrocalcinosis in post-meniscectomy knees. Lancet 1:1207, 1982.
90. Bjelle, A.: The glycosaminoglycans of articular cartilage in calcium pyrophosphate dihydrate (CPPD) crystal deposition disease (chondrocalcinosis articularis or pyrophosphate arthropathy). Calc. Tiss. Res. 12:37, 1973.
91. Hunter, G. K., Grynpas, M. D., Cheng, P. T., and Pritzker, K. P.: Effect of glycosaminoglycans on calcium pyrophosphate crystal formation in collagen gels. Calcif. Tissue Int. 41:164, 1987.
92. Lust, G., Faure, G., Netter, P., Gaucher, A., and Seegmiller, J. E.: Evidence of a generalised metabolic defect in patients with hereditary chondrocalcinosis: increased inorganic pyrophosphate in cultured fibroblasts and lymphoblasts. Arthritis Rheum. 24:1517, 1981.
93. Ryan, L. M., Wortmann, R. L., Karas, B., Lynch, M. P., and McCarty, D. J.: Pyrophosphohydrolase activity and inorganic pyrophosphate content of cultured human skin fibroblasts. Elevated levels in some patients with calcium pyrophosphate dihydrate deposition disease. J. Clin. Invest. 77:1689, 1986.
94. Tenenbaum, J., Numiz, O., Schumacher, H. R., Good, A. E., and Howell, D. S.: Comparison of phosphohydrolase activities from articular cartilage in calcium pyrophosphate deposition disease and primary osteoarthritis. Arthritis Rheum. 24:492, 1981.
95. Howell, D. S., Martel-Pelletier, J., Pelletier, J.-P., Morales, S., and Muniz, O.: NTP pyrophosphohydrolase in human chondrocalcinotic and osteoarthritic cartilage. II. Further studies on histologic and subcellular distribution. Arthritis Rheum. 27:193, 1984.
96. Muniz, O., Pelletier, J.-P., Martel-Pelletier, J., Morales, S., and Howell, D. S.: NTP pyrophosphohydrolase in human chondrocalcinotic and osteoarthritic cartilage. I. Some biochemical characteristics. Arthritis Rheum. 27:186, 1984.
97. Ryan, L. M., Wortmann, R. L., Karas, B., and McCarty, D. J.: Cartilage nucleoside triphosphate (NTP) pyrophosphohydrolase. I. Identification as an ecto-enzyme. Arthritis Rheum. 27:404, 1984.
98. Ryan, L. M., Wortmann, R. L., Karas, B., and McCarty, D. J.: Cartilage nucleoside triphosphate pyrophosphohydrolase. II. Role in extracellular pyrophosphate generation and nucleotide metabolism. Arthritis Rheum. 28:413, 1985.
99. Rachow, J. W., Ryan, L. M.: Adenosine triphosphate pyrophosphohydrolase and neutral inorganic pyrophosphatase in pathologic joint fluids: elevated pyrophosphohydrolase in calcium pyrophosphate dihydrate crystal deposition disease. Arthritis Rheum. 28:1283, 1985.
99a. Ryan, L. M., Rachow, J. W., and McCarty, D. J.: Synovial fluid ATP: A potential substrate for the production of inorganic pyrophosphate. J. Rheumatol. 18:716, 1991.
100. Ryan, L. M., Kurup, I., Rosenthal, A. K., and McCarty, D. J.: Stimulation of inorganic pyrophosphate elaboration by cultured cartilage and chondrocytes. Arch. Biochem. Biophys. 272:393, 1989.
101. Rosenthal, A. K., Cheung, H. S., and Ryan, L. M.: Augmentation of inorganic pyrophosphate elaboration in cartilage by serum factors. Arch. Biochem. Biophys. 272:386, 1989.
102. Rosenthal, A. K., Cheung, H. S., and Ryan, L. M.: Stimulation of pyrophosphate production in articular cartilage by a platelet-derived factor is independent of mitogenesis. J. Lab. Clin. Med. 115:352, 1990.
103. Rosenthal, A. K., Cheung, H. S., and Ryan, L. M.: Transforming growth factor β1 stimulates inorganic pyrophosphate elaboration by porcine cartilage. Arthritis Rheum. 34:904, 1991.
104. Ryan, L. M., Kurup, I., McCarty, D. J., and Cheung, H. S.: Cartilage inorganic pyrophosphate elaboration is independent of sulfated glycosaminoglycan synthesis. Arthritis Rheum. 33:235, 1990.
105. Pritzker, K. P., Chateauvert, J., Grynpas, M. D., Renlund, R. C., Turnquist, J., and Kessler, M. J.: Rhesus macaques as an experimental model for degenerative arthritis. P. R. Health Sci. J. 8:99, 1989.
106. Renlund, R. C., Pritzker, K. P., Cheng, P. T., and Kessler, M. J.: Rhesus monkeys (Macaca mulatta) as a model for calcium pyrophosphate dihydrate crystal deposition disease. J. Med. Primatol. 15:11, 1986.
107. Kozin, F., and McCarty, D. S.: Protein binding to monosodium urate monohydrate, calcium pyrophosphate dihydrate and silicon dioxide crystals. I. Physical characteristics. J. Lab. Clin. Med. 89:1314, 1977.
108. Kozin, F., and McCarty, D. J.: Protein absorption to monosodium urate, calcium pyrophosphate dihydrate, and silica crystals. Relationship to the pathogenesis of crystal-induced inflammation. Arthritis Rheum. 19:433, 1976.
109. Schumacher, H. R., Fishbein, P., Phelps, P., et al.: Comparison of sodium urate and calcium pyrophosphate crystal phagocytosis by polymorphonuclear leukocytes. Effects of crystal size and other factors. Arthritis Rheum. 18:783, 1975.
110. Spilberg, I., Gallacher, A., and Mandell, B.: Calcium pyrophosphate

dihydrate (CPPD) crystal–induced chemotactic factor: subcellular localization role of protein synthesis and phagocytosis. J. Lab. Clin. Med. 89:817, 1977.

111. Burt, H. M., Jackson, J. K., and Rowell, J.: Calcium pyrophosphate and monosodium urate crystal interactions with neutrophils: effect of crystal size and lipoprotein binding to crystals. J. Rheumatol. 16:809, 1989.

112. Guerne, P. A., Terkeltaub, R., Zuraw, B., and Lotz, M.: Inflammatory microcrystals stimulate interleukin-6 production and secretion by human monocytes and synoviocytes. Arthritis Rheum. 32:1443, 1989.

113. Spilberg, I., Mandell, B., Mehta, J. M., et al.: Mechanism of action of colchicine in acute urate crystal–induced arthritis. J. Clin. Invest. 64:775, 1979.

114. McCarty, D. J., Solomon, S. D., Warnock, M. L., et al.: Inorganic pyrophosphate concentrations in the synovial fluid of arthritis patients. J. Lab. Clin. Med. 78:216, 1971.

115. Doherty, M., and Dieppe, P. A.: Acute pseudogout: crystal shedding or acute crystallization. Arthritis Rheum. 24:954, 1981.

116. McCarty, D. J., Palmer, D. W., and Halverson, P. B.: Clearance of calcium pyrophosphate dihydrate (CPPD) crystals in vivo. I. Studies using ^{169}Yb labelled triclinic crystals. Arthritis Rheum. 22:718, 1979.

117. McCarty, D. J., Palmer, D. W., and James, C.: Clearance of calcium pyrophosphate dihydrate (CPPD) crystals in vivo. II. Studies using triclinic crystals doubly labelled with ^{45}C and ^{85}Sr. Arthritis Rheum. 22:1122, 1979.

118. Meed, S. D., and Spilberg, I.: Successful use of colchicine in acute polyarticular pseudogout. J. Rheumatol. 8:689, 1981.

119. Alvarellos, A., and Spilberg, I.: Colchicine prophylaxis in pseudogout. J. Rheumatol. 13:804, 1986.

120. Bowles, C., Harrington, T., Zinsmeister, A., Ellman, M., Reginato, A., McCarty, D., Ryan, L., Episonsa, L., Spilberg I., and O'Duffy, D.: Colchicine prevents recurrent pseudogout: multicenter trial. Arthritis Rheum. 29(Suppl.):S38, 1986.

121. McKendry, R. J. R., Uhthoff, H. K., Sarkar, K., et al.: Calcifying tendinitis of the shoulder: prognostic value of clinical, histologic and radiologic features in 57 surgically treated cases. J. Rheumatol. 9:75, 1982.

122. Pinals, R. S., and Short, C. L.: Calcific periarthritis involving multiple sites. Arthritis Rheum. 9:566, 1966.

123. McCarty, D. J., and Gatter, R. A.: Recurrent acute inflammation associated with focal apatite crystal deposition. Arthritis Rheum. 9:804, 1966.

124. Moskowitz, R. W., Vertes, V., Schwartz, A., et al.: Crystal-induced inflammation associated with chronic renal failure treated with periodic hemodialysis. Am. J. Med. 47:450, 1969.

125. Marcos, J. C., De Benyacar, M. A., Garcia-Morteo, O., Arturi, A. S., Maldonado-Cocco, J. A., Morales, V. H., and Laguens, R. P.: Idiopathic familial chondrocalcinosis due to apatite crystal deposition. Am. J. Med. 71:557, 1981.

126. Dieppe, P. A., Crocker, P., Huskisson, E. C., et al.: Apatite deposition disease. Lancet 1:266, 1976.

127. Schumacher, H. R., Somlyo, A. P., Tse, R. L., and Maurer, K.: Arthritis associated with apatite crystals. Ann. Intern. Med. 87:411, 1977.

128. Schumacher, H. R., Miller, J. L., Ludivico, C., and Jessar, R. A.: Erosive arthritis associated with apatite crystal deposition. Arthritis Rheum. 24:31, 1981.

129. McCarty, D. J., Halverson, P. B., Carrera, G. F., Brewer, B. J., and Kozin, F.: "Milwaukee shoulder"—association of microspheroids containing hydroxyapatite crystals, active collagenase, and neutral protease with rotator cuff defects. Arthritis Rheum. 24:464, 1981.

130. Halverson, P. B., Cheung, H. S., McCarty, D. J., Garancis, J., and Mandel, N.: "Milwaukee shoulder"—association of microspheroids containing hydroxyapatite crystals, active collagenase and neutral protease with rotator cuff defects. II. Synovial fluid studies. Arthritis Rheum. 24:474, 1981.

131. Halverson, P. B., Carrera, G. F., and McCarty, D. J.: Milwaukee shoulder syndrome. Fifteen additional cases and a description of contributing factors. Arch. Intern. Med. 150:677, 1990.

132. Cheung, H. S., and McCarty, D. J.: Mitogenesis induced by calcium-containing crystals: the role of intracellular dissolution. Exp. Cell Res. 157:63, 1985.

133. Borkowf, A., and Cheung, H. S.: Basic calcium phosphate crystals stimulate mitogenesis and collagenase production by different mechanisms. Arthritis Rheum. 30(Suppl.):S133, 1987.

134. Dieppe, P. A., Doherty, M., Macfarlane, D. G., Hutton, C. W., et al.: Apatite-associated destructive arthritis. Br. J. Rheumatol. 23:84, 1984.

135. Rachow, J. W., Ryan, L. M., McCarty, D. J., and Halverson, P.: Synovial fluid inorganic pyrophosphate concentration and nucleotide pyrophosphohydrolase activity in basic calcium phosphate arthropathy and Milwaukee shoulder syndrome. Arthritis Rheum. 31:408, 1988.

136. Fam, A. G., Pritzker, K. P. H., Stein, J. L., Houpt, J. B., and Little, A. H.: Apatite-associated arthropathy: a clinical study of 14 cases and of 2 patients with calcific bursitis. J. Rheumatol. 6:461, 1979.

137. Weinstein, R. S.: Focal mineralization defect during disodium etidronate treatment of calcinosis. Calcif. Tiss. Int. 34:224, 1982.

Chapter 78

Kenneth D. Brandt
Henry J. Mankin

Pathogenesis of Osteoarthritis

INTRODUCTION

This chapter details the descriptive pathology of osteoarthritis and emphasizes the two principal morphologic changes associated with the disease: (1) progressive softening, ulceration, and focal disintegration of the articular cartilage and (2) the formation of bone and cartilage excrescences at the joint margins (osteophytes).[1] The sequence of these changes, their inter-relationship and, in fact, their pathogenesis are not yet well understood. As noted in Chapter 79, the theories proposed by most researchers in this field are that the pathologic changes of osteoarthritis are the consequence of a wide variety of etiologic factors (some possibly interactive) that ultimately lead to failure of the mechanical properties of the joint, causing a breakdown of the articular cartilage.

STRUCTURAL AND BIOCHEMICAL FEATURES OF NORMAL ARTICULAR CARTILAGE

Articular cartilage is sparsely cellular (see Chapter 1); its biochemical characteristics, therefore, reflect principally the composition of the hyaline extracellular matrix. It should be clearly noted that the biochemical composition of normal articular cartilage varies considerably from species to species, from joint to joint, from site to site within any given joint, and with depth from the surface.

Examination of Table 78–1 shows that the matrix of normal cartilage is hyperhydrated, with its water content ranging from 65 to almost 80 percent. The water appears to exist principally in the form of either a proteoglycan or a collagen gel. Hence, it is freely exchangeable with the synovial fluid, although a small portion of the cartilage water is tightly bound to matrix components.[2, 3] A small inorganic compo-

nent is present in the form of a calcium salt, but this usually accounts for less than 5 percent of the dry weight of the tissue. The bulk of the remaining material is accounted for by the complex and interactive macromolecules, proteoglycans (both subunit and aggregate), and type II collagen.

The nature of the proteoglycans of articular cartilage is described in Chapter 3. For purposes of the following discussion, particularly in attempting to compare material from pathologic tissue with that from normal cartilage, a brief review is warranted. The predominant species of proteoglycans in cartilage, named "aggrecan," contains a large protein core ($M_r = 245$ kD) to which numerous chains of chondroitin 4-sulfate, chondroitin 6-sulfate, and keratan sulfate are covalently bound before the proteoglycan is secreted into the extracellular matrix.[4-6] The structure and function of the proteoglycans in the cartilage are detailed in Chapter 3.

The glycosaminoglycans occupy an electronegative domain of enormous proportions, and the stiff-

Table 78–1. BIOCHEMICAL COMPOSITION OF ADULT ARTICULAR CARTILAGE

As Percentage of Total Weight	
Water	66–78%
Solids	22–34%
As Percentage of Dry Weight	
Inorganic	
Ash (principally hydroxyapatite)	5–6%
Organic	
Collagen (type II)	48–62%
Proteoglycan	22–38%
Noncollagenous matrix proteins	5–15%
Minor collagens	<5%
Lipid	<1%
Hyaluronate and other saccharides	<1%
Chondronectin	<1%

ness and resiliency of the tissues are the result of the relative incompressibility of the complex proteoglycan molecules.[1] Furthermore, ample evidence exists that the proteoglycans interact with the collagen fibers. This may be an important factor in resisting shear as well as compression.

The second major component of the cartilage matrix (other than the proteoglycans) is type II collagen,[8] which has been extensively studied and is the first of the genetically distinct species of cartilage collagen to have been identified.[9]

While the predominant collagen species in articular cartilage is type II, minor amounts of type IX are covalently cross-linked to the surface of type II fibrils, and type XI appears to exist centrally within the type II fibril. Experimental data suggest that a "glue" bonds intersecting type II fibers together in the matrix. Although a molecule subserving this function has not yet been identified, the type IX collagen on the surface of the type II fibril has been considered a likely candidate.[10, 11] However, there is as yet no evidence that type IX is involved in inter-fibrillar interactions, and, based on stereochemical considerations, for type IX to function in this capacity would probably require an intermediary molecule (proteoglycan).[12] Oegema and Thompson have shown that type X collagen is present in the calcified zone of normal adult articular cartilage.[13]

The collagen fibers of most mammalian cartilages are not randomly distributed but appear to have a high degree of ordering. Thick bundles of collagen fibers lying subjacent and parallel to the surface form a "skin" and possibly serve not only as a limiting membrane but also to distribute the forces associated with compression. In contrast, the fibers in the basal layer of cartilage lie perpendicular to the surface and serve as anchors, tethering the uncalcified cartilage to the calcified zone and perhaps to the subchondral bony end-plate. In the midregions the fibers are arranged more randomly but may lie in coarse oblique bundles that aid in resisting tension. As indicated earlier, the type II collagen fibers are probably maintained in position partly by the proteoglycans, but they seem also to be connected to other matrix components and cells by small amounts of fibronectin,[14, 15] chondronectin,[16] and anchorin.[17]

Of some interest is the now well-established presence of an additional component of articular cartilage—"matrix proteins" of various sizes. These have been characterized to varying degrees[4, 18] and represent a family of additional glycoproteins, the detailed composition and function of which are largely obscure.[19] They may account for as much as 15 percent of the dry weight of the matrix.

METABOLISM OF NORMAL CARTILAGE MATRIX

The collagen in normal adult joint cartilage has been considered to be extremely stable metabolically,

and although most investigators report very long half-lives for newly synthesized collagen, others have suggested that a small proportion may have a much more rapid turnover, with a half-life of only several months.[20, 21] In support of such a view is the finding of a collagenase[22] in normal cartilage that can be activated by stromelysin[23] under the influence of synovial[24] or cartilage[25] interleukin-1 and other cytokines.

Proteoglycans seem to have a much more rapid turnover than cartilage collagen, although considerable metabolic heterogeneity is present. A small proportion of the cartilage proteoglycans may have a half-life as short as 8 days[26]; other data, however, support the probability that some of the sulfated glycosaminoglycans are so stable that they exhibit half-lives of 45 days (rabbit cartilage) or 250 to 600 days (human cartilage).[27]

This normal turnover of matrix constituents presumably reflects an enzymatically mediated process directed by the chondrocyte to satisfy needs for internal remodeling. The disappearance rates for radionuclide tracers of glycosaminoglycan synthesis appear to be similar throughout the depth of normal articular cartilage,[28] denying the possible explanation that the cartilage surface is being "shed." The processes required for synthesis of collagen appear to be independent of those for proteoglycans, since interference with the synthesis of one does not affect the other.[29, 30]

Polypeptide mediators, e.g., insulin-like growth factor-1 (IGF-1) and transforming growth factor-beta (TGF-β), stimulate synthesis of aggrecan and of collagen. These growth factors function as endocrine, paracrine, and autocrine regulators of matrix metabolism in normal cartilage.[31] They can modulate both anabolic and catabolic pathways of chondrocyte metabolism; for example, they increase proteoglycan synthesis and decrease proteoglycan aggregation, thereby reducing loss of aggrecan from the matrix.

Although the control mechanisms responsible for normal degradation of matrix constituents are not well understood, the processes associated with the degradation of proteoglycans are mediated largely by cellular autolytic enzymes, chiefly lysosomal in origin and consisting of acid proteases, glycosidases, and sulfatases. These have been extensively studied and at least partially purified.[22, 32–34]

The release of collagenase and proteoglycan-degrading proteases from the chondrocyte may be mediated by interleukin-1 (IL-1), which was initially designated "catabolin" and is a low molecular weight protein produced by mononuclear cells, including those in synovium, and by the chondrocytes themselves.[25] As indicated earlier, IL-1 stimulates synthesis and release of stromelysin, which is able to activate procollagenase within cartilage. Tumor necrosis factor (TNF) has similar activities, but its effects on chondrocytes are much less potent than those of IL-1. Equally relevant to the issues surrounding the control mechanisms for matrix turnover, normal cartilage contains a tissue inhibitor of metalloproteinases (TIMP),[35, 36] which inhibits the activities of collagenase and stromelysin.

BIOMECHANICAL CONSEQUENCES OF THE MACROMOLECULAR ORGANIZATION OF NORMAL ARTICULAR CARTILAGE
(see also Chapter 99)

Weight-bearing joints are repeatedly subjected to localized high loads. Although the soft tissues (e.g., muscles) and the subchondral bone play major roles in dissipating the energy of weight bearing, considerable mechanical force is transmitted to the cartilage. Normal joint cartilage dissipates this force by virtue of its special properties (e.g., compressibility, elasticity, and self-lubrication), all of which are attributable to its chemical composition and interactions between collagen, proteoglycans, and other molecular constituents. If not for this protective effect of the cartilage, bone would be quickly worn away by the frictional forces within the joint.

Because of its high proteoglycan concentration, cartilage has low hydraulic permeability,[37] which limits the amount of interstitial fluid lost from the surface when it is loaded in compression. Thus, when load is applied, although the pressure within the cartilage rises immediately, the cartilage deforms gradually and reversibly as water is surrendered to the joint surface as a squeeze-film; when the load is removed, the layer of exuded fluid on the surface is reimbibed.

Since the high fixed negative charge density of the proteoglycans allows them to hold enormous amounts of water, constraint of the proteoglycans by the collagen meshwork creates considerable swelling pressure within the tissue.[38] This pressure has been calculated to be greater than 3 atmospheres even in the absence of load.[39] Nonetheless, normal cartilage does not swell appreciably when placed in hypotonic solution, since the high swelling pressure of the proteoglycans is counteracted by strong tensile forces within the collagen network.

During weight bearing, the collagen network is subjected to even greater tensile stresses than it is when the joint is unloaded. When a compressive load is applied to cartilage, although the flow of water is impeded by the high interstitial swelling pressure and low hydraulic permeability of the tissue, the aqueous proteoglycan gel attempts to move away from the loaded region. The pressure gradient, however, restricts upward flow while the subchondral bone opposes downward flow. Flow, therefore, occurs mainly laterally, where it is restricted by the collagen network. The network thus receives forces acting radially from the center of the applied load, whose main vector is parallel to the joint surface. It has been shown that the tensile strength of articular cartilage is greater in this direction than in a plane perpendicular to the surface.

As indicated earlier, the functional collagen net-

work of cartilage consists of not only the type II collagen fibers themselves but also substances that may "glue" them together, to help inhibit slippage of adjacent fibers over each other. Although the collagen fibers themselves are held together by very strong covalent peptide bonds that should resist the mechanical forces transmitted to the matrix, the "glue" may be vulnerable to mechanical damage or enzymatic degradation, and this may be a proximate or contributing factor in the pathogenesis of osteoarthritis.

CHANGES IN OSTEOARTHRITIC CARTILAGE

Even if the articular cartilage is not the site of the primary abnormality within the osteoarthritic joint—and most authorities agree that it is (see Chapter 79)—it is the tissue that shows the greatest aberration from normal.

Morphologic Changes. The morphologic changes in the articular cartilage of the osteoarthritic joint are well known and are described in detail in Chapter 79.[1] The articular cartilage surface that remains has lost its homogeneous nature and is disrupted and fragmented, with pitting, clefts, and ulceration. Sometimes, with advancing disease, no cartilage remains, and bare areas are seen in which the underlying bone is exposed. Histochemical staining of the matrix for proteoglycans is uneven, and the "tidemark," which separates the calcified cartilage from the radial zone, is invaded by capillaries. The cells lie in brood clusters or clones,[40] with sometimes 50 or more cells in a cluster. Osteophytes are capped by newly formed hyaline and fibrocartilage and show great irregularity in their structure.[1, 41, 42]

Biochemical Changes. The water content of the articular cartilage is significantly increased. As has been noted by Maroudas and coworkers,[2] osteoarthritic cartilage swells markedly when immersed in fluid. This suggests some weakening of the retaining collagen network.[38, 39]

As noted, normal articular cartilage contains type II collagen.[25] Although cartilage from an osteoarthritic femoral head has been reported to contain type I as well as type II[43] collagen, suggesting that collagen synthesis by the osteoarthritic chondrocyte underwent a phenotypic change, several other studies have shown only type II collagen in fibrillated osteoarthritic cartilage.[44] When an immunofluorescence technique was applied to the study of collagen in osteoarthritic cartilage, some type I collagen was found around chondrocyte clusters in fibrillated cartilage, but antibody to type I collagen did not localize to the bulk of the diseased tissue.[45] An increased concentration of type I collagen has been noted, however, in the cartilage covering osteophytes. Although the concentration of collagen is not altered in osteoarthritic cartilage,[46, 47] the fibers are smaller than normal, and the normally tight weave in the midzone is slackened and distorted.[41, 46]

The most marked change in osteoarthritic cartilage occurs in the proteoglycans. With advancing disease, the proteoglycan concentration diminishes sharply.[41, 47, 48] As the disease worsens, less aggregate is present, and the glycosaminoglycan chains become shorter.[49-51] The keratan sulfate concentration diminishes as well, and the proportion of chondroitin 4-sulfate increases in relation to that of chondroitin 6-sulfate, reflecting synthesis by the chondrocytes of a proteoglycan typical of immature cartilage.[52] The affinity of the cartilage for safranin O, a stain that reflects the proteoglycan concentration of the tissue, diminishes progressively until in the late stages of the disease only the counterstain can be identified.[53]

Metabolic Changes. The metabolism of articular cartilage in osteoarthritis has been examined extensively. Numerous studies indicate that the rates of synthesis and secretion of matrix-degrading enzymes by the chondrocyte are markedly increased. The activities of both lysosomal and extralysosomal enzymes, which are fully capable of degrading all the matrix macromolecules, are increased several-fold.[53-55] The best studied of these enzymes are the acid and neutral proteases,[22, 32, 36] which can attack the core protein of the proteoglycan.

It has become clear that the neutral metalloproteinases of cartilage are a family of molecules that includes collagenase, stromelysin, and gelatinase.[36] These enzymes are able to degrade all the components of the extracellular matrix. Each is secreted by the chondrocyte as a proenzyme that must be activated by proteolytic cleavage of its N-terminal sequence, and each is characterized by a zinc-binding catalytic sequence containing three histidine residues and a glutamine residue.

While the G1 region of aggrecan is highly resistant to proteases, a glutamate-alanine bond within the extended region between G1 and G2 is remarkably susceptible to proteolytic degradation.[56, 57] Very low concentrations of stromelysin readily cleave the region between G1 and G2, degrading the aggregate and leading to a loss of proteoglycans from the extracellular matrix. Some of the degraded proteoglycans may be removed by the chondrocytes; others are lost into the synovial fluid.

A specific hyaluronidase has not been found in articular cartilage, but evidence is strong that one or several lysosomal enzymes can cleave both hyaluronic acid and chondroitin 6-sulfate.[22] It has been suggested that the decrease in chondroitin sulfate chain length in osteoarthritic cartilage is due to digestion of chondroitin sulfate chains by synovial fluid hyaluronidase,[52] which may diffuse into the cartilage once the disease process has been initiated. This concept is consistent with data indicating that the concentration of hyaluronic acid in osteoarthritic cartilage is low[54] even though the rate of synthesis of hyaluronic acid is considerably greater than normal.[55] The consequence of the increased activities of all these enzymes in osteoarthritis is degradation of the proteoglycan aggregate and subunit, producing proteoglycans that are incapable of aggregation.

With respect to enzymatic degradation of the other major matrix macromolecule—type II collagen—it has been difficult to find evidence of collagenase in normal cartilage, presumably because it normally exists in very low concentrations and most of it is bound to inhibitors.[22] The presence of collagenase in cultures of human osteoarthritic cartilage was documented by Ehrlich and colleagues,[58, 59] whose data indicated that the concentration of this enzyme increased markedly in osteoarthritic cartilage, suggesting that it was a major factor in progression of the disease and in the ultimate destruction of the surface. Presumably, collagenase is involved in thinning of the collagen fibers, loosening of the tight collagen network, and consequent swelling of the cartilage matrix in osteoarthritis.

Many investigators consider that IL-1 is the prime mover for cartilage matrix degradation. This cytokine is produced by mononuclear cells (including synovial lining cells) in the inflamed joint and is synthesized by chondrocytes as an autocrine activity.[60, 61] It stimulates the synthesis and secretion of a number of degradative enzymes in cartilage, including latent collagenase, latent stromelysin, latent gelatinase, and tissue plasminogen activator.[62-65] Plasminogen, the substrate for tissue plasminogen activator (TPA), is presumably synthesized by the chondrocyte or enters the matrix by diffusion from the synovial fluid.

Obviously, the aforementioned enzymes are potentially very destructive to the cartilage. The balance of the system lies with at least two inhibitors: TIMP[36, 66] and plasminogen activator inhibitor-1 (PAI-1),[67] which serve to limit the degradative activity of the active neutral metalloproteinases and of plasminogen activator, respectively.

If either TIMP or PAI-1 is destroyed or is present in insufficient concentrations relative to the active enzymes, stromelysin and plasmin are able to act on matrix substrates. Stromelysin may act in two ways: first, as a protease, degrading the protein core of the proteoglycan; and second (and more important), as a component of the activation process for collagenase.[68] The second part of this "two-hit" system is the activation of prostromelysin by plasmin, yielding a very destructive matrix-degrading enzyme.[69]

What is the evidence that IL-1 may be important in driving the progression of cartilage breakdown in osteoarthritis? Intra-articular injection of recombinant human IL-1 was shown to lead rapidly to loss of proteoglycan from articular cartilage of rabbits.[70] A similar effect was seen in vitro after incubation of normal cartilage from young animals with IL-1.[65, 71] On the other hand, IL-1 has been found to have little effect on proteoglycan release from adult canine, adult porcine, or adult human articular cartilage.[72, 73] Furthermore, although proteoglycan synthesis by young porcine cartilage is inhibited by concentrations of IL-1 even lower than those needed to cause matrix degradation,[74] as noted previously, *stimulation*, not inhibition, of proteoglycan synthesis is seen in osteoarthritis. Although it could be argued that IL-1 effects in osteoarthritis are focal, rather than diffuse,[75] in the canine cruciate-deficient model, autoradiography using $^{35}SO_4$ showed that all cells exhibit enhanced biosynthetic activity.[76]

In view of the importance attached to neutral metalloproteinases in the degradation of cartilage matrix in osteoarthritis, it is of interest that intra-articular injection of ethylenediamine tetra-acetic acid (EDTA), which chelates divalent cations, such as zinc, reduced neutral proteoglycanase activity and the severity of cartilage degeneration in a rabbit model of osteoarthritis.[77] Recently, doxycycline, which is also a chelating agent, was shown to inhibit gelatinase and type XI collagenolytic activity in extracts of human osteoarthritic cartilage,[78] and in preliminary studies oral administration of doxycycline attenuated the severity of cartilage breakdown and markedly reduced the activities of collagenase and gelatinase in cartilage of dogs with experimentally induced osteoarthritis.[79]

Despite the decrease in the concentration of tissue proteoglycans in osteoarthritis, in the early stages of the disease there is increased synthesis of proteoglycans, collagen, noncollagenous proteins, hyaluronate, and deoxyribonucleic acid (DNA), indicating cell replication and accounting for the clones of chondrocytes observed histologically.[53, 55] (Thus, this disorder is by no means a "degenerative joint disease.") Furthermore, proteoglycan and collagen synthesis[41] continue to rise in proportion to the severity of the lesion—at least until the disease, by morphologic criteria, is far advanced. When the disease becomes sufficiently severe, however, proteoglycan synthesis falls off sharply; that is, the chondrocyte "fails."[41, 53]

The fall in tissue proteoglycan concentration occurring in the face of a marked increase in proteoglycan synthesis obviously reflects an even greater increase in proteoglycan catabolism. Since osteoarthritic cartilage appears to be relatively deficient in its content of TIMP,[80] a stoichiometric imbalance between the proteoglycanases and their inhibitors may be important in the pathogenesis of the cartilage breakdown.

Even though net proteoglycan synthesis is increased in osteoarthritis, the "quality" of the products may not be normal. Proteoglycans synthesized by the osteoarthritic chondrocyte are different from normal with respect to, for example, the composition and distribution of their glycosaminoglycans,[41, 52] the size of the proteoglycan subunit,[46, 52, 81] and their ability to aggregate with hyaluronic acid.[32, 41]

These observations raise several questions: Are the proteoglycans synthesized in osteoarthritis, whose structure is similar to that of proteoglycans in immature tissue, adequate to meet the biomechanical demands placed on adult cartilage?[46] Do the newly synthesized molecules have sufficient biochemical stability to survive normally in the tissue? Is the macromolecular organization of the proteoglycans

and collagen synthesized in osteoarthritis adequate for the requisite biomechanical function? If not, faulty organization of the repair molecules could even accelerate the breakdown of the cartilage. Data are available to suggest that all of these problems may occur in osteoarthritis.

EARLIEST MATRIX CHANGES IN OSTEOARTHRITIS

How does osteoarthritis begin? The early stages of osteoarthritis in humans cannot be readily studied, because insufficient opportunity is available to study the disease early in its course. Although, in general, one must be critical of animal models, the rabbit partial meniscectomy model[82] and the canine cruciate-deficient model[83] appear, to a large extent, to simulate many of the changes of naturally occurring osteoarthritis and provide material that shows early changes of the disease. Both of these models represent "secondary" osteoarthritis produced by internal derangement of the knee joint (see Chapter 79).

The initial biochemical changes in the dog model have been most closely studied. The very first alteration appears to be an increase in the water content of the cartilage, which is detectable within days after destabilization of the joint.[84, 85] Initially, the hyperhydration occurs focally in cartilage of the tibial plateau and femoral condyle, but it soon presents throughout the entire cartilage mass of the joint. A similar increase in water content has been noted in human osteoarthritic cartilage[52] and is believed to signify early—and possibly irreversible—matrix changes.

In addition, in the initial stages in the canine model the proteoglycans are more readily extractable from the matrix than normal. This is seen also in spontaneously occurring osteoarthritis in dogs[85] and steers[86] and in experimentally induced osteoarthritis in rabbits[87] and may be related to the increase in tissue water content, which permits greater permeability of the extracting solvent.

The immediate cause of the increase in water content of osteoarthritic cartilage is not known, but it implies a failure in the elastic restraint of the collagen network, enabling the hydrophilic proteoglycans to swell to a greater degree of hydration than normal.[2] Studies of cartilage ultrastructure in the early stages of osteoarthritis show a loss of orientation of the collagen fibers near the surface and abnormally wide separation of individual fibers.

Very shortly after the increase in cartilage water appears, the newly synthesized proteoglycans in the canine model show a change in their glycosaminoglycan composition and contain a higher proportion of chondroitin sulfate and a lower proportion of keratan sulfate than normal.[84] Also, proteoglycan aggregation may be impaired, even in the earliest stages.[85] These changes occur throughout the articular cartilages of the knee before fibrillation or other morphologic changes are evident and while the tissue proteoglycan concentration is normal or even increased. They provide an explanation for the generalized decrease in stiffness that occurs in grossly normal cartilage taken from sites adjacent to fibrillated areas.[88] With progression of the disease, focal cartilage ulcerations develop. Loss of proteoglycan is seen, accompanied by worsening of the aggregation defect, persistence of the abnormalities in glycosaminoglycan composition, and decreases in chondroitin sulfate chain length. As the loss of proteoglycan becomes sufficiently great, the water content, which is initially increased, falls below normal.

Although evidence of the depletion of matrix proteoglycans with the progression of osteoarthritis is overwhelming, in the early stages of osteoarthritis both the proteoglycan concentration and the proteoglycan content may be *increased*, and the cartilage may be thicker than normal and exhibit increases in its intensity of staining with safranin O, its proteoglycan concentration, and, commonly, the net rate of proteoglycan synthesis.[89]

In serial magnetic resonance imaging (MRI) studies of cruciate-deficient dogs with osteoarthritis, Braunstein and associates[90] demonstrated that articular cartilage in the unstable knee remained thicker than normal for as long as 36 months. (On the basis of comparative life spans, 1 year in the life of the dog represents approximately 7 years in the life of a human.) Nine months later, however, MRI scans showed marked thinning of the cartilage; in some cases, no cartilage remained on the femoral condyles. Pathologic examination confirmed the MRI results.[91]

Thickening of articular cartilage in association with an increase in cartilage proteoglycan concentration in this canine model had been suggested by earlier data of McDevitt and colleagues[92] and of Vignon and associates.[93] The phenomenon is not unique to the cruciate-deficient dog but is also seen in surgically induced osteoarthritis in rabbits[93] and primary (idiopathic) osteoarthritis in rhesus *(Macaca mulatta)* monkeys.[94, 95] Notably, in 1937, Bywaters[96] described thickening of articular cartilage in the early stages of human osteoarthritis. A similar observation was recorded by Johnson in 1959.[97] Thus, in the earlier stages of osteoarthritis, before cartilage thinning and proteoglycan depletion develop, thickening of the cartilage, associated with a marked biosynthetic response by the chondrocytes leading to an increase in the concentration of matrix proteoglycans, appears to be common.

The operational concept of the pathogenesis of osteoarthritis that has been held by many workers since it was proposed by Bollet in 1967[98] is that mechanical stresses injure the chondrocyte, causing it to release degradative enzymes that result in fibrillation and matrix breakdown. On the other hand, as proposed by Freeman,[99] mechanical stresses may initially damage the collagen network rather than the cell. Although fibrillated cartilage from osteoarthritic joints shows a reduction in proteoglycan concentration, it is not clear whether proteoglycan depletion precedes fibrillation or results from it.

Biomechanical Alterations. The loss of matrix proteoglycans from osteoarthritic cartilage leads to a loss of compressive stiffness and elasticity and to an increase in hydraulic permeability. The former leads, in turn, to transmission of greater mechanical stress to the chondrocytes, the latter, to greater loss of interstitial fluid during compression and to increased diffusion of solutes through the matrix. This may be particularly relevant to the diffusion of degradative enzymes and their inhibitors both into the cartilage from the synovial fluid and through the cartilage, away from the borders of chondrocytes that have synthesized them. As noted earlier, the loss of cartilage proteoglycans will also affect cartilage self-lubrication by impairing generation of the surface squeeze-film.

Osteophytes. Whereas much interest has been directed to the mechanisms of cartilage breakdown in osteoarthritis, less attention has been focused on the pathogenesis of the bony proliferation at the joint margins and in the floor of the cartilage lesions, which may be responsible for restriction of joint movement and for some of the pain in the osteoarthritic joint, respectively (Figs. 78–1 and 78–2). Osteophytes from human osteoarthritic joints synthesize cartilage that contains a significant amount of type I collagen. The sulfated proteoglycans of osteophytic cartilage are similar to those of normal adult human cartilage with respect to monomer size and their predominance of chondroitin 6-sulfate but are relatively deficient in keratan sulfate and tend not to interact with hyaluronic acid.[100]

Neither the pathophysiology of osteophytosis nor its relationship to cartilage degeneration in osteoarthritis is entirely clear. In experimentally induced osteoarthritis, osteophytes may develop while the articular cartilage seems to be grossly normal.[101] By increasing the amount of joint surface available

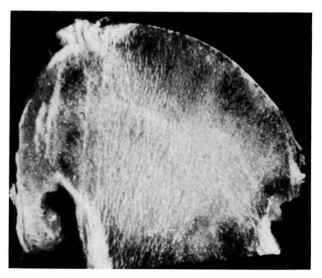

Figure 78–1. Cut section of an osteoarthritic femoral head showing the large osteophyte arising from the lateral aspect of the cartilaginous surface.

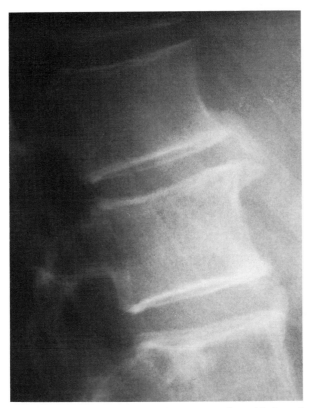

Figure 78–2. Lateral radiograph of the spine of an elderly male, showing very large anterior osteophytes. If such lesions are present posteriorly or posterolaterally, they can cause significant symptoms of cord or root compression.

for load bearing, they may be associated in some cases with regression of the early changes of osteoarthritis in the cartilage.[102]

It has been suggested that osteophytes occur as a result of the penetration of blood vessels into the basal layers of the degenerating cartilage[103] or as a result of abnormal healing of stress fractures of the subchondral trabeculae near the joint margins.[104] In experimentally induced osteoarthritis in the dog, periarticular osteophyte formation was noted to commence in the marginal zone, where synovium merges with periosteum and articular cartilage, as early as 3 days after induction of knee instability.[105] In addition to the proliferation of new cartilage, bone hyperplasia may be strikingly evident and is often associated with an increase in vascularity.[105]

Other studies have shown that bony proliferation may result from venous congestion.[106] In humans with osteoarthritis of the hip, phlebography has demonstrated a marked alteration in the pattern of venous drainage.[107] This is presumably due to changes in the medullary sinusoids, which may be compressed by subchondral cysts and thickened subchondral trabeculae, leading to formation of medullary varices.

In canine knee joints, marginal osteophytes may be produced by repeated injection of homogenates of autogenous cartilage.[108] Osteophyte formation was

preceded by thickening of the cartilage at the chondrosynovial junction, and it was suggested that the prolonged presence of cartilage debris stimulated pluripotential cells at this site to form osteophytes. By analogy, the sloughing of cartilage from the joint surface in osteoarthritis may cause osteophyte formation.

Whatever the cause of osteophytes, immobilization of the joint appears to be effective in preventing their formation.[109] Glucocorticoid administration also has been shown to markedly decrease the size and prevalence of osteophytes in experimental models of osteoarthritis.[110, 111]

THE PATHOLOGY OF OSTEOARTHRITIS

On *gross examination* of a joint affected by osteoarthritis, it is clearly evident that all of the joint structures are affected.[40, 112–114] The capsule of the joint is usually quite thickened and, at times, adherent to the deformed underlying bone[115, 116] (Fig. 78–3). The synovial lining in osteoarthritic joints often shows a moderate to marked degree of inflammatory change.[11, 28] The surface of the synovium is often hypervascular and hemorrhagic, and the lining is

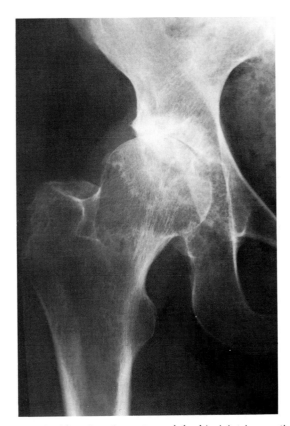

Figure 78–3. Alterations in contour of the hip joint in a patient with osteoarthritis on the basis of an old hip dysplasia. Note the shortening of the neck, the major modifications of the stress lines, and the increased density of both the femoral head and the acetabulum.

thickened and nodular and at times demonstrates hypertrophic villous folds.[114, 115] Synovial tissue in osteoarthritis of the small bones of the hand, particularly in lesions consistent with the diagnosis of "pauci-arthritis" and Heberden's nodes, may have pronounced inflammatory changes.[119-121]

Bones remote from the subchondral region in osteoarthritic joints often show remarkable changes.[40, 112-114] Considerable remodeling of the underlying bone is evident on the basis of alterations in gross structure, thickening of the cortices, and change in trabecular stress lines.[40, 114, 115, 122] The neck of the femur is almost always enlarged in patients with osteoarthritis of the hip,[112, 115, 123] and the posterior elements of the vertebrae are so hypertrophied in patients with spinal osteoarthritis as to figure prominently in the causation of lumbar claudication as a result of vertebral stenosis.[124, 125]

The pathogenesis of *osteophytes*, a cardinal feature of the disease, was detailed earlier. The size, shape, and extent of these bony excrescences vary considerably from patient to patient and from joint to joint. They are usually more extensive in the hip than the shoulder or knee.[113, 122, 123] The majority of the articular osteophytes are covered with hyaline cartilage but occasionally display only fibrous tissue or bare bone at the surface.[40, 114] Osteophytes occurring around the hip are most marked at the lateral acetabulum and the adjacent femoral head; in both locations they considerably enlarge the joint. They may also produce bony excrescences in the roof of the acetabulum and the medial neck of the femur that can lead to progressive subluxation of the hip.[112, 115, 123] Spinal osteophytes are often enormous in size, occasionally "kissing" (touching the adjacent bone), and may partially occlude the foraminal openings (see Fig. 78–2).[114]

Gross examination of a cross-section of the joint surface almost invariably shows *sclerosis* of the subchondral bony end-plate immediately subjacent to the diseased cartilage.[114] The change is most severe at the point of maximum pressure against the opposing cartilage surface. The subchondral bony shell is enlarged and very dense and displays extensions of sclerotic trabeculae descending into the old epiphyseal region.[126-128]

Osteoarthritic cysts, another cardinal feature of the disease, are frequently noted lying close to the subchondral region of the joint but occasionally appear at a considerable distance, even at times extending into the metaphyseal areas (Figs. 78–4 and 78–5).[40, 112, 114, 115, 122, 123, 128] The margins of the cysts are often sclerotic, which helps distinguish them from the cysts seen in patients with rheumatoid arthritis, in whom the bones themselves are far less dense and the cysts are usually poorly marginated.[113, 126, 128] When cysts are transected they are found to contain homogeneous clear or cloudy gelatinous material with a consistency resembling that found within ganglia adjacent to tendon sheaths[114, 115, 122] (see Fig. 78–5).

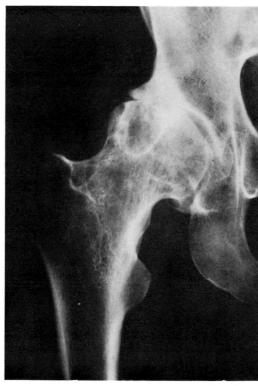

Figure 78–4. Radiograph of the femoral head of a 68-year-old woman with osteoarthritis, demonstrating an enormous cyst involving much of the weight-bearing area of the femoral head.

The surface of the joint that has been completely denuded of cartilage shows an *eburnation*, presumably on the basis of the grinding and polishing effect of rubbing against the bare bone of the adjacent joint surface. Frequently pits and tufts of fibrous tissue or fibrocartilage are noted within the eburnated, densely sclerotic surface.[122, 128]

The gross appearance of the hyaline articular cartilage in the osteoarthritic joint shows a highly variable pattern and is markedly focal in the alterations observed.[113, 114, 122, 128, 129] In some areas the cartilage shows "softening" and a yellowish or brownish discoloration, whereas in others the normally smooth glistening surface appears as a soft

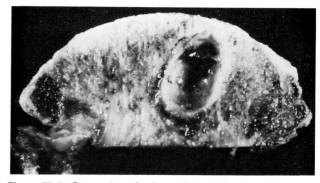

Figure 78–5. Cut section of a femoral head showing a large cyst in the weight-bearing area.

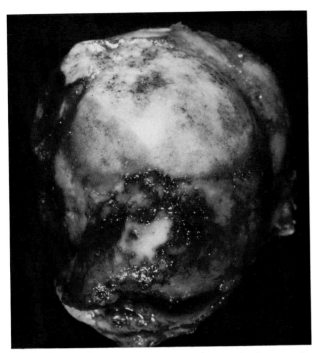

Figure 78–6. Surface of an osteoarthritic femoral head removed at the time of surgery from a 63-year-old woman. Note the irregularity of contour and marked variation in structure. Old yellowish cartilage is present along with "pebble-grained" new material. The weight-bearing area shows complete denudation of the cartilage with sclerosis and eburnation of the underlying bone.

velvety feltwork (Fig. 78–6). Ulcerations, fissures, and cracks appear on the surface and, at times, may be so extensive as to disclose the underlying sclerotic and eburnated subchondral bone. The cartilage covering osteophytes often appears thicker than that over the weight-bearing or even non–weight-bearing areas of the surface, is sometimes whiter in color, and may be either pebble-grained or smooth. In general, the sites of maximum weight bearing show the most severe changes, so that the zenith of the femoral head or the middle portions of the femoral condyles will show the most advanced alterations, whereas the marginal regions of the joints, particularly in early disease, may be relatively normal in appearance.[112–114, 122, 128, 129]

Histologic examination of the capsule, particularly in advanced disease, is likely to demonstrate thickening, focal areas of inflammatory infiltrate, neovascularity, and, in some areas, a hyalinization, amyloid deposition, and sparse cellularity.[115, 116, 123, 130] Histologic study of the synovium may show a pattern ranging from nearly normal to tissues with such severe inflammatory alterations as to suggest the diagnosis of rheumatoid arthritis (Fig. 78–7).[118–120]

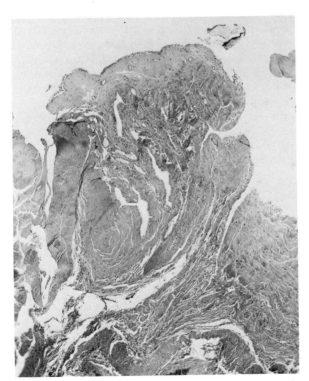

Figure 78–7. Low-power histologic study of the synovium from the hip of a patient with "standard" osteoarthritis. The synovial layers are heaped up in villi and show a moderate proliferation of the synovial cells and a modest infiltration with inflammatory cells (H & E × 150).

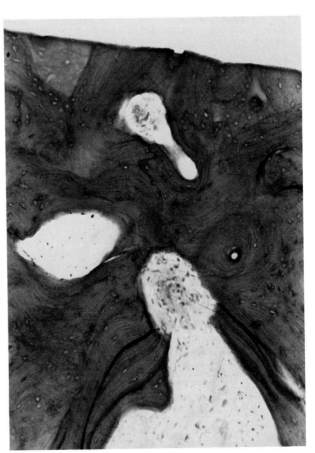

Figure 78–8. Low-power histologic section of the subchondral bone in late-stage osteoarthritis, showing the marked sclerosis, trabecular and cortical thickening, some osteogenesis, and segments of osteonecrotic bone. The marrow cavities show foci of fibrous tissue and remnants of fracture callus (H & E × 100).

Histologic examination of the bone shows considerable variation, depending on the site examined. Early in the course of the disease the subchondral area shows gross thickening of the cortex and bony sclerosis frequently with prominent cement lines and dilated vascular spaces, some of which penetrate the lower layers of the cartilage.[115, 117, 130] Later in the course, after total denudation of the cartilage occurs, one often sees a dense sclerosis with fibrous and fibrocartilaginous plugs and some evidence of new bone formation (Fig. 78–8).[40, 114, 122, 123] The marrow cavities are often replaced by fibrous tissue, and endosteal remodeling, osteoblastic rimming, and evidence of active new bone formation can be observed.[127]

The bone of the osteophytes typically shows new bone formation and, later in the course of the disease, evidence of active remodeling.[115, 127, 128] Cysts of the bone show as loose, sparsely cellular amorphous regions that stain poorly with hematoxylin and eosin.[113–115, 127, 128] Frequently, ares of new bone formation surround regions that appear to resemble microfracture callus. One major theory of the origin of cysts is that they occur as a result of degeneration of callus of stress fractures that occur in the mechanically poor bone and cannot heal because of the relative avascularity of some of the bony foci.

The cartilage histology has been the best studied.[113, 114, 122, 123, 128] The first changes seen in osteoarthritic cartilage are those of surface erosion and irregularities. At this early stage, the matrix of the cartilage shows some mild alterations in staining quality (Fig. 78–9). The tidemark, when identifiable, often shows irregularities, reduplication, discontinuous areas, and penetration by blood vessels.[114, 122, 132]

As the disorder progresses the surface layer becomes more fragmented and short vertical clefts are noted, often descending through the gliding zone of the cartilage into the transitional zone (Fig. 78–10A). The matrix shows great irregularity in staining even with hematoxylin and eosin. With metachromatic stains such as toluidine blue or Alcian blue or an orthochromatic one such as safranin O, a progressive heterogeneity with patchy depletion of color can be noted. This is seen initially in the surface areas, then deeper, and involves, first, the interterritorial areas and, subsequently, the territorial regions[41, 53, 114, 122] (see Fig. 78–9). With advancing disease, the focal fragmentation of the joint surface becomes greater, the clefts become deeper (descending now as far as the calcified zone), and the matrix stains even more irregularly (see Fig. 78–10B). Finally at end stage, only wisps of cartilage are left clinging to the denuded, eburnated, sclerotic subchondral bone (see Fig. 78–10C).

The cellular complement of the cartilage shows remarkable alterations. Pathognomonic is the increased number of cells.[40, 53, 116, 123] At first, the change is that of a diffuse mild hypercellularity, but with progression of the disease, the cells are found in "brood capsules" that sometime contain a hundred or more chondrocytes[113, 128] (see Fig. 78–10B). Eventually in moderately severe disease the majority of the cells are in such formations, some of which seem to be metabolically active, whereas others are not.[113, 134] As the disease progresses the chondrocytes become less active-looking and, in late-stage disease, show signs of cell death and autodigestion.[135, 136] These histologic studies are supported by ultrastructural observations by a number of investigators using both scanning and transmission electron microscopy[136, 137] and functional expression detailed earlier.

One of the more controversial issues regarding the pathology of osteoarthritis concerns the role of the underlying bone in the pathogenesis of the disease. A number of observations[131, 138–140] provide mechanical confirmation of the histologic findings of increased thickening of the bone. These studies have

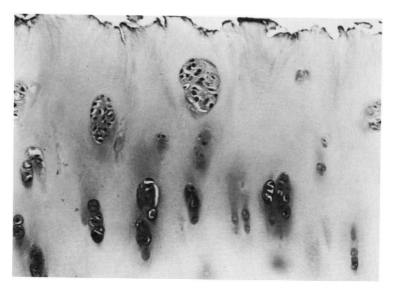

Figure 78–9. A medium-power histologic section of articular cartilage from an osteoarthritic joint stained with safranin O, a dye with special affinity for proteoglycan. Note that only the pericellular region around the clones of cells stains darkly with the dye, indicating a depletion of the proteoglycan from the tissue elsewhere (safranin O, fast green, iron hematoxylin × 200).

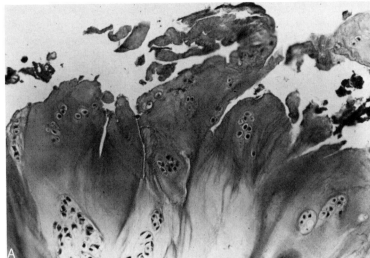

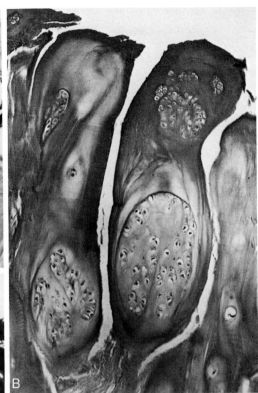

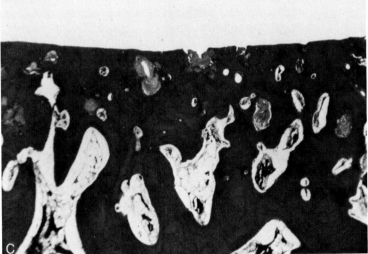

Figure 78–10. Histologic pictures of the various degrees of articular cartilage change with advancing degrees of osteoarthritis. *A,* The surface from a site on a femoral head with osteoarthritis, demonstrating surface irregularities, early cloning of the cells, and altered matrix staining (H & E × 200). *B,* The changes of more advanced disease, demonstrating deepening of the clefts to the radial zone, altered matrix staining, and large clones of cells (H & E × 200). *C,* The appearance of end-stage disease with complete denudation of the surface and eburnation and sclerotization of the underlying bone (H & E × 95).

been interpreted as displaying a "stiffening" of the subchondral plate. Radin has proposed that such a change may be part of the pathogenetic mechanism for the disease,[141] but other evidence from animal models suggests that the earliest changes seem to occur in the cartilage.[142-144] A second feature of the bone is that despite focal areas of osteonecrosis in the subchondral region,[145] a number of investigators have described the presence of increased vascularity in the epiphyseal and metaphyseal regions.[138, 146] This hypervascular state has been thought to contribute to the progression and clinical symptoms of the disease.[117] Studies by Lemperg and Arnoldi[146] have shown increased venous pressure within the femoral head of patients with osteoarthritis, and there is little question on histologic study that vascular channels are quite prominent.[40, 114, 115, 123]

ETIOLOGIC FACTORS

The previous sections have focused on the mechanisms of cartilage damage in osteoarthritis, that is,

on *pathogenetic factors.* It is likely that there is no single "cause" of osteoarthritis; that is, no *one* factor triggers the processes that result in cartilage destruction. Furthermore, since changes in any of the constituents of the joint (e.g., collagen, proteoglycans, chondrocytes, subchondral bone, synovial membrane) may affect the other constituents, the degenerative process in the articular cartilage may be initiated in a variety of ways.

Chapter 79, which deals with clinical aspects of osteoarthritis, contains a brief discussion of some of the etiologic factors that have been implicated. We have chosen to expand that discussion in this section, but the review is written from a biologic perspective and emphasizes three premises: (1) that the morphologic changes of osteoarthritis are the consequences of altered cartilage physiology; (2) that not all etiologies of osteoarthritis can legitimately be viewed as "diseases," but that some represent states of altered physiology; and (3) that, in this sense, *all* osteoarthritis is "secondary."

Aging. Of all the risk factors for primary (idiopathic) osteoarthritis, age is the strongest. Several epidemiologic studies show an increase in the presence of osteoarthritis with age. In individuals with grade 3 or grade 4 radiologic changes (i.e., those most likely to have symptoms of osteoarthritis), the increase is exponential.[147] However, even in those with clinically apparent osteoarthritis, increasing age does not necessarily lead to an increase in pain or disability,[148] the risk factors for which are largely unclear.[149]

The epidemiologic association between aging and osteoarthritis has led to the impression that osteoarthritis is a result of the aging of joint tissues. However, as indicated earlier, the data suggest that aging alone is *not* a cause of osteoarthritis, although changes in the tissues or cells that occur with aging may facilitate development of the disease. For example, with age, articular cartilage becomes increasingly susceptible to fatigue failure.[150]

There is also no basis on which to exclude the concept that development of osteoarthritis proceeds so slowly that a joint sustaining an injury early in life manifests the changes of osteoarthritis only years later. Nor do the data exclude the possibility that age-related changes in joint biomechanics may be important in the pathogenesis of osteoarthritis. It may, therefore, be relevant that with age joints become increasingly congruent with respect to their shape.[151] The cause of this increase in congruity is unknown, but it may be related to progressive diminution in blood flow, with a resulting decrease in the rate of remodeling at the osteochondral junction.[152] These changes in joint geometry may interfere with nutrition of the cartilage and alter load distribution, so that areas of cartilage that formerly were not habitually loaded are now subjected to significant compressive stresses.

Other age-related alterations in contact stresses may arise as a result of developmental changes. For example, in the human hip, a fibrocartilaginous rim at the zenith of the acetabulum may exist as a normal anatomic variant. In younger people, contact between the femoral head and the fibrocartilaginous rim does not occur; in some older people, however, contact takes place as a result of age-related remodeling, leading to pressures several-fold greater than those in younger individuals.[153] Since the biochemical composition of connective tissue is altered in response to the mechanical stresses to which it is subjected,[154] changes may be erroneously ascribed to aging when they reflect only the normal response of the tissue to a change in the functional demands placed upon it.

Aging is associated with a decrease in function of the peripheral nervous system. Reflexes are diminished; nerve conduction times are prolonged. Although deafferentation of the extremity alone produced no changes in the ipsilateral joint, and cruciate ligament transection produced only mild osteoarthritis, when the afferent nerve supply from the ipsilateral leg was surgically interrupted, dogs that were subsequently subjected to anterior cruciate ligament transection developed rapid, severe articular cartilage breakdown.[155] These findings suggest that a neurosensory disorder (perhaps related to aging) could predispose some individuals to osteoarthritis or lead to more severe osteoarthritis than would otherwise develop.

Primary Alterations in the Cartilage Matrix. Little support exists for the concept that changes in the extracellular matrix of the articular cartilage are of primary importance in most cases of osteoarthritis. However, the recent discovery of a point mutation in the complementary DNA (cDNA) coding for type II collagen in several generations of a family with chondrodysplasia and polyarticular osteoarthritis[156, 157] is an excellent example of the development of the disorder in association with a generalized defect in articular cartilage matrix. Local factors (e.g., stresses related to joint use and the degree of joint deformity) presumably influenced the appearance of osteoarthritis in certain joints but not others in affected members of the kindred.

Several other examples of cartilage matrix changes leading to osteoarthritis may be cited, including hemochromatosis, Wilson's disease, ochronotic arthropathy, gouty arthritis, and calcium pyrophosphate dihydrate (CPPD) crystal deposition disease. In these cases, hemosiderin, copper, homogentisic acid polymers, and crystals of monosodium urate of CPPD, respectively, deposit within the matrix and lead to cartilage degeneration, directly via chondrocyte injury or indirectly by increasing the stiffness of the matrix. Whether biochemical or physicochemical changes in the matrix precede the deposition of the aforementioned materials is uncertain. In view of the defect in proteoglycan aggregation that is seen in the earliest stages of osteoarthritis it is notable that proteoglycan aggregates inhibit precipitation of calcium salts[158] and of monosodium urate.[159]

The relationship of CPPD deposition disease to osteoarthritis is complex (see Chapter 77). Other metabolic disorders that serve as examples of cartilage deposition diseases (e.g., hemochromatosis, Wilson's disease, gout, ochronosis) may be associated with deposition of CPPD in articular cartilage. In addition, active calcification is common in osteoarthritic cartilage. The basal zones stain strongly for alkaline phosphatase, and matrix vesicles, indicating cartilage calcification, are seen by electron microscopy.[160] When human osteoarthritic cartilage is cultured in vitro, large quantities of alkaline phosphatase and pyrophosphate (PPi), produced by the chondrocytes during active matrix synthesis, can be recovered from the medium.[161] The level of PPi in synovial fluid from patients with osteoarthritis is very high,[162] mimicking that in CPPD, and correlates directly with the severity of osteoarthritis as judged radiographically.[163] Howell and colleagues have shown that young or proliferating chondrocytes are a major source of PPi, whereas resting chondrocytes from normal adult cartilage secrete little PPi. Thus, the increased PPi secretion in osteoarthritic cartilage may reflect the increased activity of the cells in their attempt at matrix "repair" (see earlier).

PPi is generated from adenosine triphosphate (ATP) in cartilage by the action of the exoenzyme nucleoside pyrophosphohydrolase, which is present in extracts of cartilage from patients with osteoarthritis.[164] If ATP or other nucleoside triphosphates are extensively hydrolyzed to PPi and the monophosphate by-product in vivo, increased activity of 5'-nucleotidase, which has been documented in CPPD,[165] could drive the reaction and increase the rate of PPi production. If increased removal of PPi did not occur, owing, for example, to a relative deficiency of extracellular pyrophosphatase, as shown in incubates of human osteoarthritis and CPPD cartilage, the increased PPi would be available for mineralization. The increased PPi in the osteoarthritic cartilage could then precipitate as CPPD when other factors, such as the concentration of ionized calcium and the physical state of the matrix (e.g., proteoglycan disaggregation), were favorable. By altering the physical and mechanical properties of the matrix, deposition of CPPD could then lead to accelerated cartilage breakdown.

Alterations in Chondrocyte Metabolic Activity. As indicated earlier, the anabolic and catabolic activities of the osteoarthritic chondrocyte differ from those of the normal chondrocyte. These changes are phenotypic and appear to be independent of environmental factors. Most striking in this respect is the ability of the cell to replicate its DNA, a capacity that cells in normal cartilage lose or suppress following cessation of skeletal growth.[41] The differences between osteoarthritic and normal chondrocytes with respect to their in vivo anabolic and catabolic activities persist in vitro.[81] Whether these alterations, which are presumably permanent, represent a primary change or develop after the cells are stimulated by some factor that initiates osteoarthritis is unknown.

Trauma. It is well recognized that fractures that are not well reduced and leave the joint excessively incongruent soon lead to osteoarthritis, as does recurrent dislocation of the patella, congenital dislocation of the hip, and alterations in the shape of the joint surface as a result of osteonecrosis.[166] Whether subtler degrees of trauma also lead to osteoarthritis is far less clear. For example, does repetitive impulsive loading over a lifetime initiate the sequence of metabolic, biochemical, and biomechanical events that lead to osteoarthritis? A subfracture level of trauma has been shown to accelerate remodeling in the zone of calcified cartilage, with reduplication of the tidemark, thinning of the noncalcified zone, and typical changes of osteoarthritis.[167, 168] Radin[76, 169] has suggested that repetitive trauma causes stiffening of the subchondral bone, resulting in increased wear of the overlying cartilage.

Articular cartilage is remarkably resistant to damage by shear forces.[170] In vitro, when joints are subjected to repeated oscillation, even under the maximal constant loads that can be borne by subchondral bone, the cartilage does not wear.[171] In contrast, cartilage is highly vulnerable to repetitive impact loading, which will cause the joint to wear out rapidly. It is likely that this accounts for the high frequency of osteoarthritis in shoulders and elbows of pneumatic drill operators and baseball pitchers, ankles of ballet dancers, metacarpophalangeal joints of boxers, and knees of basketball players.

Quantitatively, the major forces on articular cartilage result not from weight bearing but from contraction of the muscles that stabilize or move the joint.[172] In normal walking (an example of repetitive impact loading) four to five times the body weight may be transmitted through the knee. In squatting, the value may be as great as ten times the body weight.[40]

After force transients were eliminated by femoral nerve block, the load rate during gait in normal subjects increased approximately 2½-fold (to approximately 150 × body weight/second).[173] This suggests that a force transient can be caused by failure to decelerate the lower extremity prior to heel strike. In normal individuals, minor incoordination in muscle recruitment, resulting in failure to decelerate the leg, may generate rapidly applied impulsive forces as high as 65 × body weight/second at heel strike.[174] Forces of this magnitude were recently documented in 35 percent of normal young individuals and 100 percent of age-matched control subjects with tibiofemoral pain and normal knee radiographs who were considered to be "preosteoarthrotic." It remains to be established, however, that this microincoordination of neuromuscular control—"microklutziness"[174]—is a risk factor for osteoarthritis, although the possibility is intriguing.

Considerable attention has been directed toward understanding the mechanisms that protect the joint under physiologic conditions of impact loading, since the articular cartilage itself is too thin to be an effective shock absorber.[175] The major factors that attenuate forces delivered to the joint appear to be joint motion, with the associated lengthening of muscles under tension, and deformation of the subchondral bone.[175, 176] Seemingly minor, but unanticipated, impact loads (e.g., misstepping off a curb, slipping on a stair) have been viewed by some as a major etiologic factor in "idiopathic" joint degeneration.[177] Since the reaction time required to prepare the neuromuscular apparatus reflexively for an impact load is about 75 milliseconds,[178] unexpected falls of only about 1 inch would allow insufficient time to activate protective reflexes; under that circumstance, the load may be transmitted to the joint structure. In contrast, in a fall from a greater height, energy is absorbed by the lengthening of the muscles that surround the joint and by the motion of joint structures. Obviously, factors that lead to muscle fatigue would tend to impair this shock-absorbing mechanism, as would myopathy or muscle atrophy (as occurs in aging).

Cancellous subchondral bone, by virtue of its plasticity, functions as a major shock attenuator.[175] While most of the stiffness of the subchondral bone is attributable to the bony trabeculae, the intraosseous fluid contributes significantly; when canine femoral heads were decompressed by drilling the femoral neck, thus altering fluid boundary conditions, femoral head stiffness was reduced by more than 30 percent.[179]

Normally, the opposing surfaces of a joint are not congruous in the unloaded condition. Under loading, both the cartilage and the bone deform so that a larger proportion of the opposing surfaces comes into contact. This increase in congruity serves to distribute the load over the largest possible area.[180] Excessive loads may cause microfractures of subchondral trabeculae, which heal with callus formation and remodeling. The remodeled trabeculae may be stiffer than normal and therefore less effective as shock absorbers. Under these conditions they cannot deform normally with load, so that congruity of the joint surfaces with loading is reduced, causing forces to be concentrated at sites within the articular cartilage.

A variety of indirect evidence supports the view that physical changes in the subchondral bone may be important in osteoarthritis. An increased incidence of healing microfractures has been reported in patients with osteoarthritis,[181] although a more recent study[132] showed a reduction in the number of trabecular microfractures in osteoarthritis patients, compared with controls, and a lack of correlation between the number of microfractures and age in osteoarthritis patients. It is relevant, therefore, that approximately 30 percent of the stiffness of the subchondral region cannot be attributed to the bony trabeculae, but is due to a hydraulic factor in the trabecular tissue.[182]

Osteoporosis of the femur, which is associated with softening and greater compliance of the subchondral bone, appears to protect against osteoarthritis of the hip.[183] Conversely, in the laboratory, stiffening of the cancellous bone with methacrylate, thus reducing its deformability, leads promptly to cartilage degeneration during repetitive impact loading.[184]

Although it has been suggested[177] that trabecular microfractures may be the *primary* cause of the cartilage degeneration in osteoarthritis (i.e., that osteoarthritis is more likely to develop in individuals who have accumulated more microfractures in their lifetime than in those who have not), the evidence for this is not clear. When the articular surface was subjected to repeated impact loading in vitro, cartilage fibrillation and ultrastructural changes in the chondrocytes occurred *prior* to changes in the mechanical properties of the subchondral plate.[185]

Alterations in Regulators of Chondrocyte Metabolism. Humoral, synovial, and cartilage-derived chemical mediators as well as mechanical stimuli regulate synthetic processes of the chondrocyte. Thus, insulin and other growth factors[31] have effects on normal cartilage. Qualitative and quantitative changes in the substrates for important metabolic pathways of the chondrocyte, and in mineral and electrolyte pools, and alterations in loading all can alter the rates of synthesis or degradation of the matrix by normal chondrocytes.[32, 187, 188] Recent interest has focused on the effects on chondrocyte metabolism of prostaglandins,[187, 189, 190] heat shock proteins,[191] and IL-1 derived from synovium[24] and cartilage.[25]

As mentioned earlier, in osteoarthritis, increases in the rate of synthesis of cartilage matrix constituents may keep pace with, or even exceed, the rate of degradation for a lengthy period. Analysis of human osteoarthritic cartilage by in situ hybridization and immunolocation with probes specific for insulin-like growth factor-1 (IGF-1) message has shown that messenger ribonucleic acid (mRNA) for IGF-1 is localized in clonal clusters of chondrocytes near the fibrillated surface.[192] No difference was found between histologically normal areas of cartilage from the osteoarthritic joint and cartilage from normal individuals. Expression of the IGF-1 gene by the chondrocytes increased in proportion to the morphologic severity of the osteoarthritis. Since IGF-1 decreases both basal and IL-1–induced degradation of aggrecan and hyaluronic acid (HA) and can synergize with other growth factors to induce clonal replication of chondrocytes, local production of IGF-1 and of other growth factors (e.g., TGF-β) may contribute to matrix repair and prolong the "compensated phase" of osteoarthritis.

Recently, Schalkwijk and colleagues[193] showed that chondrocytes in articular cartilage from the inflamed joints of mice with zymosan-induced arthritis had become unresponsive to IGF-1. Whether a similar abnormality exists in osteoarthritic cartilage requires study. Notably, intra-articular administration of fibroblast growth factor has been reported to cause the healing of mechanically induced superficial cartilage defects.[194, 195]

Whether alterations in any of the aforementioned factors are etiologic in osteoarthritis or only reflect responses to changes resulting from an injury to the chondrocyte remains to be elucidated. It is apparent, however, that we need to understand better the anabolic, as well as the catabolic, pathways that act on joint cartilage in osteoarthritis.

Inflammatory Joint Disease. Osteoarthritis itself is generally not associated with much synovitis. Scattered foci of lymphocytes are present in the synovial membrane, and the synovial fluid leukocyte count is usually fewer than 2000 cells per mm³. Pannus, as seen in the rheumatoid joint, is not present. To the extent that inflammation does occur in osteoarthritis, it may be the result of crystal-induced synovitis (either calcium apatite or CPPD) or synovial clearance of cartilage breakdown products.[108] For example, chondroitin sulfate has been shown to activate Hageman factor in vitro,[196] triggering the kinin pathway. If this occurs also in vivo, it could account for the mononuclear cell infiltration and vascular hyperplasia in the synovial membrane in osteoarthritis. The low-grade synovitis leads to capsular thickening and fibrotic shortening, which may cause pain and muscle spasm.[116]

Wear particles, that is, material derived from the articular surface as a result of mechanical or enzymatic destruction of the cartilage, are present in the synovial fluid in osteoarthritis[197] and can cause the release of collagenase and other hydrolytic enzymes from synovial cells and macrophages.[198]

Although less prominent than in rheumatoid arthritis, deposits of immunoglobulin and complement can be found in the collagenous latticework of the superficial zone of the articular cartilage, suggesting that deposition of immune complexes, perhaps containing breakdown products of the cartilage as antigens, may play a role in the chronicity of the inflammatory reaction in the joint.[199]

"Milwaukee shoulder syndrome" represents a form of destructive osteoarthritis with some evidence of inflammation in the synovial membrane but minimal synovial fluid leukocytosis. Rotator cuff degeneration and severe osteoarthritis of the shoulder are present, with hydroxyapatite crystal deposition in the synovial membrane.[200] Despite high levels of active collagenase, the synovial fluid contains a paucity of cells. Presumably, crystals released from the degenerating tendons trigger the release of collagenase from synovial mononuclear cells, leading to cartilage breakdown and thus perpetuating enzyme release from the synovium.

Although the pathogenetic significance of inflammation in primary osteoarthritis receives much attention, it is clear that secondary osteoarthritis may develop as a sequela of inflammatory joint disease, such as rheumatoid arthritis, acute bacterial joint infection, and tuberculous arthritis. Initial damage to the cartilage in these cases is probably chiefly enzymatic, with breakdown of the matrix by degradative enzymes released from the synovium or leukocytes within the joint space. In addition, as indicated earlier, IL-1 suppresses proteoglycan synthesis by the chondrocyte and accelerates degradation of matrix proteoglycans.[74] Impaired chondrocyte nutrition, resulting from immobility or lack of weight bearing, may also contribute to the cartilage breakdown in inflammatory arthritis, serving as an additional factor in initiating osteoarthritis.

Obesity. Excessive body weight obviously increases the load borne by weight-bearing joints. Obesity may also cause changes in posture and gait and in overall locomotor activity, which must be taken into account in considering the joint biomechanics. In humans, obesity is associated with an increase in symptomatic osteoarthritis of the knee,[149, 201] although not of the hip.[202] Furthermore, the association has recently been shown to exist with prior, as well as concurrent, obesity,[203, 204] indicating that obesity is a risk factor for, and not merely a consequence of, osteoarthritis.

The majority of obese patients exhibit varus knee deformities.[205] This is presumably a compensatory attempt to bring the feet under the center of gravity when the thighs are separated by adiposity. In such cases, load is concentrated on the cartilage of the medial compartment, where degenerative changes most commonly develop in the knees of obese people.

Whether metabolic, genetic, or other factors, as well as mechanical factors, contribute to the osteoarthritic changes in obesity is unsettled. The data are contradictory as to whether obesity is associated with an increased prevalence of osteoarthritis in non–weight-bearing joints. In one study in which mice were fed a diet enriched with lard (a saturated fat), the frequency and severity of osteoarthritis were increased.[206] This was not confirmed in another study, however, and a diet supplemented with vegetable (unsaturated) fat did not influence the development of osteoarthritic lesions in mice, even though it led to obesity.[207] In STR/IN mice, which develop hyperlipidemia and become obese on an ordinary diet, the obesity is genetically dissociated from the osteoarthritis,[208] suggesting that other hereditary factors are etiologic for the osteoarthritis.

Immune Responses. Perhaps one of the more provocative theories related to the cause of alterations in the articular cartilages in idiopathic osteoarthritis is the suggestion that because of the aneural and avascular state of the cartilages the remainder of the body is unaware of their existence. Of perhaps greater importance is the possibility that some of the proteins of the matrix are unrecognized by the immune system as autogenous and when they or fragments of them escape from the cartilage into the synovial fluid, the local lymphocytic elements see them as antigens. This theory[209-214] provides a hypothetical explanation for the method by which even a minor injury to the cartilage may serve as the initiating event in a local (synovial) autoimmune causation or perpetuation mechanism that, over time, becomes severe enough to destroy parts of the cartilage by humoral or cellular cytotoxic antibody responses.[215]

References

1. Mankin, H. J.: Clinical features of osteoarthritis. In Kelley, W. N., et al. (eds.): Textbook of Rheumatology. 3rd ed. Philadelphia, W. B. Saunders Company, 1988.
2. Maroudas, A., Katz, E. P., Wachtel, E. J., Mizrah, J., and Soudry, M.: Physiochemical properties and functional behavior of normal and osteoarthritic human cartilage. In Keuttner, K. E., Schleyerbach, R., and Hascall, V. C. (eds.): Articular Cartilage Biochemistry. New York, Raven Press, 1986, pp. 311–330.
3. Mankin, H. J., and Thrasher, A. F.: Water binding in normal and osteoarthritic cartilage. J. Bone Joint Surg. 57A:76, 1975.
4. Oldberg, A., Antonsson, P., Hedbom, E., and Heinegård, D.: Structure and function of extracellular matrix proteoglycans. Biochem. Soc. Trans. 18:789, 1990.

5. Hardingham, T, and Bayliss, M.: Proteoglycans of articular cartilage: changes in aging and in joint disease. Semin. Arthritis Rheum. 20(Suppl. 1):12, 1990.
6. Muir, H.: The coming of age of proteoglycans. Biochem. Soc. Trans. 18:787, 1990.
7. Mak, A. F., Mow, V. C., and Lai, W. M.: Predictions of the number and strength of the proteoglycan-proteoglycan interactions from viscometric data. Trans. Orthop. Res. Soc. 10:3, 1983.
8. Mayne, R., and Irwin, M. H.: Collagen types in cartilage. In Kuettner, K. E., Schleyerbach, R., and Hascall, V. C. (eds.): Articular Cartilage Biochemistry. New York, Raven Press, 1986, pp. 23–39.
9. Miller, E. M., and Matukas, V. J.: Chick cartilage collagen: a new type of I-chain not present in bone or skin of the species. Proc. Natl. Acad. Sci. U.S.A. 64:1264, 1969.
10. Kuettner, K. E., Thonar, E. J.-M. A., and Aydelotte, M. B.: Modern aspects of articular cartilage biochemistry. In Brandt, K. D. (ed.): Cartilage Changes in Osteoarthritis. Indianapolis, Indiana University School of Medicine, 1990, pp. 3–11.
11. Eyre, D. R.: Structure and function of the cartilage collagens: role of type IX collagen in articular cartilage. In Brandt, K. D. (ed.): Cartilage Changes in Osteoarthritis. Indianapolis, Indiana University School of Medicine, 1990, pp. 12–16.
12. Smith, G. N., Jr., and Brandt, K. D.: Can type XI collagen "glue" together intersecting type II fibers in articular cartilage matrix? A proposed mechanism. J. Rheumatol. 19:14, 1992.
13. Oegema, T. R., and Thompson, R. C., Jr.: Cartilage-bone interface (tidemark). In Brandt K. D. (ed.): Cartilage Changes in Osteoarthritis. Indianapolis, Indiana University School of Medicine, 1990, pp. 43–52.
14. Engvall, E., Ruoslahti, E., and Miller, E. J.: Affinity of fibronectin to collagens of different genetic types and to fibrinogen. J. Exp. Med. 147:1584, 1978.
15. Yamada, K. M.: Cell surface interactions with extracellular materials. Annu. Rev. Biochem. 52:761, 1983.
16. Hewitt, A. T., Varner, H. H., Silver, M. H., Dessav, W., Wilkes, C. M., and Martin, V. W.: The isolation and partial characterization of chondronectin, an attachment factor for chondrocytes. J. Biol. Chem. 257:2330, 1982.
17. von der Mark, K., Hollenhaver, J., Pfaffle, M., van Menxel, M., and Muller, P. K.: Role of anchorin CII in the interaction of chondrocytes with extracellular collagen. In Kuettner, K. E., Schleyerbach, R., and Hascall, V. C. (eds.): Articular Cartilage Biochemistry. New York, Raven Press, 1986, pp. 125–138.
18. Paulsson, M., and Heinegard, D.: Noncollagenous cartilage proteins. Current status of an emerging research field. Coll. Relat. Res. 4:219, 1984.
19. Fife, R. S., and Brandt, K. D.: Extracellular matrix of cartilage. C. glycoproteins. In Woessner, J. F., and Howell, D. S. (eds.): Cartilage Degradation: Basic and Clinical Aspects. (In press.)
20. Mankin, H. J.: The structure, chemistry, and metabolism of articular cartilage. Bull. Rheum. Dis. 17:447, 1967.
21. Repo, R. U., and Mitchell, N.: Collagen synthesis in mature articular cartilage of the rabbit. J. Bone Joint Surg. 53B:541, 1971.
22. Howell, D. S., and Woessner, J. F., Jr.: Enzymes in articular cartilage. In Maroudas, A., and Holborow, E. J. (eds.): Studies in Joint Disease. Tunbridge Wells, England, Pitman Medical Publishing Company, 1980, pp. 160–169.
23. Murphy, G., Cockett, M. I., Stephens, P. E., and Smith, B. J.: Stromelysin is an activator of procollagenase. Biochem. J. 248:265, 1987.
24. Dingle, J. T.: Catabolin—a cartilage catabolic factor from synovium. Clin. Orthop. 156:219, 1980.
25. Ollivierre, F., Gubler, U., Towle, C. A., Laurencin, C., and Treadwell, B. V.: Expression of IL-1 genes in human and bovine chondrocytes: a mechanism for autocrine control of cartilage matrix degradation. Biochem. Biophys. Res. Commun. 141:904, 1986.
26. Mankin, H. J., and Lippiello, L.: The turnover of adult rabbit articular cartilage. J. Bone Joint Surg. 51A:1591, 1969.
27. Maroudas, A.: Transport through articular cartilage and some physiological implications. In Ali, S. Y., Elves, M. W., and Leaback, D. H. (eds.): Normal and Osteoarthrotic Articular Cartilage. London, Institute of Orthopaedics, 1974, pp. 33–47.
28. Mankin, H. J., and Lippiello, L.: The turnover of adult rabbit articular cartilage. J. Bone Joint Surg. 63A:131, 1981.
29. Bhatnagar, R. S., and Prockop, D. J.: Dissociation of the synthesis of sulphated mucopolysaccharides and the synthesis of collagen in embryonic cartilage. Biochim. Biophys. Acta 130:383, 1966.
30. Dondi, P., and Muir, H.: Collagen synthesis and deposition in cartilage during disrupted proteoglycan production. Biochem. J. 160:117, 1976.
31. Morales, T. I.: Cartilage proteoglycan homeostasis: role of growth factors. In Brandt, K. D. (ed.): Cartilage Changes in Osteoarthritis. Indianapolis, Indiana University School of Medicine, 1990, pp. 17–21.
32. Morales, T. I., and Kuettner, K. E.: The properties of the neutral proteinase released by primary chondrocyte cultures and its action on proteoglycan aggregates. Biochim. Biophys. Acta 705:92, 1982.

33. Sapolsky, A. I., and Howell, D. S.: Further characterization of a neutral metalloprotease isolated from human articular cartilage. Arthritis Rheum. 25:981, 1982.
34. Ehrlich, M. G.: Degradative enzyme systems in osteoarthritic cartilage. J. Orthop. Res. 3:170, 1985.
35. Dean, D. D., and Woessner, J. F., Jr.: Extracts of human articular cartilage contain an inhibitor of tissue metalloproteinases. Biochem. J. 218:277, 1984.
36. Murphy, G., and Docherty, A. J. P.: Molecular studies on the connective tissue metalloproteinases and their inhibitor TIMP. In Galuert, A. M. (ed.): The Control of Tissue Damage. Oxford, Elsevier, 1988, pp. 223–241.
37. Maroudas, A.: Physicochemical properties of cartilage in the light of ion exchange theory. Biophys. J. 8:575, 1968.
38. Maroudas, A.: Balance between swelling pressure and collagen tension in normal and degenerate cartilage. Nature 260:808, 1976.
39. Maroudas, A.: Fluid transport in cartilage. Ann. Rheum. Dis. (Suppl.) 34:77, 1975.
40. Sokoloff, L.: The Biology of Degenerative Joint Disease. Chicago, University of Chicago Press, 1969.
41. Mankin, H. J., and Brandt, K. D.: Biochemistry and metabolism of cartilage in osteoarthritis. In Moskowitz, R. W., Howell, D. S., Goldberg, V. M., and Mankin, H. J. (eds.): Osteoarthritis: Diagnosis and Management. Philadelphia, W. B. Saunders Company, 1984, pp. 43–79.
42. Brandt, K., and Fife, R. S.: Ageing in relation to the pathogenesis of osteoarthritis. Clin. Rheum. Dis. 12:117, 1986.
43. Nimni, M. E., and Deshmukh, K.: Differences in collagen metabolism between normal and osteoarthritic human articular cartilage. Science 181:751, 1973.
44. Herbage, D., Huc, A., Chabrand, D., and Chapuy, M. C.: Physicochemical study of articular cartilage from healthy and osteoarthritic human hips. Biochim. Biophys. Acta 271:339, 1972.
45. Gay, S., Muller, P. K., Lemmen, C., Remberger, K., Matzen, K., and Kuhn, K.: Immunohistological study on collagen in cartilage-bone metamorphosis and degenerative osteoarthrosis. Klin. Wochenschr. 54:969, 1976.
46. Muir, H.: Current and future trends in articular cartilage research and osteoarthritis. In Kuettner, K. E., Schleyerbach, R., and Hascall, V. C. (eds.): Articular Cartilage Biochemistry. New York, Raven Press, 1986, pp. 423–440.
47. Mankin, H. J., and Lippiello, L.: Biochemical and metabolic abnormalities in articular cartilage from osteoarthritic hips. J. Bone Joint Surg. 52A:424, 1970.
48. Bayliss, M. T.: Proteoglycan structure in normal and osteoarthritic human cartilage. In Kuettner, K. E., Schleyerbach, R., and Hascall, V. C. (eds.): Articular Cartilage Biochemistry. New York, Raven Press, 1986, pp. 295–308.
49. Brandt, K. D., Palmoski, M. J., and Perricone, E.: Aggregation of cartilage proteoglycans. Evidence for the presence of a hyaluronate binding region in proteoglycans from osteoarthritic cartilage. Arthritis Rheum. 19:1308, 1976.
50. Palmoski, M. J., and Brandt, K. D.: Hyaluronate binding by proteoglycans: Comparison of mildly and severely osteoarthritic regions of the human femoral cartilage. Clin. Chim. Acta 79:87, 1976.
51. Inerot, S., Heinegard, D., Audell, L., and Olsson, S.-E.: Articular cartilage proteoglycans in aging and osteoarthritis. Biochem. J. 169:143, 1978.
52. Bollet, A. J., and Nance, J. L.: Biochemical findings in normal and osteoarthritic articular cartilage. II. Chondroitin sulfate concentration and chain length, water and ash contents. J. Clin. Invest. 45:1170, 1966.
53. Mankin, H. J., Dorfman, H. D., Lippiello, L., and Zarins, A.: Biochemical and metabolic abnormalities in articular cartilage from osteoarthritic human hips. II. Correlation of morphology with metabolic data. J. Bone Joint Surg. 53A:523, 1971.
54. Sweet, M. B. E., Thonar, E.-J., Immelman, A. R., and Solomon, L.: Biochemical changes in progressive osteoarthrosis. Ann. Rheum. Dis. 36:387, 1977.
55. Ryu, J., Treadwell, B. V., and Mankin, H. J.: Biochemical and metabolic abnormalities in normal and osteoarthritic human articular cartilage. Arthritis Rheum. 27:613, 1984.
56. Hardingham, T., and Bayliss, M.: Proteoglycans of articular cartilage: Changes in aging and in joint disease. Arthritis Rheum. 20:12, 1990.
57. Hughes, C. E., Fosang, A. J., Murphy, G., et al.: Proteolytic digestion of cartilage proteoglycans involves destruction of the second globular domain. J. Bone Joint Surg. 57A:413, 1992.
58. Ehrlich, M. G., Mankin, H. J., Jones, H., Wright, R., Crispen, C., and Vigliani, G.: Collagenase and collagenase inhibitors in osteoarthritis and normal human cartilage. J. Clin. Invest. 59:226, 1977.
59. Ehrlich, M. G., Houle, P. A., Vigliani, G., and Mankin, H. J.: Correlation between articular cartilage collagenase activity and osteoarthritis. Arthritis Rheum. 21:761, 1978.
60. Ollivierre, F., Fubler, U., Towle, C. A., Laurencin, C., and Treadwell,

B. V.: Expression of IL-1 genes in human and bovine chondrocytes: A mechanism for autocrine control of cartilage matrix degradation. Biochem. Biophys. Res. Commun. 141:904, 1985.

61. Rath, N. C., Oronsky, A. L., and Kerwar, S. S.: Synthesis of interleukin-1–like activity by normal rat chondrocytes in culture. Clin. Immunol. Immunopathol. 47:39, 1988.

62. Kandel, R. A., Dinarello, C. A., and Biswas, C.: The stimulation of collagenase production in rabbit articular chondrocytes in interleukin-1 is increased by collagens. Biochem. Int. 15:1021, 1987.

63. Pujol, J. P., and Loyau, G.: Interleukin-1 and osteoarthritis. Life Sci. 41:1187, 1987.

64. Dodge, G. R., and Poole, A. R.: Immunohistochemical detection and immunochemical analysis of type II collagen degradation in human normal, rheumatoid, and osteoarthritic articular cartilages and in explants of bovine articular cartilage cultured with interleukin-1. J. Clin. Invest. 83:647, 1989.

65. Ratcliffe, A., Tyler, J. A., and Hardingham, T. E.: Articular cartilage cultured with interleukin-1: Increased release of link protein, hyaluronate-binding region and other proteoglycan fragments. Biochem. J. 238:571, 1986.

66. Dean, D. D., and Woessner, J. F., Jr.: Extracts of human articular cartilage contain an inhibitor of tissue metalloproteinases. Biochem. J. 218:277, 1984.

67. Yamada, H., Stephens, R. W., Nakagawa, T., and McNicol, D.: Human articular cartilage contains an inhibitor of plasminogen activator. J. Rheumatol. 15:1138, 1988.

68. Murphy, G., Cockett, M. I., Stephens, P. E., Smith, B. J., and Docherty, A. J. P.: Stromelysin is an activator of procollagenase. Biochem. J. 248:265, 1987.

69. Stephens, R. W., Ghosh, P., and Taylor, T. K.: Pathogenesis of osteoarthritis. Med. Hypotheses 5:809, 1979.

70. Pettipher, E. R., Higgs, G. A., and Henderson B.: Interleukin-1 induces leukocyte infiltration and cartilage proteoglycan degradation in the synovial joint. Proc. Natl. Acad. Sci. U.S.A. 83:8749, 1986.

71. Saklatvala, J., Pilsworth, L. M. C., Sarsfield, S. J., Gavrilovic, J., and Heath, J. K.: Pig catabolin is a form of interleukin-1: Cartilage and bone resorb, fibroblasts make prostaglandin and collagenase, and thymocyte proliferation is augmented in response to one protein. Biochem. J. 224:461, 1984.

72. Bayliss, M. T., Vilim, V., Hardingham, T. E., and Muir, H.: Age-related changes in the biosynthetic response of human articular cartilage in interleukin-1. Trans. Orthop. Res. Soc. 14:329, 1989.

73. Nietfeld, J. J., Wilbrink, B., Den Otter, W., Huber, J., and Huber-Bruning, O.: The effect of human IL-1 on proteoglycan metabolism in human and porcine cartilage explants. J. Rheumatol. 17:818, 1990.

74. Tyler, J. A.: Articular cartilage cultured with catabolin (pig interleukin-1) synthesizes a decreased number of normal proteoglycan molecules. Biochem. J. 227:869, 1985.

75. Dingle, J. T., Davies, M. E., Mativi, B. Y., and Middleton, H. F.: Immunohistochemical identification of interleukin-1–activated chondrocytes. Ann. Rheum. Dis. 49:889, 1990.

76. Radin, E. L.: Aetiology of osteoarthrosis. Clin. Rheum. Dis. 2:509, 1976.

77. Ishizue, K. K., Ehrlich, M. G., and Mankin, H. J.: Drug-induced inhibition of proteoglycanase activity in the Hulth-Telhag model. J. Orthop. Res. 7:806, 1989.

78. Yu, L. P., Jr., Smith, G. N., Jr., Hasty, K. A., and Brandt, K. D.: Doxycycline inhibits Type XI collagenolytic activity of extracts from human osteoarthritic cartilage and of gelatinase. Submitted for publication.

79. Yu, L. P., Jr., Smith, G. N., Jr., Brandt, K. D., O'Connor, B., and Brandt, D. A.: Prophylactic oral doxycycline administration reduces the severity of canine osteoarthritis. Submitted for publication.

80. Dean, D. D., Azzo, W., Martel-Pelletier, J., Pelletier, J. P., and Woessner, J. F., Jr.: Levels of metalloproteases, and tissue inhibitor of metalloproteases in human osteoarthritic cartilage. J. Rheumatol. 14 (Spec. No.):43, 1987.

81. Teshima, R., Treadwell, B. V., Trahan, C. A., and Mankin, H. J.: Comparative rates of proteoglycan synthesis and size of proteoglycans in normal and osteoarthritic chondrocytes. Arthritis Rheum. 26:1225, 1983.

82. Moskowitz, R. W., David, W., Sammarco, J., Martens, M., Baker, J., Mayor, M., Burstein, A. H., and Frankel, V. H.: Experimentally induced degenerative joint lesions following partial meniscectomy in the rabbit. Arthritis Rheum. 16:397, 1973.

83. Muir, H.: Molecular approach to the understanding of osteoarthrosis. Ann. Rheum. Dis. 36:199, 1977.

84. McDevitt, C. A., Muir, H., and Pond, M. J.: Biochemical events in early osteoarthrosis. In Ali, S. Y. Elves, M. W., and Leaback, D. H. (eds.): Normal and Osteoarthrotic Cartilage. London, Institute of Orthopaedics, 1974, pp. 207–217.

85. McDevitt, C. A., and Muir, H.: Biochemical changes in the cartilage of the knee in experimental and natural osteoarthritis in the dog. J. Bone Joint Surg. 58B:94, 1976.

86. Brandt, K. D.: Enhanced extractability of articular cartilage proteoglycans in osteoarthrosis. Biochem. J. 143:475, 1974.

87. Moskowitz, R. W., Howell, D. S., Goldberg, V. M., Muniz, O., and Pita, J. C.: Cartilage proteoglycan alterations in an experimentally induced model of rabbit osteoarthrosis. Arthritis Rheum. 22:155, 1979.

88. Kempson, G. E., Spivey, C. J., Swanson, S. A. V., and Freeman, M. A. R.: Patterns of cartilage stiffness on normal and degenerate human femoral heads. J. Biomech. 4:597, 1971.

89. Adams, M. E., and Brandt, K. D.: Hypertrophic repair of canine articular cartilage in osteoarthritis after anterior cruciate ligament transection. J. Rheumatol. 18:428, 1991.

90. Braunstein, E. M., Brandt, K. D., and Albrecht, M.: MRI demonstration of hypertrophic articular cartilage repair in osteoarthritis. Skeletal Radiol. 19:335, 1990.

91. Brandt, K. D., Braunstein, E. M., Visco, D. M., O'Connor, B., Heck, D., Katz, B., and Albrecht, M.: Cranial (anterior) cruciate ligament transection in the dog: A bona fide model of osteoarthritis, not merely of cartilage injury and repair. J. Rheumatol. 18:436, 1991.

92. McDevitt, C. A., Muir, H., and Pond, M. J.: Canine articular cartilage in natural and experimentally induced osteoarthritis. Biochem. Soc. Trans. 1:287, 1973.

93. Vignon, E., Arlot, M., Hartman, D., Moyer, B., and Ville, G.: Hypertrophic repair of articular cartilage in experimental osteoarthrosis. Ann. Rheum. Dis. 42:82, 1983.

94. Châteauvert, J., Pritzker, K. P. H., Kessler, M. J., and Grynpas, M. D.: Spontaneous arthritis in rhesus macaques. I. Chemical and biochemical studies. J. Rheumatol. 16:1098, 1989.

95. Châteauvert, J., Pritzker, K. P. H., Kessler, M. J., and Grynpas, M. D.: Spontaneous arthritis in rhesus macaques. II. Characterization of disease and morphometric studies. J. Rheumatol. 17:73, 1990.

96. Bywaters, E. G. L.: Metabolism of joint tissue. J. Pathol. Bacteriol. 44:247, 1937.

97. Johnson, L. D.: Kinetics of osteoarthritis. Lab Invest. 8:1223, 1959.

98. Bollet, A. J.: Connective tissue polysaccharide metabolism and the pathogenesis of osteoarthritis. Adv. Intern. Med. 13:33, 1967.

99. Freeman, M. A. R.: Discussion on pathogenesis of osteoarthrosis. In Ali, S. Y., Elves, M. W., and Leaback, D. H. (eds.): Normal and Osteoarthrotic Articular Cartilage. London, Institute of Orthopaedics, 1974, pp. 301–319.

100. Malemud, C. J., Goldberg, V. M., Moskowitz, R. W., Getzy, L. L., Papay, R. S., and Norby, D. P.: Biosynthesis of proteoglycan in vitro by cartilage from human osteochrondrophytic spurs. Biochem. J. 206:329, 1982.

101. Marshall, J. L., and Olsson, S. E.: Instability of the knee: a long-term study in dogs. J. Bone Joint Surg. 53A:1561, 1971.

102. Danielsson, L. G.: Incidence and prognosis of coxarthrosis. Acta Orthop. Scand. (Suppl.) 66:1, 1964.

103. Trueta, J.: Studies of the Development and Decay of the Human Frame. Philadelphia, W. B. Saunders Company, 1968.

104. Swanson, S. A. V., and Freeman, M. A. R.: The mechanics of synovial joints. In Simpson, D. C. (ed.): Modern Trends in Biomechanics. Vol. 1. London, Butterworths, 1970, p. 239.

105. Gilbertson, E. M. M.: The development of periarticular osteophytes in experimentally induced osteoarthritis in the dog. Ann. Rheum. Dis. 34:12, 1975.

106. Bernstein, M. A.: Experimental production of arthritis by artificially produced passive congestion. J. Bone Joint Surg. 15:661, 1933.

107. Phillips, R. S.: Phlebography in osteoarthritis of the hip. J. Bone Joint Surg. 48B:280, 1966.

108. Chrisman, O. D., Fessel, J. M., and Southwick, W. O.: Experimental production of synovitis and marginal articular exostoses in the knee joints of dogs. Yale J. Biol. Med. 37:409, 1965.

109. Palmoski, M. J., and Brandt, K. D.: Immobilization of the knee prevents osteoarthritis after anterior cruciate ligament transection. Arthritis Rheum. 25:1201, 1982.

110. Butler, M., Colombo, C., Hickman, K., O'Byrne, E., Steele, R., Steinetz, B., Quintavalla, J., and Yokoyama, N.: A new model of osteoarthritis in rabbits. III. Evaluation of anti-osteoarthritic effects of selected drugs administered intraarticularly. Arthritis Rheum. 26:1380, 1983.

111. Pelletier, J.-P., and Martel-Pelletier, J.: Protective effects of corticosteroids on cartilage lesions and osteophyte formation in the Pond-Nuki dog model of osteoarthritis. Arthritis Rheum. 32:181, 1989.

112. Sokoloff, L.: The pathology of osteoarthrosis and the role of ageing. In Nuki, G. (ed.): The Aetiopathogenesis of Osteoarthrosis. Tunbridge Wells, England, Pitman Medical Publishing Co. Ltd., 1980, pp. 1–15.

113. Collins, D. H.: The Pathology of Articular and Spinal Disease. London, E. Arnold and Company, 1949.

114. Jaffe, H. D.: Metabolic, Degenerative and Inflammatory Diseases of Bones and Joints. Philadelphia, Lea & Febiger, Philadelphia, 1972.

115. Ferguson, A. B., Jr.: The pathology of degenerative arthritis of the hip and the use of osteotomy in its treatment. Clin. Orthop. 77:84, 1971.

116. Lloyd-Roberts, G. C.: The role of capsular changes in osteoarthritis of the hip joint. J. Bone Joint Surg. 35B:627, 1953.

117. Arnoldi, C. C. and Reimann, I.: The pathomechanism of human coxarthrosis. Acta. Orthop. Scand. Suppl. 181:1, 1979.
118. Gordon, G. V., Villaneuva, T., Schumacher, H. R., and Gohel, V.: Autopsy study correlating degree of osteoarthritis, synovitis and evidence of articular calcification. J. Rheumatol. 11:681, 1984.
119. Ehrlich, G. E.: Inflammatory osteoarthritis. I. The clinical syndrome. J. Chronic Dis. 25:317, 1972.
120. Ehrlich, G. E.: Erosive inflammatory and primary generalized osteoarthritis. In Moskowitz, R. W., Howell, D. S., Goldberg, V. M., and Mankin, H. J., (eds.): Osteoarthritis: Diagnosis and Management. Philadelphia, W. B. Saunders Company, 1984, pp. 199–211.
121. Peter, S. B., Pearson, C. M., and Marmor, L.: Erosive osteoarthritis of the hands. Arthritis Rheum. 9:365, 1966.
122. Meachim, G., and Brooke, G.: The pathology of osteoarthritis. In Moskowitz, R. W., Howell, D. S., Goldberg, V. M., and Mankin, H. J. (eds.): Osteoarthritis: Diagnosis and Management. Philadelphia, W. B. Saunders Company, 1984, pp. 29–42.
123. Lloyd-Roberts, G. C.: Osteoarthritis of the hip. Study of the clinical pathology. J. Bone Joint Surg. 37B:8, 1955.
124. Resnick, D.: Degenerative diseases of the vertebral column. Radiology 156:3, 1985.
125. Milgram, J. W.: Osteoarthritic changes of the severely degenerative disc in humans. Spine 7:498, Sept–Oct. 1982.
126. Cameron, H. U., and Fornasier, V. L.: Fine detail radiography of the femoral head in osteoarthritis. J. Rheumatol. 6:178, 1979.
127. Jeffrey, A. K.: Osteogenesis in the osteoarthritic femoral head. J. Bone Joint Surg. 55B:262, 1973.
128. Sokoloff, L.: Osteoarthritis. In Simon, W. H. (ed.): The Human Joint in Health and Disease. Philadelphia, University of Pennsylvania Press, 1978, pp. 91–111.
129. Byers, P., Contemponi, C. A., and Farkas, T. A.: Post-mortem study of the hip joint. Ann. Rheum. Dis. 29:15, 1970.
130. Ladefoged, C.: Amyloid in osteoarthritic hip joint: deposits in relation to chondromatosis, pyrophosphate, and inflammatory cell infiltrate in the synovial membrane and fibrous capsule. Ann. Rheum. Dis. 42:659, 1983.
131. Layton, M. W., Goldstein, S. A., Goulet, R. W., Feldkamp, L. A., Kubinski, D. J., and Bole, G. G.: Examination of subchondral bone architecture in experimental osteoarthritis by microscopic computed axial tomography. Arthritis Rheum. 31:1400, 1988.
132. Fazzalari, N. L., Vernon-Roberts, B., and Barracott, J.: Osteoarthritis of the hip. Possible protective and causative roles of trabecular microfractures in the head of the femur. Clin. Orthop. Relat. Res. 216:224, 1987.
133. Hulth, A., Lindberg, L., and Telhag, H.: Mitosis in human osteoarthritic cartilage. Clin. Orthop. 88:247, 1972.
134. Telhag, H.: Nucleic acids in human normal and osteoarthritic articular cartilage. Acta Orthop. Scand. 47:585, 1976.
135. Mankin, H. J.: The articular cartilages, cartilage healing and osteoarthritis. In Cruess, R. L., and Rennie, W. R. J. (eds.): Adult Orthopaedics. Vol. 1. New York, Churchill Livingstone, 1984, pp. 163–270.
136. Weiss, C., and Mirow, S.: An ultrastructural study of osteoarthritic changes in articular cartilage of human knee. J. Bone Joint Surg. 54A:954, 1972.
137. Ghadially, F. N.: Fine structure of joints. In Sokoloff, L. (ed.): The Joints and Synovial Fluid. New York, Academic Press, 1978, pp. 105–176.
138. Radin, E. L., Ehrlich, M. G., Chernack, B. J., Abernethy, P., Paul, I. L., and Rose, R. M.: Effect of repetitive impulsive loading on the knee joints of rabbits. Clin. Orthop. 131:288, 1978.
139. Radin, E. L., and Rose, R. M.: Role of subchondral bone in the initiation and progression of cartilage damage. Clin. Orthop. 213:34, 1986.
140. Klaer, T., Pederson, N. W., Kristensen, K. D., and Starklint, H.: Intraosseous pressure and oxygen tension in avascular necrosis and osteoarthritis of the hip. J. Bone Joint Surg. 72:1023, 1990.
141. Noble, J., and Alexander, K.: Studies of tibial subchondral bone density and its significance. J. Bone Joint Surg. 67:295, 1985.
142. Takahama, A.: Histological study on spontaneous osteoarthritis of the knee in C57 black mouse. Nippon Seikeigeka Gakkai Zasshi 64:2717, 1990.
143. Mazieres, B., Blanckaert, A., and Thiechart, M.: Experimental postcontusive osteoarthritis of the knee: quantitative microscopic study of the patella and the femoral condyles. J. Rheumatol. 14:119, 1987.
144. Moskowitz, R. W., and Goldberg, V. M.: Studies of ostephyte pathogenesis in experimentally induced osteoarthritis. J. Rheumatol. 14:311, 1987.
145. Ilardi, C. F., and Sokoloff, L.: Secondary osteonecrosis in osteoarthritis of the femoral head. Hum. Pathol. 15:79, 1984.
146. Lemperg, R. K., and Arnoldi, C. C.: The significance of intraosseous pressure in normal and diseased states with special reference to intraosseous engorgement pain syndrome. Clin. Orthop. 136:143, 1978.
147. Lawrence, J. S.: Rheumatism in Populations. London, Heinemann Medical, 1977, pp. 1–572.

148. Forman, M. D., Kaplan, D. A., Muller, G. F., and Kayaalp, P.: The epidemiology of osteoarthritis of the knee. In Peyron, J. G. (ed.): Epidemiology of Osteoarthritis. Paris, Ciba-Geigy, 1980, pp. 243–250.
149. Brandt, K. D., and Flusser, D.: Osteoarthritis. In Bellamy, N. (ed.): Prognosis in the Rheumatic Diseases. Lancaster, UK, Kluwer Academic Publishers, 1991, pp. 11–35.
150. Weightman, B.: In vitro fatigue testing of articular cartilage. Ann. Rheum. Dis. 34(Suppl.):108, 1975.
151. Bullough, P. G.: The geometry of diarthrodial joints, its physiologic maintenance, and the possible significance of age-related changes in geometry to load distribution and the development of osteoarthritis. Clin. Orthop. Relat. Res. 156:61, 1981.
152. Lane, J. B., Villacin, A., and Bullough, P. G.: The vascularity and remodeling of subchondral bone and calcified cartilage in adult human femoral and humeral heads. J. Bone Joint Surg. 59B:272, 1977.
153. Swanson, S. A. V., Freeman, M. A. R., and Day, W. H.: Contact pressures in the loaded cadaver human hip. Ann. Rheum. Dis. (Suppl.) 34:114, 1975.
154. Slowman, S., and Brandt, K.: Composition and glycosaminoglycan metabolism of articular cartilage from habitually induced and habitually unloaded sites. Arthritis Rheum. 29:88, 1986.
155. O'Connor, B. L., Palmoski, M. J., and Brandt, K. D.: Neurogenic acceleration of degenerative joint lesions. J. Bone Joint Surg. 67A:562, 1985.
156. Knowlton, R. G., Katzenstein, P. L., Moskowitz, R. W., Weaver, E. J., Malemud, C. J., Pathria, M. N., Jimenez, S. A., and Prockop, D. J.: Genetic linkage of polymorphism in the type II procollagen gene (COL 2A1) to primary osteoarthritis associated with mild chondrodysplasia. N. Engl. J. Med. 322:526 1990.
157. Ala-Kokka, L., Baldwin, C. T., Moskowitz, R. W., and Prockop, D. J.: Single base mutation in tye type II procollagen gene (COL 2A1) as a cause of primary osteoarthritis associated with mild chondrodysplasia. Proc. Natl. Acad. Si. U.S.A. 87:6565, 1990.
158. Cuervo, L. A., Pita, J. C., and Howell, D. S.: Inhibition of calcium phosphate mineral growth by proteoglycan aggregate fractions in a synthetic lymph. Calcif. Tiss. Res. 13:1, 1973.
159. Perricone, E., and Brandt, K. D.: Enhancement of urate solubility by connective tissue. I. Effect of proteoglycan aggregates and buffer cation. Arthritis Rheum. 21:453, 1978.
160. Ali, S. Y., and Bayliss, M. T.: Enzymic changes in human osteoarthrotic cartilage. In Ali, S. Y., Elves, M. W., and Leaback, D. H. (eds.): Normal and Osteoarthrotic Cartilage. London, Institute of Orthopaedics, 1974, pp. 189–205.
161. Howell, D. S., Muniz, O., Pita, J. C., and Enis, J. E.: Extrusion of pyrophosphate into extracellular media by osteoarthritic cartilage incubates. J. Clin. Invest. 56:1473, 1975.
162. Altman, R. D., Muniz, O., Pita, J. C., and Howell, D. S.: Articular chondrocalcinosis. Microanalysis of pyrophosphate (PPi) in synovial fluid and plasma. Arthritis Rheum. 16:171, 1973.
163. Silcox, D. C., and McCarty, D. J., Jr.: Elevated inorganic pyrophosphate concentrations in synovial fluids in osteoarthritis and pseudogout. J. Lab. Clin. Med. 83:518, 1974.
164. Howell, D. S., Muniz, O. E., and Morales, S.: 5′-Nucleotidase and pyrophosphate (PPi)-generating activities in articular cartilage extracts in calcium pyrophosphate deposition disease (CPPD) and in primary osteoarthritis (OA). In Peyron, J. G. (ed.): Epidemiology of Osteoarthritis. Paris, Ciba-Geigy, 1980, p. 99.
165. Tenenbaum J., Muniz, O., Schumacher, H. R., Jr., Good, A. E., and Howell, D. S.: Comparison of pyrophosphohydrolase activities for articular cartilage in calcium pyrophosphate deposition disease and in primary osteoarthritis. Arthritis Rheum. 24:492, 1981.
166. Schumacher, H. R.: Secondary osteoarthritis. In Moskowitz, R. W., Howell, D. S., Goldberg, V. M., and Mankin, H. J. (eds.): Osteoarthritis: Diagnosis and Management. Philadelphia, W. B. Saunders Company, 1984, pp. 235–264.
167. Donahue, J. M., Oegema, T. R., Jr., and Thompson, R. G., Jr.: The zone of calcified cartilage: the focal point of changes following blunt trauma to articular cartilage. Trans. Orthop. Res. Soc. 11:233, 1986.
168. Oegema, T. R., Jr., Hofmeister, F., Carpenter, R. J., Chin-Purcell, M., and Thompson, R. C., Jr.: Acceleration of calcification in the zone of calcified cartilage in rabbits. Trans. Orthop. Res. Soc. 13:512, 1988.
169. Radin, E. L.: Mechanical factors in the etiology of osteoarthrosis. In Peyron, J. G. (ed.): Epidemiology of Osteoarthrosis. Paris, Ciba-Geigy, 1981, pp. 136–139.
170. Linn, F. C., and Radin, E. L.: Lubrication of animal joints. III. The effect of certain chemical alterations of the cartilage and lubricant. Arthritis Rheum. 11:674, 1968.
171. Radin, E. L., and Paul, I. L.: The response of joints to impact loading. I. In vitro wear. Arthritis Rheum. 14:356, 1971.
172. Reilly, D. T., and Mertens, M.: Experimental analysis of the quadriceps muscle force and patello-femoral joint reaction force for various activities. Acta Orthop. Scand. 43:126, 1972.
173. Collins, J. J., and Whittle, M. W.: Influence of gait parameters on the loading of the lower limb. J. Biomed. Eng. 11:409, 1989.

174. Radin, E. L., Yang, K. U., Riegger, C., Kish, V. L., and O'Connor, J. J.: Relationship between lower limb dynamics and knee joint pain. J. Orthop. Res. 9:338, 1991.

175. Radin, E. L., and Paul, I. L.: Does cartilage compliance reduce skeletal impact loads? The relative force attenuating properties of articular cartilage, synovial fluid, peri-articular soft-tissues and bone. Arthritis Rheum. 13:139, 1970.

176. Hill, A. V.: Production and absorption of work by muscle. Science 131:897, 1960.

177. Radin, E. L.: The physiology and degeneration of joints. Semin. Arthritis Rheum. 2:245, 1972–1973.

178. Jones, C. M., and Watt, D. G. D.: Muscular control of landing from unexpected falls in man. J. Physiol. 219:729, 1971.

179. Ochoa, J. A., Heck, D. A., Brandt, K. D., and Hillberry, B. M.: The effect of intertrabecular fluid on femoral head mechanics. J. Rheumatol. 18:580, 1991.

180. Bullough, P., Goodfellow, J., and O'Connor, J.: The relationship between degenerative changes and load-bearing in the human hip. J. Bone Joint Surg. 55B:746, 1973.

181. Todd, R. C., Freeman, M. A. R., and Pirie, C. J.: Isolated trabecular fatigue fractures in the femoral head. J. Bone Joint Surg. 54B:723, 1972.

182. Ochoa, J. A., Heck, D. A., Brandt, K. D., and Hillberry, B. M.: The effect of intertrabecular fluid on femoral head mechanics. J. Rheumatol. 18:580, 1991.

183. Foss, M. V. L., and Byers, P. D.: Bone density, osteoarthrosis of the hip and fracture of the upper end of the femur. Ann. Rheum. Dis. 31:259, 1972.

184. Radin, E. L.: Mechanical aspects of osteoarthrosis. Bull. Rheum. Dis. 26:862, 1975–1976.

185. Mankin, H.: Discussion of paper by L. Sokoloff. In Ali, S. Y., Elves, M. W., and Leaback, D. H. (eds.): Normal and Osteoarthrotic Articular Cartilage. London, Institute of Orthopaedics, 1974, p. 123.

186. Towle, C. A., Mankin, H. J., Avruch, J., and Treadwell, B. V.: Insulin-promoted increase in the phosphorylation of protein synthesis initiation factor eIF-2. Biochem. Biophys. Res. Commun. 121:134, 1984.

187. Treadwell B. V., and Mankin, H. J.: The synthetic processes of articular cartilage. Clin. Orthop. 213:50, 1986.

188. Lippiello, L., Kaye, C., Neumata, T., and Mankin, H. J.: In-vitro metabolic response of articular cartilage segments to low levels of hydrostatic pressure. Connect. Tissue Res. 13:99, 1985.

189. Mankin, H. J.: Current concepts review: the response of articular cartilage to mechanical injury. J. Bone Joint Surg. 64A:460, 1982.

190. Mitrovic, D., Lippiello, L., Gruson, F., Aprile, F., and Mankin, H. J.: Effects of various prostanoids on the in-vitro metabolism of bovine articular chondrocytes. Prostaglandins 22:499, 1981.

191. Madreperla, S. A., Louwerenburg, B., Mann, R. W., Towle, C. A., Mankin, H. J., and Treadwell, B. V.: Induction of heat shock protein synthesis in chondrocytes at physiological temperatures. J. Orthop. Res. 3:30, 1985.

192. Tyler, J. A., Bolis, S., Dingle, J. T., and Middleton, F. S.: Mediators of matrix catabolism. In Kuettner, K. E., Schleyerbach, R., Peyron, J. G., and Hascall, V. C. (eds.): Articular Cartilage Biochemistry and Osteoarthritis. New York, Raven Press, 1992, pp. 251–264.

193. Schalkwijk, J., Joosten, L. A. B., van den Berg, W. B., and van de Putte, L. B. A.: Chondrocyte nonresponsiveness to insulin-like growth factor I in experimental arthritis. Arthritis Rheum. 32:894, 1989.

194. Jentzsch, K. D., Wellmitz, G., Heder, G., Petzold, E., Burtrock, P., and Oehme, P.: A bovine brain fraction with fibroblast growth factor activity inducing articular cartilage regeneration in vivo. Acta Biol. Med. Germ. 39:967, 1980.

195. Cuevas, P., Burgos, J., and Baird, A.: Basic fibroblast growth factor (FGF) promotes cartilage repair in vivo. Biochem. Biophys. Res. Comm. 156:611, 1988.

196. Moskowitz, R. W., Schwartz, H. J., Michel, B., Ratnoff, O. D., and Astrup, T.: Generation of kinin-like agents by chondroitin sulfate, heparin, chitin sulfate, and human articular cartilage: possible pathophysiologic implications. J. Lab. Clin. Med. 76:790, 1970.

197. Evans, C. H., Mears, D. C., and McKnight, J. L.: A preliminary ferrographic study of the wear particles in human synovial fluid. Arthritis Rheum. 24:912, 1981.

198. Evans, C. H.: Cellular mechanisms of hydrolytic enzyme release in proteoglycan. Semin. Arthritis Rheum. 11 (Suppl. 1):93, 1981.

199. Cooke, T. D.: Significance of immune complex deposits in osteoarthritic cartilage. J. Rheumatol. 14(Spec. No.):77, 1987.

200. McCarty, D. J., Halverson, P. B., Carresa, G. F., Brewer, B. J., and Kozin, F.: Milwaukee shoulder: association of microspheroids containing hydroxyapatite crystals, active collagenase and neutral protease with rotator cuff defects. Arthritis Rheum. 24:464, 1981.

201. Kellgren, J. H., Lawrence, J. S., and Bier, F.: Genetic factors in generalized osteoarthritis. Ann. Rheum. Dis. 22:237, 1963.

202. Saville, P. D., and Dickson, J.: Age and weight in osteoarthritis of the hip. Arthritis Rheum. 11:635, 1968.

203. Felson, D. T., Anderson, J. J., Naimack, A., Swift, M., Castelli, W., and Meenan, R. F.: Obesity and symptomatic knee osteoarthritis. Results from the Framingham Study. Arthritis Rheum. 30:S130, 1987.

204. Anderson, J., and Felson, D.: Factors associated with knee osteoarthritis (OA) in a national survey. Arthritis Rheum. 29:S16, 1986.

205. Leach, R. E., Baumgard, S., and Broom, J.: Obesity: its relationship to osteoarthritis of the knee. Clin. Orthop. Relat. Res. 93:271, 1973.

206. Silberberg, M., and Silberberg, R.: Osteoarthrosis in mice fed diets enriched with animal or vegetable fat. Arch. Pathol. 70:385, 1960.

207. Sokoloff, L., and Mickelsen, O.: Dietary fat supplements, body weight and osteoarthritis in DBA/2JN mice. J. Nutr. 85:117, 1965.

208. Sokoloff, L., Crittenden, L. B., Yamamoto, R. S., and Jay, G. E.: The genetics of degenerative joint disease in mice. Arthritis Rheum. 5:531, 1962.

209. Cooke T. D.: Immune pathology in polyarticular osteoarthritis. Clin. Orthop. 213:41, 1986.

210. Moskowitz, R. W., and Kresina, T. F.: Immunofluorescent analysis of experimental osteoarthritic cartilage and synovium: evidence for selective deposition of immunoglobulin and complement in cartilaginous tissues. J. Rheumatol. 13:391, 1986.

211. Cooke, T. D.: Pathogenetic mechanisms in polyarticular osteoarthritis. Clin. Rheum. Dis. 11:203, 1985.

212. Cooke, T. D., Bennet, E. L., and Ohno, O.: Identification of immunoglobulins and complement components in articular collagenous tissues of patients with idiopathic osteoarthrosis. In Nuki, G. (ed.): The Aetiopathogenesis of Osteoarthrosis. Tunbridge Wells, England, Pitman Medical Publishing Co. Ltd., 1980, pp. 144–155.

213. Revell, P. A., Mayston, V., Lalor, P., and Mapp, P.: The synovial membrane in osteoarthritis: a histological study including the characterisation of the cellular infiltrate present in inflammatory osteoarthritis using monoclonal antibodies. Ann. Rheum. Dis. 47:300, 1988.

214. Kennedy. T. D., Plater, Z. C., Partridge, T. A., Woodrow, D. F., and Maini, R. N.: Morphometric comparison of synovium from patients with osteoarthritis and rheumatoid arthritis. J. Clin. Pathol. 41:847, 1988.

215. Goldberg, V. M.: The immunology of articular cartilage. In Moskowitz, R. W., Howell, D. S., Goldberg, V. M., and Mankin, H. J. (eds.): Osteoarthritis: Diagnosis and Management. Philadelphia, W. B. Saunders Company, 1984, pp. 81–92.

Chapter 79

Clinical Features of Osteoarthritis

Henry J. Mankin

INTRODUCTION

Osteoarthritis is a slowly progressive monoarticular (or less commonly polyarticular) disorder of unknown cause and obscure pathogenesis. The condition occurs late in life, affecting principally the hands and large weight-bearing joints, and is characterized *clinically* by pain, deformity, enlargement of the joints, and limitation of motion. *Pathologically* the disease is characterized by focal erosive lesions, cartilage destruction, subchondral sclerosis, cyst formation, and large osteophytes at the margins of the joint. The disease appears to originate in the cartilage, and the changes in that tissue, virtually pathognomonic, are progressively more severe with advancing disease; structural aberrations in the underlying bone and inflammatory alterations in the synovium are usually milder and thought to be secondary. Systemic abnormalities have not been detected. *Therapeutically,* the disorder is characterized by lack of a specific healing agent.

Historically, osteoarthritis is an "ancient" disease.[1, 2] Unlike rheumatoid disease where confirmation of the early presence of the disorder has been sought and still not confirmed, paleopathologic examination of bones from ossuaries, Egyptian mummies, or prehistoric fossils has clearly demonstrated that osteoarthritis is as old as the various mammalian species.[1-3] Every generation since recorded history has commented on the stooped posture of the tribal ancients, the slowing and awkwardness of gait of the elderly, and the gnarled hands of the octogenarian. Indeed, ancient and modern man have accepted the clinical syndrome of osteoarthritis as a sign of aging and considered the two disorders to be synonymous and comorbid.

Osteoarthritis is the most prevalent of all the joint diseases with well over fifty million U.S. citizens suffering with the pain and limitation of movement[4, 5]; the estimated costs of medical treatment and lost earnings are staggering.

CLASSIFICATION OF OSTEOARTHRITIS

Most investigators agree that osteoarthritis is not a single disease but that the observed stereotypic clinical pattern represents a "final common pathway" for a number of conditions of diverse cause.[6, 7] A classification reported in the proceedings of a workshop on etiopathogenesis of osteoarthritis held in July, 1985,[4] is depicted in Table 79–1 with only slight modifications. As can be noted, the first category is *idiopathic* which is either *localized* or *generalized*. The localized forms differ principally in anatomic location and to some extent in degree of change as seen pathologically or radiographically. Thus localized disease of the first metatarsophalangeal joint (bunion) may be a somewhat different disorder from idiopathic concentric osteoarthritis of the hip; or Forestier's disease (see Chapter 22), which some investigators classify as a form of osteoarthritis; or apophyseal posterior joint osteoarthritis of the spine,

Table 79–1. CLASSIFICATION OF OSTEOARTHRITIS (OA)

I. Idiopathic
  A. Localized
    1. Hands (Heberden's and Bouchard's nodes, erosive OA)
    2. Feet (e.g., hallux valgus, hallux rigidus)
    3. Knee (patellofemoral, medial or lateral compartment)
    4. Hip (e.g., eccentric, concentric, diffuse)
    5. Spine (e.g., apophyseal disease, intervertebral joints, spondylosis, diffuse idiopathic skeletal hyperostosis [DISH])
    6. Other single sites
  B. Generalized (GOA)
II. Secondary
  A. Trauma (acute, chronic)
  B. Congenital
    1. Localized disease (e.g., Perthes' disease, congenital dislocation of the hip [CDH], slipped capital femoral epiphysis [SCFE])
    2. Mechanical factors
    3. Bone dysplasia (e.g., dysplasia epiphysealis multiplex, spondyloepiphyseal dysplasia)
  C. Metabolic (e.g., ochronosis, hemochromatosis, calcium pyrophosphate dihydrate disease [CPPD], gout)
  D. Endocrine (e.g., acromegaly, obesity, diabetes)
  E. Other bone and joint disease (osteonecrosis, infection, Charcot's arthropathy, rheumatoid arthritis, gout)
  F. Diseases of obscure etiology (Kashin-Beck disease, Mseleni disease)

Adapted from Mankin, H. J., Brandt, K. D., and Shulman, L. E.: Workshop on etiopathogenesis of osteoarthritis. J. Rheumatol. 13:1130, 1986.

which is different from patellofemoral disease in adolescent females (chondromalacia patella).

Perhaps the most intriguing of the idiopathic group are the patients with generalized osteoarthritis (GOA).[8-14] Since the initial studies of Kellgren and Moore,[14] numerous workers have confirmed the existence of groups of epidemiologically distinct patients who have three or more sites of osteoarthritis and usually fairly extensive small joint disease.[11, 13, 14] No unique pathologic variation has been noted by study of the clinical or histologic features of the disease in this group of patients, but it seems logical that they represent some as yet unknown genetic disorder in the structure, biochemistry, or metabolism of articular cartilage.[12] Perhaps a clue lies with the observation by Knowlton et al. of a polymorphic genetic error in the gene for type II collagen in a family with primary osteoarthritis.[15]

Another area of interest among the idiopathic group of disorders is the localized disease of the hands and feet. The pathologic and biochemical characteristics of these lesions are not clear, especially their specialized forms (e.g., Heberden's nodes, Bouchard's nodes, pauciarthritis) and perhaps they should not be included with the more standard forms of the disease such as osteoarthritis of the knee in the elderly or even the simple bunion.[13, 16]

The etiologic factors linked with osteoarthritis are reviewed in Chapter 78.

The secondary causes of osteoarthritis as cited in Table 79–1 are numerous and some are only infrequently associated with the disorder. There is little doubt that osteoarthritis can occur as a result of acute or chronic trauma to the joints,[17-20] and perhaps unrecognized trauma or long-standing injury based on a malalignment may be one of the causes of the idiopathic form of the disease. Similarly, congenital or acquired variations in childhood or young adulthood can in time result in osteoarthritis (Fig. 79–1); the relationship of such entities as Legg-Calvé-Perthes disease, congenital dislocation of the hip, or slipped capital femoral epiphysis and the subsequent development of osteoarthritis of the hip is so common in occurrence as to challenge the existence of an idiopathic form of this disorder.[21-24]

An equally obvious presumptive pathogenetic mechanism may be postulated by suggesting that the variety of metabolic diseases including alkaptonuric ochronosis, hemochromatosis, and CPPD (see Chapters 77 and 84) affect the cartilage by altering the physical properties of the tissue as a result of deposition of crystalline material in the matrix or by causing some change in the collagen cross-linking.[12, 25] It is tempting to apply these same principles to other disorders in which the lesion is less certain, including the various bone dysplasias (an abnormal collagen product or three-dimensional structure?), hemoglobinopathies, or Kashin-Beck and Mseleni disease.[24, 26, 27]

Still other causes of osteoarthritic disease are those grouped under the category of *other bone and*

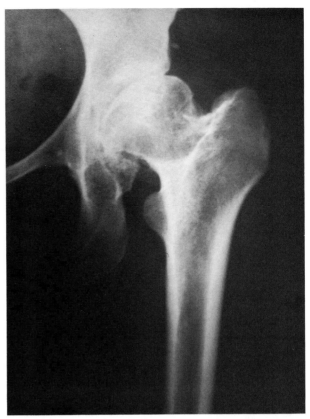

Figure 79–1. Radiograph of the hip of a 54-year-old woman who had congenital hip dysplasia and was treated for a short period with a plaster cast as a child. Over time, she developed an osteoarthritis of the hip. Radiographic changes reflect the shallow, excessively oblique acetabulum and poorly developed femoral head characteristic of old dysplasia.

joint disease, giving credence to the theory that osteoarthritis is in fact the *final common pathway* for diseased cartilage. Many patients with gout, rheumatoid arthritis, infection, Paget's disease, and osteonecrosis of various causes develop as their end-stage condition a classic osteoarthritis, indistinguishable from disorders of idiopathic or other secondary cause.[19]

EPIDEMIOLOGY OF OSTEOARTHRITIS

The *overall prevalence* of osteoarthritis varies with the population groups and with the rigor of the evaluating instrument and reporting team.[28-31] A high percentage of the population over the age of 50 have definable osteoarthritis (as described at autopsy study or on the basis of random radiographs),[1, 13, 22, 31, 32] but establishing the clinical incidence and the relationship of anatomic changes to the clinical syndrome is more difficult. The prevalence currently is believed to exceed 60 million people in the United States,[5, 28] and the number of people who retire from the work force annually as a result of osteoarthritis exceeds 5 percent,[5, 9, 29] a figure almost as high as for cardiac disease as a cause of physical impairment.[33] About 300,000 total hip replacements are performed in the United States annually and almost as many knee procedures; most of these are for osteoarthritis.[5, 34]

Some theoretical aspects of the *relationship to age* have been discussed at some length in the section on pathogenesis, but the fact of this association can be readily derived from a rather large number of studies that clearly demonstrate that the incidence of the disease is relatively low below the age of 50 but rises precipitously with advancing age[9, 35] to the point that a large percentage (estimated at over 50 percent) have some clinical signs by their sixtieth year.[36] Evidence for this contention is the finding that Heberden's nodes have a prevalence of less than 30 percent in individuals less than 70 years of age but the figure rises to almost 70 percent in people over the age of 75.[5, 35, 37] Mikkelsen et al. have shown manual or pedal osteoarthritis on radiographs in 90 percent of women and almost 80 percent of men over the age of 65.[38]

In terms of the *relationship to gender*, both males and females are equally likely to demonstrate hip disease (in fact, men appear to show this process more frequently, possibly related to the relatively high incidence of Perthes' disease and slipped capital femoral epiphysis in males[39]), but the knees and hands are more commonly affected in older women than in males at the same ages.[5, 35, 40–42] An inverse correlation has been noted between osteoarthritis (especially spinal osteophytes) and osteoporosis.[5, 41, 43, 44] In terms of the clinical syndromes of osteoarthritis and osteoporosis, however, women are predisposed to both, and the coexistence of the two disorders increases with advancing years.[33, 45]

Body habitus has long been considered to be a factor in the development of osteoarthritis although prior studies did not show conclusive evidence.[5] Some more recent studies have supported the concept that chronic significant excess body weight correlates directly with osteoarthritis.[46, 47] Both extremes of height show a correlation with osteoarthritis, but this seems more likely to be related to the presence of "Marfanoid" or acromegalic syndromes for the very tall and the various epiphyseal dysplasias in the very short.[21, 48, 49]

Heredity is unquestionably a determinant with certain types of osteoarthritis, especially those affecting the distal interphalangeal joints in women[50, 51] (Fig. 79–2), the first metatarsophalangeal joints,[5, 9, 13, 16] the somewhat obscure syndrome of generalized osteoarthritis,[10, 13, 52] and the recently described genetic defect in type II procollagen. Congenital dislocation of the hip and dysplasia epiphysealis multiplex (and spondyloepiphyseal dysplasia) are genetically transmitted disorders, and as the final joint disorder is osteoarthritis, these syndromes can be considered as hereditary causes.[21, 49, 53, 54] The same might be said for alkaptonuric ochronosis or some of the Ehlers-Danlos syndromes.[26, 55] When corrections are applied for the the cofactors of age and body habitus there is only a modest difference among the various races.[1, 5, 30, 54, 56–60]

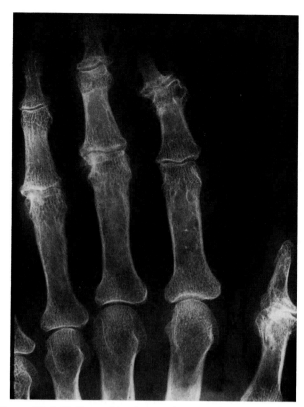

Figure 79–2. Radiographic picture of Heberden's nodes in a 64-year-old woman. Note the enlargement, sclerosis, and osteophyte formation on the distal interphalangeal (DIP) joint of the index finger and, to a lesser extent, the long fingers as well as the severe changes in the DIP joint of the thumb.

Another epidemiologic factor that may be important in the development or perpetuation of the disease is trauma.[4, 17, 61] There is little doubt that major unreduced injuries to the joint surfaces will result in osteoarthritis, and all classification systems clearly implicate such a process as a significant cause of the secondary form of the disease[4] (Fig. 79–3). The controversy lies not in the rapid appearance of osteoarthritis after such overt disorders as fractures about the wrist or ankle but with the slow development of the syndrome as a result of repetitive stereotypic movements of the extremities at the work place[9, 62, 63] or in relation to repeated trauma associated with sports activities.[20, 28, 64–66] Does chronic injury sustained by baseball pitchers lead to osteoarthritis? Do the injuries to the knees of football players lead eventually to osteoarthritis even in the absence of overt discernible fractures, dislocations, or ligamentous or meniscal tears (Fig. 79–4)? Perhaps one of the more intriguing recent findings is the tentative evidence from the Framingham study that suggests that smoking may be protective against osteoarthritis.[65] This finding is in sharp contrast with the evidence to support the detrimental effect of smoking on back problems.[67–69]

Some of the factors that do not appear to play a role in the causation or evolution of the disease include climatic conditions, occupation (with some exceptions), and other nonrheumatic disease (such as diabetes, hypertension, cardiac disorders, and cancer). The incidence of osteoarthritis in patients with chronic alcoholism is probably increased on the basis of fractures rather than for metabolic reasons.[69] As can be readily appreciated by examination of Table 79–1, the list of causes of secondary osteoarthritis is comprehensive, however, so almost all diseases that lead to fracture, osteonecrosis, metabolic abnormalities, or connective tissue alterations may be considered to be positively linked with osteoarthritis. One of the other unique features of the disease is the occasional finding that paralysis of an extremity (such as occurs with poliomyelitis and paraplegia or hemiplegia) seems to be protective.[5, 70] The nature of this protection is not known, but, partly on the basis of handedness studies,[71] it is presumed that muscle pull or the trauma associated with use of the extremity may have some role in the evolution of OA.

THE NATURAL HISTORY OF OSTEOARTHRITIS

The natural history of osteoarthritis and especially the rate at which lesions progress over a lifetime has been the subject of considerable speculation and several investigations.[1, 5, 9, 36, 41, 49, 72] Osteoarthritis may be asymptomatic for many years, and the observations of incidental findings at arthroscopy or surgery support findings at autopsy in individuals who had no history of joint abnormality during life that such alterations are lesions of "limited progression"[9]; and that certain sites such as the acetabulum are remarkably prone to develop asymptomatic and presumably stable lesions.[9] The likelihood seems high, however, that such stable lesions are rare and that osteoarthritis is almost always progressive, but at a highly variable rate. Most students of the disease consider osteoarthritis to be a disorder that is nonlinear in its evolution, so a long period of the asymptomatic disease is ultimately followed by a point at which one crosses the "threshold" of clinical sensibility. Although the rate may continue to be slow after this point, it seems more likely that the process undergoes an exponential progression to an unrelenting state of disability and crippling. (An example of this type of progression in a patient with osteoarthritis of the knee is presented in Figure 79–4.) To date there have been no correlative data that establish radiographic or even histologic markers that coincide with a "threshold."

THE CLINICAL SYNDROME

General Characteristics. Patients with osteoarthritis are in their middle or later years and according to recent data are more likely to be overweight.[46, 53, 73] Women are somewhat more frequently affected than

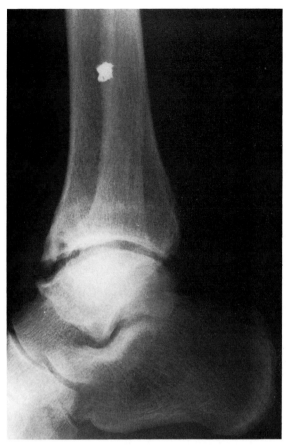

Figure 79–3. Lateral radiograph of the ankle joint of a 63-year-old male who suffered an open fracture of the ankle as a result of a shrapnel injury (note the retained metallic fragment above the ankle). The fracture was not completely reduced, and over time he developed a typical osteoarthritis of the ankle. Note the narrow joint space, subchondral sclerosis, and anterior osteophytes.

men particularly in the older age groups[5, 30, 74, 75] and especially for bone disease.[42] All races appear to be equally affected (at least in the United States) and, especially for males, a history of trauma is likely to be elicited.[42, 47]

Sites of Involvement. The most frequently affected joints are the hips, knees, spine, and small joints of the hands and feet. Patients with isolated hip disease often provide a history of early abnormality (congenital dysplasia, Legg-Calvé-Perthes disease, slipped capital femoral epiphysis, osteonecrosis).[21, 22, 49, 53, 76] Spinal osteoarthritis is frequent in the elderly, most often affecting the lumbar and cervical spines and often unrelated to prior significant disorder.[77–79] In the absence of trauma (fracture) or some form of congenital abnormality (such as dysplasia epiphysealis multiplex), the wrist, elbow, shoulder, and ankle are usually spared. Associations of osteoarthritis of the the the first metatarsophalangeal joints of the feet and the distal interphalangeal joints of the hand with female gender have been mentioned; they also appear to occur with high frequency in families.[5, 42, 51]

History. On close questioning most patients with

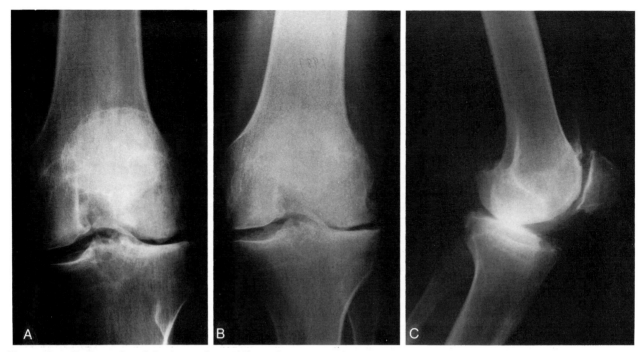

Figure 79–4. Radiographs of the knee of a middle-aged executive taken more than 3 years apart. The patient had had an open meniscectomy at the age of 16 and was asymptomatic until the first radiograph (*A*) was taken, at which time he complained of only mild swelling after vigorous athletics. The pain increased over time, and radiographs taken 3.5 years later (*B–C*) show considerably greater joint space narrowing and osteophyte formation and, on lateral view (*C*), severe osteoarthritic change.

osteoarthritis state that symptoms have been present for some time but are only very slowly progressive.[75, 80–82] Pain is the usual complaint that brings the patient to the physician. Although it may have been preceded for several years by an asymptomatic limitation of movement and deformity, it is the pain that arouses alarm and concern. The pain is almost always described as mild to moderate and dull and aching in character. However, at times it may become severe and even lancinating. One of the most constant features of the pain is its relationship to activity.[83] The pain is almost always at least partially relieved by rest and exacerbated by movement and especially by bearing weight.[7, 73, 81] Certain movements and activities are more likely to cause pain than others. In eliciting the complaints referable to osteoarthritis of the hand, it is grasp (rather than pinch), especially in such acts as opening a jar, that causes the discomfort.[51] For the hip, flexion, internal rotation, and abduction are likely to elicit pain;[41, 84] for the knee, extremes of flexion and extension; for the cervical spine, extension and rotation; and for the lumbar spine, flexion and lateral bend.[79] In terms of activities, pain with walking and especially going up or down stairs are the principal presenting complaints. In younger patients and those with milder disease, pain with athletic activities such as tennis is sometimes the principal (and only) cause for concern.

It should be noted that the pain pattern for patients with osteoarthritis may include a referred or radicular component, which may dominate the picture. Patients with osteoarthritis of the hip may have

significant referred pain that localizes to the medial side of the knee;[84] those with cervical or lumbar (or less frequently dorsal) osteoarthritis may present with all of the complaints and findings associated with discogenic disease or even cord, conus, or root compression.[79, 84, 85] In some patients with osteoarthritis of the cervical spine, pain in the shoulder, arm, forearm, or hand may be the presenting or only complaint. Similarly, in patients with even mild osteoarthritis of the lumbar spine, the pain may be principally located in the ankle or calf. Patients with spinal stenosis may have symptoms of cramping in the calves similar to those described as "intermittent claudication."

Patients with osteoarthritis almost always state that in addition to pain (and sometime preceding it) there is a gradually increasing limitation of motion. Initially this feature is not only intermittent (it may occur only after exercise) but it may be much more severe after a period of inactivity such as sitting in a chair or automobile for a long period or even after a night's sleep. Thus, "morning stiffness," long considered to be a characteristic of rheumatoid arthritis (see Chapter 52), is also a concomitant feature of osteoarthritis.[6] In early osteoarthritis, recovery from this "stiffness" is rapid—perhaps after a few steps or a few minutes in the morning. Gradually (and inexorably) it worsens and soon is present for longer periods. The patient states that he or she is less able to "work it out." Eventually the limitation becomes fixed. The degree and character of the limitation varies with the joint. For the hip, internal rotation, extension, and abduction are reduced; for the knee, flexion is lost initially and later the patient develops an extensor lag; for the cervical spine the limitation is usually concentric, while for the lumbar it more severely affects flexion. Eventually if untreated, the limitation becomes so severe as to affect gait and activities of daily living and to be a major cause of disability.

Patients with osteoarthritis often complain of crepitation, a "crackling" feeling of the affected joint (most often a knee or less commonly a hip) and may at times state that they or others in the room can hear the sound as a "creaking." Crepitation may be painless but most often it is associated with a dull aching joint pain.[5, 81]

Another major complaint of the patient who develops osteoarthritis is deformity. Patients may point out that one knee is symmetrically (or occasionally asymmetrically) larger than the other; that the bunion area is very prominent (and tender to touch); or that the distal interphalangeal joints are enlarged.[51] Frequently associated with the enlargement of the joint is a more or less severe alteration in contour such as varus deformity (bowing) of the proximal tibiae in osteoarthritis of the knees or adduction of the thumb in first carpometacarpal arthritis of the hand.

Among the most bothersome symptoms for patients with osteoarthritis is their complaint of an abnormal gait. Most people with moderate or severe osteoarthritis of the hip, knee, or ankle develop a limp, which is noticeable at first to them, but ultimately to anyone who watches them walk. The alteration will differ with site and degree of disease but is almost invariably increased with speed of the gait and exaggerated by walking on rough ground or up and down ramps. Even moderately severe osteoarthritis of a major joint (and especially when it affects two or more joints in the lower extremities) represents a great threat to the elderly patient's independence, which is already marginal in terms of physical and socioeconomic ability to maintain their status.[86]

Physical Examination. The most frequent finding is limitation of motion, which is almost universally present even in very early clinical disease. Initially this finding may be subtle, variable, and difficult to measure, but gradually with advancing severity of the disease, the limitation becomes more profound, affects more ranges, and in very severe cases, may allow only a "jog" of motion. Although sometimes described as "concentric," the limitation is usually "eccentric" in that one or another of the ranges of movement of the joint is more severely affected than others. With advancing degrees of disease, the tendency for concentricity increases, however, and the patient frequently presents with a noticeable joint contracture. The degree and nature of the contracture vary markedly with the joint and with the extent of the process. For instance, for the hip, early osteoarthritis may be detected only by a

limitation of internal rotation in extension; with advancing disease, an external rotation contracture and limitation of flexion and extension; with greater extent of the process, by a more marked limitation of flexion and a flexion contracture; and finally with "end-stage" osteoarthritis, a hip that is fixed in 30 degrees of external rotation, 10 degrees of abduction, and 45 degrees of flexion, with no further flexion possible.[84] Such a patient is able to walk, but clearly will have a profound alteration in stance and posture and a significant gait disturbance.

One of the more striking findings in osteoarthritis is crepitus.[81, 83] In early disease in which the patellofemoral joint is involved (especially in the syndrome of chondromalacia patellae) or in later disease in which the cartilage is denuded from the surface and eburnated bone articulates with a similarly irregular opposing surface, a crackling or crunching sensation is noticeable to the patient and the physician. This may be created by rubbing of the surfaces together either during motion or when the joint is passively manipulated. With increasing severity, the crepitus may be audible for some distance and the joints may be made to "creak" by putting them through a specific range of motion.

Additional findings include joint enlargement, which is often asymmetric. The increased size of the joint may be on the basis of a joint effusion, which may be quite large.[81, 87] It is not unusual to find patients with osteoarthritis of the knee in which a joint aspiration will yield 100 or more milliliters of fluid. Another reason for enlargement of the joint is the presence of osteophytes, which may significantly alter the contours of the joint. Depending on the extent of the synovitis and the degree of the osteoarthritic process, a diffuse tenderness and at times a surprising redness and warmth may be present. These latter changes are most marked on examination of the knees, elbows, ankles, and especially the small joints of the hands and feet.

Ultimately, the fixed contractures, alterations in contour of the joint, variations in station and stance, and a variety of chronic changes in the bones and joints lead to a permanent deformity of the affected extremity. Most often this takes the form of shortening and some abnormality of position in either the coronal or sagittal planes. For the hip this may consist of a short limb with a prominent trochanteric area in an externally rotated, flexed attitude; for the knee it may be either a marked bow leg or a knock knee with a flexed and usually externally rotated leg. For the ankle the abnormality may be moderate to severe eversion or inversion and an equinus or, less commonly, calcaneus deformity. The deformities associated with Heberden's nodes are well known, as is the typical hallux valgus and metatarsus primus varus, which result from osteoarthritis of the first metatarsophalangeal joint.

Gait disturbances in patients with osteoarthritis are related almost entirely to the pain associated with weight-bearing. In such a circumstance the stance phase of gait is decreased, producing an asymmetry and altered cadence.[88–90] In addition, most patients with osteoarthritis of the hip display a Trendelenburg gait (otherwise known as a "gluteus medius lurch"). Patients with this abnormality shift their trunk excessively toward the affected side during the stance phase of gait because of inability of the weakened or relatively elongated gluteus medius muscle to hold the pelvis steady.[84] Patients with knee disorders principally show a "stiff knee" gait with an alteration and asymmetry of cadence, related to their inability to fully extend the knee during heel strike or their lack of sufficient flexion to clear during swing phase.[81, 83] This abnormality gets increasingly more noticeable at faster speeds and especially during stair climbing or descent. Ultimately, in late phases of osteoarthritis of the knee, patients must ascend stairs with first the unaffected limb followed by the affected on the same step (the reverse sequence is usually used for descent) rather than using the limbs alternately. Finally, patients with "lumbar claudication" based on spinal stenosis show a slowed shuffling gait with a very limited capacity (usually measurable by them in yards) before they must stop and sit for a period of time to allow the numbness and pain in the lower extremities to subside.

Patients with foot problems usually have diminished tolerance for footwear, especially those that are tight or have pointed toes. Patients with hand osteoarthritis do surprisingly well with fine pinch, but have problems with grasp and especially such activities as opening a jar or even holding a glass. The problems of the patient with limited elbow motion are self-evident and usually, if the dominant extremity is affected, are of considerable concern to the patient particularly if they cannot bring the hand to the mouth for eating or to the head for grooming. Shoulder limitations are generally not as disabling unless the patient has pain with movement that decreases the ability to perform simple acts such as dressing, eating, or putting their hands into pockets.[91]

Imaging Studies. For the most part plain radiographs of joints affected by osteoarthritis are so highly characteristic that it is rare that more modern sophisticated technology is required to establish the diagnosis.[92–95] The combination on biplanar radiography of the affected joint of asymmetric narrowing of the joint space (more severe in the weight-bearing area), dense sclerosis of the subchondral bone, cysts adjacent to (and sometimes remote from) the joint, and the presence of large marginal osteophytes (see Chapter 37) is so highly specific for osteoarthritis that most physicians treating patients with the disease require no further studies for substantiation. A number of studies have demonstrated a modest to moderate increase in activity of the subchondral bone on ^{99m}Tc-diphosphonate bone scan[86, 92, 96] in joints affected by osteoarthritis. Sabiston et al.[97] have suggested that MRI may be helpful in early detection, and other investigators have identified cysts and

subchondral change[94] and cartilage damage and repair.[298]

If in fact a patient is suspected of having genetic or metabolic disorders such as an epiphyseal dysplasia, hemochromatosis, alkaptonuric ochronosis, hyperparathyroidism, or Paget's disease, radiographs of other joints (especially the spine and skull) and bone scans may be helpful in establishing that diagnosis. Similarly, those patients in whom the symptom complex supports the diagnosis of generalized osteoarthritis rather than the more prevalent mono- or pauciarthritic disease should be more extensively studied, also by use of examinations of multiple joints and by bone scans.[99, 100]

A second issue that can often best be clarified by more extensive or more sophisticated imaging studies is the differential diagnosis of osteoarthritis from four less prevalent but considerably more pernicious syndromes: osteonecrosis (see Chapter 97); Charcot's neuroarthropathy; pigmented villonodular synovitis (see Chapter 98); and synovial chondromatosis (see Chapter 98).[92] Osteonecrosis, usually related to some predisposing genetic or acquired disorder (fracture, dislocation, radiation, hemoglobinopathy, connective tissue disorder, dysbarism, corticosteroid administration, Gaucher's disease, alcoholism), initially affects only one side of the joint, often appears more dense on radiograph, and frequently shows a fracture in the subchondral region (the crescent sign) (Fig. 79–5).[95, 101–103] Computed tomography (CT) of the site may show significant alterations not visible on plain films, and MRI may show an infarct.[102, 104] Neuropathic arthropathy may affect any joint and on plain radiographs show changes not unlike those that one might see with severe osteoarthritis.[92, 105, 106] The alterations are often much more rapid in evolution, however, and are usually associated with a marked fragmentation of the joint and, on close inspection, a fine dusting of calcareous detritus in the enormously thickened synovium (Fig. 79–6). Neither of these findings is ordinarily seen in osteoarthritis.[105, 106] Specialized imaging studies including arthrography may show the alterations in these joints more clearly and are also helpful at times in establishing the cause (as in a patient with syringomyelia or other anatomic neurologic abnormality).

Similarly, special imaging such as arthrography or CT may be very helpful in distinguishing pigmented villonodular synovitis or synovial chondromatosis from osteoarthritis.[103, 105, 107] The former disorder is characterized by rather extensive soft tissue masses, often in nodules, which may be best seen on CT or MRI. Synovial chondromatosis, especially when most of the free bodies are not calcified or ossified occasionally masquerades as osteoarthritis,[103, 107, 108] but the two can be readily differentiated by CT, arthrography or arthroscopy.

Another reason to utilize special imaging techniques is in the diagnosis and determination of the extent of spinal osteoarthritis. Regardless of whether one is dealing with classic osteoarthritis of the facet

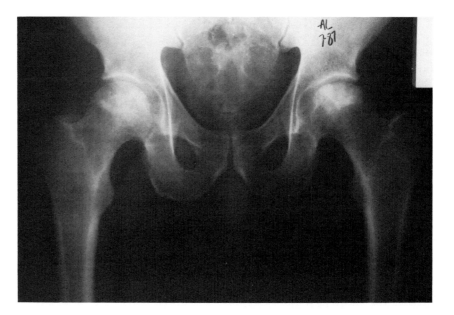

Figure 79–5. Osteonecrosis of both femoral heads in a 42-year-old male. Although the radiographs, and particularly the sclerosis, are suggestive of osteoarthritis, the absence of osteophytes and partial preservation of the joint space tend to militate against that diagnosis. The presence of a partial collapse of the femoral head on the left strongly supports the diagnosis of osteonecrosis.

joints, osteophytosis of the vertebral bodies, Forestier's disease, or post-traumatic or postsurgical osteoarthritic changes, the use of myelography, and, more recently, computerized tomography (with or without contrast) and magnetic resonance imaging (MRI) have enhanced our ability not only to make a correct diagnosis but to establish with clarity the cause of radicular or cord compressive symptoms and signs.[77, 85, 108, 109]

Arthroscopy. The technology surrounding arthroscopy has revolutionized the approach to the diagnosis of joint injury, synovial diseases, and infectious and inflammatory arthritides.[110] Osteoarthritis is one of the disorders that can be readily diagnosed by arthroscopy of the knee, shoulder,

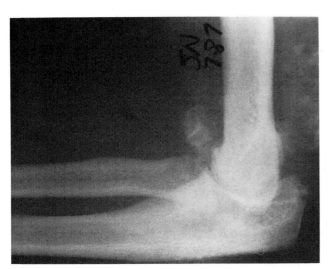

Figure 79–6. Lateral radiograph of the elbow of a 46-year-old woman with a syringomyelia and Charcot's arthropathy. Note the fragmentation of the joint and narrowing of the joint space with a fine dusting of calcareous detritus in the enlarged synovial cavity, especially posteriorly.

elbow, hip, ankle, and most recently wrist joints (see Chapter 38). Because osteoarthritis is so easily identified on the basis of clinical and radiographic findings,[83] however, there are few indications to introduce arthroscopic examination of the joint merely to establish the diagnosis. When in doubt (such as with disorders such as pigmented villonodular synovitis or synovial chondromatosis) an arthroscopic evaluation is very helpful. Occasionally, arthroscopy will help to establish the extent of the disease, which may be an important factor in planning for surgery,[110, 111] and may be effective therapy for mild to moderate disease.[111–115]

Laboratory Data. Laboratory reports about patients with osteoarthritis are usually not helpful, except perhaps in a negative sense.[83, 87] White blood cell counts and differential counts of the leukocytes are routinely normal in patients with osteoarthritis, and the sedimentation rate, although occasionally higher than normal, is probably of little value as a diagnostic aid except for patients with generalized osteoarthritis[74, 87] and as a differential diagnostic feature for the inflammatory arthritides. Similarly, tests for antinuclear antibodies, rheumatoid factor, and assessment of complement components have been found to be routinely normal.

The synovial fluid obtained from patients with osteoarthritis can be considered "noninflammatory" according to the classification established by Ropes and Bauer[87, 116–118] (see Chapter 36). Some evidence for inflammation is present, however, particularly in the form of a decrease in viscosity, mild to moderate pleocytosis, and modest elevation of synovial fluid protein.[117, 118] The fluid is almost always increased in volume and appears clear and pale yellow in color.[87, 116] Turbidity or bloody effusions are occasionally encountered, particularly in long-standing disease or in joints with a strong inflammatory component. The cell complement is usually an even mix of lymphocytes and polymorphonuclear leukocytes and the total count rarely rises above 8000 cells per ml.[116, 118, 119] Rheumatoid factor cannot be detected, complement levels are normal, and immune complexes, sometime encountered in the osteoarthritic synovium or cartilage, have not as yet been noted in synovial fluid.

"Markers". There is little doubt that a marker is an important objective for all the toilers in clinical and laboratory research in osteoarthritis. Part of the reason for the currently rather dismal suggestion that the outcome of all true osteoarthritis is the ultimate failure of the joint is that the diagnosis is made far too late to treat with simple medications, exercises, or realignment of the joint or weight reduction.

One of the first potential markers was advocated by Thonar and associates, who suggested on the basis of limited trials that a keratan sulfate epitope, circulating in the blood stream may in fact be a significant and accurate marker.[120, 121] Subsequent data have not borne this out.[122–124]

Of perhaps considerably greater current promise is the possibility that one or several synovial fluid markers may so clearly define the disease that its presence can be detected by examination of a single sample of fluid from the involved joint. A vast array of materials have been studied, including fibrillar materials such as type II collagen fragments,[125] antibodies to type I and type II,[126] and fibronectin.[127] Calcium pyrophosphate, long noted to be a finding in joint disease states (obviously including pseudogout) but also in osteoarthritis and in aged individuals, has been restudied as a potential marker.[128] The interleukins, known to play a role in cartilage degradation (see Chapter 14), have also been considered to be a likely marker, and both IL-1 and IL-6 have been implicated.[129, 130] Superoxide free radicals[131] and phospholipase[132] have also been suggested as markers, as have some of the complement pathway materials, particularly in distinguishing osteoarthritis from rheumatoid disease.[122, 133] Higher molecular weight fragments that could serve as markers include the matrix proteins,[134, 135] and recent studies have suggested that this latter material shows a greater specificity than many of the others.[135] Finally, some of the more recent efforts in molecular biology suggest that DNA probes may ultimately be of value in studying the disease, but considerably more must be known about the range of such findings in the general public and especially those affected by single joint disease.

As can readily be appreciated from the foregoing discussion there are numerous gaps in our knowledge of OA; the problem that faces the clinical investigator is that despite our obvious familiarity with the disease there remain a number of unanswered questions regarding the nature of the disorder, its epidemiology, clinical presentation, causation, and pathogenesis.

References

1. Sokoloff, L.: The Biology of Degenerative Joint Disease. Chicago, University of Chicago Press, 1969.
2. Straus, W. L., Jr., and Cave, A. J. E.: Pathology and the posture of Neanderthal man. Q. Rev. Biol. 32:348, 1957.
3. Wells, C.: Bones, Bodies and Disease: Evidence of Disease and Abnormality in Early Man. New York, Praeger Press, 1964.
4. Mankin, H. J., Brandt, K. D., and Shulman, L. E.: Workshop on etiopathogenesis of osteoarthritis. J. Rheumatol. 13:1127, 1986.
5. Peyron, J. G., and Altman, R. D.: The epidemiology of osteoarthritis. In Moskowitz, R. W., Howell, D. S., Goldberg, V. M., and Mankin, H. J. (eds.): Osteoarthritis: Diagnosis and Management. Philadelphia, W. B. Saunders Company, 1992, pp. 15–38.
6. Moskowitz, R. W., Howell, D. S., Goldberg, V. M., and Mankin, H. J. (eds.): Osteoarthritis: Diagnosis and Management. Philadelphia, W. B. Saunders Company, 1992.
7. Cooke, T. D., and Dwosh, I. L.: Clinical features of osteoarthritis in the elderly. Clin. Rheum. Dis. 12:155, 1986.
8. Ehrlich, G. E.: Erosive inflammatory and primary generalized osteoarthritis. In Moskowitz, R. W., Howell, D. S., Goldberg, V. M., and Mankin, H. J., (eds.): Osteoarthritis: Diagnosis and Management. Philadelphia, W. B. Saunders Company, 1992, pp. 329–340.
9. Peyron, J. G.: Osteoarthritis: The epidemiologic viewpoint. Clin. Orthop. 213:13, 1986.
10. Cooke, T. D.: The polyarticular features of osteoarthritis requiring hip and knee surgery. J. Rheumatol. 10:288, 1983.
11. Buchanan, W. W., and Park, W. M.: Primary generalized osteoarthritis: Definition and uniformity. J. Rheumatol. 10:4, 1983.
12. Mankin, H. J.: Speculation regarding the biochemical pathogenesis of generalized osteoarthritis. J. Rheumatol. 10:7, 1983.
13. Kellgren, J. H., Lawrence, J. S., and Bier, F.: Genetic factors in generalized osteoarthrosis. Ann. Rheum. Dis. 22:237, 1963.
14. Cooke, T. D.: Pathogenetic mechanisms in polyarticular osteoarthritis. Clin. Rheum. Dis. 11:203, 1985.
15. Knowlton, R. G., Katzenstein, P. L., Moskowitz, R. W., Weaver, E. J., Malemud, C. J., Pathria, M. N., Jiminez, S. A., and Prockop, D. J.: Genetic linkage of a polymorphism in the type II procollagen gene (COL2A1) to primary osteoarthritis associated with mild chondrodysplasia. N. Engl. J. Med. 322:526, 1990.
16. Peyron, J. G.: Inflammation in osteoarthritis: Review of its role in clinical picture, disease progress, subsets and pathophysiology. Semin. Arthritis Rheum. 11:115, 1981.
17. Chrisman, O. D., Ladenbauer-Bellis, I. M., Panjabi, M., and Goeltz, S.: 1981 Nicolas Andry Award. The relationship of mechanical trauma and the early biochemical reactions of osteoarthritic cartilage. Clin. Orthop. 161:275, 1981.
18. Bentley, G., and Dowd, G.: Current concepts of the etiology and treatment of chondromalacia patellae. Clin. Orthop. 189:209, 1984.
19. Schumacher, H. R.: Secondary osteoarthritis. In Moskowitz, R. W., Howell, D. S., Goldberg, V. M., and Mankin, H. J. (eds.): Osteoarthritis: Diagnosis and Management. Philadelphia, W. B. Saunders Company, 1992, pp. 367–398.
20. Funk, F. J.: Trauma and osteoarthritis of the knee. Some implications of change in surgical practice. In Peyron, J. G. (ed.): Epidemiology of Osteoarthrosis. Basel, Ciba-Geigy, 1981, pp. 236–242.
21. Harris, W. H.: Etiology of osteoarthritis of the hip. Clin. Orthop. 213:20, 1986.
22. Danielsson, L. Lindberg, H., and Nilsson, B.: Prevalence of coxarthrosis. Clin. Orthop. 191:110, 1984.
23. Ordeberg, G., Hansson, L. I., and Sandstrom, S.: Slipped capital femoral epiphysis in Southern Sweden. Long-term result with no treatment or symptomatic primary treatment. Clin. Orthop. 191:95, 1984.
24. Yach, D., and Botha, J. L.: Mseleni joint disease in 1981: Decreased prevalence rates, wider geographical location than before, and socioeconomic impact of an endemic osteoarthrosis in an underdeveloped community in South Africa. Int. J. Epidemiol. 14:276, 1985.
25. Howell, D. S., Treadwell, B. V., and Trippel, S. B.: Etiopathogenesis of osteoarthritis. In Moskowitz, R. W., Howell, D. S., Goldberg, V. M., and Mankin, H. J. (eds.): Osteoarthritis: Diagnosis and Management. Philadelphia, W. B. Saunders Company, 1992, pp. 233–253.
26. de Jonge Bok, J. M., and MacFarlane, J. D.: The articular diversity of early hemochromatosis. J. Bone Joint Surg. 69:41, 1987.
27. Sokoloff, L., Fincham, J. E., and du-Toit, G. T.: Pathologic features of the femoral head in Mseleni disease. Hum. Pathol. 16:117, 1985.
28. Peyron, J. G. (ed.): Epidemiology of Osteoarthritis. Symposium, Paris, June, 1980. Paris, Ciba-Geigy, 1981.
29. Lawrence, J. S.: Rheumatism in Populations. London, William Heinemann Medical Books, 1977.
30. Lawrence, J. S., and Sebo, M.: The geography of osteoarthritis. In

Nuki, G. (ed.): The Aetiopathogenesis of Osteoarthrosis. Tunbridge Wells, Pitman Medical Publishing Co., 1981, pp. 155–183.

31. Kellgren, J. H., and Lawrence, J. S.: Radiological assessment of osteoarthritis. Ann. Rheum. Dis. 16:494, 1957.

32. Valkenburg, H. A.: Clinical versus radiological osteoarthrosis in the general population. In Peyron, J. G. (ed.): Epidemiology of Osteoarthrosis. Basel, Ciba-Geigy, 1981, pp. 53–58.

33. Praemer, A., Furner, S., and Rice, D.: Musculoskeletal Conditions in the United States. Park Ridge, IL, American Academy of Orthopedic Surgeons, 1992.

34. Wilcock, J. K.: The prevalence of osteoarthritis of the hip requiring total hip replacement in the elderly. Int. J. Epidemiol. 8:247, 1979.

35. Bergstrom, G., Bjelle, A., Sorenssen, L., Sundh, V., and Svanborg, A.: Prevalence of rheumatoid arthritis, osteoarthritis, chondrocalcinosis and gouty arthritis at age 79. J. Rheumatol. 13:150, 1986.

36. Brandt, K. D., and Fife, R. S.: Ageing in relation to the pathogenesis of osteoarthritis. Clin. Rheum. Dis. 12:117, 1986.

37. Radin, E. L., and Rose, R. M.: Role of subchondral bone in the initiation and progression of cartilage damage. Clin. Orthop. 213:34, 1986.

38. Mikkelsen, W. N., Duff, I. F., and Dodge, H. J.: Age and sex specific prevalence of radiographic abnormalities of the joints of the hands, wrist and cervical spine of adult residents of the Tecumseh, Michigan community health study area, 1962–1965. J. Chronic Dis. 23:151, 1970.

39. Dingle, J. T.: Catabolin—a cartilage catabolic factor from synovium. Clin. Orthop. 156:219, 1980.

40. Bjelle, A.: Epidemiological aspects of osteoarthritis—an interview survey of the Swedish population and a review of previous studies. Scand. J. Rheumatol. (Suppl.) 43:35, 1982.

41. Nilsson, B. E., Danielsson, L. B., and Hernborg, S. A.: Clinical feature and natural course of coxarthrosis and gonarthrosis. Scand. J. Rheumatol. 43:12, 1982.

42. Cushnaghan, J., and Dieppe, P.: Study of 500 patients with limb joint osteoarthritis. I. Analysis by age, sex, and distribution of symptomatic joint sites. Ann. Rheum. Dis. 50:8, 1991.

43. Noble, J., and Alexander, K.: Studies of tibial subchondral bone density and its significance. J. Bone Joint Surg. 67:295, 1985.

44. Verstraeten A., Van Ermen H., Haghebaert, G., Nijs, J., Guesens, P., and Dequeker J.: Osteoarthrosis retards the development of osteoporosis: Observation of the coexistence of osteoarthrosis and osteoporosis. Clin. Orthop. 264:169, 1991.

45. Burr, D. B., Martin, R. B., Schaffler, M. B., Jurmain, R. D., Harner, E. J., and Radin, E. L.: Osteoarthrosis: Sex-specific relationship to osteoporosis. Am. J. Phys. Anthropol. 61:299, 1983.

46. van Saase, J. L., Vanderbroucke, J. P., van Romunde, L. K., and Valkenburg, H. A.: Osteoarthritis and obesity in the general population. A relationship calling for an explanation. J. Rheumatol. 15:1152, 1988.

47. Felson, D. T.: Osteoarthritis. Rheum. Dis. Clin. North Am. 16:499, 1990.

48. Collins, D. H.: The Pathology of Articular and Spinal Disease. London, E. Arnold and Company, 1949.

49. Dieppe, P., and Cushnaghan, J.: The natural course and prognosis of osteoarthritis of the hip. In Moskowitz, R. W., Howell, D. S., Goldberg, V. M., and Mankin, H. J. (eds.): Osteoarthritis: Diagnosis and Management. Philadelphia, W. B. Saunders Company, 1992, pp. 399–412.

50. Swanson, A. B., and Swanson, G. D.: Osteoarthritis in the hand. J. Hand Surg. 8:669, 1983.

51. Siegel, D. B., Gelberman, R. H., Smith, R.: Osteoarthritis of the hand and wrist. In Moskowitz, R. W., Howell, D. S., Goldberg, V. M., and Mankin, H. J. (eds.): Osteoarthritis: Diagnosis and Management. Philadelphia, W. B. Saunders Company, 1992, pp. 547–560.

52. Cooke, T. D.: Pathogenetic mechanisms in polyarticular osteoarthritis. Clin. Rheum. Dis. 11:203, 1985.

53. Cooperman, D. R., Wallensten, R., and Stulberg, S. D.: Acetabular dysplasia in the adult. Clin. Orthop. 175:79, 1983.

54. Hoaglund, F. T., Shiba, R., Newberg, A. H., and Leung, K. Y.: Diseases of the hip. A comparative study of Japanese Oriental and American white patients. J. Bone Joint Surg. 67:1376, 1985.

55. Schumacher, H. R.: Ochronosis, hemochromatosis and Wilson's disease. In McCarty, D. J. (ed.): Arthritis and Allied Conditions. Philadelphia, Lea & Febiger, 1979, pp. 1262–1275.

56. Blumberg, B. S., Bloch, K. J., Black, R. L., and Dotter, C.: A study of the prevalence of arthritis in Alaskan Eskimos. Arthritis Rheum. 4:325, 1961.

57. Bremner, J. M., Lawrence, J. S., and Miall, W. E.: Degenerative joint disease in a Jamaican rural population. Ann. Rheum. Dis. 27:326, 1968.

58. Solomon, L., Beighton, P., and Lawrence, J. W.: Osteoarthrosis in a rural South African Negro population. Ann. Rheum. Dis. 35:274, 1976.

59. Moskowitz, R. W.: Experimental models of osteoarthritis. In Moskowitz, R. W., Howell, D. S., Goldberg, V. M., and Mankin, H. J. (eds.): Osteoarthritis: Diagnosis and Management. Philadelphia, W. B. Saunders Company, 1992, pp. 213–232.

60. Adebajo, A. O.: Pattern of osteoarthritis in a West African teaching hospital. Ann. Rheum. Dis. 50:20, 1991.

61. Peyron, J. G.: Review of the main epidemiologic-etiologic evidence that implies mechanical forces as factors in osteoarthritis. Eng. Med. 15:77, 1986.

62. Hadler, N. M., Gillings, D. B., Imbus, H. R., et al.: Hand structure and function in an industrial setting. Influence of three patterns of stereotyped repetitive usage. Arthritis Rheum. 21:210, 1978.

63. Genti, G.: Occupation and osteoarthritis. Ballieres Clin. Rheumatol. 3:193, 1989.

64. Kannus, P., and Jarvinen, M.: Posttraumatic anterior cruciate ligament insufficiency as a cause of osteoarthritis in a knee joint. Clin. Rheumatol. 8:251, 1989.

65. Felson, D. T., Anderson J. J., Naimark A., Hannan, M. T., Kannel, W. B., and Meenan, R. F.: Does smoking protect against osteoarthritis? Arthritis Rheum. 32:166, 1989.

66. Davis, M. A., Ettinger, W. H., Neuhaus, J. M., Cho, S. A., and Hauck, W. W.: The association of knee injury and obesity with unilateral and bilateral osteoarthritis of the knee. Am. J. Epidemiol. 130:278, 1989.

67. Biering-Sorensen, F., and Thomsen, C.: Medical, social and occupational history as risk indicators for low-back trouble in a general population. Spine 11:720, 1986.

68. Kelsey, J. L., Githens, P. B., O'Conner, T., Weil, U., Calogero, J. A., Holford, T. R., White, A. A., 3d, Walter, S. D., Ostfeld, A. M., and Southwick, W. O.: Acute prolapsed lumbar intervertebral disc. An epidemiologic study with special reference to driving automobiles and cigarette smoking. Spine 9:608, 1984.

69. Typpo, T.: Osteoarthritis of the hip. Radiologic findings and etiology. Ann. Chir. Gynecol. 201:1, 1985.

70. Needs, C. J., Webb, J., and Tyndall, A.: Paralysis and unilateral arthritis: Is the association established? Clin. Rheumatol. 4:176, 1985.

71. Acheson, R. M., Chan, Y. K., and Clemmett, A. R.: New Haven survey of joint disease. XII. Distribution and symptoms in the hands with reference to handedness. Ann. Rheum. Dis. 29:275, 1970.

72. Byers, P., Contemponi, C. A., and Farkas, T. A.: Post-mortem study of the hip joint. Ann. Rheum. Dis. 29:15, 1970.

73. Hartz, A. J., Fischer, M. E., Bril, G., Kelber, S., Rupley, D., Jr., Oken, B., and Rimm, A. A.: The association of obesity with joint pain and osteoarthritis in the HANES data. J. Chronic Dis. 39:311, 1986.

74. Kellgren, J. H., and Moore, R.: Generalized osteoarthritis and Heberden's nodes. Br. Med. J. 1:181, 1952.

75. Lawrence, J. S., Bremner, J. M., and Bier, F.: Osteoarthrosis. Prevalence in the population and relationship between symptoms and x-ray changes. Ann. Rheum. Dis. 25:1, 1966.

76. Typpo, T.: Osteoarthritis of the hip. Radiologic findings and etiology. Ann. Chir. Gynaecol. (Suppl.) 201:1, 1985.

77. Resnick, D.: Degenerative diseases of the vertebral column. Radiology 156:3, 1985.

78. Milgram, J. W.: Osteoarthritic changes of the severely degerative disc in humans. Spine 7:498, 1982.

79. Emery, S. E., and Bohlman, H.: Osteoarthritis of the cervical spine. In Moskowitz, R. W., Howell, D. S., Goldberg, V. M., and Mankin, H. J. (eds.): Osteoarthritis: Diagnosis and Management. Philadelphia, W. B. Saunders Company, 1992, pp. 651–668.

80. Gresham, G. E., and Rathey, U. K.: Osteoarthritis of the knees of aged persons: Relationship between roentgenographic and clinical manifestations. J.A.M.A. 233:168, 1975.

81. Moskowitz, R. W.: Osteoarthritis—signs and symptoms. In Moskowitz, R. W., Howell, D. S., Goldberg, V. M., and Mankin, H. J. (eds.): Osteoarthritis: Diagnosis and Management. Philadelphia, W. B. Saunders Company, 1992, pp. 255–263.

82. Verbiest, H.: Radicular syndrome from developmental narrowing of the lumbar vertebral canal. J. Bone Joint Surg. 36B:230, 1954.

83. Altman, R., Asch, E., Bloch, D., et al.: Special article: Development of criteria for the classification of osteoarthritis of the knee. Arthritis Rheum. 29:1039, 1986.

84. Wilson, M. G., and Poss, R.: Osteoarthritis of the hip. In Moskowitz, R. W., Howell, D. S., Goldberg, V. M., and Mankin, H. J. (eds.): Osteoarthritis: Diagnosis and Management. Philadelphia, W. B. Saunders Company, 1992, pp. 621–650.

85. Chalmers, I. M., and Lockhead, J. A.: Neuropathic arthropathy secondary to severe degenerative spinal disease. J. Rheumatol. 9:464, 1982.

86. Badley, E. M., Lee, J., and Wood, P. H.: Impairment, disability, and the ICIDH (International Classification of Impairments, Disabilities, and Handicaps) model. II: The nature of the underlying condition and patterns of impairment. Int. Rehabil. Med. 8:118, 1987.

87. Altman, R. D.: Laboratory findings in osteoarthritis. In Moskowitz, R. W., Howell, D. S., Goldberg, V. M., and Mankin, H. J. (eds.): Osteoarthritis: Diagnosis and Management. Philadelphia, W. B. Saunders Company, 1992, pp. 313–328.

88. Khodadadeh, S.: Quantitative approach to osteoarthritic gait assessment. Eng. Med. 16:9, 1987.

89. Waters, R. L., Perry, J., Conaty, P. Lunsford, B., and O'Meara, P.: The energy cost of walking with arthritis of the hip and knee. Clin. Orthop. 214:278, 1987.

90. Brinkmann, J. R., and Perry, J.: Rate and range of knee motion during ambulation in healthy and arthritic subjects. Phys. Ther. 65:1055, 1985.

91. Curran, J. F., Ellman, M. H., and Brown, N. L.: Rheumatologic aspects of painful conditions affecting the shoulder. Clin. Orthop. 173:27, 1983.

92. Chandnani, V., and Resnick, D. L.: Roentgenologic diagnosis. In Moskowitz, R. W., Howell, D. S., Goldberg, V. M., and Mankin, H. J. (eds.): Osteoarthritis: Diagnosis and Management. Philadelphia, W. B. Saunders Company, 1992, pp. 263–312.

93. McAlindon, T. E. M., Watt, I., McCrae, F., Goddard, P., and Dieppe, P. A.: Magnetic resonance imaging in osteoarthritis of the knee: Correlation with radiographic and scintigraphic findings. Ann. Rheum. Dis. 50:14, 1991.

94. Macys, J. R., Bullough, P. G., and Wilson, P. D., Jr.: Coxarthrosis: A study of the natural history based on a correlation of clinical, radiographic and pathologic findings. Semin. Arthritis Rheum. 10:66, 1980.

95. Bonnarens, F., Hernandez, A., and D'Ambrosia, R.: Bone scintigraphic changes in osteonecrosis of the femoral head. Orthop. Clin. North Am. 16:697, 1985.

96. Christiansen, S. B., and Arnoldi, C. C.: Distribution of ^{99m}Tc-phosphate compounds in osteoarthritic femoral heads. J. Bone Joint Surg. 62A:90, 1980.

97. Sabiston, C. P., Adams, M. E., and Li, D. K.: Magnetic resonance imaging of osteoarthritis: Correlation with gross pathology using an experimental model. J. Orthop. Res. 5:164, 1987.

98. Braunstein, E. M., Brandt, K. D., and Albrecht, M.: MRI demonstration of hypertrophic articular cartilage repair in osteoarthritis. Skeletal Radiol. 19:335, 1990.

99. Ehrlich, G. E.: Inflammatory osteoarthritis. I. The clinical syndrome. J. Chronic Dis. 25:317, 1972.

100. Peter, S. B., Pearson, C. M., and Marmor, L.: Erosive osteoarthritis of the hands. Arthritis Rheum. 9:365, 1966.

101. Sarrat, P., Bouscarle, B., Felix, T., Acquaviva, P. C., Guerra, L., Kaphan, G., and Chevrot, L.: Comparative study of scintigraphy, x-ray computed tomography and magnetic resonance imaging in the diagnosis of osteonecrosis of the hip and algodystrophy. J. Radiol. 66:779, 1985.

102. Gillespy, T., 3d, Genant, H. K., and Helms, C. A.: Magnetic resonance imaging of osteonecrosis. Radiol. Clin. North Am. 24:193, 1986.

103. Kottal, R. A., Vogler, J. B., 3d, Matamoros, A., Alexander, A. H. J., and Cookson, J. L.: Pigmented villonodular synovitis: A report of MR imaging in two cases. Radiology 163:551, 1987.

104. Jergesen, H. E., Heller, M., and Genant, H. K.: Magnetic resonance imaging in osteonecrosis of the femoral head. Orthop. Clin. North Am. 16:705, 1985.

105. Ferguson, A. B., Jr.: The pathology of degenerative arthritis of the hip and the use of osteotomy in its treatment. Clin. Orthop. 77:84, 1971.

106. Norman, A., Robbins, H., and Milgram, J. E.: The acute neuropathic arthropathy—a rapid severely disorganizing form of arthritis. Radiology 90:1159, 1968.

107. Hartzman, S., Reicher, M. A., Bassett, L. W., Duckwiler, G. R., Mandelbaum, B., and Gold, R. H.: MR imaging of the knee. Part II. Chronic disorders. Radiology 162:553, 1987.

108. Sundaram, M., McGuire, M. H., Fletcher, J., Wolverson, J. K., Heiberg, E., and Shields, J. B.: Magnetic resonance imaging of lesions of synovial origin. Skeletal Radiol. 15:110, 1986.

109. Keating, J. W., Jr., Numagachi, Y., and Robertson, H. J.: Neuroimaging of the spine. Neurol. Clin. 2:797, 1984.

110. Rand, J. A.: Arthroscopic management of degenerative meniscus tears in patients with degenerative arthritis. Arthroscopy 1:253, 1985.

111. Ogilvie-Harris, D. J., and Wiley, A. M.: Arthroscopic surgery of the shoulder. A general appraisal. J. Bone Joint Surg. 68B:201, 1986.

112. Johnson, L. L.: Arthroscopic abrasion arthroplasty historical and pathologic perspective: Present status. Arthroscopy 2:54, 1986.

113. McBride, G. G., Constine, R. M., Hofmann, A. A., and Carson, R.

W.: Arthroscopic partial medial meniscectomy in the older patient. J. Bone Joint Surg. 66A:547, 1984.

114. Friedman, M. J., Berasi, C. C., Fox, J. M., DelPizzo, W., Snyder, S. J., and Ferkel, R. D.: Preliminary results with abrasion arthroplasty in the osteoarthritic knee. Clin. Orthop. 182:118, 1981.

115. Sprague, N. F., III: Arthroscopic debridement for degenerative knee joint disease. Clin. Orthop. 160:118, 1981.

116. Ropes, M. W., and Bauer, W.: Synovial Fluid Changes in Joint Disease. Cambridge, Harvard University Press, 1953.

117. Van de Putte, L. B. A., Meijer, C. J. L. M., and Lafeber, G. J. M.: Lymphocytes in rheumatoid and non-rheumatoid synovial fluids. Ann. Rheum. Dis. 35:451, 1976.

118. Fawthrop, F., Hornby, J., Swan, A., Hutton, C. Doherty, M., and Dieppe, P.: A comparison of normal and pathological synovial fluid. Br. J. Rheumatol. 24:61, 1985.

119. Wiedermann, D., and Vitulova, V.: Simultaneous analysis of eighteen proteins in the sera and knee joint effusions of patients with rheumatoid arthritis and osteoarthritis. Clin. Rheumatol. 5:416, 1986.

120. Thonar, E. J-M. A., Manicourt, D. M., Williams, J., Lenz, M. E., Sweet, M. B. E., Schnitzer, T. J., Otten, L., Glant, T., and Keuttner, K. E.: Circulating keratan sulfate: A marker of cartilage proteoglycan catabolism in OA. J. Rheumatol. 18:24, 1991.

121. Thonar, E. J-M. A., Lenz, M. E., Klintworth, G. K., et al.: Quantification of keratan sulfate in blood as a marker of cartilage catabolism. Arthritis Rheum. 28:1367, 1985.

122. Caterson, B.: Immunological aspects of markers of joint disease. J. Rheumatol. 18:19, 1991.

123. Caterson, B., Griffin, J., Mahmoodian, F., et al.: Monoclonal antibodies against chondroitin sulfate isomers: Their use as probes for investigating proteoglycan metabolism. Biochem. Soc. Trans. 18:820, 1990.

124. Ratcliffe, A., Doherty, M., Maini, R. N., et al.: Increased concentrations of proteoglycan components in the synovial fluid of patients with acute but not chronic joint disease. Ann. Rheum. Dis. 47:826, 1988.

125. Moreland, L. W., Stewart, T., Gay, R. E., Huang, G. Q., McGee, N., and Gay, S.: Immunohistologic demonstration of type II collagen in synovial fluid phagocytes of osteoarthritis and rheumatoid arthritis patients. Arthritis Rheum. 32:1458, 1989.

126. Niebauer, G. W., Wolf, B., Bashey, R. I., and Newton, C. D.: Antibodies to canine collagen types I and II in dogs with spontaneous cruciate ligament rupture and and osteoarthritis. Arthritis Rheum. 30:319, 1987.

127. Lust, G., Burton-Wurster, N., and Leipold, H.: Fibronectin as a marker for osteoarthritis. J. Rheumatol. 14:28, 1987.

128. Schumacher, H. R., Jr.: Crystals, inflammation, and osteoarthritis. Am. J. Med. 83:11, 1987.

129. Mannami, K., Mitsuhashi, T., Takeshita, H., Okada, K., Kuzuhara, A., Yamashita, T., and Sakakida, K.: Concentration of interleukin-1 beta in serum and synovial fluid in patients with rheumatoid arthritis and those with osteoarthritis. Nippon Seikeigeka Gakkai Zasshi 63:1343, 1989.

130. Hermann, E., Fleischer, B., Mayet, W. J., Poralla, T., and Meyer-zum-Buschenfelde, K. H.: Correlation of synovial fluid interleukin-6 (IL-6) activities with IgG concentrations in patients with inflammatory joint disease and osteoarthritis. Clin. Exp. Rheumatol. 7:411, 1989.

131. Chen, B. X., Francis, M. J., Duthie, R. B., Bromey, L., and Osman, O.: Oxygen free radical in human osteoarthritis. Chin. Med. J. 102:931, 1989.

132. Loeser, R. F., Smith, D. M., and Turner, R. A.: Phospholipase activity in synovial fluid from patients with rheumatoid arthritis, osteoarthritis and crystal-associated arthritis. Clin. Exp. Rheumatol. 8:379, 1990.

133. Doherty, M., Richards, N., Hornby, J., and Powell, R.: Relation between synovial fluid C3 degradation products and local joint inflammation in rheumatoid arthritis, osteoarthritis, and crystal associated arthropathy. Ann. Rheum. Dis. 47:190, 1988.

134. Heinegard D., and Saxne T.: Macromolecular markers in joint disease. J. Rheumatol. (Suppl.) 18:27:23, 1991.

135. Fife, R.: Cartilage matrix glycoprotein as a possible marker of OA. J. Rheumatol. (Suppl.) 18:27:30, 1991.

Management of Osteoarthritis

THE CORRECT DIAGNOSIS

Although osteoarthritis (OA) may be diagnosed with a high degree of sensitivity and specificity in people with chronic joint pain who fulfill clinical criteria that do not include radiographic studies,[1, 2, 3] in most cases today the diagnosis of OA is based on a combination of clinical and radiographic findings (e.g., joint space narrowing, subchondral sclerosis, osteophytes). Since these radiographic changes of osteoarthritis are common in asymptomatic individuals,[4] their clinical significance must be interpreted in light of the patient's history and physical examination. Furthermore, before the physician considers therapeutic options for the patient with joint pain and radiographic evidence of osteoarthritis, the physician must consider: Is osteoarthritis responsible for the patient's pain?

The question is not always easily answered. The issue may be confounded by the fact that rheumatic diseases are not mutually exclusive. Thus, gout, pseudogout, bacterial joint infection, or some other condition may be the proximate cause of joint pain in a patient, rather than osteoarthritis. On the other hand, the patient's symptoms may be due to soft tissue rheumatism. For example, the patient with radiographic evidence of osteoarthritis of the knee may have knee pain that is due not to the intra-articular disease, but to anserine bursitis; the patient with osteoarthritis of the acromioclavicular joint may present with shoulder pain due to coincidental bicipital tendinitis; the patient with osteoarthritis of the first carpometacarpal joint may have pain in the thumb due to an unrelated carpal tunnel syndrome or de Quervain's tenosynovitis. In each case, accurate diagnosis and treatment of the soft tissue problem may produce gratifying relief of pain, even though nothing has been done to affect the patient's osteoarthritis.

COMPONENTS AND AIMS OF THE TREATMENT PROGRAM

The components of a treatment program for the patient with osteoarthritis may include drugs, phys-ical measures, patient education (and, where appropriate, education of family members and influential others), psychosocial intervention, and surgery. Although no medical cure exists today for osteoarthritis, much can be done to relieve the patient's pain, maintain or improve mobility, and minimize disability.

How aggressively should the patient be treated? Nonsteroidal anti-inflammatory drugs are useful in producing symptomatic relief, as they are analgesic and also reduce the synovitis that is present. However, these drugs will not arrest the pathologic changes in cartilage or bone. Indeed, some may contribute to degenerative changes in cartilage and bone (see later).[5–7] Measures that protect the involved joint from mechanical damage (e.g., instructing the patient in the use of assistive devices and in patterns of joint use that avoid excessive loading of the articular cartilage; strengthening the supporting muscles to increase joint stability) are important in diminishing pain and discomfort. In many patients with osteoarthritis of the knee, isometric quadriceps exercises may eliminate the patient's pain within weeks. Although no evidence is available to indicate that such physical measures are prophylactic, it is logical to consider that they may retard or prevent progression of the disease by preventing further cartilage damage. This important question requires study.

Furthermore, the view that is widely held by patients and their doctors—that osteoarthritis is inevitably progressive—requires closer examination. In a survey of 682 elderly people, neither the prevalence nor severity of signs and symptoms suggestive of osteoarthritis of the knee increased with age, but remained constant in the seventh, eighth, and ninth decades.[8]

Although the diagnosis of OA in that survey was not confirmed radiographically, in another study of symptomatic "nonrheumatoid" individuals over age 54 with significant radiographic evidence of OA, the percentage with the most marked abnormalities similarly did not increase with age.[9] Some patients with osteoarthritis of the hip show no radiographic progression over long periods of follow-up. In some cases, radiographic improvement, with an increase in joint space, may be noted.[10, 11] In others, even in the presence of radiographic progression, pain may

Supported in part by grants (AR 20582 and AR 7448) from the National Institute of Arthritis, Diabetes, and Digestive and Kidney Diseases.

diminish, albeit usually with a loss of mobility due to biologic "splinting" of the joint by capsular fibrosis or restricting osteophytes.

Radiographic evidence of osteophytosis, in particular, is not a diagnostic criterion for osteoarthritis, or a prognostic indicator, but appears to be related to age. Thus, of patients who had osteophytes as the sole abnormality in the hip radiograph, fewer than 1 percent had developed joint space narrowing and other changes of osteoarthritis after 10 years.[10] Similar results were obtained in a study of the significance of osteophytosis in the knee; clinically important progressive cartilage damage occurred in only a minority of patients.[12]

Treatment of osteoarthritis should be tailored to fit the clinical severity of the disease. For patients with only mildly symptomatic disease, instruction in principles of joint protection, reassurance, and occasional analgesics may be all that is required. The importance of reassurance should not be minimized. Many patients with clinically mild osteoarthritis in one or two joints worry greatly that their disease will become widespread and ultimately incapacitating, dooming them to years of pain, uselessness, restricted mobility, and dependency. The physician can help considerably by pointing out that such a fate is highly unlikely. On the other hand, for the patient who has more severe disease, with impaired function and significant disability, a comprehensive, aggressive approach is warranted.

ATTENTION TO FACTORS CAUSING EXCESSIVE JOINT LOADING

Poor body mechanics may cause or aggravate osteoarthritis. Pronated feet, genu varus, and genu valgus create excessive loading on the knee, and may be corrected with orthotics, or by osteotomy. Poor posture should be corrected, and supports for the pendulous abdomen or breasts, or the excessively lordotic lumbar spine, may be helpful.

Instructing the patient in principles of joint protection is usually indicated. For patients with significant osteoarthritis of the interphalangeal or the first carpometacarpal joints, the measures listed in Table 80–1 may be helpful. They should be viewed as measures not only to diminish pain but also to prevent further joint damage.

For all patients with osteoarthritis, an analysis of the patient's vocational and avocational use of the arthritic joint is important. The pattern of use may clearly determine the development of osteoarthritis in a given joint, as shown in an interesting clinical and radiographic analysis of the hands of burlers, winders, and spinners in a worsted mill in rural Virginia.[13] Burling is a task that calls for a predominance of precision pinch in the right hand, winding is a bimanual task requiring repetitive power grip, and spinning requires predominantly precision pinch with the right hand. Results showed that the locali-

Table 80–1. MEASURES TO PREVENT FURTHER JOINT DAMAGE AND REDUCE PAIN IN THE HANDS

1. Use electric appliances (scissors, can openers, knives, mixers, power tools) whenever possible. Try to select multipurpose tools with controls that are easy to reach and operate.
2. Use lightweight utensils, such as those made of aluminum and plastic, rather than those made of glass or other heavy materials.
3. Large handles are easier to hold than small handles. Wrap a piece of foam rubber around eating utensils, toothbrushes, pens, irons, and other items with narrow handles.
4. Pinching a small zipper tab may be difficult. To pull the zipper more easily, use a ring or loop of string on the zipper tab, and place a finger through the loop.
5. Replace buttons with Velcro fasteners. Secure cuff buttons with elastic thread to eliminate the need for buttoning.
6. Use "easy-to-reach" kitchen storage to avoid the strain of reaching deeply into cupboards. Lazy Susans, slide-out shelves, and pegboard wall storage are good alternatives.
7. Allow dishes to air dry or use an automatic dishwasher.
8. Use a single-lever type of faucet, rather than one that requires twisting or turning.
9. Use a wall-mounted jar-opener that allows you to grasp the jar with both hands while twisting to open.
10. Whenever possible, slide objects to move them, instead of lifting them. To transport heavy objects, use a cart with wheels.
11. When you must lift a heavy item, do not attempt to pick it up in one hand. Get under the object and lift with the palms of both hands.

Data from form used by Occupational Therapy Department, University Hospital, Indianapolis, Indiana.

zation of impairment and radiographic evidence of osteoarthritis correlated with the demands placed on the joints by these occupational tasks.

In a similar study, the frequency of Heberden's nodes and radiographic changes of distal interphalangeal joint osteoarthritis was significantly higher in British cotton workers than in controls. Since these subjects had no greater frequency of spinal osteoarthritis and, in general, fewer musculoskeletal symptoms than the control subjects, the data suggest that the hand changes are due to repetitive occupational usage.[14]

Activities that cause excessive loading of the involved joint should be avoided, where possible. For example, for the patient with osteoarthritis of the hip or knee, modification of the workplace to permit sitting instead of standing, and elimination of requirements for kneeling or squatting will be helpful. Rest periods of 30 to 60 minutes in morning and afternoon may diminish discomfort in lower extremity joints or lumbar spine. Several shorter periods of standing or walking are more desirable than a single prolonged one. Temporary use of a cervical collar or traction may be helpful for the patient who is acutely symptomatic with cervical spondylosis, but immobilization of the painful joint, or complete bed rest, is rarely required. The practical measures listed in Table 80–2 may be helpful in reducing stress on the lumbar spine and hips and knees.

Acceptance of the recommendation to reduce

Table 80–2. MEASURES TO REDUCE STRESS TO
LUMBAR SPINE

1. Avoid lifting heavy objects.
2. Keep the back straight while lifting; lift by bending the knees.
3. Do not lift objects above waist level.
4. Avoid reaching to grasp an object, as when leaning into a car trunk.
5. Always stand close to the work surface.
6. Avoid standing for prolonged periods.
7. Push, do not pull, objects.
8. Avoid leaning over a desk or work surface for prolonged periods.
9. When driving, move the seat forward far enough to keep the knees bent and decrease the arch in the back.

Data from form used by Physical Therapy Department, University Hospital, Indianapolis, Indiana.

usage of the osteoarthritic joint is sometimes difficult for the osteoarthritic patient, who may fear that the joint will stiffen unless used continuously. The sensation of gelling that many of these individuals experience after periods of inactivity or prolonged sitting (as during an automobile or plane ride) contributes to this concern. Instructing the patient to put the involved joint through its range of motion every 15 to 20 minutes during such periods may minimize this discomfort. Also, informing the patient that prescribed exercises (see Table 80–4) are an important component of the treatment program will help reassure the individual who resists efforts to curtail activities that stress the diseased joint.

The patient with painful osteoarthritis of hip or knee may benefit from a cane (used in the contralateral hand) or, if symptoms are bilateral, crutches or a walker. These ambulation aids pose fewer problems for the patient with osteoarthritis than for the one with rheumatoid arthritis, who is more likely to encounter difficulty with their use because of concomitant involvement of hands, wrists, or shoulders. Many patients with osteoarthritis, however, are psychologically unprepared to accept an ambulatory aid. Education of the patient concerning the mechanical advantages to be derived from the device, a trial of usage to permit the patient to experience the relief of discomfort that it affords, and emphasis on the possible slowing of disease progression to be derived from its use are all warranted. The collaboration of a physical therapist in these efforts is usually desirable.

DIET

Concurrent obesity is commonly associated with osteoarthritis.[9, 15, 16] The excess weight contributes to the abnormal loading of articular cartilage in weight-bearing joints. In addition, obesity has been considered to contribute to osteoarthritis indirectly, by virtue of its association with increased bone mass.[17] Although an experimentally induced increase in the stiffness of the subchondral bone leads to breakdown of the overlying articular cartilage,[18] it remains to be

shown that the subchondral bone in obese individuals is stiffer than normal.

Despite good evidence for the association between obesity and osteoarthritis, evidence that obesity *causes* osteoarthritis, rather than resulting from the inactivity imposed by the disease when it affects weight-bearing joints, has been lacking until recently. However, data from the Framingham study show that obesity was associated with knee osteoarthritis even when obesity antedated the radiographic evaluation by 20 years.[19] Furthermore, a recent analysis of the United States Health and Nutrition Examination Survey (HANES) data demonstrated an association between osteoarthritis of the knee and self-reported minimum adult weight, which serves as an indicator of long-term obesity.[20] The association was also present in people without symptoms of knee osteoarthritis who would not have been expected to become sedentary (and therefore obese) as a result of knee pain.

Whether weight loss will reduce joint pain in the obese patient with osteoarthritis or retard the progression of joint breakdown has not been studied. It is reasonable, nonetheless, to instruct obese osteoarthritic patients in weight reduction and urge them to strive to normalize their body weight. However, this goal, although laudable, is not likely to be achieved. Because of the degree of inactivity imposed by the arthritis, and a caloric requirement that is often low, weight loss is difficult for these individuals. If the patient is sufficiently motivated, participation in a mutual support group (e.g., Weight Watchers, TOPS) can be helpful.

These measures, to the extent that they diminish joint loading, not only provide symptomatic relief but also may reduce the synovial inflammation that is attributed to cartilage breakdown. Cartilaginous wear particles, shown by ferrography to reflect cutting and rubbing wear, have been demonstrated in human synovial fluid aspirates[21] and can elicit the release from macrophages and synovial cells of neutral proteases capable of degrading proteoglycan and collagen in articular cartilage.[22]

PSYCHOLOGIC COPING AND SOCIAL SUPPORT

Yet another problem may confront the doctor who advises patients to diminish their level of physical activity. Patients with osteoarthritis often develop techniques to help maintain normality in their daily activities and in their interactions with others. These techniques are similar to those used by patients with other chronic conditions.[23] Two approaches commonly emerge: "keeping up" (i.e., maintaining the previous level of activity) and "covering up" (i.e., hiding the illness from the public).

Many patients with osteoarthritis attempt to keep up with whatever they perceive as normal activities, despite the likelihood that this may increase their joint pain. Some will seek actively to prove their ability, or to recapture their identity. For example, because they perceive a need to maintain an image of health for their coworkers or boss, patients with osteoarthritis of the knee may refuse to seek a feasible modification of their work situation by asking for a job that would permit sitting instead of standing. During work hours they may be able to keep up, but, at the end of the day, in the privacy of their home, they may collapse with pain and fatigue.

Covering up involves masking the disability and pain. Patients with osteoarthritis often relate that they will reply, "I'm fine," when someone asks how they are, even when they are experiencing considerable joint pain. They are often unwilling to reveal visible symbols of their disability, for example, a cane or a walker. They may refuse to face a trip to the shopping center because it hurts too much to walk without a cane.

For the physician to advise patients to abandon these techniques is not always helpful.[24] Through experience, most patients already know that they suffer when they overdo activities. Many know that to refuse to accept their need for a cane or walker is illogical, but they have not overcome their need to hide their physical problems from the public.

Patients with osteoarthritis who take great care to mask their discomfort or disability may wonder why their families or friends are not more helpful or sympathetic. Patients are sometimes proud because "no one knows," yet distressed because "no one cares."[23] Because osteoarthritis is often not a visible illness, and because many still consider arthritis to be only a minor disease, lack of understanding by others can be a problem even to the patient who is not keeping up or covering up. It is often useful to suggest to patients that the loss of potential support, help, and understanding is the price they may pay for covering up or keeping up. It may be pointed out that no matter how much others may care for the patient, they cannot read his or her mind. This may help the patient decide when and where to keep up or cover up.

In an analysis of NHANES I data, in which musculoskeletal impairments (not specifically OA) were considered, in comparison with those who were not disabled, those who were disabled with musculoskeletal symptoms tended to be older, nonwhite, of lower education and income, and widowed, separated, or divorced. Disability was increased in those who attributed their symptoms to an accident or injury and those who had musculoskeletal symptoms in multiple sites.[25]

The association of disability with separated or divorced marital status may be related to the lack of social support. In a randomized control trial involving chiefly black female patients of lower socioeconomic class attending a general medicine clinic, provision of health information on a regular basis resulted in improved physical health, decreased pain,

and enhanced functional status.[26] Indeed, an interaction as simple as a telephone interview appeared to provide OA patients with sufficient social support to improve their functional status;[27] in patients with knee osteoarthritis, even when the dose of analgesic or anti-inflammatory drug was held constant for the entire period of observation, improvement was as great as that seen in controlled trials of nonsteroidal anti-inflammatory drugs.[28] In similar patients with OA, "hassles" (minor stressors) were better predictors of health status than major life change events and correlated strongly with functional status.[29]

SEXUALITY

Osteoarthritis may significantly affect sexual function. This may be a particular problem for patients with osteoarthritis of the hips, knees, or spine. Results of a survey of 121 patients with osteoarthritis revealed that the most frequently mentioned causes of sexual difficulties were pain (40 percent), stiffness (75 percent), and loss of libido (22 percent).[30] Of the 81 patients who expressed sexual difficulties due to their disease, 23 percent felt these problems were the cause of marital unhappiness. Surgical treatment of osteoarthritis of the hip resulted in complete or considerable improvement in sexual function for 34 percent of the 70 patients who underwent surgery.

It is appropriate for the physician or other health care professional to initiate a discussion of sexual concerns, insofar as the patient may be reluctant to do so.[31] This may often be accomplished as a natural component of the evaluation for hip disease, during which the physician may ask about sexual problems while ascertaining the effects of the disease on other aspects of function, such as ability to arise from a sofa or toilet seat.[32] One might ask, "Has your disease caused a change in your sexual function?" and, if the answer is affirmative, "Does this change concern you?" The cause of the sexual concern should be ascertained, as well as what the patient thinks might improve the problem and how the partner feels about the problem. At times, arthritis is an excuse for, not the result of, the sexual problem. If the patient is unaware of how the partner feels about the problem, poor communication is likely to be contributory. In either case, in-depth marital counseling may be appropriate.

For the patient with limited spine or hip mobility, side-by-side position for intercourse may be preferable to one requiring the patient to be supine. Physicians should encourage couples to try a variety of positions to discover which is most comfortable for sexual activity. The Arthritis Foundation's excellent pamphlet *Living and Loving With Arthritis*, which contains suggestions for resolving a variety of sexual problems, is a valuable educational resource for arthritic patients.[33] Medical causes of sexual dysfunction in the elderly patient with arthritis, and approaches to assessment and management, have been reviewed.[34]

PHYSICAL THERAPY

Physical therapy holds a prominent position in the treatment of osteoarthritis. It involves principally the use of heat or cold, and an appropriate exercise program. It is generally useful to precede each exercise session with applications of moderate heat for 15 to 20 minutes to relieve pain and diminish stiffness. Patients should be cautioned to remove any liniment from the skin prior to heat application and to avoid lying on the heat source, as this may cause local compression of the circulation and lead to a burn. Applications of heat to joints that have undergone arthroplasty, and contain metal components, is contraindicated, as this may lead to deep thermal burns.

A variety of heat modalities may be used, for example, hydrocollator packs, electric pads, ultrasound, infrared bakers, diathermy, and paraffin baths. Patients often find moist heat more effective than dry heat. Practicality and cost should be considered in prescribing the particular modality to be employed. A warm bath or shower often proves to be the most convenient form of heat treatment. For deep-seated joints (e.g., hips, spine), ultrasound or diathermy may be particularly effective, although they often afford no greater benefit than less expensive, simpler forms of heat application.

Occasionally, heat may increase the patient's pain, and ice packs prove to be a more effective analgesic. Although controlled studies have not been performed in osteoarthritis, the efficacy of cryotherapy has been documented in patients with rheumatoid arthritis, where cryotherapy increased range of motion and decreased pain through a mechanism apparently related to endorphin release.[35]

The exercise program should be designed to preserve or improve range of motion and strengthen the involved muscles. Periarticular muscle atrophy, selective for type II fibers,[36] is common in osteoarthritis, and is presumably due to decreased activity as a consequence of joint pain. Isometric exercises are preferable to isotonic ones, since they minimize joint stress. Exercises should be initiated with three or four sessions daily. A small number of repetitions should be prescribed initially, and gradually increased to the desired maximum. Table 80–3 describes two types of isometric quadriceps exercises (quadriceps setting and straight leg raises).

In a controlled study, improvement in quadriceps strength achieved with an isometric exercise program led to a significant decrease in joint pain among subjects with knee osteoarthritis.[37] It is worth noting that the frequency with which exercises are performed by patients with osteoarthritis who are under the care of a physician for their joint pain is

Table 80–3. ISOMETRIC QUADRICEPS EXERCISES

Quadriceps Setting Exercise
1. Lie on your back, with legs stretched out straight.
2. Keeping your knee straight, press your knee down into the bed, tightening the big muscle on the front of your thigh above your knee.
3. Hold the muscle tight for 5 seconds (count: one thousand and one, one thousand and two, one thousand and three, etc.).
4. Relax the muscle for 5 seconds.
5. Repeat 10 times.
6. Perform 3 times daily (10 repetitions each time).
7. Gradually increase until you are performing this exercise 10 times daily (10–15 repetitions each time).
Note: This exercise can also be performed while sitting in a chair with legs stretched out straight. Simply press the heels into the floor, tightening the thigh muscle as above.

Straight Leg Raises
1. Lie on your back in bed.
2. To exercise the right leg, first bend the left knee, placing the left foot flat. (This will prevent any back strain during the exercise.)
3. Tighten the big muscle above the right knee and slowly lift the right leg straight up, as high as it will go. If the knee bends, do not continue to lift further.
4. Now slowly lower the leg and hold about 6 inches off the bed for 5 seconds (count: one thousand and one, one thousand and two, one thousand and three, etc.).
5. Lower the leg to the bed.
6. Repeat 5–10 times.
7. Perform 2–3 times daily.
Note: If you have severe pain during the exercise, or pain that lasts more than 15–20 minutes following the exercise, temporarily decrease the number of repetitions by one half.

Data from form used by Physical Therapy Department, University Hospital, Indianapolis, Indiana.

proportional to the amount of instruction and follow-up provided with regard to the exercise regimen.[38]

DRUG THERAPY

Drug therapy in osteoarthritis today is symptomatic. It should be recognized that many patients with this condition have only minimal symptoms and may be managed with only physical measures, without medications. However, in others, the use of analgesic or anti-inflammatory drugs is required for relief of joint pain.

The fact that drug therapy is "symptomatic" does not mean that it is not important or may not be helpful. Notably, in one study, patients with severe osteoarthritis rated their satisfaction with life lower than did patients undergoing chronic hemodialysis.[39] While this may have been related in part to such factors as living alone and duration of unemployment, chronic pain is probably a significant factor in the decreased life satisfaction among patients with osteoarthritis. Pain in osteoarthritis may be ascribed to a number of factors, for example, microfractures in subchondral trabeculae, irritation of periosteal nerve endings, ligamentous stress due to bone deformity or effusion, venous congestion caused by remodeling of subchondral bone,[40] soft tissue rheumatism, and muscle strain. Since the articular cartilage itself is aneural, pain does not arise from the degenerating cartilage.

In patients with chronic knee pain and arthroscopically proved osteoarthritis in whom the disease, on the basis of radiographic criteria, is not far advanced, the synovium may show no evidence of inflammation.[41] However, in patients with more advanced disease, synovial inflammation is common and may be a significant source of pain. A 1981 symposium dealt extensively with the topic of inflammation in osteoarthritis.[42] Usually, the synovitis in osteoarthritis is much less intense than that seen in rheumatoid arthritis, e.g., synovial fluid leukocyte counts are normal or only slightly increased (fewer than 2000 cells per mm[3]). The synovial membrane may contain foci of infiltrating lymphocytes, but pannus does not develop. Given these pathologic changes, it is not surprising that anti-inflammatory drugs have been found to afford greater symptomatic relief than simple analgesics in some patients with osteoarthritis.[43]

Analgesics

Acetaminophen, in a dose of about 650 to 1000 mg every 4 to 6 hours as needed, and propoxyphene hydrochloride (Darvon) are useful as simple analgesics in treatment of osteoarthritis. Codeine or other narcotics are rarely indicated and, if required, should be used only briefly.

A low dose of acetylsalicylic acid, for example, 650 mg every 4 to 6 hours as needed, may also provide effective analgesia in osteoarthritis. It is not superior, however, to acetaminophen or propoxyphene hydrochloride for this purpose and, in contrast to those agents, carries the risk of systemic cyclooxygenase inhibition, for example, gastropathy and renal inefficiency, especially in the elderly.[44, 45]

Since salicylate use for joint pain is widespread among patients with osteoarthritis, it should be emphasized that salicylate intoxication in the elderly may be atypical in its presentation and difficult to recognize.[46] The older individual who is salicylate-toxic may have no gastrointestinal complaints or ototoxicity (or may have decreased auditory acuity for other reasons). In such patients confusion, agitation, hyperactivity, slurring of speech, or seizures may be the presenting features of salicylate toxicity. Since these neurologic abnormalities suggest other diagnoses, it is particularly important to consider the possibility of salicylate intoxication when they are present in the elderly. Routine electrolyte determinations will be helpful, since acid-base disturbances (an anion gap) are invariably present.

Nonsteroidal Anti-inflammatory Drugs

If joint pain in the patient with osteoarthritis is not relieved by analgesics, or if clinical signs of inflammation are present (e.g., warmth, synovial effusion, erythema), treatment with a nonsteroidal anti-inflammatory drug (NSAID) may be indicated. The nonsteroidal anti-inflammatory drugs currently available (e.g., etodolac, fenoprofen, ibuprofen, Meclomen [Parke Davis], naproxen, piroxicam, sodium tolmetin, sulindac) are often effective in relieving joint pain and improving mobility and have benefited millions of patients with osteoarthritis.

When taken in the full daily dosage recommended on the package insert for rheumatoid arthritis, each of these drugs is equivalent in its anti-inflammatory effect to 12 to 15 aspirin tablets per day. Notably, however, the average daily dose required for the patient with osteoarthritis is often only one half to one third of that required for optimal management of rheumatoid arthritis.

Indomethacin is also effective in osteoarthritis. However, gastrointestinal and neurologic side effects are considerably more frequent than with the other nonsteroidal anti-inflammatory drugs, restricting its usefulness in chronic treatment of osteoarthritis. For patients with nocturnal pain, however, a single dose of 25 to 50 mg, or 75 mg of a sustained-release formulation, taken at bedtime, may produce gratifying relief. Indomethacin may be particularly effective in providing pain relief in osteoarthritis of the hip, but why it should be especially efficacious for this joint site, as opposed to others, is unknown.

Do nonsteroidal anti-inflammatory drugs modify the progression of osteoarthritis? In a double-blind study in which indomethacin was found to be superior to placebo for osteoarthritis of the hip, no effect on disease progression was noted over a 5-year period.[47] In contrast, a retrospective analysis of radiographic progression of osteoarthritis of the hip led to the conclusion that indomethacin use was associated with greater joint destruction than that seen in controls.[48]

In support of that observation, in a recent prospective study of 105 patients with advanced hip OA awaiting arthroplasty who were treated with either indomethacin or propazone, a weak inhibitor of prostaglandin synthesis, it was concluded that patients in the indomethacin group took 50 percent less time to reach arthroplasty and showed more rapid radiographic deterioration than those receiving propazone.[49] The study, however, was not fully blinded, criteria for hip arthroplasty were not stated, and the interpretation of the radiographs has been questioned.[50]

While it may be argued that the symptomatic relief produced by indomethacin and other cyclooxygenase inhibitors is sufficiently great that patients incur further damage by overusage of their osteoarthritic joints, inhibition of prostaglandin synthetase may interfere with synovial blood flow[49] or with repair of microfractures in subchondral bone,[51] increasing cyst formation and joint destruction. However, a recent study of patients whose hip radiographs were consistent with "analgesic arthropathy" (rapidly progressive atrophic change) found no basis for implicating NSAIDs in the joint disease.[52] The issue remains unresolved.

It has been widely contended that an NSAID should be the drug of choice for the elderly patient with osteoarthritis. Indeed, in a recent survey of 152 primary care practitioners, only 10 percent indicated that they would prescribe a pure analgesic as the principal drug in an uncomplicated case of osteoarthritis, while 35 percent would prescribe an NSAID in doses lower than that required for good anti-inflammatory effect. Most of the remainder indicated they would use an NSAID in a dose large enough to achieve an anti-inflammatory effect.[53]

How sound is the rationale for this approach? As indicated before, joint pain in osteoarthritis may arise from a variety of sites other than inflamed synovium. Furthermore, in patients with osteoarthritis of the knee undergoing arthroscopy because of knee instability who, notably, had *no* history of knee pain, the severity of synovitis and of degenerative changes in the articular cartilage were as great as in those with chronic joint pain due to osteoarthritis.[41]

There is no evidence that NSAIDs are superior to analgesic agents with no anti-inflammatory activity (e.g., acetaminophen) in treatment of osteoarthritis. A comparison of ketaprofen with an analgesic (dextropropoxyphene/acetaminophen) showed no difference in pain relief between the two treatment regimens.[54] Although another study reported that diclofenac was more effective than dextropropoxyphene/acetaminophen in improving pain and improving mobility in patients with osteoarthritis,[55] radiographic confirmation of the diagnosis was not obtained and soft tissue rheumatism and referred pain were not excluded. In another comparative trial in patients with osteoarthritis, no significant difference was found between flurbiprofen and the analgesic nefopam with respect to improvement in joint pain or range of joint motion after 1 month of treatment.[56] Similarly, in a 4-week randomized double-blind trial in patients with knee osteoarthritis, the efficacy of an anti-inflammatory dose of ibuprofen (2400 mg per day) was no greater than that of an essentially analgesic dose of the drug (1200 mg per day) or of acetaminophen (4000 mg per day).[57] Consistent with these findings, ibuprofen in a dose of only 1200 mg per day was equivalent to several other NSAIDs for treatment of joint pain due to osteoarthritis[58–61] even when the other drugs were used in anti-inflammatory doses.[59, 61]

These data suggest that the symptomatic relief afforded by NSAIDs may be affected by their analgesic activity independent of their actions as anti-inflammatory agents. This possibility is further suggested by recent evidence that the R- and S-enantiomers of flurbiprofen were nearly identical in their analgesic effects in two different models of inflammation-related pain, since S-flurbiprofen is a potent inhibitor of prostaglandin synthesis but the R-enantiomer is not.[62]

All of the NSAIDs mentioned earlier inhibit prostaglandin synthetase, and are thus relatively contraindicated in the patient who has an active peptic ulcer, a past history of ulcer disease, or a bleeding disorder. In such patients, nonacetylated salicylate preparations, e.g., Arthropan, Disalcid, or Trilisate, which have no effect on platelet aggregation, are more reasonable alternatives than the NSAIDs.

The renal effects of NSAIDs may also cause problems in the elderly.[45, 63] Any drug that significantly inhibits prostaglandin synthetase may diminish renal blood flow. While this is not of clinical importance in patients with normal kidneys, full doses of salicylate may lead to a rise in BUN and creatinine in patients with intrinsic renal disease, such as nephrosclerosis, which is common in the elderly. In patients who are hypertensive, or who have incipient or frank congestive heart failure, this may present a significant problem.

Disease-Modifying Drugs

Although aspirin administration was reported to prevent chondromalacia patellae in patients with recurrent dislocation of the patella,[64] the condition of the patella prior to drug administration in that study was not ascertained. A subsequent prospective double-blind study of patients with chondromalacia patellae diagnosed by arthroscopy showed no changes in signs, symptoms, or macroscopic appearance of the cartilage in either patients treated with aspirin or those given placebo.[65]

Despite a lack of clinical evidence, it has been suggested that NSAIDs may be "chondroprotective."[66] Such claims are based largely on in vitro evidence that they may modify PG or collagen metabolism, cytokine-mediated matrix degeneration, release or activity of neutral proteases, or actions of toxic oxygen metabolites.[66–76] No clinical evidence exists, however, to support the contention that NSAIDs favorably influence the progression of joint degeneration.

Indeed, salicylates and several other NSAIDs have been shown to suppress proteoglycan biosynthesis in articular cartilage in vitro.[5] Salicylates also worsen the degenerative changes in osteoarthritic[6] and atrophic[7] canine articular cartilage in vivo, although they had no effect on normal cartilage. While these effects in animals suggest that chronic administration of salicylates and some other NSAIDs may be injurious to articular cartilage, it is not possible to deduce from animal studies the effects of these drugs on the pathophysiology of osteoarthritis in humans. It is important to note, therefore, that several clinical trials are now in progress that will attempt to determine whether prolonged administration of an NSAID may modify the progression of osteoarthritis. The results of double-blind controlled comparison of naproxen sodium versus acetaminophen in patients with osteoarthritis of the knee are currently being analyzed (J. Ward: personal communication). Unfortunately, a high dropout rate in that study may limit the generalizability of the results.

Attempts are being made to design pharmacologic agents that take into account the pathophysiology of the articular cartilage in osteoarthritis. Compounds that stimulate chondrocyte metabolism or inhibit the enzymes capable of degrading articular cartilage matrix (e.g., Arteparon, Rumalon, Cartrofen) are receiving much attention.[74, 77]

No such "chondroprotective" drug (a poor term) has yet been shown in adequately controlled studies to affect the natural history of osteoarthritis in humans. However, when administered by either intra-articular or intramuscular injection for 4 to 20 weeks to dogs with OA produced by anterior cruciate ligament transection, Arteparon, a glycosaminoglycan polysulfuric acid ester, reduced the severity of histologic changes of osteoarthritis.[74, 78] When it was given by intra-articular injection 2 days after anterior cruciate ligament transection and continued twice a week for 4 weeks, cartilage degradation was less severe than in controls, suggesting the possibility of its use as a prophylactic treatment for OA.[78] In a lapine model of experimentally induced osteoarthritis, Arteparon diminished the severity of morphologic changes of osteoarthritis even when treatment was begun after initiation of the disease.[79] Unfortunately, the period of observation in these studies was relatively brief. It will be important to see if the beneficial effects are sustained.

Rumalon is a glycosaminoglycan-peptide complex derived from bovine cartilage and bone marrow extracts.[80] The available preparations are not standardized on the basis of any specific effects on cartilage. Bollet found that Rumalon increased ^{35}S-sulfate incorporation by normal and osteoarthritic human articular cartilage in vitro.[81]

Sodium pentosan polysulfate (SP54, Cartrofen) is a heparinoid that inhibits hyaluronidase, elastase, and other lysosomal enzymes, and stimulates hyaluronic acid synthesis by synovial cells.[74] In several animal models of osteoarthritis it inhibited cartilage elastase activity and decreased proteoglycan degradation. The potential advantage of this agent in comparison with Arteparon is its lack of antigenic protein constituents.

Given the in vitro data and results of in vivo studies in animal models of osteoarthritis, what are the results in humans? In a 5-year unblinded study, patients in Czechoslovakia were treated with either Arteparon or Rumalon in addition to nonsteroidal anti-inflammatory drugs.[82] Those who received either Rumalon or Arteparon were reported to show greater improvement in several parameters (e.g., knee pain and mobility, ability to climb stairs, walking time). Furthermore, radiographic progression of OA was reported to be slower in the Arteparon- and Rumalon-treated groups, and surgery was required less often, than in patients treated with NSAIDs alone.

However, failure to control for ingestion of NSAIDs and to include a placebo group has cast doubt upon the significance of these results.

In a double-blind trial of patients with OA in various joints in which, in contrast to the other study, use of NSAIDs or analgesics was not permitted, patients who were given 20 intramuscular injections of Rumalon over several months appeared to have greater symptomatic relief than placebo-treated patients.[82] In an open study of 1704 patients with osteoarthritis at various sites, those who received two series of Rumalon injections but were given neither anti-inflammatory drugs nor analgesics had fewer symptoms than those treated only with placebo.[83]

In a 1-year comparison of intramuscular Rumalon and placebo injections in 150 patients with osteoarthritis of the hip who also received NSAIDs, those with milder radiographic changes of osteoarthritis who received Rumalon reported "significantly" less pain after 48 weeks than the placebo group.[84] However, in patients with more severe radiographic findings, no decrease in pain was noted in either group.

Unfortunately, all those studies were flawed because of either uncontrolled use of NSAIDs or the lack of statistical analysis or of blinding. No conclusion about the efficacy of Rumalon in human osteoarthritis can be drawn at present. The development of such compounds is in its infancy, however, and the area warrants additional effort.

Adrenal Glucocorticoid Therapy

Systemic glucocorticoid treatment, or administration of adrenocorticotropic hormone, is not indicated in treatment of osteoarthritis. Beneficial effects are equivocal and the side effects associated with prolonged use of these agents, especially in the elderly, far outweigh any possible benefits. On the other hand, intra-articular injection of glucocorticoids may be of benefit. Hollander et al.[85] reported marked to complete relief of symptoms in 87 percent of 231 patients who received repeated injections over a 20-year period. Similar results were noted in a subsequent review of nearly 1000 patients with osteoarthritis of the knee who received intra-articular steroid injections as needed over a 9-year period.[86] In that series nearly 60 percent no longer had sufficient pain to require further injections, about 20 percent were still receiving injections, and about 20 percent had not benefited from the injections or had been lost to follow-up.

These data must be viewed alongside results of other studies, however, which have shown similar benefits following single injections of 1 percent procaine,[87] isotonic saline,[87] or the suspending vehicle.[88]

Symptomatic improvement following intra-articular steroid injection is likely to be temporary. Although pain relief after intra-articular injection was significantly greater 1 week after an injection of steroids than it was with a control injection (the suspending vehicle), by 4 weeks after the injection the response of patients who received steroid was indistinguishable from that of the controls.[89] The mechanism of pain relief with intra-articular steroids in osteoarthritis may be associated with decreases in synovial permeability,[90] even when the drug produces an increase in synovial fluid leukocytosis[91] (presumably due to postinjection synovitis caused by the microcrystalline preparation).[92] Furthermore, steroids inhibit hyaluronic acid secretion by the synovium,[93] which may help decrease the volume of synovial effusions.

Clinical experience with intra-articular steroid therapy supports its safety, although rapidly progressive joint failure has been observed after frequent, repeated injections.[94-97] The masking of pain by intra-articular steroid injections may lead to overuse, with subsequent breakdown and instability.[98, 99] Steroids may also damage cartilage directly. Weekly injections into rabbit joints for 4 to 9 weeks produced histologic evidence of cartilage degeneration,[100] and depressed synthesis of collagen and proteoglycans, leading to a decrease in proteoglycan concentration in the articular cartilage.[101] Although little histologic change was seen in non-weight-bearing joints, weight-bearing cartilage developed surface fissures and cystic degeneration. Because of the concerns stated previously, intra-articular steroids are generally employed at intervals not shorter than 4 to 6 months for a given joint.

It is of interest that intra-articular glucocorticoids may ameliorate some of the pathologic changes of osteoarthritis. Thus, repeated injections of triamcinolone acetate, 3 mg per kg, diminished osteophyte formation in rabbits with secondary osteoarthritis.[102] In another study, utilizing a somewhat different rabbit model of osteoarthritis, a single intra-articular injection of 1 mg of triamcinolone hexacetonide, a long-acting glucocorticoid, provided significant protection against articular cartilage degeneration.[103]

Oral administration of prednisone, 0.3 mg per kg per day, decreased osteophyte size and cartilage ulceration in dogs with osteoarthritis produced by transection of the anterior cruciate ligament.[104] This dose, however, would be equivalent to 17 mg per day for a 70-kg human. In a similar study in which the dose of prednisone was only one third as great, no differences were noted between treated dogs and the controls with respect to size or extent of osteophytes, severity of synovial inflammation, structural changes in the articular cartilage, or in vitro synthesis of cartilage glycosaminoglycans.[105] In humans, no evidence exists that steroids favorably influence either the pathologic changes in the articular cartilage or osteophytosis.

Some clinicians recommend weeks of joint rest (e.g., crutch walking) after intra-articular glucocorticoid therapy, while others permit an early return to usual daily activities.[106-108] The deleterious effects of intra-articular steroids on cartilage seen in rabbits after meniscectomy appeared to be potentiated by exercise,[98] arguing in favor of a period of postinjection joint rest. Neustadt reported that patients with rheumatoid arthritis who were hospitalized and placed at rest after an intra-articular injection of triamcinolone hexacetonide had a longer duration of response than ambulatory patients.[109] Similarly, patients who received prednisolone tebutate and prescribed rest had a longer period of improvement than patients treated with the same drug, or methylprednisolone, and no rest. It appears advisable to caution the patient to minimize joint loading for a period of time following the injection, even though controlled data that this is helpful in humans are not available. Injection of steroids into painful pericapsular sites and ligaments may also produce symptomatic relief and is not associated with the potential dangers of intra-articular injection.

ORTHOPEDIC SURGERY

Surgical procedures are generally reserved for patients with more severe disease, with persistent pain and significantly impaired function. Osteotomies to correct malalignment (e.g., tibial or femoral osteotomy in the patient with knee osteoarthritis and genu varus or valgus) may be of greatest benefit, however, when the disease is only moderately advanced. By altering stresses of load-bearing, and bringing more normal cartilage surfaces into opposition, such surgeries may provide effective relief of pain. Debridement of the joint, with removal of free cartilage fragments (joint mice), may prevent locking, eliminate pain, and prevent rapid wear of the joint surfaces. Surgical removal of large osteophytes may also increase range of motion, although by buttressing the joint the constraining osteophytes may, at times, serve to diminish breakdown of the articular surface. In advanced disease, arthroplasty (partial or total) or arthrodesis may be required and can generally be expected to relieve pain; often these procedures will improve range of motion as well. In weight-bearing parts, such as the hip and knee, arthrodesis is generally avoided, but in patients whose future activities will require heavy usage of the involved joint, making failure of an arthroplasty likely, arthrodesis may be the procedure of choice, even though it permanently eliminates joint motion.

The experimental application of surgical techniques to graft cells that will undergo chondroneogenesis and resurface articular cartilage defects deserves mention. For example, it has been shown that periosteal grafts could resurface large defects in the patellar groove of rabbits, especially when the joint was subjected to continuous passive motion after grafting.[110] Under these conditions, the periosteum converted from synthesis of type I collagen to synthesis almost exclusively of type II, and structural quality of the regenerated tissue at 1 year was as good as at 4 weeks after grafting, indicating the potential for long-term survival of the new cartilage.[111]

Implanted mesenchymal stem cells, containing osteochondroprogenitors derived from the bone marrow or from periosteum and incorporated into calcium phosphate porous ceramic or into a collagen gel, have been shown capable of healing large, full-thickness defects in femoral condyles of rabbits.[112]

Transplantation of intact articular growth plate cartilage or of cultured chondrocytes also has been shown to support limited repair of defects in adult rabbit articular cartilage,[113] and improved healing of full-thickness cartilage defects in rabbits was shown to occur with the use of allogeneic chondrocytes embedded in a collagen gel.[114]

TREATMENT OF OSTEOARTHRITIS AT SPECIFIC SITES

The Knee

The general measures described here will usually provide effective relief of pain and stiffness. As is the case with osteoarthritis of the hip, weight reduction is indicated if the patient is obese. Other measures to decrease joint loading should also be recommended (Table 80–4). Jogging and participation in racket sports should be discouraged. The patient should be instructed not to rest with pillows placed behind the knees, which may lead to flexion contractures. Isometric quadriceps exercises are indicated (see Table 80–3). Elastic supports or knee cages (hinged braces which lace up the front) increase stability and may protect against stress.

Flare-ups are not uncommon in osteoarthritis of the knee, and are marked by increased pain, often with joint effusion and increased warmth and tenderness of the joint. Elimination of weight-bearing is usually effective treatment for the flare-up. Aspiration of the effusion and intra-articular administration of steroid are often helpful. Steroid injections into tender periarticular ligaments may also provide relief. Often, the patient with knee osteoarthritis may be symptomatic owing to an associated anserine bursi-

Table 80–4. MEASURES TO MINIMIZE STRESS TO HIPS AND KNEES

1. Do not walk or jog as an exercise. Swimming is an excellent alternative.
2. Avoid stairs whenever possible.
3. Sit, rather than stand. Use high stools when working at a counter.
4. Use higher chairs, rather than low sofas.
5. Avoid kneeling or squatting.
6. Before arising from a chair, sit at the edge of the seat, with legs under the body. Use the arm rests to push up from the seat.

Data from form used by Physical Therapy Department, University Hospital, Indianapolis, Indiana.

tis. In this case, injection of local glucocorticoid into the tender area localizing the bursitis will often produce marked relief of pain.

Locking of the knee suggests a torn meniscus or the presence of joint mice, which should be removed surgically or arthroscopically. As described before, surgery may be of great benefit. Because of the greater complexity of the biomechanics of the knee, total knee arthroplasty has not enjoyed the same rate of success as total hip arthroplasty; nonetheless it may afford excellent pain relief, increase mobility, and improve function.

An excellent review of the current status of arthroscopic debridement, chondral shaving, and abrasion arthroplasty in management of knee osteoarthritis has recently been published.[115]

Arthroscopic debridement of the joint, with removal of loose bodies and degenerated tissue fragments, is employed in some patients with severe osteoarthritis of the knee, but controlled studies showing that it has favorable effects on pain and function in patients with OA are largely lacking. Prior to the advent of arthroscopy, it was noted that removal of loose bodies, torn menisci, and articular cartilage flaps could relieve the joint pain of patients with knee osteoarthritis—sometimes for years.[116–118] Indeed, in cases of only moderately severe osteoarthritis, not only was symptomatic relief achieved but progression of osteoarthritis was said to be favorably influenced. However, the procedure required arthrotomy with lengthy rehabilitation, significant postoperative pain, and the risk of other postsurgical complications and was not widely employed.

Arthroscopic techniques, however, now permit debridement of osteoarthritic joints without the morbidity of an arthrotomy. In uncontrolled studies, osteoarthritis patients with symptoms related to internal derangements seem to benefit most from the procedure while those with moderate OA without internal derangement benefit less frequently.[119] Those with significant joint instability without an internal derangement seem to benefit least.

The shaving of fibrillated articular cartilage, leaving a smoother surface, is also advocated as a means of achieving symptomatic relief in patients with knee osteoarthritis; no long-term clinical studies have been reported that support the efficacy of this procedure, however. In fact, in humans, shaving of damaged knee articular cartilage was considered possibly to increase fibrillation and cell necrosis in cartilage adjacent to the original defect.[120] In rabbits, shaving of normal patellar cartilage did not lead to progressive deterioration; neither, however, did it stimulate cartilage repair.[121]

Abrasion of exposed subchondral bone to cause bleeding, with formation of a fibrin clot and subsequent articular cartilage repair, is also used in treatment of knee OA. No randomized controlled trial of arthroscopic abrasion arthroplasty has been reported, but in uncontrolled studies[122–124] it decreased symptoms of OA in 60 to 83 percent of patients, while 6 to 15 percent were worse at follow-up. Furthermore, in many patients with radiographic evidence of severe osteoarthritis, the joint space increased after abrasion arthroplasty.[124] However, none of the patients became asymptomatic after treatment and the procedure was considered to be only palliative.

In the few published studies of the effects of abrasion arthroplasty in OA, follow-up periods have been brief, making it difficult to determine whether it alters progression of OA. In general, outcome measures and patient selection criteria or evaluation are not well described, and results are usually reported by the surgeon who performed the procedure.

At least part of the improvement that may occur following arthroscopy may be due to removal of debris from the joint space by the saline lavage employed during the procedure.[125, 126] Joint irrigation has been reported to reduce the pain of patients with OA who have been refractory to other medical measures,[127, 128] although, as with arthroscopy, the placebo effect may be considerable. Randomized controlled double-blind studies of this procedure with a sham lavage have not been performed.

The Hip

Diminished loading on the involved joint should be accomplished by use of an ambulatory aid (e.g., cane, crutch, walker). If a cane or crutch is prescribed, it should be used on the uninvolved side. Practical measures to reduce stress on the joint should be discussed (see Table 80–4). An obese patient should be encouraged to reduce to ideal weight. Rest periods, the use of heat, analgesic and anti-inflammatory drugs, and non-weight-bearing exercises to strengthen supporting muscles and maintain normal range of motion all are indicated. Attempts should be made to prevent flexion contractures by having the patient lie prone for periods of 30 minutes two or three times daily. Patients should be advised to utilize higher chairs, or seat cushions, rather than low chairs or sofas. Elevated toilet seats may also be helpful.

Applications of heat will help relieve muscle spasm. However, if spasm is severe, traction may be required. In many patients with osteoarthritis of the hip, limitation of motion results from capsular contractures. Exercises to strengthen adduction, extension, and external rotation are, therefore, indicated. Intra-articular injections of steroids may be helpful when pain is severe. However, they are often ineffective, perhaps owing to the difficulty in ensuring that the injection is actually placed within the joint space.

With advanced disease, surgery should be considered. Total hip arthroplasty is generally the procedure of choice and, in most cases, provides excellent pain relief and restores hip motion to a level approaching normal. Intertrochanteric osteotomy has been reported to produce lasting benefit in at least 85 percent of patients.[129, 130] Although this procedure has a role in the treatment of younger patients, later conversion to a total hip replacement may be difficult, limiting its usefulness in older patients.

The Hand

Although Heberden's nodes often develop insidiously and may be present without symptoms, in some patients they develop rapidly with localized swelling, erythema, marked tenderness, and pain. In such instances they may be particularly sensitive to pressure or to accidental trauma. Patients with Heberden's nodes require reassurance that they do not have a crippling form of arthritis, or a form that is likely to progress to involve other joints. They should be reassured that the nodes will eventually become painless, and supported in accepting the resulting cosmetic changes. Heat, in the form of contrast baths, hot soaks, or paraffin baths, is usually effective for relief of pain. If the symptoms are severe, analgesic or nonsteroidal anti-inflammatory drugs may be helpful. Local injections of glucocorticoids into or around the affected joint may be helpful, especially in the unusually painful, acutely inflamed node, which is accompanied by a large, painful, mucinous cyst. Trauma, which may aggravate pain and the deformity, should be avoided. Instructing the patient in joint protection principles (see Table 80–1) is indicated. Nylon-spandex stretch gloves, worn at night, have been reported to relieve pain and morning stiffness.[131]

Symptoms from osteoarthritis at the base of the thumb, in the first carpometacarpal joint, may also benefit from judicious use of intra-articular steroids and by splinting. A slip-on hand splint to immobilize the first carpometacarpal and metacarpophalangeal joints of the thumb can reduce pain during functional activities.[132] If severe pain persists, arthroplasty or arthrodesis may be indicated. Arthroplasty will allow retention of motion but compromise grip strength; arthrodesis will preserve good grip strength but will eliminate motion.

The Spine

Symptoms caused by osteoarthritis of the cervical spine generally respond to the measures already described, i.e., rest, heat, analgesics, and anti-inflammatory drugs. A cervical pillow may be helpful. To decrease stress on the cervical spine, the patient should be advised not to maintain the neck in extension or flexion for prolonged periods, as when shampooing or sitting near the screen in a movie theater. Prolonged periods of rotation may also increase discomfort, as when watching television while lying on a sofa, or watching a tennis match from a midcourt seat. Symptoms caused by nerve root irritation may be relieved by a cervical collar. Occasionally, severe muscle spasm or nerve root compression may require cervical traction. This may be accomplished in the home under a physician's guidance. In patients with neurologic complications whose symptoms are unresponsive to these measures, surgery may be indicated.

Symptoms resulting from osteoarthritis of the lumbar spine will also usually respond to rest, heat, and medications as described before, and simple measures for joint protection. A lumbosacral corset with abdominal support and weight reduction, if the patient is obese, may be helpful. A firm mattress or bedboards placed beneath the mattress are often beneficial. Muscle spasm may be alleviated with muscle relaxants, local heat, or massage. Exercises to strengthen the anterior abdominal muscles and to correct poor posture should be instituted when acute symptoms subside, to minimize the likelihood of recurrences. Surgery, such as laminectomy, discectomy, or fusion, may be required when symptoms are severe or neurologic deficits are present.

The Feet

Osteoarthritis of the first metatarsophalangeal joint may produce pain, limitation of motion, and marked proliferation of osteophytes in the joint margins. In early cases, relief may be obtained by metatarsal pads or metatarsal bars, or by stiffening the sole of the shoe with metal to minimize dorsiflexion at this joint during walking. If the condition is advanced and chronically painful, and these measures are ineffective, surgery may be required. Inflammation and swelling of the bursa medial to the first metatarsophalangeal joint may be treated by a local steroid injection. Osteoarthritis of the subtalar joint is often resistant to the general measures outlined here. Reduction of weight-bearing by use of a cane or crutches may be helpful. In severe cases, triple arthrodesis may be indicated.

VOCATIONAL REHABILITATION

At times, a change in occupation may be desirable. While assistance from vocational rehabilitation counselors may be helpful, a survey of 86 counselors in the Indiana Department of Rehabilitation Services, which is presumably representative of similar departments in other states, showed that 80 percent had had no on-the-job orientation about arthritis and 72 percent no formal education about arthritis in college. Seventy percent had not participated in a continuing education program about arthritis within the past 2 years.[133] It is thus incumbent on the physician to inform the counselor about the patient's limitations, disease prognosis, and so forth. Even with this information, however, the enlightened vocational rehabilitation counselor may encounter great difficulty in finding suitable employment for the arthritis patient, who is competing in a "buyer's market."

SOCIAL SECURITY DISABILITY

Disabled patients with osteoarthritis may be more concerned about their ability to provide financially for themselves and their families than about the disease itself. Patients who are unable to continue working may be eligible for Social Security Disability Insurance (DI) or Supplemental Security Income (SSI) disability benefits. Both DI and SSI disability require that the disabling condition be present, or be expected to be present, continuously for at least 12 months. To be eligible for DI, the disabled worker must have contributed to the Social Security trust

Table 80–5. SOCIAL SECURITY ADMINISTRATION'S GUIDELINES FOR DISABILITY

I. **Arthritis of a Major Weight-Bearing Joint**
With history of persistent joint pain and stiffness with signs of severe limitation of motion of the affected joint on current physical examination. With:
  A. Gross anatomic deformity of hip or knee (e.g., subluxation, contracture, bony or fibrous ankylosis, instability) with radiographic evidence of either severe joint space narrowing or significant bony destruction and severely limiting ability to walk and stand; or
  B. Reconstructive surgery or surgical arthrodesis of a major weight-bearing joint and return to full weight-bearing status did not occur, or is not expected to occur, within 12 months of onset.

II. **Arthritis of One Major Joint in Each Arm**
With history of persistent joint pain and stiffness, signs of severe limitation of motion of the affected joints on current physical examination, and radiographic evidence of either severe joint space narrowing or significant bony destruction. With:
  A. Abduction and forward flexion (elevation) of both arms at the shoulders, including scapular motion, restricted to less than 90 degrees; or
  B. Gross anatomic deformity and enlargement or effusion of the affected joints.

III. **Disorders of the Spine**
  A. Arthritis manifested by ankylosis or fixation of the cervical or dorsolumbar spine at 30 degrees or more of flexion measured from the neutral position with radiographic evidence of:
    1. Calcification of the spinal ligaments; or
    2. Bilateral ankylosis of the sacroiliac joints with abnormal apophyseal articulation.
  B. Osteoporosis, generalized (established by radiograph), manifested by pain and limitation of back motion and paravertebral muscle spasm with radiographic evidence of nontraumatic vertebral compression fracture(s).
  C. Other vertebragenic disorders (e.g., herniated nucleus pulposus, spinal stenosis) with the following persisting for at least 3 months despite prescribed therapy and expected to last 12 months. With both:
    1. Pain, muscle spasm, and significant limitation of motion in the spine; and
    2. Appropriate radicular distribution of significant muscle weakness and sensory and reflex loss.

Adapted from *Disability Evaluation Under Social Security: A Handbook for Physicians.* U.S. Department of Health and Human Services, Social Security Administration, Publication No. (SSA) 79-10089, August, 1979.

fund for a specified length of time, which is dependent on the worker's age at the onset of disability. For example, workers over age 31 must have contributed to the Social Security trust fund for 20 of the preceding 40 quarter-years. For younger workers, fewer quarters are required. SSI, in contrast to DI, is funded through general tax revenues and does not require prior contributions to the trust fund.

The Social Security Administration has published a "Listing of Impairments," which is used to determine whether the applicant's impairment significantly limits the ability to perform basic work activities. If the clinical findings meet the listed criteria (Table 80–5), the impairment will be considered severe enough to be disabling and benefits will be awarded. Since the criteria are not specific to osteoarthritis, findings that are equivalent in severity to those in Table 80–5 will also qualify for determination of disability.

If the applicant's impairment does not meet or equal the criteria mentioned in the Listing of Impairments, but is severe, he or she may still be eligible for DI or SSI disability benefits, since in determining eligibility the Social Security Administration considers also the applicant's "residual functional capacity," that is, the ability to perform work-related tasks despite physical or mental limitations. Work-related tasks that are considered include walking, standing, lifting, carrying, pushing, pulling, reaching, and handling. Pain and fatigue may be considered in determining the residual functional capacity if they are accompanied by objective medical evidence.

A booklet for physicians, prepared by the Social Security Administration, describes in detail the content of the Listing of Impairments.[134] To reduce the likelihood that patients legitimately disabled by osteoarthritis will be denied benefits, the physician must be as specific as possible about the claimant's ability to perform work-related tasks, and must document the patient's objective clinical findings.[135]

References

1. Altman, R., Asch, E., Bloch, D., Bole, G., Borestein, D., Brandt, K., Christy, W., Cooke, T. D., Greenwald, R., Hochberg, M., Howell, D., Kaplan, D., Koopman, W., Longley, S., III, Mankin, H., McShane, D. J., Medsger, T., Jr., Meenan, R., Mikkelsen, W., Moskowitz, R., Murphy, W., Rothschild, B., Segal, M., Sokoloff, L., and Wolfe, F.: Development of criteria for the classification and reporting of osteoarthritis: Classification of osteoarthritis of the knee. Arthritis Rheum. 29:1039, 1986.
2. Altman, R., Appelrouth, D., Asch, E., Bloch, D., Borenstein, D., Brandt, K. D., Brown, C., Christy, W., Cooke, T. D., Gray, R., Greenwald, R., Hochberg, M., Howell, D., Ike, R., Kapila, P., Kaplan, D., Koopman, W., Longley, S., McShane, D. J., Medsger, T., Michel, B., Murphy, W., Osial, T., Ramsey-Goldman, R., Rothschild, B., and Wolfe, F.: Criteria for classification and reporting of osteoarthritis of the hand. Arthritis Rheum. 33:1601, 1990.
3. Altman, R., Alarcon, G., Appelrouth, D., Bloch, D., Borenstein, D., Brandt, K., Brown, C., Cooke, T. D., Daniels, W., Greenwald, R., Hochberg, M., Howell, D., Ike, R., Kapila, P., Kaplan, D., Koopman, W., McShane, D. J., Medsger, T., Michel, B., Murphy, W. A., Osial, T., Ramsey-Goldman, R., Rothschild, B., Seldman, D., and Wolf, F.: Criteria for classification and reporting of osteoarthritis of the hip. Arthritis Rheum. 34:505, 1991.
4. Linholm, R. V., Koivisto, E., and Punto, L.: Radiologic signs of hip and knee joint degeneration. Postgrad. Med. 65:155, 1979.
5. Palmoski, M., and Brandt, K.: Effects of some nonsteroidal anti-inflammatory drugs on articular cartilage proteoglycan metabolism and organization. Arthritis Rheum. 23:1010, 1980.
6. Palmoski, M., and Brandt, K.: *In vivo* effect of aspirin on canine osteoarthritic cartilage. Arthritis Rheum. 26:994, 1983.
7. Palmoski, M., and Brandt, K.: Aspirin aggravates the degeneration of canine joint cartilage caused by immobilization. Arthritis Rheum. 25:1333, 1982.
8. Forman, M. D., Malamet, R., and Kaplan, D.: A survey of osteoarthritis of the knee in the elderly. J. Rheumatol. 10:282, 1983.
9. Lawrence, J. S., Brenner, J. M., and Bier, F.: Osteoarthrosis: Prevalence in the population and relationship between symptoms and x-ray changes. Ann. Rheum. Dis. 25:1, 1966.
10. Danielsson, L. G.: Incidence and prognosis of coxarthrosis. Acta Orthop. Scand. 66:9, 1964.
11. Seifert, M. H., Whiteside, C. G., and Savage, O.: A 5 year follow-up of fifty cases of idiopathic osteoarthritis of the hip. Ann. Rheum. Dis. 28:325, 1969.
12. Hernborg, J., and Nilsson, B. E.: The relationship between osteophytes in the knee joint, osteoarthritis and aging. Acta Orthop. Scand. 44:69, 1973.
13. Hadler, N. M.: The variable of usage in the epidemiology of osteoarthrosis. *In* Peyron, J. G. (ed.): Epidemiology of Osteoarthrosis. West Caldwell, NJ, Ciba-Geigy, 1981, p. 164.
14. Lawrence, J. S.: Rheumatism in cotton operatives. Br. J. Indust. Med. 18:270, 1961.
15. Acheson, R. M., and Collart, A. B.: New Haven survey of joint diseases. XVII. Relationship between some systemic characteristics and osteoarthritis in a general population. Ann. Rheum. Dis. 54:379, 1975.
16. Acheson, R. M.: Epidemiology and the arthritides. Ann. Rheum. Dis. 41:325, 1982.
17. Dequeker, J., Goris, P., and Utterhoeven, R.: Osteoporosis and osteoarthritis (osteoarthrosis): Anthropometric distinctions. J.A.M.A. 249:1448, 1983.
18. Radin, E. G.: Mechanical aspects of osteoarthrosis. Bull. Rheum. Dis. 26:862, 1975–1976.
19. Felson, D. T., Anderson, J. J., Naimack, A., et al.: Obesity and symptomatic knee osteoarthritis. Results from the Framingham Study. Arthritis Rheum. 30:S130, 1987.
20. Anderson, J., and Felson, D.: Factors associated with knee osteoarthritis (OA) in a national survey. Arthritis Rheum. 29:S16, 1986.
21. Evans, C. H., Mears, D. C., and McKnight, J. L.: A preliminary ferrographic survey of the wear particles in human synovial fluid. Arthritis Rheum. 24:912, 1981.
22. Evans, C. H., Mears, D. C., and Cosgrove, J. L.: Release of neutral proteinases from mononuclear phagocytes and synovial cells in response to cartilaginous wear particles in vitro. Biochim. Biophys. Acta 677:287, 1981.
23. Wiener, C. L.: The burden of rheumatoid arthritis: Tolerating the uncertainty. Soc. Sci. Med. 9:97, 1975.
24. Gross, M.: Psychosocial aspects of arthritis: Helping patients cope. Health Soc. Work 6:40, 1981.
25. Cunningham, L. S., and Kelsy, J. L.: Epidemiology of musculoskeletal impairments and associated disability. AJPH 74:574, 1984.
26. Weinberger, M., Hiner, S. L., and Tierney, W. M.: Improving functional status in arthritis: The effect of social support. Soc. Sci. Med. 23:899, 1986.
27. Weinberger, M., Tierney, W. M., Booher, P., and Katz, B. P.: Can the provision of information to patients with osteoarthritis improve functional status? Arthritis Rheum. 32:1577, 1989.
28. Rene, J., Weinberger, M., Mazzuca, S. A., Brandt, K. D., and Katz, B. P.: Reduction of joint pain in patients with knee osteoarthritis who have received monthly telephone calls from lay personnel and whose medical treatment regimens have remained stable. Arthritis Rheum. 35:511, 1992.
29. Weinberger, M., Hiner, S. L., and Tierney, W. M.: In support of hassles as a measure of stress in predicting health outcomes. J. Behav. Med. 10:19, 1987.
30. Currey, H. L. F.: Osteoarthrosis of the hip joint and sexual activity. Ann. Rheum. Dis. 29:488, 1970.
31. Ferguson, K., and Figley, B.: Sexuality and rheumatic disease: A prospective study. Sexuality Disability 2:130, 1979.
32. Ehrlich, G. E.: Sexual problems of the arthritic patient. *In* Ehrlich, G. E. (ed.): Total Management of the Arthritic Patient. Philadelphia, J. B. Lippincott Co., 1973, pp. 193–208.
33. Living and Loving with Arthritis. Atlanta, GA, Arthritis Foundation, 1982.
34. Brandt, K. D., and Potts, M. K.: Arthritis in the elderly: Assessment and management of sexual problems. Med. Aspects Hum. Sexuality 21:57, 1987.
35. Utsinger, P. D., Bonner, F., and Hogan, N.: Efficacy of cryotherapy

(CR) and thermotherapy in the management of rheumatoid arthritis (RA) pain: Evidence for an endorphin effect. Arthritis Rheum. 25:S113, 1982.

36. Sirca, A., and Susec-Michieli, M.: Selective type II fibre muscular atrophy in patients with osteoarthritis of the hip. J. Neurol. Sci. 44:149, 1980.

37. Chamberlain, M. A., Care, G., and Harfield, B.: Physiotherapy in osteoarthritis of the knee: A controlled trial of hospital versus home exercises. Int. Rehab. Med. 4:191, 1982.

38. Dexter, P.: Joint exercises in elderly persons with symptomatic osteoarthritis of the hip or knee: Performance patterns, medical support patterns, and the relationship between exercising and medical care. Arthritis Care Res. 5:36, 1992.

39. Laborde, J. M., and Powers, M. J.: Satisfaction with life for patients undergoing hemodialysis and patients suffering from osteoarthritis. Res. Nurs. Health 3:19, 1980.

40. Lempberg, R. K., and Arnoldi, C. C.: The significance of intraosseous pressure in normal and diseased states with special reference to intraosseous engorgement pain syndrome. Clin. Orthop. 136:143, 1978.

41. Myers, S. L., Brandt, K. D., Ehlich, J. W., Braunstein, E. M., Shelbourne, K. D., Heck, D. A., and Kalasinski, L. A.: Synovial inflammation in patients with early osteoarthritis of the knee. J. Rheumatol. 17:1622, 1990.

42. Osteoarthritis Symposium. Palm Aire, Florida, October 20–22, 1980. Howell, D. S., and Talbott, J. H. (eds.): Semin. Arthritis Rheum. XI, No. 1 (Suppl. 1), 1981.

43. Doyle, C. V., Dieppe, P. A., Scott, J., and Huskisson, E. G.: An articular index for the assessment of osteoarthritis. Ann. Rheum. Dis. 40:75, 1981.

44. Griffin, M. R., Pifer, J. M., Daughtery, Snowden, M., and Ray, W. A.: Nonsteroidal anti-inflammatory drug use and increased risk for peptic ulcer disease in elderly persons. Ann. Intern. Med. 14:257, 1991.

45. Murray, M. D., and Brater, D. G.: Adverse effects of nonsteroidal anti-inflammatory drugs on renal function. Ann. Intern. Med. 112:559, 1990.

46. Anderson, R. J., Potts, D. E., Gabow, P. A., et al.: Unrecognized adult salicylate intoxication. Ann. Intern. Med. 85:745, 1976.

47. Hodgkinson, R., and Woolf, D.: A five-year clinical trial of indomethacin in osteoarthrosis of the hip. Practitioner 210:372, 1974.

48. Ronninger, H., and Langeland, N.: Indomethacin treatment in osteoarthritis of the hip joint. Does the treatment interfere with the natural course of the disease? Acta Orthop. Scand. 50:169, 1979.

49. Rashad, S., Revell, P. Wemingway, A., Low, F., Rainsford, K., and Walker, F.: Effect of nonsteroidal anti-inflammatory drugs on the course of osteoarthritis. Lancet 2:519, 1989.

50. Lequesne, M., Lamotte, J., and Samson, M.: Conditions de démonstration radio-clinique d'un effet chondroprotecteur ou chondroagresseur. In Gaucher, A., Netter, P., Pourel, J., and Régent, D. (eds.): Actualités en Physiologie et Pharmacologie Articulaires. Paris, Masson, 1991, pp. 390–401.

51. Sudmann, E., Dregelid, E., Bessesen, A., and Morland, J.: Inhibition of fracture healing by indomethacin in rats. Eur. J. Clin. Invest. 9:333, 1979.

52. Doherty, A. M., Holt, M., Macmillan, P., Watt, I., and Dieppe, P.: Reappraisal of analgesic hip. Ann. Rheum. Dis. 45:272, 1986.

53. Mazzuca, S. A., Brandt, K. D., Anderson, S. E. and Katz, M. P.: The therapeutic approaches of community-based primary care practitioners to osteoarthritis of the hip in an elderly patient. J. Rheumatol. 18:1593, 1991.

54. Doyle, D. V., Dieppe, P. A., Scott, J., Huskisson, E. C.: An articular index for the assessment of osteoarthritis. Ann. Rheum. Dis. 40:75, 1981.

55. Parr, G., Darekar, B., Fletcher, A., and Bulpitt, C. J.: Joint pain and quality of life; Results of a randomized trial. Br. J. Clin. Pharmacol. 27:235, 1989.

56. Stamp, J., Rhind, V., and Haslock, I.: A comparison of nefopam and flurbiprofen in the treatment of osteoarthritis. Br. J. Clin. Pract. 43:24, 1989.

57. Bradley, J. D., Brandt, K. D., Katz, B. P., Kalasinski, L. A., and Ryan, S. I.: Comparison of an anti-inflammatory dose of ibuprofen, an analgesic dose of ibuprofen, and acetaminophen in the treatment of patients with osteoarthritis of the knee. N. Engl. J. Med. 325:87, 1991.

58. Breshnihan, B., Hughes, G., and Essigman, W. K.: Diflunisal in the treatment of osteoarthrosis: A double blind study comparing diflunisal with ibuprofen. Curr. Med. Res. Opin. 5:556, 1978.

59. Moxley, T. E., Royer, G. L., Hearron, M. S., et al.: Ibuprofen versus buffered phenylbutazone in the treatment of osteoarthritis: Double blind trial. J. Am. Geriatr. Soc. 23:343, 1975.

60. de Blecourt, J. J.: A comparative study of ibuprofen ("Brufen") and indomethacin in uncomplicated arthritis. Curr. Med. Res. Opin. 3:477, 1975.

61. Cimmino, M. A., Cutolo, M., Samanta, and Accardo, S.: Short term treatment of osteoarthritis: A comparison of sodium meclofenamate and ibuprofen. J. Int. Med. Res. 10:46, 1982.

62. Brune, K., Beck, W. S., Menzel-Soglowek, S., and Geisslinger, G.: Analgesia by non-opiate analgesics may not necessarily depend on prostaglandin synthesis inhibition. In Gaucher, A., Netter, P., Pourel, J., and Regent, D. (eds.): Actualités en Physiologie et Pharmacologie Articulaires. Paris, Masson, 1991, pp. 76–79.

63. Dahl, S. L., and Word, J. R.: Efficacy and tolerability of oxaprozin in the elderly. Semin. Arthritis Rheum. 15 (Suppl. 2):40, 1986.

64. Chrisman, O. D., Snook, G. A., and Wilson, T. C.: The protective effect of aspirin against degeneration of human articular cartilage. Clin. Orthop. 84:193, 1972.

65. Bentley, G., Leslie, I. J., and Fischer, D.: Effect of aspirin treatment on chondromalacia patellae. Ann. Rheum. Dis. 40:37, 1981.

66. Doherty, M.: "Chondroprotection" by non-steroidal anti-inflammatory drugs. Ann. Rheum. Dis. 48:619, 1989.

67. Ghosh, P.: Anti-rheumatic drugs and cartilage. Clin. Rheumatol. 2:309, 1988.

68. Herman, J. H., Appel, A. M., and Hess, E. V.: Modulation of cartilage destruction by select nonsteroidal anti-inflammatory drugs. In vitro effect on the synthesis and activity of catabolism-inducing cytokines produced by osteoarthritic and rheumatoid synovial fluid. Arthritis Rheum. 30:257, 1987.

69. McKenzie, L. S., Horsburgh, B. A., Ghosh, P., and Taylor, T. K. F.: Effect of anti-inflammatory drugs on sulphated glycosaminoglycan synthesis in aged human articular cartilage. Ann. Rheum. Dis. 35:487, 1976.

70. Kalbhen, D. A.: Biochemically induced osteoarthritis in the chicken and rat. In Munthe, E., and Bjelle, A. (eds.): Effects of Drugs on Osteoarthritis. Berne, Stuttgart, Huber, 1984, pp. 48–68.

71. Herman, J. H., and Hess, E. V.: Nonsteroidal anti-inflammatory drugs and modulation of cartilaginous changes in osteoarthritis and rheumatoid arthritis: Clinical implications. Am. J. Med. (Suppl.)77:16, 1984.

72. Carlin, G., Djursärd, G., and Gerdin, B.: Effect of anti-inflammatory drugs on xanthine oxidase and xanthine oxidase–induced depolymerisation of hyaluronic acid. Agents Actions 16:377, 1985.

73. Lentini, A., Ternai, B., and Thosh, P.: Inhibition of human leukocyte elastase and cathepsin G by non-steroidal anti-inflammatory compounds. Biochem. Int. 15:1069, 1987.

74. Burkhardt, D., and Ghosh, P.: Laboratory evaluation of antiarthritic drugs as potential chondro-protective agents. Semin. Arthritis Rheum. 17(Suppl. 1):3, 1987.

75. Shinmei, M., Kikuchi, T., Masuda, K., and Shimomura, Y.: Effects of interleukin 1 and anti-inflammatory drugs on the degradation of human articular cartilage. Drugs 35(Suppl. 1):33, 1988.

76. De Vries, B. J., van den Berg, W. B., Vittero, E., and van de Putte, L. B. A.: Effects of NSAIDs on the metabolism of sulphated glycosaminoglycans in healthy and post-arthritic articular cartilage. Drugs 35(Suppl. 1):24, 1988.

77. Fife, R. S., and Brandt, K. D.: Experimental modes of therapy in osteoarthritis. In Moskowitz, R. W., Howell, D. S., Goldberg, V. M., and Mankin, H. J. (eds.): Osteoarthritis, Diagnosis and Management. Philadelphia, W. B. Saunders, 1984, pp. 549–559.

78. Altman, R. D., Dean, D. D., Muniz, O. E., and Howell, D. S.: Prophylactic treatment of canine osteoarthritis with glycosaminoglycan polysulfuric acid ester. Arthritis Rheum. 32:759, 1989.

79. Dustmann, H. O., Puhl, W., and Martin, K.: Der Einflub interaartikularer Arteparoninjektionen bei Arthrose. Z. Orthop. 112:1188, 1974.

80. Bollet, A. J.: Connective tissue polysaccharide metabolism and the pathogenesis of osteoarthritis. Adv. Intern. Med. 13:33, 1967.

81. Bollet, A. J.: Stimulation of protein-chondroitin sulfate synthesis by normal and osteoarthritic cartilage. Arthritis Rheum. 11:663, 1968.

82. Rejholec, V.: Long-term studies of antiosteoarthritic drugs: An assessment. Semin. Arthritis Rheum. 17(Suppl. 1):35, 1987.

83. Wagenhauser, F. J., Amira, A., Borrachero, J., et al.: Die Behandlung der Arhrosen mit Knorpel-Knochenmark-Extrakt. Ergebnisse eines Multi-Centre-Trials. Schweiz. Med. Wochenschr. 98:904, 1968.

84. Dixon, A. S., Kersley, G. D., Mercer, R., Thompson, M., Mason, R. M., Barnes, C., and Wenley, G.: A double-blind controlled trial of Rumalon in the treatment of painful osteoarthrosis of the hip. Ann. Rheum. Dis. 29:193, 1970.

85. Hollander, J. L.: Intraarticular hydrocortisone in arthritis and allied conditions. J. Bone Joint Surg. 35A:983, 1953.

86. Hollander, J. L.: Treatment of osteoarthritis of the knees. Arthritis Rheum. 3:564, 1960.

87. Traut, E. F.: Procaine and procaine amide hydrochloride in skeletal pain. J.A.M.A. 150:785, 1952.

88. Wright, V., Chandler, G. N., Morrison, R. A. H., and Hartfall, S. J.: Intra-articular therapy in osteoarthritis. Comparison of hydrocortisone acetate and hydrocortisone tertiary butylacetate. Ann. Rheum. Dis. 19:257, 1960.

89. Friedman, D. M., and Moore, M. A.: The efficacy of intraarticular corticosteroid for osteoarthritis of the knee. Arthritis Rheum. 21:556, 1978.

90. Eymontt, M. J., Gordon, G. V., Schumacher, H. R., and Hansell, J. R.: The effects on synovial permeability and synovial fluid leukocyte

counts in symptomatic osteoarthritis after intraarticular corticosteroid administration. J. Rheumatol. 9:198, 1982.

91. Hodgkinson, R., and Woolf, D.: A five-year clinical trial of indomethacin in osteoarthrosis of the hip. Practitioner 210:372, 1974.

92. McCarty, D. J., and Hogan, J. M.: Inflammatory reaction after intrasynovial injection of microcrystalline adrenocorticosteroid esters. Arthritis Rheum. 7:359, 1964.

93. Myers, S. L.: Suppression by corticosteroid suspensions of hyaluronic acid synthesis in synovial organ cultures. Arthritis Rheum. 11:1275, 1985.

94. Zachariae, L.: Deleterious effects of corticosteroid administered topically, in particular intra-articularly. Acta Orthop. Scand. 36:127, 1965.

95. Keagy, R. D., and Keion, H. A.: Intra-articular steroid therapy: Repeated use in patients with chronic arthritis. Am. J. Med. Sci. 253:75, 1967.

96. Balch, H. W., Gibson, J. M. C., El-Ghobarey, A. F., et al.: Repeated corticosteroid injections into knee joints. Rheumatol. Rehabil. 16:137, 1977.

97. Gray, R. G., and Gottlieb, N. L.: Intra-articular corticosteroids. Clin. Orthop. 177:235, 1983.

98. Alarcon-Segovia, D., and Ward, L. E.: Marked destructive changes occurring in osteoarthritic finger joints after intraarticular injection of corticosteroids. Arthritis Rheum. 9:443, 1966.

99. Miller, W. T., and Restifo, R. A.: Steroid arthropathy. Radiology 86:652, 1966.

100. Moskowitz, R. W., Davis, W., Sammarco, J., Mast, W., and Chase, S. W.: Experimentally induced corticosteroid arthropathy. Arthritis Rheum. 134:236, 1970.

101. Behrens, F., Shepard, H., and Mitchell, N.: Alteration of rabbit articular cartilage by intra-articular injections of glucocorticoids. J. Bone Joint Surg. 58A:1157, 1976.

102. Moskowitz, R. W., Goldberg, V. M., Schwab, W., and Berman, L.: Effects of intraarticular corticosteroids and exercise in experimental models of inflammatory and degenerative arthritis. Arthritis Rheum. 18:417, 1975.

103. Butler, M., Colombo, C., Hickman, L., O'Byrne, E., Steele, R., Steinetz, B., Quintavalla, J., and Yokoyama, N.: A new model of osteoarthrosis in rabbits: III. Evaluation of antiarthrotic effects of selected drugs administered intraarticularly. Arthritis Rheum. 26:1132, 1983.

104. Pelletier, J. P., and Martel-Pelletier, J.: Protective effects of corticosteroids on cartilage lesions and osteophyte formation in the Pond-Nuki dog model of osteoarthritis. Arthritis Rheum. 32:181, 1989.

105. Myers, S. L., Brandt, K. D., and O'Connor, B. L.: "Low-dose" prednisone treatment does not reduce the severity of osteoarthritis in dogs after anterior cruciate ligament transection. J. Rheumatol. 18:1856, 1991.

106. Hollander, J. L.: Intrasynovial corticosteroid therapy in arthritis. Md. State Med. J. 19:62, 1970.

107. McCarty, D. J.: Intrasynovial therapy with adrenocorticosteroid esters. Wisconsin Med. J. 77:575, 1978.

108. Neustadt, D. H.: Intra-articular steroid therapy. In Moskowitz, R. W., Howell, D. S., Goldberg, V. M., and Mankin, H. F. (eds.): Osteoarthritis, Diagnosis and Management. 2nd ed. Philadelphia, W. B. Saunders, 1992, pp. 493–510.

109. Neustadt, D. H.: Intra-articular steroid therapy. In Moskowitz, R. W., Howell, D. S., Goldberg, V. M., and Mankin, H. J. (eds.): Osteoarthritis, Diagnosis and Management. 2nd ed. Philadelphia, W. B. Saunders, 1992, pp. 493–510.

110. O'Driscoll, S. W., Kelley, F. W., and Salter, R. B.: The chondrogenic potential of free autogenous periosteal grafts for biological resurfacing of major full-thickness defects in joint surfaces under the influence of continuous passive motion. J. Bone Joint Surg. 68-A:1017, 1986.

111. O'Driscoll, S. W., Kelley, F. W., and Salter, R. B.: Durability of regenerated articular cartilage produced by free autogenous periosteal grafts in major full-thickness defects in joint surfaces under the influence of continuous passive motion. J. Bone Joint Surg. 70-A:595, 1988.

112. Goto, T., Goldberg, V., and Kaplan, A.: Osteochondral progenitor cells enhance repair of large defects in rabbit articular cartilage. Trans. Orthop. Res. Soc. 17:598, 1992.

113. Aston, J. E., and Bentley, G.: Repair of articular surfaces by allografts of articular and growth-plate cartilage. J. Bone Joint Surg. 68(B):29, 1986.

114. Wakitani, S., Kimura, T., Hirooka, A., et al.: Repair of rabbit articular surfaces with allograft chondrocytes embedded in collagen gel. J. Bone Joint Surg. 71(B):74, 1989.

115. Buckwalter, J. A.: Arthroscopic treatment of osteoarthritic knee joints. In Brandt, K. D. (ed.): Cartilage Changes in Osteoarthritis. Indianapolis, Indiana University School of Medicine, 1991, pp. 137–141.

116. Magnuson, P. B.: Joint debridement: Surgical treatment of degenerative arthritis. Surg. Gynecol. Obstet. 73:1, 1941.

117. Haggart, G. E.: The surgical treatment of degenerative arthritis of the knee joint. J. Bone Joint Surg. 22:717, 1940.

118. Insall, J.: The Pridie debridement operation for osteoarthritis of the knee. Clin. Orthop. 101:61, 1974.

119. Stulberg, S. D., and Keller, C. S.: The principles and results of arthroscopic surgical treatment of osteoarthritis of the knee. Arthritis Rheum. 25(Suppl.):S44, 1982.

120. Schmid, A., and Schmid, F.: Results after cartilage shaving studied by electron microscopy. Am. J. Sports Med. 15:386, 1987.

121. Coventry, M. B.: Osteotomy about the knee for degenerative and rheumatoid arthritis: Indications, operative technique and results. J. Bone Joint Surg. 55A:23, 1973.

122. Friedman, M. J., Berasi, C. C., Fox, J. M., Del Pizzo, W., Snyder, S. J., and Ferkel, R. D.: Preliminary results with abrasion arthroplasty in the osteoarthritic knee. Clin. Orthop. 182:200, 1984.

123. Chandler, E. J.: Abrasion arthroplasty of the knee. Contemp. Orthop. 11:21, 1985.

124. Johnson, L. L.: Arthroscopic abrasion arthroplasty. Historical and pathologic perspective: Present status. Arthroscopy. 1980.

125. Burman, M. S., Finkelstein, F. H., and Mayer, L.: Arthroscopy of the knee joint. J. Bone Joint Surg. 16:255, 1934.

126. Jackson, R. W., Silver, R., and Marans, H.: Arthroscopic treatment of degenerative joint disease. Arthroscopy 2:114, 1986.

127. Arnold, W. J., Mather, S. E., Mostello, N., and Tongue, J.: Tidal knee lavage in patients with chronic pain due to osteoarthritis of the knee. Arthritis Rheum. 27:S66, 1984.

128. Ike, R. W., Arnold, W. J., Simon, C., and Eisenberg, G. M.: Tidal knee irrigation as an intervention for chronic pain due to osteoarthritis of the knee. Arthritis Rheum. 30:S17, 1987.

129. Mogensen, B. A., Zoega, H., and Marinko, P.: Late results of intertrochanteric osteotomy for advanced osteoarthritis of the hip. Acta Orthop. Scand. 51:85, 1980.

130. Langlais, F., Roure, J.-L., and Maquet, P.: Valgus osteotomy in severe osteoarthritis of the hip. J. Bone Joint Surg. 61B:424, 1979.

131. Ehrlich, G., and DiPierro, A. M.: Stretch gloves: Nocturnal use to ameliorate morning stiffness in arthritic hands. Arch. Phys. Med. Rehabil. 52:479, 1971.

132. Melvin, J. L.: Rheumatic Disease, Occupational Therapy and Rehabilitation. 2nd edition. Philadelphia, F. A. Davis Co., 1982, p. 345.

133. Gross, M., and Brandt, K.:Educational needs of vocational rehabilitation counselors working with clients who have arthritis. J. Appl. Rehab. Counseling 15:22, 1984.

134. Disability Evaluation Under Social Security: A Handbook for Physicians. U.S. Department of Health and Human Services, Social Security Administration, Publication No. (SSA) 79-10089, August, 1979.

135. Meenan, R. F., Liang, M. H., and Hadley, N. M.: Social Security disability and the arthritis patient. Bull. Rheum. Dis. 33:1, 1983.

Chapter 81

Jerome H. Herman

Polychondritis

INTRODUCTION

Polychondritis, a relapsing form of connective tissue disease, is primarily characterized by widespread potentially destructive inflammatory lesions involving cartilaginous structures throughout the body, the cardiovascular system, and organs of special sense. Its etiology is unknown and its pathogenesis incompletely understood. Mounting evidence suggests a select perturbation of connective structure and function incited by phlogistic and immunologic mechanisms acting in concert in organ systems perhaps enriched in a given form of connective tissue. Although physician awareness is compromised by its infrequent occurrence and often subtle modes of presentation, more than 550 cases have been reported in the world's literature.

DEMOGRAPHICS

Polychondritis occurs predominantly in whites but may affect all races. It has an equal sex prevalence. The majority of cases appear between the ages of 40 and 60 years, but onset may vary from birth to the ninth decade (Fig. 81–1). No familial predisposition is recognized. Genetic studies have failed to establish a specific class I MHC linkage. Reports of class II haplotypes are isolated and too few to enable a correlation analysis. Although an isolated instance of placental transmission has been recorded, more recent observations report uneventful labors and spontaneous delivery of healthy infants. However, the mother may continue to experience active multisystem disease.[2]

CLINICAL FEATURES

The clinical manifestations may vary considerably in location, their concurrence, severity, and duration. The reason for such variability is unknown. Table 81–1 contrasts the frequency of more common system involvement at disease onset with that appearing during the course of illness. A low-grade temperature (at times presenting with a fever of undetermined origin), malaise, fatigability, and myalgias are not uncommon symptoms.

Ears

Most prevalent is the rather sudden onset of pain, tenderness, and a violaceous erythematous swelling that is confined in a patchy or diffuse distribution to the cartilaginous portion of one or both external ears. Lobules are spared. Inflammatory encroachment may lead to narrowing of the external auditory meatus, causing a decrease in hearing. Inflammation can extend to the retroauricular soft tissues. Attacks tend to vary in severity, with duration spanning several days to weeks before subsiding spontaneously. Protracted or recurrent episodes of inflammation may lead to permanent loss of cartilage, resulting in a "cauliflower" appearance of the ears (Fig. 81–2).

Although infrequent at the onset, internal ear disease characterized by auditory or vestibular dysfunction may subsequently appear in 39 percent of patients.[3] Auditory impairment can also result from middle ear inflammation associated with eustachian tube obstruction caused by chondritis of its nasopharyngeal segment or to neurosensory abnormalities presumably secondary to vasculitis of the internal auditory artery or its cochlear branch. Symptoms may be acute or insidious in onset. Arteritis of the

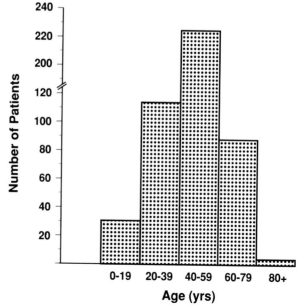

Figure 81–1. Age at onset of polychondritis in 464 patients.

1400

Table 81–1. PREDOMINANT CLINICAL MANIFESTATIONS OF RELAPSING POLYCHONDRITIS

	Frequency (Percentage of Patients)	
	Presenting	*Cumulative*
Auricular inflammation	40	84
Arthropathy (total)	38	71
Peripheral joints		67
Costochondral/manubriosternal		26
Nasal cartilage inflammation	25	64
Ocular inflammation (total)	21	54
Scleritis/episcleritis	13	35
Conjunctivitis	7	25
Iritis/Uveitis	5	17
Keratitis	3	8
Laryngotracheal-bronchial disease	21	49
Internal ear involvement (total)	11	39
Auditory		34
Vestibular		17
Cardiovascular disease (total)		28
Systemic vasculitis		14
Valvular insufficiency		10
Aneurysm		6
Cutaneous lesions	17	26

Compiled from established reviews[21, 32, 72–74] and new case presentations totaling 554 patients. The figures presented should be regarded as approximations because of incomplete reporting of case material in subspecialty journals.

internal auditory artery or its vestibular branch may result in vertigo.

Nose

Nasal chondritis is associated with symptoms of stuffiness or fullness, crusting, rhinorrhea, or occasional epistaxis. Inflammation may not be clinically evident. Repeated attacks may cause cartilage collapse, columella retraction resulting in a characteristic saddle nose deformity (Fig. 81–3).

Eyes

Ocular involvement is a common although variable feature of the disease.[4, 5] Major adnexal findings consist of unilateral or bilateral proptosis with chemosis, periorbital lid edema, and ophthalmoplegia. The most common intrinsic manifestations are scleritis/episcleritis, often associated with nongranulomatous uveitis, which may parallel inflammation elsewhere. Further findings include conjunctivitis, corneal infiltrates with associated edema or peripheral thinning, keratoconjunctivitis sicca, retinopathy (microaneurysms, hemorrhages, exudate), retinal vein or artery occlusion, retinal detachment, optic neuritis, and ischemic optic neuropathy. Corneoscleral perforation, retinal vasculitis, and optic neuritis can lead to blindness.

Joints

The arthropathy of polychondritis varies clinically from transient arthralgias to a mono-, pauci-, or polyarticular synovitis involving both large and small peripheral joints and parasternal (costochondral, sternomanubrial, sternoclavicular) articulations. Its classic presentation is that of an asymmetric, nonerosive, nondeforming arthritis of days to several weeks duration, resolving spontaneously or following response to anti-inflammatory drugs.[6] Erosive

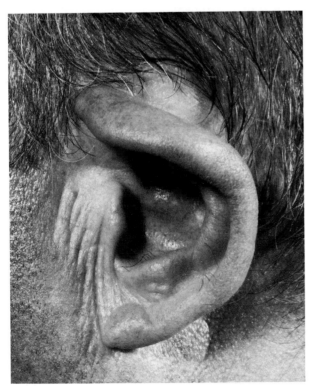

Figure 81–2. Distortion and collapse of the external ear in a patient who has polychondritis.

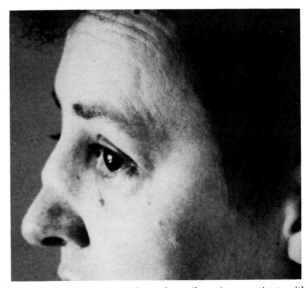

Figure 81–3. Destruction of nasal cartilage in a patient with polychondritis, creating a characteristic saddle nose deformity. (From McKay, D. A. R., et al.: Relapsing polychondritis and eye disease. Br. J. Ophthalmol. 58:600, 1974; used with permission.)

destructive disease has also been reported. Occasionally, there may be cervical, thoracic, or lumbar spine pain. Transient tenosynovitis has been described. Costochondral involvement may present with chest pain and tenderness. Destruction of these articulations is rare but can result in a flail chest. Synovial fluid in the absence of a concurrent connective tissue disease is usually noninflammatory but exceptions occur. No correlation exists between joint involvement and disease activity appearing elsewhere. Although aortitis, iritis, and rarely sacroiliitis occur in polychondritis, the frequency of HLA-B27 in these patients is no more common than in the general population.[1] Polychondritis may occur in conjunction with articular destructive processes such as adult or juvenile rheumatoid arthritis and less frequently with Reiter's disease, psoriatic arthritis, or ankylosing spondylitis.[7]

Respiratory Tract

Presenting symptoms of organ involvement may include a nonproductive cough, dyspnea, wheezing, inspiratory stridor, hoarseness, a choking sensation, or tenderness over the thyroid cartilage and anterior trachea.[8] Local airway disease may be asymptomatic. Mechanisms responsible for airway obstruction vary based on the stage of disease. These include (1) luminal encroachment secondary to glottic, subglottic, laryngeal, or tracheobronchial inflammation and edema, (2) cicatricial contractures induced by extensive fibrosis, and (3) loss of cartilaginous support with a resultant "dynamic" airway collapse during forced inspiration (larynx) or expiration (trachea). Tracheal compromise (Fig. 81–4) may necessitate tracheostomy, but even this can be ineffectual in reestablishing adequate ventilation in the presence of more distal focal or diffuse airway narrowing. Secondary infections of the upper and lower respiratory system are common. It is important to recognize that pulmonary involvement may be a forme fruste mode of presentation, occurring in the absence of other discernible features of disease. A likely chance association of polychondritis with fibrosing alveolitis has been reported in conjunction with antibodies to type II alveolar pneumocytes and bronchiolar Clara cells (progenitors of small airway ciliated cells secreting surfactant components).[9]

Heart

Most ominous is development (predominantly in males) of aortic insufficiency secondary to progressive dilatation of the aortic ring and ascending aorta or at times destruction of the valve cusps without annulus dilatation. Mitral and tricuspid valvular insufficiency occurs less frequently. Valvular involvement may be detected as early as 6 months to as late as 17 years following onset of disease and

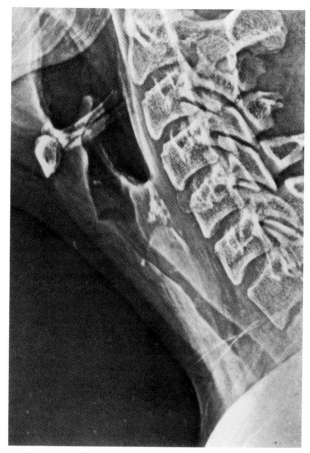

Figure 81–4. Xeroradiograph demonstrating tracheal narrowing in a 17-year-old female with polychondritis. (From Prasad, S., Grundfast, K. W., and Lipnick, R.: Airway obstruction in an adolescent with relapsing polychondritis. Otolaryngol. Head Neck Surg. 103:113, 1990; used with permission.)

bears little temporal relationship to other features. Successful valvuloplasty and valve replacement have been reported. However, failure secondary to valve dehiscence may occur due to persistent inflammation in surrounding tissue.[10] In addition, aneurysms may develop involving the ascending, thoracic, or abdominal aorta or subclavian artery (Fig. 81–5).[11] Rupture may cause death. Less frequent manifestations include pericarditis, myocarditis with conduction disturbances, endocarditis, and myocardial infarction.

Vascular System

Small, medium, and large vessel disease can occur.[12, 13] Thrombosis secondary to vasculitis may involve the descending and abdominal aorta, the subclavian, intracerebral, hepatic, superior mesenteric, and peripheral arteries. Nonvasculitic associated abdominal aortic and iliac artery thrombosis have been reported in conjunction with circulating lupus anticoagulant.[14] Cases of associated temporal arteritis, polyarteritis, Wegener's granulomatosis, allergic granulomatosis, Takayasu's disease, and leu-

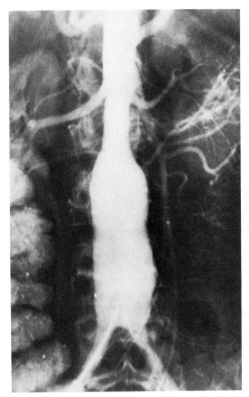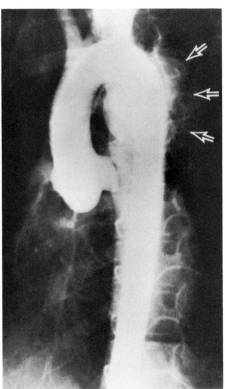

Figure 81-5. Aortograms. *Left,* An abdominal aortogram demonstrating a 9 by 3.5-cm fusiform aneurysm of the abdominal aorta below the renal arteries. *Right,* Thoracic aortogram in the left anterior oblique projection demonstrating a 5-cm saccular aneurysm in the proximal descending thoracic aorta. (From Cipriano, P. R., et al.: Multiple aortic aneurysms in relapsing polychondritis. Am. J. Cardiol. 37:1097, 1976; used with permission.)

kocytoclastic vasculitis have been described. The vasculitis may be focal or diffuse, indolent or fulminant, and rapidly fatal.

Gastrointestinal Tract

There have been few reports of gastrointestinal involvement beyond an occasional association with systemic sclerosis, diabetes, ulcerative colitis, granulomatous colitis, and systemic necrotizing vasculitis. Odynophagia and dysphagia may occur in the presence of thyroid, laryngeal, or tracheal cartilage inflammation. Esophageal manometric abnormalities have been described.[15] Minor liver function disturbances may occasionally be seen. Polychondritis has been rarely associated with primary biliary cirrhosis and sclerosing cholangitis.

Kidney

Renal disease is uncommon and when present usually reflects concurrent systemic vasculitis or other associated disease. Crescentic glomerulonephritis is being reported with increased frequency.[16]

Nervous System

Neurologic features include involvement of the second, third, sixth, seventh, eighth, or twelfth cranial nerves, hemiplegia, cerebellar signs, seizures, organic brain syndrome, and dementia.[17] Vasculitis is a presumed but unproven basis. Aseptic meningeal inflammation has been documented.[18]

Skin

No distinctive cutaneous features have been identified. Lesions have varied from biopsy-documented leukocytoclastic vasculitis to livedo reticularis, erythema multiforme, erythema nodosum, angioedema, urticaria, and keratoderma blennorrhagicum. Hyperpigmentation over sites of cartilage involvement, alopecia, and random associations with panniculitis, dermatitis herpetiformis, and psoriasis vulgaris have been reported. There has been a further description of the MAGIC syndrome (acronym for mouth and genital ulcers with inflamed cartilage) in which Behçet's disease–like features occur in conjunction with polychondritis.[19]

COEXISTENT DISEASE

As shown in Table 81-2, polychondritis can coexist with an array of connective tissue diseases. In most cases these precede the onset of polychondritis by months or years. In our present state of knowledge, it is unclear whether such associations represent the coexistence of two independent entities, connective tissue disease features arising in a

Table 81–2. CONNECTIVE TISSUE DISEASES
COEXISTENT WITH POLYCHONDRITIS (554 CASES)

Disease	No. of Reported Occurrences
Systemic vasculitis	59
Juvenile/adult rheumatoid arthritis	27
Sjögren's syndrome	15
Systemic lupus erythematosus	18
Behçet's disease	8
Ankylosing spondylitis	7
Reiter's disease	5
Systemic sclerosis	2
Polymyalgia rheumatica	2
Psoriatic arthritis	2
Retroperitoneal fibrosis	1

particular subset of polychondritis, or polychondritis appearing as a specific manifestation in a genetically distinct subset of connective tissue disease. An association has also been established with thyroid disease including Graves' disease, nontoxic goiter, and Hashimoto's disease. Ulcerative colitis and granulomatous colitis have been described, as has concurrent IgA nephropathy (Berger's disease).[20] Dysmyelopoietic and myeloproliferative syndromes culminating in acute or chronic myelogenous leukemia or aplastic anemia have been reported, as have isolated instances of carcinoma, Hodgkin's and non-Hodgkin's lymphoma.[21]

DIAGNOSIS

Laboratory Features

No laboratory tests are specific for polychondritis. Principal abnormalities are shown in Table 81–3. Most often there is an elevated sedimentation rate and modest leukocytosis, which largely correlate with disease activity. Thrombocytosis and eosinophilia may be seen. A normocytic, normochromic anemia of mild to moderate degree consistent with anemia of chronic disease frequently occurs. Hemolytic anemia is rare. Rheumatoid factor and antinuclear antibody (diffuse fluorescent pattern) may be present. Extractable nuclear antigen (ENA) reactivity and anticytoplasmic and phospholipid antibodies have been reported negative. A false-positive sero-logic test for syphilis may occur. Total hemolytic complement and C3 and C4 determinations are usually normal but on occasion elevated, reflecting an acute phase response. Transient increases of IgG, IgA, or IgE have been reported. Cryoglobulins are occasionally detected. Circulating immune complexes may be present but appear in no more than 40 percent of patients having clinically active disease. Urinary glycosaminoglycan levels may be increased.

Cartilage antibodies may be detected by indirect immunofluorescence, enzyme immunoassay (EIA), or radioimmunoassay (RIA).[22–24] Antibodies to native and denatured homologous and heterologous type II collagen have been identified in fewer than half of the patients. They lack disease specificity and are seen more frequently in early active phases. Their cyanogen bromide peptide epitope specificity appears to differ from that present in sera from rheumatoid arthritis.[25] Cell-mediated immune responses to cartilage proteoglycans can be shown with the use of peripheral blood mononuclear cells.[26] These appear to correlate with disease activity. Quantitation of serum levels of a noncollagenous 148 kD cartilage matrix protein presumably specific to tracheal, nasal septal, auricular, and xiphisternal cartilage also holds promise as a useful index of disease activity, but further studies are required to corroborate such a use.[27]

Pulmonary Assessment

A variety of measures are useful in evaluating functional and anatomic upper and lower airway disease in polychondritis.[28, 29] These include radiologic imaging (linear tomography, cinetracheography, laryngotracheography, computed tomography), fiberoptic bronchoscopy, and pulmonary function testing. Ultrafast computed tomography (providing cross-sectional images of the trachea during different phases of the respiratory cycle) and forced inspiratory and expiratory flow volume loop studies can be used to assess dynamic upper airway obstruction. Demonstration of laryngeal cartilage involvement or edema or fibrosis of surrounding tissue by computed tomography can readily provide an explanation for symptoms of hoarseness, dysphagia, or respiratory distress.

The bronchoscopic appearance of the larynx may

Table 81–3. PRINCIPAL LABORATORY ABNORMALITIES IN POLYCHONDRITIS

	No. of Reported Cases	No. Positive	Positivity (%)
Sedimentation rate elevation	350	303	87
Anemia	318	183	58
Leukocytosis	236	85	36
Antinuclear antibody	223	48	22
Rheumatoid factor	210	35	17
Eosinophilia	146	16	11
Serologic testing for syphilis	105	7	7
LE cell preparation	118	8	7

not accurately reflect results of pulmonary function testing. For instance, a normal-appearing larynx in conjunction with a decrease in maximum inspiratory flow may represent abnormal cricoarytenoid joint motion. Bronchoscopy itself poses a risk in the presence of chronic asphyxia. Death has occurred.

Further Studies

Chest radiographs may be useful in identifying aortic arch widening or prominence of the ascending or descending aorta. Computed tomography and radiographic views of the head and neck can reveal calcification of the pinna (not specific for polychondritis), nose, trachea, or larynx. Peripheral joint films may show juxta-articular bone demineralization and on occasion joint space narrowing with or without erosion. Although spine films are usually normal, there have been occasional reports of joint space narrowing, erosion of vertebral end plates and the symphysis pubis, and erosive irregularities and partial obliteration of the sacroiliac joints. Although bone scanning agents are not taken up by normal cartilage, positive scans have been reported in conjunction with cartilage calcification.

Differential Diagnosis

Conspicuous inflammatory lesions involving cartilage of the ear, nose, and laryngobronchial system distinguish polychondritis from other diseases. A variety of external auricular conditions may cause diagnostic confusion. *Infectious perichondritis* associated with external otitis may occur as a complication of mastoid surgery or trauma. An acute pyogenic process must be differentiated from chronic infections such as tuberculosis, fungal disease, syphilis, and leprosy. *Chondrodermatitis helicis nodularis*, believed to result from a developmental vascular insufficiency accentuated by aging and repetitive trauma, is characterized by circumscribed inflammatory and degenerative changes, which histologically resemble those found in long-standing polychondritis. *Cystic chondromalacia* of the auricle produces a cavitary lesion within the central area of cartilage, which may at times cause confusion. It usually occurs as a painless, nontender swelling in the upper half of the ear from which serous fluid can be readily aspirated. Auricular inflammation induced by trauma (including ear piercing), irritant chemicals, and frostbite must be excluded. The onset of chondritis following trivial burns may be delayed by weeks, occurring at sites that have long since healed. *Staphylococcus aureus* and *Pseudomonas* are frequent isolates. Required debridement often results in substantial deformity. Inflammation and destructive changes involving nasal cartilage require differentiation from *Wegener's granulomatosis, lymphomatoid granulomatosis, lethal midline granuloma, granulomatous lesions secondary to syph-*

ilis, tuberculosis and *leprosy* as well as *carcinoma* and *lymphosarcoma*. Biopsy and culture often facilitate clarification. The absence of mucosal inflammation in polychondritis is a useful differentiating feature. A saddle nose deformity may rarely be seen in rheumatoid arthritis lacking other features of polychondritis. An inherited autosomal dominant form of degenerative chondropathy has been described.[30] A saddle deformity is evident at birth, as is an associated delayed onset (9 to 12 years) of laryngeal stenosis secondary to myxoid degeneration of thyroid and cricoid cartilage.

Chronic inflammation of the tracheal wall leading to diffuse thickening and stenosis may also result from trauma associated with endotracheal intubation and infectious and noninfectious mediastinal granulomatous reactions including *tuberculosis, histoplasmosis,* and *sarcoidosis* (stenosis usually affects lobar or segmental bronchi). Mediastinal lymphadenopathy has not been described in polychondritis either radiographically or at autopsy. Further causes of tracheal stenosis include *neoplastic disease, Wegener's granulomatosis, amyloidosis,* the *saber-sheath trachea* associated with chronic obstructive pulmonary disease, and the rare entity *tracheobronchopathia osteochondroplastica,* differentiated by calcific mucosal nodules projecting into the lumen of the trachea or main stem bronchi. *Scleroma (rhinoscleroma),* a *Klebsiella rhinoscleromatis* infection endemic in Africa, Asia, and South America, may be associated with diffuse tracheal narrowing in the presence or absence of nasal or paranasal sinus disease.

Necrotizing scleritis, keratitis, polyarthritis, and *otitis media* with potential audiovestibular dysfunction may also occur in polyarteritis and Wegener's granulomatosis. Pulmonary and renal parenchymal, and central and peripheral neurologic lesions occurring in the latter help to distinguish it from polychondritis. *Cogan's syndrome* is characterized by a nonsyphilitic interstitial keratitis and audiovestibular disease but is not a generalized chondropathy. The coexistence of ocular inflammation, arthritis, and valvular or myocardial heart disease requires differentiation from rheumatoid arthritis, Behçet's disease, sarcoidosis, and the seronegative spondyloarthropathies. The mucosal lesions of Behçet's syndrome are seen in only a minority of patients with polychondritis, and the hilar adenopathy of sarcoidosis is not a component of this disease. Those patients with rheumatoid arthritis and ocular inflammation usually have erosive, symmetrical arthritis that precedes the ocular disease. Rheumatoid factor titers are usually high in these patients contrasted to polychondritis.

The lesions of aortitis and aortic aneurysms require differentiation from syphilis, Marfan's and the Ehlers-Danlos syndromes, idiopathic medial cystic necrosis, and arteriosclerosis. More benign thoracic cage syndromes such as costochondritis, Tietze's syndrome, chondrodynia costosternalis, and the xiphoid cartilage syndrome are localized processes. Costochondritis may occur secondary to infec-

Table 81–4. PROPOSED DIAGNOSTIC CRITERIA FOR POLYCHONDRITIS

Clinical Manifestations*
1. Bilateral auricular chondritis
2. Nonerosive, seronegative inflammatory polyarthritis
3. Nasal chondritis
4. Ocular inflammation (conjunctivitis, keratitis, scleritis/episcleritis, uveitis)
5. Respiratory tract chondritis (laryngeal and/or tracheal cartilages)
6. Cochlear and/or vestibular dysfunction (neurosensory hearing loss, tinnitus and/or vertigo)

PLUS†

Cartilage biopsy confirmation of compatible histologic picture

*To establish definitive diagnosis, 3 or more of the clinical manifestations are required.

†If the diagnosis is clinically obvious, it is unnecessary to obtain a biopsy for confirmation. Biopsy can be derived from the ear, nose, or respiratory tract.

Data from McAdam, L. P., et al. Medicine 55:193, 1976.

tion (tuberculosis, pyogenic organisms, fungi, viruses) with entry afforded by trauma, sternotomy incisions, drainage from infected thoracic or abdominal cavities, chest wall radiation, and deep chest wall burns, particularly of electrical origin. There has been an increased frequency of *Candida albicans* costochondral junctional infection in intravenous drug abusers associated with hematogenous seeding.[31]

McAdams and colleagues[32] have proposed the diagnostic criteria listed in Table 81–4.

PATHOLOGY

Early ear lesions contain a variable polymorphonuclear and prominent lymphocyte, monocyte/macrophage and plasma cell infiltrate in perichondrial tissue in conjunction with a focal or diffuse loss of basophilic staining consistent with matrix proteoglycan depletion[33] (Fig. 81–6). CD4+ helper/inducer lymphocytes dominate.[34] Coarse granular deposits of immunoglobulin and C3 are present at the chondrofibrous junction and may at times be seen throughout the cartilage matrix. Granulation tissue subsequently invades and replaces regions of cartilage, creating sequestered islands of degenerating cells and depleted matrix. Fibrosis eventually occurs, and cystic spaces containing gelatinous material become evident. Focal regions of calcification and bone formation may occur.

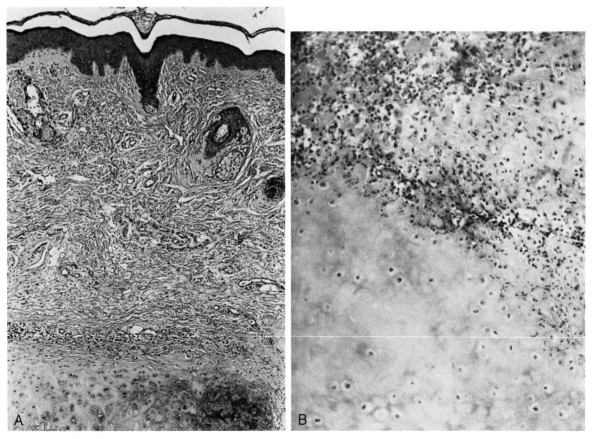

Figure 81–6. Biopsies of the external ear. *A*, Early manifestations showing narrow rim of infiltrating inflammatory cells at the chondrodermal junction in conjunction with focal proteoglycan depletion (original magnification × 20). *B*, Later stage of disease demonstrating necrotizing chondritis with inflammatory cell infiltrate, depletion of matrix proteoglycans, chondrocyte degeneration, and fibrosis (original magnification × 400). (Reproduced from Herman, J. H., and Dennis, M. V.: Immunopathologic studies in relapsing polychondritis. J. Clin. Invest. 52:549, 1973; by copyright permission of the American Society for Clinical Investigation.)

Electron microscopy studies have shown that chondrocytes in involved regions contain large quantities of lysosomes, lipid, and glycogen.[35] Cells and adjacent collagen and elastic fibers may be destroyed and replaced by small, electron-dense granules and vesicles that vary in size, shape, and density. Chondrocyte cytoplasmic processes containing such material have been observed extending into damaged regions. Viable chondrocytes may be seen phagocytosing degraded material. Diffuse, finely granular, electron-dense material has also been described on the surface of cartilage and coating elastic fibers.

Sections of involved aorta show patchy vascularization of the media with mononuclear inflammatory cell infiltration, decreased collagen and glycosaminoglycan content, and fragmentation of elastic fibers. Lymphocyte cuffing may appear around the vasa vasorum. Secondary fibrosis of the intima and adventitia occurs. The aortic ring appears stretched or dilated, whereas the valve leaflets can be normal or thickened. Endothelial proliferation observed in syphilitic aortitis is not evident, nor is there pooling in the media of periodic acid–Schiff (PAS)–positive material characteristic of medial cystic necrosis. The loss of aortic elastic tissue is similar to that encountered in Marfan's syndrome, but the glycosaminoglycan content of the aortic root is not depleted in the latter disease. Destruction of muscle fibers can lead to aneurysm formation.

The tracheal mucosa frequently appears edematous. Its cartilaginous rings show changes ranging from mild inflammation to total resorption by granulation tissue. Large and medium-sized bronchi show patchy widening of the lumina resembling bronchiectasis. There may be extensive narrowing and dissolution of these airway components. Inflammatory lesions may be discrete and localized or involve the entire upper airway.

A chronic synovitis with edematous changes, vessel dilatation, and infiltration with chronic inflammatory cells may be seen histologically.[33] An increase of phagocytic type A lining cells has been reported.

Ocular pathologic changes show a loss of basophilia and the fragmentation of elastic tissue at the scleroconjunctival angle. Scattered mast cells, plasma cells, and lymphocytes have been observed around episcleral vessels as well as vasculitis with immunoglobulin deposition in conjunctival and scleral vasculature.[5] The corneal stroma may be edematous and necrotic with an inflammatory cell infiltrate occurring in peripheral regions. Infiltration of the iris with lymphocytes, plasma cells, and granulation tissue has been described.

ETIOLOGIC AND PATHOPHYSIOLOGIC CONSIDERATIONS

The etiology of polychondritis is unknown. Its clinical and pathologic features strongly suggest a primary acquired disease in which inflammatory and immunologic responses are mounted against connective tissue constituents. Why there is selectivity for given organ involvement is unknown. Toxins have been incriminated in an intriguing case description.[36] Polychondritic features (auricular, audiovestibular, nasal, ocular, axial and peripheral joint involvement) appeared within 24 hours of the intravenous injection of a bizarre combination of materials. Unfortunately the patient exhibiting this inadvertently created model of polychondritis was lost to follow-up.

Proteinase, Oxygen Metabolite-Mediated Tissue Damage

Destructive changes occurring in the connective tissue matrix of cartilage and at other pathologic sites appear to be largely enzyme mediated. These changes reflect in part a complex local imbalance in enzyme inducer-inhibitor formation and proteinase-antiproteinase activity. Experimental studies have shown that the intravenous injection of crude papain into young rabbits can cause collapse of normally rigid ears within 4 hours.[37] Histologically, there is a diffuse loss of matrix metachromasia in ear, rib, laryngeal, tracheal, and epiphysial cartilage. Some animals show respiratory distress caused by collapse of the trachea and bronchi. Focal aortic plaque lesions have been described secondary to connective tissue alterations in the media, which may proceed to metaplastic changes. Differences from polychondritis are the absence of inflammation and the limited course of disease. Comparable histologic changes can be produced in in vivo and in vitro cartilaginous embryonic bone rudiment cultures by retinol-mediated release of chondrocyte proteinases.[38] Cytokines such as interleukin-1 (IL-1) and tumor necrosis factors (TNF), released from infiltrating mononuclear cells and local connective tissue and endothelial cells, have a similar enzyme-inducing capacity.[39–41]

Oxygen metabolites (superoxide anion, singlet oxygen, hydroxyl radical, hydrogen peroxide) produced by activated polymorphonuclear cells, monocyte/macrophages, and chondrocytes may potentially cause damage to cartilage by cleaving covalent bonds and inducing lipid peroxidation and cell membrane destruction. Radicals may also facilitate enzyme activation by inhibiting antiproteinase activity.

It is likely that tissue destruction in polychondritis is to a large measure orchestrated via the combined effects of proteinases and oxygen metabolites released within the pathologic milieu as a combined consequence of cytokine induction and attempts at phagocytic removal of degraded connective tissue matrix.

Immunologic Considerations

The predominant lymphocytic and plasma cell infiltrate observed at pathologic sites in polychondritis supports the potential role of immunologic mechanisms in its pathogenesis. Although multiple epitopes are expressed on cartilage proteoglycans, collagen, and elastin, these are to a large measure masked in the native state because of conformational structure.[42, 43] Chondrocytes also express cell surface specific and histocompatibility antigens.[44] Thus avascular cartilage may be regarded as a potential immunologically privileged tissue. Should there be a structural insult, irrespective of inciting factors, there may be release of or in situ exposure to antigenic determinants with resultant host sensitization facilitating activation of humoral and cell-mediated immunologic responses. Pathologic consequences may be widespread because of a sharing of cartilage proteoglycan antigens with the sclera, the anterior uveal tract, the endoneurium and perineurium of the optic nerve, endothelial cells, connective tissue of aortic media and intima, heart valves, myocardial sarcolemma, tracheal submucosal basement membrane, synoviocytes, and renal glomerular and tubular basement membranes.[42, 45] Of potential pathophysiologic importance is the antigenic cross-reactivity between cartilage proteoglycans, streptococcal peptidoglycans, and the purified protein derivative of *Mycobacterium tuberculosis*.[46] Vitreous collagen and the notochord also share immunogenicity with type II cartilage collagen.[47]

Older experimental animal studies have demonstrated the capacity of components of cartilage and antiproteoglycan antiserum to cause chronic synovitis, cartilage degeneration, or perichondritis (see review, ref. 42). More recently, the immunization of BALB/c mice with cartilage proteoglycans has been shown to induce a progressive destructive polyarthritis and spondylitis with accompanying humoral and cell-mediated immune reactions to the immunogen.[48] The response appeared to be sex-related and strain specific but not haplotype specific. The intra-articular injection of proteoglycans has also produced an inflammatory erosive arthritis associated with synoviocyte and chondrocyte production of collagenase and gelatinase.[49] Antiproteoglycan antibodies have been demonstrated in the sera of rabbits with antigen-induced arthritis, and following their intravenous injection, antibodies have localized to the surface of cartilage concomitant with proteoglycan loss.[50] Antibodies to chondrocyte cell surface proteins can be identified in osteoarthritic and rheumatoid sera.[51]

Native types II and XI cartilage collagen are arthritogenic in rodents and primates, ultimately inducing a destructive ankylotic process.[52–54] This is linked to immune response regions of the major histocompatibility complex (RT1 in rats and H2 in mice) and has strain specificity.[55, 56] Antibodies specific for conformational determinants on native type II collagen and cell-mediated immune responses lacking conformational or collagen type specificity occur. The specificity of antibody response (arthritogenic versus nonarthritogenic epitopes) is crucial. There

appears to be multiple gene control regulating the expression, severity, and rate of progression of disease. Passive transfer has been achieved with both cells and serum. Rats so immunized (9 to 14 percent) may develop an intense auricular chondritis with immunofluorescent localization of IgG and C3 in lesions.[57, 58] Electron-dense deposits observed in the proximity of chondrocytes correspond with IgG and C3 deposition. The specificity of the localized IgG is unknown. Auricular involvement occurs significantly later and is independent of development of arthritis. Ocular, tracheobronchial, and cardiovascular lesions do not occur. It is of interest that an auricular chondropathy characterized pathologically by focal chondrolysis and granulomatous inflammation occurs spontaneously in aging Crl:CD, fawn-hooded, and Wistar rats.[59–61] Its pathogenesis requires study.

Cartilage destruction may also be the result of an "innocent bystander" effect. In models of antigen-induced arthritis, antigen retention can be shown in the superficial layer of cartilage where it is presumed to exist in the form of immune complexes bound to collagen. Attempts to remove such fixed deposits may result in inflammatory cell release of enzymes, oxygen metabolites, prostanoids, and cytokines.

The potential importance of cell-mediated immune responses in the pathogenesis of polychondritis is suggested by studies demonstrating the capacity of lymphokines to (1) induce cartilage proteoglycan degradation via macrophage activation and (2) reversibly suppress chondrocyte synthesis of glycosaminoglycans, collagen, noncollagen protein, and nucleic acids.[62, 63] Interferon-gamma (γ) has been shown to suppress levels of procollagen mRNA and type II collagen synthesis by chondrocytes.[64]

Other Factors

Cytokines such as IL-1 and TNF-alpha (α), in addition to their catabolic-inducing potential, may further adversely affect cartilage metabolism by down-regulating proteoglycan and collagen synthesis and stimulating chondrocyte release of prostanoids and plasminogen activator.[40, 65–67] Prostaglandins of the A, B, and E series and $PGF_2\alpha$ also have a potential suppressive effect on cartilage matrix synthesis.[68] There is a growing appreciation of the importance of growth factors in not only sustaining normal cartilage metabolic homeostasis but potentially adversely affecting chondrocyte cytokine receptor expression. Thus fibroblast growth factor enhances IL-1–induced chondrocyte proteinase production by increasing the number of IL-1 receptors expressed.[69] Native and denatured components of type II collagen are able to activate the alternative pathway of complement and induce macrophage proteinase release.

Pathogenesis—A Hypothesis

Although the inciting cause may vary and the significance of genetic conditioning remains unknown, the widespread pathologic manifestations of polychondritis appear to represent a selective involvement of connective tissue. Perhaps initially there is some form of compromise to nutrient vasculature with an accompanying inflammatory response. Subsequent connective tissue matrix degradation would be largely enzymatically mediated, enzymes stemming from infiltrating cells, chondrocytes, and connective tissue fibroblasts as a consequence of immunologic and nonimmune triggering. Structural changes in connective tissue may lead to an autosensitization to proteoglycans, collagen, elastin, and perhaps chondrocyte surface proteins. One cannot dismiss the possibility that mimicry existing between a given connective tissue antigen and an infectious agent may be the inciting factor. Antibody and cell-mediated immune responses that follow may both induce and perpetuate inflammation, resulting in further tissue damage at local and more distant sites that share specific connective tissue epitopes. Released cytokines may also cause constitutional symptoms, incite an acute phase response, and adversely affect surrounding connective tissue metabolism. More comprehensive studies are required to clarify the relative significance of the observations discussed.

CLINICAL COURSE, PROGNOSIS, AND TREATMENT

Polychondritis may have a variable course. There may be episodic flares of activity, smoldering disease of ever-changing severity, or a fulminant, rapid, downhill course. Establishing a prognosis is difficult because the disease frequently is unrecognized; only the most florid cases are usually reported.

In a comprehensive analysis of 112 patients, fatalities were reported in 37 percent.[21] The median survival was 11 years from time of initial diagnosis. The 5- and 10-year probabilities of survival were 74 percent and 55 percent, respectively. The most frequent causes of death were infection, systemic vasculitis, and malignancy. Additional causes were related to airway collapse, aneurysmal rupture, valvular heart disease, and renal failure. For the group as a whole, age at diagnosis, anemia, and laryngotracheal involvement, when taken together, best predicted mortality.

Less severe manifestations can usually be controlled with nonsteroidal anti-inflammatory drugs (NSAIDs). Based on its capacity to inhibit lysosomal enzyme-mediated cartilage degradation induced by hypervitaminosis A and its immunomodulatory potential, dapsone (50 to 200 mg per day) has been used with some measure of success.

Although there is no evidence that glucocorticoids alter the natural course of disease, they are often effective in suppressing acute features and are capable of reducing the frequency and severity of recurrences. Initially, 30 to 60 mg of prednisone or its equivalent is instituted in daily divided doses, with subsequent gradual tapering to a maintenance dose of 5 to 25 mg. Daily doses as high as 80 mg to 100 mg may be required in particularly severe acute stages if laryngotracheal, bronchial, ocular, or inner ear involvement is present. Alternate-day schedules are not recommended. Pulse-therapy (1 g of methylprednisolone daily for 3 days) has anecdotally been said to moderate acute, severe, unremitting features. If disease progression occurs despite such measures, a trial of immunosuppressive agents is warranted. Chlorambucil, cyclophosphamide, 6-mercaptopurine (6-MP), azathioprine, and methotrexate (pulse-therapy) have been used with some measure of success and may provide a steroid-sparing effect. There are now sporadic reports of success being achieved with cyclosporin A[70] or monoclonal anti-CD4 antibodies in refractory patients.[70a, 70b]

The key to optimum management is individualized therapy in conjunction with a careful, prolonged follow-up. Tracheostomy may be required for relieving severe upper airway obstruction if localized to glottic or subglottic regions. Refractory stenosis or collapse of portions of the tracheobronchial tree secondary to tracheomalacia may be managed with a segmental resection if the lesion is localized. More extensive involvement may require prolonged endotracheal intubation, external tracheal splinting, or the use of a silastic tube prosthesis or metal stent. Such patients require special anesthetic considerations.[71] Although valve replacement or valvuloplasty should be considered in intractable heart failure secondary to valvular insufficiency, there is a high incidence of failure. Aortic aneurysms have been successfully resected. Ocular manifestations, particularly nodular and necrotizing scleritis, are less amenable to systemic glucocorticoids and dapsone, often requiring more potent immunosuppressive agents for successful treatment.[5]

References

1. Luthra, H. S., McKenna, C. H., and Terasaki, P. I.: Lack of association of HLA-A and B locus antigens with relapsing polychondritis. Tissue Antigens 17:442, 1981.
2. Gimvosky, M. L., and Nishiyama, M.: Relapsing polychondritis in pregnancy: A case report and review. Am. J. Obstet. Gynecol. 161:332, 1989.
3. Cody, D. T. R., and Sones, D. A.: Relapsing polychondritis: Audiovestibular manifestations. Laryngoscope 81:1208, 1971.
4. Isaak, B. L., Liesegang, T. J., and Michet, C. J., Jr.: Ocular and systemic findings in relapsing polychondritis. Ophthalmology 93:681, 1986.
5. Hoang-Xuan, T., Foster, C. S., and Rice, B. A.: Scleritis in relapsing polychondritis. Ophthalmology 97:892, 1990.
6. O'Hanlan, M., McAdam, L. P., Bluestone, R., et al.: The arthropathy of relapsing polychondritis. Arthritis Rheum. 19:191, 1976.
7. Pazirandeh, M., Ziran, B. H., Khandelwal, B. K., et al.: Relapsing polychondritis and spondyloarthropathies. J. Rheumatol. 15:630, 1988.
8. Eng, J., and Sabarathan, S.: Airway complications in relapsing polychondritis. Ann. Thorac. Surg. 51:686, 1991.
9. Raugh, G., Dorfler, H., Erunger, R., et al.: Relapsing poly(peri)chondritis associated with alveolar disease and antibodies to pneumocytes type II and Clara cells. Klin. Wochenschr. 67:784, 1989.
10. Van Decker, W., and Panidis, I. P.: Relapsing polychondritis with cardiac valvular involvement. Ann. Intern. Med. 109:340, 1988.

11. Cipriano, P. P., Alonso, D. R., Baltaxe, H. A., et al.: Multiple aortic aneurysms in relapsing polychondritis. Am. J. Cardiol. 37:1097, 1976.
12. Esdaile, J., Hawkins, D., Gold, P., et al.: Vascular involvement in relapsing polychondritis. Can. Med. Assoc. J. 116:1019, 1977.
13. Mitchet, C. J.: Vasculitis and relapsing polychondritis. Rheum. Dis. Clin. North. Am. 16:441, 1990.
14. Balsa-Criado, A., Gonzalez-Hernandez, T., Cuesta, M. V., et al.: Lupus anticoagulant in relapsing polychondritis. J. Rheumatol. 17:1426, 1990.
15. Levesque, H., Kerleau, J. M., Ducrotte, P. H., et al.: Atteinte oesophagienne au cours d'une polychondrite atrophiante. Presse Med. 19:1056, 1990.
16. Chang-Miller, A., Okamura, M., Torres, V. E., et al.: Renal involvement in relapsing polychondritis. Medicine 66:202, 1987.
17. Sundaram, M. B. M., and Rajput, A. H.: Nervous system complications of relapsing polychondritis. Neurology 33:513, 1983.
18. Brod, S., and Boss, J.: Idiopathic CSF pleocytosis in relapsing polychondritis. Neurology 38:322, 1988.
19. Orme, R. L., Nordlund, J. J., Barich, L., et al.: The MAGIC syndrome (mouth and genital ulcers with inflamed cartilage). Arch. Dermatol. 126:940, 1990.
20. Dalal, B., Wallace, A. C., and Slinger, R. P.: IgA nephropathy in relapsing polychondritis. Pathology 20:85, 1988.
21. Michet, J. M., Jr., McKenna, C. H., Luthra, H. S., et al.: Relapsing polychondritis. Survival and predictive role of early disease manifestations. Ann. Intern. Med. 104:74, 1986.
22. Ueno, Y., Chia, D., and Barnett, E. V.: Relapsing polychondritis associated with ulcerative colitis. Serial determinations of antibodies to cartilage and circulating immune complexes by three assays. J. Rheumatol. 8:456, 1981.
23. Foidart, J. M., Abe, S., Martin, G. R., et al.: Antibodies to type II collagen in relapsing polychondritis. N. Engl. J. Med. 299:1203, 1978.
24. Ebringer, R., Rook, G., Swana, G. T., et al.: Autoantibodies to cartilage and type II collagen in relapsing polychondritis and other rheumatic diseases. Ann. Rheum. Dis. 40:473, 1981.
25. Terato, K., Shimozuru, Y., Katayama, K., et al.: Specificity of antibodies to type II collagen in rheumatoid arthritis. Arthritis Rheum. 33:1493, 1990.
26. Herman, J. H., and Dennis, M. V.: Immunopathologic studies in relapsing polychondritis. J. Clin. Invest. 52:549, 1973.
27. Saxne, T., and Heinegard, D.: Involvement of nonarticular cartilage, as demonstrated by release of a cartilage-specific protein, in rheumatoid arthritis. Arthritis Rheum. 32:1080, 1989.
28. Krell, W. S., Staats, B. A., and Hyatt, R. E.: Pulmonary function in relapsing polychondritis. Am. Rev. Respir. Dis. 133:1120, 1986.
29. Wiedemann, H. P., and Matthay, R. A.: Pulmonary manifestations of the collagen vascular diseases. Clin. Chest Med. 10:677, 1989.
30. Kurien, M., Seshadri, M. S., and Raman, R.: Inherited nasal and laryngeal degenerative chondropathy. Arch. Otolaryngol. Head Neck Surg. 115:746, 1989.
31. Miro, J. M., Brancos, M. A., Abello, R., et al.: Costochondral involvement in systemic candidiasis in heroin addicts: Clinical, scintigraphic, and histologic features in 26 patients. Arthritis Rheum. 31:793, 1988.
32. McAdam, L. P., O'Hanlan, M. A., Bluestone, R., et al.: Relapsing polychondritis: Prospective study of 23 patients and a review of the literature. Medicine 55:193, 1976.
33. Mitchell, N., and Shepard, N.: Relapsing polychondritis. An electron microscopic study of synovium and articular cartilage. J. Bone Joint Surg. 54A:1235, 1972.
34. Riccieri, V., Spadaro, A., Taccari, E., et al.: A case of relapsing polychondritis: Pathogenetic considerations. Clin. Exp. Rheumatol. 6:95, 1988.
35. Hashimoto, K., Arkin, C. R., and Kang, A. H.: Relapsing polychondritis. An ultrastructural study. Arthritis Rheum. 19:91, 1977.
36. Berger, R. G.: Polychondritis resulting from intravenous substance abuse. Am. J. Med. 85:415, 1988.
37. McCluskey, R. T., and Thomas, L.: The removal of cartilage matrix in vivo by papain. J. Exp. Med. 108:371, 1958.
38. Fell, H. B., and Thomas, L.: Comparison of the effects of papain and vitamin A on cartilage. II. The effects on organ cultures of embryonic skeletal tissue. J. Exp. Med. 111:719, 1960.
39. Herman, J. H., Greenblatt, D., Khosla, R. C., et al.: Cytokine modulation of chondrocyte proteinase release. Arthritis Rheum. 27:79, 1984.
40. Saklatvala, J.: Tumour necrosis factor stimulates resorption and inhibits synthesis of proteoglycan in cartilage. Nature 322:547, 1986.
41. Arend, W. P., and Dayer, J-M.: Cytokines and cytokine-inhibitors or antagonists in rheumatoid arthritis. Arthritis Rheum. 33:305, 1990.
42. Herman, J. H., and Carpenter, B. A.: Immunobiology of cartilage. Semin. Arthritis Rheum. 5:1, 1975.
43. Baker, J. P., Caterson, B., and Christner, J. E.: Immunological characterization of cartilage proteoglycans. Methods Enzymol. 83:216, 1982.
44. Glant, T., and Mikecz, K.: Antigenic profiles of human, bone and canine articular chondrocytes. Cell Tissue Res. 244:359, 1986.
45. Poole, A. R., Pidoux, I., Reiner, A., et al.: Mammalian eyes and

associated tissues contain molecules that are immunologically related to cartilage proteoglycan and link protein. J. Cell Biol. 93:910, 1982.
46. Van Edem, W., Holoshitz, J., Nevo, Z., et al.: Arthritis induced by a T-lymphocyte clone that responds to Mycobacterium tuberculosis and to cartilage proteoglycans. Proc. Natl. Acad. Sci. U. S. A. 82:5117, 1985.
47. Stuart, J. M., Cremer, M. A., Dixit, S. N., et al.: Collagen-induced arthritis in rats. Comparison of vitreous and cartilage derived collagens. Arthritis Rheum. 22:347, 1979.
48. Mikecz, K., Glant, T. T., and Poole, R. A.: Immunity to cartilage proteoglycans in BALB/c mice with progressive polyarthritis and ankylosing spondylitis induced by injection of human cartilage proteoglycan. Arthritis Rheum. 30:306, 1987.
49. Boniface, R. J., Cain, P. R., and Evans, C. H.: Articular responses to purified cartilage proteoglycans. Arthritis Rheum. 31:258, 1988.
50. Kresina, T. F., Yoo, J. U., and Goldberg, V. M.: Evidence that a humoral immune response to autologous cartilage proteoglycan can participate in the induction of cartilage pathology. Arthritis Rheum. 31:248, 1988.
51. Mollenhauer, J., von der Mark, K., Burmester, G., et al.: Serum antibodies against chondrocyte cell surface proteins in osteoarthritis and rheumatoid arthritis. J. Rheumatol. 15:1811, 1988.
52. Trentham, D. E., Townes, A. S., and Kang, A. H.: Autoimmunity to type II collagen: An experimental model of arthritis. J. Exp. Med. 146:857, 1977.
53. Morgan, K., Evans, H. B., and Firth, S. A.: $\alpha 1 \alpha 2 \alpha 3$ Collagen is arthritogenic. Ann. Rheum. Dis. 42:680, 1983.
54. Yoo, T. J., Kim, S.-Y., Stuart, J. M., et al.: Induction of arthritis in monkeys by immunization with type II collagen. J. Exp. Med. 168:777, 1988.
55. Griffiths, M. M., Eichwald, E. J., Martin, J. H., et al.: Immunogenetic control of experimental type II collagen-induced arthritis. 1. Susceptibility and resistance among inbred strains of rats. Arthritis Rheum. 24:781, 1981.
56. Wooley, P. H., Luthra, H. S., Stuart, J. M., et al.: Type II collagen-induced arthritis in mice. 1. Major histocompatibility complex (I region) linkage and antibody correlates. J. Exp. Med. 154:688, 1981.
57. Cremer, M. A., Pitcock, J. A., Stuart, J. M., et al.: Auricular chondritis in rats. An experimental model for relapsing polychondritis induced with type II collagen. J. Exp. Med. 154:535, 1981.
58. McCune, W. S., Schiller, A. L., Dynesius-Trentham, R. A., et al.: Type II collagen-induced auricular chondritis. Arthritis Rheum. 25:266, 1982.
59. Chiu, T., and Lee, K. P.: Auricular chondropathy in aging rats. Vet. Pathol. 21:500, 1983.
60. Prieur, D. J., Young, D. M., and Counts, D. F.: Auricular chondritis in fawn-hooded rats. A spontaneous disorder resembling that induced by immunization with type II collagen. Am. J. Pathol. 116:69, 1984.
61. McEwen, B. J., and Barsoum, N. J.: Auricular chondritis in Wistar rats. Lab. Anim. 24:280, 1990.
62. Herman, J. H., Musgrave, D. S., and Dennis, M. V.: Phytomitogen-induced, lymphokine-mediated cartilage proteoglycan degradation. Arthritis Rheum. 20:922, 1977.
63. Herman, J. H., Khosla, R. C., Mowery, C. S., et al.: Modulation of chondrocyte synthesis by lymphokine-rich conditioned media. Arthritis Rheum. 25:668, 1982.
64. Goldring, M. B., Sandell, L. J., Stephenson, M. L., et al.: Immune interferon suppresses levels of procollagen mRNA and type II collagen synthesis in cultured human articular and costal chondrocytes. J. Biol. Chem. 261:9049, 1986.
65. Dingle, J. T., Page-Thomas, D. P., King, B., et al.: In vivo studies of articular tissue damage mediated by catabolin/interleukin 1. Ann. Rheum. Dis. 46:527, 1987.
66. Goldring, M. B., Birkhead, J., Sandell, L. J., et al.: Interleukin 1 suppresses expression of cartilage-specific types II and IX collagens and increases types I and III collagens in human chondrocytes. J. Clin. Invest. 82:2026, 1988.
67. Evequoz, V., Schnyder, J., Trechsel, U., et al.: Influence of macrophage products on the release of plasminogen activator, collagenase, β-glucuronidase and prostaglandin E_2 by articular chondrocytes. Biochem. J. 219:667, 1984.
68. Mitrovic D., Lippiello, L., Gruson, F., et al.: Effects of various prostanoids on the in vitro metabolism of bovine articular chondrocytes. Prostaglandins 22:499, 1981.
69. Chandrasekhar, S., and Harvey, A. K.: Induction of interleukin-1 receptors on chondrocytes by fibroblast growth factor: A possible mechanism for modulation of interleukin-1 activity. J. Cell. Physiol. 138:236, 1989.
70. Svenson, K. L. G., Homdahl, R., Klareskog, L., et al.: Cyclosporin A treatment in a case of relapsing polychondritis. Scand. J. Rheumatol. 13:329, 1984.
70a. Van der Lubbe, P. A., Miltenburg, A. M., and Breedveld, F. C.: Anti-CD4 monoclonal antibody for relapsing polychondritis. Lancet 337:1349, 1991.

70b. Choy E. H. S., Chikanza, I. C., Kingsley, G. H., et al.: Chimaeric anti-CD4 monoclonal antibody for relapsing polychondritis. Lancet 338:450, 1991.

71. Burgess, F. W., Whitlock, W., and Davis, M. J.: Anaesthetic implications of relapsing polychondritis: A case report. Anesthesiology 73:570, 1990.

72. Dolan, D. L., Lemmon, G. B., Jr., and Teitelbaum, S. L.: Relapsing polychondritis. Analytical literature review and studies on pathogenesis. Am. J. Med. 41:285, 1966.

73. Hughes, R. A. C., Berry, C. L., and Seifert, M.: Relapsing polychondritis. Three cases with a clinico-pathologic study and literature review. Q. J. Med. 61:363, 1972.

74. Arkin, C. R., and Masi, A. T.: Relapsing polychondritis: Review of current status and case report. Semin. Arthritis Rheum. 5:41, 1975.

Section XVI

Infiltrative Disorders Associated with Rheumatic Diseases

Chapter 82

Edgar S. Cathcart

Amyloidosis

INTRODUCTION

Definition. Amyloidosis is a syndrome characterized by the deposition of an insoluble proteinaceous material in the extracellular matrix of one or several organs. These deposits encroach on parenchymal tissues, compromise organ function, and produce diverse clinical manifestations. Amyloidosis is pertinent to the rheumatic diseases because it occurs as a potentially fatal complication of longstanding or poorly controlled inflammation, or it mimics more common rheumatic problems in its presentations.

Amyloidosis was formerly characterized chiefly by its histologic properties. The diagnosis was seldom made by the clinician, because it was, and in fact remains, a morphologically defined entity. The key to the modern approach to amyloidosis in all its forms has been the discovery of a characteristic and unique fibrillar ultrastructure of amyloid deposits from any source, clinical or experimental.[1, 2] The rigid, nonbranching filament, about 100 Å in diameter, became the definition of amyloidosis and provided the unifying concept of a disease that otherwise took so many forms that it was suspected of being a collection of unrelated entities. The unifying concept was further refined with the discovery that the amyloid fibril is composed of a protein arranged in a beta (β)-pleated sheet,[3] a configuration first described by Pauling and Corey. This unusual molecular arrangement is responsible for the diagnostic staining properties of amyloid, specifically the green birefringence when stained with Congo red (Table 82–1).

History of Amyloidosis Research. The history of amyloid research can be traced to 1700, when T. B. Bonet reported on two post-mortem cases of splenic infiltration with amyloid-like material. Subsequent sporadic reports were consistent with amyloid infiltration of liver or spleen, but elucidation of the morbid anatomy was not accomplished until the early nineteenth century by pathologists investigating the waxy or lardaceous enlargement of abdominal viscera. In 1842, Rokitansky distinguished lardaceous infiltrations of the liver from other types of waxy or fatty degeneration and affirmed the association of a lardaceous liver with debilitating illnesses. He further described splenic infiltration associated with hepatic disease, which implied the systemic nature of the disorder.

In 1854, Virchow initiated more than a century of controversy regarding the chemical nature of the lardaceous deposits when he called the cerebral corpora amylacea deposits amyloid (starch-like), based on their staining with iodine and acid. He similarly believed that splenic deposits of amyloid material contained starch, despite their atypical tinctorial properties. Meckel refuted the cellulose origin of amyloid but accepted amyloid as a morphologic designation. In 1859, Schmidt and Friedreich and Kekule emphasized the "albuminoid" nature of amyloid

Table 82–1. CHARACTERISTICS OF AMYLOID

Method of Study	Findings
Light microscopy	Eosinophilia
	Green birefringence with Congo red stains*
	Metachromasia with methyl violet and crystal violet stains
	Faint autofluorescence
	Fluorescence with thioflavine stains
Electron microscopy	Rigid, nonbranching fibrils of approximately 100 Å in diameter*
X-ray diffraction	Antiparallel β-pleated sheet conformation*

*Definitive criteria for amyloid.

1413

material. The proteinaceous nature of amyloid deposits has since been confirmed by numerous investigators.

Early twentieth-century amyloid research resulted in the development of experimental animal models for the disease, the recognition of the unique optical properties of amyloid deposits following Congo red staining, and the gradual incrimination of the immune system in amyloidogenesis. In 1931, Magnus Levy noted the frequent association of amyloidosis and Bence Jones proteinuria and implicated the abnormal proteins in the pathogenesis of the amyloid tissue infiltrates. In 1940, Apitz reported an atypical bone marrow plasmacytosis in amyloidosis and suggested a causal association. Osserman further strengthened the circumstantial links among bone marrow plasmacytosis, circulating paraproteinemia, and amyloidosis. These observations fell short of proving the immunologic basis of amyloidosis, however, and inconclusive immunofluorescence studies left further cause to doubt the immunoglobulin origin of amyloidosis. With the discovery of the amyloid fibril in 1959, it became possible to attempt isolation and chemical characterization of amyloid. The first proteins to be analyzed by Glenner and co-workers[4] were from patients with primary amyloidosis. Amino acid sequence data revealed these proteins to be homologous to the variable region of immunoglobulin (Ig) light chains (AL proteins). Shortly thereafter, Benditt and associates[5] discovered the extracellular protein that appears to be the major constituent of secondary amyloid deposits. This substance, now called amyloid A (AA) protein, has a molecular weight of 8500 and is composed of 76 amino acids in a sequence that is not related to that of any previously identified proteins.[6] Many classes and types of amyloid are now known to exist, with the most exciting findings emanating from studies of familial amyloid polyneuropathy (ATTR proteins) and Alzheimer's disease (Aβ protein). Thus, after many years of frustration, biochemical investigations had at least partially succeeded in determining the nature of amyloidosis, though leaving unsolved the equally important dilemmas of how and why it occurs.[6a]

Classification and Nomenclature. As new classifications based on biochemical knowledge have been developed, the older schemes retain their clinical usefulness,[3] and in fact their outlines are still visible in the new formulations (Table 82–2).

When possible, the basis for nomenclature and classification should be the fibril protein making up the amyloid deposits.[7] In many instances, the amyloid fibril proteins are identical to, or derived from, intact fragments of proteins present in serum or plasma. Such fibril protein precursors are therefore listed as a second set of data. In cases in which the given protein exists in the form of different types or variants, these forms or variants may be provided as additional information when necessary (Table 82–3). A final column provides the clinical description of the disease process affecting the patient or a family member at risk for developing amyloidosis.

Table 82–2. NOMENCLATURE AND CLASSIFICATION OF NONHEREDITARY AMYLOIDOSIS

Amyloid Protein	Amyloid Precursor	Clinical Syndrome or Association
AA	apoSAA	Secondary (reactive)
AL	Aκ, Aλ, e.g., AκIII	Primary, myeloma- or macroglobulinemia-associated
ATTR	Transthyretin	Systemic senile amyloidosis
Aβ	Amyloid precursor protein (APP)	Alzheimer's disease, Down's syndrome
Aβ2M	β₂-Microglobulin	Hemodialysis-associated
ACal	(Pro)calcitonin	Medullary carcinoma of the thyroid
AANF	Amyloid atrial natriuretic factor	Isolated atrial amyloid
AIAPP	Amyloid islet amyloid polypeptide	Insulinoma, diabetes type II
APrP	Prion protein (scrapie)	Creutzfeldt-Jakob disease

AMYLOID DEPOSITS

Examination of Amyloid

Light Microscopy. Amyloid deposits from various human and animal sources appear similar and amorphous under light microscopy. These accumulations stain eosinophilically with hematoxylin and eosin, exhibit metachromasia with crystal violet, and demonstrate an affinity for Congo red. The most useful histochemical procedure for detecting amyloid deposits involves polarization microscopy of Congo red–stained specimens, which produces a pathognomonic green birefringence. Amyloid deposits also

Table 82–3. NOMENCLATURE AND CLASSIFICATION OF HEREDITARY AMYLOIDOSIS

Amyloid Protein	Protein Precursor	Protein Type or Variant	Clinical Syndrome
AA	apoSAA		Familial Mediterranean fever
ATTR	Transthyretin	e.g., Met 30	Familial amyloid polyneuropathy (Portuguese)
		e.g., Met 111	Familial amyloid cardiomyopathy (Danish)
AApoAI	apoAI	Arg 26	Familial amyloid polyneuropathy (Iowa)
AGel	Gelsolin	Asn 187	Familial amyloidosis (Finnish)
ACys	Cystatin C	Gln 68	Hereditary cerebral hemorrhage with amyloidosis (Icelandic)
Aβ	Amyloid precursor protein (APP)	Gln 618	Hereditary cerebral hemorrhage with amyloidosis (Dutch)
APrP	Prion protein (scrapie)	Lev 102	Gerstmann-Straussler syndrome

fluoresce after staining with thioflavine dyes, but this reaction is less specific than Congo red–induced green birefringence.

Ultrastructure. Amyloid deposits have been shown by electron microscopy to contain two distinct formed elements: a fibrillar component[1, 2] and a pentagonal unit, or pentraxin (P component).[8, 9] The fibrils are characteristically thin, rigid, nonbranching, and approximately l00 Å wide. They have a tendency toward lateral aggregation to form fibers[3] (Fig. 82–1). Individual fibrils are composed of two to five filaments 25 to 30 Å wide, arranged essentially parallel to the long axis of the fibril in a twisted-ribbon fashion. This configuration produces a hollow core profile on cross-section of the fibril.

Amyloid fibrils are dispersed in the extracellular space. Fibrils distant from cellular elements are arranged almost randomly, whereas fibrils in proximity to cells may be oriented perpendicularly or parallel to the plasma membrane. Fibrils adjacent to cells often appear to merge with the membrane. The close morphologic relationship of amyloid fibrils and phagocytic cells suggests that these cells are intimately involved in the synthesis or processing of amyloid fibrils.

X-ray crystallography of amyloid fibril concentrates reveals that the fibrils consist of polypeptide chains arranged perpendicularly to the long axis of the fibril with a cross β-pleated sheet conformation. Infrared spectroscopy further indicates that the polypeptide chains are folded in an antiparallel fashion. The β-pleated sheet conformation has been found in all amyloid proteins investigated and may explain certain characteristics of amyloid deposits. Congo red–induced green birefringence of amyloid deposits implies that the dye molecules are regularly arranged with their long axes parallel to the long axes of the fibrils.

The twisted β-pleated sheet conformation of amyloid fibrils facilitates appropriate alignment of the Congo red dye molecules, which are then bound by nonionic forces to the polypeptide chains. The resistance of amyloid deposits to digestion by most mammalian enzymes may also be related to the β-pleated structure, which is rare in mammalian systems. Finally, certain polypeptides undergo a conformational change to a β-pleated sheet structure following thermal or enzymatic denaturation in vitro; with this change, they assume the tinctorial or physical properties of amyloid fibrils.

Types of Amyloid Protein

Amyloid P Component (AP Protein). P component, a member of the pentraxin family, is a normal plasma protein that was discovered by Cathcart and colleagues as a result of its cross-reactivity with antisera raised against saline extracts of human amyloid deposits.[10] No differences have yet been found between P component isolated from serum (SAP) and P component obtained from amyloid-laden tissues (AP), and their amino acid sequences are identical.[11] SAP has a doughnut-like structure composed of five globular subunits surrounding a central cavity. It is 80 Å in diameter, with a tendency to aggregate into rods with a 40 Å periodicity (Fig. 82–2). The observation that SAP and AP undergo calcium-dependent binding to agarose has greatly facilitated the isolation and purification of these proteins. AP has an intimate association with all types of amyloid deposits. AP is a normal component of basement membrane and is a major constituent of the microfibrillar network of elastic connective tissue.

In the mouse, SAP behaves as a true acute phase reactant, its concentration in the serum starting to rise 8 hours after an acute physical or chemical injury and reaching a peak after 24 to 48 hours. A remarkable homology between SAP and C-reactive protein (CRP) with respect to structure and function[12] sup-

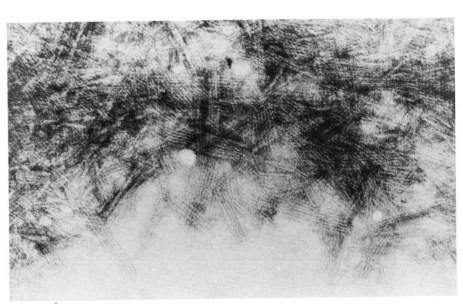

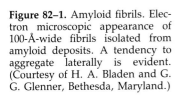

Figure 82–1. Amyloid fibrils. Electron microscopic appearance of 100-Å-wide fibrils isolated from amyloid deposits. A tendency to aggregate laterally is evident. (Courtesy of H. A. Bladen and G. G. Glenner, Bethesda, Maryland.)

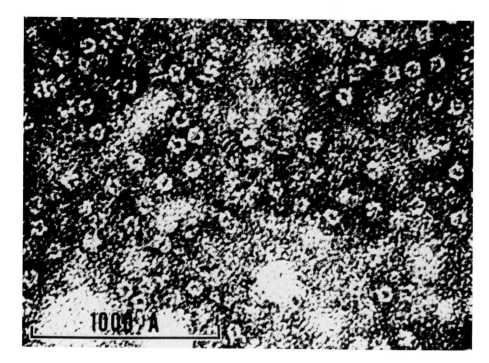

Figure 82–2. Amyloid P component. Doughnut-like structure, 80 Å in diameter, composed of five globular subunits (pentraxins).

ports the theory that SAP has been stably conserved during vertebrate evolution, possibly even to a greater extent than CRP. Complementary DNA (cDNA) isolation and complete amino acid sequencing have resulted in the localization of the human P component gene to chromosome 1.[13]

Amyloid Deposits of Immunoglobulin Light Chain Origin (AL Protein). Immunochemical studies substantiate the derivation of amyloid fibrillar proteins from immunoglobulin light chains and further demonstrate that a component antigenically related to the tissue protein can be found in the sera of many amyloidosis patients.[14] Detection of these antigenically related serum light chain components may be hampered by their low concentrations and restricted antigenicity.

Clinical observations and experimental data indicate that some but not all immunoglobulin light chains are capable of being converted to amyloid fibrils. It is postulated that the primary structure of these light chains renders them susceptible to conformational changes to a β-pleated sheet structure, that is, they are "amyloidogenic" light chains.

The two-residue variable region insertion between positions 68 and 69 that appears to be unique for lambda (λ) VI proteins[15] may provide the structural characteristics that make these Bence Jones proteins more amyloidogenic. It has also been pointed out that certain kappa (κ) III and λI, II, and III proteins may contain amyloidogenic segments.

Amyloid Deposits of Amyloid A Protein Origin (AA Proteins). A class of amyloid fibrillar proteins distinct from immunoglobulin has been isolated from tissue deposits in cases of secondary amyloidosis and familial Mediterranean fever.[6] AA proteins from different tissue and patient sources range in molecular weight from 4500 to 10,000, but they have remarkably similar amino acid compositions and sequences.

A serum component antigenically related to the AA protein (SAA) has been detected by immunodiffusion and radioimmunoassy procedures.[16] SAA has an α-β electrophoretic mobility and an apparent molecular weight of 160,000 to 180,000, resulting from an association with serum high-density lipoprotein.[17] It can be broken down with guanidine, formic acid, or sodium dodecyl sulfate to a much smaller component (SAAL or apoSAA) that contains an amino acid sequence identical to that of the smaller tissue AA protein.[18] The apoSAA proteins compose a family of amphipathic proteins, having a size of approximately 12 kD. Six major apoSAA isotypes with different solubilities and isoelectric points have been identified in humans. Recent work supports the notion that both mouse and human apoSAA isotypes may be the products of at least three different genes.[19]

There is now ample evidence that many acute phase reactants, including SAA1 and SAA2, are synthesized in the liver. SAA3 is not associated with serum high-density lipoprotein: it may be expressed by fibroblasts[20] and macrophages at sites of acute inflammation or injury. The kinetics of serum SAA production closely resemble those of another acute phase reactant, CRP, after a standard inflammatory insult in normal volunteers. The detection or quantitation of SAA has no currently recognized diagnostic or prognostic value.

Amyloid Deposits of Calcitonin Origin (ACal). The amyloid deposits found in neoplastic or degenerative disorders of endocrine glands appear to contain an amyloid fibrillar protein derived from locally synthesized polypeptides. It appears that medullary carcinoma cells synthesize an amyloidogenic procalcitonin precursor that is converted to a β-pleated sheet fibril.[21] Islet amyloid polypeptide (IAPP) has been demonstrated in the amyloid deposits of human pancreatic islets,[22] and amyloid-like fibrils can be synthesized in vitro from glucagon and insulin. Amyloid deposits are also present in bronchial carcinoid tumors, carotid body tumors, parathyroid adenomas, pheochromocytomas, pituitary adenomas, and gastrinomas. They are presumed to be locally synthesized. This class of amyloid proteins was previously called APUD (amine precursor uptake and decarboxylation) amyloid, based on the common histochemical properties of the cells involved.

Amyloid Deposits of Transthyretin Origin (ATTR). A protein obtained from a Portuguese patient with familial amyloid polyneuropathy (FAP), a syndrome first described by Andrade,[23] is immunochemically identical to plasma transthyretin (TTR). This protein differs from normal plasma TTR by a single substitution of valine for methionine at position 30.[24] Identical findings were subsequently reported for large numbers of patients belonging to affected families in Sweden, Japan, and Brazil, and at least 20 new pedigrees have been described in which variant TTR molecules occur in both type I and type II FAP.[24a] Type III (Iowa) FAP is distinctive in that the variant amyloid precursor protein is human apolipoprotein A1.[25] Type IV FAP, or Finnish hereditary amyloid, is also different from all other amyloid proteins identified so far, since it shows amino acid homology with the gelsolin gene that expresses the mutant asparagine 187 molecule.[26] Interestingly, hereditary Danish cardiac amyloidosis, which is not associated with polyneuropathy, is characterized by a plasma TTR variant that contains methionine instead of leucine at position 111.[27]

Trace deposits of amyloid can be demonstrated in the great vessels, pancreatic islets, cardiac tissue, and cerebral vessels of an aged population. These deposits are microscopic, rarely produce clinical symptoms, and are usually diagnosed at necropsy examination. Their prevalence tends to increase with age, and some authors believe they are pathogenetically related to the aging process. These are usually clinically insignificant, but extensive infiltration of myocardium and conduction tissues can occur in a minority of cases. Westermark and co-workers[28] have shown that these deposits consist of plasma nonvariant TTR fragments. A reported complete sequence of ATTR isolated from the fibrils of another patient with systemic senile amyloidosis had isoleucine substituted for valine at position 122 with no normal protein present.[29] This may represent a new hereditary form of amyloidosis that becomes clinically apparent only in old age.

Isolated deposits involving the atrium, especially the auricles, are the most common form of amyloid affecting the heart. Atrophy of muscle cells does not occur, and the clinical significance of the deposits is uncertain. The amyloid deposits in these cases are immunoreactive with atrial natriuretic factor (AANF).[30]

Amyloid Deposits of β Protein Origin (Aβ). Amyloid has been found in the neuritic plaque, the neurofibrillary tangle, and the microangiopathic lesions that occur in the brains of individuals with Alzheimer's presenile dementia and dementia of the Alzheimer's type (AD). The neuritic plaque is a complex structure consisting of a region of swollen and degenerating neuronal processes (neurites), surrounding a dense core of typical or "straight" amyloid fibrils. In contrast, the neurofibrillary tangles are intracellular fibrous bundles that can occupy most of the perinuclear cytoplasm of the affected neuronal cell bodies. They exhibit all the staining properties of amyloid, including the characteristic congophilia with birefringence, but ultrastructurally they consist of paired helical filaments, each of which is 100 Å wide, arranged in the form of a double helix and with a cross-over approximately every 800 Å. In approximately 90 percent of cases of histopathologically confirmed AD, cerebral amyloid is also found in the walls of the cortical, subcortical, and meningeal arterioles and capillaries.

Cerebral amyloid deposition at one or more of these three sites is not restricted to AD. Plaques and neurofibrillary tangles are found in the majority of patients with Down's syndrome who survive to middle age. The initial purification and partial amino acid sequence of a 4.2-kD amyloid peptide (called β protein or A4 peptide) was reported for amyloid isolated from extraparenchymal meningeal vessels in either Alzheimer's disease or Down's syndrome[31] and, subsequently, from neuritic plaque amyloid cores and neurofibrillary tangles. Based on the initial amino acid sequence, oligonucleotide probes have been synthesized, cDNA libraries have been screened, and the gene encoding the putative amyloid peptide precursor (APP) has been mapped to human chromosome 21.[32]

Amyloid Deposits of β₂-Microglobulin Origin (Aβ2M). Amyloid-laden tissue obtained at carpal tunnel release from a patient on chronic hemodialysis was subjected to chemical analysis.[33] When the protein was solubilized in guanidine, a significant amount was found to be identical to β₂-microglobulin with regard to its molecular weight of 11,000, amino acid composition, and 16 amino-terminal amino acids. Subsequently confirmed by others, these results indicated that Aβ2M is indeed a new class of amyloid, representing an intact β₂-microglobulin. β₂-Microglobulin consists of a single polypeptide chain of 99 amino acid residues. It is found in most biologic tissues both as a free monomer and as a cell membrane protein associated with class 1 HLA antigens. It has the β-pleated sheet configuration and has significant homology to the constant domain of IgG.

Amyloid Deposits of Cystatin C Origin (ACyS). Complete amino acid sequence analysis has been carried out on amyloid deposits from pooled leptomeningeal tissues and meningeal vessels of Icelandic patients with hereditary cerebral hemorrhage with amyloidosis (HCHWA).[34] The major protein is identical to residues 11 to 120 of gamma trace alkaline protein (cystatin C), except for a single amino acid substitution, glutamine for leucine, at position 68. Although HCHWA in families of Dutch rather than Icelandic origin has a similar clinical picture and pathologic findings, amyloid deposits in these patients appear to follow a single point mutation in the Aβ portion of the APP gene.[35]

Amyloid Deposits of Prion Protein Origin (APrP). A spongiform encephalopathy characterized by amyloid plaques, the proliferation of astroglial cells, and sometimes neuronal vacuolization is found in the unconventional slow virus diseases: Creutzfeldt-Jakob disease, Gerstmann-Straussler syndrome, and kuru in humans, and scrapie in animals. Whether inherited or acquired, amyloid deposits are composed of prion protein fragments that are immunoreactive with isolates from scrapie-infected hamsters. In a recent study, Prusiner and colleagues[36] inserted a mutated form of the PrP gene into mice and found that the resultant transgenic mice developed a scrapie-like spongiform encephalopathy—a disease characterized by vacuoles in brain tissue. These findings provide the most convincing evidence yet that the unnatural conformation of a precursor amyloid protein can arise through genetic mutation, and that it can be transmitted from one organism to another.

PATHOGENESIS

Besides the requirement for an appropriate primary structure, the process of amyloid formation must involve other mechanisms, such as altered expression, post-translational changes, abnormal processing of the amyloid precursor proteins, or all three.

It is generally accepted that proteolytic enzymes play a key role in the pathogenesis of primary (type AL) amyloidosis. Amyloid fibrils can form in vitro as a result of partial processing of Bence Jones proteins by human kidney lysosomal enzymes. It has also been shown that cultured bone marrow cells from a patient with multiple myeloma can cause de novo deposition of amyloid fibrils within a 14-day culture period.[37] There was morphologic evidence of Bence Jones protein synthesis by the myeloma cells (with prominent rough endoplasmic endothelium), subsequent processing of these proteins in macrophage lysosomes, and eventual secretion of the amyloid fibrils. Although the macrophages may have also ingested some amyloid material, the presence of well-oriented tufts of amyloid fibrils at the invagination sites beside packed lysosomes indicated a predominantly secretory process.

Unlike in amyloidosis of immunoglobulin origin, many steps in the genesis of secondary or type AA amyloidosis are unsettled. Human monocytes can degrade SAA protein, apparently by a surface-associated protease.[38] When normal persons and amyloid patients were compared, all amyloid patients showed an AA-sized intermediate that was noted during breakdown by monocular cells. These results have suggested that alteration in the handling of SAA protein may underlie the variable incidence of amyloidosis in different disease populations.

Polymorphonuclear neutrophils (PMNs) can also degrade SAA in vitro through a pathway that is blocked by an elastase inhibitor.[39] In these studies, PMNs and monocytes were equivalent in their ability to process SAA, demonstrating that various cell lines may be responsible for amyloid formation. Furthermore, it was shown that lysosomal enzymes capable of SAA degradation were released from PMNs by zymosan. Those results are intriguing in light of previous electron microscopic studies suggesting lysosomes as an intracellular site for deposition of amyloid. It is likely, therefore, that amyloid fibril deposition may occur at intracellular or extracellular locations, depending on local factors in various organs or sites of inflammation.

Investigations of the chemistry and pathogenesis of human amyloidosis have been paralleled by a vast body of work in experimental animals that was begun in the early years of this century. The induction of systemic amyloidosis in the mouse, rabbit, hamster, and guinea pig by serial injections of casein has been the most extensively used model. It corresponds most closely to human amyloidosis of the AA type and has permitted investigations of immune function and the role of the mononuclear phagocytic system that would not be possible in human subjects. Of the three SAA gene products discovered in mice,[20] Benditt's group has found by amino acid sequence analysis that the SAA2 isotype is the only possible precursor of murine amyloid fibril protein AA.[40]

One of the strongest clues relating the aging phenomenon to amyloidogenesis has emerged from studies of the senescence accelerated mouse (SAM), in which systemic amyloidosis is one of the most characteristic findings. The unique amyloid fibril protein has a molecular weight of 5200 and an amino acid composition differing from that of amyloid proteins of any other type, including AA. Fractionation of lipoproteins from normal mouse serum by ultracentrifugation revealed that most of the serum precursor protein (SASsam) is contained in the high-density lipoprotein fraction corresponding to apolipoprotein AII. Although the function of murine apoAII is poorly understood, it differs from the apoSAA proteins in that it does not seem to be an acute phase reactant. It now appears that identical variant apoAII molecules with a substitution of glutamine for proline at position 5 are the major constituents of amyloid proteins developing in SAMs as well as other strains of aging mice.[41] Interestingly, the SAM does not develop systemic amyloidosis if there is chronic food restriction, especially of dietary milk protein.[42] This may be interpreted as additional evidence that casein overload may play a significant role in the pathogensis of both major forms of systemic murine amyloidosis.

In 1927, Smetana[43] used India ink to effect blockage of the mononuclear phagocytic system (MPS) in experimental animals and concluded from the observed decrease in the rate of amyloid formation that reticuloendothelial cells were involved in amyloidogenesis. He further noted that, though amyloid appeared in proximity to these cells, tissue areas with the most abundant amyloid showed no uptake of India ink. He suggested that amyloid appeared as reticuloendothelial cells were altered or destroyed. More recently, extensive morphologic evidence at the electron microscopic level has also incriminated reticuloendothelial cells in the deposition of amyloid.

The concept that emerges from these and other studies is that amyloidosis is a biphasic process, both morphologically and functionally. In the animal model of secondary amyloidosis, casein or azocasein is phagocytosed by cells of the MPS, stimulating production of cytokines such as interleukin-1 (IL-1) and IL-6 and subsequently inducing an acute phase response and the production of SAA precursor proteins.[43a] Multiple injections of casein overwhelm the proteolytic capacity of the macrophage, either by inhibition of cell membrane–associated neutral serine esterase or by activation of serine protease inhibitors (i.e., serpins), one of which may be AP protein. Resistance to amyloid induction is governed by a recessive gene in A/J mouse strains[44] and is significantly affected by gender in the Syrian hamster.[45] Other factors that may affect the pathogenesis of amyloid fibril deposition include amyloid-enhancing factor(s), lipopolysaccharides (LPSs) or endotoxins, and P-component or other pentraxins (Fig. 82–3). A diet rich in n-3 polyunsaturated fatty acids (fish oil) modifies the prostaglandin profile of macrophages

and reduces the severity of amyloidosis in experimental amyloidosis.[46] Colchicine also blocks amyloid fibril deposition in casein-induced amyloidosis, presumably by depolymerization of macrophage microtubules.

Perhaps the greatest interest in the general mechanisms of amyloidogenesis has been generated by recently reported biochemical and genetic studies in Alzheimer's disease (AD) and unusual forms of familial amyloidotic polyneuropathy. For scientists studying the riddle of AD, a major unanswered question centers on the cause of neuronal dysfunction and eventual cell death. Recent data using DNA collected from families in which AD is inherited as a single dominant gene have apparently resolved part of this question. A point mutation in the gene that codes for Aβ precursor protein, APP, is found in two such families and only in those affected members.[47] The gene mutation, which does not appear to cause a dramatic change in the protein, was found in the same portion of the amyloid precursor gene in which a mutation was earlier identified by Frangione and colleagues.[35] This mutation, occurring in Dutch kindreds with HCHWA, represented the first clear data indicating that amyloid deposits could be the central event causing AD. The large amino-terminal portion of APP is identical to a proteinase inhibitor, protease nexin II (PNII). Based on a series of publications summarized by Selkoe,[49] it has been proposed that PNII is released from the holoprotein by cleavage near the cell membrane, inactivates serine proteases in the extracellular space, binds to tissue macrophages (microglia), and is internalized. This line of reasoning raises the intriguing posibility that both Aβ-type amyloidotic plaques and AA-type amyloid deposits may be caused by inappropriate secretion or imbalance of proteases and protease inhibitors.

Yankner and associates[48] have shown that Aβ protein exerts both trophic and toxic effects on neurons in cell cultures, depending on the developmental stage of the cells and the concentration of the protein. In a hippocampal neuronal cell culture, Aβ was a thousand times more neurotoxic than glutamate, a chemical long suspected of being involved in neurodegenerative diseases. These observations suggest that Aβ protein could normally function at low concentrations as a neurotropic factor during cell differentiation, but that accumulations of Aβ in the mature brain may lead to neurodegeneration.

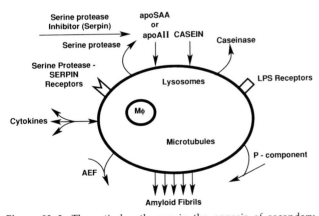

Figure 82–3. Theoretical pathways in the genesis of secondary and age-associated experimental amyloidosis. Amyloid P component (AP protein) is synthesized in the liver, as are most acute phase reactants and serine protease inhibitors (serpins). The involvement of serine protease–serpin complexes and lipopolysaccharide (LPS) receptors on the cell surface of the macrophage (Mϕ) is highly speculative. The nature of amyloid-enhancing factor (AEF) is also unknown at the present time.

CLINICAL AMYLOIDOSIS SYNDROMES

Primary and Myeloma-Associated Amyloidosis.
Primary amyloidosis best refers to those amyloidosis syndromes that occur in the absence of an associated infectious, inflammatory, neoplastic, or familial disorder. This designation implies the presence of an associated monoclonal plasma cell dyscrasia and amyloid deposits of immunoglobulin origin. Multiple myeloma–associated amyloidosis is closely related to

primary amyloidosis, except for the severity of the underlying plasma cell dyscrasia. Systemic amyloidosis also occurs in association with macroglobulinemia (Waldenström's disease), heavy chain or Franklin's disease, and agammaglobulinemia.

Primary amyloidosis is a disease of middle and advanced age, with a mean age at diagnosis of 55 years. Men are affected significantly more often than women, and whites are affected more frequently than nonwhites. Virtually all patients with primary amyloidosis demonstrate a monoclonal immunoglobulin protein in their serum or urine, or both, and a bone marrow plasmacytosis. The clinical manifestations of primary amyloidosis are protean, but certain symptom complexes suggest its presence: (1) idiopathic, sensorimotor, peripheral neuropathy with autonomic neuropathy; (2) restrictive cardiomyopathy with a low-voltage electrocardiogram and conduction disturbances in the absence of other recognized causes; (3) nonthrombocytopenic purpura with cutaneous induration, "pinch purpura," or "postproctoscopic purpura"; (4) rheumatoid-like arthritis with little inflammation and prominent large joint involvement (shoulder pad sign); (5) macroglossia; (6) hemorrhagic diathesis secondary to isolated acquired factor X deficiency; (7) idiopathic nephrotic syndrome; and (8) idiopathic carpal tunnel syndrome. Demonstration of paraproteinemia or Bence Jones proteinuria in conjunction with these clinical syndromes strongly suggests primary amyloidosis.

Multiple myeloma–associated amyloidosis closely resembles primary generalized amyloidosis in its age distribution, sex predilection, and clinical presentations.[50] Six to 15 percent of myeloma patients develop amyloidosis. The majority of patients with myeloma-associated amyloidosis demonstrate an intact immunoglobulin paraprotein in serum but also have Bence Jones proteinemia or proteinuria, or both. Excessive free light chain synthesis may be intimately related to the dissemination and formation of amyloid deposits. The ratio of κ to λ light chains in myeloma-associated amyloidosis may differ from the ratio in primary amyloidosis, in which λ Bence Jones proteins predominate.

Secondary Amyloidosis. Most rheumatologists gain first-hand knowledge of systemic amyloidosis of the AA type during the diagnostic work-up and management of patients with chronic inflammatory joint disease.[51] Historically, rheumatoid arthritis (RA) has received the most attention as a source of secondary amyloid disease, but the association merits closer scrutiny in light of recent anecdotes from the United States and several European countries. The incidence of amyloidosis in patients with RA varies from one reported series to another. The reasons for this are multiple, but, in general, most of the studies have not been systematically carried out on the population at risk. Other factors deserving consideration include age at onset of arthritis, diet, heredity, and the effects of different forms of therapy, such as glucocorticoids, gold salts, D-penicillamine,

and cytotoxic agents. Whatever the reason, amyloidosis as a complication of RA has been less commonly encountered during the last twenty years. In 1971, a careful study comparing the necropsy frequencies of amyloidosis in RA and in nonrheumatoid subjects revealed deposits typical of AA type amyloidosis in only one of 47 patients with RA: senile amyloid deposits in cerebral, aortic, cardiac, and pancreatic tissues were present in 14 of 47 arthritis patients and in 19 of 47 control subjects.[52] In juvenile rheumatoid arthritis the death rate is said to be at least four times as high in Europe as it is in the United States, and the major cause of death in Europe is renal failure due to amyloidosis. The highest frequency has been reported in Poland, where 11 percent of children with polyarthritis show secondary amyloidosis. On the other hand, lower frequencies are seen in the Americas—0.14 percent in the United States and 2 percent in Argentina.

By definition, the spondyloarthropathies share similar pathologic, radiographic, and clinical features. Among pathologic features that appear to be common to this group of diseases is amyloidosis of the AA type. Thus, numerous case reports and collected series have documented amyloid disease complicating classic cases of ankylosing spondylitis. Secondary amyloidosis has also been reported as a complication of Reiter's disease, generalized psoriasis with or without arthritis, ulcerative colitis and Crohn's disease, chronic tophaceous gout, Behçet's syndrome, and Whipple's disease. Finally, secondary amyloidosis may accompany systemic lupus erythematosus (SLE), scleroderma, dermatomyositis, polyarteritis nodosa, and Sjögren's syndrome.

The number of nonrheumatologic diseases associated with secondary amyloidosis is legion. At the present time, lepromatous leprosy probably accounts for most of the cases of amyloidosis occurring in India, Southeast Asia, Africa, and South America. In 1965, a curious but striking difference in prevalence of amyloidosis was noted in patients with leprosy in Carville, Louisiana (33 percent), versus those in Guadalajara, Mexico (3 percent). The reason for this difference in biopsy-proven disease was not known, but it was noteworthy that the Mexican patients had a significantly lower caloric intake and ate lesser amounts of saturated fat.[53]

With better treatment, amyloidosis due to tuberculosis is now seldom encountered in North America. On the other hand, 150 of 200 patients with renal amyloidosis reported from India in 1974 had underlying tuberculosis. Amyloidosis frequently complicates paraplegia, probably as a result of chronically infected decubitus ulcers and chronic pyelonephritis. Bronchiectasis, osteomyelitis, inflammatory bowel diseases, chronically infected burns, cystic fibrosis, and schistosomiasis and other parasitic infections are some of the numerous chronic inflammatory and/or infectious diseases that may predispose to AA type amyloidosis. Within the past decade, parenteral drug abuse has emerged as an important causative factor of AA secondary amyloidosis.

Familial Amyloidotic Polyneuropathy Syndromes. The first well-substantiated example of hereditary neuropathic amyloidosis came from Portugal.[23] A similar neuropathic disease has since been found in Portuguese subjects in Brazil, France, and Africa and in non-Portuguese subjects from the United States, Germany, Japan, Sweden, Italy, Greece, Turkey, Great Britain, and Ireland. This disease, designated type I polyneuropathy or Portuguese neuropathy, is inherited in an autosomal dominant manner with equal sex predilection and a high penetrance. Symptoms characteristically begin in the third or fourth decade of life with a distal sensory neuropathy in a "stocking" distribution. Upper extremity and truncal sensory deficits appear later. Motor deficits occur in advanced disease. The signs and symptoms of autonomic neuropathy (e.g., impotence, postural hypotension, gastrointestinal motility disturbances, and hypohidrosis) are prominent. Visual findings include irregular pupillary margins, sluggish light reflexes, and vitreous opacities. Renal failure, carpal tunnel syndrome, macroglossia, and heart failure are not manifestations of type I polyneuropathy. An American kindred of Swedish origin with peripheral neuropathy and systemic amyloidosis bears a phenotypic resemblance to type I polyneuropathy cases but is associated with significant renal disease.

Type II amyloid polyneuropathy is characterized by the carpal tunnel syndrome and a diffuse neuropathy that is especially prominent in the upper extremities.[54] The disease is inherited in an autosomal dominant fashion. Large kindreds have been described in Indiana (Swiss origin) and Maryland (German origin). Symptoms of carpal tunnel syndrome usually appear in the fourth or fifth decade of life, and progression of disease is slow. After several years or decades of carpal tunnel symptoms, evidence of diffuse neuropathy develops, and eventually the legs are involved. Vitreous opacities, electrocardiographic abnormalities, congestive heart failure, and hepatic, gastrointestinal, and diffuse vascular infiltration may occur, but macroglossia and uremia are rare.

Type III polyneuropathy, initially described in an Iowa family of Scottish, English, and Irish descent, is characterized by upper and lower extremity neuropathy, duodenal ulcer, and nephropathy.[55] Inherited as an autosomal dominant disease, it first becomes manifest in the third or fourth decade of life with lower extremity neuropathy. Concomitant upper extremity neuropathy is usually present. Autonomic symptoms may be prominent, and the cerebrospinal fluid protein level is usually elevated. Duodenal ulcer is apparently common, but the ulcer crater does not contain amyloid on biopsy. Renal involvement progresses at variable rates to uremia and death from renal insufficiency. No vitreous opacities have been described. Fibrils from this type of amyloidotic tissue contain apolipoprotein AI rather than TTR.[25]

Familial amyloidosis of the Finnish type, originally known as type IV polyneuropathy, is manifested by corneal lattice dystrophy, cranial nerve palsies, cutis laxa, and an autosomal dominant inheritance pattern.[26, 56] Lattice dystrophy usually appears in the third decade of life, but no vitreous opacities are detected. Visual acuity tends to be preserved to old age, but corneal ulcerations can be troublesome in patients older than 40 years of age. Upper facial paresis is a regular feature in older patients. Dermal changes begin in the fifth decade of life, with upper facial and scalp thickening. Past the seventh decade of life, the skin over the rest of the body may become atrophic and pendulous. Amyloid deposits are prominent around lattice lines and diseased peripheral nerves and in dermal appendages. Localized forms of lattice corneal dystrophy are recognized and may be distinguishable from systemic varieties by histologic and clinical criteria.

Familial Nephropathic Amyloidosis Syndromes. One of the most interesting types of secondary amyloidosis is that seen in patients with familial Mediterranean fever (FMF). In most cases of FMF the affected person is certainly of Mediterranean origin[57, 58]; for example, Jews of Sephardic ancestry, Anatolian Turks, Armenians, and Arabs of the Middle East. The tendency to develop amyloid does not appear to be linked to an autosomal dominant gene, as in the other heredofamilial amyloidosis syndromes, and seems to be a recessive trait based on studies emanating from Israel. The disease has two phenotypic manifestations that are independent of each other—amyloidosis and febrile attacks. In most patients, febrile attacks precede clinical evidence of amyloid (phenotype I), but in some, amyloidotic nephrosis has been the first indication of the disease (phenotype II). Phenotype II can be diagnosed only if another member of the patient's family is of phenotype I or if febrile attacks develop in the patient.

Those joints most frequently affected are the knee, ankle, and shoulder. Occasionally more than one joint is involved, and recurrent attacks usually involve the site affected originally. Pain, tenderness, swelling, synovial effusion, and muscle spasm are impressive. Unlike the abdominal crises, which are generally of short duration, the articular symptoms sometimes last for weeks or even months. However, despite prolonged pain and immobilization, the arthritis is not deforming, and radiographs taken during an attack show little more than juxta-articular osteoporosis. The synovial fluid initially contains increased numbers of PMNs, and the mucin clot test result ranges from poor to good.

Familial amyloidotic nephropathy with febrile urticaria and deafness (Muckle-Wells syndrome) was first described in an English family in which an autosomal dominant trait was transmitted over four generations, affecting 9 of 16 members at risk.[59] The constant feature of the disease was the "aguey bout," which lasted as long as 36 hours and was characterized by the appearance of an urticarial rash during episodes of fever with rigor, malaise, and pain in the limbs. By 1979, Muckle was able to collect or identify 63 additional cases. A protein extracted from formalin-fixed tissue obtained from a German patient at autopsy was shown by sequence analysis to be homologous with AA protein for residues 2 to 30.[60]

Amyloid nephropathy of Ostertag (AA type) is characterized by chronic nephropathy, hypertension, and hepatosplenomegaly, with amyloid deposits in kidneys, adrenal glands, and liver.[61] Several families from Massachusetts and the United Kingdom in which amyloid nephropathy is not associated with neuropathy express serum apoAI polymorphism identical to that first described in type III FAP.

Familial Cardiopathic Amyloidosis Syndromes. An amyloidotic cardiomyopathy has been reported in five members of a Danish sibship.[62] Symptoms of congestive heart failure develop in the fourth decade of life, with progression to death over 2 to 6 years. Hemodynamic studies are consistent with a restrictive cardiomyopathy. Three cases of persistent atrial standstill have been reported in another sibship. The patients have bradycardia, absent P waves, cardiac enlargement, and modest congestive heart failure. Amyloid was found in the right atrial appendage in one case.

AMYLOID INFILTRATION OF ORGAN SYSTEMS

Cutaneous Amyloid Deposits. The skin is involved in as many as 40 percent of cases of systemic amyloidosis and is more likely to be affected in primary or myeloma-associated amyloidosis than in secondary amyloidosis. Cutaneous amyloid deposition has an unexplained predilection for the face and upper trunk. Waxy, indurated papules, purpura, or tumefactions are the most frequent dermatologic signs. Excessive accumulations in the dermis occasionally produce marked skin thickening with an orange-peel effect that mimics scleroderma or myxedema. Cutaneous purpura can often be induced by gently stroking the involved skin 20 to 30 times with the examining finger or by gentle pinching. Induced purpura will be resorbed within a few days. Valsalva maneuver or proctoscopic examination will occasionally produce periorbital purpura. Alopecia can be prominent. Histologically, amyloid deposits are found in dermal and subcutaneous vessel walls or throughout the dermis, with a predilection for the dermal appendages.

Two main types of localized cutaneous amyloidosis exist, namely, lichen (including macular amyloidosis) and nodular amyloidosis. Lichen amyloidosis is a syndrome of middle-aged patients, in which coalescent papules form a lichenoid eruption that is especially prominent over the extensor surfaces of the legs and thighs. Amyloid deposits are restricted to the pericapillary areas of the papillary dermis and are not seen in vessel walls or in other organs. Papular mucinosis (scleromyxedema) is an infiltrative skin disorder of sun-exposed areas that clinically resembles cutaneous amyloidosis and is associated with a monoclonal gammopathy; however, excess proteoglycans, and not amyloid, are deposited in the dermis.

Amyloid Arthropathy
Primary Amyloid Arthropathy. One of the least common but most striking clinical manifestations of primary and myeloma-associated amyloidosis is a chronic symmetric arthropathy, mainly involving the shoulders, wrists, knees, and fingers.[63] It is often accompanied by severe constitutional symptoms of morning stiffness and fatigue. These features, plus the physical findings of joint tenderness, limitation of motion, and soft tissue swelling, may lead to an erroneous diagnosis of RA. Soft tissue contractures of the interphalangeal joints may appear rather early in the illness (Fig. 82–4). Joint swelling tends to be less inflammatory than that in rheumatoid disease, and a grittiness or unusual firmness can often be appreciated on joint examination. Subcutaneous nodules are present in more than half the cases and may be mistaken for rheumatoid nodules. Infiltration of the glenohumeral articulation and the surrounding muscles produces the characteristic "shoulder pad" sign. Microscopic amyloid deposits may be localized in articular cartilage, and macroscopic lesions in bone simulate neoplasms and may lead to pathologic fractures.

Many of the patients with amyloid arthropathy develop a carpal tunnel syndrome. Because this syndrome may also be the initial manifestation of type II familial polyneuropathy, amyloidosis should be suspected in cases of idiopathic carpal tunnel syndrome occurring in middle-aged and elderly men.

In primary amyloid arthropathy, synovial fluid analysis usually reveals a noninflammatory fluid with

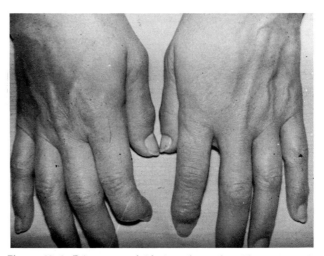

Figure 82–4. Primary amyloidotic arthropathy. There are early contractures and soft tissue swelling of the proximal and interphalangeal and metacarpophalangeal joints. Both wrists are swollen, causing median nerve compression.

predominantly mononuclear cells. The fluid may be xanthochromic, and mucin clot tests give variable results. Inspection of centrifuged, Congo red–stained sediments from synovial fluid under polarization microscopy reveals amyloid deposits in fragments of synovial villi. Radiographs show osteoporosis, lytic lesions, or soft tissue swelling. At necropsy, intracytoplasmic synovial deposition was an unusual feature of a case in which there was generalized amyloidosis in many tissues, including the synovial membrane.

Amyloid in Osteoarthritic Joints. Christensen and Sorensen first described amyloid deposits in the fibrous capsules of hips and knee joints requiring surgery for advanced osteoarthritis. Later, they found amyloid in approximately half the hip capsules in unselected autopsies,[64] and an even higher prevalence was noted in joint cartilage. The amount of amyloid was estimated histologically and was found to correlate positively with the age of the subject. These deposits are microscopic, as opposed to the dense infiltration noted in myeloma-associated arthropathy.

Amyloid in Intervertebral Joints. Calcification of the intervertebral disc associated with AL type amyloidosis is a relatively rare radiologic finding.[65] On the other hand, amyloid deposits of unknown biochemical composition are found quite frequently in the avascular, fibrocartilaginous annulus fibrosus of the discs of elderly subjects.[66] Interestingly, age-related deposition of amyloid in the intervertebral discs of an AKR strain of mice inbred for accelerated senescence (SAM) has been reported by the same group of Japanese workers. These mice also have microscopic amyloid deposits in peripheral joints similar to those seen in human forms of osteoarthritis.

Amyloid in Calcium Pyrophosphate Dihydrate Deposition Disease. In 1978, Ryan and Bernhard[67] described five patients with articular amyloid deposits, four of whom had roentgenographic chondrocalcinosis. Four of the patients had diffusely swollen hands with pitting edema and palmar tendon thickening. Three also had carpal tunnel syndrome. Amyloid deposits were later found in synovial specimens of 14 cases of crystal-proven calcium pyrophosphate dihydrate (CPPD) deposition disease.[68] The close proximity of the amyloid deposits to CPPD crystals in these and other series suggested that the amyloid deposits may stimulate local inorganic pyrophosphate (PPi) production and may bind the PPi much as amyloid binds diphosphonates, which are somewhat analogous to PP1.

Hemodialysis-Associated Amyloidosis and the Carpal Tunnel Syndrome. Median nerve compression develops in more than 70 percent of patients on long-term hemodialysis. Radiolucent cysts in the bones and joints of such patients occur with similar frequency; it is these lesions that are responsible for the erosive arthropathy and intervertebral disc destruction seen in many hemodialysis cases. The first

association of carpal tunnel syndrome and amyloid deposition as an etiologic factor was made by Assenat and coworkers[69] in 1980. Gejyo and associates[32] later isolated amyloid tissue obtained at carpal release and identified it as identical to β_2-microglobulin.

β_2-Microglobulin reaches markedly elevated serum levels in chronic renal insufficiency and appears to be even more sensitive than serum creatinine for detecting decreased glomerular filtration.[70] Dialysis membranes such as cuprophane and cellulose are incapable of clearing this protein, thus accounting for its extensive accumulation in hemodialysis patients. An important caveat to bear in mind, however, is that serum levels of β_2-microglobulin do not differ significantly in hemodialysis patients either with or without carpal tunnel syndrome. Thus, additional amyloid-"enhancing" factors must exist to explain the predilection of certain patients to developing symptomatic amyloid deposits.

The typical patient with one or all of the rheumatologic complications previously mentioned will have been on hemodialysis for 5 to 10 years. The complaints may vary from mild peripheral joint pain to severe discomfort and disability of weight-bearing joints, the spine, or both. Symmetric polyarthralgias of both shoulders and wrists are often exacerbated by dialysis. Eventual collapse of the femoral head may necessitate arthroplasty and total hip replacement. The identification of multiple cystic lesions in carpal bones, radius, and femur raises the possibility of the so-called brown tumors of osteitis fibrosa cystica seen in hyperparathyroidism. Nevertheless, differentiation between a diagnosis of hyperthyroidism and radiolucent bone cysts due to amyloid disease should not be difficult if the laboratory work-up includes serum calcium, phosphorus, and alkaline phosphatase determinations and β_2-microglobulin levels. Another entity to be considered as a cause of cysts and arthritis in a patient with renal failure is hemodialysis oxalosis. Typically, however, these patients experience arthropathy of the metacarpophalangeal joints and metatarsophalangeal joints, as well as calcification of joint capsules, tendons, cartilage, blood vessels, and skin. These unusual cases also have distinctive radiographic findings in addition to cystic erosions of bone caused by calcium oxalate accumulation.

Other conditions that may occur concomitantly in the setting of chronic renal failure include renal osteodystrophy, soft tissue calcification, avascular necrosis of bone, aluminum accumulation, septic arthritis, and crystal-induced arthritis due to sodium urate, calcium pyrophosphate, or hydroxyapatite deposition. Erosive arthritis and carpal tunnel syndrome can occur in primary arthropathy of the AL type and in type II familial polyneuropathy, but these lesions tend to be less severe and affect small joints predominantly. Amyloid arthropathy has never been reported in secondary amyloidosis, with the exception of patients with FMF and possibly severe generalized psoriasis.

Finally, it should be emphasized that hemodialysis-associated amyloidosis, as it is currently recognized, is a limited form of amyloidosis and, with a few exceptions, is generally restricted to articular and para-articular structures. Rectal biopsy specimens have occasionally shown amyloid, but abdominal fat pad aspiration for amyloid, a sensitive screening test, has been consistently negative in these patients.[71] Proper diagnostic work-up of hemodialysis patients with rheumatic complaints, therefore, depends on both an appreciation of the sundry conditions that can have an impact on articular structures and the careful choice of laboratory studies, imaging techniques, and tissue biopsy that can yield the correct diagnosis with maximum efficiency and minimal morbidity.

Amyloid Nephropathy. Renal involvement occurs in almost every type of systemic amyloidosis. Proteinuria is the commonest presentation and progresses at a variable rate to nephrotic syndrome and uremia. Hematuria is unusual in renal disease itself but can result from amyloid infiltration of the lower urinary tract. Although hypertension was once thought to be uncommon in renal amyloidosis, it has been found in 50 percent of affected patients. Renal vein thrombosis is a recognized complication of renal amyloidosis.

Amyloid deposits are most pronounced in the renal glomeruli and arteriolar walls but can also be detected along the tubular basement membrane. Peritubular deposits have been associated with nephrogenic diabetes insipidus in amyloidosis. Glomerular deposits tend to localize to the mesangial and subendothelial regions but can be seen in subepithelial locations as well. Renal involvement is suspected in cases of idiopathic proteinuria or nephrotic syndrome, especially in the presence of a chronic inflammatory disease.

Amyloid Cardiomyopathy. Cardiac infiltration occurs in primary, secondary, and familial forms of amyloidosis. The diagnosis of amyloidosis should be seriously considered in elderly patients with heart disease of unknown etiology, especially if other cardiac diseases, such as ischemic heart disease due to coronary atherosclerosis, are minimal or absent. In younger patients with multisystem diseases, amyloid cardiomyopathy should be suspected if the clinical picture closely resembles that of constrictive myocarditis. Signs and symptoms of failure of the right side of the heart may dominate the early phases of the disease, but routine radiographic findings are often within normal limits. Hemodynamic studies show a variety of patterns, including steep x and y descent, typically seen in constrictive pericarditis, or v waves typical of tricuspid regurgitation. Electrocardiograms reveal low voltage in the limb leads, conduction disturbances, arrhythmias, poor R wave progression in the precordial leads, and patterns that simulate those in acute myocardial infarction.

Echocardiography demonstrates a thick-walled ventricle with a normal or reduced cavity size. The calculated ejected fraction may be within normal limits despite clinically significant heart failure, as the predominant functional disturbance in amyloidosis is severely impaired cardiac relaxation. An unusually refractile appearance by two-dimensional echoradiographic studies termed "granular sparkling" was considered to be a highly specific finding, but similar changes have subsequently been reported in patients with chronic renal failure and hypertrophic cardiomyopathy. Several groups have confirmed that an analysis combining echocardiographic information with data obtained on a standard electrocardiogram can pinpoint the voltage abnormalities most characteristic of amyloid heart disease.

When there is echocardiographic evidence of cardiac amyloidosis, diffuse uptake of technetium-99m pyrophosphate has been used as an index of severity. Although radioisotope scans may be abnormal in patients with primary (type AL) and familial (type ATTR) cardiomyopathy, echocardiograms are said to be normal in secondary amyloidosis even when cardiac involvement is clinically apparent.

Amyloid deposits can be seen in all layers of the cardiac wall. They are most pronounced in the myocardium, at which point they encroach on muscle fibers. Although conduction and rhythm disturbances are frequent in cardiac amyloidosis, direct amyloid infiltration does not account for the majority of these disturbances. Valvular deposits are quite common in aged individuals, but they rarely produce hemodynamically significant changes. Transvenous endocardial biopsy has been employed safely in several patients to establish an ante-mortem diagnosis.

Treatment of cardiac amyloidosis is symptomatic. Digitalis is ineffective in most restrictive myocardiopathies, and it may be associated with a high incidence of sudden death in amyloidosis patients. Diuretics should be used judiciously to avoid dehydration.

Respiratory Tract Amyloid Deposits. Amyloid deposits can occur at any level of the respiratory tract, from the nasopharynx to the alveolocapillary bed. Respiratory amyloidosis is most prevalent as an isolated organ system involvement or as a component of systemic disease. Amyloid deposits in the upper nasal passages occur as mass lesions with hemorrhage or perforation. Isolated, submucosal accumulations in the vocal cord structures appear as single or multiple nodules and can cause hoarseness. These presentations usually indicate isolated disease restricted to the upper airways, without concomitant systemic amyloidosis.[72]

Five types of lower respiratory tract involvement are recognized:

1. Isolated nodular deposits of the tracheobronchial tree. They may be asymptomatic or may cause hemorrhage and signs of airway obstruction.

2. Diffuse tracheobronchial infiltration. Extensive submucosal deposits may cause wheezing and dyspnea as early manifestations. Chest radiograph

findings are usually normal. This form may be seen as a localized disease or as a component of systemic amyloidosis. Repeated bronchoscopy to remove symptomatic deposits may be necessary.

3. Hilar adenopathy.

4. Isolated nodular pulmonary amyloidosis, either solitary or multiple. Nodules are present in parenchymal tissue and often contain giant cells; these nodules cannot be differentiated radiographically from neoplastic processes. This form of disease is usually asymptomatic, and the prognosis is good with surgical removal of symptomatic nodules.

5. Diffuse pulmonary parenchymal amyloidosis. This form is usually seen with primary amyloidosis and may lead to life-threatening alveolocapillary block within months of detection.

Gastrointestinal Amyloidosis. Any level of the gastrointestinal tract may be affected by amyloid deposition. In the nonhereditary syndromes, gastrointestinal involvement can be found in approximately 50 percent of cases. Gingival and tongue infiltrations are the hallmarks of oral cavity amyloidosis. The tongue is firm to palpation and may be massively enlarged from amyloid deposits. Macroglossia may interfere with speech, deglutition, and respiration (Fig. 82–5).

The hypopharyngeal muscles and voluntary muscles of the upper third of the esophagus are prone to amyloid infiltration. Deposits may impair deglutition and cause pooling of radiographic contrast material in the piriform recess during upper gastrointestinal studies.

Amyloid deposits may also present as tumefaction in the esophagus or as diffuse infiltrates that produce a rigid, aperistaltic segment. Gastric accumulations can result in motility disturbances, hemorrhage, obstruction, achlorhydria, and vitamin B deficiency and can mimic gastric carcinoma. Radiographic findings are nonspecific in gastric amyloidosis, but findings on gastroscopic examination may

be highly suggestive of amyloid infiltration. The finding of amyloid deposits in a biopsy specimen is definitive. Small bowel amyloidosis may present as motility disturbances with diarrhea or constipation, malabsorption (which may be related to motility disorders), hemorrhage, protein-losing enteropathy, perforation, or ischemic necrosis. Radiographic changes are again nonspecific, but biopsy can be diagnostic. Amyloid deposits are most pronounced in the submucosal layer and in the vasculature. Cases of isolated intestinal amyloidosis have been reported.

Hepatic infiltration, which is present in almost 75 percent of cases of generalized, nonhereditary amyloidosis, can produce massive organomegaly but rarely causes portal hypertension or hepatic insufficiency. Liver function test results are usually normal, although sulfobromophthalein sodium retention may be increased, and alkaline phosphatase levels may be mildly elevated. In the rare case of primary amyloidosis, intrahepatic cholestasis with severe jaundice is a poor prognostic sign. Preliminary scintigraphic studies suggest that hepatic uptake of technetium or gallium isotopes may be abnormal in amyloidotic livers and inversely related to the quantity of amyloid deposits. Splenic infiltration may occasionally result in catastrophic splenic rupture.

DIAGNOSIS

Biopsy Sites. The diagnosis of amyloidosis is established by demonstration of the characteristic apple-green birefringence of Congo red–stained tissue specimens under polarization microscopy. Biopsy of virtually any organ can establish this diagnosis. As a general rule, a biopsy should be taken from an organ suspected of being infiltrated with amyloid material. If this cannot be done for any reason, rectal biopsy or abdominal fat pad aspiration[73] (or both) is the preferred technique. Rectal biopsy specimens show amyloid deposits in 75 to 85 percent of cases of generalized amyloidosis if adequate submucosal tissue is obtained for microscopic examination. Percutaneous renal biopsy is also a relatively safe, high-yield diagnostic procedure in amyloidosis. Liver biopsy has produced fatal complications but is generally safe in patients who do not have massive hepatomegaly. Biopsy of bone marrow, small bowel, skin, synovial membrane, and endomyocardium all have been used to diagnose amyloidosis.

Echography, angiography, and scintigraphy are helpful diagnostic adjuncts. After intravenous injection of iodine-123–labeled serum amyloid P component, as much as 95 percent of the specific tracer leaves the plasma, sometimes within minutes, and localizes in amyloid deposits, where it persists for prolonged periods.[74]

Immunologic Studies. All patients with systemic amyloidosis should be evaluated for evidence of an associated plasma cell dyscrasia. Evaluation includes

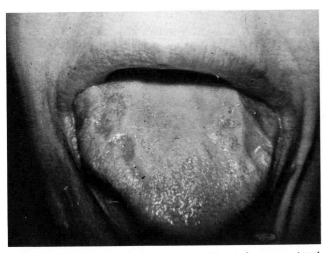

Figure 82–5. Macroglossia in a patient with myeloma-associated amyloidosis.

serum and urine electrophoresis and immunoelectrophoresis. Urine samples are tested unconcentrated and after 50- and 100-fold concentrations. Quantitative serum immunoglobulin assays are also indicated. Bone marrow aspiration and biopsy are performed to exclude multiple myeloma. Bone marrow samples are also cultured for mycobacterial and fungal agents. A skeletal radiographic survey is carried out to search for osteolytic lesions.

TREATMENT

Prognosis. Systemic forms of amyloidosis are almost invariably fatal. Renal failure and cardiac disease are the most frequent causes of death. In primary amyloidosis survival from the time of diagnosis is approximately 14 months.[50] In multiple myeloma–associated amyloidosis, survival may be even shorter, with a recent estimate of 4 months from diagnosis. Prognosis in secondary amyloidosis is dependent on the nature of the underlying disorder as well as the rate of progression of amyloidosis. In several instances in which the underlying disease could be controlled, spontaneous clinical recovery from amyloidosis has been noted.

There are sporadic case reports that suggest that primary amyloidosis occasionally responds to treatment with cytotoxic agents. This improvement may be accompanied by diminution in paraprotein levels. Cytotoxic drugs will sometimes lower paraprotein levels, although the amyloidosis progresses. Kyle and Bayrd[50] observed some improvement in patients with primary amyloidosis receiving melphalan; this has been confirmed in subsequent studies.

Despite promising results in experimental amyloidosis, colchicine has not proved to be an effective therapeutic agent in patients with primary and secondary amyloid disease. On the other hand, more than 90 percent of patients with FMF enjoy a complete remission or a marked amelioration of febrile attacks as long as they take 1 to 2 mg of colchicine daily; in the remainder, the attacks recur even on higher dosage. A recent analysis of more than 1000 patients followed for 4 to 11 years after being advised to take colchicine revealed a prevalence of amyloidosis that was one third of that observed in a comparable population of patients before the use of colchicine.[74] The drug prevented progression in more than half of the patients who had overt amyloidotic nephropathy before the trial commenced.

With respect to FMF, mention should also be made of successful attempts by Mellinkoff and co-workers[75] to reduce the number and severity of febrile episodes by use of a low-fat diet, in which the ratio of saturated to polysaturated fatty acid was reduced. Although this finding has been forgotten or ignored for more than 25 years, it surely requires follow-up in light of recent animal studies in which replacement of corn oil or coconut oil by fish oil resulted in a reduced incidence and severity of secondary amyloi-

dosis, while altering the prostaglandin profile of tissue macrophages.[47] Since fish oil contains eicosapentaenoic acid, the n-3 fatty acid precursor of the relative rare three series of prostaglandins and five series of leukotrienes, a clinical trial using the "Eskimo diet" in patients who are at risk for developing amyloidosis may be warranted.

Supportive Measures. Because amyloidosis may be a fatal disease, the patient and the family should be accorded the necessary professional counseling and psychologic support. A variety of unique problems can be encountered in systemic amyloidosis, and they demand good supportive medical care. Congestive heart failure in amyloidosis does not usually respond to digitalis. In addition, a number of reports document a high incidence of sudden death and cardiac arrhythmia in amyloidosis patients who take digitalis. Digitalis preparations should be administered in a hospital setting when other measures to manage heart failure have proved inadequate. Diuretics must also be used judiciously to avoid dehydration and cardiovascular collapse. Postural hypotension can result from volume depletion (secondary to diuretics, decreased fluid intake, or protein-osmotic diuresis), adrenal insufficiency, autonomic neuropathy, or low-output cardiac failure. Mineralocorticoids can reverse volume depletion from adrenal insufficiency. Elastic stockings may remedy neuropathic hypotension. Malabsorption syndromes, often the result of bacterial overgrowth due to visceral motility disturbances, respond to broad-spectrum antibiotics in many cases. Macroglossia may interfere with deglutition, necessitating supplemental gastrotomy feeding. Compromise of the upper airways by an enlarged tongue may necessitate tracheostomy. Hemorrhagic diatheses caused by isolated factor X deficiency do not respond to fresh-frozen plasma but may respond transiently to factor IX concentrate. Bronchoscopy with curettage of bronchial amyloid deposits can provide significant palliation in some types of respiratory tract amyloidosis.

In treating patients with end-stage renal failure resulting from amyloidosis, the choice is between maintenance dialysis and renal transplantation. The results of maintenance dialysis in such patients are not as good as in patients with nonsystemic diseases. The European experience with 212 hospital dialysis patients showed a cumulative patient survival of 76 percent for all patients at 2 years, compared with 50 percent for diabetic patients, 53 percent for patients with amyloidosis, and 65 percent for patients with SLE. Following renal transplantation in 21 patients, five patients survived for more than 3 years, and of these, one lived for 7 years and two lived for 10 years. Amyloidosis of other organ systems seems to be a slow process and probably does not influence the outcome, although cardiac involvement may be troublesome in older patients. The limiting factor in these patients appears to have been rejection rather than recurrence of amyloid disease, although recurrence did happen in one patient. In recent years, life-threatening complications and deaths after transplantation have been reduced by avoidance of an overly aggressive immunosuppressive regimen, a greater willingness to sacrifice a poorly functioning graft, and the introduction of cyclosporine.

References

1. Cohen, A. S., and Calkins, E.: Electron microscopic observation on a fibrous component in amyloid of diverse origins. Nature 183:1202, 1959.
2. Spiro, D.: The structural basis of proteinuria in man. Electron microscopic studies of renal biopsy specimens from patients with lipid nephrosis, amyloidosis, and subacute and chronic glomerulonephritis. Am. J. Pathol. 35:47, 1959.
3. Glenner, G. G.: Amyloid deposits and amyloidosis. The β-fibrilloses. N. Engl. J. Med. 302:1283, 1980.
4. Glenner, G. G., Terry, W., Harada, M., Iserksy, C., and Page, D.: Amyloid fibril proteins: Proof of homology with immunoglobulin light chains by sequence analysis. Science 172:1150, 1971.
5. Benditt, E. P., Eriksen, N., Hermodson, M. A., and Ericsson, L. H.: The major proteins of human and monkey amyloid substance: Common properties including unusual N-terminal amino acid sequences. FEBS Lett. 19:169, 1971.
6. Levin, M., Franklin, E. C., Frangione, B., and Pras, M.: The amino acid sequence of a major nonimmunoglobulin component of some amyloid fibrils. J. Clin. Invest. 51:2773, 1972.
6a. Sipe, J. D.: Amyloidosis. Annu. Rev. Biochem. 61:947, 1992.
7. Husby, G., Araki, S., Benditt, E., Benson, M. D., Cohen, A. S., Frangione, B., Glenner, G. G., Natvig, J. B., and Westermark, P.: The 1990 guidelines for nomenclature and classification of amyloid and amyloidosis. In Natvig, J. B., Forre, O., Husby, G., Husbebekk, A., Skogen, B., Slatten, K., and Westermark, P. (eds.): Amyloid and Amyloidosis, 1990. Dordrecht, Kluwer Academic Publishers, 1991, p. 7.
8. Glenner, G. G., and Bladen, H. A.: Purification and reconstitution of the periodic fibril and unit structure of human amyloid. Science 154:271, 1966.
9. Cathcart, E. S., Shirahama, T., and Cohen, A. S.: Isolation and identification of a plasma component of amyloid. Biochim. Biophys. Acta 147:392, 1967.
10. Cathcart, E. S., Comerford, F. R., and Cohen, A. S.: Immunologic studies on a protein extracted from human secondary amyloid. N. Engl. J. Med. 273:143, 1965.
11. Hawkins, P. N., Wooton, R., and Pepys, M. B.: Metabolic studies of radioiodinated serum P component in normal subjects and patients with systemic amyloidosis. J. Clin. Invest. 86:1862, 1990.
12. Osmand, A. P., Friedenson, B., Gewurtz, H., Painter, R. H., Hoffman, T., and Shelton, E.: Characterization of C-reactive protein and the complement subcomponent C1t as homologous proteins displaying cyclic pentameric symmetry (pentraxins). Proc. Natl. Acad. Sci. U.S.A. 74:739, 1977.
13. Mantzouranis, E. C., Dowton, S. B., Whitehead, A. S., Edge, M. D., Bruns, G. A., and Colton, H. R.: Human serum amyloid P component cDNA isolation, complete sequence of pre-serum P component, and localization of the gene to chromosome 1. J. Biol. Chem. 2601:7752, 1985.
14. Terry, W. D., Page, D. L., Kimura, S., Isobe, T., Osserman, E. F., and Glenner, G. G.: Structural identity of Bence Jones and amyloid fibril proteins in a patient with plasma cell dyscrasia and amyloidosis. J. Clin. Invest. 52:1276, 1973.
15. Solomon, A., Frangione, B., and Franklin, E. C.: Bence Jones proteins and light chains of immunoglobulins. J. Clin. Invest. 70:453, 1982.
16. Levin, M., Pras, M., and Franklin, E. C.: Immunologic studies of the major nonimmunoglobulin protein of amyloid. Identification and partial characterization of related serum component. J. Exp. Med. 138:373, 1973.
17. Benditt, E. P., and Eriksen, N.: Amyloid protein SAA is associated with high density lipoprotein from human serum. Proc. Natl. Acad. Sci. U.S.A. 74:4205, 1977.
18. Benditt, E. P., Eriksen, N., and Hanson, R. H.: Amyloid protein SAA is an apoprotein of mouse plasma high density lipoprotein. Proc. Natl. Acad. Sci. U.S.A. 76:4092, 1979.
19. Yamamoto, K., Shiroo, M., and Migita, S.: Diverse gene expression for isotypes of murine serum amyloid A during acute phase reaction. Science 232:227, 1986.
20. Mitchell, T. I., Coon, C. I., and Brinkerhoff, C. E.: Serum amyloid A (SAA3) produced by rabbit synovial fibroblasts treated with phorbol esters or interleukin-1 induces synthesis of collagenase and is neutralized with specific antiserum. J. Clin. Invest. 87:1177, 1991.
21. Sletten, K., Westermark, P., and Natvig, J. B.: Characterization of amyloid fibril proteins from medullary carcinoma of the thyroid. J. Exp. Med. 143:993, 1976.
22. Westermark, P., Engstrom, U., Johnson, K. H., Westermark, G. T., and Betsholtz, C.: Islet amyloid polypeptide: Pinpointing amino acid residues linked to amyloid blood formation. Proc. Natl. Acad. Sci. U.S.A. 87:5036, 1990.
23. Andrade, C.: A peculiar form of peripheral neuropathy. Familial atypical generalized amyloidosis with special involvement of the peripheral nerves. Brain 75:408, 1952.
24. Costa, P. P., Figueira, A. S., and Bravo, F. R.: Amyloid fibril protein related to pre-albumin in familial amyloidotic polyneuropathy. Proc. Natl. Acad. Sci. U.S.A. 75:4499, 1978.
24a. Jacobson, D. R., and Buxbaum, J. N.: Genetic aspects of amyloidosis. Adv. Hum. Genet. 20:69, 1991.
25. Nichols, W. C., Dwulet, F. E., Liepniks, J., and Benson, M. D.: Variant apolipoprotein AI as a major constituent of a human hereditary amyloid. Biochem. Biophys. Res. Commun. 156:762, 1988.
26. Maury, C. P.: Gelsolin-related amyloidosis. Identification of amyloid protein in Finnish hereditary amyloidosis as a fragment of variant gelsolin. J. Clin. Invest. 87:1195, 1991.
27. Nordlie, M., Sletten, K. J., Husby, G., and Ranlov, P. J.: A new prealbumin variant in familial amyloid cardiomyopathy of Danish origin. Scand. J. Immunol. 27:119, 1988.
28. Westermark, P., Sletten, K., Johansson, B., and Cornwell, G. G.: Fibril in senile systemic amyloidosis is derived from normal transthyretin. Proc. Natl. Acad. Sci. U.S.A. 87:2843, 1990.
29. Gorevic, P. D., Prelli, F. C., Wright, J., Pras, M., and Frangione, B.: Systemic senile amyloidosis: Identification of a new prealbumin (transthyretin) variant in cardiac tissue. J. Clin. Invest. 83:836, 1989.
30. Kaye, J. C., Butler, M. G., D'Ardenne, A. J., Edmondson, S. J., Camm, A. J., and Slavin, G.: Isolated atrial amyloid contains atrial natriuretic peptide: a report of six cases. Br. Heart J. 56:317, 1986.
31. Glenner, G. G., and Woo, C. W.: Alzheimer's disease and Down's syndrome: Sharing of a unique cerebrovascular amyloid fiber protein. Biochem. Biophys. Res. Commun. 120:885, 1984.
32. Goldgaber, D., Lerman, M. I., McBride, O. W., Saffiotti, U., and Gajdusek, N. C.: Characterization and chromosomal localization of a cDNA probe encoding brain amyloid of Alzheimer's disease. Science 235:877, 1987.
33. Gejyo, F., Yamada, T., Odani, S., Nakagawa, Y., Arakawa, M., Kunitomo, T., Kataoka, H., Suzuki, M., Hirasawa, Y., Shirahama, T., Cohen, A. S., and Schnid, K.: A new form of amyloid protein associated with chronic hemodialysis was identified as beta$_2$-microglobulin. Biochem. Biophys. Res. Commun. 129:701, 1985.
34. Ghiso, J., Jensson, O., and Frangione, B.: Amyloid fibrils in hereditary cerebral hemorrhage with amyloidosis of Icelandic type is a variant of gamma-trace basic protein (cystatin C). Proc. Natl. Acad. Sci. U.S.A. 83:2974, 1986.
35. Levy, E., Carman, M. D., Fernandez-Madrid, I. J., Power, M. D., Lieberburg, I., van Duinen, S. G., Bots, G. T., Luyendijk, W., and Frangione, B.: Mutation of the Alzheimer's disease amyloid gene in hereditary cerebral hemorrhage, Dutch type. Science 248:1124, 1990.
36. Hsiao, K. K., Scott, M., Foster, D., DeArmond, S. J., and Prusiner, S. B.: Spontaneous neurodegeneration in transgenic mice with mutant prion protein. Science 250:1587, 1990.
37. Durie, B. G. M., Persky, B., Soehnlen, B. J., Grogan, T. M., and Salmon, S. E.: Amyloid secretion by associated macrophages. N. Engl. J. Med. 307:1689, 1982.
38. Lavie, G., Zucker-Franklin, D., and Franklin, E. C.: Degradation of serum amyloid protein A by surface-associated enzymes of human blood monocytes. J. Exp. Med. 148:1020, 1978.
39. Silverman, S. L., Cathcart, E. S., Skinner, M., and Cohen, A. S.: The degradation of serum amyloid A protein by activated polymorphonuclear leucocytes: Participation of elastase. Immunology 46:737, 1982.
40. Meek, R. L., Hoffman, J. S., and Benditt, E. P.: Amyloidogenesis: One serum amyloid A isotype is relatively removed from the circulation. J. Exp. Med. 1631:499, 1986.
41. Higuchi, K., Yonezu, T., Tsunasawa, S., Sakiyama, F., and Takeda, T.: The single proline-glutamine substitution of position 5 enhances the potency of amyloid fibril formation of murine apo-AII. FEBS Lett. 207:23, 1986.
42. Kohno, A., Yonezu, T., Matsushita, M., Irino, M., Higuchi, K., Takeshita, S., Hosokawa, M., and Takeda, T.: Chronic food restriction modulates the advance of senescence in the senescence-accelerated mouse (SAM). J. Nutr. 7151:1259, 1985.
43. Smetana, H.: The relation of the reticulo-endothelial system to the formation of amyloid. J. Exp. Med. 45:619, 1927.
43a. Sipe, J. D., Rokita, H., and De Beer, F. C.: Cytokine regulation of the mouse SAA gene family. In Mackiewicz, A., Kushner, I., and Baumann, H. (eds.): Acute Phase Proteins: Molecular Biology, Biochemistry and Clinical Applications. Boca Raton, FL, C.R.C. Press, in press.

44. Wohlgethan, J. R., and Cathcart, E. S.: Amyloid resistance in the A/J mouse is determined by a single gene. Nature 278:453, 1979.

45. Coe, J. E., and Ross, M. J.: Amyloidosis and female protein in the Syrian hamster. Concurrent regulation by sex hormones. J. Exp. Med. 171:1257, 1990.

46. Cathcart, E. S., Leslie, C. A., Meydani, S. N., and Hayes, K. C.: A fish oil diet retards experimental amyloidosis, modulates lymphocyte function and decreases macrophage arachidonate metabolism in mice. J. Immunol. 139:89, 1987.

47. Goate, A., Chartier-Harlin, M. C., Mullan, M., Brown, J., Crawford, F., Fidani, L., Guiffra, L., Haynes, A., Irving, N., James, L., Mant, R., Newton, P., Rooke, K., Roques, P., Talbot, C., Williamson, R., Rossor, M., Owen, M., and Hardy, J.: Segregation of a missense mutation in the amyloid precursor protein gene with familial Alzheimer's disease. Nature 349(21):704, 1991.

48. Yankner, B. A., Duffy, L. K., and Kirschner, D. A.: Neurotrophic and neurotoxic effects of amyloid beta protein: reversal by tachykinin neuropeptides. Science 250(4978):279, 1990.

49. Selkoe, D. J.: Deciphering Alzheimer's disease: The amyloid precursor protein yields new clues. Science 248:1058, 1990.

50. Kyle, R. A., and Bayrd, E. D.: Amyloidosis: Review of 236 cases. Medicine 54:271, 1975.

51. Cathcart, E. S., and Wohlgethan, J. R.: Amyloidosis. In Utsinger, P. D., Zvaifler, N. J., and Ehrlich, G. E. (eds.): Rheumatoid Arthritis. Philadelphia, J. B. Lippincott Co., 1985, p. 495.

52. Ozdemir, A. I., Wright, J. R., and Calkins, E.: Influence of rheumatoid arthritis on amyloidosis of aging. Comparison of 47 rheumatoid patients with 47 controls matched for age and sex. N. Engl. J. Med. 285:534, 1971.

53. Williams, R. C., Jr., Cathcart, E. S., Calkins, E., Fite, G. L., Rubio, J. B., and Cohen, A. S.: Secondary amyloidosis in lepromatous leprosy. Possible relationship of diet and environment. Ann. Intern. Med. 62:1000, 1965.

54. Rukavina, J. G., Block, W. D., Jackson, C. E., Falls, H. F., Carey, J. H., and Curtis, A. C.: Primary systemic amyloidosis: A review and an experimental genetic and clinical study of 29 cases with particular emphasis on the familial form. Medicine 35:239, 1956.

55. Van Allen, M. W., Frolich, J. A., and Davis, J. R.: Inherited predisposition to generalized amyloidosis. Neurology 19:10, 1969.

56. Meretoja, J.: Familial systemic para-amyloidosis with lattice dystrophy of the cornea, progressive cranial neuropathy, skin changes, and various internal symptoms: A previously unrecognized heritable syndrome. Ann. Clin. Res. 1:314, 1969.

57. Heller, H., Gafni, J., Michaeli, D., Shahin, N., Sohar, E., Erlich, G., Karten, I., and Sokoloff, L.: The arthritis of familial Mediterranean fever (FMF). Arthritis Rheum. 9:1, 1966.

58. Meyerhoff, J.: Familial Mediterranean fever. Report of a large family, review of the literature, and discussion of the frequency of amyloidosis. Medicine 59:66, 1980.

59. Muckle, T. J., and Wells, M.: Urticaria, deafness and amyloidosis: A new heredofamilial syndrome. Q. J. Med. 31:235, 1962.

60. Linke, R. P., Heilman, K. L., Nathrath, W. B. J., and Eulitz, M.: Identification of amyloid A protein in a sporadic Muckle-Wells syndrome. N-Terminal amino acid sequence after isolation from formalin-fixed tissue. Lab. Invest. 48:698, 1983.

61. Weiss, S. W., and Page, D. L.: Amyloid nephropathy of Ostertag: Report of a kindred. Birth Defects 10:67, 1974.

62. Frederiksen, T., Getzche, H. J., Harboe, N., Kiaer, W., and Mellangaard, K.: Primary familial amyloidosis with severe amyloid heart disease. Am. J. Med. 33:328, 1962.

63. Wiernik, P. H.: Amyloid joint disease. Medicine 51:465, 1972.

64. Ladefogad, C., and Christensen, H. E.: Congophilic substance with green dichroism in hip joints in autopsy material. Acta Pathol. Microbiol. Scand. (A) 88:55, 1980.

65. Ballou, S. P., Khan, M. A., and Kushner, L.: Diffuse intervertebral disk calcification in primary amyloidosis. Ann. Intern. Med. 85:616, 1976.

66. Takeda, T., Sanada, H., Ishi, M., Matsushita, M., Yamamuro, T., Shimizu, K., and Hosokawa, M.: Age-associated amyloid deposition in surgically removed herniated intervertebral discs. Arthritis Rheum. 27:1063, 1984.

67. Ryan, L. M., Bernhard, G. C., Liang, G., and Kozin, F.: Amyloid arthropathy in the absence of dysproteinemia: A possible association with chondrocalcinosis. Arthritis Rheum. 21:587, 1978.

68. Teglbjaerg, P. S., Ladefogad, C., Sorenson, K. H., and Christensen, H. E.: Local articular amyloid deposition in pyrophosphate arthritis. Acta Pathol. Microbiol. Scand. (A) 87:307, 1979.

69. Assenat, H., Calemard, E., Charra, R., Laurent, G., Terrat, J. C., and Vanel, T.: Hemodialyse, syndrome du canal carpien et substance amyloide. Nouv. Presse Med. 9:1715, 1980.

70. Bardin, T., Zingroff, J., Shirahama, T., Noel, L. H., Droz, D., Voisin, N.-C., Drueko, T., Dryll, A., Skinner, M., Cohen, A. S., and Kuntz, D.: Hemodialysis-associated amyloidosis and β₂-microglobulin: A clinical and immunohistochemical study. Am. J. Med. 83:419, 1987.

71. Duston, M. A., Skinner, M., Shirahama, T., and Cohen, A. S.: Diagnosis of amyloidosis by abdominal fat aspiration. Am. J. Med. 82:412, 1987.

72. Celli, B. R., Rubinow, A., Cohen, A. S., and Brody, J. S.: Patterns of pulmonary involvement in systemic amyloidosis. Chest 74:543, 1978.

73. Stenkvist, B., Westermark, P., and Wibell, L.: Simple method of diagnostic screen for amyloidosis. Ann. Rheum. Dis. 33:75, 1974.

74. Hawkins, P. N., Lavender, J. P., and Pepys, M. B.: Evaluation of systemic amyloidosis by scintigraphy with 123I-labeled serum amyloid P component. N. Engl. J. Med. 323:508, 1990.

75. Mellinkoff, S. M., Snodgrass, R. W., Schwabe, A. D., Mead, J. F., Weimer, H. H., and Frankland, M.: Familial Mediterranean fever. Plasma protein abnormalities, low-fat diet, and possible implications in pathogenesis. Ann. Intern. Med. 56:171, 1962.

Chapter 83

William J. Arnold

Sarcoidosis

INTRODUCTION

Sarcoidosis is a puzzling, multisystem disorder of unknown etiology that primarily affects the lungs and is characterized by the presence of noncaseating granulomas in biopsy specimens from clinically involved or uninvolved organs.[1,2] While predominantly affecting young adults of either sex, sarcoidosis presents most frequently with bilateral hilar adenopathy, pulmonary infiltration, and skin and eye lesions. Peripheral lymphadenopathy, hepatosplenomegaly, cardiac, renal, and skeletal muscle involvement, and bone and joint lesions as well as central and peripheral nervous system involvement may also occur.[3-5] In the United States a higher prevalence of sarcoidosis has been noted in blacks, but individuals of any racial or ethnic origin may be affected. Histologic examination of tissue from patients with sarcoidosis reveals the presence of numerous granulomas composed primarily of epithelioid cells with occasional giant cells in the absence of caseation necrosis.[6,7] However, the earliest lesion found in the lung and also in the joints is an acute inflammatory response characterized as an alveolitis or synovitis. Once formed, the sarcoid granuloma may resolve spontaneously or slowly undergo hyaline fibrosis. Histologically similar granulomas may be found in chronic berylliosis, tuberculosis, histoplasmosis, coccidioidomycosis, lymphoma, Hodgkin's disease, bronchogenic carcinoma, foreign body granuloma, drug reactions, schistosomiasis, syphilis, and leprosy.[1,2]

CLINICAL FEATURES

Pulmonary involvement detected by chest radiograph is found in at least 90 percent of patients with sarcoidosis.[3,4] Bilateral hilar adenopathy with or without parenchymal involvement is the most frequent pulmonary finding. The prognosis of sarcoidosis is best predicted by the roentgenographic stage of the pulmonary disease at the time of diagnosis.[8] In stage 1 disease with only bilateral hilar adenopathy, total resolution occurs in approximately 60 percent of patients. With bilateral hilar adenopathy and pulmonary infiltrates concomitantly present (stage 2), there is a less favorable course with a spontaneous resolution rate of about 46 percent. In stage 3 disease in which there is dense pulmonary fibrosis and bullae often accompanied by pulmonary insufficiency and cor pulmonale, an expected resolution of only about 12 percent is found. The overall mortality in a large series of patients with sarcoidosis from several centers around the world was 6 percent.[4] Approximately 90 percent of the fatalities could be directly related to sarcoidosis.

Skin lesions other than erythema nodosum are asymptomatic and appear as hyperpigmented papules that most commonly occur around the mouth, eyes, ears, and nape of the neck (see Fig. 83–1A). Skin lesions, including erythema nodosum, are found in approximately 30 percent of patients.[3-5]

Eye involvement occurs in approximately 20 percent of patients. Although a wide spectrum of ocular abnormalities can be found, the uveal tract is affected in 75 percent of these patients. Thirteen percent of patients with uveitis may develop total blindness.

IMMUNOLOGY AND BIOCHEMISTRY

The pathogenesis of sarcoidosis is related to heightened immune processes at sites of disease activity.[6,7] During the active phase of the disease, an increased number of T helper lymphocytes are found in the lesions.[9,10] As the lesions become less active, the number of T cells decreases, and these cells are primarily T suppressor cells. Studies using bronchoalveolar lavage (BAL) have shown that the alveolitis of sarcoidosis consists principally of activated T lymphocytes and alveolar monocyte/macrophages.[9] The accumulation and activation of T cells at sites of inflammation are related to interleukin-1 (IL-1) and IL-2 production, with subsequent production of macrophage migration inhibitory factor and monocyte chemotactic factor contributing to the presence of activated macrophages. Most studies of skin and peripheral blood have found depressed indicators of cellular immunity. While cutaneous anergy to purified protein derivative (PPD) occurs in 64 percent of patients with sarcoidosis, anergy to a battery of four antigens (PPD, mumps, *Candida*, streptokinase-streptodornase [SK-SD]) occurs in no more than 20 percent of patients.[11] It is clear that studies of uninvolved tissues, such as peripheral blood, do not reflect the ongoing immune process at the site of sarcoid inflammation.

Several biochemical abnormalities have been described in patients with sarcoidosis. Hypercalcemia and hypercalciuria have been found in 3 to 28 percent of patients with sarcoidosis.[4] In vitro studies of sarcoid granuloma metabolism reveal production of 1,25-dihydroxyvitamin D and angiotensin-converting enzyme (ACE) by cells in the granuloma.[12] Hyperuricemia has been noted in from 10 to 50 percent of patients in whom it has been measured.[13, 14] Although clinical sequelae of hyperuricemia occur rarely in sarcoidosis, it has been reported that several patients have had the triad of gout, psoriasis, and sarcoidosis.[15]

Lieberman first reported elevated levels of serum ACE in patients with sarcoidosis.[16] Elevated levels occurred in 75 percent of patients and appeared to be related to active disease, whereas patients who were in remission or who were receiving steroids had normal ACE levels.[17, 18] Serum ACE levels correlate best with the amount and activity of pulmonary parenchymal involvement in sarcoidosis. The serum ACE level is elevated in most patients with acute or chronic sarcoid arthritis.[19] Although elevated serum ACE levels are found in Gaucher's disease and in leprosy, other diseases that can be confused with sarcoidosis but have normal serum ACE levels include seropositive rheumatoid arthritis (RA), Wegener's granulomatosis, lymphomatoid granulomatosis, and tuberculosis.[18, 20]

Gallium citrate binds to the surface of mononuclear cells at inflammatory sites, and gallium scans are reported to be abnormal in 97 percent of patients with active sarcoidosis.[21] Increased uptake in the pulmonary parenchyma with gallium scanning is significantly correlated with an elevated serum ACE level. Pulmonary gallium accumulation, but not serum ACE levels, correlates with the percentage of lymphocytes in BAL fluid.[22, 23]

It is possible with a high degree of specificity to arrive at a diagnosis of sarcoidosis based on noninvasive testing. Bayesian analysis of asymptomatic patients presenting with persistent bilateral hilar adenopathy has revealed that patients who are ACE positive and PPD negative have a probability of sarcoidosis of 0.95 or greater.[24] While gallium scanning may be useful both to stage the activity and to guide the therapy of sarcoidosis, it has no diagnostic role in this common clinical situation. However, while an abnormal gallium scan is not specific for sarcoidosis, if pulmonary uptake of gallium is accompanied by parotid or lacrimal gland uptake, the diagnosis of sarcoidosis is much more likely.[25] Bronchoscopic or mediastinoscopic biopsy has a limited role in asymptomatic patients who are ACE positive and PPD negative because of limited sensitivity. In patients with asymptomatic bilateral hilar adenopathy who are ACE negative and PPD negative, the probability of lymphoma is high enough to warrant an invasive biopsy.

A genetically determined predisposition to developing sarcoidosis has been noted in certain groups of patients. A significantly increased incidence of HLA-DR5 has been found in an endemic cluster of patients with sarcoidosis in Germany.[26] In addition, an increased incidence of HLA-B8, DR3 in patients with acute arthritis and sarcoidosis has been reported.[27] These observations suggest that both the occurrence and the clinical manifestations of sarcoidosis may be genetically determined.

RHEUMATOLOGIC MANIFESTATIONS

Sarcoid Arthritis

Arthritis is the most frequent rheumatic manifestation of sarcoidosis, occurring in 5 to 37 percent of patients.[14, 27] Sarcoid arthritis is two- to threefold more common in females. Two distinct clinical patterns of sarcoid arthritis have been recognized in adults.[28] The most common form of arthritis occurs acutely and is often the initial manifestation of sarcoidosis. Frequently, erythema nodosum and bilateral hilar adenopathy are associated with arthritis (Löfgren's syndrome). The clinical features of acute sarcoid arthritis are identical in patients with or without erythema nodosum.[29] Acute sarcoid arthritis is best characterized as a symmetric, migratory, additive polyarthritis most frequently involving the knees, ankles, proximal interphalangeal joints, wrists, and elbows. Monoarticular acute sarcoid arthritis is extremely unusual. The arthritis reaches maximal intensity within 3 days of onset and may last from 2 weeks to 4 months. Pain and limitation of motion are the primary signs of inflammation in acute sarcoid arthritis. Synovial effusions are usually minimal. Joint deformity or destruction does not occur in acute sarcoid arthritis.

The erythrocyte sedimentation rate (ESR) and C-reactive protein (CRP) are elevated in 80 and 60 percent of patients with acute sarcoid arthritis, respectively.[14] Approximately 15 percent of the patients will have rheumatoid factor (RF) detected in the serum by either the latex fixation technique or the sheep cell agglutination technique. In one series, hyperuricemia was noted in 25 percent of 24 patients with acute sarcoid arthritis. Chest radiographs of patients with acute sarcoid arthritis reveal bilateral hilar adenopathy, with or without interstitial changes, in more than 90 percent of the patients, while roentgenograms of involved joints reveal only soft tissue swelling.[14, 27]

Synovial biopsies of patients with acute sarcoid arthritis reveal mild inflammation with synovial lining cell hyperplasia.[27] Synovianalysis reveals a mild inflammatory fluid with a predominance of mononuclear cells. These findings are similar to BAL fluid from patients with active pulmonary sarcoidosis. Tendon sheath biopsies from patients with tenosynovitis associated with acute sarcoid arthritis have revealed noncaseating granulomas with multinucleate giant cells.[14]

Sarcoidosis should be suspected in any young adult presenting with acute polyarthritis or periarthritis, particularly in the presence of erythema nodosum. The diagnosis of rheumatoid arthritis is frequently suggested by the symmetric pattern of joint involvement and the finding of rheumatoid factor in the serum. In the early stages of acute sarcoid arthritis, acute rheumatic fever may be considered because of the migratory nature of the arthritis. Histoplasmosis may also present with bilateral hilar adenopathy and joint pain.[30] In this instance, the diagnosis is based on the isolation of Histoplasma capsulatum from blood and bone marrow cultures. Finally, the rapid development of the articular inflammation in a patient with hyperuricemia would raise the possibility of gouty arthritis. The clinical findings of bilateral hilar adenopathy, erythema nodosum, and synovianalysis with polarizing microscopy would differentiate acute sarcoid arthritis from the aforementioned possibilities. Also, the finding of an elevated level of serum ACE and a negative PPD would help confirm the diagnosis of sarcoid arthritis. While other conditions associated with arthritis may also have an elevated level of serum ACE, for example, leprosy, Gaucher's disease, and rarely osteoarthritis, this finding, together with the negative PPD, points to a diagnosis of sarcoid arthritis.[19, 20]

Chronic sarcoid arthritis may begin early or late in the course of the disease and may occur with acute exacerbations of the disease over a period of years. Rarely, chronic sarcoid arthritis may have an insidious onset and produce polyarticular joint destruction and disability, suggestive of the diagnosis of rheumatoid arthritis.[31] In chronic sarcoid arthritis, monoarticular or oligoarticular involvement in the knees and ankles is frequent.[32, 33] The diagnosis of infectious arthritis, particularly tuberculous arthritis and sporotrichosis, should be considered in patients with chronic sarcoid arthritis. Synovial fluid analysis in patients with chronic sarcoid arthritis has revealed characteristics of an inflammatory fluid. Arthroscopy of patients with chronic sarcoid arthritis has demonstrated characteristic very thin and grass-like synovial villi with biopsy specimens revealing sarcoid granulomas with little acute inflammation.[34] Therefore, the diagnosis of infectious arthritis is best excluded by arthroscopy with culture of synovial fluid and biopsy specimens.

In children, sarcoid arthritis begins before age 4 years and is manifested by painless, boggy synovial proliferation and effusions in tendon sheaths and joints.[35] Destructive articular changes and pulmonary disease are also unusual in these children with sarcoid arthritis, though skin and ocular abnormalities occur frequently.

The choice of therapy for sarcoid arthritis will depend on the severity and chronicity of the patient's symptoms. No therapy is indicated for mild, transient arthritis. In patients with moderately severe, acute sarcoid arthritis, therapy with salicylates should be attempted first. A daily total of 3.6 g of aspirin administered in divided doses has been adequate in some patients. Nonsteroidal anti-inflammatory medications may also be used in patients who

are intolerant to aspirin or in whom aspirin therapy is contraindicated. No specific information exists for the effectiveness of any one or other of the nonsteroidal anti-inflammatory agents in patients with sarcoid arthritis. However, treatment with naproxen 1000 to 2000 mg or ibuprofen 2400 to 3600 mg daily in divided doses has been anecdotally effective. Oral colchicine therapy has been reported to be effective in patients with acute or chronic sarcoid arthritis of moderate severity.[28, 36, 37] The same therapy may be effective for sarcoid periarthritis, which is characterized by warm, red, tender areas of skin overlying the joints but not involving the synovium.[38] One colchicine tablet (0.6 mg) should be administered at hourly intervals until relief is obtained or side effects such as diarrhea and nausea and vomiting occur. Although 7 mg of colchicine is the maximum recommended oral dose for an attack, it is of note that as much as 9.6 mg of oral colchicine has been required for relief.[36] In patients with severely symptomatic acute or chronic sarcoid arthritis or patients who have not responded to aspirin or colchicine, prednisone administered orally as a single daily dose of 15 to 40 mg has been effective in suppressing articular inflammation until spontaneous resolution occurs. Long-term therapy with 7.5 to 15 mg of prednisone administered on alternate days may be effective in the treatment of recurrent acute or indolent sarcoid arthritis.

Studies suggest that oral low-dose methotrexate therapy may be effective in controlling pulmonary and extrapulmonary manifestations of sarcoidosis.[39, 40] Theoretically, methotrexate can be most useful in patients with chronic sarcoid arthritis who require steroid therapy. In this situation, therapy with methotrexate (7.5 to 15.0 mg orally once a week) may lower or eliminate the necessity for chronic maintenance prednisone therapy. Anecdotal reports suggest the effectiveness of chloroquine in patients with chronic sarcoid arthritis.

Osseous Sarcoidosis

Bone lesions occur in 3 to 9 percent of patients with sarcoidosis.[3–5, 13, 41] The lesions are frequently asymptomatic and most commonly occur in the bones of the hands and feet.[13, 41] A striking association between the occurrence of bone lesions and chronic skin lesions has been noted[13] (Fig. 83–1A). When osseous sarcoid extensively involves the hands, a diffuse "spongy" thickening of the fingers and thumb may be noted (see Fig. 83–1B). Although radiographic characteristics of osseous sarcoid are variable, lytic lesions are the most common abnormality (see Fig. 83–1C). They may appear as minute cortical defects or cysts in phalangeal or metatarsal heads. Less frequent radiographic changes include thickening of cortical bone with a fine, lacy, reticular alteration of the trabecular pattern, sclerosis of the distal phalanges, or gross destructive changes of

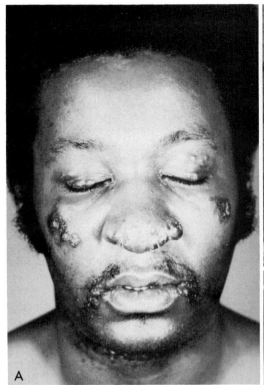

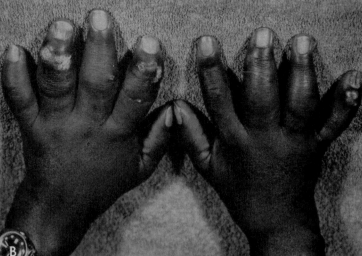

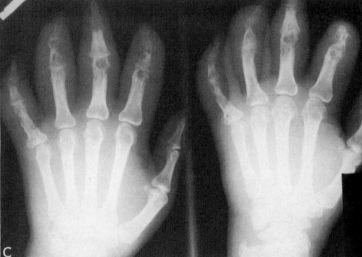

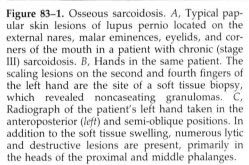

Figure 83–1. Osseous sarcoidosis. *A,* Typical papular skin lesions of lupus pernio located on the external nares, malar eminences, eyelids, and corners of the mouth in a patient with chronic (stage III) sarcoidosis. *B,* Hands in the same patient. The scaling lesions on the second and fourth fingers of the left hand are the site of a soft tissue biopsy, which revealed noncaseating granulomas. *C,* Radiograph of the patient's left hand taken in the anteroposterior (*left*) and semi-oblique positions. In addition to the soft tissue swelling, numerous lytic and destructive lesions are present, primarily in the heads of the proximal and middle phalanges.

bone that may secondarily produce joint destruction. Scanning techniques utilizing technetium (Tc-99m pyrophosphate) may be a more sensitive indicator than routine radiographs for early osseous sarcoidosis.[41]

Although osseous sarcoid is most common in the hands and feet, involvement of the skull, nasal bones, vertebrae, and long bones has been reported. Sarcoid of the skull is perhaps the rarest of all osseous involvements.[42] The lesions appear as multiple lytic defects and may be associated with overlying soft tissue masses that contain granulomas. Vertebral involvement presents radiographically as extensive lytic and sclerotic changes of one or more vertebrae in any area of the spine.[41, 43] Vertebral sarcoidosis may clinically present with either back pain or neurologic deficits resulting from spinal cord compression. Since involvement of the pedicles and disc space may occur, biopsy is needed for definitive diagnosis. Although involvement of long bones is rare, pathologic fractures have been noted secondary to osseous sarcoid. Although lytic lesions are char-

acteristic of osseous sarcoid, osteosclerotic lesions have also been reported.[41]

The diagnosis of osseous sarcoidosis is seldom difficult, since abnormal chest radiographs and chronic skin lesions are also present in greater than 70 percent of these patients. In addition, 54 percent of patients with osseous sarcoid have concomitant ocular abnormalities.

If osseous sarcoidosis is asymptomatic, therapy is not indicated. However, if pain, disability, or deformity is present, the drug of choice for osseous sarcoid at any site appears to be steroids. Documented healing of cystic and destructive lesions has occurred during steroid therapy.[13, 42–44]

Sarcoidosis of Muscle

Skeletal muscle sarcoidosis is usually asymptomatic.[46] First described by Myers and associates, involvement of skeletal muscle in patients with sarcoidosis is reliably detected only by examining serial

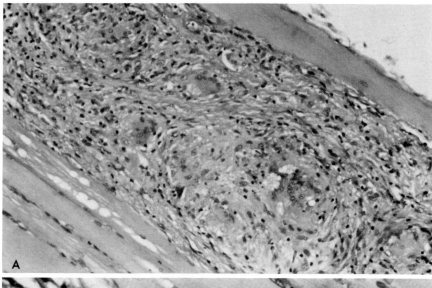

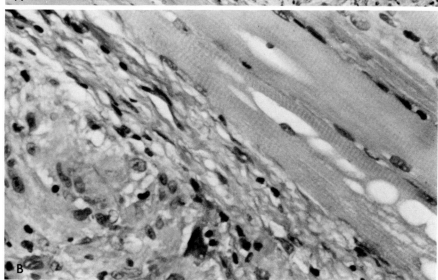

Figure 83–2. Skeletal muscle sarcoidosis. *A,* Longitudinal section of a gastrocnemius muscle biopsy specimen obtained from a patient with stage II sarcoidosis and acute muscle weakness and pain. Multiple noncaseating granulomas with giant cells and a sparse lymphocytic infiltrate are located between apparently normal muscle fibers. (Original magnification × 250.) *B,* Higher magnification demonstrates the epithelioid cells abutting a vacuolated muscle fiber that has retained its cross-striations. (Original magnification × 400.)

sections of generous muscle biopsy specimens.[47] From 50 to 80 percent of muscle biopsy specimens obtained from patients who have had sarcoidosis for less than 2 years will contain typical noncaseating granulomas[46] (Fig. 83–2). Thus, in a patient suspected of having sarcoidosis, a random muscle biopsy specimen may be useful in confirming the diagnosis.

Symptoms of skeletal muscle involvement in patients with sarcoidosis may consist of acute muscle pain and weakness or chronic muscle wasting and weakness.[46–48] Acute skeletal muscle sarcoidosis may be indistinguishable from idiopathic polymyositis, since weakness of proximal muscles is prominent and the electromyogram reveals nonspecific myositis.[49] Elevation of serum muscle enzymes such as CPK is also noted in a majority of patients. Although myopathy could occur as an isolated manifestation of sarcoidosis, the diagnosis is usually obvious because of concomitant multisystem involvement. Rarely, acute skeletal muscle sarcoidosis may be present as tender, palpable muscle nodules or pseu-

dohypertrophy of the calf muscles.[49] Biopsy of these nodules has revealed typical noncaseating granulomas. A puzzling aspect of sarcoidosis of skeletal muscle is the pathogenesis of symptomatic skeletal muscle disease. Since muscle biopsy specimens are similar in both the asymptomatic and the symptomatic forms, factors other than the presence and distribution of noncaseating granulomas must be operative.

Asymptomatic sarcoidosis of skeletal muscle requires no therapy. Administration of steroids to patients with symptomatic muscular sarcoidosis is recommended by most authors, but others have questioned the effectiveness of this therapy. Prednisone in doses of 20 to 30 mg is most effective in acute myopathy but appears to be of little benefit in chronic myopathy.[46]

References

1. Mitchell, D. N., and Scadding, J. G.: Sarcoidosis. Am. Rev. Respir. Dis. 110:774, 1974.

2. Mitchell, D. N., Scadding, J. G., Heard, B. E., and Hinson, K. F.: Sarcoidosis: Histopathological definition and clinical diagnosis. J. Clin. Pathol. 30:395, 1977.

3. Siltzbach, L. E., James, D. G., Neville, E., et al.: Course and prognosis of sarcoidosis around the world. Am. J. Med. 57:847, 1974.

4. James, D. G., Neville, E., Siltzbach, L. E., et al.: A worldwide review of sarcoidosis. Ann. N. Y. Acad. Sci. 278:321, 1976.

5. Neville, E.: Sarcoidosis: The clinical problem. Postgrad. Med. J. 64:531, 1988.

6. Thomas, P. D. and Hunninghake, G. W.: Current concepts of the pathogenesis of sarcoidosis. Am. Rev. Respir. Dis. 135:747, 1987.

7. Van Gundy, K., and Sharma, O. P.: Pathogenesis of sarcoidosis. West. J. Med. 147:168, 1987.

8. Wurm, K., and Rosner, R.: Prognosis of chronic sarcoidosis. Ann. N. Y. Acad. Sci. 278:732, 1976.

9. Hunninghake, G. W., and Crystal, R. G.: Pulmonary sarcoidosis: A disorder mediated by excess helper T-lymphocyte activity at sites of disease activity. N. Engl. J. Med. 305:434, 1981.

10. Crystal, R. G., Roberts, W., Hunninghake, G., et al.: Pulmonary sarcoidosis: A disease characterized and perpetuated by activated lung T-lymphocytes (NIH Conference). Ann. Intern. Med. 94:73, 1981.

11. Tannenbaum, H., Rocklin, R. E., Schur, P. H., and Sheffer, A. L.: Immune function in sarcoidosis. Clin. Exp. Immunol. 26:511, 1976.

12. Mason, R. S., Frankel, T., Chan, Y., et al.: Vitamin D conversion by sarcoid lymph node homogenate. Ann. Intern. Med. 100:59, 1984.

13. Neville, E., Carstairs, L. S., and James, D. G.: Bone sarcoidosis. Ann. N. Y. Acad. Sci. 278:475, 1976.

14. Spilberg, I., Siltzbach, L. E., and McEwen, C. E.: The arthritis of sarcoidosis. Arthritis Rheum. 12:126, 1969.

15. Bunim, J. J., Kimberg, D. V., Thomas, L. B., et al.: Syndrome of sarcoidosis, psoriasis and gout. Ann. Intern. Med. 57:1018, 1962.

16. Lieberman, J.: Elevation of serum angiotensin-converting enzyme (ACE) level in sarcoidosis. Am. J. Med. 59:365, 1975.

17. Rohrback, M. S., and DeRemee, R. A.: Pulmonary sarcoidosis and serum angiotensin-converting enzyme. Mayo Clin. Proc. 57:64, 1982.

18. Katz, P., Fauci, A. S., Yeager, H., and Reen, B.: Serum angiotensin-converting enzyme and lysozyme in granulomatous disease of unknown cause. Ann. Intern. Med. 94:359, 1981.

19. Sequeira, W., and Stinar, D.: Serum angiotensin-converting enzyme levels in sarcoid arthritis. Arch. Intern. Med. 146:125, 1986.

20. Lieberman, J., Nosal, A. D., Schleissner, L. A., et al.: Serum angiotensin-converting enzyme for diagnosis and therapeutic evaluation of sarcoidosis. Am. Rev. Respir. Dis. 120:329, 1979.

21. Gupta, R., Bekerman, C., Sicilian, L., et al.: Gallium 67 citrate scanning and serum angiotensin-converting enzyme levels in sarcoidosis. Radiology 144:895, 1982.

22. Rossman, M. D., Dauber, J. H., Cardello, M. E., and Daniele, R. P.: Pulmonary sarcoidosis: Correlation of serum angiotensin-converting enzyme with blood and bronchoalveolar lymphocytes. Am. Rev. Respir. Dis. 125:266, 1982.

23. Line, B. R., Hunninghake, G. W., Keogh, B. A., et al.: Gallium 67 scanning to stage the alveolitis of sarcoidosis: Correlation with clinical studies, pulmonary function studies and bronchoalveolar lavage. Am. Rev. Respir. Dis. 124:440, 1981.

24. Carr, P. L., Singer, D. E., Goldenheim, P., et al.: Noninvasive testing of asymptomatic bilateral hilar adenopathy. J. Gen. Intern. Med. 5:138, 1990.

25. Wiener, S. N., and Patel, B.: ^{67}Ga-citrate uptake by the parotid glands in sarcoidosis. Nucl. Med. 130:753, 1979.

26. Nowack, D., and Goebel, K. M.: Genetic aspects of sarcoidosis. Arch. Intern. Med. 147:481, 1987.

27. Kremer, J. M.: Histologic findings in siblings with acute sarcoid arthritis: Association with the B8, DR3 phenotype. J. Rheumatol. 13:593, 1986.

28. Kaplan, H.: Sarcoid arthritis. Arch. Intern. Med. 112:924, 1963.

29. Pennec, Y., Youinou, P., LeGoff, P., et al.: Comparison of the manifestations of acute sarcoid arthritis with and without erythema nodosum. Scand. J. Rheumatol. 11:13, 1982.

30. Thornberry, D. K., Wheat, L. J., Brandt, K. D., and Rosenthal, J.: Histoplasmosis presenting with joint pain and hilar adenopathy. Arthritis Rheum. 25:1396, 1982.

31. Boyd, R. E., and Andrews, B. S.: Sarcoidosis presenting as cutaneous ulceration, subcutaneous nodules and chronic arthritis. J. Rheumatol. 8:311, 1981.

32. Turek, S. L.: Sarcoid disease of bone at the ankle joint. J. Bone Joint Surg. 35:465, 1953.

33. Bjarnason, D. F., Forrester, D. M., and Swezey, R. L.: Destructive arthritis of the large joints. J. Bone Joint Surg. 55:618, 1973.

34. Scott, D. G. I., Porto, L. O. R., Lovell, C. R., and Thomas, G. O.: Chronic sarcoid synovitis in the caucasian: An arthroscopic and histological study. Ann. Rheum. Dis. 40:121, 1981.

35. Rosenberg, A. M., Yee, E. H., and MacKenzie, J. W.: Arthritis in childhood sarcoidosis. J. Rheumatol. 10:987, 1983.

36. Kaplan, H.: Sarcoid arthritis with a response to colchicine. N. Engl. J. Med. 263:778, 1960.

37. Kaplan, H.: Further experience with colchicine in the treatment of sarcoid arthritis. N. Engl. J. Med. 268:761, 1963.

38. Harris, E. D., Jr., and Millis, M.: Treatment with colchicine of the periarticular inflammation associated with sarcoidosis: A need for continued appraisal. Arthritis Rheum. 14:130, 1971.

39. Lower, E. E., and Baughman, R. P.: The use of low dose methotrexate in refractory sarcoidosis. Am. J. Med. Sci. 299(3):153, 1990.

40. Toews, G. B., and Lynch, J. P. III: Editorial commentary: Methotrexate in sarcoidosis. Am. J. Med. Sci. 300:33, 1990.

41. Sartoris, D. J., Resnick, D., Resnik, C., and Yaghimai, I.: Musculoskeletal manifestations of sarcoidosis. Semin. Roentgenol 20:376, 1985.

42. Franco-Saenz, R., Ludwig, G. D., and Henderson, L. W.: Sarcoidosis of the skull. Ann. Intern. Med. 72:929, 1970.

43. Baldwin, D. M., Roberts, J. G., and Croft, H. E.: Vertebral sarcoidosis. J. Bone Joint Surg. 56:629, 1974.

44. Schriber, R. A., and Firooznia, H.: Extensive phalangeal cystic lesions—limited sarcoidosis. Arthritis Rheum. 18:123, 1975.

45. Wolfe, S. M., Pinals, R. S., Aelion, J. A., and Goodman, R. E.: Myopathy in sarcoidosis: Clinical and pathologic study of four cases and review of the literature. Semin. Arthritis Rheum. 16:300, 1987.

46. Myers, G. B., Gottlieb, A. M., Mattman, P. E., et al.: Joint and skeletal muscle manifestations in sarcoidosis. Am. J. Med. 12:161, 1952.

47. Chapelon, C., Ziza, J. M., Piette, J. C., et al.: Neurosarcoidosis: Signs, course and treatment in 35 confirmed cases. Medicine. 69:261, 1990.

48. Jamal, M. M., Cilursu, A. M., and Hoffman, E. L.: Sarcoidosis presenting as acute myositis. Report and review of the literature. J. Rheumatol. 15:1868, 1988.

49. Matteson, E. L., and Michet, C.: Sarcoid myositis with pseudohypertrophy. Am. J. Med. 87:240, 1989.

Chapter 84
Iron Storage Disease

R. Elaine Lambert
James L. McGuire

INTRODUCTION

Disorders of iron overload have been recognized for more than a hundred years, beginning with Trousseau in 1865, who described an association of diabetes, cirrhosis, pancreatic fibrosis, and skin pigmentation.[1] By 1889, von Recklinghausen termed this clinical syndrome as hemochromatosis and established that the increased tissue pigment was iron.[2] Sheldon's classic monograph of 1935, which included a detailed review of 311 published cases, provided the evidence that hemochromatosis was a hereditary disease of iron overload resulting in multiple organ involvement.[3] Forty years later, Simon and colleagues provided firm evidence for genetic transmission of the disease by establishing an association between human leukocyte antigen (HLA) alleles and phenotypic disease expression.[4]

Iron storage diseases may be divided into genetic hemochromatosis (previously primary or idiopathic) and secondary iron overload states. Genetic hemochromatosis is an autosomal recessive disease characterized by inappropriately high intestinal iron absorption resulting in the pathologic deposition of iron in parenchymal cells of many organs. Secondary iron overload refers to a variety of conditions associated with increased iron availability from parenteral or oral routes, ineffective erythropoiesis, or inherited defects[5] (Table 84–1). Hemosiderosis is a term used by pathologists to describe excessive iron stain in tissues without regard to underlying etiology or to the specific target cell involved.[5]

ETIOLOGY

In genetic hemochromatosis, the excess iron is deposited in parenchymal cells with relatively little uptake by the reticuloendothelial system (RES).[6] In secondary iron overload, especially when parenterally administered, large amounts of iron are found within the RES cells, with variable deposition in other organ tissues.[5] Patients with the dyserythropoietic anemias, e.g., thalassemia major and sideroblastic anemias, may demonstrate at an early age a pattern of organ involvement indistinguishable from genetic hemochromatosis.[7] The possibility has been suggested that patients with idiopathic refractory sideroblastic anemia and pathogenic iron overload share at least one allele for genetic hemochromatosis.[8]

Patients with alcoholic cirrhosis with secondary iron overload may be difficult to distinguish from patients with genetic hemochromatosis. Both may have hepatomegaly, hypogonadism, carbohydrate intolerance, increased pigmentation, and increased intestinal iron absorption in association with elevated plasma ferritin concentrations and transferrin saturations. In comparison to genetic hemochromatosis, the histologic examination in alcoholic cirrhosis demonstrates less overall hemosiderin and a predominance of the iron stain within the Kupffer cells rather than in the parenchymal cells.[9] The excess hepatic iron found in alcoholic cirrhosis rarely exceeds 3 g, as compared with the total pool of 15 to 35 g of iron in hemochromatosis.[10]

The development of marked siderosis from excessive absorption of medicinal or dietary iron is distinctly rare. However, certain groups of black South Africans absorb excessive exogenous iron from the leaching of this metal from drums used in brewing alcoholic drinks.[10a] The iron-containing beverage produced has a low pH, thus making the iron more bioavailable than usual.[9]

About 75 percent of patients with porphyria cutanea tarda (PCT) have excessive stainable iron in the liver.[11] In PCT, heterozygosity for genetic hemo-

Table 84–1. CAUSES OF IRON STORAGE DISEASE

Genetic or hereditary hemochromatosis (primary, idiopathic)
Secondary iron overload
  Anemia due to ineffective erythropoiesis
    Thalassemia major
    Sideroblastic anemias
  Chronic liver disease
    Alcoholic cirrhosis
    Postportacaval shunt
  Increased oral intake of iron
    African dietary iron overload (Bantu siderosis)
    Medicinal iron ingestion
  Other inherited or congenital defects
    Porphyria cutanea tarda
    Congenital atransferrinemia
    Neonatal iron overload (idiopathic perinatal
      hemochromatosis)
  Parenteral iron loading
    Transfusional iron overload
    Excessive parenteral iron
    Associated with hemodialysis

Adapted from Tavill, A. S., and Bacon, B. R.: Hemochromatosis: Iron metabolism and the iron overload syndromes. *In* Zakim, D., and Boyer, T. D. (eds.): Hepatology: A Textbook of Liver Disease. Vol. 2, 2nd ed. Philadelphia, W. B. Saunders Company, 1990, p. 1274.

chromatosis may also be responsible for the associated iron overload and clinical expression of disease. The presence of the HLA-A3 haplotype is variable in PCT and the role of the yet to be identified hemochromatosis allele in this disorder remains controversial.[12, 13] Other rare congenital iron storage disorders include transferrin deficiency or atransferrinemia[14] and neonatal iron overload in which liver damage begins in utero.[15] Hemodialysis patients may be predisposed to severe hemosiderosis from repeated transfusions, chronic iron administration, hematologic abnormalities, as well as the concomitant presence of heterozygosity for genetic hemochromatosis.[16]

NORMAL IRON METABOLISM

In order to understand the altered iron metabolism in hemochromatosis, it is necessary to review normal iron metabolism. The average total body iron content is 3 to 4 g in an adult; approximately 60 percent is present as hemoglobin, 10 percent as myoglobin, 5 percent in other proteins and enzymes, and the remaining 25 percent is distributed in the storage proteins, ferritin and hemosiderin. Ferritin is the primary and most readily available iron storage protein. It is composed of an apoferritin spheric shell in which variable amounts of iron can be stored in the form of hydrated ferric oxide. Serum ferritin concentration directly reflects reticuloendothelial ferritin. As the intracellular level increases, ferritin is taken up by secondary lysosomes then denatured and hydrolyzed into relatively inert hemosiderin deposits. Despite being poorly soluble, hemosiderin can be slowly mobilized under certain circumstances.[5]

Only about 7 mg of iron is distributed within the extracellular fluid with 50 percent (3.5 mg) being bound to the primary transport protein in plasma, transferrin.[5] This single polypeptide has two iron binding sites.[17] Normally, 20 to 50 percent of transferrin is saturated with iron. Absolute levels of transferrin increase during iron deficiency and decrease during iron overload. Cellular uptake of iron involves binding of the iron-transferrin complex to specific transferrin receptors and internalization by endocytosis. Once the iron is released from its carrier protein within the endocytic vesicle, both the receptor and transferrin are recycled intact to the cell surface.[18]

The typical Western diet contains 10 to 20 mg of iron a day. Usually 1 to 2 mg of iron is absorbed daily by the duodenal mucosa, which balances the loss of iron from exfoliated gastrointestinal mucosal cells.[5] Iron homeostasis is maintained by control of intestinal iron absorption, since there is no effective physiologic mechanism to alter excretion once absorption is deranged.[10]

PATHOGENESIS

Genetic hemochromatosis is characterized by continued inappropriate gastrointestinal iron absorption in the face of expanded iron stores. Excess absorption usually ranges from 1 to 3 mg of iron per day, which results in a total accumulated pool of 15 to 35 g of iron over a 35- to 60-year period.[10] No consistent abnormality in the function of transferrin, its receptor, or ferritin has been found in hemochromatosis. Moreover, the genes for these proteins are located on chromosome 3 rather than chromosome 6, where the gene for hemochromatosis has been mapped.[19–21] In genetic hemochromatosis, levels of duodenal epithelial cell ferritin are inappropriately low[22] and regulation of the transferrin receptor is aberrant.[23] This failure in duodenal cell iron regulation may result in inappropriate iron absorption.

The precise mechanisms by which chronic iron overload leads to tissue injury are not known. Several have been proposed including: (1) increased lysosomal fragility, (2) iron-induced lipid peroxidation of organelle membranes other than lysosomes, and (3) a direct effect of iron on collagen biosynthesis, which leads to fibrosis.[24, 24a]

The hereditary nature of hemochromatosis was confirmed by studies demonstrating a close association with HLA-A3.[4] Subsequent pedigree studies also revealed an increased prevalence of HLA-B7 and HLA-B14 in patients with hemochromatosis.[25, 26] The association of HLA-A3, B7, and B14 with the disease has been explained by the linkage of the hemochromatosis locus with the major histocompatibility locus on chromosome 6.[4, 27] The hemochromatosis locus has been mapped to within 1 centimorgan of HLA-A.[27] Essentially all cases of genetic hemochromatosis result from a recessive HLA-linked gene, and thus it is possible to identify a homozygous haplotype for hemochromatosis once a proband case has been identified and HLA-typed. The homozygous state may occur in 1 per 400 individuals in white populations.[28] Heterozygotes for the hemochromatosis gene may have mild iron overload but typically have no clinical disease.[27] Thus, genetic testing allows the identification of asymptomatic homozygotes with the aim to treat prophylactically prior to the development of overt disease.

In joints as well as the other various target organs of hemochromatosis, tissue damage reflects both the amount and duration of iron deposition. The arthropathy of hemochromatosis is characterized by hemosiderin deposition found in synovium and chondrocytes.[29, 30] The presence of iron in these synthetic cells may lead to altered production of critical enzymes or substrates. For example, in the rabbit models of iron-induced arthritis, ferric iron can result in deficient collagen formation by irreversibly oxidizing ascorbic acid, which impairs proline hydroxylation.[31] Additionally, synovial fibroblasts incubated with iron have been reported to have increased production of collagenase and prostaglandin E_2.[32] Ferritin may also function as a source of iron for the promotion of superoxide-dependent lipid peroxidation, which can contribute to joint damage.[33]

Synovial hemosiderosis is not specific for disorders of iron storage. In rheumatoid arthritis, super-oxide production is increased, and iron deposition is found within macrophages localized to the area of greatest damage.[34] Chondrocalcinosis due to calcium pyrophosphate dihydrate (CPPD) or apatite deposition is a frequent finding in the arthropathy of hemochromatosis.[30, 35] Iron, as ferrous ions, inhibits synovial tissue pyrophosphatase in vitro.[35] Inhibition of this enzyme in vivo could lead to CPPD crystal formation. Additionally, the clearance of CPPD crystals from joints is inhibited in experimental synovial siderosis.[36] However, these data do not account for the progressive CPPD deposition that has occurred despite effective iron depletion by phlebotomy in some cases of hemochromatosis. Articular damage may result from iron-mediated alteration of mucopolysaccharide (proteoglycans) complexes[37] or increased lipid peroxidation resulting in membrane and lysosomal damage.[24]

CLINICAL FEATURES

Extra-articular Features

Typically, the clinical manifestations of genetic hemochromatosis appear between the age of 40 and 60, which corresponds to the 20- to 30-fold expansion of total body iron. Symptomatic disease develops at a ratio of approximately 8:1, male to female.[38] The under-representation of women has been attributed to the extra loss of iron through menstruation and pregnancies in addition to lower dietary iron intake. The pattern of organ development in hemochromatosis does not follow a predictable sequence, and the classic triad of cirrhosis, diabetes mellitus, and pigmentation (i.e., bronze diabetes) rarely occur together and are late complications.[10, 38a]

The common target organs in iron storage disease are liver, pancreas, heart, skin, joints, and pituitary. Table 84–2 lists the frequency of clinical symptoms and signs at the time of diagnosis in 163 patients with genetic hemochromatosis.[38] The liver is typically involved because it is a major site of iron storage. In addition to the hemosiderin granule deposition, hepatocyte degeneration and varying degrees of fibrosis are characteristically observed. In advanced disease, macronodular cirrhosis may be present. A strong association between heavy alcohol intake and the development of genetic hemochromatosis has long been recognized,[1, 3] possibly related to the synergistic effect of alcohol and iron on lipid peroxidation.[39] The incidence of hepatocellular carcinoma in genetic hemochromatosis is increased 200-fold.[40] Typically, hepatocellular carcinoma occurs only in cirrhotic livers, though its incidence is not altered despite successful phlebotomy therapy.[38, 41]

Hyperpigmentation of the skin is related to increased deposition of melanin and dermal iron. Coloration can vary from slate gray to brown and is most prominent in exposed areas, external genitalia, nipple areola, and flexion folds.[10] Diabetes usually

Table 84–2. FREQUENCY OF CLINICAL FEATURES AT THE TIME OF DIAGNOSIS IN PATIENTS WITH GENETIC HEMOCHROMATOSIS

	Percentage of Patients
Symptoms	
Weakness, lethargy	83
Abdominal pain	58
Diabetes mellitus	55
Arthralgia	43
Loss of libido or potency	38
Amenorrhea, secondary	22
Dyspnea on exertion	15
Neurologic symptoms*	6
Physical Findings	
Hepatomegaly	83
Pigmentation	75
Arthritis†	30
Loss of body hair	20
Splenomegaly	13
Peripheral edema	12
Jaundice	10
Gynecomastia	8
Ascites	6

*Disorientation, depression, marked lethargy, and hearing loss.
†Demonstrated by premature osteoarthritis, metacarpophalangeal joint degeneration, calcium pyrophosphate dihydrate deposition disease.[59–62]
Adapted from Niederau, C., Fischer, R., Sonnenberg, A., et al.: Survival and causes of death in cirrhotic and in noncirrhotic patients with primary hemochromatosis. N. Engl. J. Med. 313:1256, 1985. Reprinted with permission from the *New England Journal of Medicine*.

results from insulin depletion, although resistance to insulin can also occur. In the pancreas, iron is selectively deposited in islet beta cells, which impairs insulin but not glucagon secretion.[42, 43] The insulin resistance observed in some cases of hemochromatosis is likely caused by impaired hepatic insulin degradation due to iron accumulation in hepatocytes.[44] Cardiac involvement in hemochromatosis typically presents as a dilated cardiomyopathy with associated dysrhythmia and heart failure.

Impotence and loss of libido are often prominent symptoms in patients with hemochromatosis. Iron deposition in gonadotropic cells of the pituitary leads to deficient gonadotropin secretion with resultant testicular atrophy and low testosterone levels in affected men.[44] Secondary amenorrhea has been described in women with hemochromatosis.[38, 45] In some patients who have both diabetes and cirrhosis, the hypogonadism may be multifactorial.[46]

Osteoporosis has been described in patients with hemochromatosis, especially if hypogonadism is present.[47, 48] Both trabecular and cortical bone can be lost. Despite low serum 25-hydroxyvitamin D levels in hypogonadal males with hemochromatosis, osteomalacia is not found.[48, 50] Hypogonadal men not receiving phlebotomy tend to develop the lowest bone density. However, untreated eugonadal men also have diminished bone formation rates by bone histomorphometry when compared with eugonadal men undergoing treatment. In hypogonadal patients, parameters of bone resorption are elevated with inappropriately low bone formation measures. These findings suggest eugonadal untreated males have impaired osteoblastic activity, likely due to excess iron, whereas hypogonadal untreated males have the additional factor of increased resorption due to low testosterone levels.[48] Indeed, bone mineral density can be improved in some hypogonadal men with hemochromatosis by treatment with both phlebotomy and testosterone.[51]

Although there are sporadic case reports of increased susceptibility to infection in hemochromatosis, in general, infections do not constitute a major clinical problem in the disease.[52] Infections with organisms such as *Yersinia, Vibrio,* and *Listeria* have been described in diseases of iron overload.[53-55] Vertebrate hosts have evolved means of acquiring and transporting iron that effectively deprive invading organisms from access to this essential element. Thus, the increased bioavailability of iron in hemochromatosis may allow for accelerated bacterial growth and metabolism.[56] Alternatively, iron has an immunoregulatory role, as observed in various studies of iron overload, which could influence an affected host's ability to combat infection or neoplasm.[52]

Articular Features

The arthropathy of genetic hemochromatosis has been recognized as an increasingly important feature of the disease. Arthritis is present in 50 percent or more of cases of hemochromatosis[57-59] and may be the initial symptom in as many as one third of cases.[59-62] Moreover, the extent of articular disease does not correlate with severity of other organ involvement in hemochromatosis.[58, 62] The spectrum of joint disease ranges from arthralgia to symmetric polyarticular arthritis, although unilateral disease has also been described.[61, 63] Joint symptoms predominate in the hands and wrists, but knees, hips, feet, and shoulders are also common areas of involvement.[62] Progressive degenerative arthropathy with joint space narrowing, subchondral sclerosis, and cyst formation at these joints is typical of hemochromatosis.

Chondrocalcinosis has been found in 20 to 50 percent of patients diagnosed with hemochromatosis.[57, 59, 64] The location of chondrocalcinosis in hemochromatosis is primarily in the hands and wrists. Deposition in the triangular fibrocartilage above the ulnar styloid and in the metacarpal phalangeal (MCP) joints is most characteristic.[65] Widespread chondrocalcinosis may also be present in elbows, shoulders, hips, knees, ankles, feet, symphysis pubis, intervertebral discs, and periarticular soft tissues. Typically, chondrocalcinosis in hemochromatosis is associated with calcium pyrophosphate dihydrate (CPPD) or hydroxyapatite crystals. However, crystals and articular damage have been demonstrated in some joints without obvious chondrocalcinosis by radiography.[30]

The degenerative arthropathy of hemochroma-

tosis is quite similar to that of pyrophosphate arthropathy and osteoarthritis. However, the proclivity to affect MCP joints and wrists is not typical of osteoarthritis.[65] Idiopathic CPPD arthropathy and the arthropathy in hemochromatosis both commonly affect the index and middle MCP joints (so called victory or peace sign designating involvement of those MCP joints) leading to symmetric joint space narrowing, subchondral cysts, sclerosis, and squaring of the metacarpal heads. Furthermore, hemochromatosis may be distinguished from idiopathic CPPD deposition disease by: (1) the severity of MCP joint involvement, (2) likely involvement of ring and little finger MCP joints, (3) increased prevalence of hook-or beak-like osteophytes on the radial aspect of metacarpal heads, (4) minimal radiocarpal joint space narrowing, (5) presentation at an earlier age, and (6) association with juxta-articular osteopenia (Fig. 84–1).[65, 66]

The arthropathy of hemochromatosis often results in pain and stiffness prior to objective enlargement of the joint. Final stages include limitation of movement, increased pain with use, progressive deformity, and bony spur formation. Synovial thick-

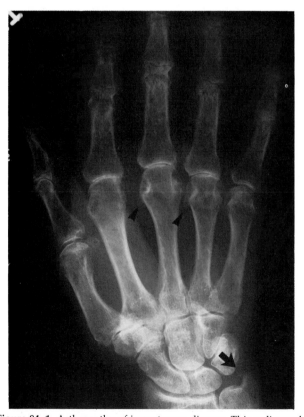

Figure 84–1. Arthropathy of iron storage disease. This radiograph demonstrates advanced arthritis present in a 66-year-old man with genetic hemochromatosis. Note the joint space narrowing and subchondral sclerosis of the metacarpophalangeal joints and hook-like osteophytes of the metacarpal heads (*arrowheads*), most pronounced in the index and middle fingers. Subtle chondrocalcinosis is present in the triangular fibrocartilage above the ulnar styloid (*arrow*).

ening, warmth, and erythema are characteristically absent. The joint effusions are noninflammatory unless acute inflammation due to CPPD or hydroxyapatite crystals occurs.[62] The involvement of MCP joints and occasional finding of subcutaneous nodules may lead to the erroneous diagnosis of rheumatoid arthritis (RA). However, the radiographic appearance as described before is atypical for RA, and the histopathology of the nodules demonstrates iron deposition within noncaseating granulomata.[59, 67, 68]

The patient who presents with unexplained chondrocalcinosis, premature osteoarthritis (<50 years old), or degenerative changes in MCP joints warrants an evaluation for hemochromatosis as well as for other diseases associated with CPPD deposition disease such as hypothyroidism, hyperparathyroidism, acromegaly, Wilson's disease, ochronosis, gout, or diabetes mellitus (see Chapter 77).

LABORATORY FEATURES

When the diagnosis of hemochromatosis is suspected, transferrin saturation and serum ferritin levels are useful screening tests. Normally, the percentage saturation of transferrin, calculated by dividing serum iron concentration by total iron-binding capacity, is 20 to 50 percent. In homozygotes with overt hemochromatosis, transferrin saturation is typically 80 to 100 percent.[5] In general, serum ferritin concentration is an accurate peripheral measure of iron stores, although acute liver injury, systemic inflammation, and neoplasia may also increase ferritin levels. Normal levels of ferritin are 20 to 300 ng per ml in men and 15 to 250 ng per ml in women, whereas levels greater than 500 ng per ml are typically found in symptomatic hemochromatosis.[5] The combination of an increased serum ferritin level and transferrin saturation of greater than 50 percent is approximately 95 percent sensitive and 85 percent specific for the diagnosis of genetic hemochromatosis.[69] Previously the measurement of urinary excretion of iron following injection of the chelator protein deferoxamine was used for screening but has been largely discarded in favor of more direct methods.[5]

Other laboratory tests may be abnormal in patients with hemochromatosis, depending on the severity of their disease. These include hyperglycemia, hepatic transaminase elevation, hypoalbuminemia, elevated alkaline phosphatase, and hyperbilirubinemia.[9]

The definitive diagnosis of hemochromatosis is made by the direct measurement of iron in a liver biopsy specimen. The extent of Prussian blue granule deposition for the identification of iron is used as a screening test and can identify the predominant cellular distribution of this metal. However, quantitative biochemical iron concentration using colorimetric or atomic absorption should also be employed.[5] As emphasized earlier, the distribution of stainable iron in genetic hemochromatosis is primarily located in the hepatocytes, whereas in alcoholic cirrhosis, iron is most prominent within the Kupffer cells.[9] The hepatic iron index, calculated by dividing hepatic iron by age, has predictive value in distinguishing homozygotes for the hemochromatosis gene from heterozygotes. It also allows for the differentiation of those patients with other liver diseases associated with increased hepatic iron, e.g., alcoholic siderosis, from patients with hemochromatosis.[70–72] The measurement of stainable hepatic iron using a microcomputerized image analysis has demonstrated a linear relationship to biochemical iron measurements. This rapid method can be accurately applied to liver biopsies, that were previously obtained and embedded in paraffin.[73] A liver biopsy can also document the extent of hepatic injury, which has prognostic value with respect to future risk of hepatocellular carcinoma.

Noninvasive hepatic imaging procedures have been proposed as alternative means of estimating the degree of iron overload in iron storage diseases. Both single- and dual-energy computed tomography (CT) may produce an increased liver attenuation coefficient that correlates with increased liver iron content.[74, 75] Although not yet widely available, dual energy CT results in the most accurate estimates of hepatic iron.[75–77] Magnetic susceptometry also appears to provide a reliable estimate of iron levels in small areas of liver but requires a specially designed superconducting-quantum-interference device, which limits its clinical availability.[78] With magnetic resonance (MR) imaging, a decrease in hepatic signal intensity occurs in presence of iron overload as shown by alterations in magnetic relaxation rates (Fig. 84–2).[79, 80] Among MR imaging measurements to determine iron overload, the ratio of second echo signal intensities of liver to paraspinous muscle is the most sensitive and specific.[77] Magnetic resonance imaging may also identify extrahepatic iron deposition in spleen, pancreas, lymph nodes, pituitary, and heart.[80, 81] The degree of correlation between single-energy CT and MR imaging with hepatic iron concentration is currently insufficient to permit prediction of hepatic iron content by these noninvasive studies alone.[77] However, these imaging techniques may be useful in patients in whom liver biopsy is contraindicated or in patients with known hemochromatosis who need to be monitored for the development of hepatocellular carcinoma or extrahepatic iron deposition.[28, 77, 81]

The synovial fluid is typically noninflammatory except in patients who develop acute inflammation due to associated CPPD or hydroxyapatite deposition disease. The synovium obtained at arthroplasty may demonstrate mild to moderate cellular proliferation, minimal to no inflammation, and occasional intracellular hemosiderin deposits.[62]

Screening

Screening of patients for hemochromatosis is aimed at making the diagnosis in the precirrhotic

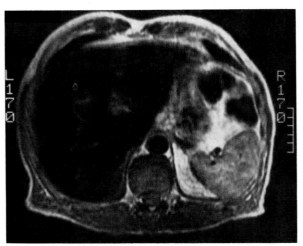

Figure 84–2. Magnetic resonance imaging in iron storage disease. This MR image is a coronal section of the abdomen of a 58-year-old man with genetic hemochromatosis who presented with CPPD arthropathy of his wrists and ankles, transferrin saturation 95 percent, and serum ferritin level 1494 ng per ml. This figure demonstrates the very low signal intensity of the liver consistent with the paramagnetic effects of excess iron deposition, which was quantitatively measured on a liver biopsy specimen as an iron concentration of 21,903 μg per g dry weight. The patient required 70 phlebotomized units to normalize his serum ferritin level. The MR image was obtained at 1.5 Tesla with echo time 20 msec and repetition time of 800 msec. (Courtesy of Dr. Lester Miller, Santa Cruz, California.)

and presymptomatic stage. Phlebotomy initiated early in the course of the disease can prevent progression and decrease mortality. Most patients with hemochromatosis do not become symptomatic until after age 40; thus, the optimal group to screen with biochemical studies would be young, asymptomatic, white adults.[28] Several studies of general populations in Sweden, England, and Australia using transferrin saturation or ferritin levels or both identified hepatic parenchymal iron overload in approximately 1 of 400 persons screened.[28, 83–86] As with all screening programs, cost and frequency of disease are major considerations.

Even though the HLA-A3 haplotype has been demonstrated in up to 75 percent of patients with hemochromatosis, HLA-A3 occurs with a prevalence of 20 percent in control white populations and thus cannot be used as a marker for the disease.[28]

Patients with any disease manifestation suggestive of hemochromatosis should be screened with transferrin saturation and serum ferritin levels. Once a case of hemochromatosis is identified, HLA typing can also be employed.[86a] Relatives having the same HLA-A and B haplotypes as the proband are presumptive homozygotes for the disease. Since hemochromatosis is inherited as an autosomal recessive trait, 25 percent of siblings of the proband would be predicted to be homozygotes with a probability of 50 percent being a heterozygote for the gene. Children of a proband and children of heterozygotes will not be affected by the disease unless the spouse is also a heterozygote for hemochromatosis. Heterozygotes

occasionally exhibit abnormal serum iron indices but are not at risk for developing the disease and therefore can be reassured. Screening is recommended for all first-degree relatives of a case of hemochromatosis with transferrin saturation, serum ferritin, and HLA typing (A and B) starting at the age of 10 years.[5] If a homozygote for the disease is identified, yearly biochemical iron testing should be followed. Then if iron overload is suggested by biochemical tests in a homozygote, a liver biopsy should be performed to confirm the diagnosis and evaluate for presence of cirrhosis.[5]

Treatment and Prognosis

The primary treatment of genetic hemochromatosis is to remove excess iron by phlebotomy. Removal of 500 ml of blood, equivalent to 250 mg of iron, on a weekly basis will eliminate 10 to 13 g of iron per year. Depletion of iron stores in advanced cases may require weekly phlebotomy for 2 or 3 years followed by maintenance phlebotomy four to six times annually to counteract continued excessive iron absorption.[10] The serum ferritin level declines progressively during phlebotomy, whereas serum iron levels and transferrin saturation remain high until iron depletion has occurred.[87, 88] Hemoglobin and hematocrit levels fall when iron deficiency develops and can be used as a monitor of adequacy of therapy during phlebotomy. Once the hemoglobin falls to 11 g per dl or the hematocrit falls to 34 percent, maintenance phlebotomy can be instituted to keep transferrin saturation at about 50 percent.[5, 89]

Phlebotomy has also been used effectively in various forms of secondary iron overload but is not feasible as treatment in diseases associated with anemia. Deferoxamine, an iron-chelating agent, may be used by subcutaneous or intravenous infusion to remove excess iron in these patients. In cases of cardiomyopathy secondary to iron overload, chelation therapy with deferoxamine combined with phlebotomy may be warranted to maximize iron removal. Although ascorbic acid can mobilize the chelatable iron pool, it must be used with caution because of its potential to cause peroxidation of intracellular lipids, which may exacerbate iron injury.[90, 91]

Effectiveness of phlebotomy therapy varies with the severity and degree of organ dysfunction in cases of hemochromatosis. Hepatic function may improve with phlebotomy, but regression of the fibrosis or cirrhosis is unusual.[41, 92] In cases of end-stage cirrhosis, liver transplantation may be a viable treatment option in certain cases.[93] Liver neoplasms, including both hepatocellular carcinoma and intrahepatic bile duct carcinoma, are life-threatening complications that occur in approximately 15 percent of patients with cirrhosis.[38] Unfortunately, the successful depletion of hepatic iron may not decrease the incidence of subsequent liver cancer.[38] Similarly, only one third of patients have improvement in their diabetes mellitus to the degree they no longer require insulin therapy.[92] With hypogonadism, iron depletion alone can occasionally restore libido, potency, or reversal of amenorrhea, but most will require supplemental hormonal therapy to replace depleted testosterone or estrogen.[45, 94, 95] Testosterone injections plus phlebotomy may also be effective therapy for improving bone mineral density in males with associated osteoporosis.[51]

Symptoms of malaise, weakness, lethargy, and right upper quadrant pain are frequently relieved with adequate phlebotomy.[5] Skin pigmentation tends to lighten with depletion of iron, but excess melanin may persist. The cardiomyopathy of hemochromatosis is potentially reversible with removal of iron; however, in severely affected cases, patients may die of heart failure during the months required for effective reduction of iron excess.[10]

In general, phlebotomy does not alleviate symptoms of arthralgia and loss of joint mobility in patients with established arthropathy associated with hemochromatosis. In fact, arthritis may progress despite phlebotomy.[57, 62, 63] Nonsteroidal anti-inflammatory drugs may be of some symptomatic benefit in managing chronic arthritis. In patients with recurrent acute episodes of calcium pyrophosphate dihydrate crystal deposition, joint aspiration, intra-articular glucocorticoids, and prophylaxis with colchicine may be beneficial. If progressive joint destruction occurs, arthroplasty may be appropriate in selected cases.

The prognosis of patients with genetic hemochromatosis depends on the amount and the duration of iron excess.[96] The presence of cirrhosis and diabetes at the time of diagnosis is a poor prognostic indicator.[38] In a 1985 study, cumulative survival of 163 patients treated with phlebotomy was 92 percent at 5 years, 76 percent at 10 years, 59 percent at 15 years, and 49 percent at 20 years.[38] Compared with normal, hemochromatosis demonstrates a liver cancer rate that is 219 times more frequent, a cardiomyopathy rate that is 306 times, a cirrhosis rate that is 13 times, and a diabetes rate that is 7 times more frequent.[38] The continued improvement in survival of patients with hemochromatosis is due in part to an increasing number of patients identified early, prior to the development of cirrhosis or diabetes.[96] In fact, the patients who are identified in the precirrhotic stage and treated with adequate phlebotomy have normal life expectancies.[38] This success rate generally reflects individuals who were diagnosed early by investigation of first-degree relatives of a proband, or those with symptoms such as fatigue or arthropathy without life-threatening organ involvement.

References

1. Trousseau, A.: Glycosurie, diabète sucré. In Clinique Médicale de l'Hotel-Dieu de Paris, 2nd ed., Vol. 2. Paris, Balliere, 1865.
2. von Recklinghausen, F. D.: Über hämochromatose. In Tagebl der Versamml Deutsch Natur und Ärtze. Heidelberg, 1889.
3. Sheldon, J. H.: Haemochromatosis. London, Oxford University Press, 1935.
4. Simon, M., Bourel, M., Genetet, B., et al.: Idiopathic hemochromatosis: Demonstration of recessive transmission and early detection by family HLA typing. N. Engl. J. Med. 297:1017, 1977.
5. Tavil, A. S., and Bacon, B. R.: Hemochromatosis: Iron metabolism and the iron overload syndromes. In Zakim, D., and Boyer, T. D. (eds.): Hepatology: A Textbook of Liver Disease. 2nd ed. Philadelphia, W. B. Saunders Company, 1990.
6. Brink, B., Disler, P., Lynch, S., et al: Patterns of iron storage in dietary iron overload and idiopathic hemochromatosis. J. Lab. Clin. Med. 88:725, 1977.
7. Modell, B., and Berdoukas, V.: Death and survival. In The Clinical Approach to Thalassemia. London, Grune & Stratton, 1984.
8. Barron, R., Grace, N. D., Sherwood, G., and Powell, L. W.: Iron overload complicating sideroblastic anemia: Is the gene for hemochromatosis responsible? Gastroenterology 96:1204, 1989.
9. Bothwell, T. H., and Charlton, R. W.: Hemochromatosis. In Schiff, L., and Schiff, E. R. (eds.): Diseases of the Liver. 6th ed. Philadelphia, J. B. Lippincott Co., 1987.
10. Smith, L. H., Jr.: Overview of hemochromatosis. West. J. Med. 153:296, 1990.
10a. Gordeuk, V., Mukiibi, J., Hasstedt, S. J., et al.: Iron overload in Africa: interaction between a gene and dietary iron content. N. Engl. J. Med. 326:95, 1992.
11. Grossman, M. E., Bickers, D. R., Poh-Fitzpatrick, M. B., et al.: Porphyria cutanea tarda: Clinical and laboratory findings in 40 patients. Am. J. Med. 67:277, 1979.
12. Edwards, C. O., Griffen, L. M., Goldgar, D. E., et al.: HLA-linked hemochromatosis alleles in sporadic porphyria cutanea tarda. Gastroenterology 97:972, 1989.
13. Beaumont, C., Fauchet, R., Nhu Phung, L., et al.: Porphyria cutanea tarda and HLA-linked hemochromatosis: Evidence against a systematic association. Gastroenterology 92:1833, 1987.
14. Goya, N., Miyazaki, S., Kodate, S., and Ushio, B.: A family of congenital atransferrinemia. Blood 40:239, 1972.
15. Knisely, A. S., Magid, M. S., Dische, M. R., et al.: Neonatal hemochromatosis. Birth Defects 22:75, 1987.
16. Hakim, R. M., Stivelman, J. C., Schulman, G., et al.: Iron overload and mobilization in long-term hemodialysis patients. Am. J. Kidney Dis. 10:293, 1987.
17. Huebers, H., Josephson, B., Huebers, E., et al.: Uptake and release of iron from human transferrin. Proc. Natl. Acad. Sci. U. S. A. 78:2573, 1981.
18. Morgan, E. H., and Baker, E.: Role of transferrin receptors and endocytosis in iron uptake by hepatic and erythroid cells. Ann. N. Y. Acad. Sci. 526:65, 1988.
19. Bothwell, T. H., Jacobs, P., and Torrance, J. D.: Studies on the behavior of transferrin in idiopathic hemochromatosis. S. Afr. J. Med. Sci. 27:35, 1962.
20. Ward, J. H., Kushner, J. P., Ray, F. A., et al.: Transferrin receptor function in hereditary hemochromatosis. J. Lab. Clin. Med. 103:246, 1984.
21. Whittaker, P., Skikne, B. S., Covell, A. M., et al.: Duodenal iron proteins in idiopathic hemochromatosis. J. Clin. Invest. 83:261, 1989.
22. Francanzani, A. L., Fargion, S., Romeno, R., et al.: Immunohistochemical evidence for a lack of ferritin in duodenal absorptive epithelioid cells in idiopathic hemochromatosis. Gastroenterology 96:1071, 1989.
23. Lombard, M., Bomford, A. B., Polson, R. J., et al.: Differential expression of transferrin receptor in duodenal mucosa in iron overload: Evidence for a site-specific defect in genetic hemochromatosis. Gastroenterology 98:976, 1990.
24. Bacon, B. R., Brittenham, G. M., Park, C. H., and Tavill, A. S.: Lipid peroxidation in experimental hemochromatosis. Ann. N. Y. Acad. Sci. 526:155, 1988.
24a. Deugnier, Y. M., Loréal, O., Turlin, B., Guyader, D., et al.: Liver pathology in genetic hemochromatosis: a review of 135 homozygous cases and their bioclinical correlations. Gastroenterology 102:2050, 1992.
25. Walters, J. M., Watt, P. W., Stevens, F. M., and Carthy, C. F.: HLA antigens in hemochromatosis. Br. Med. J. 4:520, 1975.
26. Simon, M., Bourel, M., Fauchet, R., and Genetet, B.: Association of HLA-A3 and HLA-B14 antigens with idiopathic hemochromatosis. Gut 17:332, 1976.
27. Simon, M., Yaouanq, J., Fauchet, R., et al.: Genetics of hemochromatosis: HLA association and mode of inheritance. Ann. N. Y. Acad. Sci. 526:11, 1988.
28. Adams, P. C., Halliday, J. W., and Powell, L. W.: Early diagnosis and treatment of hemochromatosis. Adv. Intern. Med. 34:111, 1989.
29. Schumacher, H. R.: Hemochromatosis and arthritis. Arthritis Rheum. 7:41, 1964.
30. Schumacher, H. R.: Articular cartilage in the degenerative arthropathy of hemochromatosis. Arthritis Rheum. 25:1460, 1982.

31. Brighton, C. T., Bigley, E. C., Jr., and Smolenski, B. I.: Iron-induced arthritis in immature rabbits. Arthritis Rheum. 13:849, 1970.
32. Okazaki, I., Brinckerhoff, C. E., Sinclair, J. F., et al.: Iron increases collagenase production by rabbit synovial fibroblasts. J. Lab. Clin. Med. 97:396, 1981.
33. Thomas, C. E., Morehouse, L. A., and Aust, S. D.: Ferritin and superoxide-dependent lipid peroxidation. J. Biol. Chem. 260:3275, 1985.
34. Blake, D. R., Gallagher, P. J., Potter, A. R., et al.: The effect of synovial iron on the progression of rheumatoid disease. Arthritis Rheum. 27:495, 1984.
35. McCarty, D. J., and Pepe, P. F.: Erythrocyte neutral inorganic pyrophosphatase in pseudogout. J. Lab. Clin. Med. 79:277, 1972.
36. McCarty, D. J., Palmer, D. W., and Garancis, J. C.: Clearance of calcium pyrophosphatase dihydrate crystals in vivo. III. Effects of synovial hemosiderosis. Arthritis Rheum. 25:706, 1981.
37. De Seye, S., Solnica, J., Mitrovic, D., et al.: Joint and bone disorders and hypoparathyroidism in hemochromatosis. Semin. Arthritis Rheum. 2:71, 1972.
38. Niderau, C., Fischer, R., Sonnenberg, A., et al.: Survival and causes of death in cirrhotic and noncirrhotic patients with primary hemochromatosis. N. Engl. J. Med. 313:1256, 1985.
38a. Adams, P. C., Kertesz, A. E., and Valberg, L. S.: Clinical presentation of hemochromatosis: a changing scene. Am. J. Med. 90:445, 1991.
39. Irving, M. G., Halliday, J. W., and Powell, L. W.: Association between alcoholism and increased hepatic iron stores. Alcoholism Clin. Exp. Res. 12:7, 1988.
40. Bradbear, R. A., Bain, C., Siskind, V., et al.: Cohort study of internal malignancy in genetic hemochromatosis and other chronic nonalcoholic liver diseases. J. Natl. Cancer Inst. 75:81, 1985.
41. Tiniakos, G., and Williams, R.: Cirrhotic process, liver cell carcinoma and extrahepatic malignant tumors in idiopathic haemochromatosis: Study of 71 patients treated with venesection therapy. Appl. Pathol. 6:128, 1988.
42. Rahier, J., Loozen, S., Goebbels, R. M., et al.: The haemochromatotic human pancreas: A quantitative immunohistochemical and ultrastructural study. Diabetologia 30:5, 1987.
43. Muller, W. A., Berger, M., Cüppers, H. J., et al.: Plasma glucagon in diabetes of haemochromatosis: Too low or too high? Gut 20:200, 1979.
44. Stremmel, W., Niederau, C., Berger, M., et al.: Abnormalities in estrogen, androgen, and insulin metabolism in idiopathic hemochromatosis. Ann. N. Y. Acad. Sci. 526:209, 1988.
45. Meyer, W. R., Hutchinson-Williams, K. A., Jones, E. E. and DeCherney, A. H.: Secondary hypogonadism in hemochromatosis. Fertil. Steril. 54:740, 1990.
46. Cundy, I., Bomford, A., Butler, J., et al.: Hypogonadism and sexual dysfunction in hemochromatosis: The effects of cirrhosis and diabetes. J. Clin. Endocrinol. Metab. 69:110, 1989.
47. Delbarre, F.: L'Osteoporose des hemochromatoses. Sem. Hop. Paris. 36:3279, 1960.
48. Diamond, T., Stiel, D., and Posen, S.: Osteoporosis in hemochromatosis: Iron excess, gonadal deficiency, or other factors? Ann. Intern. Med. 110:430, 1989.
49. Conte, D., Caraceni, M. P., Duriez, J., et al.: Bone involvement in primary hemochromatosis and alcoholic cirrhosis. Am. J. Gastroenterol. 84:1231, 1989.
50. Chow, L. H., Frei, J. V., Hodsman, A. B., and Valberg, L. S.: Low serum 25-hydroxyvitamin D in hereditary hemochromatosis: Relation to iron status. Gastroenterology 88:865, 1985.
51. Diamond, T., Stiel, D., and Posen, S.: Effects of testosterone and venesection on spinal and peripheral bone mineral in six hypogonadal men with hemochromatosis. J. Bone Miner. Res. 6:39, 1991.
52. de Sousa, M.: Immune cell function in iron overload. Clin. Exp. Immunol. 75:1, 1989.
53. Chiesa, C., Pacifico, L., Renzulli, F., et al.: Yersinia hepatic abscesses and iron overload. J. A. M. A. 257:3230, 1987.
54. Bullen, J. J., Spalding, P. B., Ward, C. G., and Gutteridge, J. M. C.: Hemochromatosis, iron, and septicemia caused by Vibrio vulniticus. Arch. Intern. Med. 151:1606, 1991.
55. van Asbeck, B. S., Verbrugh, H. A., van Oost, B. A., et al.: Listeria monocytogenes meningitis and decreased phagocytosis associated with iron overload. Br. Med. J. 284:542, 1982.
56. Weinberg, E. D.: Iron, infection, and neoplasia. Clin. Physiol. Biochem. 4:50, 1986.
57. Hamilton, E., Williams, R., Barlow, K. A., and Smith, P. M.: The arthropathy of idiopathic hemochromatosis. Q. J. Med. 37:171, 1968.
58. Dymock, I. W., Hamilton, E. B. D., Laws, J. W., and Williams, R.: Arthropathy of hemochromatosis: Clinical and radiological analysis of 63 patients with iron overload. Ann. Rheum. Dis. 29:469, 1970.
59. Huaux, J. P., Geubel, A., Koch, M. C., et al.: The arthritis of hemochromatosis: A review of 25 cases with special reference to chondrocalcinosis, and a comparison with patients with primary hyperparathyroidism and controls. Clin. Rheumatol. 5:317, 1986.
60. M'Seffar, A., Fornasier, V. L., and Fox, I. H.: Arthropathy as the major clinical indicator of occult iron storage disease. J. A. M. A. 238:1825, 1977.
61. de Jonge-Bok, J. M., and MacFarlane, J. D.: The articular diversity of early hemochromatosis. J. Bone Joint Surg. 69-B:41, 1987.
62. Schumacher, H. R., Straka, P. C., Krikker, M. A., and Dudley, A. T.: The arthropathy of hemochromatosis: Recent studies. Ann. N. Y. Acad. Sci. 526:224, 1988.
63. Askari, A. D., Muir, W. A., Rosner, I. A., et al.: Arthritis of hemochromatosis: Clinical spectrum, relation to histocompatibility antigens, and effectiveness of early phlebotomy. Am. J. Med. 75:957, 1983.
64. Dorfmann, H., Solnica, J. H., DiMenza, C., and DeSèze, S.: Les arthropathies des hèmochromatoses: Résultats d'une enquête prospective portant sur 54 malades. Sem. Hop. Paris 45:516, 1969.
65. Adamson, T. C., III, Resnik, C. S., Guerra, J., Jr., et al.: Hand and wrist arthropathies of hemochromatosis and calcium pyrophosphate deposition disease: Distinct radiographic features. Radiology 147:377, 1983.
66. Atkins, C. J., McIvor, J., Smith, P. M., et al.: Chondrocalcinosis and arthropathy: Studies in haemochromatoses and in idiopathic chondrocalcinosis. Q. J. Med. 39:71, 1970.
67. Angevine, C. D., and Jacox, R. F.: Unusual connective tissue manifestations of hemochromatosis. Arthritis Rheum. 17:477, 1974.
68. Bensen, W. G., Laskin, C. A., Little, H. A., and Fam, A. G.: Hemochromatotic arthropathy mimicking rheumatoid arthritis: A case with subcutaneous nodules, tenosynovitis and bursitis. Arthritis Rheum. 21:844, 1978.
69. Bassett, M. L., Halliday, J. W., Ferris, R. A., et al.: Diagnosis of hemochromatosis in young subjects: Predictive accuracy of biochemical screening tests. Gastroenterology 87:628, 1984.
70. Bassett, M. L., Halliday, J. W., and Powell, L. W.: Value of iron measurements in early hemochromatosis and determination of the critical iron level associated with fibrosis. Hepatology 6:24, 1986.
71. Adams, P. C.: Hepatic iron in hemochromatosis. Dig. Dis. Sci. 35:690, 1990.
72. Summers, K. M., Halliday, J. W., and Powell, L. W.: Identification of homozygous hemochromatosis subjects by measurement of hepatic iron index. Hepatology 12:20, 1990.
73. Olynyk, J., Hall, P., Sallie, R., et al.: Computerized measurement of iron in liver biopsies: A comparison with biochemical iron measurement. Hepatology 12:26, 1990.
74. Roudot-Thoraval, F., Halphen, M., Lardé, D., et al.: Evaluation of liver iron content by computed tomography: Its value in the follow-up of treatment in patients with idiopathic hemochromatosis. Hepatology 3:974, 1983.
75. Chapman, R. W. G., Williams, G., Rydder, G., et al.: Computed tomography for determining liver iron content in primary haemochromatosis. Br. Med. J. 1:440, 1980.
76. Sephton, R. G.: The potential accuracy of dual-energy computed tomography for the determination of hepatic iron. Br. J. Radiol. 59:351, 1986.
77. Bonkovsky, H. L., Slaker, D. P., Bills, E. B., and Wolf, D. C.: Usefulness and limitations of laboratory and hepatic imaging studies in iron-storage disease. Gastroenterology 99:1076, 1990.
78. Brittenham, G. M., Farrell, D. E., Harris, J. W., et al.: Magnetic-susceptibility measurement of human iron stores. N. Engl. J. Med. 307:1671, 1982.
79. Stark, D. D., Moseley, M. E., Bacon, B. R., et al.: Magnetic resonance imaging and spectroscopy of hepatic iron overload. Radiology 154:137, 1985.
80. Johnston, D. L., Rice, L., Vick, W., III, et al.: Assessment of tissue iron overload by nuclear magnetic resonance imaging. Am. J. Med. 87:40, 1989.
81. Housman, J. F., Chezmar, J. L., and Nelson, R. C.: Magnetic resonance imaging in hemochromatosis: Extrahepatic iron deposition. Gastrointest. Radiol. 14:59, 1989.
82. Olsson, K., Eriksson, K., Ritter, B., et al.: Screening for iron overload using transferrin saturation. Acta Med. Scand. 215:105, 1984.
83. Olsson, K., Ritter, B., Rosen, L. L., et al.: Prevalence of iron overload in central Sweden. Acta Med. Scand. 213:145, 1983.
84. Tanner, A., Desai, S., Lu, W., et al.: Screening for haemochromatosis in the UK: Preliminary results. Gut 26:A1139, 1985.
85. Elliott, R., Lin, B., Dent, O., et al.: Prevalence of hemochromatosis in a random sample of asymptomatic men. Aust. N. Z. J. Med. 16:491, 1986.
86. Bassett, M. L., Halliday, J. W., Bryant, S., et al.: Screening for hemochromatosis. Ann. N. Y. Acad. Sci. 526:274, 1988.
86a. Adams, P. C., and Kertesz, A. E.: Human leukocyte antigen typing of siblings in hereditary hemochromatosis: a cost approach. Hepatology 15:263, 1992.
87. Milder, M. S., Cook, J. D., Sunday, S., et al.: Idiopathic hemochromatosis: An interim report. Medicine 59:39, 1980.
88. Edwards, C. O., Cartwright, G. E., Skolnick, M. H., et al.: Homozygosity for hemochromatosis: Clinical manifestations. Ann. Intern. Med. 93:519, 1980.
89. Fox, I. H.: Iron storage disease. In Kelley, W. N., Harris, E. D., Jr., Ruddy, S., Sledge, C. B. (eds.): Textbook of Rheumatology. 3rd ed. Philadelphia, W. B. Saunders Company, 1989.

90. Mak, I. T., and Weglicki, W. B.: Characterization of iron-mediated peroxidative injury in isolated hepatic lysosomes. J. Clin. Invest. 75:58, 1985.
91. Nienhuis, A. W.: Vitamin C and iron. N. Engl. J. Med. 304:170, 1981.
92. Bomford, A., and Williams, R.: Long-term results of venesection therapy in idiopathic haemochromatosis. Q. J. Med. 45:611, 1976.
93. Dietze, O., Vogel, W., Braunsperger, B., and Margreiter, R.: Liver transplantation in idiopathic hemochromatosis. Transplant. Proc. 22:1512, 1990.
94. Kelly, T. M., Edwards, C. O., Meikle, A. W., Kushner, J. P.: Hypogonadism in hemochromatosis: Reversal with iron depletion. Ann. Intern. Med. 101:629, 1984.
95. Lufkin, E. G., Baldus, W. P., Bergstrain, E. J., and Kao, P. C.: Influence of phlebotomy treatment on abnormal hypothalamic-pituitary function in genetic hemochromatosis. Mayo Clin. Proc. 62:473, 1987.
96. Strohmeyer, G., Niederau, C., and Stremmel, W.: Survival and causes of death in hemochromatosis: Observations in 163 patients. Ann. N. Y. Acad. Sci. 526:245, 1988.

William W. Ginsburg
J. Desmond O'Duffy

Chapter 85
Multicentric Reticulohistiocytosis

Multicentric reticulohistiocytosis is a rare systemic disease of unknown etiology characterized by an infiltration of lipid-laden histiocytes and multinucleated giant cells into various tissues. Skin nodules and a destructive polyarthritis are the most common findings. There are approximately a hundred cases reported in the literature, the most comprehensive papers being reviews by Barrow and Holubar in 1969 and Chevrant-Breton in 1977.[1, 2] Various other names have been used to describe this disorder, including lipoid dermatoarthritis, reticulohistiocytosis, giant cell reticulohistiocytosis, and normocholesterolemic xanthomatosis. In 1954 Goltz and Layman introduced the term multicentric reticulohistiocytosis to describe patients demonstrating the typical skin lesions as well as definite arthritis.[3]

CLINICAL FEATURES AND COURSE

The mean age of onset is the fourth decade, but the disease has occurred from 11 to 71 years. Females seem to predominate over males by a slight margin. In approximately 60 percent of cases polyarthritis is the presenting symptom, followed by the nodular skin eruption. Diagnosis is initially very difficult without the accompanying skin nodules, which do not appear until an average of 3 years after the arthritis. In 20 percent of cases the skin eruption is the initial symptom, and in the remaining cases there is a simultaneous presentation. The skin nodules, which can range in number from a few to hundreds, are light copper to reddish brown in color. They vary in size from several millimeters to 2 cm and characteristically involve the dorsa of the fingers, including nailfolds, giving a so-called coral beads appearance. Ear, chest, and face involvement can be seen (Fig. 85–1; see color section at the front of this volume). A leonine facies can result from extensive facial and paranasal nodulation. Occasionally nodules may occur over the olecranon process, causing confusion with the subcutaneous nodules of rheumatoid arthritis (Fig. 85–2). Mucosal surfaces are also frequently involved, and lesions can occur on the lips, nasal septum, tongue, gingiva, and pharynx. In approximately 30 percent of cases severe pruritus is the first complaint, even before nodules are present.

Confluent nodules on the face or trunk may present a cobblestone texture. Some patients may experience weight loss and fever.[1, 2, 4, 5]

The polyarthritis tends to be symmetric, most commonly involving the interphalangeal joints of the fingers. Other joint involvement can include the metacarpophalangeal joints, knees, shoulders, wrists, hips, ankles, feet, elbows, and spine. Atlantoaxial and temporomandibular joints may also be affected.[1, 6] Morning stiffness occurs, and examination may reveal warm, swollen, and tender joints. Common involvement of the distal interphalangeal joints helps distinguish this from rheumatoid arthritis, but, unless the characteristic skin nodules are present, distinction is most difficult.

In 40 to 50 percent of the cases the arthritis progresses, over a 7- to 8-year period, to an arthritis mutilans. In the fingers this can produce the "main en lorgnette," or opera glass hand deformity. However, the natural history of the disease is not well defined, and an occasional patient may have mild disease, even with spontaneous remission.

Multicentric reticulohistiocytosis is not limited to involvement of the skin and joints, and cases of myositis, pleural effusions, gastric ulcers, and pericarditis secondary to histiocytic and multinucleated

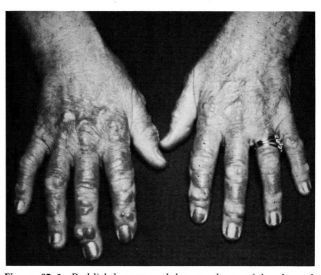

Figure 85–1. Reddish-brown nodules on dorsa of hands and around nailfolds.

1444

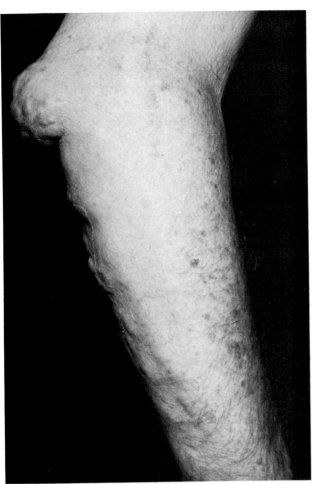

Figure 85–2. Nodular infiltrates on extensor surface of forearm can stimulate clusters of rheumatoid nodules.

giant cell infiltration have been reported. Infiltration into bronchial lymph nodes, bone marrow, hypopharynx, submandibular salivary glands, thyroid, and endocardium have also been reported.[5, 7–14]

LABORATORY AND ROENTGENOGRAPHIC FEATURES

Joint fluid analysis reveals no consistent finding. Leukocyte counts are usually below 30,000 per mm^3 with some patients having counts below 4000 and one having only 220 cells. Although monocytes are elevated in most patients, they may be normal, and polymorphonuclear cells or lymphocytes may predominate.[7, 9, 15–22] One patient had foam cells present. Synovial biopsy has revealed numerous lipid-laden histiocytes and multinucleated giant cells, such as are seen on skin biopsy.[7, 9, 17, 22]

There are no specific laboratory abnormalities in multicentric reticulohistiocytosis, although about half the patients have a slightly elevated erythrocyte sedimentation rate and a mild anemia. About 30 percent have slight to moderate hypercholesterolemia. Normal values are reported for serum uric

acid, thyroxine, glucose, triglycerides, and creatinine, as well as serologic tests for syphilis. Tests for rheumatoid factor, antinuclear antibody, serum protein electrophoresis, and LE cells are usually negative. A positive rheumatoid factor, as reported in four cases, could cause confusion in the diagnosis especially if the arthritis precedes skin manifestations.[23] Bone marrow examinations have been normal, and patients have been shown to have intact delayed hypersensitivity by skin tests to Candida, mumps, and tuberculin.[1, 5]

Roentgenographic findings may show erosive changes very similar to those of rheumatoid arthritis. As in rheumatoid arthritis, these tend to be bilaterally symmetric. However, circumscribed erosions often spread from the synovial reflections over the articular surface, resulting in widening of joint space, loss of cartilage, and resorption of subchondral bone. These changes are especially to be found in the proximal and distal interphalangeal joints. Osteoporosis is relatively mild despite the severe erosive destruction, and there is absent or minimal periosteal reaction. Hand radiographs often show well-defined extra-articular nodules (Fig. 85–3). Rarely atlantoaxial involvement, as is seen in rheumatoid arthritis, may develop.[6, 24, 25]

In one patient with involvement of pericardium, salivary glands, and mediastinum, a gallium scan demonstrated uptake in those areas.[13] Another patient had bilateral hilar uptake.[26] Gallium concentrates in granulomatous lesions with abundant histiocytes and, therefore, may be helpful to detect systemic involvement.

ASSOCIATED DISORDERS

Approximately 50 percent of patients are tuberculin positive. In one patient with both tuberculosis and multicentric reticulohistiocytosis, treatment of the tuberculosis brought a complete resolution of the multicentric reticulohistiocytosis.[15] Active tuberculosis was found in only one other case.[3] Approximately one third of the patients have xanthelasma.[1, 5]

Autoimmune diseases appear to be infrequently associated with multicentric reticulohistiocytosis. One patient had primary biliary cirrhosis and autoimmune thyroid disease, and another had Sjögren's syndrome with associated anti-Ro (SSA) antibody.[18, 27] In both patients HLA typing revealed the antigens A2 and B8. HLA studies on other patients have not been carried out.

Approximately 25 percent of patients with multicentric reticulohistiocytosis have malignant disease. The meaning of this association is unknown, but it is thought that it may represent a paraneoplastic process in certain patients. Associated malignancies have included carcinoma of the breast, stomach, cervix, ovary, colon, and lung. Hematologic malignancies, melanoma, and mesothelioma have also been reported.[1, 22, 23, 28–30] There is no predictable relationship between the onset of malignancy and multicentric reticulohistiocytosis, but in eight cases

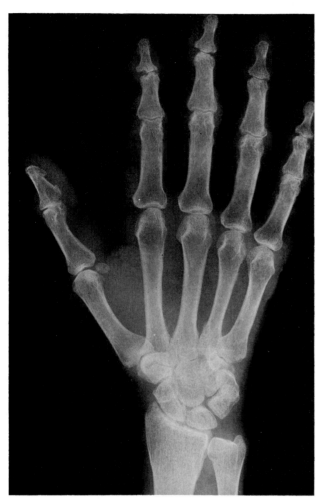

Figure 85–3. Radiograph of hand demonstrating distal interphalangeal joint erosions as well as cutaneous nodules.

the onset of both diseases was within 8 months, with the symptoms of multicentric reticulohistiocytosis usually appearing first. Treatment of the malignancy may or may not lead to improvement of the multicentric reticulohistiocytosis.[23, 28]

PATHOLOGY AND ETIOLOGY

The diagnosis of multicentric reticulohistiocytosis is made on skin or synovial biopsy demonstrating the characteristic aggregates of multinucleated giant cells and histiocytes that have a granular ground-glass appearance (Fig. 85–4). The giant cells can be as large as 50 to 100 μm in diameter, and up to 20 nuclei have been observed. In the skin the nodular infiltrate can occupy the entire dermis and is encapsulated. Histochemical staining reveals that the ground-glass cytoplasm contains a PAS reactive material. The PAS reactive material, which can be completely removed by digestion with pepsin but not with diastase, has been the subject of much investigation and conflicting opinions, but at present it is

thought to represent a mucoprotein or glycoprotein. Sudan black reactive material is also found, which suggests the presence of phospholipids, and neutral fats are present as detected by positive staining with oil red O, Nile blue, Scharlach R, and Sudan III and IV. Multicentric reticulohistiocytosis was at one time thought to represent a lipid storage disease, but no consistent abnormality of the serum or intracellular lipids has been found.[1, 4, 5, 17] Various histochemical stains are not consistently positive in all patients, and it has been suggested that the histiocytes and giant cells contain a nonspecific accumulation of lipids. It is still unclear whether the lipid accumulation is a primary or secondary event in the pathogenesis of the disease. In several reports, cells were found to contain intact and degraded collagen fibers by electron microscopy.[31–33] This has also been noted in granuloma annulare, actinic granuloma, necrobiosis lipoidica, granuloma multiforme, and syphilis and appears to be a nonspecific finding.[34, 35] Electron microscopy of the histiocytes has also shown large membrane-bound vacuoles with presumed lipid accumulation in some cases.[1, 17]

It has been postulated that multicentric reticu-

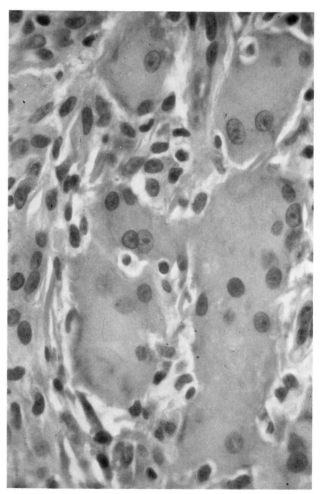

Figure 85–4. Skin biopsy demonstrating multinucleated giant cells with ground glass cytoplasm (hematoxylin and eosin, × 400).

lohistiocytosis represents a histiocytic granulomatous reaction to an unknown stimulus. Immunohistochemical studies have demonstrated that both the mononuclear and the multinucleated giant cells are monocyte/microphage in nature.[20, 36, 37] These cells express HLA class II (DR) MHC antigens.[36] The finding of elevated spontaneous production of interleukin-1 and prostaglandin E_2 by adherent cells suggests macrophage activation. Interleukin-1 has been found to cause bone resorption in vitro.[38]

Numerous cytoplasmic electron-dense granules resembling lysosomes are also seen by electron microscopy. Ultracytochemical studies demonstrate that these granules stain for acid phosphatase, which is considered an enzymatic marker for lysosomes.[33, 39] Activated macrophages contain numerous primary and secondary lysosomes. The release of neutral protease and acid hydrolase from these cells may induce tissue destruction and the inflammation seen in multicentric reticulohistiocytosis.[40, 41] Elevated levels of one of the serine proteinases, urokinase, from lesional skin and synovia have also been reported. Urokinase, presumably released by activated macrophages, is one of the major activators of latent tissue collagenase, which could contribute to cartilage and bone destruction.[42]

DIFFERENTIAL DIAGNOSIS

Besides rheumatoid arthritis, differential diagnosis includes lepromatous leprosy, sarcoidosis, xanthomatosis, generalized eruptive histiocytoma, and histiocytosis X, all of which can have skin nodules and bone changes on roentgenography.

TREATMENT

Treatment for multicentric reticulohistiocytosis has included trials of low-fat diets, clofibrate, prednisone, azathioprine, and isoniazid.[1, 15, 17, 18] None of these has consistently been shown to be of any benefit for the arthritis or skin lesions. One patient had marked improvement of skin lesions after topical nitrogen mustard therapy.[43] Several reports indicate that partial and complete remissions are consistently achieved with cyclophosphamide or chlorambucil treatment.[22, 23, 27, 29, 43-45] Several patients were able to discontinue therapy and remain in remission.[22, 29, 45] Several other patients had responses to combination chemotherapy that included cyclophosphamide.[13, 28] In patients with mild disease, symptomatic relief with salicylates or other nonsteroidal agents should first be sought. In patients with aggressive disease, treatment with cyclophosphamide or chlorambucil appears indicated. The rarity of the disease seems to preclude the possibility of a well-planned double-blind control study in one center.

References

1. Barrow, M. V. and Holubar, K.: Multicentric reticulohistiocytosis, A review of 33 patients. Medicine 48:287, 1969.
2. Chevrant-Breton, J.: La Reticulo-histiocytose multicentrique: Revue de la litterature recente (depuis 1969). Ann. Dermatol. Venereol. 104:745, 1977.
3. Goltz, R. W., and Layman, C. W.: Multicentric reticulohistiocytosis of the skin and synovia. Arch. Dermatol. Syph. 69:717, 1954.
4. Albert, J., Bruce, W., Allen, A. C., et al.: Lipoid dermatoarthritis. Am. J. Med. 28:661, 1960.
5. Orkin, M., Goltz, R. W., Good, R. A., et al.: A study of multicentric reticulohistiocytosis. Arch. Dermatol. 89:640, 1964.
6. Martel, W., Abell, M. R., and Duff, I. F.: Cervical spine involvement in lipoid dermato-arthritis. Radiology 77:613, 1961.
7. Ehrlich, G. E., Young, I., Nosheny, S. Z., and Katz, W. A.: Multicentric reticulohistiocytosis, a multisystem disorder. Am. J. Med. 52:830, 1972.
8. Fast, A.: Cardiopulmonary complications in multicentric reticulohistiocytosis. Arch. Dermatol. 112:1139, 1976.
9. Flam, M., Ryan, S. C., Mah-poy, G. L., et al.: Multicentric reticulohistiocytosis: Report of a case with atypical features and electron microscopic study of skin lesions. Am. J. Med. 52:841, 1972.
10. Waren, R. P., Evans, C. D., Hewitt, M., et al.: Reticulohistiocytosis. Br. Med. J. 1:1387, 1957.
11. Anderson, T. E., Carr, A. J., Chapman, R. S., et al.: Myositis and myotonia in a case of multicentric reticulohistiocytosis. Br. J. Med. 80:39, 1968.
12. Zeale, P. J., Miner, D., Honig, S., Waxman, M., and Bartfield, H.: Multicentric reticulohistiocytosis: A cause of dysphagia with response to corticosteroids. Arthritis Rheum. 28:231, 1985.
13. Furey, N., DiMauro, J., Eng, A., and Shaw, J.: Multicentric reticulohistiocytosis with salivary gland involvement and pericardial effusion. J. Am. Acad. Dermatol. 8:679, 1983.
14. Finelli, L. G., Tenner, L. K., Ratz, J. L., Long, B. D.: A case of multicentric reticulohistiocytosis with thyroid involvement. J. Am. Acad. Dermatol. 15:1097, 1986.
15. Gold, K. D., Sharp, J. T., Estrada, R. E., Duffy, J., and Person, D. A.: Relationship between multicentric reticulohistiocytosis and tuberculosis. J.A.M.A. 237:2213, 1977.
16. Taylor, D. R.: Multicentric reticulohistiocytosis. Arch. Dermatol. 113:330, 1977.
17. Krey, P. R., Comerford, F. R., and Cohen, A. S.: Multicentric reticulohistiocytosis, fine structural analysis of the synovium and synovial fluid cells. Arthritis Rheum. 17:615, 1974.
18. Carey, R. N., Blotzer, J. W., Wolfe, I. D., Glusman, S. M., and Arnett, F. C.: Multicentric reticulohistiocytosis and Sjögren's syndrome. J. Rheumatol. 12:1193, 1985.
19. Freemont, A. J., Jones, C. J. P., and Denton, J.: The synovium and synovial fluid in multicentric reticulohistiocytosis: A light microscopic, electron microscopic and cytochemical analysis of one case. J. Clin. Pathol. 36:860, 1983.
20. Heathcote, J. G., Guenther, L. C., and Wallace, A. C.: Multicentric reticulohistiocytosis: A report of a case and a review of the pathology. Pathology 17:601, 1985.
21. Lesher, J. L., and Allen, B. S.: Multicentric reticulohistiocytosis. J. Am. Acad. Dermatol. 11:713, 1984.
22. Coupe, M. O., Whittaker, S. J., and Thatcher, N.: Multicentric reticulohistiocytosis. Br. J. Dermatol. 116:245, 1987.
23. Catterall, M. D.: Multicentric reticulohistiocytosis: A review of eight cases. Clin. Exp. Dermatol. 5:267, 1980.
24. Gold, R. H., Metzger, A. L., and Mirra, J. M.: Multicentric reticulohistiocytosis, an erosive polyarthritis with distinctive clinical roentgenographic and pathologic features. Am. J. Roentgenol. Rad. Ther. Nucl. Med. 124:610, 1975.
25. Schwarz, E., and Fish, A.: Reticulohistiocytoma: A rare dermatologic disease with roentgen manifestations. Am. J. Roentgenol. Rad. Ther. Nucl. Med. 83:692, 1960.
26. Widman, D., Swayne, L. C., and Rozan, S.: Multicentric reticulohistiocytosis: Assessment of pulmonary disease by gallium-67 scintigraphy. J. Rheumatol. 15:132, 1988.
27. Doherty, M., Martin, M. F. R., and Dieppe, P. A.: Multicentric reticulohistiocytosis associated with primary biliary cirrhosis: Successful treatment with cytotoxic agents. Arthritis Rheum. 27:344, 1984.
28. Nunnink, J. C., Krusinski, P. A., and Yates, J. W.: Multicentric reticulohistiocytosis and cancer: A case report and review of the literature. Med. Pediatr. Oncol. 13:273, 1985.
29. Ginsburg, W. W., O'Duffy, J. D., Morris, J. L., and Huston, K. A.: Multicentric reticulohistiocytosis: Response to alkylating agents in six patients. Ann. Intern. Med. 111:384, 1989.
30. Honeybourne, D., and Kelleth, J. K.: A mesothelioma with multicentric reticulohistiocytosis. Postgrad. Med. J. 61:57, 1985.
31. Heenan, P. J., Quirk, C. J., and Spagnolo, D. V.: Multicentric reticulo-

histiocytosis: A light and electron microscopic study. Aust. J. Dermatol. 24:122, 1983.

32. Caputo, R., Alessi, E., and Berti, E.: Collagen phagocytosis in multicentric reticulohistiocytosis. J. Invest. Dermatol. 76:342, 1981.

33. Coode, P. E., Ridgway, H., and Jones, D. B.: Multicentric reticulohistiocytosis: Report of two cases with ultrastructure, tissue culture and immunology studies. Clin. Exp. Dermatol. 5:281, 1980.

34. Ragaz, A., and Ackerman, A. B.: Is actinic granuloma a specific condition? Am. J. Dermatopathol. 1:43, 1979.

35. Reed, R. J.: Connective-tissue activation. Am. J. Dermatopathol. 4:365, 1982.

36. Salisbury, J. R., Hall, P. A., Williams, H. C., Mangi, M. H., and Mufti, G. J.: Multicentric reticulohistiocytosis: Detailed immunophenotyping confirms macrophage origin. Am. J. Surg. Pathol. 14:687, 1990.

37. Green, C. A., Walker, D. J., and Malcolm, A. J.: A case of multicentric reticulohistiocytosis: Uncommon clinical signs and a repeat of T-cell marker characteristics. Br. J. Dermatol. 115:623, 1986.

38. Zagala, A., Guyot, A., Bensa, J. C., and Phelip, X.: Multicentric reticulohistiocytosis: A case with enhanced interleukin-1, prostaglandin E_2 and interleukin-2 secretion. J. Rheumatol. 15:136, 1988.

39. Tani, M., Hori, K., Nakanishi, L., Iwasaki, I., Ugawa, Y., and Jimbo, L.: Multicentric reticulohistiocytosis. Electron microscopic and ultracytochemical studies. Arch. Dermatol. 117:495, 1981.

40. Davies, P. A., and Allison, A. C.: Secretion of macrophage enzymes in relation to the pathogenesis of chronic inflammation. In Nelson, D. S. (ed.): Immunobiology of the Macrophage. New York, Academic Press, 1976, p.427.

41. Nishi, K.: Possible role of lysosomes in cells of "the epitheloid cell system." Acta Histochem. 11:252, 1978.

42. Lotti, T., Santucci, M., Casigliani, R., Fabbri, P., Bondi, R., and Panconesi, E.: Multicentric reticulohistiocytosis: Report of three cases with elevation of tissue proteinase activity. Am. J. Dermatopathol. 10:497, 1988.

43. Brandt, E., Lipman, M., Taylor, J. R., and Halprin, K. M.: Topical nitrogen mustard therapy in multicentric reticulohistiocytosis. J. Am. Acad. Dermatol. 6:260, 1982.

44. Hanauer, L. B.: Reticulohistiocytosis: Remission after cyclophosphamide therapy. Arthritis Rheum. 15:636, 1972.

45. Doherty, M., Martin, M. F. R., and Dieppe, P. A.: Multicentric reticulohistiocytosis associated with primary biliary cirrhosis: Successful treatment with cytotoxic agents. Arthritis Rheum. 27:344, 1984.

Section XVII
Infectious Arthritis

Chapter 86

Don L. Goldenberg

Bacterial Arthritis

INTRODUCTION

Bacterial arthritis continues to be the most rapidly destructive form of joint and bone disease. Despite newer, more potent antibiotics and more effective techniques of joint drainage, the morbidity and mortality from bacterial arthritis has not significantly decreased during the past two decades. Specific risk factors that have become more prominent include rheumatoid arthritis, prosthetic joint infections, and old age or immune compromised host defenses, particularly in those infected with the human immunodeficiency virus (HIV). Awareness of the potential for bacterial arthritis arising in these settings and an understanding of optimal diagnostic and therapeutic principles are of great importance.

PATHOPHYSIOLOGY

The synovium is a highly vascular, areolar connective tissue, which is not lined with a limiting basement membrane. Bacteria enter the joint hematogenously or may be introduced directly into the joint during surgery, from an adjacent osteomyelitis, or from a penetrating wound.[1] Animal models of infectious arthritis have provided a means to study the sequential histopathologic and the complex physiologic changes that occur in septic arthritis. Certain bacteria preferentially localize in joints during experimental infectious arthritis.[2] Once inside the joint, the synovial phagocytes and migrating polymorphonuclear neutrophils (PMNs) engulf the bacteria. Necrosis of chondrocytes has been noted as early as 48 hours after intra-articular bacterial injections. Abscesses form with evidence of synovial necrosis, and then granulation tissue develops. *Staphylococcus aureus* arthritis in rabbits with adjuvant arthritis demonstrated more extensive changes in the chronically arthritic joints than in previously normal joints.[2]

Proteolytic enzymes released from synovial cells and PMNs cause synovial, cartilage, and bone necrosis. Chondroitin sulfate is lost before collagen in experimental septic arthritis.[3] Intra-articular injections of *Escherichia coli* and *S. aureus* in rabbits cause a 20 to 30 percent decrease in glycosaminoglycan levels at 2 days, a 50 to 60 percent loss at 10 days, and a 65 to 80 percent decrease at 3 weeks.[3] Loss of collagen becomes significant between the second and third weeks after infection. Antibiotic treatment begun within 24 hours of infection decreases collagen loss but fails to prevent proteoglycan (PG) loss from cartilage matrix.[4]

In vitro, *S. aureus* or *S. aureus*–conditioned culture medium causes a three- to fourfold increased release of PG from cartilage explants within 48 hours.[5] The *Staphylococcus*-induced PG release is dependent on cartilage metabolism and can be blocked by inhibitors of protein synthesis.[6] There is also convincing evidence in experimental bacterial arthritis that the marked inflammatory synovitis and cartilage destruction may progress without the presence of viable bacteria.[4, 7, 8] In a model of septic arthritis induced in rabbits' knees by the injection of only 1000 *S. aureus* organisms, cartilage destruction progressed despite the fact that antibiotics sterilized 97 percent of the joints within 48 hours.[9] All these data are consistent with evidence that sepsis triggers cytokine release that in turn induces protease synthesis.

Similar pathophysiologic changes are evident in patients with septic arthritis.[1] Purulent joint effusions release proteolytic enzymes from leukocytes and promote direct pressure necrosis of cartilage. Bacteria or sterile bacterial products induce cytokines that induce chondrocytes to produce proteases. Inflammatory mediators such as tumor necrosis factor and interleukins are found in high concentrations in septic synovial fluids.[10] The local supply of proteinase inhibitors is quickly exhausted in septic arthritis, promoting rapid cartilage destruction.[11] Synovial abscess and granulation tissue eventually erode articular cartilage and bone in a fashion similar to that of

1449

Table 86–1. AFFECTED JOINT DISTRIBUTION IN ADULTS AND CHILDREN WITH NONGONOCOCCAL BACTERIAL ARTHRITIS

Joint	Percentage of Cases	
	Adults	Children
Knee	55	40
Hip	11	28
Ankle	8	14
Shoulder	8	4
Wrist	7	3
Elbow	6	11
Others	5	3
(More than one joint, usually two)	(12)	(7)

rheumatoid pannus. The process and progression of bacterial arthritis are related to local and systemic host factors as well as to microbial factors.[12] For example, inherited or isolated immunoglobulin deficiencies or impaired phagocytic activity may predispose patients to bacterial arthritis.[13, 14]

DIAGNOSIS OF NONGONOCOCCAL BACTERIAL ARTHRITIS

Clinical Manifestations. Because the clinical features and the diagnostic approaches to nongonococcal and gonococcal arthritis are distinctive, these two conditions are discussed individually. The classic presentation of nongonococcal arthritis is an abrupt onset of an acutely painful and swollen joint.[15, 16] There is usually an obvious joint effusion and marked restriction of active or passive motion. Eighty to 90 percent of nongonococcal arthritis affects a single joint, and if more than one joint is involved, the patient often has serious underlying chronic illness or a chronic arthritis such as rheumatoid arthritis (RA). The mortality of polyarticular septic arthritis is twice as great as that of monarticular arthritis.[17] The knee is the joint most often infected[15, 16]; in adults it is the site of more than 50 percent of all cases of nongonococcal bacterial arthritis (Table 86–1). Hips are more often infected in children (see Table 86–1).

Most patients are febrile, but the fever may be low grade. Shaking chills are unusual and are more common in patients with positive blood cultures. The differential diagnosis of acute nongonococcal bacterial arthritis usually includes gout, calcium pyro-phosphate dihydrate (CPPD) deposition disease, Lyme disease, viral arthritis, acute traumatic and hemorrhagic arthritis, and acute presentations of systemic rheumatic diseases such as Reiter's syndrome and RA. During the preantibiotic era and in the 1950s it was not uncommon for patients with bacterial arthritis to have a more chronic, indolent presentation.[1]

Bacteria. (See later for individual bacteria.) In adults with nongonococcal bacterial arthritis, S. aureus is responsible for 60 percent of all joint infections.[15, 16, 18] There has been relatively little change in the total number of cases of bacterial arthritis or the incidence of specific bacteria recovered from joints during the past 50 years (Table 86–2). Over the past 10 to 15 years, gram-negative bacilli and non-group A streptococci have more commonly caused bacterial arthritis, whereas pneumococci are now a rare cause of bacterial arthritis; anaerobes have been recovered more often from septic joints during the past decade.

Synovial Fluid Examination and Culture. The definitive diagnosis of bacterial arthritis can be made only by recovering the organism from the synovial fluid or by visualizing bacteria on a Gram stain smear. Therefore, whenever there is a suspicion of bacterial arthritis, the initial and most important diagnostic procedure is an arthrocentesis and examination of synovial fluid (Table 86–3) (see Chapter 35).

For optimal culture yield, the synovial fluid should be brought directly to the microbiology laboratory and immediately placed on broth and solid media.[1] Culture broths and blood culture media may give best results.[19, 14]

Specimens suspected of containing Neisseria or Haemophilus should be placed on chocolate agar and incubated in an environment of 5 to 10 percent carbon dioxide. Fluoroscopic or computed tomography (CT) guided aspirations have been helpful, but an open surgical procedure may be required to obtain synovial fluid. Arthroscopy is sometimes used diagnostically, but large volumes of lidocaine should not contact the synovial fluid because lidocaine may interfere with bacterial growth.[20]

Occasionally, the synovial fluid may be sterile, but microorganisms may be recovered from a culture of the synovial membrane, particularly when a fungus or mycobacterium is involved. A closed synovial membrane biopsy performed with a Parker-Pearson needle, arthroscopy, or open surgical biopsy will usually provide adequate synovial specimens for

Table 86–2. BACTERIA ISOLATED FROM ADULTS WITH NONGONOCOCCAL BACTERIAL ARTHRITIS

Years	Number of Cases (%)					
	S. aureus	β-Hemolytic Streptococci	Gram-neg. Bacilli	S. pneumoniae	Polymicrobial	Total
1939–1965	129(59%)	36(16%)	28(13%)	13(6%)	13(6%)	219
1965–1990	383(61%)	93(15%)	108(17%)	18(3%)	23(4%)	625

Data from Goldenberg, D. L., and Cohen, A. S.: Acute infectious arthritis. Am. J. Med. 60:369, 1976; Goldenberg, D. L., and Reed, J. I.: Bacterial arthritis. N. Engl. J. Med. 312:764, 1985; Meijers, K. A. E., Dijkmans, B. A. C., Hermans, J., van der Broek, P. J., and Cats, A.: Non-gonococcal infectious arthritis: A retrospective study. J. Infect. 14:13, 1987.

Table 86–3. SYNOVIAL FLUID EXAMINATION IN THE DIAGNOSIS OF BACTERIAL ARTHRITIS

Procedure	Important Technical Aspects	Diagnostic Yield
Culture	Plate immediately or inoculate in blood culture bottles	Nearly 100% positive in nongonococcal bacterial arthritis but only 25–50% positive in gonococcal arthritis
Gram stain smear	Best yield if centrifuge fluid. False positive gram-positive from precipitated mucin	75% positive with gram-positive cocci, 50% with gram-negative bacilli, less than 25% in gonococcal arthritis
Leukocyte count and differential leukocyte count	Generally greater than 50,000 cells/mm³ and greater than 80% PMNs	Significant overlap with noninfectious arthritis (RA, crystal-induced)
Glucose	Less than 50% of fasting, simultaneous blood sugar	Helpful but often not present and may be seen in RA
Detection of bacterial cell wall antigens	Counterimmunoelectrophoresis or similar immune test	Generally not useful, except in *H. influenzae* and *S. pneumoniae* arthritis
Concentration of fatty acids	Lactate dehydrogenase or lactic acid levels are more practical than gas liquid chromatography, which is too cumbersome	Elevated values may be of diagnostic utility in partially treated cases but are nonspecific. Low or normal values are helpful in excluding bacterial arthritis

culture when the synovial fluid is sterile. Small fragments of synovial tissue may be recovered during a "dry tap" by applying negative pressure to the arthrocentesis needle as it is slowly withdrawn through the synovium.[21]

Gram stain of synovial fluid is best performed on a centrifuged or cytocentrifuged pellet or on unspun fluid if it appears grossly purulent. Gram stain smears' positivity vary considerably (see Table 86–3).[15] Acridine orange may provide better visualization of gram-negative organisms than the standard Gram stain.[19]

Although not definitive, synovial fluid leukocyte count and differential leukocyte count provide strong support for the clinical suspicion of bacterial arthritis. Generally the synovial fluid leukocyte count is more than 50,000 cells per mm³ with more than 80 percent PMNs. However, there is considerable overlap with noninfectious effusions; 30 percent of initial synovial fluid leukocyte counts from culture-proven bacterial arthritis were less than 50,000 cells per mm³,[22] and marked synovial fluid leukocytosis is often present in crystal-induced arthritis and in RA. The synovial fluid leukocyte count may be lower than anticipated in some immunocompromised patients.[23] Synovial fluid chemistry, including glucose and lactate dehydrogenase, did not add useful diagnostic information

from that obtained simply by the leukocyte count and differential in differentiating septic from sterile inflammatory synovial fluid.[24] Rarely a "sympathetic" effusion, by definition sterile and acellular, may be aspirated from a joint adjacent to a septic bursa or a septic joint.[25, 26]

Gas liquid chromatography or less cumbersome measures of bacterial fatty acids have been used as diagnostic adjuncts to these routine synovial fluid tests.[27, 28] However, these tests lack sufficient specificity or sensitivity to be of major diagnostic utility. They may be helpful in patients who have recently been taking antibiotics and therefore are more likely to have negative synovial fluid cultures. Muramic acid, a ubiquitous bacterial cell wall component, was found at minimum levels of 250 ng per ml or approximately 40 million organisms per ml in staphylococcal septic arthritis,[29] but this test is not sensitive enough for it to be reliable.

Blood Culture and Other Tests. Approximately 50 percent of patients with nongonococcal bacterial arthritis will have a positive blood culture,[16] and sometimes the blood culture will be positive when the synovial fluid culture is negative. Any possible site of extra-articular infection (e.g., urine or skin lesions) should also be examined with a Gram stain and culture. These sites may provide a clue as to the bacteria causing the joint infection.

Most patients will have a peripheral blood leukocytosis, and almost all will manifest an elevated erythrocyte sedimentation rate (ESR) and positive C-reactive protein (CRP), but these tests provide little useful diagnostic utility in the setting of an inflammatory synovitis.

Radiologic Evaluation. Initial plain radiographs should be obtained to provide a baseline assessment of the infected joint and to rule out a possible contiguous osteomyelitis (Table 86–4). Definitive changes of bacterial arthritis usually take a number of weeks to become obvious. The earliest finding is a joint effusion with displacement of the fat pads. Periarticular osteoporosis is evident during the first week of bacterial arthritis. Joint space narrowing and erosions may be detectable within 7 to 14 days, but the rapidity of their appearance is dependent on the virulence of the organism (Fig. 86–1).

Certain unusual radiologic features of bacterial arthritis can be diagnostically useful.[30] Gas formation within the joint suggests infection, especially due to *E. coli* or anaerobes.[31] Dystrophic calcification may follow rupture of an infected joint with soft-tissue extension.[32] The radiographic features of septic arthritis secondary to extension from a contiguous osteomyelitis include prominent epiphyseal destruction or metaphyseal periostitis or osteolysis.[33] The radiologic findings in a suspected infected prosthetic joint are difficult to distinguish from mechanical loosening of the prosthesis, since both may cause zones of radiolucency at the bone-cement interface (see Chapter 112).

In joints that are particularly difficult to evaluate

Table 86–4. RADIOLOGIC EVALUATION OF SUSPECTED BACTERIAL ARTHRITIS

Technique	Utility	Findings and Comments
Plain radiographs	Baseline	To follow progressive joint changes and detect coexistent osteomyelitis
	Prosthetic joint infection	Loosening (but usually not caused by infection)
	Characteristic cartilage and bone changes usually develop after 7–14 days	Osteoporosis, marginal erosions, uniform joint space narrowing, periostitis
Nuclide bone scanning (technetium, gallium, indium)	Early changes most helpful in hip, shoulder, or axial joints. Gallium or indium more specific but less sensitive	Detects earlier changes than plain radiographs; not specific for infection
Fluoroscopy	For diagnostic aspiration of joints difficult to see such as the hip or SI joint	Inject contrast material with aspiration, useful in evaluating prosthetic joints
Computed tomography	Provides greater detail for detection of small bone and joint changes in sacroiliac and sternoclavicular joint infections	May also be useful when aspirating SI, hip, or other axial joints
Magnetic resonance	May provide earlier diagnostic utility than plain radiographs	Possible greater specificity than other techniques, especially in soft tissue extension

clinically or that have a complex anatomic structure, computed tomography (CT), radionuclide imaging, or magnetic resonance imaging (MRI) may be of diagnostic value. The hip, shoulder, sternoclavicular, and sacroiliac joints are difficult to palpate, difficult to aspirate, and are most likely to require further diagnostic evaluation radiographically. CT may demonstrate early bone erosions, reveal soft-tissue extension and facilitate arthrocentesis of shoulders, hips, and sacroiliac joints.[34, 35]

Scintigraphic abnormalities may be detected within hours or days of the onset of joint infections. However, the technetium phosphate bone scan does not adequately differentiate septic from nonseptic inflammation.[36] Gallium scan may demonstrate joint infection when the standard bone scan is negative and is particularly helpful in small children when difficulty in distinguishing normal uptake in the region of the growth plate may be encountered with technetium bone scan. Indium-labeled leukocyte scintigraphy is less sensitive than technetium bone scanning but is more specific for joint sepsis, since it

is dependent on the chemotaxis of labeled leukocytes to the infected area. It may be of particular diagnostic utility in suspected prosthetic joint infections.[37] MRI has been a useful adjunct in the diagnosis of septic arthritis.[33, 38, 39] Early detection of fluid and better definition of soft tissue extension are advantages of MRI.

IMPORTANT CLINICAL SETTINGS OF NONGONOCOCCAL BACTERIAL ARTHRITIS

Associated Arthritis. Hematogenously acquired nongonococcal bacterial arthritis often occurs in patients with compromised host defenses or prior joint damage. Bacterial arthritis is most common in young or elderly individuals in whom impaired ability to resist bacteremia is most evident. Patients with rheumatoid arthritis (RA) are prone to septic arthritis by virtue of local joint and systemic factors (Table 86–5). Animal studies of bacterial arthritis arising in arthritic joints have demonstrated marked neovas-

Table 86–5. PREDISPOSING FACTORS AND ASSOCIATED CONDITIONS IN BACTERIAL ARTHRITIS

Predisposing Factor/Condition	Possible Mechanism for Association	Important Clinical Features
Rheumatoid arthritis	Damaged joint good nidus for infection. Compromised defenses from medications (e.g., glucocorticoids, cytotoxic drugs); defective phagocytosis(?)	Usually due to *S. aureus*. Must always consider in RA. Treatment results often poor
Crystal-induced arthritis	Synovial fluid acidosis may promote crystal precipitation Enzymatic "strip-mining" of cartilage	Identification of crystals does not rule out infection
Severe osteoarthritis, Charcot's joint, hemarthrosis	Joint disorganization, chronic synovitis, and bloody effusions all provide nidus for bacteria	Always send bloody joint fluid for culture, especially in hemophiliacs
Chronic, systemic disease (e.g., SLE, sickle-cell disease, cancer)	Impaired generalized defenses due to chronic illness, phagocytic deficiencies, and medications	Often due to *S. aureus* or gram-negative bacilli
Intravenous drug use	Recurrent bacteremia	Usually due to *S. aureus* or gram-negative bacilli. Often occurs in axial joints
Intra-articular injection	Direct inoculation	Rare, usually *S. epidermidis* or *S. aureus*

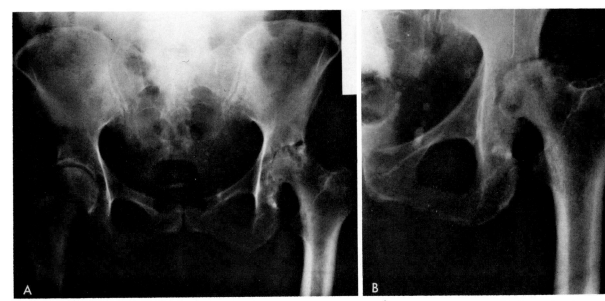

Figure 86–1. *E. coli* septic arthritis of left hip. *A,* Hip radiograph taken for mild hip pain in patient with fever of unknown source. Destruction of articular surfaces and loss of joint space are evident. *B,* Left hip radiograph 6 weeks later detailing progressive destruction of femoral head and acetabulum. The source of this infection was an intra-abdominal abscess that extended into the hip.

cularization in bones of involved joints; the vessels become plugged by bacteria, leading to osteonecrosis and osteomyelitis.[2] Defective phagocytosis has also been postulated to account for the increased incidence of septic arthritis in RA, but RA synovial fluid PMNs phagocytized *S. aureus* more effectively than peripheral blood PMNs and more efficiently than PMNs from healthy donors.[40]

The prevalence of septic arthritis complicating RA has been estimated at 0.3 to 3 percent of patients.[40] RA has usually been present for at least 10 years; most patients have had severe, seropositive RA; 50 percent have received oral or intra-articular glucocorticoids within 2 weeks prior to the infection (Table 86–6). The source of infection was most often the skin, but in 50 percent of cases no source of infection was identified.[41] Approximately one third of patients have polyarticular infection. The duration of symptoms prior to diagnosis has been longer than in other patients with septic arthritis. For example, in two reports of bacterial arthritis in patients with RA the mean duration of symptoms prior to diagnosis of a septic joint was 13.7 days and 16.4 days,[41, 42] compared with 7 days in non-RA patients.[1] *Staphylococcus aureus* has been recovered from almost 75 percent of infected RA joints, *Streptococcus* species in 15 percent, and gram-negative bacilli in 7 to 8 percent. Undoubtedly, the prolonged duration of symptoms prior to diagnosis of septic arthritis in RA delays therapy and increases morbidity and mortality (Table 86–7), and two thirds of the patients were admitted to the hospital with a diagnosis of an exacerbation of RA.[42]

Crystal-induced arthritis and coexistent septic arthritis have been reported more commonly in the recent literature.[1] There have been an equal number of cases of gout and CPPD crystal deposition disease associated with septic arthritis, and the infections have been caused by a wide spectrum of bacteria. Crystals were almost always present on the initial synovial fluid examination, but positive Gram stains were present in only 50 percent of cases.[1] Bacterial arthritis causes a decrease in synovial fluid pH, which may decrease the solubility of monosodium urate crystals (see Table 86–5).

Marked degenerative joint disease, either primary or associated with Charcot's arthropathy, has also been complicated by bacterial arthritis.[1] Patients with severely traumatized joints, or patients with recurrent hemarthrosis related to hemophilia or another bleeding disorder may develop bacterial arthritis. Any bloody synovial effusion that is aspirated should be routinely cultured, even if the index of suspicion for infection is low.

Table 86–6. DATA ON 175 PATIENTS WITH INFECTIOUS ARTHRITIS COMPLICATING RHEUMATOID ARTHRITIS (RA)

Years of RA, median (range)	12 (1–50)
Receiving corticosteroids, %	50
Peripheral leukocyte count >10,000/mm³, %	60
Infecting organisms, %	
Staphylococcus aureus	75
Others (*Streptococcus, Escherichia coli,* etc.)	25
Outcome, %	
Complete recovery	45
Poor joint outcome	36
Death	19

From Goldenberg, D. L.: Infectious arthritis complicating rheumatoid arthritis and other chronic rheumatic disorders. Arthritis Rheum. 32:496, 1989.

Table 86–7. OUTCOME OF 213 RA PATIENTS WITH PYARTHROSIS BY DECADE
COMPARED WITH THE SERIES FROM 1990

Outcome	1950s	1960s	1970s	1980s	Total	1990 Series*
Died	8(31)†	14(21)	17(25)	7(19)	46(22)	1(7)
Monoarticular, died	3(20)	4(12)	5(17)	2(14)	14(15)	0(0)
Polyarticular, died	4(42)	8(42)	5(45)	5(71)	22(47)	1(17)
Recurrence same joint	3(11)	17(25)	5(10)	4(11)	29(16)	5(36)
Joint altered	6(22)	11(16)	17(35)	10(29)	44(25)	12(92)

*From Gardner, G. C., and Weisman, M. H.: Pyarthrosis in patients with rheumatoid arthritis: A report of 13 cases and a review of the literature from the past 40 years. Am. J. Med. 88:503, 1990.
†(%).

Bacterial arthritis has also been well described in patients with systemic lupus erythematosus (SLE). In patients with bacterial arthritis, SLE had been present for an average of 6.5 years, and 95 percent of patients had been receiving glucocorticoids.[40] Encapsulated bacteria were most often recovered, including *N. gonorrhoeae*, *Salmonella* ssp., and *Proteus* ssp. SLE patients who are chronic carriers of *Salmonella* are predisposed to Salmonella bacteremia and septic arthritis.[43, 44] Selective functional hyposplenism in SLE may cause defective bacterial clearance and promote risk of severe bacteremia and septic arthritis independent of immunosuppressive medications.[45]

Intravenous Drug Use and Direct Inoculation. During the past decade, intravenous drug use has become an important predisposing factor for nongonococcal bacterial arthritis; this is especially evident at urban medical centers. Twenty-one of 28 patients with bacterial arthritis admitted to one urban hospital from 1981 to 1982 were intravenous drug users.[46] Joint sepsis in intravenous drug use abusers is most often caused by gram-negative bacilli, such as *Pseudomonas aeruginosa*. Presumably, frequent transient episodes of bacteremia during the intravenous injections of illicit drugs predispose these patients to bacterial arthritis.[47] Other predisposing conditions include the presence of indwelling venous catheters, chronic hemodialysis, and repeated skin injections. Intravenous drug users, hemodialysis patients, and diabetics receiving insulin injections often carry *S. aureus* on their skin or in their nasopharynx, and it is likely that the source of bacteria and septic arthritis arise from the patients themselves.[48]

Septic arthritis may result from therapeutic intraarticular glucocorticoid injections via four mechanisms: (1) contamination of the injectable medication, such as reports of *Pseudomonas cepacia* and *Serratia marcescens* in multidose vials of glucocorticoids; (2) from introduction of skin flora; (3) from hematogenous colonization of the puncture track; or (4) by activation of a previously quiescent joint infection.[49] The complication of postinjection infection is considered rare, and Hollander's infection rate of 1 in 16,000 is often quoted.[50] Nevertheless, 443 cases of postinjection joint bacterial arthritis have been reported.[49] *S. aureus* has been responsible for about 50 percent of cases and diagnosis is often delayed. The incidence of postarthroscopy infection has ranged from .01

percent to 1 percent.[51, 52] Factitious septic arthritis has been reported in patients who repeatedly self-administered intravenous injections of contaminated substances.[53]

Septic arthritis may also arise following joint puncture wounds.[54] This is most common in young children and usually presents soon after the puncture wound with marked joint inflammation, fever, and leukocytosis. Foreign body synovitis often is mistaken for acute septic arthritis, although most patients are not febrile and do not demonstrate elevated peripheral white blood cell counts.[55, 56] Excisional biopsy with careful microbiologic studies of the synovium may be necessary in situations where the synovial fluid is sterile or cannot be obtained.[56]

Prosthetic Joint Infection. The most important instance of bacterial arthritis associated with a sterile foreign body is that of prosthetic joint infections.[51] The overall incidence of joint infection complicating a primary arthroplasty is 0.5 to 2 percent but is much greater for revision arthroplasty.[58–60] Risk factors for early prosthetic joint infections include prolonged duration of surgery, the number of operating room personnel, an inexperienced primary surgeon, advanced age of the patient, rheumatoid arthritis or other systemic illness, and perioperative nonarticular infections[58] (Table 86–8). Staphylococci cause 70 to 80 percent of prosthetic joint infections. *S. epidermidis* is most commonly isolated from perioperative infections and *S. aureus* from later postoperative infections.[60, 61] Gram-negative bacilli, anaerobes, and non-group A streptococci are other common bacteria isolated from prosthetic joints.[60] Epidemiologic stud-

Table 86–8. RISK FACTORS FOR PROSTHETIC JOINT INFECTIONS

Early Infection	Late Infection
Prolonged duration of surgery	Type of prosthesis
Number of operating room personnel	Rheumatoid arthritis
Inexperienced primary surgeon	Nonarticular infections
Advanced age	Duration of implant(?)
Rheumatoid arthritis	Loosening of implant(?)
Perioperative nonarticular infections	

From Blackburn, W. D., Jr., Alarcón, G. S.: Prosthetic joint infections: A role for prophylaxis. Arthritis Rheum. 34:110, 1991.

ies of the operating room environment demonstrate that shorter duration of surgery, prophylactic antibiotics given immediately prior to surgery, antibiotic-impregnated methylmethacrylate cement, and cleaned and directed air flow may reduce the perioperative infection rate.[58, 59] Perioperative antibiotics, such as cephalosporins, have usually been given but they should be discontinued soon after surgery to prevent the emergence of antibiotic-resistant bacteria.[58]

The clinical presentation of prosthetic joint infections also varies with the duration of time from surgery. Most infections occurring during the first few months after surgery present with pain, swelling drainage, and sometimes fever. The major diagnostic challenge is to determine whether the infection is confined to the superficial tissues or has involved the joint. Late prosthetic joint infections often present with a prolonged indolent course of increasing joint pain. Fever is present in less than 50 percent of late prosthetic joint infections, and a peripheral blood leukocytosis occurs in only 10 percent of these patients.[57-61] Acute phase reactants such as the erythrocyte sedimentation rate (ESR) and C-reactive protein (CRP) are usually elevated in prosthetic joint infections and may be diagnostically helpful, particularly in patients with suspected prosthetic joint infections who do not have RA or another inflammatory arthritis. In patients with a noninfected hip-loosening the CRP was less than 20 mg per liter and the ESR was less than 30 mm per hr, whereas in the majority of patients with an infected hip arthroplasty, the CRP and ESR were above those values.[62]

Any drainage from a joint sinus tract should be cultured, but usually the joint will require aspiration for definitive diagnosis. A large-bore needle should be used for aspiration, usually best performed with CT guidance. If no fluid is obtained, open biopsy of the synovium and periprosthetic tissue should be performed under general anesthesia. All material should be sent for aerobic and anaerobic culture.

Treatment of the infected prosthetic joint requires prolonged antibiotics and immediate surgical intervention. If none of the prosthetic components are loose or damaged, a careful and complete débridement of all infected and abnormal tissue may rarely allow salvage of the prosthesis. However, the infection usually involves the material around the prosthesis. Less than 10 percent of prosthetic hip infections have been successfully treated without removal of the prosthesis[58-61] (see Chapter 108). Similar results have been reported for the surgical treatment of infected knee arthroplasties[63] (see Chapter 109). Mortality rates as high as 20 percent have been reported in patients with prosthetic joint infections.[58] Unusual pathogens are more commonly encountered in prosthetic joint infections including S. pneumoniae,[64] Peptostreptococcus magnus,[65] and Mycoplasma hominis.[66]

The issue of antibiotic prophylaxis in patients with prosthetic joints is still controversial.[58] Black-

burn and Alarcón estimated that the cost of possible infection or death exceeded that of antibiotic prophlyaxis.[58] They also surveyed a random sample of RA patients and found that only 10 percent had been made aware of any recommendations regarding the use of prophylactic antibiotics.

Blackburn and Alarcón suggested a set of guidelines for the prevention of prosthetic joint infections[58] (Table 86–9). All patients should be carefully screened for possible occult infection prior to surgery. Dental hygiene should be emphasized. Immunosuppressive medications should be tapered to the lowest dose possible. The question of temporarily discontinuing methotrexate has not been resolved.[69] The use of perioperative antibiotics should be timed so that bactericidal levels are present at the time of surgery. Any infection in a patient with a prosthetic joint should be quickly and aggressively eradicated. The use of prophylactic antibiotics should be based on the physician's analysis of the cost-benefit ratio for each patient, but are to be recommended for high-risk patients, such as those with RA or another chronic, medical illness, who undergo a procedure with a significant risk of bacteremia.

Other Systemic Illness. Patients with generalized systemic illness including cancer, diabetes mellitus, and alcoholism, as well as those with specific phagocytic defects, are prone to developing septic arthritis.[16] Septic arthritis, especially related to Salmonella spp. and other encapsulated bacteria, is prominent in sickle-cell disease.[70] Septic arthritis has been uncommonly reported in patients with HIV infection.[71, 73] Most cases have been caused by opportunistic pathogens, including fungal and mycobacterial arthritis. A high index of suspicion for septic arthritis and coincidental HIV infection is necessary in hemophiliacs, particularly in children who received commercial factor concentrates prior to screening for HIV.[72]

Bacterial Arthritis in Children. The bacteria that are most commonly recovered from the joints of children vary with the age of the child. In hospital-acquired neonatal septic arthritis, Staphylococcus aureus and gram-negative bacilli are the most common isolates, but streptococci are the most common in community-acquired neonatal bacterial arthritis. Group B streptococci are especially important in

Table 86–9. PREVENTION OF PROSTHETIC JOINT INFECTIONS

Careful preoperative evaluation for occult infection
Taper or discontinue immunosuppressive medications if possible
Perioperative antibiotics should be bactericidal at surgery and given briefly
Any local or systemic infection should be eradicated quickly
Prophylactic antibiotics should be given to high-risk patients undergoing a procedure associated with significant bacteremia. In less clear situations, a case-by-case cost-benefit ratio is recommended

Data from Blackburn, W. D., Jr., and Alarcón, G. S.: Prosthetic joint infections: A role for prophylaxis. Arthritis Rheum. 34:110, 1991.

neonatal septic arthritis.[74] The neonatal anatomy, with metaphyseal and epiphyseal blood vessel communication, promotes spread of bacteria from the metaphysis to the cartilaginous epiphysis. *H. influenzae* accounts for more than 50 percent of all cases in children 2 months to 2 years of age and is now the most common bacteria isolated from the joints of children.[74–77]

A bacterial etiology is found less commonly in children than in adults with suspected bacterial arthritis. In Fink and Nelson's review of 591 cases with the clinical diagnosis of septic arthritis, 34 percent had no positive cultures.[75] The 389 cases with positive cultures included 50 percent with positive synovial fluid only, 28 percent with both positive synovial fluid and blood cultures, and 10 percent with positive blood but negative synovial fluid cultures. Prior antibiotic therapy did not significantly affect the rate of positive blood cultures but decreased the synovial fluid positivity from 80 percent to 38 percent.[76] Cerebrospinal fluid cultures and counterimmunoelectrophoresis may be the only positive way to detect certain causes of bacterial arthritis in children, and are especially helpful in *Haemophilus* or meningococcal arthritis.

The clinical presentation and joints involved are similar to that in adults, with the only notable exception being a greater incidence of hip involvement (see Table 86–1).[75] Septic arthritis of the hip is a diagnostic and therapeutic challenge in children. The child usually refuses to move the leg and holds it in external rotation and abduction. There may be hip or leg edema and pain over the groin. Pain is often referred to the thigh and knee. Coexistent osteomyelitis is more often present in children and occasionally multiple simultaneous joint and bone involvement will be present.

Bacterial Arthritis in the Elderly. Elderly patients with comorbid systemic illness as well as prior joint disease or trauma are predisposed to septic arthritis.[1] As might be expected, septic arthritis in the elderly has a higher mortality and a greater risk of serious joint damage than in younger patients. For example, 4 of 21 patients older than 60 years with septic arthritis died and 11 others developed osteomyelitis or major joint damage.[78] Most patients were afebrile and had a normal peripheral blood leukocyte count. Fourteen of the infections were caused by *S. aureus* and three by *Streptococcus*. However, a report of gram-negative bacilli septic arthritis in the elderly did not find that age was a negative prognostic factor.[79] In these 22 patients the mortality was only 5 percent and 70 percent of joints had a good outcome.

Shoulder septic arthritis may be more common in the elderly.[1, 78–80] Septic arthritis of the shoulder was often misdiagnosed as tendinitis or frozen shoulder, delaying the diagnosis and appropriate treatment.[80] In 7 of 18 cases in one series septic arthritis may have been a complication of shoulder injection or arthrocentesis.[80] Each patient had an elevated ESR

and the authors recommended a high index of suspicion of septic arthritis in elderly patients with acute or subacute shoulder pathology. Unusual organisms have been recovered in recent reports of septic arthritis in the elderly, including *Morganella morganii*[81] and *Bacteroides fragilis*.[82]

SPECIFIC FORMS OF BACTERIAL ARTHRITIS

Gram-positive cocci are the most common cause of nongonococcal bacterial arthritis, and *S. aureus* causes 60 percent of such infections (see Table 86–2). During the past few years, most *S. aureus* recovered from joints have been resistant to methicillin as well as penicillin, although this varies widely in different series.[1] For example, all strains of *S. aureus* isolated from infected joints in an urban medical center from 1966 to 1977 were methicillin sensitive, but 7 of 18 strains isolated from infected joints from 1981 to 1982 were methicillin resistant.[46] Methicillin-resistant and oxacillin-resistant *S. aureus* arthritis have been especially prominent in intravenous drug users. Eighty percent of joint infections in patients with RA or any other chronic arthritis are caused by *S. aureus*. *Staphylococcus epidermidis* is an important cause of prosthetic joint infections but has also been recovered from joints of compromised hosts.[16] Rarely other coagulase-negative staphylococci, such as *S. capitis* and *S. simulans*, have caused joint infections.[1] These coagulase-negative staphylococci are often resistant to multiple antibiotics.

Beta-hemolytic streptococci continue to be an important cause of septic arthritis, accounting for 10 to 30 percent of all cases of nongonococcal bacterial arthritis.[1] Group A streptococcal septic arthritis, the most common form of streptococcal arthritis, generally results from a primary skin or soft tissue infection. There have been more reports of non-group A streptococcal arthritis during the past 10 years.[83–87] Patients with non-group A streptococcal arthritis are usually seriously ill and their joint infections are often difficult to eradicate. Many patients have associated genitourinary or gastrointestinal infections. Although group A streptococcal arthritis is most often monarticular, 20 to 40 percent of non-group A streptococcal arthritis has been polyarticular.[83–87]

The various strains of streptococci isolated must be carefully classified based on their reaction with Lancefield antisera, because treatment plan as well as the prognosis differs with various streptococcal serotypes.[83–87] Whereas the prognosis for group A streptococcal septic arthritis is generally good,[15, 16] that of non-group A streptococcal arthritis is often poor, possibly because of serious comorbidity.

Gram-negative bacilli are common causes of septic arthritis in young children, in chronically ill, elderly patients, and in intravenous drug users.[1, 15, 16, 74–76, 79] Important associated medical conditions in adults with gram-negative septic arthritis include cancer, diabetes mellitus, sickle cell anemia, connective tissue disorders, and renal transplant. Most infections are secondary to urinary tract or skin infections with subsequent bacteremic spread to a single joint. In elderly, compromised hosts, *E. coli* is the most common gram-negative bacillus isolated from joints, but *S. marcescens* and *P. aeruginosa* are the most commonly reported cause of septic arthritis in heroin users.[1] In drug users, these infections occur commonly in the sternoclavicular, sacroiliac, and vertebral joints. This unusual joint predilection is probably related to bacterial access from the injection of drugs, since the sternoclavicular joint infection tends to occur on the same side used for the drug injections.[47] Other *Pseudomonas* species,[88] *Kingella kingae*,[89] and *Klebsiella*[90] have been recovered from septic joints.

Pasteurella multocida, a gram-negative coccobacillus found in the normal oral flora of 70 to 90 percent of cats and 50 percent of dogs, has caused septic arthritis in humans following animal bites.[91–93] *Streptobacillus moniliformis*, a gram-negative, pleomorphic bacillus frequently present in the oropharynx of wild and laboratory rats, and the cause of a systemic, febrile illness termed rat-bite fever, may also cause septic arthritis.[94] The arthritis associated with *Salmonella* infection is usually reactive, but classic suppurative arthritis is well described.[95–99] *Haemophilus influenzae*, especially type b, is the most common cause of septic arthritis in children between 6 and 24 months of age.[1, 100] These children are usually healthy but have lost maternal antibodies against *H. influenzae* and have not yet generated effective levels of autologous antibodies. Many children have associated upper respiratory tract infections, otitis media, or meningitis. However, this organism rarely causes septic arthritis in adults, and when it does, it usually occurs in alcoholics or diabetics. A newly available vaccine may potentially reduce the number of infections.

The incidence of anaerobic bacterial septic arthritis has increased during the past 10 years.[101, 102] This increase probably reflects improved culture techniques and an increased awareness of anaerobic infections. *Peptococcus magnus*,[103] *Bacteroides fragilis*,[101] and various *Fusobacterium* and *Corynebacterium* have predominated. Most anaerobic joint infections have occurred as a result of postoperative wound infections, especially following joint arthroplasty, or in compromised hosts.[101–108] *Bacteroides fragilis* septic arthritis has been reported in elderly patients with rheumatoid arthritis, osteoarthritis, or prior joint damage.[82] Significant comorbid illness was present in most patients, and mortality was 50 percent. A patient with rheumatoid arthritis developed polyarticular *Clostridium perfringens* pyoarthritis.[104] Infectious arthritis caused by *Propionibacterium acnes* has been reported in prosthetic joints and following joint aspiration.[107, 108] Anaerobic bacteria require reduced oxygen tension for growth, and both synovial fluid and synovial membranes must be collected in oxygen-free, prereduced, anaerobically sterrilized containers. Foul-smelling synovial fluid or air seen in the joint on radiographs should raise the suspicion of anaerobic bacterial arthritis.[109] Anaerobic cultures should be maintained for at least 2 weeks because of the slow growth of these organisms. Antibiotic sensitivity should be routinely obtained, because many of these anaerobes are resistant to multiple antibiotics, including penicillin.[109]

Polymicrobial bacterial arthritis has been reported in 2 to 10 percent of series of nongonococcal bacterial arthritis.[15–18] Approximately 50 percent of all anaerobic joint infections are polymicrobial, and in these situations both anaerobic and aerobic bacteria are often recovered from the joint. Polymicrobial septic arthritis occurs primarily in seriously ill patients, postoperative wound infections, or as a result of direct spread, such as from an intra-abdominal or intrapelvic source into the hip.[110, 111]

Although brucellosis is not common in the United States, it is a very common and often serious infectious disease in many parts of the world. *Brucella* are small, gram-negative bacilli that grow slowly and require special media for optimal recovery.[112] In many parts of the world transmission occurs by the ingestion of unpasteurized milk or cheese, although in the United States most cases occur in farmers, meat packers, or other workers exposed to infected meat.[112–116] The most common form of chronic or relapsing brucellosis is caused by *Brucella melitensis*, and this species causes most cases of brucella arthritis. The arthritis is most often a monarthritis or asymmetric peripheral oligoarthritis. Sacroiliitis and spondylitis are common.[117–119] Arthritis occurs in 10 to 20 percent of acute brucellosis, but in 50 to 65 percent of subacute or chronic infections, especially if the infection had been present for greater than 6 months. Brucella are recovered from only 50 percent of suspected infected joints. This may relate to difficulty in growing the organisms in vitro or may represent a reactive or postinfectious arthritis. Treatment of all forms of brucella arthritis requires antibiotics, although there are few controlled studies and many opinions regarding optimal antimicrobial therapy.[120] Most authors recommend a tetracycline, such as doxycycline, 100 mg b.i.d. for 4 weeks. Rifampicin or a third-generation cephalosporin are good alternatives. Combination chemotherapy, usually with an aminoglycoside and trimethoprim, is advocated to diminish the relapse rate.

Problematic Joints. Certain joints, because of their unique anatomy, are especially difficult to diagnose and treat when they become infected. Joint effusions are difficult to detect in shoulders and hips. These joints are also difficult to aspirate or to drain adequately, and require early surgical consultation, especially in the elderly[78, 80] or in young children.[74–76]

Most patients with pyogenic sacroiliitis present with indolent back and buttock pain, which may mimic a protruded disc.[121–124] Focal tenderness over the buttock and SI area, limited straight-leg raising, and pain with pelvic compression are usually present.[124] Fever and an elevated erythrocyte sedimentation rate should raise the suspicion of septic sacroiliitis, but fever is present in only 40 to 60 percent of cases, although blood cultures are positive in 60 percent.[123] Scintigraphy and CT scans are helpful because they are abnormal long before plain radiographs reveal any changes.[33, 35, 39] The sacroiliac joint should be aspirated just above the lower border, and if the needle enters the joint but no fluid is returned, 5 ml of saline should be injected and then reaspirated.[121] If the specimen is still inadequate for bacteriologic evaluation, an open biopsy should be performed. Abscess formation within the SI joint may lead to dissection into various muscle planes, causing unusual extensions of infection, including all the way down to the ankle.[125] Septic sternoclavicular arthritis has been reported most often in intravenous drug users,[47, 126] diabetics,[126] and RA patients.[127] Most patients with septic sternoclavicular joints complain of anterior chest discomfort, have fever, and demonstrate obvious swelling over the joint and restricted range of motion of the homolateral shoulder.[126] CT scan is the most sensitive technique to visualize early changes and to document the extent of infection. Approximately 20 percent of patients with sternoclavicular joint septic arthritis develop an abscess of the chest wall or mediastinum.[127] *Staphylococcus aureus* and *P. aeruginosa*, generally in intravenous drug users, are responsible for the majority of cases of sternoclavicular septic arthritis.[127] Early surgical exploration should be undertaken in sternoclavicular septic arthritis, both to obtain adequate material for culture and to assess possible extension into the mediastinum. Septic arthritis of the temporomandibular joint[128] and pubic symphysis[129] has also been reported.

TREATMENT AND OUTCOME OF NONGONOCOCCAL BACTERIAL ARTHRITIS

Antibiotics. If nongonococcal bacterial arthritis is suspected clinically and if the synovial fluid is purulent, antibiotics should be started as soon as all specimens are obtained for culture (Table 86–10). While awaiting the culture results, antibiotics should be selected on the basis of the Gram stain and the clinical picture. If gram-positive cocci are identified, a penicillinase-resistant penicillin or, if there is a high prevalence of methicillin-resistant *S. aureus*, vancomycin should be started. Gram-negative bacilli in compromised hosts should be treated initially with an aminoglycoside and an antipseudomonal penicillin or a third-generation cephalosporin. In healthy, young adults with a negative Gram stain smear, penicillin or ceftriaxone are usually recommended. Neonates and children younger than 2 years should be started on broad-spectrum antibiotics to cover ampicillin-resistant *H. influenzae*, *S. aureus*, and group B streptococci. Possible regimens would include an antistaphylococcal penicillin and an aminoglycoside or a third-generation cephalosporin. Cephalosporins

Table 86–10. TREATMENT OF BACTERIAL ARTHRITIS

1. Aspirate any possible infected joint immediately. Remove as much fluid as possible and perform synovial fluid culture, Gram stain, leukocyte count and differential leukocyte count, glucose with simultaneous blood glucose determinations, and crystal analysis.
2. If the fluid is purulent or if organisms are seen on the Gram stain smear, start antibiotics immediately:
   a. Organisms identified on Gram stain: If gram-positive cocci, start nafcillin or (if in hospital with methicillin-resistant *S. aureus*) vancomycin. If gram-negative cocci, start ceftriaxone. If gram-negative bacilli, start an aminoglycoside and β-lactam antibiotic or third-generation cephalosporin.
   b. Negative Gram stain: In children younger than age 2, cover for penicillin-resistant *H. influenzae*, staphylococci, and gram-negative bacilli. In compromised hosts, elderly individuals, and intravenous drug users, cover for methicillin-resistant *S. aureus* and gram-negative bacilli.
3. When the specific bacterium is identified, adjust antibiotics if necessary. Administer antibiotics parenterally and in doses used to treat bacteremia.
4. Drain all purulent fluid with closed needle aspiration, arthroscopy, or arthrotomy.
5. Reassess adequacy of treatment clinically and with serial synovial fluid analysis. If inadequate therapeutic response, obtain serum and synovial fluid bactericidal concentrations and evaluate the efficacy of drainage.

are often used in possible moderate penicillin allergy, whereas vancomycin or clindamycin can be used in patients with a history of a severe penicillin allergy. Other appropriate antibiotics include imipenem, or ampicillin combined with sulbactam. Elderly and compromised patients should also have initial broad-spectrum coverage.

Once the specific bacterium is recovered from the synovial fluid or blood, antibiotics are adjusted on the basis of sensitivities, toxicity, and cost. Most antibiotics are administered intravenously for at least 2 weeks, often to be followed by 1 to 2 weeks of oral antibiotics in nongonococcal bacterial arthritis. However, there are no controlled studies of the optimal duration and route of administration. The duration of therapy is determined primarily by the patient's response. Home parenteral therapy now provides a cost-effective way of delivering high-dose antibiotics outside the hospital and is especially useful for antibiotics with a long half-life.

Most antibiotics achieve a high concentration in infected synovial fluid.[129–132] Although there is some variability according to the antibiotic tested, most antibiotics achieve synovial fluid concentrations that are much greater than the minimal inhibitory concentration necessary against the usual pathogens. In a rabbit model of *S. aureus* arthritis, parenteral administration of penicillin G, cloxacillin, clindamycin, and netilmicin achieved adequate antibacterial levels in infected joints.[132] The antibiotic concentrations were two to three times higher in infected joints compared with noninfected joints. A serum and synovial fluid antibiotic concentration or determination of bactericidal activity against the specific bacteria isolated should be obtained initially in the following situations: any gram-negative bacillary arthritis, any infection that is not responding adequately to treatment, whenever "newer" antibiotics without known efficacy in bacterial arthritis are being used, and whenever oral antibiotics are being used. Despite evidence that intra-articular instillation of antibiotics achieves joint levels comparable to parental administration,[132, 133] the combination of intra-articular and parenteral ceftazidime failed to eradicate *P. aeruginosa* septic arthritis.[34] Quinolones have been effective in gram-negative septic arthritis, but resistance may emerge early with these agents.[135] In children, early use of oral antibiotics and a shorter duration of treatment have been effective.[136–138] Oral antibiotics should be used only in maximal tolerated doses and only with careful monitoring to ensure adequate synovial fluid antibacterial concentrations. Intra-articular antibiotics should be utilized only when parenteral antibiotics are not achieving adequate bactericidal activity and with the recognition that they may cause a chemical synovitis.[1]

Joint Drainage, Open or Closed? Prompt and adequate drainage of purulent synovial effusions is an essential aspect of treatment of septic arthritis, although the optimal method of drainage is controversial.[139] Surgical intervention is generally recommended as the initial drainage procedure of choice in the following situations: (1) hip infections in children, (2) any joint that is anatomically difficult to drain or to assess the adequacy of drainage, (3) coexistent osteomyelitis requiring surgical intervention, (4) any joint that cannot be adequately drained with needle aspiration (e.g., adhesions or loculations prevent adequate drainage; a young child refusing repeated needle aspiration) and, (5) to assess possible extension of the septic arthritis into soft tissue planes, as in sternoclavicular septic arthritis. Most authors recommend initial open drainage as the procedure of choice in adults as well as in children with septic arthritis of the hip.[15, 16, 139–144] The shoulder also is difficult to drain adequately by closed-needle aspiration, although successful treatment of septic arthritis of the shoulder without open drainage has been well documented.[144, 145] However, initial needle drainage will often fail to eradicate septic arthritis of the shoulder, and delayed open surgical drainage may lead to a very poor outcome.[80]

In most other joints, there are no clear guidelines to consider one form of initial joint drainage as superior to another. The controversy of the initial drainage procedure of choice is unlikely to be resolved by a controlled, prospective trial of closed versus open joint drainage. Broy and Schmid estimated that it would require 10 years for a multi-institutional prospective study to detect a 20 percent difference in success rates in a randomized, clinical trial of open versus closed joint drainage.[144] Therefore, they pooled and analyzed all published reports of outcome of bacterial arthritis in adults from the past 25 years according to initial drainage. A total of 371 joint infections in 336 patients were analyzed.

Two hundred forty-two joints were treated medically, and 129 received initial surgical drainage. The knee was the most often involved joint and *S. aureus* the most common bacteria, with a similar distribution of joint involvement as well as bacteria in both treatment groups. There was a similar prevalence of pre-existing joint disease in both groups but a far greater prevalence of chronic debilitating illness in the medically treated patients. Sixty-six percent of the medically treated group versus 57 percent of the surgically treated group had a good outcome (P < 0.005). In all reports there has been a higher mortality in the medically treated patients, but this seems related to more serious comodbidity in these patients. The conclusion of the pooled analysis as well as our results[139] indicate that closed-needle aspiration should be the initial treatment of choice in all cases of gonococcal arthritis and in adults with nongonococcal arthritis of the knee (although arthroscopy may be very effective), wrist, ankle, and smaller joints. Hip and shoulders may be treated initially with a brief trial of needle aspiration, but unless there is a rapid and dramatic response, surgical drainage is recommended. Hips in children should be immediately drained surgically and in younger children, who are very difficult to treat with serial needle aspirations, earlier arthrotomy is appropriate.

In accessible joints, arthroscopy is an obvious alternative to either closed-needle aspiration or open surgical drainage and may have advantages over both.[146–151] However, if, after an appropriate trial of needle aspiration or arthroscopy the joint is not adequately drained, surgical drainage, exploration, and débridement should be done promptly. Serial synovial fluid cultures and leukocyte counts should be performed each time the joint is drained to help determine the response to treatment. After 7 days of antibiotics and drainage, the mean synovial fluid leukocyte count should have fallen dramatically (e.g., mean of 75,000 cells per mm^3 initially to 5000 to 25,000 cells per mm^3).[16] Thus, even if the synovial fluid is sterile, other parameters should be used to assess treatment response, and by 7 days there should be marked improvement in each parameter.

The treatment of an infected joint also includes meticulous attention to joint position, exercise, and rehabilitation. During the acute, suppurative phase, the patient will often maintain the joint in a position of slight to moderate flexion, which can lead to flexion deformities. Therefore, easily removed supporting slings, splints, or casts should be used to maintain the joint in optimal position. Even in this acute stage, muscle-tightening exercises should be initiated. Quadriceps "sets" are especially important in knee infections to help prevent muscle atrophy. Salter investigated early joint mobilization in experimental staphylococcal arthritis in rabbits.[152] The infected joints were treated with antibiotics and open drainage and either were immobilized in a cast or received intermittent active motion or continuous passive motion for 2 weeks. The immobilized knees fared the worst, and the joints that received continuous passive motion had fewer radiologic abnormalities, less loss of cartilage chondrocytes and matrix, and more normal content of collagen, keratin sulphate, chondroitin sulfate, and total hexosamine than the other knees.

Some patients will have made an uneventful recovery but, usually when beginning to ambulate, will develop a recurrent, inflammatory, but sterile effusion, a so-called postinfectious arthritis.[16] Such effusions probably represent the sequelae of a marked synovitis with the added insult of active weight-bearing, but this situation must be distinguished from an incompletely treated infection.

Results of Treatment. The therapeutic outcome of nongonococcal bacterial arthritis is related to multiple associated factors, including the duration of infection, the virulence of specific bacteria, the joints infected, host defenses, age of patient, and comorbidity as well as effective therapy. In animal studies and in patients, one of the most important correlates of outcome is the duration of time before treatment is initiated. Orchard and Stamp induced staphylococcal arthritis in rabbits and began treatment immediately, at 1 day and 2 days after infection.[153, 154] Those animals that were treated the same day as they were infected had less radiologic, gross, and histologic abnormalities than the other two groups. Sixty-four percent of 100 patients with nongonococcal bacterial arthritis treated within 1 week of initial symptoms but only 22 percent who were treated after 1 week of symptoms recovered completely.[15, 16] The specific bacteria also play an important role in outcome. In most series, essentially all patients with gonococcal arthritis recover completely, and 70 to 85 percent of patients with group A streptococcal and pneumococcal arthritis recover completely.[15, 16, 154–156] However, only 50 percent of patients with staphylococcal arthritis and gram-negative bacilli arthritis recover completely. Polymicrobial and anaerobic bacterial arthritis also generally had poor outcomes. The correlation of specific pathogens with outcome may relate as much to host factors and comorbidity as to microbial virulence.

The outcome of septic arthritis in patients with RA or another systemic connective tissue is especially poor (see Table 86–7).[40, 41, 155–158] The rate of septic arthritis in RA increased from 1 in 200 RA hospitalizations from 1976 to 1983 to 1 in 100 RA hospitalizations from 1984 to 1987.[158] The increased number of septic arthritis cases was due largely to prosthetic joint infections. The index of suspicion for septic arthritis in any patient with RA must be high. Synovial fluid should be routinely cultured whenever an RA joint is aspirated or injected. If the synovial fluid appears purulent, if the Gram stain is positive, or if the patient is clinically bacteremic, parenteral antibiotics should be started (Table 86–11). Initial antibiotics should provide broad coverage, particularly for methicillin-resistant *S. aureus.* Although there are no prospective studies regarding the opti-

Table 86–11. PROBLEMS AND RECOMMENDATIONS IN THE DIAGNOSIS AND TREATMENT OF THE INFECTED RHEUMATOID JOINT

Mimics rheumatoid arthritis exacerbation:
  Fever not prominent: absence of chills, peripheral blood leukocytosis
  Insidious onset
  More than 1 joint may be inflamed
Rheumatoid arthritis may cause a "pseudoseptic" arthritis picture
Therefore,
  1. Always think of superimposed infection
  2. Routinely culture rheumatoid synovial fluid whenever it is aspirated
  3. Never inject glucocorticoids in a rheumatoid joint unless first culturing the synovial fluid
  4. Start antibiotics immediately if the Gram stain result is positive, if there is an obvious extra-articular infection, or if the synovial fluid is purulent
  5. Drain the joint adequately; consider early arthroscopy or open drainage

Modified from Goldenberg, D. L.: Infectious arthritis complicating rheumatoid arthritis and other chronic rheumatic disorders. Arthritis Rheum. 32:496, 1989.

mal mode of drainage in infected RA joints, some authors recommend earlier surgical drainage.[40, 41] The mortality of polyarticular septic arthritis in all patients is 23 percent, but in RA patients it is 56 percent.[17, 40, 41]

Nongonococcal bacterial arthritis is a serious disease with a 5 to 15 percent mortality rate and a 25 to 60 percent rate of chronic joint damage and disability.[15, 16, 144, 155, 156] In Broy and Schmid's pooled analysis of the literature,[144] two thirds of joints were considered to have good eventual outcome. Despite modern-day antibiotics, the mortality of bacterial arthritis has not changed recently, as noted with a 12 percent mortality rate in patients with nongonococcal bacterial arthritis treated between 1970 and 1984.[156] Predictors for mortality include rheumatoid arthritis, polyarticular sepsis, positive blood cultures, and older age.[156, 157]

INFECTIOUS ARTHRITIS CAUSED BY *N. GONORRHOEAE* AND *N. MENINGITIDIS*

Disseminated Gonococcal Infection (DGI). DGI is the most common joint infection seen at many urban medical centers. Because of the clinical and demographic differences with other forms of bacterial arthritis (Table 86–12), gonococcal arthritis and DGI are usually considered a distinct entity. Patients with DGI are young, healthy, and sexually active. Instead of presenting with a characteristic acute bacterial monarthritis, DGI usually is associated with polyarthritis, tenosynovitis, and dermatitis. Blood cultures are rarely positive and even when a synovial effusion is present, *N. gonorrhoeae* are recovered from less than 50 percent of joints. The time duration from sexual contact to the onset of DGI has varied from 1

Table 86–12. CLINICAL COMPARISON OF DISSEMINATED GONOCOCCAL INFECTION (DGI) AND NONGONOCOCCAL BACTERIAL ARTHRITIS

DGI	Nongonococcal Bacterial Arthritis
Most often in young, healthy adults or compromised host	Usually occurs in small children, elderly
No pre-existing joint disease or intra-articular injections	Commonly prior arthritis, prosthetic joint
Polyarthralgia, polyarthritis	Monarthritis
Dermatitis, tenosynovitis	—
Synovial fluid culture positive <25% of cases	Synovial fluid positive in >95% of cases
Blood culture rarely positive	Blood culture positive in 40–50%
Rapid therapeutic improvement with antibiotics	Often requires prolonged treatment with antibiotics and joint drainage
Outcome good in >95%	Outcome poor in 30–50%

day to 2 months. Only 25 percent of patients with DGI have local genitourinary symptoms. Twenty-five percent of patients have a history of previous gonorrhea, but recurrent DGI is rare and should alert one to the possibility that the patient has an acquired or inherited complement component deficiency. Terminal complement deficiencies (C5-C9) are important in the gonococcal outer membrane attack and have been associated with an increased risk of *N. gonorrhoeae* and *N. meningitidis* bacteremia.[159] Women who have become infected around the time of menstruation or during pregnancy are more prone to developing DGI.[160] Microbial characteristics that promote dissemination include the presence of gonococcal pili, certain colony nutritional requirements, the presence of specific outer membrane proteins, and the ability of the gonococcal strain to resist the killing activity of normal human sera.[160, 161] Until recently, most DGI strains were very sensitive to penicillin, but more DGI strains are now penicillinase-producing or demonstrate chromosomally mediated antibiotic resistance.[162–165]

Migratory or additive polyarthralgias are the initial symptom in most patients with DGI and often have been present for 3 to 5 days prior to diagnosis. The most common findings on physical examination are tenosynovitis, dermatitis, and fever, which are present in two thirds of patients at the time of hospitalization.[160] Tenosynovitis is most often present over the dorsum of the hand, the wrist, the ankle, or the knee. Dermatitis is usually maculopapular or vesicular, but pustules, hemorrhagic bullae, erythema multiforme, and vasculitis have been reported. The skin lesions are usually present over the extremities and trunk, but they are generally asymptomatic and require careful inspection for their detection (Fig. 86–2). Sometimes new skin lesions will appear after antibiotics have been started, but the dermatitis usually disappears within a few days of treatment. Biopsy of these skin lesions demonstrates

perivascular inflammation, intraepidermal neutrophilic infiltrates, and microthrombi, but *N. gonorrhoeae* are only rarely recovered from these sites.

Purulent synovitis is present in only 25 to 50 percent of patients. Knees, ankles, wrists, and elbows are most often infected, and polyarthritis is common. The mean synovial fluid leukocyte count has ranged from 34,000 to 68,000 cells per mm^3.[160] Rarely, patients may present with a chronic, indolent monarthritis.[165] Patients with associated tenosynovitis and dermatitis may have lower synovial fluid leukocyte counts. Peripheral blood leukocytosis, elevated erythrocyte sedimentation rate, and mildly abnormal serum transaminases or other liver function tests are common but not specific. Complications may include gonococcal pericarditis and tamponade.[166]

Neisseria gonorrhoeae has been cultured from fewer than 25 percent of joints and fewer than 10 percent of blood or skin lesions in patients with DGI. However, the organism can generally be recovered from genitourinary sites. Therefore, most cases will be termed presumptive based on a typical clinical picture and a positive genitourinary or other local culture but will often have a negative synovial fluid or blood culture. In these situations, rapid improvement with antibiotics may be of further diagnostic utility.

The peripheral manifestations of DGI may involve aseptic as well as septic processes. The arthral-

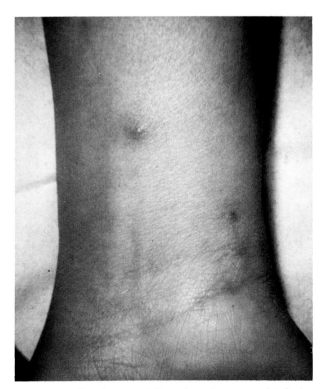

Figure 86–2. Skin lesions of disseminated gonococcal infection. The major lesion is vesicopustular, surmounting a hemorrhagic base. The other two, smaller lesions appear more necrotic and probably represent older lesions.

gias, tenosynovitis, and dermatitis characteristic of DGI are suggestive of an immune-mediated or serum-sickness condition. The inability to recover *N. gonorrhoeae* from sites of dissemination may be related to the fastidious growth requirements of this pathogen but alternatively may indicate that viable bacteria are not necessary for the evolution of DGI. Despite the absence of positive skin and synovial fluid cultures, gonococci have been identified by immunofluorescence or electron microscopy in skin and synovium.[160] Circulating immune complexes are present in DGI and are generally found in higher concentration in patients with arthralgias and tenosynovitis. Complement has been present in the blood vessel wall of DGI skin lesions, and an immune-mediated glomerulonephritis has been described. In a laboratory model of gonococcal arthritis, gonococcal lipopolysaccharide and killed gonococci caused an acute then chronic synovitis, which was indistinguishable from that following the injection of viable *N. gonorrhoeae*.[9]

The treatment of DGI is generally so effective that the therapeutic response is utilized for diagnostic purposes.[1] The differential diagnosis may include nongonococcal bacterial arthritis, bacterial endocarditis, Reiter's syndrome, hepatitis and other viral infections, acute rheumatic fever, and Lyme disease. None of these conditions responds as exquisitely to penicillin or newer cephalosporins. Patients with DGI generally become afebrile within 24 to 48 hours, and the joint and skin manifestations improve dramatically within a few days. However, patients with large, purulent joint effusions and those harboring an antibiotic-resistant DGI strain may not respond as quickly, even with appropriate antibiotics.[162–165] Because of the emergence of antibiotic-resistant DGI strains, a third-generation cephalosporin, such as ceftriaxone, should be started awaiting the culture and sensitivity results.

Meningococcal and Other Neisserial Arthritides. Meningococcal arthritis clinically resembles DGI.[167] It has been estimated that 2 to 40 percent of cases of meningococcemia have articular symptoms.[167–170] As in DGI, meningococcal arthritis may be sterile or septic, relatively acellular or purulent, and often associated with dermatitis. The articular manifestations have been considered primary when classic purulent arthritis is present and *N. meningitidis* is recovered from the synovial fluid. This accounts for only 10 to 20 percent of cases of meningococcal arthritis. Most often the arthritis is associated with acute meningococcemia and may include a sterile monarthritis, polyarthritis, or transient arthralgia. The knee is most often involved. Only 25 percent of patients have documented meningitis or another focus of infection. Chronic meningococcemia is rarely associated with positive synovial fluid cultures, but most patients do have dermatitis. Immune-mediated mechanisms are involved in the articular and dermatologic manifestations of meningococcemia.[171, 172] Antibody to *N. meningitidis*, low complement, and

meningococcal antigen have been detected in synovial fluid and synovial membrane. Circulating immune complexes have been detected in the sera and synovial fluid, and patients with complement deficiency are prone to developing meningococcemia. Most patients with acute meningococcemia and arthritis respond well to antibiotics. Joint drainage is rarely a difficult problem. The role of antibiotics in culture-negative patients is not clear, but patients generally recover completely, with fewer than 1 percent of cases developing any chronic articular complications. Rare cases of *N. catarrhalis*, now termed *Moraxella catarrhalis*,[173] and *N. mucosa*[174] arthritis have also been reported.

Septic Bursitis. Septic bursitis has become a commonly recognized form of musculoskeletal infection.[174–178] Bursae are lined by synovial membrane and contain synovial fluid that varies in composition relative to the location of the bursa.[179] The synovial fluid from deep bursae is similar in composition to joint fluid and contains a high concentration of hyaluronic acid, whereas synovial fluid from superficial bursae contains much less hyaluronic acid.

The olecranon bursa and prepatellar bursa are the sites of most septic bursitis. These bursae are superficial and overly bony sites that are constantly traumatized. Thus, most reports of septic bursitis occur in patients subjected to repeated bursal trauma, such as carpenters, laborers, and athletes. Septic olecranon bursitis may also be more common in patients with rheumatoid arthritis or gout who have chronic inflammatory bursitis and in hemodialysis patients. Septic arthritis has also been reported in deep bursa, including the deep infrapatellar bursa of the knee and the subacromial bursa.[180, 181]

In more than one half of patients, an associated skin infection is present at the time of diagnosis of septic bursitis.[176–178] The skin infection may consist of small abrasions, lacerations, or a diffuse cellulitis. These traumatic skin lesions are the usual portal of entry of the infection to the bursa from transcutaneous spread, which accounts for the predominance of *S. aureus* infections and the absence of positive blood cultures in septic bursitis. Approximately 80 percent of septic bursitis cases are caused by *S. aureus*, and another 10 percent by group A streptococci and *S. epidermidis*. Rarely patients have a positive blood culture or a nonskin pathogen is recovered from the bursal fluid, indicating hematogenous seeding of the septic bursitis. A few cases of gram-negative bacillary and pneumococcal septic bursitis have been reported.[182, 183]

The patient's symptoms usually begin abruptly with pain and swelling of the bursa. The swelling is generally confined to the bursa, but extensive soft tissue swelling and erythema are common. The patient generally will allow passive movement of the adjacent joint, but the extent of joint motion and surrounding joint tenderness are related to the intensity of soft tissue swelling. A cellulitis with edema of the entire arm, including the hand, may occur in septic olecranon bursitis. As in septic arthritis, a definitive diagnosis can be made only with aspiration and culture of the bursal fluid. An elevated bursal fluid leukocyte count and low glucose are diagnostically useful, but there is more variability in their values than in septic joints.[179]

Antibiotic levels in bursal fluid following parenteral administration have been much higher than the minimum inhibitory concentrations necessary to kill most bacteria. Until the results of the culture are known, a penicillinase-resistant semisynthetic penicillin should be started intravenously and the patient hospitalized. The length of time necessary for bursal fluid cultures to become sterile correlate with the duration of symptoms prior to diagnosis.[175–177] The average duration of time to achieve bursal fluid sterility was 4 days, and when antibiotics were continued for 5 days after culture sterility, all patients were cured. These patients can be switched to oral antibiotics once cultures become sterile. Bursal drainage is usually initiated with needle aspiration, although surgical drainage may be more effective in some situations.

Patients with prior bursal disease or compromised hosts or those with severe joint disease may not respond adequately. Such patients may require prolonged parenteral antibiotics and surgical intervention such as incision and drainage or partial or total bursectomy. However, surgical intervention may be complicated by wound-healing problems, hematoma formation, and atrophic skin. A suction-irrigation procedure was effective in patients who did not respond initially to antibiotics and needle aspiration.[184] There is a high failure rate of oral antibiotics alone, especially in those patients with fever and cellulitis.

References

1. Goldenberg, D. L.: Bacterial arthritis. In: Textbook of Rheumatology. 3rd ed. Kelley, W. N., Harris, E. D., Ruddy, S., and Sledge, C. B. (eds) Philadelphia, W. B. Saunders Company, 1989, p. 1567.
2. Mahowald, M. L.: Animal models of infectious arthritis. Clin. Rheum. Dis. 12:403, 1986.
3. Smith, L. R., Merchant, T. C., and Shurman, D. L.: In vitro cartilage degradation by E. coli and S. aureus. Arthritis Rheum. 25:441, 1982.
4. Smith, R. L., Schurman, D. J, Kajiyama, G., Mell, M., and Gilkerson, E.: The effects of antibiotics on the destruction of cartilage in experimental infectious arthritis. J. Bone Joint Surg. 69A:1063, 1987.
5. Smith, L. R, and Schurman, D. J.: Bacterial arthritis. A staphylococcal-proteoglycan releasing factor. Arthritis Rheum. 29:1378, 1986.
6. Williams, R. J. III, Smith, R. L., and Schurman, D. J.: Septic arthritis Staphylococcal induction of chondrocyte proteolytic activity. Arthritis Rheum. 33:533, 1990.
7. Schurman, D. J., Mirra, J., Ding, A., and Nagel, D. A.: Experimental E. coli arthritis in the rabbit. J. Rheumatol. 4:118, 1977.
8. Goldenberg, D. L., Reed, J. I., and Rice, P. A.: Arthritis in rabbits induced by N. gonorrhoeae, killed N. gonorrhoeae and gonococcal lipopolysaccharide. J. Rheumatol. 11:3, 1984.
9. Reigels-Nielsen, P., Frimodt-Muller, N., Sorenson, M., and Jensen, J. S.: Antibiotic treatment insufficient for established septic arthritis. Acta Orthop. Scand. 60:113, 1989.
10. Sáez-Llorens, X., Mustafa, M. M., Ramilo, O. et al.: Tumor necrosis factor α and interleukin 1 β in synovial fluid of infants and children with suppurative arthritis. Am. J. Dis. Child. 144:353, 1990.
11. Cawston, T. E., Weaver, L., Coughlan, R. J., Kyle, M. V., and Hazelman, B. L.: Synovial fluid from infected joints contain active metalloproteinases and no inhibitor activity. Br. J. Rheumatol. 28:386, 1989.
12. Shaffer, M. F., and Bennett, G. A.: The passage of type III rabbit virulent pneumococci from the vascular system into joints and certain other body cavities. J. Exp. Med. 70:293, 1939.
13. Eid, A. M., Issa, H., and Deif, A. I.: Some immunological aspects of staphylococcal hematogenous osteomyelitis. Arch. Orthop. Trauma Surg. 96:221, 1980.
14. Beard, L. J., Ferris, L., and Ferrante, A.: Immunoglobulin G subclasses and lymphocyte subpopulations and function in osteomyelitis and septic arthritis. Acta Pediatr. Scand. 79:599, 1990.
15. Goldenberg, D. L, and Cohen, A. S.: Acute infectious arthritis. Am. J. Med. 60:369, 1976.
16. Goldenberg, D. L., and Reed, J. I.: Bacterial arthritis. N. Engl. J. Med. 312:764, 1985.
17. Epstein, J. H, Zimmerman, B. III, and Ho, G., Jr.: Polyarticular septic arthritis. J. Rheumatol. 13:1105, 1986.
18. Meijers, K. A. E., Dijkmans, B. A. C., Hermans, J., van den Broek, P. L., and Cats, A.: Non-gonococcal infectious arthritis: A retrospective study. J. Infect. 14:13, 1987.
19. Von Essen, R., and Holtta, A.: Improved method of isolating bacteria from joint fluids by the use of blood culture bottles. Ann. Rheum. Dis. 45:454, 1986.
20. Dory, M. A., and Wautelet, M. J.: Arthroscopy in septic arthritis. Arthritis Rheum. 28:198, 1985.
21. Christensen, T. H., Bliddal, H., and Westh, H.: Non-suppurative bacterial arthritis diagnosed by fine-needle aspiration biopsy. Scand. J. Rheumatol. 18:235, 1989.
22. Krey, P. R., and Bailen, D. A.: Synovial fluid leukocytosis. Am. J. Med. 67:436, 1979.
23. McCutchan, H. J., and Fisher, R. C.: Synovial leukocytosis in infectious arthritis. Clin. Orthop. 257:226, 1990.
24. Shmerling, R. H, Delbanco, T. L., Tosteson, A. N. A., and Trentham, D. E.: Synovial fluid tests. What should be ordered? J. A. M. A. 264:1009, 1990.
25. Sebaldt, R. L., and Tenenbaum, J: Sympathetic synovial effusions associated with septic prepatellar bursitis. J. Rheumatol. 11:555, 1984.
26. Strickland, R. W., Raskin, R. J., and Welton, R. C.: Sympathetic synovial effusions associated with septic arthritis and bursitis. Arthritis Rheum. 28:941, 1985.
27. Borenstein, D. G., Gibbs, C. A., and Jacobs, R. P.: Gas-liquid chromatographic analysis of synovial fluid. Arthritis Rheum. 25:947, 1982.
28. Arthur, R. E., Stern, M., Galeazzi, M., Baldassare, A. R., Weiss, T. D., Rogers, J. R., and Zuckner, J.: Synovial fluid lactic acid in septic and nonseptic arthritis. Arthritis Rheum. 26:1499, 1983.
29. Christensson, B., Gilbart, J., Fox, A., and Morgan, S. L.: Mass spectrometric quantitation of muramic acid, a bacterial cell wall component, in septic synovial fluids. Arthritis Rheum. 32:1268, 1989.
30. Resnick, D., and Niwayama, G.: Osteomyelitis, septic arthritis, and soft tissue infection: The mechanism and situations. In Resnick, D., and Niwayama, G. (eds): Diagnosis of Bone and Joint Disorders. 3rd ed. Philadelphia, W. B. Saunders Company, 1988.
31. Meredith, H. C., and Rittenberg, G. M: Pneumoarthrography: An unsual radiographic sign of gram-negative septic arthritis. Radiology 128:642, 1978.
32. Arnold, S., Sty, J. R., and Starshak, R. J.: Periarticular soft tissue calcification and ossification in the septic joint. Pediatr. Radiol. 19:433, 1989.
33. Mitchell, M., Howard, B., Haller, J., Sartoris, D. J., and Resnick, D.: Septic arthritis. Radiol. Clin. North Am. 26:1295, 1988.
34. Resnick, C. S., Ammann, A. M., and Walsh, J. W.: Chronic septic arthritis of the adult hip: Computed tomographic features. Skeletal Radiol. 16:513, 1987.
35. Rosenberg, D., Baskies, A. M., and Deckers, P. J.: Pyogenic sacroiliitis. An absolute indication for computerized scanning. Clin. Orthop. 184:128, 1984.
36. Sundberg, S. B., Savage, J. P., and Foster, B. K.: Technetium phosphate bone scan in the diagnosis of septic arthritis in childhood. J. Pediatr. Orthop. 9:579, 1989.
37. Magnuson, J. E., Brown, M. L., Hauser, M. E., Berquist, T. H., Fitzgerald, R. H., Jr., and Klee, G. G.: In-III-labeled leukocyte scintigraphy in suspected orthopedic prosthesis infection: Comparison with other imaging modalities. Radiology 168:235, 1988.
38. Beltran, J., Noto, A. M., McGee, R. B., Freedy, R. N., and McCalla, M. S.: Infections of the musculoskeletal system: High-field-strength MR imaging. Radiology 164:449, 1987.
39. Wilbur, A. C., Langer, B. G., and Spigos, D. G.: Diagnosis of sacroiliac joint infection in pregnancy by magnetic resonance imaging. Magn. Reson. Imaging 6:341, 1988.
40. Goldenberg, D. L: Infectious arthritis complicating rheumatoid arthritis and other chronic rheumatic disorders. Arthritis Rheum. 32:496, 1989.
41. Gardner, G. C., and Weisman, M. H.: Pyarthrosis in patients with rheumatoid arthritis: A report of 13 cases and a review of the literature from the past 40 years. Am. J. Med. 88:503, 1990.

42. Blackburn, W. D., Jr., Dunn, T. L., and Alarcón, G. S.: Infection versus disease activity in rheumatoid arthritis: Eight years' experience. South Med. J. 79:1238, 1986.
43. Medina, E., Fraga, A., and Lavalle, C: Salmonella septic arthritis in systemic lupus erythematosus. The importance of chronic carrier state, J. Rheumatol. 16:203, 1989.
44. van de Larr, M., Meenhorst, P. L., van Soesbergen, R. M., Olsthoorn, P. G. M., and van der Korst, J. K.: Polyarticular salmonella bacterial arthritis in a patient with systemic lupus erythematosus. J. Rheumatol. 16:231, 1989.
45. Webster, J., Williams, B. D., Smith, A. P., Hall, M., and Jessup, J. D.: Systemic lupus erythematosus presenting as pneumococcal septicemia and septic arthritis. Ann. Rheum. Dis. 49:181, 1990.
46. Ang-Fonte, G. Z., Rozboril, M. B., and Thompson, G. R.: Changes in nongonococcal septic arthritis: Drug abuse and methicillin resistant Staphylococcus aureus. Arthritis Rheum. 28:210, 1985.
47. Chandrasekar, P. H., and Narula, A. P.: Bone and joint infections in intravenous drug abusers. J. Infect. Dis. 8:904, 1986.
48. Lopez-Longo, F. J., Menard, H. A., Carreño, L., Cosin, J., Ballesteros, R., and Monteagudo, I.: Primary septic arthritis in heroin users: Early diagnosis by radioisotopic imaging and geographic variations in the causative agents. J. Rheumatol. 14:991, 1987.
49. von Essen, R., and Savolainen, H. A.: Bacterial infection following intra-articular injection. Scand. J. Rheumatol. 18:7, 1989.
50. Hollander, J. L: Arthrocentesis and intrasynovial therapy. In McCarty, D. J. (ed): Arthritis and Allied Conditions. 9th ed. Philadelphia, Lea & Febiger, 1979, p. 402.
51. Montgomery, S. C., and Campbell, J.: Septic arthritis following arthroscopy and intra-articular steroids. J. Bone Joint Surg. [Br] 71:540, 1989.
52. D'Angelo, G. L., and Ogilvie-Harris, D. J.: Septic arthritis following arthroscopy, with cost/benefit analysis of antibiotic prophylaxis. Arthroscopy 4:10, 1988.
53. Elliott, T. G., Burdge, D, and Reid, G. D.: Factitious septic arthritis. Arthritis Rheum. 32:352, 1989.
54. McAllister, C. M., Zillmer, D., and Cobelli, N. J.: Clostridium perfringens and Staphylococcus epidermidis polymicrobial septic arthritis. Clin. Orthop. 241:245, 1989.
55. O'Connor, C. R., Reginato, A. L., and DeLong, W.: Foreign body reaction simulating acute septic arthritis. J. Rheumatol. 15:1558, 1988.
56. Reginato, A. L., Ferreiro, J. L., O'Connor, C. R., Barbasan, C., Arasa, J., Bednar, J., and Soler, J.: Clinical and pathologic studies of twenty-six patients with penetrating foreign body injury to the joints, bursae, and tendon sheaths. Arthritis Rheum. 33:1753, 1990.
57. Gristina, A. G.: Biomaterial-centered infection: Microbial adhesion versus tissue infection. Science 237:1588, 1987.
58. Blackburn, W. D., Jr., and Alarcón, G. S.: Prosthetic joint infections: A role for prophylaxis. Arthritis Rheum. 34: 110, 1991.
59. Haley, R. W., Culver, D. H., Morgan, W. M., White, J. W., Emori, T. G., and Hooton, T. M.: Identifying patients at high risk of surgical wound infection. Am. J. Epidemiol. 121:206, 1985.
60. Inman, R. D., Gallegeo, K. V., and Brause, B. D.: Clinical and microbial features of prosthetic joint infection. Am. J. Med. 77:47, 1984.
61. McDonald, D. J., Fitzgerald, R. H., and Ilstrup, D. M: Two-stage reconstruction of a total hip arthroplasty because of infection. J. Bone Surg. [Am] 71:828, 1989.
62. Sanzen, L., and Carlsson, A. S.: The diagnostic value of C-reactive protein in infected total hip arthroplasties. J. Bone Joint Surg. [Br] 71:638, 1989.
63. Bengtson, S., Knutson, K., and Lidgren, L.: Treatment of infected knee arthroplasty. Clin. Orthop. 245:173, 1989.
64. Sublett, K. L., and Katz, A. L.: Medical management of pneumococcal arthritis involving a knee prosthesis. Arthritis Rheum. 30:940, 1987.
65. Davies, U. M., Leak, A. M., and Davé, J.: Infection of a prosthetic knee joint with Peptostreptococcus magnus. Ann. Rheum. Dis. 47:866, 1988.
66. Nylander, N., Tan, M., and Newcombe, D. S.: Successful management of Mycoplasma hominis septic arthritis involving a cementless prosthesis. Am. J. Med. 87:348, 1989.
67. Jacobson, J. L., and Matthews, L. S.: Bacteria isolated from late prosthetic joint infections: dental treatment and chemoprophylaxis. Oral Surg. Oral Med. Oral Pathol. 63:122, 1987.
68. Tsevat, L., Durand-Zaleski, I., and Pauker, S. G.: Cost-effectiveness of antibiotic prophylaxis for dental procedures in patients with artificial joints. Am. J. Public Health 79:739, 1989.
69. Perhala, R. S., Wilke, W. S., Clough, J. D., and Segal, A. M.: Local infectious complications following large joint replacement in rheumatoid arthritis patients treated with methotrexate versus those not treated with methotrexate. Arthritis Rheum. 34:146, 1991.
70. Henderson, R. C., and Rosenstein, B. D.: Salmonella septic and aseptic arthritis in sickle-cell disease. Clin. Orthop. 248:261, 1989.
71. Goldenberg, D. L.: Septic arthritis and other infections of rheumatologic significance. Rheum. Dis. Clin. North Am. 17:149, 1991.
72. Pappo, A. S., Buchanan, G. R., and Johnson, A.: Septic arthritis in children with hemophilia. Am. J. Dis. Child. 143:1226, 1989.
73. Mesnard, W. M., Mahmood, T., and Krey, P. R.: Infectious arthritis in HIV-positive intravenous drug users. Arthritis Rheum. (Suppl) 33:R46, 1990.
74. Morrissey, R. T.: Bone and joint infection in the neonate. Pediatr. Ann. 18:33, 1989.
75. Fink, C. W., and Nelson, J. D.: Septic arthritis and osteomyelitis in children. Clin. Rheum. Dis. 12:423, 1986.
76. Speiser, J. C., Moore, T. L., Osborn, T. G., Weiss, T. D., and Zuckner, J.: Changing trends in pediatric septic arthritis. Sem. Arthritis Rheum. 15:132, 1985.
77. Welkon, C. L., Long, S. S., Fisher, M. C., and Alburger, P. D.: Pyogenic arthritis in infants and children: A review of 95 cases. Pediatr. Infect. Dis. 5:669, 1986.
78. Vincent, G. M., and Amirault, J. D.: Septic arthritis in the elderly. Clin. Orthop. 251:241, 1990.
79. Newman, E. D., Davis, D. E., and Harrington, T. M.: Septic arthritis due to gram-negative bacilli: Older patients with good outcome. J. Rheumatol. 15:659, 1988.
80. Leslie, B. M., Harris, J. Mc., and Driscoll, D: Septic arthritis of the shoulder in adults. J. Bone Joint Surg. 71-A:1516, 1989.
81. Schonwetter, R. S., and Orson, F. M.: Chronic Morganella morganii arthritis in an elderly patient. J. Clin. Microbiol. 26:1414, 1988.
82. Rosenkranz, P., Lederman, M. M., Gopalakrishna, K. V, and Ellner, J. J.: Septic arthritis caused by Bacteroides fragilis. Rev. Infect. Dis. 12:20, 1990.
83. Pischel, K. D., Weisman, M. H., and Cone, R. O.: Unique features of group B streptococcal arthritis in adults. Arch. Intern. Med. 145:97, 1985.
84. Ortel, T. L., Kallianos, J., and Gallis, H. A.: Group C streptococcal arthritis: Case report and review. Rev. Infect. Dis. 12:829, 1990.
85. Ike, R. W.: Septic arthritis due to group C streptococcus: Report and review of the literature. J. Rheumatol. 17:1230, 1990.
86. Gaunt, P. N., and Seal, D. V.: Group G streptococcal infection of joints and joint prosthesis. J. Infect. 13:115, 1986.
87. Mitchell, D., Duncan., I., Brook, A., and Collignon, P.: Streptococcus faecalis arthritis. J. Rheumatol. 16:139, 1989.
88. Matteson, E. L., and McCune, W. J.: Septic arthritis caused by treatment resistant Pseudomonas cepacia. Ann. Rheum. Dis. 49:258, 1990.
89. de Groot, R., Glover, D., Clausen, D., Smith, A. L., and Wilson, C. B.: Bone and joint infections caused by Kingella Kingae: Six cases and review of the literature. Rev. Infec. Dis. 10:998, 1988.
90. Markusse, H. M., and Timmerman, R. J.: Infectious arthritis caused by Klebsiella. Clin. Rheumatol. 8:517, 1989.
91. Nitsche, J. F., Vaugan, J. M., Williams, G., and Curd, J. G.: Septic sternoclavicular arthritis with Pasteurella mutocida and Streptococcus sanguis. Arthritis Rheum. 25:467, 1982.
92. Mitchell, H., Travers, R., and Barraclough, D.: Septic arthritis caused by Pasteurella multocida. Med. J. Aust. 1:137, 1982.
93. Chadakewitz, J., and Bia, F.: Septic arthritis and osteomyelitis from a cat bite. Yale J. Biol. Med. 61:513, 1988.
94. Holroyd, K. L., Reiner, A. P., and Dick, J. D.: Streptobacillus moniliformis polyarthritis mimicking rheumatoid arthritis: An urban case of rat bite fever. Am. J. Med. 85:711, 1988.
95. Cherubin, C. H., Neu, H., Imperato, P., Harvey, R. P., and Bellen, N.: Septicemia with non-typhoid salmonella. Medicine 53:365, 1974.
96. Brodie, T. D., and Ehresman, G. R.: Salmonella dublin arthritis: An initial case presentation. J. Rheumatol. 10:144, 1983.
97. Praet, J-P., Peretz, A., Goossens, H., van Laethem, Y., and Famaey, J-P.: Salmonella septic arthritis: Additional 2 cases with quinolone treatment. J. Rheumatol. 16:1610, 1989.
98. Miller, M. E., Fogel, G. R., and Dunham, W. K.: Salmonella spondylitis. J. Bone Joint Surg. 70-A:463, 1988.
99. Cicuttini, F. M., and Buchanan, R. R. C.: Reactive arthritis after infection with Salmonella singapore. J. Rheumatol. 16:1610, 1989.
100. Rotbart, H. A., and Glode, M. P.: Haemophilus influenzae type B septic arthritis in children. Pediatrics 75:254, 1985.
101. Rosenkranz, P., Lederman, M. M., Gopalakrishna, K. V., and Ellner, J. J.: Septic arthritis caused by Bacteroides fragilis. Rev. Infect. Dis. 12:20, 1990.
102. Nakata, M. M., and Lewis, R. P.: Anaerobic bacteria in bone and joint infections. Rev. Infect. Dis. 6:S165, 1984.
103. Hunter, T., and Chow, A. W.: Peptostreptococcus magnus septic arthritis: A report and review of the English literature. J. Rheumatol. 15:1583, 1988.
104. Lluberas-Acosta, G., Elkus, R., and Schumacher, H. R., Jr.: Polyarticular Clostridium perfringens pyoarthritis. J. Rheumatol. 16:1509, 1989.
105. Barton, L. L., Jacob, S., and Chinnadurai, S.: Septic arthritis caused by Clostridium perfringens. Am. Fam. Physician 31:135, 1985.
106. Fallon, S. M., Guzik, H. J., and Kramer, L. E.: Clostridium septicum arthritis associated with colonic carcinoma. J. Rheumatol. 13:662, 1986.
107. Yocum, R. C., McArthur, J., Petty, B. G., Diehl, A. M., and Moench, T. R.: Septic arthritis caused by Propionibacterium acnes. J. A. M. A. 248:1740, 1982.

108. Kooijmans-Coutinho, M. F., Markusse, H. M., and Dijkmons, B. A. C.: Infectious arthritis caused by *Propionibacterium acnes*: A report of two cases. Ann. Rheum. Dis. 48:851, 1989.
109. Finegold, S. M.: Anaerobic Bacteria in Human Disease. New York, Academic Press, 1977.
110. Esposito, A. L., and Gleckman, R. A.: Acute polymicrobic septic arthritis in the adult: Case report and literature review. Am. J. Med. Sci. 267:251, 1974.
111. Petty, B. G., Sowa, D. T., and Charache, P.: Polymicrobial, polyarticular septic arthritis. J. A. M. A. 249:2069, 1983.
112. Gotuzzo, E., Carrillo, C., Guerra, J., and Llosa, L.: An evaluation of diagnostic methods for brucellosis: The value of bone marrow culture. J. Infect. Dis. 153:122, 1986.
113. Buchanan, T. M., Hendricks, S. L., Patton, D. M., and Feldman, R. A.: Brucellosis in the United States, 1960–1972. Part III. Medicine 53:427, 1974.
114. Alarcón, G. S., Bocanegra, T. S., Gotuzzo, E., and Espinoza, L. R.: The arthritis of Brucellosis: A perspective one hundred years after Bruce's discovery. J. Rheumatol. 14:1083, 1987.
115. Young, E. J.: Human brucellosis. Rev. Infect. Dis. 5:821, 1983.
116. Gotuzzo, E., Alarcón, G. S., Bocanegra, T. S., Carrillo, C., Guerra, J. C., Rolando, I., and Espinoza, L. R.: Articular involvement in human brucellosis: A retrospective analysis of 304 patients. Semin. Arthritis Rheum. 12:245, 1982.
117. Hodinka, L., Gomor, B., and Meretey, K.: HLA-B27–associated spondyloarthritis in chronic brucellosis. Lancet 1:499, 1978.
118. Dawes, P. T., and Ghosh, S. K.: Tissue typing in brucellosis. Ann. Rheum. Dis. 3:526, 1985.
119. Cordero-Sánchez, M., Alvarez-Ruiz, S., López-Ochoa, J., and Garcia-Talavera, J. R.: Scintigraphic evaluation of lumbosacral pain in brucellosis. Arthritis Rheum. 33:1052, 1990.
120. Ariza, J., Guidol, E., Palares, R., Rufi, G., and Fernandes-Viladrich, P.: Comparative trial of rifampicin/doxycycline versus tetracycline/streptomycin in the therapy of human brucellosis. Antimicrob. Agents Chemother. 28:548, 1985.
121. Oka, M., and Mottonen, T.: Septic sacroiliitis. J. Rheumatol. 10:475, 1983.
122. Shanahan, M. D. G., and Ackroyd, C. E.: Pyogenic infection of the sacroiliac joint. J. Bone Joint Surg. 67-B:605, 1985.
123. Mayer, R. A., Brass, J. E., and Harrington, T. M.: Pyogenic sacroiliitis in a rural population. J. Rheumatol. 17:1364, 1990.
124. Hodgson, B. F.: Pyogenic sacroiliac joint infection. Clin. Orthop. 246:146, 1989.
125. Dangles, C. J.: Two unusual presentations of pyogenic sacroiliitis. Orthop. Rev. 16:327, 1987.
126. Muir, S. K., Kinsella, P. L., Trebilcock, R. G., and Blackstone, J. W.: Infectious arthritis of the sternoclavicular joint. Can. Med. Assoc. J. 132:1289, 1985.
127. Wohlgethan, J. R., Newberg, A. H., and Reed, J. L.: The risk of abscess from sternoclavicular septic arthritis. J. Rheumatol. 15:1302, 1988.
128. Thomson, H. G.: Septic arthritis of the temporomandibular joint complicating otitis externa. J. Larngol. Oto. 103:319, 1989.
129. Nitsche, A., Mogni, G. O., and Gorostiaga, P. E.: Septic arthritis of the pubic symphysis. Clin. Exp. Rheumatol. 7:421, 1989.
130. Parker, R. H., and Schmid, F. R.: Antibacterial activity of synovial fluid during therapy of septic arthritis. Arthritis Rheum. 14:96, 1971.
131. Schurman, D. J., Hirshman, H. P., and Nagel, D. A.: Antibiotic penetration of synovial fluid in infected and normal knee joints. Clin. Orthop. 136:304, 1978.
132. Schurman, D. J., and Kajiyama, G.: Antibiotic absorption from infected and normal joints using a rabbit knee model. J. Orthop. Res. 3:185, 1985.
133. Frimodt-Moller, N., and Riegels-Nielsen, P.: Antibiotic penetration into the infected knee. Acta Orthop. Scand. 58:256, 1987.
134. Kay, E. A., Klimiuk, P. S., Ronson, G., and Bailie, G. R.: Effect of intraarticular ceftazidime in a patient with *Pseudomonas aeruginosa* septic arthritis. Drug Intell. Clin. Pharm. 22:315, 1988.
135. Waldvogel, F. A.: Use of quinolones for the treatment of osteomyelitis and septic arthritis. Rev. Infect. Dis. 11:1259, 1989.
136. Nelson, J. D., Bucholz, R. W., Kusemiesz, H., and Shelton, S.: Benefits and risks of sequential parenteral-oral cephalosporin therapy for suppurative bone and joint infections. J. Pediatr. Orthop. 2:255, 1982.
137. Syrogiannopoulos, G. A., and Nelson, J. D.: Duration of antimicrobial therapy for acute suppurative osteoarticular infections. Lancet 2:9:37, 1988.
138. Kulhanjian, J., Dunphy, M. G., Hamstra, S., Levernier, K., Rankin, M., Petru, A., and Azimi, P.: Randomized comparative study of ampicillin/sulbactam vs. ceftriaxone for treatment of soft tissue and skeletal infections in children. Pediatr. Infect. Dis. J. 8:605, 1989.
139. Goldenberg, D. L., Brandt, K. D., Cohen, A. S., and Cathcart, E. S.: Treatment of septic arthritis. Arthritis Rheum. 18:83, 1975.
140. Mielants, H., Dhondt, E., Goethats, L., Verbruggen, G., and Veys, E.: Long-term functional results of the non-surgical treatment of common bacterial infections of joints. Scand. J. Rheumatol. 11:101, 1982.
141. Goldstein, W. M., Gleason, T. F., and Barmada, R.: A comparison between arthrotomy and irrigation and multiple aspirations in the treatment of pyogenic arthritis. Orthopedics 6:1309, 1983.
142. Ho, G., Jr., and Su, E. Y.: Therapy for septic arthritis. J. A. M. A. 247:797, 1982.
143. Bulmer, J. H.: Septic arthritis of the hip in adults. J. Bone Joint Surg. 48B:289, 1966.
144. Broy, S. B., and Schmid, F. R.: A comparison of medical drainage (needle aspiration) and surgical drainage (arthrotomy or arthroscopy) in the initial treatment of infected joints. Clin. Rheum. Dis. 12:501, 1986.
145. Master, R., Weisman, M. H., Armbuster, T. G., Slivka, J., Resnick, D., and Goergen, T. G.: Septic arthritis of the glenohumeral joint: Unique clinical and radiographic features of a favorable outcome. Arthritis Rheum. 20:1500, 1977.
146. Broy, S. B., Stulberg, S. D., and Schmid, F. R.: The role of arthroscopy in the diagnosis and management of the septic joint. Clin. Rheum. Dis. 12:489, 1986.
147. Mason, L.: Arthroscopic management of the infected knee. In Grana, S. (ed.):Update in Arthroscopic Techniques, Baltimore, University Park Press, 1984, pp. 67–77.
148. Thiery, J. A.: Arthroscopic drainage in septic arthritides of the knee: A multicenter study. Arthroscopy 5:65, 1989.
149. Stanitski, C. L., Harwell, J. C., and Fu, F. H.: Arthroscopy in acute septic knees. Clin. Orthop. 241:209, 1989.
150. Dunkle, L. M.: Towards optimum management of serious focal infections: The model of suppurative arthritis. Pediatr. Infect. Dis. J. 8:195, 1989.
151. Schurman, D. L., and Smith, R. L.: Surgical approach to the management of septic arthritis. Orthop. Rev. 16:241, 1987.
152. Salter, R. B., Bell, R. S., and Keeley, F. W.: The protective effect of continuous passive motion on living articular cartilage in acute septic arthritis. Clin. Orthop. 159:223, 1981.
153. Orchard, R. A., and Stamp, W. G.: Early treatment of induced suppurative arthritis in rabbit knee joints. Clin. Orthop. 59:287, 1968.
154. Ho, G., and Su, E. Y.: Therapy for septic arthritis. J. A. M. A. 247:797, 1982.
155. Rosenthal, J., Boles, G. G., and Robinson, W. D.: Acute nongonococcal infectious arthritis. Arthritis Rheum. 23:889, 1980.
156. Klein, R. S.: Joint infection, with consideration of underlying disease and sources of bacteremia in hematogenous infection. Clin. Geriats. Med. 4:375, 1988.
157. Yu, L. P., Jr., Bradley, J. D., Hugenberg, S., and Brandt, K. D.: Predictors of mortality in septic arthritis. Arthritis Rheum. 33(Suppl).: R32, 1990.
158. Alarcón, G. S., and Blackburn, W. D., Jr.: Is infectious arthritis occurring with increased frequency in rheumatoid arthritis? Arthritis Rheum 33(Suppl).: R45, 1990.
159. Ross, S. C., and Densen, P.: Complement deficiency states and infection. Medicine 63:243, 1984.
160. O'Brien, J. P., Goldenberg, D. L., and Rice, P. A.: Disseminated gonococcal infection: A prospective analysis of 49 patients and a review of pathophysiology and immune mechanisms. Medicine 62:395, 1983.
161. Morello, J. A., and Bohnhoff, M.: Serovars and serum resistance of *Neisseria gonorrhoeae* from disseminated and uncomplicated infections. J. Infect. Dis. 160:1012, 1989.
162. Pritchard, C., and Berney, S. N.: Septic arthritis caused by penicillinase—producing *Neisseria gonorrhoeae*. J. Rheumatol. 15:720, 1988.
163. Saraux, J. L., Vigneron, A. M., Berthelot, G., Dombret, M. C., Smiejan, J. M., and Kahn, M. F.: Disseminated gonococcal infections caused by penicillinase-producing organisms in patients with unusual joint involvement. J. Infect. Dis. 155:154, 1987.
164. Liote, F., Felten, A., and Kuntz, D.: Septic arthritis caused by chromosomally medicated penicillin—resistant gonococci. J. Rheumatol. 16:1161, 1989.
165. Livneh, A., Sewell, K. L., and Barland, P.: Chronic gonococcal arthritis. J. Rheumatol. 16:245, 1989.
166. Coe, M. D., Hamer, D. H., Levy, C. S., Milner, M. R., HoNam, M., and Barth, W. E.: Gonococcal pericarditis with tamponade in a patient with systemic lupus erythematosus. Arthritis Rheum. 33:1438, 1990.
167. Rosen, M. S., Myers, A. R., and Dickey, B.: Meningococcemia presenting as septic arthritis, pericarditis, and tenosynovitis. Arthritis Rheum. 28:576, 1985.
168. Rompalo, A. M., Hook, E. W., Roberts, P. L., et al.: The acute arthritis-dermatitis syndrome. Arch. Intern. Med. 147:281, 1987.
169. Schaad, V. B.: Arthritis in disease due to *Neisseria meningitidis*. Rev. Infect. Dis. 2:880, 1980.
170. Andersson, S., and Krook, A.: Primary meningococcal arthritis. Scand. J. Infect. Dis. 19:51, 1987.
171. Greenwood, B. M., Mohammed, I., and Whittle, H. C.: Immune complexes and the pathogenesis of meningococcal arthritis. Clin. Exp. Immunol. 59:513, 1985.

172. Adams, E. M., Hustead, S., Rubin, P., Wagner, R., Gewurz, A., and Graziano, F. M.: Absence of the seventh component of complement in a patient with chronic meningococcemia presenting as vasculitis. Ann. Intern. Med. 99:35, 1983.

173. Craig, D. B., and Wehrle, P. A.: *Branhamella catarrhalis* septic arthritis. J. Rheumatol. 10:985, 1983.

174. Abiteboul, M., Mazieres, B., Causse, B., Moatti, N., and Arlet, J.: Septic arthritis of the knee due to *Neisseria mucosa*. Clin. Rheum. 4:83, 1985.

175. Ho, G., Jr., Tice, A. D., and Kaplan, S. R.: Septic bursitis in the prepatellar and olecranon bursae. Ann. Intern. Med. 89:21, 1978.

176. Canoso, J. J., and Sheckman, P. R.: Septic subcutaneous bursitis: Report of 16 cases. J. Rheumatol. 6:96, 1979.

177. Ho, G., Jr., and Mikolich, D. J.: Bacterial infection of the superficial subcutaneous bursae. Clin. Rheum. Dis. 12:437, 1986.

178. Raddatz, D. A., Hoffman, G. S., and Franck, W. A.: Septic arthritis: Presentation, treatment and prognosis. J. Rheumatol. 14:1160, 1987.

179. Canoso, J. J.: Bursae, tendons and ligaments. Clin. Rheum. Dis. 7:189, 1981.

180. Taylor, P. W.: Inflammation of the deep infrapatellar bursa of the knee. Arthritis Rheum. 32:1312, 1989.

181. Co, D. L., and Baer, A. N.: Staphylococcal infection of the subacromial/subdeltoid bursa. J. Rheumatol. 17:849, 1990.

182. Vartian, C. V., and Septimus, E. J.: Septic bursitis caused by gram-negative bacilli. J. Infect. Dis. 160:908, 1989.

183. Gleich, S., and Fomberstein, B.: Septic olecranon bursitis due to hematogenous infection with *Streptococcus pneumoniae*. J. Rheumatol. 12:10, 1985.

184. Wright, T. W., and Sheppard, J. E.: Suction-irrigation system in refractory septic bursitis. Orthop. Rev. 14:629, 1985.

Chapter 87

Mycobacterial and Fungal Infections

Jeffery L. Meier
Gary S. Hoffman

INTRODUCTION

Mycobacteria and fungi may be responsible for chronic bone and joint infections. Involvement of skeletal structures is characterized by slow evolution of objective physical and radiographic findings. Local inflammatory processes produced by these agents are insidiously destructive and may spontaneously exacerbate and remit.[1] Systemic symptoms are often absent. Consequently, definitive or invasive diagnostic approaches tend not to be considered until roentgenographic signs of destruction and permanent injury occur. In the case of *Mycobacterium tuberculosis*, an average of 19 months has been known to elapse from the onset of symptoms (usually pain) to diagnosis.[2-5] Similar experiences abound with skeletal infections caused by atypical mycobacteria and fungi.

TUBERCULOUS SKELETAL DISEASE

From 1953 through 1984, there was a steady decline (82 percent reduction) in the incidence of tuberculosis (TB) in the United States. This rate of decline was greater for pulmonary TB than for extrapulmonary TB.[6, 7] Beginning in 1985, there has been a resurgence of tuberculosis that is associated with the emergence of human immunodeficiency virus (HIV) disease. The rate of increase in extrapulmonary tuberculosis surpasses that of pulmonary TB. These trends have produced a disproportionate increase in extrapulmonary TB: 7.8 percent of all TB was extrapulmonary in 1964, 14.1 percent in 1977, 16.2 percent in 1984, and 18.5 percent in 1989.[8-10] The reason for this increase is not entirely clear but does in part reflect a rise in prevalence of HIV and TB coinfection and a preponderant representation of minorities and immigrants, groups in which extrapulmonary TB presents with greater frequency.[8] Commensurate with the change in the incidence of extrapulmonary TB is that of osteoarticular TB, in which there was an initial decline in incidence through 1984, followed by an upward trend that continues to the present (e.g., 399 cases in 1977, 339 in 1984, 427 in 1989).[9, 10] Osteoarticular TB accounted for 1.3 and 1.8 percent of all TB in 1977 and 1989. Ostensibly, those predisposing factors that are contributing to the rise of extrapulmonary TB cases are also influencing this subgroup.

Osteoarticular TB is usually the result of lymphohematogenous spread of bacilli originating at an extraskeletal focus of infection. In some instances, bone involvement may occur as a result of contiguous spread from adjacent infected areas. Commonly, bone and joint TB will smolder or lie latent for many years before it becomes active. Reports of prosthetic joint implantation triggering reactivation of TB that was "dormant"[11] underscores the capacity of this organism to persist and reactivate. Osteoarticular TB may involve virtually any bone, joint, bursa, or tendon but has a definite predilection for the vertebrae and weight-bearing surfaces.[12-14] Multiple lesions have been reported in up to one third of cases.

Systemic symptoms may or may not be present during active osteoarticular TB. Pain is the most common presenting symptom. Chest radiographs are normal in more than half of these cases.[3, 4, 15] Tuberculin skin testing usually produces a positive reaction in this setting and remains a valuable asset in determining the cause of an undiagnosed bone or joint lesion. As an exception, a false-negative tuberculin skin test result can occur in situations of impaired cellular immunity and rarely in otherwise healthy patients.[3, 21]

Vertebral TB (Pott's disease) accounts for 50 percent of all skeletal involvement and occurs more often in the thoracolumbar spine than in the cervical or sacral spine. It usually begins at the anterior vertebral border and disc and progresses to cause disc space narrowing, vertebral end-plate destruction, and anterior vertebral body collapse.[5, 15] Consequently, an acute kyphotic angulation producing the characteristic gibbous deformity often develops. Alternatively, there may be variable involvement of the vertebral body; rarely, posterior changes are the first to be appreciated.[15-17] Infection may appear confined to a single vertebra but commonly extends by direct spread to adjoining discs and vertebrae. Skip lesions may occur by way of a hematogenous route. Multiple contiguous or interspersed sites of destruction may occur owing to direct extension from a paravertebral abscess that dissects up and down the spine. Paraspinal or psoas abscesses commonly accompany vertebral TB and may be extensive. Sinus tract formation may also occur. Neurologic complications may supervene when abscess or granulation tissue encroaches on the spinal cord. This occurs more often in the upper and mid thoracic spine where the spinal canal is narrowest.[18] The radiographic appearance of the bone lesions is variable and partly depends on the stage of infection or healing. Rarefied bone lesions or well-defined lytic lesions may later be followed by varying degrees of calcification and new bone formation, leading to a mixed lytic-sclerotic picture.[15, 16] Detection of paravertebral soft tissue calcification supports the diagnosis of TB. Computed tomographic (CT) imaging may further define the extent of vertebral and paravertebral involvement.[18] Tuberculosis of the sacroiliac joint (SIJ) constitutes 7 to 9 percent of cases of skeletal TB.[3, 19] SIJ TB is usually unilateral. Plain radiographic findings include SIJ pseudowidening owing to juxta-articular osteoporosis, erosions, and sclerosis.[19]

Appendicular TB occurs primarily within weight-bearing joints (hip, knee, ankle—in descending order of frequency) and is usually a monoarticular process.[12, 13, 20] Many months may pass before articular TB leads to focal areas of osteopenia or articular erosions. In weight-bearing joints, especially the knee and hip, subchondral erosions often precede cartilaginous destruction. Sequestration of subchondral bone may follow, and joint space narrowing tends to occur late in the course of events. Thus, infection may be advanced without significant loss of the joint space (Fig. 87–1).[22, 23] In some patients, radiographic changes may be less suggestive of TB and may be indistinguishable from other causes of chronic joint infection or even chronic noninfectious synovitis (e.g., rheumatoid arthritis).[15] With continued growth of synovial pannus and extravascular formation of fibrin, amorphous fragments—"rice bodies"—may separate from the margins of synovial granulation tissue (Fig. 87–2). Rice bodies were first described in 1895 by Riese in a case of articular TB.[22] They have since been seen in rheumatoid disease and other chronic arthritides.[3, 23] Concomitant juxta-articular osteomyelitis is often present.[3] Osteomyelitis may involve long bones secondary to a contiguous tuberculous synovitis, or conversely tuberculous osteomyelitis may lead to a septic joint.

Appendicular tuberculous osteomyelitis also occurs without joint involvement. In adults, it usually presents as a single lesion, with a predilection for metaphysis of long bones (e.g., femur, tibia, and ulna), although a wide variety of bones may be involved.[25] Contiguous sinus tracts and cold soft tissue abscesses often occur. Plain radiographs of osseous TB typically reveal lytic lesions with variable degrees of sclerosis and periosteal reaction. In children, the short tubular bones of the hands and feet may be infected (tuberculous dactylitis), a phenomenon very rarely seen in adults.[12, 15, 16] Granulomatous reaction within the diaphysis causes expansion of the medullary cavity, lytic lesions, and lamellation of periosteal bone (Fig. 87–3).

A diagnosis of osteoarticular TB is definitively established when *M. tuberculosis* is detected in synovial fluid or involved tissue obtained by either closed or open biopsy. In those cases in which microbiologic proof of extraskeletal TB is established, biopsy of bone lesions that are clinically and radiographically compatible with TB may not be essential. In tuberculous arthritis, synovial fluid analysis reveals positive acid-fast smears and cultures in 20 and 80 percent of specimens, respectively.[4] Synovial fluid chemistries and cell counts are nonspecific. The fluid is often cloudy and yellow, with elevated protein content. About 60 percent of reported cases have shown blood glucose–synovial fluid glucose differences of less than 50 mg per dl. White blood cell (WBC) counts are quite variable, ranging from fewer than 1000 cells per mm^3 to more than 100,000 cells per mm^3 and averaging between 10,000 and 20,000 cells per mm^3. Open synovial biopsies are diagnostic in more than 90 percent of cases.[4] Arthroscopic-

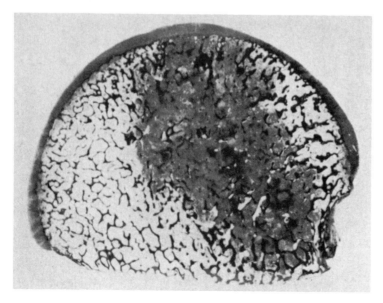

Figure 87–1. Large primary sequestrum of capitulum humeri. Articular cartilage intact. (From Luck, J. V.: Bone and Joint Diseases. Springfield, IL, Charles C Thomas, 1950, used by permission.)

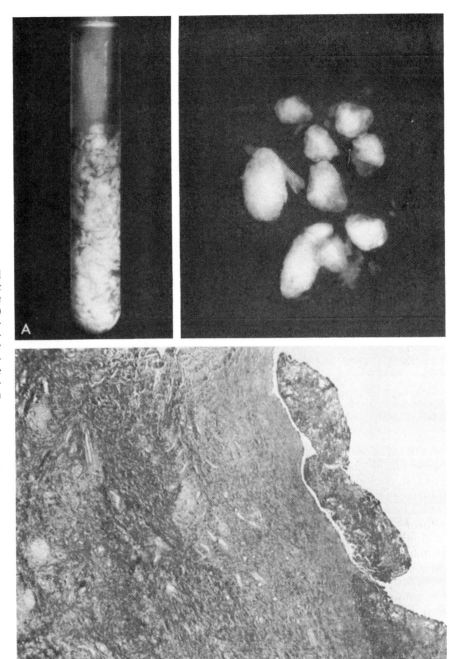

Figure 87–2. *A,* Rice bodies removed from the knee of a patient with systemic lupus erythematosus and *Mycobacterium avium* infection. *B,* Low power (× 35) microscopic view of a rice body separating from granulomatous synovial tissue. The rice body may be caused by fibrin formation in inflammatory exudate, leading to ischemic necrosis of the distal tips of synovial villi and resolution of the fibrin-cellular debris into a discrete, compact, free-floating mass.

guided synovial biopsies may be of equal diagnostic value. Tuberculous osteomyelitis is often diagnosed by histology and culture of tissue obtained by either open biopsy or percutaneous needle biopsy or aspiration. The histology of involved bone or synovial tissue usually reveals granulomata that may or may not be accompanied by caseating necrosis but occasionally may show only nonspecific inflammation, without granulomata or necrosis.[15, 27] The absence of classic granulomatous changes does not rule out fungal or mycobacterial infection. Clinical and histopathologic findings compatible with TB should prompt the initiation of presumptive antituberculous

therapy, with the caveat that atypical mycobacteria and certain fungi may produce similar findings.

Although the medical literature is replete with studies that address therapy of pulmonary TB, it contains limited studies that determine the best therapeutic approach to extrapulmonary or osteoarticular TB. Nonetheless, these studies when considered collectively establish that current improved antituberculous therapy—composed of combinations of potent bactericidal agents that penetrate well into involved tissues—results in excellent cure rates, substantially reduced duration of therapy, and improved compliance and cost-effectiveness. Isoniazid and rifampin

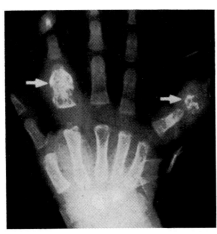

Figure 87–3. Tuberculous dactylitis (spina ventosa) of the index and fifth fingers. The fifth finger developed a sinus. Note the periosteal bone and the fusiform enlargement of the involved fingers. (From Luck, J. V.: Bone and Joint Diseases. Springfield, IL, Charles C Thomas, 1950.)

represent one such combination that is highly effective. Although many infectious disease consultants advocate prolonged treatment (1 to 2 years),[28] there is some evidence to suggest that 9 months of therapy is sufficient in uncomplicated cases.[29–31] More intensive multidrug therapies given over a 6-month period may also yield acceptable outcomes.[32–35] Surgical débridement may be an important adjunct in short-course regimens.[30, 31] Selection and subsequent adjustment of the therapeutic regimen should be based on several factors: e.g., drug resistance and side effects, infection severity, derangements of host defense, clinical and radiographic response, compliance, and socioeconomic issues. Some representative chemotherapeutic regimens are listed in Tables 87–1 and 87–2; modifications of these regimens are required if drug resistance is suspected or has been determined.

Treatment of uncomplicated vertebral TB has been evaluated by a series of controlled studies conducted by the Medical Research Council Working Party on Tuberculosis of the Spine, located in Korea, South Africa, Zimbabwe, and Hong Kong. These studies reveal that combination chemotherapy gives excellent results and that immobilization and body casting are generally unnecessary.[36, 37] Moreover, prolonged chemotherapy alone and chemotherapy plus surgery (débridement with or without anterior spinal fusion) are equally efficacious in terms of eradicating infection, sinus tracts, small to moderate-sized paravertebral abscesses, and avoiding vertebral instability or neurologic sequelae. Accordingly, surgery should be reserved for cases complicated by neurologic abnormality, spinal instability, or a large paravertebral or psoas abscess.[37, 38]

TB synovitis usually responds to chemotherapy alone. Surgery may be useful in selected cases such as those in which prior joint disease results in loculated fluid, exuberant synovial pannus, loose bodies, or progressive neurologic impairment, e.g., carpal tunnel involvement. There is a growing number of reports suggesting that quiescent tuberculous joints treated with total hip and knee arthroplasties provide a favorable outcome.[39–43] This success may hinge on improved surgical technique and prosthetic implants and on the use of perioperative antituberculous therapy (e.g., isoniazid [INH] and rifampin [RMP] given 3 weeks before and 6 to 9 months after surgery) to minimize risk of reactivation.

SKELETAL INFECTIONS CAUSED BY ATYPICAL MYCOBACTERIA

Atypical mycobacteria are ubiquitous in nature and are often isolated from soil, water, and animals. Some atypical mycobacteria are nonpathogenic in humans, and others fit within a spectrum that ranges from rare to relatively frequent causes of human disease. For many atypical mycobacteria species, it may be difficult to differentiate colonization or environmental contamination from pathogenicity. In contrast, other species when found in clinical specimens are seldom contaminants and are usually indicative of causing disease (e.g., *M. kansasii*, *M. marinum*, and *M. szulgai*). No appreciable person to person transmission of disease occurs. Atypical mycobacteria infection of bone and joint may result from percutaneous inoculation of the organism or hematogenous

Table 87–1. ANTITUBERCULOUS THERAPY*

	Initial Phase		Continuation Phase	
Regimen	*Drugs*	*Duration*	*Drugs*	*Duration*
Conventional 18–24 months	INH, RMP, ± EMB or STM (q.d.)	2 months	INH, RMP (q.d. or b.i.w.)	16–22 months
Short-course 9 months	INH, RMP (q.d.)	1 month	INH, RMP (q.d. or b.i.w.)	8 months
6 months	INH, RMP, PZA ± ETB or STM (q.d.)	2 months	INH, RMP (q.d. or b.i.w.)	4 months

*Note: These are representative regimens; other drug combinations and schedules have been used and may be required, especially in cases of drug resistance.
INH, Isoniazid; RMP, rifampin; ETB, ethambutol; STM, streptomycin; PZA, pyrazinamide; q.d., daily; b.i.w., twice weekly (supervision advised); ± optional.
Data from references 28–35, 37.

Table 87–2. RECOMMENDED DRUGS FOR INITIAL TREATMENT OF TUBERCULOSIS IN CHILDREN AND ADULTS

Drug	Dosage Forms	Daily Dose* Children	Daily Dose* Adults	Maximal Daily Dose in Children and Adults	Twice Weekly Dose Children	Twice Weekly Dose Adults	Major Adverse Reactions
Isoniazid	Tablets: 100 mg, 300 mg†‡ Syrup: 50 mg/5 ml Vials: 1 g	10 to 20 mg/kg PO or IM	5 mg/kg PO or IM	300 mg	20 to 40 mg/kg, max. 900 mg	15 mg/kg, max. 900 mg	Hepatic enzyme elevation, peripheral neuropathy, hepatitis, hypersensitivity
Rifampin	Capsules: 150 mg, 300 mg†‡ Syrup: formulated from capsules, 10 mg/ml	10 to 20 mg/kg PO	10 mg/kg PO	600 mg	10 to 20 mg/kg, max. 600 mg	10 mg/kg, max. 600 mg	Orange discoloration of secretions and urine; nausea, vomiting, hepatitis, febrile reaction, purpura (rare)
Pyrazinamide	Tablets: 500 mg‡	15 to 30 mg/kg PO	15 to 30 mg/kg PO	2 g	50 to 70 mg/kg	50 to 70, max. 3 g	Hepatotoxicity, hyperuricemia, arthralgias, skin rash, gastrointestinal upset
Streptomycin	Vials: 1 g, 4 g	20 to 40 mg/kg IM	15 mg/kg§ IM	1 g§	25 to 30 mg/kg IM	25 to 30 mg/kg IM	Ototoxicity, nephrotoxicity
Ethambutol	Tablets: 100 mg, 400 mg	15 to 25 mg/kg PO	15 to 25 mg/kg PO	2.5 g	50 mg/kg	50 mg/kg	Optic neuritis (decreased red-green color discrimination, decreased visual acuity), skin rash

PO = perorally; IM = intramuscularly.
*Doses based on weight should be adjusted as weight changes.
†Isoniazid and rifampin are available as a combination capsule containing 150 mg of isoniazid and 300 mg of rifampin.
‡A combination of isoniazid, rifampin, and pyrazinamide in a single capsule is being introduced.
§In persons older than 60 years of age, the daily dose of streptomycin should be limited to 10 mg/kg with a maximal dose of 750 mg.
Modified from American Thoracic Society: Rev. Respir. Dis. 134:355, 1986. Used by permission.

seeding. Although seemingly infrequent, various states of immunosuppression may predispose to infection.

Atypical mycobacteria infections of tendon sheaths of the hand and wrist constitute a majority of those cases involving the musculoskeletal system.[44] Articular disease most often affects digits, wrists, and knees. Infection of prepatellar and olecranon bursae are also reported.[45] The septic process is usually insidious, leading to delay in diagnosis of up to months or years. Mistaken exclusion of infection from the differential diagnosis when only routine synovial fluid cultures have been obtained has frequently led to the error of administering glucocorticoid injections.

The diagnosis of osteoarticular atypical mycobacteriosis is usually established by isolation of the organism from biopsy tissue or synovial fluid, corroborated by compatible histopathologic, clinical, and radiographic findings. Pathologic lesions produced by atypical organisms and the tubercle bacillus are usually indistinguishable; histology often reveals acid-fast bacilli, in addition to nonspecific inflammation or granulomata with or without necrosis.[46, 47] Atypical mycobacteria species that cause bone, joint, tendon sheath, and bursa infection can be categorized according to Runyon's classification, which groups species according to growth rate and colony color (Table 87–3).

Broad statements about specific therapy of musculoskeletal atypical mycobacteriosis cannot be made. In general, therapy should be selected on the basis of species, in vitro susceptibilities, host immune status, and location and extent of disease. Surgical removal of affected tissue contributes importantly to clinical resolution when the organism is relatively resistant to chemotherapy. Surgery, however, is not always necessary when treating chemotherapy-sensitive organisms. Resistance to standard antituberculous drugs is often encountered, and post-therapy recrudescence of disease is not unusual.

Mycobacterium avium–intracellulare (MAI) is distributed throughout the United States and more so in the Southeast. Infection of tendon sheaths of the hand and wrist is well described.[44–46] Bursal infection may also occur. Bones and joints[25, 47, 48] have been identified as the sole sites of involvement as well as being part of disseminated infection.[49] Therapy should be based on the extent of disease and on the immune status of the host. Surgical excision and prolonged multidrug therapy (four to five drugs given for 24 to 36 months) are usually indicated, given the relative resistance of this organism to chemotherapy. This recommendation, however, should be tempered by reports of limited MAI tenosynovitis being apparently cured by excisional therapy alone.[44] The chemotherapeutic agents are selected from a list of first-line agents[49a, 49b]: rifampin or rifabutine (investigational), ethambutol, streptomycin or amikacin, clofazimine, and possibly, ciprofloxacin. The new macrolides, clarithromycin and azithromycin, may also be of value. Isoniazid should be included in the initial therapy if *M. tuberculosis* has not been ruled out.

M. kansasii is most often found in the Southwestern United States. A wide range of bone, joint, and periarticular disease has been described: carpal tunnel syndrome, arthritis, osteomyelitis, fasciitis, tendinitis,[50–54] and reactivation infection following joint replacement.[55] Disseminated infection in an immunocompromised individual carries increased risk of multifocal musculoskeletal disease.[50] *M. kansasii* responds well to rifampin-containing regimens. The combination of isoniazid, rifampin, and ethambutol is effective and minimizes the development of secondary resistance. The usual duration of therapy is 18 to 24 months, but shorter courses may suffice when clinical response is prompt[50, 51, 53, 56]; surgery may be useful in selected cases.[57]

M. marinum is found in aquatic environments. Infection is considered an occupational (e.g., fish and crustacean handling) or hobby-associated (e.g., aquarium and swimming pool) risk. Infections are most often cutaneous. The organism's predilection for distal extremities is consonant with its requirement of a lower growth temperature, optimal growth temperature being 31 to 33°C. Infection of tendon sheaths of the hand and wrist is the most common manifestation of musculoskeletal involvement.[50] Tendons, joints, and bone may be involved as well.[58–60]

Table 87–3. ATYPICAL MYCOBACTERIA THAT HAVE CAUSED OSTEOARTICULAR OR PERIARTICULAR INFECTION

Group	Growth Rate	Color	Members
Photochromogens	3 to 4 weeks	Yellow-orange when exposed to light while being grown	*M. kansasii* *M. marinum*
Scotochromogens	3 to 4 weeks	Yellow-orange in the dark; become more reddish in light	*M. scrofulaceum, M. flavescens* *M. szulgai, M. gordonae*
Nonchromogens	3 to 4 weeks	None or light yellow	*M. xenopi* *M. avium–intracellulare* *M. triviale–terrae*
Rapid growers	1 to 3 days	Usually none, occasionally variable color	*M. fortuitum* *M. chelonei* *M. smegmatis*

Abstracted from Runyon, E. H.: Med. Clin. North Am. 43:273, 1959; and Fogan, L.: Atypical mycobacteria. Medicine 49:243, 1970, © Williams & Wilkins, 1970.

Extended treatment with the combination of rifampin and ethambutol is fairly effective.[61, 62] Surgical débridement of deep infection of the hand and wrist contributes to cure, but attendant complications of surgical wound breakdown and extensive scarring, potentially limiting function, are common. Based on the findings of an uncontrolled study, the investigators suggest that surgery can be reserved for those cases that fail chemotherapy or for those cases with adverse prognostic indicators, such as draining sinus, pain, or prior steroid injections.[63]

M. fortuitum and *M. chelonei* are commonly found in the environment. They occasionally cause osteomyelitis, usually secondary to penetrating trauma.[64] Joint and bursae involvement has been reported rarely.[65, 66] Osteomyelitis and synovitis have arisen hematogenously in immunocompromised hosts.[67, 68] Postsurgical sternum infections occur sporadically or as outbreaks.[64] Infection related to foreign bodies such as joint prostheses[64] and tympanostomy tubes (causing otitis and mastoiditis)[69] have also been reported. Treatment consists of the combination of débridement and chemotherapy. Standard antituberculous drugs are ineffective. A recommended empiric regimen includes amikacin and cefoxitin; in vitro susceptibilities guide subsequent therapy. In osteoarticular infection, it would seem prudent to administer two active parenteral drugs for approximately 6 weeks (depending on response), followed by extended therapy with a single drug to which the organism is sensitive.[70]

M. szulgai, M. xenopi, M. terrae-triviale, M. scrofulaceum, M. flavescens, M. gordonae, M. simiae, and *M. smegmatis*[45–47, 50, 71–74] rarely cause musculoskeletal infection.

MYCOTIC INFECTIONS OF BONES AND JOINTS

Osteomyelitis is the most common type of mycotic skeletal disease. The location of bone involvement is often of little differential diagnostic value. One or more sites may be involved simultaneously. Septic joints may be produced by direct extension from bone foci. Less often, synovial infections occur directly by hematogenous dissemination and seldom occur directly by traumatic or surgery-related implantation. Acute fungal arthritis is distinctly uncommon but has been reported, particularly with blastomycosis and *Candida* infection. It is the indolent course of most fungal joint infections that has led to delays in diagnosis, even for many years. The first several months of undiagnosed chronic illness are usually associated with normal radiographs, which later develop lucent and lytic changes, and still many months later show a mixed lytic-sclerotic picture.[75] Undiagnosed patients often undergo inappropriate treatment, particularly with intra-articular and systemic steroids for *nonspecific synovitis*. This is usually followed by little to no improvement, then worsening,

and finally surgery is sought for diagnostic and therapeutic assistance. In many cases, fungal arthritis may still not be considered, and synovectomy may be followed by recurrent problems.[76, 77]

Synovial fluid analyses are quite variable and depending on the stage of disease can include WBC counts ranging from noninflammatory (<1000 cells per mm³) to markedly inflammatory (>100,000 cells per mm³). Most patients have had WBC counts of 10,000 to 60,000. Either mononuclear cells or granulocytes may be predominant; granulocytes predominate at the more inflammatory end of the spectrum.

Familiarity with fungal epidemiology and extraskeletal manifestations of disease may provide vital diagnostic clues (Table 87–4). Culture of involved tissue or synovial fluid, however, remains the most reliable method of definitive diagnosis. The laboratory should be appraised that fungus might be present so noninhibitory media are used. Low colony counts are common. All mold contaminants should be fully identified because they may be a potential pathogen.

Fungi responsible for osteoarticular disease are categorized according to whether they cause deep (visceral), opportunistic deep, or rare deep infections. Although actinomycetes are bacteria, their morphology and clinical behavior resemble that of fungi. Therefore, actinomycosis is discussed at the end of this chapter.

DEEP MYCOSIS

Coccidioidomycosis

Coccidioides immitis is a dimorphic fungus that is endemic in Southwestern United States, northern Mexico, and some parts of Central and South America.[77a] The soil in arid sections of these regions supports the growth of the mycelial phase, which produces highly infectious arthrospores. Inhaled airborne arthrospores transform into the pathogenic spherule-endospore form. Skin testing with coccidioidal antigens suggests that as much as one third of the population in endemic areas have been infected.[78] Residents in endemic areas acquire infection at a rate estimated to be 2.7 percent per year.[79] Infection becomes established after inhalation or rarely after percutaneous inoculation of arthrospores. The primary pulmonary infection that ensues is symptomatic only in 40 percent of cases.[80] A mild self-limited, influenza-like illness predominates, but severe pulmonary involvement may occur. Concomitant arthralgias may occur in one third of cases, and occasional overt synovitis may appear.[80, 81] Fever and erythema multiforme or erythema nodosum often accompany arthralgias, and conjunctivitis or episcleritis may also occur. This extrapulmonary, or "acute valley fever," complex reflects a hypersensitivity response to fungal antigens. It usually resolves within days to weeks and usually portends a good prog-

Table 87–4. FUNGI CAUSING INFECTIONS OF BONES AND JOINTS

Fungus	Mode of Infection	Geographic Distribution	Frequency of Septic Bone and Joint Involvement
Deep Mycosis			
Histoplasma capsulatum	Inhalation; aerosol from soil rich in bird (especially chickens, starlings) and bat guano	Worldwide; in United States most concentrated in Midwest, Ohio and Mississippi River valleys	Rare[117]
H. duboisii	Uncertain	Africa	About 66% with disseminated disease[129]
Cryptococcus neoformans	Inhalation, often compromised host as well as normal persons	Worldwide; no regional concentration in United States	5 to 10%[111]
Coccidioides immitis	Inhalation, especially during dry, dusty months	Southwestern United States, Central and South America, especially arid dusty regions	10–50% cases of extrathoracic disease[83]
Blastomyces dermatitidis	Usually inhalation; very rarely inoculation into traumatized skin Most common among persons repeatedly exposed to soil. 9 males: 1 female[98]	United States: Mississippi and Ohio River basins, middle Atlantic states, Canada, Africa, Europe, northern South America[98]	25 to 60% disseminated blastomycoses cases[100]
Opportunistic Deep Mycosis			
Sporothrix schenckii	Postulated to arise via the lung; alcoholism and myeloproliferative diseases are predisposing factors	Worldwide	80% of cases of systemic sporotrichosis[150]
Candida species	Endogenous: in premature infants and other compromised hosts having malignancies, indwelling catheters, hyperalimentation, immunosuppressive therapies, multiple antibiotics; drug addicts (especially heroin)	Worldwide	Rare[134]
Aspergillus fumigatus	Inhalation or endogenous infection in a compromised host; dissemination via respiratory tree and blood; rarely via gastrointestinal tract	Worldwide	Rare[161]
Rare Deep Mycosis			
Maduromycoses	Fungus enters via local injury to uncovered foot	Worldwide, especially in tropical climates where inhabitants do not wear shoes; rare in United States	Usual; soft tissue infection leading to osteomyelitis[164]
Actinomycosis			
Actinomyces israelii (anaerobic bacterium)	Endogenous: host may or may not be compromised; focal cervicofacial disease or disseminated bacteremia; may follow oral trauma such as tooth extractions	Worldwide	Common in facial bones[168]

nosis. Primary intrathoracic infection may disseminate in less than 1 percent of cases. Skin, skeletal system, and meninges are common extrathoracic sites affected, but virtually any organ can be involved. Predisposing factors for dissemination include certain racial groups (Filipinos, blacks, and Hispanics), male gender, pregnancy, and immunosuppression. Reactivation of latent disease in the setting of immunosuppression (lymphomas, transplantation, acquired immunodeficiency syndrome [AIDS]) may also lead to dissemination.[82]

Coccidioidomycosis may involve bone or joint. Bone and joint involvement is present in 10 to 50 percent of cases of extrathoracic disease in non-AIDS

patients.[83] Although dissemination is usual during HIV and C. immitis coinfection, osteoarticular involvement (bone marrow excluded) is not.[79] Osseous coccidioidomycosis affects long, short, flat, and irregular bones. It often involves multiple sites and has a predilection for cancellous bone.[84] Although some authors have noted a predilection for bony prominences,[85] others found no such association.[83, 86] Osseous and articular infection commonly presents in the absence of extraskeletal stigmata.[87] Pain is the most common presenting complaint; signs of inflammation may occasionally be present. Bone and gallium scans are more sensitive than plain radiography in detecting osseous lesions,[88] but neither nuclear nor radiographic studies provide specific diagnostic features. Radiographic findings of long and flat bone involvement include irregular, well-demarcated lytic lesions with occasional sclerotic borders; sequestrum is uncommon[83, 84] (Fig. 87–4). Vertebral involvement accounts for about one fourth of cases of osseous involvement.[89] Typical radiographic features include multiple lytic lesions with ill-defined borders and paucity of sclerosis, positioned indiscriminately in the vertebral bodies and their appendages. The disc space is frequently preserved, and acute angulation deformity rarely occurs. An associated paraspinous abscess or mass may be present. Remodeling and sclerosis of bone may occur as the infection resolves with chemotherapy.[89, 91]

Articular coccidioidomycosis mostly involves the knee, wrist, and ankle joints.[92] This is usually a chronic monoarticular, and occasionally a pauciarticular, synovitis. It usually arises from extension of a contiguous osseous infection or occasionally from direct hematogenous spread.[93] Pain, effusion and restricted motion are common initial findings; signs of inflammation may occasionally be present. Early in the course of infection, there is generally no radiographic abnormality of the joint except for ef-

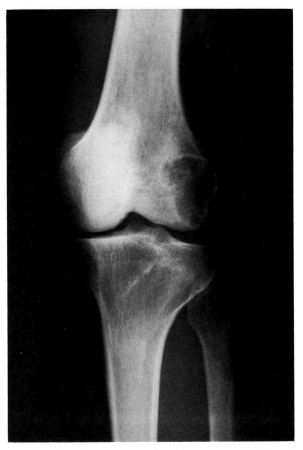

Figure 87–4. Coccidioidomycosis. Coccidioidal osteomyelitis of the lateral condyle of the femur and medial aspect of the tibial plateau in a Filipino male. Note the well-circumscribed margins of the osteolytic lesions. Inflammatory arthritis was also present. (Courtesy of John E. Bennett, M.D.)

fusion. Late radiographic changes of chronic infection may be indistinguishable from postinfectious sclerotic changes.[94]

A diagnosis of osteoarticular coccidioidomycosis is based on identification of the organism in biopsy material. Rarely is the organism seen on smear of synovial fluid. Early in the course of joint involvement, cultures of the fluid are often negative.[92] Synovial fluid analyses reveal variable inflammation with either mononuclear cell or granulocyte predominance. Histopathology of involved tissues shows granulomata, with or without necrosis, and thick-walled spherules containing endospores. The spherules can be easily detected using hematoxylin and eosin stain.[82] It is imperative that the laboratory be notified that *C. immitis* is suspected so the necessary safety measures for personnel are exercised. Serologic tests—complement fixation antibody and quantitative immunodiffusion assay—are usually positive and support the diagnosis of coccidioidomycosis.

Treatment of osteoarticular coccidioidomycosis is complicated by the infection's unpredictable natural course and variable response to therapy. Both amphotericin B and oral ketoconazole have been used with some success.[95, 96] A typical dosing regimen of amphotericin would be 0.5 to 0.7 mg per kg daily or 1 mg per kg on alternate days until the disease is subdued (e.g., 10 to 12 weeks), followed by prolonged therapy with oral ketoconazole. Alternatively, less severe disease can be treated with oral ketoconazole, 400 mg per day, for 1 year or more. Higher doses may provide a modest increase in response rate but do not result in a significant increase in sustained drug-free remission. Vertebral lesions may be more resistant to ketoconazole. An open-label trial found oral itraconazole (400 mg per day) to be a promising new therapy of osteoarticular disease, and it appears more efficacious and less toxic than ketoconazole.[97] Additionally, surgical drainage of pus in periosseous soft tissue, débridement of involved bone in select cases, and perhaps synovectomy contribute to cure.[82] The role of intra-articular amphotericin B is controversial. Articular coccidioidomycosis refractory to the above-mentioned therapies may require arthrodesis.[92, 94]

Blastomycosis

Blastomyces dermatitidis is a dimorphic fungus endemic in several regions of North America (e.g., Mississippi and Ohio river basins, Great Lakes, Midwest, southeast United States, and central Canada) and Africa. It is present in damp soil enriched in organic debris. Inhalation of mycelia-produced conidia leads to either clinically silent or apparent pulmonary infection. Like histoplasmosis and coccidioidomycosis, self-limited arthralgias and myalgias may accompany the primary infection.[98] Primary cutaneous lesions caused by percutaneous inoculation occasionally occur. Rare cases of dog bites causing

B. dermatitidis infection of digits exemplify this type of transmission.[99] Hematogenous spread from a pulmonary source affects extrapulmonary sites, usually skin and bone. Osseous and articular blastomycosis constitute 25 to 60 percent and 3 to 8 percent of systemic blastomycosis cases, respectively.[100] Conversely, about 50 to 90 percent of the cases of osteoarticular blastomycosis have had concomitant lung or skin involvement.[101–104] Osteoarticular involvement more commonly occurs in men (9:1) and is not generally associated with an immunocompromised state or other underlying medical illness.[98] This is also the case in other forms of systemic blastomycosis.

Osseous blastomycosis may involve a wide variety of bones and often occurs in more than one site. Common sites of involvement are the metaphysis of long bones; short bones, ribs, vertebrae, and skull.[104–107] Contiguous soft tissue lesions and sinus formation may occur. Bone pain rarely occurs. One study revealed about half of osseous lesions were asymptomatic; bone scans were helpful in detecting these lesions.[105] Vertebral involvement may mimic tuberculous spondylitis. Although there is no characteristic radiographic finding, osseous lesions tend to be well circumscribed and lytic, with little periosteal reaction and absence of sequestra[104, 105] (Fig. 87–5).

Articular blastomycosis involves a single joint in about 95 percent of the cases, but a polyarticular syndrome also occurs. Commonly involved joints are the knee, ankle, elbow, wrist, and hand.[100, 101, 107] In contradistinction to many other fungal arthritides, joint involvement frequently presents as an acute synovitis, often accompanied by substantial constitutional symptoms. Radiographic findings include periarticular osteomyelitis (30 percent), effusions (30 percent), or no abnormalities (40 percent).[100]

Blastomycotic arthritis can be readily diagnosed by the identification of a broad-based budding yeast with a refractile wall in synovial fluid; the yeast can be seen in more than 85 percent of cases.[100] Cytologic examination may be more sensitive than a wet mount.[108] Culture is confirmatory. In contrast to other granulomatous arthritides, the synovial fluid is often frankly purulent. Synovial biopsy is usually unnecessary. Bone involvement can be examined by histopathology and culture if the diagnosis is in question. Histology often discloses striking pyogranulomatous changes; Gomori methenamine-silver stain is useful to screen for the yeast.[107]

Ketoconazole is effective therapy for the treatment of mild to moderate severity, nonmeningeal blastomycosis involving an immunocompetent patient.[109, 110] The adult dose is 400 mg per day given for 6 to 12 months. If there is no response after about 1 month, the dose can be increased by 200 mg per day to a maximum of 800 mg per day. Severe infection is treated with intravenous amphotericin B; initial dose is 0.3 to 0.6 mg per kg per day, for a total of 1.5 to 2.0 g. Surgery is primarily adjunctive therapy

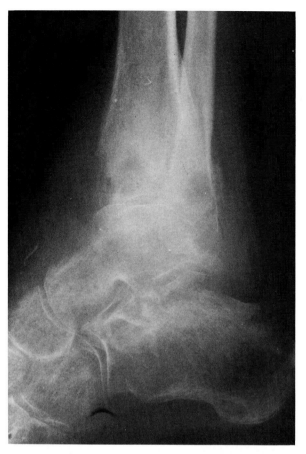

Figure 87–5. Blastomycosis. Blastomycotic osteomyelitis of the distal tibia, fibula, talus, navicula, and calcaneus. Note lucencies and loss of trabecula definition. Soft tissue swelling and erythema were also present. (Courtesy of John E. Bennett, M.D.)

and, in most situations, should be reserved for those cases not responding to medical therapy.

Cryptococcosis

Cryptococcus neoformans is a yeast-like fungus that exists worldwide. It can be isolated from several substrates in nature, particularly aged pigeon droppings and soil. Inhalation of the organism may cause either a clinically inappreciable or apparent pulmonary infection. Hematogenous dissemination may follow. About three fourths of clinically apparent cryptococcosis cases are associated with predisposing factors (e.g., lymphoreticular malignancy, sarcoidosis, glucocorticoid therapy, and AIDS). Disseminated cryptococcosis most commonly presents as meningoencephalic involvement but may affect many different organs. Skin and skeletal lesions occur in 10 and 5 percent of disseminated cases.[111] About 40 percent of cases of skeletal involvement are associated with underlying states of immunosuppression.[112] Osteoarticular involvement in the setting of AIDS is unusual.

Skeletal cryptococcosis involves a single osseous

site in three fourths of cases.[112] Multiple lesions often occur in close proximity to one another, suggesting contiguous spread. A wide variety of bones are affected, with vertebrae being the most common bones involved.[112–116] Sinus formation is uncommon. Standard radiographs reveal well-defined osteolytic or eroded lesions; periosteal reaction is infrequent (Fig. 87–6). Cryptococcal arthritis occurs rarely and is generally due to direct extension from an underlying osseous lesion.[117–119]

A diagnosis of osteoarticular cryptococcosis is based on the detection of the organism in involved material obtained by aspiration or biopsy. Culture and histopathologic examination of this material usually reveals the organism; smears are occasionally positive. Histologic findings include acute or chronic inflammation with granulomata. Joint fluid reveals inflammation with either neutrophil or lymphocyte predominance.[117] Serum cryptococcal antigen is positive in about half of skeletal cryptococcosis cases.[112]

For treatment, intravenous amphotericin B, with or without flucytosine, is effective therapy but is associated with considerable side effects.[112] Oral flu-

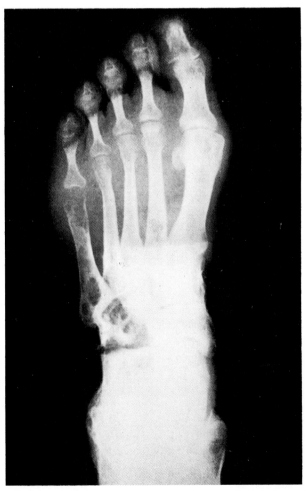

Figure 87–6. Cryptococcosis of bone. Note osteolytic lesions of the fifth metatarsal. (From Conant, N., et al.: Manual of Clinical Mycology. 3rd ed. Philadelphia, W. B. Saunders Company, 1971, used by permission.)

conazole (200 to 400 mg per day) may be efficacious but has not been thoroughly evaluated for osseous infections. The amphotericin B regimen should be used for serious forms of cryptococcosis. Drainage of purulent periosseous collections is helpful, but surgical débridement of bone lesions is usually not necessary for cure.

Histoplasmosis

Histoplasma capsulatum is a dimorphic fungus encountered in various regions of the world. It is highly endemic to the Mississippi, Missouri, and Ohio river valleys of central United States. In nature, the mold exists in moist soil, particularly when enriched in bird or bat excreta. Infection results from inhalation of mold-produced spores, which transform into budding yeast. Histoplasmin skin testing of persons living in highly endemic areas indicate that more than 80 percent of adults have experienced past infection.[120] The vast majority of these infections are subclinical. In other cases, however, histoplasmosis may present as acute pulmonary, chronic pulmonary, or disseminated disease. In the early phase of infection, about 5 to 10 percent of symptomatic cases may have concomitant rheumatologic manifestations of histoplasmosis,[121, 122] which presumably represents an immunologic reaction to the organism. These manifestations may include erythema nodosum, erythema multiforme, arthralgias, and occasionally arthritis. The arthritis may be inflammatory with synovial fluid lymphocyte predominance. Arthralgia and arthritis may involve large and small joints of the upper and lower extremities, may affect one to several joints, may have symmetric or asymmetric distribution, and may present in additive or migratory fashion. Such immunologic reactions are self-limited and generally resolve within a few weeks but rarely can lead a prolonged course.[123–125]

H. capsulatum rarely causes osteoarticular infection.[117, 126–128] Although disseminated histoplasmosis commonly involves the bone marrow, it usually does not affect skeletal structure. In rare instances, however, it may give rise to an indolent, granulomatous infection of bone, tendon sheaths, or synovium. In these cases, the organism was detected in biopsy material by either histology or culture.

African histoplasmosis (*H. capsulatum* var. *duboisii*) primarily infects bone and skin and spares lung.[128a] Osteomyelitis occurs in about two thirds of cases.[129] *H. capsulatum* var. *duboisii* is the only form of histoplasmosis with sufficient frequency of osseous involvement to comment on therapy. In those cases, amphotericin B has been effective therapy. In less severe cases, ketoconazole (400 mg per day) may also be curative.[128a, 130]

Opportunistic Deep Mycosis

Candidiasis

Candida is a yeast and a normal commensal of humans. It is commonly isolated from the oropharynx, gastrointestinal tract, and female genital tract and occasionally is isolated from skin. Superficial or deep-seated infection by endogenous *Candida* may occur when the normal system of host defense is compromised. Ten species of *Candida* (*Torulopsis glabrata* included) are regarded as important human pathogens. *C. albicans* is the most frequently encountered pathogen. The frequency of candidemia-related, deep-seated infection and disseminated candidiasis increases in tandem with increased risk factors. Malignancy, immunosuppressive therapy, abdominal surgery, central venous catheters/ parenteral nutrition, multiple antibiotics, and injection of heroin are among some of these risk factors.[131–133] The skeleton is one of the wide variety of organs that may become infected, albeit infrequently, during candidemia. Although the majority of candidal osteoarticular infections arise from hematogenous seeding, they may also occur as a result of trauma and surgery, particularly implantation of prosthetic joints.[133–135] Infection has also followed joint aspiration and intra-articular glucocorticoid injection.[134]

In most cases, appendicular *Candida* osteomyelitis involves a single long bone. Involvement of more than one osseous site and of bones of the wrist, hand, and foot occasionally occurs.[134, 136] Contiguous spread to the joint is uncommon. Vertebral *Candida* osteomyelitis often involves two adjoining vertebrae and the intravertebral disc.[137–139] In adults, the vertebrae are the most common bones infected.[134, 140] *Candida* can cause mediastinitis and sternal osteomyelitis after median sternotomy and can infect the intervertebral disc space after laminectomy.[134, 141] In general, local pain is the most common presenting symptom. Typically, constitutional symptoms are minimal or absent, and objective findings are uncommon. Osseous infection may present several months after an episode of candidemia. A course of amphotericin sufficient to treat the antecedent candidemia may not prevent osteomyelitis, particularly if the patient is immunosuppressed.[134] Radiographic findings are variable and nonspecific. These findings include lytic lesions, rarefaction, cortical destruction, and erosions.[134] In vertebral involvement, there is destruction of the end plates of adjoining vertebrae and disc space narrowing.

Candida arthritis is usually a monoarticular infection but can be polyarticular as well.[142] The knee is the most common joint involved. In infants and young children, it often presents acutely with constitutional symptoms and findings of inflammatory synovitis of the knee.[142] It may also lead a subacute or chronic course, particularly in older immunosuppressed patients.[144, 145] Effusion is the most common radiographic finding. Adjacent osteomyelitis may occur.[142]

A definitive diagnosis of osteoarticular candidiasis is usually established by culture of the involved tissue or synovial fluid. Both percutaneous needle and open biopsies effectively yield a diagnosis of *Candida* osteomyelitis. Histology often shows *Candida*

yeast and pseudohyphae. Synovial biopsies generally reveal thickening with acute and chronic inflammation. Synovial fluid analyses reveal mild to marked inflammation with predominance of granulocytes.[142, 146]

Spontaneous remission of *Candida* osteomyelitis is exceedingly rare and therefore underscores the need for therapy. Amphotericin B is the drug of choice. Intravenous amphotericin B has been effective in cure of *Candida* arthritis.[134] In the setting of joint replacement, cure requires removal of the prosthesis. The combination of flucytosine and amphotericin B may be useful in some cases.[147] *Candida* osteomyelitis may benefit by drainage of pus, such as a paravertebral abscess. Débridement of sternal osteomyelitis[134, 148] and perhaps of vertebral bodies may also be helpful.

Sporotrichosis

Sporothrix schenckii is a dimorphic fungus that grows as a mold in nature and as a yeast in host tissue. It is found worldwide and is commonly isolated from soil, plants, and plant debris. The vast majority of sporotrichosis cases are cutaneous infections, a consequence of percutaneous inoculation, that may be associated with lymphocutaneous extension. Extracutaneous sporotrichosis seldom occurs. Only five such cases occurred among 3300 sporotrichosis cases involving miners in a South African epidemic.[149] Generally, the extracutaneous sites involved are lung, bone and joint, eye, and meninges. Osteoarticular sporotrichosis is found in 80 percent of extracutaneous cases.[150] It often appears to be a result of hematogenous dissemination in a host that has alcoholism, a myeloproliferative syndrome, or other immunocompromising factors. The portal of entry is usually uncertain. A pulmonary route has been postulated although usually not evident. Osteoarticular involvement is rarely due to cutaneous inoculation; concomitant cutaneous lesions are usually at sites unrelated to osteoarticular foci, thereby supporting a hematogenous mechanism for dissemination.

Sporotrichosis involves the bone and joint and rarely the tendon sheath and bursa.[151, 152] Infection is chronic, indolent, and associated with minimal or no constitutional symptoms. Osseous sporotrichosis may occur as a solitary lesion or as multiple lesions. It typically involves the tibia, fibula, humerus, and short tubular bones of the hand and feet.[153, 154] The spine is usually spared. Concomitant arthritis and sinus formation occur frequently. Standard radiographs reveal destruction of bone without sclerosis or periosteal reaction. Articular sporotrichosis commonly involves the knee, wrist and hand, elbow, and ankle.[155–157] Monoarticular (about half the cases), pauciarticular, or polyarticular involvement may occur. Clinical findings of an inflammatory arthritis are often found. Standard radiographic studies show abnormalities in more than 90 percent,[157] including periarticular osteoporosis, poorly circumscribed patchy loss of trabeculae, and articular cartilage thinning.

Most cases of osteoarticular sporotrichosis are diagnosed by culture of involved tissue or synovial fluid. Histologically, granulomata and pyogranulomata are present in infected tissue. Organisms are best detected using methenamine silver stain.

Approximately one half to two thirds of the osteoarticular sporotrichosis cases can be cured with a single course of intravenous amphotericin B. A prolonged course of therapy may be required in cases of relapse. A role for intra-articular use of amphotericin B has not been established. Synovectomy and surgical débridement do not appear to be helpful in most cases.[158]

Aspergillosis

Aspergillus is a filamentous fungus that is ubiquitous in the environment, with worldwide distribution. It thrives on decaying matter and soil and is even recoverable from water and hospital air. Although encounters are frequent, disease is not. Factors that predispose to invasive aspergillosis are various immunocompromised states, surgery, and trauma. Several species of *Aspergillus* have been reported to cause disease; *A. fumigatus* is the most common cause. Invasive disease typically involves the lung or paranasal sinuses but may involve many different organs. The skeleton is seldom affected.

Aspergillus osteomyelitis arises from contiguous sites in the lung and paranasal sinuses as well as hematogenous spread.[140, 159–161] Sites of contiguous osseous involvement are the vertebrae, ribs, and skull. The vertebrae are the most frequent bones affected. Infection may span several vertebral bodies in association with paravertebral abscess formation, which may mimic Pott's disease and possibly lead to an epidural abscess of neurologic significance.[162] It is notable that rib involvement has occurred predominantly in the setting of chronic granulomatous disease. Isolated diskitis and articular aspergillosis has rarely been reported.[161] Intravenous amphotericin B (0.5 to 1 mg per kg per day) in conjunction with surgical débridement is the mainstay of therapy.[161, 163]

Rare Deep Mycosis

Mycetoma (Maduromycosis)

Mycetoma is a chronic destructive infection that produces a localized lesion of skin, subcutaneous tissues, and bone, which typically involves the foot (madura foot). It is caused by subcutaneous implantation, via minor trauma, of any one of many species of aerobic bacteria (*Actinomycetes*) or true fungi (*Eumycetes*). Actinomycetoma is caused by genera of *Nocardia, Streptomyces,* and *Actinomadura.* Mycetomas occur worldwide, particularly in semitropical and tropical regions, e.g., Africa and India. The most common organism encountered varies with the locality. *Pseudoallescheria boydii* is the most common cause of mycetoma in the United States.[164, 165]

A mycetoma originates in subcutaneous tissue and then by way of direct extension over a period of years may involve adjacent fascia, muscle, tendon, bone, and joints. It appears characteristically as a painless, indurated swelling with sinus tracts that intermittently extrude pus and grains. The grains contain the causative organism admixed with proteinaceous material. Diagnosis of mycetoma requires a compatible clinical presentation and demonstration of grains in extruded pus or in histologic sections of biopsy material. Culture of grains and biopsy material provides the causative species diagnosis. Culturing biopsy specimens is preferred over that of grains to avoid confounding contamination.

Actinomycetoma may respond to a combination of streptomycin and trimethoprim-sulfamethoxazole or dapsone. Except for *Madurella mycetomatis,* which may respond to ketoconazole, other causes of eumycetoma rarely respond to chemotherapy.

Actinomycosis

The actinomycetes are strictly anaerobic bacilli with gram-positive appearance. Branching properties give them a fungus-like morphology that has led to misclassification within the mycetes (actinomycosis: Greek = branching fungus). Although several species have been associated with human infections, *Actinomyces israelii* is by far the most common.[166, 167] Because its clinical behavior resembles that of the mycetes, *A. israelii* is discussed here. One of its major distinctions from the fungi is its sensitivity to antibiotics such as penicillin and tetracycline. *A. israelii* exists as a commensal in the crypts and crevices of the tonsils and gingiva. Its anaerobic requirements are particularly well supported by infected carious teeth, oral injuries associated with small necrotic foci, and breaks in the mucous membranes (e.g., dental extractions). Isolation of the bacilli from such sites is not equivalent to infection, which is best proved by demonstrating tissue invasion. The most common form of bone disease involves direct extension from the mouth to the mandible. Further extension into the maxilla, orbit, and paranasal sinuses can occur.[167–168] Abscess formation and draining sinus tracts may follow. Aggregates of branching organisms, held together by protein-polysaccharide, may form yellowish macroscopic particles ("sulfur granules") that can be found in sinus drainage.[170] Cervicofacial disease is most often mistaken for cancer[166] when classic clinical findings are absent.

Pulmonary actinomycosis may be complicated by invasion of the pleura, chest wall, and dorsal vertebrae, mimicking malignancy (Fig. 87–7). An unresolving pneumonia with contiguous bone involvement suggests malignancy or actinomycosis.

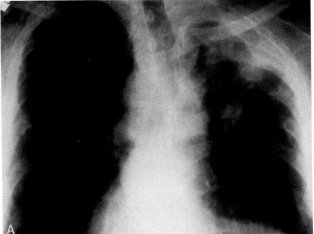
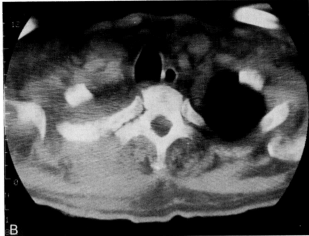
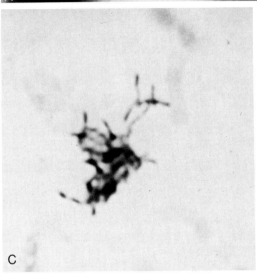

Figure 87–7. Actinomycoses. A 63-year-old man self-referred for orthopedic consultation because of upper thoracic back pain of 2 months' duration and a recently enlarging tender mass. The mass was 15 cm × 8 cm and extended from the base of the neck to approximately the level of the third thoracic vertebra. Recent past history was remarkable only for a dental procedure 6 weeks prior to onset of symptoms. *A*, Chest radiograph revealed an upper lobe density and pleural thickening. *B*, A CT scan demonstrated extension of the upper lobe density to the chest wall, causing destructive changes of the second rib and transverse process of T_2. Biopsy, Gram stain, and culture of the thoracic mass revealed gram-positive, branching bacilli, *Actinomyces myeri (C)*. The patient responded to intravenous penicillin, without requiring surgical intervention.

Although the vertebral bodies may be extensively involved and associated with paravertebral abscesses, they rarely collapse, and the disc is usually spared, helping distinguish this process from tuberculous involvement.[168, 169, 171, 172] Similar involvement of the lumbar spine may occur from direct extension of a gastrointestinal focus. Hematogenous dissemination resulting in bone or articular lesions of the extremities is extremely rare. When the limbs are involved, the initial lesion is usually in the soft tissues but may then extend to bone.[173] Remembering to include anaerobic cultures in the assessment of unusual osseous lesions, especially those of the head and neck, is essential to making a diagnosis of actinomycosis. Because actinomycetes thrive in relatively avascular regions, large doses of penicillin are required for effective treatment. Treatment may be required for several months.[166, 168, 174] The optimal duration of therapy is unknown.

References

1. LaFond, E. M.: An analysis of adult skeletal tuberculosis. J. Bone Joint Surg. 40:346, 1958.
2. Walker, G. F.: Failure of early recognition of skeletal tuberculosis. Br. Med. J. 1:682, 1968.
3. Davidson, P. T., and Horowitz, I.: Skeletal tuberculosis. A review with patient presentations and discussion. Am. J. Med. 48:77, 1970.
4. Wallace, R., and Cohen, A. S.: Tuberculous arthritis. A report of two cases with a review of biopsy and synovial fluid findings. Am. J. Med. 61:277, 1976.
5. Lifesco, R. M., Weaver, P., and Harder, E. H.: Tuberculous spondylitis in adults. J. Bone Joint Surg. 67A:1405, 1985.
6. Alvarez, S., and McCabe, W. R.: Extrapulmonary tuberculosis revisited: A review of experience at Boston City and other hospitals. Medicine 63:25, 1984.
7. Weir, M. R., and Thornton, G. F.: Extrapulmonary tuberculosis: Experience of a community hospital and review of the literature. Am. J. Med. 79:467, 1985.
8. Bloch, A. B., Rieder, H. L., Kelly, G. D. et al.: The epidemiology of tuberculosis in the United States. Semin. Respir. Infect. 4(3):157, 1989.
9. CDC: Tuberculosis statistics in the United States. U.S. Department of Health, Education, and Welfare, Public Health Service, 1988.
10. CDC: Personal communication: U.S. Department of Health, Education, and Welfare, Public Health Service, 1990.
11. Wolfgant, G. L.: Tuberculosis joint infection following total knee arthroplasty. Clin. Orthop. 201:162, 1985.
12. Luck, J. V.: Tuberculous osteomyelitis and arthritis. *In* Bone and Joint Disease. Springfield, IL, Charles C. Thomas, 1950, pp. 75–103.
13. Davies, P. D., Hunphries, M. J., Byufield, S. P., et al.: Bone and joint tuberculosis: A survey of notifications in England and Wales. J. Bone Joint Surg. 66B:326, 1984.
14. Goldberg, I., and Avidor, I.: Isolated tuberculous tenosynovitis of the Achilles tendon. Clin. Orthop. Rel. Res. 194:185, 1985.
15. Chapman, M., Murray, R. D., and Stoker, D. J.: Tuberculosis of bones and joints. Semin. Roentgenol. 14:266, 1979.
16. Nathanson, L., and Cohen, W.: A statistical and roentgen analysis of two hundred cases of bone and joint tuberculosis. Radiology 36:550, 1941.

17. Bell, D., and Cockshott, W. P.: Tuberculosis of the vertebral pedicles. Radiology 99:43, 1971.
18. Omari, B., Robertson, J. M., Nelson, R. J., et al.: Pott's disease: A resurgent challenge to the thoracic surgeon. Chest 95:145, 1989.
19. Pouchot, J., Vincenenux, P., Barge, J., et al.: Tuberculosis of the sacroiliac joint: Clinical features, outcome, and evaluation of closed needle biopsy in 11 consecutive cases. Am. J. Med. 84:622, 1988.
20. Evanchick, C. C., Davies D. E., and Harrington, T. M.: Tuberculosis of peripheral joints: An often missed diagnosis. J. Rheumatol. 13:187, 1986.
21. Goldenberg, D. L., and Cohen, A. S.: Arthritis due to tuberculous and fungal microorganisms. Clin. Rheum. Dis. 4:211, 1978.
22. Phemister, D. B.: Changes in the articular surfaces in tuberculous and pyogenic infections of joints. Am. J. Roentgenol. Rad. Ther. 12:1, 1924.
23. Golding, F. C.: Tuberculosis of joints. In Shanks, S. C., and Kerley, P. (eds.): A Textbook of X-ray Diagnosis. 4th ed. London, H. K. Lewis & Company, Ltd., 1971, pp. 307–316.
24. Riese, H.: Die Rieshorperchen in tuberculos Erkrankten. Synovalsachen. Dtsch. Z. Chir. 42:1, 1895.
25. Hoffman, G. S., Myers, R. L., Stark, F. R., and Thoen, C. O.: Septic arthritis associated with Mycobacterium avium: A case report and literature review. J. Rheumatol. 5:2, 1978.
26. Martini, M., Adjrad, A., Boudjemaa, A.: Tuberculous osteomyelitis: A review of 125 cases. Int. Orthop. 10:201, 1986.
27. Newton, P., Sharp, J., and Barnes, K. L.: Bone and joint tuberculosis in Greater Manchester 1969–1979. Ann. Rheum. Dis. 41:1, 1982.
28. Moon, M. S., Kim, I., Woo, Y. K., and Park, Y. O.: Conservative treatment of tuberculosis of the thoracic and lumbar spine in adults and children. Int. Orthop. 11:315, 1987.
29. American Thoracic Society: Treatment of tuberculosis and tuberculosis infection in adults and children. Rev. Respir. Dis. 134:355, 1986.
30. Dutt, A. K., Moers, D., and Stead, W. W.: Short-course chemotherapy for extrapulmonary tuberculosis: Nine years' experience. Ann. Intern. Med. 104:7, 1986.
31. Dutt, A. K., and Stead W. W.: Treatment of extrapulmonary tuberculosis. Semin. Respir. Infect. 4(3):225, 1989.
32. Biddulph, J.: Short course chemotherapy for childhood tuberculosis. Pediatr. Infect. Dis. J. 9:794, 1990.
33. Cohn, D. L., Catlin, B. J., Peterson, K. L., et al.: A 62-dose, 6-month therapy for pulmonary and extrapulmonary tuberculosis. Ann. Intern. Med. 112:407, 1990.
34. Hannachi, M.: Comparison of 3 chemotherapeutic regimens of short duration (6 months) in osteo-articular tuberculosis—results after 5 years. Bull. Int. Union Tuberc. 57:46, 1988.
35. Tenth Report of the Medical Research Council Working Party on Tuberculosis of the Spine: A controlled trial of six-month and nine-month regimens of chemotherapy in patients undergoing radical surgery for tuberculosis of the spine in Hong Kong. Tubercle 67:243, 1986.
36. Ninth Report of the Medical Research Council Working Party on Tuberculosis of the Spine: A ten-year assessment of controlled trials of inpatient and outpatient treatment and of plaster-of-Paris jackets for tuberculosis of the spine in children on standard chemotherapy. J. Bone Joint Surg. 67B:103, 1985.
37. Tuberculosis of the Spine: A 10-year assessment of a controlled trial comparing débridement and anterior spinal fusion in the management of tuberculosis of the spine in patients on standard chemotherapy in Hong Kong. J. Bone Joint Surg. 64B:393, 1982.
38. Louw, J. A.: Spinal tuberculosis with neurological deficit. Treatment with anterior vascularized rib grafts, posterior osteotomies and fusion. J. Bone Joint Surg. (Br.) 72-B:686, 1990.
39. Laforgia, R., Murphy J. C. M., and Redfern T. R.: Low-friction arthroplasty for old quiescent infection of the hip. J. Bone Joint Surg. (Br.) 70-B:373, 1988.
40. Eskola, A., Santavirta, S., Konttinen, Y. T., et al.: Cementless total replacement for old tuberculosis of the hip. J. Bone Joint Surg. (Br.) 70-B:603, 1988.
41. Kim, Y. Y., Ko, C. U., Ahn, J. Y., et al.: Charnley low-friction arthroplasty in tuberculosis of the hip. An eight- to 13-year follow-up. J. Bone Joint Surg. (Br.) 70-B:756, 1988.
42. Kim, Y-H: Total knee arthroplasty for tuberculous arthritis. J. Bone Joint Surg. (Am.) 70-A(9):1322, 1988.
43. Eskola A., Santavirta, S., Konttinen, Y., et al.: Arthroplasty for old tuberculosis of the knee. J. Bone Joint Surg. (Br.) 70-B:767, 1988.
44. Kelly, P. J., Karlson, A. G., Weed, L. A., et al.: Infection of synovial tissues by mycobacteria other than Mycobacterium tuberculosis. J. Bone Joint Surg. 49A:1521, 1967.
45. Wolinsky, E.: Nontuberculous mycobacteria and associated diseases. Am. Rev. Respir. Dis. 119:107, 1977.
46. Sutker, W. L., Lankford, L. L., and Tompsett, R.: Granulomatous synovitis: The role of atypical mycobacteria. Rev. Infect. Dis. 729:1, 1979.
47. Marchevsky, A. M., Damster, B., Green, S., et al.: The clinicopatho-logical spectrum of non-tuberculous/mycobacterial osteoarticular infections. J. Bone Joint Surg. 67A:925, 1985.
48. Lincoln, E. M., and Gilbert, L. A.: Disease in children due to mycobacteria other than Mycobacterium tuberculosis. Am. Rev. Respir. Dis. 105:683, 1972.
49. Blumenthal, D. R., Zucker, J. R., and Hawkins, C. C.: Mycobacterium avium complex–induced septic arthritis and osteomyelitis in a patient with the acquired immunodeficiency syndrome (letter). Arthritis Rheum. 33:757, 1990.
49a. Ellner, J. J., Goldberger, M. J., and Parenti, D. M.: Mycobacterium avium infection and AIDS: A therapeutic dilemma in rapid evolution. J. Infect. Dis. 163:1326, 1991.
49b. Wolinsky, E.: Mycobacterial diseases other than tuberculosis. Clin. Infect. Dis. 15:1, 1992.
50. Woods, G. L., and Washington, J. H., II: Mycobacteria other than Mycobacterium tuberculosis: Review of microbiologic and clinical aspects. Rev. Infect. Dis. 9:275, 1987.
51. Dillon, J., Millson, C., and Morris, I.: Mycobacterium kansasii infection in the wrist and hand. Br. J. Rheumatol. 29:150, 1990.
52. Glickstein, S. L., and Hashel, D. J.: Mycobacterium kansasii septic arthritis complicating rheumatic disease: Case report and review of the literature. Semin. Arthritis Rheum. 16:231, 1987.
53. Dixon, J. M.: Non-tuberculous mycobacterial infection of the tendon sheaths in the hand. J. Bone Joint Surg. 63B:512, 1981.
54. Minikin, B. I., Mills, C. L., Bullock, M. B., et al.: Mycobacterium kansasii osteomyelitis of the scaphoid. J. Hand Surg. 12A(6):1092, 1987.
55. Spencer, J. D.: Bone and joint infection in a renal unit. J. Bone Joint Surg. 68B:498, 1986.
56. Carroll, S. R., Newson, S. W., and Jenner, J. R.: Treatment of septic arthritis due to Mycobacterium kansasii. Br. Med. J. 289:591, 1984.
57. Sanger, J. R., Stampfl, P. A., and Franson, T. R.: Recurrent granulomatous synovitis due to Mycobacterium kansasii in a renal transplant recipient. J. Hand Surg. 12A:436, 1987.
58. Chow, S. P., Stroebal, A. B., Lau, J. H. K., et al.: Mycobacterium marinum infection of the hand involving deep structures. J. Hand Surg. 8(5):568, 1983.
59. Jones, M. W., Wahid, I. A., and Matthews, J. P.: Septic arthritis of the hand due to Mycobacterium marinum. J. Hand Surg. 13-B:333, 1988.
60. Clark, R. B., Spector, H., and Friedman, D. M.: Osteomyelitis and synovitis produced by Mycobacterium marinum in a fisherman. J. Clin. Microbiol. 28(11):2570, 1990.
61. Donta, S. T., Smith, P. W., Levitz, R. E., et al.: Therapy of Mycobacterium marinum infections. Arch. Intern. Med. 146:902, 1986.
62. Bailey, J. P., Stevens, S., Bell, W. M., et al.: Mycobacterium marinum infection. J.A.M.A. 247(9):1314, 1982.
63. Chow, S. P., Ip, F. K., Lau, J. H. K., et al.: Mycobacterium marinum infection of the hand and wrist. J. Bone Joint Surg. 69-A:1161, 1987.
64. Wallace, R. J., Swenson, J. M., Silcox, V. A., Good, R. C., et al.: Spectrum of disease due to rapidly growing mycobacteria. Rev. Infect. Dis. 5:657, 1983.
65. Gran, J. T., Eng, J., Refven, O. K., Denstad, T., et al.: Monoarthritis due to Mycobacterium chelonei. J. Rheumatol. 14:852, 1987.
66. Butarac, R., Littlejohn, G. O., and Hooper, J.: Mycobacterial disease in the musculoskeletal system. Med. J. Aust. 147:388, 1987.
67. Drabick, J. J., Duffy, P. E., Samlaska, C. P., and Scherbenske, J. M.: Disseminated Mycobacterium chelonae subspecies chelonae infection with cutaneous and osseous manifestations. Arch. Dermatol. 126:1064, 1990.
68. Lowry P. W., Jarvis, W. R., Oberle, A. D., et al.: Mycobacterium chelonae causing otitis media in an ear-nose-and-throat practice. N. Engl. J. Med. 319:978, 1988.
69. Graybill J. R., Silva, J., Fraser, D. W., et al.: Disseminated mycobacteriosis due to Mycobacterium abscessus in two recipients of renal homografts. Am. Rev. Respir. Dis. 109:4, 1974.
70. Wallace, R. J., Swenson, J. M., Silcox, V. A., et al.: Treatment of nonpulmonary infections due to Mycobacterium fortuitum and Mycobacterium chelonei on the basis of in vitro susceptibilities. J. Infect. Dis. 152:500, 1985.
71. Wallace, R. J., Nash, D. R., Tsukamura, M., et al.: Human disease due to Mycobacterium smegmatis. J. Infect. Dis. 158:52, 1988.
72. Berman, L. B.: Infection of synovial tissue by Mycobacterium gordonae (letter). Can. Med. Assoc. J. 129:1078, 1983.
73. Petrini, B., Svartengren, G., Hoffner, S. E., et al.: Tenosynovitis of the hand caused by Mycobacterium terrae. Eur. J. Clin. Microbiol. Infect. Dis. 8:722, 1989.
74. Rougraff B. T., Reeck, C. C., Jr., and Slama, T. G.: Mycobacterium terrae osteomyelitis and septic arthritis in a normal host. A case report. Clin. Orthop. 238:308, 1989.
75. Rosen, R. S., and Jacobson, G.: Fungus disease of bone. Semin. Roentgenol. 1:4, 1966.
76. Crout, J. E., Brewer, N. S., and Tompkins, R. B.: Sporotrichosis arthritis. Am. J. Med. 60:587, 1976.
77. Bayer, A. S., Yushika, T. T., Galpin, J. E., et al.: Unusual syndromes of coccidioidomycosis: Diagnostic and therapeutic considerations. Medicine 55:131, 1976.

77a. Stevens, D. A. (ed.): Coccidioidomycosis. New York, Plenum, 1980, pp. 63–85.
78. Dodge, R. R., Lebowitz, M. D., Barbee, R., and Burrows, B.: Estimates of *Coccidioides immitis* infection by the skin test reactivity in an endemic community. Am. J. Public Health 75:863, 1985.
79. Bronniamann, D. A., Adam, R. D., Galgiani, J. N., et al.: Coccidioidomycosis in the acquired immunodeficiency syndrome. Ann. Intern. Med. 106:372, 1987.
80. Bayer, A. S.: Fungal pneumonias; pulmonary coccicidioidal syndromes (part 1). Chest 79:5, 1981.
81. Resnick, D., and Niwayama, G.: Diagnosis of Bone and Joint Disorders. 2nd ed. Philadelphia, W. B. Saunders Company, 1988.
82. Ampel, N. M., Wieden, M. A., and Galgiani, J. N.: Coccidioidomycosis: Clinical update. Rev. Infect. Dis. 11(6):897, 1989.
83. Bried, J. M., and Galgiani, J. N.: *Coccidiodes immitis* infections in bones and joints. Clin. Orthop. 211:235, 1986.
84. Dalinka, M. K., Dinnenberg, S., Greendyke, W. H., et al.: Roentgenographic features of osseous coccidioidomycosis and differential diagnosis. J. Bone Joint Surg. 53-A(6):1157, 1971.
85. Carter, R. A.: Infectious granulomas of bones and joints, with special reference to coccidioidal granuloma. Radiology 23:1, 1934.
86. McGahan, J. P., Graves, D. S., Palmer, P. E. S., et al.: Classic and contemporary imaging of coccidioidomycosis. A. J. R. 136:393, 1981.
87. Winter, W. G., Larson, R. K., Honnegar, M. M., et al.: Coccidioidal arthritis and its treatment—1975. J. Bone Joint Surg. 57A:1152, 1975.
88. Moreno, A. J., Weisman, I. M., Rodriguez, A. A., et al.: Nuclear imaging in coccidioidal osteomyelitis. Clin. Nucl. Med. 12:604, 1987.
89. McGahan, J. D., Graves, D. S., and Palmer, E. S.: Coccidioidal spondylitis. Radiology 136:5, 1990.
90. Drutz, D. J., and Catanzaro, A.: Coccidioidomycosis. Part I. Am. Rev. Respir. Dis. 117:559, 1978.
91. Drutz, D. J., and Catanzaro, A.: Coccidioidomycosis. Part II. Am. Rev. Respir. Dis. 117:727, 1979.
92. Bayer, A. S., and Lucien, G. B.: Fungal arthritis. II. Coccidioidal synovitis: Clinical, diagnostic, therapeutic, and prognostic considerations. Semin. Arthritis Rheum. 8(3):200, 1979.
93. Rettig, A. C., Evanski, P. M., Waugh, T. R., et al.: Primary coccidioidal synovitis of the knee. A report of four cases and review of the literature. Clin. Orthop. 132:187, 1978.
94. Lantz, B., Selakovich, W. G., Collins, D. N., et al.: Coccidioidomycosis of the knee with a 26-year follow-up evaluation. Clin. Orthop. 234:183, 1988.
95. Graybill, J. R.: Treatment of coccidioidomycosis. Ann. N.Y. Acad. Sci. 481:544, 1988.
96. Galgiani, J. N., Stevens, D. A., Graybill, J. R., et al.: Ketoconazole therapy of progressive coccidioidomycosis. Comparison of 400- and 800-mg doses and observations at higher doses. Am. J. Med. 84:603, 1988.
97. Graybill, J. R., Stevens, D. A., Galgiani, J. N., et al.: Itraconazole treatment of coccidioidomycosis. Am. J. Med. 89:282, 1990.
98. Sarosi, G. A., and Davies, S. F.: Blastomycosis. Am. Rev. Respir. Dis. 120:911, 1979.
99. Gnann, J. W., Jr., Bressler, G. S., Bodet, C. A., et al.: Human blastomycosis after a dog bite. Ann. Intern. Med. 98:48, 1983.
100. Bayer, A. S., Scott, V. J., and Guze, L. B.: Fungal arthritis. IV. Blastomycotic arthritis. Semin. Arthritis Rheum. 9:145, 1979.
101. Fountin, F. F.: Acute blastomycotic arthritis. Arch. Intern. Med. 132:684, 1973.
102. Reeves, R. J., and Pederson, R.: Fungus infection in bone. Radiology 62:55, 1954.
103. Cush, R. G., Light, R. H. W., and George, D. B.: Clinical and roentgenographic manifestations of acute and chronic blastomycosis. Chest 69:345, 1976.
104. Gehweiler, J. A., Capp, M. P., and Chick, E. W.: Observations on the roentgen patterns in blastomycosis of bone. Am. J. Roentgenol. 108:497, 1970.
105. Macdonald, P. B., Black, G. B., and Mackenzie, R.: Orthopaedic manifestations of blastomycosis. J. Bone Joint Surg. 72-A(6):860, 1990.
106. Bassett, F. H., and Tindall, J. P.: Blastomycosis of bone. South. Med. J. 65:547, 1972.
107. Tenenbaum, M. J., Greenspan, J., and Kerkering, T. M.: Blastomycosis. CRC Crit. Rev. Microbiol. 9:139, 1982.
108. George, A. L., Jr., Hays, J. T., and Grahm, B. S.: Blastomycosis presenting as monoarticular arthritis. The role of synovial fluid cytology. Arthritis Rheum. 28(5):516, 1985.
109. NIAID Mycosis Study Group: Treatment of blastomycosis and histoplasmosis with ketoconazole. Ann. Intern. Med. 103:861, 1985.
110. Murphy, P. A.: Blastomycosis. J.A.M.A. 261(21):3159, 1989.
111. Diamond, R. D.: *Cryptococcus neoformans. In* Mandell, G. L., Douglas, R. G., Jr., and Bennett, J. E. (eds.): Principles and Practice of Infectious Diseases. 3rd ed. New York, Wiley Medical Publications, 1990, pp. 1980–1989.
112. Behrman, R. E., Masci, J. R., and Nicholas, P.: Cryptococcal skeletal infections: Case report and review. Rev. Infect. Dis. 12(2):181, 1990.
113. Collins, V. P.: Bone involvement in cryptococcosis (torulosis). A.J.R. 63:102, 1950.
114. Chelboun, J., and Nade, S.: Skeletal cryptococcosis. J. Bone Joint Surg. 59-A:509, 1977.
115. Hammerschlag, M. R., Domingo, J., Halber, J. O., and Papayanopulos, D.: Cryptococcal osteomyelitis. Report of a case and review of the literature. Clin. Pediatr. 21:109, 1982.
116. Matsushita, T., and Suzuki, K.: Spastic paraperis due to cryptococcal osteomyelitis. A case report. Clin. Orthop. 196:279, 1985.
117. Bayer, A. S., Choi, C., Tillman, D. B., and Guze, L. B.: Fungal arthritis. V. Cryptococcal and histoplasmal arthritis. Semin. Arthritis Rheum. 9(3):218, 1980.
118. Bunning, R. D., and Barth, W. F.: Cryptococcal arthritis and cellulitis. Ann. Rheum. Dis. 43:508, 1984.
119. Riccirdi, D. D., Sepkowitz, D. V., Berkowitz, L. B., et al.: Cryptococcal arthritis in a patient with acquired immune deficiency syndrome: Case report and review of the literature. J. Rheumatol. 13:455, 1986.
120. Goodwin, R. A., Loyd, J. E., and Des Prez, R. M.: Histoplasmosis in normal hosts. Medicine 60:231, 1981.
121. Rosenthal, J., Brandt, K., Wheat, L. J., and Slama, T. G.: Rheumatologic manifestations of histoplasmosis in the recent Indianapolis epidemic. Arthritis Rheum. 26:1065, 1983.
122. Friedman, S. J., Black, J. L., and Duffy, J.: Histoplasmosis presenting as erythema multiforme and polyarthritis. Cutis 34:396, 1984.
123. Thornberry, D. K., Wheat, L. J., Brandt, K. D., and Rosenthal, J.: Histoplasmosis presenting with joint pain and hilar adenopathy. Arthritis Rheum. 25:1396, 1982.
124. Sellar, T. F., Price, W. N., and Newberry, W. M.: An epidemic of erythema and erythema nodosum caused by histoplasmosis. Ann. Intern. Med. 62:1244, 1963.
125. Medeiros, A. A., Marty, S. D., Tosh, F. E., et al.: Erythema nodosum and erythema multiforme as clinical manifestations of histoplasmosis in a community outbreak. N. Engl. J. Med. 274:415, 1966.
126. Allen, J. H., Jr.: Bone involvement with disseminated histoplasmosis. Am. J. Roentgenol. 82:250, 1959.
127. Omer, G. E., Lockwood, R. S., Travis, L. O., et al.: Histoplasmosis involving the carpal joint. J. Bone Joint Surg. 45-A:1699, 1963.
128. Jones, P. G., Rolston, K., and Hopfer, R. L.: Septic arthritis due to *Histoplasma capsulatum* in a leukaemic patient. Ann. Rheum. Dis. 44:128, 1985.
128a. Kwon-Chung, K. J., and Bennett, J. E.: Histoplasmosis. In Kwon-Chung, K. J., and Bennett, J. E. (eds.): Medical Mycology. Philadelphia, Lea & Febiger, 1992, pp. 464–513.
129. Cockshott, W. P., and Lucas, A. O.: Radiologic findings in *Histoplasma duboisii* infections. Br. J. Radiol. 37:653, 1964.
130. Loyd, J. E., Des Prez, R. M., and Goodwin, R. A., Jr.: *Histoplasma capsulatum. In* Mandell, G. L., Douglas, R. G., Jr., and Bennett, J. E. (eds.): Principles and Practice of Infectious Diseases. 3rd ed. New York, Wiley Medical Publications, 1990, pp. 1980–1989.
131. Edwards, J. E., Jr., Drutz, D. J., Bennett, J. E., et al.: Disseminated candidiasis. A major problem with cancer and postoperative patients. Part 1. New York, Academy Professional Information Services, 1986.
132. Wey, S. B., Mori, M., Pfaller, M. A., et al.: Risk factors for hospital-acquired candidemia. Arch. Intern. Med. 149:2349, 1989.
133. Dupont, B., and Drouhet, E.: Cutaneous, ocular, and osteoarticular candidiasis in heroin addicts. New clinical and therapeutic aspects in 38 patients. J. Infect. Dis. 152:577, 1985.
134. Gathe, J. C., Jr., Harris, R. L., Garland, B., et al.: *Candida* osteomyelitis. Report of five cases and literature review. Am. J. Med. 82:927, 1987.
135. Levine, M., Rhehm, S. J., and Wilde, A. H.: Infection with *Candida albicans* of a total knee arthroplasty. Case report and review of the literature. Clin. Ortop. 226:235, 1988.
136. Edwards, J. E., Jr., Turker, S., Elder, H. A., et al.: Hematogenous *Candida* osteomyelitis. Report of three cases and review of the literature. Am. J. Med. 59:89, 1975.
137. Shaikh, B. S., Appelbaum, P. C., and Aber, R. C.: Vertebral disc space infection and *Candida* osteomyelitis due to *Candida albicans* in a patient with acute myelomonocytic leukemia. Cancer 45:1025, 1980.
138. Diament, M. J., Weller, M., and Bernstein, R.: *Candida* infection in a premature infant presenting as discitis. Pediatr. Radiol. 12:96, 1982.
139. Imahori, S. C., Papademetriou, T., and Ogliela, D. M.: *Torulopsis glabrata* osteomyelitis. A case report. Clin. Orthop. 219:214, 1987.
140. Simpson, M. B., Jr., Merz, W. G., Kurlinski, J. P., et al.: Opportunistic mycotic osteomyelitis: Bone infections due to *Aspergillus* and *Candida* species. Medicine 56:475, 1977.
141. Smilack, J. D., and Gentry, L. O.: *Candida* costochondral osteomyelitis. Report of a case and review of the literature. J. Bone Joint Surg. 58-A:888, 1976.
142. Bayer, A. S., and Guze, L. B.: Fungal arthritis: I. *Candida* arthritis. Diagnostic and prognostic implications and therapeutic considerations. Semin. Arthritis Rheum. 8:142, 1978.
143. Pope, T. L., Jr.: Pediatric *Candida albicans* arthritis: Case report of hip involvement and a review of the literature. Prog. Pediatr. Surg. 15:271, 1982.

144. Fainstein, V., Gilmore, C., Hopfer, R. I., et al.: Septic arthritis due to *Candida* species in patients with cancer: Report of five cases and review of the literature. Rev. Infect. Dis. 4:78, 1982.

145. Glauser, M. P., Gerster, J. C., and Delacretaz, F.: Chronic *Candida* arthritis in leukemic patients. Rev. Infect. Dis. 4:1071, 1982.

146. Katzenstein, D.: Isolated *Candida* arthritis: Report of a case and definition of a distinct clinical syndrome. Arthritis Rheum. 28:1421, 1985.

147. Smego, R. A., Perfet, J. R., and Durack, D. T.: Combined therapy with amphotericin B and 5-fluorocytosine for *Candida* meningitis. Rev. Infect. Dis. 6:791, 1984.

148. Yap, S., Ravitch, M. M., and Pataki, K. I.: En bloc chest wall resection for candidal costochondritis in a drug addict. Ann. Thorac. Surg. 31:182, 1981.

149. Lurie, H. I.: Five unusual cases of sporotrichosis from South Africa showing lesions in muscles, bones, and viscera. Br. J. Surg. 50:585, 1963.

150. Wilson, D. E., Mann, J. J., Bennett, J. E., and Utz, J. P.: Clinical features of extracutaneous sporotrichosis. Medicine 46:265, 1967.

151. Chang, A. C., Destouet, J. M., and Murphy, W. A.: Musculoskeletal sporotrichosis. Skeletal Radiol. 12:23, 1984.

152. Schwartz, D. A.: Sporothrix tenosynovitis—differential diagnosis of granulomatous inflammatory disease of the joints. J. Rheumatol. 16(4):550, 1989.

153. Altner, P. C., and Turner, R. R.: Sporotrichosis of bones and joints. Review of the literature and report of six cases. Clin. Orthop. 68:138, 1970.

154. Gladstone, J. L., and Littman, M. L.: Osseous sporotrichosis. Am. J. Med. 51:121, 1971.

155. Yao, J., Penn, P. G., and Ray, S.: Articular sporotrichosis. Clin. Orthop. 204:206, 1986.

156. Janes, P. C., and Mann, R. J.: Extracutaneous sporotrichosis. J. Hand Surg. 12A(3):441, 1987.

157. Bayer, A. S., Scott, V. J., and Guze, L. B.: Fungal arthritis. III. Sporotrichal arthritis. Semin. Arthritis Rheum. 9(1):66, 1979.

158. Bennett, J. E.: Personal communication, unpublished data, 1991. Clinical Mycology Section, Laboratory of Clinical Investigation, National Institute of Allergy and Infectious Diseases, National Institutes of Health, Bethesda, Maryland.

159. Barnwell, P. A., Jelsma, L. F., and Raff, M. I.: *Aspergillus* osteomyelitis: Report of a case and review of the literature. Diagn. Microbiol. Infect. Dis. 3:515, 1985.

160. Tach, K. J., Rhame, F. S., Brown, B., et al.: *Aspergillus* osteomyelitis. Report of four cases and review of the literature. Am. J. Med. 73:295, 1982.

161. Denning, D. W., and Stevens, D. A.: Antifungal and surgical treatment of invasive aspergillosis: Review of 1,121 published cases. Rev. Infect. Dis. 12(6):1147, 1990.

162. Mckee, D. F., Barr, W. M., Bryan, C. S., et al.: Primary aspergillosis of the spine mimicking Pott's paraplegia. J. Bone Joint Surg. 66-A:1481, 1984.

163. De Buele, K., Doncker, P., Cauwenbergh, G., et al.: The treatment of aspergillosis and aspergilloma with itraconazole: clinical results of an open international study (1982–1987). Mycoses 31:476, 1988.

164. Mahgoub, E. S.: Agents of mycetoma. *In* Mandell, G. L., Douglas, R. G., Jr., and Bennett, J. E. (eds.): Principles and Practice of Infectious Diseases. 3rd ed. New York, Wiley Medical Publications, 1990, pp. 1980–1989.

165. Tight, R. R., and Bartlett, M. S.: Actinomycetoma in the United States. Rev. Infect. Dis. 3:1139, 1981.

166. Richtsmeier, W. J., and Johns, M. E.: Actinomycosis of the head and neck. CRC Crit. Rev. Clin. Lab. Sci. 11:175, 1979.

167. Schaal, K. P., Schofield, G. M., and Pulverer, G.: Taxonomy and clinical significance of Actinomycetaceae and Proprionibacteriaceae. Infection (Suppl)8:122, 1980.

168. Goldsand, G.: Actinomycosis. *In* Hoeprich, P. (ed.): Infectious Diseases. 2nd ed. New York, Harper & Row, 1977.

169. Wang, Y.: Critical Reviews in Clinical Radiology and Nuclear Medicine. Boca Raton, Fla., CRC Press, Inc., 1975.

170. Kinderlehrer, D. A., and Reese, R. E.: Fungal infections. *In* Reese, R. E., and Douglas, R. G., Jr. (eds.): A Practical Approach to Infectious Diseases. Boston, Little, Brown & Co., 1983.

171. Rhangos, W. C., and Chick, E. W.: Mycotic infections of bone. South. Med. J. 57:664, 1964.

172. Lane, T., Goings, S., Fraser, D. W., Ries, K., Pettrozzi, J., and Abrutyn, E.: Disseminated actinomycosis with spinal cord compression: Report of two cases. Neurology 29:809, 1979.

173. Sherer, P. B., and Dobbins, J.: Actinomycosis arthritis: A case report. Med. Annu. 43:66, 1974.

174. Schaal, K. P., and Pape, W.: Special methodological problems in antibiotic susceptibility test of fermentative actinomycetes. Infection (Suppl.)8:176, 1980.

Chapter 88

Allen C. Steere

Lyme Disease

INTRODUCTION

Lyme disease, or Lyme borreliosis, was recognized as a separate entity in 1975 because of geographic clustering of children in Lyme, Connecticut, who were thought to have juvenile rheumatoid arthritis.[1] The rural setting of the case clusters and the identification of erythema migrans as a feature of the illness suggested that the disorder was transmitted by an arthropod. It soon became apparent that Lyme disease was a multisystem illness that affected primarily the skin, nervous system, heart, and joints.[2] Epidemiologic studies of patients with erythema migrans implicated certain ixodid ticks as vectors of the disease.[3] In addition to providing clues about the cause of the illness, erythema migrans, which was recognized in Sweden in 1909,[4] linked Lyme disease with certain other syndromes that had been previously described in Europe, including acrodermatitis chronica atrophicans[5] and meningopolyneuritis, or Bannwarth's syndrome.[6] These various syndromes were brought together conclusively in 1982, when a previously unrecognized spirochete, now called *Borrelia burgdorferi*, was recovered from *Ixodes dammini* ticks.[7] Soon thereafter, the spirochete was isolated from American patients with Lyme disease[8, 9] and from European patients with erythema migrans, acrodermatitis, or Bannwarth's syndrome.[10–12]

Clinically, this borrelial infection is most like syphilis in its multisystem involvement, occurrence in stages, and mimicry of other diseases.[13] Although the stages may overlap or occur alone, Lyme disease usually begins with localized infection of the skin manifested by a characteristic expanding skin lesion, called erythema migrans, that occurs at the site of the tick bite (stage 1). Within several days to weeks, the spirochete may spread to other sites (stage 2), particularly to other skin sites, the nervous system, joints, heart, or eyes. Symptoms are typically intermittent and changing at this time in the illness. After months to years, sometimes following long periods of latent infection, the spirochete may cause chronic disease (stage 3), most commonly of the joints, nervous system, or skin. Although there are regional variations, the basic outlines of the disorder are similar worldwide. Serologic testing is the most frequently used method for confirming the diagnosis. The Lyme disease spirochete is sensitive to a number of antibiotics including doxycycline, amoxicillin, and the third-generation cephalosporins.

1484

ETIOLOGIC AGENT

Borrelia species, along with the *Leptospira* and *Treponema*, belong to the eubacterial phylum of spirochetes. Of the *Borrelia* species, *B. burgdorferi* is the longest (20 to 30 μm) and narrowest (0.2 to 0.3 μm), and it has fewer flagella (7 to 11)[14] It contains many different proteins, including immunogenic membrane lipoproteins.[15] However, only a few of these proteins have been fully characterized. These include the two major outer-surface proteins, the 30- to 32-kD outer-surface protein A (OspA) and the 34- to 36-kD outer-surface protein B (OspB)[16] the 41-kD flagellar antigen[17] and the 58- to 60-kD common antigen, a heat-shock protein that is cross-reactive with an equivalent antigen in a wide range of bacteria.[18] All isolates of *B. burgdorferi* examined to date have had from four to nine pieces of extrachromosomal plasmid DNA.[19] A small 49-kb linear plasmid codes for the two major outer-surface proteins of the spirochete, OspA and B[20].

B. burgdorferi grows best at 33°C in a complex, liquid medium called Barbour-Stoenner-Kelly medium.[21] The spirochete has been cultured frequently from erythema migrans skin lesions,[22] but culture from other sites has been difficult.[8, 9] Three genomic subgroups of *B. burgdorferi* have recently been defined.[22a, 22b] To date, American isolates have been genomic subgroup 1, whereas European isolates have included all three subgroups. These differences probably account for the clinical variations in the disease in different geographic regions.

EPIDEMIOLOGY

The Lyme disease spirochete is transmitted by certain ixodes ticks that are part of the *I. ricinus* complex. These include *I. dammini* in the northeastern and midwestern United States, *I. pacificus* in the western United States, *I. ricinus* in Europe, and *I. persulcatus* in Asia. *B. burgdorferi* has been demonstrated in other tick species[23] and in mosquitoes and deer flies,[24] but only ticks of the *I. ricinus* complex seem to be important in the transmission of the spirochete to humans. The preferred host for both the larval and nymphal stages of *I. dammini* is the white-footed mouse,[25] and the preferred host for the adult stage of the tick is the white-tailed deer.[26]

Lyme disease is now the most common vector-

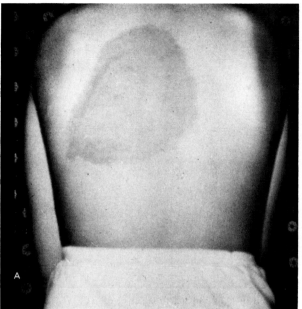
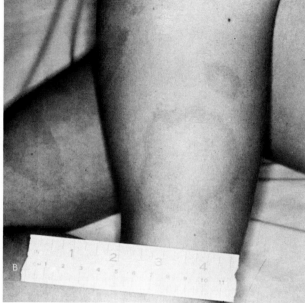

Figure 88–1. Two patients are seen, one with erythema migrans (*A*), the other with secondary annular lesions (*B*). The lesions began as red macules that expanded to form large rings. In *A*, the outer border is an intense red, the middle shows partial clearing, and the center is indurated. In *B*, the outer rims are red, and centers show nearly complete clearing. (From Steere, A. C., et al: Erythema chronicum migrans and Lyme arthritis: the enlarging clinical spectrum. Ann. Intern. Med. 86:685, 1977, used by permission.)

borne disease in the United States. From 1982 to 1991, 40,108 cases were reported to the Centers for Disease Control primarily from three areas of the country: from Massachusetts to Maryland in the Northeast, Wisconsin and Minnesota in the Midwest, and California and Oregon in the West.[47] However, sporadic cases have now been reported in 47 states. The disease also occurs in many areas of Europe, particularly in Germany, Austria, and Sweden, and in a number of eastern European countries.[28] In the countries of the former Soviet Union, cases have been recognized from the Baltic republics to the Pacific Ocean.[29] Patients with the disease have also been found in China, Japan, and Australia.

Although gene segments of *B. burgdorferi* have been identified in archival tick specimens collected during the 1940s from Montauk, Long Island,[30] the earliest known cases of Lyme disease in the United States occurred in the 1960s in residents of Cape Cod and Connecticut.[1, 31] Since then, the infection has spread and has caused focal epidemics, particularly in the northeastern United States. In Ipswich, Massachusetts, 35 percent of 190 residents of an area adjacent to a nature preserve were affected during a 7-year period.[32] Sixteen percent of the 162 residents of Great Island, Massachusetts, developed the illness during a 10-year period[31] and 7.5 percent of 200 people who participated in a study on Fire Island, New York, had the illness during a 5-year period.[33] In the United States, the great majority of affected individuals in these outbreaks had symptoms of the illness. However, in serosurveys done in Europe, the majority of patients with antibody to *B. burgdorferi* were asymptomatic. Of 346 individuals who were

studied in the highly endemic area of Liso, Sweden, 41 (12 percent) had had symptoms of the illness and 89 (26 percent) had evidence of subclinical infection.[34]

CLINICAL MANIFESTATIONS

Early Infection: Stage 1 (Localized Erythema Migrans)

After an incubation period of 3 to 32 days, erythema migrans occurs at the site of the tick bite in 60 to 80 percent of patients.[35] It usually begins as a red macule or papule that expands to form a large, annular lesion (as big as 50 cm), usually with a bright red outer border, partial central clearing, and an indurated center (Fig. 88–1*A*). Even in untreated patients, erythema migrans lesions usually fade within 3 to 4 weeks (range 1 day to 14 months).

Early Infection: Stage 2 (Disseminated Infection)

Within several days to weeks, the Lyme disease spirochete may disseminate widely. Although the list of possible manifestations is long (Table 88–1), disseminated infection is often associated with characteristic symptoms in skin, nervous system, or musculoskeletal sites.[35] Secondary annular skin lesions, which occur in about half the patients, resemble the primary erythema migrans lesion, but they are generally smaller and migrate less (Fig. 88–1*B*). Excruciating headache and mild neck stiffness are common, but they typically occur in short attacks lasting

Table 88–1. MANIFESTATIONS OF LYME DISEASE BY STAGE*

| System** | Early Infection | | Late Infection |
	Localized Stage 1	*Disseminated Stage 2*	*Persistent Stage 3*
Skin	Erythema migrans (EM)	Secondary annular lesions Malar rash Diffuse erythema or urticaria Evanescent lesions Lymphocytoma	Acrodermatitis chronica atrophicans Localized scleroderma-like lesions
Musculoskeletal		Migratory pain in joints, tendons, bursae, muscle, bone Brief arthritis attacks Myositis*** Osteomyelitis*** Panniculitis***	Prolonged arthritis attacks Chronic arthritis Peripheral enthesopathy Periostitis or joint subluxations below acrodermatitis
Neurologic		Meningitis Cranial neuritis, Bell's palsy Motor or sensory radiculoneuritis Subtle encephalitis Mononeuritis multiplex Myelitis*** Chorea*** Cerebellar ataxia***	Subtle mental disorders Axonal polyneuropathy Leukoencephalitis Encephalomyelitis Spastic parapareses Ataxic gait Dementia***
Lymphatic	Regional lymphadenopathy	Regional or generalized lymphadenopathy Splenomegaly	
Heart		AV nodal block Myopericarditis Pancarditis	Cardiomyopathy
Eyes		Conjunctivitis Iritis*** Choroiditis*** Retinal hemorrhage or detachment*** Panophthalmitis***	Keratitis
Liver		Mild or recurrent hepatitis	
Respiratory		Nonexudative sore throat Nonproductive cough Adult respiratory distress syndrome***	
Kidney		Microscopic hematuria or proteinuria	
Genitourinary		Orchitis***	
Constitutional symptoms	Minor	Severe malaise and fatigue	Fatigue

*The staging system provides a guideline for the expected timing of the different manifestations of the illness, but this may vary in an individual case.

**The systems are listed from the most to the least commonly affected.

***Since the inclusion of these manifestations is based on one or a few cases, they should be considered possible but not proven manifestations of Lyme disease.

From Steere, A. C.: Lyme disease. N. Engl. J. Med. 321:586, 1989. Reprinted by permission of *The New England Journal of Medicine.*

only hours. The early musculoskeletal pain of Lyme disease is generally migratory in joints, bursae, tendons, muscle, and bone, lasting only hours or days in a given location. At this stage, patients often appear quite ill, and they frequently have debilitating malaise and fatigue, which may be the predominant symptoms. Except for fatigue, the symptoms are typically intermittent and changing.

After several weeks, about 20 percent of the patients in the United States develop frank neurologic involvement.[36] Although there are many possible abnormalities, the triad of early neurologic abnormalities of Lyme disease consists of meningitis with superimposed cranial or peripheral neuropathy (Fig. 88–2). Cerebrospinal fluid typically has a lymphocytic pleocytosis of about 100 cells per mm³, often with elevated protein but normal glucose levels. Unilateral or bilateral facial palsy is the most common

cranial neuropathy and may be the only neurologic abnormality. The peripheral neuritis is usually an asymmetric motor, sensory, or mixed radiculoneuropathy of the limbs or trunk. These early neurologic abnormalities typically last for months, but they may recur or become chronic.

Within several weeks after the onset of the disease, about 5 percent of patients develop cardiac involvement.[37, 38] The most common abnormality is fluctuating degrees of atrioventricular block (first degree, Wenchebach, or complete heart block), but some patients have acute myopericarditis, mild left ventricular dysfunction, or rarely, cardiomegaly (Fig. 88–3) or fatal pancarditis.[39] The duration of cardiac abnormalities is usually brief (between 3 days and 6 weeks); complete heart block rarely persists for more than 1 week and the insertion of a permanent pacemaker is not necessary.[38] Rarely, patients during this

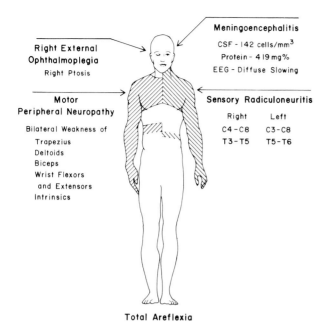

Figure 88–2. A 49-year-old man with neurologic abnormalities of Lyme disease. Five weeks after the onset of erythema migrans, the patient developed meningoencephalitis, followed by right external ophthalmoplegia, right ptosis, and bilateral motor and sensory radiculoneuropathy. The patient was totally areflexic.

period of the illness have fatal adult respiratory distress syndrome,[40] recurrent hepatitis,[41] myositis,[42] osteomyelitis,[43] panniculitis,[44] and serious involvement of the deeper tissues of the eye, including iritis followed by panophthalmitis[45] or choroiditis with exudative retinal detachments.[46]

Late Infection: Stage 3 (Persistent Infection)

A mean of 6 months after the onset of disease (range 2 weeks to 2 years), commonly after intermittent episodes of arthralgia or migratory musculoskeletal pain, about 60 percent of the patients in the United States begin to have brief attacks of asym-

metric, oligoarticular arthritis, primarily in the large joints, especially the knee (Fig. 88–4).[47] Some attacks may affect periarticular structures, including the peripheral entheses. Episodes of arthritis often become longer during the second and third years of illness, lasting months rather than weeks, and chronic arthritis—defined as 1 year or more of continuous joint inflammation—characteristically begins during this period. Typically only one or a few large joints are affected, most commonly the knee. In severe cases, chronic Lyme arthritis may lead to erosion of cartilage and bone and, rarely, to permanent joint disability. As with rubella and parvovirus-associated arthritis, Lyme arthritis seems to be milder in young children than in adults.[48] Although joint involvement is similar in the United States and Europe, it seems to be a less frequent manifestation of the illness in Europe.[49]

From months to years after disease onset, sometimes following long periods of latent infection, patients may develop chronic neurologic manifestations of the disorder.[50–52] The most common form of chronic central nervous system involvement is a subacute encephalopathy affecting memory, mood, or sleep, sometimes with subtle language disturbance. These patients often have increased cerebrospinal fluid protein levels or evidence of intrathecal production of antibody to *B. burgdorferi*; memory impairment can frequently be shown on neuropsychologic tests. In addition to encephalopathy, many of these patients have peripheral sensory symptoms, either distal paresthesias or spinal or radicular pain. Electrophysiologic testing often shows an axonal polyneuropathy, with subtle abnormalities of distal motor- or sensory-nerve conduction.

In Europe, 44 patients have been described with progressive borrelial encephalomyelitis, a severe neurologic disorder characterized by spastic paraparesis or tetraparesis, ataxia, cognitive impairment, bladder dysfunction, and cranial neuropathy, particularly deficits of the seventh or eighth cranial nerve.[53] In all cases, the diagnosis was proved by the demonstration of intrathecal production of IgG antibody to *B. burgdorferi*. One similar case with spastic diple-

Figure 88–3. Chest roentgenograms of a 22-year-old man with cardiac abnormalities of Lyme disease. Three weeks after the onset of erythema migrans, the patient developed syncopal episodes, which were found to be due to complete heart block. *Left*, On admission to the hospital, he had cardiomegaly and evidence of pulmonary venous hypertension. *Right*, Five days after treatment with intravenous penicillin and prednisone, the chest roentgenogram was normal. (Courtesy of Drs. George A. Jacoby and Theresa McLoud, Massachusetts General Hospital, Boston.)

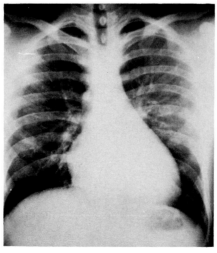
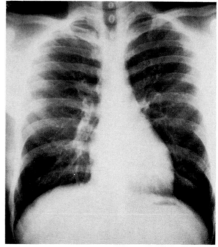

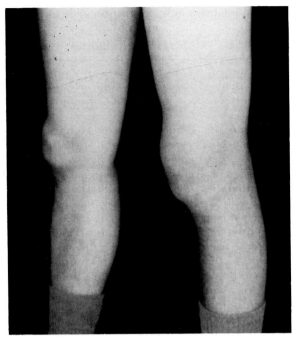

Figure 88–4. A 32-year-old man with Lyme arthritis. Fifteen months after erythema migrans, the patient began to have intermittent attacks of arthritis, primarily in his knees. At the time of this picture, the patient had had such attacks for 6 years.

gia, periventricular white matter lesions, and intrathecal antibody production to the spirochete has been reported in the United States (Fig. 88–5).[50] A few patients have been described with other neurologic abnormalities thought to be due to Lyme disease, including encephalitis, dementia, psychiatric syndromes, brain stem abnormalities, possible demyelinating disease,[54] extrapyramidal syndromes,[55] and stroke.[56] Several patients have also been described with a chronic keratitis that is similar to syphilitic keratitis.[57]

Acrodermatitis chronica atrophicans, a late skin manifestation of the disorder, has been observed primarily in Europe.[12] This skin lesion usually begins insidiously with a bluish red discoloration and swollen skin on an extremity. The inflammatory phase of the lesion may persist for years or decades, and it gradually leads to atrophy of the skin. *B. burgdorferi* has been cultured from such lesions as long as 10 years after their onset. In some patients, scleroderma-like skin lesions can occur concomitantly. In long-standing cases, chronic joint and bone involvement, including periostitis and subluxations of the small joints, may be seen underlying the cutaneous lesions.

CONGENITAL INFECTION

The transplacental transmission of *B. burgdorferi* has been reported in two infants whose mothers had Lyme borreliosis during the first trimester of pregnancy.[58, 59] Both infants died during the first week of life. In both, spirochetes were seen in various

fetal tissues stained with the Dieterle silver stain, but cultures and serologic testing were not done. In a retrospective review of 19 cases of Lyme disease during pregnancy, 5 were associated with adverse fetal outcomes.[60] Since all of the outcomes differed, they could not be linked conclusively to maternal Lyme disease. In subsequent prospective studies, no cases of congenital infection have been identified as due to the Lyme disease spirochete.[61] Although it is likely that the organism can cause an adverse fetal outcome, it seems to be rare.

PATHOGENESIS

After the spirochete is injected by the tick, it may spread locally in the skin or in the blood or lymph to practically any site. During the early stages of the illness, the spirochete has been recovered from erythema migrans lesions, blood, and cerebrospinal fluid;[8, 9, 22] and it has been seen in small numbers in specimens of myocardium, retina, muscle, bone, spleen, liver, meninges, and brain.[62] It has been shown *in vitro* that virulent strains of *B. burgdorferi* are able to resist elimination by phagocytic cells,

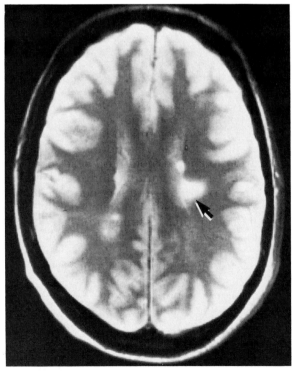

Figure 88–5. Magnetic resonance imaging (MRI) scan of the brain in a 40-year-old man with leukoencephalitis, a late neurologic manifestation of Lyme borreliosis. Six years after erythema migrans, which was followed by several brief attacks of arthritis, the patient developed spastic diplegia. MRI scan of the brain showed periventricular white matter lesions, and his cerebrospinal fluid analysis showed evidence of intrathecal antibody production to *B. burgdorferi*. (Reprinted with permission of Logigian, E. L., et al.: Chronic neurologic manifestations of Lyme disease. The *New England Journal of Medicine* 323:1444, 1990.)

thereby evading the first line in the host defense system against infection.[63] The spirochete can adhere to many different types of mammalian cells, including human epithelial cells, human umbilical vein endothelial cells, and cells derived from neonatal rat brain.[64] The organism seems to cross a cell monolayer at intercellular junctions although it can penetrate through the cytoplasm of a cell.[65] Intracellular localization of *Borrelia burgdorferi* has been demonstrated within human endothelial cells,[65a] but it is not yet clear how long the spirochete can survive there. In a rat model, permeability changes in the blood-brain barrier begin within 12 hours after inoculation of *B. burgdorferi*, and the spirochete may be cultured from cerebrospinal fluid within 24 hours.[66] Although the organism certainly has its preferred niches, such as the nervous system or joints, it is not yet known how it is able to sequester itself at these sites, in some instances for years.

Within several weeks, the peripheral blood mononuclear cells of patients begin to have heightened responsiveness to *B. burgdorferi* antigens or mitogens.[67] The specific IgM response peaks between the third and sixth week of infection[8] and often is associated with polyclonal activation of B cells, including elevated total serum IgM levels,[68] circulating immune complexes,[69] and cryoglobulins.[68] The specific IgG response develops gradually over months to an increasing array of spirochetal polypeptides.[70] Immune antibodies are required for the serum-mediated killing of the spirochete by the classic complement pathway.[71] Histologically, all affected tissues show an infiltration of lymphocytes and plentiful plasma cells.[62] Some degree of vascular damage, including mild vasculitis or hypercellular occlusion, may be seen in multiple sites, suggesting that the spirochete may have been in or around blood vessels.

Similar to the other chronic inflammatory arthritides, the synovial lesion in Lyme arthritis shows villous hypertrophy, fibrin deposition, mononuclear cell infiltrates, intense expression of HLA-DR on many cell types, and sometimes a few spirochetes in and around blood vessels.[72] In two instances, *B. burgdorferi* has been cultured from joint fluid,[73, 74] and mononuclear cell responsive to multiple polypeptide fractions of the spirochete are concentrated there.[75] In two cases of Lyme arthritis, the mean precursor frequency of *B. burgdorferi*-reactive T cells was 1/1290 in synovial fluid and 1/4250 in peripheral blood.[76] *B. burgdorferi* stimulates synovial cells grown in culture to release interleukin-1(IL-1), and IL-1 can be found in joint fluid[77] along with elevated levels of collagenase and prostaglandin E_2.[78] Joint fluid white-cell counts range from 500 to 110,000 cells per mm^3 and consist predominantly of polymorphonuclear leukocytes (PMN).[47] A novel host-derived chemoattractant for PMNs, with a calculated molecular weight of 13,900, has recently been isolated from synovial fluid.[79] Throughout the illness, C3 and C4 levels are generally normal or elevated,[68] and tests for rheumatoid factor and antinuclear antibodies are usually negative.

As with a number of rheumatic diseases, chronic Lyme arthritis appears to have an immunogenetic basis involving D-locus alleles of the major histocompatibility complex. Of 28 patients tested with chronic Lyme arthritis, 89 percent had the HLA-DR4 or HLA-DR2 specificities as compared with 27 percent of those with arthritis of short duration (relative risk, 22; $P = 0.00006$).[80] The presence of HLA-DR4 in patients with arthritis was associated with a lack of response to antibiotic therapy ($P = 0.01$). Thus, in a genetically susceptible subset of individuals, *B. burgdorferi* may trigger an immune response with autoreactive features that continues for some time after the organism has been killed.

DIAGNOSIS

Because culture and direct visualization of *B. burgdorferi* from patient specimens is difficult, serologic testing by ELISA is currently the most practical laboratory aid in diagnosis.[81, 82] However, the specific immune response in Lyme disease may be delayed, and patients with stage 1 infection are often seronegative.[83] The probability of obtaining a positive result during this stage can be increased if both acute and convalescent sera are tested.[84] In a small percentage of patients who are treated with antibiotic therapy during the first several weeks of infection, the humoral immune response to *B. burgdorferi* is aborted, but the spirochete is not completely eradicated.[85, 86] These patients may experience a subtle encephalopathy or polyneuropathy, mild joint swelling or arthralgias, and fatigue. In such patients, it may still be possible to show a cellular immune response to the spirochete by proliferative assay.[85, 86]

After the first several weeks of infection, most patients develop an antibody response to *B. burgdorferi*, particularly if the spirochete disseminates.[8, 81, 82] The highest antibody responses are often seen in patients with chronic arthritis, suggesting that the host immune response may be involved in the pathogenesis of this manifestation of the illness. Evaluation of the intrathecal antibody response by antibody-capture immunoassay is a helpful diagnostic test for neuroborreliosis.[86a] After treatment, antibody titers fall slowly, but most patients remain seropositive. The height of the titer does not tell whether the patient has active or inactive disease.[48] Patients with antibody responses that are only detectable by immunoblotting may still have active infection.[86]

False-positive results, particularly with IgM, may occur both in healthy subjects and in patients with other diseases, including syphilis, Rocky Mountain spotted fever, and autoimmune disorders.[84, 87] Immunoblotting has been advocated as a method of sorting out false positive results.[87] In general, it seems that antibody bands in the range of 21-, 28-, or 94-kD are most specific for this infection.[88] In contrast, bands at 41- and 58/60-kD are commonly found both in patients with Lyme disease and in control subjects.

In addition to the problem of false-positive laboratory results, 5 to 10 percent of patients in the United States[31, 33] and a higher percentage in Europe[34] have asymptomatic infection with *B. burgdorferi*. If these patients have symptoms caused by another disease, they may be wrongly attributed to Lyme borreliosis. Finally, serologic testing for Lyme disease is not yet standardized, and different laboratories may get different results.

DIFFERENTIAL DIAGNOSIS

Erythema migrans, an expanding skin lesion with partial central clearing, is the unique clinical marker for Lyme disease. However, this lesion may be confused with erythema annulare centrifugum or an allergic reaction to an insect bite. In some patients, erythema migrans remains an even red, as in a streptococcal cellulitis, or the center becomes vesicular and necrotic, as in tularemia. Patients with secondary annular skin lesions might be thought to have erythema multiforme; however, blistering, mucosal lesions, or involvement of the palms and soles have not been observed in Lyme disease. Especially when erythema migrans is absent, the early manifestations of Lyme disease may be confused with a viral illness.

The later manifestations of Lyme disease may mimic a number of other disorders. Like rheumatic fever, Lyme disease may be associated with sore throat followed by migratory polyarthritis and carditis. However, valvular involvement has not been seen in Lyme disease. In adults with Lyme disease, the large joint effusions, most commonly in knees, resemble those in Reiter's syndrome. In children, the attacks, though generally shorter, may be like those seen in the pauciarticular form of juvenile arthritis. Motor peripheral neuropathy due to Lyme disease may be confused with the Guillain-Barré syndrome, but Lyme disease does not seem to cause a symmetric ascending polyneuropathy. Spastic diplegia in Lyme disease may look like that in multiple sclerosis, but patients with Lyme disease have evidence of intrathecal antibody production to the spirochete. A word of caution: fibromyalgia or the chronic fatigue syndrome are commonly confused with Lyme disease. However, if these symptoms occur in Lyme disease, they are associated with objective abnormalities of the disorder.

TREATMENT

Before the cause of Lyme disease was known, studies were undertaken in which early Lyme disease was treated with oral tetracycline, penicillin, or erythromycin,[89] and the later stages of the illness were treated with parenteral penicillin.[90, 91] These regimens have now been modified because of the availability of in vitro antibiotic sensitivities to *B. burgdorferi*: they show that the spirochete is highly sensitive to the tetracyclines, ampicillin, and the third-generation cephalosporins, but it is only moderately sensitive to penicillin. Although recommendations for treatment are likely to be modified further as patient studies are completed, the current guidelines are given in Table 88–2.[10]

For early Lyme disease, oral doxycycline or amoxicillin is generally effective therapy, but doxycycline should not be given to children or pregnant women.[92, 93] Ten days of therapy is generally adequate for patients with erythema migrans alone, but 20- or 30-day courses may be necessary in patients with disseminated infection. For patients with ar-

Table 88–2. TREATMENT REGIMENS FOR LYME DISEASE

System	Regimen
Early infection*** (Local or disseminated)	
Adults	Doxycycline 100 mg orally 2 times/d for 10 to 30 d**
	Tetracycline 250 mg orally 4 times/d for 10 to 30 d**
	Amoxicillin 500 mg orally 4 times/d for 10 to 30 d**
Children (Age 8 or less)	Amoxicillin 250 mg orally 3 times/d or 20 mg/kg/d in divided doses for 10 to 30 d**
	Alternative in case of allergy to penicillin *Erythromycin 250 mg orally 3 times/d or 30 mg/kg/d in divided doses for 10 to 30 d**
Arthritis*** (Intermittent or chronic)	Doxycycline 100 mg orally 2 times/d for 30 d
	Amoxicillin and probenecid 500 mg of each orally 4 times/d for 30 d
	Ceftriaxone 2 g IV once a day for 14 d
	Penicillin 20 million U IV in 6 divided doses for 14 d
Neurologic abnormalities*** (Early or late)	Ceftriaxone 2 g IV once a day for 14 to 30 d****
	Cefotaxime 2 g IV 3 times a day for 14 to 30 d****
	Penicillin G 20 million U IV in 6 divided doses daily for 14 to 30 d****
	Alternatives in case of allergy to penicillin or cephalosporin in drugs
(Early)	Doxycycline 200 mg orally 2 times/d for 30 d
(Early or Late)	*Vancomycin 1 g bid for 14 to 30 d
Facial palsy alone	Oral regimens may be adequate
Cardiac abnormalities	
First-degree AV block (PR interval <.3S)	Oral regimens, as for early infection
High-degree AV block	Intravenous regimens, as for neurologic abnormalities
Acrodermatitis	Oral regimens for 1 month are usually adequate

*These antibiotics have not yet been tested systematically for this indication in Lyme disease.
**The duration of therapy is based upon clinical response.
***Treatment failures have occurred with any of the regimens given. Retreatment may be necessary.
****For early neurologic abnormalities, 2 weeks of therapy is generally adequate. The appropriate duration of therapy is not yet clear for patients with late neurologic abnormalities, and 4 weeks of therapy may be preferable.
From Steere, A. C.: Lyme disease. N. Engl. J. Med. 321:586, 1989. Reproduced by permission of *The New England Journal of Anatomy*.

thritis, 30-day courses of doxycycline or amoxicillin/probenecid are often adequate (see Table 88–2), but the high frequency of drug rash may limit the usefulness of the latter regimen.[92, 94] The response to treatment in patients with arthritis may be slow, and a subset of patients with chronic arthritis, primarily those with HLA-DR4, may not respond.[80] In these patients, we usually try a course of intravenous antibiotics. If the synovitis persists, we often inject intra-articular steroids. In patients who have persistent synovitis for 6 to 12 months, we generally recommend arthroscopic synovectomy.[95]

Intravenous therapy is generally necessary for patients with objective neurologic involvement (see Table 88–2), with the possible exception of those with facial palsy alone. Ceftriaxone, cefotaxime, or penicillin are most often used for this purpose.[50, 96–98] In patients with early neurologic abnormalities, the response to treatment is often rapid, but in those with late neurologic manifestations, it is frequently slow.[50] In Europe, patients with meningopolyneuritis, an early neurologic manifestation of Lyme borreliosis, have been treated successfully with doxycycline, 200 mg twice a day for 10 to 20 days,[99] but this therapy does not appear to be effective for late neurologic manifestations of the disorder. Intravenous antibiotic therapy is also standard for patients with high-degree atrioventricular node block or cardiomegaly.

Several questions about treatment remain unresolved. One concerns prophylactic antibiotic treatment of tick bites. In a small study comparing penicillin V and placebo, the risk of acquiring Lyme disease was similar to the risk of an adverse reaction to penicillin.[100] It is unclear how and whether asymptomatic infection should be treated, but such patients are often given a course of oral antibiotics. The appropriate treatment for Lyme disease during pregnancy is also unclear. A pregnant woman in Europe whose erythema migrans was treated with oral antibiotics had an infant who died of possible Lyme encephalitis,[59] and therefore, some physicians give high-dose intravenous penicillin to all women who acquire Lyme disease during pregnancy. In a murine model, immunization with the Osp A protein of the spirochete was protective against infection with the Lyme disease agent.[101] However, a vaccine for the human infection is not yet available.

References

1. Steere, A. C., Malawista, S. E., Snydman, D. R., et al.: Lyme arthritis: An epidemic of oligoarticular arthritis in children and adults in three Connecticut communities. Arthritis Rheum. 20:7, 1977.
2. Steere, A. C., Malawista, S. E., Hardin, J. A., et al.: Erythema chronicum migrans and Lyme arthritis: The enlarging clinical spectrum. Ann. Intern. Med. 86: 685, 1977.
3. Steere, A. C., Broderick, T. F., and Malawista, S. E.: Erythema chronicum migrans and Lyme arthritis: Epidemiologic evidence for a tick vector. Am. J. Epidemiol. 108: 312, 1978
4. Afzelius, A.: Erythema chronicum migrans. Acta Derm. Venereol. (Stockholm) 2:120, 1921.
5. Herxheimer, K., and Hartmann, K.: Uber Acrodermatitis chronica atrophicans. Arch. Dermatol. Syph. 61:57, 255, 1902.
6. Bannwarth, A.: Zur klinik und pathogenese der "chronischen lymphocytaren meningitis." Arch. Psychiatr. Nervenkr. 117:161, 1944.
7. Burgdorfer, W., Barbour, A. G., Hayes, S. E., et al.: Lyme disease: A tick borne spirochetosis. Science 216:1317, 1982.
8. Steere, A. C., Grodzicki, R. L., Kornblatt, A. N., et al.: The spirochetal etiology of Lyme disease. N. Engl. J. Med. 308:733, 1983.
9. Benach, J. L., Bosler, E. M., Hanrahan, J. P., et al.: Spirochetes isolated from the blood of two patients with Lyme disease. N. Engl. J. Med. 308:740, 1983.
10. Ackerman, R., Kabatzki, J., Boisten, H. P., et al.: Spirochaten-Atiologie der Erythema-chronicum-migrans-Krankheit. Dtsch. Med. Wochenschr. 109:92, 1984.
11. Preac-Mursic, V., Wilske, B., Schierz, G., et al.: Repeated isolation of spirochetes from the cerebrospinal fluid of a patient with meningoradiculitis Bannwarth. Eur. J. Clin. Microbiol. 3:564, 1984.
12. Asbrink, E., and Hovmark, A.: Early and late cutaneous manifestations of Ixodes-borne Borreliosis. Ann. N. Y. Acad. Sci. 539:4, 1988.
13. Steere, A. C.: Lyme disease. N. Engl. J. Med. 321:586, 1989.
14. Barbour, A. G., and Hayes, S. F.:Biology of Borrelia species. Microbiol. Rev. 50:381, 1986.
15. Brandt, M. E., Riley, B. S., Radolf, J. D., et al.: Immunogenic integral membrane proteins of Borrelia burgdorferi are lipoproteins. Infect. Immun. 58:983, 1990.
16. Barbour, A. G., Tessier, S. L., and Hayes, S. F.: Variation in a major surface protein of Lyme disease spirochetes. Infect. Immun. 45:94, 1984.
17. Barbour, A. G., Hayes, S. F., Heiland, R. A., et al.: A Borrelia-specific monoclonal antibody binds to a flagellar epitope. Infect. Immun. 52:549, 1986.
18. Hansen, K., Bangsborg, J. M., Fjordvang, H., et al.: Immunochemical characterization of and isolation of the gene for a Borrelia burgdorferi immunodominant 60-kilodalton antigen common to a wide range of bacteria. Infect. Immun. 56:2047, 1988.
19. Barbour, A. G.: Plasmid analysis of Borrelia burgdorferi, the Lyme disease agent. J. Clin. Microbiol. 26:475, 1988.
20. Howe, T. R., Mayer, L. W., and Barbour, A. G.: A single recombinant plasmid expressing two major outer surface proteins of the Lyme disease spirochete. Science 227:645, 1985.
21. Barbour, A. G.: Isolation and cultivation of Lyme disease spirochetes. Yale J. Biol. Med. 57:521, 1984.
22. Berger, B. W., Johnson, R. C., Kodner, C., et al.: Cultivation of Borrelia burgdorferi from erythema migrans lesions and perilesional skin. J. Clin. Microbiol. 30:359, 1992.
22a. Postic, D., Baranton, G., Saint Girons, I., et al.: Delineation of Borelia burgdorferi sensu stricto, Borrelia garinii sp. nov., and group VS461 associated with Lyme borreliosis. Int. J. Syst. Bacteriol. 42, 1992 (in press).
22b. Marconi, R. T., and Garon, C. F.: Phylogenetic analysis of the genus Borrelia: a comparison of North American and European isolates of Borrelia burgdorferi. J. Bacteriol. 174:241, 1992.
23. Schulze, T. L., Bowen, G. S., Bosler, E. M., et al.: Amblyomma americanum: A potential vector of Lyme disease in New Jersey. Science 224:601, 1984.
24. Magnarelli, L. A., and Anderson, J. F.: Ticks and biting insects infected with the etiologic agent of Lyme disease, Borrelia burgdorferi. J. Clin. Microbiol. 26: 1482, 1988.
25. Levine, J. F., Wilson, M. L., and Spielman, A.: Mice as reservoirs of the Lyme disease spirochete. Am. J. Trop. Med. Hyg. 34:355, 1985.
26. Wilson, M. L., Adler, G. H., and Spielman, A.: Correlation between abundance of deer and that of the deer tick, Ixodes dammini (Acari: Ixodidae). Ann. Entomol. Soc. Am. 172, 1986.
27. Centers for Disease Control: Lyme disease surveillance summary. 3:1, 1992.
28. Stanek, G., Pletschette, M., Flamm, H., et al.: European Lyme borreliosis. Ann. N. Y. Acad. Sci. 539:274, 1988.
29. Dekonenko, E. J., Steere, A. C., Berardi, V. P., et al.: Lyme borreliosis in the Soviet Union: A cooperative US-USSR report. J. Infect. Dis. 158:748, 1988.
30. Persing, D. H., Telford, S. R., Rys, P. N., et al.: Detection of Borrelia burgdorferi DNA in museum specimens of Ixodes dammini ticks. Science 249:1420, 1990.
31. Steere, A. C., Taylor, E., Wilson, M. L., et al.: Longitudinal assessment of the clinical and epidemiologic features of Lyme disease in a defined population. J. Infect. Dis. 154:295, 1986.
32. Lastavica, C. C., Wilson, M. L., Berardi, V. P., et al.: Rapid emergence of a focal epidemic of Lyme disease in coastal Massachusetts. N. Engl. J. Med. 320:133, 1989.
33. Hanrahan, J. P., Benach, J. L., Coleman, J. L., et al.: Incidence and cumulative frequency of endemic Lyme disease in a community. J. Infect. Dis. 150:489, 1984.
34. Gustafson, R., Svenungsson, B., Gardulf, A., et al.: Prevalence of tickborne encephalitis and Lyme borreliosis in a defined Swedish population. Scand. J. Infect. Dis. 22:297, 1990.

35. Steere, A. C., Bartenhagen, N. H., Craft, J. E., et al.: The early clinical manifestations of Lyme disease. Ann. Intern. Med. 99:76, 1983.
36. Pachner, A. R., and Steere, A. C.: The triad of neurologic manifestations of Lyme disease: Meningitis, cranial neuritis, and radiculoneuritis. Neurology 35:47, 1985.
37. Steere, A. C., Batsford, W. P., Weinberg, M., et al.: Lyme carditis: Cardiac abnormalities of Lyme disease. Ann. Intern. Med. 93:8, 1980.
38. McAlister, H. F., Klementowicz, P. T., Andrews, C., et al.: Lyme carditis: An important cause of reversible heart block. Ann. Intern. Med. 110: 339, 1989.
39. Marcus, L. C., Steere, A. C., Duray, P. H., et al.: Fatal pancarditis in a patient with coexistent Lyme disease and babesiosis: Demonstration of spirochetes in the heart. Ann. Intern. Med. 103:374, 1985.
40. Kirsch, M., Ruben, F. L., Steere, A. C., et al.: Fatal adult respiratory distress syndrome in a patient with Lyme disease. J. A. M. A. 259:2737, 1988.
41. Goellner, M. H., Agger, W. A., Burgess, J. H., et al.: Hepatitis due to recurrent Lyme disease. Ann. Intern. Med. 108:707, 1988.
42. Atlas, E., Novack, S. N., Duray, P. H., et al.: Lyme myositis: Muscle invasion by Borrelia burgdorferi. Ann. Intern. Med. 109:245, 1988.
43. Jacobs, J. C., Stevens, M., and Duray, P. H.: Lyme disease simulating septic arthritis (Letter). J.A.M.A. 256:1138, 1986.
44. Kramer, N., Rickert, R. R., Brodkin, R. H., et al.: Septal panniculitis as a manifestation of Lyme disease. Am. J. Med. 81:149, 1986.
45. Steere, A. C., Duray, P. H., and Kauffmann, D. J. H.: Unilateral blindness caused by infection with the Lyme disease spirochete, Borrelia burgdorferi. Ann. Intern. Med. 103:382, 1985.
46. Bialasiewicz, A. A., Ruprecht, K. W., Naumann, G. O., et al.: Bilateral diffuse choroiditis and exudative retinal detachments with evidence of Lyme disease. Am. J. Ophthalmol. 105:419, 1988.
47. Steere, A. C., Schoen, R. T., and Taylor, E.: The clinical evolution of Lyme arthritis. Ann. Intern. Med. 107:725, 1987.
48. Szer, I. S., Taylor, E., and Steere, A. C.: The long-term course of children with Lyme arthritis. N. Engl. J. Med. 325:159, 1991.
49. Herzer, P., Wilske, B., Preac-Mursic, V., et al.: Lyme arthritis: Clinical features, serological and radiographic findings of cases in Germany. Klin. Wochenschr. 64:206, 1986.
50. Logigian, E. L., Kaplan, R. F., and Steere, A. C.: Chronic neurologic manifestations of Lyme disease. N. Engl. J. Med. 323:1438, 1990.
51. Halperin, J. J., Little, B. W., Coyle, P. K., et al.: Lyme disease: Cause of a treatable peripheral neuropathy. Neurology 37:1700, 1987.
52. Halperin, J. J., Luft, B. J., Anand, A. K., et al.: Lyme neuroborreliosis: Central nervous system manifestations. Neurology 39:753, 1989.
53. Ackerman, R., Rehse-Kupper, B., Gollmer, E., et al.: Chronic neurologic manifestations of erythema migrans borreliosis. Ann. N.Y. Acad. Sci. 539:16, 1988.
54. Pachner, A. R., Duray, P., and Steere, A. C.: Central nervous system manifestations of Lyme disease. Arch. Neurol. 46:790, 1989.
55. Kohlhepp, W., Kuhn, W., and Kruger, H.: Extrapyramidal features in central Lyme borreliosis. Eur. Neurol. 29:150, 1989.
56. May, E. E., and Jabbari, B.: Stroke in neuroborreliosis. Stroke 21:1232, 1990.
57. Kornmehl, E. W., Lesser, R. L., Jaros, P., et al.: Bilateral keratitis in Lyme disease. Ophthalmology 96:1194, 1989.
58. Schlesinger, P. A., Duray, P. H., Burke, B. A., et al.: Maternal-fetal transmission of the Lyme disease spirochete, Borrelia burgdorferi. Ann. Intern. Med. 103:67, 1985.
59. Weber, K., Bratzke, H. J., Neubert, U., et al.: Borrelia burgdorferi in a newborn despite oral penicillin for Lyme borreliosis during pregnancy. Pediatr. Infect. Dis. J. 7:286, 1988.
60. Markowitz, L. E., Steere, A. C., Benach, J. L., et al.: Lyme disease during pregnancy. J.A.M.A. 256:3394, 1986.
61. Williams, C. L., Benach, J. L., Curran, A. S., et al.: Lyme disease during pregnancy: A cord blood serosurvey. Ann. N.Y. Acad. Sci. 539:504, 1988.
62. Duray, P. H., and Steere, A. C.: Clinical pathologic correlations of Lyme disease by stage. Ann. N.Y. Acad. Sci. 539:65, 1988.
63. Georgilis, K., Steere, A. C., and Klempner, M. S.: Infectivity of Borrelia burgdorferi correlates with resistance to elimination by phagocytic cells. J. Infect. Dis. 163:150, 1991.
64. Garcia-Monco, J. C., Fernandez-Villar, B., and Benach, J. L.: Adherence of the Lyme disease spirochete to glial cells and cells of glial origin. J. Infect. Dis. 160:497, 1989.
65. Szczepanski, A., Furie, M. B., Benach, J. L., et al.: Interaction between Borrelia burgdorferi and endothelium in vitro. J. Clin. Invest. 85:1637, 1990.
65a. Ma, Y., Sturrock, A., and Weis, J.: Intracellular localization of Borrelia burgdorferi within human endothelial cells. Infect. Immun. 59:671, 1991.
66. Garcia-Monco, J. C., Villar, B. F., Alen, J. C., et al.: Borrelia burgdorferi in the central nervous system: Experimental and clinical evidence for early invasion. J. Infect. Dis. 161:1187, 1990.
67. Sigal, L. H., Steere, A. C., Freeman, D. H., et al.: Proliferative responses of mononuclear cells in Lyme disease: Reactivity to Borrelia burgdorferi antigens is greater in joint fluid than in blood. Arthritis Rheum. 29:761, 1986.

68. Steere, A. C., Hardin, J. A., Ruddy, S., et al.: Lyme arthritis: Correlation of serum and cryoglobulin IgM with activity and serum IgG with remission. Arthritis Rheum. 22:471, 1979.
69. Hardin, J. A., Steere, A. C., and Malawista, S. E.: Immune complexes and the evolution of Lyme arthritis: Dissemination and localization of abnormal Clq binding activity. N. Engl. J. Med. 301:1358, 1979.
70. Craft, J. E., Fischer, D. K., Shimamoto, G. T., et al.: Antigens of Borrelia burgdorferi recognized during Lyme disease: Appearance of a new IgM response and expansion of the IgG response late in the illness. J. Clin. Invest. 78:934, 1986.
71. Kochi, S. K., and Johnson, R. C.: Role of immunoglobulin G in killing of Borrelia burgdorferi in the classical complement pathway. Infect. Immun. 56:314, 1988.
72. Steere, A. C., Duray, P. H., and Butcher, E. C.: Spirochetal antigens and lymphoid cell surface markers in Lyme synovitis: Comparison with rheumatoid synovium and tonsillar lymphoid tissue. Arthritis Rheum. 31:487, 1988.
73. Snydman, D. R., Schenkein, D. P., Berardi, V. P., et al.: Borrelia burgdorferi in joint fluid in chronic Lyme arthritis. Ann. Intern. Med. 104:798, 1986.
74. Schmidli, J., Hunziker, T., Moesli, P., et al.: Cultivation of Borrelia burgdorferi from joint fluid 3 months after treatment of facial palsy. J. Infect. Dis. 158:905, 1988.
75. Yoshinari, N. H., Reinhardt, B. N., and Steere, A. C.: T cell responses to polypeptide fractions of Borrelia burgdorferi in patients with Lyme arthritis. Arthritis Rheum. 34:707, 1991.
76. Neumann, A., Schlesier, M., Schneider, H., et al.: Frequencies of Borrelia burgdorferi-reactive T lymphocytes in Lyme arthritis. Rheumatol. Int. 9:237, 1989.
77. Beck, G., Benach, J. L., and Habicht, G. S.: Isolation of interleukin-1 from joint fluids of patients with Lyme disease. J. Rheumatol. 16:6, 1989.
78. Steere, A. C., Brinckerhoff, C. E., Miller, D. J., et al.: Elevated levels of collagenase and prostaglandin E₂ from synovium associated with erosion of cartilage and bone in a patient with chronic Lyme arthritis. Arthritis Rheum. 23:591, 1980.
79. Georgilis, K., Noring, R., Steere, A. C., et al.: Neutrophil chemotactic factors in Lyme disease synovial fluids. Arthritis Rheum. 34:770, 1991.
80. Steere, A. C., Dwyer, E., and Winchester, R.: Association of chronic Lyme arthritis with HLA-DR4 and HLA-DR2 alleles. N. Engl. J. Med. 323:219, 1990.
81. Craft, J. E., Grodzicki, R. L., and Steere, A. C.: The antibody response in Lyme disease: Evaluation of diagnostic tests. J. Infect. Dis. 149:789, 1984.
82. Russell, H., Sampson, J. S., Schmid, G. P., et al.: Enzyme-linked immunosorbent assay and indirect immunofluorescence assay for Lyme disease. J. Infect. Dis. 149:465, 1984.
83. Shrestha, M., Grodzicki, R. L., and Steere, A. C.: Diagnosing early Lyme disease. Am. J. Med. 78:235, 1985.
84. Berardi, V. E., Weeks, K. E., and Steere, A. C.: Serodiagnosis of early Lyme disease: Analysis of IgM and IgG antibody responses by using an antibody-capture enzyme immunoassay. J. Infect. Dis. 158:754, 1988.
85. Dattwyler, R. J., Volkman, D. J., Luft, B. J., et al: Seronegative Lyme disease: Dissociation of the specific T- and B-lymphocyte responses to Borrelia burgdorferi. N. Engl. J. Med. 319:1441, 1988.
86. Dressler, F., Yoshinari, N. H., and Steere, A. C.: The T cell proliferative assay in the diagnosis of Lyme disease. Ann. Intern. Med. 115:533, 1991.
86a. Steere, A. C., Berardi, V. P., Weeks, K. E., et al.: Evaluation of the intrathecal antibody response to Borrelia burgdorferi as a diagnostic test for neuroborreliosis. J. Infect. Dis. 161:1203, 1990.
87. Grodzicki, R. L., and Steere, A. C.: Comparison of immunoblotting and indirect enzyme-linked immunosorbent assay using different antigen preparations for diagnosing early Lyme disease. J. Infect. Dis. 157:790, 1988.
88. Zoller, L., Burkard, S., and Schafer, H.: Validity of Western immunoblot band patterns in the serodiagnosis of Lyme borreliosis. J. Clin. Microbiol. 29:174, 1991.
89. Steere, A. C., Hutchinson, G. J., Rahn, D. W., et al.: Treatment of the early manifestations of Lyme disease. Ann. Intern. Med. 99:22, 1983.
90. Steere, A. C., Pachner, A. R., and Malawista, S. E.: Neurologic abnormalities of Lyme disease: Successful treatment with high-dose intravenous penicillin. Ann. Intern. Med. 99:767, 1983.
91. Steere, A. C., Green, J., Schoen, R. T., et al.: Successful parenteral penicillin therapy of established Lyme arthritis. N. Engl. J. Med. 312:869, 1985.
92. Massarotti, E. M., Luger, S. W., Rahn, D. W., et al.: Treatment of early Lyme disease. Am. J. Med. 92:396, 1992.
93. Dattwyler, R. J., Volkman, D., Conaty, S., et al.: Amoxicillin plus probenecid versus doxycycline for the treatment of erythema migrans borreliosis. Lancet 336:1404, 1990.
94. Liu, N. Y., Dinerman, H., Levin, R. E., et al.: Randomized trial of

doxycycline vs. amoxicillin/probenecid for the treatment of Lyme arthritis: Treatment of non-responders with intravenous penicillin or ceftriaxone. Arthritis Rheum. 32:S46, 1989 (Abstract).

95. Schoen, R. T., Aversa, J. M., Rahn, D. W., et al.: Treatment of refractory chronic Lyme arthritis with arthroscopic synovectomy. Arthritis Rheum. 34:1056, 1991.

96. Pfister, H-W., Preac-Mursic, V., Wilske, B., et al.: Cefotaxime vs penicillin G for acute neurologic manifestations of Lyme borreliosis. Arch. Neurol. 46:1190, 1989.

97. Pfister, H. W., Preac-Mursic, V., Wilske, B., et al.: Randomized comparison of cenfriaxone and cefotaxime in Lyme neuroborreliosis. J. Infect. Dis. 163:311, 1991.

98. Dattwyler, R. J., Halperin, J. J., Volkman, D. J., et al.: Treatment of late Lyme borreliosis: Randomized comparison of ceftriaxone and penicillin. Lancet 1:1191, 1988.

99. Dotevall, L., and Hagberg. L.: Penetration of doxycycline into cerebrospinal fluid in patients treated for suspected Lyme neuroborreliosis. Antimicrob. Agents Chemother. 33:1078, 1989.

100. Costello, C. M., Steere, A. C., Pinkerton, R. E., et al.: Prospective study of tick bites in an endemic area for Lyme disease. J. Infect. Dis. 159:136, 1989.

101. Fikrig, E., Barthold, S. W., Kantor, F. S., et al.: Protection of mice against the Lyme disease agent by immunizing with recombinant Osp A. Science 250:553, 1990.

Chapter 89
Viral Arthritis

Thomas J. Schnitzer

INTRODUCTION

Arthritis is a frequent accompaniment to a number of common viral illnesses in humans (type B hepatitis, rubella, alphavirus infection). It also occurs, but at a lower incidence, in association with a wide range of other viral infections (mumps, enteroviruses, adenoviruses, herpesviruses). Generally, rheumatic symptoms first become apparent during the prodrome or at the onset of the clinical illness and are often temporally associated with the appearance of a characteristic skin rash. Different patterns of joint and soft tissue involvement are observed with each of the infectious agents. However, in most viral-related arthritides, joint symptoms occur suddenly, are of brief duration, and do not recur, although notable exceptions have been documented (e.g., rubella, parvovirus, and alphavirus infections). Routine laboratory studies are not helpful in establishing the etiology of the arthritis, but specific serologic tests are available to confirm the diagnosis of a viral infection. In all instances, the arthritis is nondestructive and does not lead to any currently recognized form of chronic joint disease.

Several mechanisms exist[1] by which viruses may initiate rheumatic diseases, in general, and joint signs and symptoms, in particular. The simplest and most obvious mechanism is by direct infection of synovial tissues, a process believed to occur during rubella and rubella vaccine virus infection in humans. If the interaction between the virus and the host cell is a lytic one, the attendant tissue destruction and inflammatory response may be responsible both for the joint symptoms and for the ultimate resolution of the infection. When viruses cause persistent or latent infections, however, cell destruction may be mediated by immunologic mechanisms that are directed either toward viral or host membrane–associated antigens or toward viral products released into the joint fluid or systemic circulation.[2]

Although ultimately protective, the immunologic response to viral infection can itself give rise to rheumatic manifestations.[2,3] Clearance of virus from the circulation following the onset of viremia may be associated with the development of virus-antibody complexes. In some individuals, these immune complexes may be deposited in synovial tissues, where activation of complement pathways can lead to an inflammatory response. With viruses able to cause a persistent infection in synovial tissues, immune complexes can be formed locally and released into the joint fluid, where the inflammatory response generated will give rise to the clinical signs and symptoms of arthritis.

In some persistent and latent infections, viral particles are not released from infected cells, but viral antigens are inserted into the cellular membranes, where they are recognized as foreign. Interaction at the cell surface between these viral antigens and host antigens can generate new, yet immunologically related (cross-reactive), antigenic determinants recognized by the host as "altered-self." These new determinants, as well as the original determinants found on uninfected normal host cells, will then be the target of the immunologic responses, leading to cell destruction.[4] Thus, for the initiation of autoimmune diseases, viral infection and expression of viral antigens need not persist but can occur transiently, triggering the immune response, which will be maintained by the continued presence of the original but now cross-reactive determinants of the unaltered host antigens. In the event that such antigens are tissue specific, subsequent symptoms will present as distinct syndromes or diseases.

A final mechanism that can give rise to rheumatic disease is direct viral infection of elements of the immune system.[2] Many viruses are known to be able to infect lymphocytes (e.g., Epstein-Barr virus, cytomegalovirus, measles, rubella) and can persist in such cells as well. Alteration of the immune response may arise either as a consequence of direct lysis of a particular subset of immune cells (e.g., T helper or suppressor lymphocytes, B lymphocytes) or, more likely, by a virus-induced modulation of surface components (e.g., receptors), leading to alteration in the recognition of and reaction to both host and foreign antigens.

HEPATITIS B VIRUS

Virology. The recognition by Blumberg,[5] Prince, and others of "Australia antigen" as a marker of hepatitis B virus (HBV) infection permitted identification of the etiologic agent in the sera of patients in the early 1970s.[6] Its physicochemical properties, antigenic determinants, genome structure, and protein composition have been extensively characterized, resulting in identification of HBV as the prototype of a

1494

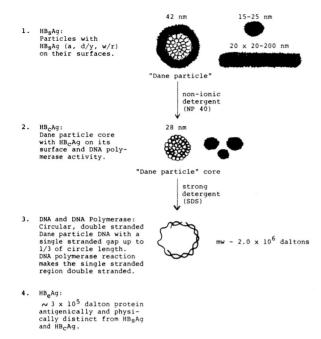

1. HB_SAg:
   Particles with
   HB_SAg (a, d/y, w/r)
   on their surfaces.

"Dane particle"

non-ionic
detergent
(NP 40)

2. HB_CAg:
   Dane particle core
   with HB_CAg on its
   surface and DNA poly-
   merase activity.

"Dane particle" core

strong
detergent
(SDS)

3. DNA and DNA Polymerase:
   Circular, double stranded
   Dane particle DNA with a
   single stranded gap up to
   1/3 of circle length.
   DNA polymerase reaction
   makes the single stranded
   region double stranded.

mw - 2.0 x 10^6 daltons

4. HB_eAg:
   ~ 3 x 10^5 dalton protein
   antigenically and physically distinct from HB_SAg
   and HB_CAg.

Figure 89–1. Composition of hepatitis B viral structures found in the blood of infected patients. (From Robinson, W. S.: Ann. N.Y. Acad. Sci. 354:372, 1980.)

new class of viruses, the "hepadenaviruses" (hepatitis-DNA-virus).[7]

The complete hepatitis B virion (Fig. 89–1) has been shown to consist of a 42-nm particle (Dane particle) composed of a 27-nm nucleocapsid surrounded by a 7-nm coat (HBsAg).[7] When the coat is synthesized in excess of nucleocapsid, HBsAg is released from infected cells and forms the 22 nm in diameter spherical and filamentous particles lacking nucleic acid that are commonly seen by electron microscopy in the sera of patients with HBV infection. The nucleocapsid is composed of a number of different elements, including two antigenically distinct constituents—the hepatitis B core antigen (HBcAg) and the hepatitis B e antigen (HBeAg), one molecule of partially double-stranded DNA, and an associated DNA polymerase activity that is capable of completing the synthesis of the shorter DNA strand.[8]

Clinical Disease. The majority of people exposed to HBV experience an acute, self-limited infection. Most often this process is not clinically apparent but does result in the development of an antibody response to HBsAg (anti-HBs). However, in 5 to 10 percent of cases, the acute HBV infection proceeds to a chronic phase that is characterized by the persistence of one or more of the serologic markers of viral presence (HBeAg, HBcAg, anti-HBcAg, anti-HBs) or the infectious virus itself.[6, 7] In approximately 30 percent of these cases, clinical illness is present (chronic active hepatitis), whereas in the remainder either evidence exists of chronic persistent hepatitis or no biochemical or pathologic abnormalities are found.[6, 8]

The clinical presentation of acute icteric HBV infection has been well described.[6–9] After an incubation period of 40 to 180 days, symptoms of headache, fatigue, anorexia, nausea, vomiting, abdominal pain, and fever appear and generally precede the development of icterus by 2 to 14 days. With the onset of jaundice these symptoms abate, and resolution of clinical disease occurs in adults over the ensuing 3 to 4 weeks. The sequence of serologic events in this type of HBV infection is shown in Figure 89–2. The earliest sign of infection is the appearance of HBsAg, which is followed by the detection of anti-HBc. Free HBcAg is not found in the serum. HBeAg appears just prior to clinical illness, is present during the period of maximum infectivity, and leads to the production of anti-HBe shortly thereafter. Anti-HBs generally appears only late in the course of the disease, not until some weeks after HBsAg has disappeared from the circulation. The reason for such a delayed appearance of anti-HBs is not known, but once present this antibody persists for years as a marker of past infection.

Hepatocyte damage is believed to occur primarily by cell-mediated immune responses directed against both HBV antigens in infected cells and tissue-specific host antigens in uninfected hepatocytes.[10]

Pathogenesis of Arthritic Symptoms. In those patients who develop joint involvement during HBV infection, an antibody response to HBsAg occurs not as shown in Figure 89–2 but earlier in the course of the disease prior to the onset of clinical symptoms.[11] Since HBsAg levels are high at this time, anti-HBs production results in the formation of soluble immune complexes. The tissue deposition of these HBsAg–anti-HBs complexes is believed to be respon-

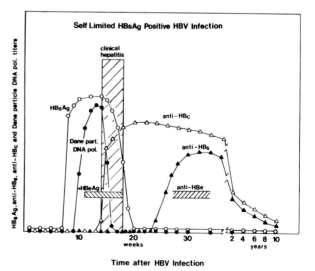

Figure 89–2. Diagrammatic representation of the temporal evolution of viral markers detectable in the blood of patients during self-limited HBsAg-positive HBV infection. (From Robinson, W. S.: Hepatitis B virus. *In* Mandell, G. L., Douglas, R. G., Jr., and Bennett, J. E. [eds.]: Principles and Practice of Infectious Diseases. New York, Churchill Livingstone, 1979, p. 1398.)

sible for the initiation of the inflammatory processes, which result in the joint manifestations observed.[12] Cryoprecipitates containing HBsAg, anti-HBs, C3, C4, and C5 have been detected in patients with arthritis associated with HBV infection,[11, 13] and longitudinal studies have confirmed the sequence of serologic events outlined in Figure 89–2 and have demonstrated complement consumption (Fig. 89–3).[11, 14]

In those people with chronic HBV infection, persistent viral antigenemia can occur,[6–9] and immune complex formation may take place later after infection. Under these circumstances not only may arthritis be apparent, but also a variety of clinical presentations may occur (see later discussion), including polyarteritis nodosa,[15] glomerulonephritis,[16] and mixed essential cryoglobulinemia.[17]

Rheumatologic Manifestations. Although first remarked on by Graves in 1843,[18] only recently has it been appreciated that joint symptoms may be a prominent manifestation during the prodromal phase of both icteric and anicteric liver disease caused by HBV.[12, 13, 19] Similar musculoskeletal involvement has not commonly been demonstrated in patients with type A or non-A, non-B hepatitis.[20] A frequency of joint symptoms (arthralgias and arthritis) of 10 to 25 percent of patients with HBV infections reflects the findings of the majority of studies.[8, 9] Occasional "outbreaks" of HBV infection have been associated with significantly higher joint attack rates, suggesting the existence of "arthritogenic" strains of HBV.[21]

The age range of patients with HBV infection who demonstrate joint manifestations is quite broad (13 to 72 years), but few cases of this association in children have been reported. Women tend to be more at risk for developing arthritis than are men, but the difference is not great and is not apparent when arthralgia is considered as well.[22] Joint symptoms are typically present during the prodromal phase of acute HBV infection and may precede clinical jaundice by days to weeks (up to 18 weeks in one report). Some of the other more commonly associated prodromal symptoms of hepatitis, such as nausea, vomiting, and abdominal discomfort, occur in only a minority (approximately 25 percent) of people with joint involvement. Fever is present in about 25 percent of patients with arthralgias and in 50 percent of those with arthritis and tends to be moderate, between 100°F and 102°F (37.8°C and 38.9°C) in most cases.[12, 13, 22] Skin involvement[22, 23] is frequently present in people having joint symptoms and often appears at the onset of the arthritis. Urticarial and maculopapular eruptions involving primarily the lower extremities are most common, but nonthrombocytopenic purpura, petechiae, and angioneurotic edema may also be seen.

The onset of articular symptoms is usually quite rapid, and joint pain may be severe. Articular involvement is generally symmetric and occurs in either an additive or a migratory fashion, but simultaneous polyarticular symptoms may also be exhibited. The small joints of the hands (metacarpophalangeal, proximal interphalangeal) and the knees are most frequently symptomatic, followed by wrists, ankles, shoulders, and elbows.[12, 22, 23] Although most patients present with both large and small joint involvement, large joint involvement alone is not uncommon. Early morning stiffness is often a prominent manifestation of this stage of the disease. Subcutaneous nodules, clinically and histologically similar to those seen in rheumatoid arthritis, have been reported[24] but are rare.

Once present, joint symptoms persist for several days to weeks, with a mean duration of 1 to 3 weeks in most reported series.[12, 22] Typically, arthralgias and arthritis resolve with the onset of jaundice, but in approximately 5 per cent of cases the two occur simultaneously. In patients who develop chronic active hepatitis (CAH) or who demonstrate chronic HBV antigenemia, arthralgias and arthritis may be present or may recur over long periods of time.[25]

Other Syndromes Associated with HBV Infection. Two other well-defined rheumatologic disorders, polyarteritis nodosa[26] and mixed essential cryoglobulinemia,[17] have been associated with HBV infection and are believed to arise as a consequence of the persistent antigenemia that occurs with subacute or chronic HBV infection. In both conditions, the deposition of immune complexes containing immunoglobulin, complement, and HBV antigen in vessel walls has been demonstrated. These two disorders differ primarily in the size of the vessels involved. This may reflect differences in the sizes or types of immune complexes formed, which, in turn,

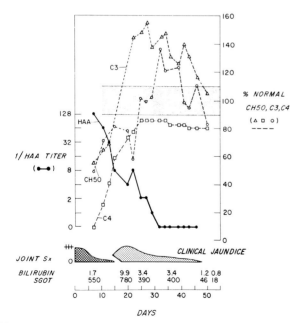

Figure 89–3. Relationship of HBsAg (HAA) titers to serum levels of C3, C4, and CH50 during the course of HBV hepatitis and associated arthritis. (From Alpert, E., Schur, P. H., and Isselbacher, K. J.: Sequential changes of serum complement in HAA-related arthritis. N. Engl. J. Med. 287:103, 1972. Used by permission.)

The joints most commonly involved are the small joints of the hands (proximal interphalangeal, metacarpophalangeal), the knees, and the wrists, followed by the ankles and the elbows. The larger joints (shoulders, hips) may also occasionally be affected.[47] Arthralgias are more common than frank arthritis, and significant stiffness is often associated with these joint complaints; often it is a presenting complaint. Periarthritis with swelling and redness around the affected joint is common, and involvement of synovial linings outside the joints themselves can lead to the development of tenosynovitis and the carpal tunnel syndrome,[48] both of which are well-recognized complications of rubella infection. Symptoms may persist for extended periods of time, with arthralgias occasionally being present for more than 1 year, but chronic joint disease or evidence of rheumatoid arthritis or other rheumatic disorders does not occur.[45, 47]

Laboratory Investigations. The laboratory values of patients with joint symptoms are not significantly different from the laboratory values of patients whose rubella infection is uncomplicated by these complaints. In general there are no distinctive laboratory abnormalities.[49, 50]

In the four cases in which joint fluid has been examined,[35, 46, 47] the synovial fluid has been described as yellow and viscous, with a protein content ranging between 1.9 and 3.8 g per dl, and containing 14,000 to 60,000 leukocytes per mm^3. The differential count has demonstrated a marked predominance of mononuclear cells. The mucin clot has been reported to be fair to poor. Isolation of rubella virus from the joint fluid has been reported only rarely.[35, 51] Synovial tissue was reported, in one case, to show active, nonspecific synovitis, whereas in another patient minimal inflammatory changes were present.

RUBELLA VACCINE VIRUS

Virology. Three vaccine strains are now licensed for use in the United States: the Cendehill strain cultured in rabbit kidney, the HP77 strain propagated in duck embryo culture, and the RA 27/3 strain grown in WI38 cells derived from human embryonic lung.[52-55] The RA 27/3 vaccine, which has been shown to be more immunogenic than either the duck-grown HP77 or the Cendehill vaccine, is the only strain available in the United States. Approximately 95 percent of individuals receiving this vaccine demonstrate serologic evidence of infection, and local antibody production is also stimulated.

Clinical Presentation. In rare instances, a rubella-like rash and lymphadenopathy occur after vaccination.[56] Fever is even less common. Transient polyneuropathies have also been reported following both rubella and rubella vaccine virus infection (see later on).[57, 58]

Rheumatologic Manifestations. A variety of musculoskeletal complaints are associated with the clinical use of rubella vaccines and include myalgias, arthralgias, arthritis, and paresthesias.[59] As with natural rubella, signs and symptoms of musculoskeletal involvement are most often observed in women. In children, the frequency of joint manifestations is about 1 to 5 percent.[60, 61]

Joint symptoms are most common; patients complain primarily of stiffness or arthralgia of involved joints, and approximately 10 to 20 percent of the latter group will have frank arthritis on examination.[62, 63] The distribution of joint involvement is generally similar to that seen in natural rubella infection, but in several studies the knee has been reported to be the most frequently involved joint, followed by the small joints of the fingers (proximal interphalangeal, metacarpophalangeal), ankles, and wrists. Symptoms first become apparent approximately 2 weeks (range 8 to 45 days) after vaccination, a time that just precedes or is coincident with seroconversion and the ability to isolate rubella from the pharynx of inoculated people.[64] Symptoms are short-lived, lasting from 1 to 5 days in general,[60-63] although more prolonged involvement does occur and has been associated on several occasions with the isolation of rubella vaccine virus from the involved joint, even as late as 3 months after inoculation.[65] Furthermore, unlike natural rubella, recurrences of joint symptoms are not uncommon,[66, 67] having been observed in approximately 1.3 percent of people with joint symptoms, a frequency that represents 0.1 percent of all children inoculated. The frequency and severity of recurrent attacks have been found to decrease with time, and despite careful long-term examination most studies have failed to demonstrate the development of any form of chronic arthritis, and rheumatoid arthritis in particular, in people demonstrating such recurrent joint symptoms.[66-68]

In addition to arthritis and arthralgias, paresthesias involving the fingers, hands, and arms have also been associated with the administration of rubella vaccine. In most instances, the clinical presentation is most compatible with carpal tunnel syndrome, but a characteristic form of brachial radiculoneuritis may also develop in recipients of rubella vaccine.[69] A second form of radiculoneuropathy involving the lumbar plexus[70] has been described after rubella vaccination and results in what has been described as the "catcher's crouch" or "catcher's leg" syndrome. Typically, affected children awake with early morning aching centered on the popliteal fossa and assume the characteristic crouching posture. Both forms of radiculoneuropathy occur 4 to 6 weeks following inoculation (range 7 to 99 days) and persist for approximately 2 weeks (range 2 to 35 days). No evidence of permanent neurologic damage has been reported.

PARVOVIRUS

Virology. Parvoviruses are among the smallest and simplest of the animal viruses. First isolated in

1975, these viruses have icosahedral symmetry and a diameter of 18 to 26 nm and are composed of only three proteins and a linear single-stranded DNA molecule.[71] Members of the parvovirus genus have a widespread distribution among animals, but their growth appears to be particularly host- and even cell-specific, suggesting the requirement for some cell factor in their replication. Additionally, viral replication appears to be dependent on cells undergoing mitosis, further supporting the role of host factors and explaining the virus's predilection for affecting rapidly dividing cells.

Clinical Presentation. Although it had been appreciated for several years that human parvovirus (HPV) infection is common (25 to 40 percent of adults have antibody to the virus), it was only in 1981 that the initial association with a clinical condition, aplastic crisis in patients with sickle cell anemia and other hemoglobinopathies, was made.[72] Not until 2 years later, in 1983, was HPV shown by seroepidemiologic data to be the cause of one of the common exanthems of childhood: "fifth" disease or erythema infectiosum.[73] Erythema infectiosum is an exanthematous disease that closely resembles rubella in its mode of clinical presentation.[73, 74] It has a peak incidence in children between the ages of 4 and 10 years and is highly contagious, with an attack rate of 90 percent reported in some outbreaks. The disease in children is generally quite mild, presenting with malaise, low-grade fever, and rash. Although the rash may resemble that of rubella, typically it presents with a "slapped-cheek" appearance. The rash may also involve the trunk and is often evanescent but has a tendency to recur over a period of several weeks. In contrast to children, adults who are infected often have no rash but more commonly present with arthritis and arthralgias that may be severe and persist, on occasion, for months to years.

Pathogenesis of Disease. The mechanism by which the joint symptoms occur has not been defined. In volunteer studies, it was found that after inoculation there was an initial viremia that cleared prior to the onset of clinical signs and symptoms of disease, suggesting an immune-complex–mediated pathogenesis.[73, 75] The time of onset of the clinical disease likewise was consistent with such an interpretation. However, actual viral infection of the joint cannot be ruled out, and virus particles have been found in the blood of at least one patient at the time of the joint symptoms.[76] Joint fluid has been examined for viral DNA with negative results,[77] but synovium itself has not been probed for evidence of viral infection. No evidence for HPV in the etiology of chronic forms of arthritis has been established, though a single report of isolation of parvovirus from the joint of a patient with rheumatoid arthritis has been made[78] but not confirmed.

Rheumatologic Manifestations. The investigation of several outbreaks of erythema infectiosum[74–76] as well as a review of patients screened at an "early synovitis" clinic[79] has enabled definition of the rheumatic signs and symptoms associated with HPV infection.[80, 81] In most respects, the rheumatologic manifestations parallel those found after rubella infection. Patients present with the sudden onset of a moderately severe symmetric peripheral polyarthropathy, initially involving the small joints of the hands and the knees but frequently spreading rapidly to involve wrists, feet, elbows, and shoulders. Often there is associated pain, swelling, and joint stiffness. The joint findings may precede the rash, but most often in adults no rash is noted, making consideration of this diagnosis more difficult. As rash is most often not present, parvovirus infection should be considered in all patients presenting with acute polyarthralgias or polyarthritis in whom rheumatoid factor is absent. Women appear to be at greater risk for developing joint symptoms than are men after HPV infection. In one outbreak[74] arthralgias were reported to occur in as many as 77 percent, and arthritis in 60 percent, of people infected. As with other viral arthropathies, no long-term joint damage or significant functional disability has been reported after HPV infection. However, joint symptoms may commonly persist for weeks to months and, in some patients, even for several years,[80, 81] raising the question of the etiologic role of this virus in chronic arthropathies such as rheumatoid arthritis. In addition, a single report[82] implicates HPV in an associated cutaneous vasculitis observed in a patient with HPV-induced arthritis.

Laboratory Findings. Laboratory findings have been surprisingly normal in the patients reported with joint symptoms. The sedimentation rate is generally within normal limits, and there is no elevation of the white blood cell count. Rheumatoid factor has been consistently absent from the sera of these patients.[77, 80] Synovial fluid analysis has demonstrated only mild inflammatory changes,[83] and synovial biopsy has shown mild edema and increased vascularity with normal synovial cells and no significant inflammatory infiltrate.[80] Diagnosis of recent infection with HPV can be confirmed by measurement of IgM antibody to the virus by enzyme-linked immunosorbent assay (ELISA). Elevated levels of viral-specific IgM antibody may persist for several months, with IgG antibody developing several weeks after infection and then being maintained over a period of years.[77, 80] Because parvovirus is endemic in most communities, the presence of high titers of IgG antibodies is of no diagnostic significance. An increased incidence of HLA-DR4 has been reported in those patients with chronic arthritis.[84]

ALPHAVIRUSES

Virology and Epidemiology. The alphaviruses, members of the Togaviridae,[85] include at least 20 serologically related but distinguishable viruses, of which five—chikungunya, O'nyong-nyong, Mayaro, Ross River, and Sindbis—cause disease in which rheumatic complaints are a major feature. Alphavirus particles are spherical and 60 to 65 nm in diameter and consist of a nucleoprotein core containing the single-stranded RNA genome surrounded by a lipoprotein envelope into which are inserted at least two viral-specified glycoproteins. The latter are the major antigens to which the host serologic response is mounted, and they permit diagnosis by standard HI, CF, and neutralization assays.

Although closely related antigenically and structurally, and in the type of clinical disease produced, the five alphaviruses associated with arthritic illnesses are found in different ecologic settings and have distinct epidemiologic features. Chikungunya virus was first isolated in East Africa.[86] Its name was derived from a local description of the illness meaning "that which bends up," and it has subsequently been reported in India, Southeast Asia, and the Philippines.[87] In rural Africa the virus is maintained in a cycle involving wild primates and forest mosquitoes; in an urban setting, transmission is likely by *Aedes aegypti*, in a human-to-mosquito-to-human cycle. The disease tends to appear suddenly, affect a large part of the susceptible population, and then disappear.[88]

O'nyong-nyong virus[89] is seen in the same area of Africa as chikungunya and produces a similar disease, as its name attests (meaning "joint breaker"). It is the only arthropod-borne virus to be transmitted by anopheline mosquitoes and was associated with a major epidemic in East Africa between 1959 and 1962 involving several million people. Since that time, only sporadic cases have been reported. Because of the similarity in geographic distribution and clinical presentation between O'nyong-nyong and chikungunya, differentiation between the two is often difficult and may require appropriate serologic testing.

Ross River virus,[90] endemic in Australia, New Zealand, and a large number of South Pacific Islands, gives rise to a disease recognized as "epidemic polyarthritis." In Australia the virus is limited primarily to rural locations, existing in a wild vertebrate–to–mosquito cycle, and affects mainly travelers to these areas during the summer and autumn. However, on various South Pacific Islands epidemics of disease have been reported, with as many as 40 to 50 percent of the local populace, as well as tourists, being affected. In these instances, human-to-mosquito-to-human transmission probably occurs.

Mayaro virus[91] has been reported from Trinidad, Surinam, Brazil, Colombia, and Bolivia, where disease is seen primarily among men working in the tropical forests. As with Ross River virus, a wild animal–to–mosquito cycle is believed to exist. Sindbis virus,[92, 93] in distinction to the preceding four alphaviruses, has a wider geographic distribution, which includes Europe, Asia, Africa, Australia, and the Philippines. Human infection is uncommon, however, and the virus is maintained primarily in a wild bird–to–mosquito cycle.

Clinical Presentation. The illnesses arising from infection by these five viruses share a great number of clinical features, of which fever, arthritis, and rash are the most constant and characteristic. However, the spectrum of disease is wide, and patients may experience any one or two of these signs in the absence of the others, making diagnosis in nonepidemic settings difficult. The incubation period ranges from 2 to 20 days and, in the case of chikungunya and O'nyong-nyong, is followed by the abrupt appearance of joint pain as the presenting manifestation of disease.[94] The other viruses result in illnesses that evolve more gradually, often with a prodromal period of 1 to 3 days that is marked by fever, malaise, and nonspecific constitutional symptoms followed by the appearance of joint manifestations.[95] Males and females are generally equally affected, although in occasional epidemics females have been affected more frequently. The peak incidence of disease has been reported in the 10- to 39-year-old age group.[88]

Fever in patients with O'nyong-nyong, Ross River, and Sindbis infections is mild, rarely exceeding 103°F (39.4°C), whereas patients with chikungunya and Mayaro infections typically appear significantly more ill, often with temperatures as high as 104°F to 105°F (40°C to 40.6°C).[95, 96] Frequently there will be a biphasic, or "saddleback," profile to the fever, with an initial temperature elevation lasting 1 to 6 days, followed by a 1- to 3-day period of normal temperature, and then the recurrence of fever for a shorter period of time. The rash seen in association with these illnesses generally appears 3 to 4 days after the onset of the joint symptoms. It is maculopapular or morbilliform in character, lasts 3 to 4 days (range 2 to 10 days), and involves predominantly the face, flexor surfaces of the extremities, and the trunk. The palms, soles, and scalp can be affected. In the case of Sindbis infection, vesicles may also be seen.[92] The rash may be mildly pruritic; desquamation does not occur, but a transient brown discoloration of the skin may remain after resolution of the exanthem.

A range of other symptoms, including headache, retro-orbital pain, mild pharyngitis, conjunctivitis, myalgias, anorexia, nausea, and vomiting, may accompany these illnesses but are not major features of the diseases. Mild lymphadenopathy is observed in all five disorders, but patients with O'nyong-nyong may demonstrate particularly striking enlargement of the posterior cervical nodes.[97] A life-threatening hemorrhagic state has been documented in patients with chikungunya from the Far East but rarely in those from Africa.[96] Other serious complications, however, have not been reported in these self-limited disorders.

Diagnosis is most often made clinically and may be confirmed either by isolation of virus from the blood of affected individuals, a procedure that is successful only during the first several days of the illness, or by demonstration in paired sera of a fourfold or greater rise in HI, CF, or neutralizing antibody titers.[88–93, 98] A number of other mosquito-borne viruses (West Nile, dengue, Bunyamwera) can also give rise to syndromes characterized by fever, rash, and arthralgias, though not arthritis. Therefore, appropriate serologic testing is indicated, particularly in nonepidemic conditions, to confirm the diagnosis.

Pathogenesis of Arthritic Symptoms. No evidence exists to implicate direct viral infection of the joints, and two studies[99, 100] have presented evidence implicating circulating immune complexes in the pathogenesis. Virus can be isolated from the blood during the first several days of illness but has never been reported in joint fluid. Complement levels have been recorded in numerous patients with Ross River virus infection, and these levels are normal or elevated rather than depressed. Recent studies have demonstrated T lymphocyte activation and depressed natural killer cell activity during clinical disease.[101]

Rheumatologic Manifestations. Arthritis can be severe, particularly in adults. The joints most frequently affected include the small joints of the hands, as well as wrists, elbows, knees, ankles, and small joints of the feet.[88–96] Previously injured joints are particularly prone to involvement. The arthritis is generally symmetric and polyarticular, although the distribution and pattern of appearance of joint symptoms are quite variable. Typically, affected joints are hot and swollen, and there may be significant periarticular soft tissue swelling and tendonitis as well. In patients with chikungunya, subcutaneous nodules clinically similar to those observed in patients with rheumatoid arthritis have been described. In the majority of alphavirus infections, joint symptoms generally resolve over a 3- to 7-day period but may recur. A variable number of patients continue to have joint pain and swelling for weeks to months, and in some patients infected by chikungunya, joint symptoms have been documented that persist for more than 1 year.[88, 102] In no instance, however, has there been evolution to a more chronic form of arthritis, and no evidence of permanent joint damage has been presented.

Laboratory Investigations. A mild leukopenia with a relative lymphocytosis is often seen during the first week of illness but need not be present. Platelet counts are usually normal, though significant thrombocytopenia has been recorded in cases of chikungunya and Mayaro infections.[88] Complement values are normal or elevated, and neither antinuclear antibodies nor rheumatoid factors are generally found. In one study of Ross River disease, a greater than expected incidence of symptomatic disease in patients with HLA-DR7 as well as the heterozygous GM phenotype a+x+b+ was observed.[103]

Joint fluids have been examined from a small number of patients with Ross River infection.[104] Synovial fluid cell counts have ranged from 1500 cells per mm^3 to 14,200 cells per mm^3, with a marked predominance of mononuclear cells. Viral antigens have been detected by immunofluorescence in these cells shortly after the onset of the arthritis, but infectious virus has never been recovered from joint fluids. Examination of skin biopsies obtained during the acute phase of the exanthem has demonstrated the presence of viral antigen and an infiltrate composed primarily of OKT8+ T cells.[105, 106]

MUMPS

Virology. Mumps virus, a member of the Paramyxoviridae family, consists of an irregular, spherically shaped particle with a mean diameter of 140 nm (range 90 to 300 nm) composed of a helical nucleocapsid containing the single-stranded RNA genome surrounded by a lipoprotein envelope covered with spikelike projections.[107] Associated with the outer coat are both the hemolytic and the neuraminidase activities of the virus as well as the viral hemagglutinin. The V (viral) antigen detected by CF has been correlated with the viral coat, whereas the S (soluble) antigen is found in the nucleocapsid.

Clinical Presentation. Subclinical infection with mumps is common (20 to 40 percent of those infected), and any of the clinical features of mumps infection may precede, follow, or occur in the absence of clinically apparent parotitis.[107] The incubation period averages 16 to 18 days (range 2 to 4 weeks) and is followed by a short prodrome of 24 to 48 hours characterized by nonspecific symptoms (low-grade fever, anorexia, malaise, headache, myalgia). Complaints of earache and tenderness over the adjacent parotid gland ensue, and parotid swelling and pain reach their peak during the next 1 to 3 days. In 75 percent of people the contralateral parotid is similarly affected 1 to 5 days later.

Although mumps is a generalized infection, the virus demonstrates a particular predilection for glandular and nervous tissues. Epididymo-orchitis[107] is the most common extrasalivary gland manifestation of mumps infection in adult men, reported in 20 to 30 percent of postpubertal males. Involvement is bilateral in 15 to 25 percent of cases, but sterility is a rare complication. Other glandular involvement includes oophoritis, seen in approximately 5 percent of postpubertal women, and less commonly mastitis, prostatitis, and thyroiditis. Central nervous system infection is common, encephalitis being reported in 1 of every 6000 cases of mumps. Clinical meningitis is seen in 1 to 10 percent of people with parotitis, although subclinical disease determined by cerebrospinal fluid pleocytosis has been reported in as many as 62 percent of those with mumps. Among patients with meningitis, a distinct male predominance has been noted. Cardiac involvement (myocarditis) may also occur and is most often subclinical, but electrocardiographic changes may be seen in as many as 15 percent of people examined.

Pathogenesis of Arthritic Symptoms.[107] Many of the manifestations occurring in close temporal relation to the onset of parotitis have been documented to be due to mumps infection of the affected tissues.

Similarly, joint inflammation may arise as a consequence of active viral replication within synovial tissues, although mumps virus has never been isolated from an involved joint. An immune complex–mediated arthropathy cannot be excluded, particularly since the joint symptoms occur at an appropriate time for immune complex formation in relation to the serologic response to infection.

Rheumatologic Manifestations. Although fewer than 50 cases of arthritis associated with mumps have been reported in the world's literature, Maisondieu[108] observed 6 people with this complication among 1334 with clinical evidence of disease. Young adult males are most commonly affected (6:1 male-to-female ratio), with the highest incidence of this complication being seen among those in the third decade of life (age range 5 to 47 years).[109] Symptoms, which include morning stiffness and arthralgias as well as the typical signs of arthritis, may precede the onset of parotitis but most commonly occur 1 to 3 weeks (mean of 10 days) after the disease becomes clinically evident. Two cases of arthritis have been reported in patients serologically shown to have been acutely infected by mumps but who failed to demonstrate parotitis.[110] Since as many as 40 percent of mumps infections may be subclinical (i.e., without parotitis), a significant number of cases of unexplained self-limited acute arthritis may occur as a consequence of infection by this virus.

Three modes of presentation of the rheumatic symptoms have been reported: (1) most commonly, patients complain of a migratory polyarthritis that involves principally the large joints (shoulders, hips, knees, and ankles), although small joints (metacarpophalangeal, proximal interphalangeal) may also frequently be symptomatic; (2) arthralgias alone may occur, without signs of arthritis; and (3) a monarticular arthritis may also be observed.[109–113] Tenosynovitis, though not common, may occur as part of this syndrome. Patients with arthritis are almost invariably febrile at the time of the onset of joint involvement, with generally modest temperature elevations (100°F to 102°F) (37.8°C to 38.9°C), but occasional patients have had temperatures in excess of 105°F (40.6°C). The duration of symptoms is highly variable (2 days to 6 months), but in the majority of patients joint involvement has cleared within 2 weeks of its onset. No residual joint damage has been observed in patients with mumps-associated arthritis. Interestingly, the incidence of orchitis (60 percent) in patients with arthritis is approximately three times the expected rate,[112] suggesting that the mechanism responsible for joint involvement (see earlier) may also lead to involvement of other organs.

Laboratory Investigations.[109–113] Patients with joint involvement during mumps infection demonstrate a moderate leukocytosis (10,000 to 15,000 white blood cells per mm³) but may have a normal white blood cell count in mild cases. The erythrocyte sedimentation rate is invariably elevated, occasionally markedly so. Rheumatoid factor is usually absent from the sera of these patients. In the only study to examine these parameters, serum complement levels were found to be normal, and immune complexes were not detectable during clinically active arthritis.[113] When positive, the CF test for antibodies to mumps virus is useful to confirm the clinical diagnosis.

Joint fluid has been examined in only two patients with mumps-associated arthritis, and in both instances the fluid was described as yellow and clear.[109, 110] One fluid specimen was said to contain numerous polymorphonuclear leukocytes, but no quantitation was provided. Virus has never been isolated from an affected joint.

ENTEROVIRUSES: COXSACKIEVIRUS AND ECHOVIRUS

Virology.[114] Coxsackieviruses and echoviruses, along with polioviruses, are members of the Enterovirus genus of the Picornaviridae family. They consist of icosahedron-shaped particles that are 20 to 30 nm in diameter and have an outer protein capsid composed of 60 capsomeres that encloses a linear, single-stranded RNA genome.

Clinical Presentation.[115–117] Infection by enteroviruses is worldwide in distribution, has a peak incidence during the summer and fall in temperate climates, and has a prevalence that varies inversely with socioeconomic levels. The prevalence of any given immunotype varies markedly, one or two types predominating each year within restricted geographic areas. Epidemics are not unusual and have provided much of the basis for our understanding of the clinical expression of infection by individual immunotypes of enteroviruses.

The spectrum of clinical disease produced by different enteroviruses is remarkably broad and shows a tremendous overlap among the different immunotypes, and the frequency of clinical disease among infected individuals is highly variable. Even though infections with the same immunotype of virus may produce an extraordinarily wide range of symptoms, certain enterovirus immunotypes are commonly associated with characteristic clinical presentations, for example, particular immunotypes of group A coxsackieviruses with herpangina and of group B coxsackieviruses with myopericarditis.

The incubation period of enterovirus infection ranges from 2 to 15 days, but generally it is 3 to 5 days. The most common clinical expression of infection with these viruses is a mild febrile illness that has an abrupt onset without a prodrome. Temperature elevations usually range from 101°F to 104°F (38.3°C to 40.0°C) and are associated with headache and malaise. Anorexia, sore throat, nausea, vomiting, and myalgias may occasionally be seen. The illness typically lasts 2 to 4 days but may be biphasic, resolving after several days, only to recur shortly thereafter. Other common manifestations of infection include mild pharyngitis, various gastrointestinal symptoms (abdominal pain, nausea, vomiting, diarrhea), conjunctivitis, and aseptic meningitis. Enterovirus infections are often accompanied by a maculopapular rash, particularly in younger individuals.

Since intercurrent infection with these viruses is common and generally asymptomatic, the finding of enterovirus in a random stool specimen, or even the observation of rising antibody titers to an enterovirus, need not be evidence of a causal relation with illness in an individual. Definitive diagnosis requires viral isolation from a site of active disease (e.g., pharynx, skin vesicle) or from more than one location (e.g., blood and stool) at the same time. Serologic screening for infection is not a particularly useful means of confirming the diagnosis of enterovirus infection because of the large number of serotypes.

Pathogenesis of Arthritic Symptoms.[114–119] The pathogenesis of the arthritis is not known. Virus has been recovered in two cases from joint fluids; one patient had X-linked agammaglobulinemia, a condition associated with persistence of virus in tissues. No evidence of the involvement of immune complexes has been presented.

Rheumatologic Manifestations.[115–118] When specifically sought, arthritis has been found to be an uncommon but definite manifestation of enterovirus infections. During one surveillance study involving 7075 individuals from whom enteroviruses were isolated, nine cases of "rheumatic disease" were reported, including six with arthritis. In a further investigation in which serologic evidence (fourfold or greater rise in neutralizing antibody titer) of infection by coxsackievirus A9 and coxsackieviruses B1 through B6 was specifically sought in individuals with the presenting complaint of acute inflammatory arthropathy, six cases of self-limited arthritis were identified.[118] The arthritis was accompanied by fever in all patients, sore throat and pleuritic pain in five patients, and rash in three patients. One had accompanying myocarditis.

In addition to these patients with coxsackievirus infection, four cases of an acute, self-limited arthritis believed to be associated with echovirus infection have been reported in adults. In these patients, both large and small joints were affected, and significant knee effusions were noted in one patient. An evanescent maculopapular rash appeared early in the course of arthritis. Joint symptoms resolved spontaneously over a 10- to 15-day period.

Laboratory Investigations.[116–118] Leukocytosis, an elevated erythrocyte sedimentation rate, and raised antistreptolysin O titers have been reported in approximately half of the patients studied. Examination of joint fluids has demonstrated cell counts ranging from 2500 to 46,900 per mm³, with 5 to 90 percent neutrophils, and a protein content of 2.9 to 4.5 g per dl. Synovial biopsy has revealed only nonspecific inflammatory changes. Virus has been recovered from synovial fluids on two occasions.[118, 119]

SMALLPOX AND VACCINIA

Virology.[120] As members of the genus Orthopoxvirus, variola virus (smallpox) and vaccinia virus, a derivative of smallpox and cowpox, share a common brick-shaped morphology and measure 250 to 300 nm × 100 nm. Each also contains a genome consisting of double-stranded DNA. Vaccinia virus is antigenically identical to variola but may be distinguished by in vitro growth properties.

Clinical Presentation.[120] Smallpox has an incubation period of 7 to 17 days that is terminated by the abrupt onset of high fever (102°F to 105°F) (38.9°C to 40.6°C), headache, and prominent myalgias. Two to 4 days later the characteristic rash appears on the face and spreads centrifugally to the trunk and extremities. The rash is initially macular and evolves in stages—first to papules, then to vesicles by day 4, to pustules by day 6, and finally to dry crusts by day 10. The mortality varies greatly by geographic location (1 to 30 percent), probably reflecting differences in the virulence of viral strains.

Pathogenesis of Arthritic Symptoms.[121] Joint involvement in all nonseptic cases arises secondary to the development of viral osteomyelitis (osteomyelitis variolosa), which involves the metaphyseal ends of the long bones, seeded at the time of the secondary viremia. The localization of virus to this growth area explains the age distribution observed (see later).

Rheumatologic Manifestations and Laboratory Investigation.[121] Joint symptoms are a well-recognized manifestation of smallpox, reported in 0.25 to 0.50 percent of patients in one smallpox epidemic. Involvement is limited almost exclusively to children younger than 10 years of age, with an incidence within this group of 2 to 5 percent of those at risk. Typically, joint pain and swelling arise 10 to 30 days after the onset of the rash. The elbows are almost invariably the first joints involved. In about 50 percent of the patients the arthritis then evolves in an additive, symmetric fashion to affect the wrists, ankles, or knees. Radiographic examination at this stage reveals changes of osteomyelitis involving the underlying metaphyseal bone. Spontaneous resolution of the arthritis ensues over the following weeks, but significant bone deformities and interference with the normal growth patterns are common sequelae. Joint aspiration during the period of acute arthritis may reveal fluid containing the characteristic elementary bodies of variola.

Arthritis has also been reported as a rare accompaniment of vaccinia infection,[122, 123] occurring 12 days after immunization in the single well-documented case.[122] The synovial fluid of the involved knee was inflammatory in nature, and vaccinia virus was recovered on culture. The swelling resolved spontaneously after 11 days, but arthralgias persisted for several months. No radiographic changes of the involved joint were observed at any time during the course of the illness.

ADENOVIRUS

Although the spectrum of disease caused by adenovirus is quite broad, arthritis is a rare manifestation of infection, reported for the first time in 1974.[124] The initial case involved a military recruit who presented with myalgias, meningeal signs, and an upper respiratory illness. Shortly thereafter, a rash, arthralgias of the hands and wrists, and frank arthritis of the knees developed. Arthrocentesis revealed a joint fluid that was straw-colored, gave a good mucin clot, and contained 4.5 g of protein per dl and 24,800 white blood cells per mm^3, with a predominance of neutrophils (89 percent). Synovial biopsy demonstrated an inflammatory synovitis. Over the next 3 weeks the joint symptoms resolved completely. The diagnosis of adenovirus type 7 infection was made serologically, but it was not possible to isolate adenovirus. Since this initial case, four additional patients[125] have been reported to have arthritis associated with serologically documented adenovirus infection. As in the initial case, arthritis developed in the majority of these patients 3 to 8 days after the onset of a nonspecific upper respiratory illness and involved both large and small joints of the upper and lower extremities. In two patients, joint fluid examination demonstrated white blood cell counts of fewer than 4000 per mm^3, with a predominance of mononuclear cells, whereas in a third patient the synovial fluid contained 8500 leukocytes per mm^3, with a predominance of neutrophils. Virus was not recovered from synovial fluid. Serum complement levels were depressed in two of three patients, and cryoproteins and immune complexes were demonstrated in both the sera and the joint fluid of all three patients.

VARICELLA-ZOSTER VIRUS

Arthritis has been reported as a rare complication of infection by each of the viruses of the Herpetoviridae family: herpes simplex virus, varicella-zoster virus (VZV), Epstein-Barr virus, and cytomegalovirus. Although arthritis has been commented on as a complication of chickenpox from as early as 1931, it was not until the 1970s that individual case reports appeared in the medical literature. Since that time, at least 21 children (ages 5 to 15 years) and one adult (age 20 years) have been observed with aseptic arthritis, and five children (age range 1.5 to 2 years) have been seen with septic arthritis complicating chickenpox.[126] Only two of the patients demonstrated an associated pericarditis; the remainder were free of the more serious systemic complications of VZV infection. In cases of aseptic arthritis, joint symptoms began from 1 day prior to 5 days after the onset of rash and were associated with swelling, significant pain, and limitation of movement. Monarticular swelling of the knee was the most common rheumatologic presentation, although two cases of polyarticular involvement have been reported. A distinct female predominance has been noted. In all instances, the joint symptoms resolved spontaneously within 1 week of onset, and no sequelae were observed.

The finding of an acute monoarthritis in a patient with chickenpox should not automatically be interpreted to represent an associated aseptic (virus-induced) arthritis because several cases of joint infection by bacteria have been reported in these patients. Patients with septic arthritis differ from those with aseptic arthritis by being younger (less than 5 years old), by displaying involvement of joints other than the knee, and by having synovial fluids with a predominance of polymorphonuclear cells rather than mononuclear cells. Distinction between these two conditions ultimately requires a culture of synovial fluid. In those instances in which the diagnosis is not apparent after examination of the joint fluid, antibiotic therapy should be initiated until the bacteriology results have been obtained. In patients with zoster, the initial presentation may mimic a septic joint, but the pain is believed to be secondary to irritation of involved nerve roots rather than true joint infection.[127]

Synovial fluid analysis has been reported in several cases of VZV-associated aseptic arthritis. In general, the fluid is clear and straw-colored and gives a fair to poor mucin clot. The synovial fluid leukocyte count is usually low but may be elevated, occasionally strikingly so (one case had more than 50,000 leukocytes per mm^3), and most often demonstrates a majority of mononuclear cells. However, early in the course of the arthritis, polymorphonuclear leukocytes may predominate. Virus has been isolated from the joint on one occasion.[128]

EPSTEIN-BARR VIRUS

True arthritis is a rare complication of Epstein-Barr (EB) virus infection, having been reported in fewer than 10 cases of either presumed or proven infectious mononucleosis.[129, 130] In contrast, arthralgias may accompany infection much more commonly. In three well-documented cases of arthritis, two patients had a monarticular arthritis involving the knee and ankle, respectively, while one developed a polyarthritis shortly after the onset of clinical disease. In all, symptoms resolved over the course of days to weeks without sequelae. Arthrocentesis revealed inflammatory joint fluids (elevated leukocyte counts with a predominance of either neutrophils or monocytes and elevated protein levels). In the one patient in whom complement levels were determined, synovial fluid C3 and C4 levels were lower than those in the serum but higher than expected for an immune complex–mediated process. Synovial tissue has been biopsied from patients with arthritis complicating infectious mononucleosis and is said to have shown a nonspecific subacute synovitis.

HERPES SIMPLEX VIRUS

Two serologically, biologically, and biochemically distinct types of herpes simplex virus (HSV) have been described: (1) HSV type 1 (HSV-1), which is associated primarily with oral infections; and (2) HSV type 2 (HSV-2), which is the predominant form in genital infections. Generalized or disseminated disease is a well-recognized, although uncommon, manifestation of HSV infection that is seen most often in immunocompromised individuals but is occasionally observed in otherwise normal people. Two cases of arthritis associated with HSV infection have been reported, and both have occurred in normal individuals with generalized HSV-1 disease.[131] In one patient, acute monarticular arthritis of the knee developed coincident with the appearance of a diffuse vesicular rash 1 week after the patient had wrestled with an individual who had similar skin lesions. The involved joint was described as warm, tender, and swollen. The synovial fluid was cloudy and had a normal viscosity, a good mucin clot, and a cell count of 10,000 per mm^3, with the majority being mononuclear leukocytes or synovial lining cells. Synovial biopsy demonstrated nonspecific inflammatory changes but no evidence of viral infection of the synovial tissues. Culture of the fluid, however, did result in isolation of HSV-1. Over the ensuing 10 days both the skin lesions and the arthritis resolved spontaneously without sequelae. In the second patient, acute monarticular arthritis of the ankle occurred in conjunction with an illness characterized by fever and a diffuse, vesicular rash. Results of throat and skin lesion cultures were positive for HSV-1. No joint fluid could be obtained for examination. Serum complement levels were reported to be normal. Joint symptoms and swelling persisted for 3 months but resolved by the fourth month.

CYTOMEGALOVIRUS

Arthritis associated with cytomegalovirus (CMV) infection has been documented in a single case.[131] In this immunosuppressed individual, generalized CMV infection occurred 12 weeks after renal transplantation and was associated with the development of an erythematous, warm, painful, and swollen knee. Initial arthrocentesis revealed a clear, yellow fluid containing fewer than 100 white blood cells per mm^3, with 40 percent neutrophils. Ten days later the joint fluid was cloudy, contained 1200 white blood cells per mm^3, with 53 percent neutrophils. A synovial biopsy at that time revealed no inflammatory response within synovial tissues, but particles morphologically consistent with CMV were observed in cells from the synovial fluid. No resolution of the arthritis occurred prior to the patient's death several months later.

HEPATITIS A VIRUS

Unlike hepatitis B virus infection, hepatitis A virus infection is not commonly associated with extrahepatic manifestations. Arthralgias and rash have been reported in as many as 10 to 14 percent of patients but have been observed only during the acute phase of the hepatitis.[132] There has been a single report of the occurrence of arthritis with an associated vasculitis in two patients who had a chronic, relapsing form of hepatitis A.[133] In these cases, a higher titer of circulating cryoglobulins, containing antibody against hepatitis A virus, was found. These cryoglobulins have been implicated in the pathogenesis of the disorder, and this presentation may represent a defined subset of what has been previously regarded as "mixed essential cryoglobulinemia" associated with liver disease.

References

1. Oldstone, M. A. B., Buchmeier, M. J., and Doyle, M. V.: Immunobiology of persistent virus infection. *In* Stevens, J. G., Todaro, G. J., and Fox, C. F.: Persistent Viruses, ICN-UCLA Symposia on Molecular and Cellular Biology. Vol. 11. New York, Academic Press, 1978.
2. Fulginiti, V. A.: Virus and virus vaccine–induced immunologic injury. *In* Talmage, D. W., Rose, B., Austen, K. F., and Vaughan, J. H.: Immunological Diseases. 3rd ed. Boston, Little, Brown & Company, 1978.
3. Editorial: Arthritis and immune complexes. Br. Med. J. 1:4, 1972.
4. Blanden, R. V., Pang, T. E., and Dunlop, M. B. C.: T cell recognition of virus-infected cells. *In* Poste, G., and Nicolson, G. L. (eds.): Virus Infection and the Cell Surface. Amsterdam, North-Holland Publishing Company, 1977.
5. Blumberg, B. S., Alter, H. J., and Visnich, S.: A "new" antigen in leukemia sera. J.A.M.A. 292:541, 1965.
6. Krugman, S., and Katz, S. L.: Viral hepatitis. *In* Infectious Diseases of Children. 7th ed. St. Louis, C. V. Mosby Company, 1981.
7. Aach, R. D.: Viral Hepatitis. *In* Feigin, R. D., and Cherry, J. D. (eds.): Textbook of Pediatric Infectious Diseases. Philadelphia, W. B. Saunders Company, 1981.
8. Robinson, W. S.: Hepatitis B virus. *In* Mandell, G. L., Douglas, R. G., Jr., and Bennett, J. E. (eds.): Principles and Practice of Infectious Diseases. New York, John Wiley & Sons, 1979.
9. Robinson, W. S., and Greenberg, H.: Hepatitis B. *In* Hoeprich, P. D. (ed.): Infectious Diseases. 2nd ed. New York, Harper & Row, 1977.
10. Thomas, H. C., Montano, L., Goodall, A., deKoning, R., Qladapo, J., and Wiedman, K. H.: Immunological mechanisms in chronic hepatitis B virus infection. Hepatology 2:116S, 1982.
11. Wands, J. R., Mann, E., Alpert, E., and Isselbacher, K. J.: The pathogenesis of arthritis associated with acute hepatitis-B surface antigen–positive hepatitis. J. Clin. Invest. 55:930, 1975.
12. Duffy, J., Lidsky, M. D., Sharp, J. T., Davis, J. S., Person, D. A., Hollinger, F. B., and Min, K. W.: Polyarthritis, polyarteritis, and hepatitis B. Medicine 55:10, 1976.
13. Shumaker, J. B., Goldfinger, S. E., Alpert, E., and Isselbacher, K. J.: Arthritis and rash. Arch. Intern. Med. 133:483, 1974.
14. Alpert, E., Schur, P. H., and Isselbacher, K. J.: Sequential changes of serum complement in HAA-related arthritis. N. Engl. J. Med. 287:103, 1972.
15. Fye, K. H., Becker, M. J., Theofilopoulos, A. N., Motsopoulos, H., Feldman, J., and Talal, N.: Immune complexes in hepatitis B antigen–associated periarteritis nodosa. Am. J. Med. 62:783, 1977.
16. Knieser, M. R., Jenis, E. H., Cowenthal, D. T., Bancroft, W. H., Burns, W., and Shalhoub, R.: Pathogenesis of renal disease associated with viral hepatitis. Arch. Pathol. 97:193, 1974.
17. Levo, Y., Gorevic, P. D., Kassab, H. J., Zucker-Franklin, D., and Franklin, E. C.: Association between hepatitis B virus and essential mixed cryoglobulinemia. N. Engl. J. Med. 296:1501, 1977.

18. Graves, R. J.: Clinical Lectures on the Practice of Medicine. Dublin, Fannin and Company, 1843.
19. Stevens, D. P., Walker, J., Crum, E., Roth, H. P., and Moskowitz, R. W.: Anicteric hepatitis presenting as polyarthritis. J.A.M.A. 220:687, 1972.
20. Chang, L. W., and O'Brien, T. F.: Australia antigen serology in the Holy Cross and football team hepatitis outbreak. Lancet 2:59, 1970.
21. Mirick, G. S., and Shank, R. E.: An epidemic of serum hepatitis studied under controlled conditions. Am. Clin. Climat. Assoc. 71:176, 1959.
22. Alarcon, G. S., and Townes, A. S.: Arthritis in viral hepatitis: Report of two cases and review of the literature. Johns Hopkins Med. J. 132:1, 1973.
23. Fernandez, R., and McCarty, D. J.: The arthritis of viral hepatitis. Ann. Intern. Med. 74:207, 1971.
24. Wenzel, R. P., and McCormick, D. P.: Arthritis and hepatitis. N. Engl. J. Med. 285:805, 1971.
25. McCarty, D. J., and Ormiste, V.: Arthritis and HB Ag–positive hepatitis. Arch. Intern. Med. 132:264, 1973.
26. Sergent, J. S., Lockshin, M. D., Christian, C. L., and Gocke, D. J.: Vasculitis and hepatitis B antigenemia. Medicine 55:1, 1976.
27. Cochrane, C. G., and Hawkins, D.: Studies on circulating immune complexes. J. Exp. Med. 127:137, 1968.
28. Kohler, P. F., Cronin, R. E., Hammon, W. S., Olin, D., and Carr, R. I.: Chronic membranous glomerulonephritis caused by hepatitis B antigen–antibody immune complexes. Ann. Intern. Med. 81:448, 1974.
29. Farivar, M., Wands, J. R., Benson, G. D., Dienstag, J. L., and Isselbacher, K. J.: Cryoprotein complexes and peripheral neuropathy in a patient with chronic active hepatitis. Gastroenterology 71:490, 1976.
30. McIntosh, R. M., Koss, M. N., and Gocke, D. J.: The nature and incidence of cryoproteins in hepatitis B antigen (HBsAg)–positive patients. Q. J. Med. 177:23, 1976.
31. Onion, D. K., Crumpacker, C. S., and Gilliland, B. C.: Arthritis of hepatitis associated with Australia antigen. Ann. Intern. Med. 75:29, 1971.
32. McKenna, P. J., O'Brian, J. T., Scheinman, H. Z., Delaney, W. E., Pellecchia, C., and Depore, J. J.: Hepatitis and arthritis with hepatitis-associated antigen in serum and synovial fluid. Lancet 2:214, 1971.
33. Top, F. H., Jr.: Rubella. In Wehrlie, P. F., and Top, F. H., Jr. (eds.): Communicable and Infectious Diseases. 9th ed. St. Louis, C. V. Mosby Company, 1981.
34. Krugman, S., and Katz, S. L.: Rubella (German measles). In Hoeprich, P. D. (ed.): Infectious Diseases of Children. 7th ed. St. Louis, C. V. Mosby Company, 1981.
35. Fraser, J. R. E., Cunningham, A. L., Hayes, K., Leach, R., and Lunt, R.: Rubella arthritis in adults. Isolation of virus, cytology and other aspects of the synovial reaction. Clin. Exp. Rheumatol. 1:287, 1983.
36. Frenkel, I. D., and Bellanti, J. A.: Immunology of measles, mumps, and rubella viruses. In Nahmias, A. J., and O'Reilly, R. J. (eds.): Immunology of Human Infection. New York, Plenum Medical Book Company, 1982.
37. Chantler, J. K., Ford, D. K., and Tingle, A. J.: Rubella-associated arthritis. Rescue of rubella virus from peripheral blood lymphocytes two years post vaccination. Infect. Immun. 32:1274, 1981.
38. Chantler, J. K., Tingle, A. J., and Petty, R. E.: Persistent rubella virus infection associated with chronic arthritis in children. N. Engl. J. Med. 313:1117, 1985.
39. Grahame, R., Armstrong, R., Simmons, N., Wilton, J. M. A., Dyson, M., Laurent, R., Millis, R., and Mims, C. A.: Chronic arthritis associated with the presence of intrasynovial rubella virus. Ann. Rheum. Dis. 41:2, 1983.
40. Phillips, P. E.: Infectious agents in the pathogenesis of rheumatoid arthritis. Semin. Arthritis Rheum. 16:1, 1986.
41. Austin, S. M., Altman, R., Barnes, E. K., and Dougherty, W. J.: Joint reactions in children vaccinated against rubella. Am. J. Epidemiol. 95:53, 1972.
42. Chambers, R. J., and Bywaters, E. G. L.: Rubella synovitis. Ann. Rheum. Dis. 22:263, 1963.
43. Smith, C. A., Petty, R. E., and Tingle, A. J.: Rubella virus and arthritis. Rheum. Dis. Clin. North Am. 13:265, 1987.
44. Miller, W. H., and Curl, O. J.: Arthritis complicating rubella in a recent epidemic. Practitioner 190:515, 1963.
45. Branch, K. G., and Taylor, J. H.: Rubella in 1962. Br. Med. J. 2:1325, 1962.
46. Johnson, I. N. L.: Complications of rubella. Br. Med. J. 2:414, 1962.
47. Green, R. H., Balsamo, R. R., Giles, J. P., Krugman, S., and Mirick, G. S.: Studies of the natural history and prevention of rubella. Am. J. Dis. Child. 110:348, 1965.
48. Heathfield, K. W. G.: Carpal-tunnel syndrome. Br. Med. J. 2:58, 1962.
49. Dresner, E., and Trombly, P.: The latex-fixation reaction in nonrheumatic diseases. N. Engl. J. Med. 261:981, 1959.
50. Robitaille, A., Cockburn, C., James, D. C. O., and Ansell, B. M.: HLA frequencies in less common arthropathies. Ann. Rheum. Dis. 35:271, 1976.
51. Grahame, R., Armstrong, R., Simmons, N. A., Mims, C. A., Wilton, J. M. A., and Laurent, R.: Isolation of rubella virus from synovial fluid in five cases of seronegative arthritis. Lancet 2:649, 1981.
52. Meyer, H. M., Parkman, P. D., and Panos, T. C.: Attenuated rubella virus. N. Engl. J. Med. 275:575, 1966.
53. DuPan, R. M., Huygelen, C., Peetermans, J., and Prinzie, A.: Clinical trials with a live attenuated rubella virus vaccine. Am. J. Dis. Child. 115:658, 1968.
54. Plotkin, S. A., Farquhar, J. D., Katz, M., and Buser, F.: Attenuation of RA 27/3 rubella virus in WI-38 human diploid cells. Am. J. Dis. Child. 118:178, 1969.
55. Fogel, A., Moshkowitz, A., Rannon, L., and Gerichter, C. B.: Comparative trials of RA 27/3 and Cendehill rubella vaccines in adult and adolescent females. Am. J. Epidemiol. 93:392, 1971.
56. Simpson, R. E. H.: Rubella and polyarthritis. Br. Med. J. 1:830, 1940.
57. Marshall, W. C.: Rubella vaccination in adult and adolescent females. Can. J. Public Health 62:58, 1971.
58. Moylan-Jones, R. J., and Penny, P. T.: Complications of rubella. Lancet 2:355, 1962.
59. Grand, M. G., Shelby, A. W., Gehlbach, S. H., Landrigan, P. J., Judelsohn, R. G., Zendel, S. A., and Witte, J. J.: Clinical reactions following rubella vaccination. J.A.M.A. 220:1569, 1972.
60. Dudgeon, A. J., Marshall, W., and Peckham, C.: Rubella vaccine trials in adults and children. Am. J. Dis. Child. 118:237, 1969.
61. Centers for Disease Control: Rubella virus vaccine. Ann. Intern. Med. 75:757, 1971.
62. Weibel, R. E., Stokes, J., Jr., Buynak, E. B., and Hilleman, M. R.: Rubella vaccination in adult females. N. Engl. J. Med. 280:682, 1969.
63. Thompson, G. R., Ferreyra, A., and Brackett, R. G.: Acute arthritis complicating rubella vaccination. Arthritis Rheum. 14:19, 1971.
64. Ogra, P. L., and Herd, J. K.: Arthritis associated with induced rubella infection. J. Immunol. 107:810, 1971.
65. Swartz, T. A., Kingberg, W., and Goldwasser, R. A.: Clinical manifestation according to age, among females given HPV-77 duck embryo vaccine. Am. J. Epidemiol. 94:246, 1971.
66. Griffiths, M. M., Spruance, S. L., Ogra, P. L., Thompson, G. R., and DeWitt, C. W.: HLA and recurrent episodic arthropathy associated with rubella vaccination. Arthritis Rheum. 20:1192, 1977.
67. Spruance, S. L., Metcalf, R., Smith, C. B., Griffiths, M. M., and Ward, J. R.: Chronic arthropathy associated with rubella vaccination. Arthritis Rheum. 20:741, 1977.
68. Deinard, A. S., and Bilka, P. J.: Joint involvement following vaccination for rubella. Minn. Med. 54:337, 1971.
69. Schaffner, W., Fleet, W. F., Kilroy, A. W., Lefkowitz, L. B., Herrmann, K. K., Thompson, R. N., and Karzon, D. T.: Polyneuropathy following rubella immunization. Am. J. Dis. Child. 127:684, 1974.
70. Kilroy, A. W., Schaffner, W., Fleet, W. F., Jr., Lefkowitz, L. B., Jr., Karzon, D. T., and Fenichel, G. M.: Two syndromes following rubella immunization. Clinical observations and epidemiological studies. J.A.M.A. 214:2287, 1970.
71. Burns, K. I., Muzyczka, N., and Hauswirth, W. W.: Replication of parvovirus. In Field, B., and Knipe, D. (eds.): Fundamental Virology. New York, Raven Press, 1986.
72. Pattison, J. R., Jones, S. E., Hodgson, J., Davis, L. R., White, J. M., Stroud, C. E., and Murtaza, L.: Parvovirus infections and hypoplastic crisis in sickle-cell anemia. Lancet 1:664, 1981.
73. Anderson, M. J., and Pattison, J. R.: The human parvovirus. Arch. Virol. 82:137, 1984.
74. Joseph, P. R.: Fifth disease and arthritis: Common immune-mediated responses to parvovirus infection. N.Y. State J. Med. 86:556, 1986.
75. Editorial: Arthritis and parvovirus infection. Lancet 1:436, 1985.
76. Reid, D. M., Brown, T., Reid, T. M. S., Rennie, J. A. N., and Eastmond, C. J.: Human parvovirus-associated arthritis: A clinical and laboratory description. Lancet 1:422, 1985.
77. Cohen, B. J., Buckley, M. M., Clewley, J. P., Jones, V. E., Puttick, A. H., and Jacoby, R. K.: Human parvovirus infection in early rheumatoid and inflammatory arthritis. Ann. Rheum. Dis. 45:832, 1986.
78. Simpson, R. W., McGinty, L., Simon, L., Smith, C. A., Godzeski, C. W., and Boyd, R. J.: Association of parvoviruses with rheumatoid arthritis of humans. Science 223:1425, 1984.
79. White, D. G., Mortimer, P. P., Blake, D. R., Woolf, A. D., Cohen, B. J., and Bacon, P. A.: Human parvovirus arthropathy. Lancet 1:419, 1985.
80. Naides, S. J., Scharosch, L. L., foto, FL., and Howard, E. J.: Rheumatologic manifestations of human parvovirus B19 infection in adults. Arthritis Rheum. 33:1297, 1990.
81. Smith, C. A., Woolf, A. D., and Lenci, M.: Parvoviruses: Infections and arthropathies. Rheum. Dis. Clin. North Am. 13:249, 1987.
82. Liloong, T. C., Coyle, P. V., Anderson, M. J., Allen, G. E., and Connolly, J. H.: Human serum parvovirus-associated vasculitis. Postgrad. Med. J. 62:493, 1986.
83. Semble, E. L., Agudelo, C. A., and Pegram, P. S.: Human parvovirus B19 arthropathy in two adults after contact with childhood erythema infectiosum. Am. J. Med. 83:560, 1987.

84. Klouda, P. T., Corbin, S. A., Bradley, B. A., Cohen, B. J., and Woolf, A. D.: HLA and acute arthritis following human parvovirus infection. Tissue Antigens 28:318, 1986.

85. Calisher, C. H., Shope, R. E., Brandt, W., Casals, J., Karabatsos, N., Murphy, F. A., Tesh, R. B., and Wiebe, M. E.: Proposed antigenic classification of registered arboviruses (Togaviridae, Alphavirus). Intervirology 14:229, 1980.

86. Lumsden, W. H. R.: An epidemic of virus disease in southern province, Tanganyika territory, in 1952-53. II. General description and epidemiology. Trans. R. Soc. Trop. Med. Hyg. 49:33, 1955.

87. Tesh, R. B., Gajdusek, D. C., Garruto, R. M., Cross, J. H., and Rosen, I.: The distribution and prevalence of group A arbovirus neutralizing antibodies among human populations in southeast Asia and the Pacific Islands. Am. J. Trop. Med. Hyg. 24:664, 1975.

88. Gear, S. H. S.: Arboviruses of Southern Africa. In Feigin, R. D., and Cherry, J. D. (eds.): Textbook of Pediatric Infectious Diseases. Philadelphia, W. B. Saunders Company, 1981.

89. Shore, H.: O'nyong-nyong fever: An epidemic virus disease in East Africa. III. Some clinical and epidemiological observations in the northern province of Uganda. Trans. R. Soc. Trop. Med. Hyg. 55:361, 1961.

90. Clarke, J. A., Marshall, J. D., and Gard, G.: Annually recurrent epidemic polyarthritis and Ross River virus activity in a coastal area of New South Wales. Am. J. Trop. Med. Hyg. 22:543, 1973.

91. Pinheiro, F. P., Freitas, R. B., Travassos da Rosa, J. F., Gabbay, Y. B., Mellow, W. A., and LeDuc, J. W.: An outbreak of Mayaro virus disease in Belterra, Brazil. Am. J. Trop. Med. Hyg. 30:674, 1981.

92. McIntosh, M., McGillivray, G. M., Dickinson, D. B., and Malherbe, H.: Illness caused by Sindbis and West Nile viruses in South Africa. S. Afr. Med. J. 38:291, 1964.

93. Skogh, M., and Espmark, A.: Ockelbo disease: Epidemic arthritis–exanthema syndrome in Sweden caused by Sindbis-virus like agent. Lancet 1:795, 1982.

94. Fraser, J. R. E., and Cunningham, A. L.: Incubation time of epidemic polyarthritis. Med. J. Aust. 1:550, 1980.

95. Fuller, C. W., and Warner, P.: Some epidemiological and laboratory observations on an epidemic rash and polyarthritis occurring in the upper Murray region of South Australia. Med. J. Aust. 2:117, 1957.

96. Nimmannitya, S., Halstead, S. B., Cohen, S. N., and Margiotta, M. R.: Dengue and chikungunya virus infection in man in Thailand. 1962–1964. I. Observations on hospitalized patients with hemorrhagic fever. Am. J. Trop. Med. Hyg. 18:954, 1969.

97. Deller, J. J., and Russell, P. K.: Chikungunya disease. Am. J. Trop. Med. Hyg. 17:107, 1968.

98. Doherty, R. L., Carley, J. G., and Best, J. C.: Isolation of Ross River virus from man. Med. J. Aust. 1:1083, 1972.

99. Julkunen, I., Brummer-Korvenkontio, M., Hautanen, A., Kuusisto, P., Lindstrom, P., Wager, O., and Penntinen, K.: Elevated serum immune complex levels in pogosta disease, an acute alphavirus infection with rash and arthritis. J. Clin. Lab. Immunol. 21:77, 1986.

100. Fraser, J. R. E., Cunningham, A. L., Muller, H. K., Sinclair, R. A., and Standish, H. G.: Glomerulonephritis in the acute phase of Ross River virus disease (epidemic polyarthritis). Clin. Nephrol. 29:149, 1988.

101. Aaskov, J. G., Fraser, J. R. E., and Dalglish, D. A.: Specific and nonspecific immunological changes in epidemic polyarthritis patients. Aust. J. Exp. Biol. Med. Sci. 59:599, 1981.

102. Mudge, R.: Epidemic polyarthritis in South Australia. Med. J. Aust. 2:823, 1974.

103. Fraser, J. R. E., Tait, B., Aaskov, J. G., and Cunningham, A. L.: Possible genetic determinants in epidemic polyarthritis caused by Ross River virus infection. Aust. N. Z. J. Med. 10:597, 1980.

104. Fraser, J. R. E., and Becker, G. J.: Mononuclear cell types in chronic synovial effusions of Ross River virus disease. Aust. N.Z. J. Med. 14:505, 1984.

105. Hazelton, R. A., Hughes, C., and Aaskov, J. G.: The inflammatory response in the synovium of a patient with Ross River arbovirus infection. Aust. N.Z. J. Med. 15:336, 1985.

106. Fraser, J. R. E., Ratnamohan, V. M., Dowling, J. P. G., Becker, G. J., and Varigos, G. A.: The exanthem of Ross River virus infection: Histology, location of virus antigen, and nature of inflammatory infiltrate. J. Clin. Pathol. 36:1256, 1983.

107. Brunell, P. A.: Mumps. In Wehrle, P. F., and Top, F. H., Jr., (eds.): Communicable and Infectious Diseases. 9th ed. St. Louis, C. V. Mosby Company, 1981.

108. Maisondieu, P.: Etude des manifestations articulaires des orcillons. Thesis Jouve, Paris, 1924.

109. Lass, R., and Shephard, E.: Mumps arthritis. Br. Med. J. 2:1613, 1981.

110. Gordon, S. C., and Lauter, C. B.: Mumps arthritis: Unusual presentation as adult Still's disease. Ann. Intern. Med. 97:45, 1982.

111. Gordon, S. C., and Lauter, C. B.: Mumps arthritis: A review of the literature. Rev. Infect. Dis. 6:338, 1984.

112. Ghosh, S. K., and Reddy, T. A.: Arthralgia and myalgia in mumps. Rheumatol. Rehabil. 12:97, 1973.

113. Magida, M. G.: Epidemic parotitis complicated by pericarditis and serositis. Ann. Intern. Med. 35:218, 1957.

114. Johnson, K. M.: Enteroviruses: Coxsackievirus and echovirus infections. In Wehrle, P. F., and Top, F. H., Jr. (eds.): Communicable and Infectious Diseases. 9th ed. St. Louis, C. V. Mosby Company, 1981.

115. Sandford, J. P., and Sulkin, S. E.: The clinical spectrum of ECHO-virus infection. N. Engl. J. Med. 261:1113, 1959.

116. Hurst, N. P., Martynoga, A. G., Nuki, G., Swell, J. R., Mitchell, A., and Hughes, G. R.: Coxsackie B infection and arthritis. Br. Med. J. 286:605, 1983.

117. Roberts-Thomson, P. J., Southwood, T. R., Moore, B. W., Smith, M. D., Ahern, M. J., Geddes, R. A., and Hill, W. R.: Adult onset Still's disease or coxsackie polyarthritis? Aust. N.Z. J. Med. 16:509, 1986.

118. Kujala, G., and Newman, H.: Isolation of echovirus type 11 from synovial fluid in acute monocytic arthritis. Arthritis Rheum. 28:98, 1985.

119. Ackerson, B. K., Raghunathan, R., Keller, M. A., Bui, Hong Dange Bui, R., Phinney, P. R., and Imagawa, D. T.: Echovirus 11 arthritis in a patient with X-linked agammaglobulinemia. Pediatr. Infect. Dis. J. 6:485, 1987.

120. Benenson, A. S.: Smallpox. In Wehrle, P. F., and Top, F. H., Jr. (eds.): Communicable and Infectious Diseases. 9th ed. St. Louis, C. V. Mosby Company, 1981.

121. Ansell, B. M.: Infective arthritis. In Scott, J. T. (ed.): Textbook of Rheumatic Diseases. 5th ed. Edinburgh, Churchill Livingstone, 1978.

122. Silby, H. M., Farber, R., O'Connell, C. J., Ascher, J., and Marine, E. J.: Acute monoarticular arthritis after vaccination. Ann. Intern. Med. 62:347, 1965.

123. Holtzman, C. M.: Postvaccination arthritis. N. Engl. J. Med. 280:111, 1969.

124. Panush, R. S.: Adenovirus arthritis. Arthritis Rheum. 17:534, 1974.

125. Utsinger, P. D.: Immunologic study of arthritis associated with adenovirus infection (abstract). Arthritis Rheum. 20:138, 1977.

126. Atkinson, L. S., Halford, J. G., Jr., Burton, O. M., and Moorhead, S. R., Jr.: Septic and aseptic arthritis complicating varicella. J. Fam. Pract. 12:917, 1981.

127. Leventhal, J. J.: Articular presentation of herpes zoster eruption (letter). Arthritis Rheum. 32:506, 1989.

128. Priest, J. R., Urick, J. J., Groth, K. E., and Balfour, H. H., Jr.: Varicella arthritis documented by isolation of virus from joint fluid. J. Pediatr. 93:990, 1978.

129. Pollack, S., Enat, R., and Barzilai, D.: Monarthritis with heterophil-negative infectious mononucleosis. Arch. Intern. Med. 140:1109, 1980.

130. Webb, J.: Infectious-mononucleosis arthritis is not rare (letter). Med. J. Aust. 149:111, 1988.

131. Friedman, H. M., Pincus, T., Gibilisco, P., Baker, D., Glazer, J. P., Plotkin, S. A., and Schumacher, H. R.: Acute monarticular arthritis caused by herpes simplex virus and cytomegalovirus. Am. J. Med. 69:241, 1980.

132. Bamber, M., Thomas, H. C., Bannister, B., and Sherlock, S.: Acute type A, B, and non-A, non-B hepatitis in a hospital population in London: Clinical and epidemiological features. Gut 24:561, 1983.

133. Inman, R. D., Hodge, M., Johnston, M. E. A., Wright, J., and Heathcote, J. H.: Arthritis, vasculitis, and cryoglobulinemia associated with relapsing hepatitis A virus infection. Ann. Intern. Med. 105:700, 1986.

Section XVIII

Arthritis as a Manifestation of Other Systemic Diseases

Chapter 90

Katherine S. Upchurch
Doreen B. Brettler

Hemophilic Arthropathy

INTRODUCTION

Any disturbance in the complex physiologic cascade of blood clotting may result in an exaggerated tendency toward traumatic hemarthrosis or, when the perturbation is severe, recurrent spontaneous hemarthrosis. Though spontaneous joint hemorrhage has been described in a variety of inherited disorders of coagulation,[1, 2] including von Willebrand's disease,[3] and in the setting of anticoagulation therapy,[4] hemophilia is the disorder in which it most frequently occurs. Bleeding into the joints is, in fact, the complication of hemophilia that most frequently requires therapeutic intervention and when recurrent can lead to chronic deforming arthritis that is independent of bleeding episodes.

The term hemophilia refers to a group of diseases in which there is a functional deficiency of a specific clotting factor. Of these, only two, hemophilia A (classic hemophilia) and hemophilia B (Christmas disease) are associated with spontaneous joint hemorrhage, the deficient factors being factor VIII and factor IX, respectively. Both are X-linked recessive disorders, though there is a spontaneous mutation rate as high as 25 percent.[5] The incidence and severity of hemorrhagic complications of hemophilia are directly related to the severity of the underlying coagulation defect.

Though the intrinsic pathway of coagulation is severely impaired in hemophilia, the extrinsic tissue-dependent pathway remains intact[6] and is probably the major hemostatic regulatory system. It is of interest that normal synovial tissue as well as cultures of synovial fibroblasts has been found to be deficient in tissue factor,[7, 8] suggesting that hemophilia patients have functional inactivity of both intrinsic and extrinsic coagulation pathways in synovium-lined joints.

CLINICAL FEATURES

The spectrum of musculoskeletal complications of hemophilia has been the subject of numerous comprehensive reviews and monographs[9-16] and includes acute hemarthrosis, subacute or chronic arthritis, and end-stage hemophilic arthropathy. Patients with hemophilia also experience soft tissue hemorrhage, which may mimic hemarthrosis, and rarely, pseudotumors and septic arthritis. The most frequently involved joints are knees, ankles, elbows, shoulders, and hips, as shown in Figure 90–1. Involvement of the small joints of the hands and feet may also occur.[17] Like the frequency of hemarthrosis and the severity of subsequent arthritis, the median number of involved joints in a given patient is directly related to the severity of the underlying disease.

Acute Hemarthrosis. Nearly all patients with severe hemophilia A or B (less than 1 percent activity of the deficient factor) and up to one half[16] of patients with moderate hemophilia (greater than 2 percent activity) experience hemarthrosis. Hemarthrosis generally first becomes manifest between the ages of 12 and 18 months when a child begins to walk and run and continues, often in a cyclical fashion,[12] into adulthood. With adulthood, however, the frequency of acute hemarthrosis diminishes, possibly owing to more prudent activity or to an undefined change in the hemostatic process.[12] Patients frequently have premonitory symptoms such as stiffness or warmth in the involved joint, followed by intense pain, which in part may be due to rapid joint capsule distension. Clinically, pain is accompanied by objective findings of warmth, a tense effusion, tenderness, limitation of motion, and a joint that is often held in a flexed position. Joint pain responds rapidly to replacement of the deficient clotting factor, as discussed below. If

Percentage Joints With:

Any Hemarthrosis	Many Hemarthrosis	Chronic Pain		Syno-vitis	Limitation of Motion	Any Radiologic Abnormality
34.5	13.3	13.9		---	16.9	21.6
54.0	38.5	13.8		9.8	27.0	52.6
28.6	8.0	5.4		---	19.8	18.8
63.1	50.9	26.8		11.6	27.0	50.2
60.8	42.8	15.2		2.2	34.2	52.4

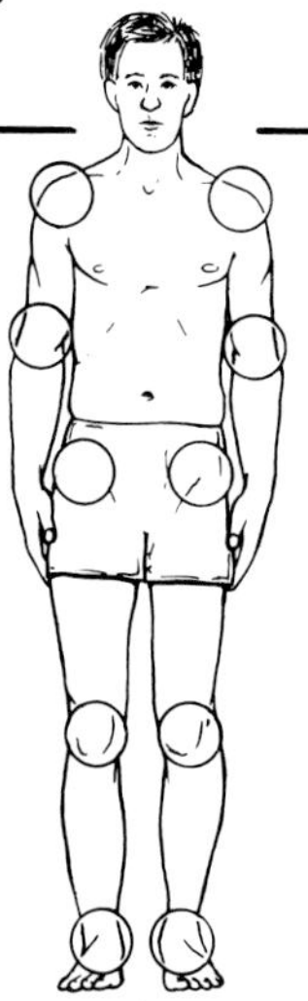

Figure 90–1. Distribution of acute hemarthrosis based on a study of 139 patients with hemophilia. Clinical and radiologic features of chronic arthritis in hemophilia. (Adapted from Steven, M. M., Madhok, S. Y., et al.: Hemophilic arthritis. Am. J. Med. 58:181, 1986, used by permission.)

hemostasis occurs rapidly, full joint function may be regained within 12 to 24 hours. If the hemorrhage is more advanced however, blood is resorbed slowly over 5 to 7 days and full joint function regained within 10 to 14 days. An episode of bleeding into a joint predisposes to further such episodes for at least two possible reasons. First, hemarthrosis stimulates proliferation, chronic inflammation, and hypervascularity of the synovial membrane. Second, hemarthrosis is accompanied by rapid atrophy of the periarticular musculature and a subsequent compromise in joint protection exerted by these muscles.

Subacute or Chronic Arthritis. Recurrent hemarthrosis may lead to a self-perpetuating condition in which joint abnormalities persist in intervals between bleeding episodes. Clinically the involved joint is chronically swollen, though painless and only slightly warm. There are findings of chronic synovitis, including prominent synovial proliferation with or without effusion. However, not all patients with a history of hemarthrosis will develop chronic synovitis or restriction of motion of involved joints, the likelihood of developing chronic arthritis being directly related to the overall severity of the clotting defect.[16] Despite an equal incidence of hemarthrosis, patients with hemophilia A more frequently have chronic arthritis than those with hemophilia B.[16]

End-stage Hemophilic Arthropathy. Long-standing end-stage hemophilic arthropathy has features in common with both degenerative joint disease and advanced rheumatoid arthritis (RA). Clinically, the joint appears enlarged and "knobby," owing to osteophytic bony overgrowth. Synovial thickening and effusion, however, are not prominent. Range of motion is severely restricted, and there frequently is fibrous ankylosis. Subluxation, joint laxity, and malalignment are common. Hemarthroses, however, decrease in frequency.

Septic Arthritis. Though many diseases such as RA and osteoarthritis (OA) confer an increased risk of bacterial infection of a previously damaged joint, septic arthritis, in the past considered rare in hemophilic arthritis, may occur more frequently than has previously been recognized and has several distinctive clinical features.[18–21] Pyogenic arthritis more commonly occurs in adult than pediatric hemophiliacs and is usually monoarticular with a predisposition for knee involvement. Compared with spontaneous hemarthrosis, septic arthritis is significantly associated with a fever greater than 38°C within 12 hours of presentation, an increased peripheral leukocyte count, and articular pain that does *not* improve with replacement therapy.[21] A predisposing factor other than hemophilic arthropathy is often identifiable, including previous arthrocentesis, arthroplasty, intravenous drug usage,[21] or HIV infection.[22] *Staphylococcus aureus* is the most frequently identified organism.

Muscle and Soft Tissue Hemorrhage. Though joint hemorrhage and subsequent arthritis are the most common clinical complications of hemophilia, bleeding into muscles and soft tissue is common and may be more insidious than hemarthrosis due to lack of premonitory symptoms. Bleeding into the iliopsoas and gastrocnemius muscles and the forearm results in well-described syndromes with which the rheumatologist should be familiar. Iliopsoas hemorrhage produces acute groin pain with marked pain on hip extension and a hip flexion contracture. Rotation is preserved, in contradistinction to intra-articular hemorrhage. If untreated, the expanding soft tissue mass may compress the femoral nerve, causing signs and symptoms of femoral neuropathy.[15, 23] Bleeding into the gastrocnemius muscle can cause an equinus deformity due to a heel corn contracture.[15] Finally, hemorrhage into closed compartments can cause acute muscle necrosis and nerve compression.[24] Of particular importance is bleeding into the volar compartment of the forearm, which can cause flexion deformities of the wrist and fingers. If a compartment syndrome is suspected, compartment pressures should be measured to confirm the diagnosis.

A large intramuscular hemorrhage may uncommonly result in the formation of a simple muscle cyst, which clinically appears to be an encapsulated soft tissue area of swelling overlying muscle. Cyst formation in this setting is confined by the muscular fascial plane and probably results from inadequate resorption of blood and clot. Subperiosteal or intraosseous hemorrhage, in contrast, may lead to a rare skeletal complication of hemophilia, a pseudotumor. Hemophilic pseudotumors are of two types: (1) the adult type that occurs proximally, usually in the pelvis or femur, and (2) the childhood type that occurs distal to the elbows or knees and carries a better prognosis than the adult type.[25, 26] Conservative early management of both muscle cysts and childhood type pseudotumors is indicated, including immobilization and factor replacement. In adult type pseudotumors, which are usually refractory to conservative therapy, and in progressive childhood pseudotumors, surgical removal is indicated[26] to avoid serious complications such as spontaneous rupture, fistula formation, neurologic or vascular entrapment, and fracture of adjacent bone. Aspiration of a pseudotumor or cyst is contraindicated.

DIAGNOSTIC IMAGING

Radiographs. The earliest radiologic changes in hemophilic arthropathy are confined to the soft tissue and reflect acute hemarthrosis. The joint capsule is distended with displacement of fat pads, and there is an increased hazy density caused by intra-articular blood. Hemarthrosis prior to epiphyseal plate closure may result in epiphyseal overgrowth and irregularity. Occasionally, premature epiphyseal closure is seen.

With the progression of chronic proliferative synovitis, irreversible radiologic changes appear. These reflect both the inflammatory and the degenerative nature of chronic hemophilic arthropathy, as summarized in Table 90–1 and illustrated in Figure 90–2A. Certain changes are unique to hemophilic arthropathy as well (see Table 90–1; Fig. 90–2B). Several radiographic systems of staging hemophilic

Table 90–1. RADIOLOGIC MANIFESTATIONS OF CHRONIC HEMOPHILIC ARTHROPATHY

Characteristic	Also seen in
Periarticular soft tissue swelling	RA
Periarticular demineralization	RA
Marginal erosions	RA
Subchondral irregularity and cyst formation	RA, OA
	RA, OA
Decreased joint space	OA
Osteophyte formation	CPPD*
Chondrocalcinosis	
Specific	
Femoral intercondylar notch widening	
Squaring of distal patellar margin (lateral view)	
Proximal radial enlargement (Fig. 90–2B)	
Talar flattening ± ankle ankylosis†	

RA, Rheumatoid arthritis; OA, osteoarthritis; CPPD, calcium pyrophosphate deposition disease.

*From Jensen, P. S., and Putnam, C. E.: Chondrocalcinosis and hemophilia. Clin. Radiol. 28:401, 1977.

†From Schreiber, R. R.: Musculoskeletal system—radiologic findings. In Brinkhous, K. M., and Hemker, H. C. (eds.): Handbook of Hemophilia. Part I. New York, American Elsevier Publishing Co., 1975.

arthropathy have been proposed,[14, 29, 30] and adherence to any one of these may prove useful in following disease progression.

Other Studies. Magnetic resonance imaging (MRI) has been suggested to be a useful, sensitive technique for following the progression of hemophilic arthropathy and aiding in early identification of candidates for synovectomy (see below).[31–33] However, because of its expense and the lack of large series correlating imaging results with surgical outcome, MRI is infrequently used. MRI[34] and ultrasonography[35, 36] are useful in both the detection and quantitation of soft tissue bleeding, cysts, and pseudotumors.

PATHOLOGIC FEATURES

Pathologic studies of human hemophilic arthropathy have been limited to synovial specimens obtained at surgery[37, 38] or at postmortem examination and thus reflect changes of advanced disease only. Studies of experimentally produced hemarthrosis in rabbits,[39] post-traumatic hemarthrosis in nonhemophilic humans,[40] and hemophilia A in dogs[91] have provided an understanding of the earliest changes induced by acute hemarthrosis and, in the latter case, their evolution to chronic arthritis.

A single hemorrhage induces changes in the synovial membrane. Early changes include focal villous synovial proliferation and subsynovial diapedesis of erythrocytes. These are followed by the appearance of perivascular inflammatory cells, including polymorphonuclear leukocytes (PMNs), lymphocytes, and mononuclear cells; patchy subsynovial fibrosis; and intracellular iron accumulation in both synovial cells and subsynovial macrophages.

With repeated hemarthroses, the synovium be-

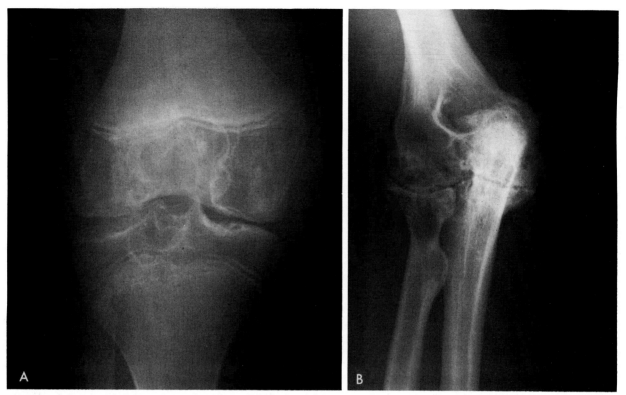

Figure 90–2. Roentgenographic changes of hemophilic arthropathy. *A,* Early arthritis of the knee, showing soft tissue swelling, widening of the femoral condyles and tibial plateau, irregularity of the distal femoral epiphysis, and a few subchondral bone cysts. *B,* More advanced arthritis involving the elbow, demonstrating almost complete loss of joint space and extensive subchondral cyst formation. The widening of the proximal radius is characteristic of hemophilic arthropathy.

comes grossly hypertrophied and hyperpigmented. Eventually the hypertrophied synovium organizes into a pannus with invasion and erosion of marginal cartilage. Histologically, there is progression of the above mentioned changes, including villous hypertrophy and subsynovial fibrosis, but inflammatory cells are scarce (Fig. 90–3). Ultrastructurally, synoviocyte hypertrophy and hyperplasia persist,[38] though studies are conflicting concerning the predominance of type A versus type B cells.[40, 42] Up to 75 percent of synoviocytes contain siderosomes (electron-dense, iron-filled deposits within lysosomes) in contrast to 10 percent in normal synovium and 25 percent in rheumatoid synovium.[42] Tissue lysis, mitochondrial destruction, and damaged endoplasmic reticulum can be seen in association with siderosomes.[42]

The articular cartilage is both grossly and microscopically abnormal in the setting of recurrent hemarthrosis.[38] There are areas of cartilage rarefaction exposing sclerotic bone, with the remaining cartilage being thin and unevenly distributed, often freely protruding into the joint cavity. Fine fissuring of cartilage can be seen. With thinning and fissuring, bony erosions appear at weight-bearing surfaces. Alcian blue staining demonstrates a loss of matrix glycosaminoglycan, as also seen in degenerative arthritis.[38, 43]

PATHOGENESIS

That recurrent hemarthrosis can duplicate the pathologic abnormalities of both synovium and cartilage seen in hemophilic arthritis was first established by Hoaglund using an experimental model of canine hemarthrosis.[44] The precise mechanisms whereby these changes occur are not firmly established.

As early as 4 days after hemarthrosis, siderosomes can be seen in the cytoplasm of synovial cells and subsynovial macrophages. These may persist for as long as 6 months in the absence of further bleeding.[40] Iron deposits likewise are prominent in articular cartilage from patients with hemophilic arthritis.[43] These observations have suggested that intracellular synovial and cartilaginous accumulations of iron may mediate tissue destruction in hemophilic arthritis. Supporting this hypothesis are studies demonstrating that (1) chondrocyte and synoviocyte iron deposits are associated with surrounding areas of cartilaginous degradation[43] and tissue lysis,[42] respectively; (2) cultured rabbit synovial fibroblasts are stimulated by the presence of iron to enhance the production of prostaglandin E_2 (PGE$_2$) and the degradative metalloproteinases;[45] and (3) iron cultured with chondrocytes or cartilage slices accumulates intracellularly, resulting in cytotoxicity.[46] In rheumatoid arthritis (RA) the importance of iron in directly mediating tissue destruction by catalyzing toxic free radical formation is becoming widely recognized,[47-50] and it seems reasonable to postulate a similar effect in hemophilia.

Hemarthrosis induces a synovial proliferative response, and the synovium itself has degradative potential in hemophilic arthritis. Both hemophilic synovium and adherent synovial cells isolated from hemophilic synovium release a neutral proteinase possibly capable of glycosaminoglycan degradation.[51] Furthermore, cultured adherent hemophilic synovial cells release collagenase in quantities equal to those reported from similar cultures of rheumatoid synovium.[51]

Hemarthrosis induces changes in cartilaginous biochemical composition through unknown means. Acute joint hemorrhage in rabbits leads to decreased cartilage compliance with proteoglycan loss.[52] These observations coupled with the above studies of the effects of iron on cartilage suggest that the biologic nature of the chondrocyte as well as biochemical composition of cartilage is altered in hemophilic arthropathy, rendering it more susceptible to mechanical stresses than normal cartilage.

Thus, current studies suggest that recurrent hemarthrosis induces joint destruction in hemophilic arthropathy through direct and indirect effects of iron on the synovium and cartilage, through the degradative effect of the proliferative synovium, and through an alteration in cartilage biochemical composition similar to that seen in degenerative arthritis.

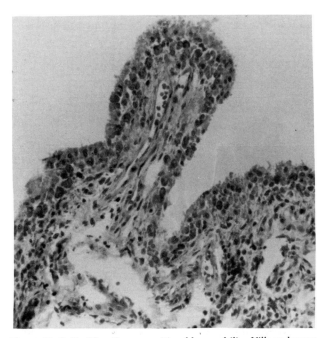

Figure 90–3. Proliferative synovitis of hemophilia. Villous hypertrophy of synovium with pigment deposition in superficial cells. The reaction is mainly synovial cell hyperplasia. Infiltrating inflammatory cells are scarce. (Hematoxylin & eosin, × 250.)

LABORATORY DIAGNOSIS

When hemarthrosis or hemophilic arthritis is suspected, diagnosis rests on the demonstration of a specific coagulopathy. Individuals with severe hemophilia A or B (defined as levels of factor VIII or IX, respectively, of 1 percent of normal) can be said to have factor VIII or IX levels of 0.01 unit per ml of plasma. The factor VIII or IX level in a normal person on a given day may range between 50 and 200 percent (0.50 to 2.00 units per ml).

Individuals with factor VIII or IX levels of equal to or less than 1 percent of normal (≤0.01 unit per ml) will have joint and muscle hemorrhages requiring therapy four or five times per month on the average, although the range is great and the episodes irregularly spaced. Individuals with factor VIII or IX levels of greater than 5 percent of normal (>0.05 unit per ml) are considered to have mild hemophilia and usually hemorrhage only with trauma or at surgery. Occasional "spontaneous" hemarthrosis may occur in such patients, especially in joints damaged by previously undertreated hemorrhage. Patients whose factor VIII or IX levels fall between these two ranges are considered to have moderately severe hemophilia, and their clinical picture falls somewhere between the two extremes. If such patients have had multiple untreated or suboptimally treated hemarthroses with subsequent joint damage, the anatomic instability of these joints will cause frequent and severe bleeding, and the condition will thus appear clinically more severe than the factor VIII or IX assay would suggest.

The treatment of each of the aforementioned disorders is unique to that disorder and generally ineffectual for the others. "A unit of fresh frozen plasma" is no longer acceptable treatment for bleeding caused by any of these conditions. For these reasons, adequate treatment requires a precise diagnosis, including (1) identification of the deficient factor (or factors), (2) precise quantitation of the factor level to allow accurate prognosis and for calculation of replacement doses, and (3) determination of the presence or absence of an acquired inhibitor antibody against factor VIII or IX in patients with hemophilia A or B.

TREATMENT

Therapy for Hemophilia

Unlike most conditions in medical practice, hemophilia should be treated at the earliest symptoms suggestive of joint hemorrhage, long before the development of any physical findings. Only in this way can the long-term disabling sequelae be prevented.

Patient Education

The keystone of therapy in hemophilia is to provide the patient with access to immediate and adequate correction of the hemostatic defect at the earliest symptom suggestive of hemorrhage. Because hemophilia treatment centers now exist in all areas of the United States and Canada, training usually takes place at a major hemophilia center.

At most centers, all patients and selected family members receive an individual half-day course on the pathophysiology, diagnosis, and therapy of hemophilia. Patients are taught the possible symptoms and signs of some of the major lesions of hemophilia and how much factor VIII or IX to give for various types of bleeding. The patient and his family are then taught intravenous technique, and family members perform several venipunctures on each other. Special attention is also paid to the indications for making contact with the physician or the hemophilia center.

Patients are instructed to raise their factor VIII or IX level via home infusion at the first suggestion of joint or muscle hemorrhage. Prophylactic infusions are used for brief periods in occasional patients, as part of a therapy program for recurrent monarticular hemarthrosis, or when a child is mastering a new physical activity such as bicycle riding.

All patients should attend yearly comprehensive evaluation sessions as a minimum mandatory requirement for continuation of the program. At this comprehensive clinic, a decision is made whether interim visits will be necessary during the ensuing year and whether changes in supportive health care measures are required. During the course of each evaluation, every patient is personally interviewed and examined by a hematologist, an orthopedic surgeon, and/or a rheumatologist. He is also usually seen by a nurse practitioner, a medical social worker, an oral surgeon, a physical therapist, a vocational counselor, and, when indicated, a genetic counselor.

Replacement Therapy

Factor VIII Replacement. The half-life of factor VIII in vivo is between 8 and 12 hours. Although the minimum plasma level necessary to achieve hemostasis will depend on the location, severity, and duration of hemorrhage, a level of 30 percent (0.30 unit per ml) is generally the goal in most acute hemorrhages. Early bleeding into muscles or joints will be arrested by a single infusion to this level in 95 percent of episodes. For advanced joint or muscle bleeding, a factor VIII level of 50 percent should be achieved.

The therapeutic material will contain a certain number of factor VIII units. One unit is equivalent to the factor VIII found in 1 ml of pooled fresh frozen plasma. For factor VIII, the replacement formula is as follows:

each unit of factor VIII infused per kilogram of body weight yields a 2 percent rise in plasma VIII level (i.e., 0.02 unit per ml)

To achieve a 50 percent level in vivo, a 70-kg man with an advanced hemarthrosis would thus require 25 × 70, or approximately 1750, units of factor VIII, assuming a starting point of essentially 0 percent factor VIII.

If a given minimum level is to be maintained over several days, this can be achieved by (1) giving an initial infusion to twice the desired minimum; (2) giving one half of this dose every 12 hours, assuming a 12-hour half-life; and (3) performing factor VIII assays every several days for more precise dose adjustments. To achieve a 20 percent level in vivo a 70-kg man with an early hemarthrosis would thus require 20 × 70, or approximately 1400, units of factor IX, assuming a starting point of essentially 0 percent factor IX. Because factor IX has a significantly longer half-life than factor VIII, and because lower in vivo minimum levels appear necessary for hemostasis, fresh frozen plasma is still sometimes used in hemophilia B. For moderately severe or severe disease, or for prolonged or major bleeding, factor IX concentrate is generally preferred, however.

If a given minimum level is to be maintained over several days, this can be achieved by methods similar to those described for factor VIII, except that the half-life of 24 hours (as compared with approximately 12 hours for factor VIII) indicates the need for either lower or less frequent subsequent doses by a factor of 50 percent. Factor IX assays should be monitored every few days for adequate control.

There are several commercially available factor IX concentrates at present. Most products contain factor II, VII, IX, and X, but because of the high hepatitis risk for individuals not previously frequently exposed to blood products, these products should probably be used only for the treatment of hemophilia B.

Wet frozen cryoprecipitate was the replacement product of choice several years ago and is still used as such in some centers. The average bag of cryoprecipitate from the average blood center should be assumed to contain approximately 70 units of factor VIII for purposes of calculation.

There are available many different commercial factor VIII concentrates, made from large pools of normal plasma and sold in lyophilized form. When the concentrate is reconstituted, one can administer 1000 units of factor VIII in 10 to 30 ml volume, depending on the product used; each vial is labeled with the number of units contained, and such figures are quite accurate. The major disadvantage is cost; current prices are in the range of 35 to 90¢ per factor VIII unit. These materials have made early and intensive home therapy possible, however, and thus overall costs of health care have greatly declined for patients treated with these materials.

Arginine vasopressin (DDAVP, desmopressin) is used in the treatment of mild hemophilia A to endogenously raise the factor VIII level in such patients. A baseline factor VIII level of at least 10 percent is required for efficacy.[54]

Factor IX Replacement. Factor IX is not found in either cryoprecipitate or factor VIII concentrate;

these two materials are totally ineffective for the treatment of hemophilia B.

The half-life of factor IX in vivo is between 20 and 24 hours. Although the plasma level necessary to achieve hemostasis will depend on the location, severity, and duration of hemorrhage, a minimum hemostatic level of 20 percent (0.20 unit per ml) is generally sought for most acute hemorrhages. Early bleeding into muscles or joints will be permanently arrested by a single infusion to this level in 95 percent of episodes. For more advanced joint or muscle bleeding a factor IX level of 40 percent should be achieved.

The therapeutic material will contain a number of factor IX units. One unit is equivalent to the factor IX found in 1 ml of pooled fresh frozen plasma. For factor IX, the replacement formula is as follows:

each unit of factor IX infused per kilogram of body weight yields a 1 percent rise in plasma IX level (i.e., 0.01 unit per ml)

Complications of Factor Replacement Therapy

Inhibitor Antibodies

The development of inhibitor antibody occurs only after exposure to factor VIII but is not related to source of replacement product or to frequency or intensity of exposure. There may be a familial predisposition to the development of this dreaded complication. Because bleeding cannot be reliably controlled in patients with inhibitor antibodies, elective surgery should not be considered in most such patients.

Inhibitor antibodies in factor VIII-deficient hemophiliacs have a highly unpredictable natural history. At times, low titer and clinically weak antibodies are easily neutralized by factor VIII and are found not to undergo anamnestic rises in titer after multiple factor VIII challenges. Such antibodies may unexpectedly become high in titer. Other patients will develop rising antibody titers after each exposure to factor VIII. Still other patients appear to have spontaneously lost their antibody despite multiple subsequent factor VIII challenges.

The type of antibody response to factor VIII infusion and the patient's clinical response will dictate therapy. The therapy of patients with inhibitor antibodies ranges from total avoidance of all exposure to factor VIII in some centers to aggressive megadose factor VIII replacement in others. Factor IX concentrate, possibly because of its variable contamination with activated factor X and procoagulant phospholipids, is often efficacious. Purposefully activated factor IX concentrates have been useful in certain patients with inhibitor antibodies who are treatment failures. Porcine factor VIII concentrate is another valuable therapy. The use of immunosuppressives or glucocorticoids has been abandoned in most centers owing to lack of efficacy in this condition and to

serious side effects. Intravenous immunoglobulin is occasionally useful,[55] and a regimen of factor VIII infusions for induction of tolerance has been proposed.[56]

In the authors' experience, patients with low titer antibodies that remain low in titer after repeated therapy often do well with standard but repeated doses of factor VIII concentrate. For those who fail to benefit, or have higher titers, factor IX concentrate is used; both groups of patients are often on home therapy, and bleeding is more likely to be arrested when treatment is applied at "aura" than if it is delayed.

Inhibitor antibody against factor IX is exceedingly rare. There is no generally accepted efficacious therapy, treatment usually including large and frequent doses of factor IX concentrate.

Human Immunodeficiency Virus (HIV). HIV was introduced into the American blood supply in the 1970s.[57] By the late 1970s factor concentrate was widely contaminated and by 1982, approximately 50 percent of persons with hemophilia were infected with HIV.[58] Currently 70 percent of American hemophiliacs are infected with HIV and over 2000 have contracted AIDS.[59–61] Since 1985, in the manufacture of concentrates, a triple barrier to viral contamination has occurred: (1) self-exclusion for donors, (2) donor screening with serologic tests for HIV, and (3) viral inactivation during concentrate production. Viral inactivation procedures include heating while the concentrate is in solution or after lyophilization and treating the concentrate with solvent/detergent to disrupt the lipid membranes of viruses.[62] Concentrates treated with a virucidal method, as are all factor concentrates in the United States, are unlikely to transmit HIV.[63]

Viral Hepatitis. A second infectious side effect of either cryoprecipitate or factor concentrate is hepatitis, which may be on the basis of parenterally transmitted hepatitis B virus (HBV), hepatitis C virus (HCV), cytomegalovirus, or other, as of yet unidentified, pathogens. In most series, the great majority of treated hemophiliacs will have plasma levels of HBV surface antibody, and a significant minority (2 to 5 percent) will carry HBV surface antigen. Presumably because of prior extensive plasma product exposure from early in life, the incidence of overt clinical hepatitis in those with moderately severe or severe hemophilia who receive pooled commercial concentrate is low.

Approximately 70 percent of hemophiliacs have antibody to HCV,[64] which, unlike HBV antibody, may be a marker for ongoing infection. Virucidal concentrate treatment methods have reduced but not eliminated parenteral transmission of HBV and HCV. Vaccination against HBV, now given to all infants with hemophilia, and donor screening are additional barriers to transmission.

Other Complications. In addition to the allergic and infectious side effects listed for factor VIII concentrate, factor IX therapy, particularly in high doses, may also predispose to deep venous and other types of thrombosis. Some physicians recommend the addition of small doses of heparin to factor IX concentrate or to the recipient in cases of high-dose factor IX replacement for surgery. Thrombosis has not been recorded in the home therapy of routine acute hemorrhage in hemophilia B.

Therapy for Musculoskeletal Complications of Hemophilia

Acute Hemarthrosis

The single most important measure in the therapy of acute hemarthrosis is prompt correction of the clotting abnormality by administration of the deficient factor. Although oral glucocorticoid therapy (5 days) has been advocated in the setting of severe or advanced acute episodes, no controlled studies support this practice.[65] Arthrocentesis, if accomplished within 24 hours of the onset of symptoms (but after factor replacement), may be symptomatically beneficial in advanced acute hemarthrosis but should be considered mandatory at any time if suspicion of infection is high, for diagnostic and potentially therapeutic purposes.[21] Analgesia and brief joint immobilization for no more than 2 days often aid in pain control. Subsequently, passive range of motion isometric exercise should be begun to reduce the likelihood of joint contracture.

Chronic Hemophilic Arthropathy

A variety of conservative measures can bring remarkable benefit in the setting of chronic hemophilic arthropathy.[66–69] These include (1) prophylactic factor infusions, (2) intensive physical therapy for muscle building and increased joint stability, (3) periods of avoidance of weight-bearing to allow regression of synovitis, (4) correction of flexion contractures by wedging casts, night splints, or the judicious use of traction, and (5) training in sports to allow future maintenance of muscle mass. In modern treatment programs, aspiration of joints with chronic synovial effusions is rarely necessary or of lasting benefit. A small study has suggested that intra-articular methylprednisolone might be of short-term value in reducing symptoms and frequency of hemarthroses in involved joints.[70] Failure of these conservative modalities to relieve symptoms or produce regression of synovitis should prompt consideration of other options, including the use of nonsteroidal anti-inflammatory drugs (NSAIDs), synovectomy, and joint replacement in the end-stage.

Despite the obvious theoretical contraindications to the usage of NSAIDs in hemophilia (namely, the antiplatelet effects typified by acetylsalicylic acid), several NSAIDs may be used safely for short periods of time. Ibuprofen, salsalate, and choline magnesium salicylate have been demonstrated in small numbers of hemophiliacs to produce no significant alterations in platelet function, bleeding time, or coagulation variables.[71–75] Ibuprofen in several studies[72–75] and choline magnesium salicylate in one study[73] have also been shown to be both safe and efficacious in reducing joint pain and analgesic dependence in patients with hemophilia.

Surgery in Hemophilic Arthropathy

Synovectomy. Synovectomy in the setting of hemophilic arthritis can be accomplished surgically, arthroscopically, or through intra-articular injections of radioactive colloids. Patients should be considered for synovectomy if, despite aggressive conservative measures, persistent repeated hemarthroses continue with ongoing chronic synovitis. In our center, specific indications for synovectomy include persistence of at least two hemathroses per month in the same joint accompanied by symptoms and signs of chronic synovitis, despite at least 4 months of conservative therapy, including intensive factor replacement. The major drawback to surgical synovectomy remains the observation, confirmed in most series, that joint motion is significantly reduced postoperatively when compared with preoperative baseline, despite intensive rehabilitation.

To overcome the reduction of joint motion, as well as the high cost of hospitalization and factor replacement therapy attendant with surgical synovectomy, arthroscopic synovectomy has been employed in chronic hemophilic arthritis in recent years (see Chapters 38 and 39). Most follow-up series report that this technique is as successful as surgical synovectomy, while resulting in less loss of motion,[76–78] particularly when continuous passive motion is used in the postoperative period.[79]

Radioisotopic synovectomy using yttrium-90[80, 81] and, by the authors in conjunction with Sledge,[82] dysprosium-165 has had some clinical success in patients with hemophilia and is especially useful in those with circulating factor inhibitors in whom surgery is absolutely contraindicated. Possible long-term carcinogenic and teratogenic effects remain the major contraindications to the use of this technique in most hemophiliacs who may have long life expectancies and are still of reproductive age. A major advantage, however, is that it is minimally invasive, resulting in low factor replacement requirements and morbidity. Radioisotopic synovectomy remains experimental in the United States.

Total Joint Replacement. Total joint replacement has been safely and successfully employed in end-stage hemophilic arthropathy;[83–86] the primary indication is pain in the involved joint refractory to all conservative measures. Of concern, however, is the fact that most hemophilic patients in need of total joint replacement are young and may, if not infected with HIV, have a long life expectancy, thus virtually insuring the need for one or more revisions during the course of their lifetime. In addition, patients are at risk for complications of surgery attributable to their underlying coagulopathy. Finally, the population of hemophilic patients who are HIV positive may have a higher than expected incidence of postoperative infections and poor results,[87] suggesting that orthopedic procedures should be reserved for the most severe cases in this setting.

References

1. Roberts, H. R., and Jones, M. R.: Hemophilia and related conditions: Congenital deficiencies of prothrombin (factor II), factor V, and factors VII to XII. In Williams, W. J., Beutler, E., Erslev, A. J., Lichtman, M. A. (eds.): Hematology. New York, McGraw-Hill, 1990.
2. Larrieu, J. M., Caen, J. P., Meyer, D. O., et al: Congenital bleeding disorders with long bleeding time and normal platelet count. II. Von Willebrand's disease (report of thirty-seven patients). Am. J. Med. 45:354, 1968.
3. Ahlberg, A., and Silwer, J.: Arthropathy in von Willebrand's disease. Acta Orthop. Scand. 41:539, 1970.
4. Wild, J. H., and Zvaifler, N. J.: Hemarthrosis associated with sodium warfarin therapy. Arthritis Rheum. 19:98, 1976.
5. Ramgren, O., Nilsson, I. M., and Blomback, M.: Haemophilia in Sweden. IV. Hereditary investigations. Acta Med. Scand. 171:759, 1962.
6. Astrup, T., and Brakman, P.: Tissue repair and vascular disease in hemophilia. In Brinkhous, K. M., and Hemker, H. C. (eds.): Handbook of Hemophilia. Part 1. New York, American Elsevier Publishing Co., Inc., 1975.
7. Astrup, T., and Sjolin, K. E.: Thromboplastic and fibrinolytic activity of the synovial membrane and fibrous capsular tissue. Proc. Soc. Exp. Biol. Med. 97:852, 1958.
8. Green, D., Ryan, C., Malandruccuolo, N., et al.: Characterization of the coagulant activity of cultured human fibroblasts. Blood 37:47, 1971.
9. Ramgren, O.: Hemophilia in Sweden. III. Symptomatology, with special reference to differences between hemophilia A and B. Acta Med. Scand. 171:237, 1962.
10. Ahlberg, A.: Hemophilia in Sweden. VII. Incidence, treatment, and prophylaxis of arthropathy and other musculoskeletal manifestations of hemophilia A and B. Acta Orthop. Scand. (Suppl.) 77:38, 1965.
11. Kisker, C. T., Perlman, A. W., and Benton, C.: Arthritis in hemophilia. Semin. Arthritis Rheum. 1:220, 1971.
12. Duthie, R. B., Matthews, J. M., Rizza, C. E., and Steel, W. M.: The management of musculo-skeletal problems in the haemophilias. Oxford, Blackwell Scientific Publications, 1972.
13. Hilgartner, M. W.: Hemophilic arthropathy. Adv. Pediatr. 21:139, 1975.
14. Arnold, W. D., and Hilgartner, M. W.: Hemophilic arthropathy. Current concepts of pathogenesis and management. J. Bone Joint Surg. 59A:287, 1977.
15. Gilbert, M. S.: Musculoskeletal manifestations of hemophilia. Mt. Sinai J. Med. 44:339, 1977.
16. Steven, M. M., Madhok, S. Y., Forbes, C. D., and Sturrack, R. D.: Hemophilic arthritis. Am. J. Med. 58:181, 1986.
17. Pavlon, H., Goldman, A. B., and Arnold, W. D.: Hemophilic arthropathy in the joints of the hands and feet. Br. J. Radiol. 52:173, 1979.
18. Rosner, S. M., and Bhogal, R. S.: Infectious arthritis in a hemophiliac. J. Rheumatol. 8:519, 1981.
19. Hofmann, A., Wyatt, R., and Bybee, S. R.: Septic arthritis of the knee in a 12-year-old hemophiliac. J. Pediatr. Orthop. 4:498, 1984.
20. Scott, J. P., Maurer, H. S., and Dias, L. D.: Septic arthritis in two teenaged hemophiliacs. J. Pediatr. 5:748, 1985.
21. Ellison, R. T., and Reller, L. B.: Differentiating pyogenic arthritis from spontaneous hemarthrosis in patients with hemophilia. West. J. Med. 144:42, 1986.
22. Ragni, M. V., and Hanley, E. N.: Septic arthritis in hemophilic patients and infection with human immunodeficiency virus (HIV) (letter). Ann. Intern. Med. 110:168, 1989.
23. Helm, M., Horoszowski, H., Seligsohn, U., et al.: Iliopsoas hematoma: Its detection, and treatment with special reference to hemophilia. Arch. Orthop. Trauma Surg. 99:195, 1982.
24. Madigan, R. P., Hanna, W. T., and Wallace, S. L.: Acute compartment syndrome in hemophilia. J. Bone Joint Surg. 63-A:1327, 1981.
25. Ahlberg, A.: On the natural history of hemophilic pseudotumor. J. Bone Joint Surg. 57A:1133, 1975.
26. Gilbert, M. S., Kreel, I., and Hermann, G.: The hemophilic pseudotumor. In Hilgartner, M. W., and Pochedly, C. (eds.): Hemophilia in the Child and Adult. New York, Raven Press, 1989.
27. Jensen, P. S., and Putman, C. E.: Chondrocalcinosis and hemophilia. Clin Radiol. 28:401, 1977.

28. Schreiber, R. R.:Musculoskeletal system—radiologic findings. In Brinkhous, K. M., and Hemker, H. C. (eds.): Handbook of Hemophilia. Part I. New York, American Elsevier Publishing Co., Inc., 1975.
29. Pettersson, H., Ahlberg, A., and Nilsson, I. M.: A radiologic classification of hemophilic arthropathy. Clin. Orthop. 149:153, 1980.
30. Greene, W. B., Yankaskas, B. C., and Guilford, W. B.: Roentgenographic classifications of hemophilic arthropathy. J. Bone Joint Surg. 71-A:237, 1989.
31. Kulkarni, M. V., Drolshagen, L. F., Kaye, J. J., et al.: MR imaging of hemophiliac arthropathy. J. Comput. Assist. Tomogr. 10:445, 1986.
32. Pettersson, H., Gillespy, T. Kitchens, C., et al.: Magnetic resonance imaging in hemophilic arthropathy of the knee. Acta Radiol. 28:621, 1987.
33. Yulish, B. S., Lieberman, J. M., Strandjord, S. E., et al.: Hemophilic arthropathy: Assessment with MR imaging. Radiology 164:759, 1987.
34. Wilson, D. A., and Prince, J. R.: MR imaging of hemophilic pseudotumors. Am. J. Roentgenol. 150:349, 1988.
35. Graif, M., Martinovitz, U., Strauss, S., et al.: Sonographic localization of hematomas in hemophilic patients with positive iliopsoas sign. Am. J. Roentgenol. 148:121, 1987.
36. Wilson, D. J., McLardy-Smith, P. D., Woodham, C. H., et al.: Diagnostic ultrasound in haemophilia. J. Bone Joint Surg. [Br.] 69:103, 1987.
37. Ghadially, F. N., Ailsby, R. L., and Yong, N. K.: Ultrastructure of the hemophilic synovial membrane and electron-probe x-ray analysis of hemosiderin. J. Pathol. 120:201, 1976.
38. Stein, H., and Duthie, R. B.: The pathogenesis of chronic hemophilic arthropathy. J. Bone Joint Surg. 63B:600, 1981.
39. Roy, S., and Ghadially, F. N.: Pathology of experimental hemarthrosis. Ann. Rheum. Dis. 25:402, 1966.
40. Roy, S., and Ghadially, F. N.: Ultrastructure of synovial membrane in human hemarthrosis. J. Bone Joint Surg. 49A:1636, 1967.
41. Swanton, M. C., and Wysocki, G. P.: Pathology of joints in canine hemophilia A. In Brinkhous, K. M., and Hemker, H. C. (eds.): Handbook of Hemophilia. Part I. New York, American Elsevier Publishing Co., Inc., 1975.
42. Morris, C. J., Blake, D. R., Wainwright, A. C., and Steven, M. M.: Relationship between iron deposits and tissue damage in the synovium: An ultrastructural study. Ann. Rheum. Dis. 45:21, 1986.
43. Hough, A. J., Banfield, W. G., and Sokoloff, L.: Cartilage in hemophilic arthropathy, Arch. Pathol. Lab. Med. 100:91, 1976.
44. Hoaglund, F. T.: Experimental hemarthrosis. J. Bone Joint Surg. 49A:285, 1967.
45. Okazaki, I., Brinckerhoff, C. E., Sinclair, J. F., Sinclair, P. R., Bonkowsky, H. L., and Harris, E. D., Jr.: Iron increases collagenase production by rabbit synovial fibroblasts. J. Lab. Clin. Med. 97:396, 1981.
46. Choi, Y. C., Hough, A. J., Morris, G. M., et al.: Experimental siderosis of articular chondrocytes cultured in vitro. Arthritis Rheum. 24:809, 1981.
47. Greenwald, R. A., and Moy, W. W.: Effect of oxygen-derived free radicals on hyaluronic acid, Arthritis Rheum. 23:455, 1980.
48. Lunec, J., Halloran, S. P., White, A. J., and Dormandy, T. L.: Free-radical oxidation (peroxidation) products in serum and synovial fluid in rheumatoid arthritis. J. Rheumatol. 8:233, 1981.
49. Fantone, J. C., and Ward, P. A.: Role of oxygen-derived free radicals and metabolites in leukocyte-dependent inflammatory reactions. Am. J. Pathol. 107:395, 1982.
50. Biemond, P., Swaak, A. J. G., vanEijk, H. G., and Koster, J. F.: Intraarticular ferritin-bound iron in rheumatoid arthritis. A factor that increases oxygen free radical-induced tissue destruction. Arthritis Rheum. 29:1187, 1986.
51. Mainardi, C. L., Levine, P. H., Werb, Z., et al.: Proliferative synovitis in hemophilia. Biochemical and morphologic observations. Arthritis Rheum. 21:137, 1978.
52. Parsons, J. R., Zingler, B. M., McKeon, J. J.: Mechanical and histological studies of acute joint hemorrhage. Orthopedics 10:1019, 1987.
53. Convery, F. R., Woo S. L. Y., Akeson, W. F., et al.: Experimental hemarthrosis in the knee of the mature canine. Arthritis Rheum. 19:59, 1976.
54. Mannucci, P. M.: DDAVP in haemophilia. Lancet 2:1171, 1977.
55. Sultan, Y., Kazatchkine, M. D., Maisonneuve, P., et al.: Anti-idiotypic suppression of autoantibodies to factor VIII by high dose intravenous gammaglobulin. Lancet 2:765, 1984.
56. van Leeuwen, E. F., Mauser-Bunschoten, E. P., van Dijken, P. J., et al.: Disappearance of factor VIII:C antibodies in patients with haemophilia A upon frequent administration of factor VIII in intermediate or low dose. Br. J. Haematol. 64:291, 1986.
57. Levine, P. H.: The acquired immune deficiency syndrome in persons with hemophilia. Ann. Intern. Med. 103:723, 1985.
58. Eyster, M. G., Goedert, J. J., Sarngadharan, M. G., et al.: Development and early natural history of HTLV-III antibodies in persons with hemophilia. J.A.M.A. 253:2219, 1985.
59. Centers for Disease Control: HIV/AIDS Surveillance Report. December 1989, pp. 1–16.

60. Jackson, J. B., Sannerud, K. J., Hopsicker, J. S., et al.: Hemophiliacs with antibody against human immunodeficiency virus are actively infected. J.A.M.A. 260:2236, 1988.

61. Eyster, M. E., Ballard, J. O., Gail, M. H., et al.: Predictive markers for the acquired immunodeficiency syndrome (AIDS) in hemophiliacs: Persistence of p24 antigen and low T4 cell count. Ann. Intern. Med. 110:963, 1989.

62. Brettler, D. B., and Levine, P. H.: Factor concentrates for treatment of hemophilia. Which one to choose? Blood 73:2067, 1989.

63. Blomback, M., Schulman, S., Berntorp, E., et al.: Survey of non-U.S. hemophilia treatment centers for HIV seroconversions following therapy with heat treated factor concentrates. MMWR 36:121, 1987.

64. Brettler, D. B., Forsberg, J. L., Dienstag, J. L., et al.: The prevalence of antibody to HCV in a cohort of hemophilic patients. Blood 76:254, 1990.

65. Kisker, C. T., and Burke, C.: Double-blind studies on the use of corticosteroids in the treatment of acute hemarthrosis in patients with hemophilia. N. Engl. J. Med. 282:639, 1970.

66. Dietrich, S. L.: Rehabilitation and nonsurgical management of musculoskeletal problems in the hemophilic patient. Ann. N.Y. Acad. Sci. 240:328, 1975.

67. Schumacher, P.: Discussion paper: Orthotic management in hemophilia Ann. N.Y. Acad. Sci. 240:344, 1975.

68. Atkins, R. M., Henderson, N. J., and Duthie, R. B.: Joint contractures in the hemophilias. Clin. Orthop. 219:97, 1987.

69. Miser, A. W., Miser, J. S., and Newton, W. A.: Intensive factor replacement for management of chronic synovitis in hemophilic children. Am. J. Pediatr. Hematol. Oncol. 8:66, 1986.

70. Shupak, R., Teitel, J., Garvey, M. B., et al.: Intraarticular methylprednisolone in hemophilic arthropathy. Am. J. Hematol. 27:26, 1988.

71. McIntyre, B. A., Phelp, R. B., and Inwood, M. J.: Effect of ibuprofen on platelet function in normal subjects and haemophilic patients. Clin. Pharmacol. Ther. 24:616, 1977.

72. Hasiba, U., Scranton, P. E., Lewis, J. H., and Spors, J. A.: Efficacy and safety of ibuprofen for haemophilic arthropathy. Arch. Intern. Med. 140:1583, 1980.

73. Thomas, P., Hepburn, B., Kim, H. C., and Saich, P.: Non-steroidal antiinflammatory drugs in the treatment of haemophilic arthropathy. Am. J. Hematol. 12:131, 1982.

74. Inwood, M. J., Kellaclley, B., and Startup, S. J.: The use and safety of ibuprofen in the haemophiliac. Blood 61:709, 1983.

75. Steven, M. M., et al.: Non-steroidal anti-inflammatory drugs in haemophilic arthritis. Haemostasis 15:204, 1985.

76. Weidel, J. D.: Arthroscopic synovectomy for chronic hemophilic synovitis of the knee. Arthroscopy 1:205, 1985.

77. Klein, K. S., Aland, C. M., Kim, H. C. et al.: Long-term follow-up of arthroscopic synovectomy for chronic hemophilic synovitis. Arthroscopy 3:231, 1987.

78. Weidel, J. D.: Arthroscopy of the knee in hemophilia. Prog. Clin. Biol. Res. 324:231, 1990.

79. Limbird, T. J., and Dennis, S. C. Synovectomy and continuous passive motion (CPM) in hemophiliac patients. Arthroscopy 3:74, 1987.

80. Menkes, C. J., et al.: Le traitement des arthropathies hemophiliques par la synoviorthese medicale. Pathol. Biol. (Paris) 23 (Suppl.): 28, 1975.

81. Rivard, G. E., et al.: Synoviorthesis in patients with hemophilia and inhibitors. Can. Med. Assoc. J. 127:41, 1982.

82. Sledge, C. B., Brigham and Women's Hospital, Boston, MA. Unpublished observations.

83. Goldberg, V. M., Heiple, K. G., Ratnoff, O. D., et al.: Total knee arthroplasty in classic hemophilia. J. Bone Joint Surg. 63-A:695, 1981.

84. Rana, N. A., Shapiro, G. R., and Green, D.: Long-term follow-up of prosthetic joint replacement in hemophilia. Am. J. Hematol. 23:329, 1986.

85. Karthaus, R. P., and Novakova, I. R. O.: Total knee replacement in haemophilic arthropathy. J. Bone Joint Surg. 70-B:382, 1988.

86. Luck, J. V., Jr., and Kasper, C. K.: Surgical management of advanced hemophilic arthropathy. An overview of 20 years' experience. Clin. Orthop. 242:60, 1989.

87. Greene, W. B., DeGnore, L. T., and White, G. C.: Orthopaedic procedures and prognosis in hemophilic patients who are seropositive for human immunodeficiency virus. J. Bone Joint Surg. 72-A:2, 1990.

Hemoglobinopathies and Arthritis

Musculoskeletal manifestations are common in the hemoglobinopathies. Problems can be seen not only in homozygous sickle cell (hemoglobin SS) disease but also in sickle C hemoglobin and sickle-thalassemia diseases. Patients with sickle cell disease and high circulating levels of hemoglobin F tend to have milder disease.[1] Rheumatic manifestations appear to be rare in sickle trait (hemoglobin AS) but have been reported in beta(β)-thalassemia.

Hemoglobin S, which is most common in blacks, results from a unique DNA base-pair substitution (β^s) in the 6th codon of the β globin gene leading to the substitution of a single amino acid in the β-chain of hemoglobin.[2] Glutamic acid, which is normally present, is replaced by valine. This change produces systemic disease, which is manifested by sickling of the erythrocytes. When this sickling occurs in small vessels it is the presumed basis for the painful crises. Abnormal interactions between sickled erythrocytes and endothelium have received emphasis.[3] Other manifestations are hemolytic anemia, hyposthenuria, leg ulcers, hyporegenerative crises, increased infections—especially with salmonellae—and the bone and joint problems to be discussed. The diagnosis is suspected when sickled cells are identified in vitro through the use of reducing agents such as metabisulfite. Diagnosis of the homozygous disease is established by starch or cellulose acetate hemoglobin electrophoresis showing 76 to 100 percent hemoglobin S. Diagnoses can now also be established with allele-specific oligonucleotide probes.[4]

Hemoglobin C disease is less common and is caused by the substitution of lysine for glutamic acid in the β-chains. The pure disease produces some hemolysis and many target cells, but this abnormal hemoglobin is most important when combined with hemoglobin S. Hemoglobin SC may be associated with a high frequency of aseptic necrosis of bone or with thromboembolic problems.[5] More than 300 human hemoglobin variants have been discovered; most are caused by mutations in single amino acids. The great majority are of no known clinical significance. Other abnormal hemoglobins can be associated with hemoglobin S, but there is little information about their musculoskeletal manifestations.

β-Thalassemia refers to another inherited disorder that is especially common in persons of Mediterranean background. A variety of mutations result in reduced or absent β-chains, producing a very unstable hemoglobin with formation of Heinz bodies. There are high levels of hemoglobin F. Patients with β-thalassemia have hemolytic anemia, which is severe and transfusion dependent in homozygotes, splenomegaly, and hyperplastic bone marrows, producing changes on skeletal radiographs. Patients with a combination of β-thalassemia and hemoglobin S often have increased hemoglobin A2. This hemoglobinopathy clinically combines features of thalassemia and homozygous sickle cell disease.

SICKLE CELL DISEASE (Table 91–1)

Bone Trabecular Changes Associated with Expansion of the Bone Marrow. Sickle cell disease and other hemoglobinopathies associated with hemolysis cause characteristic expansion of the bone marrow, producing wider intertrabecular spaces with coarser trabeculations that are most evident in the axial skeleton in which red (hematopoietic) marrow is most plentiful (Fig. 91–1). In sickle cell patients, red marrow also persists more peripherally in the long bones near joints and even in the small tarsal and carpal bones, often causing some thinning of cortical bone with widening of the medulla. Total width of the bone may be increased. Radiographic signs of marrow expansion vary widely and can be quite subtle.

In patients with SC hemoglobin, hemolysis tends to be less, and there are fewer bone trabecular changes.[6] Scattered increased densities can interrupt

Table 91–1. MUSCULOSKELETAL MANIFESTATIONS OF SICKLE CELL DISEASE

Bone trabecular changes
Hand-foot syndrome
Hyperuricemia and gout
Osteomyelitis
Septic arthritis
Joint effusions
Erosions and chronic inflammation
Bone infarctions
Avascular necrosis
Others, including muscle necrosis

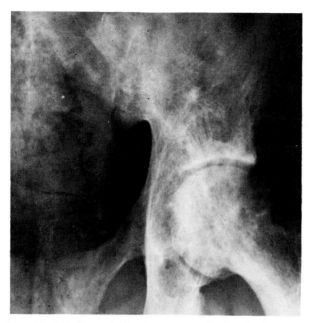

Figure 91–1. Radiograph showing coarsened trabeculae from marrow expansion in severe sickle cell anemia. Some focal densities may be a result of bone infarctions.

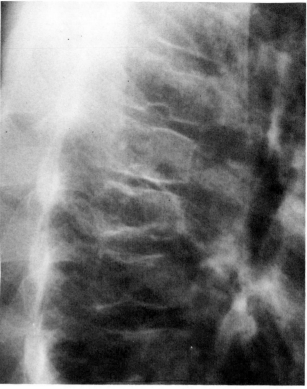

Figure 91–2. Cuplike indentation of vertebral body in radiograph in sickle cell disease.

trabecular patterns and are probably attributable to areas of marrow infarction (see later discussion).

Skull radiographs can show thickening of the diploë with a granular texture. Occasionally in severe sickle cell disease the coarse trabeculae are arranged perpendicular to the curvature of the vault, giving "hair on-end" or "porcupine quill" trabeculae. This is more common in thalassemia major than in sickle cell disease.[7]

Vertebral bodies may also have characteristic alterations. Coarsened trabeculae are most often vertical, and the bodies of the vertebrae can have a characteristic deep central cup-like indentation[8] (Fig. 91–2). Vertebral compression can occur with resulting accentuated dorsal kyphosis and lumbar lordosis. Osteophytes occasionally develop, and there can even be fusion of vertebrae.

Protrusio acetabuli has been reported in 14 of 155 adults with sickle cell disease and pelvic radiographs. This did not correlate with changes in the femoral head and was believed to be a result of softening of acetabular bone.[9]

The Hand-Foot Syndrome. Children from 6 months to 2 years of age may develop the hand-foot syndrome. This consists of dramatic, diffuse, symmetric, very tender, warm swelling of the hands, feet, or both (Fig. 91–3).[10] Hematologic signs and fever may be absent, or fever may be present with peripheral blood leukocytosis up to 55,000 cells per mm³. Swelling lasts 1 week to 3 weeks. Infarction of marrow, cortical bone, periosteum, and periarticular tissues appears most likely to be the underlying mechanism. Radiographs may be normal, especially during the first week but later show marrow densities, lytic areas, or periosteal elevation. Most of the

periosteal changes are no longer identifiable in 1 month to 4 months. Rerefaction of the medulla can occur. Hematopoiesis occurring in the small finger and toe bones of children, but not in adults even with SS hemoglobin disease, is presumably a factor in the restriction of this syndrome to childhood.

The frequency varies from 17 percent in a study of American blacks to 80 percent in a group of African children.[8] Venous stasis in the extremities of African

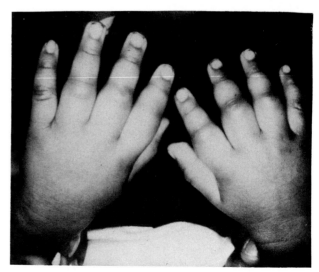

Figure 91–3. Diffusely swollen hands as seen in the hand-foot syndrome of young children with sickle cell disease.

children strapped to their mothers' backs has been suggested as a factor to explain the increased frequency in Africa. Exposure to cold is not a factor.[10] Five examples have been described in Saudi Arabians with SS hemoglobin, a reminder that the various manifestations of sickle cell disease are not restricted to blacks.[11] Although hand-foot syndrome is characteristic of SS hemoglobin disease, it has also been reported in children with SC hemoglobin disease and S thalassemia. Metatarsal lysis was seen in one case.[10] Usually only analgesics have been used for therapy. Osteomyelitis can also occur in children and must always be kept in mind.

Hyperuricemia and Gout. Approximately 40 percent of adults with sickle cell disease are hyperuricemic (most often 6.5 mg per dl to 11 mg per dl), whereas only occasionally do affected children younger than 13 years of age have elevated serum uric acid levels. Overproduction of uric acid associated with increased red cell turnover does occur and seems initially to be associated with hyperuricosuria.[12] In young people, urate clearance maintains a normal serum uric acid concentration, but in older patients uric acid excretion often diminishes and results in hyperuricemia.

Clinical diagnoses of acute gouty arthritis have been reported in patients with sickle hemoglobin.[13] Typical crystals of monosodium urate have been found less often,[11] although eight cases were found in one review.[14] Attacks may be polyarticular and associated with fever, so they could be confused with sickle cell crises unless crystals are carefully sought.

Osteomyelitis. Patients with sickle cell disease are especially susceptible to bacterial infection. The frequency of osteomyelitis, caused by a variety of organisms (but predominantly salmonellae), is more than 100 times that seen in normal populations.[15] Reasons for the increased incidence of infections may include tissue damage from sickling, increased hospital exposure to infection, impaired clearing of bacteria after splenic fibrosis, impaired phagocytosis at low oxygen tensions, impaired opsonic activity,[16, 17] and recently noted impaired production of gamma (γ)-interferon.[18] More than 80 percent of hematogenous osteomyelitis in persons without hemoglobinopathies is attributable to staphylococci, but more than 50 percent of osteomyelitis in sickle cell patients is caused by salmonellae.[15] Most other organisms have also been gram-negative.[19]

Multiple sites of osteomyelitis may be seen in infected patients. Onset may not be dramatic, and bone infection has apparently been overlooked for years. Osteomyelitis may be very difficult to distinguish radiographically from the results of bone infarction. Progression or other signs of infection are often needed for diagnosis; scans with indium-labeled leukocytes may help suggest the diagnosis.[20] Acute osteomyelitis is more common in children. The medullary cavities of diaphyses or epiphyses of long bones are often involved. Both crisis and infection may present with bone pain, fever, and leuko-

cytosis. Persistent fever must increase the concern about osteomyelitis. Infection rarely extends from bones into joints, although this seemed more common in a recent Nigerian series.[19] Abscess and sinus formation may develop. Bone destruction can occur with periosteal elevation, progressive massive longitudinal intracortical diaphyseal fissuring, and involucrum formation. Exploration or demonstration of the organism from a draining site is needed for diagnosis.

Treatment generally includes splinting severely involved bones to prevent pathologic fracture. Salmonella bone infection seems to respond well to chloramphenicol without much development of chronic osteomyelitis. Surgical drainage has not been necessary in most cases. Salmonella osteomyelitis has also been seen in sickle-thalassemia disease[21] and SC hemoglobin disease but not sickle trait.

Septic Arthritis. Septic arthritis may be seen but fortunately is not especially common[15, 22] and is much less frequent than osteomyelitis. Multiple joints are involved in some cases. A variety of organisms are seen, including staphylococci, *Escherichia coli*, *Enterobacter*, and *Salmonella*. Antibiotic therapy and drainage is usually successful. Five of six cases in one group of children had *Streptococcus* pneumonia.[23] Impaired synovial capillary flow caused by sickling has been suggested as a factor in poor responses to therapy in two patients, and exchange transfusion was suggested as an adjunct to treatment.[24]

Joint Effusions. Far more common than gout or septic arthritis are other joint effusions that appear to be attributable to sickle cell disease. Effusions are often, but not invariably, associated with fever, leukocytosis, and other manifestations of crises.[22] There is generally warmth and tenderness, which may also involve the periarticular areas. Knees have been by far the most commonly involved joints, but effusions have also often been found in elbows and other joints. Ankle effusions have occurred with leg ulcerations, suggesting a vaso-occlusive basis for both, as cultures were negative.[25] Usually only one or two joints are involved. Effusions generally subside in 2 to 14 days.

Radiographs in most of these patients at the time of effusion have shown only the results of previous cortical or medullary infarcts. The physician should not expect to see radiographic evidence of aseptic necrosis or joint space narrowing, and the acute effusions are not purely a mechanical result of severe degenerative changes. Radioisotope scans, using technetium sulfur colloid, have shown areas of decreased marrow uptake adjacent to many effused joints, suggesting small marrow infarctions.[26] Sequential radiographic and scan studies are still limited.

If the sedimentation rate (ESR) is being used in evaluation of the effusion, note that between crises the ESR is usually abnormally low. It may rise with crises or inflammation.[27]

Synovial effusions have usually been "noninflammatory," that is, clear, with most synovial fluid leukocyte counts less than 1000 cells per mm[3] and with a low percentage of polymorphonuclear leukocytes. Similar "noninflammatory" effusions have been seen in sickle-thalassemia.[22, 28]

An increasing number of reported effusions in sickle cell disease have been cloudy and have contained higher leukocyte counts in the inflammatory range.[25, 29] Effusions with leukocyte counts of 33,000[30] and 126,000[31] with 90 to 97 percent polymorphonuclear cells have been described. Crystals or organisms were not found, but some of the patients were given antibiotics. Diggs has noted "purulent exudates" in knee joints, which produced negative results for bacteria on direct examination and culture.[7] No mechanism is yet evident for these inflammatory effusions. Synovial fluid complement levels have not been depressed,[29] and synovial fluid glucose levels have been normal.[22, 30] The only inflammatory effusion studied so far by the author's group contained 29,000 leukocytes per mm[3], with 94 percent polymorphonuclear cells. No crystals were found on a careful 30-minute search with compensated polarized light. Aspiration of the same joint the next day yielded 50,100 leukocytes, with 50 percent of cells containing negatively birefringent crystals typical of monosodium urate; gout thus cannot be excluded by one synovianalysis.

Sickled erythrocytes can be seen in effusions, but this shows only that the patient has sickle hemoglobin,[22] as sickled cells can also be seen in persons with sickle cell trait and arthritis of other causes. Some effusions are dark colored because of the patient's hyperbilirubinemia.

Needle synovial biopsies[22] at the time of acute joint effusions have shown only mild focal lining cell proliferation and a few chronic inflammatory cells in two of five biopsies. Small vessels have been congested in some areas, but in four patients there has also been definite microvascular thrombosis (Fig. 91–4). Electron microscopy of synovium in the author's laboratory has confirmed the presence of occluded vessels, with some vessel lumens containing erythrocytes with the characteristic 18-nm diameter rods or "tactoids" of typical sickled hemoglobin. No electron-dense deposits have been found in vessel walls. These morphologic studies suggest synovial microvascular obstruction as a likely factor in the noninflammatory effusions.[22] Infarction of bone adjacent to joints with effusions or pain may also contribute to joint manifestations. Recent studies also have shown some phagocytosis of sickled cells, suggesting that this could be a possible mechanism for some inflammation.

No specific treatment has been required for the joint effusions. Local steroids are not useful. Treatment of crises generally involves the use of analgesics, including occasional narcotics, plus hydration. Limited exchange transfusion can eliminate many abnormal cells and help terminate prolonged crises.[32] Alkali can be given to prevent acidosis, which can

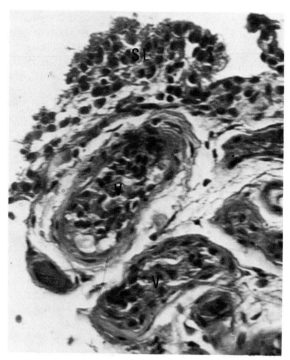

Figure 91–4. Synovium in sickle cell disease. The synovial lining layer (SL) here shows slightly increased cellularity, but, most important, the vessels (V) are occluded with cellular thrombi.

aggravate sickling. Transfusion programs and hydroxyurea therapy, which increases hemoglobin F, may decrease the frequency of crises.[33]

Bloody synovial fluid is not common in sickle cell disease, although this might be expected in some severely destroyed joints resulting from aseptic necrosis. The only hemarthrosis in the patients whom the author's group has studied proved to be due to a small fracture into the knee joint.[26] Casey and Cathcart[34] have suggested that sickle cell trait might have contributed to the development of hemarthrosis in a patient who also had rheumatoid arthritis. Hemathrosis has been briefly noted in one patient with sickle disease[35] and as a feature of inflammatory effusions.

Erosions and Chronic Inflammation. Occasional chronic synovitis with cartilage destruction or erosion has been mentioned in patients with sickle cell disease and no other evident cause for arthritis.[36, 37] Erosions have been described in uncontrolled studies at wrists, metacarpal heads, and calcanei.[37] Lymphocytic and plasma cell infiltration of synovium was seen in one report.[36] Although chronic inflammation is nonspecific and can, for example, be a response to crystals of several types, immunologic mechanisms might possibly be involved. Immune complexes have been implicated as factors in the nephropathy of sickle cell disease and in the leg ulcers.[38] Johnston and associates[39] noted an abnormality of the alternate pathway of complement activation in sickle cell disease. Defects in cell-mediated immunity have also been reported.[40] We have seen that sickle cell disease and rheumatoid (RA) or other arthritis can occur in the same patient, and cases with RA and sickle cell disease have been reported.[41, 42] Two RA patients had sickle cell crises after intra-articular steroid injections.[42]

Bone Infarctions. Bone infarctions occur most commonly in persons with SS hemoglobin, but they may also be seen in SC hemoglobin disease and S thalassemia. Localized deformities and failure of bone growth can result from infarction of the epiphyseal plate of growing children.[6] This is common in both SS hemoglobin and SC hemoglobin disease. The chronic anemia itself can cause some general retardation of growth.[43] Infarctions in cortical bone are thought to be the cause of periosteal elevation, irregular cortical thickening, and sclerosis. Infarctions in the bone marrow produce fibrosis, lysis, sclerosis, new bone formation, and calcified dense marks on radiographs. Radiographs taken at the time of acute bone pain do not show changes from that infarction; small infarcts may never produce radiographic changes.

Radioisotope studies using technetium colloid have shown areas of decreased marrow uptake at sites of bone pain, whereas radiographs were normal. This suggests decreased marrow perfusion. Strontium scans have shown increased uptake in the adjacent cortical bone. Magnetic resonance imaging now may be the most sensitive technique for detection of acute or chronic infarcts.[44] The basis for bone infarcts is presumed to be sickling and thrombosis in small vessels. The bone pains in sickle cell crises are thought to be largely a result of such infarctions. Those infarcts involving only the medulla often produce pain without local tenderness.

Aseptic Necrosis (Avascular Necrosis). When bone infarction occurs from occlusion of end arteries so that necrotic bone is at the articular margin, collapse of the periarticular bone and cartilage occurs. Although necrosis of bone in the shaft is also "aseptic" unless accompanied by infection, the term "aseptic necrosis" is usually used in reference to that necrosis associated with joint disease (see Chapter 97).

Pathologic specimens have not been obtained at the time of initial infarction, so the mechanism remains presumptive based on other findings in sickle cell disease. From pathologic studies after hip disintegration, Sherman[45] suggested that both small hemorrhages and local damage to small blood vessels were significant factors. Although most occlusion seems to be in the microvasculature, some reports suggest that large vessel obliteration can also occur.[46]

Aseptic necrosis of the head of the femur is a common finding and is the most disabling musculoskeletal complication of sickle cell disease. Incidence ranges have been from 2 to 4.5 cases per 100 patient years.[46a] Similar aseptic necrosis occurs at the humeral head, tibial condyles, and occasionally at other sites. Fragments of necrotic bone and cartilage can break loose into the joint cavity. The major joint incongruity leads to further secondary degenerative changes. Radiographs are similar to those of aseptic necrosis from other causes unless the other bony changes described are noted. Initially there is local sclerosis near the joint margin. Patchy lucencies then develop and may include a lucency between the sclerotic bone and the intact bone. Flattening, separation of the necrotic fragment, and secondary osteoarthritis may later be seen.

Radioisotope studies or magnetic resonance imaging can suggest infarction before the development of detectable aseptic necrosis.[26] Technetium pyrophosphate bone scans show increased uptake at sites of infarction. Marrow scans with colloids may show decreased uptake. Aseptic necrosis of the femoral head is rare in children, probably because the artery in the ligamentum teres femoris is patent, giving the femoral head a dual blood supply.

Early treatment can be attempted with prevention of weight-bearing, to try to allow healing without the resultant distortion of bone. Young people seem better able to replace necrotic bone. Replacement of the femoral head with a prosthesis or total hip replacement has not been performed in many patients, and this seems the treatment of choice once articular breakdown has become well established,[47] although results have been variable.[46a] Osteotomies have also been used to try to alter the line of weight-bearing. Bone marrow decompression procedures that are being tried in other types of aseptic necrosis have not been systematically evaluated in sickle cell disease. Surgical core decompression seemed helpful in a patient with aseptic necrosis of both calcanei.[48]

Aseptic necrosis of the humeral head produces much less difficulty and often needs no treatment. Shoulder prostheses have been inserted in two patients with good early results.[47] Total knee joint prosthetic replacements have rarely been required after aseptic necrosis, but good results were reported on short-term follow-up.[49] Preoperative transfusions have been used to diminish the chances of sickling. Tourniquets can be avoided to reduce anoxia and stasis. Good hydration and special efforts during anesthesia to avoid hypoxia and acidosis are merited.[49]

As noted earlier, aseptic necrosis can occur in SC hemoglobin disease and has been believed by some to be even more common than in SS hemoglobin disease.[50] This is possibly because many patients with SS hemoglobin have died at earlier ages from other complications. Diggs[7] has also explained the prominence of infarcts in SC hemoglobin disease on the basis of greater viscosity of the blood. Aseptic necrosis has also been reported in S thalassemia, with SF hemoglobin[50] as well as in sickle cell trait (see later discussion).

Other Musculoskeletal Aspects. Bony ankylosis of hips[7] and spine[51] has been reported, but it is not certain if it was caused by sickle cell disease only or whether infection also played a role. There can be incompletely explained protrusio acetabuli.[9, 52] Irregular sclerosis of sacroiliac joints superficially mimicking the changes of ankylosing spondylitis has been reported[22, 53] and is probably a result of bone infarctions at the joint.

Acute painful localized muscle swelling with necrosis can be seen with crises.[54, 55] Local intramuscular injections may be a factor in some muscle injury.[56] Myonecrosis has been demonstrated[57] and even required fasciotomy for pain relief. Fibrosis may result.[57a]

Leukemia has occasionally occurred in patients with sickle cell disease. One such patient had elbow pain owing to leukemic infiltration.[58]

Sickle Cell Trait. Sickle cell trait (hemoglobin AS) can be associated with systemic sickling under conditions of low oxygen tension.[59] Aseptic necrosis has been reported in patients with sickle cell trait,[60] but another study[61] found no greater incidence of aseptic necrosis in patients with hemoglobin AS than in age-matched controls with AA hemoglobin. There was a slightly increased history of past transient bouts of unexplained joint symptoms in the patients with sickle cell trait. Otherwise unexplained noninflammatory knee effusions were reported in a patient with sickle cell trait and diaphyseal bone infarctions.[62]

THALASSEMIA

In β-thalassemia (major, intermedia, and occasionally minor) there is increased erythrocyte destruction, causing osteopenia, wide medullary spaces, coarse trabeculations, and thin cortices, much as in sickle cell disease. However, aseptic necrosis is not characteristic. In a series of 50 thalassemic patients,[63] 25 patients (ages 5 to 33 years) had ankle pain that was exacerbated by weight-bearing and relieved by rest. There was diffuse ankle and foot tenderness and occasional ankle effusions. Radiographs of the ankles of one patient showed subchondral sclerosis suggesting microfractures. Pathologic studies on two autopsy specimens and on a specimen obtained from a femoral osteotomy showed expansion of hematopoietic marrow into the small bones, osteopenia, increased osteoid, and a striking number of microfractures, findings generally confirmed at other sites.[64] All the patients studied by Gratwick and colleagues[63] had received multiple transfusions, and iron deposition was prominent in the marrow, in osteoid, at cement lines, and in synovial lining cells. Iron was not mentioned in osteocytes or chondrocytes, but slight articular cartilage erosion was reported. Similar osseous iron deposition has been reported by deVernejoul and coworkers[65] along with signs of impaired mineralization.

The ankle problems thus appeared to be due largely to the underlying bone disease, with marrow expansion and osteomalacia also involved. Gratwick et al.[63] speculated that there might be abnormal vitamin D conversion in iron-laden tissues. Decreased 25-hydroxycholecalciferol levels, at least during the winter, have been reported in some patients.[65] More recent studies, however, showed no differences in vitamin D levels from controls in the same area.[64] No therapy has yet been found effective, although rest gives temporary relief. Transfusion therapy may decrease excessive erythropoiesis in patients with severe expansion of the marrow. In one study, 17 of 19 young Turkish patients with thalassemia major or intermedia (aged 2–17) had joint manifestations.[66] Shoulders were more prominently involved than previously noted. Periarticular bone cysts were also prominent.

One patient with thalassemia and repeated transfusions has developed an arthropathy with iron deposition in the synovium,[67] as occurs in idiopathic hemochromatosis. This degenerative arthropathy, which typically involves the second to third metacarpophalangeal joints, hips, knees, and other joints with firm swelling and stiffness, may be complicated by chondrocalcinosis or pseudogout. Other examples of secondary hemochromatosis have been seen in hypoplastic anemia, spherocytosis, and sideroblastic anemia,[68] but so far not in other hemoglobinopathies. Patients with iron overload should have chelation therapy with deferoxamine.[69] Hyperuricemia with gout[70] and septic arthritis[71] can occur in thalassemia. In patients such as these receiving multiple transfusions, the arthritis of viral hepatitis should be considered.

There are reports of aseptic necrosis in thalassemia minor,[72] but there is no evidence that this is more than coincidental. Schlumpf studied seven patients with thalassemia minor (trait) and noted pain without effusions at ankles and also at wrists and elbows.[72] Two other reports of otherwise unexplained monoarticular or oligoarticular disease in thalassemia minor have appeared. Joint effusions have been noninflammatory[73] or mildly inflammatory.[74] Large and small joints have been involved. Most patients have not had radiographic evidence of adjacent bone disease, so mechanisms of this arthropathy are still unclear. Other potentially confusing causes of leg pains in thalassemic patients include claudication-like pain when severely anemic and a postural pulsating pain believed in some cases by Finterbush and colleagues to be related to high intraosseous pressure.[75]

The sicca syndrome has been reported in thalassemia major; iron overload of the salivary gland was demonstrated and presumably resulted from repeated transfusions.[76]

Many younger patients with homozygous β-thalassemia who have HLA-identical donors will be having successful allogeneic bone marrow transplantation.[77] Some of the risks of this procedure and the attendant immunosuppression may affect muscles and joints.

References

1. Miller, B. A., Oliver, N., Salameh, M., Ahmed, M., Antognetti, G., Huisman, T. H. J., Nathan, D., and Orkin, S. H.: Molecular analysis

of the high-hemoglobin F phenotype in Saudi Arabian sickle-cell anemia. N. Engl. J. Med. 316:255, 1987.

2. Dean, J., and Schedchter, A. N.: Sickle cell anemia: Molecular and cellular bases of therapeutic approaches. N. Engl. J. Med. 299:752, 1978.

3. Klug, P. P., Kaye, N., and Jensen, W. N.: Endothelial cell and vascular damage in the sickle cell disorders. Blood Cells 8:175, 1982.

4. Saiki, R. K., Chang, C -A., Levenson, C. H., et al.: Diagnosis of sickle cell anemia and Beta thalassemia with enzymatically amplified DNA and non-radioactive allele-specific oligonucleotide probes. N. Engl. J. Med. 319:537, 1988.

5. Ballas, S. K., Lewis, C. N., Noone, A. M., et al.: Clinical, hematological and biochemical features of SC disease. Am. J. Hematol. 13:37, 1982.

6. Barton, C. J., and Cockshott, W. P.: Bone changes in hemoglobin SC disease. AJR 88:523, 1962.

7. Diggs, L. W.: Bone and joint lesions in sickle cell disease. Clin. Orthop. 52:119, 1967.

8. Lagundoye, S. B.: Radiological feature of sickle cell anemia and related hemoglobinopathies in Nigeria. Afr. J. Med. Sci. 1:315, 1970.

9. Martinez, S., Apple, J. S., Baber, C., Putman, C. E., and Rosse, W. F.: Protrusio acetabuli in sickle-cell anemia. Radiology 151:43, 1984.

10. Watson, R. J., Burko, H., Megas, H., and Robinson, M.: Hand-foot syndrome in sickle cell disease in young children. Pediatrics 31:975, 1963.

11. Perrine, R. P., Pembry, M. E., John, P., Perrine, S., and Shoup, F.: Natural history of sickle cell anemia in Saudi Arabs. A study of 270 subjects. Ann. Intern. Med. 88:1, 1978.

12. Reynolds, M. D.: Gout and hyperuricemia associated with sickle-cell anemia. Semin. Arthritis Rheum. 12:404, 1983.

13. Gold, M. S., Williams, J. C., Spivack, M., and Grann, V.: Sickle cell anemia and hyperuricemia. J.A.M.A. 206:1572, 1968.

14. Leff, R. D., Aldo-Benson, M. A., and Fife, R. S.: Tophaceous gout in a patient with sickle cell-thalassemia: Case report and review of the literature. Arthritis Rheum. 26:928, 1983.

15. Barrett-Connor, E.: Bacterial infection and sickle cell anemia. An analysis of 250 infections in 166 patients and a review of the literature. Medicine 50:97, 1971.

16. Hand, W. L., and King, N. L.: Serum opsonization of salmonella in sickle cell anemia. Am. J. Med. 64:388, 1978.

17. Wilson, W. A., Thomas, E. J., and Sissons, J. G. P.: Complement activation in asymptomatic patients with sickle cell anemia. Clin. Exp. Immunol. 36:130, 1979.

18. Taylor, S. C., Shacks, S. J., Villicana, S. M., et al.: Interferon production in sickle cell disease. Lymphokine Res. 9:415, 1990.

19. Ebong, W. W.: Acute osteomyelitis in Nigerians with sickle cell disease. Ann. Rheum. Dis. 45:911, 1986.

20. Fernandez-Ullos, M., Vasavada, P. J., and Black, R. R.: Detection of acute osteomyelitis with indium-III–labelled white blood cells in a patient with sickle cell disease. Clin. Nucl. Med. 14:97, 1989.

21. Weiss, H., and Katz, S.: Salmonella paravertebral abscess and cervical osteomyelitis in sickle thalassemia disease. South. Med. J. 63:339, 1979.

22. Schumacher, H. R., Andrews, R., and McLaughlin, G.: Arthropathy in sickle cell disease. Ann. Intern. Med. 78:203, 1973.

23. Syrogiannopoulos, G. A., McCracken, G. H., and Nelson, J. D.: Osteoarticular infections in children with sickle cell disease. Pediatrics 78:1090, 1986.

24. Palmer, D. W., and Ellman, M. H.: Septic arthritis and Reiter's syndrome in sickle cell disorders: Case reports and implications for management. South. Med. J. 69:902, 1976.

25. deCeulaer, K., Forbes, M., Roper, D., and Serjeant, G. R.: Non-gouty arthritis in sickle cell disease: Report of 37 consecutive cases. Ann. Rheum. Dis. 43:599, 1984.

26. Alavi, A., Schumacher, H. R., Dorwart, B. B., and Kuhl, D. E.: Bone marrow scan evaluation of arthropathy in sickle cell disorders. Arch. Intern. Med. 136:436, 1976.

27. Lawrence, C., and Fabry, M. E.: Erythrocyte sedimentation rate during steady state and painful crisis in sickle cell anemia. Am. J. Med. 81:801, 1986.

28. Crout, J. E., McKenna, C. H., and Petit, R. M.: Symptomatic joint effusion in sickle cell–beta-thalassemia disease. Report of a case. J.A.M.A. 235:1878, 1976.

29. Espinoza, L. R., Spilberg, I., and Osterland, C. K.: Joint manifestations of sickle cell disease. Medicine 53:295, 1974.

30. Goldberg, M. A.: Sickle cell arthropathy: Analysis of synovial fluid in sickle cell anemia with joint effusion. South. Med. J. 66:956, 1973.

31. Orozco-Alcala, J., and Baum, J.: Arthritis during sickle cell crisis. N. Engl. J. Med. 288:420, 1973.

32. Brody, J. I., Goldsmith, M. H., Park, S. K., and Soltys, H. D.: Symptomatic crises of sickle cell anemia treated by limited exchange transfusions. Ann. Intern. Med. 72:327, 1970.

33. Goldberg, M. A., Bugnara, C., Dover, G. J., et al.: Treatment of sickle cell anemia with hydroxyurea and erythropoietin. N. Engl. J. Med. 323:366, 1990.

34. Casey, D. J., and Cathcart, E. S.: Hemarthrosis and sickle cell trait. Arthritis Rheum. 13:882, 1970.

35. Saheb, F.: Arthropathy in sickle cell disease. N. Engl. J. Med. 288:971, 1973.

36. Schumacher, H. R., Dorwart, B. B., Bond, J., Alavi, A., and Miller, W.: Chronic synovitis with early cartilage destruction in sickle cell disease. Ann. Rheum. Dis. 36:413, 1977.

37. Rothschild, B. M., and Sebes, J. I.: Calcaneal abnormalities and erosive bone disease associated with sickle cell anemia. Am. J. Med. 71:427, 1981.

38. Morgan, A. G., and Venner, A. M.: Immunity and leg ulcers in homozygous sickle cell disease. J. Clin. Lab. Immunol. 6:51, 1981.

39. Johnston, R. B., Newman, S. L., and Struth, A. G.: An abnormality of the alternate pathway of complement activation in sickle cell disease. N. Engl. J. Med. 288:803, 1973.

40. Glassman, A. B., Deas, D. V., Berlinsky, F. S., et al.: Lymphocyte blast transformation and peripheral lymphocyte percentages in patients with sickle cell disease. Ann. Clin. Lab. Sci. 10:9, 1980.

41. Marino, C., and McDonald, E.: Rheumatoid arthritis in a patient with sickle cell disease. J. Rheumatol 17:970, 1990.

42. Gladman, D. D., and Bombardier, C.: Sickle cell crisis following intra-articular steroid therapy for rheumatoid arthritis. Arthritis Rheum. 30:1065, 1987.

43. Serjeant, G. R.: Delayed skeletal maturation in sickle cell anemia in Jamaica. Johns Hopkins Med. J. 132:95, 1973.

44. Rao, V. M., Fishman, M., Mitchell, D. G., et al.: Painful sickle cell crisis: Bone marrow patterns observed with MR imaging. Radiology 161:211, 1986.

45. Sherman, M.: Pathogenesis of disintegration of the hip in sickle cell anemia. South. Med. J. 52:632, 1959.

46. Stockman, J. A., Nigro, M. A., Mishkin, M. M., and Oski, F.: Occlusion of large cerebral vessels in sickle cell anemia. N. Engl. J. Med. 287:846, 1972.

46a. Milner, P. F., Kraus, A. P., Sebes, J. I., et al.: Sickle cell disease as a cause of osteonecrosis of the femoral head. N. Engl. J. Med. 325:1476, 1991.

47. Chung, S. M. K., Alavi, A., and Russell, M. O.: Management of osteonecrosis in sickle cell anemia and its genetic variants. Clin. Orthop. 130:158, 1978.

48. Allen, B. J., and Andrews, B. S.: Bilateral aseptic necrosis of calcanei in an adult male with sickle cell disease treated by a surgical coring procedure. J. Rheumatol. 10:294,1983.

49. Haberman, E. T., and Grayzel, A. I.: Bilateral aseptic necrosis of calcanei in an adult male with sickle cell disease. Clin. Orthop. 100:211, 1974.

50. Chung, S. M. K., and Ralston, E. L.: Necrosis of the femoral head associated with sickle cell anemia and its genetic variants. J. Bone Joint Surg. 51A:33, 1969.

51. Kanyerezi, B. R., Ndugwa, C., Owor, R., Singabual, S. N., Masembe, J., Nzaro, E., and Bosa, J. L.: The spinal column in sickle cell disease. J. Rheumatol. (Suppl.)1:21, 1974.

52. Martinez, S., Apple, J. S., Baber, C., Putman, C. E., and Rosse, W. F.: Protrusio acetabuli in sickle-cell anemia. Radiology 151:43, 1984.

53. Tanaka, K. R., Clifford, G. O., and Axelrod, A. R.: Sickle cell anemia (homozygous S) with aseptic necrosis of the femoral head. Blood 11:998, 1956.

54. Dorwart, B. B., and Gabuzda, T. G.: Symmetric myositis and fasciitis: Complication of sickle cell anemia during vasoocclusion. J. Rheumatol. 12:590, 1985.

55. Schumacher, H. R., Murray, W. M., and Dalinka, M. K.: Acute muscle injury complicating sickle cell crisis. Semin. Arthritis Rheum. 19:243, 1990.

56. Reynolds, M. D., and Castro, O. L.: Panniculomyositis associated with sickle cell disease. Arthritis Rheum. 33(Suppl.):S90, 1990 (abst).

57. Devereux, S., and Knowles, S. M.: Rhabdomyolysis and acute renal failure in sickle cell anemia. Br. Med. J. 290:1707, 1985.

57a. Valeriano-Marcet, J., and Kerr, L. D.: Myonecrosis and myofibrosis as complications of sickle cell anemia. Ann. Intern. Med. 115:99, 1991.

58. Ludmerer, K. M., and Kissane, J. M.: Left elbow pain and death in a young woman with sickle-cell anemia. Am. J. Med. 73:268, 1982.

59. Martin, T. W., Weisman, I. M., Zeballos, R. J., and Stephenson, S. R.: Exercise and hypoxia increase sickling in venous blood from an exercising limb in individuals with sickle cell trait. Am. J. Med. 87:48, 1989.

60. Taylor, P. W., Thorpe, W. P., and Trueblood, M. C.: Osteonecrosis in sickle cell trait. J. Rheumatol. 13:643, 1986.

61. Dorwart, B. B., Goldberg, M. A., Schumacher, H. R., and Alavi, A.: Absence of increased frequency of bone and joint disease with hemoglobin AS and AC. Ann. Intern. Med. 86:55, 1977.

62. Lally, E. V., Buckley, W. M., and Claster, S.: Diaphyseal bone infarctions in a patient with sickle cell trait. J. Rheumatol. 10:813, 1983.

63. Gratwick, G. M., Bullough, P. G., Bohne, W. H. O., Markenson, A. L., and Peterson, C. M.: Thalassemic arthropathy. Ann. Intern. Med. 88:494, 1978.

64. Rioja, L., Girot, R., Garabedian, M., and Cournot-Witmer, G.: Bone disease in children with homozygous beta-thalassemia. Bone Miner. 8:69, 1990.

65. deVernejoul, M. C., Girot, R., Gueris, J., Cancela, L., Bang, S.,

Bielakoff, J., Mautalen, C., Goldberg, D., and Miravet, L.: Calcium phosphate metabolism and bone disease in patients with homozygous thalassemia. J. Clin. Endocrinol. Metab. 54:276, 1982.

66. Arman, M. I.: Gelenk beteiligung bei Hamoglobinopathien. Akt. Rheumatol. 15:17, 1990.

67. Sella, E. J., and Goodman, A. H.: Arthropathy secondary to transfusion hemochromatosis. J. Bone Joint Surg. 55A:1077, 1973.

68. Abbott, D. F., and Gresham, G. A.: Arthropathy in transfusional siderosis. Br. Med. J. 1:418, 1972.

69. Abreu de Miani, M. S., Sanchis, M. E., and Pena Iver, J. A.: Talasemia mayor: Terapia quelante con deferoxamina. Medicina (Buenos Aires) 45:231, 1985.

70. Paik, C. H., Alavi, I., Dunca, G., and Winer, L.: Thalassemia and gouty arthritis. J.A.M.A. 213:296, 1970.

71. Schlumpf, U., Gerber, N., Bunzli, H., Elsasser, U., Pestalozzi, A., and

Boni, A.: Arthritiden bei Thalassemia minor. Schwiiz. Med. Wochenschr. 107:1156, 1977.

72. Schlumpf U.: Thalassemia minor and aseptic necrosis, a coincidence? Arthritis Rheum. 21:280, 1978.

73. Dorwart, B. B., and Schumacher, H. R.: Arthritis in beta thalassemia trait: Clinical and pathological features. Ann. Rheum. Dis. 40:185, 1981.

74. Gerster, J.-C., Dardel, R., and Guggi, S.: Recurrent episodes of arthritis in thalassemia minor. J. Rheumatol. 11:352, 1984.

75. Finterbush, A., Ferber, I., and Mogle, P.: Lower limb pain in thalassemia. J. Rheumatol. 12:529, 1985.

76. Borgna-Pignatti, C., Cammareri, V., DeStefano, P., and Magrini, V.: The sicca syndrome in thalassaemia major. Br. Med. J. 288:668, 1984.

77. Lucarelli, G., Galimberti, M., Polchi, P., et al.: Bone marrow transplantation in patients with thalassemia. N. Engl. J. Med. 322:417, 1990.

Chapter 92

James L. McGuire
R. Elaine Lambert

Arthropathies Associated with Endocrine Disorders

INTRODUCTION

The systemic manifestations of endocrine disorders reflect the diverse but specialized control that hormones exert on certain tissues. The similarities between the two systems occur at both the clinical and molecular level. The list of cells possessing various hormone receptors is rapidly expanding. Many are not in traditional target organs. The monocyte/macrophage line, lymphocyte subpopulations, fibroblasts, mast cells, and bone cells are recent additions to this list. For instance, collagenase production and bone resorption by cells of the rheumatoid synovium may be directly influenced by parathyroid hormone (PTH), calcitonin (CT), and 1,25-dihydroxyvitamin D.[1, 2] In fact, the rapidity of periarticular demineralization in RA may correlate with circulating levels of PTH and 1,25-dihydroxyvitamin D.[3]

Historically, the untreated adult endocrine disorders of acromegaly, primary hyperparathyroidism (PHP), and myxedema were initially classified within the rheumatic diseases. Moreover, the overlap of multisystem complaints, both constitutional and musculoskeletal, has served to link the endocrine syndromes with connective tissue disease. The rheumatologist usually encounters endocrine disease in one of three ways. First, a patient with a defined endocrine disorder can present with a specific rheumatologic complaint. Second, the presentation of endocrine disease as an undiagnosed systemic illness involving joints, muscles, or skin may suggest a vasculitis or connective tissue disease. Finally, a nonspecific problem such as carpal tunnel syndrome or a pseudogout attack may warrant a specific endocrine test, which may result in the early recognition of an endocrine disease. Table 92–1 is an abbreviated list of symptoms and signs that are suggestive of endocrine disease in patients seeking help from a rheumatologist.

The clinical presentation of the classic endocrine disorders such as primary hyperparathyroidism, acromegaly, and Cushing's disease has dramatically changed during the last decade because of early detection. This, in turn, results in appropriate therapeutic intervention before the complete syndrome evolves. PHP, for example, is often diagnosed by finding hypercalcemia by routine laboratory screening in a patient without "moans, groans, stones, or bones." The rheumatologist must be aware of these changing presentations of a classic disease and that nonspecific musculoskeletal signs and symptoms may represent the first manifestation of these disorders.[4]

Pediatricians constantly observe the action of hormonal regulation of skeletal growth during the evaluation of children with short stature, bone deformities, and joint hypermobility. Disorders of growth hormone (GH) production, vitamin D resistance, and PHP of childhood must be added to the differential diagnoses of abnormal skeletal growth that have included achondroplasia, osteogenesis imperfecta, and Ehlers-Danlos syndrome. In some diseases, hormonal and connective tissue abnormalities are strongly associated but are inherited independently. Patients with classic pseudohypoparathyroidism have hypocalcemia due to PTH resistance and skeletal deformities (short fourth metacarpal and stature) called Albright's hereditary osteodystrophy (AHO), which may not be related to the hypoparathyroid state. Both conditions may be inherited separately (pseudohypoparathyroidism without AHO, or AHO with normal serum calcium level). The latter

Table 92–1. CLINICAL FINDINGS COMMON TO BOTH RHEUMATOLOGIC AND ENDOCRINE DISORDERS

Skin	**Soft Tissue**
Thickening	Fibrositis
Local	Tenosynovitis
Diffuse	Bursitis
Alopecia	**Nervous System**
Vitiligo	Carpal tunnel
Easy bruisability	Depression
Blood Vessels	**Bone**
Leg ulcers	Osteopenia
Raynaud's phenomenon	Abnormal stature
Muscle	Deformities
Weakness and pain (with or	**Hand Radiograph**
without muscle enzyme	Distal tufts
elevation)	CPPD
Joints	Joint space
Pseudogout	Osteopenia
Seronegative rheumatoid	**Laboratory Tests**
arthritis	Positive rheumatoid factor
Diffusely swollen hands	Antinuclear antibody
Premature osteoarthritis	Elevated creatine kinase

is often referred to as pseudopseudohypoparathyroidism.

The appearance of an endocrine disorder during the course of an existing connective tissue disease can dramatically alter the symptoms. The concomitant development of hyperthyroidism in a patient with rheumatoid arthritis (RA) often results in joint complaints that are out of proportion to the physical findings. The dramatic aggravation or amelioration of connective tissue diseases during different stages of pregnancy has been well described. The iatrogenic Cushing's syndrome during steroid therapy results in a diagnostic dilemma when muscle weakness reappears during the clinical course of polymyositis with stable muscle enzyme levels. The appearance of PHP in a patient with active Paget's disease of bone can result in massive, rapid resorption of bone. The effects of sex and other steroid hormones on the immune response are as fascinating to the immunologist as is the "autoimmune" attack on specific endocrine glands resulting in stimulation (e.g., acanthosis nigricans and diabetes) or destruction (e.g., Hashimoto's disease) to the endocrinologist. Additionally, the immunopathologic events preceding the clinical onset of type I diabetes appear to closely parallel the genetically restricted T cell interactions with processed antigen described in other chronic disorders of the immune system.

Finally, the association of endocrine and rheumatic disorders extends beyond common autoantibodies and HLA types. For example, two new acronyms, POEMS and TASS, define syndromes that integrally link altered endocrine secretion with immune-mediated disease. POEMS (plasma cell dyscrasia with polyneuropathy, organomegaly, endocrinopathy, monoclonal protein, and skin disease) may present with scleroderma-like skin disease.[5] Diabetes hypogonadism with gynecomastia and hypothyroidism are the usual associated endocrine diseases. TASS (thyroiditis, Addison's disease, Sjögren's syndrome, and sarcoidosis) is another rare and complicated clinical syndrome, which, nevertheless, may provide some pathogenetic insights into immune regulation by hormones.[6]

DIABETES MELLITUS

Diabetes mellitus is a heterogeneous disorder that is classified according to insulin dependence to prevent ketosis, degree of insulin resistance, and age of onset. Type 1 is insulin-dependent diabetes (IDD), caused by immune-mediated destruction of pancreatic beta cells, whereas type 2 represents the majority of cases of maturity-onset diabetes that are noninsulin dependent (NIDD).

Although many reports suggest a strong association between diabetes and osteoporosis (see Chapter 96), well-controlled retrospective and prospective studies demonstrate conflicting results.[7] Nevertheless, patients with poorly controlled diabetes excrete more urinary calcium,[8] and bone formation in the growing skeleton requires insulin.[9]

The relationship of osteoarthritis to diabetes is suggested by the accelerated destruction of articular cartilage in diabetic Chinese hamsters[10] and in rats with streptozocin-induced diabetes.[11] Osteoarthritis is more common in patients with maturity-onset diabetes than in age-matched controls, but the lack of controls for obesity makes any unique association questionable.[12] Similarly, obesity is an important factor in patients with maturity-onset diabetes who have hyperuricemia and gout[13] (see Chapter 76). Controlled studies of the frequency of pseudogout in the diabetic population have not confirmed the initially reported association.[14]

The diabetic hand syndrome, or limited joint mobility (LJM), has been observed in 30 to 50 percent of IDD[15] and up to 75 percent of NIDD.[15] In both types, LJM appears to be positively correlated with duration[16] and the presence of renal or retinal microvascular disease.[15, 17] Flexion contractures in the fingers are attributed to excessive dermal collagen, which results in thickened and indurated skin around the metacarpophalangeal (MCP) and proximal interphalangeal (PIP) joints. The natural progression of the stiff hands is not well characterized. Usually it is the microvascular or associated restrictive lung disease,[18] and not the joint disease, that is functionally limiting. LJM has similarities to scleroderma, although the preservation of skin appendages on biopsies and the abnormal cross-linking of collagen (normal in scleroderma) emphasize its differences.[17, 19, 20]

LJM must be distinguished from other hand problems that complicate diabetes. Flexor tenosynovitis,[21] causing "trigger fingers," and Dupuytren's contractures of the palmar fascia occur in approximately one third of patients with IDD (type 1). Both flexor tenosynovitis and LJM have been reported to precede the onset of clinical diabetes.[22] All of these hand disorders may share a common pathogenesis involving contractile myofibroblasts, which produce increased amounts of collagen in response to microvascular ischemia.[19]

Skin disorders in diabetes mellitus have been confused with forms of scleroderma. In other patients with type 1 diabetes, abnormalities of the subcutaneous fat have been observed. Lipoatrophy at the site of repeated insulin injections is common. A rare condition called total lipodystrophy is characterized by an absence of subcutaneous fat. It is associated with severe insulin resistance, acanthosis nigricans, and the sicca syndrome.[23] A wide variety of diabetic skin changes related to vascular abnormalities can occur over the anterior tibial area. Necrobiosis lipoidica diabeticorum may suggest a small vessel vasculitis by demonstrating an obliterative endarteritis on histopathologic study.[24]

Calcific peritendinitis and bursitis of the shoulder leading to severe adhesive capsulitis are well described in patients with diabetes.[17, 25] Moreover, an association of this condition, which may be bilateral,

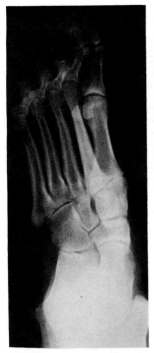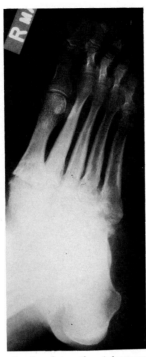

Figure 92–1. Neuropathic arthropathy involving the right tarsus in diabetes mellitus. The left tarsus is normal.

with LJM[17] and reflex sympathetic dystrophy (RSD)[26] can result in several clinical patterns of the shoulder-hand syndrome, which may be resistant to conventional therapy.

A variety of rheumatic complaints are directly related to the neuropathy of diabetes mellitus. Actual infarction of the nerve may be caused by involvement of the vasonervorum. The median nerve is particularly vulnerable to the mild compression caused by RSD or obesity. The presence of nocturnal paresthesias in any of the first four fingers or of thenar muscle wasting should suggest the carpal tunnel syndrome. RSD itself may need the background of the dysautonomia of diabetes for full expression in the setting of calcific bursitis or cervical spine osteoarthritis.[27] Peripheral neuropathies account for the high frequency of undetected foreign objects embedded in the "diabetic foot." Osteomyelitis is a common complication in this setting, especially with coexistent peripheral vascular disease.[28] An acute mononeuritis can present a confusing clinical picture. For example, involvement of the femoral nerve can cause pain and weakness in the proximal thigh and may simulate the syndromes of meralgia paresthetica, a herniated lumbar disc, or "shingles," especially prior to the vesicular eruption (herpes zoster). Moreover, pain in this region could also originate from the hip joint (osteoarthritis), the bone (avascular necrosis), or the soft tissue (greater trochanteric bursa).

In some patients with diabetes and peripheral neuropathy, a classic Charcot's arthropathy involving the tarsus and ankle results in painless deformities of the foot[29] (Figs. 92–1 and 92–2). Similar involve-

ment of the knee, with surprising preservation of function, and the spine has been described. The pathogenesis of this destructive arthropathy is not completely understood but may involve chronic calcium pyrophosphate dihydrate (CPPD) crystal shedding in the presence of altered neurogenic responses by nociceptive C type fibers.[30] A dramatic osteolysis of the bones of the forefoot is peculiar to patients with diabetes[31] (Fig. 92–3). The terms resorptive osteodystrophy, osteolysis of the forefoot, and diabetic osteopathy have been used interchangeably for this condition. The progression from patchy osteopenia to complete resorption of the distal metatarsals and proximal phalanges can be rapid. The pathophysiology of this resorptive process is largely unknown but may be preceded by loss of cortical bone induced by neuropathy that results in metatarsal fractures.[32] On the other hand, overt peripheral vascular disease and severe neuropathy are not always present.

Diffuse idiopathic skeletal hyperostosis (DISH) is associated with diabetes mellitus, especially in obese patients with maturity-onset diabetes.[33] There is some preliminary evidence that nondiabetics with DISH have an abnormal insulin response to induced hyperglycemia.[34] DISH is usually a radiographic diagnosis and is distinguished from ankylosing spondylitis by the preservation of sacroiliac joints and predominantly right-sided syndesmophytes.

An association between RA and IDD (type 1) has been made and challenged based on the shared HLA haplotypes DR4 and DR1.[35] However, DR3 is also strongly associated with IDD but not RA. The link may actually be related to common complement allotypes.[37] The rheumatologic disorders commonly described in diabetes mellitus are summarized in Table 92–2.

HYPERPARATHYROIDISM

Primary hyperparathyroidism (PHP) can first present as a vertebral body crush-fracture caused by osteopenia. The bone diseases of PHP are discussed in Chapter 96. Several additional rheumatic conditions are commonly discussed here.

First, a painless proximal muscle weakness suggestive of a myopathy has been described. Levels of the muscle enzymes creatine kinase (CK) and

Table 92–2. RHEUMATOLOGIC DISORDERS IN DIABETES MELLITUS

Direct Complications	Indirect Complications	Possible Associations
Diabetic osteolysis	Forestier's disease (DISH)	Gout
Septic arthritis	Dupuytren's contracture	CPPD crystal disease
Neuropathic joint	Frozen shoulder	Osteoporosis
Stiff hand syndrome	Carpal tunnel syndrome	Osteoarthritis
	Reflex sympathetic dystrophy	

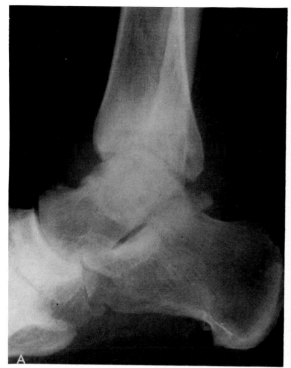

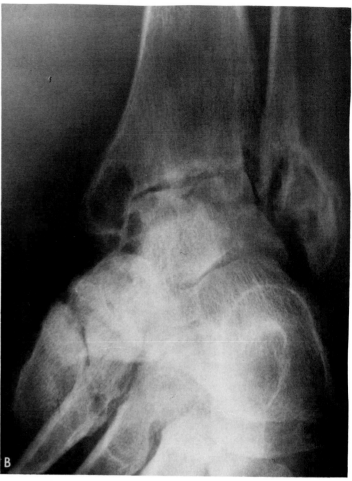

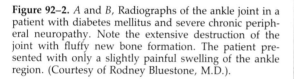

Figure 92–2. *A* and *B,* Radiographs of the ankle joint in a patient with diabetes mellitus and severe chronic peripheral neuropathy. Note the extensive destruction of the joint with fluffy new bone formation. The patient presented with only a slightly painful swelling of the ankle region. (Courtesy of Rodney Bluestone, M.D.).

aldolase are normal. The electromyogram (EMG) is characteristically abnormal; some patients have a myopathic pattern, and others demonstrate a neuropathic picture. The latter is supported by muscle biopsy findings consistent with denervation. Following the removal of the parathyroid adenoma, the neuromuscular disorder and the abnormal EMG improve dramatically.[38]

Second, an inflammatory arthritis associated with erosions and chondrocalcinosis has been described in patients with PHP.[39] One form of this arthropathy is thought to be induced by crystals. The common association of hyperuricemia and PHP supported urate as the important pathogenetic crystal, but the demonstration of CPPD crystals in synovial fluid popularized this crystal as the driving force behind the chronic inflammation. Although larger, age-matched studies are needed, the literature supports the chronic pseudogout model as a cause of the arthropathy of PHP.[40] In general, patients with PHP and chondrocalcinosis are older and have higher serum calcium levels.[41] The subsequent course of established pseudogout may be independent of the successful reversal of the hyperparathyroid state by parathyroidectomy.[42] However, the demonstration of both calcium apatite and calcium oxalate crystals[43] in

patients with secondary hyperparathyroidism due to chronic renal disease suggests that further evaluation is needed before naming any one crystal as the cause of this arthritis.

Third, the erosive arthritis in PHP described by Bywaters and associates was referred to as osteogenic synovitis to emphasize the primary role of the bone disease in the acquired articular disorder.[44] Subchondral thinning of bone resulted in collapse and eventual loss of cartilage. The resultant osteoarthritis changes were consistent with the radiographic findings (Fig. 92–4). It is interesting to note that the destructive bone disease of osteitis fibrosa cystica, the first pathologic change linking PHP and bone, has all but disappeared from the current descriptions of bone histopathologic findings in patients with PHP (see Chapter 96).

Although hyperuricemia, gout, and PHP have been reported together in some patients,[45] no strong association of gout and PHP has been confirmed. The earlier studies may reflect a different presentation of PHP than the milder disease currently being diagnosed and have generally predated the description of CPPD-induced pseudogout. The possible association of ankylosing spondylitis and PHP has not been fully confirmed in a large study.[46] Ectopic cal-

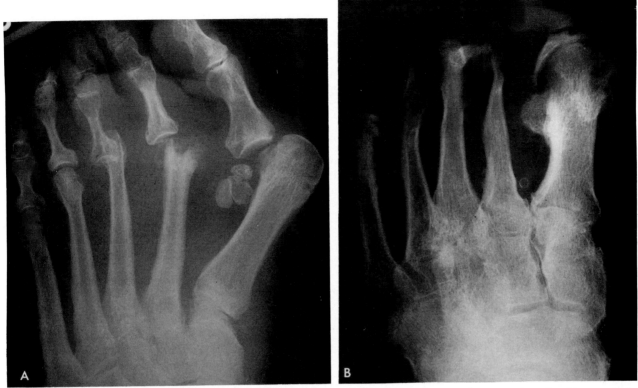

Figure 92–3. Radiograph of forefoot showing diabetic osteolysis of metatarsals and phalanges. *A,* Some sharply outlined juxta-articular erosions and early subluxations of first, second, and third metatarsophalangeal joints are evident. *B,* A variable degree of bony dissolution has resulted in tapering of bone ends and a telescoping deformity of the toes. (*B,* from Bluestone, R.: Rheumatological complications of some endocrinopathies. Clin. Rheum. Dis. 1:95, 1975.)

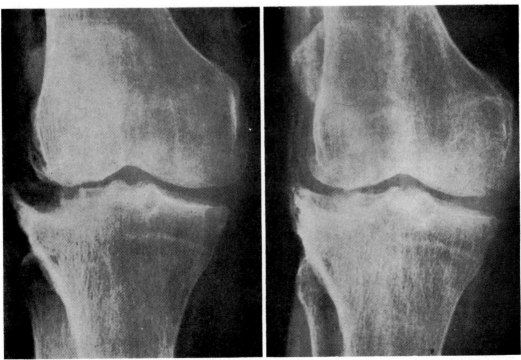

Figure 92–4. Right knee before *(left)* and 1 year after *(right)* removal of parathyroid adenoma. Collapse and erosion of lateral condyles of tibia and femur, present earlier, were partially repaired. (From Bywaters, E. G. L., et al.: Joint lesions of hyperparathyroidism. Ann. Rheum. Dis. 22:171, 1963.)

cifications in skin and tendons can present as unexplained firm nodules and acute periarticular disease, respectively.

The secondary hyperparathyroidism of chronic renal disease frequently causes bony abnormalities similar to osteitis fibrosa cystica of classic PHP. This form of renal osteodystrophy is associated with an erosive joint disease involving the hands,[47] clavicle, and axial skeleton[48] (Fig. 92–5) and may have destructive components similar to neuropathic arthropathy. The destructive spondyloarthropathy, especially of the cervical spine, can suggest a disc space infection.[49] This phenomenon is characteristically noninfectious and relates to the underlying metabolic bone disease with potential contributions from calcium crystals and beta(β)-2 microglobulin amyloidosis.[50] Moreover, neurotrophic skeletal disease has been described after renal transplantation for diabetic neuropathy[51] (see Chapter 79). The relationship to the existing secondary hyperparathyroidism is still not clear. In addition to subcutaneous calcifications,[52] calcium crystal–induced inflammation of tendon and joints has been described.

HYPOPARATHYROIDISM

Patients with hypocalcemia due to hypoparathyroidism can now be separated into groups according to the levels of immunoreactive parathyroid hormone (iPTH). Undetectable levels are found in individuals with idiopathic hypoparathyroidism (IH) and in patients who have had surgical removal of the parathyroids, whereas normal to elevated levels are found in patients with pseudohypoparathyroidism with target organ resistance.

Idiopathic hypoparathyroidism is rare. The principal muscular symptom of fatigue is directly related to the degree of hypocalcemia. A spondylitis similar to DISH has been described in patients with IH.[53] The restricted spinal movement is caused by extensive nonmarginal syndesmophytes along the anterior vertebral ligaments. There is neither sacroiliac joint narrowing nor vertebral body squaring, so ankylosing spondylitis can be excluded. A subgroup of IH has a particular susceptibility to superficial Candida infections involving the nails and skin.[54] Defects in cell-mediated immunity, including cutaneous anergy, have been described in this group.[55] IH has been associated with other endocrinopathies, such as Addison's disease, Hashimoto's disease, and hypothyroidism. The acronym HAM is used to refer to the syndrome of IH, Addison's disease, and moniliasis.[56] Interestingly, an association of IH with other connective tissue diseases usually considered "autoimmune" has not been noted.

Pseudohypoparathyroidism is generally associ-

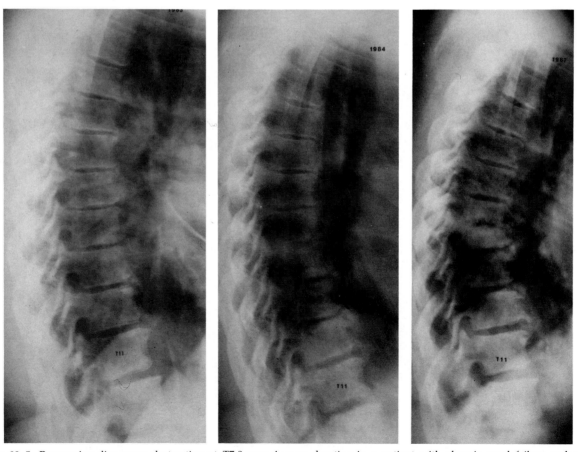

Figure 92–5. Progressive disc space destruction at T7-8 over 4 years duration in a patient with chronic renal failure and severe secondary hyperparathyroidism. Note marker for T11. (Courtesy of Burton Ellis, M.D.)

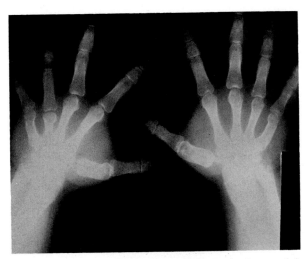

Figure 92–6. Albright's hereditary osteodystrophy in pseudohypoparathyroidism. The "knuckle-knuckle-dimple-knuckle" sign has its radiologic equivalent in the short fourth metacarpal. (Courtesy of Neil Breslau, M.D.)

ated with the skeletal deformities of a short fourth metacarpal and diminished overall stature. The condition of hormone resistance can occur independently of the somatic defects, which have been termed Albright's hereditary osteodystrophy.[57] Patients with pseudohypoparathyroidism and AHO have deficient PTH-directed cyclic AMP generation. This defect has been localized to the alpha (α) protein of the cell membrane–associated guanine(G)nucleotide stimulatory unit of adenyl cyclase.[58] This may explain the association of this endocrine disorder with other hormone-resistant states possessing the same defect in the G unit.[59]

The short metacarpals are the result of premature epiphyseal closure. AHO can be suggested by a routine examination of the hands. With a clenched fist, the so-called knuckle, knuckle, dimple, knuckle sign emphasizes the short fourth metacarpal. Defor-

mities involving the hips, pelvis, and knees have been also described in patients with AHO[60] (Fig. 92–6).

Ectopic ossifications in the subcutaneous and soft tissues are preferentially deposited around the weight-bearing joints in patients with pseudohypoparathyroidism. Whereas ectopic calcification of the basal ganglia occurs in all forms of chronic hypoparathyroidism, subcutaneous deposits of bone in the lower extremities have been described almost exclusively in patients with pseudohypoparathyroidism. However, in one case of IH, an acute calcific periarthritic attack coincided with a rapid fall in serum calcium level.[61]

VITAMIN D, RICKETS, AND OSTEOMALACIA

Patients with rickets and osteomalacia caused by renal tubular loss of phosphate and vitamin D resistance can present with distinct musculoskeletal problems. The myopathy of hypophosphatemia may result in the waddling gait of rickets. Reflex sympathetic dystrophy can be a presentation of this form of osteomalacia.[62] In X-linked hypophosphatemic rickets, extraskeletal calcification of the entheses has resulted in radiographic confusion with seronegative spondyloarthropathy and DISH[63] (Fig. 92–7). Finally, tibial bowing in rickets can cause mechanical problems that result in premature osteoarthritis (see Chapters 79, 96). The role of 1,25-dihydroxyvitamin D in the local control of the immune-response and cell differentiation, especially within the synovium, is not clear. Macrophages from synovial fluid can produce 1,25-dihydroxyvitamin D, but the regulation of this extrarenal production appears to be more influenced by interferon gamma (IFN-γ) and glucocorticoids than by traditional systemic factors such as PTH, calcium, and estrogen. In general, 1,25-dihydroxyvitamin D has an antiproli-

Figure 92–7. Hypophosphatemic osteomalacia. Calcification of the entheses can cause radiographic bridging of the sacroiliac joint (right side). The plain radiograph can simulate ankylosing spondylitis, despite computed tomography confirmation of a patent joint. (Courtesy of Marc Drezner, M.D.)

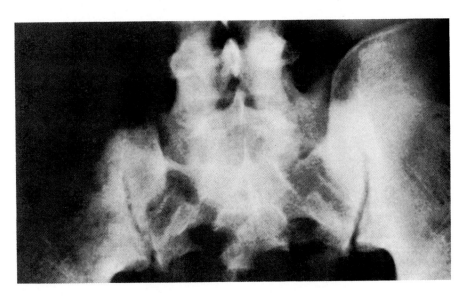

ferative effect on T cells and decreases IL-2 production.[63a]

HYPERTHYROIDISM (GRAVES' DISEASE)

The suggestion that Graves' disease, Hashimoto's thyroiditis, and hypothyroidism are not totally separate entities has often been raised. Pretibial myxedema, lymphocytic infiltration of the thyroid gland, thyroid-specific antibodies, suppressor T cell defects,[64] and eye muscle involvement[65] have been described in all three classic thyroid disorders. Moreover, the association with other "autoimmune" disorders sharing HLA-B8 and DR3 is common to both Graves' and Hashimoto's diseases. It is possible that the clinical expression of hyperthyroidism, hypothyroidism, or euthyroid goiter just reflects the predominant immunologic influence at the time. Support for this theory is based on the transition of hyperthyroid to hypothyroid stages of Hashimoto's thyroiditis and euthyroid Graves' disease with ophthalmopathy.[66]

Graves' disease is emerging as one of the best examples of endocrine autoimmunity.[67] Expression of HLA-DR (Ia) on thyroid epithelial cells (thyrocytes) may be induced by a virus or other undefined insults. Expression of Ia on thyrocytes can be readily induced by interferon gamma (IFN-γ).[68] A subsequent T cell activation in turn results in autoantibody production by B cells and glandular destruction by cytotoxic T cells.[67] The immunopathologic similarities to type 1 diabetes are obvious.

In the pathogenesis of the hyperthyroid state, thyroid-stimulating antibody (TSI) develops against the thyroid-stimulating hormone (TSH) receptor. Rather than inhibiting hormone production in a manner similar to that seen in most other antireceptor diseases such as myasthenia gravis and acanthosis nigricans with diabetes, TSI stimulates the thyrocyte to produce excessive thyroxine.[69] The role of long-acting thyroid stimulator (LATS) and other immunoglobulins in human thyrotoxicosis, acropachy, and ophthalmopathy is not fully understood.[70] The ophthalmopathy is a myopathic process generated by both cytotoxic T cells and ophthalmic immunoglobulins.[71, 71a]

Thyroid acropachy is an uncommon manifestation of Graves' disease consisting of a clinical constellation of distal soft tissue swelling, clubbing, and periostitis, especially of the metacarpals (Fig. 92–8). The symptoms may first occur after a euthyroid state is achieved and are often associated with exophthalmos and pretibial myxedema. Although unique, thyroid acropachy has obvious similarities to secondary hypertrophic osteoarthropathy (see Chapter 96).

Two skin problems described in patients with Graves' disease can be confused with other connective tissue diseases. First, onycholysis, an elevation of the nail from the nail bed, is also found in patients with Reiter's disease, psoriasis, and psoriatic arthritis. Second, pretibial myxedema can present with

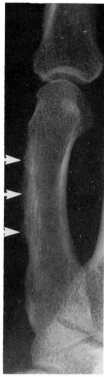

Figure 92–8. Radiograph of a fifth metacarpal from a patient with thyroid acropachy. Note the fluffy periostitis along the ulnar aspect of the bone. (From Bluestone, R.: Rheumatological complications of some endocrinopathies. Clin. Rheum. Dis. 1:95, 1975.)

nodules over the calves and shins. The pink plaques of hyaluronic acid can be confluent and simulate morphea[72] (see Chapter 66). In the nodular form, erythema nodosum enters the differential diagnosis. Pretibial myxedema is a classic component of Graves' disease. The cause is unknown, but site-specific fibroblasts, taken from the pretibial skin, were induced to produce excessive glycosaminoglycans when exposed to serum from patients with Graves' disease, whereas fibroblasts from other areas did not.[73]

Painless proximal muscle weakness without muscle enzyme level elevation has been described in approximately 70 percent of patients with hyperthyroidism. The myopathy is rapidly reversible with corrective therapy.[74]

The true incidence of adhesive capsulitis of the shoulder and fibrositis in patients with hyperthyroidism is debated. Early descriptions emphasized painful, restricted shoulders in approximately 25 percent of patients.[75] Acute calcific periarthritis of the wrist was the presentation of hyperthyroidism in one case. Similar calcium crystal–induced mechanisms may be applicable to the shoulders.[76]

The osteoporosis associated with hyperthyroidism is described in Chapter 96. Organ cultures of bone suggesting augmented bone resorption are consistent with bone histology demonstrating increased numbers of osteoclasts.[77] Additionally, impaired intestinal calcium absorption may contribute to the osteopenia.

Although the incidence of RA in patients with Graves' disease is not increased, high titers of rheumatoid factor (RF) have been described.[78] An association of Graves' disease with giant cell arteritis has been reported.[79]

Anti-DNA antibodies are found in approximately 90 percent of patients with Graves' disease,[80] yet the occurrence of systemic lupus erythematosus (SLE) has been confined to a few case reports. Rheumatic syndromes, characterized by polyarthralgia and rash, appear frequently in patients taking the antithyroid medicines propylthiouracil (PTU) and methimazole. Antinuclear antibody (ANA) positivity was not a common finding in these patients. Although drug-induced lupus has been described in patients receiving PTU,[81] it may not account for many of the rheumatic symptoms observed with this medicine (see Chapter 63).

Finally, Hashimoto's disease is a thyroiditis characterized by lymphocytic infiltration and enlargement of the gland. Eventually, primary hypothyroidism ensues, although the disease may pass through a hyperthyroid phase. The pathogenesis of Hashimoto's disease probably has close similarities to Graves' disease.[67] In addition to the presence of antimicrosomal and antithyroglobulin antibodies, specific abnormalities have been identified in cell-mediated immunity, including diminished suppressor T cell populations and increased migration inhibition factor (MIF) lymphokines in both Hashimoto's and Graves' diseases.[64] Finally, Hashimoto's disease and hypothyroidism may first appear in a patient with established connective tissue disease. The association with SLE,[82] rheumatoid arthritis, mixed connective tissue disease,[83] scleroderma,[84] Sjögren's syndrome, polymyositis, and relapsing polychondritis has been described.[85] The increased prevalence of HLA-B8, Aw30, DR3, and DR5 in patients with Hashimoto's disease is consistent with an association with other disorders having the same immunologic cluster.[86]

HYPOTHYROIDISM

In the United States, hypothyroidism is usually caused by either Hashimoto's disease or the long-term effects of thyroid ablation by radioactive iodine for Graves' disease. The rheumatic manifestations occupy a central place in the clinical picture of myxedema. Additionally, newer therapies for RA such as total lymphoid irradiation have been complicated by hypothyroidism.

Several forms of myxedematous arthropathy probably exist. The first usually affects large joints, although the MCP and metatarsophalangeal (MTP) joints can be involved. The patient presents with swelling and stiffness. The examination of the knee may produce a characteristic slow fluid wave (bulge sign). Ligamentous laxity and synovial thickening

can be prominent. The demonstration of CPPD crystals is common, but the synovial fluid is surprisingly noninflammatory (Fig. 92–9).[87, 88] Although the link between myxedema and this peculiar pseudogout form seems well established, further long-term age- and sex-matched studies need to be done. Resolution of this arthropathy with thyroid replacement is characteristic. The second type associated with Hashimoto's disease is inflammatory and can closely resemble RA.[85] One subgroup has a particularly aggressive course and rheumatoid factor positivity. The other subgroup is seronegative and has a milder clinical course. It is quite possible that the former subgroup represents both RA and Hashimoto's thyroiditis occurring in the same patient.

The myopathy of hypothyroidism may have a wide spectrum of muscle complaints, including proximal muscle pain, stiffness, and hypertrophy (Hoffmann's syndrome).[89] Moreover, despite elevations of muscle enzyme levels, weakness may not be a prominent symptom.[90] Muscle biopsy findings are usually normal, although occasional fiber destruction and mucinous infiltrates have been reported in some patients. The peculiar nature of this myopathy could suggest either polymyalgia rheumatica (when stiff, painful muscles predominate)[91] or polymyositis (when the creatine kinase (CK) level is elevated).

Carpal tunnel syndrome (CTS) has been noted in approximately 7 percent of patients with hypothyroidism. Compression of the median nerve by the extraneural accumulation of mucinous material in the tunnel has been implicated as the cause (see Chapter 101). An intrinsic neuropathy similar to that found in patients with diabetes and acromegaly may play a contributing role. Although carpal tunnel syndrome should be considered in the myxedematous patient with pain or paresthesias in any one of the first four

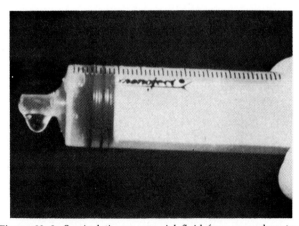

Figure 92–9. Semigelatinous synovial fluid from myxedematous patients often required several seconds to begin vertical fall from a syringe, even with greater than usual pressure on the plunger. If allowed to "string out" vertically from a Pasteur pipette, unbroken streams of greater than 45 cm occurred in these fluids. (From Dorwart, B. B., and Schumacher, H. R.: Joint effusions, chondrocalcinosis and other rheumatic manifestations in hypothyroidism. Am. J. Med. 159:780, 1975.)

fingers, other causes, such as flexor tenosynovitis, should be ruled out.

Osteonecrosis of the hip has been described in patients with myxedema (see Chapter 97).[92] Whether this mechanism accounts for some patients who experience collapse of the tibial plateau is not clear. Additionally, the hypercholesterolemia associated with hypothyroidism has been proposed as a contributing factor for both the avascular necrosis of bone and the arthropathy.[93]

The diagnosis of hypothyroidism should be entertained in all patients with unexplained CTS, seronegative RA, polymyalgia rheumatica with a normal erythrocyte sedimentation rate (ESR), and polymyositis with a normal muscle biopsy finding. The dramatic reversal of all of these rheumatic manifestations with thyroxine therapy emphasizes the importance of including myxedema in the differential diagnosis.

GLUCOCORTICOIDS, CUSHING'S SYNDROME, AND ADDISON'S DISEASE

Cushing's syndrome due to excess glucocorticoids can be either idiopathic or iatrogenic. The advanced syndrome is easily diagnosed by the characteristic moon facies, buffalo hump, abdominal stria, hypertension, and osteoporosis.

Proximal muscle weakness without muscle enzyme level elevation occurs in some patients with the natural disease. Additionally, the fluorinated steroid preparations have a greater propensity to cause the myopathy.[94] Osteoporosis is characteristic of both well-established disease and long-term daily steroid administration. Poor wound healing, easy bruisability, and blue striae have all been attributed to inhibition of collagen, elastin, and matrix synthesis by fibroblasts.

Iatrogenic Cushing's syndrome is generally associated with daily dosages of prednisone of 10 mg or greater. At lower doses, preservation of the hypothalamic-pituitary-adrenal axis and the intestinal calcium absorption is maintained.[95] The symptoms of the iatrogenic syndrome parallel the idiopathic disease, except for the higher frequencies of avascular necrosis (see Chapter 97) and cataract formation (see Chapter 32).

The appearance of new symptoms in a patient with active connective tissue disease who is receiving high doses of glucocorticoids poses a difficult diagnostic problem. Two common situations illustrate this point. First, the reappearance of weakness in a patient with polymyositis (PM) on steroid therapy could mean either reactivation of the disease or steroid-induced myopathy. This differential diagnosis is especially difficult if abnormal muscle enzyme levels persist unchanged or no further increments are observed. Attempts to evaluate this dilemma by urinary creatine levels have not been satisfactory.[96] Second, when psychotic behavior is apparent in a patient with SLE receiving steroids, steroid-induced psychosis or central nervous system (CNS) lupus must be considered.

The tapering of glucocorticoids after the desired therapeutic effect has been achieved can be associated with a withdrawal syndrome. Low-grade fever, lethargy, intense myalgias, and arthralgias are common. Moreover, these symptoms can occur when absolute levels of cortisol are within the normal range. The withdrawal syndrome can be confused with the reactivation of the primary disease[97] or the unmasking of a new "autoimmune" syndrome. In a case of RA, steroid withdrawal precipitated polyendocrine failure, which was almost totally reversible with steroid resumption.[98] Finally, a rare but somewhat specific syndrome of panniculitis has been described that occurs in patients with acute rheumatic fever who have been tapered quickly off steroids.[99]

Addison's disease itself is usually not associated with specific rheumatic complaints. Muscle weakness is common and usually related to the degree of hyperkalemia. Addison's disease has been associated with Sjögren's syndrome and other endocrinopathies.[100] The role of relative steroid deficiency in the development of chronic arthritis has been advanced by data that suggest that certain rat strains that respond to stress with blunted ACTH secretion may be more susceptible to inflammatory stimuli.[101] The role of glucocorticoids in the maintenance of the normal immune system in humans is less clear.[102]

Muscle complaints, particularly cramping, weakness, and fatigability, are common in primary hyperaldosteronism. In this disease, hypokalemia is responsible for the reversible muscle problems. The muscle enzyme levels are normal.

ACROMEGALY

The role of growth hormone in the normal adult is not clear. The effects on bone, muscle, and the immune system are currently being evaluated. It is clear that growth hormone levels tend to decline with age, and replacement therapy with recombinant growth hormone may increase muscle and bone mass in the elderly.[103] It is tempting to further postulate that the decline of growth hormone levels relates to the altered immune response associated with aging. The insidious progression of symptoms over several years characteristically escapes clinical detection.

The skeletal effects of growth hormone, mediated by production of somatomedins in the liver, are responsible for the well-coordinated growth of the epiphyseal plate during puberty. Acromegaly is the result of oversecretion of growth hormone by an adenoma, usually involving somatotropic (acidophilic) cells of the anterior pituitary gland. The chronic overstimulation of bone cells, fibroblasts, and chondrocytes in the adult skeleton can cause a variety of musculoskeletal manifestations. Serum levels of

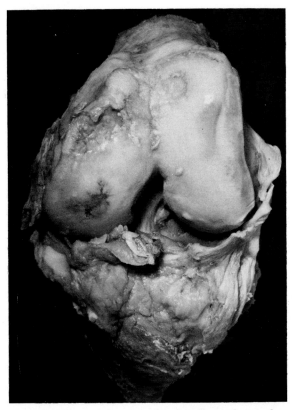

Figure 92–10. Femur in acromegaly, showing undercut ulcer on weight-bearing area of medial condyle. (From Bluestone, R., et al.: Acromegalic arthropathy. Ann. Rheum. Dis. 30:243, 1971.)

The simultaneous response of fibroblast proliferation in periarticular tissue often results in ligamentous laxity. The osteoarthritic process in the knee can be aggravated by chronic shedding of CPPD crystals, which can generate attacks of pseudogout. Moreover, the rapid enlargement of components of this joint may predispose to internal derangements, especially tears in the meniscus. Finally, osteoarthritis involvement of the temporomandibular joint (TMJ) has been described.[105]

Joint space widening, caused by overgrowth of articular cartilage, can be observed radiographically (Figs. 92–12 and 92–13). As the osteoarthritis progresses, joint space narrowing, eburnation, osteophytes, and chondrocalcinosis make the radiographic changes of acromegaly indistinguishable from those produced by other causes of osteoarthritis, including early neuropathic arthropathy. The acquired bowing of the tibia and femur in patients with acromegaly must be differentiated from Paget's disease, rickets, and postfracture repair.

The proposed pathophysiology of acromegalic arthropathy emphasizes the role of both cartilage and bone (Table 92–3). The altered cartilage growth results in easy fissuring, CPPD crystal accumulation, and, ultimately, loss of cartilage. The bone produced by activated osteoblasts may explain the subchondral rigidity and osteophyte formation (see Chapters 78 and 79).

Approximately one half of patients with acro-

type III procollagen propeptide (PIIIP), a reliable index of collagen synthesis, are markedly increased in patients with acromegaly. Monitoring of PIIIP levels during therapy appears to be a useful indicator of disease activity.[104]

Premature osteoarthritis has been described in the weight-bearing joints of patients with acromegaly. The overgrowth of cartilage may cause a particular susceptibility to fissuring and ulceration and the development of osteophytes (Figs. 92–10 and 92–11).

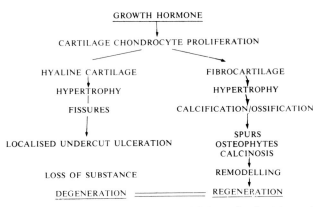

Figure 92–11. Schematic representation of the pathophysiology of acromegalic arthropathy. (From Bluestone, R.: Rheumatological complications of some endocrinopathies. Clin. Rheum. Dis. 1:95, 1975.)

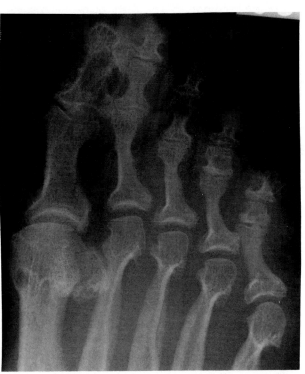

Figure 92–12. Radiograph of the forefoot in a patient with acromegaly. Note the greatly widened metatarsophalangeal joint spaces, reflecting cartilage hyperplasia; there is remodeling of metatarsal and phalangeal bones. (Courtesy of Rodney Bluestone, M.D.)

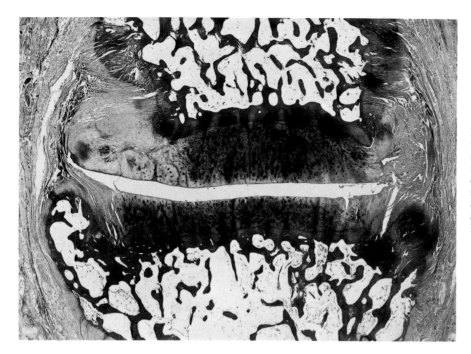

Figure 92–13. Histology of distal interphalangeal joint in acromegaly, showing hypertrophied cartilage, marginal fibrocartilage calcification of capsular insertion, and, on the other side, ossification of this. Hematoxylin & eosin × 6. (From Bluestone, R., et al.: Acromegalic arthropathy. Ann. Rheum. Dis. 30:243, 1971.)

megaly have nonradiating low back pain. The physical examination characteristically reveals normal reversal of the lumbar lordosis and an intact neurologic system. In addition, hypermobility of the spine has been described in some patients. Radiographically the intervertebral disc spaces may be increased, and large anterior osteophytes with ligamentous calcification are common.[106] The roles of osteopenia (see Chapter 96) and the acquired kyphoscoliosis in the evaluation of this symptom must be considered. The back pain of patients with acromegaly is probably the result of mechanical, metabolic, and degenerative processes. This complex interaction may explain the disappointing results often obtained with conservative measures such as physical therapy, rest, and nonsteroidal anti-inflammatory drugs (NSAIDs). On the other hand, some patients with the arthropathy of acromegaly may respond to lowering of the growth hormone levels by a long-acting somatostatin analogue.[107]

Carpal tunnel syndrome has been described in approximately one half of patients with acromegaly.

Table 92–3. PATHORADIOGRAPHIC FEATURES OF ACROMEGALIC ARTHROPATHY

Pathologic	Radiographic
Cartilage hypertrophy	Widened joint/disc space
Capsular calcification	Periarticular calcinosis
Exuberant marginal new bone formation	Large bridging osteophytes
New bone formation at tendinous/membranous insertions	Bone and joint remodeling Loss of joint space
Eventual cartilage fragmentation and ulceration	

Neural enlargement and excessive soft tissues contribute to the compression of the median nerve at the flexor retinaculum of the wrist.

Painless proximal muscle weakness is well documented in acromegaly. Muscle enzyme levels and EMG are characteristically normal. Muscle biopsies demonstrate wide variations in muscle fiber size without inflammation or destruction. This myopathic pattern was noted in half the patients. The cause of the myopathy is largely unknown but may reflect the direct action of GH on the enlarging muscle mass.[108]

The exaggerated skin folds, deep furrows, and hyperelasticity should suggest the diagnosis of acromegaly in patients with characteristic acral changes. In the early phases of the disease, some of the facial features can simulate myxedema. Later, differentiating acromegaly from pachydermatoperiostitis becomes difficult.[109] Finally, approximately one third of patients with acromegaly have Raynaud's phenomenon.[106]

The diagnosis of acromegaly can be confirmed by a lack of GH level suppression during the early phases of a glucose tolerance test (GTT). When available, comparison photographs taken a decade apart can dramatize the changes in facial features. Despite all the clinical manifestations of acromegaly, in some cases diagnosis is not made until the enlarging pituitary adenoma causes neurologic symptoms. Headaches and visual loss (usually bitemporal hemianopsia) are the most common.

For the rheumatologist, hand roentgenograms can suggest the diagnosis. Four signs are common: (1) the soft tissues are greatly increased; (2) the distal tufts are characteristically spade-like: (3) the well-described joint space widening is noted; and (4)

chondrocalcinosis of the wrist and ligamentous calcification appear.

SEX HORMONES AND PREGNANCY

The interaction of hormones with the immune and musculoskeletal systems during pregnancy results in several rheumatic conditions. Moreover, the course of existing connective tissue disease may be dramatically altered.

The immunobiology that prevents maternal-fetal rejection is complex. Elevated levels of estrogen, progesterone, prolactin, and cortisol have each been implicated to explain the marked depression of cell-mediated immunity[110, 111] and of neutrophil chemotaxis,[112] which characterizes the last trimester and early postpartum period.[113] Assignment of specific immune-modulating roles for each sex hormone remains difficult.

Levels of two rediscovered proteins, relaxin and pregnancy-associated alpha(α)-2-glycoprotein (PAG), are dramatically increased during gestation.[114] Relaxin has structural similarities to insulin but plays a collagenolytic role through enhanced plasminogen activation and collagenase production.[115] The striking effects of relaxin on collagen metabolism potentially make this hormone an attractive therapy for scleroderma.[116] Although maternal-fetal disparity for HLA-DQ antigen appears to be important for the improvement in disease activity of RA during pregnancy, PAG has a variety of immunosuppressive properties and may be relevant in combination with other hormones to the remission.[113, 117] Complement and other serum proteins that affect the sedimentation rate gradually increase during the last two trimesters.[118]

Carpal tunnel syndrome, presenting with nocturnal paresthesias of the first four digits, is common during the last trimester. Wrist splints and local steroid injections usually produce an excellent result, thus prolonged oral medicines or decompressive surgery can be avoided.

Some degree of low back pain in the last trimester is almost universal. The pain has been attributed to the multifactorial interaction of posture abnormalities (lordosis) caused by the enlarging fetus with the excess mobility of the synarthrial joints of the pelvis. Third trimester relaxin levels were significantly elevated in 35 women with severe pelvic pain and ligamentous laxity when compared with a control group of pregnant women with mild or no back pain.[119] The condition osteitis condensans ilii, which radiographically can be confused with sacroiliitis, is more common in women who have had multiple pregnancies.

The appearance of a new autoimmune disease during pregnancy and the early postpartum period is not unusual. The onset of RA,[113, 113a] scleroderma,[120] dermatomyositis,[121] mixed connective tissue disease (MCTD),[122] Raynaud's phenomenon,[123] and SLE[122]

during gestation, or in the early postpartum period, is well documented. Finally, a myriad of musculoskeletal complaints and autoantibodies that characterize postpartum thyroiditis can simulate connective tissue disease.[124]

Exacerbation and remissions in certain patients with existing arthritis are common during pregnancy. Approximately three quarters of patients with RA have improvement in their symptoms. Close correlations of PAG levels with this amelioration of joint activity have suggested a direct role for this protein in the induction of the remission. Whereas RA improves during pregnancy, patients with ankylosing spondylitis had worsening of disease activity despite elevated PAG levels.[125] The mechanism of action of PAG remains contradictory, although it may have the capacity to inhibit proteases. After delivery, RA usually returns to pregravid disease activity and the remission is not sustained.

Patients with SLE present with a different problem (see Chapter 61). Classically, exacerbation of the disease during the last trimester was the rule, but recent studies reflect the complexity of this generalization.[126] First, assessment of disease activity can be difficult. Elevations of serum complement levels and ESR are usual during gestation in normal women.[118] In lupus, the appearance of new proteinuria, hypocomplementemia, and thrombocytopenia may be a false indicator of a flare-up of the disease. Moreover, these variables do not characteristically respond to glucocorticoid therapy. Second, remissions have been described in all trimesters but at a slightly lower rate than exacerbations. Careful age-matched control studies with nonpregnant patients with SLE may confirm the prevalent conclusion that pregnancy does not increase disease activity[127] (see Chapter 61). Nevertheless, patients with active SLE should be advised that persistent disease is expected throughout gestation and fetal wastage is higher than normal, even if fertility rates are comparable to those in the general population.[122]

The skin disease of SLE must be differentiated from the common dermatologic problems of pregnancy. The butterfly rash can be confused with melasma, the so-called mask of pregnancy, in the malar region. Melasma can be caused by both estrogen and progesterone. Dramatic hair loss due to the telogen phase predominance during the postpartum period must be distinguished from the alopecia of SLE.[128] Palmar erythema is common in both but preferentially affects the fingertips in SLE.

The available studies of case reports from patients with dermatomyositis,[121] Raynaud's phenomenon,[123] scleroderma, MCTD,[122] and Takayasu disease[129] suggest that pregnancy carries some degree of risk for both mother and fetus. Successful pregnancies have been achieved but more numbers will be necessary to assign relative risk (see Chapters 61 and 63).

Sex hormones have a major role in nonpregnant patients with musculoskeletal disorders. In general, estrogens inhibit suppressor T cells, which results in B cell release and autoantibody production. Androgens inhibit certain T cell subsets and increase interleukin 2 (IL-2) production in autoimmune susceptible mice.[130] Although androgens seem to have opposing effects to estrogen, it is probably the relative concentrations and the amount of conversion of androgen to estrogen that determine net immunostimulation or immunosuppression.[131] Progesterone exerts its own anti-inflammatory effects, which may be different from those of estrogens.[132] The role of other less well known sterols on the course of immune-complex disease is being investigated. For instance, dehydroepiandrosterone (DHEA) is an adrenal androgen that can dramatically reverse the clinical features of murine lupus, possibly by improving the defective IL-2 production.[133]

The strong sex predominance of certain connective tissue diseases, both in terms of frequency and severity, is well described in RA and SLE (female) and spondylarthropathy (male). Moreover, males with Klinefelter's syndrome (XXY) demonstrate a female pattern of susceptibility to and severity of connective tissue disease. The clinical course of ankylosing spondylitis was typically mild in a Klinefelter's case, contrasting with the severe spondylitis affecting the genetically normal father.[134] The association of this genetic disorder with SLE has also been described.[135]

In lupus, murine and human studies confirm that excess estrogens, deficient androgens, or both can result in more severe immune complex disease and glomerulonephritis[130] (see Chapter 60).

RA may have dramatic changes in synovial inflammation during the menstrual cycle.[136] The pattern of postovulatory reduction of joint swelling and exacerbation just prior to menses closely reflects the wide variations of estrogen and progesterone levels during the cycle.

Birth control pills, especially those with high estrogen content, can cause effects similar to those of pregnancy, such as melasma and carpal tunnel syndrome. Rheumatoid arthritis may be ameliorated by the use of birth control pills (see discussion in Chapter 52).[137] The suggestion that oral contraceptives can prevent RA has been supported by several studies.[138–140] In SLE, disease activity may be lessened if a progesterone-only birth control pill is used. Additionally, erythema nodosum and a soft tissue tenderness similar to fibromyalgia have been described with birth control usage.[141]

Estrogen deficiency states, especially natural menopause, are associated with osteoporosis[142] (see Chapter 96). The X chromosome monosomy (XO) of Turner's syndrome results in gonadal dysgenesis. Invariably, these females have short stature and progressive osteoporosis. Whereas the osteopenia is the result of estrogen lack and is improved with conjugated estrogen, the short stature and other somatic stigmata are not dependent on estrogen for their expression.[143]

Sexual dysfunction, especially in males, has been described in patients with scleroderma, ankylosing spondylitis, or rheumatoid arthritis.[144–146] The role of testosterone levels and concomitant medications, such as MTX, is being evaluated.

AMYLOIDOSIS AND ENDOCRINE GLAND

Deposits of amyloid are commonly found within the thyroid gland in medullary carcinoma of the thyroid (MCT) and in the islet of the pancreas in type 2 diabetes. In each case the main constituent of the amyloid relates to the hormones. In MCT, it is calcitonin, whereas it is islet amyloid polypeptide (IAPP) in type 2 diabetes.[147] IAPP has some structural homology with the neuropeptide calcitonin gene-related protein (CGRP) and is not related to insulin itself.

SUMMARY

The endocrine disorders occupy a central position in the differential diagnosis of many common rheumatic conditions. This may seem surprising, because the specific cellular mechanisms and target organ of each hormone can differ so widely. The immune and endocrine systems interact at the molecular, cellular, and clinical levels. The role of numerous hormones in the local control of the immune response is being emphasized increasingly. The interesting observations, in rodents and humans, of growth hormone,[103] DHEA,[133] and relaxin[116] can now be added to 1,25-dihydroxyvitamin D[148] and the sex hormones[149] as potential therapeutic agents (Table 92–4). Despite these recent advances, cortisone remains the most important immunomodulatory agent of the last 30 years.

Carpal tunnel syndrome has been well described in hypothyroidism, acromegaly, diabetes, pregnancy, and primary hyperparathyroidism. A component of neural entrapment is common to all. Additionally, an intrinsic neuropathy may contribute to the first three.

Muscle weakness without enzyme level elevation is common to the endocrinopathies. Cushing's syndrome, steroid therapy, hyperthyroidism, acromegaly, and primary hyperparathyroidism share this presentation. On the other hand, the myopathy of hypothyroidism is often associated with moderate to marked elevations of creatine kinase. The weak, myxedematous patient has many clinical features in common with the patient with dermatomyositis.

The pathogenetic association of CPPD crystal deposition and premature (secondary) osteoarthritis has been described in a variety of metabolic disorders. Inborn errors of metabolism (ochronosis, Wilson's disease), increased urate synthesis (gout), and iron overload states (hemochromatosis) can be added to the endocrinopathies as probable causes. The

Table 92–4. TREATMENT OF CONNECTIVE TISSUE DISEASE WITH HORMONES

	Potential Mechanisms	Disorder Pathogenesis or Treatment
Established Hormone		
Glucocorticoids	Broad immuno-suppression (Chapters 7, 48)	RA, SLE, PM Vasculitis (including PMR)
Estrogen	↓ Bone resorption ↑ Intestinal calcium Absorption (Chapter 96)	Osteoporosis Prevention of RA[138]
Calcitonin	↓ Bone resorption (Chapter 96)	Paget's disease Osteoporosis
Experimental		
1,25-dihydroxy vitamin D	↓ IL-2, IFN-γ production	Psoriatic arthritis[148]
Relaxin	Monocyte differentiation ↓ Collagen synthesis[116]	Scleroderma
DHEA (dehydro-epiandrosterone)	↑ IL-2 production[133]	SLE
HCG (human chorionic gonadotropin)	↑ Testosterone levels?	Ankylosing spondylitis[149]
GH (growth hormone)	↑ Thymic function	Aging
(Growth hormone)	↑ Bone formation	Osteoporosis[103]

RA, Rheumatoid arthritis; SLE, systemic lupus erythematosus; PM, polymyositis; IL-2, interleukin-2; IFN-γ, interferon gamma.

association of acromegaly, PHP, and hypothyroidism with CPPD seems more certain than in patients with diabetes (see Chapter 77).

In a similar fashion, some patients with diabetes and primary hypoparathyroidism meet the radiologic criteria for DISH, whereas the spinal hyperostosis of acromegaly and X-linked hypophosphatemic osteomalacia does not.

The growing list of diseases associated with avascular necrosis includes Cushing's syndrome, myxedema, and hyperlipidemia. The "osteogenic synovitis" of primary hyperparathyroidism may have some component of avascular necrosis (see Chapter 97).

The changes in the soft tissues and blood vessels produced by endocrine disorders can be confused with classic connective tissue syndromes. Onycholysis is well described in thyrotoxicosis and must be added to the differential diagnoses of Reiter's disease, psoriatic arthritis, and fungal dermatoses when this nail finding is encountered. The distal nail changes of primary hypoparathyroidism may also be confused with onycholysis. Second, a variety of subcutaneous nodules are present in the endocrinopathies. Calcific nodules are described in pseudohypoparathyroidism and PHP. The firm nodules of pretibial myxedema are found in some patients with hyperthyroidism. A lobular panniculitis is associated with acute and chronic disorders of the exocrine pancreas. Third, Raynaud's phenomenon may be a

component of the vasomotor symptoms of acromegaly. Finally, hyperextensible joints have been described in acromegaly and primary hyperparathyroidism of childhood. In certain clinical settings, confusion with Ehlers-Danlos and Marfan's syndromes may be noted.

In addition to the edematous phase of scleroderma and RSD, the differential diagnosis of the unilateral or bilateral diffusely swollen hand or hands must include certain endocrine disorders and their articular sequelae. Moreover, RSD is associated with soft tissue calcifications (periarthritis) in both diabetes and renal tubular osteomalacia. The stiff hand syndrome of juvenile diabetes characteristically has swollen hands with flexed finger contractures. Subacute pseudogout of the wrist can simulate reflex sympathetic dystrophy. Finally, in myxedema and acromegaly, the soft tissues of the hands can be dramatically increased.

References

1. Amento, E. P., Bhalla, A. K., Kurnick, J. T., Kradin, R. L., Clemens, T. L., Holick, S. A., Holick, M. F., and Krane, S. M.: 1,25 Dihydroxy-vitamin D, induces maturation of the human monocyte line U937, and, in association with a factor from human T lymphocytes, augments production of the monokine, mononuclear cell factor. J. Clin. Invest. 73:731, 1984.
2. Amento, E. P., Kurnick, J. T., Epstein, A., and Krane, S. M.: Modulation of synovial cell products by a factor from a human cell line: T lymphocyte induction of a mononuclear cell factor. Proc. Natl. Acad. Sci. U.S.A. 79:5307, 1982.
3. Sambrook, P. N., Shawe, D., Hesp, R., Zanelli, J. M., Mitchell, R., Katz, D., Gumpel, J. M., Ansell, B. M., and Reeve, J.: Rapid periarticular bone loss in rheumatoid arthritis: Possible promotion by normal circulating concentrations of parathyroid hormone or calcitriol (1,25-dihydroxvitamin D₃). Arthritis Rheum. 33:615, 1990.
4. McGuire, J. L.: The endocrine system and connective tissue disorders. Bull. Rheum. Dis. 39:1, 1990.
5. Fam, A. G., Rubenstein, J. D., and Cowan, D. H.: POEMS syndrome. Arthritis Rheum. 29:233, 1986.
6. Seinfeld, E. D., and Sharma, O. P.: TASS syndrome: Unusual association of thyroiditis, Addison's disease, Sjögren's syndrome and sarcoidosis. J. R. Soc. Med. 76:883, 1983.
7. Hui, S. L., Epstein, S., and Johnston, C. C.: A prospective study of bone mass in patients with type I diabetes. J. Clin. Endocrinol. Metab. 60:74, 1985.
8. Raskin, P., Stevenson, M. K. M., Barilla, D. E., and Pak, C. Y. C.: The hypercalciuria of diabetes mellitus: Its amelioration with insulin. Clin. Endocrinol. 9:329, 1978.
9. Wettenhall, R. E. H., Schwartz, P. L., and Bornstein, J.: Actions of insulin and growth hormone on collagen and chondroitin sulfate synthesis in bone organ culture. Diabetes 18:280, 1969.
10. Silberberg, R., Gerritsen, G., and Hasler, M.: Articular cartilage of diabetic Chinese hamsters. Arch. Pathol. Lab. Med. 100:50, 1976.
11. Silberberg, R., Hirshberg, G. E., and Lesker, P.: Enzyme studies in the articular cartilage of diabetic rats and of rats bearing transplanted pancreatic islets. Diabetes 26:732, 1977.
12. Caterson, B., Baker, J. R., Christner, J. E., Pollok, B. A., and Rostand, K. S.: Diabetes and osteoarthritis. Alabama J. Med. Sci. 17:292, 1980.
13. Buchanan, K. D.: Diabetes mellitus and gout. Semin. Arthritis Rheum. 2:157, 1972.
14. McCarty, D. J., Silcox, D. C., and Coe, F.: Diseases associated with calcium pyrophosphate dihydrate crystal deposition. Am. J. Med. 56:704, 1974.
15. Starkman, H. S., Gleason, R. E., Rand, L. I., Miller, D. E., and Soeldner, J. S.: Limited joint mobility (LJM) of the hand in patients with diabetes mellitus: Relation to chronic complications. Ann. Rheum. Dis. 45:130, 1986.
16. Pal, B., Anderson, J., Dick, W. C., and Griffiths, I. D.: Limitation of joint mobility and shoulder capsulitis in insulin- and non-insulin-dependent diabetes mellitus. Br. J. Rheumatol. 25:147, 1986.
17. Fisher, L., Kurtz, A., and Shipley, M.: Association between cheiroar-

thropathy and frozen shoulder in patients with insulin-dependent diabetes mellitus. Br. J. Rheumatol. 25:141, 1986.

18. Schnapf, B. M., Banks, R. A., Silverstein, J. H., Rosenbloom, A. L., Chesrown, S. E., and Loughlin, G. M.: Pulmonary function in insulin-dependent diabetes mellitus with limited joint mobility. Am. Rev. Respir. Dis. 130:930, 1984.

19. Kapoor, A., Sibbit, W. L., Jr.: Contractures in diabetes mellitus: The syndrome of limited joint mobility. Semin. Arthritis Rheum. 18:168, 1989.

20. Gonzalez, T., Gantes, M., and Diaz-Flores, L.: Digital sclerosis and juvenile diabetes. Arthritis Rheum. 27:478, 1984.

21. Mackenzie, A. H.: Final diagnosis in 63 patients presenting with multiple palmar flexor tenosynovitis (MPFT). Arthritis Rheum. 18:415, 1975.

22. Leden, I., Jonsson, G., Larsen, S., Rank, F., Schersten, B., Svensson, B., and Thorngren, K.: Flexor tenosynovitis (FTS): A risk indicator of abnormal glucose tolerance. Scand. J. Rheumatol. 14:293, 1985.

23. Ipp, M. M., Howard, N. J., Tervo, R. C., and Gelfand, E. W.: Sicca syndrome and total lipodystrophy: A case in a fifteen-year-old female patient. Ann. Intern. Med. 85:443, 1976.

24. Ullman, S., and Dahl, M. V.: Necrobiosis lipoidica: An immunofluorescence study. Arch. Dermatol. 113:161, 1977.

25. Kaklamanis, P., Rigas, A., Giannatos, J., Matsas, S., and Economou, P.: Calcification of the shoulders and diabetes mellitus. N. Engl. J. Med. 293:1266, 1975.

26. Lequesne, M., Dang, N., Benasson, M., and Mery, C.: Increased association of diabetes mellitus with capsulitis of the shoulder and shoulder-hand syndrome. Scand. J. Rheumatol. 6:53, 1977.

27. Holt, P. J.: Rheumatological manifestations of diabetes mellitus. Clin. Rheum. Dis. 7:723, 1981.

28. Meltzer, A. D., Skversky, N., and Ostrum, B. J.: Radiographic evaluation of soft tissue necrosis in diabetics. Radiology 90:300, 1968.

29. Sinha, S., Munichoodoppa, C. S., and Kozak, G. P.: Neuropathic (Charcot) joints in diabetes mellitus (clinical study of 101 cases). Medicine (Baltimore) 51:191, 1972.

30. Jacobelli, S., McCarty, D. J., Silcox, D. C., et al.: Calcium pyrophosphate dihydrate crystal deposition in neuropathic joints: Four cases of polyarticular involvement. Ann. Intern. Med. 79:340, 1973.

31. Bluestone, R.: Rheumatological complications of some endocrinopathies. Clin. Rheum. Dis. 1:95, 1975.

32. Cundy, T. F., Edmonds, M. E., and Watkins, P. J.: Osteopenia and metatarsal fractures in diabetic neuropathy. Diabetic Med. 2:461, 1985.

33. Resnick, D., Shapiro, R. F., Wiesner, K. E., et al.: Diffuse idiopathic skeletal hyperostosis (DISH): Ankylosing hyperostosis of Forestier and Rotes-Querol, Semin. Arthritis Rheum. 7:153, 1978.

34. Julkunen, H., Heinonen, O. P., and Pyorala, K.: Hyperostosis of the spine in an adult population: Its relationship to hyperglycemia and obesity. Ann. Rheum. Dis. 30:605, 1971.

35. Rudge, S. R., Baron, F. M., and Drury, P. L.: Lack of association between rheumatoid arthritis and type I (insulin-dependent) diabetes. J. Rheumatol. 9:343, 1982.

36. Sinha, A. A., Lopez, M. T., and McDevitt, H. O.: Autoimmune diseases: The failure of self tolerance. Science 248:1380, 1990.

37. Kay, P. H., McCluskey, J., Christiansen, F. T., Feeney, D., McCann, V. J., Zilko, P. J., Dawkins, R. L., and O'Neil, G. J.: Complement allotyping reveals new genetic markers in rheumatoid arthritis and diabetes mellitus. Tissue Antigens 21:159, 1983.

38. Frame, B., Heinze, E. G., Block, M., and Manson, G. A.: Myopathy in primary hyperparathyroidism: Observations in 3 patients. Ann. Intern. Med. 68:1022, 1968.

39. Resnick, D. L.: Erosive arthritis of the hand and wrist in hyperparathyroidism. Radiology 110:263, 1974.

40. Alexander, G. M., Dieppe, P. A., Doherty, M., and Scott, D. G. I.: Pyrophosphate arthropathy: A study of metabolic associations and laboratory data. Ann. Rheum. Dis. 41:377, 1982.

41. McGill, P. E., Grange, A. T., and Royston, C. S. M.: Chondrocalcinosis in primary hyperparathyroidism. Scand. J. Rheumatol. 13:56, 1984.

42. Crisp, A. J., Helliwell, M., and Grahame, R.: The effect of hyperparathyroidism on the course of rheumatoid arthritis. Br. J. Rheumatol. 22:22, 1983.

43. Hofmann, G. S., Schumacher, H. R., and Paul, H.: Calcium oxalate microcrystalline-associated arthritis in end stage renal disease. Ann. Intern. Med. 97:36, 1982.

44. Bywaters, E. G. L., Dixon, A. S. J., and Scott, J. T.: Joint lesions of hyperparathyroidism. Ann. Rheum. Dis. 22:171, 1963.

45. Scott, J. T., Dixon, A. St. J., Bywaters, E. G. L.: Association of hyperuricemia and gout with hyperparathyroidism. Br. Med. J. 1:1070, 1964.

46. Goldin, R., Brickman, A. S., Massry, S. G., and Bluestone, R.: Ankylosing spondylitis and hyperparathyroidism. J.A.M.A. 240:759, 1978.

47. Rubin, L. A., Fam, A. G., Rubenstein, J., Campbell, J., and Saiphoo, C.: Erosive azotemic osteoarthropathy. Arthritis Rheum. 27:1086, 1984.

48. Resnick, D., Dwosh, J. L., and Niwayama, G.: Sacro-iliac joint in renal

osteodystrophy: Roentgenographic-pathologic correlation. J. Rheumatol. 2:287, 1975.

49. Kuntz, D., Navean, B., Bardin, T., Drueke, T., Treves, R., Dryll, A.: Destructive spondylarthropathy in hemodialysed patients. Arthritis Rheum. 27:369, 1984.

50. Hurst, N. P., Van Den Berg, R., Disney, A., Alcock, M., Albertyn, L., Green, M., and Pascoe, V.: Dialysis related arthropathy: A survey of 95 patients receiving chronic haemodialysis with special reference to β_2 microglobulin related amyloidosis. Ann. Rheum. Dis. 48:409, 1989.

51. Thompson, R. C., Havel, P., and Goetz, F.: Presumed neurotrophic skeletal disease in diabetic kidney transplant recipients. J.A.M.A. 249:1317, 1983.

52. Kuzela, D. C., Hoffer, W. E., Conger, J. D., Winter, S. D., and Hammond, W. S.: Soft tissue calcification in chronic dialysis patients. Am. J. Pathol. 86:403, 1977.

53. Chaykin, L. B., Frame, B., and Sigler, J. W.: Spondylitis: A clue to hypoparathyroidism. Ann. Intern. Med. 70:995, 1969.

54. Hung, W., Migeon, C. J., and Parrott, R. H.: A possible autoimmune basis for Addison's disease in three siblings, one with idiopathic hypoparathyroidism, pernicious anemia and superficial moniliasis. N. Engl. J. Med. 269:658, 1963.

55. Chilgren, R. A., Quie, P. G., Meuwissen, H. J., Good, R. A., and Hong, R.: The cellular immune defect in chronic mucocutaneous candidiasis. Lancet 1:1286, 1969.

56. DiGeorge, A. M., and Paschkis, D.: The syndrome of Addison's disease, hypoparathyroidism, and superficial moniliasis. Am. J. Dis. Child. 94:476, 1957.

57. Mann, J., Allerman, S., and Hills, A. G.: Albright's hereditary osteodystrophy comprising pseudohypoparathyroidism and pseudopseudohypoparathyroidism. Ann. Intern. Med. 56:315, 1962.

58. Pattern, J. L., and Levine, M. A.: Immunochemical analysis of the α-subunit of the stimulatory G-protein of adenylcyclase in patients with Albright's hereditary osteodystrophy. J. Clin. Endocrinol. Metab. 71:1208, 1990.

59. Levine, M. A., Downs, R. W., Moses, A. M., Breslau, N. A., Marx, S. J., Lasker, R. D., Rizzoli, R. E., Aurbach, G. D., and Spiegel, A. M.: Resistance to multiple hormones in patients with pseudohypoparathyroidism: Association with deficient activity of guanine nucleotide regulatory protein. Am. J. Med. 74:545, 1983.

60. Poznanski, A. K., Werder, E. A., Giedion, A., Martin, A., and Shaw, H.: The pattern of shortening of the bones of the hand in PHP and PPHP: A comparison with brachydactyly E, Turner syndrome, and acrodysostosis. Radiology 123:707, 1977.

61. Walton, K., and Swinson, D. R.: Acute calcific periarthritis associated with transient hypocalcemia secondary to hypoparathyroidism. Br. J. Rheumatol. 22:179, 1983.

62. Huaux, J. P., Malghem, J., Maldague, B., Devogelaer, J. P., Esselinckx, W., Withofs, H., Nagant de Deuxchaisnes, C.: Reflex sympathetic dystrophy syndrome: An unusual mode of presentation of osteomalacia. Arthritis Rheum. 29:918, 1986.

63. Polisson, R. P., Martinez, S., Khoury, M., Harrelson, J. M., Reisner, E., and Drezner, M. K.: Calcification of entheses associated with X-linked hypophosphatemic osteomalacia. N. Engl. J. Med. 313:1, 1985.

63a. Rigby, W. F. C., and Waugh, M. G.: Decreased accessory cell function and costimulatory activity by 1,25-dihydroxyvitamin D_3–treated monocytes. Arthritis Rheum. 35:110, 1992.

64. Okita, N., Row, V. V., and Volpe, R.: Suppressor T-lymphocyte deficiency in Graves' disease and Hashimoto's thyroiditis. J. Clin. Endocrinol. Metab. 52:528, 1981.

65. Gamblin, G. T., Galentine, P., Chernow, B., Smallridge, R. C., and Eil, C.: Evidence of extraocular muscle restriction in autoimmune thyroid disease. J. Clin. Endocrinol. Metab. 61:167, 1985.

66. Strakosch, G. R., Wenzel, B. E., Row, V. V., and Volpe, R.: Immunology of autoimmune thyroid diseases. N. Engl. J. Med. 307:1499, 1982.

67. Bottazo, G. F., Pujol-Borrell, R., and Hanafusa, T.: Role of aberrant HLA-DR expression and antigen presentation in induction of endocrine autoimmunity. Lancet 2:1115, 1983.

68. Matsunage, M., Eguchi, K., Fukuda, T., Otsubo, T., Ishikawa, N., Ito, K., and Nagataki, S.: Class II major histocompatibility complex antigen expression and cellular interactions in thyroid glands of Graves' disease. J. Clin. Endocrinol. Metab. 62:723, 1986.

69. Strakosch, C. R., Joyner, D., and Wall, J. R.: Thyroid-stimulating antibodies in patients with autoimmune disorders. J. Clin. Endocrinol. Metab. 47:361, 1978.

70. Shillinglaur, J., and Uttiger, R. D.: Failure of retro-orbital tissue to neutralise the biological activity of the long-acting thyroid stimulator. J. Clin. Endocrinol. Metab. 28:1069, 1968.

71. Kadlubowski, M., Irvine, W. J., and Rowland, A. C.: The lack of specificity of ophthalmic immunoglobulins in Graves' disease. J. Clin. Endocrinol. Metab. 63:990, 1986.

71a. Utiger, R. D.: Pathogenesis of Graves' ophthalmopathy. N. Engl. J. Med. 326:1727, 1992.

72. Gorman, C. A.: Unusual manifestations of Graves' disease. Mayo Clin. Proc. 47:926, 1972.

73. Cheung, H. S., Nicoloff, J. T., Kamiel, M. B., Spotler, L., and Nimni, M. E.: Stimulation of fibroblast biosynthetic activity by serum of patients with pretibial myxedema. J. Invest. Dermatol. 71:12, 1978.

74. Ramsey, I. D.: Muscle dysfunction in hyperthyroidism. Lancet 2:931, 1966.

75. Skillern, P. G.: The association of periarthritis of the shoulder with hyperthyroidism. In Transactions of the American Goiter Association. Springfield, IL, Charles C. Thomas, 1953, p. 100.

76. Doherty, M.: Triggering of acute calcific periarthritis by thyrotoxicosis. Br. J. Rheumatol. 23:76, 1984.

77. Mundy, G. R., Shapiro, J. L., Bandelin, J. G., Canalis, E. M., and Raisz, L. G.: Direct stimulation of bone resorption by thyroid hormone. J. Clin. Invest. 58:529, 1976.

78. Silverberg, J., and Volpe, R.: Rheumatoid factors in Graves' disease. Ann. Intern. Med. 88:216, 1978.

79. Thomas, R. D., and Croft, D. N.: Thyrotoxicosis and giant cell arteritis. Br. Med. J. 2:408, 1974.

80. Katakura, M., Yamada, T., Aizawa, T., Hiramatsu, K., Yukimura, Y., Ishihara, M., Takasu, N., Maruyama, K., Kameko, M., Kanai, M., and Kobahashi, I.: Presence of antideoxyribonucleic acid antibody in patients with hyperthyroidism of Graves' disease. J. Clin. Endocrinol. Metab. 64:405, 1987.

81. Amrheim, J. A., Kenny, F. M., and Ross, D.: Granulocytopenia, lupus-like syndrome and other complications of propylthiouracil therapy. J. Pediatr. 76:54, 1970.

82. Miller, F. W., Moore, G. F., Weintraub, B. D., and Steinberg, A. D.: Prevalence of thyroid disease and abnormal thyroid function test results in patients with systemic lupus erythematosus. Arthritis Rheum. 30:1124, 1987.

83. Withrington, R. H., and Seifert, M. H.: Hypothyroidism associated with mixed connective tissue disease and its response to steroid therapy. Ann. Rheum. Dis. 40:315, 1981.

84. Medsger, T. A., Jr., and Farrell, D. A.: Trigeminal neuropathy in progressive systemic sclerosis. Am. J. Med. 73:57, 1982.

85. Leriche, N. G. H., and Bell, D. A.: Hashimoto's thyroiditis and polyarthritis: A possible subset of seronegative polyarthritis. Ann. Rheum. Dis. 43:594, 1984.

86. Torfs, C. P., King, M., Huey, B., Malmgren, J., and Grumet, F. C.: Genetic interrelationship between insulin-dependent diabetes mellitus, the autoimmune thyroid diseases, and rheumatoid arthritis. Am. J. Hum. Genet. 38:170, 1986.

87. Dorwart, B. B., and Schumacher, H. R.: Joint effusions, chondrocalcinosis and rheumatic manifestations of hypothyroidism. Am. J. Med. 59:780, 1975.

88. Alexander, G. J. M., Scott, D. G. I., and Dieppe, P. A.: Pyrophosphate arthropathy: A study of metabolic associations and laboratory data. Ann. Rheum. Dis. 4:377, 1981.

89. Klein, I., Parker, M., Shebert, R., Ayyar, D. R., and Levey, G. S.: Hypothyroidism presenting as muscle stiffness and pseudohypertrophy: Hoffmann's syndrome. Am. J. Med. 70:891, 1981.

90. Hochberg, M. C., Edwards, C. Q., Barnes, H. V., Arnette, F. C., and Koppes, G. M.: Hypothyroidism presenting as a polymyositis-like syndrome. Arthritis Rheum. 19:1363, 1976.

91. How, J., Bowsher, P. D., and Walker, W.: Giant cell arteritis and hypothyroidism. Br. Med. J. 2:99, 1977.

92. Seedat, Y. K., and Randeree, M.: Avascular necrosis of the hip joint in hypothyroidism. S. Afr. Med. J. 49:2071, 1975.

93. Rubinstein, H. M., and Brooks M. H.: Aseptic necrosis of bone in myxedema. Ann. Intern. Med. 87:580, 1977.

94. Lane, R. J., and Mastaglia, F. L.: Drug-induced myopathies in man. Lancet 2:562, 1978.

95. Danowski, T. S., Boness, J. V., Sabeh, G., Sulton, R. O., Webster, M. V., and Sarver, M. E.: Probabilities of pituitary-adrenal responsiveness after steroid therapy. Ann. Intern. Med. 61:11, 1964.

96. Askari, A., Vignos, P. J., and Moskowitz, R. W.: Steroid myopathy in connective tissue disease. Am. J. Med. 61:485, 1976.

97. Dixon, R. B., and Nicholas, P. C.: On the various forms of corticosteroid withdrawal syndrome. Am. J. Med. 68:224, 1980.

98. Kabadi, U. M.: Onset of type I diabetes mellitus, hypothyroidism, and hypogonadism on withdrawal of glucocorticoid therapy and remission on its resumption in a patient with rheumatoid arthritis. Am. J. Med. 80:139, 1986.

99. Smith, R. T., and Good, R. A.: Sequelae of prednisone treatment of acute rheumatic fever. Clin. Res. Proc. 4:156, 1956.

100. Williamson, J., Patterson, R. W. W., and McGavin, D. D. M.: Sjögren's syndrome in relation to pernicious anemia and idiopathic Addison's disease. Br. J. Ophthalmol. 54:31, 1970.

101. Sternberg, E. M., Hill, J. M., Chrousos, G. P., Kamilaris, T., Listwalk, S. J., God, P. W., and Wilder, R. L.: Inflammatory mediator-induced hypothalamic-pituitary-adrenal axis activation is defective in streptococcal cell wall arthritis-susceptible Lewis rats. Proc. Natl. Acad. Sci. U.S.A. 86:2374, 1989.

102. Lane, L., Lotze, M. T., Chrousos, G. P., Barnes, K., Loriaux, D. L., and Fleisher, T. A.: Effect of chronic treatment with the glucocorticoid

103. Rudman, D., Feller, A. G., Nagraj, H. S., Gergans, G. A., Lalitha, P. Y., Goldberg, A. F., Schlenker, R. A., Cohn, L., Rudman, I. W., and Mattson, D. E.: Effects of human growth hormone in men over 60 years old. N. Engl. J. Med. 323:1, 1990.

104. Verde, G. G., Santi, I., Chiodini, P., Cozzi, R., Dallabonzana, D., Oppizzi, G., and Liuzzi, A.: Serum type III procollagen propeptide levels in acromegalic patients. J. Clin. Endocrinol. Metab. 63:1406, 1986.

105. Sledge, C. B.: Growth hormone and articular cartilage. Fed. Proc. 30:243, 1971.

106. Holt, P. J. L.: Locomotor abnormalities in acromegaly. Clin. Rheum. Dis. 7:689, 1981.

107. Layton, M. W., Fudman, E. J., Barkan, A., Braunstein, E. M., and Fox, I. H.: Acromegalic arthropathy: Characteristics and response to therapy. Arthritis Rheum. 31:1, 1990.

108. Khaleeli, A. A., Levy, R. D., Edwards, R. H. T., McPhail, G., Mills, K. R., Round, J. M., and Betteridge, D. J.: The neuromuscular features of acromegaly: A clinical and pathological study. J. Neurol. Neurosurg. Psychiatry 47:1009, 1984.

109. Mills, J. A.: Connective tissue disease associated with malignant neoplastic disease. J. Chronic Dis. 16:797, 1963.

110. Sridima, V., Pancini, F., Yank, S. L., Moawad, A., Reilly, M., and DeGroot, L. J.: Decreased levels of helper T cells: A possible cause of immunodeficiency in pregnancy. N. Engl. J. Med. 307:353, 1982.

111. Fugisaki, S., Mori, N., Sasaki, T., and Maeyama, M.: Cell mediated immunity in human pregnancy. Microbiol. Immunol. 23:899, 1979.

112. Persellin, R. H., and Liebforth, J. K.: Studies of the effects of pregnancy serum on polymorphonuclear leukocyte functions. Arthritis Rheum. 21:316, 1978.

113. Persellin, R. H.: The effect of pregnancy on rheumatoid arthritis. Bull. Rheum. Dis. 27:922, 1977.

113a. Silman, A., Kay, A., and Brennan, P.: Timing of pregnancy in relation to the onset of rheumatoid arthritis. Arthritis Rheum. 35:152, 1992.

114. Eddie, L. W., Bell, R. J., Lester, A., Geier, M., Bennett, G., Johnston, P. D., and Niall, H. D.: Radioimmunoassay of relaxin in pregnancy with an analogue of human relaxin. Lancet 1:1344, 1986.

115. Koay, E. S. C., Too, C. K. I., Greenwood, F. C., and Bryant-Greenwood, G. D.: Relaxin stimulates collagenase and plasminogen activator secretion by dispersed human amnion and chorion cells in vitro. J. Clin. Endocrinol. Metab. 56:1332, 1983.

116. Unemori, E. N., and Amento, E. P.: Relaxin modulates synthesis and secretion of procollagenase and collagen by human dermal fibroblasts. J. Biol. Chem. 265:10681, 1990.

117. Nelson, J. L., Nisperos, B. B., Hughes, K. A., and Hansen, J. A.: Maternal-fetal disparity for HLA-DQ antigens is associated with the pregnancy induced remission of rheumatoid arthritis. Arthritis Rheum. 33:S10, 1990.

118. Cecere, F. A., and Persellin, R. H.: The interaction of pregnancy and the rheumatic diseases. Clin. Rheum. Dis. 7:747, 1981.

119. MacLennan, A. H., Nicolson, R., Green, R. C., and Bath, M.: Serum relaxin and pelvic pain of pregnancy. Lancet 2:243, 1986.

120. Ballou, S. P., Morley, J. J., and Kushner, I.: Pregnancy and systemic sclerosis. Arthritis Rheum. 27:295, 1984.

121. Gutierrez, G., Dagnino, R., and Mintz, G.: Polymositis/dermatomyositis and pregnancy. Arthritis Rheum. 27:291, 1984.

122. Kaufman, R. L., and Kitridou, R. C.: Pregnancy in mixed connective tissue disease: Comparison with systemic lupus erythematosus. J. Rheumatol. 9:549, 1982.

123. Kahl, L., Blair, C., Ramsey-Goldman, R., and Steen, V.: Pregnancy outcomes in women with primary Raynaud's phenomenon. Arthritis Rheum. 33:1249, 1990.

124. Jansson, R., Bernander, S., Karlsson, A., Levin, K., and Nilsson, G.: Autoimmune thyroid dysfunction in the postpartum period. J. Clin. Endocrinol. Metab. 58:681, 1984.

125. Ostensen, M., von Schoultz, B., and Husby, G.: Comparison between serum α-2-pregnancy-associated globulin and activity of rheumatoid arthritis and ankylosing spondylitis during pregnancy. Scand. J. Rheumatol. 12:315, 1983.

126. Lockshin, M. D., Harpel, P. C., Druzin, M. L., Becker, C. G., Klein, R. F., Watson, R. M., Elkon, K. B., Reinitz, E.: Lupus pregnancy. II. Unusual pattern of hypocomplementemia and thrombocytopenia in the pregnant patient. Arthritis Rheum. 28:58, 1985.

127. Fine, L. G., Barnett, E. V., and Danovitch, G. B.: Systemic lupus erythematosus in pregnancy. Ann. Intern. Med. 94:667, 1981.

128. Schiff, B. L., and Kern, A. B.: A study of postpartum alopecia. Arch. Dermatol. 35:323, 1960.

129. Ishikawa, K., and Matsuura, S.: Occlusive thromboaortopathy (Takayasu's Disease) and pregnancy. Am. J. Cardiol. 50:1293, 1982.

130. Talal, N., Dauphinee, M. J., and Wofsy, D.: Interleukin-2-deficiency, genes, and systemic lupus erythematosus. Arthritis Rheum. 25:838, 1982.

131. Lahita, R. G., Bradlow, H. L., Ginzler, E., Pang, S., and New, M.:

Low plasma androgens in women with systemic lupus erythematosus. Arthritis Rheum. 30:241, 1987.

132. Latman, N. S., Kishore, V., and Bruot, B.: Progesterone secretion in the rat in response to an adjuvant arthritis challenge. Arthritis Rheum. 29:411, 1986.

133. Daynes, R. A., Araneo, B. A., Dowell, T. A., Huang, K., and Dudley, D. J.: Regulation of murine lymphokine production in vivo: III. The lymphoid tissue microenvironment exerts regulatory influences over T helper cell function. J. Exp. Med. 171:979, 1990.

134. Armstrong, R. D., MacFarlane, D. G., and Panayi, G. S.: Ankylosing spondylitis and Klinefelter's syndrome: Does the X chromosome modify disease expression? Br. J. Rheumatol. 24:277, 1985.

135. Marshall, J. W.: Systemic lupus erythematosus and Klinefelter's Syndrome. Am. J. Med. 84:180, 1988.

136. Latman, N. S.: Relation of menstrual cycle phase to symptoms of rheumatoid arthritis. Am. J. Med. 74:957, 1983.

137. Bole, G. G., Jr., Friedlander, M. H., and Smith, C. K.: Rheumatic symptoms and serological abnormalities induced by oral contraceptives. Lancet 1:323, 1969.

138. Hazes, J. M. W., Dijkmans, B. A. C., Vandenbrouche, J. P., de Vries, R. R. P., and Cats, A.: Reduction of the risk of rheumatoid arthritis among women who take oral contraceptives. Arthritis Rheum. 33:173, 1990.

139. Vandenbroucke, J. P., Valkenburg, H. A., Boersma, J. W., Cats, A., Festen, J. J. M., Huber-Brunig, O., and Rasker, J. J.: Oral contraceptives and rheumatoid arthritis: Further evidence for a preventive effect. Lancet 2:839, 1982.

140. Vandenbroucke, J. P., Witteman, C. M., Valkenburg, H. A., Boersma, J. W., Cats, A., Festen, J. J. M., Hartman, A. P., Huber-Bruning, O., Rasker, J. J., and Weber, J.: Noncontraceptive hormones and rheumatoid arthritis in perimenopausal and postmenopausal women. J.A.M.A. 255:1299, 1986.

141. Blomgren, S. E.: Erythema nodosum. Semin. Arthritis Rheum. 4:1, 1974.

142. Praeger, L., et al.: Roentgenographic abnormalities in phenotypic females with gonadal dysgenesis: A comparison of chromatin positive patients and chromatin negative patients. Am. J. Roentgenol. Rad. Ther. Nucl. Med. 104:899, 1968.

143. Grumbach, M. M., and Conte, F. A.: Disorders of sex differentiation. In Wilson, J. D., and Foster, D. W. (eds.): Williams Textbook of Endocrinology. 7th ed. Philadelphia, W. B. Saunders Company, 1985, p. 341.

144. Cutolo, M., Balleari, E., Giusti, M., Intra, E., and Accardo, S.: Androgen replacement therapy in male patients with rheumatoid arthritis. Arthritis Rheum. 34:1, 1991.

145. Gordon, B., Beastall, G. H., Thompson, J. A., and Sturrock, R. D.: Prolonged hypogonadism in male patients with rheumatoid arthritis during flares in disease activity. Br. J. Rheumatol. 27:440, 1988.

146. Conte, C., Steen, V., Schwentker, F. N., and Reynolds, C. F.: Sexual dysfunction in male systemic sclerosis patients. Arthritis Rheum. 33:S62, 1990.

147. Johnson, K. H., O'Brien, T. D., Betsholtz, C., and Westermark, P.: Islet amyloid, islet-amyloid polypeptide, and diabetes mellitus. N. Engl. J. Med. 321:513, 1989.

148. Huckins, D., Felson, D. T., and Holick, M.: Treatment of psoriatic arthritis with oral 1,25 dihydroxyvitamin D3: A pilot study. Arthritis Rheum. 33:1723, 1990.

149. Jimenez-Balderas, F. J., Tapia-Serrano, R., Murrieta, S., Bravo, C., and Mintz, G.: Testicular function in active ankylosing spondylitis (AS). Response to therapy with human chorionic gonadotrophin (HCG). Arthritis Rheum. 33:S158, 1990.

Chapter 93

Hypertrophic Osteoarthropathy

Roy D. Altman
Jerry Tenenbaum

INTRODUCTION

Hypertrophic osteoarthropathy (HPO) is a syndrome of (1) chronic proliferative periostitis of the long bones; (2) clubbing of fingers, toes, or both; and (3) oligosynovitis or polysynovitis.

Clubbing was described in the writings of Hippocrates, circa 400 B.C.; hence the label "Hippocratic fingers."[1] The association of clubbing and arthritis with chronic lung and chronic heart disease was noted by von Bamburger (1890)[2] and Marie (1890).[3] A familial form of HPO was subsequently described.[4] More recently, the triad of periostitis, clubbing, and arthritis has been associated with numerous extrathoracic diseases.

CLASSIFICATION

HPO may be classified as either the primary form, most often hereditary but with occasional idiopathic cases in adults, or the secondary form, most often associated with neoplastic or infectious diseases and most often bilaterally symmetric (Table 93–1).[5–26]

Isolated clubbing, not associated with periostitis or polyarthritis, can occur.[7] This familial condition may be a separate entity or an incomplete expression of HPO. Clubbing alone may be associated with chronic bronchitis, pneumoconiosis, and bacterial endocarditis.

Thyroid acropachy is a rare and unique form of HPO associated with long-standing hyperthyroidism.[25, 26]

CLINICAL SYNDROMES

Pachydermoperiostosis. Primary HPO (pachydermoperiostosis or Touraine-Solente-Golé syndrome) occurs most often within families. Symptoms usually begin at about age 1 year or in adolescence, either before or after puberty, more commonly in males.[27] It is probably transmitted by an autosomal dominant gene with variable expression. Symptoms often decline within 1 or 2 decades.

There is insidious development of clubbing with

"spade-like" enlargement of hands and feet.[28] Complaints are of cosmetic unsightliness and decreasing dexterity or awkwardness when using the fingers. Symptoms may include vague pains in the joints and along the bones.[5] Joint pain and swelling may be exacerbated by alcohol.[29]

Examination reveals marked clubbing with cylindrical thickening of forearms and legs, corresponding with radiographic periosteal changes.[4, 5] Recurrent joint effusions are mildly symptomatic.[30] Acro-osteolysis occurs with resorption of the distal phalanges of the hands and feet.[31] There is thickening and furrowing of the facial features with deep nasolabial folds and a corrugated scalp (Fig. 93–1), giving coarse, "leonine-like" features. The skin of the face and scalp is "greasy" with excessive sweating, which also particularly affects the hands and feet. The latter features are uncommon in secondary HPO. Some patients demonstrate gynecomastia, female hair distribution, striae, acne vulgaris, and cranial suture defects.[32]

Clubbing. Clubbing describes the appearance of

Table 93–1. CLASSIFICATION OF HYPERTROPHIC OSTEOARTHROPATHY

I. Primary
  A. Pachydermoperiostosis[5]
  B. Idiopathic[5]
  C. Clubbing (e.g., familial,[6] idiopathic[7])
II. Secondary
  A. Pulmonary
    1. Neoplasms (e.g., bronchogenic carcinoma[8])
    2. Infections (e.g., chronic bronchitis,[7] bronchiectasis[9])
    3. Other (e.g., cystic fibrosis,[10] pulmonary fibrosis,[11] pneumoconiosis[7])
  B. Cardiovascular
    1. Bacterial endocarditis[12]
    2. Cyanotic congenital heart disease[13]
    3. Patent ductus arteriosus[14]
    4. Other (e.g., aortic aneurysm,[15] aortic prosthesis[16])
  C. Gastrointestinal
    1. Neoplasms (e.g., carcinoma of esophagus,[17] liver,[18] colon[7])
    2. Infections (e.g., amebic dysentery[7])
    3. Hepatobiliary (e.g., biliary cirrhosis,[7] cirrhosis[19])
    4. Other (e.g., inflammatory bowel disease[20])
  D. Neoplasms (often with intrathoracic metastases) (e.g., lymphomas[21, 22, 22a])
  E. Miscellaneous (e.g., connective tissue diseases[23, 24])
  F. Thyroid acropachy[25, 26]

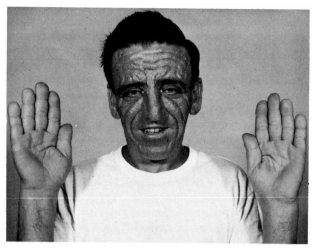

Figure 93–1. Facies and hands in pachydermoperiostosis.

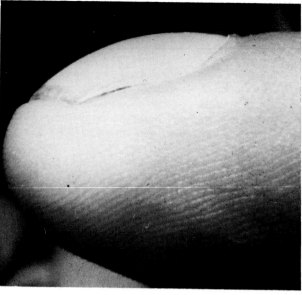

Figure 93–3. Clubbing. On lateral view, the index finger demonstrates loss of the normal 15-degree angle between the nail and the cuticle, accentuated convexity of the nail, enlargement of the distal finger pad, and shininess of the nail and adjacent skin.

the fingers or toes (Figs. 93–2 and 93–3). The presence of clubbing does not separate familial from idiopathic. Clubbing may be a feature of HPO, but periostitis and polysynovitis do not invariably accompany clubbing.

Clinically, clubbing presents as follows:

1. Initially there is a fluctuance and *softening of the nail bed*. A "rocking" sensation to palpation of the nail bed accompanies periungual erythema and telangiectasia.

2. There is *loss of the normal 15-degree angle* between the nail and the soft tissue of the nail bed (cuticle).

3. There is *accentuated convexity* of the nail.

4. The fingertip develops a *clubbed* appearance with local warmth and sweating.

5. Finally, the *nail and adjacent skin* develop a shiny or glossy change with longitudinal striations of the nail. Eponychia, paronychia, "hangnails," and breaking of the nail with accelerated nail or cuticle growth develop. Distal interphalangeal joints may become hyperextensible.

Congenital clubbing most often causes no symptoms or cosmetic unsightliness. Similar changes occur in the toes. Familial clubbing is common and may reflect an incomplete expression of pachydermoperiostosis.[6, 7] No genetic pattern has been established. Idiopathic or secondary clubbing may be a forme fruste of HPO but more likely is unrelated.

Clubbing frequently emerges insidiously over a period of months or years. Most cases of isolated clubbing are idiopathic and may simply be hereditary with delayed expression. More rapid onset of clubbing is often associated with chronic infections, such as bacterial endocarditis.[12]

Unilateral clubbing is reported with aneurysmal dilatation of large thoracic arteries in addition to apical lung neoplasms, axillary neoplasms, recurrent subluxation of the shoulder, aortic insufficiency with venous incompetence of the arm, and hemiplegia.[7] Unidigital clubbing is most often related to trauma.[7]

Secondary Hypertrophic Osteoarthropathy. Secondary HPO is most often present in adults, with age and sex distributions corresponding to those of the underlying disease.

Disease progression is often more rapid in secondary HPO. The underlying disease is usually already apparent. However, clinical manifestations of

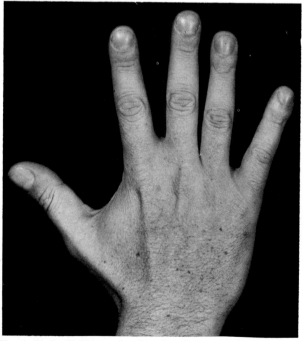

Figure 93–2. Clubbing. On this dorsal view of the hand, the fingertips are widened, replacing the normally tapered appearance of the digits.

HPO may precede symptoms of the underlying associated disease by more than a year.[8]

Periostitis usually causes relatively acute, increasing, and often severe burning and deep-seated pain of the distal extremities. The pain is particularly severe in the legs and is characteristically accentuated by dependency; relief of pain is achieved through elevation. It is not uncommon to observe the patient reversed in the hospital bed with feet elevated at the head of the bed.[33] The patient may complain of heat and swelling over the feet and legs. There may be occasional dysesthesia of the fingers with heat, sweating, clumsiness, and stiffness of the hands. Joint symptoms range from mild arthralgia to severe joint pain that is symmetric and involves metacarpophalangeal joints, wrists, elbows, knees, and ankles.[32] There is occasional pain over the temporomandibular joints or clavicles. The patient may have a low-grade fever and muscular weakness.

On examination, a broadened appearance of the distal extremities is often related to a firm, mildly pitting edema. There is often warmth and tenderness to pressure over the feet and legs, the distal shin (tibia), the radius, and the ulna. Glistening thickened skin, perspiration, and erythema are often observed. The clinical appearance of clubbing is readily apparent (see Figs. 93–2 and 93–3). The periungual tissues become edematous, erythematous, and warm. There may be a dusky discoloration of the tips of the digits. The nails may rock, loosen, or break as clubbing progresses. Severely clubbed fingers and toes resemble drumsticks. Mildly symptomatic joints are cool, with small effusions and no palpable pannus. More symptomatic joints may be warm, tender, and swollen, with definite effusions and limited range of motion. The symmetric involvement of hands, wrists, knees, and ankles with insidious onset is somewhat like rheumatoid arthritis.[34] In far advanced cases, ankylosis of joints may occur. The subcutaneous tissue around the active joints may be thickened and indurated, with hypopigmented skin suggestive of scleroderma.[35] Functional assessment often reveals clumsiness of hand function and an awkward gait. Occasional patients have gynecomastia.[36]

The insidious emergence of clubbing over months or years, with asymptomatic or mildly symptomatic bone and joint pain, is more often associated with the infectious diseases. Rapid progression of clubbing accompanied by fairly severe bone and joint symptoms is more commonly associated with malignant disease. However, because signs and symptoms of HPO may precede any symptoms of neoplasia, an assessment must include a chest radiograph.

In childhood, secondary HPO is often related to pulmonary infections,[37] congenital heart disease,[13] or osteosarcoma metastatic to the lungs. HPO caused by cyanotic congenital heart disease has been reported in as many as 31 percent of cases and is directly related to the degree of bypass of the lungs.[38]

In the adult, infections or neoplastic intrathoracic conditions are most common. HPO was observed in 9.2 percent of 1879 patients with pulmonary neoplasms, with bronchogenic carcinoma being the most common.[8, 39] In a series of localized pleural mesotheliomas, HPO and clubbing were noted only in the benign variant.[40] Relatively few case reports associate hepatobiliary and gastrointestinal diseases with HPO. Symptoms may flare with alcohol abuse.[40a]

Clubbing alone or HPO only in the lower extremities occurs in patients with patent ductus arteriosus who have developed right-to-left shunting of blood flow secondary to pulmonary hypertension,[14] infected aortic grafts,[41] or intra-abdominal fistula formation.[42] HPO can begin during pregnancy and remit post partum, most often in patients with other illnesses.[43] Clubbing has been associated with diffuse interstitial pulmonary fibrosis and rheumatoid arthritis–related fibrosing alveolitis and has been seen in the immunocompromised host with pneumonitis (e.g., AIDS).[44–46]

Thyroid Acropachy. Thyroid acropachy is an uncommon condition characterized by clubbing of the fingers and asymptomatic periosteal proliferation of the bones of the hands and feet.[25, 26] It is associated with prior (or active) hyperthyroidism, pronounced exophthalmos, and pretibial myxedema. It occurs concomitantly with exophthalmos, pretibial myxedema, and localized myxedema (nonpitting soft tissue swelling of the extremities).

LABORATORY FINDINGS

The laboratory findings in primary and secondary HPO are similar. Blood and urine tests are normal with the exception of the erythrocyte sedimentation rate (ESR), which may be increased in pachydermoperiostosis. The ESR is also often elevated in secondary HPO as well. Serum complement levels (total complement, C3, C4) are normal.[47] The latex fixation test for rheumatoid factor and the fluorescent antinuclear antibody test are negative.[30, 48] The serum alkaline phosphatase level may be increased with considerable periosteal new bone formation. Synovial fluid in pachydermoperiostosis and secondary HPO is noninflammatory (i.e., clear, yellow, normal viscosity, and low leukocyte count), demonstrating predominant lymphocytes and monocytes. The total protein in the synovial fluid is low, and complement levels (C3, C4) are normal.[30, 47]

RADIOGRAPHS AND RADIONUCLIDE SCANNING

The radiographic findings of HPO may occur in the absence of any clinical findings in both primary and secondary forms. Periosteal thickening occurs along the shafts of long and short bones, appearing first in the area of musculotendinous insertion and the distal diaphyseal regions of the long bones. It appears less often in the phalanges (Fig. 93–4). Periosteal changes appear as a continuous, thin, sclerotic line of new bone at the distal end of the diaphysis of the long bones. This finding is separated from the bony cortex by a narrow, radiolucent line. The periosteal new bone formation then becomes thicker and fuses with the cortex. This involvement progresses proximally and symmetrically with prominence of subperiosteal new bone. Still later, the cancellous portion of the involved bone may become osteoporotic with cortex thinning. These changes most often occur in the tibia, radius, ulna, fibula, femur, and occasionally the clavicles.[7]

Radiographs of the hands may reveal tufting of the terminal process and osteophytosis in more advanced stages of clubbing. Acro-osteolysis may be seen in younger patients.[49] On rare occasions, radiographs are normal in the presence of florid clinical disease.[50] Angiography demonstrates hypervascularization of the fingerpads associated with anteriovenous anastomoses and rapid filling of veins.[51]

Radionuclide bone scan utilizing a polyphosphate bone scanning agent is often helpful in documenting HPO[52] (Fig. 93–5). Scans demonstrate a pericortical linear concentration of nuclide along the radial, femoral, and tibial shafts along with periarticular uptake of the radionuclide, emphasizing the presence of synovitis. The clubbed phalanges may also accumulate nuclide, giving the digital tips a "string of lights" appearance. Unusual sites of periosteal activity may be revealed, such as the mandible, scapula, patella, and clavicle.[53] The bone scan may be positive prior to the development of symptoms.

PATHOLOGY

Periosteum. The basic lesion is subperiosteal cancellous new bone formation at the level of the distal diaphysis of tubular bones. Initially there is subperiosteal edema with resultant periosteal elevation. Subsequently there is deposition of new osteoid beneath the periosteum. This osteoid mineralizes, causing a new layer of bone predominantly around the distal portions of the long bones. With time, the process advances proximally. There is associated increased osteoclastic activity and weakening of the subperiosteal bone. Pathologic fractures occur uncommonly. These pathologic changes occur at the distal ends of the metacarpals, metatarsals, tibiae, fibulae, radii, ulnae, femora, humeri, and clavicles. Similar round cell infiltration and edema occur in the adjacent subcutaneous tissues.

Synovium. Synovial involvement is often continuous with the subperiosteal changes. Light microscopy shows normal synovium to pannus with erosion and destruction of cartilage. Synovial tissues may reveal thickening of the subsynovial blood vessels and mild synovial cellular hyperplasia.[31] The synovium becomes edematous and mildly infiltrated with lymphocytes, plasma cells, and occasional polymorphonuclear leukocytes,[30, 47, 48] but immunohistologic studies are negative.[47] Electron microscopic studies reveal occasional electron-dense subendothelial deposits in vessel walls[47, 48] with hyaline-like material on the synovial surface, in the interstitium, and in some of the dense deposits.[48] Many endothelial cells exhibit swollen cytoplasm. There is a concentric increase in basement membrane–like lamellae with intervening pericytic cytoplasmic processes and occasional endothelial cell gaps. Thickened and concentric multilamination of capillary basement membranes[47] is more often observed in pachydermoperiostosis.[30] In pachydermoperiostosis no electron-dense deposits are found in vessel walls.[30]

Clubbing. The clubbed distal portion of the digits results from an increase in the connective tissue of the nail bed as well as a proliferation of all the distal digital soft tissues. The collagen bundles in the dermis are swollen with enlargement of the rete pegs and narrowing of the epidermal papillae. There are round cell infiltrates and fibroblastic proliferation with dilatation and thickening of blood vessel walls.[7]

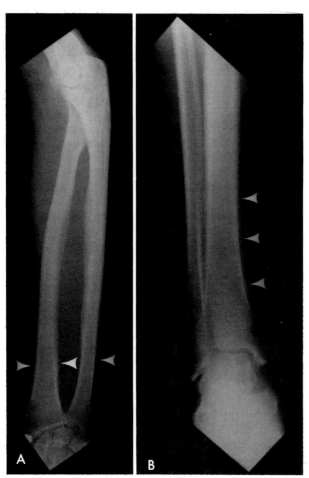

Figure 93–4. Radiograph in hypertrophic osteoarthropathy. Periosteal new bone formation is demonstrated by arrowheads at the distal portions of the radius and ulna (A) as well as the tibia (B).

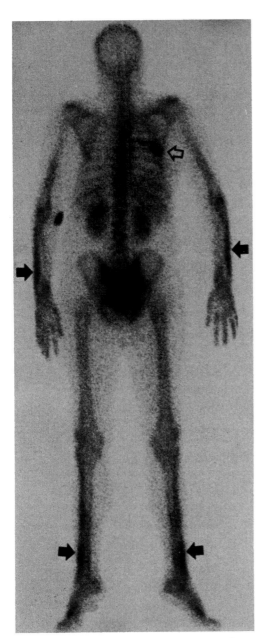

Figure 93–5. Total-body radionuclide bone scan in hypertrophic osteoarthropathy. Note localization of the nuclide to the periosteal area of the tibiae and ulnae *(closed arrows)*. The primary lesion, a bronchogenic carcinoma, also accumulated the nuclide *(open arrow)*.

DIFFERENTIAL DIAGNOSIS

Whenever HPO is diagnosed, it is crucial to search for an associated disease. This process should begin with a chest roentgenogram. Evaluation should include assessment of the cardiopulmonary and gastrointestinal systems. When clubbing, periostitis, and arthritis are present in association with a primary pulmonary lesion, the disorder is easily recognized. However, these features may appear in different combinations separated by intervals of time.

As mentioned, isolated clubbing may present as

a prodrome of HPO or may represent a separate entity. Spooning of the nails associated with hypochromic anemia should be differentiated from clubbing. Clubbing should also be differentiated from acromegaly. Calcific deposits in the distal digital pads may give the finger a clubbed appearance in the patient with scleroderma.[33]

The periostitis of HPO is usually characteristic, but one should consider periostitis of other causes such as bone tumor, osteomyelitis, subperiosteal hemorrhage, juvenile polyarthritis, syphilis, Reiter's syndrome, psoriasis, lymphagitis, and scurvy. Leg pain may suggest peripheral neuritis, Paget's disease of bone, or radiculopathy. The pretibial edema may suggest thrombophlebitis, venous stasis, or pretibial myxedema. Simultaneous presentation of synovial metastases with HPO has been reported.[54]

When the primary presenting complaint is polyarthritis, the picture may resemble rheumatoid arthritis. Pachydermoperiostosis can usually be differentiated from secondary HPO because of family history, age and sex at onset, and the nature of the periostitis. In Pachydermoperiostosis the periostitis is less symptomatic and is radiographically more thick, smooth, and dense than in HPO.

Thyroid acropachy is associated with findings of long-standing hyperthyroid such as exophthalamos. Periostitis is limited to the phalanges, in spite of the associated pretibial myxedema.

ETIOLOGY AND PATHOGENESIS

The etiology of HPO is unknown. Intrathoracic lesions of malignant or infectious nature comprise the majority of the associated systemic diseases. The most commonly related disease is bronchogenic carcinoma. The role that these conditions play in precipitation or production of HPO is speculative. The success of vagotomy in reversing or improving HPO suggests a role for reflex vagal stimulation in pathogenesis.[55] A growth factor,[56] hormonal,[36] and immune mechanisms have also been proposed.[48] Recently, platelet-endothelial interaction with production of von Willebrand factor antigen has been implicated in the pathogenesis of HPO.[56a]

MANAGEMENT

The most effective therapy for the pain and discomfort of secondary HPO is ablation or cure of the underlying condition. Infectious diseases most often can be controlled by antibiotics or drainage. Removal or effective suppressive therapy (e.g., chemotherapy) for a primary tumor most often results in prompt remission of symptoms, sometimes within hours or days.[8] Radiotherapy to a primary tumor[57] or to the metastatic lesion[58] may result in relief of joint symptoms. Joint symptoms may not recur after initial relief even with tumor progression and recurrent metastases. Vagotomy has been successful in some instances,[55] and percutaneous block of the vagus nerve was also successful in a series of patients.[59] Chemical vagotomy by atropine[60] and possibly with propantheline bromide are of benefit.[61] Anti-inflammatory agents have been quite beneficial in reducing the discomfort of HPO. Aspirin[62] and anti-inflammatory agents such as indomethacin are of possible benefit.[63] Adrenocortical steroids have been used with beneficial results.[34] Symptoms may resolve with successful treatment of bacterial endocarditis.[64] Colchicine is of potential benefit.[65]

Familial HPO and clubbing are most often asymptomatic and rarely require therapy. Salicylates should be sufficient if therapy is needed.

COURSE AND PROGNOSIS

The course of primary HPO is one of adolescent onset and self-limited disease, though recurrent joint effusions are possible.[30] The course of secondary HPO varies greatly, reflecting the activity of the underlying disease and depending on the nature of the primary condition. Symptoms may wax and wane with exacerbations and remissions of the primary condition. After resection of a lung tumor (or in some cases, after palliative treatment by resection of metastases in the lung) or a lung abscess, the symptoms and signs of arthropathy may subside rapidly over several hours or within a day. Radiographic abnormalities usually remit more slowly over weeks or months.[66] Without treatment of the primary condition, symptoms of HPO may result in a chronically painful demise.

References

1. Hippocrates: The Book of Prognostics. In The Genuine Works of Hippocrates, Vol. 1. translated by F. Adams. London, Sydenham Society, 1849.
2. von Bamburger, E.: Über Knochenveränderungen bei chronischen Lungenund Herzkrankenheiten. Ztschr. Klin. Med. 18:193, 1890–1891.
3. Marie, P.: De l'osteo-arthropathie hypertrophiante pneumique. Rev. Med. (Paris) 10:1, 1890.
4. Touraine, A., Solente, G., and Golé, L.: Un syndrome osteodermopathique: La pachydermie plicaturee avec pachyperiostose des extremites. Presse Med. 43:1820, 1935.
5. Vogl, A., and Goldfischer, S.: Pachydermoperiostosis: Primary or idiopathic hypertrophic osteoarthropathy. Am. J. Med. 33:166, 1962.
6. Seaton, D. R.: Familial clubbing of fingers and toes. Br. Med. J. 1:614, 1938.
7. Mendlowitz, M.: Clubbing and hypertrophic osteoarthropathy. Medicine 21:269, 1942.
8. Vogl, A., Blumenfeld, S., and Gutner, L. B.: Diagnostic significance of pulmonary hypertrophic osteoarthropathy. Am. J. Med. 18:51, 1955.
9. Wierman, W. H., Clagett, O. T., and McDonald, J. R.: Articular manifestations in pulmonary diseases: Analysis of their occurrence in 1,024 cases in which pulmonary resection was performed. J.A.M.A. 155:1459, 1954.
10. Matthay, M. A., Matthay, R. A., Mills, D. M., Lakshiminarayan, S., and Cotton, E.: Hypertrophic osteoarthropathy in adults with cystic fibrosis. Thorax 31:572, 1976.
11. Galko, B., Grossman, R. F., Day, A., Tenenbaum, J., Kirsh, J., and Rebuck, A. S.: Hypertrophic pulmonary osteoarthropathy in four patients with interstitial pulmonary disease. Chest 88:94, 1985.
12. Cotton, T. F.: Clubbed fingers as a sign of subacute infective endocarditis. Heart 9:347, 1921–1922.
13. McLaughlin, G. E., McCarty, D. J., and Downing, D. F.: Hypertrophic osteoarthropathy associated with cyanotic congenital heart disease. Ann. Intern. Med. 67:579, 1967.
14. Williams, B., Ling, J., Leight, L., and McGaff, C. J.: Ductus arteriosus arteriosus and osteoarthropathy. Arch. Intern. Med. 111:346, 1963.
15. Shapiro, S.: Hypertrophic osteoarthropathy. Arch. Intern. Med. 98:700, 1956.
16. Pascuzzi, C. A., Parkin, T. W., Bruwer, A. J., and Edwards, J. E.: Hypertrophic osteoarthropathy associated with primary rhabdomyosarcoma of the heart. Mayo Clin. Proc. 32:30, 1957.
17. Peirce, T. H., and Weir, D. G.: Hypertrophic osteoarthropathy associated with a non-metastasizing carcinoma of the oesophagus. J. Ir. Med. Assoc. 66:160, 1973.
18. Morgan, A. G., Walker, W. C., Mason, M. D., Herlinger, H., and Lowsowsky, M. S.: A new syndrome associated with hepatocellular carcinoma. Gastroenterology 63:340, 1972.
19. Epstein, O., Dick, R., and Sherlock S.: Prospective study of periostitis and finger clubbing in primary biliary cirrhosis and other forms of chronic liver disease. Gut 22:203, 1981.
20. Kitis, G., Thompson, H., and Allan, R. N.: Finger clubbing in inflammatory bowel disease: Its prevalence and pathogenesis. Br. Med. J. 2:825, 1979.
21. Lofters, W. S., and Walker, T. M.: Hodgkin's disease and hypertrophic pulmonary osteoarthropathy. West Indian Med. J. 28:227, 1978.
22. McNeil, M. M., Sage, R. E., and Dale, B. M.: Hypertrophic osteoarthropathy complicating primary bone lymphoma: Association with invasive Phycomyosis and Aspergillus infections. Aust. N.Z. J. Med. 11:71, 1981.
22a. Vico, P., Delcorde, A., Rahier, I., Treille de Grandsaigne, S., Famaey, J.-P., and Body, J.-J.: Hypertrophic osteoarthropathy and thyroid cancer. J. Rheumatol. 19:1153, 1992.
23. Armstrong, R. D., Crisp, A. J., and Grahame, R.: Hypertrophic osteoarthropathy and purgative abuse. Br. Med. J. 282:1836, 1981.
24. Mackie, R. M.: Lupus erythematosus in association with finger-clubbing. Br. J. Dermatol. 89:533, 1973.
25. Kinsella, R. A., and Back, D. K.: Thyroid acropachy. Med. Clin. North Am. 52:393, 1968.
26. Rothschild, B. M., and Yoon, B. H.: Thyroid acropachy complicated by lymphatic obstruction. Arthritis Rheum. 25:588, 1984.
27. Martinez-Lavin, M., Pineda, C., Valdez, T., Cajigas, J-C., Weisman, M., Gerber, N., and Steigler, D.: Primary hypertrophic osteoarthropathy. Semin. Arthritis Rheum. 17:156, 1988.
28. Diren, H. B., Kutluk, M. T., Karabent, A., Gocmen, A., Adalioglu, G., and Kenanoglu, A.: Primary hypertrophic osteoarthropathy. Pediatr. Radiol. 16:231, 1986.
29. Mueller, M., and Trevarthen, D.: Pachydermoperiostosis: Arthropathy aggravated by episodic alcohol abuse. J. Rheumatol. 8:862, 1981.
30. Lauter, S. A., Vasey, F. B., Huttner, I., and Osterland, C. K.: Pachydermoperiostosis: Studies on the synovium. J. Rheumatol. 5:85, 1978.
31. Fam, A. G., Chin-Sang, O. H., and Ramsay, C. A.: Pachydermoperiostosis: Scintigraphic, plethysmographic, and capillarscopic observations. Ann. Rheum. Dis. 42:98, 1983.
32. Reginato, A., Jr., Schinpachasse, Y., and Guerrero, R.: Familial idiopathic hypertrophic osteoarthropathy and cranial suture defects in children. Skeletal Radiol. 8:105, 1982.
33. Altman, R. D.: Personal observation.
34. Sega, A. M., and MacKenzie, A. H.: Hypertrophic osteoarthropathy: A ten year retrospective analysis. Semin. Arthritis Rheum. 12:220, 1982.
35. Gray, R. G., and Gottlieb, N. L.: Pseudoscleroderma in hypertrophic osteoarthropathy. J.A.M.A. 246:2062, 1981.
36. Ginsburg, J., and Brown, J. B.: Increased oestrogen excretion in hypertrophic pulmonary osteoarthropathy. Lancet 2:1274, 1961.
37. Cavanaugh, J. J. A., and Holman, G. H.: Hypertrophic osteoarthropathy in childhood. J. Pediatr. 66:27, 1965.
38. Martinez-Lavin, M., Bobadilla, M., Casanova, J., Attie, F., and Martinez, M.: Hypertrophic osteoarthropathy in cyonotic congenital heart disease. Arthritis Rheum. 25:1186, 1982.
39. Calabro, J. J.: Cancer and arthritis. Arthritis Rheum. 10:553, 1967.
40. Okike, N., Bernatz, P. E., and Woolner, L. B.: Localized mesothelioma of the pleura: Benign and malignant variants. J. Thorac. Cardiovasc. Surg. 75:363, 1968.
40a. Mueller, M. N., and Trevarthen, D.: Pachydermoperiostosis: Arthropathy aggravated by episodic alcohol abuse. J. Rheumatol. 8:862, 1981.
41. Sorin, S. B., Askari, A., and Rhodes, R. S.: Hypertrophic osteoarthropathy of the lower extremities as a manifestation of arterial graft sepsis. Arthritis Rheum. 23:768, 1980.
42. Stein, H. B., and Little, H. A.: Localized hypertrophic osteoarthropathy in the presence of an abdominal aortic prosthesis. Can. Med. Assoc. J. 118:947, 1978.
43. Borden, E. C., and Holling, H. E.: Hypertrophic osteoarthropathy and pregnancy. Ann. Intern. Med. 71:577, 1969.
44. Walker, W. C., and Wright, V.: Pulmonary lesions and rheumatoid arthritis. Medicine 47:501, 1968.
45. Bhat, S., Heurich, A. E., Vaquer, R. A., Dunn, E. K., Strashun, A. M.,

and Kamholz, S. L.: Hypertrophic osteoarthropathy associated with *Pneumonocystis carinii* pneumonia in AIDS. Chest 96:1208, 1989.

46. Beluffi, G., Monafo, V., Terracciano, L., Arrigoni, S., Martin, A., and Fiori, P.: Secondary hypertrophic osteoarthropathy in two children with humoral immunodeficiencies. J. Belge Radiol. 71(1):99, 1988.

47. Vidal, A. F., Altman, R. D., Pardo, D., and Schultz, D.: Structural and immunologic changes of synovium of hypertrophic osteoarthropathy. Arthritis Rheum. 20:139, 1977.

48. Schumacher, H. R.: Articular manifestations of hypertrophic pulmonary osteoarthropathy in bronchogenic carcinoma. Arthritis Rheum. 19:629, 1976.

49. Pineda, C., Fonseca, C., and Martinez-Lavin, M.: The spectrum of soft tissue and skeletal abnormalities of hypertrophic osteoarthropathy. J. Rheumatol. 17:626, 1990.

50. Horn, C. R.: Hypertrophic osteoarthropathy without radiographic evidence of new bone formation. Thorax 35:479, 1980.

51. Jajic, I., Pecina, M., Kostulovic, B., Kovacevic, D., Pavicic, F., and Spaventi, S.: Primary hypertrophic osteoarthropathy (PHO) and changes in the joints. Scand. J. Rheumatol. 9:89, 1980.

52. Rosenthall, L., and Kirsh, J.: Observations on radionuclide imaging in hypertrophic pulmonary osteoarthropathy. Radiology 120:359, 1976.

53. Ali, A., Tetalman, M. R., Fordham, E. W., Turner, D. A., Chiles, J. T., Patel, S. L., and Schmidt, K. D.: Distribution of hypertrophic pulmonary osteoarthropathy. Am. J. Radiol. 34:771, 1980.

54. Fam, A. G., and Cross, E. G.: Hypertrophic osteoarthropathy phalangeal and synovial metastases associated with bronchogenic carcinoma. J. Rheumatol. 6:680, 1979.

55. Yacoub, M. H.: Cervical vagotomy for pulmonary osteoarthropathy. Br. J. Dis. Chest 59:28, 1965.

56. Martinez-Lavin, M.: Digital clubbing and hypertrophic osteoarthropathy: A unifying hypothesis. J. Rheumatol. 14:6, 1987.

56a. Matucci-Cerinic, M., Martinez-Lavin, M., Rojo, F., Fonseca, C., and Kahaleh, B. M.: von Willebrand factor antigen in hypertrophic osteoarthropathy. J. Rheumatol. 19:765, 1992.

57. Steinfeld, A. D., and Munzenrider, J. E.: The response of hypertrophic pulmonary osteoarthropathy to radiotherapy. Radiology 113:709, 1974.

58. Rao, G. M., Gurupoakash, G. H., Poulose, K. P., and Blaskar, G.: Improvement in hypertrophic pulmonary osteoarthropathy after radiotherapy to metasasis. Am. J. Radiol. 133:944, 1979.

59. Dam, W. H., and Hagelsten, J. O.: Blocking of the vagus nerve relieving osteoarthropathy in lung disease. Dan. Med. Bull. 11:131, 1964.

60. Lopez-Enriquez, E., Morales, A. R., and Robert, F.: Effect of atropine sulfate in pulmonary hypertrophic osteoarthropathy. Arthritis Rheum. 23:822, 1980.

61. Deal, C. C., and Canoso, J. J.: Mineral response to propantheline bromide therapy in hypertrophic pulmonary osteoarthropathy: A double blind controlled case study. J. Rheumatol. 10:165, 1983.

62. Lokich, J. J.: Pulmonary osteoarthropathy; association with mesenchymal tumor metastases to the lungs. J.A.M.A. 238:37, 1977.

63. Leung, F. W., Williams, A. J., and Fan, P.: Indomethacin therapy for hypertrophic pulmonary osteoarthropathy in patients with bronchogenic carcinoma. West. J. Med. 142:345, 1985.

64. Shapiro, C. M., and Mackinnon, J.: The resolution of hypertrophic pulmonary osteoarthropathy following treatment of subacute bacterial endocarditis. Postgrad. Med. J. 56:513, 1980.

65. Matucci-Cerinic, M., Fattorini, L., Gerini, G., Corbardi, A., Pignone, A., Petrini, N., and Lotti, T.: Colchicine treatment in a case of pachydermoperiostosis with acroosteolysis. Rheumatol. Int. 8:185, 1988.

66. Shulman, L. E.: Hypertrophic osteoarthropathy. Bull. Rheum. Dis. 7:135, 1957.

Chapter 94

David S. Caldwell

Musculoskeletal Syndromes Associated with Malignancy

An estimated 15 percent of patients hospitalized with advanced malignancy will have a clinically apparent paraneoplastic syndrome—a constellation of signs and symptoms developing in association with the malignancy but not believed to be a direct result of the presence of the neoplasm. The chance of a paraneoplastic syndrome arising over the life span of a patient with cancer may reach 50 to 75 percent.

Endocrine syndromes secondary to ectopic hormone production account for one third of all paraneoplastic syndromes, while connective tissue, hematologic, and neuromuscular syndromes account for the majority of the remaining syndromes.

The existence of a causal relationship between malignancy and connective tissue disease is firmly established for some entities, such as hypertrophic osteoarthropathy, in which resection of the primary process leads to dramatic resolution of the presenting musculoskeletal symptoms. Conversely, malignancy in the setting of a preexisting connective tissue disease may occur. Whether a true relationship exists in all such cases is uncertain, as the close temporal occurrence of two common disorders may be by chance. It is also possible that the common feature is not that one produces the other, but that they share the same unknown etiology. Whether the relationship is casual or causal, it would seem that the importance of the possible relationship is twofold: (1) the awareness that an underlying malignancy may produce musculoskeletal symptoms may allow for earlier recognition of an otherwise occult, potentially curable malignancy. Conversely, knowledge that a connective tissue process may predispose to cancer may provide early recognition of a predictable malignancy; (2) the association of cancer and musculoskeletal syndromes may ultimately provide insight regarding the causation of rheumatic disorders and malignancy. Abnormal immunoregulation and immunogenetics, important determinants of host susceptibility to the development of neoplasia, may also predispose to connective tissue syndromes. Tumor-associated antigen CA 19–9 reportedly with excellent diagnostic sensitivity and specificity for identifying adenocarcinoma has been described in connective tissue disease patients with no evidence of malignancy at the time of study.[1]

Rarely situations may arise where the rheumatic disease complications may mimic malignancy: i.e., pathologic costal fracture induced by an osseous rheumatoid nodule or discogenic vertebral sclerosis or insufficiency fractures of the pelvis mimicking metastatic disease.[2, 2a, 2b]

DIRECT ASSOCIATIONS BETWEEN MUSCULOSKELETAL SYNDROMES AND MALIGNANCY

The mechanisms by which malignant disease may simulate a musculoskeletal syndrome by direct involvement are depicted in Table 94–1. Tumors involving joints are discussed in more detail in Chapter 98.

Metastatic Disease. Arthritis associated with metastatic carcinoma is most commonly monoarticular, most frequently involving the knee. Patellar metastases may resemble a septic arthritis. Involvement of the hip, ankle, wrist, hand, and foot occurs less frequently. Shoulder region metastases may

Table 94–1. DIRECT PATHOLOGIC MECHANISMS BY WHICH MALIGNANCY MAY PRESENT AS A MUSCULOSKELETAL SYNDROME

I. Metastatic disease
  A. Bone
  B. Synovium
  C. Meninges
  D. Muscle
II. Primary malignant disease
  A. Synovium
    1. Primary involvement
    2. Systemic tumor with synovial infiltration
      a. Leukemia
      b. Lymphoma
  B. Bone (juxta-articular)
    1. Primary lymphoma
    2. Osteogenic sarcoma
    3. Chondrosarcoma
    4. Giant cell tumor

mimic shoulder monoarthritis or a rotator cuff tear. Carcinomas of the breast and lung are the primary neoplasms in the majority of patients.[3] Polyarthritis resulting from metastatic skeletal invasion is usually asymmetric in distribution.

While bone metastases occur in 33 percent of cases of bronchogenic carcinoma, they rarely involve the small bones. Most unusual is the situation where small bone metastases herald underlying bronchogenic carcinoma. Approximately half the cases of metastatic hand lesions reported have had a pulmonary primary neoplasm, the other half originating from a primary source within the breast, kidney, colon, or parotid glands. Metastases should be considered when radiographs suggest a particularly destructive process.

Symmetric metastatic finger deposits may resemble the findings of rheumatoid arthritis. That rheumatoid factor occurs in up to 20 percent of patients with malignancy as well as in 42 percent of the elderly with no obvious illnesses may further obscure the malignant origin. Conversely, upon the development of malignancy, rheumatoid factor may disappear from the serum. A speckled antinuclear antibody may also be noted in elderly individuals without apparent illnesses and in patients with malignancy.[4]

Phalangeal metastases may also simulate the clinical appearance of an acute synovitis such as gout, osteomyelitis, tenosynovitis, or acro-osteolysis, a destructive process involving one or more terminal phalanges, seen in a variety of rheumatic disorders. This clinical picture can occur by direct synovial implantation or involvement of the juxta-articular or subchondral bone. The Sézary syndrome can result in terminal phalangeal infiltration with neoplastic cells and subsequent erosion of terminal tufts. Malignant bursal involvement rarely occurs. A constellation of clinical features should suggest possible underlying metastasis (Table 94–2).

Although the majority of patients with metastatic disease simulating a primary musculoskeletal disorder have had pulmonary malignancies, a variety of nonpulmonary neoplasms have been reported, including melanoma.[5] The diagnosis of underlying malignancy can generally be made by appropriate studies, including radiographs, bone scans, and local biopsy. Synovial fluid exfoliative cytology may also be of value in the early recognition of metastatic carcinomatous arthritis.[5a]

Table 94–2. FREQUENT FEATURES OF ARTHRITIS RESULTING FROM METASTATIC CARCINOMA

Presence of constitutional symptoms
Prior history of malignancy
Protracted clinical course
Negative culture results, negative crystal analysis
Medical therapeutic failure
Rapid reaccumulation of hemorrhagic noninflammatory effusion
Radiologic evidence of destructive process

Involvement of the axial skeleton by tumor may mimic spondylosis with or without radiculopathy. Radiographic evidence of tumor may be lacking. Metastatic bone lesions may also mimic other traditional radiologic diagnoses such as osteitis condensans ilii.

Metastatic tumor deposits within skeletal muscle are very rare, found in only four patients with cancer out of 500 necropsies. Nevertheless skeletal muscle metastases may occur during the course of disease, and on occasion be the presenting feature. Although carcinoma of the lung, colon, and pancreas are frequent primary sites, metastases related to leukemia, lymphoma, carcinoma of the thyroid, prostate, kidney, and breast have been observed. Forearm muscle metastases may simulate a Volkmann's type contracture.[6]

Leukemia. The musculoskeletal manifestations of leukemia include symmetric or migratory polyarthritis-arthralgias, and bone pain and tenderness. Sternal tenderness may occur in chronic myelogenous leukemia. The frequency of articular manifestations in acute leukemia is about 4 percent in adult patients and about 14 percent in children, although in some series it may be the presenting feature in as high as 13.5 percent overall.[7, 8] Leukemic synovitis may also be the initial manifestation of relapse of acute leukemia, even though it was not present when leukemia was first diagnosed.[7]

Polyarthritis may be the presenting complaint in childhood leukemia. Joint manifestations have been attributed to leukemic synovial infiltration; hemorrhage into joint or periarticular structures; synovial reaction to adjacent bony, periosteal, or capsular lesions; and crystal-induced synovitis. Leukemic arthritis, usually polyarticular, may have an additive or migratory pattern. Knee and ankle joints are most commonly involved. Back pain mimicking a radiculopathy may be caused by diffuse leukemic infiltrate of the meninges.

Distinguishing points in patients with leukemic polyarthritis include hematologic abnormalities and severe joint pain disproportionate to the degree of arthritis. The initial peripheral blood smear is often diagnostic. Synovial fluid and biopsy specimens have been examined infrequently. Synovial effusions have been described as only mildly inflammatory, rarely revealing leukemic cells even when leukemic infiltration has been seen in synovial tissue. Because focal leukemic lesions may be missed on synovial biopsy, immunocytologic analysis of joint fluid may facilitate early diagnosis of leukemic arthritis.[8a] Less often, radiographic changes suggestive of leukemia (metaphyseal rarefaction, osteolytic or periosteal reactions) may occur. In those patients without radiographic changes, bone scintigraphy utilizing the triple-phase technique may be helpful, demonstrating local abnormalities on both early and delayed images, even in the very early stages of articular disease. This is not specific, however, and will not distinguish between septic and leukemic arthritis.[7]

The sedimentation rate may be of no help in distinguishing this group of patients. Rheumatoid factor and rheumatoid-like nodules have been reported in patients with leukemia. Response to therapy may also confuse the diagnosis, as joint complaints in leukemic patients may be partially or temporarily relieved by salicylates or nonsteroidal anti-inflammatory drugs.

Because leukemic synovitis is likely a manifestation of systemic disease, either the initial event or relapse, immediate and aggressive systemic chemotherapy should begin even when there are no signs of bone marrow involvement. Adjunctive local irradiation of affected joints may reduce symptoms within days. Disappearance of bone and joint involvement often occurs promptly after the induction of therapy for leukemia and may be one of the first indications of the drug's effectiveness.

Lymphoma. Patients with lymphoma may present with musculoskeletal manifestations.[8b] Bone pain is the most common symptom attributable to osseous involvement. Synovial reaction, rarely caused by direct invasion, is most often attributed to adjacent bone disease. When arthritis has been caused by direct involvement of the synovium, a surgical procedure has been required for diagnosis except in a rare situation where arthrocentesis yielded the diagnosis through cytologic and immunologic findings. Although non-Hodgkin's lymphomas rarely present in joint tissues, neoplastic growth may originate from the synovium and locally invade surrounding structures resulting in arthritic symptoms.[9] Knee pain exacerbated by recumbency, however, may relate to lymphomatous spinal cord involvement. Articular symptoms are less frequent than might be expected in view of the frequency of skeletal invasion. Both monoarticular and polyarticular involvement attributed to lymphoma may occur.

When confronted with a chronic, nonerosive polyarthritis associated with diffuse erythroderma, cutaneous T cell lymphoma should be considered. This includes mycosis fungoides, Sézary syndrome, and other skin T cell disorders. Although the arthritis associated with cutaneous T cell lymphoma is most likely a reactive phenomenon, analysis of synovial fluid may show almost exclusively T helper cells.[10] T cell–type lymphoproliferative disorders can be divided into distinct clinicopathologic types based on membrane phenotype as CD4 and CD8. Until recently only the CD8 lymphocytosis patients had had an associated polyarthritis.[11]

Synovial Reaction to Juxta-articular Bone Tumors. Synovial reaction produced by adjacent tumor should be considered in the evaluation of patients with monoarticular arthritis. This reaction is nonspecific and may occur with malignant or benign tumors such as osteoid osteoma. Although the synovial fluid is characteristically noninflammatory, inflammatory synovial fluid as well as synovial tissue may be encountered.[12] If radiographs of a monoarticular arthropathy suggest any irregularity of adjacent bone,

tomography or radionuclide scans and serum enzyme studies should determine whether an independent bone lesion exists.

INDIRECT ASSOCIATIONS BETWEEN MUSCULOSKELETAL SYNDROMES AND MALIGNANCY

The indirect associations between musculoskeletal syndromes and malignancy are depicted in Table 94–3. The true paraneoplastic syndromes are divided into myopathies, arthropathies, and a host of miscellaneous presentations. The myopathies are reviewed extensively in Chapter 69. Hypertropic osteoarthropathy (Chapter 93), amyloidosis (Chapter 82), and secondary gout (Chapter 76) are also reviewed elsewhere. Because both acquired connective tissue disease and malignancy are common in older populations, it is often impossible to tell whether the occurrence of both in the same individual is coincidental or causally related.

Carcinoma Polyarthritis. Polyarthritis, generally resembling rheumatoid arthritis, may be the presenting manifestation of malignancy.[13] This is a distinct entity not to be confused with hypertrophic osteoarthropathy or with symmetric metastatic implants. Although most often confused with rheumatoid disease, this polyarthritis has been mistaken for adult Still's disease when associated with unexplained fever. The cause is unknown, but alterations in cellular immunity and circulating immune complexes have been considered. The possibility that the arthritis and the malignancy share a common but unknown etiologic basis exists.

Table 94–3. INDIRECT ASSOCIATIONS BETWEEN MUSCULOSKELETAL SYNDROMES AND MALIGNANCY: PARANEOPLASTIC SYNDROMES

   I. Myopathy (dermatomyositis-polymyositis)
  II. Arthropathy
      A. Hypertrophic osteoarthropathy
      B. Amyloidosis
      C. Secondary gout
      D. Carcinoma polyarthritis
      E. Jaccoud's-type arthropathy
 III. Miscellaneous presentations
      A. Lupus-like syndrome
      B. Necrotizing vasculitis
      C. Cryoproteins
      D. Immune complex disease
      E. Reflex sympathetic dystrophy syndrome
          1. Shoulder-hand syndrome
          2. Palmar fasciitis and arthritis
      F. Scleroderma (progressive systemic sclerosis)
      G. Polyarteritis
      H. Polymyalgia rheumatica
      I. Panniculitis
      J. Polychondritis
      K. Lupus antibody syndrome
      L. Pyogenic arthritis
      M. Osteomalacia
      N. Digital necrosis
      O. Erythromelalgia

Determining the true frequency of carcinoma polyarthritis is difficult and made more so by early reports that did not always exclude hypertrophic pulmonary osteoarthropathy. It is quite possible that periosteal reaction, diagnostic of the latter condition, was not detected. Carcinoma polyarthritis may occur in association with malignancy with a frequency similar to that of hypertrophic osteoarthritis and dermatomyositis. Although not diagnostic, several typical features suggest the possibility of malignancy underlying this musculoskeletal syndrome (Table 94–4). No predominant type of malignancy has been reported in association with carcinoma polyarthritis; however, 80 percent of the women with this syndrome have had breast carcinoma. In addition to solid tumor–related arthritis, joint symptoms have been reported in several hematologic neoplasms.

Serologic studies in carcinoma polyarthritis generally yield negative results. Usually, when the antinuclear antibody titer is significantly elevated, there appears to be a definite inflammatory connective tissue disease unrelated to the malignancy. Antinuclear antibodies, however, have been described in association with malignancy. A "lupus-antibody syndrome" including not only positive antinuclear antibody but also elevated anti-double-stranded DNA antibody has been described in association with several tumors.[14] The detection of antinuclear antibody in serosal fluid has been proposed as the most sensitive and specific test for determining if an effusion is caused by systemic lupus erythematosus. However, antinuclear antibody has been detected in pericardial fluid from a patient with primary cardiac lymphoma and no evidence of systemic lupus, suggesting as with serum antinuclear antibody, antinuclear antibody and serosal effusions cannot be considered pathognomonic for systemic lupus.[15] Similarly, lupus erythematosus (LE) cells have been noted in patients with lymphoma. Sedimentation rate is often markedly increased in malignancy, but this is nonspecific and not helpful diagnostically. While a characteristic noninflammatory synovial fluid is described in patients with hypertrophic osteoarthropathy, comprehensive data on synovial fluid analysis in carcinoma polyarthritis are lacking. Distinctive radiographic features for carcinoma polyarthritis have not been described.

Table 94–4. FEATURES OF CARCINOMA POLYARTHRITIS

Close temporal relationship (10 months) between onset of
  arthritis and malignancy
Late age at onset of arthritis
Asymmetric joint involvement
Explosive onset
Predominant lower extremity involvement with sparing of wrists
  and small joints of hands
Absence of rheumatoid nodules
Absence of rheumatoid factor
No family history of rheumatoid disease
Nonspecific histopathologic appearance of synovial lining

Jaccoud's-type Arthropathy. Jaccoud's-type arthropathy characterized as a rapidly developing, nonerosive, deforming, yet painless arthropathy may be the initial manifestation of carcinoma of the lung. With the exception of no history of rheumatic fever, the clinical picture is that of Jaccoud's arthropathy. The lack of pain and swelling and symmetric small joint involvement with upper extremity predominance would distinguish this from carcinoma polyarthritis.[16]

Available data indicate that when the cancer is successfully treated, the connective tissue symptoms frequently resolve. Conversely, relapse of the articular symptoms often heralds recurrence of primary or metastatic tumor. Several observations would suggest that the association of malignancy and polyarthritis is more than fortuitous: (1) a close temporal relationship between the onset of a low-grade, seronegative polyarthritis and discovery of the malignancy, (2) improvement in the connective tissue syndrome with treatment of the underlying tumor, and (3) recurrence of the connective tissue syndrome when the tumor reappears.

Definite proof of a causal relationship is lacking, as is the mechanism or mechanisms to explain the association. Tumors may synthesize mediators that provoke a connective tissue reaction. The possibility of cross-reactivity with shared determinants between synovium and immunologically foreign neoplastic tissue or its products is speculative. Equally plausible is the possibility of autoimmune phenomena arising in lymphocytes that originate in hyperplastic nodes that drain tumor sites. Other host factors in reaction to tumor may play a role in damaging natural barriers, allowing for the evolution of a connective tissue process. A common host defect may exist, the expression of which results in neoplasia and rheumatic disease. A specific antigen-antibody system may be operative in the pathogenesis of the rheumatic disease, with antigen being either tumor-associated antigen, re-expressed fetal antigen, viral antigen, or autologous nontumor antigen. Circulating immune complexes have been demonstrated in association with a variety of malignancies and may contain tumor-specific antibodies. However, other factors must be considered in view of the relatively high incidence of circulating immune complexes and the infrequent occurrence of immune complex–mediated disease in this particular setting.

Lupus-Like Syndrome. A lupus-like illness may occur in association with various malignancies such as Hodgkin's disease, myeloma, and lung, colon, and breast carcinoma. Hairy-cell leukemia has produced a variety of paraneoplastic syndromes, particularly rheumatic syndromes including polyarteritis nodosa, rheumatoid arthritis, amyloidosis, oligoarthritis, leukocytoclastic vasculitis, as well as a lupus-like illness. A syndrome compatible with SLE may develop in response to tumor recurrence, characterized by nondeforming polyarthritis, pneumonitis, pleural effusion, positive antinuclear antibody titer, and positive LE cell preparation. When patients with a history of malignancy have presenting findings of pleural effusions, pericarditis, and respiratory distress, the possibility of a potentially reversible, malignancy-induced, lupus-like illness should be considered along with the more common possibilities of metastatic tumor and radiation-induced changes.

The connective tissue disease may respond to the treatment given for the underlying primary malignancy. Ovarian adenocarcinoma has been associated with a lupus-like paraneoplastic syndrome characterized by serositis, rapidly progressive Raynaud's phenomenon, and accompanied by an unusual antinuclear antibody pattern of non-nucleolar sparse speckles. The antibodies did not appear to be directed against the common non-nucleolar antigens, DNA or histones, anticentromere, or extractable nucleolar antigen. This particular finding suggests a more causal, true paraneoplastic relationship.[17]

Necrotizing Vasculitis. Vasculitis as a paraneoplastic syndrome is more often associated with leukemias and lymphomas but may also occur with other malignancies. Vasculitides associated with malignancy are predominantly cutaneous but may involve medium-sized vessels and may be granulomatous. An acute abdomen due to vasculitis may be seen. Vasculitis may precede discovery of tumor, develop after or with the diagnosis of malignancy, or herald its recurrence. Henoch-Schönlein-type purpura has been reported in diffuse large-cell lymphoma.[18] A systemic vasculitis often resembling polyarteritis nodosa is the most common associated rheumatologic manifestation of hairy-cell leukemia.[19] Earlier studies had noted the occasional association of erythema nodosum with lymphoreticular malignancy, but some of those patients with atypical forms of erythema nodosum possibly had vasculitis.

Acute febrile neutrophilic dermatosis (Sweet's syndrome) is characterized by fever, neutrophilia, and the abrupt appearance of painful, erythematous, cutaneous plaques, primarily on the upper extremities, head, and neck (Fig. 94–1). Histologically a dense dermal infiltrate of neutrophils is noted. This syndrome clinically may resemble vasculitis. Approximately 10 to 15 percent of patients with Sweet's syndrome have a malignancy, most commonly acute myelogenous leukemia. Other malignancies have been observed and Sweet's syndrome may herald new or recurrent tumor. Anemia, abnormal platelets, immature cells in the differential or severe vesiculobullous or ulcerative cutaneous lesions, uncommon in idiopathic Sweet's syndrome, should alert the physician to serious underlying pathology. Another remote effect of cancer related to vasculitis may be mononeuritis multiplex.

Although a definite causal relationship between lymphoreticular malignancy and vasculitis cannot be established, and the possibility of a drug-induced reaction presenting with vasculitis is often difficult to exclude, substantial evidence suggests that vasculitis can be a feature of this group of malignancies.

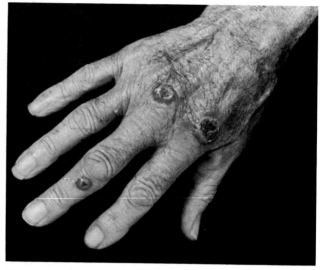

Figure 94–1. Acute febrile neutrophilic dermatosis (Sweet's syndrome). Inflammatory lesions resembling vasculitis. (Courtesy of Dr. Claude Burton.)

Mechanisms whereby vasculitis may occur as a paraneoplastic syndrome include: (1) immune complex formation composed of tumor-associated antigen/antibody, (2) direct vascular injury by antibodies to endothelial cells, possibly with cross-reactivity to leukemic cells, and (3) direct effect of leukemic cells (such as hairy cells) on the vascular wall.[18] The patient with a chronic unexplained necrotizing vasculitis should be observed for malignancy, particularly of the lymphoreticular type. When systemic vasculitis develops in the patient who has apparently had a successfully treated malignancy, tumor recurrence should be considered.

Cryoproteins. Cryoproteins may contribute to vascular injury. Peripheral gangrene secondary to circulating cryoglobulins or cryofibrinogens may occur prior to recognition of tumor. Cryoglobulinemia, with Raynaud's phenomenon, purpura, circulatory impairment, and occasionally cold-induced gangrene, is frequently associated with plasma cell dyscrasias, particularly plasma cell myeloma. Purpura (often cold-induced), thromboembolic phenomena, hemorrhagic diathesis, retinal hemorrhage, and retinal vein thrombosis may be seen with high levels of cryofibrinogen. Most commonly, this is associated with metastatic malignancy.

Immune Complex Disease. More than 50 percent of patients with cancer appear to have circulating immune complexes. Ten percent of patients with various cancers may be hypocomplementemic. The quantity of complexes may be as great as those detected in patients with SLE. Circulating immune complexes have been reported in Hodgkin's disease. Further study of immune complexes in cancer patients may improve our understanding of the immune response to tumor antigens and of immunotherapy and possibly lead to early detection of recurrence of tumor. It is also tempting to postulate the existence of a pathogenic mechanism for a variety of musculoskeletal manifestations on the basis of circulating immune complexes.

Reflex Sympathetic Dystrophy Syndrome (RSDS). RSDS, particularly two of its clinical variants, shoulder-hand syndrome and the syndrome of palmar fasciitis and polyarthritis, has been associated with various internal malignancies.[21, 22] The "palmar fasciitis and polyarthritis syndrome" appears distinct, owing to the dramatic progression and extent of symptoms. The fasciitis is more severe and the arthritis more inflammatory, and both are more rapidly progressive. The presence of fasciitis and arthritis carries a poor prognosis. Although ovarian cancer is the most frequently associated malignancy, other tumors are described.[23] While palmar fasciitis and polyarthritis are truly paraneoplastic, direct tumor involvement of the affected extremity may cause reflex sympathetic dystrophy to develop, presumably through involvement of nerve tissue. RSDS has been associated with gynecologic tumors involving the lumbosacral plexus.[24] The development of reflex sympathetic dystrophy syndrome, particularly these two variants, or failure of RSDS to respond to conventional therapy should alert the clinician to the possibility of an early malignancy. Successful removal of an otherwise asymptomatic carcinoma may be followed by dramatic improvement in pain and vasomotor disturbances in the immediate postoperative period although the contractures of RSDS have been predictably much slower to improve. Although palmar fasciitis and polyarthritis syndrome is considered a somewhat peculiar form of RSDS, the finding of IgG deposits in the palmar fascia suggests an immunopathologic mechanism rather than the traditional sympathetic nervous system alteration explanation given to account for RSDS.[24a]

Upper extremity pain simulating cervical nerve root irritation or the painful phase of shoulder-hand syndrome may also be seen with tumors of the lung that are localized to the superior sulcus, the so-called Pancoast's syndrome. This entity should always be considered in a setting of unilateral shoulder girdle–arm pain.

Scleroderma. Scleroderma may appear as the initial manifestation of malignancy. Sclerodermatous changes occasionally supervene in patients with dermatomyositis associated with cancer. In a series of 125 patients with systemic sclerosis and 235 patients with localized scleroderma, eight malignancies were found in the first group and four in the second.[25] Of the eight patients with systemic sclerosis and carcinoma, seven were women. Four of these seven women had carcinoma of the breast and two had carcinoma of the uterus.[25]

In an analysis of patients with coexisting scleroderma and malignant disease, the majority of neoplasms were of two varieties: adenocarcinoma and carcinoid tumors. Women were affected three times as often as men, and although all patients had cutaneous manifestations of scleroderma, less than half had proven systemic sclerosis.[26] In those patients with carcinoid tumors and scleroderma, serotonin may stimulate fibrous tissue proliferation. A rare form of plasma cell dyscrasia characterized by polyneuropathy, organomegaly, endocrinopathy, monoclonal protein, and skin changes (POEMS syndrome) may bear a striking resemblance to scleroderma.[27]

Polyarteritis. Polyarteritis may be seen in Hodgkin's disease, hairy-cell leukemia,[19] and various solid tumors. In hairy-cell leukemia, the vasculitis is usually typical of polyarteritis clinically and radiologically. Histologically the vasculitis is characterized by arterial wall necrosis and infiltration with mononuclear cells. Although the precise cause of vasculitis in hairy-cell leukemia is unclear, vasculitis may be associated with infection. Infiltration of hairy cells into the arterial wall may also play a pathogenic role, or autoantibodies to hairy cells may cross-react with endothelial cells, with resultant damage.[19] The connective tissue manifestations of leukemia may include recurrent infiltrations into muscles that may occasionally mimic the localized tender swellings found in polyarteritis.

Polymyalgia Rheumatica. In a series of 42 patients with temporal arteritis, cause of death was attributed to carcinoma of the breast in two patients.[28] In another series of six patients with polymyalgia rheumatica and malignancy, malignancy occurred within 3 months of the onset of polymyalgia rheumatica symptoms in five patients, whereas in one patient, the onset of polymyalgia rheumatica coincided with the appearance of metastases. Cranial arteritis has also been described as the initial manifestation of malignant histiocytosis. Follicular small cleaved cell lymphoma may simulate polymyalgia rheumatica–temporal arteritis by extensive temporal artery perivascular infiltration.

Panniculitis. Panniculitis has been associated with carcinoma in several reports since the initial description of its association with carcinoma of the pancreas appeared in 1908.[29] Subcutaneous nodules and arthritis may develop simultaneously and may precede abdominal pain or other signs and symptoms suggestive of pancreatic disease (Fig. 94–2).[30] The arthropathy, which is secondary to periarticular fat necrosis, may be monoarticular or polyarticular.[30] Eosinophilia (5 to 20 percent) occurred three times more often in the pancreatic cancer group than in the pancreatitis group. The subcutaneous fat necrosis has been attributed to the local action of blood-borne trypsin and lipase.[29] Histopathologic features consisting of foci of fat necrosis with "ghost-like" cells, with thick, shadowy walls and no nuclei, are pathognomonic.[31]

Therapy for this process with a variety of anti-inflammatory drugs, including glucocorticoids, is ineffective.[30] The possibility of subcutaneous fat necrosis should be considered in otherwise unexplained cases of polyarthritis or monoarticular arthritis with subcutaneous nodules particularly when occurring in older men. Diagnostic studies should include nodule biopsy and serum lipase determinations.[29, 30]

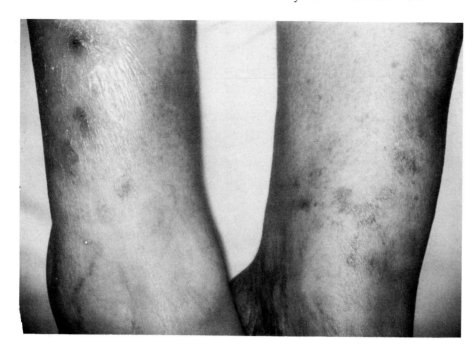

Figure 94–2. Subcutaneous fat necrosis of the lower extremity in a patient with pancreatic carcinoma. (Courtesy of Dr. Robert Gilgor.)

Erythema nodosum may also be seen in Hodgkin's disease, leukemia, as well as non-Hodgkin's lymphoma. Pathologically this could be a lymphomatous lesion simulating erythema nodosum, or true panniculitis characteristic of erythema nodosum. Hypersensitivity reaction to medication administered for the malignancy must also be considered.[32]

Polychondritis. Relapsing polychondritis has rarely been associated with malignancy. In each case, polychondritis preceded the diagnosis of malignancy.[33]

Pyogenic Arthritis. While pyogenic arthritis caused by intestinal flora may be a late complication in patients with advanced neoplastic disease, it may also be the presenting feature of carcinoma of the colon. Isolation of *Clostridium septicum* from an infected joint warrants careful search for an underlying malignant disease.[34] Whenever an unusual enteric bacteremia or its complications develop, the clinician should consider the possibility of a malignant source. Likewise, a rare cause of primary septic arthritis such as *Neisseria meningitidis* warrants careful evaluation for immunocompromise such as may occur in multiple myeloma.[34a]

Osteomalacia. Osteomalacia, characterized by bone pain, muscle weakness, and failure of newly formed bone matrix to calcify, may be associated with solid tissue tumors. Osteomalacia secondary to neoplasia, or oncogenous osteomalacia, has the unique feature of resolution after complete tumor removal. Tumors associated with this condition are characteristically benign; however, malignant tumors have been reported.[35]

Digital Necrosis. Malignancy must be considered in patients with occlusive digital artery disease. Raynaud's phenomenon may be observed and is often severe and of short duration. Its occurrence with high ANA titer though often associated with

evolving connective tissue disorder may be seen in malignancy.[36] Manifestations may range from splinter hemorrhages and pulp atrophy to digital gangrene. The latter is typically fulminant and rapidly progressive (Fig. 94–3).[37] A variety of tumors have been associated. Mechanisms proposed include cryoglobulinemia, immune complex–induced vasospasm, hypercoagulable state, marantic endocarditis with emboli, and necrotizing vasculitis.[37]

Erythromelalgia. Erythromelalgia, characterized by attacks of severe burning pain, erythema, and warmth of the extremities, involving the feet more often than the hands, exists in both primary (59 percent) and secondary (41 percent) forms. Twenty percent of those with the secondary form have had a myeloproliferative syndrome. The only nonhematologic malignant neoplasm described has been an astrocytoma. Symptoms of erythromelalgia may pre-

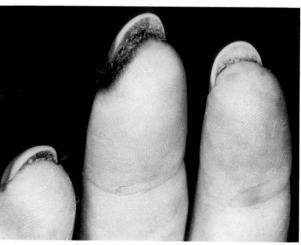

Figure 94–3. Digital necrosis in patient with malignancy.

cede the onset of a myeloproliferative disorder by a median of 2.5 years, suggesting that patients with this disorder be monitored with periodic complete blood counts. An abnormal hemoglobin level, WBC or platelet count, or presence of immature cells on the differential count should alert the clinician to the possibility of a more serious underlying disease. Treatment with single, daily-dose aspirin or of the underlying disorder will often alleviate the symptoms. Erythromelalgia may closely resemble reflex sympathetic dystrophy or one of its variants.[38] The various miscellanous presentations of the paraneoplastic syndromes associated with underlying malignancy are summarized in Table 94–5.

PREEXISTING CONNECTIVE TISSUE DISEASE

The association of musculoskeletal syndrome with malignancy also includes the development of malignancy in the setting of preexisting connective tissue disease (Table 94–6). The type of connective tissue disorder and the organ system involved often dictate the type of malignancy expected. Several mechanisms should be considered: (1) the initial event may be tissue alteration induced by the connective tissue disorder, (2) therapy for the connective tissue disorder may provoke malignancy, (3) specific HLA antigens could predispose to both conditions or an immunologic disorder may induce both, (4) environmental factors such as radiation, chemicals, or infective agents may make the host susceptible to both autoimmune disease and malignancy. In nearly all autoimmune diseases an increased incidence of malignancy has been noted.[39] The concept of oncogene activation has been proposed to explain a relationship between autoimmunity and malignancy. When overexpressed, oncogene regulation is altered or a mutation occurs inducing structural change with resultant possibility of neoplastic transformation.[40]

Systemic Lupus Erythematosus. The incidence of malignancy is increased in patients with SLE. This may relate to an immune dysfunction secondary to the disease or be a consequence of drug therapy. The most commonly reported malignancy in this situation is lymphoma, usually arising in the peripheral lymph nodes and less frequently in the lung, intestine, or CNS. Primary lymphoma of the liver as well as of the spleen has also been described.[41–43] It is possible that defective immune surveillance in the setting of chronic immune stimulation, as seen in SLE, results in emergence of a neoplastic clone of cells. Emergence of lymphoma may mimic exacerbation of SLE with adenopathy, malaise, fever, and splenomegaly with definitive diagnosis further hindered by the masking effects of steroid therapy. Striking clinical and serologic remission may ensue post radiotherapy and chemotherapy for the lymphoma.

Discoid Lupus Erythematosus. Epitheliomas of the squamous cell variety occasionally may appear in healed scars of discoid lupus erythematosus. These are usually found in the oldest plaques, developing 20 years or more after the onset of the discoid lesion. They occur primarily in men between the ages of 30 and 60 years. The pathogenesis is unclear, but it possibly relates to the chronic inflammation or scarring. Although skin cancer is relatively uncommon in black individuals, sun exposure of the hypopigmented lesions of discoid lupus may predispose to cancer. A poorly healing skin lesion in discoid LE should be evaluated.[44]

Sjögren's Syndrome. Sjögren's syndrome is a chronic inflammatory process affecting principally the exocrine glands, frequently associated with a connective tissue disorder, most often rheumatoid disease. It may closely resemble the NZB mouse model with development of salivary gland lymphoid infiltrates, generalized lymphoproliferation, autoantibodies, monoclonal IgM, and lymphoma. The risk of developing lymphoma in Sjögren's syndrome is said to be 44 times normal risk, the increased risk of lymphoma being independent of the presence of rheumatoid arthritis.[45] Patients with a history of parotid gland enlargement, splenomegaly, and lymphadenopathy are at particular risk. Other predisposing factors may include prior low-dose parotid irradiation as well as chemotherapy. As pulmonary involvement is common in patients with lymphoma in the setting of Sjögren's syndrome, lymphoma should be considered in the evaluation of Sjögren's syndrome patients with pulmonary lesions.[46] Marked gammaglobulin elevation may mimic multiple myeloma. A spectrum of lymphoproliferation occurs in the setting of Sjögren's syndrome from benign lymphoid infiltration that is confined to glandular tissue to widespread lymphoreticular malignancy. In the middle of these extremes exists a condition characterized by nonmalignant extraglandular extension of lymphoproliferation. This "pseudolymphoma" may regress in response to appropriate therapy or may progress to frank neoplasia, either macroglobulinemia or lymphoma.[47] Clues to the progression from so-called pseudolymphoma to lymphoma may be a decline in the level of serum IgM and the disappearance of rheumatoid factor, both of which may be elevated in pseudolymphoma.[47] Detection of urinary monoclonal free light chains may serve as an early diagnostic clue to the development of lymphoma and as a means of tumor monitoring.[48]

Although most studies have demonstrated that lymphomas in these patients are usually B cell in character, T cell lymphoma has been described. The fact that malignancy is a rare and late event in many of these situations is consistent with the concept that malignancy develops only after a long sequence of transitions and selection of mutant populations.

Rheumatoid Arthritis. Patients with RA develop malignancy at least comparable to the general population. They share with other autoimmune disease patients an increased risk of developing lymphoproliferative malignancies. The risk appears to be inde-

Table 94–5. MISCELLANEOUS PRESENTATIONS OF PARANEOPLASTIC SYNDROMES

Connective Tissue Syndrome	Malignancy	Clinical Setting	Clinical Alert
Lupus-like syndrome (polyarthritis, serositis, pleural effusion, positive ANA)	Various types, primary or recurrent with occult recurrence	May occur in setting of previously treated malignancy	Patient with history of malignancy and therapy for same presenting with pleural effusions, pericarditis, respiratory distress, simulating lupus. Consider local recurrence, radiation injury, or metastasis. Novel antinuclear antibody
Necrotizing vasculitis	Lymphoreticular disorders predominate	—	Chronic unexplained necrotizing vasculitis should be observed for malignancy; particularly lymphoreticular type
Cryoglobulinemia	Plasma cell dyscrasia	—	Refractory Raynaud's syndrome possibly progressing to occlusion and gangrene
Immune-complex disease	Hodgkin's disease	Nephrotic syndrome	Probable mechanism for a variety of musculoskeletal manifestations on basis of circulating immune complexes
Reflex sympathetic dystrophy syndrome / Shoulder-hand syndrome / Palmar fasciitis and polyarthritis	Ovarian cancer most frequent	Palmar fasciitis and polyarthritis dramatic in progression and extent of symptoms	Rapid development of RSDS particularly these 2 variants and/or failure of RSDS to respond to conventional therapy, consider underlying malignancy
Scleroderma	Adenocarcinoma carcinoid tumor	Sclerodermatous changes may overlap with DM	Scleroderma-like changes confined to the anterior tibial area suggest carcinoid
Polyarteritis	Hairy-cell leukemia	Polyarteritis-like clinically and radiologically	—
Polymyalgia rheumatica	—	Questionable relationship as malignancy and PMR share similar features and both associated with elevated sedimentation rate	—
Panniculitis	Pancreatic cancer	Subcutaneous nodules and arthritis, both due to fat necrosis. May precede detection of pancreatic disease. Eosinophilia 5–20%. Simulates erythema nodosum	Possibility of pancreatic cancer should be considered in patients, particularly older males, with monoarthritis or polyarthritis in association with subcutaneous nodules
Polychondritis	Hodgkin's disease	Rarely associated with malignancy	—
Pyogenic arthritis	Colon carcinoma	Intestinal flora cultured	When an unusual enteric bacteremia or its complications develop, consider possible malignant source
	Multiple myeloma	Rare cause of primary septic arthritis (N. meningitidis)	When a rare cause of septic arthritis is cultured, consider immunocompromise
Oncogenic osteomalacia	Usually benign, mesenchymal in origin	Bone pain, muscle weakness	Diligent careful search for tumor indicated in all patients with late onset apparent idiopathic osteomalacia
Digital necrosis	Variety reported. Renal cell carcinoma most common?	Severe Raynaud's phenomenon of short duration	Consider underlying malignancy when digital gangrene is fulminant and rapidly progressive
Erythromelalgia	Myeloproliferative disorders	Severe burning pain, erythema, warmth. Primarily feet, lesser extent hands involved	Any abnormality in the blood count—especially increased hemoglobin, leukocytosis, thrombocytosis, or immature cells in the differential

Table 94–6. CLINICAL SETTINGS OF PREEXISTING CONNECTIVE TISSUE DISEASE ASSOCIATED WITH MALIGNANCY

I. Disease related
    A. Lupus erythematosus
        1. Systemic
        2. Discoid
    B. Sjögren's syndrome
    C. Rheumatoid arthritis
    D. Scleroderma (progressive systemic sclerosis)
    E. Sarcoidosis
    F. Osteomyelitis
    G. Paget's disease
    H. Eosinophilic fasciitis
    I. Lymphomatoid granulomatosis
II. Complications of therapy
    A. Immunosuppressive therapy
    B. Radiation therapy
    C. Tumor formation at site of orthopedic implant

pendent of prior cytotoxic therapy. That such therapy may enhance the risk of neoplasia in RA is likely.[50] The association between lymphoma and RA seems to relate to duration of disease rather than severity, with the mean interval between onset of RA and development of lymphoma being 17 years.[51] Two clinical situations are noteworthy. The patient with long-standing RA who develops a rapidly progressive, refractory flare may have an underlying malignancy. Pulmonary nodules in patients with rheumatoid arthritis should be approached as possible carcinomas. Therapy of the associated malignancy may lead to sustained remission of long-standing rheumatoid disease.

Scleroderma (Progressive Systemic Sclerosis [PSS]). Although a variety of tumors have been associated with scleroderma, the question of a relationship between PSS and malignancy remains.[52, 53] Among malignancies reported, lung neoplasia (particularly alveolar cell carcinoma) has predominated. Alveolar cell carcinoma has accounted for 50 percent of lung tumors reported in this setting, compared with the general incidence of less than 4 percent of all primary lung neoplasms (Figs. 94–4 and 94–5). Alveolar cell carcinoma and PSS may be the result of metaplasia following, or superimposed on, fibrosis rather than a direct consequence of systemic sclerosis. The fact that inhaled oncogenic factors are poorly eliminated by a sclerodermatous lung may be an added stimulus to malignant transformation in regenerating cells. The naturally occurring disease *jaagsiekte*, or "drive sickness," provides an interesting animal model. Long-standing pulmonary interstitial fibrosis may be the initial step in the sequence of events to malignancy of any cell type.

Two case studies and an epidemiologic study have revealed the development of breast cancer at or near the onset of scleroderma.[54, 55] The close temporal sequence suggests a pathophysiologic relationship. Barrett's metaplasia and adenocarcinoma of the esophagus have now been described in scleroderma, making it necessary to evaluate constricting lesions of the lower esophagus more carefully.[56] The following guidelines for cancer screening in scleroderma have been proposed: (1) breast examination and mammography every 6 months for the first 5 years after the first onset of symptoms attributable to PSS; (2) annual chest radiographs in the fifth and all subsequent years after radiographic evidence of pulmonary fibrosis has been documented; (3) esophagoscopy and biopsy, if indicated, of distal esophageal constricting lesions; and (4) careful medical and he-

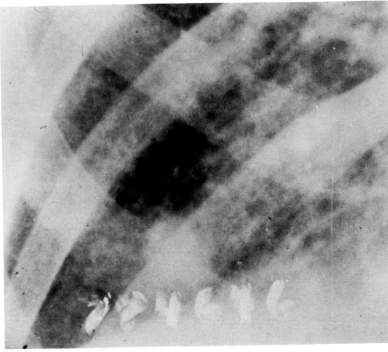

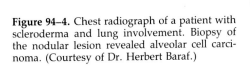
Figure 94–4. Chest radiograph of a patient with scleroderma and lung involvement. Biopsy of the nodular lesion revealed alveolar cell carcinoma. (Courtesy of Dr. Herbert Baraf.)

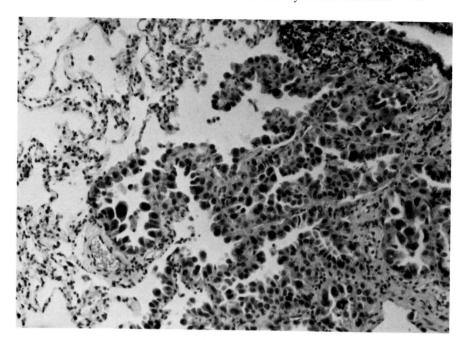

Figure 94–5. Alveolar cell carcinoma. Characteristic low-power "papillary" appearance along the periphery of an alveolar cell carcinoma (*right*) invading normal lung tissue. (Courtesy of Dr. Michael Ehrie.)

matologic follow-up of any scleroderma patient who has received immunosuppressive therapy.[52]

Werner's syndrome, a rare autosomal recessive connective tissue disorder characterized by juvenile cataracts, scleroderma-like skin changes, and accelerated aging, has a high incidence of neoplasm, often of connective tissue origin. The syndrome should not be confused with PSS but should be regarded as a cutaneous marker for internal malignancy.[56a]

Sarcoidosis. Impairment of cell-mediated hypersensitivity is a well-recognized characteristic of sarcoidosis. A consequence of this impairment may be decreased immunologic surveillance, resulting in an increase in neoplasia. Noncaseating granulomas can occur in numerous settings and are not necessarily pathognomonic for sarcoidosis. Noncaseating granulomas resembling those of sarcoidosis may be found in lymph nodes that drain sites with malignancy. Tumor-related tissue reactions resulting in granuloma formation have been described with many types of malignant lesions including cervical, bladder, gastric, lung, breast, and renal cancers as well as cutaneous and pulmonary squamous cell carcinoma. Sarcoid reactions occur in 4.4 percent of carcinomas, 13.8 percent of Hodgkin's lymphoma, and 7.3 percent of non-Hodgkin's lymphomas, and rarely in sarcomas. This reaction may be seen not only in draining lymph nodes but also in the tumor itself as well as in nonregional tissues, suggesting that tumor-derived antigenic factors provoke a hypersensitivity reaction.[57–59]

Osteomyelitis. Squamous cell carcinoma is a complication of chronic osteomyelitis with an estimated frequency of between 0.2 and 1.7 percent. Fitzgerald and colleagues, reviewing the Mayo Clinic experience, reported 25 patients with squamous cell carcinoma and 3 patients with sarcoma at the site of chronic osteomyelitis.[60] The squamous cell carcinoma

probably arises in the proliferating edges of the cutaneous ulcer and then invades the bone.[60]

Paget's Disease of Bone. Persistent, severe pain may alert the clinician to a serious complication of Paget's disease—the development of osteogenic sarcoma.[61] The frequency of this process is probably less than 1 percent. Conversely, in osteogenic sarcoma patients older than 40 years of age, the rate of occurrence of sarcoma arising from pagetic bone was 19 percent. Tumors most frequently involve the femur, humerus, skull, face, and pelvis. Survival after diagnosis is usually less than 1 year. Swelling and bone destruction in the setting of Paget's disease may be caused by other types of malignancy as well, both primary and metastatic.[62] Although several clinical signs have been noted to distinguish bone malignancy from Paget's disease, the ultimate diagnosis may require biopsy.[61]

Eosinophilic Fasciitis. Diffuse fasciitis with eosinophilia is characterized by scleroderma-like skin changes, hypereosinophilia, hypergammaglobulinemia, elevated sedimentation rate, and characteristic findings on biopsy. Eosinophils may or may not be present. Serious hematologic complications, including aplastic anemia and thrombocytopenia, have been reported during long-term follow-up. Eosinophilic fasciitis may be the result of an abnormal lymphoplasmacytic proliferation. Thus, these patients should be followed closely for development of serious hematologic disorders, including lymphoid malignancies.[63]

Lymphomatoid Granulomatosis. Lymphomatoid granulomatosis is an unusual form of vasculitis with a granulomatous reaction that is characterized by an angiotropic and angiodestructive infiltration of various tissues, particularly the lung. The cellular infiltrate composed of atypical lymphocytoid and plasmacytoid cells has lymphoproliferative characteristics. Lymphomas evolve in at least 13 percent of patients.[64]

Preexisting connective tissue disease associated with malignancy is summarized in Table 94–7.

MALIGNANCY AS A COMPLICATION OF TREATMENT

Immunosuppressive Therapy. Because of clinical evidence supporting their efficacy, immunosuppressive drugs are increasingly used to treat rheumatic diseases. The drugs in common use include the alkylating agents cyclophosphamide and chlor-

ambucil; a purine analogue, azathioprine; and methotrexate, a folic acid analogue. Sustained therapy is usually required, as months of therapy may be necessary to achieve maximal effects, and short courses usually do not induce a lasting remission. Of the adverse effects attributed to these drugs, perhaps the most alarming is the potential oncogenic effect. This effect has been best demonstrated in long-term survivors of certain malignancies treated with chemotherapy in whom second malignancies have occurred more frequently than expected. Prolonged daily therapy of rheumatoid arthritis with cyclophosphamide is clearly associated with an increased risk of urinary bladder, cutaneous, and hematologic malignancies.

Table 94–7. PREEXISTING CONNECTIVE TISSUE DISEASE ASSOCIATED WITH MALIGNANCY

Connective Tissue Disease	Malignancy	Clinical Setting	Clinical Alert
Systemic lupus erythematosus	Lymphoreticular disorders	—	Non-Hodgkin's lymphoma should be considered in SLE patients who develop adenopathy or masses. Lymphoma of the spleen is another cause of splenic enlargement in SLE
Discoid lupus erythematosus	Squamous cell epithelioma	Found in oldest plaques, 20 years or more after onset of discoid lesion primarily in males ages 30–60	A poorly healing skin lesion within discoid lupus should be evaluated
Sjögren's syndrome	Lymphoreticular disorders	Sjögren's syndrome may be associated with systemic rheumatologic disorder, most often RA. Pseudolymphoma, nonmalignant, extraglandular extension of lymphoproliferation	Clues to progression from pseudolymphoma to lymphoma: disappearance of RF and decline in IgM
Rheumatoid arthritis	Lymphoreticular disorders	—	Rapidly progressive, refractory flare in long-standing rheumatoid disease may suggest an underlying malignancy
Scleroderma (PSS)	Alveolar cell carcinoma	Pulmonary fibrosis	Annual chest radiograph in the 5th and all subsequent years after fibrosis detected
	? Breast cancer	Reports describe breast cancer at or near onset of scleroderma	Breast examination and mammography every 6 months for first 5 years after onset PSS symptoms
	Adenocarcinoma of esophagus	Barrett's metaplasia	Esophagoscopy and biopsy if indicated of distal esophageal constricting lesions
Sarcoidosis	Chest malignancy predominant	Highest incidence of "malignancy" during first 4 years after detection of granulomas	Malignant tumors can cause sarcoid-like tissue reactions leading to mistaken diagnosis of sarcoidosis prior to recognition of malignancy
Osteomyelitis	Squamous cell carcinoma	Chronic osteomyelitis with cutaneous ulcer	Lesion arises in proliferating edges of cutaneous ulcer and then invades bone
Paget's disease	Osteogenic sarcoma	Increasing incidence with advancing age	Swelling and bone destruction in preexisting Paget's disease may be sarcoma. Diagnosis may require biopsy
Eosinophilic fasciitis	Lymphoid malignancy	Serious hematologic complications: aplastic anemia, thrombocytopenia, Hodgkin's disease	Long-term follow-up may be important regarding diagnosis of malignancy
Lymphomatoid granulomatosis	Lymphoma	—	At least 13% of patients will develop lymphoma

The greatest risk occurs in those receiving the highest cumulative dose and this risk persists for years after the drug is discontinued. The calculated relative risk for the development of malignancy in this setting is 2.3. It remains to be determined if parenteral pulse therapy will reduce the risk, but preliminary results with SLE nephritis are encouraging.[65, 66] The increased lymphoproliferative risk from using high-dose azathioprine in patients with rheumatoid arthritis is about twice that due to RA alone.[67] The antimetabolites, in particular methotrexate, seem to be relatively safe with regard to oncogenic potential.[67a]

Although malignancy develops in patients with connective tissue disease treated with immunosuppressive therapy, the actual frequency of a neoplastic complication is difficult to determine because the number of patients receiving such drugs is not available. Because impairment of immune surveillance with subsequent proliferation of mutant malignant clones may already occur in the altered immune state, immunosuppressive therapy in this setting may be a very serious therapeutic maneuver, possibly further enhancing the potential for malignant growth.

The increased frequency of cervical atypia in women with SLE who receive chemotherapy suggests that such patients should have cervical smears taken regularly.[68] Glucocorticoids have been implicated in the development of cutaneous Kaposi's sarcoma, with regression of the malignancy on discontinuation of steroid therapy.[69]

The decision to use immunosuppressive drugs in a patient with a nonmalignant disease must be made carefully, given the increased risk of malignancy. Informed consent in such a situation obviously places a great burden on the patient faced with the alternatives of morbid and mortal complications of the underlying disease.

Radiation Therapy. Deep radiation therapy in the treatment of ankylosing spondylitis has drastically decreased in the last 20 years owing in large part to increasing awareness that such therapy could result in leukemia and, to a lesser extent, the availability of other therapies.[70] Basal cell carcinoma in the lumbosacral area may be a late complication of radiotherapy for ankylosing spondylitis. The skin at sites of previous irradiation should be examined carefully.

More recently, total lymphoid irradiation and total body irradiation have been implemented in the treatment of refractory rheumatoid arthritis. Although the latter is more convenient for the patient and therapist, two of four patients reported in one series developed a myeloproliferative disorder. Cytotoxic drugs before or after irradiation (or both before and after) may have contributed.[71] Osteonecrosis and pathologic fractures represent bone complications of radiation therapy. When radiation therapy is given as tumor therapy, the resultant osteitis must be distinguished from either tumor recurrence or secondary (radiation-induced) sarcoma.[72]

Orthopedic Implants. The vast majority of patients in whom metallic implants are used never experience harmful effects relating to their presence. Increasingly the greatest long-term concern in such patients is induction of carcinogenesis, which may occur by either of two mechanisms. A "solid state" mechanism has been proposed whereby a large, foreign, implanted object stimulates mutagenesis of local cells, creating tumor merely by its presence. The other possibility is that particulate metal matter (disseminated to surrounding tissues) has an innate capacity to induce cancer. This is supported by well-documented cases of carcinoma and sarcoma in refinery workers exposed to nickel, chromium, and iron as well as in animal studies showing a direct correlation between initiation of sarcomas and injection of particulate metal debris. Since 1984, a number of reports have appeared with increasing frequency describing sarcoma in the vicinity of total hip replacement. Higher concentrations of metal particulate debris (cobalt, chromium, nickel) were noted within the tumor than in surrounding normal tissue. The effects of silicone may also have to be considered. More reviews from institutions that frequently perform such surgery are needed.[73–75a]

References

1. Shimomura, C., Eguchi, K., Kawakami, A., et al.: Elevation of a tumor associated antigen CA 19–9 levels in patients with rheumatic diseases. J. Rheumatol. 16:11, 1989.
2. Garcia-Vicuna, R., Diaz-Gonzalez, F., Castaneda, S., et al.: Rheumatoid disease resembling lung neoplasia. J. Rheumatol. 17:12, 1990.
2a. Pope, T. L., Wang, G., and Whitehill, R.: Discogenic vertebral sclerosis: A potential mimic of disc space infection or metastatic disease. Orthopedics 13:1389, 1990.
2b. Hauge, M. D., Cooper, K. L., and Litin, S. C.: Insufficiency fractures of the pelvis that simulate metastatic disease. Mayo Clin. Proc. 63:807, 1988.
3. Murray, G. C., and Persellin, R. H.: Metastatic carcinoma presenting as monarticular arthritis: A case report and review of the literature. Arthritis Rheum. 23:95, 1980.
4. McCarty, G. A.: Autoantibodies and their relation to rheumatic diseases. Med. Clin. North Am. 70:237, 1986.
5. Newton, P., Freemont, A. T., Noble, J., et al.: Secondary malignancy synovitis: Report of three cases and review of the literature. Q. J. Med. 53:135, 1984.
5a. Chakravarty, K. K., and Webley, M.: Monarthritis: An unusual presentation of renal cell carcinoma. Ann. Rheum. Dis. 51:681, 1992.
6. Hazeltine, M., Duranceau, L., and Gariepy, G.: Presentation of breast carcinoma as Volkmann's contracture due to skeletal muscle metastases. J. Rheumatol. 17:1097, 1990.
7. Holdrinet, R. S. G., Corstens, F., van Horn, J. R., et al.: Leukemic synovitis. Am. J. Med. 86:123, 1989.
8. Cawley, M. I. D.: Arthritic manifestations of leukemia. Intern. Med. 7:202, 1986.
8a. Fam, A. G., Voorneveld, C., Robinson, J. B., et al.: Synovial fluid immunocytology in the diagnosis of leukemic synovitis. J. Rheumatol. 18:293, 1991.
8b. Gaudin, P., Juvin, R., Rozand, Y., et al.: Skeletal involvement as the initial disease manifestation in Hodgkin's disease: A review of 6 cases. J. Rheumatol. 19:146, 1992.
9. Haase, K. L., Dürk, H., Baumbach, A., et al.: Non-Hodgkin's lymphoma presenting as knee monarthritis with a popliteal cyst. J. Rheumatol. 17:1252, 1990.
10. Seleznick, M. J., Aguilar, J. L., Rayhack, J., et al.: Polyarthritis associated with cutaneous T cell lymphoma. J. Rheumatol. 16:1379, 1989.
11. Handel, M. L., Dodds, A. J., and Cohen, M. L.: Coexistence of RA and a monoclonal CD4 T cell lymphoproliferative disorder. J. Rheumatol. 17:84, 1990.
12. Gerster, J-C., Jaquier, E., and Ribaux, C.: Nonspecific inflammatory

monoarthritis in the vicinity of bony metastases. J. Rheumatol. 14:844, 1987.
13. Caldwell, D. S.: Carcinoma polyarthritis: Manifestations and differential diagnosis. Med. Grand Rounds 1:378, 1982.
14. Salem, N. B.: Lupus antibody syndrome with intestinal lymphoma. Arthritis Rheum. 23:613, 1980.
15. Leventhal, L. J., DeMarco, D. M., and Zurier, R. B.: Antinuclear antibody in pericardial fluid from a patient with primary cardiac lymphoma. Arch. Intern. Med. 150:1113, 1990.
16. Johnson, J. J., Leonard-Segal, A., and Nashel, D. J.: Jaccoud's-type arthropathy: An association with malignancy. J. Rheumatol. 16:1278, 1989.
17. Freundlich, B., Makover, D., and Maul, G. G.: A novel antinuclear antibody associated with a lupus-like paraneoplastic syndrome. Ann. Intern. Med. 15:295, 1988.
18. Sanchez-Guerrero, J., Gutierrez-Urena, S., Vidaller, A., et al.: Vasculitis as a paraneoplastic syndrome. Report of 11 cases and review of the literature. J. Rheumatol. 17:1458, 1990.
19. Gabriel, S. E., Conn, D. L., Phyliky, R. L., et al.: Vasculitis in hairy-cell leukemia: Review of literature and consideration of possible pathogenic mechanisms. J. Rheumatol. 13:1167, 1986.
20. Cohen, P. R., and Kurzrock, R.: Sweet's syndrome and malignancy. Am. J. Med. 82:1220, 1987.
21. Michaels, R. M., and Sorber, J. A.: Reflex sympathetic dystrophy as a probable paraneoplastic syndrome: Case report and literature review. Arthritis Rheum. 27:1183, 1984.
22. Pfinsgraff, J., Buckingham, R. B., Killian, P. J., et al.: Palmar fasciitis and arthritis with malignant neoplasms: A paraneoplastic syndrome. Semin. Arthritis Rheum. 16:118, 1986.
23. Shiel, W. C., Jr., Prete, P. E., Jason, M., et al.: Palmar fasciitis and arthritis with ovarian and non-ovarian carcinomas: New syndrome. Am. J. Med. 79:640, 1985.
24. Ameratunga, R., Daly, M., and Caughey, D. E.: Metastatic malignancy associated with reflex sympathetic dystrophy. J. Rheumatol. 16:406, 1989.
24a. Valverde-Garcia, J., Juanola-Roura, X., Ruiz-Martin, J. M., et al.: Paraneoplastic palmar fasciitis-polyarthritis syndrome associated with breast cancer. J. Rheumatol. 14:1207, 1987.
25. Christianson, H. B., Brunsting, L. A., and Perry, H. D.: Dermatomyositis: Unusual features, complications and treatment. Arch. Dermatol. 74:581, 1956.
26. Basten, A., and Bonnin, M.: Scleroderma in carcinoma. Med. J. Aust. 1:452, 1966.
27. Viard, J-P., Lesavre, P., Boitard, C., et al.: POEMS syndrome presenting as systemic sclerosis. Clinical and pathologic study of a case with microangiopathic glomerular lesions. Am. J. Med. 84:524, 1988.
28. Huston, K. A., Hunder, G. G., Lie, J. T., et al.: Temporal arteritis. A 25-year epidemiologic, clinical and pathologic study. Ann. Intern. Med. 88:162, 1978.
29. Hughes, P. S. H., Apisarnthanarax, P., and Mullins, J. F.: Subcutaneous fat necrosis associated with pancreatic disease. Arch. Dermatol. 111:506, 1975.
30. Virshup, A. M., and Sliwinski, A. J.: Polyarthritis and subcutaneous nodules associated with carcinoma of the pancreas. Arthritis Rheum. 16:388, 1973.
31. Szymanski, F. J., and Bluefarb, S. M.: Nodular fat necrosis and pancreatic disease. Arch. Dermatol. 83:224, 1961.
32. Thomson, G. T. D., Keystone, E. C., Sturgeon, J. F. G., et al.: Erythema nodosum and non-Hodgkin's lymphoma. J. Rheumatol. 17:383, 1990.
33. Miller, S. B., Donlan, C. J., and Roth, S. B.: Hodgkin's disease presenting as relapsing polychondritis. A previously undescribed association. Arthritis Rheum. 17:598, 1974.
34. Fallon, S. M., Gukzik, H. J., and Kramer, L. E.: Clostridium septicum arthritis associated with colonic carcinoma. J. Rheumatol. 13:662, 1986.
34a. Miller, M. I., Hoppmann, R. A., and Pisko, E. J.: Multiple myeloma presenting with primary meningococcal arthritis. Am. J. Med. 82:1257, 1987.
35. Ryan, E. A., and Reiss, E.: Oncogenous osteomalacia. Review of the world literature of 42 cases and report of 2 new cases. Am. J. Med. 77:501, 1984.
36. Tolosa-Vilella, C., Ordi-Ros, J., and Vilardell-Tarres, M.: Raynaud's phenomenon and positive antinuclear antibodies in a malignancy. Ann. Rheum. Dis. 49:935, 1990.
37. Petri, M., and Fye, K. H.: Digital necrosis: A paraneoplastic syndrome. J. Rheumatol. 12:800, 1985.
38. Kurzrock, R., and Cohen, P. R.: Erythromelalgia and myeloproliferative disorders. Arch. Intern. Med. 149:105, 1989.
39. Sela, O., and Shoenfeld, Y.: Cancer in autoimmune diseases. Semin. Arthritis Rheum. 28:77, 1988.
40. Williams, R. C., Sibbet, W. L., and Husby, G.: Oncogenes, viruses or rheumogenes? Am. J. Med. 80:1011, 1986.
41. Buskila, D., Gladman, D. D., Hannah, W., et al.: Primary malignant lymphoma of the spleen in SLE. J. Rheumatol. 16:993, 1989.
42. Sutton, E., Malatjalian, D., Hayne, O. A., et al.: Liver lymphoma in systemic lupus erythematosus. J. Rheumatol. 16:1584, 1989.
43. Posner, M. A., Gloster, E. S., Bonagura, V. R., et al.: Burkitt's lymphoma in a patient with systemic lupus erythematosus. J. Rheumatol. 17:380, 1990.
44. Caruso, W. R., Stewart, M. L., Nanda, V. K., et al.: Squamous cell carcinoma of the skin in black patients with discoid lupus erythematosus. J. Rheumatol. 14:156, 1987.
45. Kassan, S. S., Thomas, T. L., Moutsopoulos, H. M., et al.: Increased risk of lymphoma in Sjögren's syndrome. Ann. Intern. Med. 89:888, 1978.
46. Hansen, L. A., Prakash, U. B. S., and Colby, T. V.: Pulmonary lymphoma in Sjögren's syndrome. Mayo Clin. Proc. 64:920, 1989.
47. Anderson, L. G., and Talal, N.: The spectrum of benign to malignant lymphoproliferation in Sjögren's syndrome. Clin. Exp. Immunol. 9:199, 1971.
48. Walters, M. T., Stevenson, F. K., Herbert, A., et al.: Lymphoma in Sjögren's syndrome: Urinary monoclonal free light chains as a diagnostic aid and a means of tumor monitoring. Scand. J. Rheumatol. (Suppl.)61:114, 1986.
49. Isenberg, D. A., Griffiths, M. H., Rustin, M., et al.: T-cell lymphoma in a patient with long-standing rheumatoid arthritis and Sjögren's syndrome. Arthritis Rheum. 30:115, 1987.
50. Symmons, D. P. M.: Neoplasia in rheumatoid arthritis. J. Rheumatol. 15:9, 1988.
51. Kelly, C., and Sykes, H.: Rheumatoid arthritis, malignancy, and paraproteins. Ann. Rheum. Dis. 49:657, 1990.
52. Medsger, T. A., Jr.: Systemic sclerosis and malignancy—are they related? J. Rheumatol. 12:1041, 1985.
53. Peters-Golden, M., Wise, R. A., Hochberg, M., et al.: Incidence of lung cancer in systemic sclerosis. J. Rheumatol. 12:1136, 1985.
54. Roumm, A. D., Medsger, T. A., Jr.: Cancer and systemic sclerosis: An epidemiologic study. Arthritis Rheum. 28:1336, 1985.
55. Lee, P., Alderdice, C., Wilkinson, S., et al.: Malignancy in progressive systemic sclerosis: Association with breast carcinoma. J. Rheumatol. 10:665, 1983.
56. Katzka, D. A., Reynolds, J. C., Saul, S. H., et al.: Barrett's metaplasia and adenocarcinoma of the esophagus in scleroderma. Am. J. Med. 82:46, 1987.
56a. Khraishi, M., Howard, B., and Little, H.: A patient with Werner's syndrome and osteosarcoma presenting as scleroderma. J. Rheumatol. 19:810, 1992.
57. Israel, H. L.: Sarcoidosis, malignancy, and immunosuppressive therapy. Arch. Intern. Med. 138:907, 1978.
58. Brincker, H.: Sarcoid reactions in malignant tumors. Cancer Treat. Rev. 13:147, 1986.
59. Moder, K. G., Litin, S. C., and Gaffey, T. A.: Renal cell carcinoma associated with sarcoid-like tissue reaction. Mayo Clin. Proc. 65:1498, 1990.
60. Fitzgerald, R. H., Jr., Brewer, N. S., and Dahlin, D. C.: Squamous cell carcinoma complicating chronic osteomyelitis. J. Bone Joint Surg. 58A:1146, 1956.
61. Harris, E. D., and Krane, S. M.: Paget's disease of bone. Bull. Rheum. Dis. 18:506, 1968.
62. Nicholas, J. J., Srodes, C. H., Herbert, D., et al.: Metastatic cancer in Paget's disease of bone: A case report. Orthopaedics 10:725, 1987.
63. Michaels, R. M.: Eosinophilic fasciitis complicated by Hodgkin's disease. J. Rheumatol. 9:473, 1982.
64. Da Silva, A. M. T., Weiner, J., Dean, P., et al.: Lymphomatoid granulomatosis beginning as adult respiratory distress syndrome and rapidly progressing to lymphoma. South. Med. J. 76:805, 1983.
65. Baker, G. L., Kahl, L. E., Zee, B., et al.: Malignancy following treatment of rheumatoid arthritis with cyclophosphamide. Long-term case-control follow-up study. Am. J. Med. 83:1, 1987.
66. Gibbons, R. B., and Westerman, E.: Acute nonlymphocytic leukemia following short-term, intermittent, intravenous cyclophosphamide treatment of lupus nephritis. Arthritis Rheum. 31:1552, 1988.
67. Silman, A. J., Petrie, J., Hazleman, B., et al.: Lymphoproliferative cancer and other malignancy in patients with rheumatoid arthritis treated with Azathioprine: A 20 year follow-up study. Ann. Rheum. Dis. 47:988, 1988.
67a. Ellman, M. H., Hurwitz, H., Thomas, C., et al.: Lymphoma developing in a patient with rheumatoid arthritis taking low-dose weekly methotrexate. J. Rheumatol. 18:1741, 1991.
68. Nyberg, G., Eriksson, O., and Westberg, N. G.: Increased incidence of cervical atypia in women with systemic lupus erythematosus treated with chemotherapy. Arthritis Rheum. 24:648, 1981.
69. Erban, S. B., and Sokas, R. K.: Kaposi's sarcoma in an elderly man with Wegener's granulomatosis treated with cyclophosphamide and corticosteroids. Arch. Intern. Med. 148:1201, 1988.
70. Darby, S. C., Doll, R., Gill, S. K., et al.: Long-term mortality after a single course with x-rays in patients treated for ankylosing spondylitis. Br. J. Cancer 55:179, 1987.
71. Urowitz, M. B., and Rider, W. D.: Myeloproliferative disorders in patients with rheumatoid arthritis treated with total body irradiation. Am. J. Med. 78:60, 1985.

72. Csuka, M., Brewer, B. J., Lynch, K. L., et al.: Osteonecrosis, fractures, and protrusio acetabuli secondary to x-irradiation therapy for prostatic carcinoma. J. Rheumatol. 14:165, 1987.
73. Rock, M. G., and Unni, K. K.: Iatrogenic bone malignancy and pseudomalignancy. Curr. Opinion Rheum. 2:138, 1990.
74. Visuri, T., and Koskenvuo, M.: Cancer risk after McKee-Farrar total hip replacement. Orthopaedics 14:137, 1991.
75. Murakata, L. A., and Rangwala, A. F.: Silicone lymphadenopathy with concomitant malignant lymphoma. J. Rheumatol. 16:1480, 1989.
75a. Berkenstock, O. L.: Issues concerning possible cobalt-chromium carcinogenicity: A literature review and discussion. Contemp. Orthop. 24:265, 1992.

Section XIX

Disorders of Bone and Structural Proteins

Chapter 95

David W. Rowe
Jay R. Shapiro

Heritable Disorders of Structural Proteins

INTRODUCTION

The heritable disorders of connective tissue are a consequence of defects in the quantity or structure of collagen, elastin, and other extracellular matrix proteins. Advances in molecular biology and protein chemistry have now identified the major components of the extracellular matrix and a variety of mutations in their corresponding genes. The challenge in the ensuing years will be to relate the mutation of a specific gene to the resulting phenotype, with the hope that understanding the pathophysiologic impact of the mutation will lead to rational therapeutic strategies. The goal of this chapter is to relate how principles of connective tissue biology help explain the resulting clinical disorders that are observed when a mutation disrupts function of a component of the extracellular matrix. It is assumed that the readers will have familiarized themselves with the basic elements of collagen and elastin biochemistry in gene structure presented in Chapter 2.

BIOCHEMICAL AND MOLECULAR ASPECTS OF HERITABLE DISORDERS OF CONNECTIVE TISSUE

Relationship of Matrix Molecules and Clinical Disease

Structural Components of Connective Tissue. Currently 14 distinct collagen types are recognized, representing 21 separate genes.[1,2] This bewildering array of proteins, which is further diversified through mechanisms of alternative splicing of segments of the transcribed gene or through the use of alternative promoters that transcribe a separate ribonucleic acid (RNA), makes it difficult to relate each gene to its corresponding clinical disease. The reader may find it helpful to group the individual collagens into families of extracellular matrix proteins that provide a specific connective tissue function: tensile strength, resistance to compressive forces, and barrier-filtration (Table 95–1). To meet these structural requirements, the properties of the major collagen protein within the family are modified by the presence of minor collagens and noncollagenous proteins. This concept, that the primary protein is modified by specialized or minor collagens, portrays the connective tissue as an alloy of a number of components that are added or varied to meet the specialized demands of a specific connective tissue.

Connective tissues providing the tensile strength of skin, tendons, and ligaments are represented by the type I collagen family. Within the fibers of type I collagen are small amounts of type V collagen,[17] while type XII collagen is distributed on the surface of the fiber bundles.[18] In addition, collagen type VI is distributed throughout this matrix and is thought to help anchor interstitial collagen to surrounding structures.[19] The diversity of structural properties within this family of collagens is achieved by interaction with noncollagenous proteins.[20] In bone the presence of noncollagen matrix proteins, such as phosphoprotein[21] and osteocalcin,[22] permits the accumulation of a calcified structure with the properties of reinforced concrete. The presence of type III collagen in visceral tissue is associated with connective

Table 95–1. COLLAGEN TYPES GROUPED INTO FAMILIES OF PROTEINS WITH COMMON STRUCTURAL PROPERTIES*

Functional Component	Type I Family (Tensile CT)	Type II Family (Compressive CT)	Type IV Family (Barrier CT)
Primary collagen	I(2^3)	II(1,as^4)	IV(5^{5-7})
Integral with primary protein	V(3)	XI(3)	
Surrounding the primary protein	XII(1^8)	IX(2,ap^9)	
Anchoring	VI(3,as^{10,11})	VI(as)	VII(1)
Specialized tissue distribution	III(1)—in viscera and blood vessels	X(1^{13})—in hypertrophic chondrocytes	VIII(1^{14})—in blood vessels, neural tissue
	Elastin (as^{12})—microfibrilin		
Uncertain	XIII(as^{15})		Short chain^{16}

*The number within the parentheses is the number of genetically distinct chains that compose the collagen molecule; (as) indicates that the mRNA is alternatively spliced, while (ap) indicates an alternative promoter.

CT, collagen type.

tissue of smooth muscle cells. The interaction of the type I collagen family with elastic tissue gives blood vessels the properties of a belted automobile tire.

The second structural demand of connective tissue is resistance to compressive forces, like those that occur in joints. Type II collagen is the major constituent of cartilage, and its fibers are modified by type XI and type IX collagens.[23] In specialized cartilaginous tissues, such as hypertrophic chondrocyte, type X collagen is specifically produced.[24] Similar to members of the type I collagen family, type VI collagen is distributed throughout cartilage, allowing anchoring of this tissue to surrounding structures.[25] The alloy nature of type II collagen can be appreciated by its distribution in articular surfaces, the nose and auricle, the nucleus pulposus, and the vitreous of the eye.

The third function of connective tissue is to provide a barrier between cell types and yet allow the passage of molecules (filtration function). This function is met by the basement membrane, which is composed primarily of type IV collagen. This collagen interacts with a variety of noncollagenous components, including laminin and heparan sulfate proteoglycan.[26] A short-chain collagen has been identified in basement membrane, and it may be analogous to the minor collagens that interact with the fibrillar collagen types I and II. Type VII collagen has the important function of anchoring basement membrane to adjacent tissues.[27] Type VIII collagen may represent a specialized component that is present primarily in blood vessels and neural tissue.[28, 29] The functions of these collagens underscore the alloy nature of connective tissues within the basement membrane with their occurring in tissues as diverse as the cornea of the eye, the endothelium of a blood vessel, and the glomerulus of the kidney, where they are involved in filtration.

Beyond the structural properties of each collagen family, the extracellular matrix responds to the environment of tissue and the cells that it supports. The important aspects of this interaction are detailed in Chapter 3 and include the noncollagenous components such as fibronectin,[30] tenascin,[31] and pro-

teoglycans[32] present in the interstitial space and the family of cell surface receptors, the integrins. In a yet undefined manner, the extracellular matrix changes to meet growth and repair of tissue by relaying signals back to the cells that synthesize the necessary components.[33] Furthermore, biologic function is encoded within the primary sequence of the structural proteins. The complexity of function represented in the connective tissue proteins includes, for example, short protein sequences within an extracellular matrix protein interacting with cell surface integrins to alter the state of differentiation of the cells, growth factor–like signals to specific cells,[34] or components of the blood-clotting cascade.[35, 36] It can be anticipated that mutations within genes that encode such diversity of structural and biologic functions can only present a highly pleotrophic clinical picture. However, as the domains essential for structural function and for biologic activity are mapped through the study of mutations in humans and animal models, a more rational understanding of heritable diseases will emerge.

Relationship of Collagen Biosynthesis to Clinical Disease

The synthesis of type I collagen and the diseases that result from defects in this pathway have become the paradigm for studying mutations affecting all the fibrillar collagens and will be useful in approaching mutations of those collagens with a more complex and interrupted structure.

Collagen Synthesis. The type I collagen genes that code for the α1 and α2 collagen chains are present as one allele per haploid set of chromosomes (see Chapter 2).[37] In comparison with other mammalian genes, both type I collagen genes are large and complex, being distributed throughout 50 or 51 exons.[1] Both alleles of the collagen gene appear to be active, because in dominantly inherited disorders both normal and abnormal populations of collagen chains are observed. The level of activity of the collagen gene is determined by its promoter, which

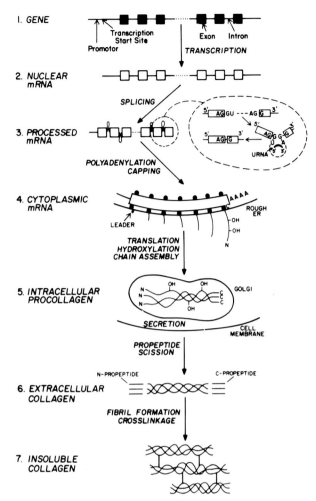

1. GENE

Transcription
Start Site
Promotor
Exon   Intron
TRANSCRIPTION

2. NUCLEAR
mRNA

SPLICING

3. PROCESSED
mRNA

5' AG GU ---AG G 3'

5' AG G 3'

AG G G

URNA

POLYADENYLATION
CAPPING

4. CYTOPLASMIC
mRNA

ROUGH
ER

LEADER

—OH

—OH

N

TRANSLATION
HYDROXYLATION
CHAIN ASSEMBLY

5. INTRACELLULAR
PROCOLLAGEN

OH   OH

N   C
N   C
N   C

GOLGI

OH

SECRETION

CELL
MEMBRANE

PROPEPTIDE
SCISSION

N-PROPEPTIDE   C-PROPEPTIDE

6. EXTRACELLULAR
COLLAGEN

FIBRIL FORMATION
CROSSLINKAGE

7. INSOLUBLE
COLLAGEN

Figure 95–1. Steps of collagen biosynthesis relevant to the heritable diseases of collagen. The structure of the gene *(step 1)* is represented by darkened squares for the exons and by a line for the introns. The RNAs *(steps 2 to 4)* are represented by open squares. See text for the narrative description of the figure.

contains deoxyribonucleic acid (DNA) elements responsive to a wide variety of transcriptional factors (Fig. 95–1, *step 1*). These elements are located at the distal end of the coding region of the gene (5' upstream region) and within the body of the gene (intron sequence).[38, 39] These sequences respond to general transcription factors present in a wide variety of cells and factors that control their synthesis in highly specialized tissue such as bone and cartilage.[40, 41] Mutations in these sequences have been observed in an experimentally derived form of osteogenesis imperfecta, the MOV13 mouse. In this disorder, a domain within the promoter has been disrupted so that the collagen is expressed in fibroblasts and blood vessel cells[42] but is not expressed in osseous tissue.[43]

The initial collagen messenger RNA (mRNA) that is transcribed is an exact copy of the gene containing both introns and exons (see Fig. 95–1, *step 2*). Twice as much α1(I) as α2(I) mRNA is transcribed from each gene.[44] The intervening sequences are removed through a splicing mechanism similar to

other eukaryotic mRNAs.[45] There are recognition sequences at the boundaries of the intron-exon junction that are complementary to a small nuclear RNA (U$_1$ RNA) that identify each exon[46] and act to bring the ends of the introns into alignment for removal and subsequent joining of the adjacent exons (see Fig. 95–1, *step 3*). The entire intron sequence must be removed because its presence would alter the reading frame of the RNA or substitute inappropriate amino acids into the encoded protein. In many cases in which the reading frame is altered, the abnormally spliced product is retained within the nucleus of the RNA and is degraded.[47, 48] The net result is a reduction of normal mRNA productively synthesized from the affected allele. Such a defect is considered a "regulatory" mutant because it results in a nonfunctional, or *null, allele* (Table 95–2). Low amounts of collagen are synthesized, but the collagen that is produced from the remaining normal allele is structurally normal.[49, 50] Other examples of regulatory mutations include those altering sequences in the promoter and large gene deletions.

On reaching the rough endoplasmic reticulum, mRNA is translated into a polypeptide chain (see Fig. 95–1, *step 4*). Abnormalities in the primary sequence of the mRNA that would result in a translationally inactive RNA include a base change that codes for a stop codon prior to the end of the coding region, and one that shifts the reading frame. In the former case, the mRNA codes for a truncated protein,[51] whereas in the latter case all the amino acids beyond the frame shift mutations would be inappropriate.[52] In both cases the amount of normal protein produced would be reduced, rendering the mutant allele null.

Post-translational Modification and Chain Assembly. As the collagen mRNA is translated, certain prolyl residues become hydroxylated, and specific lysines are hydroxylated and then glycosylated[53] (see

Table 95–2. CLASSIFICATION OF MUTATIONS OF TYPE I COLLAGEN BASED ON FUNCTIONAL CONSEQUENCE TO THE PRODUCTION OF COLLAGEN PROTEIN*

Null Mutations	Helix-Disrupting Mutations
Inactivation of transcription control sequences	Gene deletion removing complete exons and producing a truncated chain
Gene deletion or duplication of partial exons producing a frameshift	Gene duplication adding complete exons
Splicing that results in an RNA that is out of frame or contains premature stop codons	Exon skipping secondary to abnormal splicing
Increased rate of collagen mRNA degradation	Activation of cryptic splice sites that produce a retained in-frame intron sequence
Mutations that prevent incorporation of the α1(I) chain into the molecule	Point mutation of first position *gly* codons of the Gly-X-Y triplet

*Null mutations produce a reduced quantity of a structurally normal product, while mutations within the coding domains of the gene can result in a protein with abnormal structure or function.

Fig. 95–1, *steps 4 and 5*). The function of the hydroxy-proline residues appears to enhance the stability of the collagen triple helix at physiologic temperatures.[54, 55] The fact that mutants of prolylhydroxylase have not been described may imply that a half-normal level of the enzyme is sufficient to mediate normal hydroxylation, whereas a complete deficiency of the enzyme is lethal. The enzyme has two subunits, and its activity parallels the rate of collagen synthesis.[56] Lysyl hydroxylation is important for the formation of stable interchain cross-links in bone. The function of the glycosylated hydroxylysine or the heterosaccharide unit of the C-terminal propeptide is uncertain.[57, 58] Both prolyl and lysyl hydroxylase act on nascent procollagen chains and are unable to hydroxylate once the procollagen chain assumes the helical conformation. Excessive lysyl hydroxylation is observed in association with mutations that impair the rate of the helix formation.[59]

Within the Golgi apparatus, the individual procollagen chains initiate self-assembly from the C-terminal propeptide toward the N-terminal (see Fig. 95–1, *step 5*).[60] There is a highly conserved region within the C-terminal propeptide in all the collagen α-chains.[61] This region is essential for initial chain alignment and subsequent assembly. A defect in this region of the molecule inhibits incorporation of the abnormal chain into the triple helix and thus reduces total collagen synthesis (null mutation).[52, 62]

The commonest mutation of the collagen gene associated with a clinical disease is a single base change, particularly that affecting first position glycine residues of the gly-X-Y triplet. Glycine residues permit the polypeptide chain to maintain the tight helical conformation. The replacement of this glycine molecule as a result of a point mutation in the glycine codon will interfere with the formation of the triple helix[63, 64] or will induce a kink within the helical domain.[65] Molecules containing such a defect are slow to assemble, are poorly secreted,[66] and have an increased susceptibility to tissue proteases.[67] Mutations of this type can lead to enhanced intracellular or interstitial degradation of collagen α-chains and thus a lower net rate of collagen production. The term "protein suicide" has been used to characterize these types of mutations.[68] The presence of the mutant α-chain compromises the function of the normal chains that associate with the mutant chain. All molecules that interact with molecules containing the defective chain are compromised, which greatly amplifies the destructive effect of the mutant chain. Other examples of mutations that have similar adverse effects on helix stability and, subsequently, lead to protein suicide include deletion of a small region of the helical domain due to either a small gene deletion[69] or exon skipping,[70] and an insertion of an extraneous helical[71] or nonhelical sequence due to a partial gene duplication or a mutation of splicing that retains a small sequence of intron[72] (see Table 95–2).

Fiber Formation and Cross-Linking. The assem-

bled procollagen molecule is secreted, followed by removal of the N- and C-terminal propeptides (see Fig. 95–1, *step 6*).[73] Genetic defects involving the N-terminal propeptide region have been defined both in man and in animals. In this situation, failure to cleave the N-terminal propeptide interferes with the organization of the collagen fiber.[74, 75, 76] Genetic defects involving removal of the C-terminal propeptide have not been defined.

The final step in the formation of a stabilized collagen fiber is the assembly of the individual molecules into the collagen polymer[77, 78] and its subsequent stabilization by intermolecular and intramolecular cross-links (see Fig. 95–1, *step 7*). The assembly process appears to be directed by information within exposed areas of the triple helical molecule, since fiber formation can occur in vitro.[79, 80] The proper alignment of microfibrils is essential for the enzyme lysyl oxidase to initiate cross-link formation between adjacent molecules by converting the epsilon (ε) amino group of exposed lysine residues to a chemically reactive aldehyde group.[81, 82] Mutations that disrupt helix alignment further weaken the connective tissue because of a deficiency in collagen cross-linking.[83] Agents that block cross-link formation (e.g., penicillamine, or β-aminopropionitrile) result in enhanced tissue friability, bowing of the bones, and aortic aneurysms (lathyrism).[84] Besides genetic defects affecting lysyl oxidase, the absence of appropriately placed lysine residues might prevent the formation of a particularly important intermolecular cross-link. Cross-links are initially bifunctional but become trifunctional with age, leading to a highly cross-linked structure.[85] Nonenzymatic ligation of ε amino groups from glucose can further increase the cross-linkage and insolubility of the connective tissue, which may account for the fibrosis and endothelial changes associated with diabetes mellitus.[86]

Genetic Aspects of Connective Tissue Diseases

Pattern of Inheritance. Dominant traits are recognized as a result of one allele's being affected, while recessive traits require that both alleles are affected. This separation becomes less distinct as individual traits are examined more closely, and heterozygous carriers of recessive traits can be shown to have minor consequences. In general for the connective tissue proteins, mutations that affect the structure or the amount of the extracellular matrix protein are inherited as *dominant traits*. The severity of the mutation, and thus how obvious the disease is, is a reflection of how mutation compromises the function of the normal components. In many cases a strong dominant pedigree can be discerned within a family, and when this is present it is an asset to diagnosis. However, similar mutations can arise spontaneously and, in this case, will present in a *sporadic manner* without a prior dominant pedigree. Subsequent offspring, if biologically possible, would reveal the dominant character of the mutation. There is increasing realization that one normal parent can produce two or more severely affected individuals, suggesting a recessive inheritance. However, molecular analysis has shown that in most cases such a pedigree is due to *germinal mosaicism* in one parent rather than a recessively expressed co-dominant trait.[87, 88] It is still not clear why individuals who are mosaic for a severe connective tissue disease do not appear to show the connective tissue findings of their offspring.

Relation of Mutation to Mode of Inheritance. (Table 95–3). The goal of defining mutations that underlie heritable disorders is to appreciate the pathobiologic consequences of mutation. The primary defects of major collagen within a collagen family always appear to be inherited in a dominant manner or to occur sporadically. Those mutations affecting structure seem to be severer and thus are readily recognized as a defect of the protein. Mutations that affect the quantity of protein produced rather than its structure (null mutations) are less severe and may not always be appreciated as a heritable trait. However, with improved sensitivity of ascertainment a dominant pedigree should be evident.

Mutations of genes that modify the rate at which the collagen genes are transcribed probably exist. Examples of excessive fibrotic activity, such as keloids[89] or Dilantin (phenytoin) gingival hyperplasia, may reflect the presence of a mutant gene that either fails to curtail a fibrotic response or that stimulates in an uncontrolled manner the fibrotic response to certain stimuli.[90] On the other hand, diminished gene activity may underlie forms of familial osteoporosis or ligamentous laxity and may represent a relative deficiency of a gene transcription factor. Since growth factors, cytokines, and other cellular signals are transmitted through complex pathways, heritable traits that result from mutations in the pathway are likely to be complex and difficult to recognize. However, they do exist and probably are not uncommon. How mutations of these putative genes might present clinically will remain unclear until they are identified and their biology is better characterized.

In contrast, two potential mutations of gene modifiers, gene products that modify the synthesis of the collagen chain, are well described. The enzymes prolyl and lysyl oxidase, which modify the nascent collagen chains intracellularly prior to helix formation, have been isolated and studied in significant detail. Since sufficient activity can be provided from one allele, mutations of these genes are inherited in a recessive manner. The same is true for the extracellular modifiers, the procollagen peptidases, and lysyl oxidase. Finally, there are the mutations of other genes that code for proteins that interact with collagen fibers either to modify their structural properties (as in the case of the minor collagens and elastin) or to assist in the interaction with other components of the extracellular matrix and with the cells of the extracellular matrix. It can be anticipated that mutations of these structural proteins with strong interactive function will be inherited as dominant traits and probably represent the largest component of the dominantly inherited connective tissue diseases not yet understood at the molecular level.

Table 95–3. SITES OF MUTATIONS THAT AFFECT THE QUANTITY OR QUALITY OF THE EXTRACELLULAR MATRIX

	Functional Consequence of the Mutation	Clinical Example (Recognized or Suspected)	Anticipated Inheritance
Primary gene defects	Abnormal structure	Small deletions or point mutations that disrupt the collagen fiber (OI and EDS IV)	Dominant or sporadic
	Decreased production	Reduced synthesis, but the product has normal structure (OI)	Dominant or sporadic, heritability often missed
Modifiers of gene activity	Excessive activity	?Keloids, gingival hyperplasia	Dominant or sporadic, but heritability may not be recognized
	Diminished activity	?Familial osteoporosis	?Probably only recognized in a recessive manner
Modifiers of collagen chains	Intracellular modifiers	Prolyl and lysyl hydroxylase (EDS VI)	Recessive
	Extracellular modifiers	Procollagen peptidases (EDS VII), lysyl oxidase (cutis laxa)	Recessive
Proteins that interact with collagen fibers	Collagen-like	Minor collagens	?Dominant
	Noncollagenous	Proteoglycans, fibronectin, elastin	?
	Cell-associated	Integrins	?

EDS, Ehlers-Danlos syndrome; OI, osteogenesis imperfecta.

Dominant forms of Ehlers-Danlos syndrome and Marfan syndrome are examples of this class of mutation.

Another aspect of mutations of structural protein is the range of severity that results from different mutations of the same gene (Table 95–4).[91] For example, mutations of type I collagen can produce the full range of severity from lethal osteogenesis imperfecta to its mildest form, which presents as familial osteoporosis. The same spectrum has recently been demonstrated for type II collagen, in which severe forms result in lethal chondrodystrophy and spondyloepiphyseal dysplasia and yet the mildest form is a familial type of osteoarthritis. Type III collagen, which is present in high amounts in blood vessels and other tissues rich in smooth muscle, shows a similar spectrum of severity. The severest form, Ehlers-Danlos syndrome type IV, is characterized by rupture of blood vessels and viscera. Mild forms of mutations of type III collagen have recently been associated with familial aneurysms. It can be expected that a similar spectrum of severity will be found with the other collagens and potentially noncollagenous proteins of the extracellular matrix. Knowledge of the precise location of the mutations and the resulting clinical consequences provides insight into the functional domains of the various proteins and provides a way of predicting clinical severity based on the site of the mutation within the gene.

Application of Molecular Genetics to Heritable Diseases of Connective Tissue

As the techniques of mutation identification are applied to an expanding number of extracellular matrix genes, it can be anticipated that the molecular basis of many heritable disorders will become appreciated. Still remaining will be diseases not yet known to be due to a characterized gene or diseases due to an as yet undiscovered connective tissue gene. It is progress in this sphere of research that will produce the greatest excitement in the coming years.

DNA Linkage to Specific Candidate Genes. Application of molecular techniques for identifying specific mutations of structural proteins gives important information on structural function. However, prior to applying these methods to specific genes, it is necessary to identify which gene should be investigated. This is accomplished through linkage studies of DNA polymorphism in affected individuals within a given pedigree. In this procedure, genomic DNA is cut with a variety of restriction enzymes, and the DNA from a Southern blot is hybridized with DNA probes that include or are adjacent to the collagen (candidate) gene (Fig. 95–2). This strategy recognizes a pattern of bands, indicating changes in restriction sites that normally are present within the normal population. These restriction patterns are allelic, and the haplotype can be followed through generations within a specific family. The presence or absence of a restriction site is scored as (+) or (−), so that the genotype of an individual at a specific site is either +/+, +/−, or −/−. When the restriction site is within or close to the gene responsible for a dominant trait, it is possible to demonstrate coincidence of a + or − allele with the disease. The two pedigrees in the illustration demonstrate linkage and exclusion of linkage of a trait to a restriction site. It is important to realize that the linkage of the restriction site to a disease does not identify the specific mutation but does identify the allele bearing the mutation. Since many of the connective tissues diseases are dominantly inherited, one can determine whether or not the disease is linked to a specific collagen gene if there is segregation of a specific polymorphic haplotype (restriction enzyme cleavage pattern) with those individuals manifesting the disease. A mathematical analysis is performed yielding a lod (logarithm of the odds) score, which indicates the statistical probability that there is cosegregation of the polymorphism with the disease and strongly suggests that the candidate gene encodes the protein responsible for the disease process. Useful polymorphisms are now known for all the fibrillar collagen genes and elastin. Linkage polymorphism has been important in deciding whether a collagen gene or the gene for another structural protein is or is not causative in a dominantly inherited connective tissue disease.

DNA Linkage with Anonymous Probes. The second approach of linkage utilized DNA probes to single copy DNA fragments scattered throughout the entire human chromosome. Known as anonymous DNA probes, a panel of these hybridization fragments can be used to eventually locate the region of the chromosome containing the mutant locus causing a specific disorder. Subsequent finer mapping of the chromosome with highly technical molecular methods eventually can identify the precise gene. This approach, referred to as reverse genetics,[97] was first dramatically demonstrated in Duchenne's muscular dystrophy[98] and more recently in cystic fibrosis.[99] It is now being applied actively to achondroplasia.

Animal Models. Naturally occurring mutations of connective tissue proteins and, more recently,

Table 95–4. SPECTRUM OF CLINICAL SEVERITY RESULTING FROM DIFFERENT MUTATIONS OF COLLAGEN GENES*

Structural Protein	Severest Form	Mildest Form
Type I	OI	Osteoporosis[92]
Type II	Lethal Chondrodystrophy[93]	Osteoarthritis[94]
Type III	EDS type IV	Familial aneurysms[95]
Type IV	Alport's syndrome[96]	?

*The documented cases for collagen types I to III can be anticipated for the other collagen types.

EDS, Ehlers-Danlos syndrome.

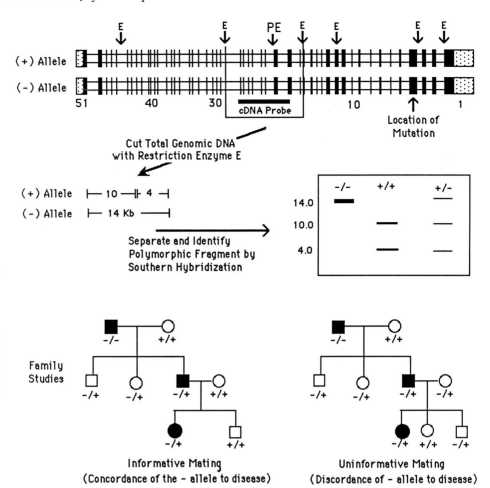

Figure 95–2. Restriction fragment length polymorphism (RFLP) analysis. Total genomic DNA is cut with a restriction enzyme E, which cuts the collagen gene at E in all individuals and in a proportion of individuals at PE. The presence or absence of PE is determined by the Southern hybridization by one band at 14 kilobases (kb) or two of 10 kb and 4 kb. Then the genotype of an individual for the PE site within the collagen gene is +/+, +/−, or −/−. The pedigree on the left demonstrates that the (−) allele always migrates with the disease (*filled symbol*). However in the pedigree on the right, the (−) allele is not associated with the disease, so linkage to the collagen gene is excluded. The confidence that a candidate gene is linked to a particular trait is increased when a number of informative matings (−/+ vs. +/+) can be examined.

mutations induced by laboratory manipulations are other ways in which the structure and function of a connective tissue protein can be explored. Because mouse genetics is so highly defined and the animal is so manipulable to genetic experimentation, it will prove to be a most informative area of research. Ectopic expression of mutant collagen genes has demonstrated the strong dominant nature of structural mutations of type I[100, 101] and type II[102] collagen. The ability to target and inactivate endogenous genes has the potential for revealing the function of minor collagen or noncollagen components of the extracellular matrix through the use of embryonic stem cells.[103] The ultimate goal in understanding the pathophysiologic basis of a disease and evaluating strategies of treatment is to create exact replicas of the human disease in mice by manipulating the mouse genome.

CLINICAL EVALUATION OF HERITABLE CONNECTIVE TISSUE DISORDERS

In view of the complexity of connective tissue proteins, it is not surprising that the variety of disorders that fall under this broad heading can be overwhelming. In an effort to present this informa-

tion in an organized fashion, the disorders have been grouped based on the family of connective tissue proteins that are affected by the underlying mutation (Table 95–5). The type I collagen family will be emphasized, since it is the best characterized, but similar advances can be anticipated for the other two families.

Ehlers-Danlos Syndrome

The connective tissue disorders grouped as the different types of Ehlers-Danlos syndrome (EDS) illustrate the genetic and clinical variability that is so characteristic of this disease. The types of EDS will be presented based on the mode of inheritance, to emphasize the character and site of the putative gene defects (Table 95–6).

Dominantly Inherited EDS

The autosomal dominant forms of the disease account for 90 percent of the reported cases.[104] Clinically, they are the most difficult to separate because of a sizable overlap in phenotype. It should be pointed out that as many as 50 percent of individuals

Table 95–5. DISEASES AFFECTING THE FAMILY OF TENSILE CONNECTIVE TISSUES

Family Subtypes	Tissue Distribution	Associated Heritable Diseases
Unmodified	Skin, tendon	Ehlers-Danlos syndrome, all types except IV
Modified by type III collagen	Blood vessel and viscera	Ehlers-Danlos syndrome type IV
Modified for mineralization	Bone	Osteogenesis imperfecta
Modified for elasticity	Blood vessel, skin	Marfan syndrome, cutis laxa, pseudoxanthoma elasticum

with clinical signs of EDS do not fit into any current classification.

EDS I and II. These prototypic forms of EDS (Fig. 95–3) are characterized by severe or mild hyperextensibility of large and small joints and are the classic forms of EDS. Large joint hyperextensibility is marked in EDS I and is mild and limited to the hands and feet in EDS II. At times, it may be difficult to decide whether limited hyperextensibility is present in an older sibling or parent, since joint laxity decreases with increasing age. Recurrent joint dislocations, periodic joint effusion related to trauma, and the eventual appearance of osteoarthritis pose significant management problems.[105–108] Bilateral synovial thickening has been observed in EDS along with the accumulation of small masses of crystalline material in synovial villi. Osborn and co-workers observed that EDS types II and III were found to constitute 5 percent of cases in a pediatric arthritis clinic population.[109] Infants may be born prematurely to affected mothers because of early rupture of membranes and are found to be hypotonic and floppy, with articular hyperextensibility. As these children grow, their muscle strength tends to improve, although decreased strength can be demonstrated in many adults.

Patients with EDS have parrot-like facies, a broad nasal root, and epicanthal folds. They may be floppy-eared, and traction on the ears or elbow will reveal skin hyperextensibility. Their skin is warm and has a velvety smooth texture. A gaping "fish-mouth" wound may appear when skin is traumatized. Thin, atrophic, corrugated, and hyperpigmented scars are found on the forehead and lower extremities (papyraceous, or "cigarette paper," scars). Typically, skin lesions heal slowly after surgery or trauma. The ability to touch the tip of the tongue to the nose (Gorlin's sign) is also evidence of tissue hyperelasticity. Molluscoid pseudotumors (violaceous subcutaneous tumors ranging in size from 0.5 to 3 cm) may be palpated in the tissue over the forearms and lower extremities. Pseudotumors are calcified fat-containing cysts that are found over pressure points and may be visualized on radiograph. Although many patients claim to bruise easily, ecchymoses distributed over the extremities are found only in patients with the severer forms of the disease. Severe bilateral varicose veins are a common problem. Systemic findings may reveal evidence of spontaneous pneumothorax, pneumomediastinum, and subpleural blebs.[110] Mitral valve prolapse and tricuspid valve insufficiency may complicate EDS I.[111, 112] The spectrum of skeletal findings in EDS I and II has been summarized by Coventry.[113] These include thoracolumbar kyphoscoliosis, a long giraffe-like neck,

Table 95–6. EHLERS-DANLOS SYNDROME

		Distinguishing Clinical Features	Molecular Abnormality	General Comments
Autosomal dominant	I	Excessive joint laxity and skin hyperextensibility	Unknown	Fraying of collagen fibers
	II	Less severe than type I	Unknown	Differentiation between milder forms of EDS can be difficult
	III	Lax joints with normal skin	Unknown	
	IV	Thin skin, rupture of blood vessels and viscera	Mutations of type III collagen gene affecting structure or synthesis of the protein	New mutations or germinal mosaicism probably account for sporadic cases
	VII	Recurrent joint dislocation in childhood	Mutation of type I collagen that inactivates the N-terminal procollagen cleavage site; procollagen accumulates in tissues	Overlap with mild osteogenesis imperfecta
	VIII	Periodontitis	Unknown	Skin and joint findings similar to EDS I or EDS II
Autosomal recessive	VI	Scoliosis, ocular rupture	Lysyl hydroxylase deficiency	Clinical and biochemical heterogeneity
	X	Bruising	Possible fibronectin abnormality	Single cases never confirmed by molecular studies
X-linked recessive	V	Hyperextensible skin	Unknown	Reports of lysyl oxidase deficiency not confirmed
	IX	Occipital horns and bladder neck obstruction	Low lysyl oxidase activity; low serum copper levels	This form may overlap with X-linked cutis laxa

EDS, Ehlers-Danlos syndrome.

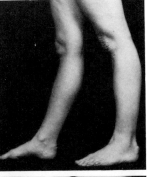
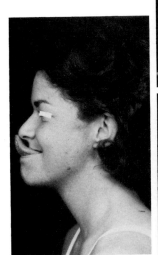
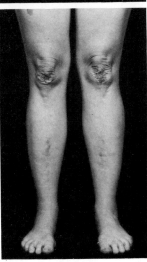

Figure 95–3. EDS I. Tissue elasticity, joint hypermobility, and tissue fragility are demonstrated by the patient's ability to extend her tongue to the tip of the nose (Gorlin's sign), by hyperextensibility at the knee (genu recurvatum), and by characteristic "cigarette paper" or papyraceous scars of the knees and tibial skin. (Courtesy of V. McKusick, M.D.)

downward sloping of the ribs of the upper part of the thorax, and a tendency to reversal of the normal cervical, thoracic, and lumbar curves. Anterior wedging of thoracic vertebral bodies occasionally may be seen; however, there has been no systematic study of bone mineral content in EDS.

EDS III (Benign Hypermobility Syndrome). In 1967, Kirk and colleagues[114] applied the term "hypermobility syndrome" to patients having generalized joint laxity associated with musculoskeletal complaints. Also apparent was a strong familial tendency, with dominant inheritance and variable expression. Although the majority of individuals with this syndrome are asymptomatic, there are many with rheumatologic complaints that pose problems in diagnosis and therapy. There is also the added anxiety about the relationship of physical activity to joint trauma, a factor that may adversely limit a patient's lifestyle.

The extent of joint laxity may be measured in terms of the following criteria:[115] (1) passive approximation of the thumb toward the forearm with the wrist in flexion, (2) passive hyperextension of digits, (3) active hyperextension of the knee more than 10 degrees, (4) passive and excessive dorsiflexion of the ankle and eversion of the foot, and (5) the ability to touch the floor with the palms without bending the knees (Fig. 95–4). Generalized hyperextensibility may be considered present if three of six joint pairs test positive. It may be diagnostically important in evaluating the heritable disorders of connective tissue to carefully differentiate small joint extensibility as opposed to both large and small joint extensibility. Using a goniometer, Boone and Azen[116] measured the arcs of active joint motion in males between the ages of 18 months and 54 years and found that joint laxity diminishes with age in the normal population. Others have found mobility of the upper limb joints to be a continuously distributed variable subject to age, ethnic factors, and the particular joint being tested.[117, 118]

By definition, patients with the hypermobility syndrome lack the excessive skin laxity and the other stigmata of EDS or Marfan syndrome. Although hypermobility is usually apparent in early childhood, patients generally become symptomatic and seek medical advice during their 20s and 30s. Finsterbush and Pogrund[119] documented musculoskeletal complaints in 100 patients with generalized joint hypermobility, of whom 51 were female and 49 were male. Fifty-six patients had localized complaints, and 44 patients had more generalized musculoskeletal complaints, including episodic acute knee pain, patellar dislocation, and patellofemoral arthritis with effusion. Bilateral ankle instability, progressive scoliosis with back pain, and pain due to hyperextension at the elbow were also seen. Recurrent dislocation at several joints—sternoclavicular, shoulder, and hip—was particularly frequent in infants. Hypermobile joints were found in 65 percent of first-degree relatives. In the severely affected kindred described by Horton and colleagues[120] as exhibiting "familial joint instability," chronic sequelae included hypoplasia of the femoral heads and acetabula with the formation of pseudoacetabula. An association between hypermobility and osteoarthritis has been suggested.[121] A relationship between joint hypermobility and mitral valve prolapse remains unresolved.[122–124]

EDS VIII. The characteristics of this dominantly inherited syndrome, as reported by McKusick[125] and others,[126] include (1) a severe resorptive periodontitis that leads to early loss of teeth and (2) marked fragility of the skin in the absence of hyperelasticity, which leads to dystrophic scarring. Joint hypermobility is mild. Even the limited number of cases reported, to date, suggests that clinical variability as occurs in the other types will also be seen in EDS VIII. The dental findings, however, have been rather uniform.

Molecular Pathology of EDS I to EDS III and VIII. Little progress has been made in understanding the underlying molecular basis of dominantly inherited EDS.[127, 128] Abnormally large or small or frayed dermal collagen fibrils and disordered elastic fibers have been noted, but these findings may not be

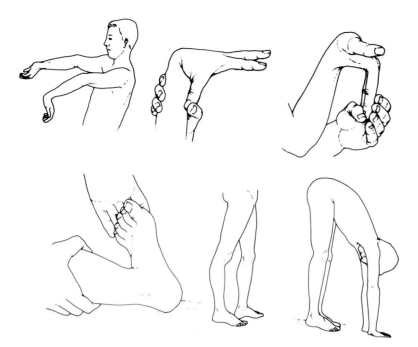

Figure 95–4. Maneuvers that may be used to establish the presence of clinically significant joint laxity. Examples of joint laxity found in the Ehlers-Danlos syndrome. It is not unusual to find extreme laxity of the small joints and less laxity in large joints. Laxity decreases with age, so that the dominant nature of most of these syndromes may not be appreciated when examining older family members. (Redrawn and modified from Wynne-Davies, R.: Acetabular dysplasia and familial joint laxity: Two etiological factors in congenital dislocation of the hip. A review of 589 patients and their families. J. Bone Joint Surg. 52B:704, 1970.)

specific.[129–131] Factors involved in the orientation and lateral growth of collagen and elastin fibers are areas of active investigation. Of primary importance may be the hydrophilic and charge differences on the surface of these molecules, which are determined by the primary sequence of the chains and are probably modified by other extracellular substances, such as glycosaminoglycans.[132] Since primary protein studies of collagen from EDS fibroblasts have not shown an abnormality, the approach in the future will be directed to linkage polymorphism of minor collagen and the noncollagen matrix genes within dominant families.[133]

Therapy. Obviously, there is no specific therapy directed at the molecular defect in the dominantly inherited forms of EDS. Supportive therapy, however, is essential to preserve normal joint function. Planned exercise programs and muscle-strengthening exercises are useful and do much to maintain a positive outlook in these individuals, who may have a poor prognosis if joint stability and articular surfaces are compromised by excessive activity or chronic trauma.[134, 135] The presence of multiple ecchymoses will raise concern about a bleeding diathesis, particularly at the time of elective surgery. Although no consistent basis for the hemorrhagic tendency in EDS I has been identified, caution is advised in the patient with a strong history of easy bruisability.[136] The recent discovery of von Willebrand–like protein sequences within certain matrix proteins lends credence to the clinical impression of a mild defect in hemostasis.[35, 36, 137]

EDS VII (Arthrochalasis Multiplex Congenita Form). This form of EDS (Fig. 95–5) is marked by pronounced joint hypermobility, moderate cutaneous elasticity, moderate brusing, round facies, and short stature. These patients experience multiple dislocations involving large joints, such as the hips.

Their tissues are very friable, a factor that complicates orthopedic procedures.

Molecular Pathology. EDS VII, along with the bovine and ovine homologue dermatosparaxis,[138, 139] has provided insight into the process of normal fiber formation. The initial observation was an accumulation of procollagen within the dermis of affected children.[140] With subsequent recognition that procollagen had both N- and C-terminal extension propeptides and that there were separate enzymes respon-

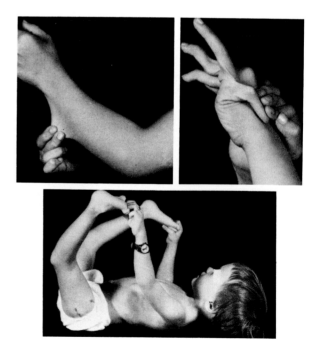

Figure 95–5. EDS VII. This variant is marked by the presence of short stature and round facies. Joint hypermobility and skin laxity are severe, and recurrent dislocations may require surgical repair. (Courtesy of V. McKusick, M.D.)

sible for their removal,[69] the syndrome has become more sharply defined as an accumulation of procollagen with the N-terminal peptides still attached (pN collagen). Interference of the extension propeptide with normal fiber formation probably accounts for the clinical disorder.[141-143] At present, two distinctly different genetic abnormalities result in procollagen accumulation. The first (VIIA) is an inactive N-terminal procollagen peptidase, a condition that has recessive inheritance.[140] The extent of procollagen accumulation is a reflection of the degree of enzyme inactivity. The second (VIIB) and probably commoner abnormality is the resistance of a procollagen chain to the action of the N-terminal procollagen peptidase. The resistance probably results from an amino acid substitution or deletion in the pro-α1- or pro-α2-chain, leading to half of the pro-α-chains containing an abnormal N-terminal extension[144, 145] or deletion of the region due to exon skipping.[146-150] Thus, one dose of the abnormal gene deranges collagen structure sufficiently to be recognized as a dominant trait. Overlapping syndromes of EDS VII and mild osteogenesis imperfecta may be explained by mutations within the helical domain of the collagen chain, placing the N-terminal cleavage site out of register for enzymatic cleavage of the propeptide.[151]

Recessively Inherited EDS

Although the recessive forms of EDS represent only a small portion of the spectrum of EDS, these variants are sufficiently well characterized to be recognized as distinct syndromes. The recessive forms tend to be severer than those that are dominantly inherited.

EDS VI (Ocular Form). The first description of a biochemical defect related to collagen biosynthesis was described in 1972 by Pinnell and colleagues.[152] Their report described hydroxylysine-deficient collagen in two sisters with severe scoliosis, recurrent joint dislocation, and hyperextensible skin and joints. Premature rupture of fetal membranes had occurred at the birth of one of the children. Both were floppy at birth, with poor respiratory movements and subsequent bouts of pneumonia. Spinal deformity was apparent, as was easy bruisability. Early growth and motor development were delayed, and muscle mass was diminished. Their skin was described as pale, translucent, and velvety, and it showed the typical gaping, fish-mouth wound after trauma.

The range of clinical manifestations of EDS VI (Fig. 95–6) is broadly representative of that of EDS. One exception has been involvement of the ocular tissues, with microcornea, retinal detachment, and glaucoma. The eye is particularly susceptible to trauma, often leading to enucleation. A recent survey of patients with this disorder did not find abnormalities of the eye other than myopia.[153] Mild arachnodactyly, chest wall deformity associated with narrow shoulders, molluscoid pseudotumors, thin atrophic

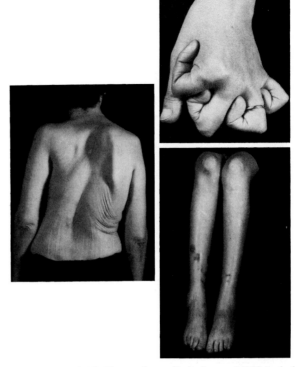

Figure 95–6. EDS VI. The ocular-scoliotic form of EDS includes severe scoliosis at an early age, thin hyperelastic skin (tibial scars), and hyperextensible joints with recurrent dislocations. (Courtesy of V. McKusick, M.D.)

scars, and easy bruisability also occur. Hyperextensibility of joints is marked.

Molecular Pathology. In the original description of EDS VI, it was found that the hydroxylysine content of collagen in skin and tendons was less than 1 residue per 1000 total amino acids, in contrast with 4 residues per 1000 in control tissue.[152] The hydroxylysine content was somewhat less than normal in bone and was normal in cartilage. Subsequently, a number of investigators demonstrated low lysyl hydroxylase activity in fibroblasts obtained from individuals with this form of EDS.[137, 154] Enzyme levels in amniotic fluid fibroblasts may be useful in prenatal diagnostic studies.[155] The mechanism of the low activity was shown to result from an altered affinity (K_m) for ascorbic acid, the cofactor of the enzyme.[156] Although these studies suggested that at higher levels of ascorbic acid, enzyme activity would increase, there is no systematic study demonstrating the effectiveness of ascorbic acid in this disease. In fact there are a number of inconsistencies that may represent heterogeneity within this syndrome. Now that the human enzyme has been purified, it will be possible to combine immunologic, biochemical, and molecular studies from various patients and in this way differentiate among different mutations within the lysyl hydroxylase enzyme complex.[157]

The consequence of deficient hydroxylysine content of collagen is related to the role of this amino acid in cross-link formation. Hydroxylysine-containing cross-links are able to undergo a stabilizing change (Amadori rearrangement), which is particularly common to the types of cross-links found in bone. Although individuals with EDS VI do form reducible cross-links, a significant proportion appear to lack the hydroxylysine residue,[158] which enters into the formation of the hydroxypyridinium cross-links.[85, 159]

EDS X. In the original case report of EDS X[160] the proband had hypermobile joints, easy bruising, fish-mouth scars on her extremities, and mitral valve prolapse. Although this presentation clinically resembled EDS II or III, the characteristic velvety feel of the skin was absent, as were striae. Platelets obtained from this patient revealed resistance to aggregation in response to collagen and adenosine diphosphate (ADP), whereas the responses to serotonin, thrombin, and epinephrine were diminished. Since normal plasma or cryoprecipitate was found to correct the clotting defect, it was suggested that a qualitative deficiency of fibronectin caused the abnormality. Molecular confirmation of this suggestion is still lacking.

X-Linked EDS: EDS V and EDS IX (Occipital Horn Syndrome). These forms of EDS are the least well characterized, but they are distinguished by their X-linked inheritance pattern.[161, 162] These patients had strikingly extensible skin and bruisability, with molluscoid pseudotumors. Although joint hypermobility was mild, they experienced recurrent dislocation.

EDS IX is characterized by skeletal dysplasia, occipital horns, diarrhea, and obstructive uropathy.[163, 164] The propositus had an unusual facial appearance and had undergone repair of bladder neck obstruction at age 5 years. Mild hyperextensibility of the small joints was present, but cutaneous elasticity was normal. A remarkable finding was the presence of two symmetric bony spurs projecting inferiorly from the occiput. Skeletal dysplasia was also evident by virtue of modeling defects seen in the distal ulna, fusion of the capitate-hamate, and generalized osteoporosis.

Molecular Pathology. The recent observation that biglycan, a minor noncollagenous glycoprotein, is located on the X-chromosome provides the first candidate structural gene for these disorders.[165] Mutations of structural genes on the X-chromosome should be inherited as X-linked dominants, while mutations of enzymes (see the discussion on Menkes' kinky hair syndrome) should be inherited as X-linked recessives.

Disorders of Specialized Tensile Connective Tissue: EDS IV

EDS IV (Ecchymotic or Arterial Form). The clinical characteristic in EDS IV is repeated arterial rupture, commonly involving iliac, splenic, or renal arteries or the aorta, resulting in either massive hematomas or death.[166] These patients have thin, soft, and transparent skin, through which a prominent venous pattern is seen. They are also susceptible to rupture of internal viscera and may experience repeated rupture of diverticula on the antimesenteric border of the large bowel. Uterine rupture may complicate pregnancy, although in many instances delivery may be uneventful.[167] The causes of death in eight families included gastrointestinal rupture in three cases, peripartum uterine rupture in two cases, and rupture of the hepatic artery in one case.[166]

In contrast with the other forms of EDS, these patients do not have hyperextensible joints, and although their skin is thin, it is not hyperelastic. EDS IV includes, as a subgroup, patients who have been described as acrogyric.[168] These individuals have a characteristic thin facies, prominent eyes, and extremities that lack subcutaneous fat, giving the appearance of premature aging. Peripheral joint contractures and acro-osteolysis have been described.[169] Spontaneous pneumothorax and mitral valve prolapse occur frequently.[170] Periodontitis with tooth loss can suggest overlap with EDS VIII.[171]

Surgical repair of ruptured vessels or internal viscera is extremely difficult because of friable tissues.[172] Both anesthetic and surgical difficulties related to intubation, spontaneous arterial bleeding during surgery, and the ligation of vessels that tear under pressure complicate surgical maneuvers. Arteriography may be dangerous.[173]

Molecular Pathology. Although EDS IV was clinically recognized as a disorder distinct from the other forms of EDS, the finding by Pope and colleagues[174] that tissues from these individuals were deficient in type III collagen clearly distinguished this as a separate form of EDS. Subsequent studies have shown both clinical and biochemical heterogeneity.[166, 175] Most of the patients studied have a dominant pedigree consistent with a primary defect in one of the type III collagen alleles. Restriction fragment length polymorphism (RFLP) has been used to provide genetic counseling to families with this disease.[176] The types of biochemical defects are similar to those found with type I collagen in association with osteogenesis imperfecta (see later). The first defect is decreased or absent production of an electrophoretically normal type III procollagen molecule, suggestive of a null allele due to abnormal RNA splicing. This defect is associated with a milder phenotype.[88] The second category of defects includes mutations that interrupt the helical domain of α1 (III) molecules and result in severe disease. Fibroblastic cells derived from these individuals contain dilated rough endoplasmic reticulum with retained type III procollagen that is inefficiently secreted and is more susceptible to proteolytic digestion.[177] Glycine mutations of the Gly-X-Y triplet,[178, 179] small deletions due to exon skipping[180] or gene deletions,[181] and insertion of nonhelical sequences secondary to improper splicing of introns[72] are most frequently found to account for these abnormalities.

Disorders of Specialized Tensile Tissue: Osteogenesis Imperfecta

Osteogenesis imperfecta (OI) refers to a generalized disorder of connective tissue that predominantly affects the skeletal system.[182–185] It is estimated to affect approximately 10,000 persons in the United States. The gene prevalence of OI is calculated as 4 to 5 per 100,000.[186] These estimates may fall short of its true prevalence because of the number of very mild cases that are either undiagnosed or diagnosed late in life. The traditional designations of OI congenita and OI tarda should be discarded. In the discussion that follows, the clinical classification of Sillence[187, 188] has been merged with more recent information concerning the locus of the molecular defect in each clinical variant (Table 95–7) and is presented in the order of decreasing severity.

Lethal OI (Sillence Type II). About 10 percent of OI patients have this form of the disease, which is incompatible with survival. Most cases result from new mutations, although cases suggesting recessive inheritance have been observed and probably represent germinal mosaicism in one of the parents.[87, 88] Infants are born with severe bone fragility and experience multiple intrauterine fractures. Radiographs of these children reveal a characteristic beading of the ribs, representing callus over multiple fractures, and an "accordion type" deformity of the extremities, which appear crumpled, foreshortened, and broad.[189, 190] There is little ossification of the cranium (wormian bones), and the skull appears large in comparison with the short and deformed extremities.[191] Respiratory reserve is very limited, and death ensues usually within a week. Prenatal diagnosis by ultrasound is possible starting at about the sixteenth week of pregnancy[192] and should be used in families with a previously affected infant.

Molecular Pathology. The biochemical abnormality common to the lethal form of OI appears to be an impaired ability to synthesize and secrete type I collagen.[183] As a result, the amount of type I collagen of bone is low, whereas the quantity of the minor collagen types, III and V, is relatively high.[193–195] Bone collagen fibers are distinctly smaller than the fibers from age-matched normal infants, and retained collagen is observed within dilated endoplasmic reticulum.[127]

The biochemical basis of the lack of collagen secretion appears to reside within the primary structures of either the α1(I)- or the α2-chains. In the best studied case, which resulted from a partial gene deletion encoding three exons,[196, 197] the shortened α1(I)-chains compromised helix formation of all molecules containing the shortened α-chain.[198, 199] In this manner, a defective α-chain can lead to impaired secretion,[66] decreased helical stability,[63, 64, 67] abnormal fiber formation,[65, 200] impaired interactions with other matrix molecules,[201] and defective cross-link formation.[202] This cascade of events that results from the incorporation of one mutant chain into an interactive supramolecular structure has been aptly termed protein suicide.[68] Small helical deletions that result from mutations that impair splicing of the collagen mRNA, leading to exon skipping, have a similar outcome.[203, 204] Furthermore, a single glycine substitution with the Gly-X-Y triplet is equally severe.[64, 205–212] There appears to be a correlation between the length of the helix that is destabilized and the severity of the phenotype[213] when the α1 chain is involved, although inconsistencies with this rule are seen with the α2 chain.[214]

Severe Deforming OI (Sillence Type III). This

Table 95–7. CHARACTERISTICS OF OSTEOGENESIS IMPERFECTA

Sillence Type	Clinical Features	Frequency (%)	Inheritance	No. of Fractures	Scleral Color	Presence of DI	Biochemical Abnormality
I	No major skeletal deformities	50	Dominant, occasionally sporadic	5–15	Blue	Infrequent	Null mutation of α1(I) gene
II	Lethal; severely deformed	5	Dominant new mutation or germinal mosaicism	Multiple in utero and at birth	Blue or gray	Occurs, but prevalence is uncertain	Mutations of α1(I) or α2(I) that disrupt the integrity of the helical domain of collagen
III	Major skeletal deformities; very osteopenic; usually not ambulatory	20	Dominant new mutation or germinal mosaicism; possible genetic compound	30–60	Usually gray, occasionally blue	25%	Mutations of α1(I) or α2(I) that disrupt the integrity of the helical domain of collagen
IV	Moderate osteopenia and bony deformity; usually ambulatory but with mechanical support	25	Dominant, occasionally sporadic	10–25	White or gray	25%	Mutations of the α2(I) gene affecting the stability of the helical domain

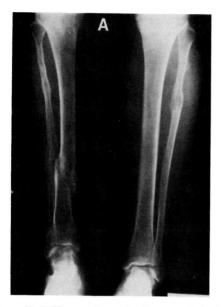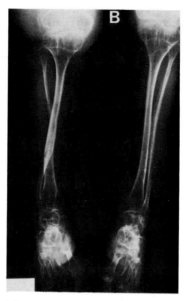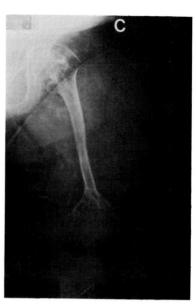

Figure 95–7. These radiographs illustrate skeletal differences among variants of osteogenesis imperfecta (OI). *A*, Dominant, mild, with minimal deformity; *B*, moderate OI, mild epiphyseal dysplasia; *C*, severe OI, marked diaphyseal narrowing and widening of the metaphysis with severe epiphyseal dysplasia. Lethal OI is not illustrated.

variant is the classic form of OI and accounts for about 20 percent of cases. The disease usually appears sporadically, although several families have now been reported with more than one affected child, normal parents, and an absence of consanguinity. This variant is characterized by severe deformity of the limbs, marked kyphoscoliosis, and marked growth retardation. Although termed progressive deforming by Sillence, the deformities are fully established by the age of 5 years and remain relatively unchanged until the middle years, when kyphoscoliosis may worsen.[215] The extent of growth retardation is remarkable in that many patients may not surpass 3 feet (90 to 100 cm in height). Molding occurs in utero and during infancy, producing frontal bossing and a characteristic occipital "overhang" termed the helmet deformity. Wormian bones and delayed closure of fontanelles may be observed. Platybasia may cause the external ear canals to slant upward as the base of the skull, softened by defective ossification, sinks on the cervical vertebrae.[216] This may lead to hydrocephalus, cranial nerve palsy, and upper and lower motor neuron lesions.[217, 218] The majority of patients have white sclerae as adults, although bluish discoloration is apparent in childhood. Approximately 25 percent of these patients have dentinogenesis imperfecta (DI) (see earlier), necessitating constant dental care throughout childhood. Severe hearing impairment occurs in 10 percent of patients, although milder degrees of hearing loss are commoner. An unusual and characteristic feature of individuals in this group is a high-pitched voice.

The skeleton is quite soft and deforms easily, particularly prior to puberty, leading to scoliosis and severe deformity of the sternum and limbs. Sponta-

neous fractures occur with little stress, so that the infant may experience 20 or more fractures during the first 1 to 3 years of life. These children tend to be hypotonic and have lax joints so that head control and motor development are delayed. Patients with this variant are usually wheelchair-bound for most of their lives. Radiographs of the skeleton reveal marked osteopenia, narrowing of the diaphysis, and widening of the metaphysis, which merges into a dysplastic epiphyseal zone filled with whorls of partially calcified cartilage (popcorn deformity) (Fig. 95–7C).[219] Osteopenia causes collapse of vertebral endplates. Lack of weight-bearing increases the severity of osteoporosis and increases the risk of fracture. In spite of this, spontaneous fractures do not occur as frequently after puberty. However, a trauma, such as an automobile accident or falling from a wheelchair, can have disastrous results. In spite of these multiple complications, we have seen patients survive, with gainful employment, into their 60s. Pulmonary function is diminished because of distortion of the spine and chest cage and may worsen in adulthood. Prenatal diagnosis in the second trimester has been achieved.[220]

Molecular Pathology. The best studied case has demonstrated a complete deficiency of $\alpha2(I)$-chain synthesis, producing a collagen molecule of three $\alpha1(I)$-chains.[221] This structure is unstable relative to the $[\alpha1(I)]_2 \alpha2$ molecule[222] but illustrates the fact that the abnormalities in the $\alpha2(I)$-chain are better tolerated than those in the $\alpha1(I)$-chain. The absence of $\alpha2(I)$-chains in the collagen molecule results from a four-base deletion in the $\alpha2(I)$ gene that "frameshifts" the C-terminal propeptide,[62] so that synthesized chains fail to get incorporated into a triple helical structure.[223] Other cases are the result of helix destabilization by mutations in the molecule similar to those of lethal OI.[224–226] It is not clear whether all defects in this group are collagen related or are mutations in other bone-related proteins.

OI of Moderate Severity (Sillence Type IV). Clinically, these patients overlap with those having mild disease; however, occasional patients may be more severely affected. Inheritance in this group is dominant, with sporadic cases representing new mutations. Their sclerae tend to be white, although others have observed families in which sclerae are blue at birth but lighten to white with age. In our limited series, they appear to have more molding of the skull, and an occipital overhang may be palpable. Kyphoscoliosis is present, and during adolescence progressive spinal deformity may occur. As a corollary, one sees hyperextensible joints and pes planus. The majority of fractures occur during childhood and recur during the postmenopausal period in women. Following each fracture there tends to be long bone deformity, a difficulty not typically encountered in mildly affected (OI type I) subjects. Radiographs of the long bones and vertebral bodies demonstrate marked osteopenia and vertebral collapse. Although there is marked cortical thinning, bowing, and coarsening of trabeculae, the overall architecture of the bone remains intact (Fig. 95–7B). The presence of moderate degrees of skeletal deformity eventually requires that these patients resort to the use of a cane or a walker; at times they may be forced to use a wheelchair.

Dentiogenesis imperfecta (DI) has been used as one of the criteria in separating individual patients within categories I and IV.[227] DI is inherited as a dominant trait. The relationship between OI and DI has not yet been precisely defined. Both deciduous and permanent teeth have an opalescent and translucent appearance, which tends to darken with age. Primary teeth are more severely affected. The enamel is normal; however, the dentin is dysplastic so that chipping of enamel occurs and the teeth are thus subjected to erosion and breakage. On radiograph there is an exaggerated constriction at the coronal junction and obliteration of pulpal spaces. Early consideration should be given to capping affected teeth to minimize wear and breakage.

Molecular Pathology. This form of OI represents a heterogeneous grouping both clinically and biochemically. RFLP analysis has demonstrated linkage of OI type I to both the α1(I) and the α2(I) genes[228–230] and has been employed in prenatal diagnosis of OI type IV.[231] The first structural abnormality of the α2(I)-chain to be demonstrated in this form of OI was a 15 amino acid deletion in the N-terminal helical region of the α2(I)-chain,[232] which proved to be due to a splicing abnormality that skipped exon 12.[233] An alteration in molecular stability, analogous to that observed in lethal OI from mutations in the α2(I)- or the α1(I)-chain, has been observed,[234–237] which results from glycine point mutations within the helical domain.[238]

Mild OI (Sillence Type I). Affected individuals have OI of mild to moderate severity in terms of both the clinical course and the radiologic appearance of the peripheral skeleton (Fig. 95–7A). The disease is usually inherited as an autosomal trait but may occur in a sporadic manner. These patients have a characteristic triangular facial shape caused by mild prominence of the frontal bones. Sclerae are blue, with the tint varying from a deep hue to pale blue-gray. Patients have reported that the color of their sclerae may vary over time; in general, deeper hues are seen in children. Arcus senilis not related to lipid abnormalities occurs in many patients during the middle years. Although the authors have not observed the occurrence of DI in this group, a subgroup of patients having DI has been noted by Levin.[227] During the second and third decades of life, a characteristic high-frequency, sensorineural or mixed hearing loss can be detected.[239, 240] Hypermetabolism with diaphoresis is a frequent and unexplained clinical observation. The incidence of mitral valve prolapse is not increased in these patients, but individual kindreds with increased diameter of the aortic root have been found on echocardiography.[241] The skin of the patient with mild OI has normal elasticity but is occasionally thin and somewhat smooth in texture. Although many patients complain of easy bruising, detailed studies of clotting function in OI patients have not revealed a consistent abnormality.[242] Many patients are found to have had hyperextensible joints as children, but this tends to be less marked in adults.[118]

Mildly affected patients usually do not have fractures at birth, although there is occasionally a fracture of a clavicle or of an extremity during delivery. Prenatal diagnosis by ultrasound is not helpful in the mild form because intrauterine fractures are uncommon. The first fracture may occur either in the newborn nursery with daily handling or as the infant starts to crawl. The frequency of fracture thereafter depends, in part, on the child's activity, the need for immobilization, and the attitude of the family toward independent activity. In general, these patients have approximately 5 to 15 fractures prior to puberty, although they may experience several minor traumatic fractures of the digits or the small bones of their feet. Poor alignment or repeated immobilization leads to recurrent fractures, which may induce bowing, shortening of a limb, or subsequent disturbance of gait. Osteopenia is observed in both the spine and the peripheral skeleton and progresses with age to early-onset postmenopausal osteoporosis.[243] It is remarkable that in spite of multiple fractures, the long bones usually heal with no significant deformity. These children almost never require the insertion of intramedullary rods and almost never develop nonunion at a fracture site. Mild scoliosis is frequently present. As occurs in other variants, the frequency of fractures diminishes markedly after puberty, an observation that is not explained by the level of activity or the child's ability to protect against trauma.

While osteopenia, moderate coarsening of trabeculae, and cortical thinning are observed in radiographs, many cases are so mild as to be missed on routine examination. In fact, the diagnosis may be first suspected when a parent with unrecognized disease is found to have an affected child. This situation has led to the accusation of child abuse.[244–246]

Molecular Pathology. Cultured fibroblasts from these individuals synthesize low amounts of type I collagen, whereas type III collagen production is normal. Therefore, the ratio of type III to type I collagen is elevated in both cultured cells[48, 247] and in collagens extracted from skin biopsies.[248, 249] The underproduction of a normal type I collagen molecule may explain the recurrent fractures that are seen during periods of rapid growth and bone remodeling, when the demand for collagen production is high. The fall in fracture rates after puberty would then be explained by the ability of the osteoblasts to match the decreased demand for collagen production.

The molecular basis of the low production of type I collagen appears to be related to diminished activity of one of the $\alpha 1(I)$ collagen alleles, since the rate of $\alpha 1(I)$ production is half that expected. Because collagen molecules composed of more than one $\alpha 2$-chain are unstable, the rate of $\alpha 1$-chain synthesis determines the rate of type I collagen production. The unincorporated $\alpha 2$-chains are degraded.[49, 236] The level of $\alpha 1(I)$ collagen mRNA is also half that expected, suggesting a nonfunctional $\alpha 1$ collagen gene or instability of its mRNA.[48] Recent examination of $\alpha 1(I)$ mRNA in the nuclear compartment of cultured fibroblasts demonstrated excessive accumulation of an $\alpha 1(I)$ mRNA containing an unspliced intron.[50] Another mechanism for a null $\alpha 1(I)$ gene is a frameshift mutation that alters the initial incorporation of the pro$\alpha 1(I)$-chain into the triple helix.[250, 251] Consistent with a null mutation of the $\alpha I(I)$ gene is the recent demonstration that the heterozygous (and visually normal) MOV13 mouse has osteopenia, reduced bone strength, and a hearing deficit similar to patients with OI type I.[252] Mutations near or within the helical domain can also result in OI that is mild and nondeforming. It represents the mildest spectrum of mutations that can alter normal triple helical interactions,[253] forming the bridge between OI and familial osteoporosis.[254, 255]

Therapy. There have been multiple attempts at treatment with a variety of hormones and drugs, none of which has been successful. The list includes administration of mineral supplements, fluoride, calcitonin, androgenic steroids, ascorbic acid, and vitamin D.[256, 257] The rationale for the use of each of these has not always been clear, and as a result many of these trials have been inconclusive. Unless therapy is directed at modification of the abnormal gene or gene product, merely enhancing production of defective collagen chains may have little beneficial effect on bone strength. Agents that increase collagen production[258] may be of benefit in null mutations of collagen genes by stimulating the production from the remaining normal allele. The heterozygous MOV13 mouse may provide a valuable model to test this hypothesis.

The use of surgery to correct deformities and to facilitate weight-bearing has been the subject of several reviews.[259, 260] Intramedullary rods have been placed in many children with salutary effects, both cosmetic and functional. Every child with OI will benefit from appropriate rehabilitative therapy.[261] Bracing with new light-weight plastics can be accomplished as the child begins to walk in order to minimize microfracture and bowing of the upper femurs.[262] Muscle-strengthening exercises are essential as primary care and following immobilization for fracture. Perhaps the most beneficial programs have been developed around swimming, preferably in heated pools, and as part of a planned program of rehabilitative medical care.

Disorders of Specialized Tensile Tissue: The Elastomeric Complex

The inclusion of the following disorders as elastin-related diseases is somewhat artificial, since collagen also may be abnormal. However, the prominent clinical and pathologic features of these disorders are centered on tissues whose function requires elastic strength. The overlap between the collagen and the elastin abnormalities in these diseases probably relates to the interaction of common matrix molecules and enzymes that modify these structural proteins.

Marfan Syndrome and Related Variants

In its most typical form, Marfan syndrome includes dislocation of the lens (ectopia lentis), dilation of the ascending aorta with aortic regurgitation, tall stature, and arachnodactyly. The syndrome is heterogeneous, with patients having either asthenic or nonasthenic habitus who are distinct from subjects with the marfanoid hypermobility syndrome and congenital contractural arachnodactyly. The assumption is that a separate gene defect underlies each clinical phenotype.[263]

Classic (Asthenic) Form of Marfan Syndrome. The nonasthenic form refers to subjects with excessive tallness, with long, thin extremities (dolichostenomelia) and diminished subcutaneous fat. It has been reported in 2 to 6 persons per 100,000.[264] However, the real prevalence may exceed these numbers if mild cases go unrecognized. Since Marfan syndrome is inherited as an autosomal dominant trait, 50 percent of offspring are at risk, with equal prevalence in males and females.

Patients with the classic form of the syndrome tend to be excessively tall. Arm span frequently is 8 cm or more in excess of height. Disproportionately long limbs cause the lower truncal segment (LS, pubis to heel) to be more than 2 inches longer than the upper segment (US, pubis to crown), producing a US:LS ratio of less than 0.85. However, both arm and leg length discrepancies are present in as many as 10 percent of the normal population and may be normal for blacks.[265] Therefore, neither excessive height nor lengthened arm span and longer lower segment can be relied on to confirm the diagnosis of Marfan syndrome.

Arachnodactyly occurs in 90 percent of patients with the asthenic form, but this is not diagnostic, since elongation of hands and feet may occur in otherwise normal individuals. Confirmation of arachnodactyly may be sought using the following: (1) the thumb, or Steinberg, test, which is positive when the thumb, enclosed in the clenched fist, extends beyond the hypothenar border;[266] (2) the wrist (Walker-Murdoch) sign, in which there is overlap of the thumb and fifth digit as they encircle the opposite wrist;[267] and (3) the metacarpal index, which is the mean value of the lengths divided by the midpoint widths of the second, third, and fourth metacarpals. In normal subjects, the metacarpal index ranges from 5.4 to 7.9, whereas in patients with Marfan syndrome it ranges from 8.4 to 104.[265]

Skeletal abnormalities include dolichocephaly (long, narrow face with prognathism), a high arched palate, loss of normal cervical curve, kyphoscoliosis, pectus excavatum or carinatum, funnel-shaped deformities of the chest, and spondylolisthesis. These patients are subject to slipped epiphyses, talipes equinovarus, and long, unstable feet with pes planus.[268] Hallux valgus and contractures of the toes are common. Joint laxity tends to be variable but may appear marked in some patients, causing genu recurvatum and recurrent dislocations. Hyperextensibility leads to joint pain and effusion. Although the prevalence of osteoporosis is unknown, there are reports of vertebral rarefaction or collapse.[265]

Spinal abnormalities include increased interpeduncular distance of nonrotated vertebrae, vertebral inversion (flattening of the normal kyphosis at the dorsal level and kyphosis or disappearance of the physiologic lordosis at the lumbar level), and vertebral dysplasia (dolichospondylia, elongated vertebral bodies with increased concavity). Scoliosis constitutes one of the major management problems in Marfan syndrome. In one series the average age of onset was 10.5 years (range 3 to 15 years), with rapid progression during adolescence.[269] If mechanical bracing or physical therapy fails to halt progression, spinal fusion should be considered, particularly when the curvature exceeds 45 to 50 degrees.

Ectopia lentis occurs in 50 to 80 percent of patients with Marfan syndrome. Subluxation of the lens is usually bilateral and appears by the age of 5 years. Although the lens is typically displaced upward, displacement into any quadrant may occur. Visual acuity is diminished in many patients because of lens subluxation or secondary acute glaucoma.[270]

Cardiovascular abnormalities are responsible for the majority of deaths from Marfan syndrome. The average life span of these patients is approximately 32 years. Mitral valve prolapse, with mitral regurgitation, and aneurysmal dilatation of the ascending aorta, with regurgitation and aortic rupture, are the primary lesions. Auscultatory evidence of mitral and aortic valve disease exists in approximately 60 percent of affected individuals. Widespread use of echocardiography shows valve involvement to be more frequent (80 percent). Therefore, the chest radiograph should not be relied on to establish the presence of aortic root disease. Involvement of the aortic root may be discovered at any age, from the first[271, 272] to the sixth decades of life, and is gradually progressive. The diameter of the aorta slowly increases, giving the ascending aorta a characteristic "sausage shape" on angiography. Roberts and Honig[273] have provided excellent clinicopathologic correlation of the cardiovascular lesions. There are three groups of patients: (1) those with chronic aortic regurgitation, (2) those with aortic dissection, and (3) those with isolated mitral regurgitation. Aortic regurgitation, dissection, and rupture occur most commonly when the aorta dilates to 6 cm or more in adults. To monitor gradual enlargement of the aorta, echocardiography is recommended once a year until the size exceeds 50 percent of normal for the body surface area, at which time studies are repeated every 6 months. The use of propranolol to retard aortic dilatation is currently recommended.[274] Although vigorous activity should be discouraged, pregnancy appears to be safe if aortic dilatation is not present.[275] Antibiotic prophylaxis should be instituted in all patients with mitral or triscuspid valve prolapse because of an increased incidence of infective endocarditis. The outlook for surgical correction of Marfan syndrome defects of the aortic root has improved considerably during the past decade.[276]

Pulmonary function may be compromised by kyphoscoliosis and malformations of the sternum and ribs.[277] The spectrum of pulmonary lesions in Marfan syndrome includes congenital malformations, cystic disease, emphysema, spontaneous pneumothorax, and increased susceptibility to respiratory infections.[278, 279]

Asthenic versus Nonasthenic Forms of Marfan Syndrome. This distinction was proposed by McKusick[186] to draw attention to an obvious difference in phenotype within families and among isolated patients. Although the nonasthenic patient may be considered as representing a forme fruste of the syndrome,[280] it has been emphasized that those with few or mild signs of the disease harbor the same gene as do more severely affected relatives.[182]

Marfanoid Hypermobility Syndrome. Patients in this category have many stigmata of classic Marfan syndrome plus the added feature of hyperelastic skin and hyperextensible joints, suggestive of Ehlers-Danlos syndrome. The patient reported by Cotton and Brandt[281] was tall, with arachnodactyly, ectopia lentis, and a history of spontaneous pneumothorax. Since these patients have features of both Ehlers-

Danlos and Marfan syndromes, they are considered to represent a distinct entity.[282–284]

Congenital Contractural Arachnodactyly (CCA). This syndrome includes an autosomal dominant inheritance, tall stature, arachnodactyly, dolichostenomelia, and multiple contractures involving large joints.[285] There is a characteristic "crumpled ear" deformity due to a flattened helix with partial obliteration of the concha.[286] Osteopenia occurs frequently. Marked deformity of the chest cage also occurs, and scoliosis may be progressive and severe. For unknown reasons, the contractures tend to become less severe with age. The ocular and typical cardiac lesions of classic Marfan syndrome are absent. The observation that dolichostenomelia and arachnodactyly may occur in relatives lacking the marfanoid habitus suggests variable expression of the CCA gene.[287, 288]

Molecular Pathology. Despite scattered data suggesting an abnormality in the cross-linking of collagen,[289, 290] elastin,[291, 292] or both, no primary defect in the structure of these proteins[293] or lysyl oxidase[294] could be demonstrated. Since Marfan syndrome is inherited as a dominant trait with relatively large pedigrees, DNA linkage analysis has clearly demonstrated that the disease is not a mutation of the major fibrillar proteins or of elastin.[295, 296] Since a candidate gene was lacking, linkage with anonymous DNA probes was utilized first to exclude chromosomes[297] that did not harbor the Marfan locus and, subsequently, to localize at least certain forms of the disease to a region of chromosome 15.[298]

At the same time that the DNA linkage studies were being conducted, Godfrey and associates[299] demonstrated immunofluorescent abnormalities of the elastin-associated microfibrillar protein segregated to individuals with Marfan syndrome. While inconsistencies of this finding clearly existed, this observation provides another candidate gene to be evaluated. The microfibrillar proteins are widely distributed in skin, blood vessel, pleura, perichondrium, and periosteum.[300] They are the major support proteins for the suspensory ligament of the lens. It is likely that the microfibrillar structure is composed of a number of structural proteins, one of which may be located on chromosome 15.[301] This suspicion was confirmed with linkage studies utilizing probes for the microfibrillin gene,[302, 303] and mutations were demonstrated in the gene in association with the Marfan phenotype.[304] The structural aspects of the protein are not yet known, and so the significance of the mutations is yet to be appreciated, but this is an active area of investigation.

Cutis Laxa

This term refers to a group of generalized connective tissue disorders in which the common clinical feature is lax, redundant, and inelastic skin. The skin in these patients is wrinkled and sags in loose folds, imparting a prematurely aged appearance.[305–307] Ac-

quired cutis laxa may follow penicillamine ingestion,[308] inflammatory skin disease, or a nonspecific febrile illness.[309]

The autosomal dominant form is mild, largely limited to the dermis, and thus compatible with a normal life span. Dermal changes may be present in infancy but usually are not marked until the second or third decade, when tissues loosen and become redundant on the face and extremities. Unlike EDS, the skin in cutis laxa does not recoil when stretched. Several patients have been found to harbor bronchiectasis or mild pulmonary emphysema.[310] Aside from pulmonary infections in childhood and the occurrence of inguinal hernias, these patients remain in good health. The joints are not hyperextensible in this disease.

The recessive variety is severer, as evidenced by diagnosis at birth or shortly thereafter and the early development of severe cardiopulmonary complications.[311, 312] The X-linked variety of cutis laxa appears to be intermediate in severity between the autosomal recessive and the autosomal dominant forms[313] and, in some classifications, is included as another X-linked form of EDS.

Molecular Pathology. Microscopic examination of the dermis reveals alterations in both elastic fibers and collagen. Fine elastic fibers that normally rise into the dermal papillae may be absent. Individual elastic fibers that vary greatly in diameter are short, globular in outline, and less compact; the elastica may be more abundant at deeper levels of the dermis.[314] Globular, fragmented, and clumped elastic fibers have also been observed in the lung and aorta. Although no information regarding the abnormality in elastin structure and biosynthesis is currently available, the autosomal dominant form should yield to techniques of molecular biology, now that human elastin complementary DNA (cDNA) and genomic probes are available.

Therapy. Treatment is limited to plastic surgery, which can significantly improve the patient's appearance. Unlike EDS, surgery is not complicated by excessive bleeding or tissue fragility.

Menkes' Kinky Hair Syndrome

First described by Menkes in 1962, this is a sex-linked disorder of copper metabolism that involves connective tissue by affecting metalloenzymes essential to collagen and elastin synthesis.[315] The disease begins in utero and is apparent at birth. The syndrome derives its name from the kinky (pili torti), beaded, and brittle sparse hair, which is evident by the first month of life. Poor head control, reflex abnormalities, seizures, and spasticity occur in association with mental retardation.[316, 317]

Infants with Menkes' syndrome have low serum copper, low serum ceruloplasmin, and diminished white cell cytochrome-C oxidase activity.[318] Trace mineral analysis of post-mortem specimens reveals marked reductions in hepatic and brain copper content but elevated renal, skeletal muscle, and placental copper content.[319, 320] Attempts to increase longevity with administrations of oral or intravenous copper have not been successful.[319]

Molecular Pathology. Although the X-linked connective tissue syndromes have little clinical similarity with Menkes' syndrome, there may be a common biochemical link. Lysyl oxidase and its cofactor, copper,[321] are important in the initial steps of collagen cross-linking.[82] From studies of the mouse homologue, the aneurysm-prone mottled mouse,[322] and Menkes' kinky hair syndrome, either the enzyme or the copper transport (or both) is linked to the X-chromosome. Byers and colleagues[306] studied fibroblasts from two male cousins with the X-linked form of cutis laxa. Lysyl oxidase activity was found to be low, whereas collagen extractability was enhanced, and the amount of lysyl-derived aldehydes and collagen cross-links was diminished.[306] X-linked cutis laxa has been shown to have low immunologic and enzymatic activity for lysyl oxidase. Now that this enzyme has been cloned,[323] progress should be expected in understanding the molecular basis of the defect. Recent chromosomal localization of lysyl oxidase to chromosome 5 excludes this gene as primary to any X-linked connective tissue disease.[324]

In Menkes' syndrome, abnormal cellular copper transport results in low levels of serum copper. In contrast, a high intracellular copper content is present in cultured fibroblasts. High levels of zinc and cadmium plus the protein that binds these metals, metallothionein, are also found in these cells.[325] Thus, the putative lesion may lead to an inability to transfer copper to cellular enzymes, resulting in the neurologic and connective tissue syndromes.[326–328] Initial reports of decreased lysyl oxidase activity in EDS V were not verified with the use of more specific enzyme assays.[81] Furthermore, a reduction in the cross-link content was not demonstrated. However, low lysyl oxidase activity, increased collagen solubility,[329] and decreased amounts of immunologic reactive enzyme protein[330] have been found in cultured fibroblasts from individuals with EDS IX.

Pseudoxanthoma Elasticum (PXE)

A rare disorder, PXE is characterized by degeneration and calcification of elastic fibers in the skin, retina, and blood vessels.[331, 332] PXE is inherited primarily as an autosomal recessive trait, less frequently as an autosomal dominant trait.[333–335] In its classic form, PXE is recognized by the presence of asymptomatic, symmetric, yellowish-white xanthomatoid papules in flexural skin folds, which, in the dominant variant, appear during the second or third decade of life but, in recessive forms, appear earlier. These initially involve the skin of the neck and axilla and progress to other areas, where they coalesce to give a redundant, thickened appearance.[336] Mucocutaneous lesions may also occur.[337]

Angioid streaks of the retina, radially oriented and resembling vessels, are the result of a break in Bruch's membrane.[336] Retinal lesions may be demonstrated with fluorescence angiography. Visual loss in PXE, which varies from mild loss to legal blindness, is the result of maculopathy and retinal hemorrhage. In the lung, lesions are associated with dyspnea and include vascular calcification and intimal fibrosis due to damage of the elastic laminae in arteries, arterioles, and venules. Calcific deposits occur in alveolar lumina and may be visualized in radiographs.[338] Involvement of the heart may cause angina, dyspnea, and arrhythmias, suggestive of a cardiomyopathy.[339, 340] Endomyocardial biopsy and post-mortem specimens have revealed fragmented and mineralized elastic fibers similar to those seen in the skin. Intimal fibrosis may compromise the coronary circulation. Mitral valve prolapse was found in 71 percent in one series of 14 patients, but there was no association between the severity of skin lesions and valve dysfunction.[341] Both genitourinary and uterine bleeding complicate the clinical course of PXE. Arteries of the gastrointestinal tract are particularly susceptible to rupture, which occurred in 14 percent of patients in one series.[342, 343] Wound healing is generally normal in PXE until late in the course of the disease, when dermal calcification may be extensive. Hyperextensibility may lead to dislocations of both large and small joints.

Molecular Pathology. Dermal elastic fibers are frayed, swollen, and clumped and appear to be increased in number. The centers of elastin fibers are replaced by an electron-dense material, which appears to disrupt the fiber, leading to calcification. Nonaffected skin in PXE has also been shown to contain increased quantities of this dense material, and elastic fibers are microscopically normal in PXE.[344] No information regarding the nature of the abnormality of elastic structure or synthesis is currently available.[345] Since heterogeneity is present in this syndrome, a wide spectrum of structural or regulatory defects of elastin or its modifying proteins can be anticipated.[346]

References

1. Vuorio, E., and deCrombrugghe, B.: The family of collagen genes. Annu. Rev. Biochem. 59:837, 1990.
2. Burgeson, R. E.: New collagens, new concepts. Annu. Rev. Cell Biol. 4:551, 1988.
3. Kuhn, K.: The classical collagens: Types I, II and III. *In* Mayne, R., and Burgeson, R. (eds.): Structure and Function of Collagen Types. New York, Academic Press, 1987, p. 1.
4. Bennett, V. D., and Adams, S. L.: Identification of a cartilage-specific promoter within intron 2 of the chick alpha 2(I) collagen gene. J. Biol. Chem. 265:2223, 1990.
5. Fagg, W. R., Timoneda, J., Schwartz, C. E., Langeveld, J. P. M., Noelken, M. E., and Hudson, B. G.: Glomerular basement membrane: Evidence for collagenous domain of the alpha 3 and alpha 4 chains of collagen IV. Biochem. Biophys. Res. Commun. 170:322, 1990.
6. Gunwar, S., Saus, J., Noelken, M. E., and Hudson, B. G.: Glomerular basement membrane. Identification of a fourth chain, alpha 4, of type IV collagen. J. Biol. Chem. 265:5466, 1990.
7. Hostikka, S. L., Eddy, R. L., Byers, M. G., Höyhtyä, M., Shows, T. B., and Tryggvason, K.: Identification of a distinct type IV collagen alpha chain with restricted kidney distribution and assignment of its

gene to the locus of X chromosome–linked Alport syndrome. Proc. Natl. Acad. Sci. U.S.A. 87:606, 1990.

8. Dublet, B., Oh, S., Sugrue, S. P., Gordon, M. K., Gerecke, D. R., Olsen, B. R., and Van der Rest, M.: The structure of avian type XII collagen: alpha 1(XII) chains contain 190-kDa non–triple helical amino-terminal domains and form homotrimeric molecules. J. Biol. Chem. 264:3150, 1989.

9. Nishimura, I., Muragaki, Y., and Olsen, B. R.: Tissue-specific forms of type IX collagen-proteoglycan arise from the use of two widely separated promoters. J. Biol. Chem. 264:20033, 1989.

10. Saitta, B., Stokes, D. G., Vissing, H., Timpl, R., and Chu, M.-L.: Alternative splicing of the human alpha 2(VI) collagen gene generates multiple mRNA transcripts which predict three protein variants with distinct carboxyl terminal. J. Biol. Chem. 265:6473, 1990.

11. Doliana, R., Bonaldo, P., and Colombatti, A.: Multiple forms of chicken alpha 3(VI) collagen chain generated by alternative splicing in type A repeated domains. J. Cell Biol. 111:2197, 1990.

12. Indik, Z., Yeh, H., Ornstein-Goldstein, N., Kucich, U., Abrams, W., Rosenbloom, J. C., and Rosenbloom, J.: Structure of the elastin gene and alternative splicing of elastin mRNA: Implications for human disease. Am. J. Med. Genet. 34:81, 1989.

13. LuValle, P., Ninomiya, Y., Rosenblum, N. D., and Olsen, B. R.: The type X collagen gene. Intron sequences split the 5'-untranslated region and separate the coding regions for the non-collagenous amino-terminal and triple-helical domains. J. Biol. Chem. 263:18378, 1988.

14. Yamaguchi, N., Benya, P. D., Van der Rest, M., and Ninomiya, Y.: The cloning and sequencing of alpha 1(VIII) collagen cDNAs demonstrate that type VIII collagen is a short chain collagen and contains triple-helical and carboxyl-terminal non–triple-helical domains similar to those of type X collagen. J. Biol. Chem. 264:16022, 1989.

15. Pihlajaniemi, T., and Tamminen, M.: The alpha1 chain of type XIII collagen consists of three collagenous and four noncollagenous domains, and its primary transcript undergoes complex alternative splicing. J. Biol. Chem. 65:6922, 1990.

16. Dixit, S. N.: Short-chain basement membrane collagen: Further characterization and its biosynthesis by F-9 embryonal carcinoma cells. Eur. J. Biochem. 186:411, 1989.

17. Birk, D. E., Fitch, J. M., Babiarz, J. P., and Linsenmayer, T. F.: Collagen type I and type V are present in the same fibril in the avian corneal stroma. J. Cell Biol. 106:999, 1988.

18. Gordon, M. K., Gerecke, D. R., Dublet, B., Van der Rest, M., and Olsen, B. R.: Type XII collagen. A large multidomain molecule with partial homology to type IX collagen. J. Biol. Chem. 264:19772, 1989.

19. Keene, D. R., Engvall, E., and Glanville, R. W.: Ultrastructure of type VI collagen in human skin and cartilage suggests an anchoring function for this filamentous network. J. Cell Biol. 107:1995, 1988.

20. Cidadao, A. J.: Interactions between fibronectin, glycosaminoglycans and native collagen fibrils: An EM study in artificial three-dimensional extracellular matrices. Eur. J. Cell Biol. 48:303, 1989.

21. Gotoh, Y., Pierschbacher, M. D., Grzesiak, J. J., Gerstenfeld, L., Glimcher, M. J.: Comparison of two phosphoproteins in chicken bone and their similarities to the mammalian bone proteins, osteopontin and bone sialoprotein II. Biochem. Biophys. Res. Commun. 173(1):471, 1990.

22. Doi, Y., Okuda, R., Takezawa, Y., Shibata, S., Moriwaki, Y., Wakamatsu, N., Shimizu, N., Moriyama, K., and Shimokawa, H.: Osteonectin inhibiting de novo formation of apatite in the presence of collagen. Calcif. Tissue Int. 44:200, 1989.

23. Mendler, M., Eich-Bender, S. G., Vaughan, L., Winterhalter, K. H., and Bruckner, P.: Cartilage contains mixed fibrils of collagen types II, IX, and XI. J. Cell Biol. 108:191, 1989.

24. Chen, Q., Gibney, E., Fitch, J. M., Linsenmayer, C., Schmid, T. M., and Linsenmayer, T. F.: Long-range movement and fibril association of type X collagen within embryonic cartilage matrix. Proc. Natl. Acad. Sci. U.S.A. 87:8046, 1990.

25. Ayad, S., Marriott, A., Morgan, K., and Grant, M. E.: Bovine cartilage types VI and IX collagens. Characterization of their forms in vivo. Biochem. J. 262:753, 1989.

26. Grant, D. S., Leblond, C. P., Kleinman, H. K., Inoue, S., and Hassell, J. R.: The incubation of laminin, collagen IV, and heparan sulfate proteoglycan at 35°C yields basement membrane–like structures. J. Cell Biol. 108:567, 1989.

27. Kirkham, N., Gibson, B., Leigh, I. M., and Price, M. L.: A comparison of antibodies to type VII and type IV collagen laminin and amnion as epidermal basement membrane markers. J. Pathol. 159:5, 1989.

28. Jander, R., Korsching, E., and Rauterberg, J.: Characteristics and in vivo occurrence of type VIII collagen. Eur. J. Biochem. 189:601, 1990.

29. Kittelberger, R., Davis, P. F., and Greenhill, N. S.: Immunolocalization of type VIII collagen in vascular tissue. Biochem. Biophys. Res. Commun. 159:414, 1989.

30. Ruoslahti, E.: Fibronectin and its receptors. Annu. Rev. Biochem. 57:375, 1988.

31. Lightner, V. A., Gumkowski, F., Bigner, D. D., and Erickson, H. P.: Tenascin, hexabrachion in human skin: Biochemical identification and localization by light and electron microscopy. J. Cell Biol. 108:2483, 1989.

32. Ruoslahti, E.: Proteoglycans in cell regulation. J. Biol. Chem. 264:13369, 1989.

33. Gulberg, D., Terracio, L., Borg, T. K., and Rubin, K.: Identification of integrin-like matrix receptors with affinity for interstitial collagens. J. Biol. Chem. 264:12686, 1989.

34. Baldwin, C. T., Reginato, A. M., and Prockop, D. J.: A new epidermal growth factor–like domain in the human core protein for the large cartilage-specific proteoglycan. Evidence for alternative splicing of the domain. J. Biol. Chem. 264:15747, 1989.

35. Chu, M.-L., Pan, T.-C., Conway, D., Kuo, H.-J., Glanville, R. W., Timpl, R., Mann, K., and Deutzmann, R.: Sequence analysis of alpha 1(VI) and alpha 2(VI) chains of human type VI collagen reveals internal triplication of globular domains similar to the A domains of von Willebrand factor and two alpha 2(VI) chain variants that differ in the carboxy terminus. EMBO J. 8:1939, 1989.

36. Chu, M.-L., Zhang, R.-Z., Pan, T., Stokes, D., Conway, D., Kuo, H.-J., Glanville, R., Mayer, U., Mann, K., Deutzmann, R., and Timpl, R.: Mosaic structure of globular domains in the human type VI collagen alpha3 chain: Similarity to von Willebrand factor, fibronectin, actin, salivary proteins and aprotinin type protease inhibitors. EMBO J. 9:385, 1990.

37. Retief, E., Parker, M. I., and Retief, A. E.: Regional chromosome mapping of human collagen genes α2(I) and α1(I) (COL1A2 and COL1A1). Hum. Genet. 69:304, 1985.

38. Bornstein, P., McKay, J., Liska, D. J., Apone, S., and Devarayalu, S.: Interactions between the promoter and first intron are involved in transcriptional control of α1(I) collagen gene expression. Mol. Cell. Biol. 8:4851, 1988.

39. Karsenty, G., and deCrombrugghe, B.: Two different negative and one positive regulatory factors interact with a short promoter segment of the alpha 1(I) collagen gene. J. Biol. Chem. 265:9934, 1990.

40. Raghow, R., and Thompson, J. P.: Molecular mechanisms of collagen gene expression. Mol. Cell. Biochem. 86:5, 1989.

41. Ramirez, F., and Di Liberto, M.: Complex and diversified regulatory programs control the expression of vertebrate collagen genes. FASEB J. 4:1616, 1990.

42. Hartung, S., Jaenisch, R., and Briendl, L. M.: Retrovirus insertion inactivates mouse α1(I) collagen gene by blocking initiation of transcription. Nature 320:365, 1986.

43. Kratochwil, K., Von der Mark, K., Kollar, E. J., Jaenisch, R., Mooslehner, K., Schwarz, M., Haase, K., Gmachl, I., and Harbers, K.: Retrovirus-induced insertional mutation in Mov13 mice affects collagen I expression in a tissue-specific manner. Cell 57:807, 1989.

44. Sandmeyer, S., Gallis, B., and Bornstein, P.: Coordinate transcriptional regulation of type I procollagen genes by Rous sarcoma virus. J. Biol. Chem. 256:5022, 1981.

45. Aebi, M., and Weissmann, C.: Precision and orderliness in splicing. Trends Genet. 3:102, 1987.

46. Robberson, B. L., Cote, G. J., and Berget, S. M.: Exon definition may facilitate splice site selection in RNAs with multiple exons. Mol. Cell. Biol. 10:84, 1990.

47. Fukumaki, Y., Ghosh, P. K., Benz, E. J., Reddy, V. B., Lebowitz, P., Forget, G., and Weissman, S. M.: Abnormally spliced messenger RNA in erythroid cells from patients with b+ thalassemia and monkey cells expressing a cloned b+ thalassemic gene. Cell 28:585, 1982.

48. Genovese, C., Brufsky, A., Shapiro, J., and Rowe, D.: Detection of mutations in human type I collagen mRNA in osteogenesis imperfecta by indirect RNase protection. J. Biol. Chem. 264:9632, 1989.

49. Barsh, G. S., David, K. E., and Byers, P. H.: Type I osteogenesis imperfecta: A nonfunctional allele for proα1(I) chains of type I procollagen. Proc. Natl. Acad. Sci. U.S.A. 79:3838, 1982.

50. Rowe, D. W., Shapiro, J. R., Poirier, M., and Schlesinger, S.: Diminished type I collagen synthesis and reduced α1(I) collagen mRNA in cultured fibroblasts from patients with dominantly inherited (type I) osteogenesis imperfecta. J. Clin. Invest. 71:689, 1985.

51. Atweh, G. F., Brickner, H. E., Zhu, X.-X., Kazazian, H. H., Jr., and Forget, B. G.: New amber mutation in a β-thalassemic gene with nonmeasurable levels of mutant messenger RNA in vivo. J. Clin. Invest. 82:557, 1988.

52. Bateman, J. F., Lamande, S. R., Dahl, H. H., Chan, D., Mascara, T., and Cole, W. G.: A frameshift mutation results in a truncated nonfunctional carboxyl-terminal proalpha 1(I) propeptide of type I collagen in osteogenesis imperfecta. J. Biol. Chem. 264:10960, 1989.

53. Kivirikko, K. K., and Myllya, R.: Post-translational enzymes in the biosynthesis of collagen: intracellular enzymes. Methods Enzymol. 82A:245, 1982.

54. Jimenez, S. A., Harsch, M., Murphy, L., and Rosenbloom, J.: Effects of temperature on confrontation, hydroxylation, and secretion of chick tendon procollagen. J. Biol. Chem. 29:4480, 1974.

55. Nemethy, G., and Scheraga, H. A.: Stabilization of collagen fibrils by hydroxyproline. Biochemistry 25:3184, 1986.

56. Helaakoski, T., Pajunen, L., Kivirikko, K. I., and Pihlajaniemi, T.:

Increases in mRNA concentrations of the alpha and beta subunits of prolyl 4-hydroxylase accompany increased gene expression of type IV collagen during differentiation of mouse F9 cells. J. Biol. Chem. 265:11413, 1990.

57. Kivirkko, K. I., and Myllyla, R.: Collagen glycosyltransferases. Int. Rev. Connect. Tissue Res. 8:23, 1979.
58. Clark, C. C., and Kefalides, N. A.: Localization and partial composition of the oligosaccharide units on the propeptide extension of type I procollagen. J. Biol. Chem. 253:47, 1978.
59. Rao, V. H., Steinmann, B., De Wet, W., and Hollister, D. W.: Decreased thermal denaturation temperature of osteogenesis imperfecta mutant collagen is independent of post-translational overmodifications of lysine and hydroxylysine. J. Biol. Chem. 264:1793, 1989.
60. Rosenbloom, J., Endo, R., and Harsch, M.: Termination of procollagen chain synthesis by puromycin: Evidence that assembly and secretion require a COOH-terminal extension. J. Biol. Chem. 241:2070, 1976.
61. Yamada, Y., Kühn, K., and deCrombrugghe, B.: A conserved nucleotide sequence, coding for a segment of the C-propeptide, is found at the same location in different collagen genes. Nucl. Acid Res. 11:2733, 1983.
62. Pihlajaniemi, T., Dickson, L. A., Pope, F. M., Korhonen, V. R., Nicholls, A., Prockop, D. J., and Myers, J. C.: Osteogenesis imperfecta: cloning of a proα2(I) collagen gene with a frameshift mutation. J. Biol. Chem. 259:12941, 1984.
63. Bonadio, J., Holbrook, K. A., Gelinas, R. E., Jacob, J., and Byers, P. H.: Altered triple helical structure of type I procollagen in lethal perinatal osteogenesis imperfecta. J. Biol. Chem. 260:1734, 1985.
64. Baker, A. T., Ramshaw, J. A. M., Chan, D., Cole, W. G., and Bateman, J. F.: Changes in collagen stability and folding in lethal perinatal osteogenesis imperfecta. The effect of α1(I)-chain glycine-to-arginine substitutions. Biochem. J. 261:253, 1989.
65. Vogel, B. E., Doelz, R., Kadler, K. E., Hojima, Y., Engel, J., and Prockop, D. J.: A substitution of cysteine for glycine 748 of the α1 chain produces a kink at this site in the procollagen I molecule and an altered pN-proteinase cleavage site over 225 nm away. J. Biol. Chem. 263:1924, 1988.
66. Barsh, G. S., and Byers, P. H.: Reduced secretion of structurally abnormal type I procollagen in a form of osteogenesis imperfecta. Proc. Natl. Acad. Sci. U.S.A. 78:5142, 1981.
67. Constantinou, C. D., Vogel, B. E., Jeffrey, J. J., and Prockop, D. J.: The A and B fragments of normal type I procollagen have a similar thermal stability to proteinase digestion but are selectively destabilized by structural mutations. Eur. J. Biochem. 163:247, 1987.
68. Prockop, D. J.: Osteogenesis imperfecta: phenotypic heterogeneity, protein suicide, short and long collagen. Am. J. Hum. Genet. 36:499, 1984.
69. Willing, M. C., Cohn, D. H., Starman, B., Holbrook, K. A., Greenberg, C. R., and Byers, P. H.: Heterozygosity for a large deletion in the alpha 2(I) collagen gene has a dramatic effect on type I collagen secretion and produces perinatal lethal osteogenesis imperfecta. J. Biol. Chem. 263:8398, 1988.
70. Bonadio, J., Ramirez, F., and Barr, M.: An intron mutation in the human alpha 1(I) collagen gene alters the efficiency of pre-mRNA splicing and is associated with osteogenesis imperfecta type II. J. Biol. Chem. 265:2262, 1990.
71. Byers, P. H., Starman, B. J., Cohn, D. H., and Horwitz, A. L.: A novel mutation causes a perinatal lethal form of osteogenesis imperfecta: an insertion in one alpha 1(I) collagen allele (COL1A1). J. Biol. Chem. 263:7855, 1988.
72. Kuivaniemi, H., Kontusaari, S., Tromp, G., Zhao, M., Sabol, C., and Prockop, D. J.: Identical G+1 to A mutations in three different introns of the type III procollagen gene (COL3A1) produce different patterns of RNA splicing in three variants of Ehlers-Danlos syndrome IV. An explanation for exon skipping with some mutations and not others. J. Biol. Chem. 265:2067, 1990.
73. Peltonen, L., Halila, R., and Ryhanen, L.: Enzymes converting procollagens to collagens. J. Cell. Biochem. 28:15, 1985.
74. Dombrowski, K. E., and Prockop, D. J.: Cleavage of type I and type II procollagens by type I/II procollagen N-proteinase. Correlation of kinetic constants with the predicted conformations of procollagen substrates. J. Biol. Chem. 263:16545, 1988.
75. Hulmes, D. J. S., Kadler, K. E., Mould, A. P., Hojima, Y., Holmes, D. F., Cummings, C., Chapman, J. A., and Prockop, D. J.: Pleomorphism in type I collagen fibrils produced by persistence of the procollagen N-propeptide. J. Mol. Biol. 210:337, 1989.
76. Weil, D., D'Alessio, M., Ramirez, F., and Eyre, D. R.: Structural and functional characterization of a splicing mutation in the pro-alpha2(I) collagen gene of an Ehlers-Danlos type VII patient. J. Biol. Chem. 265:16007, 1990.
77. Birk, D. E., Southern, J. F., Zycband, E. I., Fallon, J. T., and Trelstad, R. L.: Collagen fibril bundles: A branching assembly unit in tendon morphogenesis. Development 107:437, 1989.
78. Birk, D. E., Zycband, E. I., Winkelmann, D. A., and Trelstad, R. L.: Collagen fibrillogenesis in situ: Fibril segments are intermediates in matrix assembly. Proc. Natl. Acad. Sci. U.S.A. 86:549, 1989.

79. Kadler, K. E., Hojima, Y., and Prockop, D. J.: Assembly of type I collagen fibrils de novo. Between 37 and 41°C the process is limited by micro-unfolding of monomers. J. Biol. Chem. 263:10517, 1988.
80. Na, G. C., Phillips, L. J., and Freire, E. I.: In vitro collagen fibril assembly: Thermodynamic studies. Biochemistry 28:7153, 1989.
81. Kuivaniemi, H.: Partial characterization of lysyl oxidase from several human tissues. Biochem. J. 15:639, 1985.
82. Cronlund, A. L., Smith, B. D., and Kagen, H. M.: Binding of lysyl oxidase to fibrils of type I collagen. Connect. Tissue Res. 14:109, 1985.
83. Prockop, D. J.: Mutations that alter the primary structure of type I collagen. The perils of a system for generating large structures by the principle of nucleated growth. J. Biol. Chem. 265:15349, 1990.
84. Barron, M. W., Simpson, C. F., and Miller, E. S.: Lathyrism: A review. Q. Rev. Biol. 49:101, 1974.
85. Eyre, D. R., and Oguchi, H.: The hydroxypyridinium cross-links of skeletal collagens: their measurement, properties and a proposed pathway of formation. Biochem. Biophys. Res. Comm. 92:403, 1980.
86. Buckingham, B., and Reiser, K. M.: Relationship between the content of lysyl oxidase–dependent cross-links in skin collagen, nonenzymatic glycosylation, and long-term complications in type I diabetes mellitus. J. Clin. Invest. 86:1046, 1990.
87. Constantinou, C. D., Pack, M., Young, S. B., and Prockop, D. J.: Phenotypic heterogeneity in osteogenesis imperfecta: The mildly affected mother of a proband with a lethal variant has the same mutation substituting cysteine for alpha I-glycine 904 in a type I procollagen gene (COL1A1). Am. J. Hum. Genet. 47:670, 1990.
88. Cohn, D. H., Starman, B. J., Blumberg, B. H., and Byers, P. H.: Recurrence of lethal osteogenesis imperfecta due to parental mosaicism for a dominant mutation in a human type I collagen gene (COL1A1). Am. J. Hum. Genet. 46:591, 1990.
89. Russell, S. B., Trupin, J. S., Myers, J. C., Broquist, A. H., Smith, J. C., Myles, M. E., and Russell, J. D.: Differential glucocorticoid regulation of collagen mRNAs in human dermal fibroblasts. Keloid-derived and fetal fibroblasts are refractory to down-regulation. J. Biol. Chem. 264:13730, 1989.
90. Bocchieri, M. H., and Jimenez, S. A.: Animal models and fibrosis. Rheum. Dis. Clin. North Am. 16:153, 1990.
91. Kuivaniemi, H., Tromp, G., and Prockop, D. J.: Mutations in collagen genes: Causes of rare and some common diseases in humans. FASEB J. 5:2052, 1991.
92. Prockop, D. J.: Osteogenesis imperfecta—a model for genetic causes of osteoporosis and perhaps several other common diseases of connective tissue. Arthritis Rheum. 31:1, 1988.
93. Vissing, H., D'Alessio, M., Lee, B., Ramirez, F., Godfrey, M., and Hollister, D. W.: Glycine to serine substitution in the triple helical domain of pro-alpha 1(II) collagen results in a lethal perinatal form of short-limbed dwarfism. J. Biol. Chem. 264:8265, 1989.
94. Ala-Kokko, L., Baldwin, C. T., Moskowitz, R. W., and Prockop, D. J.: Single base mutation in the type II procollagen gene (COL2A1) as a cause of primary osteoarthritis associated with a mild chondrodysplasia. Proc. Natl. Acad. Sci. U.S.A. 87:6565, 1990.
95. Kontusaari, S., Tromp, G., Kuivaniemi, H., Ladda, R. L., and Prockop, D. J.: Inheritance of an RNA splicing mutation (G+1 IVS20) in the type III procollagen gene (COL3A1) in a family having aortic aneurysms and easy bruisability: Phenotypic overlap between familial arterial aneurysms and Ehlers-Danlos syndrome type IV. Am. J. Hum. Genet. 47:112, 1990.
96. Barker, D. F., Hostikka, S. L., Zhou, J., Chow, L. T., Oliphant, A. R., Gerken, S. C., Gregory, M. C., Skolnick, M. H., Atkin, C. L., and Tryggvason, K.: Identification of mutations in the COL4A5 collagen gene in Alport syndrome. Science 248:1224, 1990.
97. Orkin, S. H.: Reverse genetics and human disease. Cell 47:845, 1986.
98. Koenig, M., Monaco, A. P., and Kunkel, L. M.: The complete sequence of dystrophin predicts a rod-shaped cytoskeletal protein. Cell 53:219, 1988.
99. Koshland, D. E.: The cystic fibrosis gene story (editorial). Science 245:1029, 1989.
100. Altschuler, R. A., Hawkins, J. E., Jr., Bateman, J. F., Mascara, T., and Jaenisch, R.: Transgenic mouse model of the mild dominant form of osteogenesis imperfecta. Proc. Natl. Acad. Sci. U.S.A. 87:7145, 1990.
101. Khillan, J. S., Olsen, A. S., Kontusaari, S., Sokolov, B., and Prockop, D. J.: Transgenic mice that express a mini-gene version of the human gene for type I procollagen (COL1A1) develop a phenotype resembling a lethal form of osteogenesis imperfecta. J. Biol. Chem. 266:23373, 1991.
102. Vandenberg, P., Khillan, J. S., Prockop, D. J., Helminen, H., Kontusaari, S., and Ala-Kokko, L.: Expression of a partially deleted gene of human type II procollagen (COL2A1) in transgenic mice produces a chondrodysplasia. Proc. Natl. Acad. Sci. U.S.A. 88:7640, 1991.
103. Capecchi, M. R.: Altering the genome by homologous recombination. Science 244:1288, 1989.
104. Hollister, D. W.: Heritable disorders of connective tissue: Ehlers-Danlos syndrome. Pediatr. Clin. North Am. 25:575, 1978.
105. Beighton, P., and Horan, F.: Orthopedic aspects of the Ehlers-Danlos syndrome. J. Bone Thorac. Surg. 51B:444, 1969.

106. Bird, H. A., Tribe, C. R., and Bacon, P. A.: Joint hypermobility leading to osteoarthrosis and chondrocalcinosis. Bull. Rheum. Dis. 37:203, 1978.

107. Kornberg, M., and Aulicino, P.: Hand and wrist joint problems in patients with Ehlers-Danlos syndrome. J. Hand Surg. 10:193, 1985.

108. Moore, J., Tolo, V., and Weiland, A.: Painful subluxation of the carpometacarpal joint of the thumb in Ehlers-Danlos syndrome. J. Hand Surg. 10:6611, 1985.

109. Osborn, T. G., Lichenstein, J. R., Moore, T. L., Weiss, T., and Zuckner, J.: Ehlers-Danlos syndrome presenting as rheumatic manifestations in the child. J. Rheumatol. 8:79, 1981.

110. Ayres, J., Pope, P., Reidy, J., and Clark, T.: Abnormalities of the lungs and thoracic cage in Ehlers-Danlos syndrome. Thorax 40:300, 1985.

111. Leier, C. V., Call, T. D., Tulkerson, P. K., and Woolery, C. F.: The spectrum of cardiac defects in the Ehlers-Danlos syndrome types I and III. Ann. Intern. Med. 92:171, 1980.

112. Cupo, L. N., Pyeritz, R. E., Olson, J. L., McPhee, S. J., Hutchins, G. M., and McKusick, V.: Ehlers-Danlos syndrome with abnormal collagen fibrils, sinus of Valsalva aneurysms, myocardial infarction, panacinar emphysema and cerebral heterotopia. Am. J. Med. 71:1051, 1981.

113. Coventry, M. B.: Some skeletal changes in the Ehlers-Danlos syndrome. J. Bone Joint Surg. 13A:855, 1961.

114. Kirk, J. A., Ansell, B., and Bywaters, E. G.: The hypermobility syndrome. Ann. Rheum. Dis. 26:419, 1967.

115. Wynne-Davies, R.: Acetabular dysplasia and familial joint laxity: Two etiological factors in congenital dislocation of the hip. A review of 589 patients and their families. J. Bone Surg. 52B:704, 1970.

116. Boone, D. C., and Azen, S. P.: Normal range of motion of joints in male subjects. J. Bone Joint Surg. 61A:756, 1979.

117. Green, F. A., Wood, P. H. N., and Sackett, D. L.: The effect of age, body weight, and use on joint movement in a random population study. Arthritis Rheum. 8:444A, 1965.

118. Wordsworth, P., Ogilvie, D., Smith, R., and Sykes, R.: Joint mobility with particular reference to racial variation and inherited connective tissue disorders. Br. J. Rheumatol. 26:9, 1987.

119. Finsterbush, A., and Pogrund, H.: The hypermobility syndrome. Clin. Orthop. 168:124, 1982.

120. Horton, W. A., Collins, D. L., De Smet, A. A., Kennedy, J. A., and Schimke, R. N.: Familial joint instability syndrome. Am. J. Med. Genet. 6:2221, 1980.

121. Lewkonia, R.: Does generalized articular hypermobility predispose to generalized osteoarthritis? Clin. Exp. Rheumatol. 4:115, 1986.

122. Grahame, R., Pitcher, E. D., Gabell, A., and Harvey, W.: A clinical and echocardiographic study of patients with hypermobility syndrome. Am. Rheum. Dis. 40:541, 1981.

123. Pitcher, D., and Grahame, R.: Mitral valve prolapse and joint hypermobility: evidence for a systemic connective tissue abnormality. Ann. Rheum. Dis. 41:352, 1982.

124. Jessee, E. F., Owen, D. S., and Sagar, K. B.: The benign hypermobile joint syndrome. Arthritis Rheum. 23:1053, 1980.

125. Stewart, R. E., Hollister, P. W., and Rimoin, D. C.: A new variant of Ehlers-Danlos syndrome: An autosomal dominant disorder of fragile skin, abnormal scarring and generalized periodontis. Birth Defects 13(38):85, 1977.

126. Hartsfield, J. K., Jr., and Kousseff, B. G.: Phenotypic overlap of Ehlers-Danlos syndrome types IV and VIII. Am. J. Med. Genet. 37:465, 1990.

127. Byers, P. H., and Holbrook, K. A.: Molecular basis of clinical heterogeneity in the Ehlers-Danlos syndrome. Ann. N.Y. Acad. Sci. 460:298, 1985.

128. Biesecker, L. G., Erickson, R. P., Glover, T. W., and Bonadio, J.: Molecular and cytologic studies of Ehlers-Danlos syndrome type VIII. Am. J. Med. Genet. 41:284, 1991.

129. Holbrook, K. A., and Byers, P. H.: Skin is a window on heritable disorders of connective tissue. Am. J. Med. Genet. 34:105, 1989.

130. Holbrook, K. A., and Byers, P. H.: Structural abnormalities in the dermal collagen and elastic matrix from the skin of patients with inherited connective tissue disorders. J. Invest. Dermatol. 79:7S, 1982.

131. Junqueira, L., and Roscoes, J.: Reduced collagen content and fibre bundle disorganization in skin biopsies of patients with Ehlers-Danlos syndrome. Histochem. J. 17:197, 1985.

132. Uamakage, A., Uchigama, Y., Nihei, Y., and Ishikawa, H.: Glycosaminoglycan alteration in the skin of children with classical Ehlers-Danlos syndrome. Acta Derm. Venereol. 65:489, 1985.

133. Wordsworth, P., Ogilvie, D., Smith, R., and Sykes, B.: Exclusion of the alpha 1(II) collagen structural gene as the mutant locus in type II Ehlers-Danlos syndrome. Ann. Rheum. Dis. 44:431, 1985.

134. Bilkey, W. J., Baxter, T. L., Kottke, F. J., and Mundale, M. D.: Muscle function in Ehlers-Danlos syndrome. Arch. Phys. Med. Rehabil. 62:444, 1981.

135. Sheon, R. P., Kursner, A. B., Farber, S. V., and Finkel, R. I.: The hypermobility syndrome. Arch. Phys. Med. Rehabil. 62:444, 1981.

136. Uden, A.: Collagen and bleeding diathesis in Ehlers-Danlos syndrome. Scand. J. Haematol. 28:425, 1982.

137. Takagi, J., Kasahara, K., Sekiya, F., Inada, Y., and Saito, Y.: A collagen-binding glycoprotein from bovine platelets is identical to propolypeptide of von Willebrand factor. J. Biol. Chem. 264:10425, 1989.

138. Lenaers, A., Ansay, M., Nusgens, B. V., and Lapiere, C. M.: Collagen made of extended α chains, procollagen, in genetically defective dermatosparaxic calves. Eur. J. Biochem. 23:533, 1971.

139. Becker, U., Timpl, R., Hjelle, O., and Prockop, D.: NH_2-terminal extensions on skin collagen from sheep with a genetic defect in conversion of procollagen into collagen. Biochemistry 15:2853, 1976.

140. Lichtenstein, J. R., Martin, G. R., Kuhn, L. D., Byers, P. H., and McKusick, A. A.: Defect in conversion of procollagen to collagen in a form of Ehlers-Danlos syndrome. Science 183:298, 1973.

141. Wirtz, M. K., Keene, D. R., Hori, H., Glanville, R. W., Steinmann, B., Rao, V. H., and Hollister, D. W.: In vivo and in vitro nonconvalent association of excised alpha 1(I) amino-terminal propeptides with mutant pN alpha 2(I) collagen chains in native mutant collagen in a case of Ehlers-Danlos syndrome, type VII. J. Biol. Chem. 265:6312, 1990.

142. Halila, R., Seinmann, B., and Peltonen, L.: Processing of type I and III procollagens in Ehlers-Danlos syndrome type VII. Am. J. Hum. Genet. 39:222, 1986.

143. Minor, R. R., Sippola-Thiele, M., McKeon, J., Berger, J., and Prockop, D. J.: Defects in the processing of procollagen to collagen are demonstrable in cultured fibroblasts from patients with the Ehlers-Danlos and osteogenesis imperfecta syndromes. J. Biol. Chem. 261:10006, 1986.

144. Steinmann, B., Tuderman, L., Peltonen, L., Martin, G. R., McKusick, V. A., and Prockop, D. J.: Evidence for a structural mutation of procollagen type I in a patient with the Ehlers-Danlos syndrome type VII. J. Biol. Chem. 255:8887, 1980.

145. Eyre, D. R., Shapiro, F. D., and Aldridge, J. F.: A heterozygous collagen defect in a variant of the Ehlers-Danlos syndrome type VII. J. Biol. Chem. 260:11322, 1985.

146. Weil, D., Bernard, M., Combates, N., Wirtz, M. K., Hollister, D. W., Steinmann, B., and Ramirez, F.: Identification of a mutation that causes exon skipping during collagen pre-mRNA splicing in an Ehlers-Danlos syndrome variant. J. Biol. Chem. 263:8561, 1988.

147. Weil, D., D'Alessio, M., Ramirez, F., De Wet W., Cole, W. G., Chan, D., and Bateman, J. F.: A base substitution in the exon of a collagen gene causes alternative splicing and generates a structurally abnormal polypeptide in a patient with Ehlers-Danlos syndrome type VII. EMBO J. 8:1705, 1989.

148. Weil, D., D'Alessio, M., Ramirez, F., and Eyre, D. R.: Structural and functional characterization of a splicing mutation in the pro-alpha 2(I) collagen gene of an Ehlers-Danlos type VII patient. J. Biol. Chem. 265:6007, 1990.

149. Nicholls, A. C., Oliver, J., Renouf, D. V., McPheat, J., Palan, A., and Pope, F. M.: Ehlers-Danlos syndrome type VII: A single base change that causes exon skipping in the type I collagen alpha2(I) chain. Hum. Genet. 87:193, 1991.

150. D'Alessio, M., Ramirez, F., Blumberg, B. D., Wirtz, M. K., Rao, V. H., Godfrey, M., and Hollister, D. W.: Characterization of a COL1A1 splicing defect in a case of Ehlers-Danlos syndrome type VII: Further evidence of molecular homogeneity. Am. J. Hum. Genet. 49:400, 1991.

151. Kuivaniemi, H., Sabol, C., Tromp, G., Sippola-Thiele, M., and Prockop, D. J. A.: 19-base pair deletion in the pro-a2(I) gene of type I procollagen that causes in-frame RNA splicing from exon 10 to exon 12 in a proband with atypical osteogenesis imperfecta and in his asymptomatic mother. J. Biol. Chem. 263:11407, 1988.

152. Pinnell, S. R., Krane, S. M., Kenzora, J. E., and Glimcher, M. J.: A heritable disorder of connective tissue: hydroxylysine-deficient collagen disease. N. Engl. J. Med. 286:1013, 1972.

153. Wenstrup, R. J., Murad, S., and Pinnell, S. R.: Ehlers-Danlos syndrome type VI: Clinical manifestations of collagen lysyl hydroxylase deficiency. J. Pediatr. 115:405, 1989.

154. Krane, S. M., Pinnell, S. R., and Erbe, R. W.: Lysyl-protocollagen hydroxylase deficiency in fibroblasts from siblings with hydroxylysine-deficient collagen. Proc. Natl. Acad. Sci. U.S.A. 69:2899, 1972.

155. Demture, P. P., Priest, J. H., Snoddy, S. C., and Elsas, L. J.: Genotyping and prenatal assessment of collagen lysyl hydroxylase deficiency in a family with Ehlers-Danlos syndrome type VI. Am. J. Hum. Genet. 36:783, 1984.

156. Quinn, R. S., and Krane, S. M.: Abnormal properties of collagen lysyl hydroxylase from skin fibroblasts of siblings and hydroxylysine-deficient collagen. J. Clin. Invest. 57:83, 1976.

157. Turpeenniemi-Hujanen, T. M., Puistola, U., and Kivirikko, K. I.: Human lysyl hydroxylase: Purification to homogeneity, partial characterization and comparison of catalytic properties with those of a mutant enzyme from Ehlers-Danlos syndrome type VI fibroblasts. Coll. Relat. Res. 1:355, 1981.

158. Eyre, D. R., and Glimcher, M. J.: Reducible cross-link in hydroxylysine-deficient collagens of a heritable disorder of connective tissue. Proc. Natl. Acad. Sci. U.S.A. 69:2594, 1972.

159. Black, D., Farquharson, C., and Robins, S. P.: Excretion of pyridinium cross-links of collagen in ovariectomized rats as urinary markers for increased bone resorption. Calcif. Tissue Int. 44:343, 1989.

160. Arneson, M. A., Hammerschmidt, D. E., Furcht, L. T., and King, R. A.: A new form of Ehlers-Danlos syndrome. J.A.M.A. 244:144, 1980.

161. DiFerrante, N., Leachman, R. D., Angelini, P., Donnelly, P. V., Francis, G., Almazan, A., Guiseppe, S., and Franzblau, C.: Ehlers-Danlos Type V (X-linked form): A lysyl oxidase deficiency. Connect. Tissue Res. 3:49, 1975.

162. Beighton, P., and Curtis, D.: X-linked Ehlers-Danlos syndrome type V: The next generation. Clin. Genet. 27:474, 1985.

163. Hollister, D. W.: Clinical features of Ehlers-Danlos syndrome types VIII and IX. In Akeson, W. H., Bornstein, P., and Glimcher, V. M. J. (eds.): AAOS Symposium on Heritable Disorders of Connective Tissue. St. Louis, C. V. Mosby Company, 1982, p. 102.

164. Lazoff, S. G., Rybak, J. H. J., Parker, B. R., and Lyzzatti, L.: Skeletal dysplasia, occipital horns, diarrhea and obstructive uropathy—a new hereditary syndrome. Birth Defects 9:71, 1975.

165. Fisher, L. W., Termine, J. D., and Young, M. F.: Deduced protein sequence of bone small proteoglycan I (biglycan) shows homology with proteoglycan II (decorin) and several nonconnective tissue proteins in a variety of species. J. Biol. Chem. 264:4571, 1989.

166. Byers, P. H.: Inherited disorders of collagen gene structure and expression. Am. J. Med. Genet. 34:72, 1989.

167. Peaceman, A. M., and Cruikshank, D.: Ehlers-Danlos syndrome and pregnancy: Association of type IV disease with maternal death. Obstet. Gynecol. 69:428, 1987.

168. Pope, F. M., Narcisi, P., Nicholls, A. C., Liberman, M., and Oorthuys, J. W. E.: Clinical presentations of Ehlers-Danlos syndrome type IV. Arch. Dis. Child. 63:1016, 1988.

169. Lewkonia, R. M., and Pope, F. M.: Joint contractures and acroosteolysis in Ehlers-Danlos syndrome. J. Rheumatol. 12:140, 1985.

170. Jaffe, A. S., Getman, E. M., Rodney, G. E., and Uitto, J.: Mitral valve prolapse: a consistent manifestation of type IV Ehlers-Danlos syndrome. Circulation 64:121, 1981.

171. Hartsfield, J. K., Jr., and Kousseff, B. G.: Phenotypic overlap of Ehlers-Danlos syndrome types IV and VIII. Am. J. Med. Genet. 37:465, 1990.

172. Gertsch, P., Loup, P. W., Lochman, A., and Anani, P.: Changing patterns in the vascular form of Ehlers-Danlos syndrome. Arch. Surg. 121:1061, 1986.

173. Cikrit, D., Miles, J. H., and Silver, D.: Spontaneous arterial perforation: The Ehlers-Danlos specter. J. Vasc. Surg. 5:248, 1987.

174. Pope, F. M., Martin, G. R., Lichtenstein, J. R., Penttinen, R., Gerson, B., Rowe, D. W., and McKusick, V. A.: Patients with Ehlers-Danlos syndrome type IV lack type III collagen. Proc. Natl. Acad. Sci. U.S.A. 72:1314, 1975.

175. Superti-Furga, A., Steinmann, B., Ramirez, F., and Byers, P. H.: Molecular defects of type III procollagen in Ehlers-Danlos syndrome type IV. Hum. Genet. 82:104, 1989.

176. Tsipouras, P., Byers, P., Schwartz, R., Chu, M. -L., Weil, D., Pepe, G., Cassidy, S. B., and Ramirez, F.: Ehlers-Danlos syndrome type IV: Cosegregation of the phenotype to a CO3A1 allele of type III procollagen. Hum. Genet. 74:41, 1986.

177. Stolle, C. A., Pyeritz, R., Myers, J., and Prockop, D.: Synthesis of an altered type III procollagen in a patient with type IV Ehlers-Danlos syndrome. J. Biol. Chem. 260:1937, 1985.

178. Tromp, G., Kuivaniemi, H., Shikata, H., and Prockop, D. J.: A single base mutation that substitutes serine for glycine 790 of the α1(III) chain of type III procollagen exposes an arginine and causes Ehlers-Danlos syndrome IV. J. Biol. Chem. 264:1349, 1989.

179. Tromp, G., Kuivaniemi, H., Stolle, C., Pope, F. M., and Prockop, D. J.: Single base mutation in the type III procollagen gene that converts the codon for glycine 883 to aspartate in a mild variant of Ehlers-Danlos syndrome IV. J. Biol. Chem. 264:19313, 1989.

180. Cole, W. G., Chiodo, A. A., Lamande, S. R., Janeczko, R., Ramirez, F., Dahl, H. H., Chan, D., and Bateman, J. F.: A base substitution at a splice site in the COL3A1 gene causes exon skipping and generates abnormal type III procollagen in a patient with Ehlers-Danlos syndrome type IV. J. Biol. Chem. 265:17070, 1990.

181. Vissing, H., D'Alessio, M., Lee, B., Ramirez, F., Byers, P. H., Steinmann, B., and Superti-Furga, A.: Multiexon deletion in the procollagen III gene is associated with mild Ehlers-Danlos syndrome type IV. J. Biol. Chem. 266:5244, 1991.

182. Smith, R., Francis, J. M. O., and Houghton, G. R.: The Brittle Bone Syndrome. London, Butterworth, 1983.

183. Byers, P. H.: Brittle bones—fragile molecules: Disorders of collagen gene structure and expression. Trends Genet. 6:293, 1990.

184. Rowe, D. W., and Shapiro, J. R.: Osteogenesis Imperfecta. In Avioli, L., and Krane, S. (eds.): Metabolic Bone Disease. 2nd ed. Philadelphia, W. B. Saunders, 1990, p. 659.

185. Rowe, D. W.: Osteogenesis Imperfecta. In Heersche, J. N., and Kanis, J. A. (eds.): Bone and Mineral Research. Vol. 7. Amsterdam, Elsevier Science Publication, 1991, p. 209.

186. McKusick, V. A.: The classification of heritable disorders of connective tissue. Birth Defects 11(6):7, 1975.

187. Sillence, D. O., and Danks, D. M.: Genetic heterogeneity in osteogenesis imperfecta. J. Med. Genet. 16:101, 1979.

188. Sillence, D.: Osteogenesis imperfecta: an expanding panorama of variants. Clin. Orthop. Rel. Res. 159:11, 1981.

189. Byers, P. H., Tsipouras, P., Bonadio, J. F., Starman, B., and Schwartz, R. C.: Perinatal lethal osteogenesis imperfecta (OI type II): a biochemically heterogeneous disorder due to new mutations in the genes for type I collagen. Am. J. Hum. Genet. 42:237, 1988.

190. Sillence, D. O., Barlow, K. K., Garber, A. P., Hall, J. G., and Rimoin, D. L.: Osteogenesis imperfecta type II: delineation of the phenotype with reference to genetic heterogeneity. Am. J. Med. Genet. 17:407, 1984.

191. Cremin, B., Goodman, H., Prax, M., Spranger, J., and Beighton, P.: Wormian bones in osteogenesis imperfecta and other disorders. Skeletal Radiol. 8:35, 1982.

192. Shapiro, J. E., Byers, P. H., Levin, S. L., Barsh, G. S., and Goldstein, P.: Prenatal diagnosis of lethal perinatal osteogenesis imperfecta (OI type II). J. Pediatr. 100:127, 1982.

193. van der Rest, M., Hayes, A., Marie, P., Desbarats, M., Kaplan, P., and Glorieux, F. H.: Lethal osteogenesis imperfecta with amniotic band lesions: collagen studies. Am. J. Med. Genet. 24:433, 1986.

194. Pope, F. M., Nicholls, A. C., Eggleton, C., Narcissi, P., Heg, E. N., and Parkin, J. M.: Osteogenesis imperfecta (lethal) bones contain types III and V collagen. J. Clin. Pathol. 33:534, 1980.

195. Bonaventure, J., Zylberberg, L., Cohen-Solal, L., Allain, J.-C., Lasselin, C., and Maroteaux, P.: A new lethal brittle bone syndrome with increased amount of type V collagen in a patient. Am. J. Med. Genet. 33:299, 1989.

196. Chu, M. L., Willams, C. J., Pepe, G., Hirsch, J. L., Prockop, D. J., and Ramirez, F.: Internal deletion in a collagen gene in perinatal lethal form of osteogenesis imperfecta. Nature 304:78, 1984.

197. Barsh, G. S., Roush, C. L., Bonadio, J., Byers, P. H., and Gelinas, R. E.: Intron-mediated recombination may cause a deletion in an α1(I) collagen chain in a lethal form of osteogenesis imperfecta. Proc. Natl. Acad. Sci. U.S.A. 82:2870, 1985.

198. Williams, C. J., and Prockop, D. J.: Synthesis and processing of a type I procollagen containing shortened pro α1(I) chains by fibroblasts from a patient with osteogenesis imperfecta. J. Biol. Chem. 258:5915, 1983.

199. Bonadio, J., Holbrook, K. A., Gelinas, R. E., Jacob, J., and Byers, P. H.: Altered triple helical structure of type I procollagen in lethal perinatal osteogenesis imperfecta. J. Biol. Chem. 260:1734, 1985.

200. Kobayashi, K., Hata, R., Nagai, S., Niwa, J., and Hoshino, T.: Direct visualization of affected collagen molecules synthesized by cultured fibroblasts from an osteogenesis imperfecta patient. Biochem. Biophys. Res. Commun. 172:217, 1990.

201. Nogami, H., and Oohira, A.: Defective association between collagen fibrils and proteoglycans in fragile bone of osteogenesis imperfecta. Clin. Orthop. Rel. Res. 232:284, 1988.

202. Petrovic, O. M., and Miller, J.: An unusual pattern of peptide-bound lysine metabolism in collagen from an infant with perinatal osteogenesis imperfecta. J. Clin. Invest. 73:1569, 1984.

203. Tromp, G., and Prockop, D. J.: Single base mutation in the proα2(I) collagen gene that causes efficient splicing of the RNA from exon 27 to exon 29 and synthesis of a shortened but in-frame proα2(I) chain. Proc. Natl. Acad. Sci. U.S.A. 85:5254, 1988.

204. Bonadio, J., Ramirez, F., and Barr, M.: An intron mutation in the human alpha1(I) collagen gene alters the efficiency of pre-mRNA splicing and is associated with osteogenesis imperfecta type II. J. Biol. Chem. 265:2262, 1990.

205. Cohn, D. H., Byers, P. H., Steinmann, B., and Gelinas, P. E.: Lethal osteogenesis imperfecta resulting from a single nucleotide change in one human proα1(I) collagen allele. Proc. Natl. Acad. Sci. U.S.A. 83:6045, 1986.

206. Vogel, B. E., Minor, R. R., Freund, M., and Prockop, D. J.: A point mutation in a type-I procollagen gene converts glycine-748 to the α1 chain to cysteine and destabilizes the triple helix in a lethal variant of osteogenesis imperfecta. J. Biol. Chem. 262:4737, 1987.

207. Bateman, J. F., Chan, D., Walker, I. D., Rogers, J. G., and Cole, W. G.: Lethal perinatal osteogenesis imperfecta due to the substitution of arginine for glycine at residue 391 of the α1(I) chain of type I collagen. J. Biol. Chem. 262:7021, 1987.

208. Bateman, J. F., Lamande, S. R., Dahl, H. H., Chan, D., and Cole, W. G.: Substitution of arginine for glycine 664 in the collagen α1(I) chain in lethal perinatal osteogenesis imperfecta. Demonstration of the peptide defect by in vitro expression of the mutant cDNA. J. Biol. Chem. 263:11627, 1988.

209. Baldwin, C. T., Constantinou, C. D., Dumars, K. W., and Prockop, D. J.: A single base mutation that converts glycine 907 of the α2(I) chain of type I procollagen to aspartate in a lethal variant of osteogenesis imperfecta. The single amino acid substitution near the carboxyl terminus destabilizes the whole triple helix. J. Biol. Chem. 264:3002, 1989.

210. Kadler, K. E., Torre-Blanco, A., Adachi, E., Vogel, B. E., Hojima, Y., Prockop, D. J.: A type I collagen with substitution of a cysteine for

glycine-748 in the alpha1(I) chain copolymerizes with normal type I collagen and can generate fractal-like structures. Biochemistry 30:5081, 1991.

211. Steinmann, B., Westerhausen, A., Constantinou, C. D., Superti-Furga, A., and Prockop, D. J.: Substitution of cysteine for glycine-alpha1-691 in the proalpha1(I) chain of type I procollagen in a proband with lethal osteogenesis imperfecta destabilizes the triple helix at a site C-terminal to the substitution. Biochem. J. 279:747, 1991.

212. Tsuneyoshi, T., Westerhausen, A., Constantinou, C. D., and Prockop, D. J.: Substitutions for glycine alpha1–637 and glycine alpha2–694 of type I procollagen in lethal osteogenesis imperfecta. The conformational strain on the triple helix introduced by a glycine substitution can be transmitted along the helix. J. Biol. Chem. 266:15608, 1991.

213. Starman, B. J., Eyre, D., Charbonneau, H., Harrylock, M., Weis, M. A., Weiss, L., Graham, J. M., Jr., and Byers, P. H.: Osteogenesis imperfecta. The position of substitution for glycine by cysteine in the triple helical domain of the proalpha1(I) chains of type I collagen determines the clinical phenotype. J. Clin. Invest. 84:1206, 1989.

214. Wenstrup, R. J., Shrago-Howe, A. W., Lever, L. W., Phillips, C. L., Byers, P. H., and Cohn, D. H.: The effects of different cysteine for glycine substitutions within alpha2(I) chains. Evidence of distinct structural domains within the type I collagen triple helix. J. Biol. Chem. 266:2590, 1991.

215. Sillence, D. O., Barlow, K. K., Cole, W. G., Dietrich, S., Garber, A. P., and Rimoin, D. L.: Osteogenesis imperfecta type III. Delineation of the phenotype with reference to genetic heterogeneity. Am. J. Med. Genet. 23:821, 1986.

216. Frank, E., Berger, T., and Tew, J. M.: Basilar impression and platybasia in osteogenesis imperfecta tarda. Surg. Neurol. 17:116, 1982.

217. Tsipouras, P., Barbas, G., and Mathews, W.: Neurological correlates of osteogenesis imperfecta. Arch. Neurol. 43:150, 1986.

218. Pauli, R. M., and Gilbert, E. F.: Upper cervical cord compression as a cause of death in osteogenesis imperfecta type III. J. Pediatr. 108:579, 1986.

219. Bullough, P. G., Davidson, D. D., and Lorenzo, J. C.: The morbid anatomy of the skeleton in osteogenesis imperfecta. Clin. Orthop. 159:42, 1981.

220. Robinson, L. P., Worthen, W. J., Lachman, R. S., Adormian, G. E., and Rimoin, D. R.: Prenatal diagnosis of osteogenesis imperfecta type III. Prevent. Diagn. 1:7, 1987.

221. Nicholls, A. C., and Pope, F. M.: Biochemical heterogeneity of osteogenesis imperfecta: A new variant. Lancet 1:1193, 1979.

222. Deak, S. B., van der Rest, M., and Prockop, D. J.: Altered helical structure of a homotrimer of α1(I) chains synthesized by fibroblasts from a variant of osteogenesis imperfecta. Coll. Rel. Res. 5:305, 1985.

223. Chu, M. L., Nicholls, A. R., Pope, F. M., Rowe, D. W., and Prockop, D. J.: Presence of mRNA for proα2(I) chains in fibroblasts from a patient with osteogenesis imperfecta whose type I collagen does not contain α1(I) chains. Coll. Relat. Res. 4:389, 1984.

224. Valli, M., Tenni, R., and Cetta, G.: Moderately severe osteogenesis imperfecta: Biochemical studies showing variable defect localization in the triple-helical domain of type I collagen. Matrix 10:200, 1990.

225. Pack, M., Constantinou, C. D., Kalia, K., Nielsen, K. B., and Prockop, D. J.: Substitution of serine for alpha1(I)-glycine 844 in a severe variant of osteogenesis imperfecta minimally destabilizes the triple helix of type I procollagen. The effects of glycine substitutions on thermal stability are either position or amino acid specific. J. Biol. Chem. 264:19694, 1989.

226. Cohen-Solal, L., Bonaventure, J., and Maroteaux, P.: Dominant mutations in familial lethal and severe osteogenesis imperfecta. Hum. Genet. 87:297, 1991.

227. Levin, L. S.: The dentition in the osteogenesis imperfecta syndromes. Clin. Orthop. 159:64, 1981.

228. Tsipouras, P., Myers, J. C., Ramirez, F., and Prockop, D.: RFLP associated with the proα2(I) gene of human type I procollagen. J. Clin. Invest. 72:1262, 1983.

229. Groflor-Rabic, A. F., Wallis, G., Brebner, D. K., Beighton, P., Bester, A. J., and Mathew, C. G.: Detection of a high frequency Rsal polymorphism in the human proα2(I) collagen gene which is linked to an autosomal dominant form of osteogenesis imperfecta. EMBO J. 4:1745, 1985.

230. Sykes, B., Ogilvie, D., Wordsworth, P., Wallis, G., Mathew, C., Beighton, P., Nicholls, A., Pope, F. M., Thompson, E., Tsipouras, P., Schwartz, R., Jensson, O., Arnason, A., Borresen, A.-L., Heiberg, A., Frey, D., and Steinmann, B.: Consistent linkage of dominantly inherited osteogenesis imperfecta to the type I collagen loci: COL1A1 and COL1A2. Am. J. Hum. Genet. 46:293, 1990.

231. Tsipouras, P., Swartz, R., Goldberg, J. D., Berkowitz, R. L., and Ramirez, F.: Prenatal prediction of osteogenesis imperfecta (OI type IV): exclusion of inheritance using a collagen gene probe. J. Med. Genet. 24:406, 1987.

232. Byers, P. H., Shapiro, J. R., Rowe, D. W., David, K. E., and Holbrook, K. A.: Abnormal α2 chain in type I collagen from a patient with a form of osteogenesis imperfecta. J. Clin. Invest. 71:689, 1983.

233. Liu, S.-C., Stover, M. L., McKinstry, M., Angilly, J., Shapiro, J., and Rowe, D. W.: Errors in type I collagen mRNA splicing in osteogenesis imperfecta. In Cohn, D. V., Glorieux, F., and Martin, T. J. (eds.): Calcium and Bone Metabolism: Basic and Clinical Aspects. Vol. 10. Amsterdam, Elsevier, 1990, pp. 207–213.

234. Wenstrup, R. J., Hunter, A. G. W., and Byers, P. H.: Osteogenesis imperfecta type IV: evidence of abnormal triple helical structure of type I collagen. Hum. Genet. 74:47, 1986.

235. Brenner, R. E., Vetter, U., Nerlich, A., Wörsdorfer, O., Teller, W. M., and Müller, P. K.: Biochemical analysis of callus tissue in osteogenesis imperfecta type IV. Evidence for transient overmodification in collagen types I and III. J. Clin. Invest. 84:915, 1989.

236. Wenstrup, R. J., Willing, M. C., Starman, B. J., and Byers, P. H.: Distinct biochemical phenotypes predict clinical severity in nonlethal variants of osteogenesis imperfecta. Am. J. Hum. Genet. 46:975, 1990.

237. Valli, M., Mottes, M., Tenni, R., Sangalli, A., Gomez, L., Rossi, A., Antoniazzi, F., Cetta, G., Pignatti, P. F.: A de Novo G to T transversion in a pro-alpha1(I) collagen gene for a moderate case of osteogenesis imperfecta. Substitution of cysteine for glycine 178 in the triple helical domain. J. Biol. Chem. 266:1872, 1991.

238. Wenstrup, R. J., Cohn, D. H., Cohen, T., and Byers, P. H.: Arginine for glycine substitution in the triple-helical domain of the products of one α2(I) collagen allele (COL1A2) produces the osteogenesis imperfecta type IV phenotype. J. Biol. Chem. 263:7734, 1988.

239. Shapiro, J. R., Pikus, A., Weiss, G., and Rowe, D. W.: Hearing and middle ear in function in osteogenesis imperfecta. J.A.M.A. 247:2120, 1982.

240. Pedersen, U.: Osteogenesis imperfecta clinical features, hearing loss, and stapedectomy. Biochemical osteodensitometric, corneometric and histological aspects in comparison with otosclerosis. Acta Otolaryngol. 415(S):1, 1985.

241. Hortop, J., Tsipouras, P., Hanley, J., Maron, B., and Shapiro, J.: Cardiovascular involvement in osteogenesis imperfecta. Circulation 73:54, 1986.

242. Evensen, S. A., Myhre, L., and Storworken, H.: Haemostatic studies in osteogenesis imperfecta. Scand. J. Hematol. 33:77, 1984.

243. Paterson, C. R., McAllion, S., and Stellman, J. L.: Osteogenesis imperfecta after the menopause. N. Engl. J. Med. 310:1694, 1984.

244. Paterson, C. R., and McAllion, S. J.: Osteogenesis imperfecta in the differential diagnosis of child abuse. Br. Med. J. 299:1451, 1989.

245. Taitz, L. S.: Child abuse and metabolic bone disease: Are they often confused? Br. Med. J. 302:1244, 1991.

246. Gahagan, S., and Rimsza, M. E.: Child abuse or osteogenesis imperfecta: How can we tell? Pediatrics 88:987, 1991.

247. Brenner, R. E., Vetter, U., Nerlich, A., Wörsdorfer, O., Teller, W. M., and Müller, P. K.: Altered collagen metabolism in osteogenesis imperfecta fibroblasts: A study on 33 patients with diverse forms. Eur. J. Clin. Invest. 20:8, 1990.

248. Sykes, B., Francis, N. J., and Smith, R.: Altered relation of two collagen types in osteogenesis imperfecta. N. Engl. J. Med. 296:1200, 1977.

249. Oxlund, H., Pedersen, U., Danielson, G. C., Oxlund, I., and Elfrond, O.: Reduced strength of skin in osteogenesis imperfecta. Eur. J. Clin. Invest. 15:408, 1985.

250. Willing, M. C., Cohn, D. H., and Byers, P. H.: Frameshift mutation near the 3' end of the COL1A1 gene of type I collagen predicts an elongated proalpha1(I) chain and results in osteogenesis imperfecta type I. J. Clin. Invest. 85:282, 1990.

251. Bateman, J. F., Lamande, S. R., Dahl, H. H., Chan, D., Mascara, T., and Cole, W. G.: A frameshift mutation results in a truncated nonfunctional carboxyl-terminal proalpha1(I) propeptide of type I collagen in osteogenesis imperfecta. J. Biol. Chem. 264:10960, 1989.

252. Bonadio, J., Saunders, T. L., Tsai, E., Goldstein, S. A., Morris-Wiman, J., Brinkley, L., Dolan, D. F., Altschuler, R. A., Hawkins, J. E., Jr., Bateman, J. F., Mascara, T., and Jaenisch, R.: Transgenic mouse model of the mild dominant form of osteogenesis imperfecta. Proc. Natl. Acad. Sci. U.S.A. 87:7145, 1990.

253. Steinmann, B., Nicholls, A., and Pope, F. M.: Clinical variability of osteogenesis imperfecta reflecting molecular heterogeneity: cysteine substitutions in the α1(I) collagen chain producing lethal and mild forms. J. Biol. Chem. 261:8958, 1986.

254. Spotila, L. D., Constantinou, C. D., Sereda, L., Ganguly, A., Riggs, B. L., and Prockop, D. J.: Mutation in a gene for type I procollagen (COL1A2) in a woman with postmenopausal osteoporosis: Evidence for phenotypic and genotypic overlap with mild osteogenesis imperfecta. Proc. Natl. Acad. Sci. U.S.A. 88:5423, 1991.

255. Shapiro, J., Stover, M.-L., Burn, V., McKinstry, M., Burshell, A., and Chipman, S.: An osteopenic nonfracture syndrome with features of mild osteogenesis imperfecta associated with a substitution of a cysteine for glycine at triple helix position 43 in the proα1(I) chain of type I collagen. J. Clin. Invest. 89:567, 1992.

256. Albright, J. A.: Systemic treatment of osteogenesis imperfecta. Clin. Orthop. 159:88, 1981.

257. Pedersen, U., Charles, P., Hansen, H. H., and Elbrond, O.: Lack of

effects of human calcitonin in osteogenesis imperfecta. Acta Orthop. Scand. 56:260, 1985.
258. Jorgensen, P. H., Andreassen, T. T., and Jorgensen, K. D.: Growth hormone influences collagen deposition and mechanical strength of intact rat skin. A dose-response study. Acta Endocrinol. (Copenh.) 120:767, 1989.
259. Moorefield, W. G., and Miller, G. R.: Aftermath of osteogenesis imperfecta, the disease of adulthood. J. Bone Surg. 62A:113, 1980.
260. Rodriquez, R. P., and Bailey, R. W.: Internal fixation of the femur in patients with osteogenesis imperfecta. Clin. Orthop. 159:126, 1981.
261. Bleck, E. E.: Nonoperative treatment of osteogenesis imperfecta. Clin. Orthop. 159:111, 1981.
262. Binder, H., Hawks, L., Graybill, G., Gerber, N. L., and Weintrab, J. C.: Osteogenesis imperfecta: rehabilitation approach with infants and young children. Acta Phys. Med. Rehab. 65:532, 1984.
263. Pyeritz, R. E., and McKusick, V. A.: Basic defects in the Marfan syndrome. N. Engl. J. Med. 305:1011, 1981.
264. Pyeritz, R., and McKusick, V. A.: The Marfan syndrome: diagnosis and management. N. Engl. J. Med. 300:772, 1978.
265. Sinclair, R. J. G., Kitchen, A. H., and Turner, R. W. D.: The Marfan syndrome. Q. J. Med. 113:19, 1960.
266. Steinberg, I.: A simple screening test for the Marfan syndrome. Am. J. Roentgenol. 97:118, 1966.
267. Walker, B. A., and Murdock, J. L.: The wrist sign: A useful physical finding in the Marfan syndrome. Ann. Intern. Med. 126:276, 1970.
268. McKusick, V. A.: The classification of heritable disorders of connective tissue. Birth Defects (Original Article Series) 11(6):1, 1975.
269. Savini, R., Cervellati, S., and Beroaldo, E.: Spinal deformities in Marfan's syndrome. Ital. J. Orthop. Traumatol. 1:19, 1980.
270. Maumenee, I. H.: The eye in the Marfan syndrome. Trans. Am. Ophthalmol. Soc. 79:684, 1981.
271. Gross, D. M., Robinson, L. K., Smith, L. T., Glass, N., Rosenberg, H., and Duvic, M.: Severe perinatal Marfan syndrome. Pediatrics 84:83, 1989.
272. Vetter, U., Mayerhofer, R., Lang, D., Bernuth, G. V., Ranke, M. B., and Schmaltz, A. A.: The Marfan syndrome: Analysis of growth and cardiovascular manifestation. Eur. J. Pediatr. 149:4526, 1990.
273. Roberts, W. C., and Honig, H. S.: The spectrum of cardiovascular disease in the Marfan syndrome: a clinicomorphologic study of 18 necropsy patients. Am. Heart J. 104:115, 1982.
274. Pyeritz, R. E.: The Marfan syndrome. Am. Fam. Physician 34:83, 1986.
275. Pyeritz, R. E.: Maternal and fetal complications of pregnancy in the Marfan syndrome. Am. J. Med. 71:784, 1981.
276. Kouchoukos, N. T., Marshall, W. G., and Wedige-Stecher, T. A.: Eleven-year experience with composite graft replacement of the ascending aorta and aortic valve. J. Thorac. Cardiovasc. Surg. 92:691, 1986.
277. Arn, P. H., Scherer, L. R., Haller, J. A., Jr., and Pyeritz, R. E.: Outcome of pectus excavatum in patients with Marfan syndrome and in the general population. J. Pediatr. 115:954, 1989.
278. Streeten, E. A., Murphy, E. A., and Pyeritz, R. E.: Pulmonary function in the Marfan syndrome. Chest 91:408, 1987.
279. Berliner, S., Dean, H., and Pinkhas, J.: Spontaneous penumothorax in a patient with Marfan syndrome. Respiration 42:127, 1981.
280. Emanuel, R., Marcomichelakis, E., Mores, C., Jefferson, K., Macfaul, P. A., and Withers, R.: Formes frustes of Marfan's syndrome presenting with severe aortic regurgitation: clinicogenetic study of 18 families. Br. Heart J. 39:190, 1977.
281. Cotton, D. J., and Brandt, K.: Cardiovascular abnormalities in the Marfanoid hypermobility syndrome. Arthritis Rheum. 19:763, 1976.
282. Walker, B. A., Beighton, P., and Murdoch, J. L.: The Marfanoid hypermobility syndrome. Ann. Intern. Med. 71:349, 1969.
283. Schuttle, J. E., Gaffney, F. A., Blend, L., and Blumquist, C. G.: Distinctive anthropometric characteristics of women with mitral valve prolapse. Am. J. Med. 71:533, 1981.
284. Goodman, R. M., Baba, W., and Wooley, C.: Observations on the heart in a case of combined Ehlers-Danlos and Marfan's syndromes. Am. J. Cardiol. 24:734, 1969.
285. Ramos-Arroyo, M. A., Weaver, D. D., and Beak, R. K.: Congenital contractural arachnodactyly. Clin. Genet. 27:570, 1985.
286. Epstein, C. J., Graham, C. B., Hodgkin, W. F., Hecht, F., and Motulsky, A. G.: Hereditary dysplasia of bone with kyphoscoliosis, contractures, and abnormally shaped ears. J. Pediatr. 73:379, 1968.
287. Meinecke, P.: Marfan-like features and congenital contractural arachnodactyly. J. Pediatr. 100:1006, 1982.
288. Bass, H. N., Sparkes, R. S., Crandall, B. F., and Marcy, M. S.: Congenital contractural arachnodactyly, keratoconus and probably Marfan syndrome in the same pedigree. J. Pediatr. 94:591, 1981.
289. Priest, R. E., and Moinuddin, J. F.: Collagen of Marfan syndrome is abnormally soluble. Nature 245:264, 1973.
290. Boucek, R. J., Noble, N. L., Gunja-Smith, Z., and Butler, W. T.: The Marfan syndrome: A deficiency in chemically stable collagen cross-links. N. Engl. J. Med. 305:989, 1982.
291. Abraham, P. A., Perejda, A. J., Carnes, W. H., and Uitto, J.: Marfan syndrome: demonstration of abnormal elastin in aorta. J. Clin. Invest. 70:1245, 1982.
292. Halme, T., Savunen, T., Aho, H., Vihersaari, T., and Penttinen, R.: Elastin and collagen in the aorta wall: changes in the Marfan syndromes and annuloaortic ectasia. Exp. Mol. Pathol. 43:1, 1985.
293. Harley, V. R., Chan, D., Rogers, J. G., and Cole, W. G.: Marfan syndrome: Absence of type I or III collagen structural defects in 25 patients. J. Inherited Metab. Dis. 13:219, 1990.
294. Halme, T., Vikersaari, T., and Penttinen, R.: Lysyl oxidase activity and synthesis of desmosines in cultured human aortic cells and skin fibroblasts. Scand. J. Clin. Lab. Invest. 46:31, 1986.
295. Tsipouras, P.: Marfan syndrome: Light at the end of the tunnel. Am. J. Hum. Genet. 46:643, 1990.
296. Kainulainen, K., Savolainen, A., Palotie, A., Kaitila, I., Rosenbloom, J., and Peltonen, L.: Marfan syndrome: Exclusion of genetic linkage to five genes coding for connective tissue components in the long arm of chromosome 2. Hum. Genet. 84:233, 1990.
297. Blanton, S. H., Sarfarazi, M., Elberg, H., deGroote, J., Farndon, P. A., Kilpatrick, M. W., Tsipouras, P., et al.: An exclusion map of Marfan syndrome. J. Med. Genet. 27:73, 1990.
298. Kainulainen, K., Pulkkinen, L., Savolainen, A., Kaitila, I., and Peltonen, L.: Location on chromosome 15 of the gene defect causing Marfan syndrome. N. Engl. J. Med. 23:935, 1990.
299. Godfrey, M., Menashe, V., Weleber, R. G., Koler, R. D., Bigley, R. H., Lovrien, E., Zonana, J., and Hollister, D. W.: Cosegregation of elastin-associated microfibrillar abnormalities with the Marfan phenotype in families. Am. J. Hum. Genet. 46:652, 1990.
300. Sakai, L. Y., Keene, D. R., and Engvall, E.: Fibrillin, a new 350-KD glycoprotein, is a component of extracellular microfibrils. J. Cell. Biol. 103:2499, 1986.
301. Maslen, C. L., Corson, G. M., Maddox, B. K., Glanville, R. W., and Sakai, L. Y.: Partial sequence of a candidate gene for the Marfan syndrome. Nature 352:334, 1991.
302. Lee, B., Godfrey, M., Vitale, E., Hori, H., Mattei, M.-G., Sarfarazi, M., Tsipouras, P., Ramirez, F., and Hollister, D. W.: Linkage of Marfan syndrome and a phenotypically related disorder to two different fibrillin genes. Nature 352:330, 1991.
303. Kainulainen, K., Steinmann, B., Collins, F., Dietz, H. C., Francomano, C. A., Child, A., Kilpatrick, M. W., Brock, D. J. H., Keston, M., Pyeritz, R. E., and Peltonen, L.: Marfan syndrome: No evidence for heterogeneity in different populations, and more precise mapping of the gene. Am. J. Hum. Genet. 49:662, 1991.
304. Dietz, H. C., Cutting, G. R., Pyeritz, R. E., Maslen, C. L., Sakai, L. Y., Corson, G. M., Puffenberger, E. G., Hamosh, A., Nanthakumar, E. J., Curristin, S. M., Stetten, G., Meyers, D. A., and Francomano, C. A.: Marfan syndrome caused by a recurrent de novo missense mutation in the fibrillin gene. Nature 352:337, 1991.
305. Beighton, P.: The dominant and recessive forms of cutis laxa. J. Med. Genet. 9:216, 1972.
306. Byers, P. H., Siegel, R. C., Holbrook, K., Narayanan, S. A., Bornstein, P., and Hall, J. G.: X-linked cutis laxa; defective cross-link formation due to decreased lysyl oxidase activity. N. Engl. J. Med. 202:61, 1980.
307. Uitto, J., Ryhanen, L., Abraham, P. A., and Perejda, A. J.: Elastin in diseases. J. Invest. Dermatol. 79:1605, 1982.
308. Linares, A., Zarranz, J. J., Rodriquez-Alarcon, J., and Diaz-Perez, S. L.: Reversible cutis laxa due to maternal D-penicillamine treatment. Lancet 2:43, 1974.
309. Marshall, J., Heyl, T., and Weber, H.: Postinflammatory elastolysis and cutis laxa. S. Afr. Med. J. 40:1016, 1966.
310. Merten, D. F., and Roonery, R.: Progressive pulmonary emphysema associated with generalized elastolysis (cutis laxa). Radiology 13:691, 1974.
311. Weir, K. E., Jaffe, H. S., Blaufuss, A. H., and Beighton, P.: Cardiovascular abnormalities in cutis laxa. Eur. J. Cardiol. 5:253, 1977.
312. Hajjer, B. A., and Jayner, E. N.: Congenital cutis laxa with advanced cardiopulmonary disease. J. Pediatr. 73:116, 1968.
313. Ogur, G., Yuksel-Apak, M., and Demiryont, M.: Syndrome of congenital cutis laxa with ligamentous laxity and delayed development: report of a brother and sister from Turkey. Am. J. Med. Genet. 37:6, 1990.
314. Marchase, P., Holbrook, R., and Pinnell, S. R.: A familial cutis laxa syndrome with ultra-structural abnormalities of collagen and elastin. J. Invest. Dermatol. 75:399, 1980.
315. Menkes, J. H., Alter, M., Steigleder, G. K., Weakley, D. R., and Sung, J. H.: A sex-linked recessive disorder with retardation, peculiar hair, and focal cerebral and cerebellar degeneration. Pediatrics 29:764, 1962.
316. Wheeler, M. E., and Roberts, P. F.: Menkes' steely hair syndrome. Arch. Dis. Child. 51:269, 1976.
317. Troost, D., Van Rossum, A., Straks, W., and Willemse, J.: Menkes' kinky hair disease. II: a clinicopathologic report of three cases. Brain Rev. 4:115, 1982.
318. Willemse, J., Van deu Hamer, C., Prins, H. W., and Jonker, P. L.: Menkes' kinky hair disease. I. Comparison of classical and unusual clinical and biochemical features in two patients. Brain Rev. 4:105, 1982.

319. Williams, D. M., and Arthur, C. L.: Tissue copper concentrations of patients with Menkes' kinky hair disease. Am. J. Dis. Child. 135:375, 1981.
320. Camakaris, J., Danks, D., Ackland, L., Cartwright, E., Borger, P., and Colton, R. G. H.: Altered copper metabolism in cultured cells from human Menkes' syndrome and mottled mouse mutants. Biochem. Genet. 18:117, 1980.
321. Gacheru, S. N., Trackman, P. C., Shah, M. A., O'Gara, C. Y., Spacciapoli, P., Greenaway, F. T., and Kagan, H. M.: Structural and catalytic properties of copper in lysyl oxidase. J. Biol. Chem. 265:19022, 1990.
322. Rowe, D. W., McGoodwin, E. B., Martin, G. H., and Grahn, D.: Lysyl oxidase activity in the aneurysm-prone mottled mouse. J. Biol. Chem. 252:939, 1977.
323. Trackman, P. C., Pratt, A. M., Wolanski, A., Tang, S.-S., Offner, G. D., Troxler, R. F., and Kagan, H. M.: Cloning of rat aorta lysyl oxidase cDNA: Complete codons and predicted amino acid sequence. Biochemistry 29:4863, 1990.
324. Hämäläinen, E.-R., Jones, T. A., Sheer, D., Taskinen, K., Pihlajaniemi, T., and Kivirikko, K. I.: Molecular cloning of human lysyl oxidase and assignment of the gene to chromosome 5q23.3-31.2. Genomics 11:508, 1991.
325. Labadie, G. V., Hirschhorn, K., Katz, S., and Beratis, N.: Increased copper metallothionein in Menkes' cultured skin fibroblasts. Pediatr. Res. 15:257, 1981.
326. Prohaska, J. R.: Genetic diseases of copper metabolism. Clin. Physiol. Biochem. 4:87, 1986.
327. Carner, W. H.: Copper and connective tissue metabolism. Int. Rev. Connect. Tissue Res. 4:197, 1968.
328. Danks, D. M.: Of mice and men: metals and mutations. J. Med. Genet. 23:99, 1986.
329. Kuivaniemi, H., Peltonen, L., Palotie, A., Kaitila, I., and Kivirikko, K. I.: Abnormal copper metabolism and deficient lysyl oxidase activity in a heritable connective tissue disorder. J. Clin. Invest. 69:730, 1982.
330. Kuivaniemi, H., Peltonen, L., and Kivirikko, K. I.: Type IX Ehlers-Danlos syndrome and Menkes' syndrome: The decrease in lysyl oxidase activity is associated with a corresponding deficiency in the exzyme protein. Am. J. Hum. Genet. 37:798, 1985.
331. McKusick, V.: Pseudoxanthoma elasticum. In Akeson, W. H., Bornstein, P., and Glimcher, J. J. (eds.): Heritable Disorders of Connective Tissue. St. Louis, C. V. Mosby Company, 1972, p. 475.
332. Goodman, R. M., Smith, E. W., and Paton, D.: Pseudoxanthoma elasticum: a clinical and histopathological study. Medicine 42:297, 1963.
333. Berlyne, G. M., Bulmer, M. G., and Platt, R.: The genetics of pseudoxanthoma elasticum. Q. J. Med. 30:201, 1961.
334. Pope, F. M.: Historical evidence for the genetic heterogeneity of pseudoxanthoma elasticum. Br. J. Dermatol. 92:493, 1985.
335. DePaepe, A., Viljoen, D., Matton, M., Beighton, P., Lenaerts, V., Vossaert, K., DeBie, S., Voet, D., DeLaey, J.-J., and Kint, A.: Pseudoxanthoma elasticum: Similar autosomal recessive subtype in Belgian and Afrikaner families. Am. J. Med. Genet. 38:16, 1991.
336. Altman, L. K., Fialkow, P. J., Parker, F., and Sagebiel, R. W.: Pseudoxanthoma elasticum. Arch. Intern. Med. 134:1048, 1974.
337. Goette, D. K., and Carpenter, W. M.: The mucocutaneous marker of pseudoxanthoma elasticum. Oral Surg. 51:68, 1981.
338. Jackson, A., and Loh, C.: Pulmonary calcification and elastic tissue damage in pseudoxanthoma elasticum. Histopathology 4:607, 1980.
339. Przybojewski, J. Z., Maritz, F., Tiedt, F. A. C., and Van der Walt, J. J.: Pseudoxanthoma elasticum with cardiac involvement. S. Afr. Med. J. 59:268, 1981.
340. Navrro-Lopez, E., Llorian, A., Ferrer-Roca, O., Betriv, A., and Sanz, G.: Restrictive cardiomyopathy in pseudoxanthoma elasticum. Chest 78:113, 1980.
341. Lebwohl, M., DiStefano, K., Prioleau, P. G., Uram, M., Yannuzzi, L. A., and Fleischmajer, R.: Pseudoxanthoma elasticum and mitral prolapse. N. Engl. J. Med. 307:228, 1982.
342. Meislik, J., Neldner, K., Reever, E., and Ellis, P.: Laser treatment in the maculopathy of pseudoxanthoma elasticum. Can. J. Ophthalmol. 13:210, 1978.
343. Cunningham, J. R., Lippman, S. M., Reine, W. A., Francomano, C. A., Maumenee, I. H., and Pyeritz, R. E.: Pseudoxanthoma elasticum: Treatment of gastrointestinal hemorrhage by arterial embolization and observations on autosomal dominant inheritance. Johns Hopkins Med. J. 147:168, 1980.
344. Huang, S. N., Steele, H. D., Kumar, G., et al.: Ultrastructural changes of elastic fibers in pseudoxanthoma elasticum: A study of histogenesis. Arch. Pathol. 83:108, 1967.
345. Uitto, J., Christiano, A. M., Kähäri, V.-M., Bashir, M. M., and Rosenbloom, J.: Molecular biology and pathology of human elastin. Biochem. Soc. Trans. 19:824, 1991.
346. Uitto, J.: Biochemistry of the elastic fibers in normal connective tissues and its alterations in diseases. J. Invest. Dermatol. 72:1, 1979.

Chapter 96

Theodore J. Hahn

Metabolic Bone Disease

INTRODUCTION

Although the functioning of all organ systems is regulated by local and systemic factors, bone is almost unique in the degree to which it is responsive to these influences. Its mass, shape, chemical composition, and mechanical properties are in large part the product of the coordinated effects of multiple hormonal and local factors that act on it. In simplest terms, metabolic bone diseases are generalized skeletal disorders caused by alterations in bone cell metabolism as a result of abnormal systemic or local stimuli. This chapter discusses the methods for evaluating metabolic bone disorders and then examines the major metabolic bone diseases in detail. The cellular, hormonal, and local factors that regulate bone metabolism are discussed in Chapter 4.

CLINICAL EVALUATION OF OSTEOPENIC BONE DISORDERS

History and Physical Examination

The age of onset, location, and frequency of fractures should first be determined to establish the duration and severity of the disorder. Severe vertebral osteopenia is often accompanied by loss of height. In advanced cases, a loss of 2 to 6 inches is common. This loss is the result of both vertebral compression fractures and altered posture owing to kyphosis. Questioning should be directed toward determining the presence of risk factors for specific osteopenic disorders. These include a family history of osteoporosis; a history of treatment with supraphysiologic doses of glucocorticoids or other agents that adversely influence bone metabolism; premature gonadal hormone deficiency; disorders of thyroid, parathyroid, or adrenal function; juvenile-onset diabetes; gastrointestinal or renal disorders; cigarette smoking or alcohol abuse; a childhood history of deficient calcium intake; prolonged physical inactivity; and evidence of multiple myeloma or other neoplastic disorders that adversely influence bone cell function.

Confirmatory evidence for osteopenia and its various specific etiologies should be sought on physical examination. Dorsal kyphosis may be the first clinical indication of loss of spinal bone mass. With advanced bone loss, severe kyphosis is combined with loss of vertebral height to reduce the volume of the thoracic and abdominal cavities. This can result in respiratory difficulties, abdominal protuberance, early satiety owing to increased pressure on the stomach, and pain caused by the pressure of the lower costal margins abutting on the pelvic brim. Specific areas of spinal tenderness and paravertebral muscle spasm may indicate recent vertebral fractures. Proximal myopathy may suggest a vitamin D or phosphate deficiency state, thyrotoxicosis, or a neoplastic disorder. Subtle cushingoid features may hint of a previously undetected state of glucocorticoid excess, and testicular atrophy could suggest hypogonadism in an otherwise normal osteopenic male. Occasionally, blue sclerae may signal osteogenesis imperfecta tarda in a young adult with severe osteopenia.

Radiologic Quantitation of Osteopenia

Radiologic quantitation of the degree of bone loss involves variable degrees of uncertainty, depending on the technique employed.[1, 2] No currently available technique is entirely satisfactory.

Routine radiographic techniques are capable of detecting generalized osteopenia only after a 30 to 50 percent loss of bone mass.[3] Trabecular bone has a higher rate of metabolic activity and hence is more sensitive to imbalances in bone formation and resorption. Therefore, in generalized osteopenia, radiologic evidence of bone loss is usually observed first in areas of the skeleton with the highest content of trabecular bone. These regions include the vertebrae, pelvis, ribs, and metaphyseal ends of long bones. Among the earliest radiologic signs of osteopenia in the vertebra are decreased radiodensity of the body of the vertebra and a relative increase in density of the upper and lower end plates owing to loss of trabecular bone in the vertebral body (Fig. 96–1). With more advanced bone loss, there may be biconcave compression of the vertebral end plates owing to the pressure of the intervertebral discs (Fig. 96–2) or herniation of the nucleus pulposus into the body of the vertebra, producing a mushroom-shaped defect in the upper or lower vertebral surface (Schmorl's node). Anterior wedge compressions give rise to kyphotic deformity, e.g., the dowager's hump.

The progressive loss of groups of trabeculae in the upper femur form the basis of the semiquantitative Singh index of bone loss. The reproducibility and prognostic value of this technique, however, are

1593

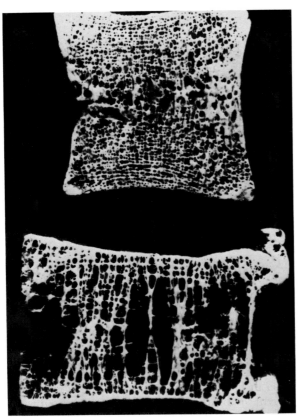

Figure 96–1. Midsagittal view of a lumbar vertebra of a young *(upper)* and an elderly *(lower)* female. Note marked loss of trabeculae with age. (From Avioli, L. V., and Krane, S. M. [eds.]: Metabolic Bone Disease. Vol I. New York, Academic Press, 1977. Used by permission.)

questionable.[4] In regions of predominantly cortical bone such as the shafts of the clavicle, femur, humerus, or metacarpals, decreased cortical thickness and increased porosity may be observed. This is the basis of the metacarpal index, which is calculated on the basis of cortical bone loss in the second metacarpal. If the combined thickness of the two cortices at the midshaft point is less than 45 percent of total bone width, this is considered to be evidence of significantly decreased bone mass.[5] This technique, however, is insensitive to trabecular bone loss, a major factor in most forms of osteopenia.

The *photon absorption bone mass measurement technique* is capable of detecting a less than 5 percent loss of bone mass and represents a major technical advance in the quantitation of osteopenia. Single-beam photon absorption (SPA) measurements of bone mass in the appendicular skeleton, typically in the distal radius or ulna, have been widely used for the past 20 years and have been shown to predict fracture risk in population studies.[1] SPA is relatively insensitive in the early detection of most forms of osteopenia in an individual patient, however, because it measures an area of primarily cortical (compact) bone. Cortical bone, in contrast to the more cellular trabecular (spongiosa) bone found in the ribs, vertebrae, and ends of long bones, is relatively slow to

respond in most osteopenic disorders. On the other hand, SPA bone mass measurement of the forearm may be a useful adjuvant assessment in certain situations in which there can be disproportionate loss of cortical bone, such as in primary hyperparathyroidism.[6]

Dual-beam photon absorptiometry (DPA) techniques have been developed that can measure bone density in the lumbar spine and femoral neck. DPA techniques are particularly useful because the spine and femoral neck contain a high proportion of trabecular bone, show a greater percentage decrease in mass in metabolic bone disorders, and are high-risk areas for fracture.[7] Thus, it is now possible to detect osteopenia routinely in its very early stages. Earlier DPA instruments, which used an isotopic source to generate the photon beam, were capable of detecting a 3 to 5 percent loss of bone mass. Although this degree of accuracy represented a major advance over standard radiographic techniques, it was not sufficient to permit reliable annual monitoring of therapeutic responses in patients with postmenopausal and other forms of osteoporosis, in which the rate of bone loss is on the order of 1 to 2 percent per year.

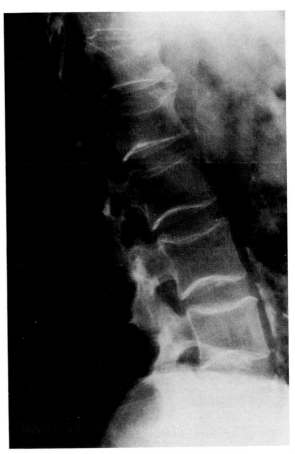

Figure 96–2. Lumbar vertebrae in moderately severe osteoporosis. Note the distinct cortices on the upper and lower borders of the vertebrae, in contrast to the "washed out" appearance of the central portions of the vertebral bodies. Varying degrees of early compression are seen in the lower three vertebrae, while the upper two vertebrae demonstrate partial collapse.

The development of *dual-energy x-ray–based absorptiometry* (DEXA) technology, however, now permits measurement of spine and hip bone density with a reproducibility error of approximately 1 and 2 percent, respectively, under optimal circumstances.[1, 2] This is sufficient sensitivity to permit meaningful annual follow-up measurements in most osteopenic disorders.

Quantitative computed tomography (QCT) measurement of vertebral trabecular bone mass is also useful for quantitating bone mass in the spine and has the special advantage of being capable of separately determining cortical and trabecular bone mass in the vertebrae.[8, 9] In expert hands, this technique can reliably detect a 5 percent loss of spine bone mass. The reproducibility of QCT measurements, however, is usually considerably less than that of DEXA techniques.

DEXA and QCT vertebral mass measurements each have their individual advantages and disadvantages[1, 8, 9] (Table 96–1). DEXA measurements can be done rapidly (15 to 20 minutes for both spine and hip), are highly reproducible, and impart a total absorbed dose of radiation, which is 0.5 to 1 percent that of QCT. On the other hand, DPA and DEXA measurements of the spine are subject to artifacts produced by overlying aortic calcifications and extensive osteophytic disease. These latter disorders increase in frequency with age and may invalidate DPA and DEXA spine bone mass measurements in patients over age 70. QCT is not subject to these artifacts but has a lower degree of reproducibility. Thus, for the majority of patients, DEXA bone mass measurement is the current technique of choice for routine clinical monitoring.

The *indications for clinical bone mass measurement* (Table 96–2) have been a point of considerable controversy. The accuracy of SPA and earlier DPA techniques was not sufficient to detect early osteopenia or to monitor the response to treatment over reasonable intervals of time. With the advent of highly accurate DEXA techniques, however, it has become generally accepted that there are at least four specific indications for routine DEXA measurement of bone mass: (1) perimenopausal or recent postmenopausal status in women who are potential candidates for estrogen replacement therapy, (2) vertebral abnormalities on routine radiography that suggest osteopenia, (3) a history of long-term glucocorticoid therapy, and (4) asymptomatic primary hyperparathyroidism.[1, 10] In addition, it seems advisable to screen certain other individuals at high risk for osteopenia, including patients with biliary cirrhosis, gastrointestinal malabsorption, partial gastrectomy, prolonged immobilization, chronic treatment with other agents known to affect bone adversely (anticonvulsant drugs, cyclosporin A, high-dose heparin), a history of prolonged thyroid hormone excess, or a strong family history of osteoporosis (see appropriate sections following).

Biochemical Testing

Serum biochemistries, particularly calcium and phosphate concentration, should be determined in the morning after an overnight fast to avoid variations caused by dietary intake and normal circadian rhythms.

Serum calcium is approximately 50 percent ionized (free), 40 percent complexed to proteins (mainly albumin), and 10 percent complexed to citrate, phosphate, and bicarbonate.[11] Determination of the serum ionized calcium directly measures the biologically active calcium fraction. The total serum calcium concentration can be roughly corrected for changes in serum protein concentration by adding or subtracting 0.8 mg per dl calcium for each 1 g per dl change in serum albumin relative to the mean normal value. *Serum phosphate* concentration must always be determined in the fasting state because serum phosphate levels routinely increase by 1 to 2 mg per dl after a meal.[12] Only about 10 percent of the serum inorganic phosphate is bound to plasma proteins.[11]

Although *alkaline phosphatase* is a marker of osteoblastic activity, serum total alkaline phosphatase level is a relatively insensitive index of bone turnover owing to the presence of hepatobiliary, intestinal, and other isoenzymes.[13] Accordingly, the serum specific bone alkaline phosphatase isoenzyme level is a more accurate index of osteoblastic activity. Marked elevations of serum alkaline phosphatase occur most commonly in osteomalacia and Paget's disease. Following a major bone fracture, however, increased osteoblastic activity can elevate the serum alkaline phosphatase level by as much as twofold to threefold for a period of several months. Serum levels of the osteoblast-specific protein *osteocalcin* (bone Gla protein) provide a similar index of osteoblast activity independent of bone resorption.[14–16] Osteocalcin levels exhibit a marked diurnal variation, however, being highest at about 4:00 A.M. and falling by as much as 50 percent to a nadir in the afternoon. Hence, to use osteocalcin measurements to follow bone responses, use of carefully timed early morning determinations is mandatory. Moreover, osteocalcin levels may change postprandially, are increased by decreasing renal function, may be induced by vitamin D metabolites, and may vary throughout the menstrual cycle.[16a] Thus, osteocalcin measurements are useful only when employed under carefully controlled conditions.

Urinary calcium excretion reflects primarily the filtered calcium load. Changes in serum ionized calcium concentration are usually accompanied by parallel changes in urinary calcium excretion. The normal range of 24-hour urinary calcium excretion is 1.5 to 4 mg per kg ideal body weight.[17] Subnormal values are seen in hypocalcemia and disorders associated with reduced intestinal calcium absorption. Hypercalcemic disorders, increased bone resorption, and states of increased intestinal calcium absorption pro-

Table 96–1. RADIOLOGIC TECHNIQUES FOR QUANTITATING BONE MASS

Technique	Bone Loss Detection Threshold	Radiation Dose (mrem)	Advantages	Disadvantages
Standard radiograph Vertebrae	30–50%	400–1000	Simple, relatively inexpensive, routinely available	Very insensitive, highly variable
Metacarpal index Phalanx	20–30%	40–70	Simple, inexpensive, accurate for cortical mass	Relatively insensitive, does not detect trabecular bone loss
Single-beam photon absorptiometry Forearm	4–6%	10–20	Low radiation dose, accurate for appendicular cortical mass	Poor correlation with vertebral mass, arm repositioning is source of error in longitudinal studies, poor correction for differences in surrounding soft tissues
Dual-energy photon absorptiometry, isotope-based (DPA) Vertebrae	5–7%	5–8	Sensitive, low radiation dose, good correlation with risk of vertebral fracture, corrects for soft tissue differences	Aortic calcifications and osteophytes may interfere, measures combined cortical and trabecular bone
Femoral neck	7–9%	5–8	Sensitive, low radiation dose, good correlation with risk of hip fracture, corrects for soft tissues, can measure areas of primarily trabecular or mixed cortical/trabecular bone	More time-consuming, repositioning is potential source of error
Dual-energy x-ray absorptiometry (DEXA) Vertebrae	1–3%	1–3	As for DPA, except more accurate, faster, lower radiation dose	As for DPA
Femoral neck	2–5%	1–3		
Quantitative computed tomography	5–7%	200–1000	Sensitive, good correlation with risk of vertebral fractures, can measure both pure trabecular and mixed cortical/trabecular mass, no interference from aortic calcifications or spinal osteophytes	Higher radiation dose, results may vary with instrument, vertebral fat infiltration may produce artifactually low readings in osteoporosis

Table 96–2. INDICATIONS FOR BONE DENSITY MEASUREMENT

Definite
Perimenopausal and postmenopausal status in women who are potential candidates for estrogen replacement therapy
Vertebral abnormalities on routine radiograph that suggest osteopenia
Long-term glucocorticoid therapy
Asymptomatic primary hyperparathyroidism
Possible
Biliary cirrhosis
Gastrointestinal malabsorption or partial gastrectomy
Prolonged near-total immobilization
Prolonged treatment with other agents known or suspected to affect bone adversely (anticonvulsant drugs, cyclosporin A, high-dose heparin, methotrexate)
Strong family history of osteoporosis

duce hypercalciuria. In addition, the fasting morning urinary calcium/creatinine ratio obtained after a 12-hour overnight fast reflects the rate of bone resorption relative to formation. This test is performed on a morning spot urine obtained after the bladder has been emptied of the overnight urine. A fasting urinary calcium/creatinine ratio of greater than 0.30 suggests increased bone resorptive activity.[18, 19] The usefulness of the fasting urinary calcium/creatinine ratio declines after menopause because estrogens promote renal tubular resorption of calcium.[20] Because urinary calcium excretion is influenced by the filtered sodium load, a somewhat more accurate, sodium-corrected value for urinary calcium excretion can also be employed.[18] The influence of diuretic agents should also be considered; thiazide diuretics markedly decrease urinary calcium excretion, whereas furosemide and other loop diuretics increase calcium excretion.

Urinary phosphate excretion is primarily determined by dietary phosphate intake. Hence, measurement of 24-hour urinary phosphate excretion is of little diagnostic value. On the other hand, fasting fractional phosphate excretion is regulated by parathyroid hormone (PTH) and renal transport mechanisms. Therefore, increased levels of PTH or primary renal tubular phosphate resorption defects result in a decreased renal tubular resorption of filtered phosphate. This is best quantitated by determining the renal maximal transport capacity for phosphate ($TmPO_4$) expressed in terms of glomerular filtration rate (GFR), i.e., the $TmPO_4/GFR$.[21] This is a simple measurement performed by obtaining a morning fasting urine sample for phosphate and creatinine concentration, with blood phosphate and creatinine concentration measured at the same time. The urinary $C_{PO4}/C_{creatinine}$ ratio is then calculated by the equation:

$$\frac{(U_{PO4} \times S_{Creat})}{(S_{PO4} \times U_{Creat})}$$

Using the nomogram in Figure 96–3, the $TmPO_4/GFR$ can then be determined. When creatinine and phos-

phate concentrations are expressed in mass units (milligram per deciliter), the normal range for $TmPO_4/GFR$ is 2.5 to 4.0 mg per dl. Subnormal values indicate either increased PTH activity, as in hyperparathyroidism, or a primary defect in the renal phosphate resorption mechanism.

Serum PTH assays can be directed toward the COOH-terminal or NH_2-terminal segments, the midportion, or the intact PTH molecule.[22] Since biologic activity resides in amino acids 1 through 34 at the NH_2-terminal end, serum immunoreactive and bioactive PTH levels do not necessarily correlate. Only 5 to 30 percent of the circulating immunoreactive hormone is intact PTH; the remainder consists primarily of inactive COOH-terminal fragments.[23] The proportion of inactive fragments is further increased in renal insufficiency, in which clearance of the biologically inactive COOH-terminal fragments is markedly reduced. Hence, in patients with renal failure, COOH-terminal directed PTH assays give markedly elevated values, which do not accurately reflect the status of PTH biologic activity. COOH-terminal directed PTH assays were the first to be widely applied and were the clinical standard during the past decade. Midmolecule and intact molecule PTH assays, however, are not subject to artifactual elevations in renal insufficiency. Although both are suitable for detection of primary hyperparathyroidism and other states of chronic increased PTH secretion, the two-site intact molecule assay is the current measurement of choice.[22] Although measurement of circulating NH_2-

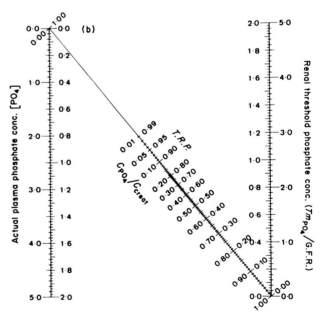

Figure 96–3. Nomogram for estimation of $TmPO_4/GFR$. The C_{PO4}/C_{creat} ratio (or tubular resorption of phosphate) is first calculated. Then a line drawn intersecting the value on the far-left vertical line for serum phosphate concentration (in either mg/dl *[outside scale]* or S.I units *[inside scale]*) and the value for C_{PO4}/C_{creat} on the middle vertical gives the $TmPO_4/GFR$ when extended to the far-right vertical line. (From Walton, R. J. and Bijvoet, O. L. L.: Nomogram for derivation of renal threshold phosphate concentration. Lancet 2:309, 1975, used by permission.)

terminal fragments theoretically offers a more direct index of PTH biologic activity, NH_2-terminal fragment levels are subject to more frequent fluctuations and hence are not as reliable in detecting chronic increases in PTH secretion.

Serum 25-hydroxyvitamin D [25(OH)D] assay is the most reliable and sensitive index of overall vitamin D status, since the hepatic production of this metabolite is in large part a function of vitamin D availability. Thus, significant vitamin D deficiency is associated with a reduced serum 25(OH)D level. In contrast, the serum 1,25-dihydroxyvitamin D [1,25(OH)$_2$D] concentration is tightly regulated and declines only in the most advanced stages of vitamin D deficiency.[24] Hence, use of 1,25(OH)$_2$D measurements should be limited to documenting reduced renal 25(OH)D-1a-hydroxylase activity such as occurs in renal insufficiency and tumor-induced osteomalacia.[23, 24]

Bone Biopsy

Bone biopsy may occasionally be useful in evaluating patients with metabolic bone disorders when the diagnosis is in doubt. To be of value, however, the biopsy must be performed in standardized fashion and interpreted by an expert bone histologist. The biopsy is obtained from the iliac crest under local anesthesia, using a Bordier needle or similar trochar.[25] Undecalcified sections are then examined to determine indices of osteoblast and osteoclast activity and to assess the degree of mineralization of newly formed bone matrix (osteoid) (Fig. 96–4). The rate of bone formation can be measured by taking advantage of the fact that tetracycline compounds localize in regions of newly forming bone and fluoresce under ultraviolet light. Before biopsy, the patient is given two 3-day courses of tetracycline (1 g per day) separated by an interval of 14 to 21 days. This ordinarily results in two bands of fluorescence when the bone biopsy is examined by fluorescent microscopy. The distance between the fluorescent bands divided by the number of days between the courses of tetracycline gives the bone formation rate. In normal adults, this value averages 1 μ per day. In patients with osteomalacia, there is a characteristic pattern of impaired bone uptake of tetracycline and delayed mineralization.

In most routine cases, the pathogenesis of the

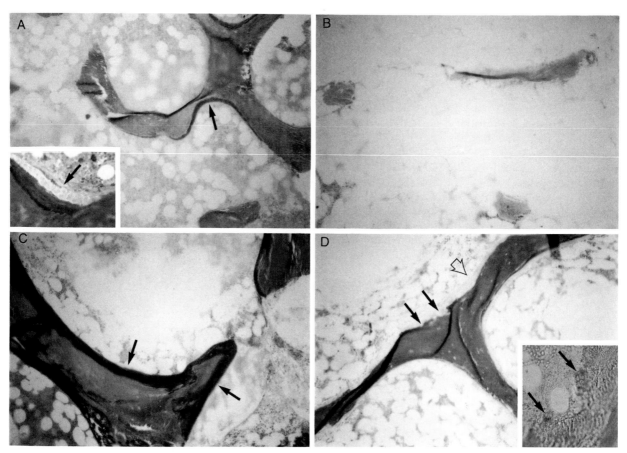

Figure 96–4. Bone histology in osteopenic disorders (undecalcified iliac crest bone biopsies). *A,* Normal bone. *B,* Osteoporosis. Note decreased size and fragmentation of bone trabeculae, reduced numbers of bone cells on the trabecular surface. *C,* Osteomalacia. Note marked increase in thickness and number of osteoid seams on the surface of mineralized bone. *D,* Osteitis fibrosa cystica (hyperparathyroidism). Note increased number of multinucleated osteoclasts, increased number of active osteoblasts, and fibrous tissue replacement of bone and marrow. (Courtesy of Dr. William G. Goodman, Nephrology Section, Sepulveda VA Medical Center, Los Angeles, CA.)

osteopenic disorder can be established with sufficient certainty on the basis of clinical data alone, and bone biopsy is not required. Primary indications for bone biopsy include determining the presence of osteomalacia in patients in whom the diagnosis is uncertain and evaluating the cellular response to therapy in patients with disorders such as renal osteodystrophy. Bone biopsy is far less sensitive than DPA, DEXA, and QCT in assessing changes in bone mass.

OSTEOPENIC BONE DISORDERS

Osteopenia is a purely clinical diagnosis indicating a decrease in bone mass relative to normal values for persons of identical age, sex, and race. This diagnosis can be presumed on the basis of a history of frequent bone fractures following minimal trauma but must be confirmed by documenting decreased bone mass radiographically.

The bone histologic changes seen in patients with osteopenia are of three main types: (1) osteoporosis, in which there is a parallel loss of bone mineral and matrix; (2) osteomalacia, characterized by deficient mineralization of bone and a resultant accumulation of unmineralized osteoid; and (3) osteitis fibrosa, in which there is increased PTH-stimulated osteoclastic resorption of bone mineral and matrix, with replacement by fibrous tissue (Table 96–3). Many patients with osteopenia exhibit a mixture of histologic changes with one form predominating.

Osteoporosis

Primary (Involutional) Osteoporosis

Pathogenesis. Osteoporosis (Table 96–4) is characterized by a parallel loss of bone mineral and matrix. With age, bone formation decreases to a greater extent than does resorption, resulting in a gradual loss of bone.[26] It is useful to classify age-related (physiologic) osteoporosis into two basic types. *Type I osteoporosis* is associated with estrogen loss in women owing to surgical or natural menopause and androgen loss in men. Its characteristic features include an increased rate of bone turnover with resorption exceeding formation and a relatively rapid rate of bone loss. Trabecular bone (which comprises a high proportion of the vertebrae, ribs, and pelvic bones) is especially affected, as demonstrated by the increase in vertebral fractures that occurs in women shortly after menopause. Rapid

Table 96–3. HISTOLOGIC CLASSIFICATION OF OSTEOPENIC DISORDERS

Osteoporosis	Decreased bone mineral and matrix
Osteomalacia	Decreased bone mineralization with normal or increased matrix
Osteitis fibrosa	PTH-stimulated bone resorption with replacement by fibrous elements

Table 96–4. CAUSES OF OSTEOPOROSIS

Physiologic
Postmenopausal estrogen deficiency (type I)
Primary age-related (involutional) (type II)
Secondary
Endocrine
  Glucocorticoid excess
  Premature ovarian failure
  Testicular insufficiency
  Thyroid hormone excess
  Diabetes mellitus (insulin-dependent)
Immobilization
Neoplastic disorders producing osteoclast-activating factors (OAFs): myeloma, lymphomas, leukemias
Chronic inflammatory disorders: rheumatoid arthritis, primary biliary cirrhosis
Treatment with cyclosporin A, methotrexate, or high-dose heparin
Chronic calcium or protein deficiency
Lipid storage disorders—Gaucher's disease
Congenital
Osteogenesis imperfecta tarda
Miscellaneous disorders—homocystinuria, Marfan's syndrome

type I bone loss in women occurs for 5 to 10 years following menopause. *Type II osteoporosis* is the result of the more gradual age-related decline in bone mass that occurs in both men and women after the fourth decade of life. The basic cause of this bone loss is unknown. Type II osteoporosis affects cortical bone and is associated with an increased incidence of hip fracture. Thus, the majority of hip fracture patients are over 70 years of age.[27]

Among the most important *risk factors for primary osteoporosis*, gender plays a predominant role (Table 96–5). Males and females have similar bone mass through early childhood. After puberty, however, males have a consistently greater bone mass, presumably owing to the anabolic effects of androgens.[28] Accordingly, age-related osteoporosis is far more common in women. By extreme old age, however, a marked loss of bone mass usually occurs in men as well.[29] Premature menopause in women and hypogonadism in men are major causes of accelerated bone loss leading to osteoporosis.[30–32] Genetic factors are also important determinants of bone mass. Whites and Asians have a consistently lower bone mass throughout life than do blacks and accordingly

Table 96–5. RISK FACTORS FOR AGE-RELATED OSTEOPOROSIS

Female gender
Premature loss of gonadal function
White or Asian ancestry
Family history of osteoporosis
Small bone structure
Thin body habitus
Decreased physical activity
Low calcium intake
Cigarette smoking
Alcohol abuse
Nulliparity

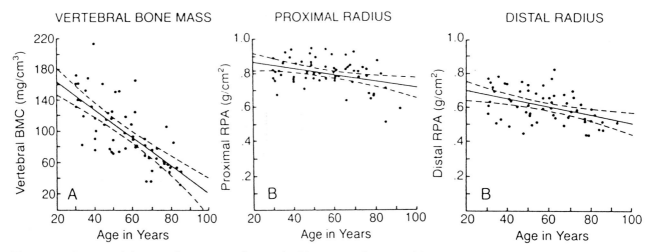

Figure 96–5. Patterns of change in bone mass with age in healthy men (with 95% confidence interval of the estimates) in the vertebrae *(A)* as measured by computed tomography, and the proximal radius *(B)* and distal radius *(C)* as measured by photon absorptiometry. (Modified from Meier, D. E., Orwoll, E. S., and Jones, J. M.: Marked disparity between trabecular and cortical bone loss with age in healthy men. Ann. Intern. Med. 101:605–612, 1984. Used by permission.)

have a much higher incidence of osteoporosis.[33] A study in the western United States demonstrated that vertebral and hip fracture incidence was highest in whites, followed by Asian Americans, and then black and Hispanic Americans.[34] Certain populations have an especially high incidence of osteoporosis, including Scandinavians and Eskimos.[35] In addition, osteoporosis exhibits a strong familial pattern.[30] There is a positive correlation between body weight and bone mass,[33, 36] and slim body habitus is associated with increased risk of osteoporosis, perhaps in part owing to a decreased rate of formation of estradiol in adipose tissue.[37] Increased hepatic oxidation of estrogens and androgens may similarly play a role in the increased incidence of osteoporosis in cigarette smokers.[38] The effects of alcohol abuse are probably multifactorial and may include direct toxic effects on bone cells.[30, 39]

Starting at about age 40, there is a progressive decline in bone mass that continues throughout life. The rate of bone loss initially averages 0.5 percent per year, increases somewhat with age to 1 to 2 percent annually, and then declines in extreme old age.[30, 40, 41] Loss is more rapid in vertebral bone, relative to appendicular sites, owing to the higher content of trabecular bone in the axial skeleton (Figs. 96–5 and 96–6). In addition, women at menopause undergo a marked acceleration of bone loss to rates of 2 to 4 percent per year for a period of 5 to 8 years, owing to loss of estrogen inhibition of bone resorption and turnover rate. This type I loss is initially most marked in the trabecular bone in vertebrae, ribs, pelvis, and the ends of long bones.

A variety of hypotheses have been advanced to attempt to explain the progressive loss of bone that normally occurs with age in both men and women (type II osteoporosis). These include reduced stimulation of osteoblasts owing to decreased muscle mass and a more sedentary lifestyle, increased PTH levels

owing to decreased efficiency of intestinal calcium absorption and increased urinary calcium loss, decreased renal mass leading to reduced 1,25(OH)$_2$D production, increased sensitivity of bone to PTH owing to declining gonadal hormone production, and reduced production of osteoblasts owing to decreased osteogenic stem cell function.[30, 42, 43] Probably most of these factors play a role in the pathogenesis of age-related osteoporosis. Certainly age-related bone loss is often a mixed process. For example, histologic evidence of concurrent osteoporosis and osteomalacia can be observed in postmenopausal women.[44] Moreover, histologic findings in patients

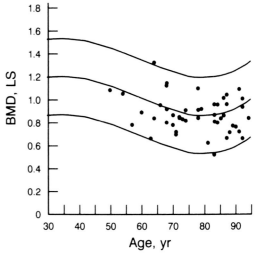

Figure 96–6. Pattern of change in bone mineral density (BMD) of the lumbar spine (LS) with age among women in Rochester, Minnesota. Women over age 50 years with one or more vertebral fractures are also indicated (●). (From Melton, L. J., III, Kan, S. H., Frye, M. A., Wahner, H. W., O'Fallon, W. M., and Riggs, B. L.: Epidemiology of vertebral fractures in women. Am. J. Epidemiol. 129:1000–1011, 1989. Used by permission.)

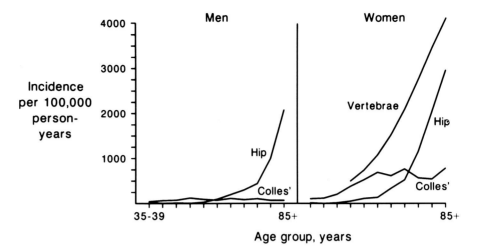

Figure 96–7. Age-related incidence of Colles' hip and vertebral fractures in men and women. (From Riggs, B. L., and Melton, L. J., III: Involutional osteoporosis. N. Engl. J. Med. 314:1676, 1986. Reprinted with permission from *The New England Journal of Medicine.*)

with osteoporosis range from a pattern of increased osteoclastic activity with moderate bone forming activity *(high turnover osteoporosis)* to virtually quiescent bone *(low turnover osteoporosis).*[45]

Clinical Features. Osteoporosis is a common disorder of late middle age and old age, affecting women approximately five times more frequently than men. Osteoporosis accounts for at least 1.2 million fractures annually in the United States, roughly distributed by site as vertebrae, 44 percent; hip, 20 percent; distal forearm, 14 percent; and other limb sites, 23 percent.[30, 46] The incidence of vertebral fractures in women increases soon after menopause and continues to rise with age. In contrast, hip fracture incidence rises gradually with age until late in life, when it increases rapidly to a very high rate, starting at about age 70[27] (Fig. 96–7). One third of women older than 65 years of age will have vertebral fractures, and by extreme old age one third of women and one sixth of men will have had a hip fracture. Hip fracture is frequently a catastrophic occurrence, carrying an associated mortality of 12 to 20 percent and necessitating long-term nursing home care for up to half of the survivors. Osteoporosis morbidity is not, however, limited to women. Twelve percent of all vertebral compression fractures and 20 to 25 percent of all hip fractures occur in men.[32]

The typical patient with osteoporosis is a light-framed white or Asian female between 50 and 70 years of age whose female relatives have a similar history of osteoporosis. The initial complaint is often spontaneous onset of severe back pain owing to a vertebral compression fracture. In other cases, progressive asymptomatic kyphosis is the first clinical indication of decreased bone mass. There are few characteristic physical findings in patients with primary osteoporosis. As a group, such patients are generally thinner and less muscular than their non-osteoporotic counterparts. Vertebral compression fractures with anterior wedging of the vertebral bodies lead to the typical "dowager's hump" and a pronounced downward angulation of the rib cage. A loss of 2 to 6 inches in height is common in advanced

cases with multiple vertebral compression fractures. Multiple vertebral compressions and progressive kyphosis lead to reduced lung capacity and increased pressure on the abdominal cavity, resulting in abdominal protuberance (Fig. 96–8). Recent vertebral fractures are associated with tenderness over the involved vertebra and local paravertebral muscle spasm. Radicular pain and neurologic abnormalities are uncommon, since the compression process generally spares the neural arch.

It is not possible to diagnose primary osteoporosis definitively by means of radiography alone. All that can be ascertained radiologically is that the bone mass is reduced. The degree of osteopenia can be quantitated radiologically as discussed earlier in the

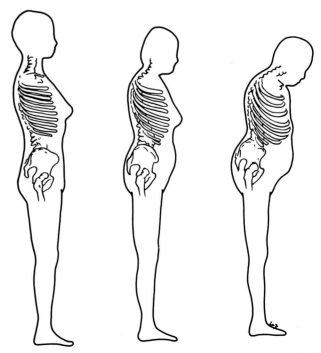

Figure 96–8. Sequence of spinal changes in osteopenia. Vertebral compression fractures cause sharp kyphosis (dowager's hump), loss of height, and a compression of the abdominal cavity that leads to abdominal protuberance.

Table 96–6. LABORATORY FINDINGS IN METABOLIC BONE DISEASES

Disorder	Serum					Urine	
	Ca	PO₄	Alkaline Phosphatase	iPTH	25(OH)D	Ca	TmPO₄/ GFR
Primary osteoporosis	N	N	N	N	N	N	N
Secondary osteoporosis							
Glucocorticoid excess	N	N	N, ↓	N, ↑	N	N	N, ↓
Estrogen deficiency	N	N	N	N	N	N	N
Testosterone deficiency	N	N	N	N	N	N	N
Osteomalacia							
Vitamin D deficiency	↓	↓	↑	↑	↓	↓	↓
Phosphate depletion	N	↓	↑	N	N	↑	N
Primary hyperparathyroidism	↑	↓	N, ↑	↑	N	↑	↓
Renal osteodystrophy	N, ↑, ↓	↑, N	↑, N	↑	N	↓	↓
Paget's disease	N	N	↑	N	N	N	N

N, Normal; ↑, increased; ↓, decreased.

section on radiologic quantitation of osteopenia. In typical involutional osteoporosis, routine serum and urinary biochemical values are entirely normal (Table 96–6), and the diagnosis is therefore based largely on the clinical situation and exclusion of other generalized demineraling disorders including endocrinopathies, osteomalacia, and multiple myeloma. When the diagnosis is in doubt, iliac crest bone biopsy may occasionally be useful.

A specific small subset of older women with osteoporosis is characterized by elevated serum PTH levels and a marked reduction of 24-hour urine calcium excretion.[47] Histologically, these patients have high turnover osteoporosis as manifested by increased osteoclastic activity superimposed on severe osteoporosis. The basis of this disorder is not well defined but probably represents an extreme manifestation of the usual age-related decline in intestinal calcium absorption.

An additional subset of osteoporosis that occurs in young and middle-aged men is characterized by hypercalciuria and bone histologic evidence of increased osteoclastic activity.[48] All standard hormonal and vitamin D metabolite measurements are normal, and serum iPTH is in the low to normal range. The increased osteoclastic activity in these individuals presumably reflects the effects of an as yet unidentified humoral osteoclast-stimulating factor.

Management. The treatment of osteoporosis is currently far from satisfactory. Much of the problem lies in the fact that the majority of patients are in the older age groups and consequently have reduced bone turnover rates. Therefore, any manipulations that reduce bone resorption or increase bone formation require an extended period of time before improvement is manifested clinically.

Prophylaxis is the most effective form of management because there are currently no treatment regimens proved to produce a major, clinically useful reversal of bone loss in advanced osteoporosis (Table 96–7). There has been increased interest in the potential importance of *peak bone mass*. It appears likely that achieving the highest possible peak bone mass in early adulthood will reduce the ultimate degree of

osteoporosis produced by age-related bone loss in later life.[49, 50] Peak bone mass is achieved by about age 35, after which bone density starts a downward trend.[51] In women, 90 percent or more of this peak value may be reached by age 16.[49] Hereditary and racial factors are probably the most important determinants of peak bone mass. Black children have higher bone density than do white children,[52–54] bone density in teenage girls correlates to that of their mothers and fathers,[49] and bone density in monozygotic twins is better correlated than in dizygotic

Table 96–7. REGIMENS FOR MANAGEMENT OF OSTEOPOROSIS*

Prophylaxis
Identify high-risk individuals on basis of risk factors
General measures
  Maintain regular program of weight-bearing physical activity
  Maintain adequate calcium intake (800 mg/day premenopausal and 1500 mg/day postmenopausal)
  Eliminate adverse health habits—smoking, alcohol excess
Strongly consider estrogen replacement in high-risk women at menopause
Established Osteoporosis
Rule out endocrine disorders, osteomalacia, and multiple myeloma
Quantitate bone mass by DEXA measurement and follow at 12-month intervals to monitor response to treatment
General measures as for prophylaxis
Reduce risk of falling by minimizing use of sedatives and psychoactive drugs, and "fall-proofing" patient's home environment
If 24-hour urine calcium is less than 1 mg/kg body weight (off of thiazide therapy), supplement cautiously with vitamin D plus calcium to maintain urine calcium at 2–3 mg/kg/24 hours
Strongly consider estrogen replacement in women less than 5 years after menopause or if there is evidence of high bone turnover (increased serum osteocalcin, fasting urinary Ca/Cr >0.30); estrogen is also of benefit in older individuals
Calcitonin may be of benefit in patients with high bone turnover in whom estrogens cannot be used
Sodium etidronate given *cyclically* for 2 weeks out of every 3 months may be of benefit. At present, treatment should not be continued more than 2 years until further long-term data are available

*See text for dosages and side effects.
DEXA, Dual-energy x-ray absorptiometry.

twins.[53] Hormonal status is important, since there are significant correlations between bone mass and both serum estrogen and androgen levels in young women.[55] Also, preliminary studies indicate that calcium balance correlates with calcium intake in teenage girls,[49] and recent twin studies indicate that calcium supplementation in prepubertal children can significantly enhance the rate of increase in bone mineral density.[49a]

Finally, physical activity also has an important influence on bone mass in young adults.[55a] Compressive forces increase bone mass in animals,[56] and prospective studies have shown that military recruits can increase their tibial bone density by 8 to 12 percent following 14 weeks of intensive basic training.[57] In addition, muscle-building and weight-bearing exercise produces a greater increase in bone density than does aerobic exercise.[58] On the other hand, in young women strenuous training to a degree that causes amenorrhea is usually associated with a decrease in bone mass to subnormal levels owing to estrogen deficiency. Bone mass in amenorrheic athletes, however, is generally greater than that in amenorrheic nonathletes,[59–61] indicating that estrogen status and physical activity have separate, additive effects on bone mass. Therefore, achieving maximal peak bone mass in young women requires maintenance of optimum calcium intake, menstrual status, and exercise levels.

It is currently a matter of controversy as to whether women should undergo routine bone density screening for osteoporosis. It seems reasonable, however, to screen most high-risk women, especially light-framed white and Asian females with a family history of osteoporosis, at the onset of menopause, using a highly sensitive technique such as DEXA. If bone mass at menopause is within normal limits, no specific intervention regimen may be warranted, whereas individuals with subnormal bone mass should be identified early and specific preventive measures started as soon as possible. All high-risk individuals, however, regardless of bone density level, should be started on a general preventive program. This should include proper nutrition, appropriate calcium intake, and a regular regimen of weight-bearing physical activity, such as walking for 30 to 60 minutes three or more times each week. Also, risk factors such as cigarette smoking and excessive alcohol intake should be eliminated.

In women who are already osteoporotic, measures should be taken to minimize the risk of falling. The major risk factors for falls in the elderly are also determinants of risk for hip fracture.[62–64] Such factors include arthritis and other forms of lower limb dysfunction, neurologic disorders, visual impairment, poor cognitive function, and use of psychoactive drugs. High mobility also correlates with fracture risk, presumably owing to an increased risk of experiencing severe trauma. Management should include efforts to limit the potential adverse influence of these factors and to eliminate factors from the patient's environment that increase the risk of falling.

However, although 90 percent of hip fractures are associated with a fall, less than 5 percent of falls result in a fracture. Hence, bone strength plays a major role in fracture prevention.

The role of calcium supplementation in preventing bone loss is currently controversial. In most women, calcium intake is considerably less than the recommended level required to maintain calcium balance.[65] Dietary calcium intake in individuals with poor intake of dairy products can be as low as 400 mg per day. The current recommendation for total calcium intake (diet plus supplements) is 1200 mg per day for ages 10 to 25, 800 to 1000 mg per day for ages 30 to 40, 800 to 1000 mg per day for postmenopausal women receiving estrogen replacement, and 1000 to 1500+ mg per day for postmenopausal women not on estrogens.[66] Often only an inordinately high calcium intake, however, on the order of 1500 to 2500 mg per day, can overcome the decline in intestinal calcium absorption that occurs in older postmenopausal women not receiving estrogens,[66] and the amount of calcium supplementation required to achieve this total intake is often poorly tolerated.

The form in which calcium supplementation is taken is of some importance. In achlorhydric patients, calcium citrate is preferable to calcium carbonate or other compounds, owing to its better solubility at high pH.[67] In all other patients, calcium carbonate is the generally preferred form, owing to considerations of tablet size and cost. Calcium carbonate is best absorbed when taken with meals, when tablet gastric retention time is greater and acidity is higher. Because calcium carbonate tablets from various manufacturers vary considerably in their solubility owing to differences in manufacturing techniques,[68] the patient should test the solubility of the particular tablet being used by determining whether it flakes into a particulate state after 30 minutes in a glass of vinegar.

Several studies have reported that a 2-year course of calcium supplementation in women at menopause does not produce a detectable decrease in the rate of bone loss.[69, 70] Also, a study of 400 elderly white women showed no relationship between calcium intake and bone loss over a 5-year period.[71] There is a considerable body of evidence, however, that suggests a beneficial long-term effect of calcium supplementation on the rate of appendicular cortical bone loss in postmenopausal women. The calcium effect appears greatest when baseline calcium intake is low (less than 800 mg per day).[72] Adequate calcium intake may be of greatest importance during childhood and adolescence, to promote maximal peak bone mass in early adulthood.[49, 72a] An increased incidence of lactose intolerance has been observed in osteoporotic patients, suggesting that life-long calcium deprivation owing to avoidance of dairy products may accelerate the development of osteoporosis.[73] Therefore, it is recommended that premenopausal women have a calcium intake of at least 800 to 1000 mg per day, increasing to 1200 to 1500 mg per day after menopause. This level of calcium intake has been shown to maintain calcium balance.[65] Twenty-four hour urinary calcium excretion should be determined before starting calcium supplements to exclude pre-existing hypercalciuria (urinary excretion of >4 mg calcium per kg body weight per 24 hours). In the subset of osteoporotic patients with clinical evidence of deficient calcium absorption and bone biopsy evidence of increased PTH activity, vitamin D and calcium intake should be increased to a level sufficient to maintain urinary calcium excretion in the normal range.

It appears likely that *exercise* can help maintain bone mass in adults.[74] Perimenopausal women who performed 3 hours per week of the President's Council on Fitness exercises showed an increase in total body calcium.[75, 76] There is current controversy as to the relative merits of simple weight-bearing exercise such as walking or jogging, as opposed to resistance exercise such as weight training, with each approach having its proponents.[77–80] Current data indicate that optimal results seem to require skeletal weight bearing and some resistive muscle activity.[80] The exercise program must be maintained, however, because all bone mass benefits are lost if the exercise is discontinued. At present, it is reasonable to recommend a program of walking for 30 to 60 minutes three to four times per week as a general exercise program for maintaining bone mass and lower extremity muscle tone in perimenopausal and postmenopausal women.

Estrogen replacement starting at the menopause should be considered the mainstay of osteoporosis prevention. This approach has been shown to be of definite benefit in reducing the rate of bone loss and the incidence of bone fractures and should be considered in all high-risk women (see under Gonadal Hormone Deficiency later).

Calcitonin inhibits bone resorption by suppressing osteoclast activity and can be used for the treatment of senile or postmenopausal osteoporosis in situations in which estrogen cannot be employed. Injectable and intranasal calcitonin can inhibit bone loss both at the menopause and in established osteoporosis.[81–83] A typical effective regimen would be calcitonin, 50 to 100 units subcutaneously 3 days a week.[81] At this time, intranasal calcitonin is not available in the United States. Responses are most marked in patients with a high bone turnover rate.[81, 82] As is the case with other antiresorptive agents such as estrogen and diphosphonates, calcitonin may produce a 4 to 8 percent increase in vertebral bone mass over the first 12 to 18 months of therapy. This appears to be due to an initial continuation of bone forming activity in the presence of suppressed bone resorption.[84] Formation and resorption, however, subsequently establish a new equilibrium, albeit at a lower bone turnover rate. Thus, the long-term effect is a diminished rate of bone loss. When therapy is discontinued, the rate of bone loss returns to previous levels.[82] Calcitonin has not yet been conclusively shown to reduce fracture rates, although the bone density response suggests that

this will be the case. There is also a mild, apparently central, analgesic effect of calcitonin, which may provide some additional benefit.[85] The current use of calcitonin in osteoporosis is limited by the inconvenience of the need for injections, frequent troublesome physiologic side effects (flushing, nausea), and high cost. With the general introduction of intranasal calcitonin, some of these problems may be overcome. Calcitonin has also proved useful in the treatment of the syndrome of high turnover osteoporosis associated with hypercalciuria and osteoclastosis in middle-aged men.[48]

Diphosphonates are slowly hydrolyzable diphosphate analogues that inhibit osteoclastic bone resorption. Data suggest that these antiresorptive agents may prove useful in the treatment of postmenopausal osteoporosis.[85a] Diphosphonates have the advantage of oral administration and minimal side effects limited to the gastrointestinal tract (indigestion, mild abdominal bloating). Studies have shown that in patients with postmenopausal osteoporosis, a 2-year course of cyclical treatment with oral sodium etidronate, given in a dose of 400 mg once daily for 2 weeks out of every 3 months, produced a 4 to 6 percent increase in spinal bone density relative to control subjects (Fig. 96–9). Moreover, the occurrence of new vertebral fractures was significantly reduced.[86, 87] Sodium etidronate *must* be used cyclically, however, since it has mineralization-inhibiting effects, which can reduce bone strength and actually increase fracture incidence if the drug is used on a

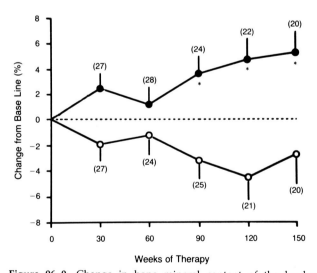

Figure 96–9. Change in bone mineral content of the lumbar vertebrae (L-2 to L-4) in postmenopausal women with osteoporosis who received intermittent cyclic therapy with sodium etidronate *(solid circles)* or placebo *(open circles).* The bars indicate the SEM for each value; values in asterisks are the numbers of patients evaluated at each time point. Asterisk denotes values significantly different from basal and control group values (p < 0.01). (From Storm, T., et al.: Effect of intermittent cyclical etidronate therapy on bone mass and fracture rate in women with postmenopausal osteoporosis. N. Engl. J. Med. 322:1265, 1990. Reprinted with permission from *The New England Journal of Medicine.*)

daily basis in high doses.[88] The longer-term effects of sodium etidronate on fracture incidence have not been examined, and decreased bone mineralization must be considered a potential adverse side effect of long-term therapy. This agent has not yet received approval from the Food and Drug Administration for use in osteoporosis. Newer diphosphonate analogues, such as pamidronate (APD), have minimal effects on osteoblast function and may therefore prove more suitable for long-term therapy.[89] These agents, however, are not yet available in the United States. Patients should receive calcium supplementation of 500 to 1000 mg per day during etidronate treatment.

Fluoride therapy has been used for a number of years on an experimental basis for the treatment of osteoporosis. Fluoride stimulates bone formation and can substantially increase vertebral bone mass.[90, 91] The basis of these effects appears to be direct stimulation of osteoblast replication and function.[92] A 4-year prospective, controlled, double-blind study examined the effects of sodium fluoride, 75 mg per day, plus calcium, 1500 mg per day, versus calcium alone on bone mass and fracture incidence in women with postmenopausal osteoporosis.[93] Although bone density increased by 35 percent in the spine and 12 percent in the femoral neck, there was a 4 percent decrease in cortical bone in the forearm. Moreover, fluoride therapy did not reduce the incidence of new vertebral fractures, and the treatment group had a threefold higher rate of nonvertebral fractures, primarily in the lower extremities (Fig. 96–10). Thus, the fluoride-stimulated new bone appeared to lack normal strength. It has been suggested that the lack of improved bone strength may have been due to toxic effects of the high dose of fluoride used in these studies, and others using slow-release fluoride cyclically in lower doses have reported reduced vertebral fracture incidence, in concert with evidence of improved bone matrix structure.[94, 95] Until the efficacy of these regimens is proved in larger controlled studies, however, fluoride therapy must be considered experimental and without proved benefit in osteoporosis.

Other Regimens. *Thiazides* reduce urinary calcium excretion and produce a mild systemic alkalosis, both of which effects should favor increased bone mass. There have been contrasting findings with regard to clinical efficacy, however, with various groups reporting increased bone mass and decreased fracture incidence[96, 97] and others findings no beneficial effect.[98] Therefore, thiazides cannot be currently recommended for osteoporosis prevention. Loop diuretics, however, such as furosemide increase urinary calcium excretion, have been associated with increased hip fracture incidence,[98] and should not be routinely used in patients with osteoporosis. *Coherence therapy* attempts to induce synchronous functioning of all bone remodeling units by the repeated sequential administration of agents that should first activate bone-forming units and then depress osteo-

clastic activity. This should theoretically both enhance the number of active bone remodeling units and stimulate bone formation in excess of resorption. Examples of such regimens are the sequential administration of phosphate followed by a diphosphonate[99] or growth hormone followed by calcitonin.[100] Although preliminary results have been encouraging, longer-term studies in larger population groups are required to establish coherence therapy as a useful approach to osteoporosis. The efficacy of *calcitriol* therapy to enhance bone mass by increasing intestinal calcium absorption is controversial[101, 102] and must be considered as being of no proved benefit. *Anabolic steroids* such as nandrolone deconate, given in a dose of 50 mg intramuscularly every 2 to 3 weeks, can significantly increase vertebral bone mass in postmenopausal osteoporosis.[103] Treatment may be associated with masculinizing side effects, how-

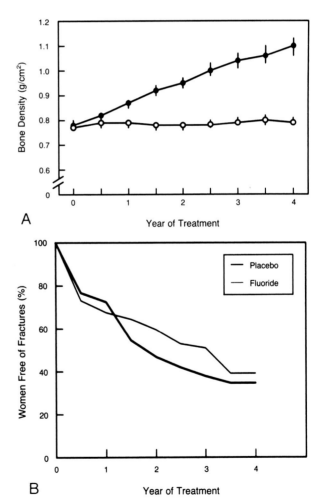

Figure 96–10. Response to treatment with sodium fluoride, 75 mg per day, plus calcium, 1500 mg per day, in postmenopausal women with osteoporosis. The upper panel illustrates the change in lumbar spine bone density in the fluoride-treated group (*solid circles*) and the placebo group (*open circles*). The lower panel shows the proportion of patients who did not have new vertebral fractures. (From Riggs, B. L., et al.: N. Engl. J. Med. 322:802, 1990. Reprinted with permission from *The New England Journal of Medicine.*)

ever, including possible adverse effects on low-density lipoprotein (LDL) and high-density lipoprotein (HDL) cholesterol, and gains in bone mass regress when therapy is discontinued. Reduction of fracture incidence has not yet been demonstrated.

Endocrine Disorders

Glucocorticoid Excess. Cushing's disease or long-term treatment with supraphysiologic doses of glucocorticoids frequently produces a severe osteopenia, which resembles idiopathic osteoporosis.[104, 105] Occasionally, the typical features of Cushing's syndrome may not be apparent, and osteopenia can be the major presenting problem. The osteopenia is considerably more severe in those regions of the skeleton with a high content of trabecular bone.[106] Hence, fractures are particularly common in the vertebrae, ribs, and ends of long bones. The reported incidence of bone fractures in glucocorticoid-treated patients ranges from 8 to 18 percent and is at least twofold to threefold greater than in similar patients treated with other agents.[105–108]

A number of risk factors for the development of steroid-induced osteopenia have been identified (Table 96–8). A direct relationship has been demonstrated between the cumulative glucocorticoid dose, the degree of bone loss, and the incidence of bone fractures. There is no correlation, however, between the current daily steroid dose and any of these parameters.[106, 108] Also, relative to other steroid-treated individuals, patients with inflammatory arthritis exhibit a greater degree of bone loss.[106] This may reflect the additive effects of relative immobilization and increased production of inflammatory cytokines.[106, 109] The basic predisposition to lose bone in response to glucocorticoid administration is independent of age, sex, race, menopausal status, or level of physical function.[108] The occurrence of clinically significant reductions in bone mass, however, leading to increased fracture incidence is greatest in children, postmenopausal women, patients of both sexes over the age of 50, and relatively immobilized individuals.[106–108] In older, immobilized, and postmenopausal individuals, pre-existing low bone mass values permit a rapid further reduction to a clinically significant degree of osteopenia. In younger individuals, a high initial rate of bone turnover predisposes to more rapid bone loss.

The bone loss produced by glucocorticoid excess appears to be due to two primary mechanisms: (1) suppression of osteoblast function and (2) inhibition of intestinal calcium absorption.[104] In addition, glucocorticoids also promote bone loss by directly stimulating PTH secretion and enhancing urinary calcium excretion[110, 111] (Fig. 96–11). Suppression of osteoblastic bone-forming activity appears to play the predominant role[112] and is apparently a direct effect of glucocorticoids, mediated in part by suppression of osteoblast function and osteoblast precursor maturation.[113, 114] Moreover, the marked reduction in

Table 96–8. RISK FACTORS FOR GLUCOCORTICOID-INDUCED OSTEOPENIA

Major
High total cumulative dose of glucocorticoids
Age less than 15 or greater than 50 years
Postmenopausal status
Secondary
Long duration of glucocorticoid therapy
Disorders associated with markedly increased production of inflammatory cytokines (e.g., rheumatoid arthritis)
General osteoporosis risk factors
Female gender
White or Asian ancestry
Relative immobilization
Small body build

serum testosterone levels seen in men on glucocorticoid therapy probably contributes significantly to loss of bone mass.[115]

Glucocorticoids were originally thought to decrease intestinal calcium absorption by altering the conversion of vitamin D to its active metabolites. Serum 25OHD and 1,25(OH)$_2$D levels, however, are essentially normal in steroid-treated individuals.[116, 117] Hence, the inhibitory effect of glucocorticoids on intestinal calcium absorption appears to be a direct effect on the mucosal cell. As a result of the decreased calcium absorption, a secondary increase in PTH levels may occur, which tends to increase osteoclastic bone resorption.[117] This may be further aggravated by glucocorticoid stimulation of PTH secretion and urinary calcium loss.

Bone histology in glucocorticoid osteopenia characteristically demonstrates suppressed bone formation and increased osteoclastic activity, and trabecular wall thickness is decreased.[117, 118] These changes in trabecular bone can occur quite rapidly. Patients started on treatment with prednisone in a dose of 10 to 25 mg per day have been reported to show a 27 percent decrease in trabecular bone volume by iliac crest bone biopsy after 6 months.[119] Only minimal further change was observed in a subgroup of these patients restudied after 19 months. Also, QCT studies have demonstrated a 15 percent decrease in spine bone density 12 months after initiation of treatment with similar doses of prednisone.[120]

The biochemical changes in patients with glucocorticoid-induced osteopenia are generally not striking. Fasting serum calcium, phosphate, PTH, and vitamin D metabolite levels are generally within normal limits. Serum alkaline phosphatase and osteocalcin levels decline progressively after the initiation of steroid therapy, reflecting a rapid decrease in osteoblastic activity.[121–123] Alkaline phosphatase values, however, usually remain within the normal range and increase significantly after bone fracture. Urinary calcium excretion is often elevated during the first several years of therapy.[111, 121] This hypercalciuria, which occurs despite decreased intestinal calcium absorption, reflects both a "spillover" of calcium not assimilated into bone owing to decreased

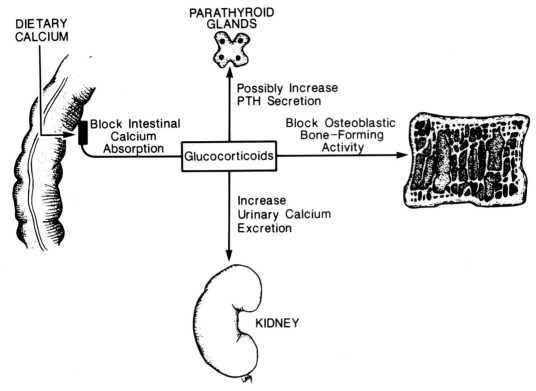

DIETARY CALCIUM

PARATHYROID GLANDS

Possibly Increase PTH Secretion

Block Intestinal Calcium Absorption

Glucocorticoids

Block Osteoblastic Bone-Forming Activity

Increase Urinary Calcium Excretion

KIDNEY

Figure 96–11. Mechanisms by which glucocorticoids promote bone loss in man.

osteoblastic activity and the direct calciuric effect of glucocorticoids. In patients maintained on moderate doses of steroids for several years, however, 24-hour urinary calcium excretion is frequently within the normal range.[117]

Management. Improved bone density, together with histologic evidence of both increased bone formation and decreased resorption, has been observed in patients with Cushing's disease following adrenalectomy.[124, 125] Moreover, we have observed a striking "rebound" increase in new bone formation in patients following the cessation of steroid therapy. This presumably reflects a normal osteoblastic response to increased stress stimulation from weakened bone, following removal of glucocorticoid inhibition. However, bone mass does not return to levels observed before the period of glucocorticoid excess.

Maintaining *glucocorticoid doses* at the lowest possible levels should be of benefit (Table 96–9). Significant osteopenia, however, has been observed in patients treated for prolonged periods with steroid doses as low as 7.5 to 10 mg of prednisone per day.[106, 108] Animal studies have suggested that alternate-day glucocorticoid regimens may produce less severe bone loss.[126] Clinical studies of the severity of bone loss and fracture incidence in patients treated with alternate-day regimens, however, have failed to demonstrate any significant advantage.[127] The use of short-acting glucocorticoids where possible should theoretically be of benefit. Deflazacort, a recently developed oxazoline derivative of prednisolone, has

been reported to have reduced deleterious effects on bone relative to its anti-inflammatory actions.[128] Longer-term controlled studies, however, are required to confirm these properties. Moreover, this agent is currently not available in the United States.

It would be highly desirable to have a means of directly *stimulating bone formation.* Weight-bearing

Table 96–9. MANAGEMENT OF GLUCOCORTICOID-INDUCED OSTEOPENIA*

Prophylaxis
Maintain glucocorticoid dose at lowest possible level
General measures
Maintain regular program of weight-bearing physical activity
Maintain adequate intake of calcium (800–1200 mg/day premenopausal and 1500–2000 mg/day postmenopausal) and vitamin D (400–800 units/day)
Eliminate adverse health habits—smoking, alcohol excess
Reduce urinary calcium loss with hydrochlorothiazide
Consider prophylactic estrogen replacement, calcitonin, or diphosphonate therapy in high-risk patients
Follow serum testosterone levels in men, and start testosterone replacement therapy when indicated
Established Osteopenia
Rule out endocrine disorders, osteomalacia, and multiple myeloma
Maintain glucocorticoid dose at lowest possible level
General measures as for prophylaxis
Reduce urinary calcium loss with hydrochlorothiazide
Maintain normal gonadal hormone status—estrogen replacement therapy in postmenopausal or amenorrheic women and testosterone replacement where indicated in men
Start calcitonin or diphosphonate therapy

*See text for dosages and side effects.

physical activity should be helpful, but there are obvious limits to this modality. Sodium fluoride administration has been suggested to be of potential benefit on the basis of its ability to stimulate increased bone density and histologic evidence of increased trabecular bone volume in steroid-treated patients.[129, 130] Also, short-term studies have shown a stimulatory effect of nandrolone deconate on bone density in postmenopausal women on glucocorticoids.[131] These regimens, however, remain unproved in glucocorticoid osteopenia. On the other hand, reduced serum testosterone levels in steroid-treated males should be treated with appropriate testosterone supplementation (e.g., 50 to 200 mg testosterone enantate intramuscularly every 3 weeks) to help maintain bone and muscle mass.

Inhibiting bone resorption is more easily accomplished and appears to be of benefit. Earlier studies demonstrated that the reduced intestinal calcium absorption in patients on glucocorticoids could be reversed by administration of *vitamin D*, 50,000 units two to three times weekly, or 25-hydroxyvitamin D, 40 to 50 µg per day, in combination with calcium, 500 mg per day.[117, 132] This produced a suppression of PTH levels and an increase in bone mass relative to controls and improved bone histology. Bone mass values, however, remained below normal levels. Similar results have been obtained by other investigators.[133, 134] 1,25-Dihydroxyvitamin D (calcitriol) also increased calcium absorption but was ineffective in increasing bone mass, possibly owing to suppressive effects on osteoblast function.[135] Vitamin D metabolite therapy, however, carries with it a significant risk of hypercalciuria and hypercalcemia[102, 136] and requires biochemical monitoring at monthly intervals. On the other hand, supplementation with *calcium*, 1000 mg per day, can reduce bone resorption and decrease the loss of bone mass[137] and is a relatively safe regimen. A complementary approach is to reduce urinary calcium loss with *hydrochlorothiazide*, 25 mg twice daily. Thiazide therapy has been shown to reduce serum PTH levels in glucocorticoid-treated patients[111] and also reduces the risk of hypercalciuria. In perimenopausal or postmenopausal women, estrogen replacement therapy should be instituted where possible to reduce bone loss.

Calcitonin is a potent inhibitor of bone resorption, but its effects in steroid osteopenia have not been extensively examined. Short-term studies of parenteral calcitonin in steroid-treated patients have reported reduction of bone loss.[138, 139] Moreover, in one study, patients treated prophylactically with calcitonin intramuscularly (100 units daily for 1 month, then every other day) or intranasally in equivalent dose had no significant loss of vertebral bone mass over a period of 2 years after the initiation of moderate-dose prednisone therapy, in contrast to a 15 percent loss in the control group.[140] *Diphosphonates* have a potentially major role in glucocorticoid osteopenia. In patients treated chronically with glucocor-

ticoids, oral pamidronate (APD) administration produced an initial increase in appendicular and vertebral bone density followed by stabilization over a subsequent period of 18 months.[141, 142] Biochemical indices of bone resorption were markedly reduced.[143] Sodium etidronate, the only diphosphonate currently available in the United States, has not been examined for its efficacy in steroid osteopenia.

The general approach to minimizing glucocorticoid-induced bone loss involves maintaining an intake of 400 to 800 units of vitamin D and 1500 to 2000 mg of calcium per day. Hydrochlorothiazide is a useful adjuvant to reduce urinary calcium losses. Weight-bearing exercise, particularly walking, should be encouraged to stimulate bone-forming activity, and gonadal hormone deficiencies should be corrected. Calcitonin and the disphosphonates appear to be potentially useful agents for preventing or partially reversing bone loss. The efficacy of all of these regimens in reducing fractures, however, remains to be demonstrated.

Gonadal Hormone Deficiency. *Estrogen deficiency* after natural or surgical menopause or in association with amenorrhea or ovulatory disturbances is almost invariably associated with significant loss of bone mass.[144–146] Indeed, premature menopause is a major risk factor for the development of involutional osteoporosis in women.[30, 31] Following loss of ovarian function, there is a marked acceleration of the rate of bone loss for a period of 5 to 8 years.[144, 147] Bone histology in estrogen deficiency demonstrates increased bone turnover characterized by increased osteoclastic bone resorption in combination with a relative reduction in bone formation rate. Estrogen administration reduces the rate of bone resorption and thereby decreases the rate of bone loss.[30] This effect is accompanied by a reduction in indices of bone turnover, including serum osteocalcin and alkaline phosphatase levels and fasting urinary calcium/creatinine ratios.[148]

The precise mechanisms of estrogen effects on bone remain undefined. Estrogen receptors have been demonstrated on osteoblasts, and estrogens directly affect osteoblast function in vitro.[149, 150] The primary effect of estrogen, however, is to decrease bone resorption, perhaps by altering osteoblast or marrow cell regulation of osteoclast development and function.[150a] Estrogen decreases the sensitivity of bone to resorption-stimulating agents such as PTH in vivo,[151] and estrogen administration is useful in reducing bone resorption in postmenopausal women with primary hyperparathyroidism.[152] It has also been variously suggested, but not proved, that the effects of estrogens on bone may be in part mediated via regulation of calcitonin, insulin-like growth factor, or vitamin D metabolism.[153] Estrogen deficiency is associated with mildly reduced levels of serum PTH and 1,25(OH)$_2$D, which revert to normal after estrogen administration. These changes, however, appear to be secondary to estrogen-related effects on the rate of calcium release from bone.[30] The osteopenia produced by estrogen deficiency is clinically indistinguishable from that produced by various other disorders. Serum and urinary chemistries are generally within normal limits, and the bone histology is not diagnostic. Thus, the diagnosis of estrogen deficiency osteoporosis is based on the clinical picture, a history of premature loss of ovarian function, and the exclusion of other disorders.

Estrogen replacement therapy is a mainstay in the prevention of estrogen deficiency bone loss. Estrogen administration for 5 to 10 years starting at the menopause is sufficient to produce an approximately 50 percent decrease in hip fractures and a 90 percent decrease in vertebral fracture incidence.[154, 155] To be most effective, therapy should be started within 3 years of menopause during the accelerated phase of bone loss. Estrogen replacement, however, also reduces bone loss in older women[156, 157] (Fig. 96–12). Although as with all antiresorptive agents estrogen may produce an initial small increase in bone mass while the equilibrium between bone formation and resorption rates is being re-established, estrogen administration will not restore bone mass to normal. The rate of further loss, however, is reduced. Cessation of estrogen replacement results in an acceleration of bone loss similar to that which occurs at menopause.[158]

The minimal daily dose of estrogen effective in inhibiting bone loss is 25 μg of ethinyl estradiol or 0.625 mg of conjugated estrogens given 25 days each month.[159, 160] Estradiol delivered transdermally by patch appears to offer similar protection, with a reduced risk of undesirable side effects, such as hypertension and increased coagulability,[161, 162] associated with estrogen effects on hepatic protein production. In patients with an intact uterus, a progestin such as medroxyprogesterone acetate, 10 mg per day, must be given for the last 11 to 12 days of each cycle to reduce the risk of endometrial carcinoma.[162] The C-21 progestins (such as medroxyprogesterone acetate) appear to have an antiresorptive effect on bone similar to that of estrogen, whereas the androgenic progestins (such as norethisterone) may increase trabecular bone mass.[163] The latter, however, may also be more likely to reverse the beneficial effects of estrogen on lipid metabolism. Many women who would benefit from estrogen replacement do not wish to take it, a major disincentive being the return of regular menses.[164] In this situation, continuous treatment with premarin, 0.625 mg per day, plus medroxyprogesterone acetate, 2.5 mg per day, has the advantage of affording similar protection without causing menstrual cycles in most women.[156]

In addition to reducing bone loss, estrogen replacement has major beneficial effects on lipid metabolism and the cardiovascular system.[165, 166] In postmenopausal women, estrogen replacement reduces the risk of stroke and heart attack by up to 50 percent. This major benefit potentially outweighs even that of protection against bone fractures. Although use of estrogen unopposed by progestins in women

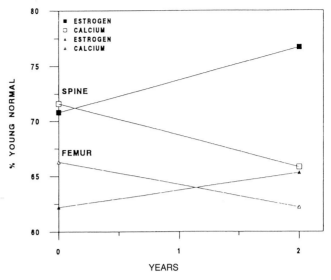

Figure 96–12. Comparative effects of estrogen replacement therapy versus calcium supplementation alone on bone density in the lumbar spine and femoral neck in women with established postmenopausal osteoporosis. (From Lindsay, R., and Tohme, J. F.: Estrogen treatment of patients with established postmenopausal osteoporosis. Obstet. Gynecol. 72:290–295, 1990. Reprinted with permission from The American College of Obstetricians and Gynecologists.)

with an intact uterus leads to an increased risk of uterine cancer, the addition of a progestin reduces the risk to below control levels.[162] In addition, postmenopausal estrogen replacement therapy appears to confer minimal or no increased risk of breast cancer. Studies suggest a maximum potential relative risk on the order of 1.3 after 10 to 20 years of therapy, with a rapid decline to normal once estrogen is discontinued.[167, 168] Because this risk appears to be far outweighed by the major benefits, most authorities recommend estrogen/progestin replacement for women at high risk for osteoporosis. Estrogen can stimulate the growth of pre-existing breast cancer, however, and a screening mammogram is therefore required before starting estrogen replacement therapy.

Androgen Deficiency. Hypogonadism is a major risk factor for osteoporosis in males,[32] and osteopenia is commonly observed in both primary and secondary testicular failure.[169–172] Testosterone exerts an anabolic effect on bone growth during puberty.[173] Thus, the severity of the osteopenia in hypogonadal males may reflect both the absence of the formation-stimulating effects of testosterone and the resorption-inhibiting effects of estrogens. The possible role of decreased gonadal functioning in producing the marked bone loss observed in older men remains controversial.[29, 174]

Other than for the clinical signs of androgen deficiency, reduced serum testosterone levels, and eunuchoidism in the case of primary gonadal failure, there are no distinguishing features of androgen deficiency osteopenia. Serum and urinary biochemistries are generally within normal limits. Bone biopsy reveals variable osteoblastic bone-forming activity and slightly increased bone resorption[170, 172]; however, these findings are nonspecific. The appropriate treatment is standard replacement doses of testosterone (e.g., testosterone enanthate, 200 to 300 mg intramuscularly every 3 weeks) once bone growth has ceased in late adolescence. There is preliminary evidence that such therapy can normalize bone metabolism by decreasing bone resorption and increasing bone formation.[170–172]

Hyperthyroidism. Hyperthyroidism produces a marked increase in bone turnover rate, with resorption exceeding formation. The result is bone loss, which is radiologically indistinguishable from involutional osteoporosis.[175, 176] Evidence indicates that chronic thyroid hormone replacement with greater than physiologic doses (100 to 125 μg 1-thyroxine per day) can lead to an acceleration of bone loss.[175] Even thyroid replacement in the physiologic range can accelerate bone loss,[177, 178] and serum triiodothyronine (T_3) levels show an inverse correlation with bone mass.[179] Thus, thyroid replacement doses should be carefully maintained in the normal range, as assessed by lack of suppression of ultrasensitive thyroid-stimulating hormone (TSH) assay levels. Bone histologic changes in endogenous hyperthyroidism are those of high turnover osteoporosis.[176] Serum PTH levels in overt hyperthyroidism are suppressed owing to the increased efflux of bone calcium into the extracellular fluid (ECF), and $1,25(OH)_2D$ production is secondarily decreased. Urinary calcium excretion is often increased, and mild hypercalcemia may occur, especially in younger individuals. Appropriate management includes early mobilization to stimulate bone formation, hydration, and treatment of the hyperthyroidism.

Diabetes Mellitus. There is an increased incidence of osteopenia in patients with diabetes mellitus, primarily of the juvenile-onset, insulin-dependent type.[153, 180] Osteopenia is relatively uncommon in adult-onset (type II) diabetes, possibly because such individuals characteristically have increased body mass and adipose tissue, both of which are protective against bone loss. The basis for the association between insulin-deficiency diabetes and osteopenia is unclear; however, decreased insulin and insulin-like growth factor I (IGF-I) stimulation of bone collagen synthesis may be important factors. There is no specific therapy other than to optimize insulin dosage.

Acromegaly. Significant osteopenia has been occasionally reported in acromegaly. Evidence suggests, however, that acromegaly not complicated by hyperparathyroidism (the MEA I syndrome) is not associated with bone loss. Indeed, increased bone mass is usually observed.[181]

Other Disorders

Immobilization Osteoporosis. Partial or total immobilization produces a rapid decrease in bone formation in the immobilized portion of the skeleton. Because bone resorption is initially unaffected, a rapid net loss of bone mineral occurs, especially in younger individuals with high bone turnover rates. In near-total immobilization, markedly increased urinary calcium excretion and hypercalcemia may occur.[182] Complete immobilization can produce as much as a 20 percent loss of bone mass over 4 months.[74] Mechanical compressive therapy, although of theoretical benefit, does not improve calcium balance.[183] Similarly, calcium and phosphate supplements are of no benefit and may worsen the hypercalciuria. General therapeutic measures include maintenance of water and electrolyte balance and mobilization where possible. In extreme situations, severe hypercalcemia may be controlled with calcitonin, intravenous sodium etidronate, or mithramycin.

Miscellaneous Disorders. Generalized osteopenia mimicking osteoporosis may occur in a number of other disease states, such as hyperparathyroidism, multiple myeloma, carcinomatosis, sickle cell diseases, and lipid storage disorders such as Gaucher's disease.[184] Multiple myeloma should always be considered as a cause of osteopenia in older patients, especially in the presence of anemia, since up to one third of cases present as generalized bone loss. The decrease in bone mass appears to be due to increased local production of osteoclast-activating factors such as tumor necrosis factor-beta (TNF-β).[185] Many nutritional deficiency syndromes have been associated with osteopenia of diverse histologic types. Osteoporosis has also been observed in patients receiving large doses of heparin (15,000 to 40,000 units per day) for 6 months or more, but the basis for the demineralization is unclear.[186] Long-term cyclosporine therapy produces a high turnover osteopenia often accompanied by an elevated serum alkaline phosphatase level.[187] Although experimental cyclosporine osteopenia in animals responds to calcitonin administration,[188] calcitonin efficacy in the human disorder remains to be determined.

Osteogenesis Imperfecta Tarda. This disorder can produce severe osteopenia in adults.[189] The adult-onset form of osteogenesis imperfecta should be considered in young adults with severe osteopenia and a history of multiple fractures, especially of the long bones of the legs. This disorder can be produced by a variety of mutations in the type I collagen gene that result in the formation of unstable collagen helices.[190] Platybasia of the skull and bone islands in the cranium may be observed. The diagnosis of the adult disorder can be confirmed by demonstrating typical thin-shaft deformities in the long bones, typically in the metacarpals and metatarsals, and by excessive osteocyte numbers and diminished osteoid on bone biopsy. Classic blue sclerae are present in less than one half of cases. Treatment with sodium fluoride, gonadal hormones, and calcitonin has been advocated, but it is not clear whether any of these agents can reduce fracture rate.

Osteomalacia and Rickets

Osteomalacia is characterized by the accumulation of increased amounts of unmineralized bone matrix (osteoid) and a decrease in the rate of bone formation.[191, 192] The normally closely coupled process of bone matrix deposition and mineralization is disturbed. In contrast to the normal 5- to 10-day lag between osteoid synthesis and mineralization, in severe cases of osteomalacia there may be a delay of 3 months or more. Histologically, excess osteoid is present. These osteoid seams differ from those often seen in states of increased bone turnover in that they lack a mineralization front, a feature that can be demonstrated by bone biopsy after tetracycline labeling. Rickets is a characteristic form of osteomalacia that occurs in children before closure of the epiphyses and is marked by defective mineralization and maturation of the epiphyseal cartilage.

Osteomalacia can be caused by a wide variety of disorders that produce skeletal calcification defects. It was previously thought that physical-chemical solubility factors, as reflected by the serum calcium X phosphate product, were the important determinants in the development of osteomalacia. It now seems more likely, however, that osteomalacia is the result of direct adverse effects of phosphate or vitamin D deficiency on osteoblast function.

Clinical Features

The rarely seen, full-blown clinical syndrome of osteomalacia is easily recognized and consists of severe bone pain, skeletal deformity, and fractures. Skeletal pain and tenderness are particularly marked in the pelvis and lower extremities and are aggravated by weight bearing. Often there is marked muscle weakness. This is especially true in the hip-girdle muscles, resulting in a waddling gait. Children with rickets have the added features of retarded growth, bowing of long bones, and abnormal proliferation of the epiphyseal cartilage plate. The last-mentioned results in epiphyseal widening and associated periarticular pain. The more common subtle forms of osteomalacia, however, are less easily recognized since the patient may be relatively asymptomatic. A history of a disorder that predisposes to osteomalacia is helpful in this setting.

In rickets, the principal radiologic changes are bowing of the long bone and widening, fraying, and cupping of all active growth plates[191] (Fig. 96–13). These changes are most apparent in sites of active growth, such as the sternal ends of the ribs and the metaphyseal ends of long bones. Craniosynostosis occurs occasionally.

In adults, epiphyseal changes do not occur, since bone growth has ceased. The radiographic findings

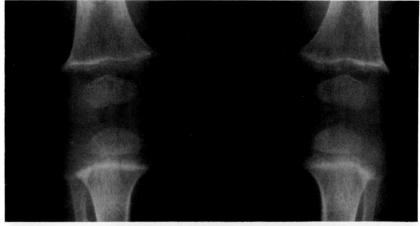

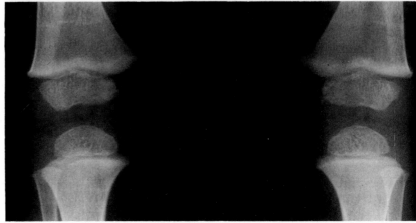

Figure 96–13. *A*, Radiographs of the knees of a 13-month-old child with rickets due to vitamin D deficiency. Note the widened growth plates, frayed epiphyses, and irregular widened metaphyses. *B*, Almost complete healing of rickets after 5 months of treatment with vitamin D.

in osteomalacia in adults are those of generalized demineralization with increased trabecular markings. The only diagnostic radiologic findings are pseudo-fractures (Looser's zones), which are linear radiolucencies that are perpendicular to the bone surface and most commonly found symmetrically distributed in the ribs, long bones, lateral scapular margins, and pelvic rami (Fig. 96–14). In contrast to true fractures, these lesions are painless, usually do not extend through both cortices, and do not have associated callus formation. Histologically, pseudofractures are regions of fibrous tissue containing trabeculae of immature bone. The pathogenesis of these lesions has been variously attributed to local pressure from nutrient arteries or to muscle attachments, which cause increased local stress.[191] Pseudofractures are infrequently observed, however, even in moderately severe cases of osteomalacia.

When the full-blown picture of osteomalacia is present, the diagnosis is easily established. In less clear-cut cases, however, diagnostic uncertainty can be resolved by performing a bone biopsy following tetracycline labeling. The number and thickness of osteoid seams per unit area of bone provide a sensitive index of osteomalacia, and tetracycline labeling allows microscopic confirmation of deficient osteoid mineralization, the ultimate criterion of osteomalacia.

Etiologies of Osteomalacia

Table 96–10 summarizes the various causes of osteomalacia. Categories 1 through 3 all have reduced serum phosphate levels or vitamin D deficiency as a

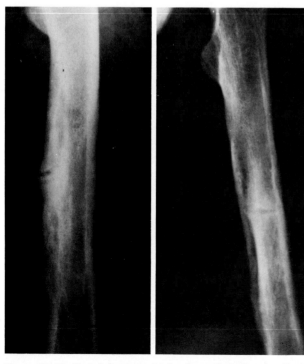

Figure 96–14. Pseudofractures in the femoral shafts of patients with familial hypophosphatemic rickets.

Table 96–10. CAUSES OF OSTEOMALACIA

Vitamin D Deficiency
Decreased absorption
  Nutritional deficiency (rare)
  Fat malabsorption states
    Celiac disease
    Pancreatic insufficiency
    Hepatobiliary disorders
Defective metabolism
  Anticonvulsant drugs, sedatives, rifampin
  Chronic renal failure
  Vitamin D–dependency rickets
Impaired action
  Deficient tissue receptors
Chronic Hypophosphatemia (with Normal Vitamin D)
Primary renal phosphate wasting syndromes
  Familial hypophosphatemic rickets
  Inherited or acquired mixed renal tubular defects
    Fanconi's syndrome, type I renal tubular acidosis
Chronic phosphate depletion
  Antacid abuse
  Chronic parenteral nutrition
Defective Mineralization with Normal Calcium, Phosphate, and Vitamin D
Aluminum toxicity
Hypophosphatasia
Fibrogenesis imperfecta ossium

common factor; category 4 disorders have in common defective hydroxyapatite crystal formation.

Vitamin D Deficiency. Vitamin D deficiency osteomalacia is characterized by reduced intestinal calcium absorption, low serum calcium concentration, hypophosphatemia, elevated serum alkaline phosphatase, reduced serum 25(OH)D, and increased serum PTH. Owing to tight regulation by PTH, the serum $1,25(OH)_2D$ remains within normal limits in all but the most advanced cases. Hence, it is of little diagnostic value. The $TmPO_4/GFR$ is reduced, reflecting the phosphaturic effect of PTH. Twenty-four-hour calcium excretion is usually markedly decreased (less than 1 mg per kg body weight).[191, 192] Proximal muscle weakness may be observed. All abnormalities are resolved by restoration of normal vitamin D status.

In the United States, dietary vitamin D deficiency is relatively rare owing to widespread vitamin D supplementation of foods.[193] When dietary vitamin D intake is chronically less than 70 IU per day, however, as in strict vegetarian or fat-free diets, and sunlight exposure is minimal, osteomalacia can occur. Elderly patients are particularly susceptible to nutritional osteomalacia, owing to dietary deficiencies and limited sunlight exposure. Nutritional vitamin D deficiency characteristically responds to vitamin D in doses of 400 to 1000 IU per day; however, doses four to ten times higher are generally employed.[191]

Moderately severe vitamin deficiency is seen most commonly in disorders associated with intestinal fat malabsorption: hepatobiliary disease, pancreatic insufficiency, gluten-sensitive enteropathy, blind-loop syndromes, visceral scleroderma, and following jejunoileal bypass for obesity.[194, 195] Vitamin D absorption correlates inversely with fecal fat excretion. Dietary calcium may also combine with fatty acids to form insoluble soaps, further decreasing calcium absorption. Osteomalacia and reduced serum 25(OH)D levels are also seen in gastrectomy patients; however, since vitamin D absorption appears to be normal in these individuals, reduced vitamin D intake owing to altered dietary habits may be at fault.[196] Bone biopsy can reveal significant osteomalacia even in the absence of definite clinical manifestations. Osteoporosis, possibly owing to chronic calcium deficiency, often occurs concomitantly. Treatment consists of management of the underlying disorder, in addition to vitamin D and calcium administration. Vitamin D is given orally in doses of 50,000 to 200,000 units per day, depending on the severity of the malabsorption. 25(OH)D (40 to 100 μg per day) is useful in this situation because it is more readily absorbed and more rapid in its onset of action. Parenteral preparations vary considerably in potency and must be considered unreliable.[197] It is not appropriate to treat vitamin D deficiency with 1,25(OH)$_2$D, since suppression of osteoblast function may occur. Calcium supplementation of 1000 to 2000 mg per day should be provided. The response to therapy is monitored by following serum and urine calcium values at 1- to 2-week intervals. The bone response is usually heralded by a transient further increase in the serum alkaline level, reflecting increased osteoblastic activity. Improvement in the underlying disease can be associated with markedly reduced vitamin D requirements, so patients must be followed carefully.

Defective Vitamin D Metabolism or Action

Vitamin D–Dependent Rickets. Pseudo vitamin D–deficiency rickets (vitamin D–dependent rickets) is a rare sporadic disorder that clinically mimics nutritional rickets but requires higher doses of vitamin D (10,000 to 30,000 units per day) or physiologic doses of 1,25(OH)$_2$D to reverse the clinical and biochemical abnormalities.[198] The basis of this disorder appears to be defective renal production of 1,25(OH)$_2$D. The diagnosis is based on characteristic somatic abnormalities, normal 25(OH)D and reduced 1,25(OH)$_2$D levels, and failure to respond to vitamin D in physiologic doses of 400 to 1000 units per day.

Another group of disorders characterized by partial vitamin D resistance is caused by an end-organ resistance to 1,25(OH)$_2$D.[199] This heterogeneous group of inherited disorders, originally termed vitamin D–dependent rickets type II, is characterized by the biochemical and radiologic features of osteomalacia in association with increased serum 1,25(OH)$_2$D levels. Alopecia occurs in some but not all kindreds. Resistance to the tissue effects of 1,25(OH)$_2$D is due to varying combinations of impaired cytosol binding and decreased nuclear translocation of 1,25(OH)$_2$D.

Drug-Induced Osteomalacia. Chronic treatment with drugs that induce the hepatic mixed-function oxidase enzyme system produces an increased incidence of rickets and osteomalacia. This is particularly true for agents such as phenobarbital, diphenylhydantoin, and rifampin.[106, 193] Hypocalcemia, hypophosphatemia, increased serum PTH, elevated serum bone alkaline phosphatase, and reduced serum 25(OH)D levels occur in 4 to 60 percent of such individuals, with the incidence and severity of the disorder determined by the patient's level of vitamin D intake, degree of sunlight exposure, and total drug dose. Osteomalacia is present on bone biopsy. The basis of the disorder appears to be an accelerated rate of hepatic microsomal degradation of vitamin D and 25(OH)D. Diphenylhydantoin also further impairs mineral metabolism by direct inhibitory effects on intestine and bone.[200] Severe cases may require 4000 to 20,000 units per day for a year or longer to correct all abnormalities. Routine prophylaxis consists of maintaining a vitamin D intake of 800 to 1000 units per day.

Tumor-Associated Osteomalacia. Osteomalacia that resolves after the resection of a tumor of mesenchymal origin has occasionally been described.[201] In these cases, typical biochemical and histologic features of osteomalacia occur in association with normal serum 250HD levels. Serum 1,25(OH)$_2$D concentrations, however, are markedly reduced. Administration of physiologic amounts of 1,25(OH)$_2$D results in resolution of the biochemical abnormalities and healing of the osteomalacia. It is presumed that the tumor elaborates substances that inhibit renal 25(OH)D-1-hydroxylase activity.

Chronic Hypophosphatemia

Primary Renal Phosphate Wasting Syndromes. *Familial hypophosphatemic rickets (FHR)*, previously known as vitamin D–resistant rickets, is one of the most common forms of osteomalacia and rickets. Most cases are familial, usually transmitted as an X-linked dominant trait. The trait is variably expressed, with clinical manifestations that range from asymptomatic mild hypophosphatemia to marked hypophosphatemia associated with severe bone disease.[191, 202] Males are affected more severely than females. In severe cases, the diagnosis is usually established by the second year of life. The clinical picture is that of severe rickets with generalized demineralization, pseudofractures, bowing of the long bones, growth retardation, and an increased propensity to fracture. The characteristic biochemical findings in FHR include normal serum calcium concentration, a variable but often marked hypophosphatemia, elevated serum alkaline phosphatase levels, and marked renal phosphate wasting (reduced TmPO$_4$/GFR). Intestinal calcium absorption and urinary calcium excretion are often slightly reduced. Adults with FHR frequently have symptomatic osteomalacia, short body habitus, and symptoms of degenerative joint disease owing to lower extremity deformities.[203] Bone density in adult FHR patients is often increased in the axial skeleton owing to hyperosteoidosis but is decreased in the extremities.[204]

The basis of the disorder appears to be a primary

defect in phosphate transport in kidney and intestine. Serum 25(OH)D levels are normal. Serum 1,25(OH)$_2$D concentrations, however, are in the low-normal range, inappropriate to the marked hypophosphatemia. Thus, renal 1,25(OH)$_2$D production appears to be functionally subnormal. Long-term treatment with pharmacologic doses of 1,25(OH)$_2$D (1.0 to 3.0 µg per day), phosphate (1.0 to 2.0 g per day), and calcium, 1000 mg per day, has been shown to improve renal phosphate retention, promote positive phosphate balance, improve bone mineralization, and produce growth acceleration.[202]

A sporadic form of *adult-onset hypophosphatemic osteomalacia* owing to an acquired, isolated renal phosphate leak is occasionally observed.[205] The clinical presentation may be marked by the gradual onset of generalized myalgias and arthralgias mimicking a rheumatic disorder. Pseudofractures are often observed. This syndrome must be differentiated from other disorders associated with acquired renal phosphate leaks, such as mesenchymal tumors, multiple myeloma, glycogen storage disease, Wilson's disease, and heavy metal poisoning. The sporadic adult-onset form of hypophosphatemic osteomalacia responds to treatment with phosphate, calcium, and 0.5 to 1.5 µg per day of 1,25(OH)$_2$D.

Other Renal Tubular Defects. Osteomalacia may occur in association with a variety of renal tubular defects. The most widely recognized renal tubular disorders associated with osteomalacia or rickets are distal renal tubular acidosis (RTA) and Fanconi's syndrome.[191, 206] Both syndromes have familial and sporadic forms. Both RTA and Fanconi's syndrome can be associated with defects in the renal handling of phosphate, hydrogen ion, glucose, amino acids, sodium, and potassium. Sporadic forms of renal tubular defects may also be caused by dysproteinemias, heavy metal poisoning, or other toxins. Hypophosphatemia owing to renal phosphate loss plays a primary role in the pathogenesis of the osteomalacia. Treatment is as for the other renal phosphate wasting syndromes. In RTA, acidosis may also play an important role, since correction of the acidosis alone may reverse the osteomalacia. This may reflect the effect of pH on renal 1-hydroxylase activity.[207] RTA is commonly associated with hypercalciuria and sometimes with secondary parathyroid hyperplasia. Treatment consists of correction of the acidosis and, when bone disease is severe, supplementing with vitamin D (50,000 to 300,000 units per day), calcium, and phosphate.

Chronic Phosphate Depletion. Phosphate deficiency with bone pain, osteomalacia, muscle weakness, and hypercalciuria has been reported in patients chronically taking large doses of nonabsorbable magnesium or aluminum hydroxide antacids, which interfere with intestinal phosphate absorption.[208] Treatment consists of discontinuing the antacids and supplementing with phosphate and calcium.

Defective Mineralization Without Associated Abnormalities of Calcium, Phosphate, or Vitamin

D. *Aluminum bone disease* occurs most commonly in patients with chronic renal insufficiency (see under Renal Osteodystrophy). In addition, in patients receiving long-term total parenteral nutrition (TPN) therapy with aluminum-contaminated solutions, a syndrome of bone pain, osteopenia, increased bone fractures, and histologic evidence of osteomalacia has occasionally been reported. These changes occur in association with normal serum 25(OH)D levels, decreased serum iPTH, and a tendency toward increased serum calcium concentration.[209] Osteoblast activity is reduced, and bone formation is markedly decreased. The tendency to hypercalcemia apparently reflects the decreased ability of bone to accumulate calcium rapidly. This syndrome has virtually disappeared with increased awareness of the importance of strict standards for low aluminum content in parenteral solutions.

Hypophosphatasia is a rare inherited metabolic bone disorder characterized by decreased circulating and tissue levels of bone alkaline phosphatase, defective bone mineralization, and increased urinary excretion of the alkaline phosphatase substrates, phosphoethanolamine, and pyrophosphate.[210] The adult form, which is transmitted as an autosomal dominant disorder, is associated with residual rachitic deformities, premature loss of teeth, and osteopenia with recurrent fractures. The disorder may be more common than is currently recognized, since a mild reduction in serum bone alkaline phosphatase levels may not be readily apparent. There is currently no treatment for this disorder other than for surgical repair of fractures and pseudofractures.[211]

Fibrogenesis imperfecta ossium is a rare disorder caused by a primary defect in the synthesis or maturation of collagen, leading to impaired mineralization.[212] The few patients who have been reported have developed progressive skeletal pain after age 50. The entire skeleton shows thickened trabeculae and an overall appearance of increased bone density. Bone cortical thickness, however, is reduced, and pseudofractures are observed. A marked reduction in bone collagen content and a disordered collagen fiber pattern are characteristic of the disorder.

Osteitis Fibrosa

Primary Hyperparathyroidism

Clinical Features

Prevalence. Primary hyperparathyroidism is the most common cause of hypercalcemia in the general population. Its prevalence has been reported to range from one in 400 to one in 1000 patients, and the peak incidence is in the sixth or seventh decades.[213–216] More than 75 percent of patients are 40 to 70 years of age, and the female/male ratio is approximately 2.5:1.

The syndrome of primary hyperparathyroidism can be caused by single or multiple benign adenomas, hyperplasia of all four glands, or parathyroid carcinoma (Table 96–11). The reported relative incidence of these various types is single adenoma, 60 to 88 percent; two to three gland involvement, 5 to 26 percent; generalized hyperplasia, 6 to 17 percent; and parathyroid carcinoma, 0.2 to 1 percent.[214, 215] Serum calcium and PTH concentrations correlate roughly with tumor size. More than 90 percent of adenomas are of the chief cell variety. Chief cell hyperplasia accounts for the vast majority of hyperplastic glands and is especially common in familial hyperparathyroidism and multiple endocrine adenomatosis.[217] Parathyroid carcinoma is a rare cause of hyperparathyroidism. Patients with this disorder tend to have higher serum calcium levels and an increased incidence of skeletal and renal involvement, and a neck mass is palpable in up to 50 percent of cases.[218] The pathogenesis of primary hyperparathyroidism remains undefined. It has been suggested that the disorder may be caused by reduced expression of a parathyroid cell calcium receptor mechanism.[219]

The clinical spectrum of hyperparathyroidism has shifted, owing to the increased detection of earlier and milder cases as a result of the routine use of blood biochemical profiles. In contrast to the severe renal and skeletal manifestations, which previously characterized the presentation, mild constitutional symptoms now predominate. Nearly 50 percent of patients present asymptomatically, manifesting only mild biochemical abnormalities detected on routine biochemical screening.[213–215] On the other hand, patients may occasionally present with so-called acute hyperparathyroidism, a syndrome characterized by severe symptomatic hypercalcemia and markedly elevated serum PTH levels.[220] The severity of the hypercalcemia in acute hyperparathyroidism appears to be in part aggravated by immobilization and dehydration associated with intercurrent illnesses.

Renal disorders remain a relatively common manifestation of primary hyperparathyroidism. Hypercalcemia and hypercalciuria lead to an impaired ability to concentrate the urine. As a result, polyuria and nocturia can be early manifestations. Nephrolithiasis is a relatively common complication and may occur in up to 20 percent of patients.[213–215] The stones are usually composed of calcium oxalate or calcium phosphate. Nephrocalcinosis can produce a variety of tubular defects including renal tubular acidosis and when extensive can lead to progressive renal failure. Marked hypercalciuria and kidney stones may occur primarily in those patients whose renal 1,25(OH)$_2$D production is highly responsive to PTH.[221]

Bone disease is clinically evident in 5 to 10 percent of patients. Osteitis fibrosa cystica, the classic bone disease of hyperparathyroidism, is characterized by (1) generalized demineralization, (2) subperiosteal resorption, (3) bone pain, and (4) bone cysts or "brown tumors." However, this is now an extremely rare presentation. Although routine radiographs may reveal diffuse demineralization indistinguishable from other forms of osteopenia, there are frequently no readily apparent skeletal abnormalities. Sensitive radiologic techniques, however, such as DPA or QCT measurement of vertebral bone mass, demonstrate trabecular bone loss in many patients, and cortical bone mass in the extremities is frequently reduced[6] (Fig. 96–15). The most common specific radiologic finding of hyperparathyroidism is subperiosteal resorption (Fig. 96–16). This lesion is characterized by erosions and irregular demineralization of the bone cortex and is seen most commonly in the middle phalanges and clavicles.[222] It is rarely observed, however, other than in the severe secondary hyperparathyroidism associated with chronic renal failure. Histologically, osteitis fibrosa is characterized by increased numbers of osteoclasts in the bone cortex and trabeculae, reduced trabecular size, and variable fibrous replacement of bone and marrow elements.[223]

Joint symptoms may be caused by a variety of lesions[224] (Table 96–12). Chondrocalcinosis, owing to

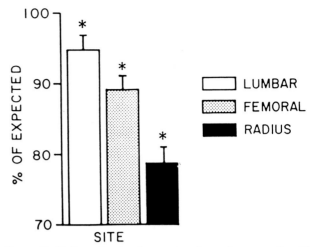

Figure 96–15. Bone density changes in primary hyperparathyroidism. Bone density values at three different sites—radius, femoral neck, and lumbar spine—are shown as a percentage of expected values for age-, sex-, and ethnicity-matched normal subjects. The divergence from expected values is different at each site (p = 0.0001). (From Silverberg, S. J., Shane, E., de la Cruz, L., et al.: Skeletal disease in primary hyperparathyroidism. J. Bone Miner. Res. 4:283–291, 1989. Used by permission.)

Table 96–11. CAUSES OF OSTEITIS FIBROSA

Primary hyperparathyroidism
Secondary hyperparathyroidism
  Vitamin D deficiency
    Decreased absorption
    Defective metabolism
  Chronic renal failure
    Defective vitamin D metabolism
    Phosphate retention
  Decreased calcium absorption
  Renal resistance to PTH
    Pseudohypoparathyroidism

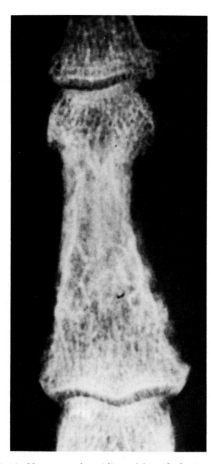

Figure 96–16. Hyperparathyroidism. Magnified view of middle phalanx demonstrating marked subperiosteal resorption on both the medial and the lateral surfaces.

an increased serum calcium X phosphate product, can produce pseudogout. In addition, there is an increased incidence of true gout owing to an elevation of serum uric levels caused by PTH inhibition of renal urate excretion.[225] Increased resorption of articular bone leading to a deformity of the joint cartilage may suggest rheumatoid arthritis. Joint pain may also be caused by metastatic periarticular calcification with calcium deposition in tendons. *Muscle weakness* is a common manifestation of primary hyperparathyroidism and is occasionally accompanied by muscle atrophy or other features of myopathy. These abnormalities are reversed by surgical correction of the hyperparathyroidism.

Gastrointestinal symptoms are caused primarily by the effects of hypercalcemia and include anorexia, nausea, vomiting, constipation, and vague abdominal pain. In addition, peptic ulcers occur with increased frequency,[216] probably owing to increased calcium stimulation of gastrin secretion, which leads to increased gastric acid production. In addition, patients with hyperparathyroidism associated with the syndrome of multiple endocrine neoplasia type I (MEN I) have an increased incidence of peptic ulcer owing to associated gastrin-secreting pancreatic tumors. Pancreatitis also occurs with increased fre-

quency in patients with hyperparathyroidism and is often associated with pancreatic calculi. During an acute attack of pancreatitis, the serum calcium may be deceptively low, but serial determinations eventually uncover the hypercalcemia.

Cardiovascular manifestations include hypertension in up to 50 percent of cases.[216] However, there is usually no significant improvement in the blood pressure following parathyroid surgery.[226] Hypercalcemia causes shortening of the Q-T interval and may produce PR interval prolongation, which can predispose to arrhythmias.

Central nervous system manifestations are primarily caused by the hypercalcemia and can include malaise, fatigue, apathy, and depression. Mental obtundation and coma are fairly predictable signs of marked hypercalcemia.[216] Occasionally, severe anxiety or psychotic behavior may occur. There have been sporadic reports of marked improvement in psychiatric disorders following parathyroidectomy,[227] but this is the exception rather than the rule.[228]

Ectopic calcification in the skin, eyes, and other soft tissues is occasionally seen in patients with hyperparathyroidism. Band keratopathy is a rare finding caused by calcium deposition within the cornea. These grayish lesions are concentric with the limbus and are most noticeable in the nasal and temporal areas but may require slit lamp confirmation. Calcium deposits in the bulbar and palpebral conjunctiva can cause burning and lacrimation. Severe pruritus occurs occasionally but rapidly disappears after parathyroidectomy.

MEN syndromes frequently have hyperparathyroidism as a prominent feature. The MEN I syndrome is characterized by parathyroid hyperplasia, functioning pancreatic adenomas, and pituitary adenomas. Other endocrine tumors may also be encountered.[229] This syndrome occurs sporadically, but it may also be transmitted as an autosomal dominant trait. The MEN II syndrome is characterized by the triad of parathyroid chief cell hyperplasia, medullary thyroid carcinoma, and pheochromocytoma.[230] In both MEN syndromes, hyperparathyroidism is usually the first abnormality noted.

Biochemical Findings and Differential Diagnosis. The combination of fasting hypercalcemia, hypophosphatemia, and increased serum iPTH concen-

Table 96–12. BONE AND JOINT MANIFESTATIONS OF PRIMARY HYPERPARATHYROIDISM

Osteitis fibrosa cystica
Diffuse demineralization
Subperiosteal resorption
Phalanges, distal clavicles
Brown tumors
Fractures
Diffuse bone pain
Articular disorders
Pseudogout
Gout
Resorption of articular bone
Periarticular metastatic calcification

tration is diagnostic of primary hyperparathyroidism. Several serum calcium determinations may be required, since calcium concentrations may fluctuate. Intact or mid-molecule PTH assay[22] is the diagnostic procedure of choice. Detection of hypophosphatemia is improved by measurements made in the fasting state because serum phosphate concentration rises postprandially. Serum alkaline phosphatase may be slightly elevated when there is extensive bone involvement.[216] The serum chloride is frequently elevated above 102 mEq per liter, reflecting the mild metabolic acidosis caused by increased proximal renal tubular bicarbonate excretion. Mean serum uric acid levels are increased by 1 to 2 mg per dl, owing to decreased distal tubular urate secretion. The serum $1,25(OH)_2D$ concentration is often mildly increased owing to the renal effects of PTH. Despite the calcium-retaining renal tubular effects of PTH, 24-hour urinary calcium excretion is usually increased (>4 mg per kg body weight) owing to the increased filtered calcium load. Calcium excretion is never decreased except in the presence of renal insufficiency. $TmPO_4/GFR$ is decreased, reflecting the phosphaturic effects of PTH.

The *differential diagnosis* of primary hyperparathyroidism includes all other causes of hypercalcemia. Those hypercalcemic disorders associated with either increased intestinal calcium absorption (e.g., vitamin D intoxication, sarcoidosis) or with a local factor–mediated increase in bone resorption rate (e.g., metastatic carcinoma, multiple myeloma) are characterized by suppressed PTH levels, however, and a consequent increase in serum phosphate and urinary $TmPO_4/GFR$ values.[231] Rarely, hypophosphatemia can be observed in nonhyperparathyroid hypercalcemia, either owing to decreased intake causing phosphate depletion or to dysproteinemias, which produce a proximal tubular phosphate leak syndrome. The ectopic PTH syndrome caused by lung, renal, and various other cancers produces hypercalcemia and hypophosphatemia, owing to the production of a *PTH-like peptide*, which activates the normal PTH receptor.[23, 233] Although PTH-related peptide has some homology with PTH at the amino-terminal portion of the molecule, it is not detected in standard PTH assays; hence, the serum iPTH is characteristically depressed.[234]

Familial hypocalciuria hypercalcemia (FHH) is an inherited, autosomal dominant disorder that closely resembles mild primary hyperparathyroidism, in that it is characterized by mild hypercalcemia and hypophosphatemia.[235, 236] In contrast to primary hyperparathyroidism, however, serum iPTH levels are usually within the normal range, and renal calcium clearance is markedly reduced; 24-hour urinary calcium excretion is usually less than 1 mg per kg body weight, and fasting urinary Ca/Cr is less than 0.10. It is important to distinguish FHH from primary hyperparathyroidism because FHH is an essentially benign disorder not associated with renal or skeletal disease. Moreover, parathyroid surgery is contraindicated in FHH because subtotal parathyroidectomy does not reverse the hypercalcemia. Screening of other family members usually uncovers additional asymptomatic individuals and confirms the diagnosis.

Treatment

Medical Management. Because primary hyperparathyroidism is usually not a relentlessly progressive disorder, many patients may not require surgery. Currently accepted criteria for neck exploration in primary hyperparathyroidism include a mean serum calcium concentration greater than 1 mg per dl above the upper limit of normal radiologic evidence of bone disease including severe osteopenia, decreased renal function, metabolically active (enlarging or new) renal calculi, infected nephrolithiasis, poorly controlled peptic ulcer disease, pancreatitis, and clinical situations in which prolonged observation is impractical.[214, 215, 237] In addition, surgery is generally warranted in all patients presenting before age 40.

Patients who do not fulfill any of the operative criteria or who have coexisting medical problems that increase the risk of surgery may be followed medically.[213] In one group of 147 such patients followed for 5 years, fewer than 20 percent subsequently progressed to meet one or more operative criteria, and only 3 percent developed decreased renal function.[238] Medical management consists of enforced hydration, a high salt intake to promote calcium excretion, and a low calcium diet (less than 400 mg per day). Weight-bearing exercise such as walking should be encouraged to promote bone formation. The use of thiazide diuretics should be avoided because these agents decrease urinary calcium excretion[111] and thereby aggravate the hypercalcemia. Treatment with estrogens is often of benefit in reducing hypercalcemia, hypercalciuria, and bone resorption in postmenopausal women with hyperparathyroidism.[239] Neutral phosphate supplementation (1.5 to 2.5 g per day in four divided doses) may reduce urine calcium levels and inhibit stone formation. Owing to the increased risk of ectopic calcification and reduced renal function, however, phosphate therapy must be employed with extreme caution. In addition, phosphate therapy should not be used in patients with recurrent urinary tract infections and an alkaline urine because this situation is associated with increased risk of formation of (alkaline-insoluble) calcium phosphate stones.

Surgical Management

Localization of Abnormal Parathyroid Tissue. Various techniques have been used to aid in the preoperative localization of abnormal parathyroid glands.[214, 215, 240] The combination of selective angiography and venous sampling for PTH assay offers a relatively high success rate but is technically difficult and expensive. CT is particularly useful before the reoperation of patients with previously failed parathyroid surgery. The combination of technetium-thallium subtraction scanning and ultrasonography has also been employed.[240] Under most circumstances, however, there is a significant incidence of false-positive results. None of these localization techniques is an adequate substitute for surgical expertise. An experienced surgeon familiar with parathyroid anatomy can almost always successfully locate and excise the involved glands without extensive use of localization techniques. On the other hand, in reoperation for previously unsuccessful parathyroid surgery, the combination of angiography, venous sampling for PTH assay, technetium-thallium scanning, and CT should be routinely employed.

The definitive therapy for primary hyperparathyroidism is removal of the abnormal parathyroid tissue. Although most abnormal parathyroid glands are in the neck, some occur in the mediastinum. Of the latter, most are in the anterior mediastinum, usually in association with the thymus. More than 75 percent of these mediastinal parathyroids are accessible through a neck incision, and therefore only about 5 percent of all patients require mediastinotomy.[214, 215] The standard surgical approach has been to explore the neck initially, remove any obviously enlarged parathyroid glands, and obtain a biopsy of the normal glands. Because of the difficulty in identifying hyperplasia at the time of surgery, however, it has been advocated that 3½ parathyroid glands should routinely be removed regardless of their gross appearance.[214]

Following successful surgery, the serum calcium falls to normal levels within 24 hours. Patients with extensive bone disease may rapidly deposit calcium into their demineralized skeleton, resulting in transient hypocalcemia and tetany. In these cases, serum calcium usually reaches its nadir between the fourth and tenth postoperative days. This phenomenon is commonly referred to as the "hungry bone" syndrome. Tetany may also occur if the parathyroids are totally excised or if the remaining glands have been injured. In this case, serum calcium should be maintained at slightly subnormal levels (7.5 to 8.5 mg per dl) by intravenous or oral calcium supplementation.[214] If serum calcium cannot be maintained without calcium supplements by 1 week postoperatively, permanent hypoparathyroidism is likely.

Successful surgery results in eventual regression of the bone lesions of osteitis fibrosa. It has not yet been determined, however, whether bone mass routinely returns to normal. Renal disease is also arrested but may not be totally reversed. The long-term outlook for renal function in advanced cases may be poor despite adequate surgical correction of the hyperparathyroidism.[241]

Secondary Hyperparathyroidism

A variety of disorders, summarized in Table 96–13, are characterized by resistance to the action of PTH. The factor common to all of these disorders is

Table 96–13. CAUSES OF SECONDARY HYPERPARATHYROIDISM

Vitamin D deficiency
  Decreased absorption
    Nutritional deficiency
    Fat malabsorption states
  Defective metabolism or action
    Chronic renal failure
    Anticonvulsant drug therapy
    Tissue receptor deficiency
Decreased calcium absorption (normal vitamin D)
  Age-related "primary" decreased absorption
  Glucocorticoid excess
  High phosphate intake
Increased urinary calcium loss
  Renal tubular acidosis
  Renal leak type idiopathic hypercalciuria
Hypocalcemia owing to increased serum phosphate
  Renal insufficiency
  Acute tissue destruction
Target-organ resistance to PTH
  Vitamin D deficiency
  Renal insufficiency
  Pseudohypoparathyroidism

hypocalcemia leading to increased PTH release. Vitamin D deficiency results in decreased intestinal calcium absorption with a secondary increase in PTH secretion. Osteopenia occurs commonly in this situation (see under Osteomalacia). In renal failure, increased phosphate retention and decreased $1,25(OH)_2D$ production lead to marked hyperparathyroidism and a characteristic group of bone disorders (see under Renal Osteodystrophy). Pseudohypoparathyroidism is a genetic disorder characterized by hypocalcemia, hyperphosphatemia, and somatic abnormalities.[242] The basis of the disorder is renal resistance to the effects of PTH, and bone changes of osteitis fibrosa are occasionally observed.

Renal Osteodystrophy

Renal osteodystrophy is a mixture of osteitis fibrosa, osteomalacia, osteoporosis, and osteosclerosis caused by chronic renal failure.[243, 244] Any combination of these disorders may occur in uremic patients. The radiographic picture of advanced renal osteodystrophy is characteristically a patchy mixture of osteopenic and osteosclerotic changes (Fig. 96–17).

Osteomalacia often occurs early in renal failure. Its pathogenesis is not completely understood but is almost certainly multifactorial, owing both to decreased $1,25(OH)_2D$ production and to increased aluminum deposition in bone. A significant number of renal patients with pure osteomalacia show no histologic response to vitamin D metabolite treatment and indeed are unusually prone to develop hypercalcemia. Evidence suggests that this syndrome is caused by the toxic effects of aluminum accumulation in bone.[209, 245, 246] Aluminum deposition in such individuals is the result of increased absorption of alu-

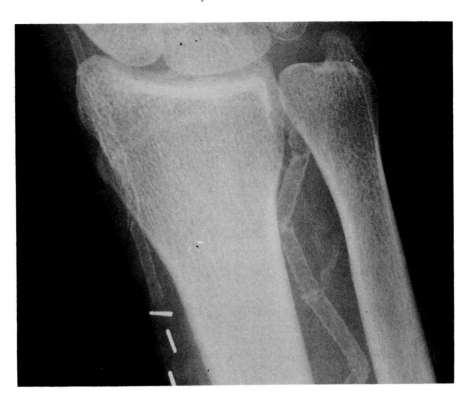

Figure 96–17. Renal osteodystrophy with severe arterial calcification.

minum derived from aluminum-containing, phosphate-binding antacids and decreased aluminum excretion owing to impaired renal function. Previously, aluminum contamination of dialysate solutions played the primary role in the pathogenesis of aluminum bone disease, but increased awareness of the problem and stricter standards for the permissible aluminum content of parenteral solutions has virtually eliminated this source of aluminum overload. Moreover, calcium carbonate is rapidly replacing aluminum-containing antacids as the primary phosphate-binding agent used for controlling serum phosphate levels in patients with renal insufficiency.[246] Established aluminum bone disease can be managed by aluminum chelation with deferoxamine.[209]

Osteitis fibrosa often becomes evident in more advanced renal disease. PTH hypersecretion occurs in response to the hypocalcemic stimulus produced by decreased renal phosphate clearance and reduced $1,25(OH)_2D$ production. Marked parathyroid hyperplasia can ultimately occur, and in the absence of vitamin D deficiency or aluminum overload, extensive osteitis fibrosa then becomes the dominant skeletal lesion. Treatment with $1,25(OH)_2D$ (0.5 to 1.0 μg per day) in combination with calcium supplementation and serum phosphate control produces substantial improvement in bone symptoms, a decrease in serum iPTH and alkaline phosphatase levels, and improved bone mineralization.[247] Serum calcium levels should not be normalized before correcting the serum phosphate concentration, to avoid the risk of metastatic calcification.

Osteoporosis occurs in combination with other bone changes in chronic renal failure. Possible predisposing factors include chronically reduced calcium and elevated PTH levels, acidosis, and malnutrition. Osteosclerosis appears in local areas of the skeleton in many uremic individuals. It is usually most obvious in the lumbar vertebrae, where bands of osteosclerosis alternate with less dense bone to produce the so-called "rugger-jersey spine."

PAGET'S DISEASE OF BONE

Paget's disease of bone is a chronic skeletal disorder of unknown cause that occurs in 3 percent of the population over 40 and 10 percent of persons in their ninth decade.[248–250] Familial patterns of inheritance have been occasionally reported.

The disorder is characteristically not symptomatic or only minimally so. Bone pain and skeletal deformity are the most common complaints. Commonly, there is only local skeletal involvement with perhaps one or two vertebrae involved. In contrast, extensive multifocal forms can be associated with considerable pain, deformity, and disability. Although the lumbosacral spine, skull, pelvis, femur, and tibia are the areas most frequently affected, the disease has been described in all parts of the skeleton. The course is unpredictable; the disease may remain localized, be rapidly progressive, or wax and wane.

The earliest phase of Paget's disease is an increase in osteoclastic bone resorption, which is manifested radiologically as a localized osteolytic area, often in the skull (*osteoporosis circumscripta*), or as a flame-shaped radiolucency in the ends of long bones[251] (Fig. 96–18). In time, a compensatory in-

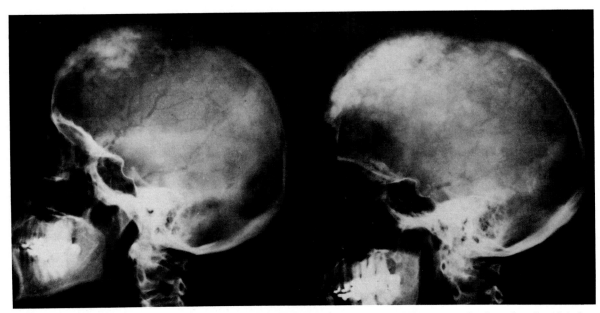

Figure 96–18. Paget's disease of the skull. Early phase *(left)* demonstrates areas of radiolucency in the frontal and occipital regions ("osteoporosis circumscripta") with a patchy increase in osteoblastic activity in the frontal region. More advanced phase *(right)* demonstrates increased osteoblastic activity with thickening and deformity of the skull, and involvement of the facial bones.

crease in osteoblastic activity occurs, characterized by disorganized formation of new bone, which lacks the normal trabecular pattern. In chaotic fashion, new bone is formed, destroyed, and reconstituted at abnormally rapid rates. An involved bone may increase in size, yet be susceptible to deformity or fracture owing to its abnormal structure (Fig. 96–19). Pain in Paget's disease can be due to (1) osteoarthritis (most commonly in the hip or knee) owing to altered joint architecture or altered posture as a result of leg deformities; (2) impingement on nerve roots, especially in the lumbar spine; and (3) direct involvement of bone. The most common deformities are kyphosis, bowing of the extremities, and enlargement of the skull. When the disease involves the skull, development of platybasia can lead to impingement on the long tracts of the spinal cord, and cranial nerve compression can lead to nerve deafness, vestibular dysfunction, and optic atrophy. High output congestive heart failure is a rare complication seen when there is extensive involvement of the skeleton and appears to be due to greatly increased blood flow to bone. Osteogenic sarcoma is a uniformly lethal complication but occurs in fewer than 1 percent of cases. It usually originates in the metaphyseal regions of long bones, particularly the proximal portion of the humerus.

The diagnosis of Paget's disease is based primarily on the characteristic radiographic findings and an elevated serum alkaline phosphatase level. Radionuclide bone scans provide the most sensitive means of determining the location of active Paget's lesions. The characteristic biochemical abnormalities are an elevated serum alkaline phosphatase and increased urinary hydroxyproline excretion. Both of these parameters parallel the course of the bone disease.

Serum and urine calcium levels and other biochemical parameters are usually within normal limits. In patients with extensive involvement, however, immobilization can lead to hypercalciuria and hypercalcemia owing to the markedly increased bone turnover rate.

In most cases, treatment of mild pain with aspirin or nonsteroidal anti-inflammatory agents is adequate. Treatment with osteoclast-inhibiting agents is indicated in more severe cases in which there is impingement on cranial or spinal nerves or extensive involvement of the skull, pelvis, or lower extremities, which could lead to serious complications. Calcitonin (50 to 100 M.R.C. units per day) can decrease bone pain, reduce high outpatient failure, and decrease indices of disease activity. Clinical and biochemical responses are generally seen after several months of therapy. Calcitonin is frequently effective in doses as low as 50 to 100 M.R.C. units three times weekly, and treatment can be continued indefinitely. Occasionally, development of high-titer neutralizing antibodies can produce resistance to calcitonin. Diphosphonates may also be effective. Sodium etidronate given orally at a dose of 5 μg per kg per day (typically 200 mg twice daily) can decrease alkaline phosphatase and hydroxyproline by 50 percent over a 6-month period, often with a period of continuing remission after discontinuation of therapy. Higher doses of sodium etidronate suppress osteoblast function and can produce osteomalacia, bone pain, and increased fracture incidence. Sodium etidronate is commonly used in 6- to 9-month courses, alternating with 6 or more months without treatment. In severe cases, a combination of calcitonin and etidronate treatment can be employed. Current experience with APD indicates that this

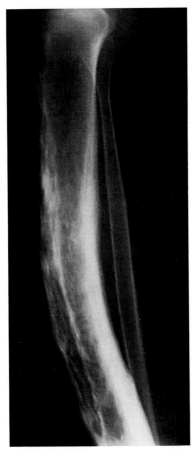

Figure 96–19. Paget's disease in the tibia. Note the disorganized trabecular pattern, thickening of the shaft, and bowing.

second-generation bisphosphonate can produce prolonged remission with minimal risk of side effects.[257] Mithramycin (15 to 25 μg per kg body weight per day) rapidly decreases all indices of activity. Hepatic, renal, and hematologic toxicities, however, limit the usefulness of this drug.

Despite biochemical improvement and evidence of improved bone remodeling after treatment with these various agents, bone deformity and neurologic defects generally persist or are only minimally reversed. The major goals of drug therapy are to reduce pain and limit further deformity.

MISCELLANEOUS DISORDERS

Osteopetrosis

Osteopetrosis (Albers-Schonberg disease, marble bone disease) is a rare inherited disorder characterized by increased skeletal density owing to decreased osteoclast function.[253] The severe form is inherited as an autosomal recessive trait, and common features include an enlarged head, optic atrophy, hearing loss, impaired growth, fractures, osteomyelitis, hepatosplenomegaly, lymphadenopathy, and anemia. The mild form is usually inherited as an autosomal

dominant trait. About half of these patients are asymptomatic, although fractures, cranial nerve palsies, bone pain, and osteomyelitis occur in some patients. Serum calcium, phosphorus, and alkaline phosphatase concentrations are usually normal, but hypocalcemia, hypophosphatemia, and elevated alkaline phosphatase levels can occur. A recently recognized syndrome of autosomal recessive osteoporosis, type I RTA, and basal ganglia calcification has been found to be associated with carbonic anhydrase II deficiency.[253]

The radiologic features of osteopetrosis include a markedly increased skeletal density, absent marrow cavities, "club-like" deformities of the long bones, and a "bone within a bone" appearance of the vertebral bodies (Fig. 96–20). Bone histology reveals remnants of fetal calcified cartilage and woven bone. Numerous osteoclasts may be present but are not actively engaged in bone resorption.

Studies in patients with osteopetrosis and genetic osteopetrotic mice have demonstrated that normal bone resorption can be restored by transplantation of normal bone marrow.[254] Macrophage colony stimulating factor has been shown to reverse the bone lesions in osteopetrotic mice.[258] These findings suggest that decreased osteoclast function in osteopetrosis may be the result of defective production of

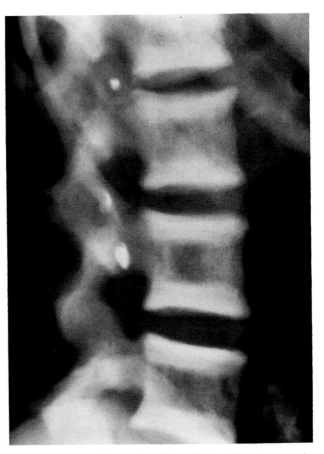

Figure 96–20. Lumbar spine of a patient with osteopetrosis. Marked osteosclerosis in the vertebral end plates gives a "rugger jersey" appearance.

certain cells of the monocyte-macrophage series or their regulatory factors.

Fibrous Dysplasia

Fibrous dysplasia of bone is a disorder of unknown cause that does not appear to have a genetic basis. The classic triad of abnormal findings includes bone lesions, precocious puberty (primarily in girls), and café au lait skin lesions with serrated edges. The disorder usually becomes clinically apparent between the ages of 3 and 10, and it is more common in girls.[256-258]

The bone lesions of fibrous dysplasia have a characteristic "ground-glass" radiologic appearance and may be multiloculated (Fig. 96–21). Focal cortical thinning and expansion of the diaphysis are observed.[258, 259] These lesions may involve the femur, tibia, pelvis, hands, feet, humerus, skull, and facial bones. Gross deformities such as shepherd's-crook deformity of the femur, coxa vara, tibial bowing, and protrusio acetabuli are common. Increased radiodensity of the base of the skull, thickening of the occiput, and involvement of the facial bones are also observed. Pain, deformity, and pathologic fractures are the primary manifestations of the underlying bone disease. A variety of malignant tumors may arise in the bone lesions.

Serum calcium and phosphorus concentrations are usually normal in patients with this disorder, but serum alkaline phosphatase activity and urinary hydroxyproline excretion are often considerably elevated, reflecting increased bone turnover. Bone histology demonstrates the presence of fibrous tissue within the bone trabeculae. A woven bone pattern is observed, with random distribution of collagen fibers, which appear to extend into the surrounding fibrous tissue. Numerous osteoblasts are seen in areas of active new bone formation, and large numbers of osteoclasts occur in adjacent regions. Occasional islands of cartilage may be found, and fluid-filled cysts can develop in areas of previous surgery or trauma. Following fracture, callus formation is often deficient.

The pathogenesis of fibrous dysplasia remains undefined. It is not clear whether the disorder has an underlying metabolic basis, since monostotic forms occur. Although the histologic finding of increased osteoclasts suggests that calcitonin might be an effective therapy, the few patients so treated have not experienced significant improvement.

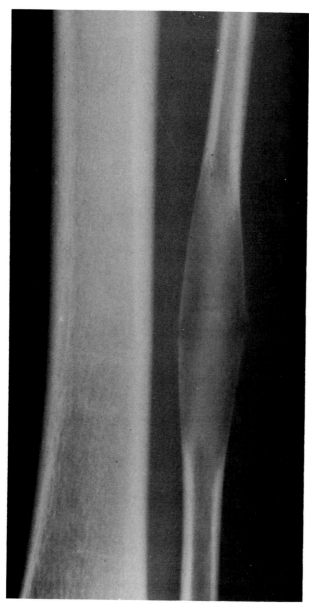

Figure 96–21. Fibrous dysplasia in the lower extremity. Note the expansion of the diaphysis of the fibula, the ground glass appearance, and the cortical thinning.

References

1. Johnston, C. C., Jr., Slemenda, C. W., and Melton, L. J., III.: Clinical use of bone densitometry. N. Engl. J. Med. 324:1105, 1991.
2. Orwoll, E. S., Oviatt, S. K., and the Nafarelin/Bone Study Group: Longitudinal precision of dual-energy x-ray absorptiometry in a multicenter study. J. Bone Miner. Res. 6:191–197, 1991.
3. McFarland, W.: Evaluation of bone density from roentgenograms. Science 119:810, 1955.
4. Khairi, M. R. A., Cronin, J. H., Robb, J. A., et al.: Femoral trabecular index and bone mineral content measured by photon absorption in senile osteoporosis. J. Bone Joint Surg. 58A:221, 1976.
5. Garn, S. M., Pozanski, A. K., and Nagy, J. M.: Bone measurement in differential diagnosis of osteopenia and osteoporosis. Radiology 100:509, 1971.
6. Parisien, M., Silverberg, S. J., Shane, E., Dempster, D. W., and Bilezikian, J. P.: Bone disease in primary hyperparathyroidism. Endocrinol. Metab. Clin. North Am. 19:19, 1990.
7. Wahner, H. W.: Measurements of bone mass and bone density. Endocrinol. Metab. Clin. North Am. 18:995, 1989.
8. Sartoris, D. J., and Resnick, D.: Current and innovative methods for noninvasive bone densitometry. Radiol. Clin. North Am. 28:257, 1990.
9. Steiger, P., Block, J. E., Steiger, S., Heuck, A. F., Friedlander, A., Ettinger, B., Harris, S. T., Gluer, C. and Genant, H. K.: Spinal bone mineral density measured with quantitative CT: Effect of region of interest, vertebral level, and technique. Radiology 175:537, 1990.
10. Tosteson, A. N. A., Rosenthal, D. I., Melton, L. J., III, and Weinstein, M. C.: Cost effectiveness of screening perimenopausal white women for osteoporosis: Bone densitometry and hormone replacement. Ann. Intern. Med. 113:594, 1990.
11. Marshall, R. W.: Plasma fraction. In Nordin, B. E. C. (ed.): Calcium,

Phosphate and Magnesium Metabolism. Edinburgh, Churchill Livingstone, 1976, p. 162.

12. Jaun, D.: The causes and consequences of hypophosphatemia. Surg. Gynecol. Obstet. 153:589, 1981.

13. Schiele, F., Henny, J., Hitz, J., Petitclerc, C., Geuguen, R., and Siest, G.: Total bone and liver alkaline phosphatases in plasma: Biological variations and reference limits. Clin. Chem. 29:634, 1983.

14. Price, P.: Osteocalcin. In Peck, W. A., (ed.): Bone and Mineral Research, Annual 1. Amsterdam, Excerpta Medica, 1983, p. 157.

15. Lian, J. B., and Gunberg, C. M.: Osteocalcin: Biochemical considerations and clinical applications. Clin. Orthop. 262:267, 1988.

16. Hauschka, P. V., Lian, J. B., Cole, D. E. C., and Grundberg, C. M.: Osteocalcin and matrix Gla protein: Vitamin K-dependent protein in bone. Phys. Rev. 60:990, 1988.

16a. Delmas, P. D.: Biochemical markers of bone turnover: methodology and clinical use in osteoporosis. Am. J. Med. 91(Suppl. 5B):59S, 1991.

17. Robertson, W. G.: Urinary excretion. In Nordin, B. E. C. (ed.): Calcium, Phosphate and Magnesium Metabolism. Edinburgh, Churchill Livingstone, 1976, p. 113.

18. Need, A. G., Guerin, M. D., Pain, R. W., Hartley, T. F., and Nordin, C.: The tubular maximum for calcium reabsorption: Normal range and correction for sodium excretion. Clin. Chim. Acta. 150:87, 1985.

19. Need, A. G., Philcox, J. C., Hartley, T. F., and Nordin, B. E.: Calcium metabolism and osteoporosis in corticosteroid-treated postmenopausal women. Aust. N.Z. J. Med. 16:341, 1986.

20. Nordin, B. E. C., Need, A. G., Morris, H. A., Horowitz, M., and Robertson, W. G.: Evidence for a renal calcium leak in postmenopausal women. J. Clin. Endocrinol. Metab. 72:401, 1991.

21. Walton, R. J., and Bijvoet, O. L. M.: Nomogram for derivation of renal threshold phosphate concentration. Lancet 2:309, 1975.

22. Endres, D. B., Villanueva, R., Sharp, C. F., Jr., and Singer, F. R.: The measurement of parathyroid hormone. Endocrinol. Metab. Clin. North Am. 18:611, 1989.

23. Habener, J. F., Rosenblatt, M., and Potts, J. T., Jr.: Parathyroid hormone: Biochemical aspects of biosynthesis, secretion, action, and metabolism. Physiol. Rev. 64:985, 1984.

24. Bell, N. H.: Vitamin D–endocrine system. J. Clin. Invest. 76:1, 1985.

25. Malluche, H. H., and Fuagere, M-C.: Bone biopsies: Histology and histomorphometry. In Avioli, L. V., and Krane, S. M. (eds.): Metabolic Bone Disease and Clinically Related Disorders. 2nd ed. Philadelphia, W. B. Saunders Company, 1990, pp. 283–328.

26. Raisz, L. G., and Smith, J.: Pathogenesis, prevention and treatment of osteoporosis. Annu. Rev. Med. 40:251, 1989.

27. Cummings, S. R., Kelsey, J. L., Nevitt, M. C., and O'Dowd, K. J.: Epidemiology of osteoporosis and osteoporotic fractures. Epidemiol. Rev. 7:178, 1985.

28. Thomas, K. A., Cook, S. D., Bennett, J. T., Whitecloud, T. S., and Rice, J. C.: Femoral neck and lumbar spine densities in a normal population 3–20 years of age. J. Pediatr. Orthop. 11:48, 1991.

29. Meier, D. S., Orwoll, E. S., Keenan, E. J., and Fagerstrom, F.: Marked decline in trabecular bone mineral content in healthy men with age: Lack of association with sex steroid levels. J. Am. Geriatr. Soc. 35:189, 1987.

30. Riggs, B. L., and Melton, L. J., III.: Involutional osteoporosis. N. Engl. J. Med. 314:1676, 1986.

31. Aloia, J. F., Cohn, S. H., Vaswani, A., Yeh, J. K., Kapo, Y., and Kenneth, E.: Risk factors for postmenopausal osteoporosis. Am. J. Med. 78:95, 1985.

32. Jackson, J. A., and Kleerekoper, M.: Osteoporosis in men: Diagnosis, pathophysiology, and prevention. Medicine 69:137, 1990.

33. Liel, Y., Edwards, J, Shary, J., Spicer, K. M., Gordon, L., and Bell, N. H.: The effects of race and body habitus on bone mineral density of the radius, hip and spine in premenopausal women. J. Clin. Endocrinol. Metab. 66:1247, 1988.

34. Silverman, A. L., and Madison, R. E.: Decreased incidence of hip fracture in Hispanics, blacks and Asians. Am. J. Public Health 78:1482, 1988.

35. Mazees, R. B., and Mather, W. B.: Bone mineral content in Canadian Eskimos. Hum. Biol. 47:45, 1975.

36. Dawson-Hughes, B., Shipp, C., Dadowski, L., and Dallal, G.: Bone density of the radius, spine, and hip in relation to per cent of ideal body weight in postmenopausal women. Calcif. Tiss. Int. 40:310, 1987.

37. Kley, H. K., Deselaers, T., Peerenboom, H., and Kruskemper, H. L.: Enhanced conversion of androstenedione to estrones in obese males. J. Clin. Endocrinol. Metab. 51:1128, 1980.

38. Michnovicz, J. J., Hershcopf, R. J., Naganuma, H., Bradlow, H. L., and Fishman, J.: Increased 2-hydroxylation of estradiol as a possible mechanism for the anti-estrogen effect of cigarette smoking. N. Engl. J. Med. 315:1305, 1986.

39. Spencer, H., Rubio, N., Rubio, E., Indreika, M., and Seitam, A.: Chronic alcoholism: Frequently overlooked cause of osteoporosis in men. Am. J. Med. 80:393, 1986.

40. Cann, C. E., Genant, H. K., Kolb, F. O., and Ettinger, B.: Quantitative computed tomography for prediction of vertebral fracture risk. Bone 6:1, 1985.

41. Riggs, B. L., Wahner, H. W., Melton, J., Richelson, L. S., Judd, H. L., and Offord, K. P.: Rates of bone loss in the appendicular and axial skeletons of women. J. Clin. Invest. 77:1487, 1986.

42. Bab, I., Passi-Even, L., Gazit, D., Sekeles, E., Ashton, B. A., Peylan-Ramu, N., Ziv, I., and Ulmansky, M.: Osteogenesis in in vivo diffusion chamber cultures of human marrow cells. Bone Miner. 4:373, 1988.

43. Tsuji, T., Hughes, F. J., McCulloch, C. A. G., and Melcher, A. H.: Effects of donor age on osteogenic cells of rat bone marrow in vitro. Mech. Age. Dev. 51:121, 1990.

44. Aaron, J. E., Stasiak, L., Gallagher, J. C., et al.: Frequency of osteomalacia and osteoporosis in fractures of the proximal femur. Lancet 1:7851, 1974.

45. Whyte, M. P., Bergfeld, M. A., Murphy, W. A., Avioli, L. V., and Teitelbaum, S. L.: Postmenopausal osteoporosis: A heterogeneous disorder as assessed by histomorphometric analysis of iliac crest bone from untreated patients. Am. J. Med. 72:193, 1982.

46. Avioli, L. V.: Significance of osteoporosis: A growing international health care problem. Calcif. Tiss. Int. 49(Suppl.):S5, 1991.

47. Teitelbaum, S. L., Rosenberg, E. M., Richardson, C. A., and Avioli, L. V.: Histological studies of bone from normocalcemic postmenopausal osteoporotic patients with increased circulating parathyroid hormone. J. Clin. Endocrinol. Metab. 42:537, 1976.

48. Perry, H. M., III, Fallon, M. D., Bergfeld, M., Teitelbaum, S. L., and Avioli, L. V.: Osteoporosis in young men: A syndrome of hypercalciuria and accelerated bone turnover. Arch. Intern. Med. 142:1295, 1982.

49. Matkovic, V., Fontana, D., Tominac, C., Goel, P., and Chesnut, C. H., III: Factors that influence peak bone mass formation: A study of calcium balance and the inheritance of bone mass in adolescent females. Am. J. Clin. Nutr. 52:878, 1990.

50. Ott, S. M.: Editorial: Attainment of peak bone mass. J. Clin. Endocrinol. Metab. 71:1082A, 1990.

51. Rodin, A., Murphy, B., Smith, M. A., Caleffi, M., Fentiman, I., Chapman, M. G., and Fogelman, I.: Premature bone loss in the lumbar spine and neck of femur: A study of 225 Caucasian women. Bone 211:1, 1990.

52. Pollitzer, W. S., and Anderson, J. J. B.: Ethnic and genetic differences in bone mass: A review with hereditary vs. environmental perspective. Am. J. Clin. Nutr. 50:1244, 1990.

53. Pocock, N. A., Eisman, J. A., Hopper, J. L., Yeates, M. G., Sambrook, P. N., and Eberi, S.: Genetic determinants of bone mass in adults. J. Clin. Invest. 80:706, 1987.

54. Seeman, E., Hopper, J. L., Bach, L. A., Cooper, M. E., Parkinson, E., McKay, J., and Jerums, G.: Reduced bone mass in daughters of women with osteoporosis. N. Engl. J. Med. 320:554, 1989.

55. Buchanan, J. R., Myers, C., Lloyd, T., Leuenberger, P., and Demers, L. M.: Determinants of peak trabecular bone density in women: The role of androgens, estrogen, and exercise. J. Bone Miner. Res. 3:673, 1988.

55a. Eisman, J. A., Sambrook, P. N., Kelly, P. J., and Pocock, N. A.: Exercise and its interaction with genetic influences in the determination of bone mineral density. Am. J. Med. 91(Suppl. 5B):5S, 1991.

56. Lanyon, L. E.: Strain-related bone modeling and remodeling. Top. Geriatr. Rehabil. 4:13, 1989.

57. Margulies, J. Y., Simkin, A., Leitcher, I., Bivas, A., Steinberg, R., Giladi, M., Stein, M., Kashtan, H., and Milgrom, I.: Effect of intense physical activity on the bone-mineral content in the lower limbs of young adults. J. Bone Joint Surg. 68A:1090, 1986.

58. Davee, A. M., Rosen, C., and Adler, R. A.: Exercise patterns and trabecular bone density in college women. J. Bone Miner. Res. 5:245, 1990.

59. Drinkwater, B. L., Nilson, K., Ott, S., and Chesnut, C. H.: Bone mineral density after resumption of menses in amenorrheic athletes. J.A.M.A. 256:380, 1986.

60. Marcus, R., Cann, C., Madvig, P., Minkoff, J., Goddard, M., Bayer, M., Martin, M., Gaudiani, L., Haskell, W., and Genant, H.: Menstrual function and bone mass in elite women distance runners. Ann. Intern. Med. 102:158, 1985.

61. Jones, K. P., Ravinikar, V. A., Tulchinsky, D., and Schiff, I.: Comparison of bone density in amenorrheic women due to athletics, weight loss, and premature menopause. Obstet. Gynecol. 66:5, 1985.

62. Kelsey, J. L., and Hoffman, S.: Risk factors for hip fracture. N. Engl. J. Med. 316:404, 1987.

63. Grisso, J. A., Kelsey, J. L., Strom, B. L., Chiu, G. Y., Maislin, G., O'Brien, L. A., Hoffman, S., Kaplan, F., and the Northeast Hip Fracture Study Group: Risk factors for falls as a cause of hip fracture in women. N. Engl. J. Med. 324:1326, 1991.

64. Porter, R. W., Miller, C. G., Grainger, D., and Palmer, S. B.: Prediction of hip fracture in elderly women: A prospective study. Br. Med. J. 301:638, 1990.

65. Heaney, R. P., Recker, R. R., and Saville, P. D.: Calcium balance requirements in middle-aged women. Am. J. Clin. Nutr. 30:1603, 1977.

66. Arnaud, C. D., and Sanchez, S. D.: The role of calcium in osteoporosis. Annu. Rev. Nutr. 10:397, 1990.

67. Recker, R. R.: Calcium absorption and achlorhydria. N. Engl. J. Med. 313:70, 1985.

68. Shangraw, R. F.: Factors to consider in the selection of a calcium supplement. Public Health Rep. Suppl. 104:46, 1989.
69. Riis, B., Thomsen, K., and Christiansen, C.: Does calcium supplementation prevent postmenopausal bone loss? N. Engl. J. Med. 316:173, 1987.
70. Ettinger, B., Genant, H. K., and Cann, C. E.: Postmenopausal bone loss is prevented by treatment with low-dosage estrogen with calcium. Ann. Intern. Med. 106:40, 1987.
71. Anderson, J. J. B., Reed, J. A., Tylavsky, F. A., Lester, G. E., Talamage, R. V., and Taft, T. N.: Lack of an effect of dietary calcium in preventing the loss of radial bone mass in high-calcium consuming elderly white women. In Christiansen, C., and Overgaard, K. (eds.): Osteoporosis 1990. Copenhagen, Osteoporess APS, 1990, pp. 981–984.
72. Cumming, R. G.: Calcium intake and bone mass: A quantitative review of the literature. Calcif. Tiss. Int. 47:194, 1990.
72a. Johnston, C. C., Jr., Miller, J. Z., Slemenda, C. W., Reister, T. K., Hui, S., Christian, J. C., and Peacock, M.: Calcium supplementation and increases in bone mineral density in children. N. Engl. J. Med. 327:82, 1992.
73. Finkenstedt, G., Skrabal, F., Gasser, R. W., and Braunsteiner, H.: Lactose absorption, milk consumption, and fasting blood glucose concentrations in women with idiopathic osteoporosis. Br. Med. J. 292:161, 1986.
74. Birge, S. J., and Dalsky, G.: The role of exercise in preventing osteoporosis. Public Health Rep. Suppl. 104:54, 1989.
75. Aloia, J. F., Cohn, S. H., Ostuni, J. A., Cane, R., and Ellis, K.: Prevention of involutional bone loss by exercise. Ann. Intern. Med. 89:356, 1978.
76. President's Council on Fitness: Adult Physical Fitness: A program for men and women. United States Government Printing Office, 1965.
77. Dalsky, G., Stocke, K. S., and Ehsani, A. A.: Weight-bearing exercise training and lumbar spine bone mineral content in postmenopausal women. Ann. Intern. Med. 108:824, 1988.
78. Rockwell, J. C., Sorenson, A. M., Baker, S., Leahey, D., Stock, J. L., Michaels, J., and Baran D. T.: Weight training decreases vertebral bone density in postmenopausal women: a prospective study. J. Clin. Endocrinol. Metab. 71:988, 1990.
79. Cavanaugh, D. J., and Cann, C. E.: Brisk walking does not stop bone loss in postmenopausal women. Bone 9:201, 1988.
80. Marcus, R.: Understanding osteoporosis. West. J. Med. 155:53, 1991.
81. Civitelli, R., Gonnelli, S., Zacchei, F., Bigazzi, S., Vattimo, A., Avioli, L. V., and Gennari, C.: Bone turnover in postmenopausal osteoporosis: Effect of calcitonin treatment. J. Clin. Invest. 82:1268, 1988.
82. Overgaard, K., Hansen, M. A., Nielsen, V. H., Riis, B. J., and Christiansen, C.: Discontinuous calcitonin treatment of established osteoporosis—effects of withdrawal of treatment. Am. J. Med. 89:1, 1990.
83. Macintyre, I., Stevenson, J. C., Whitehead, M. I., Wimalawansa, S. J., Banks, L. M., and Healy, M. J. R.: Calcitonin for prevention of postmenopausal bone loss. Lancet 1:900, 1988.
84. McDermott, M. T., and Kidd, G. S.: The role of calcitonin in the development and treatment of osteoporosis. Endoc. Rev. 8:377, 1987.
85. Ljunghall, S., Gardsell, P., Johnell, O., Larsson, K., Lindh, E., Obrant, K., and Sernbo, I.: Synthetic human calcitonin in postmenopausal osteoporosis: A placebo-controlled, double-blind study. Calcif. Tiss. Int. 49:17, 1991.
85a. Parfitt, A. M.: Use of bisphosphonates in the prevention of bone loss and fractures. Am. J. Med. 91(Suppl. 5B):42S, 1991.
86. Storm, T., Thamsborg, G., Steiniche, T., Geneant, H. K., and Sorensen, O. H.: Effect of intermittent cyclical etidronate therapy on bone mass and fracture rate in women with postmenopausal osteoporosis. N. Engl. J. Med. 322:1265, 1990.
87. Watts, N. B., Harris, S. T., Genant, H. K., Wasnich, R. D., Miller, P. D., Jackson, R. D., Licata, A. A., Ross, P., Woodson, G. C., Yanover, M. J., Mysiw, W. J., Kohse, L., Rao, M. B., Steiger, P., Richmond, B., and Chestnut, C. C., III: Intermittent cyclical etidronate treatment of postmenopausal osteoporosis. N. Engl. J. Med. 323:73, 1990.
88. Johnston, C. C., Altman, R. D., Canfield, R. E., Finerman, G. A. M., Taubee, J. D., and Ebert, M. L.: Review of fracture experience during treatment of Paget's disease of bone with sodium etidronate. Clin. Orthop. 172:186, 1983.
89. Valkema, R., Vismans, F. J., Papaoulos, S. E., Pauwels, E. K., and Bijvoet, O. L.: Maintained improvement in calcium balance and bone mineral content in patients with osteoporosis treated with the bisphosphonate APD. Bone Miner. 5:183, 1989.
90. Riggs, B. L.: Treatment of osteoporosis with sodium fluoride: An appraisal. In Peck, W. A. (ed.): Bone and Mineral Research Annual 2. New York, Elsevier, 1984, pp. 366–393.
91. Hansson, T., and Roos, B.: The effect of fluoride and calcium on spinal bone mineral content: A controlled, prospective (3 years) study. Calcif. Tissue Int. 40:315, 1987.
92. Farley, J. R., Wergedal, J. E., and Baylink, D. J.: Fluoride directly stimulates proliferation and alkaline phosphatase activity of bone-forming cells. Science 222:330, 1983.
93. Riggs, B. L., Hodgson, S. F., O'Fallon, M., Chao, E. Y. S., Wahner,

H. W., Muhs, J. M., Cedel, S. L., and Melton, L. J., III: Effect of fluoride treatment on the fracture rate in postmenopausal women with osteoporosis. N. Engl. J. Med. 322:802, 1990.
94. Pak, C. Y. C., Sakhaee, K., Zerwekh, J. E., Parcel, C., Peterson, R., and Johnson, K.: Safe and effective treatment of osteoporosis with intermittent slow release sodium fluoride: Augmentation of vertebral bone mass and inhibition of fractures. J. Clin. Endocrinol. Metab. 68:150, 1989.
95. Zerwekh, J. E., Antich, P. P., Sakhaee, K., Gonzales, J., Gottschalk, F., and Pak, C. Y. C.: Assessment by reflection ultrasound method of the effect of intermittent slow-release sodium fluoride calcium citrate therapy on material strength of bone. J. Bone Miner. Res. 6:239, 1991.
96. Transbol, I., Christensen, M. S., Jensen, G. F., Christiansen, C., and McNair, P.: Thiazides for the postponement of postmenopausal bone loss. N. Engl. J. Med. 309:344, 1983.
97. LaCroix, A. Z., Wienpahl, J., White, L. R., Wallace, R. B., Scherr, P. A., George, L. K., Cornoni-Huntley, J., and Ostfeld, A. M.: Thiazide diuretic agents and the incidence of hip fracture. N. Engl. J. Med. 322:286, 1990.
98. Heidrich, F. E., Stergachis, A., and Gross, K. M.: Diuretic use and risk for hip fracture. Ann. Intern. Med. 115:1, 1991.
99. Anderson, C., Cape, R. D., Crilly, R. G., Hodsman, A. B., and Wolf, B. M.: Preliminary observations of a form of coherence therapy for osteoporosis. Calcif. Tiss. Int. 36:341, 1984.
100. Aloia, J. F., Vaswani, A., Meunier, P. J., Edouard, C. M., Arlot, M. E., Yeh, J. K., and Cohn, S. H.: Coherence treatment of postmenopausal osteoporosis with growth hormone and calcitonin. Calcif. Tiss. Int. 40:253, 1987.
101. Gallagher, J. C., and Goldbar, D.: Treatment of postmenopausal osteoporosis with high doses of synthetic calcitriol. A randomized controlled study. Ann. Intern. Med. 113:649, 1990.
102. Ott, S. M., and Chesnut, C. H., III: Calcitriol treatment is not effective in postmenopausal osteoporosis. Ann. Intern. Med. 110:267, 1989.
103. Need, A. G., Horowitz, M., Bridges, A., Morris, E. A., and Nordin, B. E. C.: Effects of nandrolone deconate and antiresorptive therapy on vertebral density in osteoporotic postmenopausal women. Arch. Intern. Med. 149:57, 1989.
104. Lukert, B. P., and Raisz, L. G.: Glucocorticoid-induced osteoporosis: Pathogenesis and management. Ann. Intern. Med. 112:352, 1990.
105. Reid, I. R.: Steroid osteoporosis. Calcif. Tiss. Int. 45:63, 1989.
106. Hahn, T. J.: Drug-induced disorders of vitamin D and mineral metabolism. Clin. Endocrinol. Metab. 9:107, 1980.
107. Adinoff, A. D., and Hollister, J. R.: Steroid-induced fractures and bone loss in patients with asthma. N. Engl. J. Med. 309:265, 1983.
108. Dykman, T. R., Gluck, O. S., Murphy, W. A., Hahn, T. J., and Hahn, B. H.: Evaluation of factors associated with glucocorticoid-induced osteopenia in patients with rheumatic diseases. Arthritis Rheum. 28:361, 1985.
109. Thomson, B. M., Saklatvala, J., and Chambers, J.: Osteoblasts mediate interleukin 1 stimulation of bone resorption by rat osteoclasts. J. Exp. Med. 164:104, 1986.
110. Au, W. Y. W.: Cortisol stimulation of parathyroid hormone secretion by rat parathyroid glands in organ culture. Science 193:1015, 1976.
111. Suzuki, Y., Ichikawa, Y., and Homma, M.: Importance of increased urinary calcium excretion in the development of secondary hyperparathyroidism patients under glucocorticoid therapy. Metabolism 32:151, 1983.
112. Prummel, M. F., Wiersinga, W. M., Lips, P., Sanders, G. T. B., and Sauerwein, H. P.: The course of biochemical parameters of bone turnover during treatment with corticosteroids. J. Clin. Endocrinol. Metab. 72:382, 1991.
113. Dietrich, J. W., Canalis, E. M., Maina, D. M., and Raisz, L. G.: Effects of glucocorticoids on fetal rat bone collagen synthesis. Endocrinology 104:715, 1979.
114. Chyun, Y. S., Kream, B. E., and Raisz, L. G.: Cortisol decreases bone formation by inhibiting periosteal cell proliferation. Endocrinology 114:477, 1984.
115. Reid, I. R., France, J. T., Pybus, J., and Ibbertson, H. K.: Low plasma testosterone levels in glucocorticoid-treated male asthmatics. Br. Med. J. 291:574, 1985.
116. Hahn, T. J., Halstead, L. R., and Baran, D. T.: Effects of short-term glucocorticoid administration on intestinal calcium absorption and circulating vitamin D metabolite concentrations in man. J. Clin. Endocrinol. Metab. 52:111, 1981.
117. Hahn, T. J., Halstead, L. R., Teitelbaum, S. L., and Hahn, B. H.: Altered mineral metabolism in glucocorticoid-induced osteopenia: Effect of 25-hydroxyvitamin D administration. J. Clin. Invest. 64:655, 1979.
118. Dempster, D. W., Arlott, M. A., and Meuniwer, P. J.: Mean wall thickness and formation of trabecular bone packets in corticosteroid-induced osteoporosis. Calcif. Tiss. Int. 35:410, 1983.
119. LoCascio, V., Bonucci, E., Imbimbo, B., Ballanti, P., Tartarotti, D., Galvanni, G., Fucella, L., and Adami, S.: Bone loss after glucocorticoid therapy. Calcif. Tiss. Int. 36:435, 1984.
120. Grecu, E., Gordan, G., Simmons, R., and Weinshelbaum, L.: Medroxy-

progesterone acetate as an antagonist of adverse effects on calcium metabolism. In Christiansen, C., Johansen, J. S., and Riis, B. J. (eds.): Osteoporosis 1987. Kobenhavn, Osteopress, pp. 1077–1080.

121. Hahn, T. J., Halstead, L. R., Strates, B., Imbimbo, B., and Baran, D. T.: Comparison of subacute effects of oxazacort and prednisone on mineral metabolism in man. Calcif. Tiss. Int. 31:109, 1980.

122. Reid, I. R., Chapman, G. E., Fraser, T. R. C., Davies, A. D., Surus, A. S., Meyer, J., Huq, N. L., and Ibbertson, H. K.: Low serum osteocalcin levels in glucocorticoid-treated asthmatics. J. Clin. Endocrinol. Metab. 62:379, 1986.

123. Neilsen, H. K., Charles, P., and Mosekilde, L.: The effect of single oral doses of prednisone on the circadian rhythm of serum osteocalcin in normal subjects. J. Clin. Endocrinol. Metab. 67:1025, 1988.

124. Breessot, C., Meunier, P. J., Chapuy, M. C., Lejeune, E., Edouard, C., and Darby, A. J.: Histomorphometric profile, pathophysiology and reversibility of corticosteroid-induced osteoporosis. Metab. Bone Dis. Rel. Res. 1:303, 1979.

125. Pocock, N. A., Eisman, J. A., Dunstan, C. R., Evans, R. A., Thomas, D. H., and Huq, L. N.: Recovery from steroid-induced osteoporosis. Ann. Intern. Med. 107:319, 1987.

126. Sheagren, J. N., Jowzey, J., Bird, D. C., et al.: Effect on bone growth of daily versus alternate-day corticosteroid administration: An experimental study. J. Lab. Clin. Med. 89:120, 1977.

127. Gluck, O. S., Murphy, W. A., Hahn, T. J., and Hahn, B. H.: Bone loss in adults receiving alternate day glucocorticoid therapy: A comparison with daily therapy. Arthritis Rheum. 24:892, 1981.

128. Villareal, D. T., Civitelli, R., Gennari, C., and Avioli, L. V.: Is there an effective treatment for glucocorticoid-induced osteoporosis? Calcif. Tiss. Int. 49:141, 1991.

129. Spector, S., Greenwald, M., and Silverman, S. A.: Successful treatment of osteoporosis due to steroid-dependent COPD and asthma. Am. Rev. Respir. Dis. 139:A16, 1989.

130. Meunier, P. J., Briancon, D., Chavassieux, P., Edouard, C., Boivin, G., Conrozier, T., Marcelli, C., Pastoureau, P., Delams, P., and Casez, J. P. In Christiansen, C., Johansen, J. S., and Riis, B. J. (eds.): Osteoporosis 1987. Kobenhavn, Osteopress, 1987, pp. 1074–1076.

131. Need, A. G.: Corticosteroids and osteoporosis. Aust. N.Z. J. Med. 17:267, 1987.

132. Hahn, T. J., and Hahn, B. H.: Osteopenia in patients with rheumatic disease: Principles of diagnosis and therapy. Semin. Arthritis Rheum. 6:165, 1976.

133. Muenier, P. J., Briancon, D., Chavassieux, P., et al.: Treatment with fluoride: Bone histomorphometric finds. In Christiansen, C., Johansen, J. S., and Riis, B. J. (eds.): Osteoporosis 1987. Kobenhavn, Osteopress, 1987, pp. 824–828.

134. Munno, O. D., Beghe, F., Favini, P., di Giuseppe, P., Pontrandolfo, A., Occhipinti, G., and Pasero, G.: Prevention of glucocorticoid-induced osteopenia: Effect of oral 25-hydroxyvitamin D and calcium. Clin. Rheumatol. 2:202, 1989.

135. Dykman, T. R., Haralson, K. M., Gluck, O. S., Murphy, W. A., Teitelbaum, S. L., Hahn, T. J., and Hahn, B. H.: Effect of 1,25-dihydroxyvitamin D and calcium on glucocorticoid-induced osteopenia in patients with rheumatic diseases. Arthritis Rheum. 27:336, 1984.

136. Davies, M.: High dose vitamin D therapy: Indications, benefits and hazards. Int. J. Vitamin Nutr. Res. Suppl. 30:81, 1989.

137. Reid, I. R., and Ibbertson, H. K.: Calcium supplements in the prevention of steroid-induced osteoporosis. Am. J. Clin. Nutr. 44:287, 1986.

138. Ringe, J. D., and Welzel, D.: Salmon calcitonin in the therapy of corticoid-induced osteoporosis. Eur. J. Clin. Pharmacol. 33:35, 1987.

139. Luengo, M., Picado, C., del Rio, L., Guanabens, N., Montserrat, J. M., and Setoain, J.: Treatment of steroid-induced osteopenia with calcitonin in corticosteroid-dependent asthma. Am. Rev. Respir. Dis. 142:104, 1990.

140. Montemurro, L., Schiraldi, G., Fraioli, P., Tosi, G., Riboldi, A., and Rizzato, G.: Prevention of corticosteroid-induced osteoporosis with salmon calcitonin. Calcif. Tiss. Int. 49:71, 1991.

141. Reid, I. R., King, A. R., Alexander, C. J., and Ibbertson, H. K.: Prevention of steroid-induced osteoporosis with (3-amino-1-hydroxypropylidene)-1,1-bisphosphonate (APD). Lancet 1:143, 1988.

142. Reid, I. R., Heap, S. W., King, A. R., and Ibbertson, H. K.: Two-year followup of bisphosphonate (APD) treatment in steroid osteoporosis (letter). Lancet 2:1144, 1988.

143. Reid, I. R., Schooler, B. A., and Stewart, A. W.: Prevention of glucocorticoid-induced osteoporosis. J. Bone Miner. Res. 5:619, 1990.

144. Lindsay, R.: Prevention of spinal osteoporosis in oophorectomised women. Lancet 2:1152, 1980.

145. Richelson, L. S., Wahner, H. W., Melton, L. J., III, and Riggs, B. C.: Relative contributions of aging and estrogen deficiency to postmenopausal bone loss. N. Engl. J. Med. 311:1273, 1984.

146. Prior, J. C., Vigna, Y. M., Schechter, M. T., Burgess, A. E.: Spinal bone loss and ovulatory disturbances. N. Engl. J. Med. 323:1221, 1990.

147. Mazess, R. B.: On aging bone loss. Clin. Orthop. 165:239, 1982.

148. Stock, J. L., Coderre, J. A., and Mallette, L. E.: Effects of a short course of estrogen on mineral metabolism in postmenopausal women. J. Clin. Endocrinol. Metab. 61:595, 1985.

149. Eriksen, E. F., Colvard, D. S., Berg, N. J., Graham, M. L., Mann, K. G., Spelsberg, T. C., and Riggs, B. L.: Evidence of estrogen receptors in normal human osteoblast cells. Science 241:84, 1988.

150. Benz, D. J., Haussler, M. R., and Komm, B. S.: Estrogen binding and estrogenic responses in normal human osteoblast-like cells. J. Bone Miner. Res. 6:531, 1991.

150a. Jilka, R. L., Hangoc, G., Girasle, G., Passeri, G., Williams, D. C., Abrams, J. S., Boyce, B., Broxmeyer, H., and Manolagas, S. C.: Increased osteoclast development after estrogen loss: mediation by interleukin-6. Science 257:88, 1992.

151. Orimo, H., Fujita, T., and Yoshikawa, M.: Increased sensitivity of bone to parathyroid hormone in ovariectomized rats. Endocrinology 90:760, 1972.

152. Selby, P. L., and Peacock, M.: Ethinyl estradiol and norethindrone in the treatment of primary hyperparathyroidism in postmenopausal women. N. Engl. J. Med. 314:1481, 1986.

153. Raisz, L. G., and Kream, B. E.: Regulation of bone formation (2 parts). N. Engl. J. Med. 309:29, 1983.

154. Lindsay, R.: Estrogen/progestogen therapy: Prevention and treatment of postmenopausal osteoporosis. Proc. Soc. Exp. Biol. Med. 191:275, 1989.

155. Barzel, U. S.: Estrogens in the prevention and treatment of postmenopausal osteoporosis: A review. Am. J. Med. 85:847, 1988.

156. Christiansen, C., and Riis, B. J.: 17β-Estradiol and continuous norethisterone: A unique treatment for established osteoporosis in elderly women. J. Clin. Endocrinol. Metab. 71:836, 1990.

157. Lindsay, R., and Tohme, J. F.: Estrogen treatment of patients with established postmenopausal osteoporosis. Obstet. Gynecol. 72:290, 1990.

158. Lindsay, R., Maclean, A., Kraszewski, A., Hart, D. M., Clark, A. C., and Garwood, J.: Bone response to termination of estrogen treatment. Lancet 1:325, 1978.

159. Horsman, A., Jones, M., Francis, R., and Nordin, C.: The effect of estrogen dose on postmenopausal bone loss. N. Engl. J. Med. 309:1405, 1983.

160. Lindsay, R., Hart, D. M., and Clark, D. M.: The minimum effective dose of estrogen for prevention of postmenopausal bone loss. Obstet. Gynecol. 63:759, 1984.

161. Chetkowski, R. J., Meldrum, D. R., Steingold, K. A., Randle, D., Lu, J. K., Eggena, P., Hershman, J. M., Alkjaersig, N. K., Fletcher, A. P., and Judd, H. L.: Biologic effects of transdermal estradiol. N. Engl. J. Med. 314:1615, 1986.

162. Judd, H. L., Meldrum, D. R., Deftos, L. J., and Henderson, B. E.: Estrogen replacement therapy: Indications and complications. Ann. Intern. Med. 98:195, 1983.

163. Gallagher, J. C., Kable, W. T., and Goldgar, D.: Effect of progestin therapy on cortical and trabecular bone: Comparison with estrogen. Am. J. Med. 90:171, 1991.

164. Cauley, J. A., Cummings, S. R., Black, D. M., Mascioli, S. R., and Seeley, D. G.: Prevalence and determinants of estrogen replacement therapy in elderly women. Am. J. Obstet. Gynecol. 163:1438, 1990.

165. Stampfer, M. J., Willett, W. C., Colditz, G. A., Rosner, B., Speizer, F. E., and Hennekens, C. H.: A prospective study of postmenopausal hormones and coronary heart disease in U. S. women. N. Engl. J. Med. 313:1044, 1985.

166. Barrett-Conner, E. L.: The risks and benefits of long-term estrogen replacement therapy. Public Health Rep. Suppl. 104:62, 1989.

167. Bergkvist, L., Adami, H., Persson, I., Hoover, R., and Schairer, C.: The risk of breast cancer after estrogen and estrogen-progestin replacement. N. Engl. J. Med. 321:293, 1989.

168. Colditz, G. A., Stampfer, M. J., Willett, W. C., Hennekens, C. H., Rosner, B., and Speizer, F. E.: Prospective study of estrogen replacement therapy and risk of breast cancer in postmenopausal women. J.A.M.A. 264:2648, 1990.

169. Greenspan, S. L., Neer, R. M., Ridgway, E. C., and Klibanski, A.: Osteoporosis in men with hyperprolactinemic hypogonadism. Ann. Intern. Med. 104:777, 1986.

170. Francis, R. M., Peacock, M., Aaron, J. E., Selby, P. L., Taylor, G. A., Thompson, J., Marshall, D. H., and Horsman, A.: Osteoporosis in hypogonadal men: Role of decreased plasma 1,25-dihydroxyvitamin D, calcium malabsorption, and low bone formation. Bone 7:261, 1986.

171. Finkelstein, J. S., Klibanski, A., Neer, R. M., Greenspan, S. L., Rosenthal, D. I., and Crowly, W. F.: Osteoporosis in men with idiopathic hypogonadotropic hypogonadism. Ann. Intern. Med. 106:354, 1987.

172. Jackson, J. A., Kleerekoper, A., Parfitt, M., Rao, D. S., Villanueva, A. R., and Frame, B.: Bone histomorphometry in hypogonadal and eugonadal men with spinal osteoporosis. J. Clin. Endocrinol. Metab. 65:53, 1987.

173. Cassorla, F. G., Skerda, M. C., Valk, I. M., Hung, W., Cutler, G. B., and Loriaux, D. L.: The effects of sex steroids on ulnar growth during adolescence. J. Clin. Endocrinol. Metab. 58:717, 1984.

174. Foresta, C., Ruzza, G., Mioni, R., Guarneri, G., Gribaldo, R., and Meneghello, A.: Osteoporosis and decline of gonadal function in the elderly male. Hormone Res. 19:18, 1984.

175. Perry, H. M., III: Thyroid replacement and osteoporosis. Arch. Intern. Med. 146:4, 1986.
176. Mosekilde, L., Eriksen, E. F., and Charles, P.: Effects of thyroid hormones on bone and mineral metabolism. Endocrinol. Metab. Clin. North Am. 19:35, 1990.
177. Ross, D. S., Neer, R. M., Ridgway, E. C., and Daniels, G. H.: Subclinical hyperthyroidism and reduced bone density as a possible result of prolonged suppression of the pituitary-thyroid axis with L-thyroxine. Am. J. Med. 82:1167, 1987.
178. Terri, L. P., Kerrigan, J., Kelly, A. M., Braverman, L. E., and Baran, D. T.: Long-term thyroxine therapy is associated with decreased bone density in premenopausal women. J.A.M.A. 259:3137, 1988.
179. Schoutens, A., Laurent, E., Markowicz, E., Lisart, J., and de Maertelaer, V.: Serum triiodothyronine, bone turnover, and bone mass changes in euthyroid pre- and post-menopausal women. Calcif. Tiss. Res. 49:95, 1991.
180. Wiske, P. S., Wentworth, S. M., Norton, J. A., Jr., Epstein, S., and Johnston, C. C., Jr.: Evaluation of bone mass and growth in young diabetics. Metabolism 31:848, 1982.
181. Wahner, H. W., Dunn, W. L., and Riggs, L.: Assessment of bone mineral. Parts 1 and 2. J. Nucl. Med. 25:1136, 1984.
182. Wolf, A., Chuinard, R., Riggens, R., et al.: Immobilization hypercalcemia: A case report and review of the literature. Clin. Orthop. 118:124, 1976.
183. Hamtman, D. A., Vogel, J. M., Donaldson, C. L., et al.: Attempts to prevent disease osteoporosis with calcitonin, longitudinal compression and supplementary calcium and phosphate. J. Clin. Endocrinol. Metab. 36:845, 1973.
184. Avioli, L. V., and Lindsay, R.: The female osteoporotic syndrome(s). In Avioli, L. V., and Krane, S. M. (eds.): Metabolic Bone Disease and Clinically Related Disorders. 2nd ed. Philadelphia, W. B. Saunders Company, 1990, pp. 397–451.
185. Mundy, G. R.: The hypercalcemia of malignancy. Kidney Int. 31:142, 1987.
186. Griffith, H. T., and Liu, D. T. Y.: Severe heparin osteoporosis in pregnancy. Postgrad. Med. J. 60:424, 1984.
187. Aubia, J., Masarom, J., Serrano, S., Lloveras, J., and Marinoso, L. L.: Bone histology in renal transplant patients receiving cyclosporin. Lancet 1:1048, 1988.
188. Stein, B., Takizawa, M., Katz, I., Joffee, I., Berlin, J., Fallon, M., and Epstein, S.: Salmon calcitonin prevents cyclosporin-A-induced high turnover bone loss. Endocrinology 129:92, 1991.
189. Whyte, M. P.: Heritable metabolic and dysplastic bone diseases. Endocrinol. Metab. Clin. North Am. 19:133, 1990.
190. Prockop, D. J., Baldwin, C. T., and Constantinou, C. D.: Mutations in type I procollagen genes that cause osteogenesis imperfecta. Adv. Hum. Genet. 19:105, 1990.
191. Mankin, H. J.: Rickets, osteomalacia and renal osteodystrophy. An update. Orthop. Clin. North Am. 21:81, 1990.
192. Marel, G. M., McKenna, M. J., and Frame, B.: Osteomalacia. In Peck, W. A. (ed.): Bone and Mineral Research 4. New York, Elsevier, 1986, p. 335.
193. Hahn, T. J., Hendin, B. A., Sharp, C. R., et al.: Serum 25-hydroxycalciferol levels in children on chronic anticonvulsant therapy. N. Engl. J. Med. 292:550, 1975.
194. Haddad, J.: Vitamin D economy in gastrointestinal disease. Ann. Intern. Med. 87:629, 1977.
195. Halverson, J. D., Teitelbaum, S. L., Haddad, J. G., and Murphy, W. A.: Skeletal abnormalities after jejunoileal bypass. Ann. Surg. 189:785, 1979.
196. Eddy, R. L.: Metabolic bone disease after gastrectomy. Am. J. Med. 50:442, 1971.
197. Whyte, M. P., Haddad, J. G., Jr., Walters, D. D., et al.: Vitamin D bioavailability: Serum 25-hydroxyvitamin D levels in man after oral, subcutaneous, intramuscular, and intravenous vitamin D administration. J. Clin. Endocrinol. Metab. 48:906, 1979.
198. Delvin, E. E., Glorieux, F. H., Marie, P. T., and Pettifor, J. M.: Vitamin D dependency. Replacement therapy with calcitriol. J. Pediatrics 99:26, 1981.
199. Liberman, U. A., Eil, C., and Marx, S. J.: Resistance to 1,25-dihydroxy-vitamin D: Association with heterogeneous defects in cultured skin fibroblasts. J. Clin. Invest. 71:192, 1983.
200. Hahn, T. J., Scharp, C. R., Richardson, C. A., et al.: Interaction of diphenylhydantoin and phenobarbital with hormonal mediation of fetal rat bone resorption in vitro. J. Clin. Invest. 62:406, 1978.
201. Nuovo, M. A., Dorfman, H. D., and Chalew, S. A.: Tumor-induced osteomalacia and rickets. Am. J. Surg. Pathol. 13:588, 1989.
202. Rasmussen, H., and Tennenhouse, H. S.: Hypophosphatemias. In Scriver, C. R., Beaudet, A. L., Sly, W. S., and Valee, D. (eds.): The Metabolic Basis of Inherited Disease. 6th ed. New York, McGraw-Hill, 1989, pp. 2581–2604.
203. Reid, I. R., Hardy, D. C., Murphy, W. A., Teitelbaum, S. L., Bergfeld, M. A., and Whyte, M. P.: X-linked hypophosphatemia: A clinical, biochemical, and histopathologic assessment of morbidity in adults. Medicine 68:336, 1989.
204. Reid, I. R., Murphy, W. A., Hardy, D. C., Teitelbaum, S. L., Bergfeld, M. A., and Whyte, M. P.: X-linked hypophosphatemia: Skeletal mass in adults assessed by histomorphometry, computed tomography, and absorptiometry. Am. J. Med. 90:63, 1991.
205. Burnett, V., Baker, R. K., and Wallach, S.: Primary hypophosphatemic rickets in an elderly woman. Arch. Intern. Med. 131:581, 1973.
206. Bergeron, M., and Gougoux, A.: The renal Fanconi syndrome. In Scriver, C. R., Beaudet, A. L., Sly, W. S., and Valee, D. (eds.): The Metabolic Basis of Inherited Disease. 6th ed. New York, McGraw-Hill, 1989, pp. 2569–2580.
207. Reddy, G. S., Jones, G., Kooh, S. W., and Fraser, D.: Inhibition of 25-hydroxylase D$_3$-1-hydroxylase by chronic metabolic acidosis. Am. J. Physiol. 243:E265, 1982.
208. Chines, A., and Pacifici, R.: Antiacid and sucralfate-induced hypophosphatemic osteomalacia: A case report and review of the literature. Calcif. Tiss. Int. 47:291, 1990.
209. Sherrard, D. J., and Andress, D. L.: Aluminum-related osteodystrophy. Adv. Intern. Med. 34:307, 1989.
210. Whyte, M.: Hypophosphatasia. In Scriver, C. R., Beaudet, A. L., Sly, W. S., and Valee, D. (eds.): The Metabolic Basis of Inherited Disease. 6th ed. New York, McGraw-Hill, 1989, pp. 2843–2855.
211. Coe, J. D., Murphy, W. A., and Whyte, M. P.: Management of femoral fractures and pseudofractures in adult hypophosphatasia. J. Bone Joint Surg. 68-A:981, 1986.
212. Frame, B., Frost, H. M., Pak, C. Y. C., et al.: Fibrogenesis imperfecta ossium: A collagen defect causing osteomalacia. N. Engl. J. Med. 285:769, 1971.
213. Potts, J. T., Jr.: Management of asymptomatic hyperparathyroidism. J. Clin. Endocrinol. Metab. 70:1489, 1990.
214. Petti, G. H., Jr.: Hyperparathyroidism. Otolaryngol. Clin. North Am. 23:339, 1990.
215. Clark, O. H., and Duh, Q. Y.: Primary hyperparathyroidism. A surgical perspective. Endocrinol. Metab. Clin. North Am. 18:701, 1989.
216. Mallette, L. E., Bilezikian, J. P., Heath, D. A., and Aurbach, G. D.: Primary hyperparathyroidism: Clinical and biochemical features. Medicine 53:127, 1974.
217. Marc, S. J., Powell, D., Shimkin, P. M., et al.: Familial hyperparathyroidism. Ann. Intern. Med. 78:371, 1973.
218. Shane, E., and Bilezikian, J. P.: Parathyroid carcinoma: A review of 62 patients. Endocrine Rev. 3:218, 1983.
219. Akerstrom, G., Rastad, J., Ljunghall, S., and Johansson, H.: Clinical and experimental advances in sporatic primary hyperparathyroidism. Acta Chir. Scand. 156:23, 1990.
220. Fitzpatrick, L. A., and Bilezikian, J. P.: Acute primary hyperparathyroidism. Am. J. Med. 82:275, 1987.
221. Broadus, A. E., Horst, R. L., Lang, R., Littledike, E. T., and Rasmussen, H.: The importance of circulating 1,25-dihydroxyvitamin D in the pathogenesis of hypercalciuria and renal-stone formation in primary hyperparathyroidism. N. Engl. J. Med. 302:421, 1980.
222. Genent, H. K., Heck, L. L., Lanzl, L. H., et al.: Primary hyperparathyroidism: A comprehensive study of clinical, biochemical and radiographic manifestations. Radiology 109:513, 1973.
223. Habener, J. F., and Potts, J. T., Jr.: Primary hyperparathyroidism. In Avioli, L. V., and Krane, S. M. (eds.): Metabolic Bone Disease and Clinically Related Disorders. 2nd ed. Philadelphia, W. B. Saunders Company, 1990, pp. 475–545.
224. Bhalla, A. K.: Musculoskeletal manifestations of primary hyperparathyroidism. Clin Rheum. Dis. 12:691, 1986.
225. Scott, J. T., Dixon, A. S., and Bywaters, E. G. L.: Association of hyperuricemia and gout with hyperparathyroidism. Br. Med. J. 1:1070, 1964.
226. Madhavan, T., Frame, B., and Block, M. A.: Influence of surgical correction of primary hyperparathyroidism on associate hypertension. Arch. Surg. 100:212, 1970.
227. Joborn, C., Hetta, J., Frisk, P., Palmer, M., Akerstrom, G., and Ljunghall, S.: Primary hyperparathyroidism in patients with organic brain syndrome. Acta Med. Scand. 219:91, 1986.
228. Primary hyperparathyroidism and delirium in the elderly. J. Am. Geriatr. Soc. 36:157, 1988.
229. Ballard, H. S., Frame, B., and Hartsock, R. J.: Familial multiple endocrine adenoma: Peptic ulcer complex. Medicine 43:481, 1964.
230. Steiner, A. L., Goodman, A. D., and Powers, S. R.: Study of a kindred with pheochromocytoma, medullary thyroid carcinoma, hyperparathyroidism and Cushing's disease: Multiple endocrine neoplasia, Type 2. Medicine 47:371, 1968.
231. Muggia, F. M.: Overview of cancer-related hypercalcemia: Epidemiology and etiology. Semin. Oncol. 17:3, 1990.
232. Stewart, A. F., and Braodus, A. E.: Parathyroid hormone-related proteins: Coming of age in the 1990s. J. Clin. Endocrinol. Metab. 71:1410, 1990.
233. Martin, T. J., Allan, E. H., Caple, I. W., Care, A. D., Danks, J. A., Diefenbach-Jagger, H., Ebeling, P. R., Gillespie, M. T., Hammonds, G., Heath, J. A., et al.: Parathyroid hormone-related protein: Isolation, molecular cloning, and mechanism of action. Recent Prog. Horm. Res. 45:467, 1989.

234. Lufkin, E. G., Koa, P. C., and Heath, H., III: Parathyroid hormone radioimmunoassays in the differential diagnosis of hypercalcemia due to primary hyperparathyroidism of malignancy. Ann. Intern. Med. 106:559, 1987.
235. Heath, H., III: Familial benign (hypocalciuric) hypocalcemia. A troublesome mimic of mild primary hyperparathyroidism. Endocrinol. Metab. Clin. North Am. 18:723, 1989.
236. Marx, S. J., Attie, M. R., and Spiegel, A. M.: An association between neonatal severe primary hyperparathyroidism and familial hypocalciuric hypercalcemia in three kindreds. N. Engl. J. Med. 306:257, 1982.
237. Consensus Development Conference Panel: Diagnosis and management of asymptomatic hyperparathyroidism: Consensus development conference statement. Ann. Intern. Med. 114:593, 1991.
238. Purnell, D. C., Scholz, D. A., Smith, L. H., et al.: Treatment of primary hyperparathyroidism. Am. J. Med. 56:800, 1974.
239. Marcus, R.: Estrogens and progestins in the management of primary hyperparathyroidism. Endocrinol. Metab. Clin. North Am. 18:715, 1989.
240. Foster, G. S., Bekerman, C., Blend, M. J., Byrom, E., and Pinsky, S. M.: Preoperative imaging in primary hyperparathyroidism. Role of thallium-technetium subtraction scintigraphy. Arch. Otolaryngol. Head Neck Surg. 115:1197, 1989.
241. Britton, D. C., Thompson, M. H., Johnston, I. D. A., and Fleming, L. B.: Renal function following parathyroid surgery in primary hyperparathyroidism. Lancet 2:74, 1976.
242. Speigel, A. M.: Pseudohypoparathyroidism. In Scriver, C. R., Beaudet, A. L., Sly, W. S., and Valee, D. (eds.): The Metabolic Basis of Inherited Disease. 6th ed. New York, McGraw-Hill, 1989, pp. 2013–2027.
243. Malluche, H., and Fuagere, M. C.: Renal bone disease 1990: An unmet challenge for the nephrologist. Kidney Int. 38:193, 1990.
244. Tzamaloukas, A. H.: Diagnosis and management of bone disorders in chronic renal failure and dialyzed patients. Med. Clin. North Am. 74:961, 1990.
245. Gokal, R.: Renal osteodystrophy and aluminum bone disease in CAPD patients. Clin. Nephrol. 30(Suppl. 1):S64, 1988.
246. Salusky, I. B., Foley, J., Nelson, P., and Goodman, W. G.: Aluminum accumulation during treatment with aluminum hydroxide and dialysis in children and young adults with chronic renal disease. N. Engl. J. Med. 324:527, 1991.
247. Delmez, J. A., and Slatopolsky, E.: Recent advances in the pathogenesis and therapy of uremic secondary hyperparathyroidism. J. Clin. Endocrinol. Metab. 72:735, 1991.
248. Nagant de Deuxchaisnes, C. N., and Krane, S.: Paget's disease of bone: Clinical and metabolic observations. Medicine 43:233, 1964.
249. Singer, F. R.: Paget's Disease of Bone. New York, Plenum Medical Book Company, 1977.
250. Rebel, A. (ed.): Symposium on Paget's Disease. Clin. Orthop. Rel. Res. 217:1, 1987.
251. Whyte, M. P., Daniels, E. H., and Murphy, W. A.: Osteolytic Paget's bone disease in a young man. Am. J. Med. 78:326, 1985.
252. Hosking, D. J.: Advances in the treatment of Paget's disease. Drugs 40:829, 1990.
253. Harinck, H. I. J., Bijvoet, O. L. M., Blanksma, D., and Dahlinghaus-Nienhuys, P. J.: Efficacious management with aminobisphosphonate (APD) in Paget's disease of bone. Clin. Orthop. Rel. Res. 217:79, 1987.
254. Bollerslev, J.: Autosomal dominant osteopetrosis: Bone metabolism and epidemiological, clinical and hormonal aspects. Endocrine Rev. 10:45, 1989.
255. Marks, S. C., Jr.: Osteoblast biology; lessons from mammalian mutations. Am. J. Med. Genet. 34:43, 1989.
256. Felix, R., Cecchini, M. G., and Fleisch, H.: Macrophage colony stimulating factor restores in vivo bone resorption in the Op/Op osteopetrotic mouse. Endocrinology 127:2592, 1990.
257. Harris, W. H., Dudley, H. R., Jr., and Barry, R. J.: The natural history of fibrous dysplasia. An orthopaedic, pathologic, and roentgenographic study. J. Bone Joint Surg. 44A:207, 1962.
258. Stompro, B. E., Wolf, P., and Haghighi, P.: Fibrous dysplasia of bone. Am. Fam. Phys. 39:179, 1989.
259. Kransdorf, M. J., Moser, R. P., Jr., and Gilkey, F. W.: Fibrous dysplasia. Radiographics 10:519, 1990.
260. Barat, M., Rybak, L. P., and Mann, J. L.: Fibrous dysplasia masquerading as chronic maxillary sinusitis. Ear Nose Throat J. 68:44, 1989.

Chapter 97
Osteonecrosis

Marvin E. Steinberg
David R. Steinberg

INTRODUCTION

The terms *osteonecrosis, avascular necrosis* (AVN), and *ischemic necrosis* of bone are synonymous and refer to a condition in which there has been a circulatory impairment of an area of bone, leading to its eventual death. This may be caused by a number of factors, often acting alone, but at times acting in concert with each other. Frequently, the cause cannot be determined, and the condition is referred to as idiopathic.

There are a few specific areas of the skeleton for which this condition seems to have a predilection. These include the femoral and humeral heads, the femoral condyles, the proximal tibia, and some of the small bones of the foot and ankle and of the wrist. The development of AVN is determined at least in part by the anatomy of the vascular supply to the region. In some instances, only one specific area is involved, whereas in others, there may be multiple sites of involvement. The clinical picture may be quite variable and depends on the size and location of the necrotic segment, the etiologic factors, and the age of the patient. This has led to speculation that AVN may not be a single disease entity but may actually be the end point for a number of unrelated disorders, all of which cause vascular impairment of bone.

There are different forms of AVN, which affect children, younger adults, and the elderly. There are significant differences among them, especially in regard to treatment and prognosis. These are described in detail later. Our emphasis here is on the nontraumatic variety seen generally in the younger adult. This condition affects primarily the hip, knee, and shoulder and is often bilateral. Especially in the hip, the area most frequently affected, it usually progresses to collapse of the articular surface if untreated and eventually leads to significant pain and disability. Surgical replacement of the joint is frequently required, an approach that has certain consequences in the younger patient. Our goal is therefore to diagnose this condition as early as possible and to institute a regimen of management designed to encourage revascularization of bone and prevent collapse. Unfortunately, we do not yet have a completely satisfactory method to accomplish this.

The methods for diagnosing AVN in its earliest phases, notably magnetic resonance imaging (MRI), have improved dramatically. It is essential that all clinicians dealing with patients who are at high risk for developing AVN be aware of these developments. Whichever method of treatment is elected, the results will be better when it is instituted early in the course of the disorder.

This chapter discusses the etiology, pathogenesis, and clinical picture of AVN. It emphasizes the advances that now enable us to make an early diagnosis. The various treatment options are described objectively. Although trauma is the most frequent cause of AVN, the post-traumatic variety is well covered in standard works on fractures and trauma and therefore is mentioned only briefly here.

POST-TRAUMATIC AVASCULAR NECROSIS

By far the most common cause of AVN is a displaced fracture adjacent to a joint. The condition is encountered most frequently in the subcapital or transcervical region of the hip (Fig. 97–1). It is also seen in comminuted fractures of the humeral head, displaced fractures of the talus, and fractures through the scaphoid bone at the wrist. It results from a disruption to the major blood supply to the affected region. If the collateral circulation is not sufficient, the involved area of bone dies. It is also seen occasionally with dislocations of the hip.

In most instances, the die is cast at the time of the initial injury. Although prompt anatomic reduction and stabilization of the fracture or dislocation is certainly desirable, there is little evidence that this will significantly alter the development of AVN except in certain types of dislocation.

In most cases, the history of trauma is quite clear cut, and the diagnosis of fracture or dislocation can be made immediately with appropriate radiographs. Occasionally, as with pathologic fractures that develop through regions of abnormal bone and sites of major weight bearing, there is no history of a single major traumatic event. The most frequent site for this is perhaps the hip. In other instances, it has been postulated that relatively minor or repeated trauma to an area can result in AVN without a clinically diagnosable fracture. This occurs in the small bones of the wrist and occasionally the knee.

The exact incidence of AVN following fracture is difficult to determine because it varies with the severity of the fracture, amount of displacement, and to some extent the method of treatment. Boyd and

1628

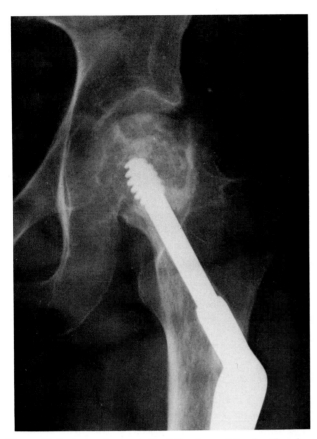

Figure 97–1. Avascular necrosis of the femoral head with subsequent collapse following a displaced transcervical fracture treated with open reduction and internal fixation.

George[1] found that 34 percent of displaced transcervical fractures showed x-ray evidence of AVN within 3 years, and 14 percent did not unite. There is a definite correlation between AVN and delayed union and nonunion. Because of the poor prognosis for certain types of fractures, these are often treated by primary prosthetic replacement, particularly in the hip and shoulder.

When AVN occurs after open reduction and internal fixation of a fracture, its development is often insidious. The fracture per se, the operative procedure, and the presence of mechanical devices used to hold the fracture fragments often make early diagnosis of AVN difficult or impossible. Eventual collapse of the affected region of the joint usually leads to pain and decreased motion. The diagnosis is confirmed by routine radiographic examination. Bone scans and MRI are not as useful here as they are in the diagnosis of nontraumatic AVN.

If a small area of bone is involved, revascularization and healing may take place, and the articular surface may not collapse. If a large segment is involved, it will usually collapse and lead to significant pain and disability. In these instances, prosthetic replacement of the affected region may be required. This is especially true in the hip and the shoulder. In areas not amenable to replacement, such as the talus, a bone fusion or stabilization may be required.

Because the majority of these fractures, especially those involving the hip, occur in older individuals, prosthetic replacement is usually a satisfactory solution. The case is somewhat different, however, in the younger individual. Because of the longer life expectancy and the greater physical demands placed on the involved joint, prosthetic replacement is usually not a permanent solution to the problem. Even in the younger patient, however, it may still be the best alternative.[2–6, 8]

NONTRAUMATIC AVASCULAR NECROSIS

Etiology

Nontraumatic AVN of bone is not a single disease. It is rather a localized pathologic event that results when there has been an impairment of the circulation to a specific region of bone of sufficient magnitude to cause death of bone cells and marrow. Several etiologic factors have been identified, as listed in Table 97–1. It is often found in association with a number of medical disorders or conditions, as listed in Table 97–2.

In certain instances, the cause and effect relationship seems reasonably clear. For example, in sickle cell anemia, it is generally accepted that clumps of abnormal red cells form emboli that physically block the arteries and arterioles.[7, 9–11] In caisson disease or dysbaric osteonecrosis, the etiologic factor is nitrogen bubbles that form microemboli within the vessels and perhaps in the perivascular fat and marrow as well, thus increasing the intraosseous pressure and causing extraluminal compression of the vessels.[12–15]

In other instances, a cause and effect relationship may not be so direct. For example, in cases of prolonged glucocorticoid administration and exces-

Table 97–1. ETIOLOGIC FACTORS IN AVASCULAR NECROSIS

Gross disruption of vessels
    Displaced femoral neck fractures
    Dislocation
External vascular occlusion
    Marrow hypertrophy
    Marrow infiltration or replacement
    Increased intraosseous pressure
    Joint effusion
    Dislocation
Thrombosis
    Vascular disorders
    Altered coagulation
Embolization
    Blood clot
    Lipid droplets
    Sickle cells
    Nitrogen bubbles
Osteopenia with microfractures
Cytotoxicity
Multifactorial
Idiopathic

Table 97–2. CONDITIONS ASSOCIATED WITH AVASCULAR NECROSIS

Traumatic
Fracture of the femoral neck
Traumatic dislocation of the hip
Trauma to the hip without fracture or dislocation
Reconstructive hip surgery (including cup arthroplasty, surface replacement arthroplasty, cuneiform osteotomy of the femoral neck, and synovectomy)
Hip manipulation (including treatment of congenital dysplasia of the hip and use of traction in the correction of slipped epiphysis)
Nontraumatic
Juvenile
    Slipped capital femoral epiphysis
    Legg-Calvé-Perthes disease
    Idiopathic juvenile avascular necrosis
Adult
    Systemic steroid administration
    Excessive alcohol intake
    Chronic liver disease
    Renal transplantation
    Lupus erythematosus and other collagen vascular disorders
    Caisson disease or decompression sickness
    Exposure to high altitude
    Sickle cell disease and sickle cell variants
    Miscellaneous hemoglobinopathies and coagulopathies
    Ileitis and colitis
    Pancreatitis
    Metabolic bone disease
    Hyperlipidemias
    Burns
    Pregnancy
    Gout
    Gaucher's disease
    Sarcoidosis
    Tumors
    Chemotherapy and other toxic agents
    Fabry's disease
    Arteriosclerosis and other vascular occlusive disorders
    Radiation
    Smoking

sive alcohol use, it has been proposed that there is an alteration in the circulating lipids that results in vascular obliteration by microemboli of fat.[16–20] There may be a number of other factors implicated, however. Alcoholics are prone to repeated trauma and to a number of medical problems. Glucocorticoids are most frequently administered to chronically ill patients with disease processes that may affect blood vessels, marrow, and bone in other ways. Thus, in the patient with systemic lupus erythematosus (SLE), there is often a concomitant vasculitis. In the patient with chronic renal disease, who may also have undergone renal transplantation, metabolic factors including renal osteodystrophy also affect the bone. In such circumstances, it has been proposed that the etiology of the AVN is "multifactorial" and is not related to a single factor.[11, 21–29] However, in our own prospective study of 73 renal transplant patients, we found that no patient with renal osteodystrophy developed AVN unless they were on high doses of steroids; a number of patients without documented osteodystrophy who were on high doses of steroids did develop AVN.[30]

The role of osteopenia or osteoporosis in the steroid-treated patient has also been implicated as a possible cause for AVN. It is theorized that the osteopenia leads to microfractures, which in turn lead to avascularity of bone. In our opinion, osteopenia per se does not play a major role in the development of AVN. We have only to point to the fact that a large percentage of elderly patients have severe osteopenia, often with vertebral compression fractures, yet very few of these develop AVN.

If one reviews the list of conditions for which high doses of glucocorticoids have been administered, one finds that they are so diverse that the only common denominator seems to be the steroid itself. These include, for example, central nervous system trauma, skin disorders, asthma and other allergies, gastrointestinal disorders, renal transplantation, and SLE.

There also seems to be a definite relationship between the development of AVN and both the dose and the duration of steroid administration. In the patient with rheumatoid arthritis who has been on low doses of steroid for quite some time, the incidence of AVN is low, whereas in patients with SLE who have been treated with high doses for a much shorter period, the incidence is considerably higher. On the other hand, in renal transplant patients, we found no direct correlation between the dose or duration of steroid administration and AVN. It should be noted, however, that all of these patients received a high dose of steroid for a prolonged period of time.[30] It would thus appear that once a certain threshold has been reached, increasing the dose of steroid further may not add significantly to the incidence of vascular impairment.

It is therefore our opinion that in the patient on long-term high dose steroid administration, the steroid itself is the most important but perhaps not the only etiologic factor in the production of AVN. Although the mechanism or mechanisms have not been conclusively established, we agree that the most reasonable explanation is that steroid administration causes an alteration in circulating lipids, which in turn cause mircoemboli to the arteries of the affected region.

In many series, the second most common association is with excessive alcohol intake. In some patients, chronic consumption of two or more alcoholic drinks per day may lead to AVN. The mechanism has not been completely established, but alteration in circulating lipids with microembolus formation may once again be implicated.

It is not surprising that patients exhibit differing degrees of sensitivity to steroids or alcohol. For example, in rheumatoid arthritis, the development of AVN is significantly higher in patients who develop cushingoid features than in those who do not, even though the dose of steroid may be similar. Chronic alcohol consumption is quite common, yet only a very small percentage of users develop AVN.

Other conditions have been mentioned occasionally in connection with AVN. These include miscellaneous hyperlipidemias, gout,[31] arteriosclerosis,[11] Gaucher's disease,[11, 21] burns, and pelvic irradiation.[33] The limited number of these cases prevents a clear delineation of the etiology and pathogenesis.

In many instances, no specific etiologic factor can be identified. Patients who fit into this category have been referred to as having idiopathic AVN[32, 34, 60] and constitute approximately 20 percent of our own series. These patients as well as those in other categories may have a marginal circulation to the involved area, which requires only the smallest of insults to render it inadequate to sustain the viability of the tissues in the area supplied. They may also have a propensity for microembolization, perhaps by lipid droplets, without a clearly identifiable etiologic factor. As our clinical awareness increases and our diagnostic tools improve, the numbers of patients being placed into the idiopathic category will most likely diminish.

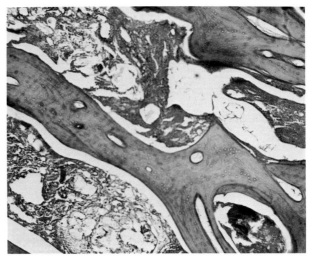

Figure 97–2. Photomicrograph through the center of the avascular region showing necrotic marrow and dead trabeculae. (50×)

Pathogenesis

The pathogenesis may vary from patient to patient, depending in part on the etiology, the size and anatomic location of the necrotic segment, and the age of the patient. This condition occurs most commonly in the femoral head, and this is the region from which most of the data have been collected. Except in the case of post-traumatic AVN, a common series of events takes place despite the etiologic factors involved. The following description applies primarily to nontraumatic AVN of the femoral head in the adult. It must be kept clearly in mind that the area initially involved is the cancellous bone beneath the weight-bearing surface. Later the articular surface itself may become involved, and eventually secondary changes may appear in the acetabulum. Thus, AVN should rarely be confused with the many types of arthritis that involve the articular cartilage on both sides of the joint simultaneously.

Although there may be a single massive vascular insult, it is more likely that there is a series of lesser insults spread out over a period of weeks to months. At a certain point, the remaining circulation is no longer sufficient to sustain viability of the cells in the region, and death of marrow elements occurs. Later, osteocytes die, and microscopic examination of the tissue shows empty lacunae devoid of cells (Fig. 97–2). Initially the patient is asymptomatic and may remain asymptomatic until well after the condition is diagnosed by radiograph or imaging. In other instances, however, the patient may develop a significant amount of pain before evidence of collapse of the articular surface or other radiographic abnormalities. It has been proposed that this is due to increased intraosseous pressure, which has been documented in a number of cases, and to tissue ischemia. In many instances, this pain can be markedly relieved by a simple surgical decompression of the affected area. This increased intraosseous pressure does play a role in the pathogenesis of the condition, although its exact role is uncertain.[35, 36]

Soon after the initial vascular insult, the normal physiologic processes of repair are set into motion. If the involved area is small, spontaneous healing may occur, and the whole process may remain subclinical. This undoubtedly does take place frequently and may result in sclerotic areas noted on subsequent radiographs and referred to as "bone infarcts" or "bone islands." If the involved area is large, the repair process is usually unable to replace it completely. At the periphery of the lesion, vascular ingrowth occurs, and some of the necrotic marrow and bone is replaced. In other areas, new, living bone is laid down on the remnants of old, dead trabeculae. This leads to a marked thickening of trabeculae, which accounts for the sclerotic margins

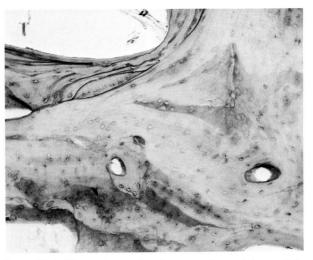

Figure 97–3. Photomicrograph taken near the periphery of the avascular region showing markedly thickened trabeculae composed of new, living bone laid down on old dead bone. (100×)

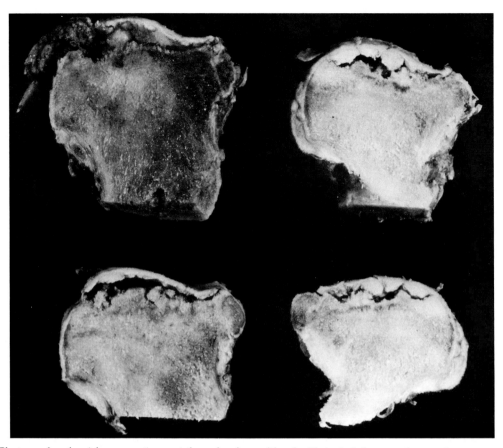

Figure 97–4. Photographs of serial cross-sections cut through a femoral head with typical changes of avascular necrosis. Note collapse of the cancellous bone beneath the articular cartilage and its attached subchondral plate.

seen on radiographs (Fig. 97–3). The front of vascularized granulation tissue is unable to project completely into the depths of the avascular area, and the repair processes come to a halt. With continued stress on the nonviable bone, microfractures occur that cannot be repaired. Eventually, the cancellous bone beneath the major weight-bearing region collapses. The articular surface is supported by a strong subchondral bone plate and may maintain the normal configuration of the joint for a while longer. The space left between this plate and the collapsed trabeculae accounts for the radiolucent "crescent sign" often seen on radiographs. As the process continues, flattening of the articular surface eventually occurs, and symptoms increase (Figs. 97–4 and 97–5). It should be noted that the articular cartilage itself remains viable and mechanically intact until late (Fig. 97–6). This is because it is not dependent on the circulation of the underlying bone but is nourished by the synovial fluid that bathes its articular surface (see Chapter 1). With progressive collapse of the articular surface, the cartilage is subjected to abnormal stresses and eventually undergoes a gradual process of degeneration. Eventually secondary changes in the opposite side of the joint occur. Thus, in the latter stages of AVN, joint line narrowing may be seen, often in conjunction with cystic and sclerotic

changes in the acetabular bone. It must be stressed that on the acetabular side, these are secondary to the pathology in the femoral head and are not due to the AVN per se. Eventually, advanced degenera-

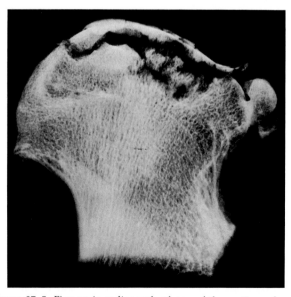

Figure 97–5. Fine grain radiograph of one of the sections shown in Figure 97–4.

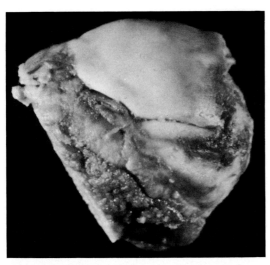

Figure 97–6. Photograph of a femoral head with avascular necrosis removed at the time of total hip replacement. The subchondral bone has collapsed causing the articular surface to wrinkle. The cartilage, however, remains relatively intact.

tion of both the acetabulum and the femoral head occur with almost complete destruction of the joint.

It should be noted that this progression is not inevitable. In our own series, approximately 10 to 15 percent of those patients with clinically diagnosed AVN did not show progression over a period of up to ten years. In some, a large radiolucent lesion with a sclerotic border remained unchanged for several years. In others, a certain degree of collapse occurred initially but then seemed to stabilize with little further progression. In many cases, the involved area is quite small and heals spontaneously without clinical symptoms or radiologic evidence of disease.

The course of events may vary significantly. If the avascular area is not near an articular surface, it usually remains asymptomatic and is of little consequence. In the distal femur and proximal tibia, repair is much more likely to occur, and joint collapse is seen less frequently than in the femoral and humeral heads and talus. In the childhood forms of AVN, such as Legg-Calvé-Perthes disease, the picture is quite different. It is not at all uncommon to see revascularization and remodeling in even large areas of aseptic bone.[2, 4, 5, 27, 29, 37-40] This is discussed in more detail later.

Clinical Picture

The area most commonly affected is the femoral head, followed by the humeral head, the femoral condyles, and the proximal tibia. In the hips, it is bilateral in more than 50 percent of patients. Once it has been diagnosed in the hip, it will appear in other regions in approximately 15 percent of patients. Bilateral involvement is not simultaneous, and if both hips or shoulders become involved, they are often at different stages of development of the lesion. It will

usually become apparent in the second hip or shoulder within 1 year after it is diagnosed in the first. When there is a specific and limited predisposing event, such as a relatively short course of steroid, the diagnosis is usually made within 3 months to 2 years.

The clinical findings in AVN are nonspecific. In many instances, patients remain asymptomatic. This is especially true if the lesion is small or the area of involvement is not near a joint. When symptoms do occur, the initial complaint is pain. This may develop either before or after changes are noted on plain radiographs. The pain may be related to increased intraosseous pressure and tissue ischemia or to microfractures and eventual collapse of an articular surface. This is accompanied by a progressive increase in pain, and a limp may develop when the lower extremity is involved. Limitation of motion follows. In general, symptoms are at least partially relieved by rest and exacerbated by activity and weight bearing.

Most patients with atraumatic AVN are relatively young, with the peak incidence occurring in the thirties and forties. Not infrequently it will be seen in the twenties and even in the late teens. An exception to this is the type of osteonecrosis of the knees that occurs in an elderly population. This is discussed later. There are also forms of AVN that affect youngsters, such as idiopathic juvenile AVN and Legg-Calvé-Perthes disease. These are also discussed separately.

In the young adult with nontraumatic AVN, a careful history usually elicits a predisposing factor or an associated condition in approximately 80 percent of patients. One should therefore ask specifically about systemic steroid administration, alcohol ingestion, sickle cell disease and other hematologic problems, and abnormalities of lipid metabolism. Less commonly encountered factors should also be kept in mind, such as local irradiation, exposure to hyperbaric environments, and the other conditions listed in Table 97–2.

Physical findings are nonspecific. In the early stages, examination of the affected part may be within normal limits. Later a limp may be detected if the lower extremity is involved. Range of motion of the affected region may be limited and may cause pain.[41-44]

Laboratory Tests

In most cases, routine laboratory tests are within normal limits. In certain instances, however, they may be quite helpful, such as in diagnosing sickle cell disease. Although a common theory concerning the cause of AVN involves fat emboli, routine testing for altered circulating lipids rarely reveals any abnormalities. Perhaps one of the most important aspects of serologic testing is to rule out other disorders that might cause hip pathology and might mimic the symptoms of AVN.

Miscellaneous Studies

A special study that may be helpful in the diagnosis of AVN is a direct measurement of the intraosseous pressure in the affected region.[35, 36] This requires that a trochar be inserted directly into bone. A radiopaque agent may also be injected and the vascular pattern examined by radiographs. These procedures are most often done in the operating room and usually require a general anesthetic. Although the finding of elevated intraosseous pressure may help to make the diagnosis of AVN in the preradiologic stage, many believe that this is non-specific and does not distinguish between AVN and other disorders affecting the region. With the development of noninvasive imaging techniques, such as MRI, this procedure has a very limited application at the present time.[45, 46]

Because of the sensitivity and specificity of MRI, biopsy is now rarely used as an isolated diagnostic test, and a biopsy specimen usually becomes available only when treatment involves either a "core decompression" or decompression and grafting.

Imaging Modalities

The various imaging modalities currently available are the mainstay in the diagnosis of AVN. These include routine radiographs, tomograms or laminograms, computed tomography (CT), technetium bone scans, single photon emission computed tomography (SPECT), and MRI.

Radiography

Routine radiographs are the simplest and best means for diagnosing AVN. They must be of extremely high quality and must include both anteroposterior and lateral projections because early changes are often subtle. Initially, radiographs are normal. Later, they may show generalized osteopenia, although this is a nonspecific finding and may reflect the general metabolic state of the bone and not AVN per se. Still later, the bone presents a mottled appearance composed of adjacent areas of radiolucency and radiodensity (stage II) (Fig. 97–7). This often reflects the presence of "cysts" and sclerosis. The cystic lesions are, in fact, areas of dead bone that have undergone resorption and replacement with fibrous tissue or amorphous material, whereas the sclerotic areas represent thickened trabeculae formed when new bone is laid down on old, dead bone. In some instances, the picture is one of a uniform increase in density rather than mottling. This is particularly true in post-traumatic AVN. This may represent not a true increase in bone density

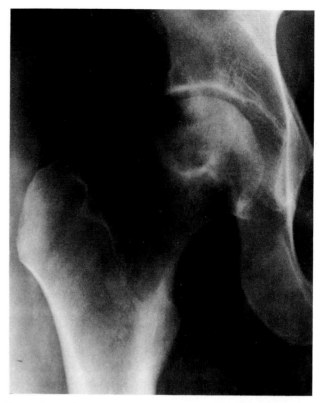

Figure 97–7. Characteristic radiographic picture of avascular necrosis. The center of the involved area is radiolucent with a sclerotic margin. Collapse has not yet occurred. (Stage II)

but a relative increase that results when the adjacent, vascularized areas become osteopenic secondary to osteoporosis of disuse. At this stage, the x-ray picture may be pathognomonic of AVN, provided that other conditions have been ruled out.

When there has been collapse of the cancellous bone beneath the subchondral plate, there is often seen a radiolucent line on radiographs, described as a "crescent sign" (stage III) (Fig. 97–8). Eventually the subchondral plate and the articular surface also collapse (stage IV) (Fig. 97–9). At this point, degeneration of the opposing articular cartilage begins and later appears as narrowing of the joint space (stage V) (Fig. 97–10). Eventually advanced degenerative changes in the entire joint result (stage VI) (Fig. 97–11).

It must be kept in mind that the earliest changes are confined to the subchondral bone of the femoral head. Narrowing of the joint line and involvement of the bone on the opposite side of the joint are late findings. If this is kept in mind, there will be little tendency to confuse AVN with the many other forms of arthritis that generally involve both sides of the joint more or less simultaneously.

Radionuclide Bone Scan

Bone scanning today is done primarily with technetium 99m diphosphonate. This agent has been

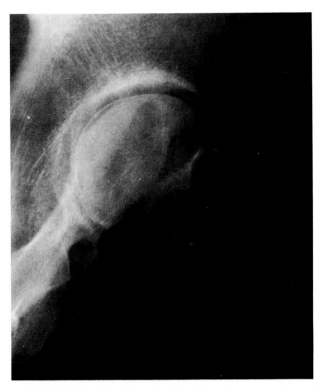

Figure 97–8. Lateral radiograph of a hip with more advanced avascular necrosis showing a typical crescent sign, indicating collapse of cancellous bone beneath the articular cartilage and its attached subchondral plate. (Stage III)

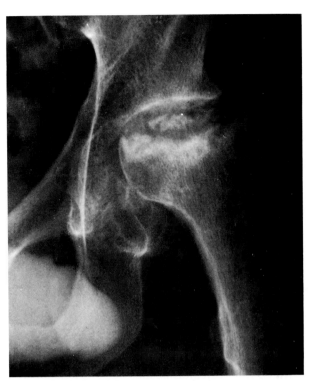

Figure 97–10. More extensive collapse of the femoral head has occurred and has led to narrowing of the joint space. The bony acetabulum remains relatively intact. (Stage V)

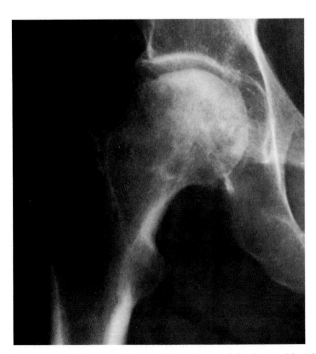

Figure 97–9. Collapse of the cancellous bone of the femoral head has led to flattening of the articular surface. (Stage IV)

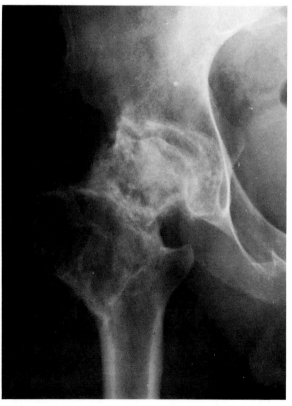

Figure 97–11. An end-stage hip with advanced degenerative changes in both the femoral head and the acetabulum. Note that a previous intertrochanteric osteotomy had been performed. (Stage VI)

in use for the past several years and is extremely sensitive, although nonspecific, in identifying various disorders of bone. It has been helpful in diagnosing AVN because the technetium scan will frequently be abnormal before changes appear on routine radiographs. The picture seen most frequently is that of decreased uptake over the femoral head resulting in a "hot" spot on the film (Fig. 97–12). This increased uptake of isotope reflects a region of increased vascularity or increased new bone formation, which are part of the attempted repair process surrounding the avascular region.

If the avascular area is large enough, a "cold" spot may appear at the center of the lesion where isotope uptake is decreased or absent (Fig. 97–13). Usually, however, this is surrounded by the "hot" area. Because the scan depicts a three-dimensional object in a two-dimensional image, the cold central area is often obliterated on the film.

Increased uptake of isotope on a bone scan is a nonspecific finding that may be seen in many other conditions. Only if these have been ruled out is it reasonable to assume that the positive scan indicates AVN. The presence of the cold central area surrounded by the region of increased uptake is, however, much more specific and is usually diagnostic of AVN even in the presence of a normal radiograph. As with any other test, both false-negative and false-positive results may occur with technetium scans.[45, 47, 48]

With the development of MRI, bone scans are being used less frequently in the diagnosis of AVN. They may serve a useful role if MRI is not available or if a relatively quick and less expensive method is desired to scan the entire skeleton.

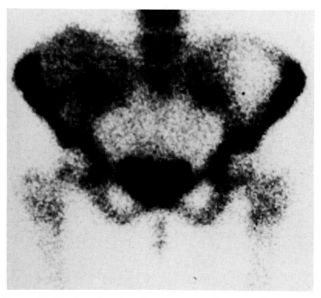

Figure 97–13. A technetium bone scan at the time of a normal radiograph showed a decreased uptake in both femoral heads, leading to the diagnosis of avascular necrosis. This was confirmed by biopsy.

Magnetic Resonance Imaging

MRI is being used with increasing frequency for the early diagnosis of AVN. It is sensitive to the earliest changes that take place in this condition and can detect abnormalities in the fat and bone marrow well before changes occur in the bone itself. MRI is both more specific and more sensitive than bone scanning. It does not subject the patient to harmful radiation. It often detects AVN before abnormalities appear on plain films and occasionally before they appear on bone scans (Figs. 97–13 and 97–14). It is therefore useful when there is clinical suspicion of AVN despite normal radiographs. MRI of both hips should be obtained when the diagnosis has been made in one hip because the incidence of bilaterality is more than 50 percent. It should also be considered when shoulders or knees are involved.

At the present time, MRI is perhaps the best single method for the early diagnosis of AVN. It has largely replaced bone scans, tomograms, and CT.[42, 45, 46]

Other Imaging Modalities

Tomograms or laminograms have been used for quite some time to supplement plain radiographs. They usually show the architectural detail of the bone better than routine radiographs and may be of some value in questionable cases, especially where CT or MRI is not readily available. They may occasionally show small degrees of articular collapse that do not appear on plain films. At the present time, however, we rarely use them.

CT may enable one to diagnose AVN before routine radiographs or laminograms. Because CT

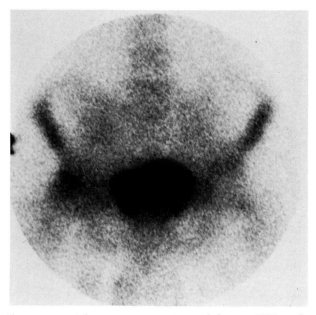

Figure 97–12. A bone scan in a patient with known AVN on the right and a normal radiograph on the left, despite pain, showed an increased uptake of isotope on the right, whereas the uptake on the left was within normal limits.

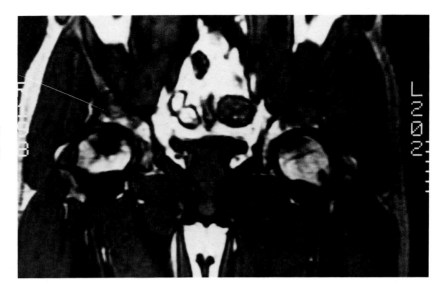

Figure 97–14. The MRI showed areas of decreased signal intensity in both femoral heads, consistent with the diagnosis of bilateral avascular necrosis (coronal views).

abnormalities depend on changes in bone density, they cannot be relied on to diagnose this condition in its very earliest stages. CT scanning therefore has only a limited role in the early diagnosis of AVN.

There has been some interest in the role of SPECT as another modality for the early diagnosis of AVN. This study combines the advantages of CT and bone scanning. On theoretical grounds it should prove valuable and should give us a much better three-dimensional representation of the involved area. Experience with this technique is limited, and we are uncertain as to its future role.

There are certain angiographic techniques that may also be useful in diagnosing and evaluating AVN. These include superselective angiography as described by Theron[49] and intraosseous venography as described by Arlet and Ficat[35] and Hungerford.[36] These techniques, however, are not in general use in most institutions.

At the present time, we use good quality anteroposterior and lateral radiographs as our basic diagnostic tool. If these are not diagnostic or show only unilateral involvement, we obtain an MRI. In most instances, the use of these two modalities coupled with a careful clinical assessment of the patient leads to an early diagnosis of AVN.

Radiographic Staging

It is extremely useful to describe the extent of involvement by a staging system. A few such systems have been used both in the United States and abroad for the past several years. Although of significant value, these are generally overly simple and not quantitative. Accordingly, we have developed a quantitative staging system that is particularly effective in evaluating the femoral and humeral heads. It is based in part on these older systems but has added earlier stages that allow us to describe the status of the involved bone before changes appear on routine radiographs. It also includes a precise and objective

quantification of the extent of involvement, both of the bone as a whole and of the articular surface (Table 97–3). This system has been used to evaluate approximately 1000 femoral and humeral heads and has proved extremely valuable in following progression of the condition and determining the best method of treatment.[50, 51]

Management

At this time, we do not have a completely satisfactory method for treating AVN of the major

Table 97–3. STAGING OF AVASCULAR NECROSIS OF THE FEMORAL HEAD

Stage	Criteria
0	*Normal* radiograph, bone scan, and MRI
I	Normal radiograph, *abnormal* bone scan, and/or MRI Mild (<15%) Moderate (15–30%) Severe (>30%)
II	Sclerosis and/or cyst formation in femoral head Mild (<15%) Moderate (15–30%) Severe (>30%)
III	Subchondral collapse (crescent sign) without flattening Mild (<15%) Moderate (15–30%) Severe (>30%)
IV	Flattening of head without joint narrowing or acetabular involvement Mild (<15% of surface and <2 mm depression) Moderate (15–30% of surface or 2–4 mm depression) Severe (>30% of surface or >4 mm depression)
V	Flattening of head *with* joint narrowing and/or acetabular involvement* Mild Moderate Severe
VI	Advanced degenerative changes

*The overall grade is the average of the femoral head involvement, which is determined as in stage IV, and the acetabular involvement, which is estimated.

weight-bearing joints in adults. Several different approaches have been described. These depend in part on the area of involvement, the stage of the condition, and the personal preference of the treating physician. Unfortunately, definitive data concerning the effectiveness of each of these approaches are not available. AVN of the femoral head in adults is the area most commonly affected and the one that is perhaps the most difficult to treat effectively. An outline of its management follows. The management of AVN in other locations and at other ages is discussed later.

Because this condition affects primarily young adults and is bilateral in more than 50 percent of the cases, our goal is to preserve rather than to replace the femoral head. Whichever method of treatment is selected, results are generally best if therapy is instituted early in the course of the disease.

Nonoperative Management

A number of physicians continue to treat AVN of the femoral head with limited weight bearing or non–weight bearing in the hope that spontaneous healing will occur. Although the treatment may be effective in the pediatric population with Legg-Calvé-Perthes disease, it is usually not effective in the adult. As mentioned, there are certainly many cases of AVN that involve either a small area of bone or an area away from a weight-bearing surface that remain asymptomatic and are never diagnosed. These either may heal spontaneously or may remain as small abnormal areas with no clinical consequences. If a lesion is adjacent to an articular surface and large enough either to produce symptoms or to appear on radiographs or other images, spontaneous healing is much less likely. In our own series of 48 cases of hip involvement treated nonoperatively, we found that only 10 percent of clinically diagnosed lesions did not show progression. Ninety percent went on to collapse of the femoral head, and 80 percent required partial or total joint replacement within the first 2 to 3 years after diagnosis (Fig. 97–15).[52] Therefore, limited weight bearing or non–weight bearing is not advocated if the goal is to save the femoral head. This approach is reserved for the patient in whom prophylactic measures are not indicated, such as the individual with an advanced stage of the disease, the older patient, and the patient with a poor general prognosis and limited life expectancy. In such cases, the use of a cane or crutches may serve as a palliative measure until such time as hip arthroplasty is indicated.

Prophylactic Procedures

The current methods being used to retard or reverse the progression of this disorder include drilling or decompression, bone grafting, osteotomy, and electrical stimulation. Unfortunately, none of these

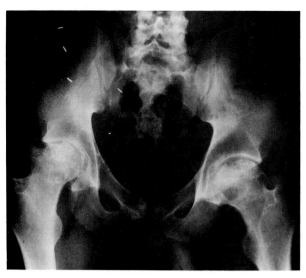

Figure 97–15. AP radiograph of the pelvis of a 26-year-old man taken 3½ years after a renal transplant. The patient had severe pain in both hips. Radiographs show early collapse on the left and late collapse with joint narrowing on the right.

has yet been able to achieve the desired degree of effectiveness.

Drilling or Decompression. One of the simplest procedures used in an attempt to retard or reverse the progression of AVN is drilling or decompression of the involved area. This procedure was introduced many years ago and at that time involved drilling a series of small channels from the lateral cortex of the femur into the avascular region of the femoral head. The goal was to open up channels for the ingrowth of new blood vessels. It was known as "forage." Arlet and Ficat[35] and Hungerford[36] have renewed interest in this approach. They have referred to it as a "core decompression" because they remove a large central core of bone as well as two smaller cores from the femoral head and neck. These cores are examined histologically to confirm the diagnosis. Their basic goal was to provide a mechanical decompression to the area because they had documented that there was a marked increase in the intraosseous pressure both within and adjacent to the lesion of AVN. Early reports indicated up to 80 to 90 percent good-to-excellent results when the procedure was performed early in the course of the disease. Later reports have been more conservative but still claim that progression can be retarded and prognosis improved in at least 50 to 60 percent of cases.[1, 53, 55, 56]

Bone Grafting. Many types of grafting procedures have been described for the treatment of AVN. These include the use of cancellous bone, cortical bone, muscle-pedicle bone grafts, bone grafts with a microvascular anastomosis, and osteochondral allografts. It should be noted that in virtually any bone grafting procedure to the femoral head that is done through the lateral approach, a decompression is also effected.

In 1949, Phemister[57] reported the use of a cortical

graft inserted from a lateral approach into the femoral head and neck. This technique has been used by a number of surgeons since its introduction. Bonfiglio and colleagues reported up to 78 percent satisfactory long-term results.[3, 58, 59] Other authors, however, have generally not been able to duplicate this high degree of success.[60] We are currently using a combination of decompression and bone grafting, employing cancellous rather than cortical bone. The graft is obtained from the operative site by the use of a Michele trephine rather than a solid drill to prepare the central channel. Two additional smaller channels are directed into the lesion. The cancellous graft is then placed very loosely into the central channel and extends from the avascular area down to relatively normal, vascularized bone in the femoral neck.[61, 62] Satisfactory results have been obtained in 50 to 60 percent of 300 hips on which we have performed the procedure. At a mean follow-up of 3 years, 70 percent of hips are still functioning without replacement, as compared with only 31 percent of hips treated non-operatively. At the present time, this is our standard approach for the younger patient with early AVN.[61–63]

Opening up a channel into the center of the lesion provides a mechanical decompression to an area that has been shown to be under increased pressure. Some believe that this increased pressure itself is an important component in the propagation of the disease process and that relieving the pressure aids in its resolution. The fact that many patients do report immediate relief of pain following the surgery indicates that at least some symptomatic effect has been derived from this procedure. The channels opened through the dense barriers that wall off the avascular segment from the adjacent living bone also act as pathways for vascular ingrowth, which in turn contributes to the removal and revitalization of the necrotic tissue. In addition, the use of a cortical strut of bone as a graft may provide a mechanical buttress to retard collapse of the articular surface, and the use of a loose-fitting cancellous graft may serve as a scaffold to expedite the ingrowth of both vascular and bone tissue.

Meyers and others have employed a bone graft with an intact muscle-pedicle in an attempt to provide immediate and direct revascularization to the necrotic area. Although they have been satisfied with their results, others have had less success with this technique.[64, 65]

Gilbert et al.,[66] Urbaniak,[67, 68] Richards,[68a] and Rubash[68b] have used a grafting technique that employs a microvascular anastomosis between the graft and regional vessels to bring an immediate blood supply into the avascular region; this should hasten the process of repair. Preliminary results with this technically difficult procedure have been encouraging, and it may prove to be a useful although demanding approach.

There has also been interest in removing the necrotic segment of bone with its overlying articular cartilage and replacing it with an osteochondral allograft.[69] Not only is this surgery itself technically demanding, but also there are many problems yet to be solved in regard to obtaining the appropriate graft material, ensuring its mechanical fit, and preserving its viability. At the present time, this technique must be considered experimental.

Osteotomy. A number of different osteotomies have been described for the treatment of AVN of the femoral head. These involve cutting through the bone of the proximal femur and changing the relationship between the femoral head and the shaft. Osteotomies have been performed in various planes, including flexion, extension, varus, valgus, and rotation. The reported results vary considerably.[70–73] Of the various osteotomies described, the transtrochanteric rotational osteotomy, described by Sugioka in 1973,[74, 75] is perhaps the most promising. With this technique, the head can be rotated a full 90 degrees, thus bringing a relatively uninvolved segment of the articular surface into the major weight-bearing region, formerly occupied by the necrotic segment. Although Sugioka has reported excellent long-term results in a large series of cases, not all investigators have been able to duplicate them.[76] The role of the osteotomy in treatment of early AVN of the femoral head thus requires further refinement and evaluation.

Electrical Stimulation. Because of the osteogenic effect of certain types of electrical stimulation and their value in promoting the healing of established nonunions, there has been interest in applying this technique to the treatment of AVN. Good results have been reported with the use of pulsing electromagnetic fields applied externally without supplemental surgery.[1, 77, 78] At our own institution, direct current stimulation has been used as an adjunct to decompression and bone grafting in approximately 80 patients[61] and capacitive coupling in another 20.[63] Direct current seemed to improve somewhat the results obtained by decompression and grafting alone, whereas capacitive coupling had no effect.

The role of electrical stimulation in the treatment of AVN, either alone or as an adjunct to surgery, is promising. This technique, however, is still in a stage of evaluation and refinement and should not be considered as a standard approach to the treatment of AVN at this time.

Arthroplasty

The prophylactic measures described have as their goal the preservation of the spherical and structurally intact femoral head. These procedures work best in the early stages of the disease. Once collapse has occurred, the chance of salvaging the femoral head is extremely small. When radiographs demonstrate anything beyond a minimal degree of collapse or when the patient has developed even moderate discomfort, limp, or decreased motion, such preventive measures are generally no longer indicated. At that point, the patient is usually continued on symptomatic care until pain and disability warrant reconstructive surgery. An arthroplasty of the hip is then generally advised. This usually involves replacement of the femoral head alone with an endoprosthesis; replacement of the entire joint with a total hip; or, rarely, a cup arthroplasty or a surface replacement arthroplasty.

Cup Arthroplasty. Before the development of total hip replacement, cup arthroplasty was the mainstay for reconstruction of the badly involved hip. For many reasons, this procedure was almost completely abandoned once total hip replacement became established. There has been a renewed interest, however, in the cup arthroplasty for the treatment of AVN. The original approach has been modified. Two groups in France have used what they refer to as the "adjusted" cup arthroplasty, primarily as a temporizing procedure in this condition.[72, 79] Rather than allowing the cup free motion on both the femoral and the acetabular sides of the joint, it is fitted tightly over the femoral head so little motion occurs here. Virtually all of the motion then occurs between the cup and the acetabulum. They have reported satisfactory 5- to 7-year results. A modification of this approach has been reported by Nelson,[80] who modified the classic cup arthroplasty by cementing the cup onto the femoral head, which is then placed into the relatively normal acetabulum. He, too, has reported good short-term results in a relatively small number of patients.[80] Both of these approaches merit consideration in the young patient with a relatively normal acetabulum in whom an arthroplasty other than total hip replacement is desired.

Surface Replacement Arthroplasty. At one time it was thought that surface replacement arthroplasty might prove to be a useful alternative to total hip replacement in the young adult. A number of patients with AVN underwent surface replacement. Unfortunately, the 5-year failure rate was unacceptable, and this approach has by and large been abandoned in most centers.[81] There are certain theoretical advantages to this technique, however, and investigators are still working to eliminate some of the problems originally encountered. If this can, in fact, be accomplished, surface replacement arthroplasty might once again be considered a viable alternative in the treatment of AVN of the hip.[82]

Femoral Endoprosthetic Replacement. Before the advent of total hip replacement, the classic treatment for advanced AVN was replacement of the femoral head using an endoprosthesis. At that time, these prostheses were inserted into the femoral canal without the use of bone cement. Long-term results were not satisfactory, and a high number of failures occurred. These were attributed to motion within the femoral canal, protrusio acetabuli, or both.[83] With the advent of total hip replacement, the number of endoprostheses inserted for AVN diminished significantly. In the past several years, however, there has been increasing concern about the relatively high

failure rate of total hip replacement in the young, heavy, active adult. Accordingly, interest has focused on other alternatives, especially the femoral endoprosthesis. It was reasoned that if the prosthesis could be fixed rigidly within the shaft, either by the use of cement or biologic ingrowth, problems related to femoral stem motion and migration could be virtually eliminated. It was also presumed that with the newer type of bipolar prosthesis, degeneration of the articular cartilage of the acetabulum and protrusio acetabuli could be diminished. When component failure eventually did occur, it was further suggested that revision would be easier than with a conventional total hip replacement.

Although there are many who still favor the use of a bipolar endoprosthesis rather than a total hip replacement, most series with follow-up periods greater than 5 years have shown that the results with endoprostheses, both bipolar and unipolar, are less predictable and less satisfactory than with total hip replacement.[84, 85] Even normal articular cartilage cannot be expected to withstand articulating against a metal prosthesis for a prolonged period without undergoing significant deterioration, and in cases of AVN that are symptomatic enough to require arthroplasty, secondary degenerative changes have usually already developed in the acetabular cartilage. Therefore, despite the theoretical appeal of this approach, we advise against the use of a femoral endoprosthesis, whether solid or bipolar, for most patients with AVN who have a reasonable life expectancy.

Total Hip Replacement. In the older population, total hip replacement remains the arthroplasty of choice for the treatment of the severely involved hip. Its role in the younger patient is open to a greater difference of opinion.

Some years ago, a series of disturbing reports appeared describing poor results with total hip replacement in young, active, healthy patients, including many with AVN. Since that time, both the components for total hip replacement and the techniques for fixing them to bone have improved considerably. This has led to a significant improvement in their results and in their durability.

Before criticizing the use of total hip replacement in the younger patient, we must stop to consider the alternatives. No replacement arthroplasty will function as well in the younger, active patient as it will in the older, less active patient. Comparing these two groups serves little purpose. The question is which of the various arthroplasties is best for the patient with AVN. In most cases, the answer will be that total hip replacement is still the best procedure for the patient with advanced AVN whose pain and disability can no longer be managed satisfactorily with conservative methods.[84, 85]

Miscellaneous Procedures

Two other procedures that might be considered under special circumstances are hip fusion and Girdlestone pseudarthrosis or resection arthroplasty. A fusion is a surgical procedure that obliterates the joint and promotes a solid bone union between the adjacent bones that formerly articulated with each other. It has certain advantages in the young, heavy, active male. It must, however, be restricted to the patient with unilateral hip disease and with normal knees and a normal spine. Once a fusion is established, it is quite durable.

The Girdlestone pseudarthrosis is a procedure that surgically removes the femoral head and neck as well as the protruding margins of the acetabulum. The patient is treated postoperatively in such a manner that fibrocartilage forms on the opposing bone surfaces, which then eventually form a false joint or pseudarthrosis. Although the patient is left with considerable shortening and instability, an excellent range of motion is preserved, and pain is generally relieved.

Either the fusion or the pseudarthrosis might be considered in selected cases in which an arthroplasty is contraindicated.

Summary

There are thus many options available for the treatment of AVN of the femoral head. These depend in large part on the stage of the disorder at the time that the diagnosis is made. The advantages and disadvantages of each have been described. They are summarized in Table 97–4.

OTHER FORMS OF AVASCULAR NECROSIS

There are a number of other conditions of undetermined etiology that presumably represent variants of AVN. Different areas of the body are affected, the age of onset differs, and the treatment and prognosis often vary considerably from AVN of the femoral head in the adult. In certain circumstances, other areas of the skeleton may be affected by the classic form of AVN, usually in addition to but

Table 97–4. TREATMENT OF NONTRAUMATIC AVASCULAR NECROSIS OF THE HIP IN THE ADULT

Nonoperative management
　Limited weight bearing
　Electrical stimulation
Prophylactic surgery
　Drilling or decompression
　Bone grafting
　Osteotomy
Arthroplasty
　Cup arthroplasty
　Surface replacement arthroplasty
　Femoral endoprosthetic replacement
　Total hip replacement
Miscellaneous procedures
　Fusion
　Resection arthroplasty

occasionally without involvement of the femoral head. This most frequently occurs with the head of the humerus, the femoral condyles, and occasionally the talus. Other forms of this disorder seem to involve predominantly children and include Legg-Calvé-Perthes disease, Köhler's disease, Freiberg's disease, and osteochondritis dissecans. Still other forms involve the small bones of the wrist or foot and may be related to unrecognized trauma. These conditions are described here.

Legg-Calvé-Perthes Disease

Legg-Calvé-Perthes disease is a condition that many believe is the juvenile counterpart of idiopathic AVN in the adult. It affects children between the ages of 4 and 12. One or both hips may be involved. Although the cause has not been definitely established, it is presumably related in some way to an altered blood supply to the femoral head. Trauma has not been seriously implicated. There are considerable variations in age of onset, duration of the disease process, degree of involvement, and end result.

The prognosis is generally best when the disease occurs early in life because the processes of repair are then most active. The prognosis also varies with the size of the involved segment, smaller areas of involvement having a better prognosis. In many instances, an entire necrotic femoral head may be gradually replaced by viable bone. The remodeling process may lead to a femoral head that is virtually normal in some instances, whereas in others, there may be flattening and enlargement of the head and broadening of the neck (Figs. 97–16 and 97–17). The more residual distortion, the more likely is the patient to develop progressive degenerative changes in subsequent years. These symptoms, however, may not appear until adulthood.

Because of the propensity for spontaneous healing of Legg-Calvé-Perthes disease, nonoperative management is usually the treatment of choice. Remodeling of the femoral head is best if it can be contained within the acetabulum during the healing process. Therefore, in most instances, the affected limb should be maintained in a moderate degree of abduction by the use of any one of a number of different splinting or bracing devices. In this position, full weight bearing is often allowed. Under certain circumstances, surgical procedures might be indicated relatively early in the course of the disease. These procedures include osteotomies of the pelvis and of the proximal femur and are designed to provide better coverage and containment of the femoral head within the acetabulum. In addition to improving the anatomic relationships, they may also eliminate the need for years of bracing in abduction. For this reason, some authorities believe that the surgical approach is preferred over the nonsurgical in many instances.[86–88]

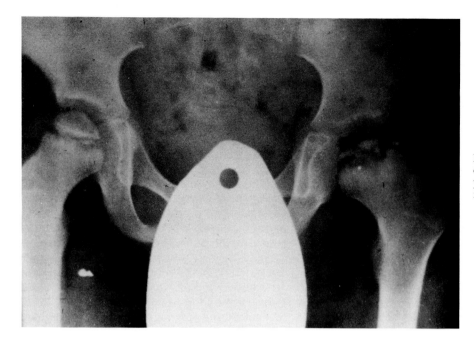

Figure 97–16. Legg-Calvé-Perthes disease in the left femoral head of a 5-year-old boy. Note the sclerosis and fragmentation.

Avascular Necrosis of the Humeral Head

AVN of the humeral head is seen most commonly following comminuted fractures of the head itself, especially those treated by open reduction and internal fixation.[89]

Atraumatic AVN of the humeral head is seen in the same patient population that develops femoral head involvement. Cruess[90] reported an incidence of 20 percent, and in our own series, patients with hip involvement had a 15 percent incidence of shoulder involvement. In most cases, this developed in patients on prolonged steroid administration, but there was also a high incidence in those with sickle cell anemia. In our series of 55 shoulders with AVN, the average age at the time of diagnosis was 44 years. Men and women were affected equally, and bilaterality was observed in 72 percent. Ninety percent had involvement of one or both hips. The clinical status was quite variable, ranging from asymptomatic to severely disabled. Most patients had moderate pain and loss of motion. The disability in general was less than with a similar degree of involvement of the hip. Because the shoulder is a non–weight bearing joint, it is easier to eliminate the stresses on it than it is in the hip or the knee. In addition, motion that is lost at the true shoulder joint, the glenohumeral joint, can in part be compensated for by motion at the scapulothoracic joint.

The radiographic picture is similar to that seen

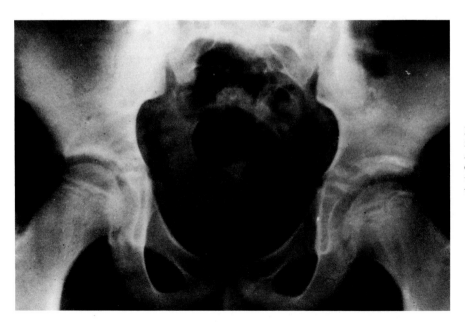

Figure 97–17. Film taken 6 years later, following conservative management. Almost complete remodeling has occurred, although slight broadening of the head and neck remain. The patient was asymptomatic.

in AVN of the femoral head (Fig. 97–18). Involvement is limited to the humeral head itself until quite late in the disease, when secondary degenerative changes may develop in the glenoid. We have found bone scans to be confirmatory but rarely positive before either radiographic changes or clinical findings. Early involvement is best diagnosed by MRI. At some point, the lesion usually reaches a plateau, although most patients are left with a considerable degree of flattening of the humeral head.

Most shoulders may be treated with conservative management. This includes range of motion exercises, anti-inflammatory agents, analgesics, and limitation of physical stress. Prophylactic surgery is rarely undertaken. Those shoulders that fail to respond to this routine and in which pain and loss of function are significant might be considered for surgery. In these instances, shoulder arthroplasty is the procedure of choice and involves either a hemiarthroplasty (replacement of the humeral head alone) or a total shoulder joint replacement. The experience with these procedures is more limited than with arthroplasty of the hip and the knee, but the results are improving steadily[90] (see Chapter 107).

Avascular Necrosis of the Knee

AVN of the knee may involve either the distal femur or the proximal tibia and may involve one or

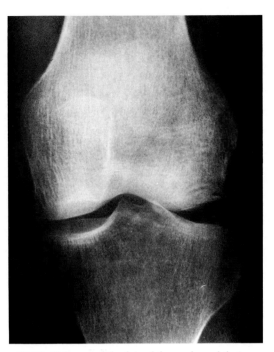

Figure 97–19. Collapse of the lateral femoral condyle in a young woman on chronic steroid treatment following renal transplantation. Both knees and hips were involved.

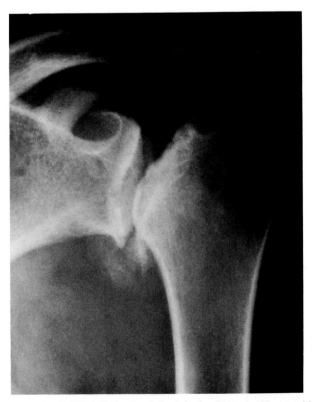

Figure 97–18. AP radiograph of the left shoulder of a 30-year-old woman on chronic steroid treatment for severe lupus erythematosus. The humeral head has collapsed secondary to avascular necrosis and calcific debris is present within the joint.

both condyles or plateaus. There seem to be at least two distinct forms of this condition. The first occurs in those patients who are also prone to develop AVN of the femoral head and usually develops in conjunction with femoral head involvement. It is found most often in association with steroid administration but has also been seen in sickle cell anemia and in dysbaric osteonecrosis. It has been detected in fewer than 10 percent of our own patients with hip involvement.

The lateral femoral condyle is affected in more than 60 percent of patients, with or without concomitant involvement of the medial condyle. Proximal tibial involvement is less common. Bilaterality occurs in more than 50 percent of patients (Fig. 97–19).[91–93]

A second form of this condition has been referred to in the literature primarily as osteonecrosis rather than AVN. It generally afflicts an older age group, the average patient being over 50 years of age at the time of onset. Women are affected three times more than men. The medial side of the joint is most commonly involved, with the lesion occurring more often in the femoral condyles than in the tibial plateaus (Fig. 97–20). Less frequently the lateral femoral condyle is affected. The onset of pain is usually sudden and is often associated with increased physical activity. Examination reveals tenderness over the involved area. There may be an associated synovitis and joint effusion, and occasionally a flexion contracture is seen. In the younger individual, this lesion has been confused with a tear of the medial meniscus or pes anserine bursitis. In the older patient, it may be difficult to distinguish it from osteoarthritis. The

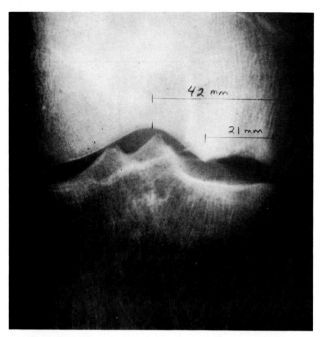

Figure 97–20. Collapse of the medial femoral condyle in a 66-year-old woman with idiopathic osteonecrosis. Note the method for determining the extent of involvement of the articular surface.

cause of this condition is uncertain, although it has been suggested that it may be secondary to multiple small stress fractures occurring in the subchondral region of osteoporotic bone.[91, 94–97]

The radiographic appearance of both forms of this condition may be quite similar. Initially, plain films are within normal limits, and the diagnosis may depend on technetium bone scanning or MRI.[98–100] Later, radiographs may demonstrate a subchondral radiolucency of variable size with a surrounding sclerotic rim. In more advanced cases, there is collapse of the articular surface, and later secondary degenerative changes take place in the opposite side of the joint.

The prognosis depends most often on the size of the lesion as it appears in the initial anteroposterior radiograph.[101] Those patients with small lesions occupying less than 45 percent of condylar width as seen in the anteroposterior view will rarely go on to collapse. There is usually spontaneous healing and a decrease in symptoms. Over the course of the next several years, degenerative arthritis of the knee often develops, however. Patients with lesions larger than 50 percent of the condyle width usually develop more rapid collapse and have a poor prognosis.

Conservative management is advocated for those patients with normal radiographs and those with smaller lesions. This consists of limited weight bearing, quadriceps strengthening, and anti-inflammatory agents. If a satisfactory symptomatic response occurs during the first several weeks, no further therapy may be required. In the younger patient with a significant amount of pain, core decompression has given symptomatic relief in some instances.

It is uncertain whether it will affect the eventual outcome of the condition. With more advanced lesions in the younger patient, a high tibial osteotomy has been recommended to transfer weight from the affected compartment. Satisfactory results have been reported by several authors.[102, 103] Results have varied considerably, with débridement, drilling, and curettage done either through the arthroscope or as an open procedure.[104, 105] For advanced unicompartmental disease, especially in the older patient, hemiarthroplasty has been advised. When degenerative changes have involved both compartments of the joints and symptoms warrant, a total knee replacement is the treatment of choice. Grafting with osteochondral allografts has been done in a limited number of cases but must not be considered a standard approach at this time.[92, 106]

Avascular Necrosis of the Carpal Bones

Lunate (Kienböck's Disease)

AVN of the lunate bone is seen occasionally (Fig. 97–21). It usually occurs in the dominant wrist of younger adults. It may be associated with an anatomic variation in the relationship of the distal radius to the distal ulna. It is believed by many to result from an unrecognized stress fracture or repeated minor trauma to the wrist. It has been seen in sickle

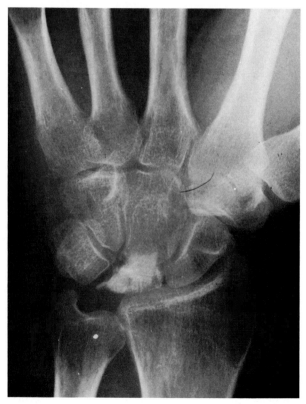

Figure 97–21. Avascular necrosis of the lunate bone (Kienböck's disease).

cell anemia. Treatment options include immobilization and symptomatic management, radial shortening or ulnar lengthening, limited intercarpal fusion, proximal row carpectomy, and wrist fusion.[107]

Scaphoid (Preiser's Disease)

Although post-traumatic AVN of the scaphoid is a well-recognized condition, an atraumatic presentation of this process is much less common. The condition affects primarily the proximal pole of the scaphoid because its only blood supply comes from the distal portion of the bone. Often the trauma is relatively minor, and the fracture goes unrecognized until AVN becomes well established. This condition may remain asymptomatic but usually presents with wrist pain, limitation of motion, tenderness in the snuffbox, and reproduction of pain with passive dorsiflexion of the thumb. Initially, plain radiographs may be normal, and a bone scan may be required to make the diagnosis. Later, the picture is one of sclerosis, cyst formation, fragmentation, and eventually degenerative arthritis of the entire wrist. In addition to a fracture of the scaphoid, etiologic factors include repetitive microtrauma and steroid administration. In some, no etiologic agent can be identified. Treatment is similar to that for Kienböck's disease.[108–110]

Capitate

Only a small number of cases of idiopathic AVN of the capitate have been reported. The clinical and radiologic features, etiologic factors, and treatment are similar to those described for the scaphoid and lunate bones.[111, 112]

Avascular Necrosis of the Foot and Ankle

Tarsal Navicular (Köhler's Disease)

This rare form of AVN occurs in the pediatric population, age 4 through 10. It is three times as common in males as in females. The child presents with an antalgic gait and localized tenderness and swelling over the navicular. The susceptibility of the tarsal navicular to ischemia is thought to be due to the late ossification of this important weight-bearing bone. Ischemia may result from excessive shear forces occurring at the chondro-osseous junction.

Radiographic changes consist of sclerosis and eventual fragmentation and flattening. Irregular ossification of the navicular is often a normal variant and must not be confused with this condition.

Symptoms usually last from 3 to 15 months, and the healing process can be hastened considerably by cast immobilization. In virtually all instances, this is a self-limiting process, and the navicular will eventually regain a normal radiographic appearance (Figs. 97–22 and 97–23). The youngster is normally left with little or no disability.[113–115]

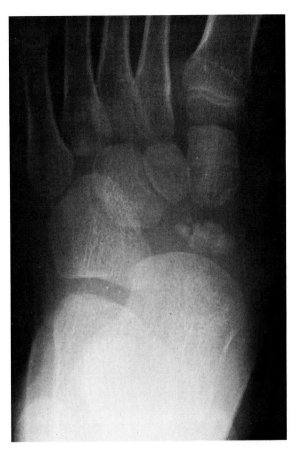

Figure 97–22. Avascular necrosis with fragmentation of the tarsal-navicular in a 6-year-old boy without history of trauma.

Talus

AVN of the talus results most frequently from trauma, with a reported incidence of up to 91 percent in severe fracture dislocations.[116, 117] Atraumatic AVN is rare;[118, 119] it was noted in fewer than 10 percent of our own patients with AVN of the hips. Age, sex, and associated conditions were similar. Symptomatic management has occasionally been successful, especially if the lesion is small. If a significant portion of the talus is affected, the articular surface will eventually collapse and will lead to a significant degree of pain and disability (Fig. 97–24). Ankle motion may become severely restricted. Bracing may be required, and in cases of extreme disability, ankle fusion or pantalar arthrodesis may be indicated. Unfortunately, total ankle replacement has not proved successful in these cases.

Metatarsals (Freiberg's Disease)

AVN of a metatarsal head, usually the second, is known as Freiberg's infraction or Freiberg's disease. It is usually seen in adolescents, with females predominating over males in the ratio of 3:1. The cause is unclear, although trauma has been implicated.

This condition presents as localized pain and

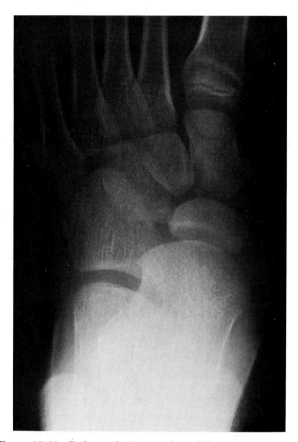

Figure 97–23. Radiograph 2 years later following conservative management. Note that there is almost complete resolution of the process with a normal appearing navicular.

swelling under the metatarsal head with decreased motion of the metatarsophalangeal joint. Radiographs may be within normal limits or may show sclerosis, fragmentation, or flattening of the distal metatarsal. Bone scans are useful in the early diagnosis.

Freiberg's disease is generally a self-limiting condition in the adolescent and is initially treated nonoperatively. If symptoms warrant, a short leg cast may be used for 3 to 4 weeks, followed by a metatarsal arch support. In some cases, pain persists for a prolonged period or occurs in adult life. In such instances, surgery may be required if nonoperative methods are ineffective. Osteotomy of the affected bone or resection of the metatarsal head may alleviate symptoms.[120–122]

Osteochondritis Dissecans

Osteochondritis dissecans is a condition in which a fragment composed of articular cartilage and subchondral bone demarcates and often separates from the surrounding bone and cartilage. The cause has not been established, but local ischemia and trauma have been implicated, thus its inclusion in the section on AVN. There may be a hereditary component to this disorder.

The most common site affected is the distal femur, but it has also been reported in the talus, hip, and elbow. Males are involved more frequently than females. Although it can occur in many age groups, it predominates in adolescents and young adults.

The patient usually presents with joint pain and may demonstrate decreased motion, effusion, and a limp. Radiographically, osteochondritis dissecans appears as a well-circumscribed sclerotic lesion, which is separated from the surrounding bone by a radiolucent line. The osteochondral fragment may remain in situ with intact articular cartilage overlying it, or it may be partially or completely separated from the subchondral bone and displaced into the joint (Fig. 97–25).

The prognosis and treatment depend on the joint involved, the size of the lesion, and the age of the patient. In general, when this occurs in the young, skeletally immature patient, there is an excellent chance of spontaneous healing.[123, 124] Conservative management including immobilization may hasten the process. In the older patient with closed epiphyses, the prognosis is much poorer, and the segment is much more likely to break loose and cause degenerative changes in the joint.[125] Tomograms, arthrography, and arthroscopy may be useful in evaluating the extent of the involvement. Drilling of the lesion may be required to promote vascular ingrowth and healing (Figs. 97–26 and 97–27). If the fragment has already broken loose and is small, it may be removed and the bed drilled to promote the ingrowth of fibrocartilage. If the fragment is large and the overlying cartilage seems viable, it may be replaced into

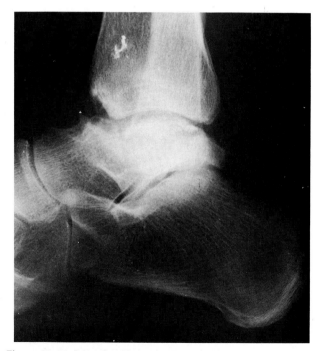

Figure 97–24. Lateral ankle radiograph of a patient with steroid-dependent lupus erythematosus showing collapse of the articular surface of the talus.

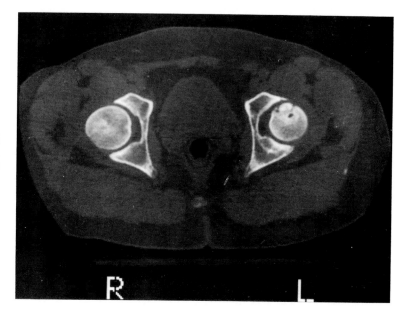

Figure 97–25. CT scan of both hips in a 30-year-old patient with spontaneous onset of pain on the left. The typical lesion of osteochondritis dissecans is seen in the left femoral head.

its bed after débridement and held in place until healing occurs. Occasionally, replacement by an osteochondral allograft is required.[126]

SUMMARY AND CONCLUSIONS

AVN of bone is not a single disease but is a common end point for a number of pathologic con-ditions, all of which result in impairment of the circulation to a specific area of the skeleton. Several joints may be affected, most frequently the hip, knee, and shoulder, and less frequently, the wrist, ankle, and foot. There appear to be several different variants of this condition. The most common cause is a displaced fracture, generally involving a joint. Al-

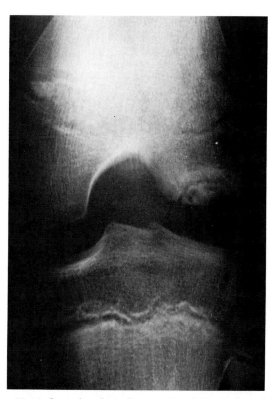

Figure 97–26. Osteochondritis dissecans involving the lateral femoral condyle of a 14-year-old boy. Symptoms developed following minimal trauma.

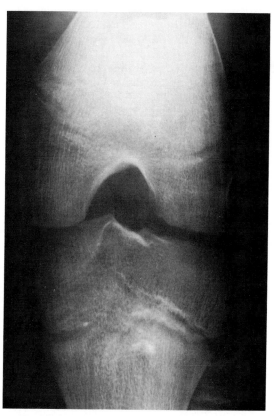

Figure 97–27. Radiographs taken 9 months after arthroscopic drilling of the lesion show significant healing with a nearly normal articular silhouette.

though this form of AVN has been touched on briefly here, it is covered in greater detail in fracture texts. Our attention has been focused on the nontraumatic varieties.

Most of the cases that we encounter involve younger adults and are associated with a variety of conditions that cause circulatory impairment. Most common among these are prolonged glucocorticoid administration and excessive alcohol intake. Although the course of the condition does vary somewhat with anatomic location and etiologic factors, a general series of events usually occurs. If a small area of bone is involved, the condition may remain asymptomatic and escape detection. Spontaneous healing usually occurs. With a larger area of involvement, however, progressive changes usually occur and result in collapse of the articular surface. This in turn leads to pain, disability, and eventual degenerative arthritis. In the major weight-bearing joints, specifically the hip and the knee, this often necessitates a surgical arthroplasty with partial or total joint replacement. Prophylactic procedures, if instituted early, may help to retard and even reverse this progression. At the present time, however, the prophylactic procedures available are not as effective as we would desire.

Methods for the early diagnosis of AVN have improved considerably over the past several years. These include a heightened clinical awareness of this condition and the use of various imaging modalities, including good quality radiographs, bone scanning, and especially MRI. The earlier the diagnosis is made, the better will be the results of treatment. This will become increasingly important as methods for treatment improve. It should be emphasized that in most instances, spontaneous healing does not occur, and the results of symptomatic management or partial weight bearing are poor.

There are other forms of AVN that have different clinical and radiographic patterns. These include osteonecrosis about the knee, generally seen in older individuals, and lesions presumed to be variants of AVN, which most often affect the small bones about the wrist, foot, and ankle. These latter are often seen in children and young adults, respond well to conservative management, and have a good prognosis.

Much remains to be done to increase our understanding of the etiology of this condition or group of conditions and to improve the methods available for its management. At the present time, a number of newer procedures are undergoing evaluation. It is hoped that at least some of these will prove effective and will increase our ability to treat this most frustrating disorder.

References

1. Boyd, H. B., and George, I. L.: Complications of fractures of the neck of the femur. J. Bone Joint Surg. 29B:13, 1947.
2. Bohr, H., and Larsen, E. H.: On necrosis of the femoral head after fracture of the neck of the femur. J. Bone Joint Surg. 47B:330, 1965.
3. Bonfiglio, M., and Voke, E. M.: Aseptic necrosis of the femoral head and nonunion of the femoral neck. J. Bone Joint Surg. 50A:48, 1968.
4. Catto, M.: A histological study of avascular necrosis of the femoral head after transcervical fracture. J. Bone Joint Surg. 47B:749, 1965.
5. Catto, M.: The histological appearances of late segmental collapse of the femoral head after transcervical fracture. J. Bone Joint Surg. 47B:777, 1965.
6. Jacobs, B.: Epidemiology of traumatic and non-traumatic osteonecrosis. Clin. Orthop. 130:51, 1978.
7. Sennara, H., and Gorry, F.: Orthopedic aspects of sickle cell anemia and allied hemoglobinopathies. Clin. Orthop. 130:154, 1978.
8. Sevitt, S.: Avascular necrosis and revascularization of the femoral head after intracapsular fractures. J. Bone Joint Surg. 46B:270, 1964.
9. Chung, S. M. K., Alavi, A., and Russell, M. O.: Management of osteonecrosis in sickle-cell anemia and its genetic variants. Clin. Orthop. 130:158, 1978.
10. Chung, S. M. K., and Ralston, E. L.: Necrosis of the femoral head associated with sickle-cell anemia and its genetic variants. J. Bone Joint Surg. 51A:33, 1969.
11. Jones, J. P., Jr., and Engleman, E. P.: Osseous avascular necrosis associated with systemic abnormalities. Arthritis Rheum. 9:728, 1966.
12. Jones, J. P., Jr., and Behnke, A. R., Jr.: Prevention of dysbaric osteonecrosis in compressed-air workers. Clin. Orthop. 130:118, 1978.
13. Chryssanthou, C. P.: Dysbaric osteonecrosis: Etiological and pathogenetic concepts. Clin. Orthop. 130:94, 1978.
14. Kawashima, M., Torisu, T., Hayashi, K., and Kitano, M.: Pathological review of osteonecrosis in divers. Clin. Orthop. 130:107, 1978.
15. Markham, T. N.: Ann Arbor case reports: Aseptic necrosis in a high-altitude flier. J. Occup. Med. 9:123, 1967.
16. Fisher, D. E.: The role of fat embolism in the etiology of corticosteroid-induced avascular necrosis: Clinical and experimental results. Clin. Orthop. 130:68, 1978.
17. Lee, K. C., Corcoran, S. F., and Parsons, J. R.: Hyperlipidemia and idiopathic aseptic necrosis of the femoral head in adults. Orthopaedics 3:651, 1980.
18. Wang, G., Moga, D. B., Richemer, W. G., et al.: Cortisone-induced bone changes and its response to lipid clearing agents. Clin. Orthop. 130:81, 1978.
19. Jones, J. P., Jr.: Alcoholism, hypercortisonism, fat embolism and osseous avascular necrosis. In Zinn, W. M. (ed.): Idiopathic Ischemic Necrosis of the Femoral Head. Stuttgart, Thieme Verlag, 1971.
20. Jones, J. P., Jr., and Sakovich, L.: Fat embolism of bone. J. Bone Joint Surg. 48A:149, 1966.
21. Boettcher, W. G., Bonfiglio, M., Hamilton, H. H., et al.: Non-traumatic necrosis of the femoral head. I. Relation of altered hemostasis to etiology. J. Bone Joint Surg. 52A:312, 1970.
22. Cruess, R. L., Blennerhassett, J., MacDonald, F. R., et al.: Aseptic necrosis following renal transplantation. J. Bone Joint Surg. 50A:1577, 1968.
23. Dubois, E. L., and Cozen, L.: Avascular (aseptic) bone necrosis associated with systemic lupus erythematosus. J.A.M.A. 174:108, 1960.
24. Hall, M. C., Elmore, S. M., Bright, R. W., et al.: Skeletal complications in a series of human renal allografts. J.A.M.A. 208:1825, 1969.
25. Johnson, R. L., Smyth, C. J., Holt, G. W., et al.: Steroid therapy and vascular lesions in rheumatoid arthritis. Arthritis Rheum. 2:224, 1959.
26. Kenzora, J. E., and Glimcher, M. J.: The role of renal bone disease in the production of transplant osteonecrosis. Orthopaedics 4:305, 1981.
27. Steinberg, M. E., Koh, J. K., Alavi, A., et al.: Non-traumatic avascular necrosis of the femoral head in adults. Orthop. Digest, March, 5:17, 1977.
28. Kenzora, J. E., and Glimcher, M. J.: Accumulative cell stress: The multifactorial etiology of idiopathic osteonecrosis. Orthop. Clin. North Am. 16:667, 1985.
29. Cruess, R. L.: Osteonecrosis of bone: Current concepts as to etiology and pathogenesis. Clin. Orthop. 130:151, 1978.
30. Spence, R. K., Alavi, A., Barker, C. F., et al.: Osteonecrosis in the renal transplant recipient—a prospective study. In Arlet, J., Ficat, R. P., and Hungerford, D. S. (eds.): Bone Circulation. Baltimore, Williams & Wilkins, 1984, pp. 246–249.
31. Hunder, G. G., Worthington, J. W., and Bickel, W. H.: Avascular necrosis of the femoral head in a patient with gout. J.A.M.A. 203:101, 1968.
32. Mankin, H. J., and Brower, T. D.: Bilateral idiopathic aseptic necrosis of the femur in adults: "Chandler's disease." J. Hosp. Joint Dis. 23:42, 1962.
33. Fries, G.: Zur Rontgen-Diagnostik Osteoradionekrotischer Huftveranderugen nach Rontgen-Radiumbestrahlung weiblicher Genitalkarzinome. Strahlentherapie 132:113, 1967.
34. Hamilton, H. E., Bonfiglio, M., Sheets, R. F., and Connor, W. E.: Relation of altered hemostasis to idiopathic aseptic necrosis of the femoral head. J. Clin. Invest. 44:1058, 1965.
35. Ficat, R. P., and Arlet, J.: In Hungerford, D. S. (ed.): Ischemia and Necrosis of Bone. Baltimore, Williams & Wilkins, 1980, pp. 131–171.
36. Hungerford, D. S.: Bone marrow pressure, venography, and core

decompression in ischemic necrosis of the femoral head. *In* Sledge, C. B. (ed.): The Hip: Proceedings of the Seventh Open Scientific Meeting of the Hip Society. St. Louis, C. V. Mosby, 1979, pp. 218–237.
37. Bobechko, W. P., and Harris, W. R.: The radiographic density of avascular bone. J. Bone Joint Surg. 42B:626, 1960.
38. Glimcher, M. J., and Kenzora, J. E.: The biology of osteonecrosis of the human femoral head and its clinical implications. I. Tissue biology. Clin. Orthop. 138:284, 1979.
39. Glimcher, M. J., and Kenzora, J. E.: Osteonecrosis: The pathobiology, clinical manifestations, therapeutic dilemmas. Instructional Course 103, American Academy of Orthopaedic Surgeons, Annual Meeting, Atlanta, 1980.
40. Phemister, D. B.: Changes in bones and joints resulting from interruption of circulation. I. General consideration and changes resulting from injury. Arch. Surg. 41:436, 1940.
41. Steinberg, M. E.: Avascular necrosis of the femoral head. *In* Tronzo, R. G. (ed.): Surgery of the Hip Joint. Vol. II. New York, Springer-Verlag, 1987, pp. 1–29.
42. Steinberg, M. E., and Steinberg, D. R.: Avascular necrosis of the femoral head. *In* Steinberg, M. E. (ed.): The Hip and Its Disorders. Philadelphia, W. B. Saunders Company, 1991, pp. 623–647.
43. Glimcher, M. J., and Kenzora, J. E.: The biology of osteonecrosis of the human femoral head and its clinical implications. II. The pathological changes in the femoral head as an organ and in the hip joint. Clin. Orthop. 139:283, 1979.
44. Glimcher, M. J., and Kenzora, J. E.: The biology of osteonecrosis of the human femoral head and its clinical implications. III. Discussion of the etiology and genesis of the pathological sequelae; comments on treatment. Clin. Orthop. 140:273, 1979.
45. Mitchell, M. D., Kundel, H. L., Steinberg, M. E., Kressel, H. Y., Alavi, A., and Axel, L.: Avascular necrosis of the hip: Comparison of M. R., C. T., and scintigraphy. A.J.R. 147:67, 1986.
46. Steinberg, M. E., Thickman, D., Chen, H. H., et al.: Early diagnosis of avascular necrosis by magnetic resonance imaging. *In* Arlet, J., and Mazieres, B., (eds.): Bone Circulation and Bone Necrosis. New York, Springer-Verlag, 1990, pp. 281–285.
47. Alavi, A., McCloskey, J. R., and Steinberg, M. E.: Early detection of avascular necrosis of the femoral head by 99m technetium diphosphonate bone scan: A preliminary report. Clin. Orthop. 127:137, 1977.
48. D'Ambrosia, R. D., Shoji, H., Riggins, R. S., et al.: Scintigraphy in the diagnosis of osteonecrosis. Clin. Orthop. 130:139, 1978.
49. Theron, J.: Superselective angiography of the hip. Radiology 124:649, 1977.
50. Steinberg, M. E., Hayken, G. D., and Steinberg, D. R.: A new method for evaluation and staging of avascular necrosis of the femoral head. *In* Arlet, J., Ficat, R. P., and Hungerford, D. S. (eds.): Bone Circulation. Baltimore, Williams & Wilkins, 1984, pp. 398–403.
51. Steinberg, M. E., and Steinberg, D. R.: Evaluation and staging avascular necrosis of the femoral head. Semin. Arthroplasty 2(3):175, 1991.
52. Steinberg, M. E., Hayken, G. D., and Steinberg, D. R.: The "conservative" management of avascular necrosis of the femoral head. *In* Arlet, J., Ficat, R. P., and Hungerford, D. S. (eds.): Bone Circulation. Baltimore, Williams & Wilkins, 1984, pp. 334–337.
53. Warner, J. J., Philips, J. H., Brodsky, G. L., and Thornhill, T. S.: Studies of nontraumatic osteonecrosis: The role of core decompression in the treatment of nontraumatic osteonecrosis of the femoral head. Clin. Orthop. Rel. Res. 225:104, 1987.
54. Aaron, R. K., Lennox, D. W., Bunce, G. E., and Eert, T.: The conservative treatment of osteonecrosis of the femoral head: A comparison of core decompression and pulsing electromagnetic fields. Clin. Orthop. 249:209, 1989.
55. Hungerford, D.: Personal communication, 1991.
56. Stulberg, B. N., Bauer, T. W., and Belhobek, G. H.: Making core decompression work. Clin. Orthop. Rel. Res. 261:186, 1990.
57. Phemister, D. B.: Treatment of the necrotic head of the femur in adults. J. Bone Joint Surg. 31A:55, 1949.
58. Bonfiglio, M.: Aseptic necrosis of the femoral head in dogs: Effect of drilling and bone grafting. Surg. Gynecol. Obstet. 98:591, 1954.
59. Boettcher, W. G., Bonfiglio, M., and Smith, K.: Nontraumatic necrosis of the femoral head. II. Experiences in treatment. J. Bone Joint Surg. 52A:322, 1970.
60. Marcus, N. D., Enneking, W. F., and Massam, R. A.: The silent hip in idiopathic aseptic necrosis—treatment by bone grafting. J. Bone Joint Surg. 55A:1351, 1975.
60a. Petty, W.: Personal communication, July 1992.
61. Steinberg, M. E., Corces, A., Steinberg, D. R., et al.: Osteonecrosis of the femoral head: Results of core decompression and grafting, with and without electrical stimulation. Clin. Orthop. Rel. Res. 249:199, 1989.
62. Steinberg, M. E., Brighton, C. T., Steinberg, D. R., et al.: Treatment of avascular necrosis of the femoral head by a combination of bone grafting, decompression, and electrical stimulation. Clin. Orthop. 186:137, 1984.
63. Steinberg, M. E., Brighton, C. T., Bands, R. E., and Hartman, K.:

Capacitive coupling as an adjunctive treatment for avascular necrosis. Clin. Orthop. Rel. Res. 271:11, 1990.
64. Chen, Z. W.: Iliac crest graft with vascular pedicle. Orthop. Trans. 9(3):401, 1985.
65. Meyers, M. H.: The treatment of osteonecrosis of the hip with fresh osteochondral allografts and with the muscle-pedicle graft technique. Clin. Orthop. 130:202, 1978.
66. Gilbert, A., Judet, H., Judet, J., and Agatti, A.: Microvascular transfer of the fibula for necrosis of the femoral head. Orthopaedics 9:885, 1986.
67. Urbaniak, J. R.: Avascular necrosis of the femoral head treated by vascularized fibular graft. Orthop. Trans. 9(3):401, 1985.
68. Urbaniak, J. R.: The treatment of aseptic necrosis of the femoral head by free vascularized fibular graft. Presented at the 18th Open Scientific Meeting of the Hip Society, New Orleans, 1990.
68a. Richards, R. R.: Bone grafting with microvascular anastomosis in osteonecrosis of the femoral head. Semin. Arthroplasty 2(3):198, 1991.
68b. Rubash, H.: Personal communication, June 1992.
69. Meyers, M. H.: Resurfacing of the femoral head with fresh osteochondral allografts—long term results. Clin. Orthop. 197:111, 1985.
70. Maistrelli, G. L., Fusco, U., Avai, A., and Bombelli, R.: Osteonecrosis of the hip treated by intertrochanteric osteotomy—a four to fifteen year follow-up. J. Bone Joint Surg. 70:761, 1988.
71. Jacobs, M. A., Hungerford, D. S., Krackow, K. A., and Lennox, D. W.: Intertrochanteric osteotomy for avascular necrosis of the femoral head. J. Bone Joint Surg. (Br.) 71:200, 1989.
72. Kerboul, M., Thomine, J., Postel, M., and Merle D'Aubigne, R.: The conservative surgical treatment of idiopathic aseptic necrosis of the femoral head. J. Bone Joint Surg. 56B:291, 1974.
73. Merle d'Aubigne, R., Postel, M., Mazabraud, A., et al.: Idiopathic necrosis of the femoral head in adults. J. Bone Joint Surg. 47B:612, 1965.
74. Sugioka, Y.: Transtrochanteric rotational osteotomy in the treatment of idiopathic and steroid-induced femoral head necrosis, Perthes disease, slipped capital femoral epiphysis, and osteoarthritis of the hip. Clin. Orthop. 184:12, 1984.
75. Sugioka, Y., Hotokebuchi, T., and Tsutsui, H.: Transtrochanteric anterior rotational osteotomy for idiopathic and steroid-induced necrosis of the femoral head. Clin. Orthop. Rel. Res. 277:111, 1992.
76. Tooke, S. M. T., Amstutz, H. C., and Hedley, A. K.: Results of transtrochanteric rotational osteotomy for femoral head osteonecrosis. Clin. Orthop. Rel. Res. 224:150, 1987.
77. Bassett, C. A. L., Schink-Ascani, M. M., and Lewes, S. N.: Treatment of femoral head osteonecrosis with pulsed electromagnetic fields (PEMFs). *In* Arlet, J., Ficat, R. P., and Hungerford, D. S. (eds.): Bone Circulation. Baltimore, Williams & Wilkins, 1983, pp. 343–354.
78. Eftekhar, S. A., Schink-Ascani, M. M., Mitchell, S. N., et al.: Osteonecrosis of the femoral head treated by pulsed electromagnetic fields (PEMFs): A preliminary report. *In* Hungerford, D. S. (ed.): The Hip. St. Louis, C. V. Mosby, 1983, pp. 306–330.
79. Sedel, L.: Personal communication, 1989.
80. Nelson, C. L.: Personal communication, June 1992.
81. Steinberg, M. E.: Symposium on Surface Replacement Arthroplasty of the Hip. Summary and conclusions. Orthop. Clin. North Am. 13:895, 1982.
82. Amstutz, H. C., Kabo, M., Dorey, F., and Kilgus, D. J.: Porous surface replacement of the hip with Chamfer cylinder design. Presented at the Annual Meeting of the American Orthopaedic Association, Hot Springs, VA, 1986.
83. Steinberg, M. E., and Unger, A. S.: Femoral endoprosthetic replacement in younger patients. Presented at the 52nd Annual Meeting of the American Academy of Orthopaedic Surgeons, Las Vegas, 1985.
84. Lachiewicz, P. F., and Desman, S. M.: The bipolar endoprostheses in avascular necrosis of the femoral head. J. Arthroplasty 3(2):131, 1988.
85. Cabanela, M. E.: The bipolar prosthesis in avascular necrosis of the femoral head. Semin. Arthroplasty 2(3):228, 1991.
85a. Kirschenbaum, I. K., Vernace, J. V., Booth, R. E., Balderston, R. A., and Rothman, R. H.: Total hip arthroplasty for osteonecrosis. Semin. Arthroplasty 2(3):234, 1991.
85b. Harris, W. H.: Personal communication, July 1992.
86. Ralston, E. L.: Legg-Calve-Perthes disease—factors in healing. J. Bone Joint Surg. 43A:249, 1961.
87. Menelaus, M. B.: Lessons learned in the management of Legg-Calve-Perthes disease. Clin. Orthop. 209:41, 1986.
88. Chung, S. M. K.: Legg-Calve-Perthes disease. *In* Chung, S. M. K. (ed.): Hip Disorders in Infants and Children. Philadelphia, Lea & Febiger, 1981, pp. 235–253.
89. Sturzenegger, M., Fornaro, E., and Jakob, R. P.: Results of surgical treatment of multifragmented fractures of the humeral head. Arch. Orthop. Trauma Surg. 100(4):249, 1982.
90. Cruess, R. L.: Corticosteroid-induced osteonecrosis of the humeral head. Orthop. Clin. North Am. 16(4):789, 1985.
91. Aglietti, P., Insall, J. N., Buzzi, R., and Deschamps, G.: Idiopathic osteonecrosis of the knee—aetiology, prognosis and treatment. J. Bone Joint Surg. 65B:588, 1983.

92. Bayne, O., Langer, F., Pritzker, K. P. H., Houpt, J., and Gross, A. E.: Osteochondral allografts in the treatment of osteonecrosis of the knee. Orthop. Clin. 16(4):727, 1985.
93. Sasaki, T., Yagi, T., Monju, J., Masuda, T., Fukazawa, M., and Konno, H.: Steroid-induced osteonecrosis of the femoral condyle—a clinical study of 18 knees in 10 patients. Nippon Seikeigeka Gakkai Zasshi 60(3):361, 1986.
94. Lotke, P. A., Abend, J. A., and Ecker, M. L.: The treatment of osteonecrosis of the medial femoral condyle. Clin. Orthop. 171:109, 1982.
95. Lotke, P. A., and Ecker, M. L.: Osteonecrosis of the medial tibial plateau. Contemp. Orthop. 10(2):47, 1985.
96. Lotke, P. A., and Ecker, M. L.: Osteonecrosis of the knee. Orthop. Clin. North Am. 16(4):797, 1985.
97. Rozing, P. M., Insall, J., and Bohne, W. H.: Spontaneous osteonecrosis of the knee. J. Bone Joint Surg. 62A(1):2, 1980.
98. Burk, D. L., Jr., Kanal, E., Brunberg, J. A., Johnstone, G. F., Swensen, H. E., and Wolf, G. L.: 1.5-T surface coil magnetic resonance imaging of the knee. A. J. R. 147(2):293, 1986.
99. Pollack, M. S., Dalinka, M. K., Kressel, H. Y., Lotke, P. A., and Spritzer, C. E.: Magnetic resonance imaging in the evaluation of suspected osteonecrosis of the knee. Skeletal Radiol. 16(2):121, 1987.
100. Reicher, M. A., Bassett, L. W., and Gold, R. H.: High-resolution magnetic resonance imaging of the knee joint: Pathologic correlation. A. J. R. 145(5):903, 1985.
101. Muheim, G., and Bohne, W. H.: Prognosis in spontaneous osteonecrosis of the knee. J. Bone Joint Surg. 52B(4):605, 1970.
102. Koshino, T.: The treatment of spontaneous osteonecrosis of the knee by high tibial osteotomy with and without bone grafting or drilling of the lesion. J. Bone Joint Surg. 64A(1):47, 1982.
103. Insall, J. N., Joseph, D. M., and Msika, C.: High tibial osteotomy for varus gonarthrosis. J. Bone Joint Surg. 66A(7):1040, 1984.
104. Miller, G. K., Maylahn, D. J., and Drennan, D. B.: The treatment of idiopathic osteonecrosis of the medial femoral condyle with arthroscopic debridement. Arthroscopy 2(1):21, 1986.
105. Weidel, J. D.: Arthroscopy in steroid-induced osteonecrosis of the knee. Arthroscopy 1(1):68, 1985.
106. Gross, A. E., McKee, N. H., Pritzker, K. P. H., and Langer, F.: Reconstruction of skeletal deficits of the knee—a comprehensive osteochondral transplant program. Clin. Orthop. 174:966, 1983.
107. Almquist, E. E.: Kienböck's disease. Clin. Orthop. 202:69, 1986.
108. Allen, P. R.: Idiopathic avascular necrosis of the scaphoid—a report of two cases. J. Bone Joint Surg. 65B:333, 1983.
109. Aptekar, R. G., Klippel, J. H., Becker, K. E., Carson, D. A., Seaman, W. E., and Decker, J. L.: Avascular necrosis of the talus, scaphoid, and metatarsal head in systemic lupus erythematosus. Clin. Orthop. 101:127, 1974.
110. Harper, P. G., Trask, C., and Souhami, R. L.: Avascular necrosis of bone caused by combination chemotherapy without corticosteroids. Br. Med. J. (Clin. Res.) 288(6413):267, 1984.
111. Bolton-Maggs, B. G., Helal, B. H., and Revell, P. A.: Bilateral avascular necrosis of the capitate—a case report and a review of the literature. J. Bone Joint Surg. 66B(4):557, 1984.
112. James, E. T. R., and Burke, F. D.: Vibration disease of the capitate. J. Bone Joint Surg. 9B(2):169, 1984.
113. Ippolito, E., Ricciardi-Pollini, P. T., and Falez, F.: Kohler's disease of the tarsal navicular: Long-term follow-up of twelve cases. J. Pediatr. Orthop. 4:416, 1984.
114. Waugh, W.: The ossification and vascularization of the tarsal navicular and their relation to Kohler's disease. J. Bone Joint Surg. 40B(4):765, 1958.
115. Williams, G. A., and Cowell, H. R.: Kohler's disease of the tarsal navicular. Clin. Orthop. 158:53, 1981.
116. Hawkins, L. G.: Fractures of the neck of the talus. J. Bone Joint Surg. 52A(5):991, 1970.
117. Morris, H. D.: Aseptic necrosis of the talus following injury. Orthop. Clin. North Am. 5(1):177, 1974.
118. Baron, M., Paltiel, H., and Lander, P.: Aseptic necrosis of the talus and calcaneal insufficiency fractures in a patient with pancreatitis, subcutaneous fat necrosis, and arthritis. Arthritis Rheum. 27(11):1309, 1984.
119. Miskew, D. B., and Goldflies, M. L.: Atraumatic avascular necrosis of the talus associated with hyperuricemia. Clin. Orthop. 148:156, 1980.
120. Braddock, G. T. F.: Experimental epiphyseal injury and Freiberg's disease. J. Bone Joint Surg. 41B:1549, 1959.
121. Mandell, G. A., and Harcke, H. T.: Scintigraphic manifestations of infraction of the second metatarsal (Freiberg's disease). J. Nucl. Med. 28(2):249, 1987.
122. Smillie, I. S.: Freiberg's infraction (Kohler's second disease). J. Bone Joint Surg. 39B:580, 1957.
123. Pappas, A. M.: Osteochondritis dissecans. Clin. Orthop. 158:59, 1981.
124. Linden, B.: Osteochondritis dissecans of the femoral condyles. J. Bone Joint Surg. 59A:769, 1977.
125. McCullough, C. J., and Venugopal, V.: Osteochondritis dissecans of the talus—the natural history. Clin. Orthop. 144:264, 1979.
126. Alexander, A. H., and Lichtman, D. M.: Surgical treatment of transchondral talar-dome fractures (osteochondritis dissecans). J. Bone Joint Surg. 62A:646, 1980.

Section XX
Tumors Involving Joints

Chapter 98

Andrew E. Rosenberg
Alan L. Schiller

Tumors and Tumor-Like Lesions of Joints and Related Structures

INTRODUCTION

The joint is a common site for the development of reactive tumor-like lesions such as loose bodies; however, it is infrequently involved by benign or malignant neoplasms. Neoplasms of the joint usually involve the synovium and may arise de novo or may secondarily invade it from neighboring bone or soft tissue structures and from distant sites via the vascular system. Theoretically, any type of mesenchymal neoplasm can arise in a joint; however, the majority recapitulate the phenotype of periarticular tissues, including synovial lining cells, fat, blood vessels, fibrous tissue, and cartilage. Overall, primary benign lesions of the joint are much commoner than their malignant counterparts.

Recent advances in cell biology have increased our understanding of synovial neoplasia. Important among these are the identification of cytogenetic aberrations in certain lesions that prove their neoplastic nature and the use of immunohistochemistry to further define and subclassify particular tumors. This latter development has helped resolve some of the controversial issues regarding the ·concept of "tenosynovial" sarcomas that were generated by not having the technology to show that this group is actually composed of tumors of unrelated phenotypes. This chapter discusses some of the non-neoplastic tumor-like lesions and benign and malignant neoplasms of the synovium.

LOOSE BODIES

Loose bodies, or "joint mice," are generic terms for free-floating structures within a joint cavity. They may be exogenous, such as fragments of a bullet, or endogenous, such as pieces of articular cartilage, menisci, ligaments or bone.[1] When not otherwise specified, "loose bodies" refers to pieces of articular cartilage and or subchondral bone that have become detached and lie free within the joint or that have become secondarily embedded in the synovium. Loose bodies are the commonest tumor-like lesion of the joint.

Osteoarticular loose bodies result from fractures or destruction of the joint in the setting of osteoarthritis or other arthritides. The detached articular cartilage remains viable because it receives its nourishment from the synovial fluid; the bone dies because it is supplied only by blood vessels. As the loose body tumbles in the joint, its edges become round and smooth, and eventually it becomes embedded within the synovium. At this stage it may either be resorbed or stimulate a proliferative response in which the loose body serves as scaffolding for the deposition of newly formed fibrous and hyaline cartilage, which may secondarily undergo enchondral ossification.[2] The newly formed cartilage and bone surround the loose body like the cambium layers of a tree (Fig. 98–1). As the loose body enlarges, the deeper portions of the cartilage can no longer be supported by diffusion of synovial fluid and it dies and becomes calcified. This combination of events produces the dense, speckled, ring-like calcifications seen on radiograph (Fig. 98–2). It is also in this fashion that loose bodies become larger than the initial osteochondral defect from which they originated (Fig. 98–3). Loose bodies can be painful and limit the range of joint motion. Radiographically and histologically the differential diagnosis includes

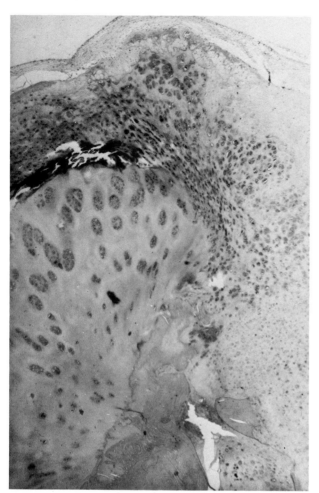

Figure 98–1. Osteoarticular loose body embedded within synovium. Note that the piece of articular cartilage and attached subchondral bone are surrounded by newly formed layers of metaplastic cartilage and bone. (× 23.)

synovial chondromatosis. Treatment is simple excision.

FATTY LESIONS OF THE SYNOVIUM

Although the subsynovial connective tissue of diarthrodial joints is rich in fat, a true lipoma of the synovium is rare. Lipomas have been described in the knee and ankle joints[3-5] and tendon synovial sheaths of the hands, ankles, and feet, in which they affect the extensor more frequently than the flexor synovial sheaths.[6] Synovial lipoma can be sessile or pedunculated and, similar to a lipoma arising in the subcutis, is composed of lobules of mature adipocytes delineated by a thin fibrous capsule. Pedunculated lipomas may produce pain if they twist on their stalks and become ischemic.

A commoner but still unusual fatty lesion of the joint is lipoma arborescens, also known as villous lipomatous proliferation of the synovium.[7-9] This disorder is characterized by a diffuse increase in the quantity of subsynovial fat, which bulges the over-

lying synovial lining and produces a villous architecture. It is not certain whether the proliferating fat is neoplastic or a manifestation of a hyperplastic or reactive process. Lipoma arborescens usually involves the suprapatellar portion of the knee joint (Fig. 98–4); however, it has also been observed in the hip, ankle, and wrist.[8] Although the process is usually localized to one joint, several cases of bilateral knee involvement have been reported.[9] Affected patients tend to be middle-aged males who usually present with a history of variable pain, swelling, and limitation of motion.[8, 9] The duration of symptoms is long, and symptoms may be present for as long as 30 years.[9] Plain films typically show joint fullness and changes of osteoarthritis of the involved joint. This combination of findings produces speculation regarding the relationship between these two disease processes. Arthrography reveals multiple, lobulated filling defects[10] and computed tomography (CT) scans show a low-density villonodular mass.[8] Laboratory studies are unremarkable, and the joint effusions consist of clear, yellow fluid, free of crystals.[9] At surgery, the affected synovium has a prominent villous or villonodular architecture and is tan-yellow (Fig. 98–5). Histologically, the lesion is composed of

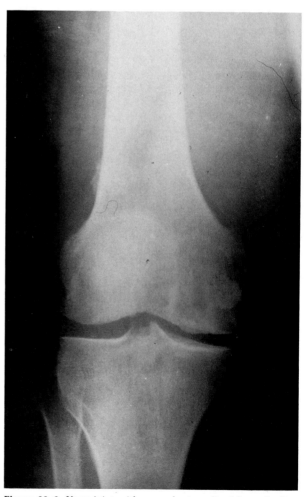

Figure 98–2. Knee joint with several mineralized loose bodies.

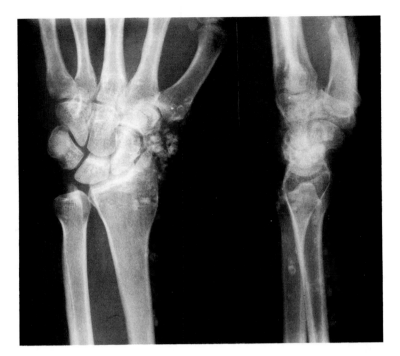

Figure 98–11. Radiographs of the wrist with prominent multiple calcified bodies of varying sizes present in the soft tissues of the wrist and extending along the forearm. These bodies have a smooth surface and a lucent center, some of which have a trabeculated pattern rather than an amorphous, densely calcified center. The diagnosis is synovial osteochondromatosis.

Symptoms and Signs

Patients present complaining of joint pain, swelling, stiffness, crepitation, and limitation of motion, with a locking or grating feeling on movement.[34, 52] The symptoms are usually long-standing, recurrent, and progressive.[52]

Radiographic Features

The plain radiographic findings depend largely on whether the cartilage nodules are calcified or ossified and whether they erode the adjacent bony structures. Visible calcifications may not be present in 5 to 33 percent of cases; however, in the majority there are multiple, oval intra-articular radiodensities that range in size from a few millimeters to several centimeters.[53] The pattern of mineralization varies and may appear as irregular flecks that represent calcified cartilage or demonstrate a trabecular architecture that is a manifestation of enchondral ossification (Figs. 98–11 and 98–12). Lesions that are not mineralized are best visualized on an arthrogram, where they produce multiple filling defects.[53] In approximately 11 percent of cases the nodules erode the neighboring skeleton, especially along the anterior aspect of the distal femur.[34] CT examination shows mass-like areas in the synovium that have a density similar to that of skeletal muscle. CT can also

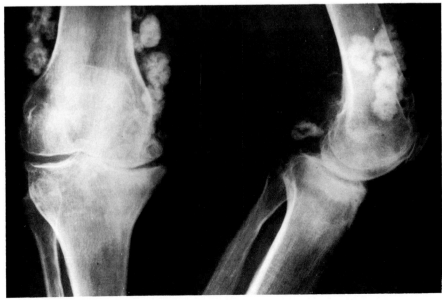

Figure 98–12. Synovial osteochondromatosis of the knee with narrowing of the joint space and multiple large calcified bodies filling the joint space and suprapatellar pouch.

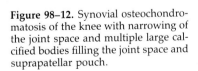

detect small calcifications and erosions before they are apparent on plain films.[40] MRI shows that the nodules of cartilage have low signal intensity on T_1-weighted sequences and high intensity on T_2-weighted sequences.[40] This reflects the high water content typical of cartilage. Areas of calcification or mineralized bone have a low signal intensity on both T_1- and T_2-weighted sequences.[40] Both CT and MRI scans are helpful in identifying the intra-articular source of the lesion and its anatomic extent. In long-standing disease the involved joints may show juxta-articular osteoporosis and changes of secondary osteoarthritis.

The cartilage in extra-articular synovial chondromatosis has identical radiographic changes. However, the nodules of cartilage are more frequently mineralized and can appear as a linear arrangement of small calcific densities that extend along the sheath and span a number of joints.

The radiographic differential diagnosis of synovial chondromatosis includes osteochondritis dissecans, osteoarthritis with loose bodies, tuberculosis, hemopathic arthropathies, pseudogout with extensive synovial calcification, and synovial tumors.[54] In many instances, the clinical story and radiographic picture should lead to the correct diagnosis. There are, however, a significant number of cases in which the radiographs and clinical picture are so vague that only a biopsy will remove all doubts about the patient's condition.

Gross Pathology

Characteristic of synovial chondromatosis is a thickened synovium containing numerous opalescent firm nodules of cartilage that bulge from the surface in a cobblestone pattern (Fig. 98–13). The nodules are usually less than 5 cm in size and frequently lose

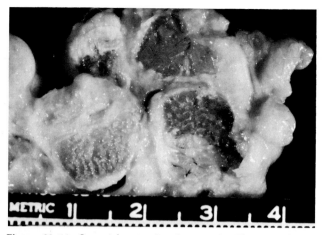

Figure 98–14. Synovial osteochondromatosis. The smooth-surfaced nodules are seen merging with the synovium rather than appearing as implanted pieces of cartilage that may easily separate from the synovium and have irregular roughened surfaces. Prominent bone trabeculae and a fatty marrow are easily seen within each nodule.

their attachment to the synovium and form loose bodies, sometimes hundreds of them. The calcified cartilage is white, and areas of ossification manifest as gritty, tan trabeculae that may house fatty marrow (Fig. 98–14). The synovium adjacent to the cartilage may demonstrate reactive changes, such as edema, hyperemia, and villous transformation.

Microscopic Features

The cartilage develops in the connective tissue of the subsynovial compartment. The mesenchymal cells give rise to small to medium-sized, round chondrocytes that produce the hyaline matrix and eventually form individual nodules that blend peripherally with the surrounding tissues (Figs. 98–15 and 98–16). This process has been divided into three

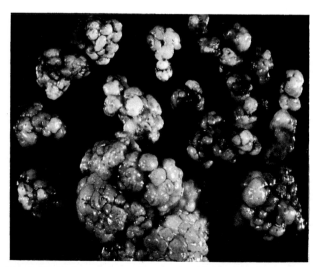

Figure 98–13. Synovial chondromatosis with innumerable cartilage nodules forming a cobblestone-like appearance of the synovial lining. (Courtesy of Dr. C. Campbell.)

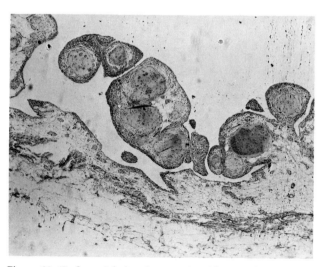

Figure 98–15. Synovial chondromatosis with metaplastic hyaline cartilage nodules in the synovium. The adjacent noncartilaginous synovium is normal. (Hematoxylin & eosin × 36.)

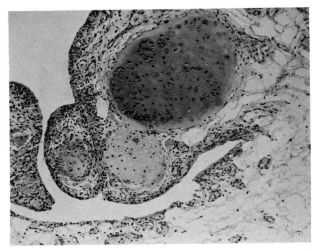

Figure 98–16. A higher view of chondromatosis illustrating the continuity between synovial tissue and metaplastic hyaline cartilage nodules. (Hematoxylin & eosin × 160.)

stages: (1) an early active phase characterized by the formation of cartilage that is confined to the synovium, (2) a transition phase in which both synovial cartilage and loose bodies are present, and (3) a quiescent phase in which most or all of the cartilage nodules have been shed into the joint and no new cartilage develops in the synovium. In some cases the cartilage may be hypercellular, and the chondrocytes binucleate, large, and hyperchromatic, similar to a chondrosarcoma (Fig. 98–17). However, in the absence of necrosis, myxoid cartilage, spindle cells, and mitotic activity, experience has shown that these lesions with atypical chondrocytes behave in a benign fashion. Infrequently, the disease manifests as a single extremely large nodule of cartilage that may undergo partial enchondral ossification. This giant intra-articular osteochondroma can severely limit joint motion and may be clinically confused with a neoplasm.[55, 56]

Ultrastructurally, the chondrocytes in synovial chondromatosis have abundant rough endoplasmic reticulum, prominent Golgi structures, and peripheral aggregates of glycogen.[57] These features are very similar to those present in the chondrocytes of normal articular cartilage and other benign cartilaginous tumors and have supported the interpretation that synovial chondromatosis, even with atypical cartilage, is benign.[56]

Over time the nodules of cartilage attached to the synovium are invaded by blood vessels. This results in enchondral ossification with woven and lamellar bone formation and even the development of a medullary cavity with fatty marrow (Fig. 98–18). If these nodules lose their synovial attachments and become free-floating, they may continue to increase in size. Growth continues because the cartilage derives its nourishment from synovial fluid, although the osseous portion and marrow die.

Clinical Course and Prognosis

The treatment of choice for synovial chondromatosis is excision of the involved synovium and removal of all loose bodies. The prognosis is very good, although there may be recurrences if removal is incomplete. Most recurrences are in the setting of diffuse involvement of the synovium[34] or in the active or transition phases of the disease. More rarely, when chondromatosis is associated with cartilage nodules embedded in fat or muscle, spontaneous regression of the disease has been seen even after incomplete excision. The cartilage nodules in these cases are thought to have herniated through a capsular defect or to have been implanted during a previous surgical procedure rather than to be the result of extra-articular or capsular cartilage metaplasia.[58]

Synovial chondromatosis rarely undergoes malignant transformation into a chondrosarcoma.[59–62]

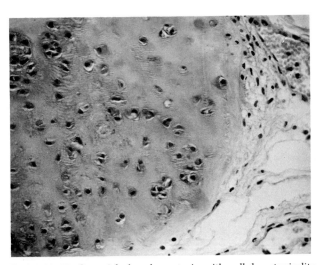

Figure 98–17. Synovial chondromatosis with cellular atypicality and binucleate cells. (Hematoxylin & eosin × 400.)

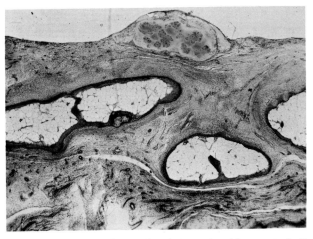

Figure 98–18. Synovial osteochondromatosis with a metaplastic hyaline cartilage nodule near the synovial surface and bony nodules deeper in the synovium. Note the fatty marrow inside the osseous nodules. (Hematoxylin & eosin × 23.)

However, it should be noted that a significant percentage of the reported synovial chondrosarcomas showed evidence of underlying synovial chondromatosis.[61, 62]

CHONDROMA OF TENDON SHEATH AND PERIARTICULAR STRUCTURES

The solitary soft tissue chondroma is considered to be a true benign neoplasm. It commonly arises in tendon sheaths and infrequently involves joint capsules or other periarticular structures.

Tendon sheath chondromas usually arise in the flexor tendon sheaths of the distal extremities[63] and are about three times commoner in the hands than in the feet.[63, 64] They affect the sexes equally and are detected in early to middle adulthood,[65] as they present as a painless, slowly growing, firm mass. Radiographically they appear as extraosseous, well-delineated soft tissue lesions. They contain calcifications that are either punctate or ring-like in 33 to 70 percent of cases.[66] Grossly the tumors are ovoid, firm, blue-white, well-circumscribed masses of hyaline cartilage. They are usually 1 to 2 cm in dimension and, unlike synovial chondromatosis, are solitary. Histologically the hyaline cartilage is well formed, with occasional small foci of myxoid change. The cartilage can be cellular and the chondrocytes may demonstrate cytologic atypia that causes confusion with chondrosarcoma.[67, 68] The treatment of choice is simple excision. Although these tumors may recur in a minority of cases, they are benign and do not metastasize.[63–65, 69]

The intracapsular, periarticular, or para-articular regions are uncommon sites for soft tissue chondromas. When they occur, they usually originate in the anterior infrapatellar region of the knee[70] (Fig. 98–19). In this location the chondroma can achieve large size (8 cm) and mechanically interfere with knee motion. The morphology and biologic behavior are similar to those of soft tissue chondromas that arise elsewhere. Interestingly, intracapsular chondromas have been reported in the knees of three members of a family with familial dysplasia epiphysealis hemimelica.[71] There have been two other cases described in which cartilaginous hamartomas of the volar plates of the proximal and distal interphalangeal joints of the hands and feet were associated with peculiar hypertrophic skin lesions of the hand and hemihypertrophy of the limb.[72, 73] It is possible that these peculiar cartilaginous lesions represent an abnormality in which primitive cartilage tissue persists in joint sites, much akin to the involvement of bones in multiple enchondromatosis (Ollier's disease).

VILLONODULAR SYNOVITIS

Villonodular synovitis comprises a group of benign tumors that affect the synovial lining of joints,

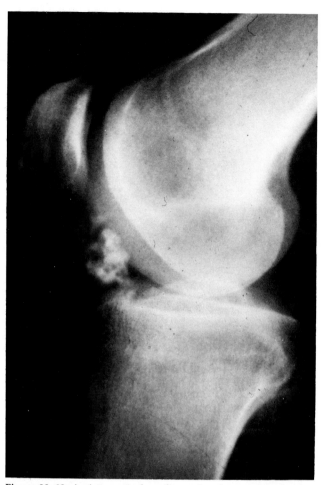

Figure 98–19. An intra-articular solitary chondroma of the knee in the infrapatellar region, represented as a well-delineated mass with amorphous dense calcification, suggesting mineralized cartilage. (Courtesy of Dr. C. Campbell.)

tendon sheaths, and bursae. Included in this group are pigmented villonodular synovitis (diffuse), localized nodular tenosynovitis, and the rare localized nodular bursitis. Some variants may be locally aggressive and invade bone, joint capsules, tendons, and adjacent soft tissues. However, despite the destructive potential of these tumors, they never metastasize.

The common histologic denominator of these lesions is the exuberant proliferation of synovial lining cells, which may spread along the synovial surface and invade downward into the subsynovial connective tissue. The growing cells expand the subsynovial compartment, producing finger-like extensions, villi, and redundant folds. These projections often fuse into nodules and form convoluted lobulated masses admixed with a tangle of hair-like villi. The process may be a local phenomenon involving only part of the synovial lining, or it may be extensive with the whole synovial surface affected.

Until recently, the etiology of villonodular synovitis was a mystery. Experimental animal models produced lesions that morphologically resembled the human condition but biologically were self-limited and resolved when the inducing factor, usually a blood serum component or iron, was stopped.[74, 75] Therefore, the role of trauma and repeated episodes of hemorrhage is probably not important. Also, neither hemophilic patients nor those people with other bleeding disorders are prone to developing villonodular synovitis, despite frequent bouts of intra-articular hemorrhage and resultant secondary osteoarthritis and joint destruction.

Cytogenetic studies have recently shown the aberrant findings of trisomy 7 in two cases of pigmented villonodular synovitis and six consistent chromosome rearrangements in one case of localized nodular tenosynovitis.[76, 77] These results suggest that each member of this family of lesions develops from a clonal proliferation of cells; hence, these lesions should be considered benign neoplasms.[76, 77]

Pigmented Villonodular Synovitis

The prototype of the villonodular synovitis group is pigmented villonodular synovitis that diffusely involves the synovial lining of a joint or tendon sheath (synonyms: synovial xanthoma, synovial fibroendothelioma, synovial endothelioma, benign fibrous histiocytoma, xanthomatous giant cell tumor). The term localized nodular synovitis (see later) is used if the disease is confined to one clearly delineated focus of the synovium.

Age and Sex. Although pigmented villonodular synovitis may occur in all age groups, spanning childhood to old age, most affected patients are young adults in the third to fourth decades of life.[78] The sexes tend to be equally affected, although some series have reported a predominance of either males or females.[78–80]

Sites. Unilateral involvement of the knee is most commonly seen and occurs in about 80 percent of cases.[80, 81] The next commonest sites are the hip, ankle, calcaneocuboid joints, elbow, and the tendon sheaths of the fingers and sometime the toes. Occasionally involvement is seen in the hand, soles of the feet, and unusual locations such as the temporomandibular joint[82] and the posterior elements of the spine. Bursal involvement is rare, but when it occurs it usually develops in the popliteal and iliopectineal bursae and the bursa anserina.[11] There are two reported cases involving the temporomandibular joint[83] and the hip[84] in which synovial chondromatosis coexisted with pigmented villonodular synovitis. Occasionally, the disease affects large tendon sheaths proximal to the ankle and wrist and masquerades as a soft tissue mass adjacent to a large joint.[85] It is thought that these lesions dissect through either a joint capsule or tendon sheath and extend along fascial planes to produce a soft tissue mass.

In the vast majority of the cases pigmented villonodular synovitis is monoarticular. Bilaterality or involvement of multiple separate sites has been infrequently reported.[80] Interestingly, some patients with polyarticular disease have also had significant congenital anomalies.[86]

Invasion of bone on either side of a joint can be seen with intra-articular, bursal, or tendon sheath involvement.[87] This most frequently occurs when the tumor involves "tight" joints, such as the hip, elbow, wrist, and feet.[46] Rarely, only one bone may be invaded by an intra-articular lesion, which may mimic a primary bone tumor.[88]

Symptoms and Signs. Pigmented villonodular synovitis usually presents as a monoarticular arthritis. The main complaints include pain and mild intermittent or repeated bouts of swelling. The symptoms develop insidiously and slowly progress over a long period of time, ranging from months to years.[80] The involved area may be stiff, swollen, and warm, and a palpable mass can sometimes be appreciated. Point tenderness can be detected in approximately 50 percent of patients.[80] Anatomic instability of the involved joint is uncommon.[89]

Joint aspiration frequently yields blood-tinged, brown fluid that lacks diagnostic abnormalities.[90] Synovial fluid analysis may show a low glucose content, a minimally elevated protein level, and a fair mucin clot.[80] The inflammatory cell count is usually low but may be elevated.[80] Similar findings can also be seen in trauma, Charcot's joint, bleeding disorders, sickle cell disease, and Ehlers-Danlos syndrome.[80]

Radiographic Features. In at least two thirds of cases, a soft tissue density due to the tumor, effusion, or both can be visualized on a plain film.[91] Joint narrowing or calcification is uncommon. Arthrography may demonstrate numerous nodular filling defects that extend into an expanded joint space.[92] Arteriograms are unusually striking owing to the prominent vascularity of the tumor. There tends to be an inverse correlation between the degree of vascularity and the amount of fibrosis or scarring of the lesion.[93] CT scans and MRI are useful in delineating the extent of disease and can detect both intralesional lipid and hemosiderin deposits, which are important diagnostic features.[94–96] Extension into the bone manifests radiographically as multiple subchondral, well-marginated, cyst-like lucencies or juxtacortical oval pressure erosions[95] (Figs. 98–20 and 98–21). In the knee, the intercondylar region of the femur is the most frequently invaded location, as the tumor grows along ligamentous insertions. Periarticular osteopenia, joint destruction, and periosteal reactions are unusual. The joint space is preserved until late in the course of the disease.[95] The differential diagnosis of a given case might include tuberculosis, which generally has more osteopenia and joint destruction; hemophilia, which is also associated with more extensive joint destruction; synovial chondromatosis, which frequently has calcified radiopaque bodies; and rheumatoid arthritis, which demonstrates severer osteopenia and joint narrowing.

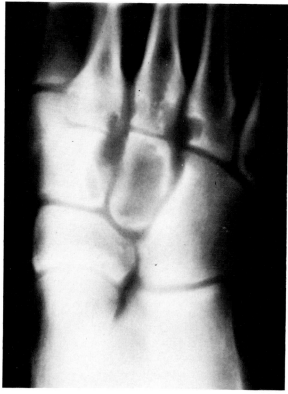

Figure 98–20. Pigmented villonodular synovitis involving the small joints of the foot with multiple bone erosion. There is no calcification present in the lesion.

Arthroscopic Findings. Although arthroscopy is not a required procedure in evaluating patients with pigmented villonodular synovitis, the lesion has been identified unexpectedly. In these instances the synovium is red-brown and distorted by numerous hypertrophic villi and nodular projections.[97, 98]

Gross Pathology. Grossly, the synovium in pigmented villonodular synovitis is red-brown to mottled orange-yellow and looks like a plush angora rug. Matted masses of villous projections and synovial folds are prominent and are admixed with sessile or pedunculated, rubbery to soft nodules (0.5 to 2 cm in diameter) enmeshed within the synovial tissue (Fig. 98–22). The synovial membrane is thick and succulent and is often coated with a fibrinous exudate. Red-brown or golden-brown tissue may extend deep into subsynovial structures or invade the joint capsule. When the joint capsule is transgressed, adjacent soft tissue structures, including nerves and vessels, may be coated by wispy, red-brown tissue. Extensive soft tissue invasion produces a soft to rubbery, red-brown mass with hemorrhagic cysts. Similar tissue may be present near the chondroosseous junction or may be wrapped around vascular and ligamentous attachments to bone surfaces, which represent entrance points into the bone interior. If a tendon sheath is involved, a sausage-shaped mass may be evident as the sheath is distended by the proliferating tumor. Although other conditions such as hemochromatosis and hemosiderosis may simi-

larly stain the synovium brown, the nodular component is usually absent, and, in addition, microscopic features are definitive for separating these entities (see later).

Microscopic Features. Microscopic examination reveals marked synovial cell hyperplasia with surface proliferation and, more important, subsynovial invasion by masses of polygonal or round cells with pink cytoplasm and round vesicular nuclei (Fig. 98–23). Included among the invading synovial cells are multinucleated giant cells, hemosiderin-laden macrophages, and fibroblasts (Fig. 98–24). Hemosiderin can also be seen between cells and in synovial lining cells, and polygonal cells. Foci of hemorrhage are common and are surrounded peripherally by the giant cells and macrophages. Scattered collections of foamy macrophages (xanthoma cells) filled with lipid are also common. The previously described cell populations fill the distended synovial villi and cause them to fuse with adjacent ones, forming nodules. In some nodules, there may be massive fibrosis with interlacing bands of hyalinized collagen with little cellular activity except for a few scattered giant cells and macrophages. Often a scant, diffuse, chronic inflammatory component is seen, particularly near foci of hemorrhage. Occasional mitoses may be present in the proliferating cells, but cytologic criteria

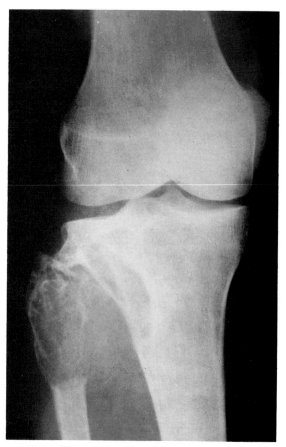

Figure 98–21. Pigmented villonodular synovitis involving the tibiofibular joint with an adjacent extensive soft tissue mass and eccentric erosion of both bones. The knee joint is normal.

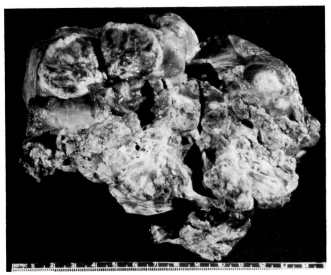

Figure 98–22. The gross specimen of this case shows a large, bulky, soft tissue mass that is mottled from red to yellow, soft, and focally hemorrhagic. The lesion totally obscures the fibular head and pushes into the soft tissue as a lobulated mass.

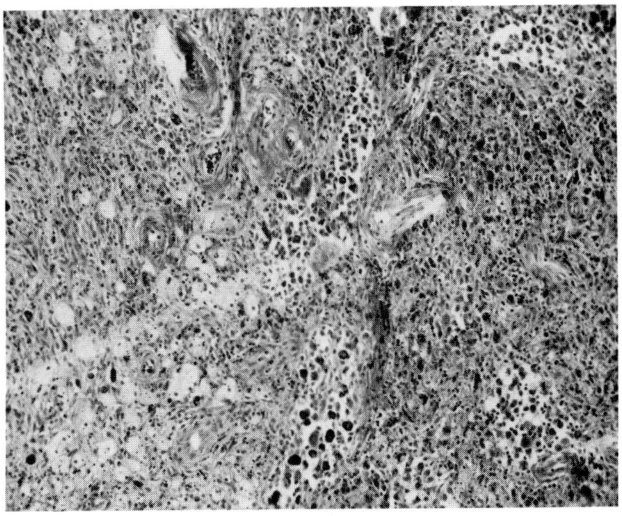

Figure 98–24. Pigmented villonodular synovitis with polygonal and round synovial-type cells, hemosiderin-laden macrophages, prominent vascularity, and scattered foam cells (macrophages). (Hematoxylin & eosin × 160.)

for malignancy are absent. The differential microscopic features include the fact that in synovial hemochromatosis and hemosiderosis, pigment is found mainly in the synovial lining cells or macrophages. However, in pigmented villonodular synovitis, the pigment is usually found in most cell types throughout the tumor. Furthermore, collections of foam cells, giant cells, and, most important, the invasive synovial cells are absent in hemosiderosis and hemochromatosis. Rarely, extensive hemorrhage into soft tissue components of pigmented villonodular synovitis has been confused with vascular hamartomas.[99]

If there is bone erosion, the tumor enters the bone along vascular foramina or ligamentous and synovial attachments. A biopsy taken from an intraosseous focus may cause much confusion, since giant cell tumor of bone may be offered as a diag-

nostic possibility. This diagnosis should be ruled out by clinical suspicion coupled with the absence of the histologic features typical of giant cell tumor such as random distribution of osteoclastic-type giant cells, the characteristic stromal cells, and the similarity of the nuclei of the giant cells and stromal cells.

Treatment. The treatment of pigmented villonodular synovitis has not been standardized and has included radiation therapy, total synovectomy, arthrodesis, bone-grafting, and primary arthroplasty.[80] This situation may exist because no single therapy has been consistently successful. Currently, wide synovectomy is the recommended treatment. However, it is difficult to perform an actual complete synovectomy, and residual involved synovium frequently remains, causing a local recurrence rate of 16 to 48 percent.[80, 81] Rarely, recurrent disease may require more radical surgery, such as ray resection or even amputation.

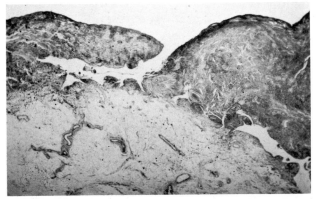

Figure 98–23. A low-power view of a synovium that is thickened and thrown into papillary folds by invading synovial lining cells, a characteristic feature of pigmented villonodular synovitis. (Hematoxylin & eosin × 16.)

Localized Nodular Synovitis

Localized nodular synovitis is the localized or focal expression of pigmented villonodular synovitis in which only a discrete area of the synovium is involved (*synonyms:* benign giant cell synovioma, benign synovioma). Histologically, it is identical to the nodules of pigmented villonodular synovitis. The main difference is that the prominent synovial villi present in pigmented villonodular synovitis are absent or sparse. The localized variant usually consists of a single sessile or pedunculated, sometimes lobulated, nodule or mass that ranges from 1 to 8 cm in diameter (Fig. 98–25). Most commonly it is unilateral, arises in the knee, between the meniscus and joint capsule or intercondylar fossa[11] (Fig. 98–26), and is equally distributed between the sexes.[100]

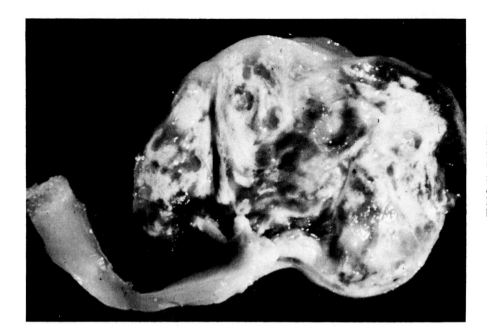

Figure 98–25. Localized nodular synovitis on cross-section with mottled hemorrhagic and yellow soft tissue, similar to a nodule of pigmented villonodular synovitis, with a long stalk. This is typical for this lesion. (Courtesy of Dr. C. Campbell.)

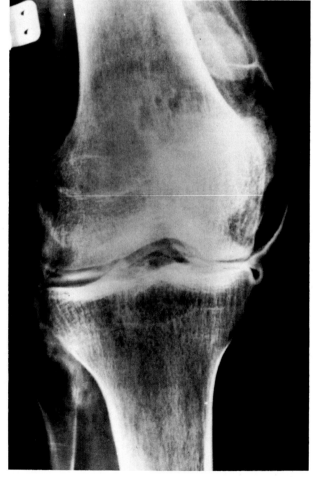

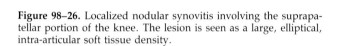

Figure 98–26. Localized nodular synovitis involving the suprapatellar portion of the knee. The lesion is seen as a large, elliptical, intra-articular soft tissue density.

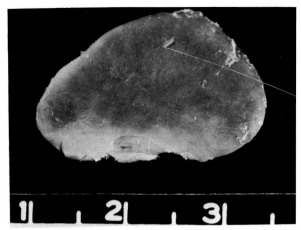

Figure 98–27. An infarcted localized nodular synovitis that twisted on its stalk. Histologically it was of dense collagen and necrotic hemorrhagic tissue. Grossly the lesion was bright red.

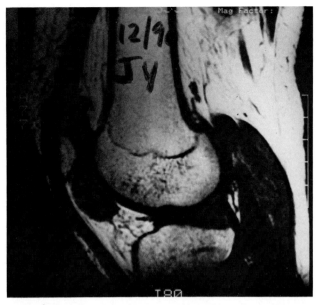

Figure 98–28. MRI of knee showing localized nodular synovitis.

The symptoms are similar to those of pigmented villonodular synovitis except that in the localized variant there is a lower incidence of pain and stiffness[79] and a higher frequency of joint locking as the mass interferes with motion. A minority of patients may present with acute severe joint pain caused by torsion and infarction of the tumor (Fig. 98–27). Effusions are common, but the synovial fluid tends to be less bloody than that in pigmented villonodular synovitis and may even be clear. Imaging studies show a heterogeneous nodular mass that contains lipid and hemosiderin deposits (Fig. 98–28). There is usually no bone invasion. Marginal excision is usually curative,[78, 101] and small lesions can be extirpated arthroscopically.

Localized Nodular Tenosynovitis

Localized nodular tenosynovitis arises from the tendon sheath and usually involves the hand or wrist and less frequently the foot or ankle[79] (*synonyms:* giant cell tumor of tendon sheath, fibroxanthoma of tendon sheath). In fact, localized nodular tenosynovitis is the commonest soft tissue tumor of the hand. In the hand, it usually develops from the flexor tendon sheaths of the fingers. The index finger is most commonly affected and is followed, in descending order of frequency, by the middle finger, ring finger, little finger, and thumb.[78] Finger tumors predominate in females, with a ratio of at least 2:1,[79, 102] and tumors of the toes have an equal sex distribution.[79] On average, patients are in the third to fifth decades of life and present with a painless, palpable, firm mobile mass. Clinically, the mass is usually solitary and located on the flexor surface but may bulge into the extensor or lateral aspects of the digits (Fig. 98–29). The tumors are slow-growing, and the interval between detection and surgical treatment has ranged from several weeks to more than a decade, with an average of slightly more than 2 years.[79, 102] Radiographically they appear as well-circumscribed soft tissue masses, and in about 25 percent of cases there is adjacent extrinsic excavation of the bone cortex that is bounded by a sclerotic margin[79, 102] (Fig. 98–30).

The gross pathology is that of a multinodular,

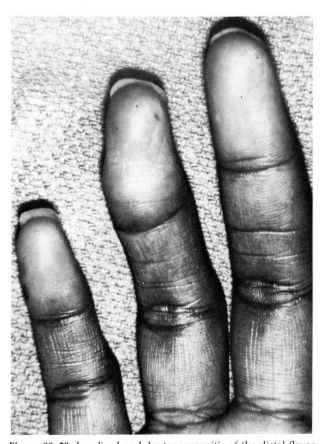

Figure 98–29. Localized nodular tenosynovitis of the distal flexor surface of the fourth finger. Note the distended, flattened, overlying skin. The mass straddles the distal interphalangeal joint. (Courtesy of Dr. C. Campbell.)

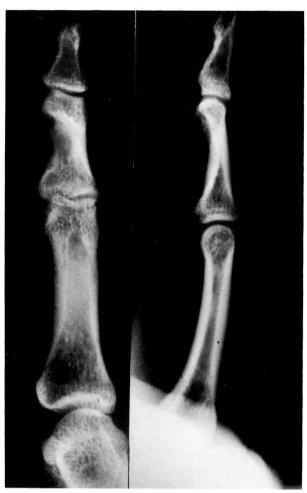

Figure 98–30. A localized nodular tenosynovitis of the middle second phalanx with pressure erosion of the flexor aspect of the middle phalanx. There is a scalloped, well-margined bone lesion, including a more distal subcortical cyst.

round, rubbery mass, generally not larger than 5 cm in diameter, which is firmly attached but easily peeled off the involved tendon. At surgery the lesion may "pop out" of the incision as an encapsulated mass. Careful attention should be paid to the external surface of the mass because the lesion may infiltrate the adjacent structures and not be truly encapsulated. The cut surface ranges from hues of yellow to orange-brown, depending on the amount of lipid and blood pigments present. Often there are bands or septa of white fibrous tissue that divide the lesion. Cystic spaces are unusual. Microscopically, the cell types present are identical to those in pigmented villonodular synovitis (Fig. 98–31). Ultrastructurally, the proliferating cells have features similar to both type A and type B synovial lining cells.[102–104] Their antigenic and enzymatic profiles suggest that they have a monocyte-macrophage lineage similar to that of osteoclasts.[102, 105]

These tumors are benign and do not metastasize. Rarely have malignant giant cell tumors of tendon sheath been reported.[106] The treatment of choice is

conservative surgical excision, which is usually curative. There may be local recurrence if the tumor is incompletely excised.[79, 102]

MALIGNANT TUMORS OF THE JOINT

Malignant tumors of the joint are uncommon and are subclassified into primary and secondary types. Primary joint malignancies are sarcomas, and they commonly arise in large diarthrodial joints and usually originate from synovium. Potentially any sarcoma can develop in the synovium, but those that do so most commonly are chondrosarcoma and synovial sarcoma. Other types that have arisen in the synovium are extraordinarily rare and, in the authors' experience, have included malignant fibrous histiocytoma and angiosarcoma[107] (Fig. 98–32). Secondary malignant tumors of the synovium include extension of sarcomas from the adjacent skeleton or soft tissues and metastases. Although the subsynovial connective tissue is very vascular, metastases or involvement of the synovium by lymphoma or leukemia is relatively infrequent.

Primary Sarcomas of the Joints

The sarcomas that arise in joints are the same as those that develop in the soft tissues and are treated similarly. The treatment of choice is by a team approach using surgery consisting of either a wide en bloc local excision or an amputation, radiation therapy, and sometimes chemotherapy. The most important factor influencing prognosis is the initial treatment of the tumor. Unfortunately, there is a common trap that leads to an all-too-familiar pattern

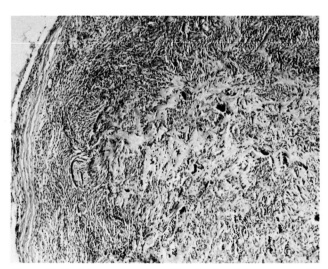

Figure 98–31. A low-power view of localized nodular tenosynovitis to emphasize the relatively good delineation of the mass from adjacent soft tissue and the broad bands of collagen traversing the lesion. Note the scattered osteoclast-type giant cells. (Hematoxylin & eosin × 160.)

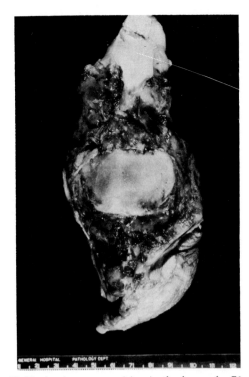

Figure 98–32. Angiosarcoma arising in the knee of a 76-year-old man as friable red-tan tissue replacing the synovium, crawling over the patella, and filling up all synovial recesses. The patient died 8 months later with microscopic lung metastases.

Table 98–1. SURGICAL STAGES

Stage	Grade	Site
IA	Low (G_1)	Intracompartmental (T_1)
IB	Low (G_1)	Extracompartmental (T_2)
IIA	High (G_2)	Intracompartmental (T_1)
IIB	High (G_2)	Extracompartmental (T_2)
III	Any (G) regional or distant metastasis	Any (T)

Reprinted from Enneking, W. F., Spanier, S. S., and Goodman, M. A.: A system for the clinical staging of musculoskeletal sarcoma. Clin. Orthop. Rel. Res. 153:106, 1980.

grade), anatomic site (intracompartmental, T_1; or extracompartmental, T_2), and presence of metastases (M0, no metastases; or M1, metastatic disease). Therefore, a low-grade, intracompartmental tumor without metastases is a stage IA tumor. However, if it extends into another anatomic compartment, it becomes a stage IB lesion. All high-grade tumors are a stage II lesion, and if any lesion has metastatic foci, it becomes a stage III tumor regardless of grade or site.

The surgical procedures for soft tissue tumors are divided into four categories based on the surgical margin to the neoplasm. These are summarized in Table 98–2. This systematic approach has standardized surgical procedures and has linked them to the appropriate use of radiotherapy and chemotherapy.

Chondrosarcoma

Chondrosarcoma arising in the synovium is unusual, and only 23 cases have been reported in the English language.[60, 61, 108–112] In approximately 50 percent of the cases, the chondrosarcoma arose in association with pre-existing synovial chondromatosis.[112] The patients are usually in the fifth to seventh decade of life, and there is an equal sex distribution.[112] Patients present with a progressively enlarging joint mass that may be associated with mechan-

of inadequate initial therapy. Namely, the lesion is frequently incompletely excised during the initial operation because it looks very innocuous, often being well delineated and easily "shelled out" from its site. It is only after surgery that the diagnosis is made by the pathologist and it is realized that tumor tissue has been left behind that should necessitate further treatment. However, some clinicians may delay any further treatment; the patient is followed until the appearance of recurrences, which will invariably develop, and only then will more extensive surgery be performed. Therefore, most soft tissue sarcomas have had initially incomplete surgical therapy, which condemns the patient to recurrent tumor and a poor prognosis. Ideally, a soft tissue tumor should be biopsied soon after its appearance in such a manner that the biopsy tract can be excised with the tumor. After the pathologist makes the diagnosis, radiation therapy and early definitive surgery should be carried out. The surgeon's suspicion and awareness of the existence of such tumors before any therapy is administered are likely to be the best insurance for a better prognosis.

The surgical staging of soft tissue sarcomas is now standardized. Incorporated in the system are pretreatment features such as the grade of tumor (degree of cytologic atypicality), site of lesion, and biologic behavior (presence or absence of metastases) and the type of surgery that is to be performed. As illustrated in Table 98–1, all tumors are graded according to their histologic grade (low grade or high

Table 98–2. SURGICAL MARGINS*

Type	Plane of Dissection	Result
Intralesional	Piecemeal debulking or curettage	Leaves macroscopic disease
Marginal	Shell out en bloc through pseudocapsule or reactive zone	May leave either "satellite" or "skip" lesions
Wide	Intracompartmental en bloc with cuff of normal tissue	May leave "skip" lesions
Radical	Extracompartmental en bloc with entire compartment	No residual lesions

*The plane of dissection used to achieve a particular margin is shown as well as the result of that margin in terms of residual lesion remaining in the wound.

Reprinted from Enneking, W. F., Spanier, S. S., and Goodman, M. A.: A system for the clinical staging of musculoskeletal sarcoma. Clin. Orthop. Rel. Res. 153:106, 1980.

ical dysfunction, pain, and stiffness. In patients with pre-existing synovial chondromatosis, the duration of symptoms is usually long-standing, and in some cases symptoms have been present for as long as 25 years.[112] The majority of the chondrosarcomas have arisen in the knee, followed by the hip and elbow. Radiographic studies usually demonstrate a periarticular soft tissue mass that may show dense irregular or ring-like calcifications. Occasionally, invasion into the medullary cavity of adjacent bone is present. The radiographic differential diagnosis varies according to the presence of calcification and includes synovial chondromatosis, synovial sarcoma, pigmented villonodular synovitis, and chronic synovitis.[112]

Grossly, the involved joint is filled with synovium that is massively thickened by innumerable variously sized nodules of opalescent blue-white cartilage. Some of the nodules may be free-floating in the joint cavity. The tumor may extend into the adjacent soft tissue and bone.

Microscopically the tumor is composed predominantly of hyaline cartilage. Rarely, the matrix is entirely myxoid.[113] The neoplastic cartilage is cellular and contains cytologically malignant chondrocytes. Characteristically the periphery of the lobules of cartilage is the most cellular, and it is in this region that some of the tumor cells are spindled. Other findings include myxoid change of the matrix, necrosis, and permeation of invaded bone.[112] Coexisting synovial chondromatosis can be identified by the presence of well-formed nodules of hyaline cartilage that is less cellular, cytologically less atypical, and frequently mineralized.

Treatment is usually surgical extirpation, with consideration given to chemotherapy in high-grade lesions or those that have metastasized. Inadequate surgical removal virtually ensures local recurrence, which may necessitate future radical excision. Metastases have occurred in approximately one third of reported patients, with the lung being the commonest site of systemic spread.[112]

Synovial Sarcoma

Synovial sarcoma (*synonym:* malignant synovioma) is a relatively common sarcoma, accounts for approximately 6 to 10 percent of soft tissue sarcomas, and was the fourth commonest sarcoma diagnosed at the Soft Tissue Branch of the Armed Forces Institute of Pathology between 1970 and 1979.[114, 115] Its morphology is reminiscent of early joint development with large polygonal cells that secrete hyaluronic acid and form a microscopic "joint space." These polygonal cells resemble synovial lining cells and are surrounded by spindle cells that simulate subsynovial mesenchymal cells. Since either one of these two cell populations may predominate, synovial sarcoma has been subtyped into biphasic, monophasic spindle cell, and monophasic epithelioid types. Earlier descriptions of this tumor attest to its wide spectrum of morphology—such names as adenosarcoma and

synovial fibrosarcoma were used until the term "synovial sarcoma," which was first introduced in 1936,[116] became commonplace.

Age and Sex. Synovial sarcoma commonly affects adolescents and young adults. In a series of 134 cases 83.6 percent of the tumors occurred in patients between 10 and 50 years of age, with a median age of 31.3 years.[117] Synovial sarcoma is slightly more common in males than in females. The occurrence of synovial sarcoma in children younger than 15 years is unusual.[118]

Sites. Although the term "synovial sarcoma" implies that the tumor originates from the synovium, fewer than 10 percent of cases actually are intra-articular or in continuity with a synovial lining.[119] The fact that many synovial sarcomas arise near joints was also misconstrued as supporting the tumor's synovial origin.[120] Approximately 60 to 70 percent of synovial sarcomas arise in the extremities, especially the lower limb, in the vicinity of large joints, particularly the popliteal area of the knee, and in the foot.[114, 117] Regions of the thigh, leg, hand, and digits may be affected, and in the distal extremities the tumors often are adjacent to joint capsules, tendon sheaths, or both. In the upper limb, distal involve-

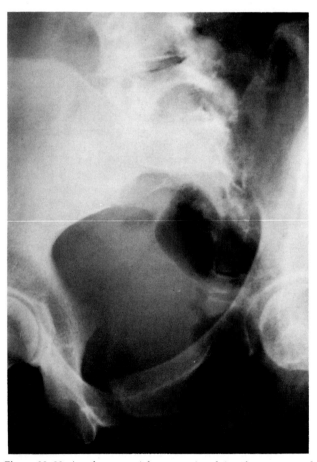

Figure 98–33. Another synovial sarcoma involving the sacrum and ilium on both sides of the sacroiliac joint. The large soft tissue component is not well seen. In contrast with the previous case, there are no soft tissue calcifications.

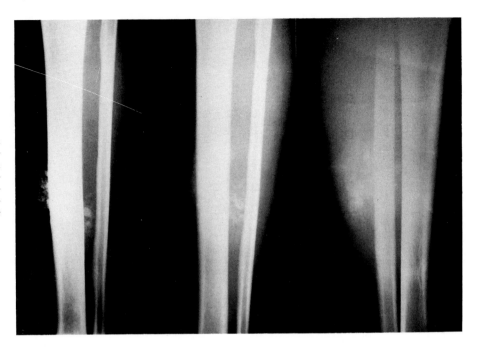

Figure 98–34. Synovial sarcoma in the soft tissues of the calf represented in these multiple views as a large soft tissue density with amorphous speckled and nodular calcifications. There is slight pressure erosion of the medial aspect of the fibula.

ment is commoner than in arm or elbow sites. Tumors have been reported in the neck,[121, 122] torso, craniofacial region,[123] retroperitoneum,[124] orbit,[122] tongue,[122] mediastinum,[125] and soft palate.[126] These rarer sites suggest an undifferentiated mesenchymal cell origin for synovial sarcoma, since the sites are not near joints or synovium.

Symptoms and Signs. There are no clinical features related to synovial sarcoma that distinguish it from other sarcomas. The commonest complaint is the development of a slowly enlarging, deep-seated, palpable mass that is painful in little more than 50 percent of the cases.[117] Symptoms may be present before medical evaluation is sought for unusually long periods of time, ranging from months to 20 years,[114] with an average of about 2.5 years.[117] Delay in diagnosis is more frequent with tumors that are located in the deep soft tissues in comparison with those based in the more superficial and clinically noticeable regions. In some cases involving the knee region, vague mild pain may be present for several months before a mass is appreciated, and if the tumor reaches a large size, limitation of motion may finally occur. Head and neck lesions produce symptoms related to their specific sites, such as hoarseness and difficulty in breathing or swallowing. Rarely, a patient may present with symptoms secondary to pulmonary metastases, such as hemoptysis.[117]

Radiographic Features. Classically, the plain film findings of synovial sarcoma are a well-circumscribed, deep-seated soft tissue mass (Fig. 98–33). It is one of the few primary soft tissue tumors that frequently calcifies. Approximately 30 to 50 percent of cases will have radiographic detectable calcifications that can have a fine, stippled, or dense appearance[128] (Fig. 98–34). The calcification may be focal or present throughout most of the tumor.[129]

Adjacent periosteal reaction is elicited in approximately 20 percent of cases,[128] but the tumors infrequently erode into bone. CT scanning is important in delineating the anatomic extent of the tumor and is more sensitive in demonstrating calcification or periosteal reaction. Angiography is not very helpful because synovial sarcomas may be hypervascular or hypovascular[127]; however, it does show the relation of the tumor to important vessels.[128] The radiographic differential diagnosis includes hemangioma, lipoma, synovial chondromatosis, soft tissue chondrosarcoma or osteosarcoma, myositis ossificans, aneurysms, and other sarcomas.

Pathology. The gross pathology of synovial sarcoma is invariably a well-demarcated, pink to yellow, rather fleshy mass that easily detaches, or "shells out," from its tumor bed. The cut surface is usually uniform, gray-yellow, and rubbery. If calcification is present, the tumor may be gritty. In larger tumors, areas of hemorrhage, necrosis, or both with cystification and gelatinous breakdown of tissue may also be seen. Occasionally the tumors interdigitate between tendons, muscle, and fascial planes or wrap around neurovascular bundles (Fig. 98–35). Extension into a joint is very uncommon.

Synovial sarcoma is subtyped into three patterns based on the morphology of the tumor cells. These types are monophasic spindle cell, monophasic epithelial-like or pseudoglandular, and biphasic synovial sarcoma. Obviously, there is some subjectivity in the use of such a classification system, since many of these tumors have a variable histologic picture. Furthermore, some pathologists will not make the diagnosis of monophasic synovial sarcoma, particularly since the spindle cell type is often indistinguishable from a fibrosarcoma by light microscopy. A useful differential observation is that marked cellular pleo-

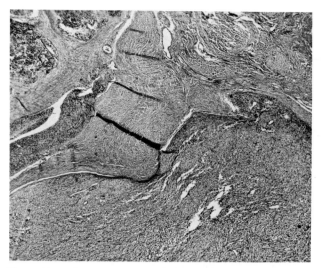

Figure 98–35. Low-power view of a synovial sarcoma to point out the highly cellular tongues of tumor that push out into the soft tissue. If this lesion were "shelled-out," a recurrence surely would follow. (Hematoxylin & eosin × 36.)

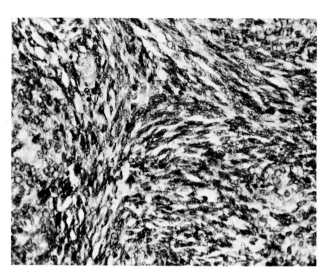

Figure 98–37. Synovial sarcoma, monophasic spindle cell type, with interdigitating fascicles of spindle cells. The cells have plump nuclei, little cytoplasm, and very little collagen production. (Hematoxylin & eosin × 400.)

morphism and atypia are usually not present in synovial sarcoma; when these findings are present, they tend to point to some other type of neoplasm, such as a high-grade, malignant fibrous histiocytoma. Microscopically the hallmark of the commoner biphasic synovial sarcoma is the two different populations of neoplastic cells consisting of epithelioid and spindle cells (Fig. 98–36). The epithelioid cells may be cuboidal or columnar and, like true epithelium, have well-defined cytoplasmic borders and intercellular junctions. These cells may form gland-like spaces, line papillae or cleft-like spaces, or grow in solid sheets. The epithelioid cells are usually surrounded by the small and plump spindle cells. The spindle cells grow in dense fascicles that may be arranged in a "herringbone" pattern. In most bi-

phasic synovial sarcomas, the spindle cell component predominates. Also, it is in the spindle cell regions that calcification of hyalinized stroma most frequently occurs. In the monophasic variants, either the spindle or the epithelioid cells predominate (Figs. 98–37 and 98–38).

Electron microscopy and tissue culture observations indicate some unifying and common features of both cell types composing synovial sarcoma.[130, 131] These include a distinct basal lamina between epithelioid and spindle cells and specialized cell junctions, such as desmosomes and maculae adherens, which are present mostly between the epithelioid cells but also between some spindle cells. The epithelioid cells may also have microvilli, intercellular spaces, free ribosomes, arrays of endoplasmic retic-

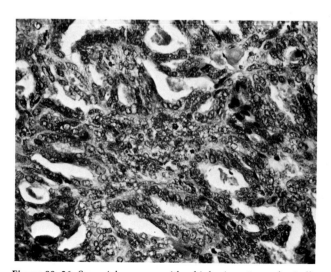

Figure 98–36. Synovial sarcoma with a biphasic pattern of spindle cells and epithelial-like cells arranged around gland-like spaces. Mitoses are evident and the lumina of the pseudoglands contain hyaluronic acid. (Hematoxylin & eosin × 400.)

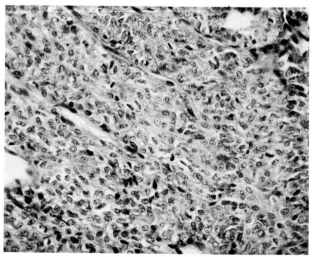

Figure 98–38. Synovial sarcoma, monophasic epithelial-like cells with sheets of polygonal or oval cells with indistinct cytoplasmic borders. There is slight nuclear pleomorphism. (Hematoxylin & eosin × 400.)

ulum, prominent Golgi apparatuses, and small vesicles (Figs. 98–39 and 98–40). The spindle cells secrete amorphous extracellular fibrils without periodicity and possess microfibrils. There are usually few recognizable collagen fibrils. Since most of these features are nonspecific and may be found in many cells of the body, they do not necessarily support the view that synovial sarcoma represents a neoplasm of a primitive ancestor cell committed to modulate into synovial tissue. In tissue culture, both cell types make proteoglycans, a feature that synovium shares with other mesenchymal tissues.

Immunohistochemistry has shown that both the epithelioid and the spindle cell components stain with antibodies to keratin, epithelial membrane antigen, and carcinoembryonic antigen, features usually associated with epithelial neoplasms.[132, 133] This pattern of reactivity has helped make it possible to separate synovial sarcoma from other morphologically similar tumors, such as fibrosarcoma and malignant schwannoma. It has also provided evidence that synovial sarcoma does not arise from or recapitulate the synovium, since normal synovial cells do not stain with these antibodies.[134]

Cytogenetic studies of synovial sarcomas have detected a consistent translocation involving chromosome X and 18.[135] This finding may lend insight into the genesis of synovial sarcoma as well as be used as a diagnostic feature.

Prognosis and Treatment. The prognosis of synovial sarcoma is not very good. The 5-year survival rates range from 25[134] to 55 percent,[136] with only 11 to 38 percent[136] of patients surviving 10 years. There is some evidence to suggest that more modern modes of therapy improve outcome.[137]

There are a number of factors that influence prognosis. Tumors that are small (less than 5 cm)

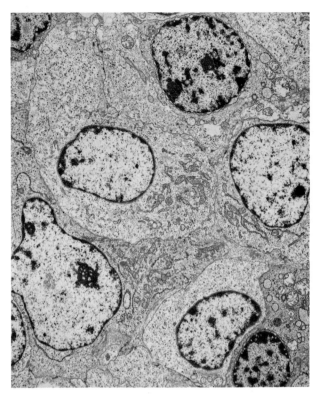

Figure 98–40. Higher power electron microscopic print of synovial sarcoma. The abutting cell borders have frequent junctions. The cytoplasm contains a background of free ribosomes and scattered microfilaments. Moderate numbers of mitochondria and cisternae of rough endoplasmic reticulum are usually localized in one end of the cell, and cisternae are slightly dilated and contain a material of medium electron density. (× 4300.)

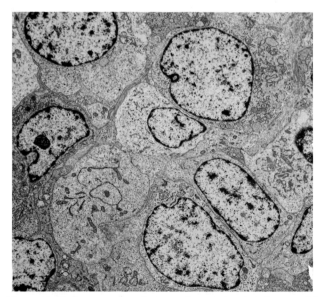

Figure 98–39. Lower power electron microscopic print of a synovial sarcoma. The neoplastic cells are polygonal and slightly elongate and have abutting cell borders. There is a high nuclear-cytoplasmic ratio, and prominent nucleoli are sometimes visible. (× 3260.)

and distally located have a lower probability of metastasizing. High mitotic rates, large areas of necrosis, aneuploidy, vascular invasion, and local recurrence are foreboding findings.[138] The impact of histologic subtype has been controversial. Some studies have indicated that the monophasic spindle cell variant behaves the most aggressively and that those tumors that have a predominant glandular component,[139] are heavily calcified,[129] or have a diploid pattern by flow cytometry[140] do the best.

The natural history of synovial sarcoma is local recurrence, which may be repetitive. Most recurrences manifest within 2 years after initial treatment; however, intervals longer than 10 years are not exceptional.[114] Ultimately, metastases develop in most patients and involve regional lymph nodes in 10 to 23 percent of patients,[141, 142] with other common sites being the lungs and skeleton. About 10 percent of patients die with metastatic disease within 1 year of diagnosis, and 90 percent of these patients have massive pulmonary metastases.

Treatment must contend with issues involving both local and systemic therapy. Successful local control can usually be achieved by limb salvage surgery combined with radiation. Because the regional lymph nodes are commonly involved, their status should be carefully evaluated, and they should be treated if enlarged.[115] Systemic treatment consists of various chemotherapy regimens, none of which is particularly successful.

Secondary Malignant Tumors of the Joint

Sarcomas

Primary bone sarcomas such as chondrosarcoma and osteosarcoma infrequently invade the joint capsule or articular surface and involve the synovium. When this occurs, it may be difficult to distinguish, on histologic features alone, some forms of synovial chondromatosis from a low-grade intraosseous chondrosarcoma that has secondarily spread into the joint.

Primary soft tissue sarcomas rarely destroy joint capsules and invade the synovium. However, certain soft tissue sarcomas have a propensity to grow along tendon sheaths for significant distances from the main mass. Because of this pattern of spread and certain microscopic features, these sarcomas, namely, clear cell sarcoma, epithelioid sarcoma, chordoid sarcoma, and synovial sarcoma, were believed to have a common histogenesis and were lumped together to form the entity "tendosynovial sarcoma." However, subsequent clinical, immunohistochemical, and ultrastructural studies have shown these tumors to be distinct clinicopathologic entities. For instance, clear cell sarcoma is now known to be a malignant melanoma that arises in the soft tissues,[143] and chordoid sarcoma an extraskeletal form of myxoid chondrosarcoma. Epithelioid sarcoma appears to be unique, and its normal tissue counterpart has not yet been identified. Therefore, the term "tendosynovial sarcoma" is no longer appropriate.

Metastatic Carcinoma

The synovium, unlike other richly vascular tissues, is rarely the site of metastatic carcinoma. This may reflect the fact that only clinical cases in which joint symptoms prevail are reported, since at autopsy joints are not routinely examined. Most of the carcinomas that have metastasized to the synovium originate in the lung, followed by the gastrointestinal tract and breast.[144–148] The affected patients are usually elderly, and the joint most frequently involved is the knee. In many of the reported cases, the underlying bone has also contained metastatic deposits.

Malignant Lymphoproliferative Disease

The various different types of malignant lymphoproliferative diseases, including leukemia, lymphoma, and myeloma, all may involve the synovium and produce osteoarticular symptoms.[149–151] Joint symptoms are more frequent in the setting of acute leukemia and have been observed in 3 percent of adult patients and 10 to 15 percent of children.[150, 151] Both large and small joints can be affected, and the arthritis is often asymmetric, migratory, and severe. The symptoms may result from leukemic infiltration of the synovium or irritation of the juxta-articular periosteum. When arthritis is a presenting symptom, there may be confusion with septic arthritis, rheumatic fever, subacute bacterial endocarditis, or rheumatoid arthritis.[151]

References

1. Milgram, J. W.: The classification of loose bodies in human joints. Clin. Orthop. 124:282, 1977.
2. Milgram, J. W.: The development of loose bodies in human joints. Clin. Orthop. 124:292, 1977.
3. Lichtenstein, L.: Bone Tumors. 2nd ed. St. Louis. C. V. Mosby Co., 1959.
4. Pudlowsky, R. M., Gilula, L. A., and Kyriakos, M.: Intra-articular lipoma with osseous metaplasia: Radiographic-pathologic correlation. Am. J. Roentgenol. 132:471, 1979.
5. Coventry, M. B., Harrison, E. G., and Martin, J. F.: Benign synovial tumors of the knee: A diagnostic problem. J. Bone Joint Surg. 48(A):1350, 1966.
6. Rodman, G. P.: Tumors of synovial joints, bursa, and tendon sheaths. In Hollander, J. E. (ed.): Arthritis and Allied Conditions. A Textbook of Rheumatology. 7th ed. Philadelphia. Lea & Febiger, 1966.
7. Allen, P. W.: Lipoma arborescens. In Tumors and Proliferations of Adipose Tissue. Chicago, Year Book Medical Publishers, Inc., 1981, p. 129.
8. Noel, E. R., Tebib, J. G., Dumontet, C., Colson, F., Carret, J. P., Vauzelle, J. L., and Bouvier, M.: Synovial lipoma arborescens of the hip. Clin. Rheumatol. 6:92, 1987.
9. Hallet, T., Lew, S., and Bansal, M.: Villous lipomatous proliferation of the synovial membrane (lipoma arborescens). J. Bone Joint Surg. 70(A):264, 1988.
10. Burgan, D. W.: Lipoma arborescens of the knee: Another cause of filling defects on a knee arthrogram. Diagn. Radiol. 101:583, 1971.
11. Jaffe, H. L.: Tumors and Tumorous Conditions of the Bones and Joints. Philadelphia, Lea & Febiger, 1958.
12. Hoffa, A.: The influence of the adipose tissue with regard to the pathology of the knee joint. J.A.M.A. 43:795, 1904.
13. Gozal, D., Soudry, M., Arad, P., Jaffe, M., and Boss, J. H.: Arteriovenous hemangioma of the joint capsule of the knee in a child. Eur. J. Pediatr. 148:198, 1988.
14. Lichtenstein, L.: Tumors of synovial joints, bursae, and tendon sheaths. Cancer 8:816, 1955.
15. Bennett, G. E., and Cobey, M. C.: Hemangioma of joint: report of 5 cases. Arch. Surg. 38:487, 1939.
16. Atkinson, T. J., Wolf, S., Anavi, Y., and Wesley, R.: Synovial hemangioma of the temporomandibular joint: Report of a case and review of the literature. J. Oral Maxillofac. Surg. 46:804, 1988.
17. Resnick, D., and Oliphant, M.: Hemophilia-like arthropathy of the knee associated with cutaneous and synovial hemangioma. Diagn. Radiol 114:323, 1975.
18. Zvantseva, V. A.: Hemangioma of the synovial membrane of the knee joint. Vestn. Khir. 1178:52, 1976.
19. Mulder, J. W.: Hemangioma of the knee joint. Arch. Chir. Neerl. 24:135, 1972.
20. Larsen, E.: Synovial hemangioma in the elbow joint. Ugeskr. Laeger 137:1199, 1975.
21. Burman, M. S., and Milgram, J. E.: Hemangioma of tendon and tendon sheath. Surg. Gynecol. Obstet. 50:397, 1930.
22. Cobey, M. C.: Hemangioma of joints. Arch. Surg. 46:465, 1943.
23. Choong, P., and Baker, C.: Arthrocutaneous hemangiomatosis with destructive arthritis. Aust. N. Z. J. Surg. 60:725, 1990.
24. Osgood, R. B.: Tuberculosis of the knee joint. Angioma of the knee joint. Surg. Clin. North Am. 1:681, 1921.
25. Ryd, L., and Stenstrom, A.: Hemangioma mimicking meniscal injury. A report on 10 years of knee pain. Acta Orthop. Scand. 60:230, 1989.
26. Tudisco, C., Conteduca, F., and Puddu, G.: Synovial hemangioma of the meniscal wall simulating a meniscal cyst. A case report. Am. J. Sports Med. 16:191, 1988.
27. Geschickter, C. F., and Copeland, M. M.: Tumors of Bone. 3rd. ed. Philadelphia. J. B. Lippincott, 1949, p. 693.
28. Chung, E. B., and Enzinger, F. M.: Fibroma of tendon sheath. Cancer 44:1945, 1979.
29. Pulitzer, D. R., Martin, P. C., and Reed, R. J.: Fibroma of tendon sheath. A clinicopathologic study of 32 cases. Am. J. Surg. Pathol. 13(6):472, 1989.
30. Southwick, G. J., and Karamoskos, P.: Fibroma of tendon sheath with bone involvement. J. Hand Surg. 15B:373, 1990.

31. Lundgren, L. G., and Kindbloom, L. G.: Fibroma of tendon sheath: A light and electron microscopic study of 6 cases. Acta Pathol. Microbiol. Immunol. Scand. 92:401, 1984.

32. Cooper, G., and Schiller, A. L.: Anatomy of the Guinea Pig. Cambridge, MA, Harvard University Press, 1975.

33. Symeonides, P. P., and Ioannides, G.: Ossicles in the knee menisci. Report of 3 cases. J. Bone Joint Surg. 54(A):1288, 1972.

34. Maurice, H., Crone, M., and Watt, I.: Synovial chondromatosis. J. Bone Joint Surg. 70(B):807, 1988.

35. Wilson, W. J., and Parr, T. J.: Synovial chondromatosis. Orthopedics 11:1179, 1988.

36. Jacob, R. A., Campbell, W. P., and Niemann, K. M. W.: Synovial chondrometaplasia. A case report. Clin. Orthop. 109:152, 1975.

37. Giustra, P. E., Furman, R. S., Roberts, L., and Killoran, P. J.: Synovial osteochondromatosis involving the elbow. Am. J. Roentgenol. 127:347, 1976.

38. Varma, B. P., and Ramakrishna, Y. J.: Synovial chondromatosis of the shoulder. Aust. N. Z. J. Surg. 46:14, 1976.

39. Gudmundsen, T. E., and Siewers, P. B.: Synovial chondromatosis of the shoulder. Acta Orthop. Scand. 58:419, 1987.

40. Burnstein, M. I., Fisher, D. R., Yandow, D. R., Hafez, G. R., and DeSmet, A. A.: Case Report 502. Skeletal Radiol. 17:458, 1988.

41. Holm, C. L.: Primary synovial chondromatosis of the ankle. A case report. J. Bone Joint Surg. 58A:878, 1976.

42. Szepesi, J.: Synovial chondromatosis of the metacarpophalangeal joint. Acta Orthop. Scand. 46:926, 1975.

43. Lewis, M., Marshall, J. L., and Mirra, J. M.: Synovial chondromatosis of the thumb. J. Bone Joint Surg. 56(A):180, 1974.

44. Milgram, J. W.: Synovial osteochondromatosis in the foot. Bull. Hosp. Joint Dis. Orthop. Inst. 47:245, 1987.

45. Blankestijn, J., Panders, A. K., Vermey, A., and Scherpbier, A. J.: Synovial chondromatosis of the temporomandibular joint: Report of 3 cases and review of the literature. Cancer 55:479, 1985.

46. Forssell, K., Happonen, R. P., and Forsell, H.: Synovial chondromatosis of the temporomandibular joint. Report of a case and review of the literature. Int. J. Oral Maxillofac. Surg. 17:237, 1988.

47. Von Arx, D. P., Simpson, A. M., and Batman, P.: Synovial chondromatosis of the temporomandibular joints. Br. J. Oral Maxillofac. Surg. 26:297, 1988.

48. Sim, F. H., Dahlin, D. C., and Ivins, J. C.: Extra-articular synovial chondromatosis. J. Bone Joint Surg. 59(A):492, 1977.

49. Jones, W. A.: Tenosynovial chondroma of the hand. J. Hand Surg. (Br.) 11:276, 1986.

50. Milgram, J. W., and Hadesman, W. M.: Synovial osteochondromatosis in the subacromial bursa. Clin. Orthop. 236:154, 1988.

51. Bertoni, F., Pignatti, G., Bacchini, P., and Compartacci, M.: Miscellaneous synovial lesions. Curr. Opin. Rheumatol. 2:120, 1990.

52. Murphy, F. P., Dahlin, D. C., and Sullivan, R.: Articular synovial chondromatosis. J. Bone Joint Surg. 44(A):77, 1962.

53. Madewell, J. E., and Sweet, D. E.: Tumors and tumor-like lesions in or about joints. In Resnick, D., and Niwayama, G. (eds.): Diagnosis of Bone and Joint Disorders. 2nd ed. Philadelphia, W. B. Saunders Co., 1988.

54. Ellman, M. H., Krieger, M. I., and Brown, N.: Pseudogout mimicking synovial chondromatosis. J. Bone Joint Surg. 57(A):863, 1975.

55. Sarmiento, A., and Elkins, R. W.: Giant intra-articular osteochondroma of the knee. J. Bone Joint Surg. 57(A):560, 1975.

56. Leeson, M. C., Wilcox, P., Greenberg, B., and Ewing, J. W.: Giant intra-articular loose bodies of the knee. Orthop. Rev. 15:393, 1986.

57. Allred, C. D., and Gondos, B.: Ultrastructure of synovial chondromatosis. Arch. Pathol. Lab. Med. 106:688, 1982.

58. Dunn, A. W., and Whisler, J. H.: Synovial chondromatosis of the knee with associated extracapsular chondromas. J. Bone Joint Surg. 55(A):1747, 1973.

59. Milgram, J. W., and Addison, R. G.: Synovial osteochondromatosis of the knee. Chondromatous recurrence with possible chondrosarcomatous degeneration. J. Bone Joint Surg. 58(A):264, 1976.

60. Goldman, R. L., and Lichtenstein, L.: Synovial chondrosarcoma. Cancer 17:1233, 1964.

61. Manivel, J. C., Dehner, L. P., and Thompson, R.: Case report 460. Skeletal Radiol. 17:66, 1988.

62. Bertoni, F., Unni, K. K., Beabout, J. W., and Sim, F. H.: Chondrosarcomas of the synovium. Cancer 67:155, 1991.

63. Dahlin, D. C., and Salvador, A. H.: Cartilaginous tumors of the soft tissues of the hands and feet. Mayo Clin. Proc. 49:721, 1974.

64. Chung, E. B., and Enzinger, F. M.: Chondroma of soft parts. Cancer 41:1414, 1978.

65. Fletcher, C. D. M., and Krausz, T.: Cartilaginous tumors of soft tissue. Appl. Pathol. 6:208, 1986.

66. Zlatkin, M. B., Lander, P. H., Begin, L. R., and Hadjipavlou, A.: Soft tissue chondromas. Am. J. Roentgenol. 144:1263, 1985.

67. Reiman, H., and Dahlin, D. C.: Cartilage and bone-forming tumors of the soft tissues. Semin. Diagn. Pathol. 3:288, 1988.

68. Lichtenstein, L., and Goldman, R. L.: Cartilage tumors in soft tissues, particularly in the hand and foot. Cancer 17:1203, 1964.

69. Someren, A., and Merritt, W. H.: Tenosynovial chondromas of the hand. A case report with a brief review of the literature. Hum. Pathol. 9:476, 1978.

70. Nuovo, M. A., Desai, P., Shankman, S., and Present, D.: Intracapsular para-articular chondroma of the knee. Bull. Hosp. Joint Dis. Orthop. Inst. 50:189, 1990.

71. Hensinger, R. N., Cowell, H. R., Ramsey, P. L., and Leopold, R. G.: Familial dysplasia epiphysealis hemimelica associated with chondromas and osteochondromas. Report of a kindred with variable presentations. J. Bone Joint Surg. 56(A):1513, 1974.

72. Heiple, K. G., and Elmer, R. N.: Multiple chondromatous hamartomas. Report of a case. J. Bone Joint Surg. 54(A):393, 1972.

73. Hensinger, R. N., and Rhyne, D. H.: Multiple chondromatous hamartomas. Report of a case. J. Bone Joint Surg. 56(A):1068, 1974.

74. Young, J. M., and Hudacek, A. G.: Experimental production of pigmented villonodular synovitis in dogs. Am. J. Pathol. 30:799, 1954.

75. Singh, R., Grenal, D. S., and Chakravarti, R. N.: Experimental production of pigmented villonodular synovitis in the knee and ankle joints of rhesus monkeys. J. Pathol. 98:137, 1969.

76. Ray, R. A., Morton, C. C., Lipinski, K. K., Corson, J. M., and Fletcher, J. A.: Cytogenetic evidence of clonality in a case of pigmented villonodular synovitis. Cancer 67:121, 1991.

77. Fletcher, A. J., Henkle, C., Atkins, L., Rosenberg, A. E., and Morton, C. C.: Trisomy 5 and trisomy 7 are non-random aberrations in pigmented villonodular synovitis: Confirmation of trisomy 7 in uncultured cells. Genes Chromosomes Cancer 4:264, 1992.

78. Docken, W. P.: Pigmented villonodular synovitis: A review with illustrative case reports. Semin. Arthritis Rheum. 9:1, 1979.

79. Roa, A. S., and Vigorita, V. J.: Pigmented villonodular synovitis. (Giant cell tumor of the tendon sheath and synovial membrane.) A review of 81 cases. J. Bone Joint Surg. 66A:76, 1984.

80. Flandry, F., and Hughston, J. C.: Pigmented villonodular synovitis. J. Bone Joint Surg. 69(A):942, 1987.

81. Byers, P. D., Cotten, R. E., Deacon, D. W., Lowy, M., Newman, P. H., Sissons, H. A., and Thomas, A. D.: The diagnosis and treatment of pigmented villonodular synovitis. J. Bone Joint Surg. 50(B):290, 1968.

82. Miyamoto, Y., Yani, T., and Hamaya, K.: Pigmented villonodular synovitis of the temporomandibular joint. Case report. Plast. Reconstr. Surg. 59:283, 1977.

83. Raibley, S. O.: Villonodular synovitis with synovial chondromatosis. Oral Surg. 44:279, 1977.

84. Janssens, X., Veys, E. M., and Cuvelier, C.: Pigmented villonodular synovitis of the hip—association with osteochondromatosis. Clin. Exp. Rheumatol. 5:329, 1987.

85. Arthand, J. B.: Pigmented nodular synovitis. Report of 11 lesions in non-articular locations. Am. J. Clin. Pathol. 58:511, 1972.

86. Leszcynski, J. R., Hucknell, J. S., Percy, J., LeRiche, J. C., and Lentle, B. C.: Pigmented nodular synovitis in multiple joints, occurrence in a child with cavernous hemangioma of the lip and pulmonary stenosis. Ann. Rheum. Dis. 34:269, 1975.

87. Kindbloom, K. G., and Gunterverg, B.: Pigmented villonodular synovitis involving bone. Case report. J. Bone Joint Surg. 60(A):830, 1978.

88. Jergensen, H. E., Mankin, H. J., and Schiller, A. L.: Diffuse pigmented villonodular synovitis mimicking a primary bone neoplasm. A report of 2 cases. J. Bone Joint Surg. 60(A):830, 1978.

89. Larmon, W. A.: Pigmented villonodular synovitis. Med. Clin. North Am. 49:141, 1965.

90. Myers, B. W., Masi, A. T., and Feingenbaum, S. L.: Pigmented villonodular synovitis and tenosynovitis. A clinical epidemiologic study of 100 cases and literature review. Medicine 59:223, 1980.

91. Smith, J. H., and Pugh, D. G.: Roentgenographic aspects of articular pigmented villonodular synovitis. Am. J. Roentgenol. 87:1146, 1962.

92. Wolf, R. D., and Giuliano, V. J.: Double contrast arthrography in the diagnosis of pigmented villonodular synovitis of the knee. Am. J. Roentgenol. 110:793, 1970.

93. Rosenthal, D. I., Coleman, P. P., and Schiller, A. L.: Pigmented villonodular synovitis. Correlation of angiographic and histologic findings. Am. J. Roentgenol. 135:581, 1980.

94. Butt, W. P., Hardy, G., and Ostlere, S. J.: Pigmented villonodular synovitis of the knee: computed tomographic appearances. Skeletal Radiol. 19:191, 1980.

95. Goldman, A. B., and DiCarlo, E. P.: Pigmented villonodular synovitis. Diagnosis and differential diagnosis. Radiol. Clin. North Am. 26:1327, 1988.

96. Burke, D. L., Jr., Mitchell, D. G., Rifkin, M. D., and Vinitski, S.: Recent advances in magnetic resonance imaging of the knee. Radiol. Clin. North Am. 28:379, 1990.

97. Dorfmann, H.: Arthroscopic detection of synovial disorders. Contemp. Orthop. 10:19, 1985.

98. Flandry, F. C., Hughston, J. C., Barrack, R. L., Kurtz, D., McCann, S., and Jacobson, K. E.: Pigmented villonodular synovitis of the knee. Orthop. Trans. 10:599, 1986.

99. Burnett, R. A.: A cause of erroneous diagnosis of pigmented villonodular synovitis. J. Clin. Pathol. 29:17, 1976.

100. Fraire, A. E., and Fechner, R. E.: Intra-articular localized nodular synovitis of the knee. Arch. Pathol. 93:473, 1972.
101. Granowitz, S. P., and Mankin, H. J.: Localized pigmented villonodular synovitis of the knee. Report of five cases. J. Bone Joint Surg. 49(A):122, 1967.
102. Ushijima, M., Hashimoto, H., Tsuneyoshi, M., and Enjoji, M.: Giant cell tumor of the tendon sheath (nodular tenosynovitis). Cancer 57:875, 1986.
103. Schumacher, H. R., Lotke, P., Athreya, B., and Rothfuss, S.: Pigmented villonodular synovitis: Light and electron microscopic studies. Semin. Arthritis Rheum. 12:32, 1982.
104. Alguacil-Garcia, A., Unni, K. K., and Goellner, J. R.: Giant cell tumor of tendon sheath and pigmented villonodular synovitis: An ultrastructural study. Am. J. Clin. Pathol. 69:6, 1978.
105. Wood, G. S., Beckstead, J. S., Medeiros, L. J., Kempson, R. L., and Warnke, R. A.: The cells of giant cell tumor of tendon sheath resemble osteoclasts. Am. J. Surg. Pathol. 12:444, 1988.
106. Carstens, P. H. B., and Howell, R. S.: Malignant giant cell tumor of tendon sheath. Virchows Arch. (Pathol. Anat.) 382:237, 1979.
107. Case Records of the Massachusetts General Hospital. N. Engl. J. Med. 309:1042, 1983.
108. Case Records of the Massachusetts General Hospital. N. Engl. J. Med. 266:725, 1964.
109. Goldman, R. L., and Lichtentenstein, L.: Synovial chondrosarcoma. Cancer 17:1233, 1964.
110. Hamilton, A., Davis, R. I., and Nixon, J. R.: Synovial chondrosarcoma complicating synovial chondrosarcoma. J. Bone Joint Surg. 69(A):1084, 1987.
111. Perry, B. E., McQueen, D. A., and Lin, J. J.: Synovial chondromatosis with malignant degeneration to chondrosarcoma. J. Bone Joint Surg. 70(A):1259, 1988.
112. Bertoni, F., Unni, K. K., Beabout, J. W., and Sim, F. H.: Chondrosarcomas of the synovium. Cancer 67:155, 1991.
113. Kindblom, L.-G., and Angervall, L.: Myxoid chondrosarcoma of the synovial tissue: A clinicopathologic, histochemical and ultrastructural analysis. Cancer 52:1886, 1983.
114. Enzinger, F. M., and Weiss, S. W.: Soft Tissue Tumors. St. Louis. C. V. Mosby Co., 1988.
115. Russel, W. O., Cohen, H. J., Enzinger, F. M., Hajdu, S. I., et al.: A clinical and pathological staging system for soft tissue sarcomas. Cancer 40:1562, 1977.
116. Moberger, G., Nilsonne, U., and Friberg, S.: Synovial sarcoma. Acta Orthop. Scand. Suppl. No. 11, 1968.
117. Cadman, N. L., Soule, E. H., and Kelly, P. J.: Synovial sarcoma. An analysis of 134 tumors. Cancer 18:613, 1965.
118. Crocker, D. W., and Stout, A. P.: Synovial sarcoma in children. Cancer 12:1123, 1959.
119. Dardick, I., O'Brien, P. K., Jeans, M. T. D., and Massiah, K. A.: Synovial sarcoma arising in an anatomical bursa. Virchows Arch. (Pathol. Anat.) 397:93, 1982.
120. DeSanto, D. A., Tennant, R., and Rosahn, P.: Synovial sarcomas in joints, bursae and tendon sheaths. Surg. Gynecol. Obstet. 72:951, 1961.
121. Roth, J. A., Enzinger, F. M., and Tannenbaum, M.: Synovial sarcoma of the neck. A follow-up study of 24 cases. Cancer 13:1243, 1975.
122. Jacobs, L. A., and Weaver, A. W.: Synovial sarcoma of the head and neck. Am. J. Surg. 128:527, 1974.
123. Scmookler, B. M., Enzinger, F. M., and Brannon, R. B.: Orofacial synovial sarcoma. A clinicopathologic study of 11 new cases and review of the literature. Cancer 50:269, 1982.
124. Ariel, I. M., and Pack, G. T.: Synovial sarcoma. Review of 25 cases. N. Engl. J. Med. 268:1272, 1963.
125. Witkin, G. M., Miettinen, M., and Rosai, J.: A biphasic tumor of the mediastinum with features of synovial sarcoma. A report of 4 cases. Am. J. Surg. Pathol. 13:490, 1989.
126. Massarelli, G., Tanda, F., and Salis, B.: Synovial sarcoma of the soft palate. Report of a case. Hum. Pathol. 9:341, 1978.
127. Mackenzie, D. H.: Synovial sarcoma. Cancer 19:169, 1966.
128. Scialabba, F. A., and Deluca, S. A.: Synovial cell sarcoma. Am. Fam. Physician 41:1211, 1990.
129. Varela-Duran, J., and Enzinger, F. M.: Calcifying synovial sarcoma. Cancer 50:345, 1982.
130. Gabbiani, G., Kaye, G. I., Lattes, R., and Majno, G.: Synovial sarcoma. Electron microscopy of a typical case. Cancer 28:1031, 1971.
131. Mickelson, M. R., Brown, G. A., Maynard, J. A., Cooper, R. R., and Bonfiglio, M.: Synovial sarcoma. An electron microscopic study of monophasic and biphasic forms. Cancer 45:2109, 1980.
132. Corson, J. M., Weiss, L. M., Banks-Schlegel, S. P., and Pinkus, G.: Keratin proteins and carcinoembryonic antigen in synovial sarcoma. An immunohistochemical study of 24 cases. Hum. Pathol. 15:615, 1984.
133. Miettinen, M.: Immunohistochemistry of soft tissue tumors: possibilities and limitations in surgical pathology. Pathol. Ann. 25(Part 1):1, 1990.
134. Miettinen, M., and Virtanen, I.: Synovial sarcoma—a misnomer. Am. J. Pathol. 117:1825, 1984.
135. Wang-Wuu, S., Soukup, S. W., and Lange, B. J.: Another synovial sarcoma with t(x;18). Cancer Genet. Cytogenet. 29:179, 1987.
136. Soule, E. H.: Synovial sarcoma. Am. J. Pathol. 10(Suppl. 1):78, 1986.
137. Wright, P. H., Sim, F. H., Soule, E. H., and Taylor, W. F.: Synovial sarcoma. J. Bone Joint Surg. 64(A):112, 1982.
138. Rooser, B., Willen, H., Hugoson, A., and Rydholm, A.: Prognostic factors in synovial sarcoma. Cancer 63:2182, 1989.
139. Cagle, L. A., Mirra, J. M., Storm, F. K., Roe, D. J., and Eilber, F. R.: Histologic features relating to prognosis in synovial sarcoma. Cancer 59:1810, 1989.
140. El-Naggar, A. K., Ayala, A., Abdul-Karim, F. W., McLemore, D., Ballance, W. W., Garnsey, L., Ro, J. Y., and Batsakis, J. G.: Synovial sarcoma. A DNA flow cytometric study. Cancer 65:2295, 1990.
141. Pack, G. T., and Ariel, I. M.: Synovial sarcoma (malignant synovioma): A report of 60 cases. Surgery 28:1042, 1950.
142. Hajdu, S. I., Shiu, M. H., and Fortner, J. G.: Tendosynovial sarcoma: A clinicopathological study of 136 cases. Cancer 39:1201, 1977.
143. Chung, E. B., and Enzinger, F. M.: Malignant melanoma. Am. J. Surg. Pathol. 7(5):405, 1983.
144. Khan, F. A., Garterhouse, W., and Khan, A.: Metastatic bronchogenic carcinoma: An unusual case of localized arthritis. Chest 67:738, 1975.
145. Moutsopoulos, H. M., Fye, K. H., Pugay, P. I., and Shearn, M. A.: Monoarthritic arthritis caused by metastatic breast carcinoma. Value of cytologic study of synovial fluid. J.A.M.A. 234:75, 1975.
146. Goldenberg, D. L., Kelley, W., and Gibbons, R. B.: Metastatic adenocarcinoma of synovium presenting as an acute arthritis. Diagnosed by closed synovial biopsy. Arthritis Rheum. 18:107, 1975.
147. Newton, P., Freemont, A. T., Noble, J., Scott, N., Greenan, D. M., and Hiltan, R. C.: Secondary malignant synovitis: Report of three cases and review of the literature. Q. J. Med. 53:135, 1984.
148. Benhamon, C. L., Tourliere, D., Brigant, S., Maitre, F., and Cauderlier, P.: Synovial metastasis of an adenocarcinoma presenting as a shoulder monoarthritis. J. Rheumatol. 15:1031, 1988.
149. Mintz, G., Robles-Saavedra, E. J., Enriquez, R. D., Jimenez, F. J., and Juan, M. L.: Hemarthrosis as the presenting manifestation of true myeloma joint disease. Arthritis Rheum. 21:148, 1978.
150. Rogalsky, R. J., Black, G. B., and Reed, M. H.: Orthopaedic manifestations of leukemia. J. Bone Joint Surg. 68(A):494, 1986.
151. Marsh, W. L., Bylund, D. J., Heath, V. C., and Anderson, M. J.: Osteoarticular and pulmonary manifestations of acute leukemia. Case report and review of the literature. Cancer 57:385, 1986.

Section XXI

Medical Orthopedics and Rehabilitation

Chapter 99

Sheldon R. Simon
Eric L. Radin

Biomechanics of Joints

BIOMECHANICS OF NORMAL JOINTS

Joint Stability. There are six possible types of joint motion about three perpendicular axes: three rotational and three translational (Fig. 99–1). In general, most joint motion is minimally translational and primarily rotational.[1] If motions were solely rotational, at any instant, the center of the radius of the arc of motion would repeatedly be at the same point. Usually, a small component of translational movement exists, and the deviation from absolute rotatory motion may be noted by the changes in the path of the joint's "instantaneous centers of rotation" (Fig. 99–2). These centers have been measured for the shoulder, elbow, wrist, knee, and ankle and were found to vary only slightly from true arcs of rotation.[2–6]

Joint stability is created by bony configurations, ligaments, and muscles,[7] with different joints using different combinations of these constructs. Although each joint is characterized by its own unique bony contour, one side is usually concave, and the other convex.[8] Since bone is the most rigid anatomic structure, the greater the arc of motion enclosed by the bone, the greater the amount of inherent stability that exists. For example, at the hip the spherical head of the femur is almost enclosed by a hemispherical arc of bony acetabulum.[9] By contrast, the shoulder, with a flatter radius of curvature and less enclosed humeral head, is easier to dislocate or sublux (Fig. 99–3). In such circumstances, ligaments may provide some stability, but ligaments provide stability only in circumstances of modest loading, as they can tear.

A ligament resists motions in the plane in which it lies (Fig. 99–4). In resisting displacement, ligaments have some stretch.[10] For example, the cruciate ligaments of the knee complement bony contours by defining the translation of the tibia on the femur.[11]

The muscle-tendon complexes are similar to ligaments in the way they stabilize joints. Muscles have the added advantage of active shortening. Since ligaments are only passive stabilizers, the advantage of muscles, which are active, in controlling joint motion is obvious. Muscle action, in fact, protects ligaments from tearing.[7, 12–14]

The spine illustrates the intricate balance between the three structural stabilizers. To protect the spinal cord while allowing rotatory motions of the trunk, a sophisticated stabilizing arrangement has evolved. The intervertebral "unit" (vertebra–intervertebral disc–vertebra) is composed of (1) one amphiarthrodial joint (the intervertebral disc) and two diarthrodial intervertebral facet joints; (2) multiple ligaments (anterior and posterior longitudinal, ligamentum flavum and interspinous); and (3) paraspinal muscles (Fig. 99–5). The disc is the major supporting

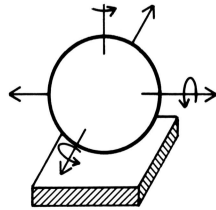

Figure 99–1. All motions of two adjacent bodies relative to each other consist of translational motions along three mutually perpendicular axes and three rotational motions about these same three axes.

1675

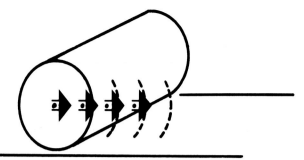

Figure 99–2. If a body rotates in place, the center of its rotation does not move. If the body translates as it rotates, movement of the center of rotation reflects this motion.

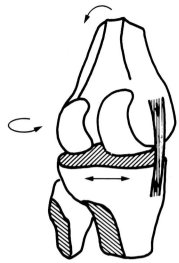

Figure 99–4. At the knee the medial collateral ligament can restrict only the valgus rotational motions, that is, motions parallel to the ligament's length. It cannot restrict anteroposterior or mediolateral translational or flexion-extension rotational motions of the joint, motions that are perpendicular to its axis.

unit between the vertebral bony units and helps maintain the vertical rigidity of the system.[15, 16] Although the disc will stabilize vertical loads and prevent vertical translation, it does not stabilize horizontal translation.[17] For example, when a person bends to tie a shoelace, the body's weight is located anterior to the spine. This configuration compresses the disc and tends to topple the spine by creating forces that tilt and slide one vertebral unit over the one below it. To prevent these slipping motions, each vertebral body overhangs, posteriorly, the one below it. This arrangement is provided by posterolateral intervertebral facet joints. They prevent anteroposterior and mediolateral translational motions. The ligaments and muscles limit the extent of motion, control the degree of and speed with which motions occur, and act as the major source of stability in rotation (Fig. 99–6). When all is said and done, control of the position of the loaded spine ultimately depends on the paraspinal muscles.[18]

Joint Motions. The types of motions and the degree to which each motion is allowed is distinct in each joint.[19] In the human, the primary function of the upper extremities is to carry and manipulate objects; the primary function of the lower extremities is locomotion. To provide for the wide sphere of function that an extremity can encompass, the most proximal joint must have the widest range of motion. It must allow for rotatory motions of large degrees in all three planes (Fig. 99–7).[20] Because most external forces on the extremity are exerted at some distance

from the joint, stabilizing forces around the most proximal joint must be high.

The joint configuration established to suit these demands at the shoulder is a ball on a relatively flat surface, requiring significant muscular and ligamen-

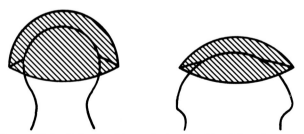

Figure 99–3. Both the hip and the shoulder joints have no rotational restrictions and have similar ball-in-socket shapes. The glenoid socket does not stabilize the humeral head as well as the acetabulum stabilizes the femoral head.

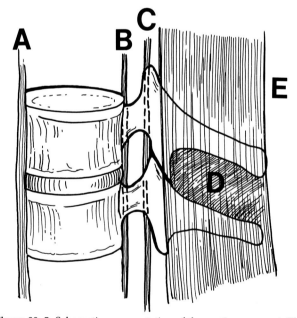

Figure 99–5. Schematic representation of the motion segment. The vertebral bodies are separated by the intervertebral disc. Each vertebral body is connected to its posterior elements and spinous process. The anterior-longitudinal ligament (A) and posterior-longitudinal ligament (P) run up the front and back of the vertebral bodies. The ligamentum flavum (C) runs behind the spinal canal, which is the space between B and C. The interspinous ligament (D) joins the spinous processes. Muscles are applied to the posterior surfaces of the bones and vertical surfaces of the spinous processes (E).

Figure 99–6. The intervertebral unit of the spine has multiple structures contributing to its stability. The disc *(A)* prevents vertical translational motions, like a balloon placed in a coffee can. The facet joints *(B)* prevent forward translation, permitting the more proximal vertebrae only to rotate about the more distal one in a prescribed arc. Multiple ligaments and paraspinal muscles control the speed and extent of motion within this arc of movement through their "clamping" effect on the posterior elements *(C)*.

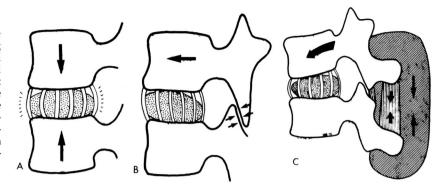

tous stability, with minimal bony constraint.[21] The hip, which functions to balance body mass, needs greater stability to prevent translational motions and a smaller range of rotational motion. It derives much of its stability from encapsulating bony contours; it is a ball and socket, with muscles playing an important role. Paralyzed individuals are more likely to dislocate their hips.[22]

In order for an extremity to function at all locations within its range, a means is provided to alter the length of the limb. Rotational motion of the elbow and knee joints allows overall length changes as adjacent limb segments move (Fig. 99–8). For example, at the initiation of the swing phase of walking, hip flexors flex the hip while the knee flexes passively; this creates a relative shortening of the limb's length to provide floor clearance. It is most efficient to provide such control with a single muscle that

spans two joints. One joint moves in a direction to stretch the muscle, and the other rotates in an opposite direction, lessening the degree of active contraction necessary (Fig. 99–9). Of necessity, muscle-tendon systems must span the periphery of rotational joints to control their actions and stabilize them in all directions.

Joint Forces. The force causing joint rotation about an axis is not merely the contractile or stretching force produced in the muscle but is the product of this force multiplied by the distance between the joint's center of rotation and the tendon (see Fig. 99–7; Fig. 99–10). The tendon placed at the periphery of the joint gives the muscle a mechanical advantage in creating the greatest torque with the least effort.[23]

Muscle contraction produces compressive forces across the joint tending to squeeze the joint together (Fig. 99–11). This force also maintains stability against forces that might pivot a joint open (see Figs. 99–6C, 99–7, and 99–10; Fig. 99–12). Muscle forces create high forces that the joint surface must withstand.[7] In some movements, if the joint is rotated into certain positions, the muscles become more parallel to the joint surface (Fig. 99–13). The muscles

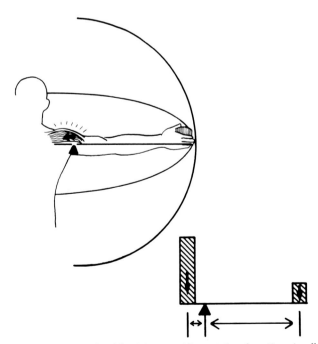

Figure 99–7. The shoulder joint provides rotational motions in all planes, allowing the arm to be placed in many locations. To provide such freedom while still maintaining joint stability, shoulder muscles must be large; they are situated close to the fulcrum of balance, whereas the weight that they control is far away.

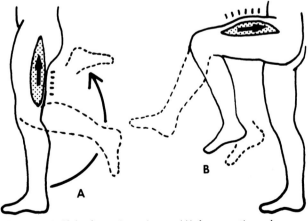

Figure 99–8. If the femur is stationary *(A)*, knee motions alone are not an effective means of producing limb shortening. Under such circumstances the foot can move only in a single prescribed 180-degree arc behind the knee. However, if at the same time the thigh is allowed to move by rotatory motions produced about the hip *(B)*, the limb can be shortened or placed within a wide spherical volume.

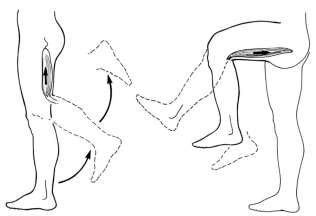

Figure 99–9. The hamstring muscles originate above the hip and insert below the knee. With the hip straight, considerable contraction of the hamstrings is necessary to bend the knee. However, with the hip flexed, the hamstrings are stretched behind the hip, and a relatively modest contraction is all that is necessary to bend the knee in that circumstance.

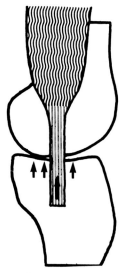

Figure 99–11. The force that a muscle produces tends to squeeze or compress the joint it spans.

then lose their mechanical advantage and must increase the force applied to maintain the applied torque. In most of the weight-bearing joints in the lower extremities, the intra-articular force can be up to three to four times body weight.[24]

In some cases the shear force or rotational torque parallel to the joint line is helpful in stabilizing the joint against inertial or weight-bearing forces that tend to translate the two sides of the joint. In some situations, as in the fingers' flexor tendons, pulleys are provided to maintain a constant direction of pull across the joint (Fig. 99–14). In some cases, shear forces can be detrimental.[25]

Joint Control. The magnitude of the interarticular forces depends on what the functional activity is, how the activity is performed, and how fast it is performed.[26–29] For example, while walking, the knee

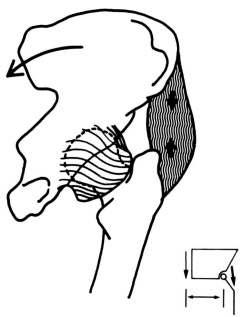

Figure 99–10. When one-legged support is required, the abductor muscles contract to produce a rotational force about the hip joint opposite to that produced by body weight. The farther away the muscle-tendon complex is from the center of the joint, the lower the muscle force needs to be to create the same rotational force. In most cases the distance of the muscle-tendon complex from the center of the joint is less than that of the weight it is trying to counteract. This produces a larger force in the muscles than the weight it balances. As a consequence, during the functional activities of daily living the major muscles about the hip typically produce forces two to four times body weight.

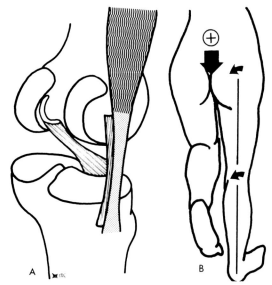

Figure 99–12. Being eccentrically placed, a muscle will produce compressive force that will prevent a joint from pivoting open. At the knee the vastus lateralis assists knee ligaments (A), preventing body weight medially placed from opening up the lateral side of the joint during one-legged support (B).

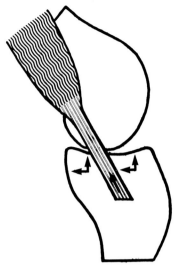

Figure 99–13. In many areas, the muscles placed on the concave, medial, or lateral sides of the joint become more parallel to the surface of the joint as the joint is flexed. Joint compressive forces are reduced, but shear forces arise.

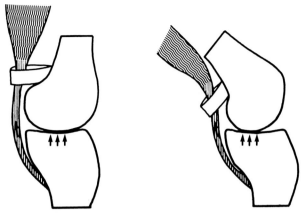

Figure 99–14. At certain joints, pulleys located proximal to the joint maintain flexor tendons at fixed distances and orientation to the joint's surface.

flexes 15 to 20 degrees during the early stance phase. The quadriceps muscle attempts to prevent collapse of the leg under the body's weight as the leg is decelerating; most of the force exerted is compressive. If the individual walks faster, greater muscle activity is needed for deceleration, creating higher compressive loads across the joint (Fig. 99–15). Quadriceps activity increases even further during running, where it is needed for acceleration.[30] In contrast, during the swing phase of walking most of the forces are internal, no significant muscle activity is needed, and knee joint forces are minimal.[29]

Quadriceps and other muscle activity at all joints during common activities appears to be dictated by fixed, preprogrammed neurologic responses. Activities requiring involvement of the low back region also require the participation of one or more joints of the upper and lower extremities.

The ability of an individual to perform a task in a chosen manner depends on the strength of various relevant muscle groups. For example, if a person has strong enough back muscles, he or she may pick something up by keeping the legs straight and bend-

ing over (Fig. 99–16A). Or, the person may bend at the hips, knees, and ankles, keeping the back straight, and lift the object mainly with the leg muscles, (see Fig. 99–16B) if there is sufficient strength in the leg muscles.[31, 32] A person might elect to use a combination of these two methods, employing both back and lower extremity muscles (see Fig. 99–16C). Overall temperament and manner may dictate how a person will perform a specific task (Figs. 99–16 to 99–18).[33] Using a combination of upper and lower extremity efforts plus the paraspinal muscles places less stress on the lumbar region. Proper form utilizes various joints and also relates to the speed with which the movement at the joint occurs (Figs. 99–17 and 99–18).

Joint Structure. It is estimated that each year the joints of our lower extremities undergo approximately 2 million oscillatory cycles solely in the act of walking. Even under this extreme loading condition, for up to 80 years, most of our lower extremity joints do not wear out.[34] The joint lubricant, synovial fluid, and articular cartilage are built to withstand the interarticular frictional forces created. The biochemical composition and geometric distribution of water and organic matrix within the articular cartilage provide conformational load-bearing. The subchondral trabecular bony bed that the cartilage sits on absorbs

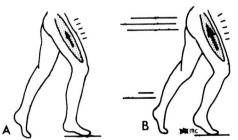
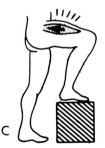
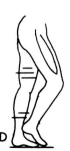

Figure 99–15. The muscle activity of the quadriceps depends on the type of activity that is being performed, that is, the early stance phase of walking (A), running (B), and going up stairs (C), and the early swing phase of walking or running (D).

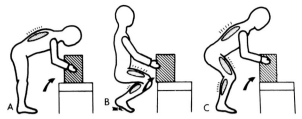

Figure 99–16. A person attempting to lift a box off the floor may utilize hip, trunk, and arm motions (A); hip, knee, and ankle motions (B); or a combination of all of these (C). Muscles needed, and the magnitude of the force from each that is required, depend on which method the individual chooses.

some of the shock of impulsive loading.[35] Each aspect of the joint structure is optimized to allow joint movement to occur, reduce the mechanical forces that it must withstand, and provide nourishment and protection.

Minimization of Frictional Forces. Rotational movements of a joint create a sliding motion of one articular surface on another. Such motion could create shear or frictional forces between the two surfaces, causing joint breakdown; yet joints do not wear down by rubbing.[36]

Frictional force is defined as the resistance one moving surface exerts on the other to impede its progress.[37] Such resistance depends on compressional load, the composition of the materials, and the characteristics of the lubricant interposed between the two surfaces (Fig. 99–19). The resistance to movement may be quantified by a dimensionless number called the "coefficient of friction." The lower this number, the more slippery is the movement of

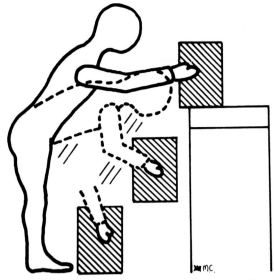

Figure 99–18. Whatever method a person chooses to utilize when lifting a box off the floor, different speeds may be employed during different intervals of the act. Changes in speeds require muscles to control both weight and inertial acceleration and deceleration, creating additional, often unnecessary forces and stresses across the joints if "improper form" is used.

the two surfaces, and the lower the shear forces created between them. Good man-made joints, such as steel-on-steel lubricated by oil, operate at coefficients of friction between 0.1 and 0.5. Biologic diarthrodial joints operate at coefficients of friction of approximately 0.002, nearly one hundredth that of what humans can at present design![38, 39] Thus, if a walking 70-kg man creates a 200-kg compressive force across the lower extremity joint, the shear or frictional force at the joint would be only 0.4 kg. The low frictional forces that minimize surface wear ap-

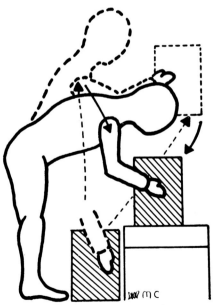

Figure 99–17. Whatever muscles a person chooses to utilize when lifting a box off the floor, nonpurposeful movement may be employed, such as overshooting the table and then setting the box back down. Muscles needed for such unnecessary movements create forces and stresses across respective joints.

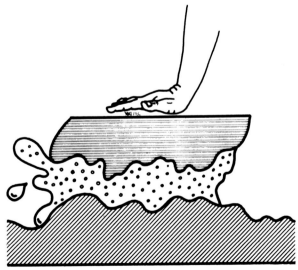

Figure 99–19. The ease with which one surface may be slid over another is dependent on the compressive load, the characteristics of the two opposing materials and their surfaces, and the nature of the material interposed between the two surfaces.

pear to be related to a number of biologic constructs of the joint. The porous deformable collagen surface is arranged with its surface fibers parallel to the surface of the joint. This orientation is ideal for preserving surface integrity as it strongly resists shear forces tending to disrupt the surface by pulling the fibers apart.[40, 41]

Articular cartilage, with an intact surface layer but without any fluid imbibed within it, has a coefficient of friction of 0.3.[42] If saline is added, the cartilage imbibes the fluid like a sponge; and when the wet cartilage surfaces slide against each other, the coefficient of friction is reduced to as much as 0.010.[38] If glycoprotein molecules, called "lubricin," which naturally occur in synovial fluid, are added to the saline, the coefficient of friction is further reduced to 0.002.[43] The self-pressurized fluid squeezed out of the fluid-soaked cartilage,[44] and the lubricin in the synovial fluid, are the major features that reduce the frictional forces so effectively that the articular surface sees little shear stress at its surface. How the various lubricating mechanisms interact to produce low levels of frictional resistance is still a matter of controversy. Many theories have been proposed[45–47]; common to all is the movement of fluid in and out of the porous cartilage. McCutchen[44] postulated that as the cartilage is compressed, the fluid from within seeps out and forms a self-pressurized layer separating the two surfaces. Theoretical evidence and in vitro tests from Mow and associates[47, 48] suggest that in the trailing area of compression, fluid is imbibed into articular surface, while at the leading edge where compression is developing, fluid is expressed (Fig. 99–20).

The lubrication mechanisms in joints are so efficient that in normal joints frictional forces do not appear to be a cause of articular cartilage breakdown.

Maximization of Contact Area. The breakdown of any mechanical structure depends on the total force and the area over which it is loaded. For

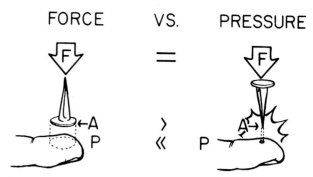

Figure 99–21. An individual's response to a tack pressed into a finger is dependent on the pressure of stress that the tack exerts at the skin. The force may be the same whether the point of the tack or the head of the tack is pressed against the skin, but the skin will feel worse when the same force is exerted over a small area (point).

example, if a tack is pressed into a person's finger, the person's reaction will depend on whether the point or the flat part of the tack is being pushed into the skin (Fig. 99–21). Joint structures are designed to provide an increasing contact surface with increasing forces to keep articular compressive stress minimal.

Joints provide this contact area in different ways.[49–51] In all joints, under load, the articular cartilage under contact is squeezed down (i.e., it compresses). The load-bearing contact area of the knee becomes greater with increasing loads because the menisci come into play and increase the contact area.[52–54] The contact area of the tibiotalar joint increases with load-sharing of the fibulotalar joint.[55] Articular cartilage and subchondral bone can withstand only so much pressure. Physiologic joint pressure approximates 5.0 MN per square meter,[56] and pressures in all joints are equivalent. Even though the contact areas of the small joints of the hands and feet are smaller, so are their compressive loads.

Resistance to Compressive Stresses. Cartilage is constructed in an ideal way to withstand compressive stresses.[57] It has two components: a liquid and a solid. The liquid is a dialysate of synovial fluid and is incompressible but can flow.[58, 59] However, for this fluid to withstand the compressive loads that joints sustain, it must be contained. The cartilage matrix grossly resembles a sponge with multiple pores. The small diameter[60] of these functional pores and their arrangement in circuitous "tunnels," created by the hydrophilic collagen and proteoglycan matrix components, prevent large molecules from entering the cartilage and offer considerable resistance to interstitial fluid flow (Fig. 99–22).[61, 62] These characteristics provide adequate containment for the fluid to support the load.

At any instant, only a part of the joint is load-bearing or compressed. If one part is in compression, the adjacent area is being stretched and pulled apart. This places high compressive and tensile stresses on the organic matrix of cartilage.

Although there is agreement as to the tangential parallel arrangement of the collagen fibers on the

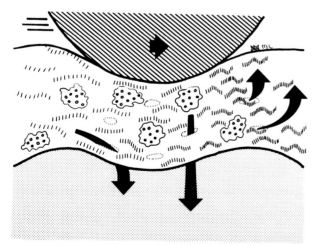

Figure 99–20. To minimize the resistance of moving one cartilage surface over another, the porous cartilaginous surface is layered with viscous macromolecules but primarily weeps synovial fluid dialysate at the leading edge, absorbs this fluid in the trailing area, and deforms in the "area of contact," allowing the two cartilaginous surfaces to be kept apart.

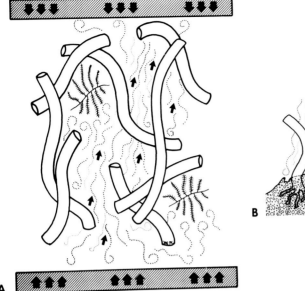

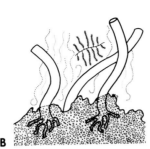

Figure 99–22. Cartilage is composed of a liquid and a multicomponent solid consisting of collagen and hydrophilic proteoglycan molecules. In the middle layer *(A)* the mechanical and electrical properties and architectural design of the solid "contain" the fluid, preventing it from being compressed while still allowing fluid flow, providing nourishment for cartilage cells. In the deepest zone *(B)*, although the content of proteoglycans decreases, the collage is secured tightly to subchondral bone similar to liquid-solid properties.

surface of the articular cartilage and the perpendicular ones at its base, controversy about the arrangement of the collagen in the middle zone of articular cartilage persists. Some say the arrangement is random and when the joint is loaded it becomes more parallel to the surface.[63] Others claim that the midzone collagen is mainly vertical, as Benninghoff originally suggested almost 100 years ago.[64, 65] In either case, the midzone fibers alter their alignment under compression to provide maximal resistance against load. Such changes allow the matrix to accommodate the imposed loads, decrease the pore size, and increase resistance to fluid flow through the cartilage, with the permeability of the tissue (ease of flow) decreasing exponentially.[62] The mechanical strength of cartilage increases as greater loads are imposed.[66] The greater the depth of the cartilage layer examined, the larger the importance of these relationships.[67, 68]

The electrical properties of proteoglycans and their interaction with the surrounding substances contribute to the material properties of the articular cartilage. The carboxyl and sulfate groups of the glycosaminoglycan are endowed with highly polyionic charge characteristics.[66, 69] The charge correlates with the fixed negative charge density found in articular cartilage, which increases with depth from the surface. The large, fixed proteoglycan molecules are highly charged and attract a large volume of water, which tends to neutralize the fixed negative charge. Under compressive loads, water is pushed out of the zone of highest pressure, allowing the cartilage to compress and increasing its fixed charge density. This increases the resistance to the flow of such fluid away from it, increasing the mechanical strength of the cartilage. When the pressure is removed, the fixed negative charge osmotically attracts water, and the cartilage regains its precompressed thickness. Under most circumstances this fluid flow, under pressure, allows articular cartilage to compress

under load without permanent damage to its matrix.[66]

In light of the preceding discussion, it is easy to understand how enzymatic destruction of cartilage matrix in arthritic (primarily inflammatory) joint conditions can lead to cartilage destruction.[70] In osteoarthritic (primarily mechanical) joint deterioration, it is believed that repetitive impulsive-loading damages the matrix.[71] In this circumstance, the compressive load is applied too rapidly for the interstitial cartilage water to have the time to flow, and the cartilage matrix is then subjected to compression and fails in fatigue.[72]

Additional Resistance to Compressive Loads. The articular cartilage rests on a layer of calcified cartilage, supported by a subchondral bone plate. This plate is supported by subchondral trabecular bone whose lattice arrangement follows the major stress trajectories of the transmitted load.[73] The trabecular bone density is related to the quantity of the habitually transmitted load. The articular ends of the joints are expanded to increase their potential contact area and thus diminish the articular stress. Trabecular bone is ten times more compliant than cortical bone,[74] and micromotion of the subchondral trabecular bone and subchondral plate aids in joint conformation under load[75] and can probably help absorb impulsive loads if they are not applied too quickly.[76]

As an example, at the hip (Fig. 99–23) the concave acetabulum, under low loads, contacts with the head of the femur about its periphery. As the load increases, the surface tends to flare out for maximum joint confinement under load.[77] Movement of the marrow and some bending of the acetabular and femoral head trabeculae allow subchondral deformation without matrix damage.[78] However, at very high rates of loading, there is insufficient time for the marrow to flow, and the trabecular bone can be subjected to microdamage. This microdamage, with

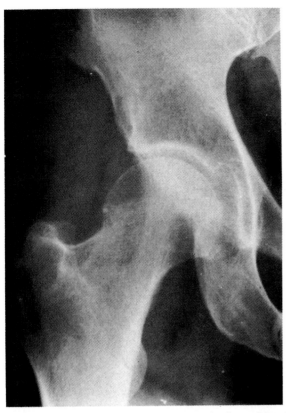

Figure 99–23. At the hip, trabecular bone in the femoral head is concentrated along an axis 160 degrees to the vertical, where the greatest concentration of forces occurs. In contrast, the trabecular bone on the acetabular side flares out to occupy an area greater than the joint's contacting surface, distributing the same forces over a wide area and thereby reducing the stresses and allowing some of the stresses to be absorbed by bone deformation.

repetitive impulsive-loading, can accumulate and lead to fatigue failure.[72] The repair of the subchondral bone damage stiffens the trabecular structure. This process also turns on once dormant endochondral ossification, which duplicates or widens the tidemark base on which the articular cartilage rests. The articular cartilage is thinned at the expense of ossification. This thinning of the articular cartilage increases the shear stress, particularly in its depth, which can lead to fragmentation[79] (see Chapter 78).

The ability of the subchondral bone to absorb compressive loads provides added protection for the cartilage under most circumstances. Although cartilage is very compliant, even in its normal state it is not thick enough to deform adequately to absorb impulsive loads.[80] It is felt that idiopathic mechanically induced progressive cartilage loss requires subchondral plate thickening and cartilage thinning as a prerequisite.[81] (see Chapter 78).

BIOMECHANICS OF JOINT DEGENERATION

Under normal conditions, joints last. Nature's marvelous mechanical architecture allows most in-dividuals years of good service from their joints. Yet, under certain circumstances, these structures can wear out. This loss is remarkably disabling. Proper restoration requires therapeutic modalities that consider the joint as an organ and that respect the physiologic inter-relationships of its tissue.

Normal function of any joint requires that all structures (cartilage, bone, ligaments, synovium, capsule, and muscle) act in combination to allow smooth steady motion while maintaining stability. Alteration of any individual component alters the delicate balance and can lead to mechanical breakdown of the joint. Although many factors may initiate cartilage damage, by definition it is mechanical factors that lead to the progressive joint dysfunction known as osteoarthrosis (see Chapter 78).

Coxarthrosis. More than 1 million people older than 60 years of age have impaired locomotion because of osteoarthritis of the hip (coxarthrosis). Symptoms are often present for many years before the dysfunction becomes disabling.[82–84]

At the hip, the greatest muscle forces in walking arise during the stance phase. These forces are needed to balance the body's weight and inertial forces as the trunk moves over the hip. The body weight is medial to the hip joint on a long fulcrum (see Fig. 99–10). To balance this weight, the trunk shifts laterally to bring the weight closer to the center of the fulcrum.[85, 86] With hip discomfort, an individual tends to reduce walking speed and minimize the muscular effort about the hip. This slowed gait increases the duration of the muscle's action in the gait cycle, unless the stance phase on that side is shortened; thus, an asymmetric gait (limp) is produced (see Chapter 108).

Trunk shift, pelvic drop, slower walking speed, and a shortened stance phase on the involved side are characteristics of the Trendelenburg antalgic gait. In order to reduce forces effectively, the entire body weight cannot be transmitted through the leg. A substitute "peg leg" must be utilized via the use of a cane or crutch.[86]

Such aids to walking can reduce the forces, motions, and pain. Altering gait, however, and the use of a cane may not be enough if the joint is subjected to repetitive impulsive-loading. In most individuals, musculoskeletal protective mechanisms, mainly instantaneous deceleration of the limb just before impact (e.g., just before the heel strikes the floor in gait, or the finger strikes the key in typing) prevent such high loading rates from occurring.[87] Subgroups of individuals have been identified who lack this important protective mechanism. In these individuals, minor incoordination allows the potential impulsive-loading inherent in many activities of daily living to be transmitted to the joints.[88] It is hypothesized that such individuals will go on to progressive joint deterioration in spite of other protective mechanisms.

Secondary coxarthrosis due to congenital, developmental, traumatic, infectious, and other abnormalities can lead to intolerably high compressive stresses on the joint, or shear stresses. Secondary coxarthrosis is thought to be more common than primary coxarthrosis.[89]

Gonarthrosis and Ligamentous Injury. Osteoarthrosis of the knee, gonarthrosis, accounts for almost as great an incidence of locomotion disability as does coxarthrosis.[90] A comparison of the biomechanics of the hip and the knee illustrates how different joints have different safety factors in the balance between the stresses imposed on them and their structural resistance to these stresses. In addition, dysfunction in joint components other than its articular cartilage can cause joint deterioration.

The knee, like the hip, is more frequently involved in secondary osteoarthrosis than in primary osteoarthrosis. The two most common causes of secondary gonarthrosis are malalignment of the lower extremity and instability of the knee. Stability of the knee, under impulsive loads, is the function primarily of the muscles that span the knee joint. Ligaments can act as checkreins but, at the extremes of joint excursion, will be subject to tearing and rupture. Appropriate, timely antagonistic muscle contraction, that is, synchronous coordinated quadriceps and hamstring contraction, can prevent the knee from being impulsively loaded at its extremes of motion, except when the external forces are enormous (e.g., a foot caught in a fixed position while a person is being tackled in American football while deforming pressures are being applied to the knee). The reaction of the muscles to prevent ligamentous rupture must involve a very quick response, too quick for reflexive action to be implicated.[91] Such neuromuscular protection must be preprogrammed and would be effective in situations in which the activity is anticipated, such as in running. It is transient, rapidly applied, unexpected loads that would tend to supersede this preprogrammed muscular control. For example, isolated anterior cruciate rupture occurs in cases of significant anterior sliding of the tibia under the femur. Timely hamstring contraction would prevent such subluxation. It would seem that some patients with isolated anterior cruciate ligament rupture can accommodate for the instability it potentially creates by neuromuscular training.[92]

The knee rotates as it flexes. Decoupling this obligatory flexion-rotation movement by restraining one of the motions while forcing the other will tear a meniscus.[93] As the menisci are load-bearing, significant tears decrease the joint contact area,[94] locally increasing the interarticular stress. If the local stress is too high for the joint tissues to bear, they will fail and osteoarthrosis will result.[95] Although isolated anterior cruciate ligament tears have not been shown to lead to gonarthrosis,[96–99] they do create a circumstance in which it is easier to decouple knee flexion and rotation. Combined anterior cruciate ligament rupture and meniscal tear, frequently associated with stretching or rupture of the medial collateral liga-

ment, are associated with a high incidence of gonarthrosis.[100]

Malalignment of the lower extremity can also lead to interarticular stress concentrations. Knock knees put increased stress on the tibiofemoral compartment; bow legs concentrate stress in the medial compartment. These deformities do not invariably lead to gonarthrosis; other factors such as loss of joint parallelism may also be involved.[88] With an oblique rather than horizontal knee joint, vertical body loads tend to sublux the joint sideways, creating impulsive shear stresses. These will be very damaging to the joint.

An individual can attempt to compensate for knee joint deterioration by reducing the joint load. Decreasing walking speed decreases quadriceps activity.[101, 102] Joint stability (maintenance of knee extension) may be retained by leaning the trunk forward over the knee in the stance phase instead of by contracting the quadriceps. In the coronal plane, the major compensatory action would be a shift of the trunk away from the most involved compartment of the joint.

On the concave side of a varus-valgus angulation (medial collateral ligament when the joint goes into varus, lateral collateral ligament when it goes into valgus), a contracture may result. This contracture further limits the individual's attempt to redistribute joint forces more appropriately.[103, 104] If sufficiently severe, the lack of compensatory mechanisms, along with the other factors previously mentioned, may be accompanied by rapid, unremitting joint deterioration.

Patellofemoral Osteoarthrosis. The most common cause of osteoarthrosis of the patellofemoral joint is recurrent lateral subluxation of the patella. The patella articulates in the femoral trochlear groove, which faces forward. The patella is a sesamoid bone that is part of the quadriceps expansion. It inserts on the tibia through the patellar tendon, which attaches to the anterior tibial tubercle. In a knock knee deformity, the proximal tibia is angled in a lateral direction, and the anterior tibial tubercle is lateral to its usual position, tending to pull the patella laterally out of its groove as the knee flexes (Fig. 99–24). On extension, the patella pops back into its groove. Osteoarthrosis, from repetitive impulsive-loading secondary to this recurrent subluxation, frequently follows.

There is a subtler anatomic cause of patellofemoral osteoarthrosis—rotatory malalignment of the lower extremity. The most common form is associated with anteversion of the femoral neck, a congenital deformity in which the femoral neck is angled further forward than usual. External rotation of the hip, especially in extension, is markedly limited by this deformity. Growing children, while walking, try to compensate for their pigeon-toed internally rotated lower extremities by trying to put their feet straight ahead. Sometimes this compensation is aided by the prescription of shoe wedges or torsional braces. As

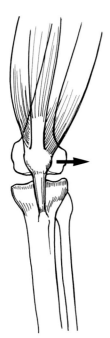

Figure 99–24. In a knock knee (genu valgum) situation, the insertion of the patellar tendon is lateral to the centerline of the limb. This tends to sublux the patella laterally when the quadriceps is contracted.

a child grows, tibial growth compensates with an external rotational deformity, taking the anterior tibial tubercle with it. That means that the insertion of the patellar tendon is lateral to where it usually is, and recurrent lateral subluxation of the patella results.[105]

Arthrosis Secondary to Inflammatory Arthritis. Many factors can contribute to secondary osteoarthrosis. A common cause can be joint destruction from inflammatory causes, such as rheumatoid arthritis. In these conditions, articular destruction may become severe enough to cause loss of joint contact surface or ligamentous failure. These provoke stress concentrations, either in compression or shear, and secondary arthrosis, joint deterioration from mechanical factors, is superimposed. It is of interest that primary mechanical joint deterioration, osteoarthrosis, can itself cause a secondary inflammatory process, particularly in the synovium, as the result of cartilage fragmentation within the intra-articular space.[106]

Low Back Pain. Low back pain epitomizes how difficult it is for the body to compensate for joint damage and mechanical dysfunction. When one considers how each component of this articular system— vertebral bodies, discs, facet joints, ligaments, and muscles—is so specifically designed to control joint stability and motion, it is easy to appreciate why back problems are so difficult to manage. Many different conditions cause low back problems; one of these, "spondylosis," will be used as an illustration (see also Chapter 27).

Spondylosis, osteoarthrosis of the spine, constitutes the leading cause of morbidity in middle age.[107–115] The initial symptom is back pain.[116] The patient compensates for this by trying to reduce the forces across the spinal motion segment (vertebral body–disc–vertebral body) and to reduce spinal movements. Again, as in all joints, the major load is not from body weight but from muscle action. To reduce interarticular force, the use of paraspinal muscles must be decreased in frequency, lessened in magnitude, or both. However, to splint the spine, except while recumbent, the paraspinal and abdominal muscles must function as an internal brace.[117] As long as the patient attempts to function, a vicious cycle is established. Any position, other than lying flat, requires paraspinal muscle contracture, which increases the interarticular pressure and provokes back pain. Back pain leads to additional muscle spasm in an attempt to hold the back still.

The patient's ability to compensate for back pain is extremely limited because if the paraspinal muscle spasm is severe enough even recumbency may not relieve it. Medications, bed rest, heat, and traction can be used to break the cycle. Once the spasm has subsided, the patient can be ambulated with support, such as a back brace or cast. Support applied chronically, however, can cause muscle atrophy, producing more spinal instability and spasm, making it very difficult to wean the patient off the support. Patients with muscle atrophy whose support is taken away have difficulty in stabilizing the intervertebral motion segments,[118] and that creates high strains on the intervertebral disc, facet joints, and ligaments, all of which are innervated with pain fibers.

CONCLUSION

Joint physiology and pathophysiology depend on interactions of tissue biology and biomechanics. Osteoarthritis, mechanically induced joint failure, can be fully understood and treated only if the mechanics of the joints and their compensating mechanisms are appreciated.

References

1. MacConaill, M. A.: The movements of bones and joints. J. Bone Joint Surg. 31B:100, 1949.
2. Poppen, N. K., and Walker, P. S.: Normal and abnormal motion of the shoulder. J. Bone Joint Surg. 58A:195, 1976.
3. Chao, E. Y. S., and Morrey, B. F.: Three-dimensional rotation of the elbow. J. Biomech. 11:57, 1978.
4. McMurty, R. Y., Youm, Y., Flatt, A. E., et al.: Kinematics of the wrist, II. Clinical applications. J. Bone Joint Surg. 60A:955, 1978.
5. Walker, P. S., Shoji, J., and Erkman, M. J.: The rotational axis of the knee and its significance to prosthesis design. Clin. Orthop. 89:160, 1972.
6. Laurin, C., and Mathiev, J.: Sagittal mobility of the normal ankle. Clin. Orthop. 108:99, 1975.
7. O'Connor, J., Shercliff, T., and Goodfellow, J.: The mechanics of the knee in the sagittal plane. Mechanical interactions between muscles, ligaments, and articular surfaces. In Muller, W., and Hackenbruch, W. (eds.): Surgery and Arthroscopy of the Knee. New York, Springer-Verlag, 1988.
8. Simkin, P. A., Graney, D. O., and Fiechtner, J. J.: Roman arches, human joint, and disease: differences between convex and concave sides of joints. Arthritis Rheum. 23:1308, 1980.

9. Radin, E. L.: The physiology and degeneration of joints. Semin. Arthritis Rheum. 2:245, 1973.
10. Benedict, J. V., Walker, L. B., and Harris, E. H.: Stress-strain characteristics and tensile strength of unembalmed human tendon. J. Biomech. 1:53, 1968.
11. Menschik, A.: The axes of the knee-joint in motion. Manuscript, 1975.
12. White, A. A., III, and Raphael, I. G.: The effect of quadriceps loads and knee position on strain measurements of the tibial collateral ligament. An experimental study on human amputation specimens. Acta Orthop. Scand. 43:176, 1972.
13. Sylvia, L. E.: A more exact measurement of the sagittal stability of the knee joint. Acta Orthop. Scand. 46:1008, 1975.
14. Marshall, J. L., Girgis, F. G., and Zelko, R. R.: The biceps femoris tendon and its functional significance. J. Bone Joint Surg. 54A:1444, 1972.
15. Parke, W. W., and Schiff, D. C. M.: The applied anatomy of the intervertebral disc. Orthop. Clin. North Am. 2:309, 1971.
16. Markolf, K. L., and Morris, J. M.: The structural components of the intervertebral disc. A study of their contributions to the ability of the disc to withstand compressive forces. J. Bone Joint Surg. 56A:675, 1974.
17. MacNab, I.: The traction spur. An indicator of segmental instability. J. Bone Joint Surg. 53A:663, 1971.
18. Morris, J. M.: Biomechanics of the spine. Arch. Surg. 107:418, 1973.
19. Kapandji, I. A.: The Physiology of Joints. 2nd ed. Edinburgh, E. R. S. Livingstone, 1970.
20. Cleland, J.: The shoulder-girdle and its movements. Lancet 1881, p. 293.
21. Saha, A. K.: Theory of Shoulder Mechanism. Springfield, IL, Charles C. Thomas, 1961.
22. Somerville, E. W.: Paralytic dislocation of the hip. J. Bone Joint Surg. 41B:279, 1959.
23. Dec, J. B., Inman, V. T., and Eberhart, M. S.: The major determinants in normal and pathological gait. J. Bone Joint Surg. 35A:543, 1953.
24. Denham, R. A.: Hip mechanics. J. Bone Joint Surg. 41B:550, 1959.
25. Flatt, A. E.: The pathomechanics of ulnar drift. Social and Rehabilitation Services Final Report. Grant No. RD, 226m, 1971.
26. Johns, R. J., and Draper, I. T.: The control of movement in normal subjects. Bull. Johns Hopkins Hosp. 115:447, 1964.
27. Basmajian, J. V., and Latif, A.: Integrated actions and functions of the chief flexors of the elbow. J. Bone Joint Surg. 39A:1106, 1957.
28. Barnett, C. H., and Harding, D.: The activity of antagonist muscles during voluntary movement. Ann. Phys. Med. 2:290, 1955.
29. Elftman, H.: Biomechanics of muscle with particular application to studies of gait. J. Bone Joint Surg. 48A:363, 1966.
30. Bigland, B., and Lippold, O. J. C.: The relation between force, velocity, and integrated activity in human muscles. J. Physiol. 123:214, 1954.
31. Farfan, H. F.: Muscular mechanism of the lumbar spine and the position of power and efficiency. Orthop. Clin. North Am. 6:135, 1975.
32. Davis, P. R.: Posture of the trunk during the lifting of weights. Br. Med. J. 5114:87, 1959.
33. Davis, P. R., Troup, J. D., and Barnard, J. H.: Movements of the thoracic and lumbar spine when lifting: A chondrocyclophotographic study. J. Anat. 99:13, 1965.
34. Sokoloff, L.: The Biology of Degenerative Joint Disease. Chicago, University of Chicago Press, 1969.
35. Radin, E. L., and Paul, I. L.: Importance of bone in sparing articular cartilage from impact. Clin. Orthop. 78:342, 1971.
36. Radin, E. L., and Paul, I. L.: Response of joints to impact loading. I. In vitro wear. Arthritis Rheum. 14:356, 1971.
37. Naylor, H.: Bearings and lubrication. Chart. Mech. Eng. 12:642, 1965.
38. Linn, F. C., and Radin, E. L.: Lubrication of animal joints, III: the effect of certain chemical alterations of the cartilage and lubricant. Arthritis Rheum. 2:674, 1968.
39. Simon, S. R., Paul, I. L., Rose, R. M., and Radin, E. L.: "Stiction-friction" of total hip prostheses and its relationship to loosening. J. Bone Joint Surg. 57A:226, 1975.
40. Muir, H., Bullough, P., and Maroudas, A.: The distribution of collagen in human articular cartilage with some of its physiological implications. J. Bone Joint Surg. 52B:554, 1970.
41. Kempson, G. E., Freeman, M. A. R., and Swanson, S. A. V.: Tensile properties of articular cartilage. Nature 220:1127, 1968.
42. Jones, E. S.: Joint lubrication. Lancet 226:1426, 1934.
43. Radin, E. L., Swann, D. A., and Weisser, P. A.: Separation of a hyaluronate-free lubricating fraction from synovial fluid. Nature 228:377, 1970.
44. McCutchen, C. W.: Mechanism of animal joints. Sponge-hydrostatic and weeping bearings. Nature 184:1284, 1959.
45. Walker, P. S., Dowson, D., Longfield, M. D., et al.: Boosted lubrication in synovial joints by fluid entrapment and enrichment. Ann. Rheum. Dis. 27:512, 1968.
46. MacConaill, M. A.: The movements of bones and joints. J. Bone Joint Surg. 31B:100, 1949.
47. Mansour, J. M., and Mow V. C.: On the natural lubrication of synovial joints: normal and degenerate. J. Lubr. Technol. 99:163, 1977.
48. Torzilli, P. A., and Mow, V. C.: On the fundamental fluid transport mechanisms through normal and pathological articular cartilage during function. II. The analysis, solution and conclusions. J. Biomech. 9:587, 1976.
49. Bullough, P. G., Goodfellow, J. B., Greenwald, A. S., et al.: Incongruent surfaces in the human joint. Nature 217:1290, 1968.
50. Oberlander, W.: On biomechanics of joints. The influence of functional cartilage swelling on the congruity of regular curved joints. J. Biomech. 11:151, 1978.
51. Simon, W. H., Friedenberg, S., and Richardson, S.: Joint congruence. A correlation of joint congruence and thickness of articular cartilage in dogs. J. Bone Joint Surg. 55A:1614, 1973.
52. Kettelkamp, D. B., and Jacobs, A. W.: Tibiofemoral contact area: determination and implications. J. Bone Joint Surg. 54A:349, 1972.
53. Maquet, P. G., Van de Berg, A. J., and Simoret, J. C.: Femorotibial weight-bearing areas. Experimental determination. J. Bone Joint Surg. 57A:766, 1975.
54. Walker, P. S., and Erkman, J. J.: The role of the menisci in force transmission across the knee. Clin. Orthop. 109:184, 1975.
55. Greenwald, A. S., and Matejczyk, M.-B.: A contact area study of the human ankle joint. Orthop. Rev. 6:85, 1967.
56. Walker, P. S.: Human Joints and Their Artificial Replacements. Springfield, IL, Charles C. L. Thomas, 1977.
57. Freeman, M. A. R.: Articular Cartilage. New York, Grune & Stratton, 1974.
58. MacConaill, M. A.: The movement of bones and joints. IV. The mechanical structure of articulating cartilage. J. Bone Joint Surg. 33B:251, 1951.
59. Linn, F. C., and Sokoloff, L.: Movement and composition of interstitial fluid of cartilage. Arthritis Rheum. 8:481, 1965.
60. McCutchen, C. W.: The frictional properties of animal joints. Wear 5:1, 1962.
61. Hayes, W. C., and Mockros, L. F.: Viscoelastic properties of human articular cartilage. J. Appl. Physiol. 31:562, 1971.
62. Mansour, J. M., and Mow, V. C.: The permeability of articular cartilage under compressive strain and at high pressures. J. Bone Joint Surg. 58A:509, 1976.
63. McCall, J.: Load deformation response of the microstructure of articular cartilage. In Wright, V. (ed.): Lubrication and Wear in Joints. London, Sector Publishing Limited, 1969.
64. Benninghoff, A.: Form und bau der gelenkknorpel in ihren beziehungen zur funktion. I. Die modellierenden und formerhaltenden faktoren des knorpelfeliefs. Zeit. Gest. Anat. 76:43, 1925.
65. Bullough, P. G., Yawitz, P. S., Tafra, L., and Boskey, A. L.: Topographical variations in the morphology and biochemistry of adult canine tibial plateau articular cartilage. J. Orthop. Res. 3:1, 1985.
66. Maroudas, A.: Physico-chemical properties of articular cartilage. In Freeman, M. A. R. (ed.): Adult Articular Cartilage. New York, Grune & Stratton, 1974.
67. Bullough, P. G., and Goodfellow, J.: The significance of the fine structure of articular cartilage. J. Bone Joint Surg. 50B:852, 1968.
68. Roth, V., Wirth, C., Mow, V. C., et al.: Variation of tensile properties of articular cartilage with age. Transactions, 24th Annual Meeting of the Orthopedic Research Society, Dallas, TX, 1978, Vol. 3, p. 9.
69. Rosenberg, L.: Cartilage proteoglycans. Fed. Proc. 32:1467, 1973.
70. Smith, R. L.: Soluble mediators of articular cartilage degradation in juvenile rheumatoid arthritis. Clin. Orthop. 259:31, 1990.
71. Simon, L. R., Radin, E. L., Paul, I. L., and Rose, R. M.: Response of joints to impact loading. II. In vivo behavior of subchondral bone. J. Biomech. 5:267, 1972.
72. Radin, E. L., Parker, H. G., Pugh, J. W., Steinberg, R. S., Paul, I. L., and Rose, R. M.: Response of joints to impact loading. III. Relationship between trabecular microfractures and cartilage degeneration. J. Biomech. 6:51, 1973.
73. Wolff, J.: Virchows Arch. 50:389, 1870.
74. Radin, E. L., Paul, I. L., and Lowy, M.: A comparison of the dynamic force-transmitting properties of subchondral bone and articular cartilage. J. Bone Joint Surg. 52A:444, 1970.
75. Radin, E. L., and Paul, I. L.: The biomechanics of congenital dislocated hips and their treatment. Clin. Orthop. 98:32, 1974.
76. Pugh, J. W., Rose, R. M., and Radin, E. L.: Elastic and viscoelastic properties of trabecular bone: dependence on structure. J. Biomech. 6:475, 1973.
77. Goodfellow, J. W., and Bullough, P. G.: Studies of age changes in the human hip joint. J. Bone Joint Surg. 50B:222, 1968.
78. Ochoa, J. A., Heck, D. A., Brandt, K. D., and Hillberry, B. M.: The effect of intertrabecular fluid on femoral head mechanics. J. Rheumatol. 18:580, 1991.
79. Radin, E. L., and Fyhrie, D.: Joint physiology and biomechanics. In Mow, V. C., Woo, S. Y. L., and Ratcliffe, T. (eds.): Symposium on Biomechanics of Diarthrodial Joints. Vol. II. New York, Springer-Verlag, 1990.
80. Radin, E. L., and Paul, I. L.: Importance of bone in sparing articular cartilage from impact. Clin. Orthop. 78:342, 1971.
81. Radin, E. L., Burr, D. B., Fyhrie, D., Brown, T. D., and Boyd, R. D.:

Characteristics of joint loading as it applies to osteoarthrosis. *In* Mow, V. C., Woo, S. Y. L., and Ratcliffe, T. (eds.): Symposium on Biomechanics of Diarthrodial Joints. Vol. I. New York, Springer-Verlag, 1990.

82. McAndrew, M. P., and Weinstein, S. L.: A long-term follow-up of Legg-Calvé-Perthes disease. J. Bone Joint Surg. 66A:860, 1984.
83. Ordeberg, G., Hansson, L. I., and Sandstrom, S.: Slipped capital femoral epiphysis in southern Sweden: long-term result with closed reduction and hip plaster spica. Clin. Orthop. 220:148, 1987.
84. Crawford, A. W., and Slovek, R. W.: Fate of the untreated congenitally dislocated hip. Orthop. Trans. 2:73, 1978.
85. Johnston, R. C., Brand, R. A., and Crowinshield, R. D.: Reconstruction of the hip. A mathematical approach to determine optimum geometric relationships. J. Bone Joint Surg. 61A:639, 1979.
86. Blount, W.: Don't throw away the cane. J. Bone Joint Surg. 38A:695, 1956.
87. Radin, E. L., Yang, K. H., Whittle, M. W., Jefferson, R. J., and O'Connor, J. J.: The generation and transmission of heelstrike transient and the effect of quadriceps paralysis. *In* Gait Analysis and Medical Photogrammetry. Oxford, Oxford Orthopaedic Engineering Center, 1987.
88. Radin, E. L., Yang, K. H., Reigger, C., Kish, V. L., and O'Connor, J. J.: Relationship between lower limb dynamics and knee joint pain. J. Orthop. Res. 9:398, 1991.
89. Murray, R. O.: The aetiology of primary osteoarthrosis of the hip. Br. J. Radiol. 38:810, 1965.
90. Cracchiolo, A.: Statistics of total knee replacement. Clin. Orthop. Rel. Res. 120:2085, 1976.
91. Sjolander, P.: A Sensory Role for the Cruciate Ligaments. Umea University Medical Dissertations, Umea, 1989.
92. Nicholas, J. A.: Personal communication, 1970.
93. Radin, E. L., Simon, S. R., Rose, R. M., and Paul, I. L.: Practical Biomechanics for the Orthopaedic Surgeon. New York, John Wiley & Sons, 1979.
94. Radin, E. L., Maquet, P., and DeLamotte, F.: Role of the menisci in the distribution of stress in the knee. Clin. Orthop. 185:290, 1984.
95. Freeman, M. A. R.: Pathogenesis of Osteoarthrosis: A Hypothesis in Modern Trends in Orthopaedics. London, A. G. Apley, 1972.
96. Hughston, J. C., Cross, M. J., and Andrews, J. R.: Classification of lateral ligament instability of the knee. J. Bone Joint Surg. 56A:1539, 1974.
97. Hughston, J. C., Andrews, J. R., Cross, M. F., et al.: Classification of knee ligament instabilities. Part I: The medial compartment and cruciate ligaments. J. Bone Joint Surg. 58A:159, 1976.
98. Hughston, J. C., Andrews, J. R., Cross, M. J., et al.: Classification of knee ligament instabilities. Part II: The lateral compartment. J. Bone Joint Surg. 58A:173, 1976.

99. Radin, E. L.: Factors influencing the progression of osteoarthrosis. *In* Ewing, J. W. (ed.): Basic Science and Clinical Symposium on Articular Cartilage. New York, Raven Press, Ltd., 1989.
100. Fairbanks, T. J.: Knee joint changes after meniscectomy. J. Bone Joint Surg. 30B:665, 1948.
101. Reilly, D. T., and Martens, M.: Experimental analysis of the quadriceps muscle force and patello-femoral joint reaction force for various activities. Acta Orthop. Scand. 43:126, 1972.
102. Zdravkovic, D., and Damholt, V.: Knee and quadriceps function after fracture of the femur. Acta Orthop. Scand. 42:460, 1971.
103. Kostuik, J. P., Schmidt, O., Harris, W. R., and Wooldridge, C.: A study of weight transmission through the knee joint with applied varus and valgus loads. Clin. Orthop. 108:95, 1975.
104. Kettelkamp, D. B.: Clinical implications of knee biomechanics. Arch. Surg. 107:406, 1973.
105. Radin, E. L.: Anterior tibial tubercle elevation in the young adult. Orthop. Clin. North Am. 17:297, 1986.
106. Chrisman, O. D., Fessel, J. M., and Southwick, W. O.: Experimental production of synovitis and marginal articular exostoses in the knee joints of dogs. Yale J. Biol. Med. 37:409, 1965.
107. Snook, S. H., and Ciriello, V. M.: Low back pain in industry. ASSE J. 17:17, 1972.
108. Bond, M. B.: Low back injuries in industry. Indust. Med. Surg. 39:204, 1970.
109. National Center for Health Statistics: Prevalence of Chronic Skin and Musculo-skeletal Conditions, United States 1969. Series 10, No. 92.
110. Rowe, M. L.: Low back pain in industry. J. Occup. Med. 11:161, 1969.
111. National Center for Health Statistics: Limitation of Activity Due to Chronic Conditions, United States 1969 and 1970. Series 10, No. 80, 1973.
112. National Center for Health Statistics: Types of Injuries. Incidence and Associated Disability, United States 1965–1967. Series 10, No. 57, 1969.
113. Rowe, M. L.: Low back disability in industry: updated position. J. Occup. Med. 13:476, 1971.
114. Horal, J.: The clinical appearance of low back disorders in the city of Gothenburg, Sweden. Acta Orthop. Scand. Suppl. 118:1, 1969.
115. Kosiak, M., Aurelius, J. R., and Hatfield, W. F.: Backache in industry. J. Occup. Med. 8:51, 1966.
116. Hirsch, C.: Etiology and pathogenesis of low back pain. Isr. J. Med. Sci. 2:362, 1966.
117. Morris, J. M., Lucas, D. B., and Bresler, B.: Role of the trunk in stability of the spine. J. Bone Joint Surg. 43A:327, 1961.
118. Lucas, D. B., and Bresler, B.: Stability of the ligamentous spine. Technical Report Series 11, No. 40, Biomechanics Laboratory, University of California, Berkeley and San Francisco. The Laboratory, December 1960.

Chapter 100
Sports Medicine

Arthur L. Boland
Jonathan T. Deland

Injuries resulting from recreational activities are common clinical problems confronting physicians in their offices and hospital emergency rooms. Acute traumatic injuries to ligaments and musculotendinous units may occur in any age group and lead to functional disability if not promptly diagnosed and appropriately treated. Likewise, repetitious athletic activities may insidiously cause damage to periarticular tissues, especially tendons and bursae, producing pain, gradual restriction of motion, and troublesome limitation of function. To recognize and manage accurately these traumatic and overuse syndromes, one must be familiar with the specific anatomic features of the involved joints, the common mechanisms of injury, the physical demands of specific athletic activities, the relevance of the clinical signs and symptoms, and the acceptable treatment options. It is important to realize that pain experienced near one joint may be referred from an adjacent joint or the spine. Musculotendinous or capsular contractures about the hip, for example, may elicit discomfort in the thigh or knee; similarly, tightness of the gastrocnemius–soleus muscle complex may result in symptoms about the foot and ankle. These observations necessitate that care be taken to regain flexibility and strength throughout the body, not just at the level of injury. Following immobilization, potentially troublesome weaknesses and contractures may develop not only in the involved extremity, but also in the contralateral limb. These changes, when either overlooked or unsuspected, can lead to recurrent or related problems as the patient attempts to return to preinjury activity. Thus, adequate rehabilitation is a important aspect of the treatment of musculoskeletal injuries.

GENERAL ANATOMIC CONSIDERATIONS

Joint function is dependent on a number of complex inter-related factors. These include (1) the specific bone joint geometry and associated intra-articular structures (meniscus, labrum), (2) the static ligamentous support, (3) the dynamic musculotendinous units, (4) the neurovascular structures, and (5) developmental abnormalities.[1–7] Each joint has a degree of static stability determined by its bone geometry plus its capsular and ligamentous support. Thus, the hip and elbow joints with their relatively stable articulations are less prone to ligamentous strain and subsequent instability than are the loosely

constrained shoulder and knee joints. The major ligaments about joints are oriented to guide joints through a functional range of motion, resisting applied distraction, rotation, and shearing forces. Unfortunately, the collagen structure of these ligaments allows only a few millimeters of elongation before their fibers become taut and fail. Forces applied to these ligaments beyond their tensile strength result in ligamentous sprains, from minor to complete disruption. An appreciation of which specific ligaments resist which forces applied to a joint is essential to diagnose joint laxities and estimate potential functional loss. The examining physician must know not only where to locate these ligaments, but also in which position to place the joint when applying clinical stress to assess the degree of ligamentous damage. The evaluation of ligamentous injuries is one of the most difficult clinical tasks for physicians examining patients with acute athletic injuries.

Damage to intra-articular structures, such as the menisci and glenoid labrum, results in significant functional disabilities. These structures assist not only in stabilizing joints, but also in reducing joint compressive loads by distributing the impact uniformly over a larger surface area.[8, 10] Thus, they protect the articular cartilage from unphysiologic loads. During joint motion, they also assist in lubrication by dispersing the joint fluid uniformly over the articular surface. Consequently, joint stability, nutrition, and biomechanics are adversely affected by injuries to these important intra-articular structures.

The musculotendinous units dynamically control joint motion. Sudden overloads to these structures produce disruption of their fibers, most frequently at the musculotendinous junction. Classified as strains, they result in hemorrhage and necrosis, followed by an inflammatory repair process. Severe muscle strains can cause residual muscle weakness and fibrous contractures, which significantly affect joint function during strenuous activities.[11] Loss of flexibility, for example, in the hamstrings or the quadriceps muscle may result in abnormal loads through the patellofemoral joint, producing degenerative changes in the articular cartilage, increased subchondral pressure, and patellofemoral pain. Repetitious activities such as rowing, running, and throwing can produce acute tenosynovitis and bursitis. The subsequent inflammatory response results in swelling, tenderness, and crepitus. Among the major causative factors leading to bursitis and tendinitis are the lack of flexibility and inadequate muscle strength to withstand repeated athletic demands.[12]

Neurovascular injuries resulting from direct trauma or entrapment are troublesome diagnostic problems.[13, 24] A thorough evaluation of these conditions may require electromyography (EMG), determination of nerve conduction times, compartment pressure evaluations, and arteriography.

Finally, joint function can be significantly affected by unrecognized developmental congenital malformations.[15, 16] Scoliosis, leg length inequality, rotational deformities of the extremities, subtalar coalitions, and pronated feet may go undetected until symptoms develop following strenuous athletic or occupational activities. These conditions, which significantly alter joint biomechanics, must be considered in evaluating individuals with acute or chronic pain syndromes. To avoid diagnostic errors, one must therefore be aware of the intra-articular, ligamentous, musculotendinous, neurovascular, and developmental factors that affect joint function. Most importantly, one must examine the entire patient, assessing carefully the alignment of the spine and extremities in both stance and gait.

SHOULDER INJURIES

Specific Injuries

Glenohumeral Subluxation

History. Glenohumeral subluxations occur commonly in young adults and frequently lead to significant disability.[17, 19] The mechanism of injury is similar to that of an anterior shoulder dislocation, often from a fall or contact injury with the arm in abduction and external rotation. The patient describes a "slipping" in the shoulder accompanied by sudden pain. Frequently the patient does not seek medical advice after this initial injury. When the pain subsides, the individual has little trouble until again required to use the arm with force in the abducted, externally rotated position. Activities such as throwing, serving a tennis ball, and swimming lead to recurrent sub-

luxation, pain, and more capsular laxity. The glenohumeral capsular ligaments are the major restraints that prevent subluxation (Fig. 100–1). Laxity of the shoulder results in a sensation of instability and lack of confidence in the shoulder. This has been referred to as "dead arm syndrome."[166-167]

Physical Examination. If the patient is seen shortly after an episode of subluxation, there will be tenderness anteriorly over the joint capsule. As the arm is passively brought into abduction and external rotation, the patient experiences apprehension and resists further motion in that plane. Pain and weakness are often found on resisted contraction of the external rotator cuff muscles. Crepitus in the anterior capsule is often noted when the shoulder is abducted. The crepitus may be caused by the humeral head and by tears in the anterior glenoid labrum. One must be careful to evaluate the axillary nerve to rule out neuropraxia. Injuries to the axillary nerve result in weakness of the deltoid and loss of sensation over the lateral surface of the shoulder.

Diagnostic Tests. Routine radiographs are frequently normal. Occasionally, however, a small avulsion fracture is noted along the anterior inferior rim of the glenoid (Fig. 100–2). An arthrogram[20-22] may show enlargement of the capsular recesses anteriorly and inferiorly to the coracoid process. Computed tomography (CT) scan may be helpful in detecting injuries to the glenoid labrum.[168, 169] Magnetic resonance imaging (MRI) of the shoulder has been helpful in detecting post-traumatic damage in the rotator cuff tendons.

Treatment. Treatment of the acute primary subluxation is immobilization of the arm in a sling to allow the capsular tissues to heal. Following immobilization, a rehabilitation program should be initiated to strengthen the rotator cuff muscles, especially the subscapularis muscle. Because the rate of recurrence is extremely high even when proper treatment has been given, the patient should be advised to avoid strenuous activities with the arm in the abducted and externally rotated position. Those individuals who have functional disability from recurrent subluxation may require surgical correction. At the time of the surgery, damage to the glenoid labrum,

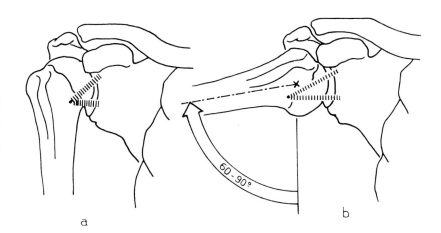

Figure 100–1. The anterior inferior and anterior middle glenohumeral ligaments are relaxed when the shoulder is in neutral (*a*) and become taut in abduction (*b*). (Reproduced with permission from Kapandji, I. A.: Physiology of the Joint. Paris, Editions Maloine, 1970.)

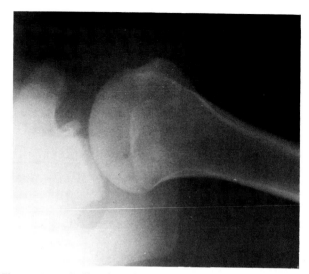

Figure 100–2. Axillary lateral view of the shoulder, demonstrating bony changes along the anterior rim of the glenoid in a patient with recurrent anterior subluxations.

loose bodies, and attenuation of the anterior capsule are commonly encountered. Results of surgical correction are predictably good, although the patient may have some restriction of external rotation postoperatively, depending on the specific procedure carried out.[18]

One must also recognize that after repeated overhead activities, especially in those individuals with generalized ligamentous laxity, multidirectional instability may develop. This condition has been described[146] and requires careful evaluation because stabilizing only the anterior capsule may make this condition worse. At times one may encounter an individual who subluxes primarily posteriorly.[23] This occurs when the arm is forced into an adducted and internally rotated position. Young people who lift weights in the bench press position may aggravate this condition by forcing the humeral head out into the capsule posteriorly. Avoiding the position and strengthening the external rotators are advised.

Acromioclavicular Separations

History. Acromioclavicular (AC) separations result from a fall or a blow on the top of the shoulder.[24–26] As the shoulder girdle descends, the clavicle is restrained by the first rib, resulting in damage to the AC and coracoclavicular ligaments. The first-degree or mild AC separation is characterized by injury only to the AC capsule and no detectable separation of the joint clinically or radiographically. There is marked tenderness and soft tissue swelling over the AC joint. When the involved arm is adducted, pain is reproduced at the injury site. In the more severe injuries, the coracoclavicular ligaments as well as the AC capsule are disrupted. In these second-degree and third-degree separations, the distal end of the clavicle is elevated. These

deformities are noted when compared with the uninjured side. Careful assessment of the neurovascular structures around the shoulder should be conducted to exclude potential complications such as brachial plexus injuries.

Diagnostic Tests. Radiographs should always be obtained to rule out a fractured clavicle. Comparison films of the uninjured shoulder are necessary to detect minor subluxations. Stress films taken with weights attached to the wrists may be helpful to define the severity of the injury.

Treatment. Treatment of the first-degree AC separation is symptomatic and includes ice, compression pad, and a sling. When the pain and swelling have begun to subside in 5 or 6 days, the patient can begin a rehabilitation program. This initially consists of range of motion exercises, begun in a supine position to avoid the force of gravity. When motion is regained, a strengthening program can be initiated to restore power to the entire shoulder region.

The more severe second-degree and third-degree AC separations require a more prolonged period of immobilization or surgery.[26, 27] If the separation can be reduced by depression of the clavicle, immobilization may be continued using a shoulder harness. If the reduction cannot be maintained or if the patient remains symptomatic, surgical correction may be indicated. Many orthopedists favor a nonoperative approach to second-degree and third-degree AC separations, with a functional rehabilitation program before deciding on the need for surgery.[30, 31] Symptomatic degenerative changes can develop in the AC joint following even minor AC separations.[28, 29] Follow-up radiographs may show joint narrowing or erosive changes in the distal clavicle (Fig. 100–3).[32, 33] When chronic pain is experienced as the arm is used in the adducted and forward flexed position, excision of the distal portion of the clavicle is indicated and successful.

Overuse Syndromes

Anatomic Considerations. The strenuous and repetitious shoulder motions required to throw, serve a tennis ball, and swim frequently result in damage to the capsule, the rotator cuff tendons, and bursa in the subdeltoid region of the shoulder.[16, 35–42] Impingement syndromes, rotator cuff injuries, bicipital tendinitis, and chronic subdeltoid bursitis have been discussed in Chapter 26. These pathologic changes also occur in athletes who are involved in sports in which the arm is repeatedly brought first into abduction, extension, and external rotation followed by a forceful acceleration into forward flexion, adduction, and internal rotation. The throwing mechanism is divided into the cocking, acceleration, and follow-through phases[19, 46, 64] (Fig. 100–4). In the initial cocking motion, the external rotators, deltoid, and rhomboids abduct, extend, and externally rotate the

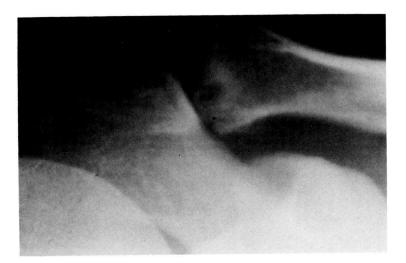

Figure 100–3. Radiograph demonstrating AC joint narrowing and subchondral cystic changes in the distal clavicle.

shoulder. Injuries to the infraspinatus and teres minor musculotendinous unit can occur as the arm is brought suddenly back into this position. The anterior capsule and subscapularis muscle are elongating during the cocking phase and are placed under considerable passive stretch. As this motion is repeated, the anterior capsule may become attenuated, allowing the shoulder to sublux anteriorly.[44] Injuries to the glenoid labrum and to the intra-articular portion of the biceps tendon, which assists in stabilizing the humeral head in the glenoid, can occur with these transient subluxations. As the arm comes rapidly forward during the later acceleration phase of

throwing, the subscapularis muscle actively contracts to bring the arm into forward flexion, adduction, and internal rotation. The posterior rotator cuff muscles are under considerable stress as they contract to decelerate the arm during the follow-through phase. Posterior capsular as well as anterior capsular laxity may result from these rigorous motions. The subtle subluxations that occur during the throwing motion may cause damage to the intra-articular labrum and articular cartilage. Consequently, injuries to the capsular attachment, the musculotendinous units, and the intra-articular components of the joint can result from this vigorous throwing activity.

Another mechanism of injury to the arm as it is brought from the abducted, externally rotated position into forward flexion and internal rotation is the impingement of the subdeltoid bursa and rotator cuff tendons, particularly the supraspinatus, under the overlying coracoacromial arch.[36, 39] The anterolateral aspect of the acromion and the firm coracoacromial ligament form the superior restraints above the humeral head. Repeated impingement on these structures may produce recurrent microtrauma causing hemorrhage and edema, followed by an inflammatory reaction, fibrosis, and eventually rupture of the rotator cuff tendons. Throwing and swimming the freestyle and butterfly strokes produce a forceful adduction motion. During this phase, the blood supply to the distal attachment of the rotator cuff tendons is impaired.[37] Vascular injection studies of the supraspinatus muscle reveal that it receives its blood supply from vessels coming from the muscle proximally and extending distally into its tendinous component.[47, 48] These studies suggest that when the arm is in the adducted position, pressure from the humeral head below produces an obstruction to normal blood flow into the distal tendinous segment. Consequently, in swimming and throwing there is not only repeated impingement of the supraspinatus and subdeltoid bursa under the coracoacromial arch, but also a repetitious ischemia to these vulnerable tendons. These mechanical and vascular factors contribute significantly to the pathologic changes that

THE PITCHING ACT

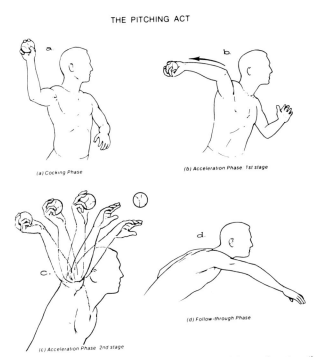

(a) Cocking Phase

(b) Acceleration Phase 1st stage

(c) Acceleration Phase 2nd stage

(d) Follow-through Phase

Figure 100–4. Diagram depicting the cocking (a), acceleration (b and c), and follow-through (d) phases of the throwing act. (Reproduced with permission from Woods, G. W., Tullos, H. S., and King, J. W.: The throwing arm: Elbow joint injuries. J. Sports Med. 1:43, 1973.)

result in these painful shoulder syndromes in athletes.

History. The overuse shoulder injuries are usually characterized by the insidious onset of pain. The symptoms are experienced initially after practice or participation in the activity. As the changes become more severe, the pain is present during the activity and eventually becomes disabling, preventing participation. Characteristically, the patient has difficulty localizing the exact site of the pain. Not infrequently the discomfort is experienced over the anterior/superior aspect of the shoulder and later appears in the posterior capsule. At other times, it may radiate down toward the humeral attachment of the deltoid. Occasionally the athlete perceives a clicking or crepitation within the shoulder from labral tears or subluxation. Attempts should be made, by questioning the individual, to determine in which phase of motion the pain is most severe. This may give the physician a clue as to the exact location of the inflammatory response.

Physical Examination. On physical examination the shoulder should be inspected for asymmetry, especially about the scapulothoracic and infraspinatus muscles. Occasionally, axillary[13] suprascapular[14] nerve entrapments can result in obvious weakness and wasting of the deltoid and infraspinatus muscles (see Chapter 26). A careful palpation of the anterior and posterior capsules of the shoulder and of the attachment of the specific rotator cuff muscles while gently rotating the humerus is tedious but rewarding in localizing tenderness. There is typically a painful arc between 70 and 120 degrees of abduction and

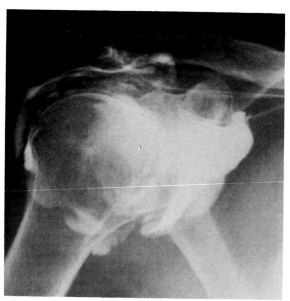

Figure 100–6. Arthrogram of a patient with chronic impingement and rotator cuff tear demonstrating extension of contrast material into the subacromial space.

forward flexion.[36, 37] Resistance to abduction and forward flexion exacerbates the pain. Moving the arm passively into forward flexion and internal rotation frequently elicits pain and occasionally crepitus as the subdeltoid structures impinge on one another under the coracoacromial arch. One should examine the shoulder in the upright and supine positions, looking for instability. A frequent clinical finding is weakness and pain on resisted external rotation in abduction. A careful neurologic examination should be carried out to exclude referred pain or weakness from cervical spine injuries and to determine whether there is any specific weakness in rotator cuff units.

Diagnostic Tests. Routine radiographs are frequently normal, especially in younger age groups. In middle-aged and older athletes, however, degenerative changes in the AC joint, osteophytes under the acromion, sclerosis at the humeral tuberosities, and traction spurs or avulsion fracture around the glenoid may be observed[49] (Fig. 100–5). Double-contrast arthrography[20–22] can help define partial or complete rotator cuff tears (Fig. 100–6), and tomographic[50] studies performed with arthrography can assist in detecting loose bodies or degenerative changes within the glenohumeral joint (Fig. 100–7). CT scans can outline intra-articular pathology such as labrum tears and cartilaginous loose bodies.[51]

Treatment. The treatment of overuse syndromes about the shoulder is symptomatic and dictated by the extent of the injury. In first-degree and mild second-degree injuries in which symptoms occur only after practice and do not affect performance during participation, the treatment should consist primarily of rest, with a reduction of the offending motion. These individuals may be able to tolerate shorter practice sessions with a less vigorous work-

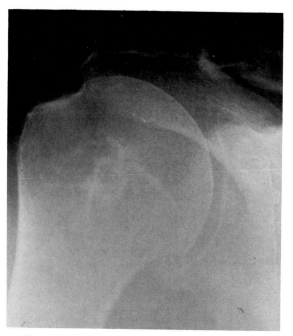

Figure 100–5. Radiograph demonstrating degenerative changes in the AC joint, osteophytes inferiorly on the acromion, and sclerosis of the humeral tuberosities in a patient with symptoms of chronic impingement syndrome.

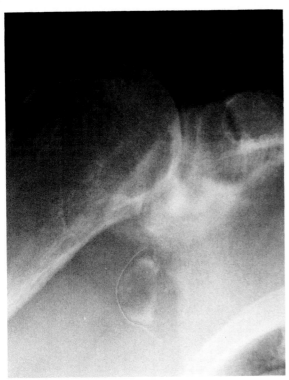

Figure 100–7. Arthrogram demonstrating narrowing of the anterior glenohumeral joint and a large loose fragment with inferior capsule.

out. Ice should be applied for 15 to 20 minutes following each practice, and oral nonsteroidal anti-inflammatory drugs (NSAIDs) are recommended. In the more severe second-degree and third-degree injuries in which the pain is disabling, total rest from the offending activities is necessary. In addition to NSAIDs and ice, ultrasound treatments and injections of local anesthetics and steroids are helpful. It is important to realize that steroid injections into tendons produce local tissue necrosis.[52, 56] Therefore, following injections, athletes should be required to rest for at least 2 weeks to allow adequate regeneration of the tissue. It is much safer and therapeutically more beneficial to inject the subdeltoid bursa rather than the tendons.

Most often these conditions respond to conservative management, especially if the treatment can be started early. An important part of the rehabilitation is strengthening of the shoulder musculature, particularly the rotator cuff group.[57, 58] Many swimmers and throwers exhibit relative weakness in the external rotator muscle group, a finding that may be a significant etiologic factor. Gentle pendulum exercises are initiated first, followed by progressive resistance exercises to the rotator cuff group, the deltoid, and the scapulothoracic muscles (trapezius, rhomboids, latissimus dorsi, and serratus anterior). Because poor swimming, throwing, and serving technique may contribute to the onset of the problem, a coach or instructor should be consulted before allowing the participant to return to practice. Correction of potentially harmful techniques is necessary to avoid recurrences.

In patients who do not respond to conservative treatment, arthroscopy can be helpful in locating rotator cuff tears, and advanced impingement syndromes may require corrective arthroscopic or open surgery.[39, 59, 60] Excision of the coracoacromial ligament, partial anterior acromionectomy, repair of the rotator cuff lesions, and occasionally arthrotomy of the glenohumeral joint for removal of the loose bodies and correction of subluxation may be necessary.

ELBOW INJURIES

Humeral Epicondylitis ("Tennis Elbow")

Anatomic Considerations. Athletic[61–64] and occupational activities may produce painful injuries to the soft tissues about the elbow. Lateral epicondylitis, or "tennis elbow," is perhaps the most common syndrome encountered by physicians treating recreational athletes. Direct trauma or repetitive activities, however, such as using a screwdriver, may also initiate these complaints. Similar pathologic changes and symptoms may also develop on the medial epicondyle from repetitious throwing activities that produce valgus force through the elbow.

The various etiologic factors responsible for tennis elbow are still unclear and controversial.[65–72] The most widely accepted theory is that there is a mechanical overload placed on the common extensor muscle tendon at its attachment on the lateral epicondyle. Repeated contraction of these muscles, producing wrist extension and supination, causes small tears of the extensor aponeurosis followed by inflammatory response. Although some authors believe that the diagnosis is periostitis, routine radiographs rarely reveal periosteal reaction around the lateral epicondyle. Entrapment of the recurrent branch of the radial nerve to the joint has also been considered as a possible cause of lateral epicondylitis.[71, 72]

Mechanism of Injury. Many recreational tennis players note that the backhand stroke reproduces their pain.[65] Improper technique, particularly leading with a flexed elbow, has therefore been incriminated as a major cause of lateral epicondylitis. Poor tennis hitting techniques, improper size of the racquet grip, excessive tension on the racquet strings, and improper weight of the racquet are all factors that have been discussed and are difficult to analyze and evaluate objectively. Most recreational tennis players, however, have relative weakness of their extensor muscle groups compared with the flexor mass, making overload of the extensors more likely in these inadequately conditioned players. Evaluation of the experienced professional tennis players, on the other hand, reveals a much higher incidence of medial epicondylitis.[77] Medial injuries are associated with the serve, which resembles the throwing motion. In both of these activities, there is a significant valgus force through the elbow, placing the medial collateral ligament and the flexor musculotendinous units under considerable tension.

History. Epicondylitis may develop insidiously or from an acute overload. The pain is clearly localized to either the medial or the lateral epicondyles, with occasional radiation into the forearm. Shaking hands, opening doors, and direct contact all reproduce the pain.

Physical Examination. On examination there is localized tenderness over the involved medial or lateral epicondyle. When the lateral side is involved, resistance to wrist extension and supination reproduces the pain. When the medial epicondyle is involved, resistance to wrist flexion and pronation often produces pain. Because there is an inflammatory response within the extensor aponeurosis resulting in contracture of the muscle unit, passive extension of the elbow when the wrist is held in flexion and pronation will maximally stretch the extensor group and produce pain. Similarly, extension of the elbow with the wrist supinated and extended will often reproduce symptoms of medial epicondylitis.

A careful neurologic examination should be performed to rule out entrapment of either the medial or the ulnar nerves. Pronator teres syndrome can be encountered, in which the median nerve is entrapped as it passes through that muscle. This condition often produces sensory and motor changes distally in the hand similar to those noted with carpal tunnel syndrome. EMG and nerve conduction studies may be required to confirm this diagnosis. Throwing and serving at tennis may lead to damage to the ulnar nerve on the medial side of the elbow.[77, 78] The valgus overload may produce subluxation of the ulnar nerve from its groove or simply mechanical impingement and inflammation without subluxation. There may be local tenderness over the ulnar groove with dysesthesias extending into the forearm and hand. An examination should be made for weakness of the intrinsic hand muscles and sensory changes in the fourth and fifth fingers. Although collateral ligament injuries of the lateral side of the elbow are uncommon, repeated valgus forces through the elbow in throwing and serving a tennis ball may produce an acute or a chronic strain of the medial collateral ligament. It is difficult to diagnose this injury because the flexor muscle mass overlies the medial collateral ligament. If the tenderness appears to be deep to the flexor mass and if there is pain on valgus stress of the elbow, one can more confidently entertain a diagnosis of medial collateral ligament injury. The injuries may coexist and should be suspected.

Diagnostic Tests. Radiographic examination for lateral epicondylitis is most frequently normal. In cases of medial epicondylitis in growing children, however, one must look carefully for widening or separation of the medial epicondylar apophysis. "Little League elbow" is characterized by separation of this medial epicondylar apophysis from valgus forces (Fig. 100–8) and chondral and osteochondral defects in the radial capitellar joint from compressive loads.[73–76] In the mature individual with chronic medial epicondylitis, particularly the baseball pitcher, degenerative changes may be noted in the elbow joint, with loose bodies near the olecranon and traction spurs along the medial side of the trochlea. Arthrotomograms and CT scans may be helpful in localizing loose bodies and chondral injuries within the joint.

Treatment. The treatment of tennis elbow is conservative, with rest being the most important component initially. When the pain is severe, splinting the elbow in 90 degrees of flexion for 3 to 5 days will help reduce the acute inflammation and pain. Prolonged immobilization, however, should be discouraged. Oral NSAIDs, ultrasound, and ice will also assist in relieving the inflammatory response. Ultrasound with 10 percent hydrocortisone cream (phonophoresis) may also be helpful. Local injections of bupivacaine hydrochloride and steroids can be useful when the pain is acute and well localized. One should again keep in mind the complications of steroid injections. Subcutaneous fat necrosis can result in unsightly and painful scars around the elbow.

When local pain and tenderness have subsided, a muscle strengthening and flexibility program is

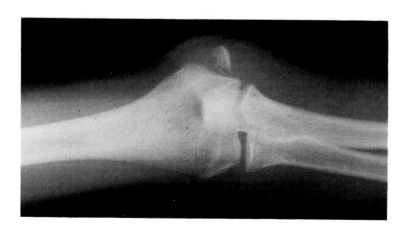

Figure 100–8. Radiograph demonstrating an avulsion fracture of the medial epicondyle in a skeletally immature baseball pitcher.

essential to avoid recurrence.[65] Isometric wrist extension and flexion exercises should be initiated as soon as they can be performed painlessly. Passive stretching of the extensor groups by extending the elbow with the wrist flexed and pronated is also essential. Gradual progressive resistance exercises should be continued with weights until the extremity has returned to a normal functional level of strength. The patient should return to activity gradually, first hitting against the backboard for 5 to 10 minutes and then progressively increasing this time over the next several days until the patient is confident that he or she can hit all strokes comfortably to avoid recurrence. Application of ice after participation is encouraged along with a conscientious stretching program.

Because poor technique and improper equipment may be related to tennis injuries, patients with these injuries who want to resume these sports should consult with an instructor to determine if their tennis racquet and techniques are correct. The use of a forearm band may be helpful in reducing the tension through the extensor muscle mass.[65] With early and proper conservative treatment of tennis and throwing injuries of the elbow, there is rarely need for surgery. It is not uncommon, however, for chronic epicondylitis to take 6 to 12 months to become asymptomatic. In the occasional incapacitating chronic epicondylitis that is unresponsive to conservative treatment, release of the extensor aponeurosis, exploration of the joint with removal of loose bodies, or partial synovectomy may be indicated.

Olecranon Bursitis

Acute traumatic olecranon bursitis may develop from a direct blow to the elbow, resulting in marked swelling from hemorrhage within the bursal sac. Aspiration will often relieve acute pain and swelling but must be done with proper sterile technique. When the aspirant is not bloody, cell counts and cultures should be obtained. One must consider gout, rheumatoid arthritis (RA), and sepsis in the differential diagnosis of acute or chronic bursitis. Following aspiration, a compressive elastic (Ace) bandage is usually sufficient to keep the bursa decompressed. Special pads may be constructed to protect the elbow and prevent recurrences. Cases of recurrent chronic olecranon bursitis with fibrosis of the bursa may require surgical excision.

Trochanteric Bursitis

Anatomic Considerations. Acute trochanteric bursitis produces pain over the lateral side of the hip and proximal thigh. This bursa lies over the lateral aspect of the greater trochanter and under the tensor fasciae latae. The gluteus maximus muscle posteriorly and the tensor fasciae latae muscle anteriorly com-bine to form a bipennate muscle mass, which then extends distally as the iliotibial band.[2] This band eventually attaches to the lateral aspect of the tibia.

History. With prolonged sitting or repeated hip flexion and extension, the tensor fasciae latae is compressed over the greater trochanter, producing a mechanical inflammation of the underlying bursa. At times it is associated with a snapping sensation as the band slips over the bony prominences of the trochanter. Sitting in a deep chair or car seat often exacerbates the pain. The discomfort often radiates along the lateral aspect of the thigh, producing symptoms suggestive of sciatica. In acute severe cases, motion of the hip is so painful that the condition can mimic an acute septic arthritis or synovitis of the hip.

Physical Examination. Examination reveals maximum tenderness laterally over the greater trochanter with extension of the tenderness distally for a few inches below the trochanter. With the hip in extension, gentle internal and external rotation of the hip is less painful than that experienced with a septic hip or acute synovitis of the hip. Hip flexion and rotation are painful in trochanteric bursitis, and the patient experiences pain walking.

Diagnostic Tests. A normal white blood cell count, erythrocyte sedimentation rate (ESR), and temperature help exclude an infectious process. Routine anteroposterior and lateral radiographs of the hip may show some soft tissue swelling lateral to the trochanter, but the hip capsule should not appear distended, as is seen in intra-articular conditions of sepsis or synovitis. In young children, one must always consider early osteomyelitis developing in the metaphyseal bone near the trochanter. Appropriate laboratory tests and the clinical course are helpful in diagnosing this condition.

Stress fractures[79-81] (Fig. 100–9) and avulsion fractures (Fig. 100–10) should be considered in athletes with hip pain. Discomfort in the anterior hip and groin in runners can be caused by stress fractures of the femoral neck, pubic rami, or subtrochanteric region of the femur. Radiographs are typically normal during the first 4 to 6 weeks after the onset of symptoms. Bone scans,[82] however, are abnormal early in the clinical course and should be ordered if this diagnosis is suspected. Children sustain avulsion fractures of the lesser trochanter, anterior iliac spine, and ischial apophysis more frequently during running and jumping activities. The diagnosis of a slipped femoral capital epiphysis must be considered whenever an adolescent develops the sudden or gradual onset of hip, thigh, or knee pain. This is a serious injury, which requires prompt diagnosis and treatment. These patients have painful limitation of hip motion, especially internal rotation, and often complain of pain extending down toward the knee. Comparison radiographs of the asymptomatic hip may be necessary to detect these conditions. Frog lateral films are most helpful diagnostically.

Treatment. The treatment of acute trochanteric bursitis is rest, application of ice, NSAIDs, and often

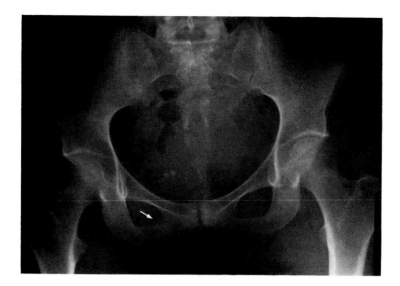

Figure 100-9. Radiograph of a jogger demonstrating a stress fracture of the inferior pubic ramus.

an intrabursal injection of a local anesthetic agent and steroid. Ultrasound treatments may also be helpful in relieving inflammation. A partial weight-bearing crutch gait is suggested until the patient can walk comfortably without assistance.

One must be diligent in looking for an underlying biomechanical cause of the trochanteric bursitis. Leg length inequalities, producing a pelvic obliquity and prominence of the trochanter on the long side, result in increased mechanical pressure from the overlying fascia lata. Jogging can cause contractures of the tensor fasciae latae muscle, resulting in snapping of the iliotibial band over the trochanter. These contractures must be stretched out with a proper physical therapy program to avoid recurrence of the bursitis. Leg length discrepancies should be balanced by a lift placed in the shoe on the short side. With prompt and proper symptomatic treatment, combined with the correction of any contractures with physical therapy, patients with trochanteric bursitis recover satisfactorily. On rare occasions, however,

surgical release of the tight fascia over the trochanter may be indicated.

KNEE INJURIES

The common knee injuries sustained in athletics involve the menisci, the articular cartilage, the ligamentous structures, and the musculotendinous units. By careful history taking and examination, the injured structures can most often be isolated. In significant trauma, it is important to note that more than one structure may be injured. Examination should therefore include consideration of all the various possibilities.

Meniscal Tears

Anatomic Considerations. The menisci are attached to the tibia peripherally by the coronary

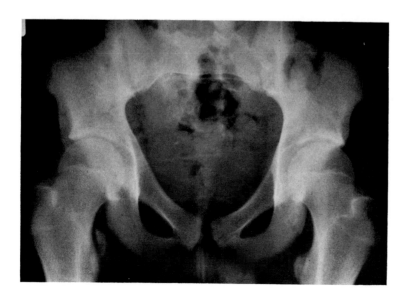

Figure 100-10. Radiograph of a young soccer player demonstrating an avulsion fracture of the lesser trochanter.

ligament in the deep meniscal component of the capsular ligaments. Although the anterior and posterior horns of the menisci of the intercondylar notch are firmly attached, the peripheral fixation allows enough laxity for the menisci to move forward and backward in flexion and extension. The menisci have several important functions. They act to distribute a load evenly over a wide surface. Their wedge shape and capsular attachment also help them function as stabilizers for the knee. Finally, they assist in dispersing the synovial fluid over the articular cartilage and thereby add to joint lubrication and nutrition. These multiple functions underline the importance of the menisci.[8-10]

Mechanism of Injury. The menisci are torn by compressive, rotational, and shearing forces in the knee.[16, 84] These forces can result in different types of tears. A common type is a vertical tear in the meniscal substance or its capsular attachment. Such a tear can be produced by twisting into a deep knee position. Distraction causes peripheral separation of the meniscus from its capsular attachment. This type of tear occurs in varus or valgus type injury. Horizontal cleavage type tears occur with an increased incidence in patients who are middle-aged or older. These tears often occur in a setting of a mild arthritis and can result from a relatively trivial compressive and rotational injury.[85] A combination of these different types of tears is not uncommon. Double tears as well as complex tears can occur. Such tears present a challenge to the orthopedist who is trying to preserve as much meniscal function as possible.

History. The history can range from a description of a tearing or popping sensation in the knee during a period of physical stress to no recall of the original incident. Swelling within 6 to 10 hours indicates bleeding into the knee. If the meniscus is responsible for this, a tear at the peripheral vascular portion of the meniscus should be suspected. An acute hemarthrosis can also be caused by tear of the anterior cruciate ligament, partial tear of the medial collateral ligament, subluxation of the patella, or osteochondral fractures. The swelling, which starts well after the acute incident, is not uncommon and is more consistent with a nonperipheral meniscal tear. Swelling causes the patient to complain of fullness in the knee or loss of flexibility. Specifically, the physician should ask about intermittent painful buckling of the knee, true locking, and inability to extend the knee fully. These are all suggestive but not diagnostic of a meniscal tear. The patient may have one of these symptoms or only vague pain. It is important to note that locking or painful buckling may have other causes. Loose bodies or the stump of an anterior cruciate ligament tear can cause such mechanical symptoms. Thus, although helpful, history alone does not necessarily make the diagnosis of a meniscal tear.

Physical Examination. An appropriate history with specific joint line tenderness is the hallmark of a meniscal tear. This is particularly true of medial meniscal tears. The examiner should palpate precisely along the joint line with the knee flexed at 90 degrees and compare the tenderness to that on the opposite knee. The same procedure is done on the lateral side, noting particularly tenderness anterior or posterior to the fibular collateral ligament. Unfortunately, with the presence of the popliteal tendon as well as the fibular collateral ligament, tenderness is not as frequently elicited in the lateral meniscal tear. Swelling and any small decrease in the range of motion should be noted. A decrease in motion not attributable to swelling is suggestive of a meniscal tear. Two dynamic tests can be used to help make the diagnosis of a tear. With the lower leg hanging over the side of the table, a forceful external rotation of the lower leg will often cause pain in the case of the medial meniscal tear. This test is not appropriate in the setting of a medial collateral ligament injury, which would also cause pain. A click palpated at the joint line while the knee is spontaneously rotated, flexed, and compressed by the foot is known as a McMurray's sign. Although a true McMurray's sign is not present in the majority of cases, when present, it is highly suggestive of a tear.

Diagnostic Tests. Routine radiographs should be taken. These include anteroposterior, lateral, and tunnel views as well as a 30 degree sunrise view of the patellofemoral joint. The radiographs can help exclude osteochondral fractures of the patella, loose bodies, avulsion of the tibial spines, osteochondritis dessicans, or in the case of considerable trauma, a tibial plateau fracture. Although arthroscopy has become a popular diagnostic tool, arthrography[21, 22] is still useful and less expensive (Figs. 100–11 through 100–14). It can locate peripheral tears or aspects of a complex tear that may be missed at

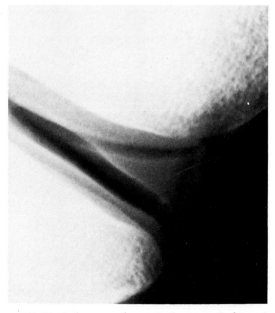

Figure 100–11. Arthrogram demonstrating a vertical tear in the vascular peripheral portion of the medial meniscus.

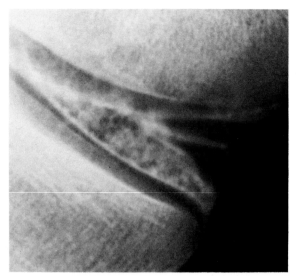

Figure 100–12. Arthrogram demonstrating a horizontal tear extending into the avascular portion of the medial meniscus.

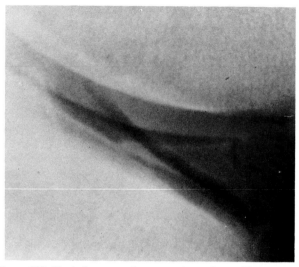

Figure 100–14. Arthrogram demonstrating a long oblique tear in the medial meniscus.

arthroscopy. Arthrography should be arranged electively after the patient has started to rehabilitate the knee and after swelling and pain have begun to subside. Accuracy of this test is dependent on the technique and experience of the radiologist. In expert hands, accuracy is more than 90 percent, with accuracy for lateral meniscal tears being somewhat less than for medial meniscal tears. MRI may in the future prove as useful as arthrography in meniscal tears. Diagnostic arthroscopy[86, 87] may be indicated when routine radiographs and arthrograms are inconclusive and the knee remains symptomatic.

Treatment. Because of motion and lack of blood supply, meniscal tears usually do not heal. The tears that are likely to heal are small tears in the peripheral vascular portion of the meniscus. Thus, a patient who is having symptoms after an injury should have an arthrogram or be referred to a specialist. The treatment of a meniscal tear is nonemergent except

for the locked knee. If the knee has a sizable limitation to the range of motion that is not attributable to swelling, the knee should be arthroscoped within 7 to 14 days of the injury. A sizable limitation is considered not being able to reach within 10 degrees of full extension in a knee with no or minimal effusion. A knee that is left in flexion for weeks can develop a flexion contracture that is difficult to eliminate. In such a locked knee, an arthrogram need not be done. If a near full range of motion is present and other injuries have been adequately checked for, the immediate treatment can be a knee immobilizer and crutches. The presence of a meniscal injury need not be confirmed at this time. Rehabilitation can be started. It should include active range of motion exercises, isometric quadriceps strengthening, and progressive weight bearing as tolerated. If symptoms improve over time, the patient can slowly return to activities as long as he or she is having no pain and has regained full muscle strength. The persistence of symptoms should raise the question of a meniscal injury and indicate arthrography or surgical referral.

When surgery is performed, proper technique retains as much of the meniscus as possible. Arthroscopic evaluation is performed, and only the torn, unstable portion of the meniscus is removed.[93, 95] Thus, a total meniscectomy is no longer common. Long-term follow-up studies of patients who have had meniscectomies indicated that 60 percent of such patients have some type of symptoms by 10 to 15 years after their surgery.[91, 92, 96] At present less of the meniscus is removed, but the long-term follow-up has not been documented. It is anticipated that these patients will be less symptomatic. It has been shown that meniscal tears are related to the development of degenerative arthritis in animal studies and in the clinical setting.[88, 92] In a tear in the peripheral third of the meniscus, meniscal repair, either open or arthroscopic, can be considered.[97–99] The success rate of this procedure declines remarkably in knees that

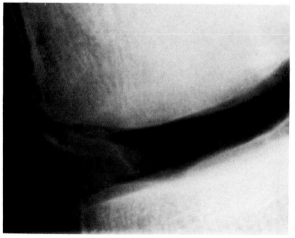

Figure 100–13. Arthrogram demonstrating a vertical tear in the avascular portion of the medial meniscus (bucket handle tear).

are unstable from injuries such as anterior cruciate ruptures. Thus, a meniscal repair is recommended when the type of tear is appropriate and when the knee is stable or being stabilized.

Ligamentous Injuries

Anatomic Considerations. The classification of knee ligament injuries is complex and still undergoing evolution. A detailed classification system is cumbersome, can be confusing, and is presented elsewhere.[85, 100, 101, 185] A more simplified version of simple instabilities is presented here. By being familiar with at least this simplified version, the physician is better able to diagnose injuries.

There are four major ligaments that provide stability in four anatomic directions.[102] These are the cruciate and collateral ligaments and can be called the primary restraints.[149] They are the primary restraints to anterior, posterior, varus, and valgus instability. Secondary restraints are those structures that are next to rupture if force in that particular direction continues. The anterior cruciate ligament provides primary restraint to anterior motion of the tibia on the femur. When ruptured, the lateral and to a lesser extent the medial tibial plateau can be subluxed forward on the femur. The posterior cruciate ligament provides the primary restraint for posterior instability. The medial collateral ligament provides the restraint on the medial side. It thereby is the first line of defense if valgus stress is placed on the knee (i.e., when the lower leg is forced laterally putting tension on the medial side). The lateral collateral ligament protects the lateral side of the knee and is ruptured by varus force.

Unfortunately, most injuries are not sustained in one straight direction. Thus, more than one structure and more than one ligament can be injured at the same time. Other important ligamentous structures include the popliteal-arcuate complex in the posterolateral corner and the semimembranosus complex and posterior oblique ligament in the posteromedial corner. When the primary restraint has been identified as being ruptured, the examiner should consider the possibility of injury to the remaining primary restraints, capsule, and the structures just mentioned. The mechanism of injury, tenderness, and instability tests help guide the physician to injured structures. It is important after examining a patient to be able to identify which structures have sustained injury.

Mechanism of Injury. Valgus force such as may occur in a contact injury to the outside of the knee is a common mode of failure. The medial collateral ligament is the first to fail and then its deeper capsular portion.[103-105] The anterior cruciate ligament is next to rupture. Thus, a combination of a medial collateral ligament and anterior cruciate ligament tear is not uncommon. The other common mode of anterior cruciate ligament failure does not involve the medial collateral ligament.[106, 107] Internal rotation in hyperextension forces the anterior cruciate to be wound tightly around the posterior cruciate and impinge in the intercondylar notch, often resulting in isolated damage to the anterior cruciate ligament. Varus injuries affect not only the fibular collateral ligament, but also the posterolateral corner and finally the cruciate ligaments. The posterior cruciate ligament is most commonly torn in one of two different ways: by hyperextension or by a blow to the anterior tibia when the knee is flexed.

History. The history should include the mechanism of the injury and notation of any previous injury to the knee. The presence of a tearing or popping obviously indicates significant injury to a ligament or possibly the meniscus. Contact injuries to the medial or lateral side frequently result in collateral ligament injury with a possible cruciate ligament tear. Noncontact pivoting and jumping injuries commonly produce an "isolated" tear of the anterior cruciate ligament. The timing of swelling after the injury should be noted. If the swelling occurs within the first 8 to 10 hours, one should consider a hemarthrosis. This is consistent with a diagnosis of an anterior cruciate ligament tear, an incomplete tear of the medial collateral ligament, subluxation of the patella, peripheral separation of the meniscus, or an osteochondral fracture. Swelling that develops later is most often an effusion associated with a tear in the avascular portion of the meniscus, a condylar injury, or a mild sprain of the medial collateral ligament.

Physical Examination. The injured knee should always be compared to the uninvolved knee. The knees should be evaluated for full range of motion and ligamentous laxity. With a healthy knee as a baseline, subtle changes on the injured side can be noted. The degree of swelling and the range of motion should be documented. Next, any tenderness over the collateral ligaments should be located. These structures are directly palpable, and tenderness is easily elicited. On the medial side, the femoral attachment is frequently tender in a mild sprain, whereas in severe sprains the tenderness may be over the tibial portion of the ligament or the entire ligament. On the lateral side, the ligament is best felt in the figure-of-four position with the knee flexed at 90 degrees and a slight varus stress applied. Ligamentous injuries can be simply graded; the following grading system is frequently used for collateral ligament injuries: A grade I injury is without any demonstrable increase in laxity of the ligament. A grade II injury is with an increase in laxity but still with a firm end point. A grade III injury has no good end point attributable to the ligament in question. Grade III injuries of the medial collateral ligament often have less intra-articular swelling as the fluid escapes via the tear. Without a tense hemarthrosis, these more severe injuries can be less painful as well as having less intra-articular swelling.

Each of the primary restraints should be tested

in a position that does not allow the secondary restraints to deceive the examiner.[152] In certain positions, the secondary restraints can make the examiner think the primary restraint is intact when it is not. For example, the medial collateral ligament should be tested for 30 degrees of flexion where the capsule and the cruciate ligaments are more relaxed. In this position, valgus stress is applied by holding the lateral knee and gently forcing the lower leg out to the lateral side. The amount of medial opening felt should be compared with that in the uninjured knee. If medial instability is also noted in full extension, tear of the posterior cruciate ligament and capsule should be suspected as well. The lateral collateral ligament is also tested in 30 degrees of flexion. The lower leg is over the side of the table, so the table as well as the examiner's hand restrains the femur while varus stress is placed in the lower leg. One should watch for opening on the lateral side. The cruciate ligaments are the most difficult to assess. They are not directly palpable, and in the setting of increased anteroposterior motion, it can be hard to label the increased motion as anterior versus posterior. The test for anterior cruciate instability in an acutely injured knee is Lachman's test.[107, 108] With the knee flexed 15 degrees, the hamstrings are palpated to make certain they are lax. With one hand grasping the distal femur and the other the proximal tibia, the tibia is gently pulled anteriorly. Motion significantly more than that of the injured knee or motion of a centimeter or more indicates an anterior cruciate ligament rupture. A pivot shift is used to demonstrate the functional instability and can be difficult to elicit in an acutely injured knee. The posterior cruciate ligament is best tested in 90 degrees of flexion with the posterior capsule relaxed. The drop back of the tibia on the femur should be noted (Fig. 100–15). Palpation anteriorly on the medial femoral condyle down to the prominent anterior lip of the medial tibial plateau is also done. If this lip is dropped back or its absence is not attributable to swelling, a posterior rather than an anterior cruciate injury should be suspected. Again the other knee is used for comparison. In posterior cruciate injuries or knee

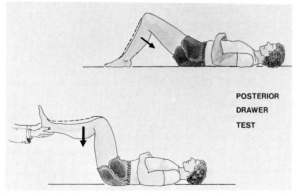

Figure 100–15. Inspection of the knee from the side reveals a posterior drawer or posterior sag, indicating damage to the posterior cruciate ligament.

dislocations, neurovascular examination is essential to exclude damage to the popliteal vessels. Neuropraxia of the peroneal nerves is frequently associated with lateral collateral ligament injury.

Diagnostic Tests. Routine anteroposterior, lateral, tunnel, and 30 degree sunrise radiographic views should be obtained. Both the anterior and the posterior cruciate can be torn off with a fragment of bone from the tibia.[109] A small avulsion fracture of a chip of bone along the lateral tibial plateau (Segond's fracture) is consistent with an anterior cruciate injury. Stress films are not routinely done because the physical examination (if done intelligently) is reliable. Aspiration of the knee joint may be used to decompress a tense hemarthrosis and make a patient more comfortable. Arthrography[21, 22] is generally not used for a diagnosis of ligamentous injuries, although it can visualize structures such as the anterior cruciate ligament. MRI studies are the most accurate nonoperative way to detect damage to the anterior and posterior cruciate ligaments. Examination under anesthesia and arthroscopy are the definitive procedures used to define the extent of intra-articular and ligamentous damage.

Treatment. Incomplete injuries to the medial collateral ligament can be successfully treated conservatively.[111] After 3 to 5 days of immobilization in 30 degrees of flexion in a splint or knee support, the soft tissue swelling and tenderness will begin to recede. Early range of motion exercises and protective weight bearing may be allowed. Crutches should be continued until the patient can fully bend the knee and flex at least to 95 degrees. Ice is applied during the first 48 to 72 hours. During the rehabilitation period, warm whirlpools may be beneficial. It is essential to regain adequate strength in the hamstrings and quadriceps muscles in addition to a full range of motion. Return to participation in sports should not be allowed until pain and tenderness have receded and muscle strength has been regained.[11] Weakness and contractures of the ipsilateral hip can occur after periods of immobilization for knee injury, and the hip must be rehabilitated along with the injured joint.

A complete, isolated medial collateral ligament injury should at least have an appropriate surgical referral. An injury to the lateral collateral ligament is more uncommon. It may be associated with an injury to the posterolateral corner, and surgical consideration should also be given. In general, knees with a complete rupture of a primary restraint or rupture of more than one ligament should be given a surgical referral for evaluation.[101]

Isolated posterior cruciate injuries may be treated conservatively. Unfortunately, good and excellent results from posterior cruciate surgery have not been the rule. The cruciate ligaments, when torn, are usually too disrupted to be repaired successfully by suturing alone but require augmentation with autogenous grafts, allografts, or synthetic supports. Over the next several years, techniques that use stronger, precisely placed grafts may be developed.[153] This may improve the results from posterior cruciate ligament repair or reconstruction.

Repairs with augmentation or reconstruction of an anterior cruciate ligament injury have in the last 5 years shown consistently good to excellent results.[154, 155] The placement of stronger grafts according to isometric principles has produced good results. Despite these results, not every injury should receive surgical treatment. Recreational athletes who are willing to alter their activities need not undergo reconstruction. Activities that put the knee at risk for a giving-way episode of instability include pivoting, jumping, or stopping on the injured leg. Bracing can be helpful but should not be used as a guarantee to a stable knee in sports. In a significant percentage of patients, bracing does not eliminate episodes of giving way in sports. Thus, athletes who want to return to their previous level of function in sports with pivoting and jumping should consider surgical treatment. Because reconstruction has good results, loss of the 7- to 10-day interval for repair with augmentation is not critical. The patient may choose to wait and see how well the knee does after appropriate rehabilitation. If conservative treatment is chosen, the patient should be started on a rehabilitation program that includes muscle strengthening and the use of a brace in sports. Patients should be warned of the possibility of unsuspected meniscal tears or chondral fractures, which if symptomatic, require arthroscopy.[107] If after maximal strengthening and use of a brace, the patient experiences giving way, consideration should be given to reconstruction. In this way, episodes of giving way and possible meniscal tears from instability can be minimized. Perhaps the worst form of treatment is to allow the patient to play sports in a manner that brings about giving-way episodes and thereby puts the patient at further risk for injury to the menisci.

Patellar Tendinitis

History. Patellar tendinitis (jumper's knee)[112, 113] is a disabling inflammation of the attachment of the patellar tendon at the inferior pole of the patella. Commonly seen in young recreational or competitive athletes, it is precipitated by jumping, hurdling, and running. Climbing or descending stairs and deep knee bends may exacerbate the pain. The pain is localized to the area immediately below the patella.

Examination. With the knee in full extension, there is local tenderness at the inferior pole of the patella. This is best identified by depressing the superior pole of the patella and then palpating the inferior pole. This tilts the inferior pole up and allows the tenderness to be more easily located. This tenderness should be compared with that on the opposite knee. These patients often have tight hamstrings, as evidenced by limitation of straight leg raising. The quadriceps mechanism can also be contracted. This

is best noted by placing the patient prone on the examining table, flexing the knee, and demonstrating limited knee flexion. Although routine radiographs are usually normal, irregular calcifications at the inferior pole of the patella may be present. This is similar to the changes noted at the tibial tubercle in Osgood-Schlatter disease.

Treatment. Treatment consists of application of ice and restriction of activity, with particular avoidance of climbing or descending stairs and jumping. Immobilization in a splint is helpful if the lesion is symptomatic with walking. Oral anti-inflammatory drugs are suggested; however, glucocorticoid injections are generally not recommended. If glucocorticoid injections are employed, one must realize these substances produce focal tissue necrosis of the tendon and render the tendon subject to spontaneous rupture if the quadriceps mechanism is stressed.[52]

The most important component of the treatment of the patellar tendinitis is adequate rest until the tenderness has subsided. Stretching of the contracted musculature such as the quadriceps and hamstrings is also particularly important. Persistent contractures in these areas will lead to recurrence of pain when the athlete resumes participation. The patient should not return to sports until pain and tenderness have dissipated. Early return to sports makes the condition all the more difficult to eradicate. The patient should be warned of this and the fact that treatment of the problem can last for several months. When the patient does return to sports, a gradual warm-up period with adequate stretching and the application of ice compresses for 15 to 20 minutes following competition can be helpful. For those resistant to this therapy, if a bone scan is abnormal at the inferior pole of the patella, operative therapy to remove fragments of bone or degenerated tendon can be helpful.

Prepatellar Bursitis ("Housemaid's Knee")

Prepatellar bursitis is commonly seen in contact sports such as wrestling.[114] Traumatic in origin, the swelling of the prepatellar bursa produces the sensation of stiffness and limitation of motion. The swelling is localized to the bursa and does not involve the knee joint itself. When marked swelling occurs, aspiration, followed by compression with a foam rubber pad and elastic (Ace) bandage, is indicated. Compression should be maintained for 3 to 5 days because reaccumulation of fluid in a bursa is common. Protective padding should be worn when the individual resumes participation.

Pes Anserinus Tendinitis Bursitis

The medial hamstring group consists of the sartorius, gracilis, and semitendinosus tendons. These are attached below the flare of the medial metaphysis approximately four fingerbreadths from the joint line. The pes anserinus bursa surrounds these tendons and allows them to glide smoothly over the bony prominence of the tibial metaphysis. Running and jogging activities may result in an acute inflammation of these tendons.[79] The pain is felt along the medial side of the knee, and it can radiate along the posteromedial aspect of the thigh. This is often seen in individuals just after beginning a jogging program. It is also frequently seen in middle-aged or older women who are heavy and have valgus knees. In addition to the local tenderness over the tendons and bursa, the patient often experiences pain when hamstring contractions are resisted and the tendons palpated. This is a helpful diagnostic test. One should look for predisposing factors such as hamstring contractures with limited straight leg raising; genu valgum; an out-toeing gait (external tibial torsion); and the history of beginning a jogging program without adequate time to build up endurance, strength, and flexibility. Occasionally, the semimembranosus, which attaches to the posteromedial aspect of the tibia, is involved and produces pain that can mimic a meniscal injury.

The treatment is symptomatic, using oral anti-inflammatory agents, local application of ice, reduction of activity, and occasionally ultrasound treatments. Local glucocorticoid injections may be helpful in the acute stages. An alternate form of application is to use 10 percent hydrocortisone cream with ultrasound (phonophoresis) for a treatment program involving ten treatments over 3 to 4 weeks. Gentle stretching of any hamstring contractures should also be done. When the pain and tenderness have subsided, a formal rehabilitation program to regain full flexibility and strength of the hamstrings is essential.

Iliotibial Band Syndrome

Recreational athletes frequently develop disabling pain in the lateral aspect of the knee as the result of friction from a tight iliotibial band.[79, 83, 115] This is a particularly common injury in runners. The iliotibial band is a thick fibrous structure and is an extension of the fascia lata in the lateral thigh. It courses over the lateral femoral condyle and attaches to the tibia at Gerdy's tubercle. With repeated knee flexion and extension, the tight band produces rubbing and inflammation of the tissues at the lateral femoral epicondyle (Fig. 100–16). Predisposing factors include tightness of the hip abductor muscles, bowlegs, running regularly on sloping surfaces, and excessive pronation of the feet. The tenderness is localized in the area of the lateral femoral epicondyle.

Treatment. Treatment consists of oral anti-inflammatory agents, application of ice, ultrasound treatment, and stretching of the iliotibial band and hip abductors. In the case of pronated feet, longitudinal arch supports are used. Stretching of the iliotibial band is a particularly important part of the program and can be done under the guidance of a physical therapist. Local injections of glucocorticoids or phonophoresis may be helpful, but correction of any biomechanical factors or training errors is essential to prevent recurrence.

Summary. These various overuse syndromes about the knee are particularly difficult to treat. They develop insidiously and may be the result of several factors. Careful neurologic evaluation should be carried out to exclude the possibility of sciatica from chronic disc disease or spondylolisthesis. Leg length inequalities, contractures about the hip, tightness of

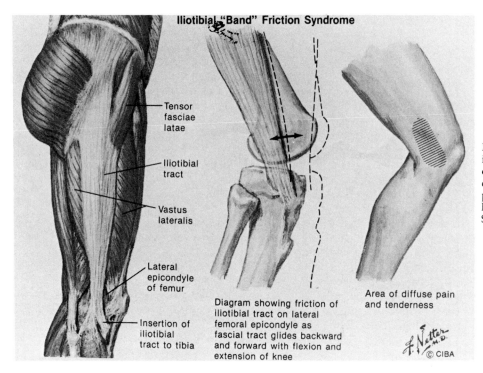

Iliotibial "Band" Friction Syndrome

Tensor fasciae latae

Iliotibial tract

Vastus lateralis

Lateral epicondyle of femur

Insertion of iliotibial tract to tibia

Diagram showing friction of iliotibial tract on lateral femoral epicondyle as fascial tract glides backward and forward with flexion and extension of knee

Area of diffuse pain and tenderness

Figure 100–16. Diagram of how the iliotibial band produces mechanical inflammation of the lateral femoral epicondyle. (Reproduced with permission from Brody, D. M.: Running injuries. CIBA Clinical Symposia 32, No. 4, 1980.)

the hamstrings and quadriceps muscle groups, valgus and varus malalignments of the knee, excessive tibial torsion, and foot deformities may all help produce the abnormal forces that cause so-called runner's knees. One can certainly localize the site of tenderness by examining the knee only. A complete examination of the entire lower extremity and spine, however, is necessary to evaluate the etiologic factors.

Patellofemoral Pain Syndrome

Patellofemoral pain can be one of the most perplexing and difficult knee problems. The complexity of this problem should not be underestimated. Larson[156] has pointed out that the cause of the patellofemoral pain can be divided into three categories. These are (1) abnormalities of the patellofemoral configuration, (2) deficiencies of the supporting muscles or soft tissues, and (3) malalignment of the extremity relating to the knee mechanics. A patient with patellofemoral pain may have any one or a combination of these etiologic factors.[117, 118] Chondromalacia of the patella does not constitute a diagnosis. It describes a softening or destruction of the cartilage on the undersurface of the patella either felt as crepitus on physical examination or seen on direct visualization. Chondromalacia is an end-stage pathologic entity, which has various causes noted previously. A patient should be first described as having patellofemoral pain syndrome. If changes on the undersurfaces of the patella are noted, the term chondromalacia can be used but may not necessarily be related to symptoms. More important, the examiner should then describe the anatomic reasons for the patellofemoral pathology.

Anatomic Considerations. The patella is a large sesamoid bone that articulates with the femur in a groove formed by the trochlea and femoral condyles. The contact areas and the amount of compressive forces through this joint increase with flexion and with contraction of the quadriceps muscle.[117] Different portions of the patella contact the femur at different levels of flexion.[157] Activities performed in flexion, such as running, ascending and descending stairs, squatting, and jumping all dramatically increase the load through this joint to several times body weight. Factors that produce malalignment of the joint cause improper tracking of the patella and eventual pathologic change. These factors can be divided into the patellofemoral configuration, soft tissue support, and extremity alignment categories mentioned earlier. For example, developmental abnormalities such as a shallow trochlear groove, small patella, or patella alta can result in instability of the patella as it enters the trochlear groove. The dynamic control of the patella is through the quadriceps muscles. The vastus medialis, particularly its distal oblique fibers, is the most important stabilizing component of this muscle group because only they pull the patella medially. Weakness of the vastus medialis coupled with overdeveloped vastus lateralis or tightened lateral retinaculum produces a lateral subluxation of the patella. Excessive genu valgum or external tibial torsion also places the patellar tendon attachment lateral to the normal axis of alignment and can contribute to lateral subluxation and abnormal compressive forces. Finally, a hyperextension deformity of the knee can cause patellar instability.

Symptoms. Early in the clinical course, patellofemoral pain syndrome is characterized by a vague, poorly localized discomfort or ache. Often it is difficult to implicate the patella as the cause of the problem. The discomfort is characteristically made worse, however, by prolonged sitting (positive "theater sign") and by descending and ascending stairs. The discomfort is relieved by placing the knees in extension. Clicking and crepitus can be noted by the patient, particularly in such activities as rising from a chair or climbing stairs. Buckling or pseudolocking, resulting from patellofemoral pain or transient subluxation of the patella, is also a common symptom. Pivoting motions may precipitate buckling and pain and make one entertain the diagnosis of meniscal tear. Swelling can occur with an acute lateral subluxation from injury to the medial soft tissues. Chronic swelling with the sensation of stiffness and limitation of motion, however, strongly suggest that there are degenerative changes in the patellofemoral joint. In this setting, the disruption of the cartilage structure and subsequent ingestion of debris by synovial macrophages may cause a synovitis.

Physical Examination. Although the history often definitively localizes the cause of the patient's pain as patellofemoral, confirmation should be sought in the physical examination. Tenderness is often noted while attempting to palpate the medial facet of the patella. Sensitivity can be generalized and noted in the medial and lateral patella retinaculum. With chondromalacia, crepitus is detected with flexion and extension. To detect crepitus, one should place the palm over the patella and passively flex and extend the knee. Pain can often be produced by compression of the patella in extension or during manual resistance to knee extension. In cases of gross patellar subluxation, pressing the patella laterally often produces apprehension as the patient experiences sensation of impending subluxation. If the patient has buckling or pseudolocking symptoms, one must examine for a meniscal problem and check the integrity of the knee ligaments.

When location of the pathologic process in the patellofemoral joint has been confirmed, the cause should be ascertained. The alignment of the patellofemoral joint with the knee in extension can be measured by using a Q angle. This is accomplished by estimating a line along the quadriceps tendon intersected by a line marking the axis of the patellar tendon from the tibial tubercle to the patella.[158] Values of more than 15 degrees indicate an excessive angle and can contribute to a lateral compression syndrome. With the patient sitting and the lower leg flexed 90 degrees over the side of the table, the examiner checks for lateral tilting of the patella and an upward facing patella (patella alta). The tracking of the patella is noted as the knee is actively brought into full extension. Lateral tracking or lateral facing of the patella may be observed. Next, the soft tissues are checked by looking for atrophy of the vastus medialis. A tight lateral retinaculum can be identified by the inability to tip the lateral edge of the patella above the horizontal with the knee in extension. Contractures of the hamstrings and quadriceps are evidenced by limitation of straight leg raising and limitation of passive knee flexion with the patient lying prone. Finally, the examiner checks the overall alignment of the extremity. Contour of the lower extremity should be inspected in supine position, while standing, and during gait. One should look for the presence of genu valgum, external tibial torsion, and hyperextension of the knee.

Radiographic Examination. Although not helpful in every case, a standing anteroposterior radiograph, a lateral view with the knee flexed at 30 degrees, and a patella sunrise view with the knee flexed at 20 to 30 degrees are helpful. On the anteroposterior view, the varus/valgus alignment of the extremity should be measured. On the lateral view, the presence of patella alta or patella baja can be noted. Insall's technique of determining the height of the patella on a lateral view at 30 degrees of knee flexion is a reliable method. The length of the patella on the lateral view versus the length of the patellar tendon from the inferior pole to the tip of the tibial tubercle is measured. The tendon length should be within 80 to 120 percent of the first length.[122] The sunrise view is used to examine the contour of the patellofemoral joint and to look for evidence of unequal wear.[119, 120] In chronic lateral compression of the patella, there may be excessive lateral tilt with sclerosis noted in the subchondral bone of the lateral facet and osteoporosis evident in the medial portion of the patella (Fig. 100–17). Chronic subluxation of the patella may result in avulsion fractures or traction spurs on the medial facet of the patella. Tomograms can be helpful in defining osteochondral fractures or irregularities of the patella and femoral surfaces. Although not in routine clinical use, CT scans of the patellofemoral joint at various flexion angles have been helpful in identifying subtle malalignment problems.[159] Although arthrography can visualize the patellofemoral joint, it is not routinely used. Arthroscopy provides direct visualization of the pathologic changes on the undersurface of the patella. Such changes are noted more frequently than the crepitus on physical examination would indicate. Some surgeons have attempted to use direct visualization of the patellofemoral joint under local anesthesia to document any abnormalities in dynamic tracking.

Treatment. Most patients with patellofemoral disease have minimal radiographic changes and can be treated conservatively. This is particularly true of

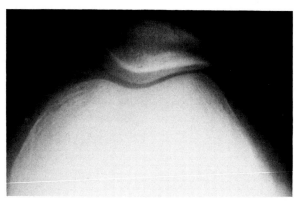

Figure 100–17. Tangential view of the patella, demonstrating lateral patellar subluxation, narrowing of the lateral patellofemoral joint, subchondral sclerosis of the lateral facet, and relative osteoporosis of the medial facet in a patient with patellofemoral pain syndrome.

the young woman with patellofemoral pain. Although bone malalignment is not correctable by a conservative program, rest from certain activities and a change in muscular forces can be helpful. Reduction in activities such as stair climbing, running, bending at the knees, and sitting in a deep knee position should be emphasized. In the rehabilitation program one should seek to correct all musculotendinous contractures noted in the hamstrings, quadriceps, or hip abductors. Quadriceps strengthening exercises are particularly important. They should be done isometrically in full extension with the use of progressive ankle weights up to 15 to 20 pounds. Such a program provides strengthening of the quadriceps with emphasis on the vastus medialis obliquus. Oral anti-inflammatory agents are also helpful. Restraining braces providing support along the side of the patella can minimize symptoms from lateral subluxation.[123] Patients should be warned that the condition is often not quickly alleviated and may take months to improve. Follow-up studies indicate that 80 percent of patients with this condition can be managed successfully by these conservative measures.[121, 122, 160] With minimal radiographic changes, the young patient should have a 6- to 12-month trial of adequate conservative therapy before surgery is considered.

Patients with associated displaced osteochondral fractures of the patella or femoral condyle will require prompt surgical intervention to reduce or excise these fragments and prevent incongruity. Patients who have minimal radiographic changes and who have failed to improve with a good conservative program should be referred for consideration of surgical debridement of the patella and realignment of the extensor mechanism. It is important that the patient has cooperated in the rehabilitation program to show that such a program has been adequately tried and that the patient will cooperate with postoperative rehabilitation. Operative therapy is not uniformly successful and should not be described as a guaranteed solution to the problem.[158] Improvement is gained in 70 to 80 percent of properly selected individuals. Patients should be carefully selected according to identifiable anatomic abnormalities, failure of a conservative program, and ability to cooperate and respond to a postoperative rehabilitation program.

LOWER LEG PAIN

With the present interest in fitness and running, physicians are called on to diagnose troublesome leg pains. The most common problems include shin splints, stress fractures, Achilles tendinitis, and compartment syndromes. Differentiating among these entities is not always easy. Finding the most tender area is important. It is sometimes helpful to see the patient directly after the offending physical activity when the tenderness is most pronounced.

Shin Splints

This condition is more accurately termed posterior tibial stress syndrome.[124, 125] Although the exact cause is debated, the pain and tenderness appear to be localized over the medial border of the tibia at the junction of its proximal two thirds and distal one third. This area is directly in the course of the posterior tibial tendon. Whether this entity represents tendinitis or a periostitis is unknown. It is often associated with excessive pronation of the feet, which during running will place greater stress on the posterior tibial tendon. Many of these patients have associated tight Achilles tendons. Radiographs and bone scans are normal but should be performed in those with persistent pain to rule out stress fractures. The treatment consists of oral anti-inflammatory agents, rest, and proper orthotics to correct any excessive pronation of the feet. Ultrasound treatments and heel cord stretching exercises are helpful. When the tenderness and pain are resolved, the patient can gradually return to activity but should do so with a careful training program. Proper running shoes and training techniques are important. The patient should be referred to one of the many books that describe acceptable training and conditioning programs.

Stress Fractures

Stress fractures are the result of excessive demands coupled with insufficient conditioning.[79, 80] Stress fractures are often seen in the individual who has increased his or her mileage too quickly and not allowed time for the bone to adapt. Given enough time, bone density and strength increase in response to progressive increases in physical training (Wolff's law). Stress fractures commonly occur in the proximal tibia and distal fibula and can also occur in the metatarsals. Direct bony tenderness is noted over the fracture site and is the key to suspecting the diagnosis. Induration may occur. In addition to improper training, other etiologic factors include a tight heel cord and limitation of flexibility in the subtalar joint (cavovarus deformities). Adequate subtalar motion is essential for absorption of compression weight-bearing forces in gait.

Radiographic Examination. Routine radiographs usually do not demonstrate this fracture for at least 4 to 6 weeks following onset of symptoms. Bone scans are the most helpful and are abnormal early in the clinical course.[82, 161, 162]

Treatment. Although no immobilization is necessary, rest is essential. Usually within 6 to 8 weeks, the individuals are comfortable and their tenderness has resolved. At this time, they can resume training in a gradual manner. The underlying biomechanical problems must be corrected with stretching exercises or orthotics and the training modified with a more gradual increase in distance to prevent recurrence of injury.

Achilles Tendinitis

Achilles tendinitis is characterized by pain and swelling along the tendon sheath proximal to its insertion on the os calcis. The condition encompasses a spectrum of pathologic changes, from simple tenosynovitis involving the peritenon to interstitial disruption of the Achilles tendon fibers.[127, 128] Usually gradual in onset, at times it can appear suddenly. The patient notes stiffness with ankle motion and pain with attempts to push off on the ball of the foot. The pain may be noticed during or directly after the activity. On physical examination, there is tenderness and crepitus along the distal third of the Achilles tendon in those patients with acute tenosynovitis. In chronic injuries, an indurated nodule in the tendon may be palpable. Routine radiographs are normal; however, CT or MRI scan may show soft tissue thickening of the tendon.

If the patient is symptomatic when walking, treatment should include crutches with minimal weight bearing or a period of immobilization in a short-leg cast. Oral anti-inflammatory agents, ultrasound treatments, and contrast ice and warm whirlpools may be helpful. Glucocorticoid injections, which may be given around the tendon sheath but not within the tendon, are infrequently recommended. Subcutaneous atrophy and scarring as a result of these injections can be particularly severe complications in this area. A temporary heel lift can be helpful in relieving pain, but this should be combined with a stretching program to regain flexibility in the gastrocnemius–soleus complex. Stretching is an essential part of the rehabilitation program. Finally, a strengthening exercise, performed by lowering the heel over the edge of a stair and then raising on the toes, is helpful in regaining both power and flexibility.

Compartment Syndrome

The muscles of the anterior, lateral, and posterior superficial and deep compartments of the lower leg are surrounded by a tight fascia sheath and buttressed by the tibia, fibula, and intramuscular septum. Although the four compartments just listed are those that have been classically described, the posterior compartment can be even further subdivided.[162] With the repeated muscular activity in an athletic event, the muscles in any one of these compartments may hypertrophy beyond the normal volume and cause increased pressure. This increased pressure results in venous obstruction with edema and subsequently ischemia of the muscles and nerves.[129, 131] The ischemic pain subsides when the individual stops running but recurs when the activity is repeated. When these individuals are examined directly after running, there is tenderness and induration over the involved compartment. If the patient attempts to run through the pain, there may be severe pain with associated dysesthesias and paresthesias, suggesting neurologic involvement. The anterior compartment is most frequently involved. Routine radiographs are normal. A definitive diagnosis can be made by measuring the compartment pressure, using the technique described by Whitesides and Mubarak.[132, 133]

Unfortunately, this condition is difficult to treat conservatively. Rest and a change in the training program should be tried. Those individuals who insist on continuing with their present athletic activities may require surgical decompression by fasciotomy. A less common form of claudication can occur in runners as the result of entrapment of branches of the popliteal artery as they course through the muscles and fascial layers in the back of the calf. These conditions are rare and require arteriography for diagnosis.

Achilles Tendon Rupture

Middle-aged individuals involved in running, jumping, and racquet sports are at risk for an acute disruption of the Achilles tendon. Most commonly this occurs in the distal portion of the Achilles tendon above its attachment to the os calcis. The sensation at the time of injury can mimic the feeling of an object striking the back of the lower leg. This is followed by inability to stand on the ball of the foot or to toe off in normal gait. On physical examination, the patient should be placed prone and the tendon palpated in search of a palpable defect. Such a defect is not always felt. With the patient still prone, one should squeeze the calf (gastrocnemius–soleus complex) and watch for plantar flexion of the foot. If there is no plantar flexion movement of the foot, disruption of the Achilles tendon is confirmed. This is known as a positive Thompson's sign. Acceptable treatment for acute ruptures of the Achilles tendon includes surgical reattachment or immobilization in a long-leg cast in plantar flexion. Both these methods will give satisfactory results, and the choice depends on the personal preferences of the physician. Our preference for competitive athletes is reattachment of the tendon.

Gastrocnemius Tear

This injury is also characterized by a sudden pain in the calf, although it is more proximal than the site of the classic Achilles tendon rupture. This may be as dramatic and painful as a ruptured Achilles tendon, but it is considerably less serious. This injury has been frequently referred to as a torn plantaris muscle. It actually consists, however, of a disruption at the musculotendinous junction of the medial head of the gastrocnemius.[134, 152] There is tenderness and swelling along the medial portion of the gastrocnemius. The defect may be palpable if the patient is seen before the swelling occurs or after it has subsided. These patients are also unable to walk on their toes because of pain and weakness. The Thompson's test is negative. The treatment does not include surgery or prolonged immobilization. A posterior short-leg splint for 3 to 5 days followed by partial weight-bearing gait is recommended. When the pain and swelling have subsided sufficiently to allow a rehabilitation program to begin, the patient should start by gentle stretching and strengthening of the gastrocnemius complex. Although it takes several more weeks to regain full strength and flexibility, the patient can anticipate a good functional result.

ANKLE SPRAINS

Ankle sprains may be the most neglected recreational musculoskeletal injury. Unfortunately, patients who have sustained significant injuries to the lateral ligaments of the ankle may have residual disability from inadequate treatment and rehabilitation.

Anatomic Considerations. The lateral ankle ligaments are much more commonly injured than the medial deltoid ligament. There are three major ligaments on the lateral side. The anterior talofibular ligament crosses anteriorly from the fibula to attach to the talus. This ligament is tight in plantar flexion and is most frequently torn with plantar flexion and inversion. The anterior talofibular ligament prevents the anterior translation of the talus on the tibia. The calcaneofibular ligament runs distally from the fibula to attach to the calcaneus. It is tight in dorsiflexion and may be disrupted in this position in combination with inversion. The posterior talofibular ligament is rarely torn except in total dislocations of the ankle. Proximal to these ligaments, there is the anterior inferior tibiofibular ligament, which stabilizes the fibula to the tibia. It is disrupted as the talus forces the fibula laterally with eversion or less commonly inversion stress. On the medial side of the ankle, the medial deltoid ligament is disrupted with eversion and dorsiflexion injuries and is most often, although not always, associated with a fracture of the fibula.[1, 2, 163] Predisposing factors to ankle sprains are muscle weakness, previous sprains, and developmental limitation of subtalar motion.

History. A sudden inversion injury is the most common mechanism of lateral ligament injuries. Normally the first ligament to rupture is the anterior talofibular ligament or the deltoid ligament may be involved. The pain is initially severe in all of the injuries and is often associated with a popping or tearing sensation. Swelling over the site of the injury occurs within a few hours, and the patient has difficulty bearing weight.

Physical Examination. Although there may be a diffuse hemarthrosis, there is generally more swelling over the site of the ligamentous damage. The examiner should gently palpate each of the ankle ligaments described for areas of maximal tenderness. In addition, the examiner should be careful to palpate the medial malleolus and the entire length of the fibula from the knee to the ankle. Ankle sprains may be associated with proximal fibular fractures, and such a fracture may alter treatment. In addition, conditions that can be mistaken for common lateral ankle sprain must be excluded. Subluxation of the peroneal tendons should be confirmed by tenderness directly over the tendon with minimal or no tenderness over the individual ankle ligaments. The base of the fifth metatarsal should also be palpated to exclude a fracture, which can cause lateral foot and

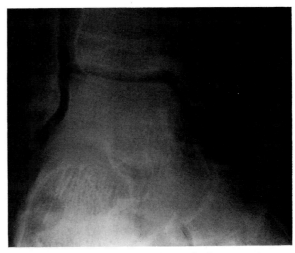

Figure 100–19. Anteroposterior radiograph, demonstrating an osteochondral injury to the superior lateral aspect of the talus following an ankle injury.

ankle pain. The active range of motion should be checked. There will be some limitation of dorsiflexion and plantar flexion secondary to joint swelling and pain. Tests for instability are painful in the acute setting and must be done under adequate anesthesia, either local or general, to be useful.[136, 139] Ankle sprains are commonly graded.[165] A grade I sprain includes partial tears, most often of the anterior talofibular ligament; a grade II sprain is a complete tear of the anterior talofibular ligament; and a grade III sprain is rupture of at least the anterior talofibular and the calcaneofibular ligaments. If the patient is seen soon after the injury and there was not much swelling, maximal tenderness in each of these areas can be helpful in assessing a significant injury to each of these ligaments.

Radiographic Examination. Although not required in the patient with a minimal sprain in the anterior talofibular ligament, routine radiographs should be performed in significant ankle sprains. These should include anteroposterior, lateral, and mortise views. In addition to fractures of the distal and proximal fibula and the medial malleolus, one should look for fractures at the distal tibia or talus (Figs. 100–18 and 100–19). Stress films are not commonly obtained with an acute injury. In evaluating a patient with a chronic ankle instability, an anterior stress film and an inversion stress film are used to assess the anterior talofibular and the calcaneofibular ligaments (Fig. 100–20). An abnormal anterior stress film indicates damage to at least the anterior talofibular ligament.[136, 137] A positive finding on inversion tilt film is indicative of disruption of the calcaneofibular ligament.[138, 139] It is important to obtain comparative stress films of the normal ankle because it is the degree of change compared with the injured ankle that is significant. For the anterior stress test view, 3 mm or more of talar displacement compared with the normal side is significant. For the inversion test, a talar tilt more than 5 degrees in comparison

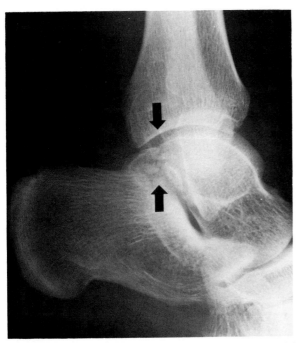

Figure 100–18. Lateral radiograph demonstrating a fracture of the posterior aspect of the talus following a plantar flexion injury to the ankle.

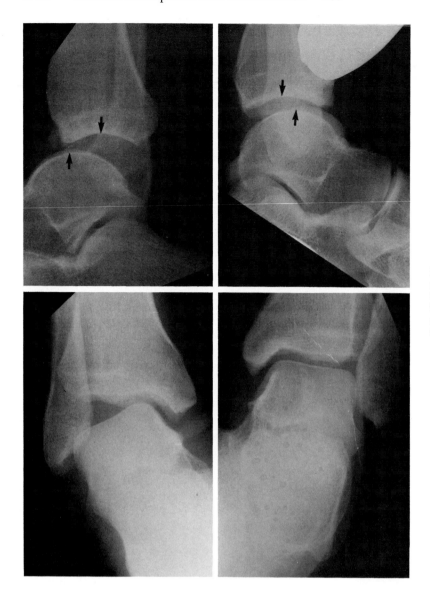

Figure 100–20. Stress radiograph of the ankle, revealing excessive anterior subluxation of the talus in the lower left film and instability on inversion in the lower right film. The normal contralateral ankle is depicted under stress in the upper two films.

with the normal side indicates significant damage to the calcaneofibular ligament. Ankle arthrography will identify the presence of a ligament tear of a medial or lateral side of the ankle.[21, 22, 164] It is particularly useful in defining chondral fractures of the talus and loose bodies (Fig. 100–21). In the setting of chronic pain, an arthrogram or arthrotomogram may uncover a chondral or bone injury that had not been detected.

Treatment. Ankle sprains of primarily the anterior talofibular ligament are treated conservatively. However, conservative treatment should not mean neglect. The use of ice during the first 48 hours and elevation in a compression bandage for several days are critical in decreasing the morbidity of this injury. Crutches and early mobilization with weight bearing and progressive strengthening exercises are used. The patient should begin with range of motion exercises for dorsiflexion and plantar flexion and when more comfortable, should begin strengthening the peroneal muscles. With prompt and proper treatment, most patients are off crutches within 1 week

and returning to good function in activities of daily living. The prevention of swelling with compression and ice and the use of early rehabilitation prevent stiffness and weakness. These are the major disabilities of ankle injuries. Patients with an eversion injury to the anterior inferior tibiofibular ligament should be warned that recovery time can be longer than for a routine lateral ankle sprain.

The treatment of severe combined sprains of the anterior talofibular ligament and calcaneofibular ligament is controversial. The choices include early functional mobilization and rehabilitation, cast mobilization, and surgical repair. No one method has given uniformly good and excellent results.[140, 142] Professional athletes and dancers have been recommended to have surgical repair of grade III injuries.[165] Patients, however, may still have pain and even functional instability after surgical repair. Patients with prolonged immobilization in plaster with or without operative procedures can have troublesome joint contractures and residual weakness of the per-

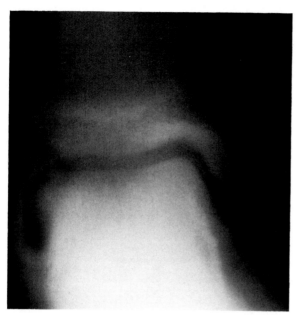

Figure 100–21. Arthrotomogram of the ankle demonstrating a defect in the articular cartilage on the superior lateral aspect of the talus following an ankle sprain.

oneal muscles. The authors' preference is for early rehabilitation and functional bracing in the cases of severe sprains in most individuals. A careful rehabilitation program should begin with range of motion exercises and progress to strengthening exercises of the peroneal muscles and dorsiflexors. It should finally include proprioceptive exercises with a device such as a tilt board.[141, 145] Flexibility and strengthening exercises for the Achilles tendon and gastrocnemius–soleus complex should not be neglected.[143] The patient should not be allowed to return to athletics until not only the pain has resolved, but also good strength and proprioceptive use of the ankle have returned. Flexibility and strengthening exercises for the Achilles tendon and gastrocnemius–soleus complex should not be neglected. To help prevent reinjury, protective taping or bracing should be used when the patient returns to full participation.[144] In the small number of patients with residual functional instability, operative procedures for chronic instability are successful.[163]

Complete deltoid ligament injuries without fractures are uncommon. Special care should be taken to exclude other injuries such as a proximal fibula fracture. It is possible to sustain a complete tear in the medial collateral ligament, the tibiofibular ligament, and the interosseous membrane without a fibula fracture. In these patients, the ankle mortise is disrupted. They have widening of the ankle at the syndesmosis located between the distal tibia and the fibula. Such widening may be seen on mortise or anteroposterior views of the ankle. Alternatively, an external rotation stress view with some form of anesthesia may be necessary to confirm the diagnosis. In contrast to the lateral and pure medial ankle sprains, these injuries of the syndesmosis should have strong consideration given to operative therapy.[163]

SUMMARY

A wide variety of acute, traumatic, and chronic overuse athletic injuries have been discussed. Unfortunately, treatment failures result not only from improper diagnosis, but also from failure to rehabilitate a patient completely. Physicians must be reminded of the importance of patient education and rehabilitation. Restoration to adequate strength, endurance, and flexibility is essential for a safe return to recreational or competitive athletics. The practicing physician must give this goal as much dedication and interest as formulating an accurate diagnosis and treatment plan.

References

1. Kapandji, I. A.: Physiology of the Joint. Vols. I and II. Edinburgh, E&S Livingstone, 1970.
2. Goss, C. M.: Gray's Anatomy of the Human Body. 28th ed. Philadelphia, Lea & Febiger, 1966.
3. Noyes, F. R., Torvik, P. J., Hyde, W. B., and Delucas, J. L.: Biomechanics of ligament failure. J. Bone Joint Surg. 56A:1406, 1974.
4. Noyes, F. R., DeLucas, J. L., and Torvik, P. J.: Biomechanics of anterior cruciate failure. J. Bone Joint Surg. 56A:236, 1974.
5. Tipton, C. M., James, S. L., Mergner, W., et al: Influence of exercise on strength of medial collateral ligament of dogs. Am. J. Physiol. 218:894, 1970.
6. Tipton, C. M., Matthes, R. D., Maynard, J. A., et al: The influence of physical activity on ligaments and tendons. Med. Sci. Sports 7:165, 1975.
7. Weisman, G., Pope, M. H., and Johnson, R. J.: Cyclic loading in knee ligament injuries. Am. J. Sports Med. 8:24, 1980.
8. Walker, P. S., and Erkman, M. J.: The role of the menisci in force transmission across the knee. Clin. Orthop. 109:184, 1975.
9. Maquet, P. G., and VanDeBerg, A. J.: Femorotibial weight bearing areas. J. Bone Joint Surg. 57A:766, 1978.
10. Kurosawa, H., et al.: Load-bearing mode of the knee joint: Physical behavior of the knee joint with and without menisci. Clin. Orthop. 149:283, 1980.
11. Allman, F. L., Jr.: Rehabilitation of the injured athlete. In Ryan, A. J., and Allman, F. L., Jr. (eds.): Sports Medicine. New York, Academic Press, 1974.
12. Clancy, W. G.: Tendinitis and plantar fasciitis in runners. In D'Ambrosia, R., and Drez, D. (eds.): Prevention and Treatment of Running Injuries. Thorofare, NJ, Slack Inc., 1982.
13. Cahill, B. R.: Quadrilateral space syndrome. In Omer, G. E., Jr., and Spinner, M. D. (eds.): Management of Peripheral Nerve Injuries. Philadelphia, W. B. Saunders Company, 1980.
14. Drez, D., Jr.: Suprascapular neuropathy in the differential diagnosis of rotator cuff injuries. Am. J. Sports Med. 4:43, 1976.
15. Snyder, R. B., Lipscomb, A. B., and Johnston, R. K.: The relationship of tarsal coalitions to ankle sprains in athletes. Am. J. Sports Med. 9:313, 1981.
16. O'Donoghue, D. H.: Treatment of Athletic Injuries. 3rd ed. Philadelphia, W. B. Saunders Company, 1976.
17. Blazina, M. E., and Saltzman, J. S.: Recurrent subluxations of the shoulder in athletes. Proceedings of the American Academy of Orthopedic Surgeons. J. Bone Joint Surg. 51A, 1969.
18. Rowe, C. R., and Zarins, B.: Recurrent subluxation of the shoulder. J. Bone Joint Surg. 63A:863, 1981.
19. Bateman, J. E.: The Shoulder and Neck. 2nd ed. Philadelphia, W. B. Saunders Company, 1978.
20. Neviaser, J. S.: Arthrography of the Shoulder. Springfield, IL, Charles C. Thomas, 1975.
21. Freiberger, R. H., and Kaye, J.: Arthrography. New York, Appleton-Century-Crofts, 1979.
22. Arndt, R. D., Horns, J. W., and Gold, R. H.: Clinical Arthrography. Baltimore, Williams & Wilkins, 1981.

23. Fowler, P. J.: Posterior Subluxation of the Shoulder in Swimmers. Presented at the Annual Meeting of the American Orthopedic Society for Sports Medicine, Lake of the Ozarks, Missouri, 1982.
24. Hoyt, W. A., Jr.: Etiology of shoulder injuries in athletes. J. Bone Joint Surg. 49A:755, 1967.
25. Moseley, H. F.: Shoulder Lesions. 3rd ed. Baltimore, Williams & Wilkins, 1969.
26. Allman, F. L., Jr.: Fractures and ligamentous injuries of the clavicle and its articulation. J. Bone Joint Surg. 49A:744, 1967.
27. Vrist, M. R.: Complete dislocations of the acromioclavicular joint. J. Bone Joint Surg. 45A:1750, 1963.
28. Bergfeld, J. A., Andrish, J. T., and Clancy, W. G.: Evaluation of the acromioclavicular joint following first and second degree sprains. Am. J. Sports Med. 6:153, 1978.
29. Cox, J. S.: The fate of the acromioclavicular joint in athletic injuries. Am. J. Sports Med. 9:50, 1981.
30. Browne, J. E., Stanley, R. F., and Tullos, H. S.: Acromioclavicular joint dislocations: Comparative results following operative treatment with and without primary clavisectomy. Am. J. Sports Med. 5:258, 1977.
31. Glick, J. M., Milburn, L. J., Haggerty, J. F., et al.: Dislocated acromioclavicular joint: Follow-up study of 35 unreduced acromioclavicular dislocations. Am. J. Sports Med. 5:264, 1977.
32. Alexander, O. M.: Radiology of the acromioclavicular articulation. Med. Radiogr. Photogr. 30:34, 1954.
33. Jacobs, P.: Post-traumatic osteolysis of the outer end of the clavicle. J. Bone Joint Surg. 46B:705, 1964.
34. Mumford, E. B.: Acromioclavicular dislocation: A new operative treatment. J. Bone Joint Surg. 23:799, 1941.
35. Bennett, G. E.: Shoulder and elbow lesions distinctive of baseball players. Ann. Surg. 126:107, 1947.
36. Hawkins, R. J., and Kennedy, J. C.: Impingement syndromes in athletes. Am. J. Sports Med. 3:151, 1980.
37. Kennedy, J. C., and Hawkins, R. T.: Swimmer's shoulders. Physician Sports Med. 2:35, 1974.
38. Priest, J. D., and Nagel, D. A.: Tennis shoulder. Am. J. Sports Med. 4:28, 1976.
39. Jackson, D. W.: Chronic rotator cuff impingement in the throwing athlete. Am. J. Sports Med. 4:231, 1976.
40. Bateman, J. E.: Cuff tears in athletes. Orthop. Clin. North Am. 4:721, 1973.
41. Neer, C. S., and Welsh, R. P.: The shoulder in sports. Orthop. Clin. North Am. 8:583, 1977.
42. Richardson, A. B., Jobe, F. W., and Collins, H. R.: The shoulder in competitive swimming. Am. J. Sports Med. 8:159, 1980.
43. Barnes, D. A., and Tullos, H. S.: An analysis of 100 symptomatic baseball players. Am. J. Sports Med. 6:62, 1978.
44. Norwood, L. A., DelPizzo, W., Jobe, F. W., and Kerland, R. K.: Anterior shoulder pain in baseball pitchers. Am. J. Sports Med. 6:103, 1978.
45. Lombardo, S. J., Jobe, F. W, Kerlan, R. K., et al.: Posterior shoulder lesions in throwing athletes. Am. J. Sports Med. 5:106, 1977.
46. Tullos, H. S., and King, J. W.: Throwing mechanism in sports. Orthop. Clin. North Am. 4:709, 1973.
47. Rathbun, J. B., and MacNab, I.: The microvascular pattern of the rotator cuff. J. Bone Joint Surg. 52B:540, 1970.
48. Moseley, H. F., and Goldie, I.: The arterial pattern of the rotator cuff. J. Bone Joint Surg. 45B:780, 1963.
49. Weiner, D. S., and MacNab, I.: Superior migration of the humeral head: A radiological aid in the diagnosis of tears of the rotator cuff. J. Bone Joint Surg. 52B:524, 1970.
50. Braunstein, E. M., and O'Connor, G.: Double contrast arthrotomography of the shoulder. J. Bone Joint Surg. 64A:192, 1982.
51. Danzig, L., Resnick, D., and Greenway, G.: Evaluation of shoulders by computed tomography. Am. J. Sports Med. 10:138, 1982.
52. Kennedy, J. C., and Willis, R. B.: The effects of local steroid injections on tendons: A biomechanical and microscopic correlative study. Am. J. Sports Med. 4:11, 1976.
53. Ismail, A. M., Balakishnan, R., and Rajakumar, M. K.: Rupture of patellar tendon after steroid infiltration. J. Bone Joint Surg. 51B:503, 1969.
54. Malmed, E. P.: Spontaneous bilateral rupture of the calcaneal tendon during steroid injection. J. Bone Joint Surg. 47B:104, 1965.
55. Unverferth, L. J., and Olix, M. L.: The effects of local steroid injections on tendons. J. Sports Med. 1:31, 1973.
56. Wrem, R. N., Goldner, J. L., and Markee, J. L.: An experimental study of the effects of cortisone on the healing process and tensile strength of tendons. J. Bone Joint Surg. 36A:588, 1954.
57. Jobe, F. W., and Moynes, D. R.: Delineation of diagnostic criteria and a rehabilitation program for rotator cuff injuries. Am. J. Sports Med. 10:336, 1982.
58. Boland, A. L.: Rehabilitation of the injured athlete. In Strauss, R. H. (ed.): Sports Medicine and Physiology. Philadelphia, W. B. Saunders Company, 1979.
59. Neer, C. S.: Anterior acromioplasty for the chronic impingement syndrome in the shoulder: A preliminary report. J. Bone Joint Surg. 54A:41, 1972.
60. Codman, E. A.: The Shoulder-Rupture of the Supraspinatous Tendon and Other Lesions in and About the Subacromial Bursa. Boston, Thomas Todd Company, 1934.
61. Bennett, G. E.: Elbow lesions of baseball players. Am. J. Surg. 98:484, 1959.
62. Slocum, D. B.: Classification of elbow injuries from baseball pitching. Tex. Med. 64:48, 1968.
63. King, J. W., Brelsford, H. J., and Tullos, H. S.: Analysis of the pitching arm of the professional baseball pitcher. Clin. Orthop. 67:116, 1969.
64. Woods, G. W., Tullos, H. S., and King, J. W.: The throwing arm: Elbow joint injuries. Am. J. Sports Med. 4:43, 1977.
65. Nirschl, R. P.: The etiology and treatment of tennis elbow. J. Sports Med. 2:308, 1975.
66. Goldie, I. G.: Epicondylitis lateralis humeri. Acta Chir. Scand. Suppl. 339:1, 1961.
67. Conrad, R. W., and Hooper, W. R.: Tennis elbow: Its course, natural history, conservative and surgical management. J. Bone Joint Surg. 55A:1177, 1973.
68. Garden, R. S.: Tennis elbow. J. Bone Joint Surg. 43B:100, 1961.
69. Stack, J. K.: Acute and chronic bursitis in the region of the elbow joint. Surg. Clin. North Am. 29:155, 1949.
70. Trethowan, W. H.: Tennis elbow. Br. Med. J. 2:1218, 1929.
71. Kaplan, E. B.: Treatment of tennis elbow (epicondylitis) by denervation. J. Bone Joint Surg. 41A:147, 1959.
72. Roles, N. C., and Maudsley, R. H.: Radial tunnel syndrome: Resistant tennis elbow as a nerve entrapment. J. Bone Joint Surg. 54B:499, 1972.
73. Gugenheim, J. J., Stanley, R. T., Woods, G. W., and Tullos, H. S.: The Little League survey: The Houston Study. Am. J. Sports Med. 4:189, 1976.
74. Larson, R. L., Singer, K. N., and Nagel, D. A.: The Little League survey: The Eugene study. Am. J. Sports Med. 4:201, 1976.
75. Adams, J. E.: Bone injuries in the very young athlete. Clin. Orthop. 58:129, 1968.
76. Tullos, H. S., and King, J. W.: Lesions of the pitching arm in adolescents. J.A.M.A. 220:264, 1972.
77. Priest, J. D., Jones, H. H., and Nagel, D. A.: Elbow injuries in the highly skilled tennis players. Am. J. Sports Med. 2:137, 1974.
78. Delpizzo, W., Jobe, F. W., and Norwood, L.: Ulnar nerve entrapment syndrome in baseball players. Am. J. Sports Med. 5:182, 1977.
79. D'Ambrosia, R., and Drez, D.: Prevention and Treatment of Running Injuries. Thorofare, N. J., Slack, Inc., 1982.
80. McBryde, A. M., Jr.: Stress fractures in athletes. J. Sports Med. 3:212, 1975.
81. Kaltsas, D. S.: Stress fractures of femoral neck in young adults. Report of 7 cases. J. Bone Joint Surg. 63B:33, 1981.
82. Siddiqui, A. R.: Bone scans for early detection of stress fractures. N. Engl. J. Med. 298:1033, 1978.
83. Brody, D. M.: Running injuries. CIBA Clinical Symposia 32(4), 1980.
84. Smillie, I. S.: Injuries of the Knee Joint. 4th ed. Baltimore, Williams & Wilkins, 1970.
85. Miller, W.: The Knee. Form, Function and Ligament Reconstruction. New York, Springer-Verlag, 1983.
86. Dandy, D. J.: Arthroscopic Surgery of the Knee. London, Churchill Livingstone, 1981.
87. Johnson, L. L.: The Comprehensive Examination of the Knee. St. Louis, C. V. Mosby, 1977.
88. King, D.: The function of semilunar cartilages. J. Bone Joint Surg. 18:1069, 1936.
89. Cox, J. S., Nye, C. E., et al.: The degenerative effects of partial and total resection of the medial meniscus in dog's knees. Clin. Orthop. 109:178, 1975.
90. Shapiro, F., and Glimcher, M. J.: Induction of osteoarthritis in the rabbit knee joint. Clin. Orthop. 147:287, 1980.
91. Tapper, E. M., and Hoover, N. W.: Late results after meniscectomy. J. Bone Joint Surg. 51A:517, 1969.
92. Johnson, R. J., Kettlekamp, D. B., Clark, W., and Leaverton, P.: Factors affecting late results after meniscectomy. J. Bone Joint Surg. 56A:719, 1974.
93. McGinty, J. B., Geuss, L. F., and Marvin, R. A.: Partial or total meniscectomy. J. Bone Joint Surg. 59A:763, 1977.
94. Jackson, R. W.: The results of partial arthroscopic meniscectomy in patients over 40 years of age. J. Bone Joint Surg. 64B:481, 1982.
95. Dandy, D. J., and Jackson, R. W.: The diagnosis of problems after meniscectomy. J. Bone Joint Surg. 57B:349, 1975.
96. Fairbank, T. J.: Knee joint changes after meniscectomy. J. Bone Joint Surg. 30B:664, 1948.
97. Cabaud, H. E., Rodkey, W. G., and Fitzwater, J. E.: Medial meniscus repairs: An experimental and morphologic study. Am. J. Sports Med. 9:3, 129, 1981.
98. Cassidy, R. E., and Shaffer, A. J.: Repair of peripheral meniscus tears: A preliminary report. Am. J. Sports Med. 9:209, 1981.

99. DeHaven, K. E.: Selective approach to meniscectomy. Presented at the American Academy of Orthopaedic Surgeon's Knee Injury Course. Boston, 1983.

100. Slocum, D. B., and Larson, R. L.: Rotary instability of the knee. J. Bone Joint Surg. 50A:211, 1968.

101. Hughston, J. C., Andrews, J. R., et al.: Classification of knee ligament instabilities. J. Bone Joint Surg. 58A:159, Part I; 58A:665, 1974.

102. Brantigan, O. C., and Voshell, A. F.: Ligaments of the knee joint. J. Bone Joint Surg. 28:66, 1946.

103. Warren, L. F., Marshall, J. L, and Girgis, F.: The prime static stabilizer of the medial side of the knee. J. Bone Joint Surg. 56A:665, 1974.

104. Kennedy, J. C., and Fowler, P. J.: Medial and anterior instability of the knee: An anatomical and clinical study using stress machines. J. Bone Joint Surg. 53A:1257, 1971.

105. Kennedy, J. C., et al.: Tension studies of human knee ligaments, yield point, ultimate failure and disruption of the cruciate and tibial collateral ligaments. J. Bone Joint Surg. 58A:350, 1976.

106. DeHaven, J. C., et al.: Diagnosis of acute knee ligament injuries with hemarthrosis. Am. J. Sports Med. 8:9, 1980.

107. Noyes, F. R., Bassett, R. W., Grood, E. S., and Butler, D. L.: Arthroscopy in acute traumatic hemarthrosis of the knee: Incidence of anterior cruciate tears and other injuries. J. Bone Joint Surg. 62A:687, 1980.

108. Torg, J. S., Conrad, W., and Kalen, V.: Clinical diagnosis of anterior cruciate ligament instability in the athlete. Am. J. Sports Med. 4:84, 1976.

109. Kennedy, J. C.: The Injured Adolescent Knee. Baltimore, Williams & Wilkins, 1979.

110. Noyes, F. R., and Spievack, E. S.: Extraarticular fluid dissection in tissue during arthroscopy. Am. J. Sports Med. 10:346, 1982.

111. Clancy, W. G., Bergfeld, J., O'Connor, G. A., and Cox, J. A.: Symposium: Functional rehabilitation of medial collateral ligament sprains. Am. J. Sports Med. 7:206, 1979.

112. Blazina, M.: Jumper's knee. Orthop. Clin. North. Am. 4:665, 1973.

113. Roels, J., Martens, M., et al.: Patellar tendinitis (jumper's knee) Am. J. Sports Med. 6:362, 1978.

114. Estwanik, J. J., Bergfeld, J., and Canty, T.: Report of injuries sustained during the Olympic wrestling trials. Am. J. Sports Med. 6:335, 1978.

115. Renne, J. W.: The iliotibial band friction syndrome. J. Bone Joint Surg. 57A:1110, 1975.

116. James, S. L., Bates, B. T., and Osternig, L. R.: Injuries to runners. Am. J. Sports Med. 6:40, 1978.

117. Ficat, R. P., and Hungerford, D. S.: Disorders of the Patellofemoral Joint. Baltimore, Williams & Wilkins, 1977.

118. Outerbridge, R. E.: The etiology of chondromalacia patella. J. Bone Joint Surg. 43B:752, 1961.

119. Laurin, C. A., et al.: The abnormal lateral patellofemoral angle. J. Bone Joint Surg. 60A:55, 1978.

120. Merchange, A. C., Mercer, R. L., et al.: Roentgenographic analysis of patellofemoral congruence. J. Bone Joint Surg. 56A:139, 1964.

121. Insall, J., and Salvati, E.: Patella position in the normal knee joint. Radiology 101:101, 1971.

122. Henry, J. H., and Crosland, J. W.: Conservative treatment of patellofemoral subluxations. Am. J. Sports Med. 7:12, 1979.

123. Palumbo, P. M.: Dynamic patellar brace: A new orthosis in the management of patellofemoral disorders. Am. J. Sports Med. 9:45, 1981.

124. Slocum, D. B.: The shin splint syndrome: Medical aspects and differential diagnosis. Am. J. Surg. 114:875, 1967.

125. Mubarak, S. J., Gould, R. N., et al.: The medial tibial stress syndrome: A cause of shin splints. Am. J. Sports Med. 10:201, 1982.

126. Baker, J., Frankel, V. H., et al.: Fatigue fractures: Biomechanical considerations. J. Bone Joint Surg. 54A:1345, 1972.

127. Clancy, W. G., Neidhart, D., and Brand, R. L.: Achilles tendinitis in runners: A report of five cases. Am. J. Sports Med. 4:46, 1976.

128. Puddu, G., Ippolito, E., and Postacchini, F.: A classification of Achilles tendon disease. Am. J. Sports Med. 4:145, 1976.

129. Reneman, R. S.: The anterior and the lateral compartmental syndrome of the leg due to intensive use of muscles. Clin. Orthop. 113:69, 1975.

130. Mubarak, S. J., Owen, C. A., Garfin, S. R., et al.: Acute exertional superficial posterior compartment syndrome. Am. J. Sports Med. 6:287, 1978.

131. Snook, G. A.: Intermittent claudication in athletes. Am. J. Sports Med. 3:71, 1975.

132. Whitesides, T. E., Haney, T. C., et al.: Tissue pressure measurements as a determinant for the need of fasciotomy. Clin. Orthop. 113:43, 1975.

133. Mubarak, S. J., Hargens, A. R., Owen, C. A., et al.: The wick catheter technique for measurement of intramuscular pressure: A new research and clinical tool. J. Bone Joint Surg. 58A:1016, 1976.

134. Miller, W. A.: Rupture of the musculotendinous junction of the medial head of the gastrocnemius muscle. Am. J. Sports Med. 5:191, 1977.

135. Thompson, T. C.: A test for rupture of the tendon Achilles. Acta Orthop. Scand. 32:461, 1962.

136. Seligson, D., Gassman, J., and Pope, M.: Ankle instability: Evaluation of the lateral ligaments. Am. J. Sports Med. 8:39, 1980.

137. Frost, H. M., and Hanson, C. A.: Technique for testing the drawer sign in the ankle. Clin. Orthop. 123:49, 1977.

138. Laurin, C., and Mathiew, J.: Sagittal mobility of the normal ankle. Clin. Orthop. 108:99, 1975.

139. Cox, J. S., and Hewes, T. F.: "Normal" talar tilt angle. Clin. Orthop. 140:37, 1979.

140. Freeman, M. A.: Treatment of ruptures of the lateral ligaments of the ankle. J. Bone Joint Surg. 47B:661, 1965.

141. Freeman, M. A.: The etiology and prevention of functional instability of the foot. J. Bone Joint Surg. 47B:678, 1965.

142. Staples, O. S.: Ruptures of the fibular collateral ligaments of the ankle: Result study of immediate surgical treatment. J. Bone Joint Surg. 57A:101, 1975.

143. McClusky, G. M., et al.: Prevention of ankle sprain. Am. J. Sports Med. 4:151, 1976.

144. Garrick, J. C., and Reque, R. K.: Role of external supports in the prevention of ankle sprains. Med. Sci. Sports 5:200, 1973.

145. Glich, J. M., Gordon, R. B., and Nishimoto, D.: The prevention and treatment of ankle injuries. Am. J. Sports Med. 4:136, 1976.

146. Neer, C. S., and Foster, C. P.: Inferior capsular shift for involuntary inferior and multidirectional instability of the shoulder. J. Bone Joint Surg. 62A:897, 1980.

147. Pappas, A., et al.: Biomechanics of baseball pitching. Am. J. Sports Med. 13:216, 1985.

148. Jobe, F. N., et al.: EMG analysis of the shoulder in throwers. Am. J. Sports Med. 13:216, 1985.

149. Butler, D. S., Noyes, F. R., and Grood, E. S.: Ligamentous restraints to anterior-posterior drawer in the human knee. J. Bone Joint Surg. 62A:259, 1980.

150. Grood, E. S., Noyes, F. R., Butler, D. L., and Suntay, W. J.: Ligamentous and capsular restraints preventing straight medial and lateral laxity in intact human cadaver knees. J. Bone Joint Surg. 63A:1257, 1981.

151. Noyes, F. R., and Grood, E. S.: Classification of ligament injuries: Why an anterolateral laxity or anteromedial laxity is not a diagnostic entity. In Griffin, P. P. (ed.): Instructional Course Lectures. Chicago, American Academy of Orthopaedic Surgeons, 1987.

152. Peterson, L., and Renstrom, P.: Sports Injuries. Chicago, Year Book Medical Publishers, 1986.

153. Clancy, W. G., et al.: Treatment of knee joint instability secondary to rupture of the posterior cruciate ligament. J. Bone Joint Surg. 65A:310, 1983.

154. Clancy, W. G., et al.: Anterior cruciate ligament reconstruction using one-third of the patellar ligament, augmented by extra-articular tendon transfers. J. Bone Joint Surg. 64A:352, 1982.

155. Jackson, D. W., and Drez, D.: The Anterior Cruciate Deficient Knee, New Concepts in Ligament Repair. St. Louis, C. W. Mosby, 1987.

156. Larson, R. L.: The unstable patella in the adolescent and preadolescent. Orthop. Rev. 14:156, 1985.

157. Huberti, H. H., and Hayes, W. C.: Patellofemoral contact pressures. J. Bone Joint Surg. 66A:715, 1984.

158. Insall, J. N.: Surgery of the Knee. New York, Churchill Livingstone, 1984.

159. Schutzer, S. F., Rambsby, G. R., and Fulkerson, J. P.: The evaluation of patellofemoral pain using computed tomography. Clin. Orthop. 204:286, 1986.

160. Fisher, R. L.: Conservative treatment of patellofemoral pain. Orthop. Clin. North Am. 17:269, 1986.

161. Holder, L. E.: Current concepts review: Radionuclide bone imaging in the evaluation of bone pain. J. Bone Joint Surg. 64A:1391, 1982.

162. Detmer, D. E.: Chronic compartment syndrome: Diagnosis, management and outcomes. Am. J. Sports Med. 13:162, 1985.

163. Rockwood, C. A., and Green, D. P.: Fractures in Adults. Vol. 2. Philadelphia, J. B. Lippincott, 1984.

164. Yablon, P., Isadore, G., Segal, D., and Leach, R. E.: Ankle Injuries. New York, Churchill Livingstone, 1983.

165. Hamilton, W. G.: Foot and ankle injuries in dancers. Clin. Sports Med. 7:143, 1988.

166. O'Brien, S. J., et al.: The anatomy and histology of the glenohumeral ligament complex of the shoulder. Am. J. Sports Med. 18:449, 1990.

167. O'Connell, P. W., et al.: The contribution of the glenohumeral ligament to anterior stability of the shoulder joint. Am. J. Sports Med. 18:579, 1990.

168. Burk, D. L., et al.: Rotator cuff tears: Prospective comparison of MR imaging with arthrography, sonography and surgery. A.J.R. 153:87, 1989.

169. Evancho, A. M., et al.: MR imaging diagnosis of rotator cuff tears. A.J.R. 151:751, 1988.

Chapter 101

Entrapment Neuropathies and Related Disorders

Peripheral nerve entrapment may result from a number of mechanisms, including pressure (compression), stretch, friction, and angulation. The pathophysiology of the nerve entrapment syndromes differs owing to this variety. Additional clinical circumstances influence these disorders, including the patient's age and the presence of underlying systemic diseases (e.g., diabetes mellitus). Compression on a nerve within a closed space can occur wherever a peripheral nerve passes through an opening in fibrous tissue or through an osseofibrous canal (e.g., carpal tunnel), soft tissue swelling (e.g., rheumatoid arthritis), an anomalous or hypertrophied muscle (e.g., the pronator teres syndrome), a constricting scar or ligament, a bony deformity, or a tumor or mass (e.g., soft tissue tumor or ganglion) (Table 101–1). Damage to a peripheral nerve may result from high pressure exerted for a short time (e.g., acute radial nerve palsy) or from moderate or low pressure exerted for long periods of time or intermittently (e.g., certain cases of ulnar neuropathy at the elbow).

Peripheral nerve entrapment syndromes are most often characterized physiologically by focal slowing and histologically by a segmental demyelination and remyelination. Entrapment syndromes appear to result from direct mechanical injury, such as chronic low pressure or friction (e.g., the carpal tunnel syndrome). Additional minor roles in the production of nerve damage may be played by ischemia, damage to the blood-brain barrier, and fibrosis.

In addition to the clinical examination (Table 101–2), the evaluation of patients with peripheral nerve entrapments should include various electrophysiologic studies (Table 101–3). Electrodiagnostic procedures are valuable under four circumstances: (1) when the clinical diagnosis is uncertain; (2) to follow the course of patients with entrapment neuropathies being treated conservatively; (3) to detect or exclude coexisting conditions, such as a radiculopathy or subclinical polyneuropathy; and (4) prior to operation. In some orthopedic office practices, a simple digital neurometer has been utilized to measure peripheral nerve motor latencies[1]; however, it should be cautioned that in the initial evaluation of patients with entrapment syndromes, detailed electrophysiologic studies should be performed in a well-established clinical neurophysiology laboratory.

Recent neuroimaging computerized technology

Table 101–1. PERIPHERAL ENTRAPMENT NEUROPATHIES

Nerve	Entrapment Syndrome
Upper Limbs	
Median	Carpal tunnel
	Pseudo–carpal tunnel (sublimis)
	Digital nerve
	Anterior interosseous nerve
	Pronator teres
	Ligament of Struthers
	Double crush
Ulnar	Guyon's canal
	Digital nerve
	Cubital canal
	Tardy ulner palsy
	Double crush
Radial	Saturday night palsy
	Posterior interosseous nerve
	Tennis elbow
Musculocutaneous	Coracobrachialis
Suprascapular	Suprascapular foramen
	Infraspinatus branch
Dorsal scapular	Scalenus medius
Brachial plexus	Thoracic outlet
	Scalenus anticus
	Costoclavicular
	Hyperabduction
Lower Limbs	
Sciatic	Pinformis
	Popliteal (Baker's) cyst
Common peroneal	Hereditary compression neuropathy
	Ganglion
	Leprosy
	Popliteal (Baker's) cyst
Posterior tibial	Popliteal (Baker's) cyst
	Tarsal tunnel
	Medial and lateral plantar nerve
	Interdigital nerve
Femoral	Pressure by space limiting process
Saphenous	Subsartorial (Hunter's) canal
Lateral femoral cutaneous	Meralgia paresthetica
Obturator	Obturator canal
	Osteitis pubis
Ilioinguinal	Anterior superior iliac spine
Genitofemoral	Adhesions after surgery

From Nakano, K. K.: Neurology of Musculoskeletal and Rheumatic Disorders. Boston, Houghton Mifflin, 1979. Copyright © 1979 John Wiley & Sons, Inc. Reprinted by permission of John Wiley & Sons, Inc.

has assisted in the diagnosis and planning of surgical approaches to certain peripheral entrapment syndromes (Figs. 101–1 and 101–2).[2–5]

Neurologists, neurosurgeons, orthopedic sur-

Table 101–2. SYMPTOMS AND SIGNS OF CARPAL TUNNEL SYNDROME IN 1016 PATIENTS

Symptom or Sign	%
Median paresthesias	100
Nocturnal paresthesias	71
Proximal extension of pain	38
Tinel's sign	
Positive	55
Negative	29
Unknown	17
Phalen's test	
Positive	53
Negative	23
Unknown	24
Sensation on sensory examination	
Decreased	28
Normal	36
Unknown	36
Thenar muscle strength	
Decreased	18
Normal	42
Unknown	41
Thenar muscle bulk	
Wasted	18
Normal	31
Unknown	50

From Spinner, R. J., Bachman, J. W., and Amadio, P. C.: The many faces of carpal tunnel syndrome. Mayo Clin. Proc. 64:829, 1989.

geons, hand surgeons, rheumatologists, and internists with specific interest in neurologic diseases deal with the peripheral nerve entrapment syndromes on a daily basis. Peripheral nerve entrapments occur commonly, and the clinician must have a method of evaluating, assessing, and treating patients with these syndromes (Fig. 101–3).[6, 7] Entrapment neuropathies produce focal disturbances of nerve function. The differential diagnosis of peripheral nerve entrapments therefore revolves around other conditions that may damage nerves in a focal manner; these disorders include degenerative, vascular, inflammatory, and metabolic diseases. The clinician must be alert to the possibilities of diagnostic confusion; the following conditions may resemble entrapment neuropathies: polyneuropathies (symmetric, asymmetric, demyelinating), brachial plexopathy,[8–12]

radiculopathy, amyotrophic lateral sclerosis, and vasospastic conditions (Raynaud's phenomenon, peripheral neuropathies with vasomotor changes, reflex sympathetic dystrophy).[13, 14] The different entrapment neuropathies will be discussed herein according to the peripheral nerves that they involve.

UPPER LIMB

Median Nerve

Carpal Tunnel Syndrome (CTS). The commonest entrapment neuropathy occurs in the carpal tunnel of the hand, at the point where the median nerve passes in company with the flexor tendons of the fingers (see Figs. 101–1 and 101–2). In the majority of the cases the physical findings will be specific, and the diagnosis easily established.[15, 16] Various disorders that may be associated with CTS include rheumatoid arthritis, hypothyroidism, amyloid,[17] gout, acromegaly, lactation,[18] renal failure with chronic hemodialysis,[19, 20] lipoma of the flexor digitorum superficialis,[21] fascia of the flexor digitorum superficialis,[22] ganglion cysts,[23] the paraplegic's daily activities,[24] gonococcal tenosynovitis,[25] pigmented villonodular synovitis,[26] Lyme borreliosis,[27, 28] arterial anomalies,[29] repetitive use of the hands in certain occupations,[30] and other previously known inflammatory reactions involving tendons and connective tissues of the wrist. Early diagnosis and treatment become important because delay can result in irreversible median nerve damage with persistent symptoms and permanent disability. In addition to standard electrodiagnostic tests[31] and, on occasion, magnetic resonance imaging (MRI),[2–4] other clinical tests (e.g., tethered median nerve stress test,[32] provocative work simulation machines,[33] and pressure measurements within the carpal tunnel)[34–37] have been advocated in the diagnosis and management of CTS.

Nonsurgical treatment would be advised for patients with mild symptoms, intermittent symptoms, or an acute flare-up of CTS from a specific injury.

Table 101–3. SUMMARY OF THE EMG-NCV FINDINGS BY LOCATION OF DISEASE IN THE MOTOR UNIT

	Location						
		Nerve Root					
Study	Spinal Cord: Anterior Horn Cell	ANTERIOR MOTOR ROOT	DORSAL GANGLION Pre-	Post-	Peripheral Nerve	Neuromuscular Junction	Muscle
MNCV	N	N	N	N	+	N	N
SNAP	N	N	N	±	+	N	N
EMG	+	+	N	N	+	±	+
Repetitive stimulation	±	N	N	N	±	+	N
F wave	+	+	N	N	+	N	N
H reflex	+	+	+	+	+	N	N
SER	N	N	+	+	+	N	N

N = normal; + = abnormal; ± = occasional abnormality; MNCV = motor nerve conduction velocity; SNAP = sensory nerve action potential; EMG = electromyography; SER = somatosensory evoked response.
From Nakano, K. K.: Neurology of Musculoskeletal and Rheumatic Disorders, Houghton Mifflin, 1979. Copyright © 1979 John Wiley & Sons, Inc. Reprinted by permission of John Wiley & Sons, Inc.

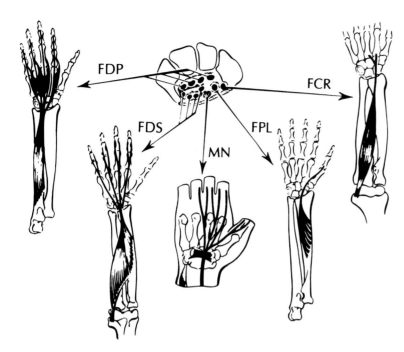

Figure 101–1. Cross-sectional appearance of the carpal tunnel at the level of hamate. (Used with permission from Middleton, W. D., Kneeland, J. B., Kellman, G. M., Cates, J. D., Sanger, J. R., Jesmanowicz, A., Froncisz, W., and Hyde, J. S.: MR imaging of the carpal tunnel: Normal anatomy and preliminary findings in the carpal tunnel syndrome. Am. J. Roentgenol. 148:307–316, 1987. © 1987 by American Roentgen Ray Society.)

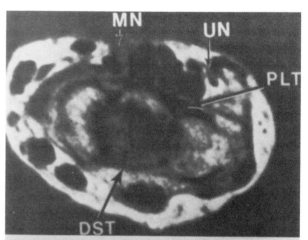

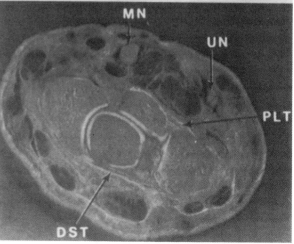

Figure 101–2. MR images through the proximal carpal tunnel. (From Mesgarzadeh, M., Schneck, C. D., and Bonakdarpour, A.: Carpal tunnel: MR imaging. Part I. Normal anatomy. Radiology 171:743–748, 1989. Used by permission.)

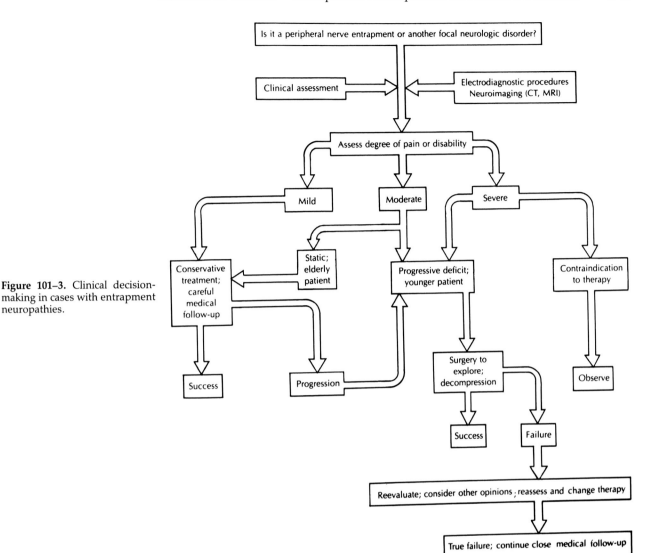

Figure 101–3. Clinical decision-making in cases with entrapment neuropathies.

Five types of nonsurgical therapy are (1) avoiding the activities that precipitate the condition (e.g., hammering), (2) splinting the wrist in the neutral position, (3) local steroid injection, (4) a brief course of either oral steroids or nonsteroidal anti-inflammatory medications, and (5) a trial of diuretics, particularly when the CTS symptoms appear premenstrually. For the mild night CTS symptoms a removable volar wrist splint with the wrist in a neutral position will often alleviate all symptoms. This type of splint should be used for a few weeks and then discarded. If symptoms persist or recur, additional treatment is indicated. Local steroid injections or a trial of oral medication would be recommended for mild persistent symptoms or in the elderly or poor surgical risk patients who complain of pain from the CTS. Local steroid injections often relieve the pain but may not change the other symptoms of CTS. Those patients with any thenar atrophy or muscle weakness or those with advanced sensory loss should not receive local steroid injections to relieve the CTS.

Surgical treatment of CTS demands care and skill and is one of the most successful operations that can be performed on the hand. Complications of the operation and poor results are usually related to poor surgical technique.[38, 39] Indications for surgical therapy for CTS include (1) failure of nonoperative treatment or clinical evidence of thenar atrophy, (2) persistent sensory loss, and (3) re-exploration when the patient fails to respond to carpal tunnel release or for recurrent CTS. Surgery with a CO_2 laser may offer an alternative technique in the treatment of CTS.[40]

Anterior Interosseous Nerve Syndrome (AINS). The AIN is a purely motor branch of the median nerve that supplies the flexor pollicis longus (FPL), the pronator quadratus (PQ), and the flexor digitorum profundus (FDP) of the index and middle fingers.[1, 2]

Treatment of AINS depends on the cause.[38, 41, 42] Penetrating wounds require immediate exploration and surgical repair. Impending Volkmann's contracture demands immediate surgical decompression. In spontaneous AINS cases associated with specific occupations, a trial of nonsurgical therapy should be the initial step in management and includes the patient's avoiding the activity that exacerbates the symptoms, resting the affected upper limb, and taking anti-inflammatory medications. If no improvement occurs within 8 to 12 weeks, surgical exploration should be considered. However, in the presence of known direct extrinsic compression or in cases of partial lesions of AINS, a longer trial of nonsurgical therapy would be suggested.

Pronator Teres Syndrome (PTS). The PTS is a relatively rare entrapment of the median nerve that occurs at the level of the pronator teres.[43]

Nonsurgical treatment is indicated in those cases of PTS with mild, intermittent symptoms associated with strenuous use of the involved limb (especially repeated elbow flexion and pronation). Use of anti-inflammatory medications and splints on the elbow and wrist often proves beneficial in conjunction with avoidance of exacerbating activities.

Surgical therapy is indicated in those PTS cases with persistent or progressive symptoms. Exploration, with release of a potential compressive band, may be necessary.

Rarely, median neuralgia can be caused by a brachial pseudoaneurysm.[44] This entity has been reported in a case of intermittent hemodialysis in which an unusual neurovascular complication of an antebrachial arteriovenous fistula occurred in a 15-year-old boy. Neurosurgical resection of the pseudoaneurysm in the forearm provided relief from the neuralgia.

Ligament of Struthers Compression. On rare occasions, the median nerve may become entrapped by a ligament of Struthers on the anteromedial surface of the humerus about 5 cm above the medial epicondyle.

The diagnosis of this entrapment neuropathy can be made on discovery of a supracondylar process on radiograph. Surgical exploration of the median nerve above the elbow with release of the aberrant ligament, and neurolysis when indicated, should alleviate the condition.

Median Nerve Compression in the Region of the Shoulder. High median nerve compression in the region of the shoulder or proximal humerus is uncommon. Most cases of high median nerve compression result from trauma.

Treatment of high median nerve compression is conservative, especially when the condition is caused by extrinsic trauma (e.g., crutch palsy). The time for full return of neurologic function varies, depending on the severity of the compression. In rare situations of a spontaneous onset without known injury, a complete evaluation including angiography, and in some cases surgical exploration, may be necessary to establish the source of the compression.

Digital Nerves in the Hand. Digital neuropathies result from acute or chronic trauma, a mass (cysts, tumors, osteophytes), or an area of localized inflammation (flexor tenosynovitis, Dupuytren's contracture).

Treatment of a digital nerve compression due to a cyst or tumor within the palm or digit is surgical. Furthermore, chronic trauma to the hands, as seen in woodchoppers, musicians, laborers, and staplers, should be avoided.

Ulnar Nerve

Entrapment in the Region of the Elbow. Ulnar nerve entrapment in the region of the elbow is the second most frequent upper limb compression neuropathy. In contrast with CTS, in which sensory impairment generally exists as the most significant disability, in ulnar nerve entrapment motor loss is usually the most important problem. Clinically, patients with ulnar neuropathy at the elbow (cubital tunnel) experience onset of or increase in one or more of the symptoms of pain, numbness, or tingling with the elbow flexion test (full elbow flexion with full extension of the wrists for 3 minutes).[45] Early diagnosis and treatment results in complete cure, whereas delayed therapy leads to incomplete return of function in the small intrinsic muscles of the hand.

Treatment depends on the cause and severity of the ulnar nerve compression, and on the length of time the symptoms have been present. *Nonsurgical treatment* appears to be indicated for the patient with intermittent symptoms, acute or chronic mild neuropathy, or mild neuropathy associated with an occupational cause. Therapy entails avoidance of repetitive flexion and extension of the elbow, resting the elbow, or splinting the elbow in extension. For intermittent symptoms associated with repetitive flexion-extension, change of activity may alleviate the condition. For a mild neuropathy produced by a blow or chronic pressure, splinting the elbow in an extended position may prove helpful. A bivalved long-arm cast can be fabricated for a more prolonged period. Splinting may be continued for 2 or 3 months, especially if the symptoms remain intermittent or show improvement. As long as symptoms do not progress, and particularly as long as there exists no motor involvement or objective sensory loss, then surgical intervention is not necessary. Careful clinical follow-up is important, and the patient should be checked for development of motor deficit, atrophy, or weakness, since development of any of these findings calls for a change in the therapeutic program.

Surgical techniques in the treatment of ulnar neuropathies at the elbow remain controversial[46, 47]; however, the best results of surgery occur in patients with mild signs and symptoms, while poor results develop in patients with severe atrophy. Medial epicondylectomy for ulnar neuropathy at the elbow provided symptomatic improvement in 98 percent of 46 patients undergoing this operation, while only 54 percent showed improved motor strength.[48] In patients with an ulnar neuropathy at the elbow and an associated anconeus epitrochlearis muscle, surgical treatment with excision of the anconeus epitrochlearis and cubital tunnel release without anterior transposition of the ulnar nerve has been successful.[49] According to the authors, anterior transposition of the ulnar nerve appears unnecessary in such cases.

Entrapment at the Wrist. Compressions of the ulnar nerve within or distal to Guyon's canal result from trauma; prolonged bicycling[50]; masses, including ganglions[51-53] and rarely a tuberculoma[54]; anomalies[55-57]; or inflammation.

Treatment of ulnar nerve compression in this location depends on the origin and duration of the condition. For mild compressions associated either with a single traumatic event or with chronic trauma, conservative treatment should be initially prescribed. Avoidance of the trauma, with or without splinting, often results in complete return of function. In cases not responding to nonsurgical care, surgical exploration, decompression, and neurolysis should be done. If the hook of the hamate bone is fractured, it should be excised along with decompression and neurolysis of the nerve. Ganglia and other soft tissue masses should be removed.[51, 52, 54]

Dorsal Sensory Branch Compression. Isolated neuropathy of the dorsal sensory branch of the ulnar nerve is associated with either blunt trauma or lacerations.

Treatment in most cases of blunt trauma includes protecting the area of injury, and symptoms will subside within a few weeks. In conditions of painful neuromas following a laceration, surgical exploration may be considered. If the involved nerve is entrapped in scar tissue, neurolysis may be beneficial.

Digital Nerves in the Hand. Mechanisms and treatment are similar to those discussed under the median nerve digital nerve syndromes.

Radial Nerve

High Radial Nerve Compressions. High radial nerve compressions occur proximal to the elbow prior to the division into the posterior interosseous branch and the sensory branch. Most of these radial nerve lesions are traumatic. Recently a 20-year-old male laborer was found to have a high radial nerve palsy following strenuous muscular activity.[58] At surgery he had a nerve constricture from the lateral head of the triceps muscle.

Treatment of traumatic radial nerve compression is generally conservative, as most patients with radial nerve paresis secondary to compression recover spontaneously. Treatment of a compression lesion of the radial nerve at a high level should include a cockup splint made of plaster or plastic for the wrist joint. This should be applied if the paresis lasts longer than a week. In long-lasting weakness, a spring-loaded extensor brace for the fingers may be used. In humeral fractures requiring surgical exploration,

the radial nerve should also be explored at the time of surgery, and in displaced fractures of the distal part of the humerus early exploration is necessary because of the high frequency of radial nerve entrapment between the fracture fragments.

Posterior Interosseous Nerve Syndrome (PINS). The PINS is an entrapment of the deep branch of the radial nerve just distal to the elbow joint.[59] Motor weakness of the extensors of the wrist and fingers (sparing the extensor carpi radialis longus and brevis) is seen. Infrequently, PINS occurs after excision of the radial head,[60] as an isolated paralysis of the descending branch,[61] or in association with congenital hemihypertrophy.[62]

Treatment of most cases of PINS is surgical. Ganglia, tumors, and lipomas should be removed surgically, and the PIN should be freed from any compressive bands or other structures.

Resistant Tennis Elbow. The PIN may be entrapped and mimic lateral epicondylitis in resistant tennis elbow.[63-65]

Treatment includes surgical exploration with release of the extensor carpi radialis tendon origin and release of any constricting vascular or fibrous band. In 30 percent of 111 cases of tennis elbow in Finland there appeared relief of PIN symptoms following surgery.[65]

Superficial Radial Nerve Lesions. The superficial radial nerve can be damaged by lacerations or compression around the wrist because of its superficial position. Infrequently, this nerve can be compressed by handcuffs, a wristwatch, or other straps and bandages around the wrist.

Treatment in cases of a compressive band or cast includes removal of the offending compression. In conditions of traction neuropathy as a result of surgery, symptoms often subside but may persist for 6 to 8 weeks. For persistent symptoms, surgical exploration is advisable. If there exists entrapment of the nerve by scar tissue, neurolysis will be helpful. If the superficial radial nerve shows a complete laceration, with neuroma of the stump, the prognosis for resolution of the symptoms is guarded.

Thoracic Outlet Syndromes (TOS)

The paresthesias of the TOS commonly precede the development of persistent pain, atrophy, or muscle weakness. The anatomic territories affected include those of the ulnar nerve and the medial cutaneous nerve of the forearm. Bony, fascial, and muscular structures can interfere with the functions of the neurovascular bundle located in the thoracic outlet.

Two types of *nonsurgical therapy* for TOS include (1) a corset and restraints to prevent elevation of the arms or the hands placed behind the head, and (2) a set of exercises designed to correct slumping shoulder posture. These exercises consist of full range of motion of the shoulder girdle, similar lateral and rotational movements of the neck, and exercises to strengthen rhomboid and trapezius muscles and to induce an erect posture.

Surgical treatment of TOS should be considered according to the following criteria: (1) signs of muscle wasting appear in the involved hand; (2) intermittent paresthesias are replaced by sensory loss; and (3) pain becomes incapacitating. First-rib resection through the transaxillary approach has been commonly used. Alternatively, exploration from above, usually with removal of the anterior scalene muscle, and exploration of the thoracic outlet has been utilized. This latter supraclavicular procedure possesses the advantage that a cervical rib, if present, will be directly within the field. Additionally, constricting bands may be found passing from a rudimentary rib, or from the transverse process of C7, to attach to the first rib. Disadvantages of the supraclavicular approach include (1) the surgical scar is cosmetically less acceptable; (2) temporary damage to the phrenic nerve or to the long thoracic nerve from retraction during the extensive dissection may result; and (3) more surgical dissection may be required with this procedure.

Suprascapular Nerve

A suprascapular nerve entrapment is characterized by pain and atrophy of the supraspinous and infraspinous muscles.[66–69]

Treatment depends on the cause and duration of the symptoms. Observation and conservative care are indicated in cases of acute blunt trauma with or without scapular fracture. In the case of a severe comminuted fracture of the scapula with obvious involvement of the scapular notch, earlier surgical exploration may be considered. In those cases experiencing repetitive minor trauma, avoiding the trauma generally corrects the problem. Whenever there exist persistent signs and symptoms, or in cases of spontaneous onset without a known cause, surgical exploration may be indicated.

Dorsal Scapular Nerve

In dorsal scapular nerve entrapments there is weakness of the rhomboideus major and minor and the levator scapulae as well as a tendency of the scapula to wing on wide abduction movements of the arm.

Treatment should be directed toward the cervical spine and includes sedation, muscle relaxants, analgesics, and physical therapy, since this syndrome is secondary to scalene hyperactivity caused by inadequacy of the spinal stabilization system. In severe cases, surgical neurolysis may be considered.

Long Thoracic Nerve

Because of the long thoracic nerve's straight anatomic course and fixation, it can be stretched. This occurs most often in heavy laborers or after direct trauma. In this condition the shoulder girdle displaces slightly backward, while the lower scapula demonstrates undue winging. Recovery from this syndrome usually occurs within 6 months of the original stretch injury.

Musculocutaneous Nerve

Very occasionally, the musculocutaneous nerve may become entrapped by the coracobrachial muscle, or it may even be ruptured by violent extension of the forearm. Surgical exploration may be necessary to differentiate a nerve entrapment from a nerve rupture. If coracoid mobilization becomes necessary during surgery, the musculocutaneous nerve and its branches should be identified and protected, keeping in mind the variations in anatomy and the level of penetration.[70]

Axillary Nerve

Most lesions of the axillary nerve are traumatic (a blow on the tip of the shoulder after a motor vehicle accident or a football injury). The treatment and prognosis of axillary nerve injury depend on the cause. A poor prognosis for full recovery may result from stretch injuries of the distal portions of the brachial plexus as the shoulder sags with deltoid atrophy.

LOWER LIMB

Sciatic Nerve

Sciatic nerve entrapments are uncommon, and most patients complaining of symptoms traceable to the sciatic nerve possess disease of the intervertebral discs or other structures of the lumbosacral spine (spinal stenosis, degenerative disease, rheumatoid or osteoarthritis, ankylosing spondylitis, intravertebral tumor,[71] and metastatic disease). A variation in the course of the sciatic nerve involves its passage between parts of the piriform muscle (the division of the nerve that becomes the peroneal trunk is usually the one that deviates). True compression of the sciatic nerve may occur from the piriform muscle, a myofascial band in the distal portion of the thigh between the biceps femoris and the abductor magnus, Baker's cyst, muscle fibrosis after intramuscular injections, and anticoagulation complications and after trauma (e.g., hip operation or needle biopsy[72] or sitting on hard surfaces.[73]

Treatment of the piriformis syndrome consists of

operating on the piriform muscle, removing one of the heads of origin, and releasing any constriction. Other causes of slowly progressive sciatic palsy should be treated according to the condition that caused the symptoms.[72] The iatrogenic symptoms related to damage to the sciatic nerve from hip surgery or from fracture in the pelvis or hip joint area have not usually been approached surgically.

Peroneal Nerve

The most frequent mechanism of damage to the peroneal nerve at the head of the fibula is acute compression of the nerve, causing a neuropraxic lesion. Fractures and other acute traumatic lesions may damage the nerve. Compressive causes of peroneal nerve damage include improperly applied plaster casts, tight stockings, bandages, other constrictive garments, and rarely cysts.[74] Unconsciousness from drug overdosage, anesthesia, or acute illness with stupor or coma will render patients susceptible to a peroneal compressive neuropathy.

Treatment in the majority of cases is *nonsurgical.* With motor disturbance, bracing with a plastic orthosis molded to the posterior calf and projecting in the shoe onto the plantar surface of the foot provides stability. With this type of brace, a compressive lesion of the peroneal nerve can be watched for several months before any consideration of a surgical approach need be considered.

Surgical therapy should be considered in those patients with a slowly progressive disturbance of peroneal nerve function in whom there is pain and progressive motor and sensory loss, entrapment neuropathy, ganglion, cyst, or other tumor. In such conditions relatively early exploration is indicated, since little would be gained by further delay and a simple entrapment is unlikely.

Anterior Tarsal Tunnel Syndrome. This syndrome involves an entrapment of the terminal portion of the deep peroneal nerve where it runs below the dense superficial fascia of the ankle.

Nonsurgical therapy includes a comfortable foot position, by splint, rest, or a combination of both, and then treating the patient conservatively, obtaining slow and gradual relief. Local steroid injection may provide temporary relief.

Surgical release of the entrapment may be needed, and it is necessary to trace the nerve far enough proximally to exclude a lesion in the ankle under the extensor retinaculum.

Posterior Tibial Nerve

Tarsal Tunnel Syndrome (TTS). In the TTS, the posterior tibial nerve becomes entrapped at the level of the medial malleolus, the point from which the nerve supplies sensory innervation to the sole of the foot and motor innervation to the intrinsic muscles

of the foot (Figs. 101–4 and 101–5).[75] Pain in the sole of the foot is the primary symptom of TTS.

Nonsurgical therapy begins with removal of any irritating process and bracing the foot with a medial arch support. Anti-inflammatory medications work against local phlebitis or tenosynovitis.

Surgery may be needed in as many as 60 percent of cases of TTS. The surgical approach involves a curved incision below the medial malleolus, extending beyond the distal limit of the retinaculum. The laciniate ligament and the retinaculum are opened, and the nerve is freed. The release and dissection of the nerve must be carried as far distally as possible, typically to the level of its bifurcation into the plantar nerves.[75]

Medial and Lateral Plantar Nerve Syndrome. A partial TTS (either a medial or a lateral plantar nerve deficit in the foot) alerts the clinician to the possibility of a process distal to the flexor retinaculum. Symptoms include weakness and burning of the feet. Conservative measures, including rest and local steroid injection into the appropriate area, should be done initially. Surgery should be considered if the symptoms or signs progress, or if the exact level of compression is not certain.

Interdigital Nerves. The medial and lateral plantar nerves terminate in the interdigital nerves. Morton's neuroma may occur at the region of the interdigital nerve in the third and fourth interspaces of the foot and become a source of lower limb pain.

Initial conservative management consists of pad-

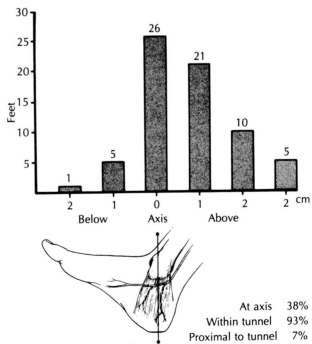

At axis   38%
Within tunnel   93%
Proximal to tunnel 7%

Figure 101–4. Distribution of posterior tibial nerve branching. (With permission from Havel, P. E., Elbraheim, N. A., Clark, S. E., Jackson, T., and DiDio, L.: Tibial nerve branching in the tarsal tunnel. Foot Ankle 9:117–119, 1988. © 1988, American Orthopaedic Foot Society.)

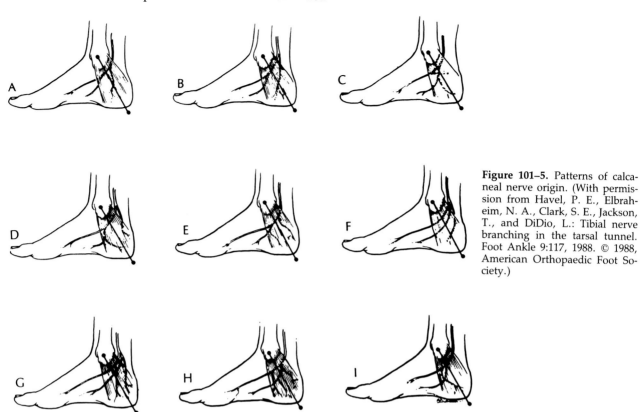

Figure 101–5. Patterns of calcaneal nerve origin. (With permission from Havel, P. E., Elbraheim, N. A., Clark, S. E., Jackson, T., and DiDio, L.: Tibial nerve branching in the tarsal tunnel. Foot Ankle 9:117, 1988. © 1988, American Orthopaedic Foot Society.)

ding the metatarsal head or changing to shoes that cause less lateral pinching. Commonly, a surgical excision of the nerve is required. This is done by an incision over the web space between the toes; the branch of the nerve is identified and tracked proximally until the branch point at which the two digital nerves are formed from the proper interdigital nerve.

Sural Nerve

The sural nerve is subject to laceration or compressive lesions primarily at the level of its exit through fascia, with subsequent paresthesias radiating into the lateral part of the foot. Since the sural nerve can be a site for nerve biopsy, clinical symptoms similar to lacerations and compressive lesions may ensue after biopsy. If initial avoidance of continued irritation, and rest of the area, do not produce resolution of the symptoms, surgical exploration may be considered.

Lateral Femoral Cutaneous Nerve

Meralgia Paresthetica (MP). The usual cause of MP is entrapment of the lateral femoral cutaneous nerve where it passes underneath or through the inguinal ligament at its origin on the anterior iliac spine.

Nonsurgical therapy consists of avoiding any new or recently started exercise, and removing constrict-

ing binders, corsets, or tight belts. If pregnancy or weight gain appear to be provocative factors, the passage of time and weight reduction will improve symptoms. In certain conditions, local nerve blocks may be beneficial.

Surgical procedures should be considered if the symptoms are relatively long-lasting or very painful. Surgery consists of release of the entrapment at the level of the nerve's exit under the inguinal ligament. If the lateral femoral nerve is cut, unpleasant paresthesias may increase.

Femoral Nerve

Femoral nerve lesions may produce weakness and atrophy of the quadriceps muscle, reduction in the knee reflex on the affected side, and a sensory loss over the anterior thigh and medial calf.

Treatment usually does not require surgery. Most pelvic lesions in the femoral triangle at the region of the inguinal ligament are treated by waiting if a vascular process is suspected, or by medical management if a tumor or other mass lesion is the cause. Treatment of a femoral neuropathy may necessitate a long leg brace, including a spring-loaded knee assist to produce knee extension so the patient may walk safely. Alternatively, if the lesion is expected to be of short duration, assistance with a crutch will suffice.

Saphenous Nerve. The saphenous nerve, one of three sensory branches of the femoral nerve, has a long course through the adductor canal, penetrating fascia above the level of the knee and supplying the medial calf, the medial malleolus, and a small portion of the medial part of the arch of the foot. Entrapments, trauma, or surgical procedures may produce a saphenous neuropathy. Treatment is usually symptomatic (i.e., rest, anti-inflammatory medication, and physical therapy).

Ilioinguinal Nerve

The point of entrapment of the ilioingual nerve often is located slightly medial to the anterior iliac spine, and clinically the patient complains of burning pain over the lower abdomen, radiating down into the inner portion of the upper thigh and into the scrotum or labia majora. Often the cause of this syndrome is trauma (blow to the abdominal wall, a surgical incision, or a scar). Conservative measures include rest and anti-inflammatory medications. Neurolysis is indicated in severely affected patients who are experiencing pain.

Genitofemoral Nerve

The genitofemoral nerve supplies the skin over the upper thigh below the femoral triangle and the lower lateral scrotum or labia, and descends through the pelvis over the iliac muscle near the obturator nerve. In retroperitoneal processes, such as tumor and hemorrhage, the genitofemoral nerve may be involved. Relief of symptoms can be provided by surgery to free adhesions entrapping the nerve.

Obturator Nerve

The clinical symptoms of obturator neuropathy are sensory, including paresthesias, sensory loss, and radiating pain in the medial thigh. Most obturator nerve lesions are traumatic, resulting from pelvic fracture, gunshot wound, or other major trauma. Initial therapy includes rest, appropriate analgesics, and anti-inflammatory medications. Rarely, surgical intrapelvic section of the nerve may become necessary.

MISCELLANEOUS ENTRAPMENT SYNDROMES

Double-Crush Syndromes

Degenerative cervical spine disease, with variable degrees of spondylosis, is a common clinical condition. When a patient becomes symptomatic from the cervical spine process and develops a concomitant entrapment neuropathy (especially CTS and ulnar neuropathies), one conveniently refers to the entire clinical picture as the *double-crush syndrome*.

With the use of electrodiagnostic studies and CT scans this syndrome can be readily discerned. The patient with the double-crush syndrome responds only if treatment is directed toward both processes—that is, if a cervical collar, exercises, and anti-inflammatory medications are utilized for the cervical spine symptoms and if specific therapy is instituted for the specific entrapment neuropathy.

Rectus Abdominis Syndrome

Any of the branches of intercostal nerves T7 to T12 may be entrapped within the substance of the rectus muscle, leading to localized pain in the abdominal wall that becomes exaggerated by pressure over the rectus muscle or by elevating one leg while the patient is in a supine position. Conservative measures including local steroid injections often provide relief of symptoms.

Pseudoradicular Syndrome

In undiagnosed persistent leg pain, the pseudoradicular syndrome should be considered.[76] Of about 4000 patients with lower extremity pain referred to a medical center for evaluation of suspected lumbar radiculopathy, 36 patients were found to have peripheral nerve entrapments as the sole cause of their leg pain (nine patients had femoral nerve entrapments proximal to the inguinal ligament; seven had saphenous nerve entrapments about the knee; 20 had peroneal nerve entrapments at or above the popliteal fossa; and nine had tibial nerve entrapments in the popliteal space).[76] The diagnosis was made on the basis of selective spinal and peripheral nerve blocks as well as electrophysiologic studies. Thirty-two patients underwent surgical exploration and external neurolysis (12 with peroneal, nine with tibial, seven with saphenous, and four with femoral nerve lesions). Prior to lumbar spine surgery, peripheral nerve lesions should be ruled out.

Compartment Syndromes

Compartment syndromes (CS) occur in specific clinical situations in which locally increased tissue pressure within a closed muscle compartment compromises local circulation and neuromuscular function.[77-84] The increased frequency of CS correlates with prevalence of limb trauma, drug and alcohol abuse, limb surgery, limb ischemia, and physical exertion of limb muscles. Factors that reduce the tolerance of limbs for increased tissue pressure include hypotension, hemorrhage, arterial occlusion, and limb elevation. The clinical features of CS include (1) tense compartment envelope, (2) severe pain in excess of that clinically expected for the specific condition, (3) pain on passive stretch of the muscles

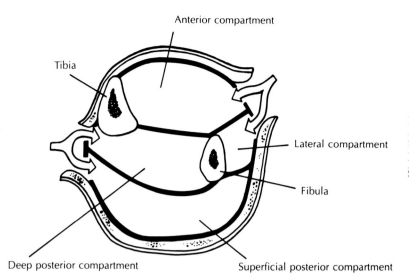

Figure 101–6. Cross-section through the upper third of the left calf. (From Lagerstrom, C. F., Reed, R. L., II, Rowlands, B. J., and Fischer, R. P.: Early fasciotomy for acute clinically evident post-traumatic compartment syndrome. Am. J. Surg. 158:36–39, 1989. Used by permission.)

in the compartment, (4) muscle weakness within the compartment, and (5) altered sensation in the distribution of the nerves coursing through the compartment. Anatomic locations within the body in which the CS may occur include (1) *leg* (Fig. 101–6), anterior, lateral, and posterior (superficial and deep); (2) *thigh* (Fig. 101–7), quadriceps muscle; (3) *buttock,* gluteal muscles; (4) *hand,* interosseous muscles; (5) *forearm,* dorsal and volar; and (6) *arm,* deltoid and biceps muscles.

Treatment of the CS aims at minimizing neurologic deficits by promptly restoring local blood flow. *Nonsurgical measures* include eliminating external en-velopes and maintaining local arterial pressures and preserving peripheral nerve function. The objective of *surgery* is to decompress limiting envelopes and débride nonviable tissue (Fig. 101–8).[77, 78, 80–83]

Other medical conditions that may be confused with CS include (1) infection or inflammation, (2) arterial occlusion, and (3) primary nerve injury, entrapment, or both. Careful clinical examination, tissue pressure measurements,[77, 82, 85] direct nerve stimulation, electrodiagnostic studies, Doppler sonography, and arteriography and venography will assist in differentiating between these conditions and the various true CS.

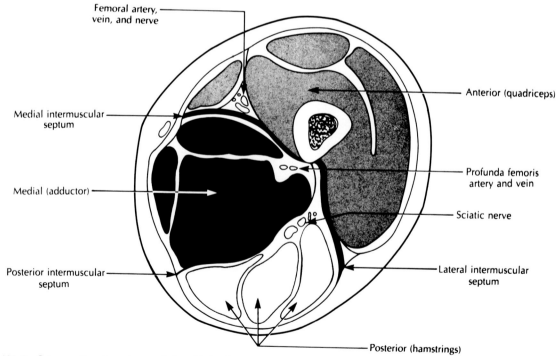

Figure 101–7. Cross-sectional anatomy of the thigh, demonstrating the anterior (quadriceps), posterior (hamstrings), and medial (adductor) compartments. (From Schwartz, J. T., Brumback, R. J., Lakatos, R., Poka, A., Bathon, G. H., and Burgess, A. R.: Acute compartment syndrome of the thigh. A spectrum of injury. J. Bone Joint Surg. 71A:392, 1989. Used by permission.)

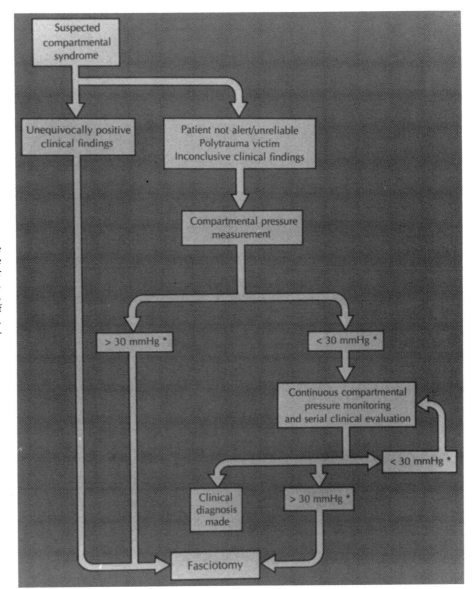

Figure 101–8. Algorithm used in the diagnosis and treatment of an acute compartment syndrome of the lower leg, secondary to a tibial fracture. (From Bourne, R. B., and Rorabeck, C. H.: Compartment syndromes of the lower leg. Clin. Orthop. Rel. Res. 240:97, 1989. Used by permission.)

Repetitive Strain Disorder and Occupation-Related Syndromes

Three categories of patients in whom this type of diagnosis can be considered were proposed by Barton in an editorial of the British Medical Journal.[86]

The first category includes patients in whom the diagnosis of repetitive strain disorder is beyond doubt; for example, peritendinitis crepitans (de Quervain's disease), a tender swelling where the radial wrist extensors cross under the abductor pollicis longus and extensor pollicis brevis, described in washerwomen and autoworkers in England. Also included in the first group, but having a less defined pathophysiology, are musicians,[86–91] dancers,[92, 93] keyboard operators,[94] and avid athletes (joggers,[95, 96] cross-country skiers,[97] sailboard enthusiasts,[98] rock climbers,[99] and those participating in other sport activities[100]). When the pain arises in the arm and shoulder in this last group of individuals it is best conceptualized as a form of fatigue.[101]

Within the second category of patients are those who have "genuine" problems that are mistakenly believed to be caused by their employment, but that, in fact, are just part of many of the natural processes that affect the human body. In fact, some forms of usage can exacerbate the symptoms of some regional musculoskeletal illness (e.g., carpal tunnel syndrome).[102] Apparently, sociopolitical phenomena allow some of these patients to attribute symptoms to their work.[86]

The third, and apparently the smallest, category includes those who realize that their symptoms, if indeed they exist, are not caused by their work but hope to establish such a relation in order to get a financial reward.

An optimal approach to treatment of repetitive strain disorders combines physical and psychologic techniques.[103]

Overuse Syndromes. Overuse syndromes are symptom complexes defined as injuries caused by the cumulative effects on tissues of repetitive physical stresses that exceed physiologic limits.[88] Among musicians and dancers the overuse syndromes originate in the constant repetition of intense practice of a musical instrument or dancing, respectively.[88-93] This situation most commonly affects the muscle-tendon units, and the usual symptom is pain while playing the instrument or dancing and, not long thereafter, disability. In the initial stages, the pain subsides when the activity stops. During later advanced stages (after severe or prolonged injury to the muscle-tendon unit) pain persists, and if injury continues accurate performance may become impossible.

Musicians on keyboard instruments must repeat movements of extension, flexion, and rotation of their fingers. Overuse (or misuse) problems with the extensors of the fingers and wrist, the lumbrical muscles, and the interosseous muscles of the dominant hand can easily develop. Viola and violin players can develop problems in the fingers, hands, and wrists compounded by the awkward position in which the instrument must be held. Rotation of the neck to the left and abduction and external rotation of the left shoulder predispose the cervical spine and left shoulder to pain in these joints. Viola and cello players may have the same digital and manual difficulties, and they have the added risk of developing paresthesias in the legs. Wind instrument players may suffer overuse that affects the embouchure (position of the lips), the soft palate, and the muscles of the pharynx, leading to inadequate volume, imperfect control, and, at times, inaccuracy of intonation.[88]

It appears that overuse leads to muscle-fiber injury. Muscle biopsy studies from players with overuse syndromes show glycogen depletion and acute degenerative changes in muscle fibers, edema of the perimysium and areolar tissues, interstitial hemorrhage, thrombosis of venules, and margination of leukocytes around arterioles.[88] Additional changes include hypertrophy of the type 2 muscle fibers, increase in the number of central nuclei, and mitochondrial abnormalities.

Overuse syndromes and peripheral nerve entrapments may overlap because hypertrophy of small muscle groups can cause compression of nerves at various anatomic sites. An important clinical difference between entrapment neuropathies and overuse syndromes is that the former produce weakness, sensory changes, or both in addition to discomfort, pain, and loss of ability to play or dance accurately. Among the entrapment syndromes, CTS is the one most often seen in musicians. Other rare entrapment syndromes include entrapment of the median nerve in the pronator teres (PTS) or in the forearm (AIN). The ulnar nerve can be entrapped at the elbow or wrist (especially in flute players). Rarely will the radial nerve become involved among musicians.

Most authorities recommend rest for the overuse syndrome.[88] Penneys[91] notes that in order to play a musical instrument well, one must stress the importance of respecting the body and the soul, and stay within the normal biologic limitations of the motor units and ligaments.

Dystonias. Dystonia has been defined as a movement disorder characterized by sustained muscle contractions, frequently causing repetitive movements, twisting, or abnormal postures.[104, 105] A classic example of a focal dystonia is "writer's cramp"; neurophysiologic electrodiagnostic studies have demonstrated abnormalities of muscle control, with concurrent contraction of both agonist and antagonist muscle groups, and abnormalities in the normal reflex inhibition of antagonist muscles.[104] As many as 15 percent of instrumental performers experience focal dystonias in one form or another.[88] These people initially report loss of coordination while playing an instrument, often accompanied by curling or extension of fingers during passages that require rapid and forceful finger movements. Once the disorder develops, the loss of motor control progresses slowly over years and is not accompanied by sensory symptoms. There exists no firm evidence that relates focal dystonias to an overuse injury preceding the dystonia. When a physician is confronted by a painless hand problem suggesting some features of an entrapment syndrome, focal dystonia should be considered when loss of motor function is characterized by some loss of voluntary motor control. A diagnosis of hysteria should be excluded in these patients.

Perioperative Nerve Lesions

Perioperative nerve lesions (PONL) refer to focal neuropathies that are the result of acute trauma during surgical procedures.[106] In the differential diagnosis, events that are only indirectly related to a medical procedure as well as others that are only coincidental will be included. There appears to be no specific pattern of pathophysiologic mechanisms in PONL. The syndromes can be discussed according to the clinical setting in which they occur.

Brachial Plexus Palsy in Surgery. The brachial plexus appears to be the most susceptible of all nerve groups to damage from poor positioning during anesthesia. Stretching appears to be the usual cause of injury; the plexus has a relatively long course, traveling from the vertebral foramina to the axilla, and it lies in close proximity to a number of mobile bony structures. In brachial plexus stretch injuries, most patients recover within 3 months; recovery, however, may be prolonged for more than a year. Although surgery is not indicated in most cases, some studies suggest improvement in motor function after certain types of brachial plexus injury.[107] MRI evaluation may provide clinical information of distal as well as proximal lesions of the brachial plexus and assist in defining both the nature and the extent of injury.[108]

Open heart surgery by a median sternotomy approach can give rise to a brachial plexus palsy. In this clinical situation, it is not clear that improper positioning always produces the palsy.

Serious neurologic complications can develop from a surgical procedure for TOS. Patients may develop causalgia with relatively few neurologic deficits on clinical examination.

Ulnar Nerve Palsy. Among the commonest focal peripheral neuropathies are those involving the ulnar nerve. Intraoperative positional damage to the ulnar nerve in anatomic variants has been reported.[109] In case of increased mobility of the ulnar nerve at the elbow, it has been recommended that the arm should be placed in supination with the elbow extended and carefully padded at the time of surgical procedures. Other cases occur during the postoperative period, or symptoms that previously had been mild or transient may abruptly become obvious and disabling. As ulnar nerve disorders are often heterogeneous, some reflecting long-standing trauma, some entrapment in the cubital tunnel, it appears that various factors play a role in postoperative ulnar neuropathies. Ulnar nerve lesions during surgical procedures may reflect the additive effects of positioning as well as a subclinical compression of pre-existing neuropathy at the cubital tunnel. Furthermore, diabetic patients may be more susceptible to compressive neuropathies.

Included among the ulnar neuropathies associated with medical procedures are two patients who sustained mild ulnar mononeuropathies at the level of the upper arm after injections by the same nurse.[110] In these cases, the nurse attempted to inject the middle deltoid; the ulnar nerve was reached by standing at the patient's side and injecting "sidearm" into the upper arm.

Peroneal Nerve. Peroneal nerve palsies can occur with knee arthroplasties, and this complication appears most commonly in those with severe knee deformities. Positioning or use of certain appliances may also produce a peroneal neuropathy.

Sciatic Nerve, Obturator Nerve, and Femoral Nerve. Sciatic, obturator, or femoral nerve injury may occur with total hip arthroplasty, and, rarely, patients have had one or more nerves embedded in methacrylate. Sciatic nerve palsy may occur more often in diabetic patients undergoing surgical procedures than in normal individuals. Hematoma formation may be a potential source of femoral neuropathy during renal transplantation.

Lateral Femoral Cutaneous Nerve. Meralgia paresthetica may occur after iliac bone grafting and as a complication of a groin flap. In these instances there appears to be injury to the lateral femoral cutaneous nerve where it passes close by the iliac crest.

Iliohypogastric Nerve, Ilioinguinal Nerve, and Genitofemoral Nerve. Hernial repair, lower abdominal surgery, or gynecologic surgery may injure these three nerves as they traverse the lower abdominal wall.

The ilioinguinal nerve can be injured at the time of inguinal herniorrhaphy; this nerve has a retroperitoneal course after its origin from T12 and L1 nerve roots and becomes extraperitoneal after it passes medial to the anterior iliac crest, and runs along the inguinal canal with the spermatic cord. Patients who have injury to the ilioinguinal nerve complain of pain and may report sensory loss in a strip of skin extending along the inguinal canal to the base of the penis and scrotum, or to the labia.

The iliohypogastric nerve has a course and distribution slightly rostral to the ilioinguinal nerve. Its sensory supplies are to the region of the skin over the greater trochanter and the lower abdominal wall just above the pubis.

The genitofemoral nerve remains retroperitoneal and much more medial in the pelvis and eventually supplies the femoral triangle (a small area of skin on the medial thigh) and most of the scrotum and penis or labia.

In patients suffering long-lasting pain, paresthesias as a result of injury to one of these nerves of the lower abdomen, a surgical exploration is often the best choice of treatment.

Obstetric Injuries. During vaginal delivery a woman may develop infrequently a painless unilateral lower limb weakness; often this is a footdrop, suggesting a partial sciatic nerve injury. Other clinical presentations include weakness of knee extension and reduction of knee reflex, indicating a femoral neuropathy. Although these disorders may be due to pressure on the lumbosacral plexus by the fetal head, the cause may be multivariate.

CONCLUSIONS

In addition to a careful clinical neurologic examination, the evaluation of any patient with a suspected peripheral nerve entrapment syndrome, perioperative nerve injury, compartment syndrome, or overuse syndrome should include electrodiagnostic studies (especially electromyography and nerve conduction studies), appropriate radiographs, use of current neuroimaging technologies (i.e., MRI and CT) when indicated, and laboratory studies in patients suspected of having systemic illnesses. In most patients with compresson neuropathies, focal nerve injuries, and the compartment syndromes, diagnosis and therapy can be effected early if a thorough clinical evaluation commences when the patient initially complains of symptoms. It is vitally important to distinguish the correct categories of repetitive strain disorders so that appropriate diagnosis and therapy can be rendered. As more knowledge accumulates, additional information concerning the mechanisms of and therapy for the entrapment neuropathies, focal nerve lesions, and overuse syndromes will become available.

References

1. Feierstein, M. S.: The performance and usefulness of nerve conduction studies in the orthopedic office. Orthop. Clin. North Am. 19:859, 1988.
2. Middleton, W. D., Kneeland, J. B., Kellman, G. M., Cates, J. D., Sanger, J. R., Jesmanowicz, A., Froncisz, W., and Hyde, J. S.: MR imaging of the carpal tunnel: Normal anatomy and preliminary findings in the carpal tunnel syndrome. Am. J. Radiol. 148:307, 1987.
3. Mesgarzadeh, M., Schneck, C. D., and Bonakdarpour, A.: Carpal tunnel: MR imaging. Part I. Normal anatomy. Radiology 171:743, 1989.
4. Mesgarzadeh, M., Schneck, C. D., Bonakdarpour, A., Mitra, A., and Conaway, D.: Carpal tunnel: MR imaging. Part II. Carpal tunnel syndrome. Radiology 171:749, 1989.
5. McCollam, S. M., Corley, F. G., and Green, D. P.: Posterior interosseous nerve palsy caused by ganglions of the proximal radioulnar joint. J. Hand Surg. 13A:725, 1988.
6. Nakano, K. K.: Entrapment neuropathies. In Kelley, W. N., Harris, E. D., Jr., Ruddy, S., and Sledge, C. B. (eds.): Textbook of Rheumatology. 3rd ed. Philadelphia, W. B. Saunders, 1989, pp. 1844–1859.
7. Dawson, D. M., Hallett, M., and Millender, L. H.: Entrapment Neuropathies. Boston, Little, Brown and Co., 1990, pp. 1–434.
8. Tebib, J. G., Bascoulergue, J., Dumontet, C., Paupert-Ravault, A., Prallet, B., Colson, F., and Bouvier, M.: Brachial plexus compression by an iatrogenic arteriovenous fistula. Clin. Rheumatol. 6:593, 1987.
9. Redmond, J. M. T., Cros, D., Martin, J. B., and Shahani, B. T.: Relapsing bilateral brachial plexopathy during pregnancy. Report of a case. Arch. Neurol. 46:462, 1989.
10. Katirji, M. B.: Brachial plexus injury following liver transplantation. Neurology 39:736, 1989.
11. LeQuang, C.: Postirradiation lesions of the brachial plexus. Results of surgical treatment. Hand Clin. 5:23, 1989.
12. Berwick, J. E., and Lessin, M. E.: Brachial plexus injury occurring during oral and maxillofacial surgery: A case report. J. Oral Maxillofac. Surg. 47:643, 1989.
13. Seale, K. S.: Reflex sympathetic dystrophy of the lower extremity. Clin. Orthop. Rel. Res. 243:80, 1989.
14. Werner, R., Davidoff, G., Jackson, M. D., Cremer, S., Ventocilla, C., and Wolf, L.: Factors affecting the sensitivity and specificity of the three-phase technetium bone scan in the diagnosis of reflex sympathetic dystrophy syndrome in the upper extremity. J. Hand Surg. 14A:520, 1989.
15. Greenspan, J.: Carpal tunnel syndrome. A common but treatable cause of wrist pain. Postgrad. Med. 84:34, 1988.
16. Spinner, R. J., Bachman, J. W., and Amadio, P. C.: The many faces of carpal tunnel syndrome. Mayo Clin. Proc. 64:829, 1989.
17. Kyle, R. A., Eilers, S. G., Linscheid, R. L., Gaffey, T. A.: Amyloid localized to tenosynovium at carpal tunnel release. Natural history of 124 cases. Am. J. Clin. Pathol. 91:393, 1989.
18. Wand, J. S.: The natural history of carpal tunnel syndrome in lactation. J. R. Soc. Med. 82:349, 1989.
19. Chanard, J., Bindi, P., Lavaud, S., Toupance, O., Maheut, H., and Lacour, F.: Carpal tunnel syndrome and type of dialysis membrane. Br. Med. J. 298:867, 1989.
20. Ullian, M. E., Hammond, W. S., Alfrey, A. C., Schultz, A., and Molitris, B. A.: Beta$_2$-microglobulin-associated amyloidosis in chronic hemodialysis patients with carpal tunnel syndrome. Medicine 68:107, 1989.
21. Brand, M. G., and Gelberman, R. H.: Lipoma of the flexor digitorum superficialis causing triggering at the carpal canal and median nerve compression. J. Hand Surg. 13A:342, 1988.
22. Shimizu, K., Iwasaki, R., Hoshikawa, H., and Yamamuro, T.: Entrapment neuropathy of the palmar cutaneous branch of the median nerve by the fascia of flexor digitorum superficialis. J. Hand Surg. 13A:581, 1988.
23. Kerrigan, J. J., Bertoni, J. M., and Jaeger, S. H.: Ganglion cysts and carpal tunnel syndrome. The J. Hand Surg. 13A:763, 1988.
24. Gellman, H., Chandler, D. R., Petrasek, J., Sie, I., Adkins, R., Waters, R. I.: Carpal tunnel syndrome in paraplegic patients. J. Bone Joint Surg. 70:517, 1988.
25. DeHertogh, D., Ritland, D., and Green, R.: Carpal tunnel syndrome due to gonococcal tenosynovitis. Orthopedics 11:199, 1988.
26. Chidgey, L. K., Szabo, R. M., and Wiese, D. A.: Acute carpal tunnel syndrome caused by pigmented villonodular synovitis of the wrist. Clin. Orthop. Rel. Res. 228:254, 1988.
27. Steere, A. C.: Lyme disease. N. Engl. J. Med. 321:586, 1989.
28. Halperin, J. J., Volkman, D. J., Luft, B. J., and Dattwyler, R. J.: Carpal tunnel syndrome in Lyme borreliosis. Muscle Nerve 12:397, 1989.
29. Widder, S., and Shons, A. R.: Carpal tunnel syndrome associated with extra tunnel vascular compression of the median nerve motor branch. J. Hand Surg. 13A:926, 1988.
30. Margolis, W., and Kraus, J. F.: The prevalence of carpal tunnel syndrome symptoms in female supermarket checkers. J. Occup. Med. 29:953, 1987.
31. Nathan, P. A., Meadows, K. D., and Doyle, L. S.: Sensory segmental latency values of the median nerve for a population of normal individuals. Arch. Phys. Med. Rehabil. 69:499, 1988.
32. LaBan, M. M., MacKenzie, J. R., and Zemenick, G. A.: Anatomic observations in carpal tunnel syndrome as they relate to the tethered median nerve stress test. Arch. Phys. Med. Rehabil. 70:44, 1989.
33. Braun, R. M., Davidson, K., and Doehr, S.: Provocative testing in the diagnosis of dynamic carpal tunnel syndrome. J. Hand Surg. 14:195, 1989.
34. Okutsu, I., Ninomiya, S., Hamanaka, I., Kuroshima, N., and Inanami, H.: Measurement of pressure in the carpal canal before and after endoscopic management of carpal tunnel syndrome. J. Bone Joint Surg. 71A:679, 1989.
35. Szabo, R. M., and Chidgey, L. K.: Stress carpal tunnel pressures in patients with carpal tunnel syndrome and normal patients. J. Hand Surg. 14A:624, 1989.
36. Rojviroj, S., Sirichatrivapee, W., Kowsuwon, W., Wongwiwattananon, J., Tamnanthong, N., and Jeeravipoolvarn, P.: Pressures in the carpal tunnel. J. Bone Joint Surg. (Br.) 72:516, 1990.
37. Winn, E. J., Jr., and Habes, D. J.: Carpal tunnel area as a risk factor for carpal tunnel syndrome. Muscle Nerve 13:254, 1990.
38. Crandall, R. E., and Weeks, P. M.: Multiple nerve dysfunction after carpal tunnel release. J. Hand Surg. 13A:584, 1988.
39. McConnell, J. R., and Bush, D. C.: Intraneural steroid injection as a complication in the management of carpal tunnel syndrome. Clin. Orthop. 250:181, 1990.
40. Bergman, R. S., Murphy, B. J., and Foglietti, M. A.: Clinical experience with the CO$_2$ laser during carpal tunnel decompression. Plast. Reconstr. Surg. 81:933, 1988.
41. Serner, C. O.: The anterior interosseous nerve syndrome. Int. Orthop. 12:193, 1989.
42. Geissler, W. B., Fernandez, D. L., and Graca, R.: Anterior interosseous nerve palsy complicating a forearm fracture in a child. J. Hand Surg. 15A:44, 1990.
43. Jones, N. F., and Ming, N. L.: Persistent median artery as a cause of pronator syndrome. J. Hand Surg. 13A:728, 1988.
44. Ergungor, M. F., Kars, H. Z., and Yalin, R.: Median neuralgia caused by brachial pseudoaneurysm. Neurosurgery 24:924, 1989.
45. Buehler, M. J., and Thayer, D. T.: The elbow flexion test. A clinical test for the cubital tunnel syndrome. Clin. Orthop. Rel. Res. 233:213, 1988.
46. Dellon, A. L.: Review of treatment results for ulnar nerve entrapments at the elbow. J. Hand Surg. (Am.) 14:688, 1989.
47. Gabel, G. T., and Amadio, P. C.: Reoperation for failed decompression of the ulnar nerve in the region of the elbow. J. Bone Joint Surg. 72A:213, 1990.
48. Goldberg, B. J., Light, T. R., and Blair, S. J.: Ulnar neuropathy at the elbow: Results of medial epicondylectomy. J. Hand Surg. 14A:182, 1989.
49. Masear, V. R., Hill, J. J., and Cohen, S. A.: Ulnar compression neuropathy secondary to the anconeus epitrochlearis muscle. J. Hand Surg. 13A:720, 1988.
50. Hankey, G. J., and Gubbay, S. S.: Compressive mononeuropathy of the deep palmar branch of the ulnar nerve in cyclists. J. Neurol. Neurosurg. Psychiatry 51:1588, 1988.
51. Cavallo, M., Poppi, M., Martinelli, P., and Gaist, G.: Distal ulnar neuropathy from carpal ganglia: A clinical and electrophysiological study. Neurosurgery 22:902, 1988.
52. Kuschner, S. H., Gelberman, R. H., and Jennings, C.: Ulnar nerve compression at the wrist. J. Hand Surg. 13A:577, 1988.
53. Giuliani, G., Poppi, M., Pozzati, E., and Forti, A.: Ulnar neuropathy due to a carpal ganglion: The diagnostic contribution of CT. Neurology 40:1001, 1990.
54. Nucci, F., Mastronardi, L., Artico, M., Ferrante, L., and Acqui, M.: Tuberculoma of the ulnar nerve: Case report. Neurosurgery 22:906, 1988.
55. Dodds, G. A., III, Hale, D., and Jackson, W. T.: Incidence of anatomic variants in Guyon's canal. J. Hand Surg. 15A:352, 1990.
56. Zook, E. G., Kucan, J. O., and Guy, R. J.: Palmar wrist pain caused by ulnar nerve entrapment in the flexor carpi ulnaris tendon. J. Hand Surg. 13A:732, 1988.
57. Milek, M. A., and Thompson, J. D.: Compression of the deep branch of the ulnar nerve at the adductor hiatus producing pain without muscle atrophy. J. Hand Surg. 13A:283, 1988.
58. Mitsunaga, M. M., and Nakano, K. K.: High radial nerve palsy following strenuous muscular activity. A case report. Clin. Orthop. Rel. Res. 234:139, 1988.
59. Papadopoulos, N., Paraschos, A., and Pelekis, P.: Anatomical observations on the arcade of Froshse and other structures related to the deep radial nerve. Anatomical interpretation of deep radial nerve entrapment neuropathy. Folio Morphol. 37:319, 1989.
60. Crawford, G. P.: Late radial tunnel syndrome after excision of the radial head. J. Bone Joint Surg. 70A:1416, 1988.
61. Hirayama, T., and Takemitsu, Y.: Isolated paralysis of the descending

branch of the posterior interosseous nerve. J. Bone Joint Surg. 70A:1402, 1988.

62. Dumitru, D., Walsh, N., and Visser, B.: Congenital hemihypertrophy associated with posterior interosseous nerve entrapment. Arch. Phys. Med. Rehabil. 69:696, 1988.

63. Chard, M. D., and Hazelman, B. L.: Tennis elbow—a reappraisal. Br. J. Rheumatol. 28:186, 1989.

64. Nirschl, R. P.: Prevention and treatment of elbow and shoulder injuries in the tennis player. Clin. Sports Med. 7:289, 1988.

65. Jalovaara, P., and Lindholm, R. V.: Decompresion of the posterior interosseous nerve for tennis elbow. Arch. Orthop. Trauma Surg. 108:243, 1989.

66. Kaspi, A., Yanai, J., Pick, C. G., and Mann, G.: Entrapment of the distal suprascapular nerve. An anatomical study. Int. Orthop. 12:273, 1988.

67. Lang, C., Druschky, K. F., Strum, U., Neundörfer, B., and Fahlbusch, R.: Suprascapular nerve entrapment syndrome. Dtsch. Med. Wochenschr. 113:1349, 1988.

68. Alon, M., Weiss, S., Fishel, B., and Dekel, S.: Bilateral suprascapular nerve entrapment syndrome due to an anomalous transverse scapular ligament. Clin. Orthop. Rel. Res. 234:31, 1988.

69. Kiss, G., and Komar, J.: Suprascapular nerve compression at the spinoglenoid notch. Muscle Nerve 13:556, 1990.

70. Flatow, E. L., Bigliani, L. U., and April, E. W.: An anatomic study of the musculocutaneous nerve and its relationship to the coracoid process. Clin. Orthop. Rel. Res. 244:166, 1989.

71. Bourque, P. R., and Dyck, P. J.: Selective calf weakness suggests intraspinal pathology, not peripheral neuropathy. Arch. Neurol. 47:79, 1990.

72. Papadopoulos, S. M., McGillicuddy, J. E., and Messina, L. M.: Pseudoaneurysm of the inferior gluteal artery presenting as sciatic nerve compression. Neurosurgery 24:926, 1989.

73. Crisci, C., Baker, M. K., Wood, M. B., Litchy, W. J., and Dyck, P. J.: Trochanteric sciatic neuropathy. Neurology 39:1539, 1989.

74. Rondepierre, P., Martini, L., Wannib, G., and Floquet, J.: Intraneural cyst: An unusual cause of peroneal nerve palsy. Rev. Neurol. 146:375, 1990.

75. Havel, P. E., Ebraheim, N. A., Clark, S. E., Jackson, W. T., and DiDio, L.: Tibial nerve branching in the tarsal tunnel. Foot Ankle 9:117, 1988.

76. Saal, J. A., Dillingham, M. F., Gamburd, R. S., and Fanton, G. S.: The pseudoradicular syndrome. Lower extremity peripheral nerve entrapment masquerading as lumbar radiculopathy. Spine 13:926, 1988.

77. Bourne, R. B., and Rorabeck, C. H.: Compartment syndromes of the lower leg. Clin. Orthop. Rel. Res. 240:97, 1989.

78. Schwartz, J. T., Brumback, R. J., Lakatos, R., Poka, A., Bathon, G. H., and Burgess, A. R.: Acute compartment syndrome of the thigh. A spectrum of injury. J. Bone Joint Surg. 71A:392, 1989.

79. Lehto, M., Rantakokko, V., Kormano, M., and Järvinen, M.: Flexor hallucis longus muscle atrophy due to a chronic compartment syndrome of the lower leg. Br. J. Sports Med. 22:41, 1988.

80. Ziv, I., Mosheiff, R., Zeligowski, A., Liebergal, M., Lowe, J., and Segal, D.: Crush injuries of the foot with compartment syndrome: Immediate one-stage management. Foot Ankle 9:185, 1989.

81. Lagerstrom, C. F., Reed, R. L., II, Rowlands, B. J., and Fischer, R. P.: Early fasciotomy for acute clinically evident posttraumatic compartment syndrome. Am. J. Surg. 158:36, 1989.

82. Rorabeck, C. H., Fowler, P. J., and Nott, L.: The results of fasciotomy in the management of chronic exertional compartment syndrome. Am. J. Sports Med. 16:224, 1988.

83. Almdahl, S. M., and Samdal, F.: Fasciotomy for chronic compartment syndrome. Acta Orthop. Scand. 60:210, 1989.

84. Styf, J.: Diagnosis of exercise-induced pain in the anterior aspect of the lower leg. Am. J. Sports Med. 16:165, 1988.

85. Rorabeck, C. H., Bourne, R. B., Fowler, P. J., Finlay, J. B., and Nott, L.: The role of tissue pressure measurement in diagnosing chronic anterior compartment syndrome. Am. J. Sports Med. 16:143, 1988.

86. Barton, N.: Repetitive strain disorder. Br. Med. J. 299:405, 1989.

87. Bird, H.: Overuse injuries in musicians. Br. Med. J. 298:1129, 1989.

88. Lockwood, A. H.: Medical problems of musicians. N. Engl. J. Med. 320:221, 1989.

89. Fry, H. J. H.: Overuse syndromes in instrumental musicians. Semin. Neurol. 9:136, 1989.

90. Revak, J. M.: Incidence of upper extremity discomfort among piano students. Am. J. Occup. Ther. 43:149, 1989.

91. Penneys, R.: Motion and emotion: A discussion of the interaction between physical motion and human emotion. Semin. Neurol. 9:122, 1989.

92. Bejjani, F. J., Halpern, N., Pio, A., Dominguez, R., Voloshin, A., and Frankel, V. H.: Musculoskeletal demands on flamenco dancers: A clinical and biomechanical study. Foot Ankle 8:254, 1988.

93. Bowling, A.: Injuries to dancers: prevalence, treatment, and perceptions of causes. Br. Med. J. 298:731, 1989.

94. Green, R. A., and Briggs, C. A.: Effect of overuse injury and the importance of training on the use of adjustable workstations by keyboard operators. J. Occup. Med. 31:557, 1989.

95. Paty, J. G.: Diagnosis and treatment of musculoskeletal running injuries. Semin. Arthritis Rheum. 18:48, 1988.

96. Marti, B., Vader, J. P., Minder, C. E., and Abelin, T.: On the epidemiology of running injuries. The 1984 Bern Grand-Prix study. Am. J. Sports Med. 16:285, 1988.

97. Steinbrück, K.: Frequency and aetiology of injury in cross-country skiing. J. Sports Sci. 5:187, 1987.

98. McCormick, D. P., and Davis, A. L.: Injuries in sailboard enthusiasts. Br. J. Sports Med. 22:95, 1988.

99. Bollen, S. R.: Soft tissue injury in extreme rock climbers. Br. J. Sports Med. 22:145, 1988.

100. Rowell, S., and Rees-Jones, A.: Injuries treated at a sports injury clinic compared with a neighbouring accident and emergency department. Br. J. Sports Med. 22:157, 1988.

101. Järvholm, U., Palmerud, G., Styf, J., Herberts, P., and Kadefors, R.: Intramuscular pressure in the supraspinatus muscle. J. Orthop. Res. 6:230, 1988.

102. Hadler, N. M.: The roles of work and of working in disorders of the upper extremity. Baillieres Clin. Rheumatol. 3:121, 1989.

103. Stokes, M. J., Cooper, R. G., and Edwards, R. H. T.: Normal muscle strength and fatigability in patients with effort syndromes. Br. Med. J. 297:1014, 1988.

104. Fry, H., and Hallett, M.: Focal dystonia (occupational cramp) masquerading as nerve entrapment or hysteria. Plast. Reconstr. Surg. 82:908, 1988.

105. Jankovic, J., and Shale, H.: Dystonia in musicians. Semin. Neurol. 9:131, 1989.

106. Daswon, D. M., and Krarup, C.: Perioperative nerve lesions. Arch. Neurol. 46:1355, 1989.

107. Tsai, T. M.: Improvement in motor function after brachial plexus surgery. J. Hand Surg. 15A:30, 1990.

108. Gupta, R. K., Mehta, V. S., Banerji, A. K., and Jain, R. K.: MR evaluation of brachial plexus injuries. Neuroradiology 31:377, 1989.

109. Haupt, W. F.: Intraoperative positional damage to the ulnar nerve in anatomic variants. Dtsch. Med. Wochenschr. 114:1789, 1989.

110. Geiringer, S. R., and Leonard, J. A.: Injection-related ulnar neuropathy. Arch. Phys. Med. Rehabil. 70:705, 1989.

Chapter 102

John J. Nicholas

Rehabilitation of Patients with Rheumatic Diseases*

INTRODUCTION

A current definition of the *rehabilitation* process is

... the development of a person to the fullest physical, psychological, social, vocational, avocational, and educational potential consistent with his or her physiological or anatomical impairment and environmental limitations. Realistic goals are determined by the persons concerned with patient care. Thus, one is working to obtain optimal functioning despite residual disability, even if the impairment is caused by a pathological process that cannot be reversed with the best of modern medical treatment.[1]

In addition, there are patients who, following an illness, accident, or surgical procedure, recover entirely and have no residual physical impairment. They can perform exercise and other therapies and improve their condition so they reach the level of functioning that existed *prior* to the onset of their disability. Examples of such patients are those recovering from arthroplasties, hip fractures, and multiple trauma. Rehabilitation practice will include *both* types of patients.

One survey shows that physiatrists in training do not receive many hours of instruction in the treatment of rheumatic diseases;[2] and a second survey reveals that rheumatologic teaching programs provide rheumatology fellows with little instruction in the principles and practice of rehabilitation care.[3] A major goal of this chapter is to describe what rehabilitation health professionals do and what appropriate treatments consist of so proper referrals can be made and the rehabilitation process can be provided and monitored by the treating physician.

Rehabilitation techniques must be delivered by teamwork.[4] This is a commonly asserted principle, and the success of team treatment on an arthritis unit has been demonstrated.[5] However, in order for a *group* of therapists to form a *team*, there must be close cooperation among all members, with leadership and clearly defined goals. The leader of a treatment team must know what each team member can do and whether he or she is doing it; in addition,

the team leader must be involved with monitoring the results of team treatment.

EVALUATION

A careful evaluation must be performed to assess the rehabilitation treatment needs (functional deficits) and potential for improvement. Most of the health-related disciplines perform an evaluation, but for the present, treating physicians must rely ultimately on their evaluations to prescribe therapy. Discrepancies between findings on multiple evaluations should be reconciled with mutual consideration and repeated evaluation. In addition to a history of the Present Illness and a Review of Systems, certain historical data must be obtained so the examining physician can get a clear picture of what the patient can and cannot do (how he or she functions). Some of this information must be corroborated by observations from the treating health professionals, as well as the physician, but much important data may be obtained by appropriate questions. The physician should inquire about and get a description of the difficulty with which the patient performs various activities of daily living (ADL) and vocational activities. These should include toilet hygiene; dressing; daily hygiene; performing tasks in the home such as meal preparation, cleaning, and care of children; working activities such as transferring in and out of an automobile or using public transportation; and any difficulties at work. Vocational information should include the use of heavy equipment, the performance of tasks requiring strength and manual dexterity, the need to perform tasks requiring dexterous movements, and the ability of the patient to get to the place of work and return. A compassionate physician should also include questions about the patient's avocational and sexual activities and should inquire about pain and fatigue and the ability to sleep.

In addition, the physician needs to respond to the patient's assertion, "I hurt all over." Usually, patients do not hurt all over. And while it is senseless to argue this point, it is important for the physician to discover which areas hurt more than others. In this way, a therapeutic approach can be tailored to

*The author wishes to acknowledge the contributions of Lynn Gerber, M.D., and Jeanne Hicks, M.D., to the writing of this chapter.

each patient's needs. There is no way to treat "all over" pain other than with psychiatric medications or systemic medications. However, pain in particular joints or regions of the musculoskeletal system may be treated successfully by some of the numerous rehabilitation modalities, which include splints, casts, joint injections, hot packs, cold packs, TENS equipment, etc.

The physician must perform a general and rheumatologic physical examination. In evaluation for rehabilitation programs, specific attention must be paid to measurements of range of motion. Musculoskeletal diseases commonly limit the normal range of motion (ROM) of an involved joint. It is important, therefore, to discover which joints are limited. Because there is insufficient time during an evaluation to record the ROM of the joints that have *normal* values, one should examine all joints but consider recording only abnormal values.[6] The normal values with which to compare abnormal ones can be easily, and usually accurately, obtained from the corresponding contralateral joint (see Chapter 21). Published normal values for range of motion frequently vary greatly with age and are too wide-ranging to be satisfactory for an individual patient's evaluation. When patients have bilateral joint involvement, the physician should use an estimate of normal that has developed through experience. One must keep in mind that some patients have hypermobile joints. This phenomenon can usually be discovered by testing uninvolved joints. The ROM of these patients may be compromised, but values for them will remain in the "normal" range[7] and can be quantitated using a goniometer (see Chapter 21).

The physician must also determine the difference between *active* and *passive* motion deficits. If a patient cannot move a joint through the ROM but the physician is able to do so (an active ROM deficit), there is evidence of guarding due to pain or weakness or failure to cooperate. If neither the physician nor the patient can move the joint (lack of passive motion), there is likely a mechanical block or a great deal of pain. The physician must distinguish the cause of the active/passive motion discrepancy.

In addition, the physician must determine what is causing the loss of motion. Is it joint pain and inflammation? Is it bony enlargement or encroachment upon the joint? Is it stiffening and contracture of the capsule or surrounding muscle and ligaments, or is it fluid within the joint? A change in joint ROM of between 5 and 10 degrees may be significant, but a change of motion between 10 and 15 degrees usually indicates genuine pathology and not simply a variation due to measurement error.[8–11] It helps to repeat the measurement. When measuring painful joints, it is appropriate to determine whether the patient has had a recent joint injection, pain medication, or an exacerbation of disease, or whether it is early morning and the patient still has overnight stiffness.

MANUAL MUSCLE TESTING FOR MOTOR STRENGTH

The most convenient and reasonably reliable method of measuring strength is the manual muscle test (MMT). In this test, the physician measures the patient's strength by comparison with standard criteria (see Chapters 21 and 24). A scale of one to five is used: grade one strength is "trace" movement of a muscle; grade two (or *poor* grade) is obvious movement of the muscle, but not through the complete range of joint motion; grade three (or *fair* grade) is movement through the full ROM against gravity; grade four (or *good* grade) is movement through the full ROM against gravity with some resistance added; and grade five (*normal* grade) is movement through the full ROM taking normal resistance.

It is obvious that grade three (movement voluntarily by the patient through the full ROM against gravity) is an objective standard of measurement. A reliable measurement of the difference between grades four and five (good and normal) depends on the experience of the physician. Muscle testing devices are of greatest value for measuring good and normal grade muscles.

Whether a patient has normal muscle strength is a matter of considerable interest. This is true with patients with joint pain as well as those with muscle disease. If a patient has greater than grade three (fair grade) strength, it will be difficult for the physician to estimate strength accurately. The clinician's opinion must be based on several features, including whether the patient is giving *maximum* effort.

In addition, the amount of effort the patient puts out even when trying maximally will be modified by age (older patients are weaker); sex (female patients are weaker per pound body weight); weight (heavier patients seem to provide stronger muscle force); or lack of understanding.[12] The patient who does not understand what the physician wants will not be able to provide a maximum contraction. Physicians must, therefore, give explicit instructions, usually by *demonstrating* to the patient just what muscle contraction is being elicited. One must not ask a patient to "contract your biceps" and be confident that he or she will obtain maximal contraction. "Make a muscle," "Try your hardest," "Harder, harder, harder," are typical terms used to elicit maximal strength from patients during a muscle examination.

The anatomic posture and position of a patient during testing is also important.[13] If you wish to test for greater than fair (grade three) grade muscle strength of the triceps muscle, the patient must be in such a position that the triceps is being contracted against, not with, gravity. In addition, if one wishes to test the strength of the gluteus maximus muscle and it is felt that the strength will be less than fair or only fair, the patient must lie prone. In addition, when testing hip flexion, the patient must be supine, or one will not be able to see whether the patient can move the leg through the full ROM against gravity.

It is worth noting that disuse atrophy from lying in bed during an illness is usually not a focal problem. The patient, therefore, who has weakness of one shoulder or weakness of both legs must have the cause for the weakness investigated. However, if the patient has a single joint or multiple joints involved, it is likely that the muscles around those joints will promptly become weak and atrophic due to pain and inflammation. Weakness of noninflamed joints may be due to local pressure palsies, trauma to nerves (stretch injuries or inadvertent surgical section), or systemic neuropathy.

At the present time, there are various devices that may be used to measure a patient's muscle strength. These include the hand-held dynamometer,[14–16] which appears to be more reliable for measuring upper-extremity strength than lower-extremity strength.

ENDURANCE

It has been demonstrated on many occasions that the strength, endurance, and aerobic capacity of individual arthritic patient's muscles are diminished.[17–19] Inflammatory disease may also affect nutrient arteries, nerves, and the muscle fibers themselves. There is agreement that the VO_2 max is the best measurement of a patient's condition or aerobic ability. Endurance (aerobic capacity) can therefore be tested by running or walking on a treadmill or ergometer. Modern muscle testing machines can measure *both* the single repetition maximum strength of individual muscles and the *endurance* of individual muscles on repeat contractions. Endurance testing is usually not necessary, unless the physician wishes to institute a program of aerobic exercise, or to test a patient's aerobic capacity. Testing muscle strength will likely reveal greater deficits than anticipated and may stimulate prescription of exercises to be taught by a physical therapist and diligent monitoring of muscles, e.g., prior to or following arthroplasty or during a remission of disease.

EVALUATION OF PAIN AND TENDERNESS

Patient pain is a subjective emotion but attempts have been made to design reproducible measures. Chief among these is the visual analogue scale.[20–22] Patient reporting reliability has been fairly constant, and changes occur following therapeutic procedures.

In addition, tenderness, or patient assessment of pain after an examiner has palpated his or her joints, has also been measured. McCarty et al. devised a "dolorimeter," which has been demonstrated to have reproducibility and to respond to therapeutic measures.[23] Both the patient's diagnosis and the response to therapy may be evaluated by an examination of joint pain and joint tenderness.

Joint pain and tenderness are also to be distinguished from pain with motion and joint stiffness.[24] Joint stiffness is a measurable quality that often occurs after resting a joint (e.g., morning stiffness) and diminishes with use or motion. Pain on motion from a diseased joint will often increase with use or motion, unlike stiffness.

EVALUATION OF FUNCTION

In order to improve patient function, it is important to evaluate the extent to which a patient can perform a job or other ADL. Function consists of both impairment and disability. *Impairment* describes physical abnormalities that can be measured, and *disability* describes the inability to perform important functions as a result.[25] Physical impairment may not always cause a patient to be disabled; however, some patients may be greatly disabled through minor physical impairments. An example of the latter would be the loss of a finger on the hand of a professional violinist. It is obvious, therefore, that disability depends on what the patient must do in normal life as well as the measurable physical limitations.

Information about disability can usually *not* be adequately obtained from the medical history, the physical examination, and the laboratory evaluation. Abnormalities of function, or disability, usually require further investigation. Many of these observations are performed routinely in the occupational therapy suite. Scales are available in which patients are asked to *report* what activities they can and cannot perform, and there are scales where the patient is asked to demonstrate many of these activities.

There are also functional scales that physicians use. Although the physician may not feel the need for a comprehensive, repeatable measurement, some items that are important in each patient's life should be selected and historical information and demonstrations obtained to determine whether the patient has improved. This assessment of the patient's progress is important both to demonstrate a treatment effect and to demonstrate to third party payors that there is improvement and, thus, the need for continued care. A comprehensive description and evaluation of standard scales of functional measurement are readily available.[26–31]

REHABILITATION TREATMENT METHODS

When is it appropriate to apply rehabilitative treatment methods for the patient with arthritis? For years, the therapeutic "pyramid" was the standard analogy.[32–34] More recently a therapeutic model has been described as a "therapeutic target."[35] In this model, treatment is started in the center of the target with family, physician, and patient interaction while cytotoxic medicines and surgery are relegated to the outer rings. In other approaches, rehabilitation treatment methods are consistently recommended *early* in the course of the patient's disease, and some treatment methods have specific times and appropriate sites of use, as described in the following sections.[36-38]

MODALITIES—HEAT AND COLD

Heat. Moist heat, including baths and spas, has traditionally been the first modality for rehabilitative treatment of arthritic joints.[39] Nevertheless, the application of these modalities (treatment methods) is still in large part guided by the historic principle of cost, custom, and convenience rather than scientific data. In fact, scientific data suggest that some of the methods of heat application are not clinically beneficial.[40]

Lehmann et al. have demonstrated an increase in temperature in soft tissue structures at depths of 5 to 7 cm with short-wave diathermy.[41] Microwave (900 or 2456 MHz)[42] and ultrasound[43] diathermy have been shown to heat deep muscles and soft tissue interfaces, respectively, at 3 to 4 cm or more below the surface. Ultrasound weakens collagen in vitro.[44, 45] Patients cannot tolerate microwave, and ultrasound has not been very effective.[46-48]

Hollander has demonstrated that simple moist heating pads *decreased* the temperature in knee joints as much as 2.2°F while relieving pain.[49] An explanation for the relief from ineffective heating modalities and lack of improvement or actual exacerbation from deep, effective heating modalities is explained in the work of Harris et al.,[40] who demonstrated that collagenase becomes increasingly active as temperatures rise equivalent to those found within the joints of patients with RA. Thus, there might be an increase in joint destruction and inflammation as the temperature rises from treatment with effective deep heat methods.

Pain relief in joints can be obtained from superficial heating through total body immersion (Hubbard tanks, therapeutic pools, spas, hydrotherapy) or electric lights, infrared heating, and paraffin wax. The optimal duration of superficial heating of soft tissues from moist heating packs has been demonstrated by Lehmann et al. to be about 20 to 30 minutes, dependent on the extent of the circulation in the area.[50] No increase in juxta-articular erosions was seen following hand and wrist joint heating.[51] The duration of pain relief may be somewhat brief, but the patient may also demonstrate an increased ROM and an increased ability to contract muscles following treatment.

The physician will most likely prescribe moist heating pads to affected joints and paraffin wax to the hands or wrists. The duration of the treatment will be guided by the cooling of the heating pad (15 to 20 minutes). The frequency of applications, guided by convention, is once or twice daily.

The physician should be aware, however, of certain harmful effects associated with modalities of heat. Moist heating pads, electric heating pads, short-wave, and microwave diathermy may produce severe burns, especially in denervated skin or in patients with peripheral neuropathies. Microwave will also cause increased heating over metallic implants.[52] Ultrasound is reflected by the interface between materials of different densities, thus its use in ultrasound diagnostics, and will, therefore, heat selectively the interface between joint capsules, muscles, etc. It is, however, reflected from metallic implants and does not cause a hot spot there.

Cold. Ice packs are preferred by some patients with muscular pain or joint disease, and they decrease the swelling around acutely injured joints or soft tissue. The mechanism may be that cold decreases both skin and superficial muscle temperatures and decreases muscle spindle activity.[53, 54]

Ethyl chloride or fluromethane sprays[55] cool the skin and relieve pain when applied to "trigger points" and "tender points" of patients with the fibrositis syndrome and regional myofascial pain syndromes. One should avoid cold in patients with Raynaud's phenomenon, cryoglobulinemia, and cold hypersensitivity.[56] Cold packs also provide pain relief to some RA joints.[57]

OTHER MODALITIES

TENS. TENS (transcutaneous neuromuscular stimulation) treatment is currently provided through the use of a portable battery pack that is worn by the patient. Four electrodes are attached to the battery pack, which has multiple settings to adjust, by trial and error, the shape of the stimulus curve, the frequency, and the intensity of stimulation. The electrodes are applied directly over the painful area. The current is applied continuously as long as the pain is present and is restarted when the pain recurs. The location of the electrodes is changed if there is skin irritation or if the pain location changes.

TENS has been used with success in the case of frozen shoulders and adhesive capsulitis, fibromyalgia, herpes zoster,[58] and chronic back pain.[59] It is probably not helpful for routine use over rheumatoid joints. It is thought that TENS causes pain relief by supplying impulses that divert the brain's attention from impulses transmitted by other fibers (the Gate theory of pain relief).[60]

Acupuncture. Acupuncture is thought to function much as does TENS. However, the skin must be punctured and the modality must be applied to more *precise* locations. The increased risk of hepatitis and the increased costs of the expert acupuncturist are offset by the cost of a TENS unit. Acupuncture has been applied to patients with arthritis with little success to inflammatory arthritis,[61-64] but it probably will provide relief in some cases of musculoskeletal pain and even OA if persistently employed.[65]

EXERCISE

When joints cannot be moved vigorously because of arthritic pain, the surrounding muscles will probably become weak and a patient's aerobic capacity will decrease. Exercise is, therefore, of interest to the physician and patient with arthritis. Furthermore, patients and physicians have observed that use of inflamed joints or arthritic joints may cause an increase in the pain and other signs of inflammation. Patients with OA frequently notice an increase in pain when the joint is used, and, conversely, there is relief of pain when the joint is rested. The physician, therefore, is on the horns of dilemma: to treat the arthritic patient with exercise to maintain strength/endurance or to rest the involved joints and obtain relief from pain and inflammation.[66]

Types of Exercise. *Passive exercise* occurs when the patient does not contract the muscles and a therapist or machine moves the muscles for the patient.[67] *Assisted exercise* occurs when the patient contracts the muscles but is also assisted by a therapist or a machine. *Active exercise* occurs when the patient contracts the muscles.

Types of Active Exercise. *Isometric exercise* occurs when the patient contracts a muscle without joint motion (for example, pushing your head against a wall). *Isotonic exercise* (active exercise, dynamic exercise) is a term applied when the patient contracts the muscles and the joints move. *Isotonic* is now applied interchangeably with *active* to any active or dynamic exercise.

Isokinetic exercise (active exercise) does not occur in daily activity, but occurs when one contracts muscles against a resistance moving at a *maximally limited rate*. If the rate set by the machine is slow, the patient may push very hard (and register many foot pounds of effort), but the resistance will not move any faster. If the resistance is set to move very rapidly, the patient will push but be unable to catch up with the high speed and thus apply very little force.

Active exercise is commonly thought of as a muscular shortening/contraction to bring the resistance closer to the origin of the muscle (*concentric* contraction). Alternatively, muscles may contract while the origin and insertion are becoming farther apart (*eccentric* contraction). During eccentric contraction, more force is generated. Examples include the stabilizing contraction of the quadriceps while the leading leg steps *down* to the next step, and lowering a heavy object as the biceps lengthens.

Furthermore, exercise is divided into exercise for increasing strength or for increasing endurance. Muscle contraction against high resistance when performed with relatively few repetitions is followed by an increase in muscle strength and hypertrophy of muscle fibers. Contraction of muscles against a relatively low resistance can be performed with many repetitions, and it regularly is followed by an increase in endurance. Also, strength is related to the cross-sectional area of muscles—the larger a muscle becomes, the more strength it has. Initially, muscle strength may increase while there is no hypertrophy.[68]

Machover and Sapecky have demonstrated that patients with RA can increase the strength in their quadriceps muscles with isometric exercise.[69] Ekblom and colleagues also demonstrated that patients with RA can increase their ADL, both type 1 and type 2 muscle fiber size, and their strength and aerobic capacity after performing endurance training on treadmills or bicycles.[70-73]

Exercise has other effects on arthritic patients. Clinically it has been known for years that patients with gout, OA, RA, and hemiplegia, peripheral nerve damage, and polio develop *unilateral* arthritis. That is, the arthritis occurs with more severity on the side that is exercised (not involved with the neurologic deficit) and with much less severity on the rested (neurologically involved) side.[74-79] Merritt and Hunder demonstrated that in crystalline-induced arthritis in rats, the amount of fluid and the white count in those joints that were exercised were greater than in the joints that were rested.[80] Agudelo demonstrated the same phenomenon in dogs.[81] Merritt also demonstrated that isometric exercise did not increase the amount of synovial fluid or white count, whereas passive range-of-motion exercises did. Animal experiments have confirmed these findings.[82, 83]

In addition, clinicians can often obtain histories of excessive exercise or use of joints (e.g., preparing the home for holiday visits, excessive shopping, increased work on the job) from patients suffering exacerbations or "flare-ups" of their joint disease. These clinical and laboratory data seem to support the assertion that exercise of an arthritic joint—OA or inflamed—will cause an exacerbation of pain and inflammation. They also support the contention that isometric exercise will cause the least increase in inflammation.

Perlman and colleagues,[84] Kay and colleagues,[85] and Banwell and colleagues[86, 87] have shown that aerobic exercise on treadmills or bicycles is followed by an increase in aerobic capacity and ADL capacity, and an enthusiastic response from their patients. Danneskiold-Samsøe and colleagues demonstrated an increase in strength and endurance following underwater exercise.[88] While these reports are encouraging, more time is required before the physician should unhesitatingly prescribe aerobic exercise for arthritic patients. Even in RA or OA patients who have mild disease, there exists the possibility that exercise will eventually lead to premature joint damage. For the present, therefore, isometric exercise can be prescribed to tolerance to maintain strength around involved joints, but endurance training should probably be viewed with cautious skepticism.

Additionally, there is recent evidence that patients with OA can perform isometric exercise followed by an increase in strength and a diminution of pain.[89, 90]

Isometric exercise is dull, and compliance is difficult to obtain. The use of rubber bands (Therabands) provides a means of inexpensive isometric exercise equipment that can be used at home. The devices can be utilized to obtain tension in many directions so that various exercises can be performed with different muscles.

If isometric or other types of exercise are dull and boring, the peer pressure of recreational exercise may provide the stimulation to continue. Local Arthritis Foundation chapters have arranged aquatic aerobic and strengthening exercise groups and Tai Chi groups.

Passive ROM exercise also has a role in postoperative joint treatment. Originally developed to increase nourishment of postoperative joint cartilage, the passive constant range of motion machine now regularly increases ROM after surgery and may even decrease joint contractures if joint surfaces are intact.

The use of functional electric stimulation (FES) provides aerobic exercise for the paralyzed muscles of spinal cord injury patients. FES can help the arthritic patient regain the ability to contract a muscle after surgery, when the patient may have forgotten how to produce a maximum contraction owing to the long period of pain prior to the operation.

REST

Systemic and Local. The effect of rest is more clearly defined than exercise. Prolonged systemic rest causes well-known deconditioning effects, and prolonged systemic rest also rests individual inflamed joints and causes diminution of inflammation. Local rest causes deterioration in both joint surfaces and surrounding tissues, but also a decrease in inflammation and pain.[91-97] The physician should carefully observe the effect of rest on the patient's joints to provide *balanced* rest and exercise for the patient.

Systemic Rest. Rest causes diminution in balance, orthostatic hypotension, decreased cardiac output, decreased muscular strength, and negative nitrogen balance. In the late nineteenth century, patients with joint disease were confined to prolonged bed rest with "good results."[98] Partridge and Duthie much later showed that patients confined to bed with casts on their elbows and knees for 14 days did not suffer a diminution in ROM, and their hematocrit rose and sedimentation rate fell.[99] Mills et al. hospitalized patients with RA for 4 weeks and compared them with a control group who were up and around ad lib[100] but found no signs of decreased inflammation in the rested group. However, patients had been selected so that those with involved hips and knees who were most likely to improve with rest in bed were excluded from the study.

Lee and colleagues rested a group of patients with RA for 4 weeks and compared them without advantage with outpatients who did not have as much rest.[101] Alexander observed patients with RA

and compared them with a group of outpatients[102] and concluded that the patients with the most severe involvement, and specifically the joints most involved, improved the most from rest.

One can conclude that inflamed individual joints in patients with RA and probably OA will benefit if the patient and joint are rested for as long as 14 days.

Local Rest. Individual joints can also be rested with splints or casts.[103, 104] There is anecdotal evidence of pain relief in nearly every case. Hugh Owen Thomas placed many patients with arthritis of the hip, knee, and ankle in devices similar to the Thomas splint, which now bears his name, for as long as 6 months.[105] He claimed invariable success. More recently, in a classic study, Gault and Spyker reported that the unilaterally casted hands of a group of patients from the Minneapolis Veteran's Administration Hospital exhibited diminished inflammation when compared with the used or uncasted hand.[106]

Knee casts have also been shown to decrease joint pain, without markedly decreasing strength or decreasing the sedimentation rate; these are not widely accepted by patients, however, because they are awkward and lack style.[107, 108]

MOBILIZATION TECHNIQUES

One type of gentle mobilization technique, described by Maigne, consists of mild manipulation and movement of joints through an ROM just beyond that which can be accomplished by the patient's active muscle contraction.[109] These gentle manipulations are felt to improve pain for various noninflammatory musculoskeletal disorders but not those in RA.

The manipulation of frozen shoulders under anesthesia has not been uniformly followed by marked improvement. The manipulation of knees and probably other joints following total knee arthroplasty is often necessary and *is* followed by an increase in ROM.

Spinal manipulations as practiced by chiropractors, osteopaths, and physical therapists are often followed by immediate but temporary relief. The physician must be careful of the diagnosis in the patient and the technique of the therapist before recommending or allowing this type of therapy. As long as no harm is done, mobilization therapy probably provides prompt and temporary relief while the patient, especially one with an acute back injury, is improving.

TRACTION

Traction includes applying force in a manner to distract the cervical or lumbar vertebral bodies. Whether traction exerts its effect by significant separation of one vertebral body from the next is controversial; however, it appears that the lordotic curve of both the cervical and lumbar spines diminishes when traction is applied and the intervertebral foramina can be seen to increase in area. The increase allows more space for a nerve root compressed by extruded disc material. When applying cervical traction, one position, usually anterior flexion forward and laterally flexed away from the side of root impingement, relieves pain the best. Traction should be set up in this position with weight from 10 to 15 lb or more, sufficient to relieve pain. Traction can be applied with the patient erect or supine.

Lumbar traction requires more force and is more awkward. Traction is usually applied with the patient supine and both the hips and the knees flexed 90 degrees. The chest must be stabilized while the pull is applied to the legs—sufficient weight is "enough"—often 40 to 80 lb.

Both cervical traction and lumbar traction should be applied two to three times a day or the more often the better. It should be continued until pain relief has been present for some time. Continuous cervical traction is usually intolerable and the proper posture cannot be maintained.

AIDS AND APPLIANCES TO FACILITATE FUNCTION

Devices to help walking are the most common aids prescribed and supplied to patients with arthritis. Patients use canes, crutches, and walkers to diminish the weight on the hips, knees, ankles, and feet.

Canes provide the least relief from weight-bearing on the legs and the least amount of stability. However, they allow greater mobility and ease of use. Canes should be held in the contralateral hand when attempting to limit the weight on the hip, but it is not at all clear in which hand the cane should be held to relieve pain of the knee, foot, and ankle. The style of cane that resembles a shepherd's crook and places the weight above the shaft of the cane provides greater stability than the traditional cane.

Crutches are much more mobile but less stable than walkers and more stable than a cane. Axillary crutches are to be fitted so that the arm rest is 1.5 to 2 inches below the axilla so the patient will not bear weight there and develop a brachial plexus palsy. Handle grips may be enlarged to fit patients' arthritic hands. The axillary supports may be padded to prevent rubbing against the chest wall, and rubber caps may be placed on the tips for greater stability. Canadian or Loftstrand or forearm crutches eliminate some of the weight at the wrist joint. Platform crutches, which totally remove the stress and weight from the wrists, are much heavier and more awkward but highly suitable for patients with arthritis of the wrist joint.

Walkers give more stability and can fold up and be placed in the trunk of a car. They can be provided with wheels on the anterior legs so they can be pushed. Usually, however, they are of the "pickup" style, which requires that the whole walker be lifted and moved from place to place. A platform walker is available that allows the patient to rest the elbows and forearms on a platform.

All walkers, canes, and crutches transmit weight through the shoulders to the floor. If the shoulders and arms cannot tolerate the weight or the legs are unstable or experience pain, a wheelchair will be required. The chair must be fitted to the patient's body habitus—large, small, tall, etc. Leg rests should be adjustable and swing aside or even be removable. Arm rests can be standard or desk type and should be removable to make transfers easier. Hand spokes may be added to help propel the wheels. To add speed and endurance and diminish the patient's energy requirement, a motor-driven wheelchair or an Amigo-like vehicle—a three-wheeled machine—may be provided. With any type of wheelchair, special seating can increase the patient's tolerance and diminish localized pain.

Automobiles may be fitted with door openers, adaptive ignition switches, and overhead transfer slings. Adaptable car seats can be adjusted—some electrically.

The occupational therapist evaluates and provides devices that help patients cut and prepare food, open cans and jars, and lift heavy pots and pans.[110-112] Cleaning can be made easier with lightweight vacuum cleaners and brushes with enlarged and specially angled handles. Pans can be lined with foil to save scrubbing.

The practical application of the theories of *energy conservation* and *joint protection* (Cordery) must be taught.[113] Meal preparation and trips to the store should be carefully planned to diminish their frequency. The goal is to help the patient change those lifelong work habits that the patient can no longer maintain but finds difficult to modify.

Toilet and other self-care hygiene is often a problem for the arthritic patient with deformed hands and painful hips or knees. An occupational therapist can provide advice and aids such as long-handled reachers, button hooks, zipper pulls, shoe horns, and sock pullers. Clothing should be lightweight and easy to put on. Velcro fasteners should replace buttons and zippers. Stretch straps and waists are generally easier to use than rigid straps or hooked or belted waists. Outerwear such as capes, ponchos, and down jackets are also easier to don and are warm and lightweight.

Elevated toilet seats help patients who have difficulty getting up from chairs. Grab bars also assist arising. A portable commode chair may be a necessity for patients who cannot get in and out of their bathrooms.

SPLINTING

Splints (orthotic devices) are frequently used in treating patients with rheumatic diseases to immobilize a painful body part, mobilize a stiff joint, support a body part in a functional position, and maintain alignment to reduce deformity and to preserve function. Splints are most commonly prescribed for the feet, hands, and wrists.

The Foot. The foot in RA develops very characteristic anatomic abnormalities and associated dynamic ones. Commonly, the forefoot undergoes subluxation of the MTP joints, with development of callosities and pain, hallux valgus, and cock-up toe deformities, while the hindfoot usually develops a pronation position with an everted calcaneus. Pain occurs during weight-bearing, especially as weight is transferred from the forefoot onto the MTP joints. There may be a loss of the heel-toe transfer of weight and a tendency to slow the gait to almost a shuffle. The foot begins to function as a *pedestal* rather than as an aid to the forward propulsion of body weight.

The aims of treatment are to provide a comfortable foot upon which to stand and to provide a dynamic assist for walking. Functional footwear is recommended with shoes sufficiently wide to accommodate the spread-out forefoot without too much pressure, deep enough to clear the tops of the toes, and firm enough to support the medial arch. A heel less than 1.5 inches is best to minimize stress across the MTP joints. Materials should be soft and pliable, and the sole should be able to at least partly absorb the ground reaction force. The shoe must be large enough for any orthotic devices.

Metatarsalgia may be relieved by providing an internal pad placed proximal to the MTP joints or an external bar placed proximal to the MTP joint on the sole of the shoe (Fig. 102–1). Adding a rocker bottom to the sole of the shoe will assist in weight transfer from posterior to anterior and reduce the amount of force needed to propel the body over the MTP joints. It also limits motion at the tibiotalar joint.

The *hindfoot* may also be involved and is usually associated with medial arch collapse. Functionally, when the arch collapses, there is a decrease in the ability of the foot to supinate, and the foot strikes the floor with a flattened arch, absorbing ground reaction forces at the midfoot instead of at the heel and toe. A total contact orthosis designed to support the medial arch using a soft pad (scaphoid pad) or rigid plastic medial arch may help. Occasionally a hindfoot orthosis or UCBL (University of California at Berkeley Laboratory) orthotic to control the calcaneus and reduce it from valgus to neutral is required (Fig. 102–2).[114, 115]

A variety of materials are available for use in fabricating these splints. These include Spenco, Aliplast, Plastizote, Pelite, and polypropylene.

The Hand and Wrist. Orthotic devices for the wrist and hand must be lightweight and permit the individual to use the hand in functional activities. They must be cosmetically acceptable. The most commonly used splints for the hand and wrist include the functional wrist splint, which can be used with and without a thumb post to support an unsta-

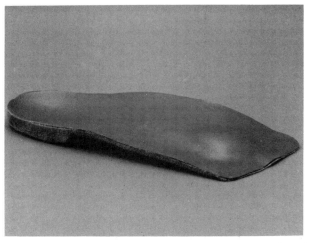

Figure 102–1. Custom-molded shoe insert to support arch and relieve MT weight-bearing.

ble MCP joint. Also, a CMC joint support splint and Bunnell-type ring splints to reduce PIP hyperextension (swan neck deformities) or PIP flexion (boutonniere deformities) (Fig. 102–3) may be helpful—some resemble silver rings.

A variety of dynamic splints have been used to preserve alignment and provide a gentle stretch to the intrinsic muscles of the hands (see Fig. 102–3). These splints have small cuffs on the proximal PIP joints and an elastic band attached to help pull the finger into extension. This design allows for a gentle stretch on the intrinsic muscle and supports the MCP so they remain in neutral alignment.

To date, no data are available to demonstrate that splinting prevents the progression of deformity of the wrist, fingers, hands, or feet.

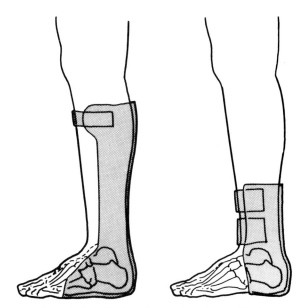

Figure 102–2. Custom-designed hindfoot orthosis.

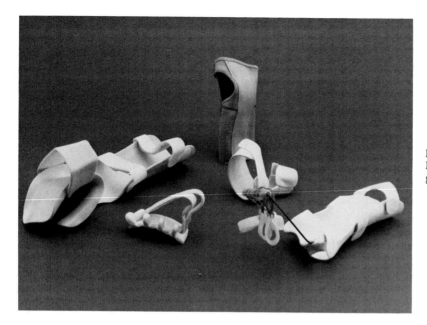

Figure 102–3. Custom-designed resting splints, MCP extension splint, dynamic ulnar deviation guard, and CMC joint spica.

NECK BRACES

Cervical spine orthoses perform several functions, the chief of which is to provide stability and changes in posture and rest for the posterior muscles. Patients who have had an extension flexion injury generally find pain relief when held in a neutral, or at least not hyperextended, position. A plastic Mayo-type collar or a Plastizote collar is usually sufficient. A sponge collar is not very effective in providing support. Patients who have soft herniated discs need to be held in a position in which the pressure on the nerve root is eliminated, and plastic Mayo-type collars are generally suitable; often these collars must be turned around and worn backward.

Patients with RA and atlantoaxial subluxation or subluxation at lower levels will often remain asymptomatic. However, these patients must be carefully followed with neurologic examinations and lateral flexion-extension views of the cervical spine to detect any progression.

The occurrence of compression fractures in the thoracic spine is not uncommon, and generally a Knight-Taylor brace (Fig. 102–4) will relieve pain. These patients do not generally need hyperextension or reduction of these fractures, so a Jewett hyperextension brace, which is uncomfortable, is not necessary. A plastic TLSO (thoraco-lumbar-sacral orthosis), which stabilizes the spine by spreading weight to all areas of contact and then places the weight on the iliac crests so the lumbosacral joint is partially bypassed, is very effective and more readily accepted.

These devices may cause increased motion of the muscles that are being stabilized, and they may also cause atrophy of the spinal musculature. Therefore, a weaning process should be followed so the spinal stabilizing muscles will gradually resume their old tasks.

REHABILITATION TREATMENT OF SPECIFIC DISEASES

Rheumatoid Arthritis (RA)

RA is the most destructive and complicated form of arthritis to treat with rehabilitation: there are more types of treatments, and the application of these treatments is more complicated.

It may be helpful to divide RA into acute and

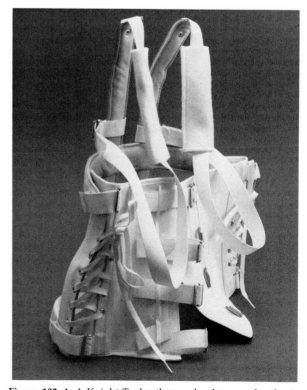

Figure 102–4. A Knight-Taylor thoraco-lumbar-sacral orthosis.

chronic forms in order to consider how to apply rehabilitation treatment methods.

Acute Rheumatoid Arthritis. The patient with acute RA has multiple inflamed joints. There may be deformities or not, and there is muscle wasting. Steinbrocker radiographic changes are generally Steinbrocker I, II.

Range of Motion. The loss of ROM is readily predictable (Table 102–1).[116] When loss of ROM (deformity) occurs, the physician and patient must try to correct it by practicing active ROM and strengthening exercises at the affected joints.

Moist Heat. The patient will immediately obtain pain relief from moist heat. This may be in the form of moist hot packs, paraffin wax to the hands and wrists, spa therapy, Hubbard tanks, therapeutic pools, electric lights, infrared bakers, etc. The prescription is usually twice daily application for approximately 20 to 30 minutes. Active ROM exercises should be instituted to strengthen weakened muscles.

Isometric exercises with elastic bands should be prescribed. Small ankle or hand-held weights are probably too heavy, and the patient cannot be expected to exercise all multiple joints. Those joints that have the most marked muscle atrophy and weakness should be selected for exercises. These usually are the shoulder abductors, the knee extensors, the hip extensors, and the muscles of the hands.

The occupational therapist should teach the patient the ADL he or she cannot now do, and teach *energy conservation.* Splints may be provided for pain-

Table 102–1. PREDICTED DEFORMITIES

Joint	Deformity	Position of Splinting
Head and neck	Flexion, rotation	Full extension, cervical spine, chin forward
Dorsal spine	Flexion, chest flat	Full extension
Shoulder	Adduction, internal rotation	90 degrees abduction, neutral rotation
Elbow	Flexion, pronation	90 degrees flexion, 10 degrees supination
Wrist	Palmar flexion	30 degrees dorsiflexion
Thumb	Flexion	Extension, apposition
Finger	Flexion, ulnar deviation	Extension, no lateral deviation
Hips	Flexion, adduction, external rotation	Extension. In line with body. Foot pointing upward
Knee	Flexion	Extension
Ankle	Plantar flexion	Right angle to leg
Foot	Valgus, spread of forefoot	No varus or valgus, upward pressure beneath second, third, and fourth metatarsal bones
Toe	Plantar flexion in phalangeal joints, flexion at metatarsophalangeal joints	In line with plantar surface of foot

From Steinbrocker, O.: Arthritis in Modern Practice. Philadelphia, W. B. Saunders Company, 1947.

ful, inflamed wrists to protect them while lifting and to wear at night if there is significant inflammation and pain upon arising in the morning. They can decrease flexion deformities.

Shoes should relieve pressure on the metatarsal heads, support the longitudinal arches, allow space for swollen toes, be wide enough for the foot to spread, and grip the heel so a valgus deformity will not occur. Inserts will help (see Fig. 102–1). Patients often select slippers and soft shoes because their feet are painful, but these soft shoes or slippers do not support the foot and allow the deformities to progress.

Patients should also be counseled at this time in many ways. There may be marital/sexual problems. The patient's family and spouse may not realize how fatigued and miserable the patient feels and will expect more than he or she can produce. The patient should be advised not to become overly fatigued on the job and not to perform activities that, in the long run, will destroy the integrity of various joints. A less strenuous vocation may be required.

Whether the patient should be hospitalized is a question not always answered by the patient's needs, but often by the patient's insurance carrier. If the patient has many joints involved with several joints quite severely affected and ready relief has not been obtained by systemic medication or injections, it is reasonable that the patient be hospitalized for rest and comprehensive treatment. Patients especially with disease in the hips, knees, ankles, and feet will benefit from bed rest and instruction. DRG-exempt rehabilitation units have a diagnostic category of polyarthritis, which makes patients with RA eligible for services. Spiegel et al.[117] have shown that hospitalization on an average of 13 days per year in an arthritis rehabilitation unit is correlated with better scores in compliance, knowledge, patient pain assessment, physician assessment, tender joints, local activity, manual dexterity, and ADL.

Chronic Rheumatoid Arthritis. Patients with chronic RA may have multiple joints showing signs of inflammation, but they usually are less inflamed, and with more frequent deformities. The deformities that occur are highly predictable. Steinbrocker listed these deformities as early as 1942 (see Table 102–1).[116] Many of these can be prevented if the patient assiduously adheres to a program of splints, exercises, and shoe modifications. The physician must offer these recommendations to the patient even if the physician thinks the patient will not comply. The patient should perform isometric exercises and active ROM in an effort to extend the wrist, abduct the shoulder, and extend the knee and hip. Serial casts at the knee or turnbuckle casts or even cloth knee immobilizers can be applied. As long as the patient wears them a significant amount of the time, the knee flexor muscles will "give," and the knee will become straighter; that is, it will extend unless the joint surfaces are extremely irregular and destroyed. While undergoing ROM exercising, the patient may find application of heat and joint injections particularly helpful.

At this time, the patient's and the family's social, vocational, and personal situation must again be reviewed by appropriate counselors and steps taken to modify the patient's life and vocation if needed.[118]

If surgery is required for the patient's joints, both preoperative and postoperative muscle strengthening should be prescribed. The muscles have probably lost the ability to respond maximally or they have lost control because pain or fluid in joints reflexively inhibits their activity. Patients, therefore, should be taught to contract the muscle to prepare for increased postoperative ROM. Functional electric stimulation (FES) can be used to assist in this task as well as biofeedback with surface electrodes.

Studies have demonstrated that patients with RA cannot continue performing physically demanding vocational tasks.[119] The patient, therefore, should complete a Social Security application, and the physician should carefully fill in the required information when the forms are required.

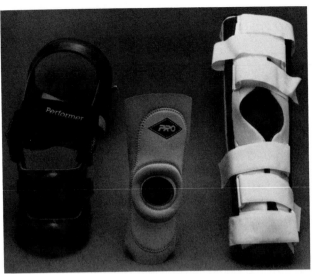

Figure 102–5. Examples of mild *(center)*, moderate *(left)*, and marked *(right)* limiting and stabilizing knee braces.

Osteoarthritis

The patient with osteoarthritis (OA) should be taught to perform range-of-motion exercises; the first physical impairment is that involved joints lose motion. Muscles atrophy around involved joints. The patient should be taught multiple-angle isometric exercises to keep up strength. This is a tedious and boring task, and must be promoted enthusiastically.

Other therapies include the application of spicas for the CM and MCP joints of the thumbs. By immobilizing this joint, patients can obtain pain-free function and relatively little loss of dexterity in their hands. In addition, canes, walkers, and crutches will be appropriate for patients with hip, knee, foot, and ankle pain. It has been shown that a cane held in the contralateral hand reduces hip pain.[120] The patient should try holding a cane in either hand to relieve knee pain (see section on walking aids). Knee braces are difficult because the better the pain relief, the more restriction of motion occurs with their use. A simple sleeve (Fig. 102–5) is the least expensive and least limiting. Knee cages and complex braces designed to provide mediolateral stability may be prescribed for strenuous activities but are often found too cumbersome and activity-limiting for daily use by patients.

A rocker bottom shoe can be prescribed for patients with rigid toes, and shoes with a SACH heel and soft, spongy sole also relieve toe pain. In addition, patients with painful knees will benefit from wearing shoes with SACH heels and soft soles. An example is the Rockport Walker shoe with Vibram sole.

The cervical spine is another region in which pain commonly comes from problems other than the underlying cervical OA that is nearly ubiquitous. If the patient has pain on extension of the cervical spine or radicular symptoms are present, then perhaps a Plastizote or plastic cervical collar (Mayo) that diminishes extension will help limit symptoms.

Psoriatic Arthritis

Joint swelling, often quite severe, and tendinitis or tenosynovitis as well as enthesitis are characteristic of psoriatic arthritis (PsA). Ice, moist heat, and joint injections, and the use of canes, crutches, or walkers to relieve weight-bearing joints have been shown to be helpful. Once pain is relieved and the swelling is reduced, more normal motion, weight-bearing, and ADL training can be resumed.

In addition to splinting to diminish pain, joints may be supported with splints in a position of maximal function. The wrist and fingers are involved in a high proportion of cases and often progress quite rapidly. Functional wrist splints used at the first indication of synovitis may help preserve function and alignment. Passive stretching and ring splints may help maintain posture if there is rapid progression toward ankylosis.

Sausage toes due to tenosynovitis must be accommodated by high toe box and extra-depth shoes. Metatarsal relief pads or metatarsal bars may help. A longitudinal arch orthotic is often needed to immobilize joints and provide pain relief with weight-bearing. Involvement of the hindfoot may require soft inserts to elevate the heel to relieve the pain of plantar fasciitis and more extensive orthoses to immobilize the tibiotalar and talocalcaneal joints. If there is involvement of the spine, measures similar to those appropriate in patients with ankylosing spondylitis should be applied. All in all, the prognosis for function is usually better in psoriatic arthritis than in RA because not as many joints are as severely involved. This should encourage the physician to be optimistic and vigorous in treatment.

Juvenile Rheumatoid Arthritis

One distinction between adult rheumatoid arthritis (RA) and juvenile rheumatoid arthritis (JRA) is that children continue to grow whereas adults do not; length discrepancies may occur, with bones either being lengthened or shortened because of the periarticular inflammation and shortened by the premature closure of epiphyses due to the use of steroids. Rehabilitation treatment must include examination for leg length discrepancies and the application of appropriate shoe lifts. Canes and crutches may also be provided. Often significant soft tissue stiffening and ankylosis occur, and serial casts can diminish flexion contractures at the knee and wrist. Heat may be applied to inflamed joints, and pool therapy is especially likely to induce compliance with strengthening and endurance exercises. It must be stressed that the physician must enlist the parents' aid in obtaining compliance from young patients with their splint wearing and exercises. Children are no more likely to comply than adults, but there is a built-in therapeutic assessment monitor in the family.

Ankylosing Spondylitis

Ankylosing spondylitis is commonly ignored by treatment with rehabilitation modalities. The patient should be taught exercises that consist of forced expansion of the chest and the application of pressure against the abdomen. In addition, the patient will predictably lose an erect posture and develop scoliosis and kyphoscoliosis of the cervical, thoracic, and lumbar spines. Patients normally become more stooped at the end of the day (as we all do) because our spines shrink and probably because we walk more hunched over. This habitus is exaggerated in the patient with ankylosing spondylitis, and the patient should be encouraged on annual or semiannual visits to perform exercises to extend the spine. These include push-ups, back arching when prone, and walking into a corner with the hands on top of the head, the elbows flexed, and the shoulders abducted. These exercises, of course, should be performed many times. Patients should be counseled that, even though they seem to be losing the fight to maintain a totally erect posture, they are probably winning the fight to prevent themselves from becoming disabled by kyphosis.

Outpatient treatment at least twice monthly for 4 months has been shown to increase spinal ROM and function when compared with no treatment.[121] An additional study demonstrated a positive relationship between exercise and work capacity.[122] Hospitalization for pain relief, rehabilitation, treatment,

instruction, and diagnosis of resistant pain may be required.

Progressive Systemic Sclerosis

Patients with progressive systemic sclerosis (PSS) particularly develop contractures of the fingers. These are very resistant to splinting. The patient should be encouraged to perform extension and flexion exercises with the fingers. Plaster casts may be placed on the fingers to encourage the healing of sores. The patient should be very careful with hand hygiene to keep sores from getting infected. If hands become significantly impaired, aids and devices should be prescribed.

Localized scleroderma, which invades muscles and may cause knee flexion contractures, etc., often responds to active resistive exercises and splinting to prevent flexion contractures.

Polymyositis/Dermatomyositis

The most common manifestation of polymyositis/dermatomyositis (PM/DM) is proximal muscle weakness associated with difficulty in reaching for objects, dressing, rising from low chairs, climbing stairs, and walking. About 10 to 15 percent of patients also have distal weakness of the extremities causing problems with dexterity and grasp. Patients will require bathroom equipment and assistive devices to help with reaching and dressing. Patients who have a very weak quadriceps muscle (two fifths strength) will benefit from a double upright brace locked in 5 degrees of plantar flexion to create an extension moment at the knee and stabilize it during the stance phase of gait.

ROM losses are common in patients whose weakness keeps them from putting their joints through a full arc of motion or who have been at bed rest from an acute disease flare. Children with DM quickly develop joint contractures of the shoulders, elbows, and ankles. Calcific deposits in the soft tissues surrounding the joints contribute to these contractures. Adequate ROM and stretching programs are critical in maintaining motion and preventing contractures.

Weakness and ROM deficits are less prominent in PM associated with other collagen vascular diseases. However, the weakness associated with inclusion body myositis is slow and progressive, and often these patients reach a point where ambulation with braces and a walker is no longer possible. A motorized scooter should be prescribed for them.

Patients with active, stable myositis and inactive myositis have been able to increase their muscle strength during a 4-week isometric exercise program.[123] In this program, patients perform six isometric contractions three times a week—each held for 6 seconds with a 20-second rest period between each contraction. There was no clinically significant rise in CPK values or blood pressure during the exercise program. Those patients with long-standing disease and significant muscle atrophy did not significantly increase their strength, whereas those with disease for only 1 to 2 years and less atrophy had significant strength increases.

Joint involvement with arthritis is most often seen in the PM group associated with collagen vascular disease and in DM. These patients may need appropriate splints and joint conservation techniques.

If dysphagia persists, speech pathology consultation and swallowing studies should be obtained.

Systemic Lupus Erythematosus

Patients with systemic lupus erythematosus (SLE), on occasion, have had spontaneous rupture of the Achilles and patellar tendons (especially when taking systemic steroids), and there should be gentle rather than sudden stretching of these joints.

Nonerosive hand arthritis (Jaccoud's arthritis) usually occurs after many years of SLE. The joint deformities—boutonniere, swan neck, ulnar deviation, MCP subluxation—are usually reducible. Patients, therefore, may wear splints actively to keep their fingers in the proper alignment while performing ADL. These hands usually do not demonstrate the osteoporosis that accompanies hand involvement in RA, and hand surgery will be well tolerated.

When aseptic necrosis of a joint occurs, surgery will usually ultimately be required at the hip, but the prescription of canes, walkers, and crutches is appropriate in the interim.

Progressive resistive exercises are not commonly prescribed in SLE.

Shoulder Hand Syndrome or Reflex Sympathetic Dystrophy

Reflex sympathetic dystrophy (RSD) is a mysterious, fairly common disease in which a hand, shoulder, knee, or foot/ankle becomes disabled due to exquisite pain on motion and tenderness. This is usually accompanied by swelling, mottling (livedo reticularis), and excessive cold sweat. These patients should be treated immediately with oral steroids or given stellate ganglion blocks or lumbar sympathetic blocks. The blocks should be performed so that a skin sensor demonstrates an increase in temperature of a degree Fahrenheit or so of the involved area. Under these conditions, the involved extremity usually becomes pain free, and ROM will be markedly increased. As the ROM increases, the patient's condition improves.

The ROM must be performed within a short time after the sympathetic block while pain relief is still present. A series of these blocks followed by exercise may be necessary.

Compliance

Rehabilitation modalities, exercises, aids, and devices do little good if the patient neglects to perform or use them. Unfortunately, investigators have discovered that medical[124, 125] and arthritic patients[126, 127] exhibit a similar lack of compliance.

Parker and Bender in 1957 questioned 56 patients who had been provided a "home treatment" program, and found only 54 percent were continuing it at 12 months.[128] Carpenter and Davis in 1976 questioned 54 patients about their compliance with an exercise program and discovered only 55 percent were continuing to follow instructions.[129] The reasons given for noncompliance were many and diverse and without discernible trends.

Belcon[126] reviewed studies that described compliance with splint use (Table 102–2). Compliance rates varied from 28 to 78 percent. Again there was no consistent reason or set of reasons for noncompliance common to the studies. The prevalence of noncompliance may be so high, in fact, that it becomes difficult to assess the efficacy of splint use.

Studies of compliance with prescribed medications have been more numerous. Joyce[130] studied 60 females with definite RA and found 33 to be "obedient" on the basis of collecting unused pills and analyzing for a phenol red marker that had been incorporated into the medication unbeknownst to the patients. Overall, 38 of 108 urine samples were positive for phenol red and 40 of 78 appeared to comply on pill count. They found that their "obedient" patients had fewer active joints, fewer signs of toxicity, and reported fewer side effects from their medication.

Geertsen, Gray, and Ward[131] studied 123 patients with classic or definite RA, all seen by the same physician. Compliance was measured by physician estimate according to his personal opinion, data obtained on blood salicylate levels, and clinic attendance records. The physician qualified 63 as full compliers and 60 as poor or partial compliers. They discovered that patients who felt they were kept waiting overly long, that the doctor spent very little time with them, that the doctor was not personal in his relationship to them but was more businesslike, and that there was poor communication between doctor and patient were poor compliers.

Wright and Hopkins[132] surveyed 200 "rheumatic" patients with a questionnaire that assessed patient preference. They found that patients preferred capsules to tablets, once daily administration, effectiveness, and absence of toxicity.

Lee and Tan[133] studied 100 patients with RA from New Zealand using patient report. Sixty-three and nine tenths percent of their patients claimed to be taking their antirheumatic medications *all* of the

Table 102–2. SPLINT COMPLIANCE STUDIES

Reference	n	Study Design	Intervention or Disease Feature	Compliance Measure	Compliance Result	Compliance Definition	Disease Definition	Regimen Definition	Duration of Observation
21	56	Cross-sectional analytic survey	Home physiotherapy	Interview	39%	0	0	0	+
22	218	Cross-sectional analytic survey	Home physiotherapy	Interview	65%	0	0	0	+
23	40	Cross-sectional analytic survey	a) ASA use	a) Interview + serum assay	78%	+	0	0	0
			b) Exercise	b) Interview	40%	+	0	0	0
			c) Splint wear	c) Interview	25%	+	0	0	0
24	12	Time series	Exercise/visual feedback	Electronic counter	Enhancement	+	0	+	+
25	46	Cross-sectional analytic survey	Splint wear	Weighted-index	28%	+	0	0	0
26	36	Cross-sectional analytic survey	Splint wear	Interview	50%	0	0	0	0
27	50	Cross-sectional analytic survey	Splint wear	Interview	62%	+	+	0	+
28	66	Prospective analytic survey	Splint wear	Interview	65%	0	+	+	+

*n indicates the number of study subjects; + = presence, 0 = absence of the indicated feature; ASA = acetylsalicylic acid.
From Belcon, M.C., et al.: A critical review of compliance studies in rheumatoid arthritis. Arthritis Rheum. 27:1230, 1984.

time. Twenty-eight and six tenths percent described lessening of symptoms; 23.8 percent forgetfulness; 21.4 percent side effects; 14.3 percent inconvenience; and 9.5 percent dislike of taking pills as reasons for noncompliance.

Deyo, Inouye, and Sullivan[134] studied 66 patients with RA as well as 41 with OA, 27 with gout, 14 with ankylosing spondylitis, and 24 with "other," and assessed compliance by counting the percentage of doses they obtained from their pharmacy with the percentage prescribed. They found that the more appointments that were kept, the better the patients complied, and, interestingly, the more drugs they took, the better was their compliance. They also found a variation between different types of drugs: 80 percent being the highest for prednisone and penicillamine.

Wasner et al.[135] studied 33 patients with RA and 32 patients with ankylosing spondylitis and assessed compliance by pill count at the end of each 6-week period of drug trial. They found the more pills patients took each day, the less they complied.

Bond and Monson[136] studied 81 rheumatology or renal patients from a rheumatology clinic at a veteran's hospital. They assessed compliance by pharmacy prescription filling. They found that intervention by a clinical pharmacist and nurse clinician to help educate and solve patient compliance problems enhanced compliance.

Owen, Friesen, Roberts, and Flux[137] studied 178 RA patients. Compliance was assessed by a questionnaire, and 63.5 percent of patients reported good compliance. Those patients who complied had a higher sedimentation rate, a greater duration of morning stiffness, more active disease.

There appear to be as many reasons for noncompliance as there are investigations. The various reasons would not be valid for all populations or probably even different individuals. It would seem reasonable that each physician must assess the individual patient to discover any noncompliance and the reasons for it. We suggest the physician do this whenever the patient starts doing badly and there is a question of compliance or efficacy from medication or rehabilitation treatment.

Drug studies reinforce our conclusions from the studies about rehabilitation treatments. The consensus is that there are numerous reasons for noncompliance, and at least some patient will admit nearly every reason that the investigator offers as a possible cause of noncompliance. The physician, therapist, or sensitive office staff should repeatedly inquire whether the patient *at that time* is having difficulty with compliance with exercises, aids and devices, splints, or medications. If noncompliance can be discussed, then there is the opportunity for the cause to be discovered and remedies provided. Monitoring the results of rehabilitation treatments is essential for proper patient care; treatment cannot accomplish its goals unless compliance is high.

Compliance studies have included "home treatment programs,"[128] exercise programs,[129] splint use,[126] and medication.[130–137] Many causes of noncompliance were defined in these studies with none being predominant. Therefore, it is suggested that the *particular current* cause of noncompliance (if any) be determined, possibly through a nonthreatening interview, so a remedy may be sought.

References

1. DeLisa, J., Martin, G. M., and Currie, D. M.: Rehabilitation medicine: Past, present and future. *In* Rehabilitation Medicine: Principles and Practice. Philadelphia, J. B. Lippincott, 1988, p. 3.
2. Hicks, J., and Nicholas, J. J.: Rehabilitative rheumatology content in current rehabilitation medicine training programs. Arch. Phys. Med. Rehab. 66:631, 1985.
3. Hicks, J., and Nicholas, J. J.: Rehabilitative rheumatology content in current rheumatology training programs. Arthritis Rheum. 27:1076, 1984.
4. Halstead, L. S.: Team care in chronic illness: A critical review of the literature of the past 25 years. Arch. Phys. Med. Rehab. 57:507, 1976.

5. Cosgrove, J. L., Nicholas, J. J., Barwak, J., Brewer, C., Mientus, J., McConnell, R., and Rinaldo, D.: The effects of a treatment team on a special unit. Am. J. Phys. Med. Rehab. 67:253, 1988.
6. Moll, J. M., and Wright V.: Measurement of joint motion. Clin. Rheum. Dis. 2:3, 1976.
7. Grahame, R.: The hypermobility syndrome. Ann. Rheum. Dis. 49:190, 1990.
8. Committee for the Study of Joint Motion, American Academy of Orthopedic Surgeons: Joint Motion: Method of Measuring and Recording. Chicago, American Academy of Orthopaedic Surgeons, 1965.
9. Hoppenfeld, S.: Physical Examination of the Spine and Extremities. New York, Appleton-Century-Crofts, 1976.
10. Bates, B.: Guide to Physical Examination and History Taking. 4th ed. Philadelphia, J. B. Lippincott, 1987.
11. Erickson, R. P., and MacPhee, M. C.: Rehabilitation Medicine Principles and Practice. Philadelphia, J. B. Lippincott, 1988.
12. Nicholas, J. J., Robinson, L. R., Logan, A., and Robertson, R.: Isokinetic testing in non-athletic normal subjects. Arch. Phys. Med. Rehab. 70:210, 1989.
13. Kendall, F. B., and McCreary, E. K.: Muscles: Testing and Function. Baltimore, Williams & Wilkins, 1983.
14. Bohannon, R. W.: Test-retest reliability of hand-held dynamometry during a simple session of strength assessment. Phys. Ther. 66:206, 1986.
15. Bohannon, R. W., and Andrews, A. W.: Interrater reliability of hand-held dynamometry. Phys. Ther. 67:931, 1987.
16. Bohannon, R. W.: Testing isometric limb muscle strength with dynomometers, Critical Reviews. Phys. Rehab. Med. 2:75, 1990.
17. Ekblom, B., Lovgren, O., Alderin, M., Fridstrom, M., and Satterstrom, G.: Physical performance in patients with rheumatoid arthritis. Scand. J. Rheumatol. 3:121, 1974.
18. Minor, M. A., Hewett, J. E., Webel, R. R., Dreisinger, T. E., and Kay, D. R.: Exercise tolerance and disease related measures in patients with rheumatoid arthritis and osteoarthritis. J. Rheumatol. 15:905, 1988.
19. Nordesjo, L., Nordgren, B., Wigren, A., and Kolstad, K.: Isometric strength and endurance in patients with severe rheumatoid arthritis or osteoarthrosis in the knee joints. Scand. J. Rheumatol. 12:152, 1983.
20. Anderson, K. O., Bradley, L. A., McDaniel, L., et al.: The assessment of pain in rheumatoid arthritis. Arthritis Rheum. 30:36, 1987.
21. Callahan, L. F., Brooks, R. H., Summey, J. A., and Pincus, T.: Quantitative pain assessment for routine care of rheumatoid arthritis patients, using a pain scale based on activities of daily living of a visual analogue pain scale. Arthritis Rheum. 30:630, 1987.
22. Scott, J. T., and Huskisson, E. C.: Graphic representation of pain. Pain 2:175, 1976.
23. McCarty, D. J., Gattner, R. A., and Phelps, P.: A dolorimeter for quantification of articular tenderness. Arthritis Rheum. 8:551, 1965.
24. Rhind, V. M., Unsworth, A., and Haslock, I.: Assessment of stiffness in rheumatology: The use of rating scales. Br. J. Rheumatol. 26:126, 1987.
25. Melvin, J. L.: Status report on interdisciplinary medical rehabilitation. Arch. Phys. Med. Rehab. 70:273, 1989.
26. Dictionary of the Rheumatic Diseases. Vol. III. Health Status Measurement. American College of Rheumatology, 1988, pp. 7–9, 43–45.
27. Harvey, R. F., and Jellinek, H. M.: Patient profiles: Utilization in functional performance assessment. Arch. Phys. Med. Rehab. 64:268, 1983.
28. Harvey, R. F., and Jellinek, H. M.: Functional performance assessment: A program approach. Arch. Phys. Med. Rehab. 62:456, 1981.
29. Granger, G. V., and Hamilton, B. B.: The Uniform Data System for Medical Rehabilitation Report of First Admissions for 1990. Am. J. Phys. Med. Rehabil. 71:108, 1992.
30. Moskowitz, E., and McCann, C. B.: Classification of disability in the chronically ill and aging. J. Chronic Dis. 5:342, 1957.
31. Mahoney, F. L., and Barthel, D. W.: Functional evaluation: The Barthel Index. Md. St. Med. J. 14:61, 1965.
32. Lightfoot, R. W., Jr.: Arthritis and Allied Conditions. 10th ed. Philadelphia, Lea & Febiger, 1985.
33. Kantor, T. O.: Order out of chaos—the primary mission of the pyramid. J. Rheumatol. 17:1580, 1990.
34. Pincus, T., and Callahan, L. F.: Remodelling the pyramid or remodelling paradigms concerning rheumatoid arthritis—lessons from Hodgkin's disease and coronary artery disease. J. Rheumatol. 17:1582, 1990.
35. Bensen, W. G., Bensen, W., Adachi, J. D., and Tugwell, P. X.: Remodeling the pyramid: The therapeutic target of rheumatoid arthritis. J. Rheumatol. 17:987, 1989–1990.
36. Wilske, K. R., and Healy, L. A.: Challenging the therapeutic pyramid: A new look at treatment strategies for rheumatoid arthritis. J. Rheumatol. 17:4, 1990.
37. Swezey, R.: Rheumatoid arthritis: The role of the kinder and gentler therapies. J. Rheumatol. 17:8, 1990.
38. Wand, J. R.: Earlier intervention with second line therapies. J. Rheumatol. 17(Suppl. 25):18, 1990.
39. Sukenik, S., Buskila, D., Neumann, L., Kleiner-Baumgarten, A., Zimlichman, S., and Horowitz, J.: Sulphur bath and mud pack treatment for rheumatoid arthritis at the dead sea area. Ann. Rheum. Dis. 49:99, 1990.
40. Harris, E. D., Jr., and McCroskery, P. A.: The influence of temperature and fibril stability on degradation of cartilage collagen of rheumatoid synovial collagenase. N. Engl. J. Med. 290:1, 1974.
41. Lehmann, J. F., Warren, C. G., and Scham, S. M.: Therapeutic heat and cold. Clin. Orthop. 99:207, 1974.
42. DeLatour, B. J., Lehmann, J. F., Stonebridge, J. B., Warren, C. G., and Guy, A. W.: Muscle heating in human subjects with 915 MHz microwave contact applicator. Arch. Phys. Med. Rehab. 51:147, 1970.
43. Lehmann, J. F., McMillon, J. A., Brunner, G. D., and Blumberg, J. B.: Comparative study of the efficiency of short wave, microwave and ultrasound diathermy in heating the hip joint. Arch. Phys. Med. Rehab. 40:510, 1959.
44. Warren, C. G., Lehmann, J. F., and Koblausky, J. H.: Heat and stretch procedures: An evaluation using rat tail tendon. Arch. Phys. Med. Rehab. 57:122, 1976.
45. Warren, C. G., Lehmann, J. F., and Koblausky, J. H.: Elongation of rat tail tendon. Arch. Phys. Med. Rehab. 52:465, 1971.
46. Feibel, A., and Fast, A.: Deep heating of joints: A reconsideration. Arch. Phys. Med. Rehab. 57:513, 1976.
47. Hashish, I., Harvey, W., and Harris, M.: Anti-inflammatory effects of ultrasound therapy: Evidence for a major placebo effect. Br. J. Rheumatol. 25:77, 1986.
48. Horvath, S. M., and Hollander, S. L.: Intra-articular temperature as a measure of joint reaction. J. Clin. Invest. 28:469, 1949.
49. Hollander, J. L., and Horvath, S. M.: Changes in joint temperature produced by diseases and by physical therapy. Arch. Phys. Med. Rehab. 30:437, 1949.
50. Lehmann, J. F., Silverman, D. R., Baum, B. A., Kirk, N. L., and Johnstone, V. C.: Temperature distributions in the human thigh, produced by infrared, hot pack and microwave application. Arch. Phys. Med. Rehab. 47:291, 1966.
51. Mainardi, C. M., Walter, J. M., Spiegel, P. K., Goldkamp, O. G., and Harris, E. D., Jr.: Rheumatoid arthritis: Failure of daily heat therapy to affect its progression. Arch. Phys. Med. Rehab. 60:390, 1979.
52. Lehmann, J. F.: Diathermy. In Handbook of Physical Medicine and Rehabilitation. 2nd ed. Philadelphia, W.B. Saunders Company, 1971.
53. Miglietta, O.: Action of cold on spasticity. Am. J. Phys. Med. 52:198, 1973.
54. Knutsson, E., and Martensson, E.: Effects of local cooling on monosynaptic reflexes in man. Scand. J. Rehab. Med. 1:126, 1969.
55. Travell, J.: Ethylchloride spray for painful muscle spasm. Arch. Phys. Med. Rehab. 33:291, 1952.
56. Olson, J. E., and Stravino, V. P.: A review of cryotherapy. Phys. Ther. 52:840, 1972.
57. Kirk, J. A., and Kersley, G. D.: Heat and cold in the physical treatment of rheumatoid arthritis of the knee: A controlled clinical trial. Ann. Phys. Med. 9:270, 1968.
58. Magora, F., Aladjemoff, L., Tannenbaum, J., and Magora, A.: Treatment of pain by transcutaneous electrical stimulation. Acta Anaesthesiol. Scand. 22:589, 1978.
59. Ersek, R. A.: Transcutaneous electrical neurostimulation: A new therapeutic modality for controlling pain. Clin. Orthop. 128:314, 1977.
60. Melzack, R., and Wall, P. D.: Pain mechanisms: A new theory. Science 150:971, 1965.
61. Mann, S. C., and Baragar, F. D.: Preliminary clinical study of acupuncture in rheumatoid arthritis. J. Rheumatol. 1:126, 1974.
62. Gaw, A. C., Chang, L. W., and Shaw, L. C.: Efficacy of acupuncture on osteoarthritic pain: A controlled double blind study. N. Engl. J. Med. 293:275, 1975.
63. Moore, M. E., and Berk, S. N.: Acupuncture for chronic shoulder pain: An experimental study with attention to the role of placebo and hypnotic susceptibility. Ann. Intern. Med. 84:381, 1976.
64. Godfrey, C. M., and Morgan, P.: A controlled trial of the theory of acupuncture in rheumatoid arthritis. J. Rheumatol. 5:121, 1978.
65. Melzack, R.: Acupuncture and musculoskeletal pain. J. Rheumatol. 5:119, 1978.
66. Piersol, G. M., and Hollander, J. L.: The optimum rest-exercise balance in the treatment of rheumatoid arthritis. Arch. Phys. Med. Rehab. 28:500, 1947.
67. DeLateur, B. J.: Exercise for strength and endurance. In Basmajian, J. V. (ed.): Therapeutic Exercise. 4th ed. Baltimore, Williams & Wilkins, 1984.
68. Moritani, T., and DeVries, H. A.: Neural factors vs hypertrophy in the time course of muscle strength gain. Am. J. Phys. Med. 58:115, 1979.
69. Machover, S., and Sapecky, A. J.: Effect of isometric exercise on the quadriceps muscle in patients with rheumatoid arthritis. Arch. Phys. Med. Rehab. 47:737, 1966.
70. Ekblom, B., Lovgren, O., Alderin, M., Fridstrom, M., and Satterstrom, G.: Effect of short-term physical training on patients with rheumatoid arthritis I. Scand. J. Rheumatol. 5:70, 1976.

71. Nordemar, R., Edstrom, L., and Ekblom, B.: Changes in muscle fibre size and physical performance in patients with rheumatoid arthritis after short-term physical training. Scand. J. Rheumatol. 5:70, 1976.
72. Nordemar, R., Berg, U., Ekblom, B., and Edstrom, L.: Changes in muscle fibre size and physical performance in patients with rheumatoid arthritis after 7 months' physical training. Scand. J. Rheumatol. 5:233, 1976.
73. Nordemar, R.: Physical training in rheumatoid arthritis: A controlled long term study. II. Functional capacity and general attitudes. Scand. J. Rheumatol. 10:25, 1981.
74. Stecher, R. M., and Karnash, L. J.: Heberden's nodes. VI. The effect of nerve injury upon formation of degenerative joint disease of the fingers. Am. J. Med. Sci. 213:181, 1947.
75. Thompson, M., and Bywaters, E. G. L.: Unilateral rheumatoid arthritis following hemiplegia. Ann. Rheum. Dis. 21:370, 1962.
76. Glyn, J. H., Sutherland, I., Walker, G. F., and Young, A. C.: Low incidence of osteoarthritis in hip and knee after anterior poliomyelitis: A later review. Br. Med. J. 2:739, 1966.
77. Glick, L. N.: Asymmetrical rheumatoid arthritis after poliomyelitis. Br. Med. J. 3:26, 1967.
78. Bland, J. H., and Eady, W. M.: Hemiplegia and rheumatoid arthritis. Arthritis Rheum. 11:72, 1968.
79. Glynn, J. J., and Clayton, M. L.: Sparing effect of hemiplegia on tophaceous gout. Ann. Rheum. Dis. 35:534, 1976.
80. Merritt, J. L., and Hunder, G. G.: Passive range of motion, not isometric exercise, amplifies acute urate synovitis. Arch. Phys. Med. Rehab. 64:130, 1983.
81. Agudelo, C. A., Schumacher, H. R., and Phelps, P.: Effect of exercise on urate crystal-induced inflammation in canine joints. Arthritis Rheum. 15:609, 1972.
82. Murray, D. G.: Modification of experimental arthritis in rabbits by tenotomy. J. Surg. Res. Clin. Lab. Invest. 6:488, 1966.
83. Glynn, L. E.: The chronicity of inflammation and its significance in rheumatoid arthritis. Ann. Rheum. Dis. 27:105, 1968.
84. Perlman, S. G., Connell, K. J., Clark, A., Robinson, M. S., Conlon, P., Gecht, M., Caldron, P., and Sinarone, J. M.: Dance-based aerobic exercise for rheumatoid arthritis. Arthritis Care Res. 3:29, 1990.
85. Minor, M. A., Hewett, J. E., Webel, R. R., Anderson, S. K., and Kay, D. R.: Efficacy of physical conditioning exercise in patients with rheumatoid arthritis and osteoarthritis. Arthritis Rheum. 32:1396, 1989.
86. Harkcom, T. M., Lampman, R. M., Banwell, B. F., and Castor, C. W.: Therapeutic value of graded aerobic exercise training in rheumatoid arthritis. Arthritis Rheum. 28:32, 1985.
87. Beals, C. A., Lampman, R. M., Banwell, B. F., Braunstein, E. M., Albers, J. W., and Castor, C. W.: Measurement of exercise tolerance in patients with rheumatoid arthritis and osteoarthritis. J. Rheumatol. 12:458, 1985.
88. Danneskiold-Samsøe, B., Lynsberg, K., Risum, T., and Telling, M.: The effect of water exercise therapy given to patients with rheumatoid arthritis. Scand. J. Rehab. Med. 19:3, 1987.
89. Fisher, N., Pendergast, D., Gresham, G., and Calkins, E.: Muscle rehabilitation: its effect on the muscular and functional performance of patients with knee osteoarthritis. Arch. Phys. Med. Rehab. 72:367, 1991.
90. Fisher, N., Pendergast, D. R., and Calkins, E. C.: Maximal isometric torque of knee extension as a function of muscle length in subjects of advancing age. Arch. Phys. Med. Rehab. 71:729, 1990.
91. Akeson, W. H., Amiel, D., LaViolette, D., and Secrist, D.: The connective tissue response to immobility: An accelerated aging response? Exp. Gerontol. 3:289, 1968.
92. Woo, S. L. Y., Matthews, J. V., Akeson, W. M., Amiel, D., and Convery, F. R.: Connective tissue response to immobility. Arthritis Rheum. 18:257, 1975.
93. Evans, E. B., Eggers, G. W. N., Butler, J. K., and Blumel, J.: Experimental immobilization and remobilization of rat knee joints. J. Bone Joint Surg. 47A:737, 1960.
94. Greenleaf, J. E., Bernauer, E. M., Juhos, J. T., Young, H. L., Morse, J. T., and Staley, M.: Effects of exercise on fluid exchange and body composition in man during 14-day bed rest. J. Appl. Physiol. 43:126, 1977.
95. Saltin, B., Blomqvist, G., Mitchell, J. H., Johnson, R. L., Wildenthal, K., and Chapman, C. B.: Response to exercise after bed rest and after training. Circulation 38(Suppl. 17):1, 1968.
96. Drinkwater, B. L., and Horvath, S. M.: Detraining effects on young women. Med. Sci. Sports 4:91, 1972.
97. Finsterbush, A., and Friedman, B.: Early changes in immobilized rabbits' knee joints: A light and electron microscopic study. Clin. Orthop. 92:305, 1973.
98. Sayre, L.: Orthopedic Surgery and Diseases of the Joints. (Delivered at Bellevue Hospital Medical College during the Winter Session of 1985.) New York, D. Appleton and Company, 1876.
99. Partridge, R. E. H., and Duthie, J. J. R.: Controlled trial of the effect of complete immobilization of the joints in rheumatoid arthritis. Ann. Rheum. Dis. 22:91, 1963.
100. Mills, J. A., Pinals, R. S., Ropes, M. W., Short, C. L., and Sutcliffe, J.: Value of bed rest in patients with rheumatoid arthritis. N. Engl. J. Med. 284:453, 1971.
101. Lee, P., Kennedy, A. C., Anderson, J., and Buchanan, W. W.: Benefits of hospitalization in rheumatoid arthritis. Q. J. Med. 43:205, 1974.
102. Alexander, G. J. M., Hortas, C., and Bacon, P. A.: Bed rest, activity and the inflammation of rheumatoid arthritis. Br. J. Rheumatol. 22:134, 1983.
103. Kelly, M.: The prevention of deformity in rheumatic disease. Med. J. Aust. 2:1, 1950.
104. Kelly, M.: Rheumatoid arthritis: The active immobilization of acutely inflamed joints. N.Z. Med. J. 60:311, 1961.
105. Thomas, H. O.: Diseases of the Hip, Knee and Ankle Joints with their Deformities, Treated by a New and Efficient Method. 3rd ed. London, Lewis, 1878.
106. Gault, S. J., and Spyker, J. M.: Beneficial effect of immobilization of joints in rheumatoid and related arthritides: A splint study using sequential analysis. Arthritis Rheum. 12:34, 1969.
107. Harris, R., and Copp, E. P.: Immobilization of the knee joint in rheumatoid arthritis. Ann. Rheum. Dis. 21:353, 1962.
108. Nicholas, J. J., and Ziegler, G.: Cylinder splints: Their use in the treatment of arthritis of the knee. Arch. Phys. Med. Rehab. 58:264, 1977.
109. Maigne, R.: Manipulations and mobilizations of the limbs. In Rogoff, J. B. (ed.): Manipulation, Traction and Massage. Baltimore, Williams & Wilkins, 1980.
110. Gall, E., and Riggs, G. (eds.): Arthritis patient education. In Rheumatic Diseases, Rehabilitation and Management. London, Butterworth, 1984.
111. Melvin, J. L.: Rheumatic Disease Occupational Therapy and Rehabilitation. Philadelphia, F. A. Davis Company, 1982.
112. Furst, G., Gerber, L., and Smith, C.: Rehabilitation Through Learning. Energy Conservation and Joint Protection. A Work Book for Persons with Rheumatoid Arthritis. US Department of Health and Human Services, NIH, 1982.
113. Cordery, J. C.: Joint protection: A responsibility of the occupational therapist. Am. J. Occup. Ther. 19:285, 1965.
114. Gerber, L. H., Hunt, G., and Horwitz, S.: Ankle orthosis for rheumatoid disease. Arthritis Rheum. 28:547, 1985.
115. Weist, D. R., Unters, R. L., Bontrager, E. L., et al.: The influence of heel design on a rigid ankle foot orthosis. Orthotics-Prosthetics 33:3, 1979.
116. Steinbrocker, O.: Arthritis in Modern Practice. Philadelphia, W.B. Saunders Company, 1942.
117. Spiegel, J. S., Spiegel, T. M., Ward, N. B., Paulus, H. E., Leake, B., and Kane, R. L.: Rehabilitation for rheumatoid arthritis patients. Arthritis Rheum. 29:628, 1986.
118. Creed, F.: Psychological disorders in rheumatoid arthritis: A growing consensus? Ann. Rheum. Dis. 49:808, 1990.
119. Nicholas, J. J.: Peripheral joint impairment. In Scheer, S. (ed.): Assessing the Vocational Capacity of the Impaired Worker. Rockville, Md, Aspen Publishers, 1990, p. 101.
120. Blount, W. P.: "Don't throw away the cane." J. Bone Joint Surg. 38A:695 (2), 1956.
121. Kraas, G., Stokes, B., Groh, J., Helena, A., and Goldsmith, C.: The effect of comprehensive home physiotherapy and supervision on patients with ankylosing spondylitis—a randomized controlled trial. J. Rheumatol. 17:228, 1990.
122. Fisher, L. R., Cawley, M. I. O., and Holgate, S. T.: Relation between chest expansion, pulmonary function, and exercise tolerance in patients with ankylosing spondylitis. Ann. Rheum. Dis. 49:921, 1990.
123. Hicks, J., Miller, F., Plotz, P., et al.: Strength improvement without CPK elevation in a polymyositis patient on an isometric exercise program. Arthritis Rheum. (Suppl.) 31:559, 1988.
124. Blackwell, B.: Drug therapy-patient compliance. N. Engl. J. Med. 289:249, 1973.
125. Haynes, R. B., Taylor, D. W., and Sackett, D. L. (eds.): Compliance in Health Care. Baltimore, Johns Hopkins University Press, 1979.
126. Belcon, M. C., Haynes, R. B., and Tugwell, P.: A critical review of compliance studies in rheumatoid arthritis. Arthritis Rheum. 27:1228, 1984.
127. Deyo, R. A.: Compliance with therapeutic regimens in arthritis: Issues, current status, and a future agenda. Semin. Arthritis Rheum. 12:233, 1982.
128. Parker, L. B., and Bender, L. F.: Problem of home treatment in arthritis. Arch. Phys. Med. Rehab. 38:392, 1957.
129. Carpenter, J. O., and Davis, L. J.: Medical recommendations—followed or ignored? Factors influencing compliance in arthritis. Arch. Phys. Med. Rehab. 57:241, 1976.
130. Joyce, C. R. B.: Patient co-operation and the sensitivity of clinical trials. J. Chronic Dis. 15:1025, 1962.
131. Geertsen, H. R., Gray, R. M., and Ward, J. R.: Patient non-compliance within the context of seeking medical care for arthritis. J. Chronic Dis. 26:689, 1973.

132. Wright, V., and Hopkins, R.: Administration of antirheumatic drugs. Ann. Rheum. Dis. 35:174, 1978.
133. Lee, P., and Tan, L. J. P.: Drug compliance in outpatients with rheumatoid arthritis. Aust. N.Z. J. Med. 9:274, 1979.
134. Deyo, R. A., Inouye, T. S., and Sullivan, B.: Noncompliance with arthritis drugs: Magnitude, correlates, and clinical implications. J. Rheumatol. 8:931, 1981.
135. Wasner, C., Britton, M. C., Kraines, R. G., Kaye, R. L., Bobrove, A. M., and Fries, J. F.: Nonsteroidal anti-inflammatory agents in rheumatoid arthritis and ankylosing spondylitis. J.A.M.A. 246:2168, 1981.
136. Bond, C. A., and Monson, R.: Sustained improvement in drug documentation, compliance, and disease control—a four-year analysis of an ambulatory care model. Arch. Intern. Med. 144:1159, 1984.
137. Owen, S. G., Friesen, W. T., Roberts, M. S., and Flux, W.: Determinants of compliance in rheumatoid arthritic patients assessed in their home environment. Br. J. Rheumatol. 24:313, 1985.

Section XXII

Reconstructive Surgery in Rheumatic Diseases

Chapter 103   Clement B. Sledge

Introduction to Surgical Management

The various forms of arthritis produce similar consequences in the involved joints: pain, loss of function, progressive damage, and deformity. Reconstructive surgery may be indicated to relieve any or all of these disabilities. In selected situations, surgery may be indicated to *prevent* these consequences. Although the general consequences of arthritic damage to the joint are similar, there are significant differences between osteoarthritis and rheumatoid arthritis; indeed, there are unique surgical aspects to many of the "rheumatoid variants." In some instances these unique features place the patient at risk from surgery, and in others they jeopardize the eventual result. These features will be discussed under the heading Preoperative Evaluation and serve to emphasize two philosophical points: (1) the surgeon who operates on arthritic patients, especially rheumatoid patients, should be familiar with the special technical aspects necessitated by the unusual requirements of the patient with multiple joint involvement, and (2) the surgeon should be part of a team, composed of rheumatologists, nurses, therapists, social workers, and—most important—the patient. At first glance it may seem foolish to list the patient as part of the team. To do so emphasizes that the surgical patient with rheumatoid arthritis is frequently weak and discouraged and must look forward to a series of operations before reasonable functional independence is achieved. Often the patient has excessive expectations regarding the outcome of surgery.[1, 2] By participating in the planning and staging of the surgical events, the patient can better understand the duration of treatment, the necessity of prolonged physical therapy, and the ultimate realistic goal of the procedure or procedures.

Because relief of pain is the most consistent feature of reconstructive surgery, pain is the primary indication for operative intervention. Restoration of motion and function, distinct from relief of pain, is less predictable and requires careful assessment of each patient's disability before improvement can be offered. Some surgical procedures in rheumatoid arthritis are as much prophylactic as therapeutic (e.g., synovectomy, fusion of the first and second cervical vertebrae, fusion of the base of the thumb). The patient should understand the preventive aspects so there will not be disappointment when the therapeutic result does not seem to justify the pain and inconvenience of surgery.

Additionally, societal and socioeconomic goals must be considered. The patient with rheumatoid arthritis has an average length of hospitalization of about 12 to 14 days for each surgical procedure and may require two to six or more major procedures. The economic costs are considerable even when everything proceeds without complication. If a deep infection occurs after a hip replacement, the costs may be well over $100,000. Most patients coming to multiple joint replacement surgeries either have left the work force because of disability or have postponed surgery until they are ready for retirement. The majority are women who have not worked outside the home. These factors make calculation of a cost-benefit ratio difficult. Without putting a dollar value on the "quality of life," can such extensive procedures be justified? One study of 16 patients undergoing bilateral hip and knee replacement showed that none of those patients returned to work after this expensive series of operations involving an average of 3 months of hospitalization.[3] A more

1745

recent study, however, does demonstrate that the quality of life is significantly improved by joint replacements and that this improvement can be expressed in financial terms and in "quality-adjusted life years."[4] Precise data are not available, but preliminary studies strongly suggest that society also benefits in terms of decreased need for home help, home modifications, and hospitalization or confinement to an institution because of loss of independent functional capacity. A spouse or child may be released from the helping role and thereby returned to the working force.[5] For many individual patients, however, the goal must be relief of pain, restoration of functional independence, and a qualitative improvement of life without the need for pure economic justification.[4, 6, 7] Part of the difficulty in assessing the potential benefit of a surgical procedure, to the patient or to society, is the lack of uniform measures of functional assessment before and after surgery. Few studies have reported critical assessment of the outcome in patients with rheumatoid arthritis joint replacement; further studies await adoption and general application of uniform criteria of assessment.[8, 9]

Certainly the major single advance in the care of patients with arthritis was the development of the concept of total joint replacement by Charnley.[10] The concepts initially involved in replacement of the arthritic hip have now been expanded to cover most of the other joints. In patients with osteoarthritis, there are numerous alternatives to joint replacement, many of which are preferable, especially in younger patients. In patients with rheumatoid arthritis, procedures such as arthrodesis, synovectomy, repair of ruptured tendons, and other "nonprosthetic" procedures still play an important role. For predictable relief of pain and restoration in function, however, joint replacement surgery has revolutionized the outlook for patients with multiple joint involvement. Subsequent chapters of this book will therefore emphasize joint replacement surgery in patients with rheumatoid arthritis and its variants, but, when appropriate, alternative procedures will be mentioned, as will certain features pertinent to the patient with osteoarthritis.

PREOPERATIVE EVALUATION

The first consideration is whether a painful joint in a patient with rheumatoid arthritis requires surgery. If synovitis is the cause of the patient's pain and disability, continued medical management with drugs and physical methods is appropriate. If it can be determined that structural damage to the joint is the problem, it is unrealistic to expect that medication will be sufficient. A trial of anti-inflammatory medication and physical therapy is appropriate, particularly for the weight-bearing joints, when the use of crutches may allow the acute disabling symptoms to subside to an acceptable level, even in the presence of structural damage. If these measures fail and

structural damage can be demonstrated on physical examination or by radiographic examination, arthrodesis or arthroplasty can be considered. It is better to perform surgery on each joint as it becomes structurally destroyed than to wait until the patient has multiple destroyed joints requiring prolonged hospitalization, multiple anesthetics, and a series of debilitating surgical procedures. General operative risk should be assessed, especially from the point of view of the systemic manifestations of the rheumatic diseases. The patient should be in optimal medical condition and, when on glucocorticoids, should be on the lowest possible maintenance dose. Obvious sources of infection should be identified and eradicated to prevent postoperative hematogenous seeding of the operative site. Carious teeth should be filled or extracted before surgery on the joints, and urinary tract infections should be identified and treated. Many female patients have asymptomatic bacteriuria, and urine culture before surgery is an absolute requirement. In male patients, prostatic hypertrophy, if severe, should be treated before surgery to avoid postoperative catheterization with its attendant risk of infection and bacterial seeding. It is useful to determine if the patient is able to void in the supine position. Frequently, preoperative practice at supine voiding will facilitate recovery in the postoperative period. Most difficult to evaluate is the patient's motivation and ability to participate meaningfully in the postoperative program. Patients should be evaluated by physical and occupational therapists, both to assess their ability to participate in the program and to determine what specific requirements might present in the postoperative period. Instruction in crutch ambulation before surgery shortens the postoperative instruction period. If multiple procedures are envisioned, it is often useful to perform a simple procedure first so that the ability of the patient to follow the postoperative program can be assessed. If both hips and knees require surgery, the hip can be used for this assessment. The relief of pain and improvement in function following hip arthroplasty are essentially independent of the patient's cooperation. The postoperative period is characterized by minimal pain. If the patient is unable to cooperate with a therapy program after hip replacement, it is unlikely that he or she will be able to participate in the postoperative program after a more painful arthroplasty, which requires maximal patient cooperation.

The patient with rheumatoid arthritis or its variants poses certain special problems that bear on the results and risks of surgery. The patient with rheumatoid arthritis frequently has multiple joints involved, each interfering with the function of the others. The rheumatoid patient undergoing surgery is on average 10 years younger than patients with osteoarthritis undergoing similar procedures and therefore has longer to live with a prosthetic joint than does the osteoarthritic counterpart.[11] This means that there will be more time for complications to appear, such as delayed infection, late loosening, and wear of the component parts. Much has been written of the increased susceptibility to infection in patients with rheumatoid arthritis,[12, 13] and it has been documented that the patient undergoing total hip replacement in rheumatoid arthritis does have a significantly increased risk of late hematogenous seeding of the prosthetic joint.[14] Approximately 10 per cent of patients coming to surgery at the author's institution are on maintenance glucocorticoids, and this has been shown in some studies to increase the risk of infection.[15] Aspirin, used by almost all patients, may produce difficulties with intraoperative and postoperative bleeding. Careful assessment of bleeding and clotting times is useful, but platelet transfusions are occasionally required. Some patients are on chronic immunosuppressive treatment, and the effect of these drugs, including methotrexate, on postoperative infection must be considered.[16–18] Although there is controversy regarding the relationship between penicillamine treatment and wound healing,[19–21] it is the opinion of most surgeons with experience in the field that there is a definite delay in wound healing in patients on penicillamine. This may delay the postoperative rehabilitation program until satisfactory wound healing is achieved.

There is both clinical and laboratory evidence to suggest that the rheumatoid process is perpetuated in a given joint by retention of articular cartilage.[22, 23] Whether this is because of sequestered antigen-antibody complexes, the continued release of cartilage breakdown products producing synovial inflammation, or undiscovered factors is unknown. It has been a frequent observation, however, that patients undergoing total knee replacement in whom the patellar cartilage is retained will have involvement of the prosthetic joint in systemic flare-ups, whereas patients in whom all cartilage has been removed will not experience involvement of the prosthetic knee in such flare-ups.[24] The quality of bone in patients with rheumatoid arthritis frequently is poor. This may be because of direct involvement of the subchondral trabecular bone by rheumatoid granulation tissue, or it may be related to the catabolic effects of chronic steroid use, the bone resorption related to excessive production of prostaglandins,[25] tumor necrosis factor,[26] or interleukin-6[27] by rheumatoid synovium, or an excess of parathyroid-like activity in these patients.[28] Regardless of the cause, the quality of bone is of great concern with regard to the long-term fixation of prosthetic components to bone. Many prosthetic devices transfer the enormous joint reactive forces directly to the bone-cement interface, which may be unable to withstand these forces over a long period of time. For this reason, it is desirable to use prosthetic devices that are minimally constrained and to transfer forces away from the bone-cement interface into the more compliant and forgiving soft tissues.

The patient with juvenile rheumatoid arthritis presents certain unique features that bear directly on the results to be expected from surgical intervention. As in patients with ankylosing spondylitis, there appears to be a much greater involvement of the soft tissues surrounding the joint, with the result that the ultimate range of motion achieved after joint arthroplasty is less than would be predicted from the range achieved at surgery.[29] After arthroplasty, there is a progressive loss of motion in these patients, and the effect of this loss on ultimate functional capacity must be anticipated.[30] The young age at which patients with juvenile rheumatoid arthritis undergo arthroplasty exposes their prosthetic joints both to greater functional demands and a longer period of exposure to late complications, such as infection and loosening.[31] In addition, these patients often have severe micrognathia, which may make intubation difficult or produce postoperative respiratory problems.[32]

The patient with ankylosing spondylitis has diminished chest excursion and therefore is at greater risk for postoperative pulmonary problems and requires chest physical therapy to minimize these problems. Because of rigidity of the cervical spine, intubation is extremely difficult, sometimes requiring preoperative tracheostomy before an anesthetic agent can be delivered. Ossification in the spinal ligaments can produce great difficulty in carrying out spinal anesthesia; careful assessment of the patient by the anesthesiologist is useful in choosing the appropriate type and route of anesthetic and in anticipating difficulties. After total hip replacement, the patient with ankylosing spondylitis frequently fails to achieve the same range of motion that patients with rheumatoid arthritis or osteoarthritis achieve. This is due to the increased involvement of the periarticular soft tissues seen in this disease and to an increased frequency of postoperative heterotopic ossification in the muscles and capsules surrounding the hip joint.[33] Although the range of motion achieved may be only 65 degrees of hip flexion, this often makes a significant improvement in the patient's function and independence. If warned of this preoperatively, the patient can make a more informed decision regarding the desirability of surgery and is less likely to experience disappointment in the postoperative period.[7]

Patients with gout, either as their primary diagnosis or as a secondary diagnosis, often experience painful postoperative flares that require skillful management, as these attacks of gouty arthritis are more difficult to treat postoperatively than the usual spontaneous gouty attack.

Patients with psoriatic arthritis sometimes have involvement of the skin in the area of the proposed surgical incision. Several papers report the frequent contamination of psoriatic skin with microorganisms and suggest an increased risk of infection after incision through such skin.[34–36] It is therefore desirable to clear up the skin at the operative site by appropriate local therapy before surgery. The arthropathies related to inflammatory bowel disease pose a special threat of postoperative infection because of both late hematogenous seeding from a focus of infection in the bowel and the occasional source of contamination from a colostomy in proximity to the incision for hip replacement.

Systemic lupus erythematosus presents a very difficult problem for both the patient and the physician. The patients are often young and on large doses of glucocorticoids, and they may have a near-normal life expectancy when they develop osteonecrosis.[37] To implant a prosthetic joint in a young patient invites the long-term failures related to wear and loosening; to do so in a patient on long-term glucocorticoid treatment adds the further risk of infection. The presence of renal involvement in these patients may have implications with regard to their life expectancy. In the young patient with a limited life expectancy, prosthetic replacement may well be justified to relieve pain and improve the quality of life for the remaining years. On the other hand, in the patient with a normal life expectancy, there will almost certainly be late problems after joint replacement in the third and fourth decades. These patients often present with avascular necrosis of a femoral condyle with pain, deformity, and functional loss. It may be better to accept the lesser result produced by a tibial or femoral osteotomy than to carry out joint replacement surgery with the high probability of eventual complication.

Patients with Reiter's syndrome (see Chapter 57), as well as those with ankylosing spondylitis (see Chapter 56), have a significant incidence of cardiac involvement. Careful preoperative cardiac assessment should be carried out in such patients.

In addition to the systemic problems presented by the patients with rheumatoid arthritis, the involvement of multiple joints presents special problems. As the patient will require crutches after lower extremity surgery, it is essential preoperatively to evaluate the patient's ability to use crutches. If there is extensive involvement of the shoulder, elbow, or wrist, axillary crutches may not be appropriate. Forearm crutches will sometimes be a suitable alternative, particularly if involvement of the wrist or elbow makes the use of axillary crutches painful. Occasionally, it will be necessary to carry out arthrodesis or arthroplasty of the wrist before surgery on the lower extremities so that the patient will be able to use forearm crutches in the postoperative period.[38] In addition, patients who do not have 110 degrees of knee flexion find it difficult to arise from a seated position without applying major force to the upper extremity. If the upper extremities are unable to cope with these forces, special attention must be directed to obtaining maximal hip and knee flexion after surgery to minimize the need for upper extremity assistance.[3] The major joints of the upper extremity, the elbow and shoulder, require arthroplasty less often than the weight-bearing joints of the lower extremity. Indeed, relieving the patient of the need to use crutches by performing arthroplasties of the hips and knees often diminishes shoulder pain to a tolerable level. In a few patients, pain or lack of motion of the shoulder, with the attendant difficulty in placing the hand in a functional position, requires surgical treatment.[39] In the elbow, synovectomy (with or without radial head excision) may be adequate.[40, 41] If pain relief is not adequate after synovectomy, or if motion is inadequate, elbow replacement is appropriate (see Chapter 105).[42, 43]

Patients with rheumatoid arthritis usually have involvement of both hips even though only one may require arthroplasty. Involvement of the contralateral hip will handicap the patient's postoperative recovery and may diminish the ultimate range of motion achieved in the operated hip. If it is obvious that both hips will require arthroplasty, it is preferable to carry out both during the same hospitalization to facilitate functional recovery. In some circumstances, such as difficult intubation or limitations that will interfere with postoperative hygiene, it is justifiable to carry out bilateral total hip replacements during the same period of anesthesia, and several studies report no decrease in quality of outcome or increase in complications with simultaneous procedures of the hip,[44] knees,[45] or a hip and a knee.[46]

Patients undergoing hip or knee arthroplasty are sometimes disappointed to find that painful foot deformities prevent comfortable ambulation after their extensive surgical procedures. In addition, the plantar surface of the feet and dorsum of the toes are subject to skin breakdown because of rheumatoid deformities. These may become sources of bacterial contamination after arthroplasty to more proximal joints. These areas of skin breakdown should be healed before surgery on proximal joints to prevent proximal spread of infection. This can often be achieved by satisfactory shoe modifications and protective footwear (see Chapter 28) but may require surgical correction[47] (see Chapter 110). Such surgery should be carried out before hip and knee arthroplasty so problems of skin breakdown and infection, frequent after foot surgery, will not compromise the results of arthroplasties of the proximal joint. The temporomandibular joint is frequently involved in patients with juvenile rheumatoid arthritis as well as adult rheumatoid arthritis. In juvenile rheumatoid arthritis, involvement of the temporomandibular joint combined with micrognathia may produce difficulties with intubation and respiration after extubation.[32] Careful preoperative analysis by the anesthesiologist will prevent some of these difficulties, and fiberoptic intubation will minimize trauma and postoperative laryngeal edema.

The cervical spine is significantly involved in 30 to 40 per cent of patients with rheumatoid arthritis.[48-50] Usually this is asymptomatic and unknown by the patient but it should be sought in the preoperative evaluation to avoid the potentially disastrous consequences of excessive manipulation of the neck during intubation. The patient with marked C1–2 instability may sustain damage to the medullary respiratory center and long spinal tracts when the neck is manipulated during intubation. In the presence of severe instability with neurologic deficit, surgical stabilization should precede other reconstructive procedures[51] (see Chapter 106).

In addition to these general considerations, there are specific interactions between adjacent joints that may jeopardize the technical aspects of surgery. For example, involvement of the ipsilateral hip and knee usually leads to the performance of hip arthroplasty first. The position of the flexed knee is used as a guide for insertion of the femoral component in the hip arthroplasty. In the presence of severe knee instability or valgus deformity, or both, proper placement of the hip component will be compromised.[52] If the component is placed in retroversion, postoperative dislocation of the hip becomes more frequent. Similarly, if the hip has been arthrodesed, the position of knee components must be suitably altered depending on the degree of abduction or adduction of the arthrodesed hip.

CHOICE OF PROCEDURE

In some instances, advanced age, increased risk factors, lack of patient motivation, or relatively minor pain will suggest that the patient should accept limited function rather than undergo a complex and potentially dangerous surgical procedure. In the upper extremity, the wrist is a good example of this dilemma. Three options are available: splinting, arthrodesis, or arthroplasty. Arthrodesis provides a stable, painless wrist but jeopardizes function to some extent, particularly in the performance of personal hygienic chores.[53] For that reason, patients with bilateral involvement often are advised to have an arthroplasty on one wrist, using some form of prosthetic implant or fascial interposition.[41] Some patients will be better served by the use of a wrist splint, worn at night and during work but removed when flexibility is required.[54] Similarly, in the lower extremity, painful foot and ankle deformities often are best managed by special shoes and inserts to minimize pressure points or an orthosis to splint the ankle and correct heel valgus (see Chapter 28).

Patients whose joint symptoms are unresponsive to medical management and joint protection measures should be evaluated radiographically to determine the extent of joint destruction. If the disease is still primarily limited to the synovium, with little or no loss of cartilage, synovectomy (surgical, arthroscopic, or chemical) should be considered (see Chapter 39). Although the benefits of synovectomy have been shown to be lost after 3 to 5 years,[55] some protection of the joint may be possible if this procedure is carried out early,[56] but controversy exists.[57]

POSTOPERATIVE MANAGEMENT

The role of physical therapy in the postoperative management of patients undergoing joint replacement surgery has not been clearly defined. Controlled prospective studies are notably lacking. In their place is the nearly universal acceptance of the importance of postoperative physical therapy, an acceptance based on personal experience. The requirements for such therapy appear to vary from joint to joint. For example, Charnley did not advocate postoperative physical therapy for patients undergoing hip replacements.[10] His early and late follow-up studies suggest that physical therapy may play a minimal role in the rehabilitation of these patients. At the other extreme is the clear-cut advantage of careful and prolonged therapy after surgery of the hand. Regardless of the lack of scientific evidence, essentially all surgeons with experience in the field of joint replacement surgery are convinced that the active participation of both the patient and the physical therapist in a postoperative exercise program will improve muscle strength, increase motion, and educate the patient in proper protection of the operated joint.

Orthoses are frequently useful after reconstructive surgery of the upper extremity, in which case they may function either as static devices to maintain position and prevent deformity or as dynamic devices to aid in the restoration of motion and strength.[54] In the lower extremity, the most frequently used orthotic device is the crutch. Its function is to protect weakened muscles until they become strong, prevent falls as the patient learns to function with a new prosthetic joint, and protect the bone-cement interface until healing can occur, ideally minimizing the complication of late loosening.

Radiographic evaluation, critical in the preoperative assessment of the need for surgery and proper technical approach, is the mainstay of postoperative evaluation (see Chapter 112). Parameters to be assessed are the alignment of the prosthetic components, adequacy of cement fixation, restoration of joint alignment, and detection of postoperative loosening, as indicated by the development of a radiolucent zone between the methacrylate cement and the bone. Studies of prosthetic placement in the hip have indicated the undesirability of a varus configuration to the femoral component as well as increased frequency of loosening in patients with incomplete filling of the proximal femur with methacrylate, voids in the methacrylate, and increased rates of dislocation with retroverted femoral components or excessively abducted acetabular components.[14] In the knee, late loosening has been correlated with faulty alignment of the prosthetic components, and the early development of a radiolucent line, particularly at the bone-cement interface on the tibial side, has given early warning that certain prosthetic designs are inappropriate.

As loosening is a time-related complication and infection may make its appearance late, prolonged follow-up of patients undergoing joint arthroplasty is necessary. If early signs of loosening develop, decrease in joint loading by appropriate use of crutches and avoidance of strenuous activities may prevent or slow the progress of such loosening. Because of evidence that patients with artificial joints continue to be at some increased risk for hematogenous infection, careful attention must be devoted to the prevention of infection anywhere in the body and its prompt recognition and treatment. Many surgeons recommend that patients utilize prophylactic antibiotics before dental or urologic procedures although the cost-effectiveness of that approach has been questioned.[58] Regardless of whether such prophylaxis is used, patients should be aware of the potential danger of untreated infections and seek early medical attention for even minor infections.

CONCLUSION

Despite the dramatic advances in joint replacement surgery in the last two decades, all such procedures must still be considered evolutionary. Changes in design, surgical technique, and materials continue, with improvements coming rapidly for some joints and more slowly for other joints, such as the hip. For this reason, such surgery should be delayed as long as possible in patients who continue to function at a satisfactory level with tolerable discomfort. The old and reliable procedures such as fusion and osteotomy should be utilized when appropriate, especially in younger patients. One clear lesson gained from experience with joint replacements is that the more anatomic the replacement, the greater its long-term success is likely to be. Another clear lesson is that there is a close and obvious relationship between the technical expertise with which an arthroplasty is performed and its immediate and ultimate functional result. New materials for prosthetic replacement and new techniques of fixation of prosthetic devices to bone have been developed with improvement in outcomes.[59-61] Clearer understanding of normal joint anatomy and function will result in improved anatomic designs with greater life expectancy. Functional analysis of large numbers of patients who have undergone arthroplasty will determine the appropriate indications for surgery and choice of prosthetic designs, but medical judgment in selecting patients for surgery and the use of precise surgical technique in carrying out the operation will remain the dominant aspects in the surgical management of arthritis.

References

1. Burton, K. E., Wright, V., and Richards, J.: Patient's expectations in relation to outcome of total hip replacement surgery. Ann. Rheum. Dis. 38:471, 1979.
2. Kay, A., Davison, B., Badley, E., et al.: Hip arthroplasty: Patient satisfaction. Br. J. Rheumatol. 22:243, 1983.
3. Jergesen, H. E., Poss, R., and Sledge, C. B.: Bilateral total hip and knee replacement in adults with rheumatoid arthritis. An evaluation of function. Clin. Orthop. 137:120, 1978.
4. Williams, A.: The importance of quality of life in policy decisions. In Walker, S. R., and Rosser, R. M. (eds.): Quality of Life: Assessment and Application. Lancaster, UK, MTP Press Ltd., 1988, pp. 279–290.
5. Liang, M. H., Cullen, K. E., Larson, M. G., et al.: Cost-effectiveness of total joint arthroplasty in osteoarthritis. Arthritis Rheum. 29:937, 1986.
6. Johnson, K. A.: Arthroplasty of both hips and both knees in rheumatoid arthritis. J. Bone Joint Surg. 57A:901, 1975.
7. Walker, L., and Sledge, C.: Total hip arthroplasty in ankylosing spondylitis. Clin. Orthop. 262:198, 1991.
8. Johnston, R., Fitzgerald, R., Harris, W., et al.: Clinical and radiographic evaluation of total hip replacement. J. Bone Joint Surg. 72-A:161, 1990.
9. Liang, M., Katz, J., Phillips, C., et al.: The American Academy of Orthopaedic Surgeons Task Force on Outcome Studies: The Total Hip Arthroplasty Outcome Evaluation Form of The American Academy of Orthopaedic Surgeons. J. Bone Joint Surg. 73-A:639, 1991.
10. Charnley, J.: Low Friction Arthroplasty of the Hip: Theory and Practice. Berlin, Springer-Verlag, 1979.
11. Poss, R., Ewald, F. C., Thomas, W. H., et al.: Complications of total hip replacement arthroplasty in patients with rheumatoid arthritis. J. Bone Joint Surg. 58A:1130, 1976.
12. Gristina, A. G., Rovere, G. D., and Shoji, H.: Spontaneous septic arthritis complicating rheumatoid arthritis. J. Bone Joint Surg. 56A:1180, 1973.
13. Kellgren, J. H., Ball, J., Fairbrother, R. W., et al.: Suppurative arthritis complicating rheumatoid arthritis. Br. J. Med. 1:1193, 1958.
14. Poss, R., Thornhill, T. S., Ewald, F. C., et al.: Factors influencing the incidence and outcome of infection following total joint arthroplasty. Clin. Orthop. 182:117, 1984.
15. Garner, R. W., Mowat, A. G., and Hazleman, B. L.: Wound healing after operations on patients with rheumatoid arthritis. J. Bone Joint Surg. 55B:134, 1973.
16. Foker, J. E., Schwartz, R., Smith, D. C., et al.: Surgical problems in immunodeficient and immunosuppressed children. Surg. Clin. North Am. 59:213, 1979.
17. O'Loughlin, M.: Infections in the immunosuppressed patient. Med. Clin. North Am. 59:495, 1975.
18. Perhala, R. S., Wilke, W. S., Clough, J. D., et al.: Local infectious complications following large joint replacement in rheumatoid arthritis patients treated with methotrexate versus those not treated with methotrexate. Arthritis Rheum. 34:146, 1991.
19. Burry, H. C.: Penicillamine and wound healing—a potential hazard? Postgrad. Med. J. 50(Suppl.):75, 1974.
20. Deshmukh, K., and Nimni, M. E.: A defect in the intramolecular and intermolecular cross-linking of collagen caused by penicillamine. J. Biol. Chem. 244:1787, 1969.
21. Schorn, D., and Mowat, A. G.: Penicillamine in rheumatoid arthritis: Wound healing, skin thickness and osteoporosis. Rheumatol. Rehabil. 16:223, 1977.
22. Cooke, T. D., Richer, S., and Hurd, E.: Localization of antigen-antibody complexes in intra-articular collagenous tissues. Ann. N.Y. Acad. Sci. 256:10, 1975.
23. Ohno, O., and Cooke, T. D.: Electron microscopic morphology of immunoglobulin aggregates and their interactions in rheumatoid articular collagenous tissues. Arthritis Rheum. 21:516, 1978.
24. Sledge, C. B., and Ewald, F. C.: Total knee arthroplasty experience at the Robert Breck Brigham Hospital. Clin. Orthop. 145:78, 1979.
25. Robinson, D. R., Tashjian, A. H., Jr., and Levine, L.: A possible mechanism for bone destruction in rheumatoid arthritis. J. Clin. Invest. 56:1181, 1975.
26. Bertolini, D. R., Nedwin, G. E., Bringham, T. S., et al.: Stimulation of bone resorption and inhibition of bone formation in vitro by human tumour necrosis factors. Nature 319:516, 1986.
27. Field, M., Chu, C. Q., Feldmann, M., et al.: Interleukin-6 localization in rheumatoid arthritis. Rheumatol. Int. (In press).
28. Kennedy, A. C., Allam, B. F., Rooney, P. J., et al.: Hypercalcemia in rheumatoid arthritis: Investigation of its causes and implications. Ann. Rheum. Dis. 38:401, 1979.
29. Stuart, M. J., and Rand, J. A.: Total knee arthroplasty in young adults who have rheumatoid arthritis. J. Bone Joint Surg. [Am.] 70:84, 1988.
30. Singsen, B. H., Isaacson, A. S., Burnstein, B. H., et al.: Total hip replacement in children with arthritis. Arthritis Rheum. 21:401, 1978.
31. Sledge, C. B.: Joint replacement surgery in juvenile rheumatoid arthritis. Arthritis Rheum. 20:567, 1977.
32. Conway, W., Bauer, G., and Barns, M.: Hypersomnolence and intermittent upper airway obstruction. Occurrence caused by micrognathia. J.A.M.A. 237.2740, 1977.
33. Ritter, M. A., and Vaughan, R. B.: Ectopic ossification after total hip arthroplasty: Predisposing factors, frequency, and effect on results. J. Bone Joint Surg. 59A:345, 1977.
34. Aly, R., Maibach, H. I., and Mandel, A.: Bacterial flora in psoriasis. Br. J. Dermatol. 95:603, 1976.
35. Lambert, J. R., and Wright, V.: Surgery in patients with psoriasis and arthritis. Rheumatol. Rehabil. 18:35, 1979.
36. Marples, R. R., Heaton, C. L., and Kligman, A. M.: Staphylococcus aureus in psoriasis. Arch. Dermatol. 107:568, 1973.

37. Griffiths, I. D., Maini, R. N., and Scott, J. T.: Clinical and radiological features of osteonecrosis in systemic lupus erythematosus. Ann. Rheum. Dis. 38:413, 1979.
38. Beckenbaugh, R. D.: Implant arthroplasty in the rheumatoid hand and wrist: Current state of the art in the United States. J. Hand Surg. 8:675, 1983.
39. Friedman, R. J., Thornhill, T. S., Thomas, W. H., et al.: Non-constrained total shoulder replacement in patients who have rheumatoid arthritis and class-IV function. J. Bone Joint Surg. [Am.] 71:494, 1989.
40. Tulp, N. J., and Winia, W. P.: Synovectomy of the elbow in rheumatoid arthritis. Long-term results. J. Bone Joint Surg. [Br.] 71:664, 1989.
41. Tillmann, K.: Recent advances in the surgical treatment of rheumatoid arthritis. Clin. Orthop. Sept. (258):62, 1990.
42. Ewald, F. C., Scheinberg, R. D., Poss, R., et al.: Capitellocondylar total elbow arthroplasty. J. Bone Joint Surg. 62A:1259, 1980.
43. Souter, W. A.: Surgery of the rheumatoid elbow. Ann. Rheum. Dis. 2:871, 1990.
44. Salvati, E., Hughes, H., and Lachiewicz, P.: Bilateral total hip-replacement arthroplasty in one stage. J. Bone Joint Surg. 60-A:640, 1978.
45. Stanley, D., Stockley, I., and Getty, C. J.: Simultaneous or staged bilateral total knee replacements in rheumatoid arthritis. A prospective study. J. Bone Joint Surg. [Br.] 72:772, 1990.
46. Head, W. C., and Paradies, L. H.: Ipsilateral hip and knee replacements as a single surgical procedure. J. Bone Joint Surg. 59A:352, 1977.
47. Stockley, I., Betts, R. P., Getty, C. J., et al.: A prospective study of forefoot arthroplasty. Clin. Orthop. Nov. (248):213, 1989.
48. Nakano, K. K.: Neurologic complications of rheumatoid arthritis. Orthop. Clin. North Am. 6:861, 1975.
49. Rana, N. A., Hancock, D. O., Taylor, A. R., et al.: Upward translocation of the dens in rheumatoid arthritis. J. Bone Joint Surg. 55B:471, 1973.
50. Rana, N. A., Hancock, D. O., Taylor, A. R., et al.: Atlantoaxial subluxation in rheumatoid arthritis. J. Bone Joint Surg. 55B:458, 1973.
51. Santavirta, S., Slatis, P., Kankaanpaa, U., et al.: Treatment of the cervical spine in rheumatoid arthritis. J. Bone Joint Surg. [Am.] 70:658, 1988.
52. Poss, R., and Sledge, C. B.: Symposium on Rheumatoid Disease. Orthopedic Clinics of North America, 1984.
53. Millender, L. H., and Nalebuff, E. A.: Arthrodesis of the rheumatoid wrist. An evaluation of sixty patients and a description of a different surgical technique. J. Bone Joint Surg. 55A:1026, 1973.
54. Convery, F. R., and Minteer, M. A.: The use of orthoses in the management of rheumatoid arthritis. Clin. Orthop. 102:118, 1974.
55. McEwen, C.: Multicenter evaluation of synovectomy in the treatment of rheumatoid arthritis. Report of results at the end of five years [see comments]. J. Rheumatol. 15:765, 1988.
56. Jensen, C. M., Poulsen, S., Ostergren, M., et al.: Early and late synovectomy of the knee in rheumatoid arthritis. Scand. J. Rheumatol. 20:127, 1991.
57. Doets, H. C., Bierman, B. T., and von, Soesbergen, R. M.: Synovectomy of the rheumatoid knee does not prevent deterioration: 7-year follow-up of 83 cases. Acta Orthop. Scand. 60:523, 1989.
58. Tsevat, J., Durand, Z. I., and Pauker, S. G.: Cost-effectiveness of antibiotic prophylaxis for dental procedures in patients with artificial joints. Am. J. Public Health 79:739, 1989.
59. Walker, D. J., Usher, K., O'Morchoe, M., et al.: Outcome from multiple joint replacement surgery to the lower limbs. Br. J. Rheumatol. 28:139, 1989.
60. Harris, W., and Sledge, C.: Total hip and total knee replacement. N. Engl. J. Med. 323(part 1):725; (part 2):801, 1990.
61. Mehlhoff, M. A., and Sledge, C. B.: Comparison of cemented and cementless hip and knee replacements. Arthritis Rheum. 33:293, 1990.

Chapter 104
The Hand

Barry P. Simmons
Lewis H. Millender
Edward A. Nalebuff

INTRODUCTION

Evaluating the patient with rheumatoid hand deformities and developing a rational plan of treatment can be among the more difficult aspects of rheumatoid surgery, especially considering the great number of joints and tendons that may become involved, the complexity and severity of the deformities, and the functional disabilities that can occur. In addition, patients are seen during various stages of the disease, and the progress and severity of disease will vary with different patients. A clear knowledge of the pathogenesis of hand deformities, tendon involvements, and inter-relationships of the different joints in the hand permits prediction of the types of deformity that may develop and allows treatment before serious joint destruction develops. For example, when it becomes apparent that a boutonnière deformity or a thumb deformity is occurring, better results can be obtained if surgery is carried out before loss of bone stock and destruction of soft tissue occur. At later stages, more extensive surgical procedures are required.

Because of the progressive nature of the rheumatoid process, it is helpful to consider the treatment in different categories: nonsurgical treatment, preventive or therapeutic surgery, and reconstructive or salvage surgery for specific hand deformities.

NONSURGICAL TREATMENT

Although one often thinks of rest and exercise, splinting, and steroid injections early in the management of rheumatoid hand involvement, these modalities are important during all stages of the disease.[1, 2]

Rest and Exercise. The patient with rheumatoid arthritis (RA) should understand the principles of rest and exercise and their practical application. Diseased joints require exercise to prevent stiffness and maintain motion; active motion exercise is needed to maintain tendon gliding and strong muscles. Conversely, inflamed, painful, swollen joints require rest to decrease acute synovitis. Therefore, when a joint is warm, painful, and inflamed, exercise must be reduced, and rest increased. As the inflammatory process subsides, exercise can be increased. Short, frequent periods of exercise are more beneficial than long, vigorous ones, which can activate the synovial inflammation.

One should teach patients to decide how much exercise and activity they can carry out. They must learn to monitor their activity. If after any activity, such as working in the garden, hands become more swollen, more painful, or stiff, then the activity has been too strenuous, and it should be altered.

Splinting. Resting and dynamic splints alleviate pain, may decrease the progression of deformity during the active stages of the disease, and aid in postoperative management. Resting splints are especially effective for wrist pain and allow patients to use the hand while wearing the splint.[2] Similarly, thumb splints can alleviate pain and allow function. Full hand-wrist-thumb splints also alleviate pain but restrict function. These are often used mainly at night. Various types of dynamic splints are used to stretch out fixed deformities, such as boutonnière deformities. However, dynamic splinting is used mainly after reconstructive surgery, especially after metacarpophalangeal (MCP) joint arthroplasty.[3-5]

Steroid Injections. The judicious use of local injections of steroids often reduces active synovitis and tenosynovitis. They can be used for symptomatic carpal tunnel syndrome, flexor tenosynovitis, and dorsal tenosynovitis, as well as for any joint that does not respond to medical treatment. Frequent and repeated administration to the same area may cause tendon ruptures and steroid-induced arthropathies. One should probably not inject one joint or one tendon sheath more than three times a year.[2] If there is persistence of or an increase in the local disease after this time, surgical intervention is indicated.[6]

PREVENTIVE AND THERAPEUTIC SURGERY

Dorsal Tenosynovitis. Dorsal tenosynovitis is a frequent manifestation of rheumatoid hand disease resulting from a proliferation of the tenosynovium that surrounds the extensor tendons over the dorsum of the wrist.[6-8] Dorsal tenosynovitis may be the presenting sign in RA, and RA must be the primary diagnosis to rule out when dorsal tenosynovitis is present. It produces a soft, nonpainful mass that may be located along any or all of the extensor compartments; accompanying pain should alert one to underlying radiocarpal or radioulnar involvement.[6, 8]

Dorsal tenosynovitis is significant because it may lead to extensor tendon ruptures, either from attrition or from infiltrative disease. Although one cannot predict which patients will experience ruptured tendons, there are certain helpful guidelines for predicting who may rupture. Patients with progressive disease who have not responded to medical therapy have ruptured tendons more frequently. Patients who have had a previous tendon rupture are more prone to another tendon rupture if they develop tenosynovitis. Patients with a rapidly enlarging synovial mass tend to rupture more frequently.[6, 9]

Tenosynovectomy is recommended for patients with persistent tenosynovitis who have not responded to a 4- to 6-month period of conservative therapy. Earlier tenosynovectomy is indicated for patients who are more prone to tendon ruptures.[1, 6–10]

The surgical technique is safe and effective, and the morbidity is low. The procedure can be carried out with the patient under regional anesthesia, and is generally done on an out-patient basis. Postoperative immobilization is short, and therefore patients generally have little problem regaining their range of motion. Dorsal tenosynovectomy can be carried out in conjunction with other rheumatoid hand surgical procedures, such as distal ulnar excision and wrist synovectomy, which would be performed through the same incision, or other procedures on the hand and digits. The recurrence rate after dorsal tenosynovectomy is low, being 5 to 6 percent in 73 patients reviewed.[11, 12]

Dorsal Tenosynovitis with Extensor Tendon Rupture. The complication of dorsal tenosynovitis is tendon rupture, which occurs secondary to infiltrative tenosynovitis or attrition on a bony spur, such as the distal ulnar or Lister's tubercle.[13–15] The most frequent tendons to rupture are the extensors to the ring and small fingers and the long extensor of the thumb. In severe destructive disease, multiple digital extensor tendons rupture. Even the wrist extensor tendons can rupture, with a resultant severe flexion deformity of the wrist.[16]

Single extensor tendon ruptures may cause a slight extension lag because of cross-connections between the tendons. A rupture of the extensor digiti quinti tendon may even cause a minimal extensor lag because its function is shared with the common digital extensor. When more than one tendon is ruptured, the extension lag and functional loss become obvious. When patients are examined for extensor tendon function, the extensor digit quinti should be tested independently, especially when there is a prominent distal ulna, which will frequently lead to this tendon rupture.

Because the results of tendon transfer are inversely proportional to the number of tendon ruptures, prompt diagnosis and early treatment are important. In addition, a single rupture frequently is followed by a second and even a third rupture. Therefore, an extensor tendon rupture is an indication for prompt surgery to correct the loss and to prevent further complications.[6, 11, 17, 18]

The technique for extensor tendon repair is not complicated. Dorsal tenosynovectomy is carried out, and distal ulnar excision is performed if indicated. In addition, any bony spicule of the carpus is carefully rongeured away. Wrist joint synovectomy also may be carried out. Either adjacent tendon suture or tendon transfer using extensor indicis proprius is generally used for single and double ruptures (Fig. 104–1). For more complicated ruptures, wrist extensor tendons or flexor digitorum superficialis tendons are utilized.[18, 19] In the presence of multiple ruptures with a painful subluxed wrist joint, wrist fusion is carried out in conjunction with tendon transfer. In this situation, the wrist extensor tendons can be utilized to replace the ruptured digital extensors. Because of the excursion, better motion results from use of the flexor superficialis than the wrist extensors; however, if the digital joints are severely involved, the wrist extensors can be used.

As noted, the morbidity and the results are directly proportional to the number of tendons ruptured plus the status of the adjacent joints. Because much of the hand must be immobilized for 4 weeks after surgery to allow for tendon healing, joint stiffness may develop, and therefore rehabilitation requires more time plus additional therapy. Because of this, both patients and physicians should be alerted to the complications of dorsal tenosynovitis. Ideally, early tenosynovectomy should be carried out before tendon rupture occurs.

Flexor Tenosynovitis. Flexor tenosynovitis is due to a proliferation of tenosynovium that normally lines the flexor tendons. The signs and symptoms of flexor tenosynovitis are related to the anatomic differences and can be categorized as wrist, palmar, and digital flexor tenosynovitis. As with dorsal tenosynovitis, early diagnosis and prompt treatment of flexor tenosynovitis will prevent the complications of tendon rupture and permanent damage secondary to median nerve compression.[6, 9, 20]

Wrist Flexor Tenosynovitis. Wrist flexor tenosynovitis may present with signs and symptoms of carpal tunnel syndrome because of tenosynovitis within the carpal tunnel, causing compression of the median nerve. Some patients may have limited active digital flexion owing to impairment of flexor tendon excursion. On physical examination, unless there is limited active range of motion, the signs will be minimal. Because the flexor tendons are covered by thick fascia, wrist flexor tenosynovitis does not bulge as much and therefore, in contrast with dorsal tenosynovitis, is much less apparent. If the volar surface of the wrist is observed carefully, loss of skin wrinkles and lack of venous markings can sometimes be observed. Additionally, evidence of thenar muscle atrophy will sometimes be noted, especially with long-standing median nerve compression.

The treatment for early wrist flexor tenosynovitis is steroid injection, wrist splinting, and medical management. For persistent wrist flexor tenosynovitis, carpal tunnel release and tenosynovectomy should

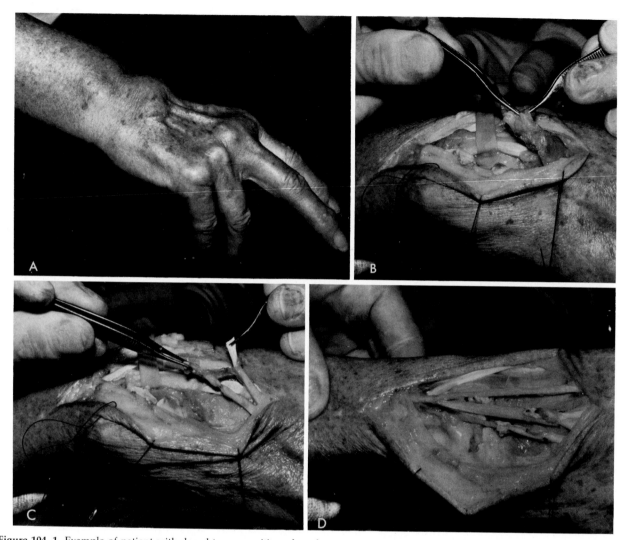

Figure 104–1. Example of patient with dorsal tenosynovitis and tendon rupture. *A*, Dorsal tenosynovitis with double tendon rupture. *B*, Dorsal tenosynovectomy. Note tenosynovium held by forceps. *C*, Dorsal tenosynovectomy. Note tenosynovium excised prior to transfer. *D*, Tendon transfer completed. Extensor indicis proprius has been transferred to ruptured extensor tendon of fifth digit, and ruptured fourth extensor tendon transferred to intact third extensor tendon.

be carried out early to prevent permanent median nerve damage, to restore active digital flexion, and to prevent tendon rupture[6, 9] (Fig. 104–2).

Palmar Flexor Tenosynovitis. Tenosynovitis proliferating within the proximal portion of the palm results in snapping and locking as the tendon slides within the tendon sheath. Patients will usually be able to flex the digit fully, but as the digit extends the nodule catches on the proximal edge of the tendon sheath, and the digit snaps into extension. Sometimes the digit will become acutely locked in flexion and cannot be extended actively. A painful snap occurs as the digit is passively extended. On examination, the flexor tendon nodule can be palpated, and one can feel a grating as the patient actively flexes and extends the digit.[6, 9]

Digital Flexor Tenosynovitis. In contrast with palmar flexor tenosynovitis, digital flexor tenosynovitis is due to proliferation of tenosynovium within the digit. The commonest finding in this condition is

loss of active digital flexion with preserved passive digital flexion. This is due to impairment of tendon excursion within the narrow tendon sheath. Additionally, grating and locking can be seen as the tendon nodule slides within the sheath, and a fullness can sometimes be felt and observed over the volar surface of the digit.[6, 9]

A less common but important manifestation of digital flexor tenosynovitis is stiffness of the proximal interphalangeal (PIP) joints. In some rheumatoid patients, especially those with PIP joint synovitis associated with pain, limited active flexion associated with digital flexor tenosynovitis can lead to PIP joint stiffness. This occurs because the patients are unable to flex the digits actively, and this, plus the associated PIP joint synovitis with pain, leads to PIP joint stiffness. The diagnosis is established by obtaining a history of flexor tenosynovitis (previous locking, snapping, or limited active range of motion prior to stiffness) and from noting PIP joint stiffness with

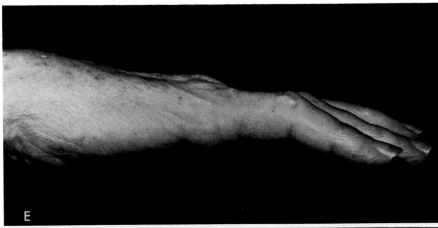

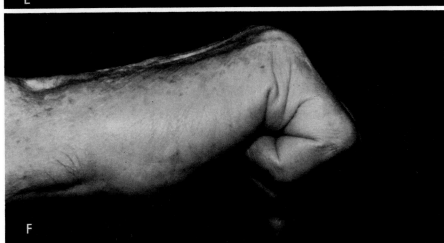

Figure 104–1 *Continued E* and *F*, Range of motion demonstrated 3 months postoperatively.

minimally involved joints by radiograph. In addition, some digits may show only loss of active motion, with preserved passive range of motion, which helps establish the diagnosis.

The treatment for early palmar and digital flexor tenosynovitis is steroid injection and medical therapy. However, palmar and digital flexor tenosynovectomy should be carried out for persistent flexor tenosynovitis that does not respond to conservative therapy. For PIP joint stiffness caused by this condition, tenosynovectomy plus PIP joint manipulation and a vigorous postoperative hand therapy program can often restore a considerable range of motion.[6, 9]

Flexor Tendon Rupture. Flexor tendon rupture can occur within the carpal tunnel, palm, or digit. Fortunately, it is not common; the results of treatment of multiple palmar and digital flexor tendon ruptures are not as good as those for their extensor counterparts.

At the wrist, attrition ruptures of the flexor pollicis longus and/or the flexors of the index finger are caused by a bony spur of the scaphoid that protrudes volarly. Additionally, flexor tendon rupture within the carpal tunnel can occur from infiltrative flexor tenosynovitis.[6–9]

Within the palm and digit, flexor tendon ruptures are less common because there are no bony spurs that lead to attrition ruptures and also because the symptoms of locking and snapping cause the patient to seek earlier medical treatment, which will result in earlier diagnosis and treatment.[6, 9]

Flexor tendon rupture in the wrist is treated with tenosynovectomy, removal of the scaphoid spur, and often a bridge graft, tendon graft, or ring superficialis tendon transfer[21] for the ruptured flexor pollicis longus and a side-to-side suture of the ruptured flexor digitorum profundus (Fig. 104–3.) If the thumb interphalangeal joint is destroyed, arthrodesis is preferable to tendon repair or graft. If a single rupture is diagnosed within the digit or palm, prompt flexor tenosynovectomy is advisable to prevent a rupture of the remaining intact tendon.[6, 9] If flexor or digitorum profundus rupture occurs, tenodesis or arthrodesis of the distal interphalangeal (DIP) joint is indicated. For flexor digitorum sublimis rupture, only tenosynovectomy is indicated to protect the intact flexor digitorum profundus.

The difficult problem arises when both flexor digitorum profundus and flexor digitorum sublimis ruptures occur within the same digit, thereby eliminating both DIP and PIP joint flexion. The results of tendon grafts, either primary or secondary after a tendon rod, are often disappointing. Therefore, in older patients or those with severe joint involvement,

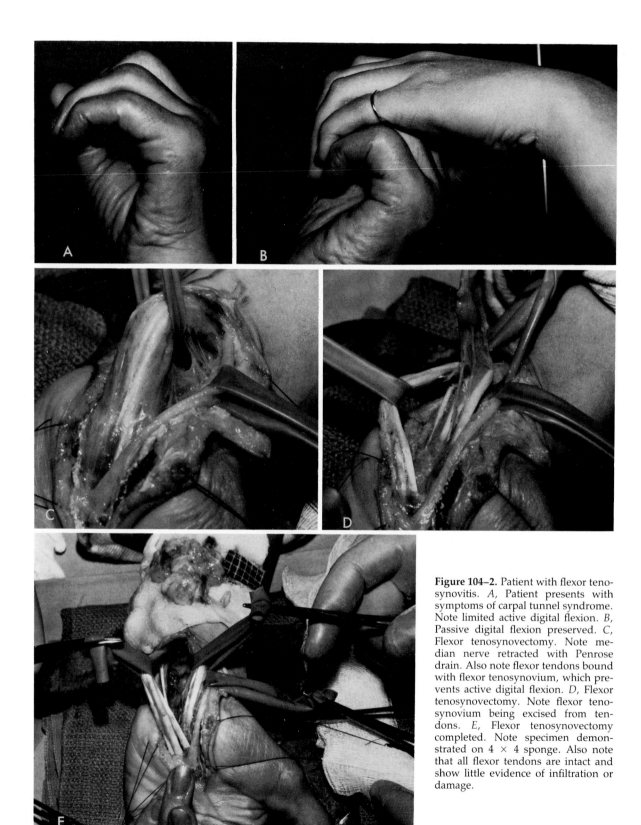

Figure 104–2. Patient with flexor teno-synovitis. *A,* Patient presents with symptoms of carpal tunnel syndrome. Note limited active digital flexion. *B,* Passive digital flexion preserved. *C,* Flexor tenosynovectomy. Note median nerve retracted with Penrose drain. Also note flexor tendons bound with flexor tenosynovium, which prevents active digital flexion. *D,* Flexor tenosynovectomy. Note flexor tenosynovium being excised from tendons. *E,* Flexor tenosynovectomy completed. Note specimen demonstrated on 4 × 4 sponge. Also note that all flexor tendons are intact and show little evidence of infiltration or damage.

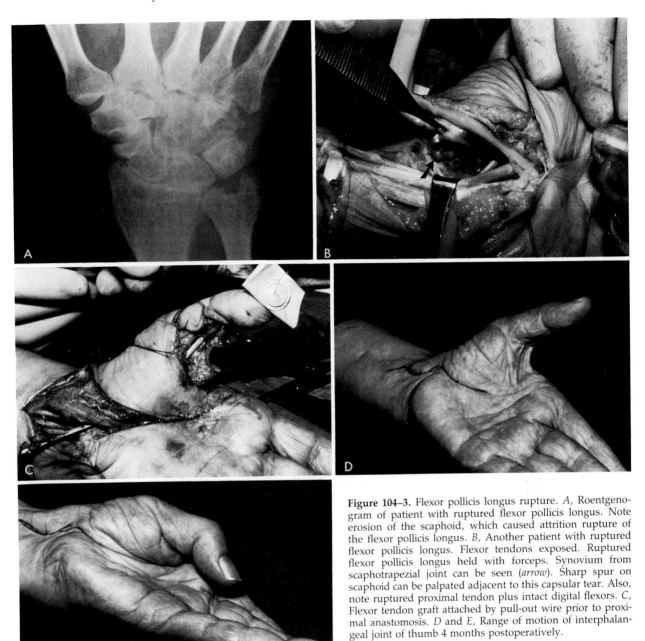

Figure 104–3. Flexor pollicis longus rupture. *A*, Roentgenogram of patient with ruptured flexor pollicis longus. Note erosion of the scaphoid, which caused attrition rupture of the flexor pollicis longus. *B*, Another patient with ruptured flexor pollicis longus. Flexor tendons exposed. Ruptured flexor pollicis longus held with forceps. Synovium from scaphotrapezial joint can be seen (*arrow*). Sharp spur on scaphoid can be palpated adjacent to this capsular tear. Also, note ruptured proximal tendon plus intact digital flexors. *C*, Flexor tendon graft attached by pull-out wire prior to proximal anastomosis. *D* and *E*, Range of motion of interphalangeal joint of thumb 4 months postoperatively.

the best approach has generally been to carry out PIP and DIP joint arthrodeses in an acceptable position of function. Active motion of the MCP joints will still be possible because of the intact intrinsic muscles. One can also suture one of the ruptured long flexor tendons into the base of the proximal phalanx to increase the strength of MCP joint flexion.

Synovectomy. In contrast with tenosynovectomy, which is an established surgical procedure, the case for synovectomy in the small joints of the wrist and hand is certainly less well defined. The reason for this is that no good data have been presented to show that synovectomy will appreciably alter the natural course of the disease. Even though the long-term results of synovectomy cannot be pre-

dicted, the procedure does have some definite, although limited, indications in the hand.[2, 8]

The primary indications for synovectomy of the wrist or digital joint are for the small group of patients with smoldering, slowly progressive disease who are responding to systemic medication but who continue to show synovitis in one or more joints. Typically, this type of patient has responded to three steroid injections over a 6- to 12-month period but continues to develop recurrent synovitis, sometimes with pain. Roentgenograms show minimal involvement with little evidence of progression. Synovectomy will alleviate pain in this patient and, ideally, delay or prevent further joint destruction. In contrast, when synovectomy is attempted in patients who show a more destructive, progressive type of disease, it is less frequently successful in preventing further joint destruction and further progression of the disease and is often followed by a loss of joint motion.

Synovectomy can be carried out in almost any joint of the hand or wrist. On the authors' service, it is more frequently carried out in the wrist to relieve pain. Synovectomy is also useful in the PIP joints, especially to prevent progressive boutonnière deformities, which are difficult to treat in the advanced stages.[22]

Synovectomy is less frequently indicated in the digital MCP joints.[23] Because of the many factors working to cause volar and ulnar deformity, progression of the deformity is frequently not altered by this procedure. Even though there is little articular cartilage or bony joint destruction within the MCP joint, if there is early subluxation or a moderate amount of ulnar drift, the authors have been reluctant to carry out synovectomy even when associated with intrinsic release and extensor tendon relocation. Under these conditions, the authors would either carry out arthroplasty or wait until there was more deformity, and then resort to arthroplasty.

Radiation synovectomy using dysprosium-165 has shown promise in the knee.[24] However, in the digital joints it has not been successful. Although the synovium has been rendered inactive, the effect on dorsal apparatus and overlying skin has been deleterious. A different isotope with less soft tissue penetration may be beneficial.

RECONSTRUCTIVE AND SALVAGE SURGERY

In spite of early recognition, splinting, and "prophylactic surgery," the natural progression of RA often leads to destructive changes in the joints of the hand and wrist. The late effects of this disease include loss of articular cartilage, stretching of the joints' supporting structures, and actual bone loss. The clinical aspects of these changes include pain, instability, and deformity with subsequent loss of function. After these changes have occurred, it is no longer possible to restore the joint to its former state. The surgeon must then resort to "salvage" surgery to relieve pain and provide stability and motion. No joint of the hand is immune to these destructive changes. The surgeon, in reality, has only two choices in the management of destroyed joints—arthrodesis or arthroplasty. Each of these procedures has benefits and drawbacks and therefore represents a compromise with full function. The surgical choice between these two operations takes judgment and experience.

Many factors must be considered in making the choice between fusion and arthroplasty. The most important factor to consider is which joint is involved. Other factors that must be taken into account at each joint level will be discussed in more detail.

Metacarpophalangeal Joints. The MCP joints of the hand are single condylar joints allowing 80 to 90 degrees of flexion as well as rotatory and lateral motions. They play an important role in positioning the fingers; if they are fixed in poor position, hand function will be greatly reduced. Unfortunately, MCP joint involvement is common in RA. The capsule laxity, which gives the joints varied mobility, makes subluxation and dislocation common late sequelae of synovitis. The extensor tendons pass precariously across the joints and, with stretching of the supporting attachments, often deviate ulnarward and then slip between the metacarpal heads. Once this has occurred, all extensor force is lost, and progressive flexion of the MCP joints occurs. As the patient tries to extend the joints, they deviate ulnarward instead. Similarly, with flexor tenosynovitis the sheath stretches, allowing a change in alignment of the flexor tendons, which now become a deforming force.[25] There is often a stretching of the radial collateral ligaments and subsequent shortening of the ulnar collateral ligaments and intrinsic muscles. The end result may appear as dislocated MCP joints with the fingers fixed in flexion or severely deviated ulnarward. The net result is a significant loss of hand function—for example, the ability to grasp large objects if the fingers are fixed in flexion. With ulnar deviation, the fingers are beyond the reach of the thumb, and precision activities requiring thumb-digit opposition are lost.

Soft tissue reconstruction for MCP joint deformity might be considered. However, there should be relatively good maintenance of a joint space. As previously noted, the tendency to recurrent deformity is sufficiently high that there is limited indication. A small series has suggested that this be considered; further follow-up on a larger series of patients is necessary.[26]

To restore function, arthroplasty is the treatment of choice at the MCP joint level. Although fusion of the MCP joints can be obtained with the finger realigned, the presence of MCP joint motion greatly enhances overall gripping ability. With the arthroplasty techniques available, this can be achieved in a predictable way. Arthroplasties to correct deformity and relieve pain while maintaining motion are best exemplified at the MCP joint level. It was here that arthroplasties of rheumatoid hands were first attempted, and the surgical lessons learned were later used at the PIP joint levels.

The initial attempts to correct MCP joint deformities while maintaining motion were made more than 30 years ago by Riordan and Fowler.[27] Their resection-type arthroplasty consisted of resecting enough of the metacarpal heads to allow digital realignment. The fingers were then held in place with Kirschner's wires for approximately a month, after which motion was allowed, using dynamic splinting to maintain alignment as motion was regained. To support the resected joint surfaces, local soft tissue structures such as the extensor tendons were sutured to the bases of the proximal phalanges.

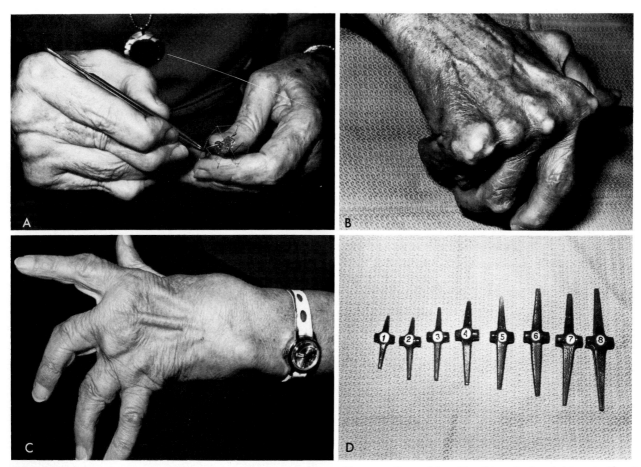

Figure 104–4. Arthroplasty of the MCP joints—indications. *A,* Even with severe finger deformities this patient maintains significant hand function. She demonstrates the ability to manipulate delicate electronic components. Arthroplasty was delayed until function decreased. *B,* This patient has dislocated MCP joints, limiting extension and the ability to grasp large objects. Metacarpophalangeal arthroplasties are indicated. *C,* A common indication for arthroplasty is severe fixed ulnar deviation, as seen in the patient's middle, ring, and small fingers. *D,* Preferred arthroplasty is the Swanson flexible hinge implant shown here.

Vaino,[28] in Finland, and Tupper,[29] in the United States, modified the resection arthroplasty using the volar plate as a supporting structure interposed between the metacarpal and proximal phalanges. Although these techniques are still being used today, most surgeons utilize an implant to help maintain digital alignment and motion. The search for the ideal implant is a continuing process. Initial attempts to improve on resection arthroplasty using a prosthetic replacement were made by Flatt,[1] who designed a hinged metallic device with double-prong stems inserted into the medullary canals of the metacarpal and proximal phalanges. These first-generation joint replacements were utilized during the early 1960s but lost popularity as a result of the frequent complications, such as implant fracture, bone resorption, and perforation of the rigid metallic stems of the prostheses. In the latter 1960s, Swanson[5, 30, 31] and Neibauer[32] independently developed a second-generation prosthesis made of silicone rubber. In both designs, the prosthesis acts as a flexible implant or spacer between the resected bone ends. The design of each implant differs in that stems of Neibauer's implant are Dacron-coated to allow bone ingrowth

into the prosthesis. Swanson's implant does not have a Dacron covering and does not become fixed to the intramedullary canals. The implant depends for support on the encapsulation that surrounds it. Motion is achieved both by implant flex and by a sliding action along the implant stem. The authors prefer the Swanson-type implant arthroplasty, and in this chapter use of the term arthroplasty at the MCP and PIP joint levels is to be construed by the reader as this type (Fig. 104–4*D*).

More recently, cemented metal to plastic implants have been developed but have experienced the same complications as Flatt's prosthesis.[1, 32–36] The biomechanics of these joints must be more clearly defined in order to develop an effective, rigid prosthesis.

Results of Arthroplasty. With the flexible implant arthroplasty, the surgeon can, in most cases, correct MCP joint subluxation, dislocations, and ulnar deviation of the fingers (Fig. 104–5). Numerous factors affect the ultimate result, including the condition of the surrounding soft tissues, the strength and mobility of the controlling muscles, the status of the adjacent joints, the use of postoperative splinting

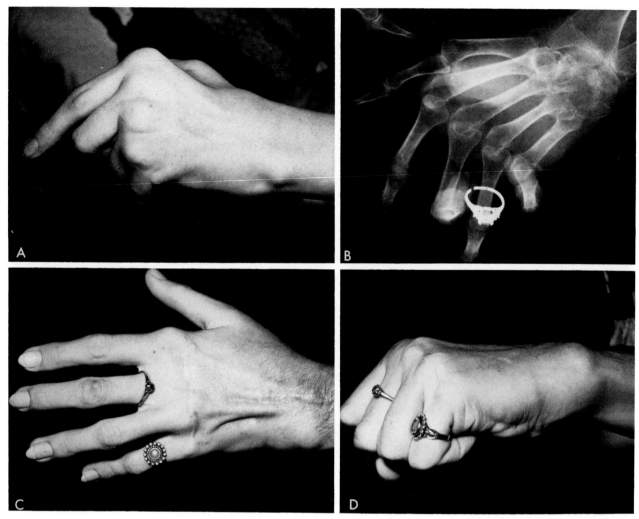

Figure 104–5. Example of MCP arthroplasty to improve joint function and the appearance of rheumatoid hand deformity. *A,* Preoperative digital extension. Note MCP joint subluxations with associated boutonnière deformity of middle finger. *B,* Preoperative radiograph shows advanced wrist involvement in addition to MCP and PIP joint deformities. *C,* Note improved function and appearance of hand and wrist following second-stage wrist fusion and MCP arthroplasties. *D,* Excellent postoperative digital flexion.

and exercises,[37] and, last but not least, the motivation of the patient. With proper surgical technique, and barring complications, the surgeon should expect to realign the digit, relieve pain originating at the MCP joint level, and maintain between 30 and 60 degrees of motion, averaging about 45 degrees.[38]

The complications of implant arthroplasty include recurrent ulnar drift, limited motion, implant fracture, dislocation, and infection.[39] In an effort to avoid recurrent ulnar drift, the surgical technique requires adequate release of the shortened ulnar structures, adequate bone resection, and good repair of the radial collateral ligament and capsule. In addition, proper postoperative splinting for 6 to 12 weeks is essential. Despite this, recurrent ulnar drift is estimated to occur approximately 30 to 45 percent of the time.[38]

In some patients, realignment of the fingers and relief of pain are obtained, but the range of motion is less than anticipated. Inadequate surgical release of contracted soft tissues may be a factor, but this

complication often occurs if the patient has limited excursion and strength of the flexor muscles and tendons. Postoperative exercises play an important role in determining the range of motion achieved.[7] If inadequate motion is obtained, revision of the arthroplasty is possible and can improve motion.

Addressing both ulnar drift and motion, Bieber and colleagues[40] followed 46 patients for an average of 5 years. Ulnar drift improved from 25 degrees preoperatively to 5 degrees postoperatively but recurred to average 12 degrees. The extension deficit decreased from 56 degrees to 10 degrees, and the range of motion increased from 17 degrees to 51 degrees. However, these deteriorated with time: the extension deficit increased to 22 degrees, and the range of motion decreased to 39 degrees. Longer follow-up, 11 years, on the Dacron-reinforced prosthesis, has shown further deterioration.[41] Whether this is due to that prosthesis or whether such deterioration will happen with Swanson's prosthesis as well has still not been determined.[41] Considering the nature of the Silastic prosthesis and the necessity for encapsulation, it is not surprising that there was some deterioration of results. However, despite this, patient satisfaction was high.[40, 42]

Implant fracture can also occur, but its frequency is low (less than 5 percent) with the high-performance silicone rubber used today. Bone response to the implant is often favorable. Remodeling results in a cortical bony shell around the stems and thickening of the cortical bone at the metacarpal and phalangeal metaphysis. The proximal phalanx maintains its length, although there is about a 9 percent decrease in metacarpal length.[43]

To decrease implant fracture even further, titanium grommets have been suggested for both the proximal phalanx and the metacarpal to shield the implant from the bone edges.[44] However, if implant fracture does occur, it is often asymptomatic and noted only on radiograph. Several months following implant insertion, encapsulation has already taken place. Once this has occurred, implant fracture may not significantly affect the result. Dislocations of the implant are rare and usually occur at the time of surgery or shortly thereafter. When this complication occurs, replacement is usually needed to restore proper digital alignment.

Infections around the implant occur in fewer than 1 percent of the joints inserted.[39] Usually an isolated joint is involved, and removal of the implant combined with appropriate antibiotic coverage is sufficient to control the infection. Removal of the implant converts the arthroplasty to a resection type, and some loss of motion is anticipated.

Earlier surgery would be considerably easier, especially in the severe cases with significant bony erosion, severe ulnar drift, and flexion contractures. However, although the Silastic prosthesis is excellent for pain relief, it not only does not restore full motion but also fails to restore any significant pinch or grip strength. Despite the drawbacks, patient satisfaction is high.[38]

Proximal Interphalangeal Joints. The PIP joints, like their distal counterparts, are mostly hinge joints allowing flexion and extension. The range of motion at this level is normally full extension to 110 degrees of flexion. This mobility, although only slightly greater than that at the distal joint, is far more important in bringing the fingertip toward the palm. Its flexion, combined with 70 or 80 degrees of MCP joint motion, is all that is required for the fingertips to reach the distal palmar crease without any additional help from the distal joints. For this reason, loss of motion at the PIP level is more of a hardship for the patient, and attempts to preserve it are more frequently indicated (Fig. 104–6). The need for lateral stability is still important. However, it is technically easier to restore collateral ligament support, and in the middle digits (ring and long fingers) the adjacent finger provides a measure of lateral support when the patient makes a fist. This lack of adjacent digital support is particularly noted in the index finger and

makes arthrodesis of the PIP joint more frequently indicated in this finger (Fig. 104–7). Unlike the distal joints, in which fusion is the procedure of choice in salvage conditions, the surgeon has a choice between an arthrodesis or a flexible implant arthroplasty at this level. Factors to consider in making this decision include the type or severity of deformity, the digit involved, the condition of adjacent joints, and the status of the extensor and flexor apparatus.

The deformities at the PIP joint are flexion, hyperextension, and lateral deformities. Flexion deformities are usually caused by a lack of extensor support at the PIP joint. The central slip of the extensor mechanism attaches to the base of the middle phalanx and is essential in maintaining or providing active extension. Unfortunately, synovitis of the PIP joints stretches out this thin structure, and the ability to extend the PIP joint actively is lost. As the joint slips into flexion, secondary changes occur. The lateral bands of the extensor mechanism are displaced volarly, and as they contract in this position, they lead to distal joint hyperextension. At first, this boutonnière deformity is passively correctable, but later the accessory collateral ligaments and volar plates shorten, and the deformity becomes fixed. As the fixed deformity increases in degree, the surgical ability to restore extension becomes less. Beyond a certain point (70 to 80 degrees of fixed flexion), it is usually not possible to restore full adequate extension at the PIP level even by a resection of bone, and one must choose fusion as the salvage procedure of choice.

Hyperextension deformities of the PIP joint can be primary or secondary. Stretching out of the volar plate by synovitis or rupture of the superficial flexor tendon can lead to secondary PIP joint hyperextension followed by a distal joint flexion. The combined PIP joint hyperextension and distal joint flexion is called a swan neck deformity. If the PIP joint surfaces are intact and nonpainful, correction of the deformity and restoration of motion can be achieved by various soft tissue procedures.[45] This should be done only if the MCP joints are acceptable. If the MCP joins are subluxed, are in significant ulnar deviation, or are associated with considerable ulnar intrinsic tightness, they must be attended to first, or soft tissue procedures at the PIP joint level will fail.

In the late stages with irregular joint surfaces, the surgeon again must resort to either fusion or arthroplasty to correct the deformity and eliminate pain. If mobility is also desired, arthroplasty must be selected as the surgical procedure. At this point, the surgeon must weigh the other factors to be considered in making this choice, including which finger is involved.

The ability to flex the PIP joints becomes increasingly important as one moves from the index to the small digit. The index finger is used in picking up objects or performing delicate tasks in opposition with the thumb. It is particularly important in lateral pinch, in which the thumb presses against this radial

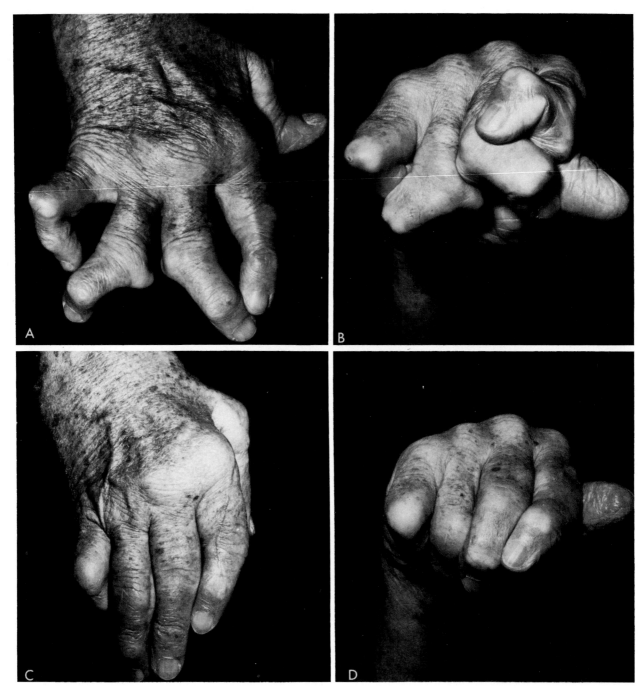

Figure 104–6. Example of PIP joint arthroplasties for severe deformities. *A,* Preoperative view of hand with fingers in extension. Note severe lateral deformities of PIP joints. *B,* Patient's fingers overlap on attempted flexion. Grasping ability is poor. *C,* Postoperative extension following PIP arthroplasties. *D,* Postoperative flexion.

surface. Most of these fusions are carried out with the PIP joint in slight to moderate flexion. For this reason, fusion of the index finger PIP joint is less of a handicap than is fusion of the more ulnar digits used in grasp. In the ring and small fingers, acute flexion of the PIP joint is needed to grasp small objects firmly. For this reason, arthroplasty is likely to be chosen over fusion in these digits, and if fusion is selected because of other factors, the position

chosen to stabilize the joint is in more flexion than that chosen for the index finger.

The condition of the adjacent joints must be taken into account in making the choice between PIP joint fusion and arthroplasty. If the distal joints have already been or must be fused, this increases the indication for arthroplasty at the PIP level. On the other hand, if one anticipates arthroplasties at the MCP joint level, the surgeon may decide on fusion

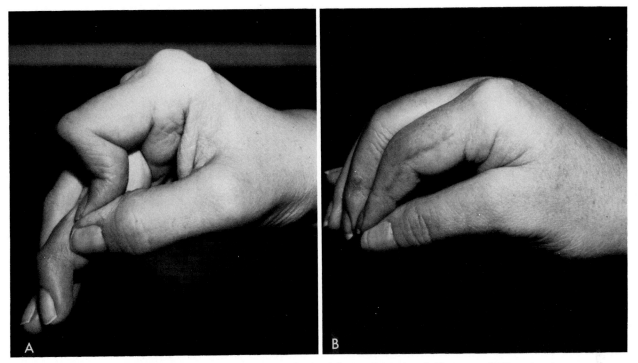

Figure 104–7. Proximal interphalangeal fusion of index finger for fixed flexion deformity. *A*, Note poor pinch posture because of severe flexion contracture of index PIP joint. *B*, Improved function obtained by fusion of PIP joint in 25-degree flexion.

for the PIP joints. If the intramedullary canals are of sufficient size and the extensor and flexor tendons are functioning well, it is possible and even desirable to perform arthroplasties at both the PIP and the MCP levels, particularly for the ulnar digits, in order to allow grasping of small objects. As noted earlier, the MCP joint condition affects the results of arthroplasty at the PIP joint. For an implant arthroplasty to function, it is necessary that the tendon muscle units controlling motion of the joints have sufficient power and amplitude. It is foolhardy to insert a joint prosthesis unless the extensor and flexor tendons are functioning or can be restored. This is particularly important with the flexor tendons. If the flexor tendons are ruptured, it is wiser to fuse a destroyed PIP joint than to try to obtain motion. On the other hand, flexor tendons with limited excursion secondary to adhesions and/or nodular tenosynovitis can usually be restored by tenosynovectomy and tenolysis. This type of tendon involvement is not, therefore, a contraindication to arthroplasty.

In general, the results of arthroplasty at the PIP joint level are better with swan neck deformity than with boutonnière deformity. However, even then the average range of motion is only 30 to 40 degrees, with long-term loss of an additional 5 to 10 degrees.

Distal Interphalangeal Joints. The DIP joints of the digits, like the PIP joints, are hinge joints, normally allowing 70 to 80 degrees of flexion from a fully extended position. With intact collateral ligaments, the joints are quite stable against lateral stresses. The volar support is provided by a thickened capsule (volar plate), which with an intact flexor

digitorum profundus tendon resists hyperextension forces. Normal extension is provided by an intact extensor mechanism attached to the base of the distal phalanges. This extensor mechanism is activated by both the digital extensor muscles and the intrinsics (lumbrical and interosseous muscles) of the hand. As a result of RA, the cartilaginous joint surfaces can be destroyed, which causes pain and limitation of motion. The loss of bone substance or collateral ligament support can lead to lateral deformities. Attenuation or rupture of the distal extensor attachment is followed by a "mallet" deformity, while stretching out of the volar plate or rupture of the long flexor tendon can result in distal joint hyperextension. As a result of these changes, either singularly or in combination, the patient develops an unsightly deformity, which not only is painful but also results in decreased function.

Unfortunately, it is not possible to restore a damaged joint to its former state, and the surgeon must then aim at a somewhat lower target—relief of pain, correction of deformity, and restoration of useful function. Of the two salvage procedures, fusion and arthroplasty, fusion is the preferred treatment at the distal joint level. There are two main reasons for this approach: (1) the difficulty involved in restoring active motion and joint stability, and (2) the relative unimportance of mobility in the distal joints. Although it is technically possible to insert a joint prosthesis, repair the extensor mechanism, reconstruct the collateral ligaments, and even restore flexor tendon function, the potential gain is not worth the inherent risks, except in highly selected cases.

Actually, the loss of motion in the distal joint is not particularly disabling if the joint is stable in good position. The best position of the distal joint is either full extension or, at most, 5 to 10 degrees of flexion. In this position, the digit has a normal appearance with the fingers extended. When the patient makes a fist, the lack of distal joint motion is not obvious and is of little functional significance. Picking up or holding objects between the thumb and the involved digit is not compromised, with the distal joint being almost straight. This position enhances "pulp-to-pulp" pinch, which is more useful than "tip pinch," which requires distal joint mobility.

Fusion of the distal joints not only achieves a beneficial effect at the operative site but also can help function at the more proximal joint level. For example, a distal joint fusion in neutral position balances the extensor and flexor forces. This can be helpful in correcting a mild swan neck deformity (PIP hyperextension) that is secondary to a distal joint mallet deformity.[22, 23, 46] In addition, fusion in the distal joint simplifies and strengthens extensor or flexor forces at the PIP joint level, where active motion is more important than at the distal joint.

The Wrist. The wrist is the foundation on which hand function is built. A painful, unstable wrist reduces hand function without digital involvement and, in fact, may be a primary factor in producing digital deformities. Deformities of the wrist result from several factors. Early synovial involvement occurs between the carpal bones, with the scapholunate being the commonest area of early synovitis. Stretching of the intercarpal and radiocarpal ligaments by synovitis leads to a disruption and subsequent shifting of the carpal bones in relation to the radius. The carpus can shift ulnarward or volarward in relation to the radius. With volar shift, the carpus can dislocate and displace proximally. A secondary phenomenon that occurs is attrition ruptures of the wrist extensor tendons, further aggravating the dislocation and leading to severe flexion deformity of the wrist. With ulnar shift of the carpus, there is often a radial deviation of the wrist. Stretching of the extensor carpi ulnaris tendon or rupture of this stabilizing force is also thought to be a significant factor in this deformity. With radial deviation of the carpus, the metacarpals become angulated radially in relation to the radius, and this, in turn, is followed by ulnar deviation of the digits at the MCP joints.[47] Patients who have this "zigzag" deformity are poor candidates for MCP arthroplasties to correct the ulnar deviation until the wrist alignment has been restored. Chronic synovitis of the distal radioulnar joint stretches the supporting ligaments, maintaining proper alignment between the radius and the ulna. Dorsal displacement of the ulna follows, and, if bony erosions have occurred, the rough edge, which protrudes dorsally, can wear away the adjacent extensor tendons to the fingers.

In advanced cases, surgical attempts to realign the wrist and alleviate pain include total or partial fusion and arthroplasty.[48] The choice between these procedures depends on many factors, including the condition of the wrist extensors, the amount of bone resorbed in the carpus, and the status of the hand, the opposite wrist, and even the lower extremities. Total wrist fusion accomplishes several things. It eliminates pain, provides stability for hand function, and corrects alignment.[49–53] Although the patient gives up flexion and extension motions, supination and pronation are preserved. The position of fusion is important. Although arthrodesis in 15 degrees to 20 degrees of dorsiflexion is preferable in traumatic arthritis, the same is not necessarily true in patients with RA.[53a] Neutral or slight flexion is acceptable and may be preferable in the severely compromised wrist-hand unit.[53] The high incidence of union, with limited immobilization, achieved by the intramedullary fixation technique, which obligates neutral or slight fixation of the wrist, is a worthwhile tradeoff.[52] The great advantage in a solid wrist fusion is stability and dependability. Disease is arrested at this site, and it no longer is a source of pain. Progression or recurrence of deformity is now halted. If the patient has lower extremity problems that require a cane or crutch support, the fused wrist provides the necessary support. The benefits of a single fused wrist far outweigh the disadvantages of the loss of flexion and extension, and even in the young vigorous patient this is a reliable solution to the problem of a destroyed wrist joint.

Although total wrist fusion has been an accepted treatment for the severely involved wrist, there are many patients in whom the major changes are limited to the radiocarpal joints with the midcarpal area still preserved. In anatomic studies, Taleisnik[54] has demonstrated the paucity of ligaments in the midcarpal region. Because the synovium is concentrated in areas with abundant ligaments, the midcarpal area often escapes destruction.[55, 56] Stretching or destruction of the radiocarpal ligaments allows ulnar translocation of the whole proximal carpal row on the radius or separation of the lunate from the scaphoid. In this latter, that is, scapholunate dissociation, the scaphoid remains in its usual place on the distal radius but, being separated from the rest of the carpus, flexes.[57] The lunate and remainder of the carpus translocate ulnarward.

In those patients with ulnar translocation of the lunate, the articulations about the capitate may be preserved. In these patients, radiolunate fusion restores the anatomy to a more normal situation and can preserve up to 50 percent of normal wrist motion (about 65 degrees). If the radioscapholunate joint is destroyed, this can be fused, but there is a greater loss of motion, leaving only between 40 and 50 degrees.[58] A further benefit of these limited arthrodeses is that, by restoring the wrist to a more normal anatomic position, there seems to be some protection of the remaining midcarpal joints. A combination of limited arthrodesis and arthroplasty is also possible. In patients with adequate preservation of the midcarpal alignment, a radioscapholunate arthrodesis and midcarpal arthroplasty allow maintenance of some motion and provide good pain relief. The head of the capitate and the proximal edge of the lunate are removed and replaced by a condylar implant with the stem in the capitate.[59]

Since this disease is usually symmetric in distribution, the loss of bilateral wrist motion can create a functional loss for the patient. In those patients whose major difficulty with the wrist is pain and in whom a significant range of motion is still present, an alternative treatment, arthroplasty, is available. Attempts to preserve motion at the wrist have paralleled those in the digits. Initial arthroplasties relied on the wrist capsule and surgical alterations of the shape of the distal radius to form a shelf.[60] Swanson[5] introduced a flexible wrist implant shaped like the digital implant. In this arthroplasty, the lunate and scaphoid are removed, and the stems of the implant are inserted into the radius proximally and the capitate and third metacarpal shaft distally. In an early series of 60 Swanson's implants, an average range of motion of over 60 degrees was obtained.[61] Patients with implants obtained relief from pain, with grip strengths equal to those of the fused side. However, although the early results with the use of this implant were excellent, long-term results have been disappointing, 25 percent to 50 percent have had further problems with pain and deformity secondary to implant subsidence or breakage.[59, 61-63, 63a] In an attempt to decrease prosthesis problems, Swanson developed a titanium grommet to shield the prosthesis from the edges of the bone.[44] To date, no studies have proved that the results are altered. Use of the Silastic implant should be limited to patients who have bilateral wrist disease, are not crutch walkers, have adequate bony alignment and bone stock, refuse to accept an arthrodesis, and realize that the goal is only 60 degrees of motion and that the failure rate is high.

With the success of metal to plastic prostheses there has been development of similar devices for the wrist.[64-72, 73] These can be inserted with or without methylmethacrylate fixation. Their early development was marked by problems with imbalance. Although these have been overcome, painful loosening has become more apparent with time. Although Volz[68] initially reported only 3 cases of loosening in 100 cases, others have shown rates as high as 30 percent.[72, 74] Furthermore, revision has been even more difficult than that with the Silastic prosthesis. The recently introduced porous coated biaxial prosthesis simulates the midcarpal joint anatomically. Long-term follow-up is still not available. Early results indicate possible problems with progressive flexion deformities, presumably due to an axis of rotation that is too far dorsal. Thus, except for patients with the qualifications noted, partial or complete wrist arthrodesis is still the procedure of choice.

As a result of renewed interest in the anatomy and function of the distal radioulnar joint, multiple surgical alternatives to the standard distal ulna resection are now available.[75-82] These include arthrodesis of the distal radioulnar joint with a proximal ostectomy of 2 to 3 cm to allow maintenance of rotation (Sauve-Kapandji procedure), resection of the articular surface of the ulna with capsular interposition (Bower's procedure), triangular fibrocartilage reconstruction, and ulnar shortening. However, these procedures all demand some maintenance of distal radioulnar joint surface cartilage integrity and/or a semblance of a triangular fibrocartilage complex. In RA this is rarely the case, and so their application is unfortunately limited. The standard procedure remains resection of the distal ulna (Darrach procedure).[83] This should be conservative, being limited to the portion that articulates with the sigmoid notch of the radius. The proximal end of the ulna must be stabilized with volar capsule and/or a strip of ulnar wrist tendons, especially if the wrist is fused. Then, the remaining ulna, although mobile, does not cause symptoms. Also, the risk of extensor tendon rupture is minimized. Swanson[84] developed a distal ulnar prosthesis that provides a Silastic cap over the distal ulna. However, because of a high incidence of loosening and breakage, it is now infrequently used.

The Thumb. The thumb of the rheumatoid patient deserves special comment. Its importance to hand function is well recognized. Unfortunately, it is frequently involved with RA and can, as a result of muscular imbalance or joint destruction, assume bizarre deformities.[85] The commonest deformity seen originates at the MCP joint, which assumes a flexed position secondary to stretching out or loss of the extensor force. As sequela of this, the distal joint assumes a hyperextended position, and the patient tends to adduct the first metacarpal to substitute for the lack of extension. This thumb deformity is made worse with each pinch force of the thumb against the other digits. The reverse deformity with MCP joint hyperextension is usually secondary to changes at the carpometacarpal joint level with synovitis. The carpometacarpal joint subluxes, and the first metacarpal adducts. The patient then hyperextends the MCP joint to substitute for the lost abduction. With the tendon imbalance produced, the distal joint often assumes a flexed position. Other deformities can occur as a result of collateral ligament or tendon ruptures occurring in combination with joint changes.

How does one treat the advanced thumb deformity? The distal joint of the thumb is treated in fashion similar to that for the distal joints of the other digits—by fusion. It is usually fused in the straight or slightly flexed position to restore a stable pinch (Fig. 104–8). At the thumb MCP joint level, as at the digital PIP joints, one can choose between fusion or arthroplasty. With isolated MCP joint disease, a fusion in 15 degrees of flexion gives excellent results with little functional loss. However, with associated interphalangeal joint disease an arthroplasty is preferred at the MCP level to avoid fusion of two adjacent joints. The silicone implant gives

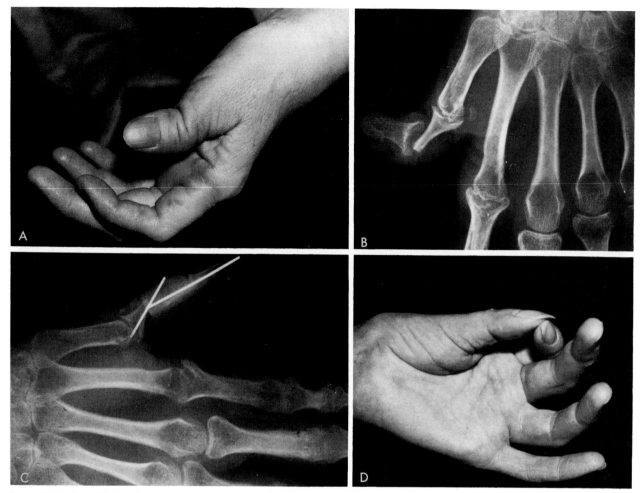

Figure 104–8. Unstable distal joint treated by fusion with bone graft. *A*, Clinical appearance of the thumb with collapse of interphalangeal joint. *B*, Radiograph shows significant absorption of the distal end of the proximal phalanx. *C*, Postoperative radiograph shows use of bone graft to restore length and facilitate joint fusion. *D*, Note stable pulp pinch between lengthened thumb and index finger. Distal joint fused in slight flexion.

excellent results with good pain relief, about 25 degrees of motion, good stability and no breakage.[86] At the carpometacarpal joint level it is important to maintain motion. A fusion here could become quite disabling if the patient developed subsequent instability and required fusions distally. Because of the loss of bone stock in the carpus, the trapezium implants found to be successful in degenerative arthritis have tended to sublux in patients with RA. For this reason, the resection-type arthroplasty has been preferred in which the trapezium is removed, with or without tendon interposition, allowing the metacarpal to be realigned properly.[87] An alternative is to use a modified prosthesis, either the single stem Silastic toe implant or the condylar implant, which has less height than the trapezium implant and thus does not dislocate. The results of either procedure appear to be similar; however, because of the report of destructive Silastic synovitis in long-term studies, it might be preferable to avoid use of the prosthesis.[89–90]

Summary. Much can be done for the rheumatoid patient with hand involvement. Early prophylactic surgery, splinting, and exercises can slow but not stop the progression of deformity. Therapeutic operations on the tendons and nerves can restore lost function, and salvage surgery such as fusion can correct deformities and eliminate pain where motion is not essential. Arthroplasties have also been developed that make it possible to maintain mobility in those joints that must move in order to maintain significant function.

OTHER ARTHRITIC CONDITIONS

Osteoarthritis

Osteoarthritis of the hand is characterized not by synovial hypertrophy but by a gradual loss of articular cartilage. This condition is most prevalent in postmenopausal women but can appear at a younger age in men, in whom previous joint trauma is thought to be a contributing factor. The onset of this condition is slow, with pain being the chief symptom. Radiographic examination of the involved joints initially shows a loss of joint space followed by the appearance of osteophytes. Sclerosis of adjacent bone is also seen. With loss of collateral ligament support or as a result of stretching of the extensor mechanism, these joints become deformed with decreased functional capacity. Although any joints in the hand or wrist can be the site of RA, there are three sites where osteoarthritis is frequently seen: the DIP and PIP joints of the fingers (and interphalangeal joint of the thumb) and the carpometacarpal joint of the thumb.

The distal joint is the commonest location of osteoarthritis. The typical patient with symptomatic involvement at this level is the postmenopausal female. These patients seek medical attention because of pain or unhappiness with the appearance of the distal joints of their fingers. Osteophyte formation at the margins of the joints (Heberden's nodes) is a typical physical finding, as is deviation, either in an ulnar or a radial direction. There is a loss of joint motion noted on clinical examination, but this is seldom of concern to the patient. In fact, as the joint loses motion, pain decreases. These patients with distal joint arthritis may develop a small cystic mass on the dorsal aspect of the distal phalanx. These mucous cysts gradually enlarge and stretch the overlying skin. Although they originate from the joint, they may appear at the base of the fingernail, where pressure against the nail matrix causes irregular nail growth (Fig. 104–9).

The treatment of arthritis of the distal joint and the interphalangeal joint of the thumb includes splinting, analgesics for mild pain, and arthroplasty or arthrodesis with spur removal for unstable and unsightly joints. The preferred position for fusion is 0 to 10 degrees of flexion. Bothersome mucous cysts are treated with local excision of the cyst but especially removal of any underlying bony spurs that are thought to be factors contributing to their development. Recurrence of mucous cysts is occasionally seen and can be eliminated by joint fusion. When distal joint fusion is contemplated in these patients, one should also carefully evaluate the PIP joint. The fusion of the distal joint puts an additional strain on the PIP joint, and the patient may develop increased symptoms in this area.

There has been some enthusiasm for DIP arthroplasty, as opposed to arthrodesis.[91, 92] The Swanson Silastic spacer is the implant of choice. Although patients often have an extensor lag of about 10 degrees, pain relief is excellent, the average active range of motion is 30 degrees, and patients feel that they have more dexterity than with arthrodesis.

At the PIP joint level, the gradual loss of joint motion assumes major significance, with the patient finding it difficult to grasp small objects. The joints enlarge with spur formation (Bouchard's nodes) and become unsightly. Pain may also be noted with loss of joint articular cartilage. Lateral deformities of this joint, mainly ulnar, are common, with stretching of the collateral ligaments and bone resorption. This leads to overlapping of the fingers and considerable loss of functional ability. The pain at this level can be controlled by splinting, but restoration of motion can be achieved only by arthroplasty. The use of flexible implants has been worthwhile in this regard in those patients who have less than 50 degrees of active motion. Although some patients regain 60 to 70 degrees of motion with arthroplasties, one cannot expect to achieve more than an average of 50 degrees with this procedure initially; long-term follow-up shows a loss of another 5 to 10 degrees. When patients are being considered for PIP joint arthroplasties because of osteoarthritis, attention should be directed toward the distal joints. If there is distal joint involvement, it is advisable to combine fusion of the distal joint with arthroplasty of the PIP joint. This eliminates pain distally and concentrates all the flexor and extensor force to the PIP joint. As in the PIP and MCP joints in the patient with RA, metal-to-plastic and metal-to-metal cemented and uncemented prostheses have been tried. They have a high incidence of painful loosening with recurrent deformity, requiring revision.[31] Their use is not recommended.

Recently, there has been interest in re-creating motion in a fused PIP joint whether the fusion has been spontaneous or surgically induced. Surprisingly, the results have been as good as those with primary arthroplasties.[93] The Swanson Silastic prosthesis has been the only implant used to date. Two technical factors must be emphasized. The dorsal apparatus must be reconstructed if it has been surgically altered, even if a tendon graft is required. After the prosthesis has been placed the excursion of the flexor tendons must be checked to make sure that they are not scarred within the fibrosseous canal. The surgeon makes a transverse incision in the palm and pulls on the flexors.

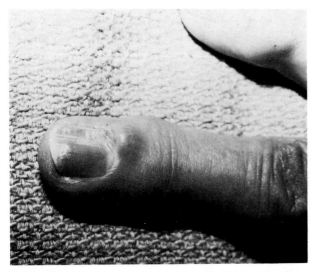

Figure 104–9. Mucous cyst associated with distal joint osteoarthritis. Note alteration in nail growth.

Discussion of surgical technique is beyond the scope of this chapter. However, it is worth pointing out that, contradictory to the usual dorsal approach for arthroplasty of the PIP joint, the volar approach offers several advantages. It avoids having to tinker with the easily scarred dorsal apparatus or even, if one uses a straight dorsal approach, having to take down the central slip. The volar approach also makes it possible to check the excursion of the flexor tendons without a separate incision. Also, the rehabilitation seems to be somewhat easier for the patient. However, to date, the final results do not seem to be any different. Obviously, if the dorsal apparatus needs reconstruction, the volar approach should not be used.

The third area of common hand involvement in osteoarthritis is the carpometacarpal joint of the thumb. This is the joint that most commonly requires surgery, usually because of pain, as a result of osteoarthritis. These patients present with increasing pain at the base of the thumb. The joint space between the first metacarpal and the trapezium narrows, with loss of articular cartilage. Rotatory motions of the joint are particularly painful. With a gradual lateral subluxation of the joint, the typical patient develops a "shoulder," or a prominence at the base of the thumb. With the first metacarpal adducted, there is a gradual development of MCP joint hyperextension. These patients have increasing difficulty in applying pressure with the thumb; any activity requiring pinch is painful. Simple activities such as opening a car door become difficult and painful. With increased adduction of the first metacarpal, the patient has difficulty in grasping large objects, as the first web space between the thumb and index finger narrows. There is a resultant hyperextension and/or radial deviation deformity that develops at the MCP joint.

Increased use and exercise cause a flare-up of pain and should be avoided. Resting and splinting are frequently helpful in relieving pain and certainly should be tried before any surgery is contemplated. Many of these patients respond to a conservative approach with relief of pain that is long-lasting in spite of advanced radiographic findings. In those patients who do not respond to conservative treatment, arthroplasty affords an excellent solution. Two surgical approaches are commonly used. In one procedure the trapezium is removed and replaced by autogenous soft tissue, such as joint capsule or tendon (resection arthroplasty). In the other, the trapezium is replaced by a prosthesis.

The resection arthroplasty gives predictable relief of pain with some loss of pinch power. In order to prevent or minimize proximal migration of the first metacarpal, a portion of rolled-up tendon "anchovy" is commonly utilized. The advantage of this technique is simplicity of surgery and consistency of satisfactory results. Other resection techniques may use a sling to prevent proximal migration and/or to preserve the proximal half of the trapezium.[94-99]

Trapezium replacement arthroplasties can also be used to maintain space and thumb alignment. The early results of this technique, mainly using the Silastic trapezial prosthesis, have been excellent in relieving pain and restoring motion and strength to a level close to normal. However, this approach requires close attention to surgical technique to prevent prosthetic subluxation, which is the major complication encountered. If only the trapeziometacarpal joint is involved, it can be selectively replaced, a hemiarthroplasty, by a condylar implant.[89] This reduces the incidence of prosthetic dislocation. However, with time there have been increasingly frequent reports of prosthetic erosion or breakage and/or Silastic synovitis and deterioration of results.[90, 100, 101] Use of a cemented, ball-and-socket prosthesis again showed excellent early results.[102] However, like the Silastic prostheses, results have deteriorated with time because of loosening of components.[103] Thus, in the vast majority of cases, complete trapezial resection with autogenous tissue interposition, with or without ligamentous reconstruction, is the procedure of choice.

With any carpometacarpal joint arthroplasty it is important to correct any MCP joint hyperextension deformity that may be present. This can be accomplished by fusion in fixed deformities and by volar capsular repair in patients with flexible joints.

Finally, carpometacarpal fusion can be successful in restoring stability and relieving pain in these patients but should be utilized only in those patients who have localized trapeziometacarpal joint involvement and in whom MCP flexion is maintained. It is currently advised only in traumatic arthritis in the young patient. This procedure requires 10 to 12 weeks of postoperative casting and has become less frequently used since the introduction of successful arthroplasties.[104]

Systemic Lupus Erythematosus

Systemic lupus erythematosus (SLE) is a multisystem connective tissue disease that often has musculoskeletal involvement.[105] This includes muscle pain and atrophy as well as various articular complaints.[106] The latter are some of the most frequent clinical manifestations of the disease.[107] The commonest joints involved are the knees, but the smaller joints of the hands and the wrists are also frequently involved.[108, 109] The most typical pattern of involvement is one of migratory arthralgias.

The hand involvement in lupus is generally more benign than that in RA. Bleifield and Inglis[110] reported that there was some hand involvement in 86 percent of 50 randomly examined lupus patients. Most patients reported evanescent arthralgias, although some described definitive evidence of swelling and synovitis. The commonest cause of symptoms in the hand is Raynaud's phenomenon, occurring in 50 percent of patients. Definite hand deformities have been reported in as many as 35 percent of lupus patients. These deformities can affect any joint in the hand and can cause any of the rheumatoid-like deformities (Fig. 104–10).

In contrast with RA or osteoarthritis, the articular cartilage in lupus is not involved, and, unless there is a secondary degenerative type of arthritis from the ligamentous laxity, the articular cartilage will be completely normal (see Fig. 104–10). However, because of the ligamentous laxity, some of the severest unstable digital deformities can be seen in these patients. Because of this, early reconstructive surgery prior to severe dislocations and severe fixed deformities is indicated.[111]

The Wrist. Wrist involvement is a frequent radiographic manifestation of the lupus hand but usually is asymptomatic. The commonest findings are those of ligamentous laxity. This results in dorsal subluxation of the distal ulna, which can result in pain and limited rotation. Ulnar translocation of the carpus is common, and intercarpal dissociation manifested by an increased scapholunate gap and rotation of the lunate is also seen. These generally are asymptomatic, and even in the more significant collapse patterns pain is unusual.

Digital Deformities. The commonest digital deformities seen in SLE are secondary to ulnar subluxation of the extensor tendons at the MCP joint and their subsequent overpull at the PIP joints. This picture of MCP flexion deformity with mild ulnar deviation combined with PIP hyperextension and DIP flexion, or swan neck deformity, is known as Jaccoud's syndrome. Initially, these deformities are passively correctable, but eventually they become fixed.

At the PIP joints, as mentioned, swan neck deformities are commonest, but boutonnière and lateral deformities also occur. Initially these deformities are supple, but with time they become fixed, and secondary degenerative changes develop.

The type of surgery performed for lupus deformities depends on whether destructive changes have occurred. In Jaccoud's syndrome, attention must be directed at both the MCP and the PIP joints. At the MCP joints the ulnar collateral ligament should be released, the dorsal hood reefed on the radial side, and a strip of the extensor tendon tenodesed to the proximal phalanx or wrapped around the radial collateral ligament. At the PIP joint, a slip of the superficialis is left on its insertion on the middle phalanx, cut proximal to the A1-A2 pulley complex, and sewed back on itself around the pulley, creating a fixed flexion contracture of about 20 degrees. Prolonged postoperative splinting is necessary.

This surgery, although extensive, has relatively good results if it is done when all the joints are fully passively correctable. Once fixed deformities occur, arthroplasty yields the best results (Fig. 104–11).

The Thumb. The lupus thumb deformity most commonly results from involvement in all three joints. Initially, one sees an extension lag at the MCP joint, with hyperextension at the interphalangeal joint. Even at this early stage, one notes an early laxity at the carpometacarpal joint. As the laxity increases to dorsal radial subluxation and ultimately dislocation, the thumb deformity abruptly changes to one with adduction of the first metacarpal and hyperextension of the MCP joint and flexion at the interphalangeal joint (Fig. 104–12).

As in other areas, surgery is most effective when carried out early. Carpometacarpal ligamentous stabilization, using a portion of the flexor carpi radialis, has been successful in maintaining stabilization of the joint. Reinforcement of the MCP joint with a rerouted extensor pollicis longus for supple flexion deformity is helpful. For dislocated carpometacarpal joints or carpometacarpal joints with articular changes, arthrodesis or arthroplasty is carried out. As discussed earlier, appropriate distal surgery such as MCP ligamentous stabilization or fusion must be included. Interphalangeal fusion is frequently needed for marked instability of the interphalangeal joint.

Psoriasis

Approximately 5 percent of patients with psoriasis develop arthritis, predominantly involving the small bones of the hands and feet. Generally, arthropathy develops in patients with severe skin involvement, although 20 percent of psoriatic patients present with arthritis prior to development of skin changes.[112] Unlike RA, psoriasis rarely presents with an exuberant proliferative synovitis, or tenosynovitis. Characteristically, there is more diffuse involvement of all soft tissues, which predisposes to scarring.

Digital Deformities. Digital stiffness from involvement of the skin is common. Patients classically present with a "sausage digit" (finger and/or toe). Articular cartilage and metaphyseal bony changes most commonly involve the DIP and PIP joints. At the DIP level, the severity of arthritis frequently parallels the degree of nail deformities; these are pitting, ridging, thickening, or detachment. Radiographically, erosive articular destruction in the interphalangeal joints (PIP more than DIP) predominates (Fig. 104–13). Pencil-and-cup deformities are characteristic. Progressive distal phalangeal osteolysis with tuft resorption is highly suggestive of psoriatic arthropathy. Severe resorption may result in an "opera-glass hand," with skin collapse over resorbed phalanges. As with other seronegative arthropathies, metaphyseal periostitis may develop with "paint-brush" or "whiskering" of the individual phalanx. Involvement of the wrist includes carpal erosions, joint-space narrowing, and spontaneous intercarpal fusions but generally is present only in patients with severe interphalangeal involvement.[113]

Frequently with psoriatic arthritis, spontaneous fusion of the DIP and intercarpal joints in a functional position occurs, and these patients do not require

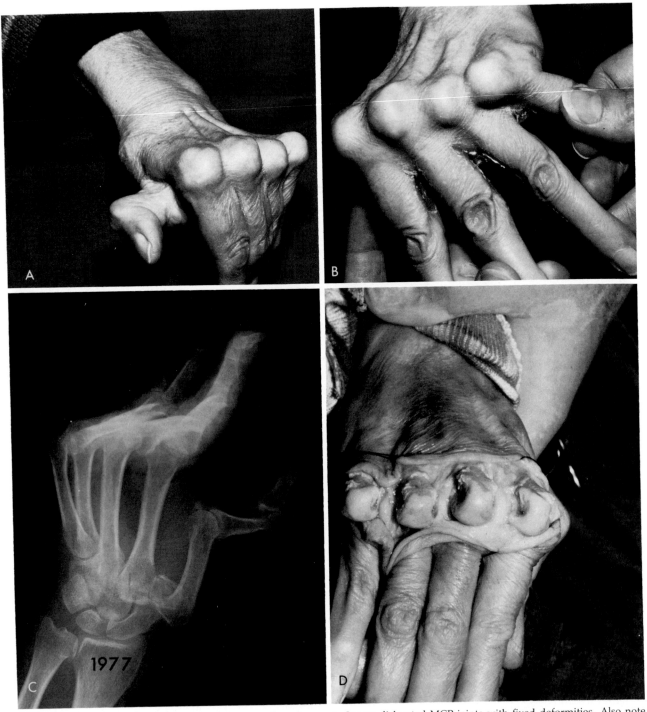

Figure 104–10. Hand deformities seen with lupus erythematosus. *A,* Severe dislocated MCP joints with fixed deformities. Also note dislocated carpometacarpal joint. *B,* Severe skin maceration associated with fixed MCP joint dislocations and poor skin hygiene. *C,* Radiograph showing dislocated MCP joints and severe thumb deformity with dislocation of carpometacarpal joint or thumb. *D,* Metacarpophalangeal joints exposed at surgery. Note minimal loss of cartilage and no evidence of any bone erosions or bony destruction.

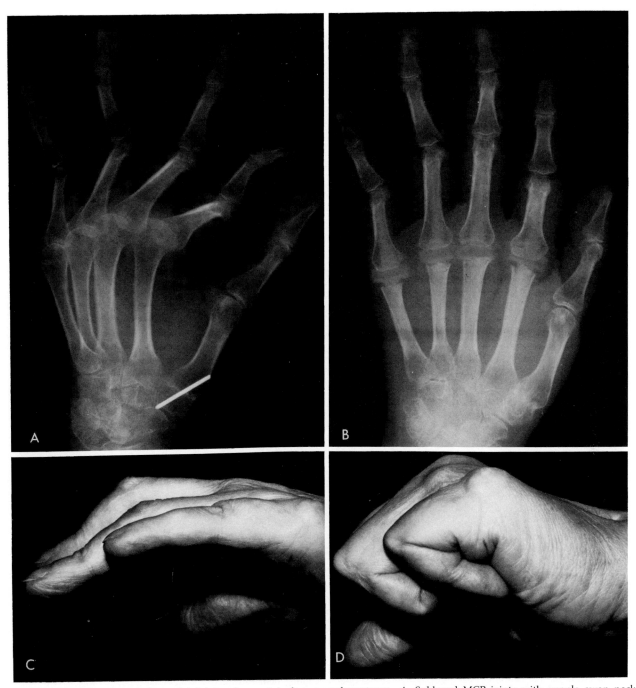

Figure 104–11. Metacarpophalangeal joint involvement in lupus erythematosus. *A*, Subluxed MCP joints with supple swan neck deformities. Also note recent arthrodesis of carpometacarpal joint of the thumb. *B*, Same patient after MCP joint arthroplasty of digits 2 to 5. *C* and *D*, Extension and flexion 4 years after MCP joint arthroplasties.

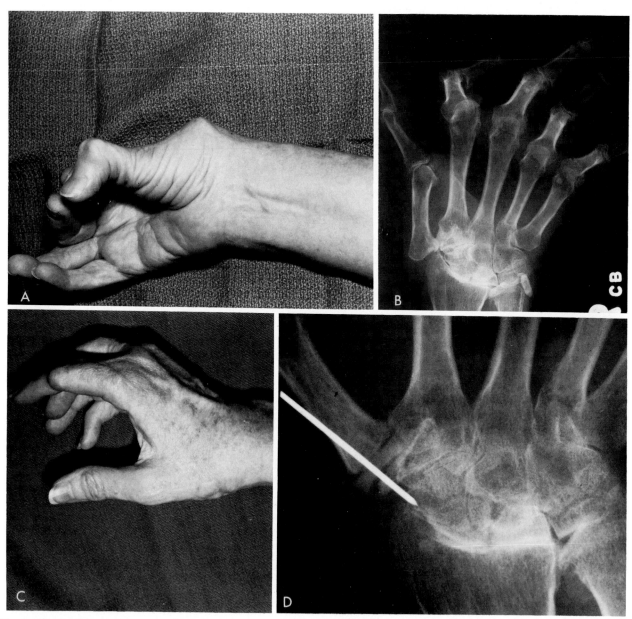

Figure 104–12. Advanced lupus erythematosus thumb deformity. *A,* Dislocated carpometacarpal joint with adduction deformity of metacarpal and hyperextension deformity of MCP joint. *B,* Radiograph of patient in *A.* Also note collapsed deformity of wrist, dislocation of MCP joints, and lateral dislocation of index PIP joint. *C,* Postoperative status: hemiarthroplasty of carpometacarpal joint and soft tissue reconstruction of MCP joint. *D,* Radiograph demonstrating hemiarthroplasty utilizing silicone prosthesis, with K-wire used for temporary prosthetic fixation.

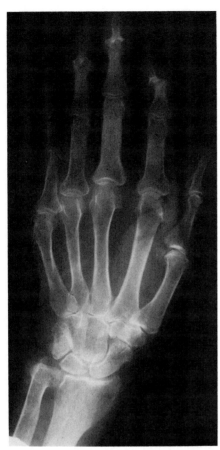

Figure 104–13. Psoriatic involvement with DIP joint erosive changes. The index and long finger DIP joints have subluxed. The MCP joints are uninvolved.

surgical intervention. The PIP joint is involved most severely, and often these patients develop flexion contractures greater than 90 degrees. The radiographs of these patients frequently show a narrowed but not completely destroyed joint space. However, the articular cartilage usually is involved more significantly than expected, and joint release usually fails. In addition, there may be an adhesive tenosynovitis that prevents good flexor tendon function, predisposing to recurrent contracture or stiffness. Unless there are significant flexion deformities and/or pain, surgery usually is not advisable. If either is present, arthrodesis in a functional position is advocated.[113]

Arthroplasty at the MCP and PIP levels is reserved for those patients with severe involvement. At the time of PIP arthroplasty, it is wise to check the excursion of the flexor tendons. This can be done by a transverse incision in the palm at the level of the A1 pulley.

MCP arthroplasties are performed for the same indications as those in RA, that is, pain, deformity, stiffness, and lack of function. However, the rate of infection is higher than that in patients with RA and lupus, and the eventual range of motion is less.[113]

The Wrist. Although surgery is required less frequently at the wrist, the indications and procedures are the same as those in RA. Arthrodesis is still the procedure of choice. There has been insufficient experience with arthroplasties to compare the results with arthrodesis.

The Thumb. Arthritic thumb involvement of the interphalangeal, MCP, and carpometacarpal joints occurs, with the carpometacarpal joint affected most severely. Carpometacarpal destruction with stiffness and decreased opposition may occur. Swan neck deformities are even rarer than in RA. At the carpometacarpal level, arthroplasty should be performed. If there is involvement of the scaphotrapezial joint, resection of the trapezium with tendon-capsule interposition is preferred. With just trapeziometacarpal disease, resection of the distal half of the trapezium can be performed with either tendon or condylar Silastic implant interposition. The trapezium implant has been avoided because of the significant rate of dislocation and/or synovitis in long-term follow-up.

At the thumb MCP level, either Silastic interposition arthroplasty or arthrodesis can be performed. We prefer arthroplasty, which may be done at the same time as carpometacarpal arthroplasty, except when a swan neck deformity is present. When swan neck deformities are present, there is a tendency toward recurrent hyperextension at the MCP level and a resultant "collapse" deformity at the carpometacarpal and interphalangeal levels. In this situation, MCP arthrodesis has yielded the best results (Fig. 104–14). Arthroplasties at the interphalangeal level yield very little motion, with a tendency toward hyperextension; joint releases result in very little motion (see Fig. 104–14). For arthrodesis, the interosseous titanium (Herbert) screw has been of great value. To date, the fusion rate has been 100 percent, with limited postoperative immobilization needed.

As in all arthritides, the results in patient satisfaction are best from thumb and wrist surgery as compared with finger surgery.

Scleroderma. Scleroderma may present as progressive systemic sclerosis or CRST/CREST (calcinosis, Raynaud's syndrome, esophageal dysfunction, sclerodactyly, telangiectasia) syndrome.[114] It is commoner in women in their third and fourth decades. Initial hand involvement is usually with Raynaud's syndrome, skin sclerosis, and decreased digital motion.[115] More than 75 percent of patients have calcinosis, usually in areas of chronic stress, such as the radial aspect of the index fingers, at bony prominences, and in the dominant hand. Sclerosis of the soft tissues is associated with distal tuft resorption in a conical shape and PIP joint contractures. There is an overlap of scleroderma with the inflammatory arthritides (30 to 40 percent rheumatoid factor positive, 35 to 90 percent antinuclear antibody positive), which may be a factor in the articular narrowing and localized osteoporosis seen in the DIP and PIP joints. Aggressive synovitis is uncommon. Thumb carpometacarpal involvement includes trapezial resorption with metacarpal dorsoradial subluxation and intra-

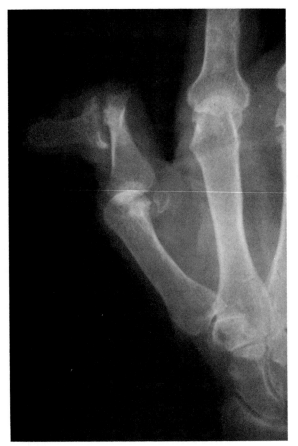

Figure 104–14. Psoriatic pencil-in-cup deformity of the thumb interphalangeal joint that has progressed to instability and subluxation.

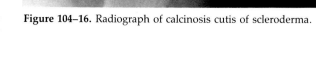

Figure 104–16. Radiograph of calcinosis cutis of scleroderma.

articular calcification.[115] Tenosynovitis is rare and predominantly is seen in patients with progressive systemic sclerosis.

Severe acrosclerosis may result in PIP flexion

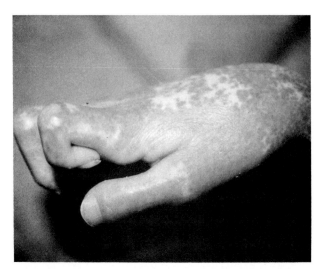

Figure 104–15. Severe acrosclerosis of scleroderma with PIP joint contractures greater than 90 degrees and dorsal skin breakdown and ulceration.

contractures and thumb metacarpal adduction contractures from sclerosis of the skin, collateral ligaments, joint capsule, and tendon sheaths (Fig. 104–15). At the PIP level, severe progressive flexion contractures may result in attenuation of the central slip and dorsal skin, which may ulcerate and potentially cause septic arthritis. In these situations PIP arthrodesis allows dorsal skin healing and improved digital function. However, the position for the arthrodesis is often as much as 60 degrees of flexion because the severe soft-tissue contracture prevents further correction. Arthroplasty has limited indications, yielding little increased range of motion because of the skin sclerosis (average 30 degrees range of motion), and carries the risk of delayed healing and infection.

Calcinosis is commoner in CREST syndrome than diffuse disease and frequently involves the volar aspect of the thumb and index and long fingers (Fig. 104–16). Colchicine may decrease the incidence of calcification. Surgical debulking is indicated when the lesions interfere with hand function or result in skin breakdown and potential infection.[116]

In scleroderma, Raynaud's syndrome may be severe and result in foci of digital ischemic necrosis (Fig. 104–17). The lesion of arterial spasm and stenosis is more commonly in the proper digital artery than in the common digital artery. If these ischemic

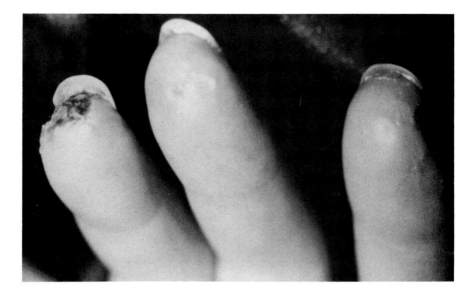

Figure 104–17. Scleroderma with distal ischemic necrosis of the index, long, and ring fingers in various stages of healing.

lesions are not infected, they can be treated with dressing changes. It may be 3 to 4 months before they heal. The patient is admonished to avoid cold exposure and to discontinue cigarette smoking. Medical therapy for severer cases has included oral nifedipine (Procardia, Adalat), prazosin (Minipress), and interarterial reserpine, with modest success.

Surgical cervical sympathectomy has been unsuccessful. Digital sympathectomy is described in limited cases[117] for relieving the pain of digital tip ulcerations.[118] It also may hasten healing, but longlasting positive results have not been proved. Microvascular reconstruction has had limited success. Attempts at skin grafting of the ulcers have been complicated by poor healing and sclerodermatous

transformation of the graft. These ulcers may progress to gangrene. Autoamputation of the distal digits is allowed to progress if there is minimal pain and no infection. During the period of autoamputation, meticulous wound care is advised. These lesions of ischemic necrosis may become secondarily infected with *Staphylococcus* and *Pseudomonas*. When there is associated severe pain, septic arthritis, or extensive gangrene, digital amputation is recommended.

Congenital scleroderma is even rarer (Fig. 104–18). Unlike scleroderma in adults, congenital scleroderma in children is less a vascular problem and more a problem of contractures. The progressive collagenization of the soft tissues in a growing child results in severe deformities. Correction is difficult

Figure 104–18. Congenital scleroderma with index finger MCP extension contracture and PIP flexion contracture. Further deformity occurred with growth; attempted surgical correction was unsuccessful.

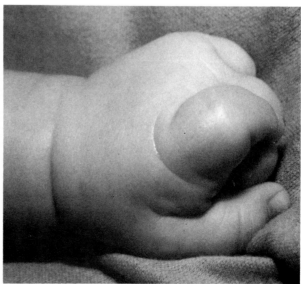

to achieve and maintain, and useful motion unlikely. Amputations often are necessary.[119, 120]

References

1. Flatt, A. E.: The Care of the Rheumatoid Hand. St. Louis, C.V. Mosby Company, 1963.
2. Millender, L. H., and Nalebuff, E. A.: Evaluation and treatment of early rheumatoid hand involvement. Orthop. Clin. North Am. 6:697, 1975.
3. Millender, L. H., and Nalebuff, E. A.: Metacarpophalangeal joint arthroplasty utilizing the silicone rubber prosthesis. Orthop. Clin. North Am. 4:349, 1973.
4. Nalebuff, E. A.: Metacarpophalangeal surgery in rheumatoid arthritis. Surg. Clin. North Am. 49:823, 1969.
5. Swanson, A. B.: Flexible Implant Resection Arthroplasty in the Hand and Extremities. St. Louis, C. V. Mosby Company, 1973.
6. Millender, L. H., and Nalebuff, E. A.: Preventive surgery—tenosynovectomy and synovectomy. Orthop. Clin. North Am. 6:765, 1975.
7. Kessler, L., and Vainio, K.: Posterior (dorsal) synovectomy for rheumatoid involvement of the hand and wrist. A follow-up study of sixty-six procedures. J. Bone Joint Surg. 48:1048, 1966.
8. Linscheid, R. L.: Surgery for rheumatoid arthritis—timing and techniques: The upper extremity. J. Bone Joint Surg. 50A:605, 1968.
9. Nalebuff, E. A., and Potter, T. A.: Rheumatoid involvement of tendons and tendon sheaths in the hand. Clin. Orthop. 59:147, 1968.
10. Lipscomb, P. R.: Surgery for rheumatoid arthritis—timing and techniques: Summary. J. Bone Joint Surg. 50A:614, 1968.
11. Millender, L. H., Nalebuff, E. A., Albin, R., Ream, J., and Gordon, M.: Dorsal tenosynovectomy and tendon transfer in the rheumatoid hand. J. Bone Joint Surg. 56A:601, 1974.
12. Brown, F. E., and Brown, M. L.: Long-term results after tenosynovectomy to treat the rheumatoid hand. J. Hand Surg. 13A:704, 1988.
13. Cracchiolo, A., III, and Marmor, L.: Resection of the distal ulna in rheumatoid arthritis. Arthritis Rheum. 12:415, 1969.
14. Vaughan-Jackson, O. J.: Attrition ruptures of tendons in the rheumatoid hand. In Proceedings of the Joint Meeting of the Orthopaedic Association of the English-Speaking World. J. Bone Joint Surg. 40A:1431, 1958.
15. Vaughan-Jackson, O. J.: Rupture of extensor tendons by attrition at the inferior radioulnar joint. Reports of two cases. J. Bone Joint Surg. 30B:528, 1948.
16. Straub, L. R., and Wilson, E. H., Jr.: Spontaneous rupture of extensor tendons in the hand associated with rheumatoid arthritis. J. Bone Joint Surg. 38A:1208, 1956.
17. Nalebuff, E. A.: Surgical treatment of finger deformities in the rheumatoid hand. Surg. Clin. North Am. 49:833, 1969.
18. Nalebuff, E. A.: Surgical treatment of tendon rupture in the rheumatoid hand. Surg. Clin. North Am. 49:811, 1969.
19. Nalebuff, E. A., and Patel, M. R.: Flexor digitorum sublimis transfer for multiple extensor tendon ruptures in rheumatoid arthritis. Plast. Reconstr. Surg. 52:530, 1973.
20. Nalebuff, E. A.: Surgical treatment of rheumatoid tenosynovitis in the hand. Surg. Clin. North Am. 49:799, 1969.
21. Posner, M. A.: Flexor superficialis tendon transfers to the thumb—an alternative to the free tendon graft for treatment of chronic injuries within the digital sheath. J. Hand Surg. 8A:876, 1983.
22. Nalebuff, E. A., and Millender, L. H.: Surgical treatment of the boutonniere deformity in rheumatoid arthritis. Orthop. Clin. North Am. 6:753, 1975.
23. Millender, L. H., and Nalebuff, E. A.: Reconstructive surgery in the rheumatoid hand. Orthop. Clin. North Am. 6:709, 1975.
24. Sledge, C. B., Zuckerman, J. D., Shortkroff, S., Zalutsky, M. R., Venkatesan, P., Snyder, M. A., and Barrett, W. P.: Synovectomy of rheumatoid knee using intra-articular injection of dysprosium-165-ferric hydroxide macroaggregates. J. Bone Joint Surg. 69A:970, 1987.
25. Simmons, B. P., and de la Caffiniere, J. Y.: Physiology of flexion of the fingers. In Tubiana, R. (ed.): The Hand. Vol 1. Philadelphia, W. B. Saunders Company, 1981, p. 377.
26. Wood, V. E., Ichtertz, D. R., and Yahiku, H.: Soft tissue metacarpophalangeal reconstruction for treatment of rheumatoid hand deformity. J. Hand Surg. 14A:163, 1989.
27. Riordan, D. C., and Fowler, S. B.: Surgical treatment of rheumatoid deformities of the hand. J. Bone Joint Surg. 40A:1431, 1958.
28. Vaino, K.: Arthrodeses and arthroplasties in the treatment of the rheumatoid hand. In La Main Rheumatismale. Paris, Expansion Scientifique Francaise, 1966, pp. 30–35.
29. Tupper, J. W.: Personal communication.
30. Swanson, A. B.: Silicone rubber implants for replacement of arthritic or destroyed joints in the hand. Surg. Clin. North Am. 48:1113, 1968.
31. Swanson, A. B.: Flexible implant arthroplasty for arthritic finger joints. J. Bone Joint Surg. 54A:435, 1972.
32. Neibauer, J. J.: Dacron-silicone prosthesis for the metacarpophalangeal and interphalangeal joints. In Cramer, L. H., and Chase, R. A. (eds.): Symposium on the Hand. Vol. 3. St. Louis, C.V. Mosby Company, 1971, pp. 96–105.
33. Flatt, A. E., and Ellison, M. R.: Restoration of rheumatoid finger joint function. III: A follow-up note after fourteen years of experience with metallic-hinge prosthesis. J. Bone Joint Surg. 54A:1317, 1972.
34. Flatt, A. E.: Restoration of rheumatoid finger-joint function. Interim report on trial of prosthetic replacement. J. Bone Joint Surg. 43A:753, 1961.
35. Beckenbaugh, R. D., and Linscheid, R. L.: Arthroplasty in the hand and wrist. In Green, D. P. (ed.): Operative Hand Surgery. New York, Churchill Livingstone, 1988, p. 167.
36. Hagert, C. G.: Advances in hand surgery: Finger joint implants. Surg. Annu. 10:253, 1978.
37. Steffee, A. D., Beckenbaugh, R. D., Linscheid, R. L., and Dobyns, J. H.: The development, technique, and early clinical results of total joint replacement for the metacarpophalangeal joint of the fingers. Orthopaedics 4:175, 1981.
38. Blair, W. F., Shurr, D. G., and Buckwalter, J. A.: Metacarpophalangeal joint implant arthroplasty with a Silastic spacer. J. Bone Joint Surg. 66A:365, 1984.
39. Millender, L. H., Nalebuff, E. A., Hawkins, R. B., and Ennis, R: Infection after silicone prosthetic arthroplasty in the hand. J. Bone Joint Surg. 57A:825, 1975.
40. Bieber, E. J., Weiland, A. J., and Volenec-Dowling, S.: Silicone-rubber implant arthroplasty of the metacarpophalangeal joints for rheumatoid arthritis. J. Bone Joint Surg. 68A:206, 1986.
41. Derkash, R. S., Niebauer, J. J., and Lane, C. S.: Long-term follow-up of metacarpophalangeal arthroplasty with silicone dacron prosthesis. J. Hand Surg. 11A:553, 1986.
42. Vahranen, V., and Viljakka, T.: Silicone rubber implant arthroplasty of the metacarpophalangeal joints in rheumatoid arthritis. J. Hand Surg. 11A:333, 1986.
43. Swanson, A. B., Poiterin, L. A., Swanson, G. DeG., and Kearney, J.: Bone remodeling phenomenon in flexible implant arthroplasty in the metacarpophalangeal joints. Clin. Orthop. 205:254, 1986.
44. Swanson, A. B., Swanson, G. DeG., and Maupin, B. K.: Flexible implant arthroplasty of the radiocarpal joint: Surgical technique and long-term study. Clin. Orthop. 187:94, 1984.
45. Gainor, B. J., and Hummel, G. L.: Correction of swan-neck deformity by lateral band mobilization. J. Hand Surg. 10A:370, 1985.
46. Nalebuff, E. A., and Millender, L. H.: Surgical treatment of swan neck deformity in rheumatoid arthritis. Orthop. Clin. North Am. 6:753, 1975.
47. Pahle, J. A., and Raunio, P.: The influence of wrist position on finger deviation in the rheumatoid hand. A clinical and radiological study. J. Bone Joint Surg. 51B:664, 1969.
48. Nalebuff, E. A., and Garrod, K. J.: Present approach to the severely involved rheumatoid wrist. Orthop. Clin. North Am. 15:369, 1984.
49. Carroll, R. E., and Dick, H. M.: Arthrodesis of the wrist for rheumatoid arthritis. J. Bone Joint Surg. 53A:1365, 1971.
50. Clayton, M. L.: Surgical treatment at the wrist in rheumatoid arthritis. A review of thirty-seven patients. J. Bone Joint Surg. 47A:741, 1965.
51. Dupont, M., and Vainio, K.: Arthrodesis of the wrist in rheumatoid arthritis. A study of 140 cases. Ann. Chir. Gynaec. Fenn. 57:513, 1968.
52. Mannerfelt, L., and Malmsten, M.: Arthrodesis of the wrist in rheumatoid arthritis. A technique without external fixation. Scand. J. Plast. Reconstr. Surg. 5:124, 1971.
53. Millender, L. H., and Nalebuff, E. A.: Arthrodesis of the rheumatoid wrist. An evaluation of sixty patients and a description of a different surgical technique. J. Bone Joint Surg. 55A:1026, 1973.
53a. O'Driscoll, S. W., Horii, E., Ness, R., Cahalan, T. D., and Richards, R. R.: The relationship between wrist position, grasp size, and grip strength. J. Hand Surg. 17A:169, 1992.
54. Taleisnik, J.: The ligaments of the wrist. J. Hand Surg. 1:110, 1976.
55. Taleisnik, J.: Wrist: Anatomy, function and injury. In AAOS Instructional Course Lecture. Vol. 27. St. Louis, C.V. Mosby Company, 1978, p. 61.
56. Taleisnik, J.: Rheumatoid arthritis of the wrist. In Strickland, J. W., and Steichen, J. B. (eds.): Difficult Problems in Hand Surgery. St. Louis, C.V. Mosby Company, 1982.
57. Linched, R. L., Dobyns, J. H., Beabout, J. W., and Bryan, R. S.: Traumatic instability of the wrist: Diagnosis, classification and pathomechanics. J. Bone Joint Surg. 54:1612, 1972.
58. Taleisnik, J.: Subtotal arthrodeses of the wrist joint. Clin. Orthop. 187:81, 1984.
59. Fatti, J. F., Palmer, A. K., and Mosher, J. F.: The long-term results of Swanson silicone rubber interpositional wrist arthroplasty. J. Hand Surg. 11A:166, 1986.
60. Albright, J. A., and Chase, R. A.: Palmar-shelf arthroplasty of the wrist in rheumatoid arthritis. A report of nine cases. J. Bone Joint Surg. 52A:89, 1970.

61. Goodman, M. J., Millender, L. H., Nalebuff, E. A., and Phillips, C. A.: Arthroplasty of the rheumatoid wrist with silicone rubber: An early evaluation. J. Hand Surg. 5:114, 1980.
62. Brase, D. W., and Millender, L. H.: Failure of silicone rubber wrist arthroplasty in rheumatoid arthritis. J. Hand Surg. 11A:175, 1986.
63. Haloua, J. P., Collin, J. P., Schernberg, F., and Sandre, J.: Arthroplasty of the rheumatoid wrist with Swanson implant. Long-term results and complications. Ann. Chir. Main 8:124, 1989.
63a. Jolly, S. L., Ferlic, D. C., Clayton, M. L., Dennis, D. A., and Stringer, E. A.: Swanson silicone arthroplasty of the wrist in rheumatoid arthritis: A long-term follow-up. J. Hand Surg. 17A:142, 1992.
64. Meuli, H. C.: Arthroplastie du poignet. Ann. Chir. 27:527, 1973.
65. Meuli, H. C.: Arthroplasty of the wrist. Clin. Orthop. 149:118, 1980.
66. Meuli, H. C.: Meuli total wrist arthroplasty. Clin. Orthop. 187:107, 1984.
67. Volz, R. G.: The development of a total wrist arthroplasty. Clin. Orthop. 116:209, 1976.
68. Volz, R. G.: The development of a total wrist arthroplasty. Clin. Orthop. 187:112, 1984.
69. Beckenbaugh, R. D., and Linscheid, R. L.: Total wrist arthroplasty. A preliminary report. J. Hand Surg. 2:339, 1977.
70. Beckenbaugh, R. D.: Implant arthroplasty in the rheumatoid hand and wrist: Current state of the art in the United States. J. Hand Surg. 8:675, 1983.
71. Ferlic, D. C.: Implant arthroplasty of the rheumatoid wrist. Hand Clin. 3:169, 1987.
72. Cooney, W. P., Beckenbaugh, R. D., and Linscheid, R. L.: Total wrist arthroplasty: Problems with implant failures. Clin. Orthop. 187:121, 1984.
73. Figgie, M. P., Ranawat, C. S., Inglis, A. E., Sobel, M., and Figgie, H. E., III: Trispherical total wrist arthroplasty in rheumatoid arthritis. J. Hand Surg. 15A:217, 1990.
74. Dennis, D. A., Ferlic, D. C., Clayton, M. L., and Volz, R. G.: Total wrist arthroplasty in rheumatoid arthritis: A long-term review. J. Hand Surg. 11A:483, 1986.
75. Palmer, A. K., and Werner, F. W.: Biomechanics of the distal radioulnar joint. Clin. Orthop. 87:26, 1984.
76. Palmar, A. K.: The distal radioulnar joint: Anatomy, biomechanics, and triangular fibrocartilage complex abnormalities. Hand Clin. 3:31, 1987.
77. Palmar, A. K., Skahem, J., Werner, F. W., and Glisson, R. R.: The extensor retinaculum of the wrist: An anatomic and biomechanical study. J. Hand Surg. 10B:11, 1985.
78. Palmar, A. K., and Werner, F. W.: The triangular fibrocartilage complex of the wrist: Anatomy and function. J. Hand Surg. 6:153, 1981.
79. Bowers, W. H.: Distal radioulnar joint. In Green, D. P. (ed.): Operative Hand Surgery. New York, Churchill Livingstone, 1982, p. 743.
80. Bowers, W. H.: Distal radioulnar joint arthroplasty: the hemiresection interposition technique. J. Hand Surg. 10A:169, 1985.
81. Bowers, W. H.: Problems of the distal radioulnar joint. Adv. Orthop. Surg. 1:289, 1984.
82. Gonsalves, D.: Correction of disorders of the distal radioulnar joint by artificial pseudarthrosis of the ulna. J. Bone Joint Surg. 56B:462, 1974.
83. Darrach, W.: Partial excision of lower shaft of ulna for deformity following Colles' fracture. Ann. Surg. 57:764, 1913.
84. Swanson, A. B.: Implant arthroplasty for disabilities of the distal radioulnar joint. Use of a silicone rubber capping implant following resection of the ulnar head. Orthop. Clin. North Am. 4:373, 1973.
85. Nalebuff, E. A.: Diagnosis, classification and management of rheumatoid thumb deformities. Bull. Hosp. Joint Dis. 29:119, 1968.
86. Figgie, M. P., Inglis, A. E., Sobel, M., Bohn, W. W., and Fisher, D. A.: Metacarpal-phalangeal joint arthroplasty of the rheumatoid thumb. J. Hand Surg. 15A:210, 1990.
87. Kvarnes, L., and Reikeras, O.: Rheumatoid arthritis at the base of the thumb treated by trapezium resection or implant arthroplasty. J. Hand Surg. 10B:195, 1985.
88. No entry.
89. Howard, F. M., Simpson, L. A., and Belsole, R. J.: Silastic condylar arthroplasty. Clin. Orthop. 195:144, 1985.
90. Smith, R. J., Atkinson, R. E., and Jupiter, J. B.: Silicone synovitis of the wrist. J. Hand Surg. 10A:45, 1985.
91. Brown, L. G.: Distal interphalangeal joint flexible implant arthroplasty. J. Hand Surg. 14A:653, 1989.
92. Zimmerman, N. B., Suhey, P. V., Clark, G. L., and Wilgis, E. F. S.: Silicone implant arthroplasty of the distal interphalangeal joint. J. Hand Surg. 14A:882, 1989.
93. Iselin, F., Pradet, G., and Gouet, O.: Conversion to arthroplasty from proximal interphalangeal joint arthrodesis. Ann. Chir. Main 7:115, 1988.
94. Eaton, R. G., Glickel, S. Z., and Littler, J. W.: Tendon interposition arthroplasty for degenerative arthritis of the trapeziometacarpal joint of the thumb. J. Hand Surg. 10A:645, 1985.
95. Burton, R. I., and Pellergrini, V. D.: Surgical management of basal joint arthritis of the thumb. Part II. Ligament reconstruction with tendon interposition arthroplasty. J. Hand Surg. 11A:324, 1986.
96. Dell, P. C., Brushart, T. M., and Smith, R. J.: Treatment of trapeziometacarpal arthritis: Results of resection arthroplasty. J. Hand Surg. 3:243, 1978.
97. Froimson, A. L.: Tendon arthroplasty of the trapeziometacarpal joint. Clin. Orthop. 70:191, 1970.
98. Eaton, R. G., and Glickel, S. Z.: Trapeziometacarpal arthritis. Staging as a rationale for treatment. Hand Clin. 3:455, 1987.
99. Amadio, P. C., Millender, L. H., and Smith, R. J.: Silicone spacer or tendon spacer for trapezium resection arthroplasty: Comparison of results. J. Hand Surg. 7:237, 1982.
100. Hoffman, D. Y., Ferlic, D. C., and Clayton, M. L.: Arthroplasty of the basal joint of the thumb using a silicone prosthesis: Long-term follow-up. J. Bone Joint Surg. 69A:993, 1987.
101. Sollerman, C., Herrlin, K., Abrahamsson, S. -O., and Lindholm, A.: Silastic replacement of the trapezium for arthrosis: A twelve-year follow-up study. J. Hand Surg. 13B:426, 1988.
102. Cooney, W. P., and Linscheid, R. L.: Total arthroplasty of the thumb trapeziometacarpal joint. Clin. Orthop. 220:35, 1987.
103. Boeckstyns, M. E. H., Sinding, A., Elholm, K. T., and Rechnagel, K.: Replacement of the trapeziometacarpal joint with a cemented (Caffiniere) prosthesis. J. Hand Surg. 14A:83, 1989.
104. Alberts, K. A., and Engkvist, O.: Arthrodesis of the first carpometacarpal joint: 33 cases of arthrosis. Acta Orthop. Scand. 60:258, 1989.
105. Ropes, M. W.: Systemic Lupus Erythematosus. Cambridge, MA, Harvard University Press, 1976, pp. 12–74.
106. Labowitz, R., and Schumaker, H. R., Jr.: Articular manifestations of systemic lupus erythematosus. Ann. Intern. Med. 74:911, 1971.
107. Dubois, E. L.: Lupus Erythematosus: A Review of the Current Status of Discoid and Systemic Lupus Erythematosus and their variants. 2nd ed. Los Angeles, University of Southern California Press, 1974, pp. 40–42, 58–61, 70–71, 232–237, 464–475, 525–536.
108. Green, N., and Osmer, J. C.: Small bone changes secondary to systemic lupus erythematosus. Radiology 90:118, 1968.
109. Weisman, B. N., Rappaport, M. B. B., Sosman, J. L., and Schur, P. H.: Radiographic findings in the hands in patients with systemic lupus erythematosus. Radiology 126:313, 1978.
110. Bleifield, C. J., and Inglis, A. E.: The hand in systemic lupus erythematosus. J. Bone Joint Surg. 56A:1207, 1974.
111. Dray, G. J., Millender, L. H., and Nalebuff, E. A.: The surgical treatment of hand deformities in systemic lupus erythematosus. J. Hand Surg. 6:339, 1981.
112. Resnick, D., and Niwayama, G: Diagnosis of Bone and Joint Disorders. Philadelphia, W.B. Saunders Company, 1988, pp. 1171–1198, 1267–1292.
113. Belsky, M., Feldon, P., et al.: Hand involvement in psoriatic arthritis. J. Hand Surg. 7:203, 1982.
114. Jones, N., Imbriglia, J., et al.: Surgery for scleroderma of the hand. J. Hand Surg. 12A:391, 1987.
115. Resnick, D., and Niwayama, G.: Diagnosis of Bone and Joint Disorders. Philadelphia, W.B. Saunders, 1988, pp. 1171–1198, 1293–1318.
116. Mendelson, B., Linscheid, R., et al: Surgical treatment of calcinosis cutis in the upper extremity. J. Hand Surg. 2:318, 1987.
117. Flatt, A.: Digital artery sympathectomy. J. Hand Surg. 5:550, 1980.
118. Wiglis, E.: Evaluation and treatment of chronic digital ischemia. Ann. Surg. 193:693, 1981.
119. Floyd, W., Simmons, B., and Griffin, P.: Focal scleroderma affecting the hand. J. Bone Joint Surg. 67A:637, 1985.
120. Waters, P., and Simmons, B.: Unusual arthritic disorders in the hand: Part II. Surgical Rounds for Orthopedics. October, 1990, pp. 27–32.

Chapter 105

B. F. Morrey

Reconstruction and Rehabilitation of the Elbow Joint

ANATOMY AND BIOMECHANICS

The anatomy and biomechanics of the elbow joint are most readily understood by considering its three elements of function: providing motion, stability, and a fulcrum for strength functions. These will be discussed in the context of clinical pathology and as it relates to surgical intervention.

Motion

The elbow is classified as a trochleo-giglemoid joint. That is, a hinged joint about a trochlea or pulley. A second degree of freedom is provided by pronation and supination motion of the forearm. The unique articular orientation of the distal humerus anteriorly and the opening of the greater sigmoid fossa of the ulna posteriorly allow the elbow to transverse an arc of flexion of about 150 degrees and yet be stable in full extension. Pronation and supination require an intact proximal and distal radioulnar joint. Normally, this arc of motion is approximately 165 to 170 degrees. Pronation is typically 75 to 80 degrees, while supination is 85 to 90 degrees.[1]

The center of elbow rotation may be approximated by a single line that passes through the center of the projected articular curvatures of the capitellum and trochlea.[2] This axis of rotation is colinear with the distal anterior cortex of the humerus in the sagittal plane.[3] In the anterior-posterior plane, the axis of rotation is approximated by a line through the middle of the lateral epicondyle to the inferior border of the medial epicondyle (Fig. 105–1). Knowledge of the location and approximation of the hinged axis is important to perform the reconstructive procedure of distraction arthroplasty.[4, 5] For total joint replacement, simple hinge motion is not an effective model. Some tolerance or play at the articulation that allows simulation of the normal complex motion has been shown to be a prerequisite to avoid long-term loosening of semiconstrained joint designs.[6]

Constraint

The elbow is one of the most congruous joints of the body and as such is inherently stable due to its articular configuration. The medial and lateral collateral ligaments provide the major contributions to varus/valgus stability. Of these, the anterior portion of the medial collateral ligament has been shown to be the most significant single ligamentous stabilizer of the joint.[7, 8] The collateral ligament must be preserved or reconstructed when performing resurfacing or interposition joint arthroplasty. In extension, the anterior capsule provides about 25 percent of the varus/valgus stability.[7] The lateral collateral ligament offers a relatively constant constraint throughout the arc of motion, whereas the posteromedial collateral ligament is taut only in flexion.[9] Furthermore, the importance of the lateral ligaments of the joint is emerging and helps explain conditions such as recurrent elbow subluxation.[10]

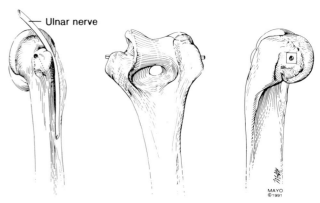

Figure 105–1. The axis of elbow flexion is through the center of the lateral condyle at the attachment of the radial collateral ligament and the undersurface of the medial epicondyle on the AP projection. The axis is through the projected arc of curvature of the capitellum and trochlea as viewed on the lateral projection. This axis is colinear with the anterior border of the distal humerus. (By permission, Mayo Foundation.)

The two articulations of the elbow joint, the ulnohumeral and radiohumeral, provide approximately 50 percent of the overall stability of this joint, leaving approximately 50 percent of stability to the soft tissue constraint. Experimental data reveal that removing the radial head reduces resistance to valgus stress by about 30 percent for small (that is, less than five degrees) displacements.[11, 12] A recent study that simulates more physiologic function and loading suggests the radial head does not provide stability if the medial ligament is intact.[13] Hence, this is termed a secondary stabilizer of the elbow (Fig. 105–2).

Forces

The forces that cross the elbow joint are considered cyclic in nature. With elbow flexion the resultant force is directed posteriorly; with extension, the resultant force is anteriorly directed.[14] This is an important concept to help understand the failure pattern of the early generation of total joint arthroplasty. The magnitude of this force approximates three times the body weight and thus there is a considerable force transmitted through a relatively small area.[15] However, the actual forces at the elbow joint are considerably more complex than can be described by the resultant vector alone. More detailed studies are required to elucidate the force distribution between the radiohumeral and ulnohumeral joints, especially during physiologic conditions. To date, the studies of Halls and Travill[16] and Walker et al.[17] indicate that up to 60 percent of a maximally applied axial force is transmitted across the radiohumeral joint in the extended elbow. During use, however, the flexed supinated elbow is the position of greatest strength and in this position less than 33 percent of body weight is transmitted across the radius.[18] With pronation the radius ''screws home'' against the capitellum, causing greater force transmission at this joint.[18] With the elbow extended and the forearm pronated, muscle contraction can cause forces of approximately one times body weight at the radial head. If the

radial head is removed for fracture or disease, the interosseous membrane and the triangular fibrocartilage at the wrist absorb the axially directed force. This accounts for the satisfactory clinical results that are usually appreciated in patients requiring radial head excision.

FUNCTION

The function of the elbow joint consists of two basic elements: that of providing a stable link and that of enough motion to position the hand in space. It is obvious that the status of the associated joints, the shoulder, the wrist, and the hand, is important when analyzing elbow function. Amis et al.[19] have studied a group of 200 patients being followed in a rheumatology clinic. Among those with elbow symptoms, 83 percent complained of shoulder involvement and 92 percent had problems with the hand and wrist. Thus, the clinician may expect the elbow to be an isolated problem in 10 percent or less of patients presenting with rheumatoid arthritis.

Compromised shoulder motion reduces the effectiveness of the elbow and places greater significance on elbow function. Similarly, wrist pathology can markedly alter the ability to pronate and supinate the hand independent of the status of the elbow joint. In some patients, particularly those with rheumatoid arthritis, the status of these additional joints should be specifically examined.

Motion

Associated motion of the neck, hip, and knee may compensate for lost elbow flexion and extension. Shoulder function has less potential than once thought to compensate for loss of elbow motion.[20] Limited forearm pronation can be compensated for to some extent by shoulder abduction, although patients may complain of fatigue with this compensatory position. The one motion loss that is not readily compensated for is supination, since the shoulder is not able to readily adduct to accommodate for this loss. It has been shown that the amount of motion required for routine daily activities is approximately 100 degrees of flexion and extension from 30 to 130 degrees and approximately 100 degrees of forearm rotation equally divided between pronation and supination (Fig. 105–3).[21]

Strength

Several characteristics of the normal strength pattern are useful to the clinician in assessing afflictions of the elbow joint (Fig. 105–4).[22] The strongest position of elbow flexion is at 90 degrees and the forearm in neutral or supination. Furthermore, strength of extension is only approximately 70 per-

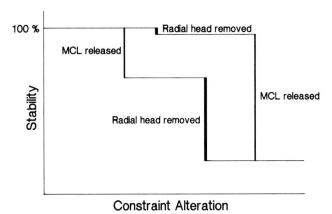

Figure 105–2. The radial head serves as a secondary stabilizer of the elbow joint.[13] (By permission, Mayo Foundation.)

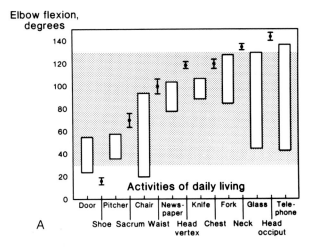

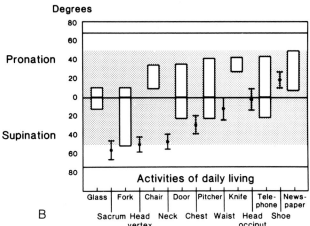

Figure 105–3. The functional arc of flexion for selected activities of daily living is about 30 to 130 degrees (A). The functional arc of pronation and supination for these activities is also 100 degrees, 50 degrees of pronation and 50 degrees of supination (B).

cent that of flexion owing to the mechanical advantage and size of the muscles in each group. Supination strength function is about 10 degrees greater than pronation strength. Males tend to be stronger than females on an average by a factor of two, and the dominant extremity is about 5 to 7 percent stronger than the nondominant extremity.[22]

Stability

The stability of the elbow joint is difficult to examine when subtle changes are present and is obvious when there is gross joint destruction, as in the patient with severe rheumatoid arthritis. Because stability is important for the elbow to serve as an effective link or fulcrum, marked instability even without associated pain, when incapacitating, is an indication for surgical intervention.

DISEASE AND PRESENTATION

Rheumatoid arthritis is the most common affliction of the elbow joint that prompts consultation with a rheumatologist. Post-traumatic sequela is an equally common presentation to the orthopedic surgeon. Because the elbow is vulnerable to sepsis, hematogenous septic arthritis, especially in patients on steroids with rheumatoid arthritis, is an occasional but serious problem. Direct spread from an infected olecranon bursa is a concern in those with rheumatoid arthritis. Hence, a swollen olecranon bursa *with pain* is assumed to be infected and is aspirated with a course of antibiotics initiated after the aspiration. In the noninfected incidence, the bursa may become quite large but is not painful, thus an important point to the differential diagnosis. Postoperative infection is also more common in patients with elbow involvement than after similar surgeries on the hip, knee, and shoulder.[23]

In addition to these conditions, the elbow may be afflicted with hemophilia and other inflammatory processes such as gout and pseudogout, but there are no particular distinguishing features concerning elbow involvement in these disease states.

Rheumatoid Arthritis

While protean in presentation, the extent of rheumatoid joint involvement has been variously classified[24, 26]; we have modified these classifications into four rather simple and readily defined groups[25] (Fig. 105–5), which follow.

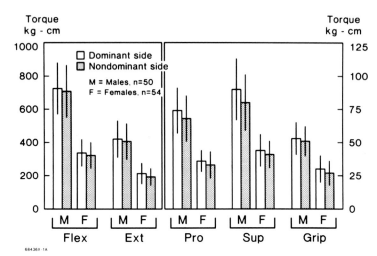

Figure 105–4. The mean strength of the various functions for male and female, including differences for dominant and nondominant extremities. Standard deviation is given. The relationship of flexion and extension strength as well as the differences between males and females and dominances are noted.

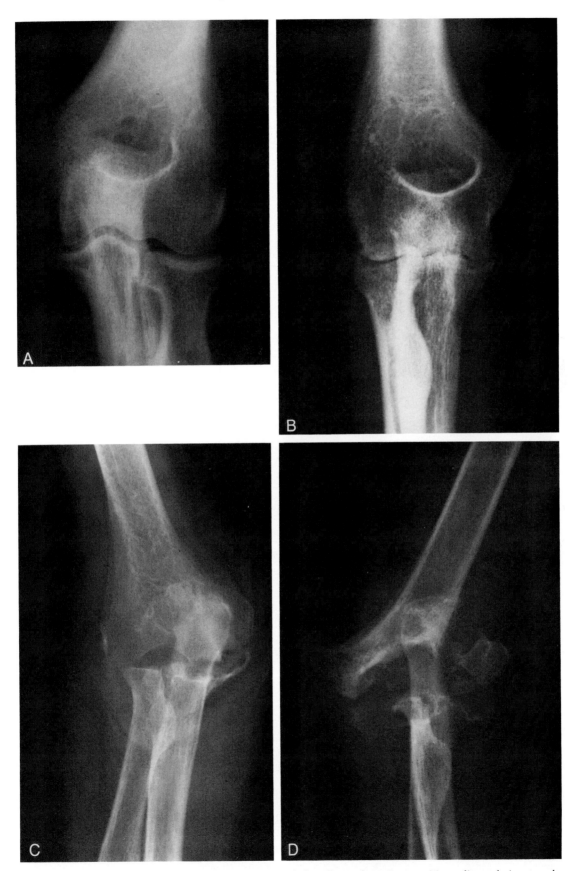

Figure 105–5. Mayo classification of rheumatoid involvement of the elbow. *Stage 1*: synovitis; radiograph is normal or shows osteoporosis only *(A). Stage 2*: synovitis; some mechanical symptoms. Radiograph shows joint narrowing and subchondral changes; the contour is not destroyed *(B). Stage 3*: less synovitis; mild to moderate instability. Radiograph shows architectural changes *(C). Stage 4*: grossly unstable; radiograph shows gross destruction *(D). (A to D,* By permission of Mayo Foundation.)

Table 105–1. TYPICAL ELBOW FUNCTIONAL INVOLVEMENT IN A POPULATION OF PATIENTS WITH RHEUMATOID ARTHRITIS

Motion	Degrees (Mean)
Flexion	20–137°
Pronation or supination	62–55°
Strength	**Percentage of Normal**
Males	53%
Females	46%
Instability	**Percent**
None	76%
Mild	8%
Moderate	8%
Severe	8%

Modified from Amis, A. A., Hughes, S. J., Miller, J. H., and Wright, Z.: A functional study of the rheumatoid elbow. Rheum. Rehabil. 21:151, 1982. Used with permission.

Stage 1. No gross articular alteration. Osteoporosis is present. Joint mechanics are normal. Synovitis is the prominent pathologic process.

Stage 2. Joint narrowing is present but the contour of the joint is not badly disrupted. Osteoporosis is usually present. Bone cysts may have developed but they are not a prominent feature.

Stage 3. The joint architecture has been altered and the contour of the joint is lost. The joint is somewhat unstable. The olecranon as viewed on the lateral projection is thinned. Cystic formation is common.

Stage 4. Gross joint destruction. The articular surface has been resorbed. Mechanical dysfunction and gross instability are characteristic (see Fig. 105–5).

The spectrum of clinical presentation has been studied by Amis et al.[19] At any given time, patients with rheumatoid involvement will demonstrate pain and functional involvement as depicted in Table 105–1. The most common indication for surgery is pain (Fig. 105–6A). Instability will justify surgical intervention in about 10 to 15 percent of patients (Fig. 105–6B). Motion is generally in the functional range, although some patients will benefit from improved motion after the arthroplasty; this is usually considered a secondary goal of the surgery. Strength loss is related to pain and instability and as such is not generally a primary indication for reconstructive surgery in this patient population.

Post-traumatic Arthritis

Unlike the patient with rheumatoid arthritis, loss of motion is a typical complaint and prompts a surgical opinion in the patient with post-traumatic arthritis (Fig. 105–7). While this limited arc of motion may be painful, this is not usually a major complaint. The stability of patients with post-traumatic arthritis is generally good as is strength of flexion and extension. Thus, the major complaint at the time of presentation for post-traumatic elbow is limitation of motion greater than is required for activities of daily living with or without significant pain.

Degenerative Arthritis

Degenerative arthritis of the elbow is not frequently diagnosed in the United States but is well

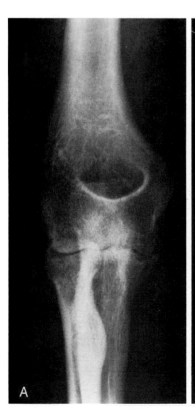 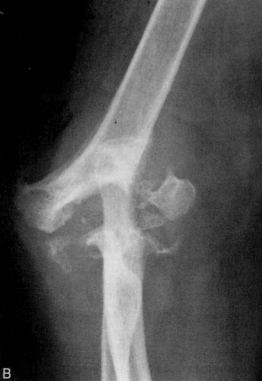

Figure 105–6. The patient with rheumatoid arthritis and a painful elbow. The joint architecture has been reasonably well maintained, but the joint space has been lost. This is classified as stage 2 involvement *(A)*. Extensive resorption and destruction of the architecture of the joint rendering the elbow unstable is an example of a grade 4 or extensive rheumatoid involvement *(B)*.

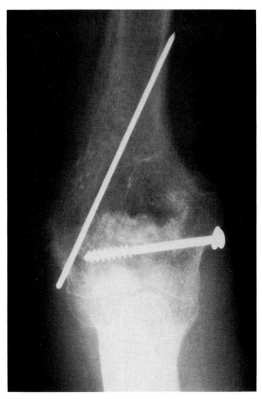

Figure 105–7. Post-traumatic arthritis is characterized by destruction of the joint architecture, which is usually painful but often presents clinically by loss of motion or joint stiffness.

recognized in Asia, particularly Japan. What little evidence is available suggests that this process is actually a form of post-traumatic, overuse arthritis.[27] The typical early presentation for the joint with primary degenerative arthritis is loss of elbow extension. Limitation of flexion is subsequently noted with complaints of pain at the extremes of flexion and extension. The patient tends to seek attention with loss of about 30 degrees of extension and 10 to 20 degrees loss of flexion. Radiographically, osteophytes are noted anteriorly and posteriorly (Fig. 105–8). Loose bodies occur in about 25 percent. Treatment to date has been symptomatic or limited arthroscopic procedures. In some instances removal of osteophytes is indicated to relieve the impingement pain that is noted at the extremes of flexion and extension.

INDICATIONS AND SURGICAL OPTIONS

The primary indication for surgery on the elbow is to restore joint function or to relieve pain.

Pain

Pain is the most common primary indication for elbow surgery, and pain relief is most predictable and complete after prosthetic replacement, especially for rheumatoid arthritis; however, interposition or distraction arthroplasty should be considered with post-traumatic arthritis. Limited resection and partial

replacement also are variably successful at achieving pain relief in selected circumstances.

Motion

Distraction and interposition arthroplasty are the two procedures specifically directed at improving motion as the primary goal. If more than 60 degrees of flexion contracture is present and if this markedly limits the patient's occupation or daily activities, surgical release is considered. Flexion of less than 100 degrees does not allow the patient to reach the mouth or head. Thus, surgical intervention is appropriate for this patient as well. In most instances, the prosthetic joint replacement is also effective at restoring a functional arc of motion but this is not generally a primary goal of such surgery.

Stability

Description of primary ligamentous reconstruction for instability of the elbow is beyond the scope of this text. However, in patients with gross instability from rheumatoid arthritis, in tumor resection, or traumatic bone loss, the articulated hinge total joint replacement is effective. In these instances, if the instability causes marked dysfunction of the extremity, restoration of functional stability is the primary goal of surgery.[5]

Strength

The prosthetic joint replacements may be effective at improving strength by virtue of the reflex inhibition associated with pain that is eliminated by

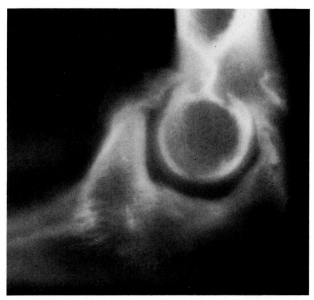

Figure 105–8. Lateral tomogram of an elbow with primary degenerative arthritis shows the characteristic osteophytes from the tip of the olecranon and the coronoid process.

the prosthetic joint replacement.[28] Strength is generally decreased in the stiff or ankylosed elbow after interposition or distraction arthroplasty.

PARTIAL RESECTION–REPLACEMENT ARTHROPLASTY

Some disease or traumatic states involve only a portion of the joint, and a limited resection or replacement procedure may be effective.

Radial Head Resection/Replacement

Radial head excision is commonly employed at the time of elbow synovectomy. Synovectomy of the knee has been performed for over 100 years,[29] and synovectomy with radial head excision has been performed in this country for more than 40 years.[30] The rationale and anticipated results of synovectomy have been dealt with in detail in Chapter 39 of this volume. This is the accepted procedure for early stages of rheumatoid arthritis (stages 1 and 2) with chronic refractory synovitis and pain. Removal of the radial head is a common feature of this procedure and is recommended by the majority of authors.[31–36] The occasional author, however, suggests leaving the radial head if it is not significantly involved.[37, 38] Currently, arthroscopic synovectomy is my treatment of choice if the removal of the radial head is not required or anticipated.

For rheumatoid arthritis, the indication for radial head resection and synovectomy is primarily relief of pain. In this regard, it has been a successful operation, at least in the short-term of 3 to 5 years, in approximately 75 percent of patients. The best results are to be anticipated in those with less architectural damage. Although the issue is debated, radial head excision and synovectomy should, in my opinion, be reserved for the patient with a reasonably intact joint (stage 2 disease). This is not an operation to be offered for limitation of motion, since motion is variably affected by the procedure. In approximately half of the patients, motion will not be changed by the operation. In approximately 30 percent, there will be some improvement, and in 20 percent, motion may be lost after the procedure.

Replacement of the radial head by a silastic implant is recommended by a few authors.[39] However, the increasing concern about silicone debris, synovitis, and lymphadenitis has lessened enthusiasm for the implant and it should not be done routinely after radial head resection.[40–43]

It has been noted that the radiographic changes of the disease process progressed even in the face of decreased symptoms after a radial head resection and synovectomy (Fig. 105–9).[34, 43] Other than technique, little has changed in the indications for this operation as a reasonable temporizing procedure, but surgery should not be offered with the anticipated results of a predictable long-lasting effect.

Distal Humerus

A search of the world literature reveals that, excluding the proximal radius, 21 custom implant

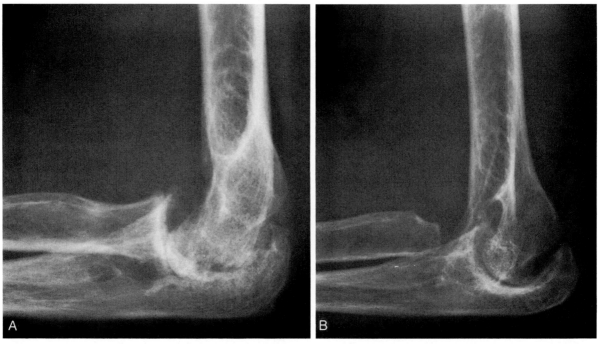

Figure 105–9. Patient with stage 2 rheumatoid involvement of the elbow and painful synovitis refractory to medical management *(A)*. Three years after radial head excision and synovectomy, patient has no pain and 120 degrees of flexion and is well pleased with the early result *(B)*.

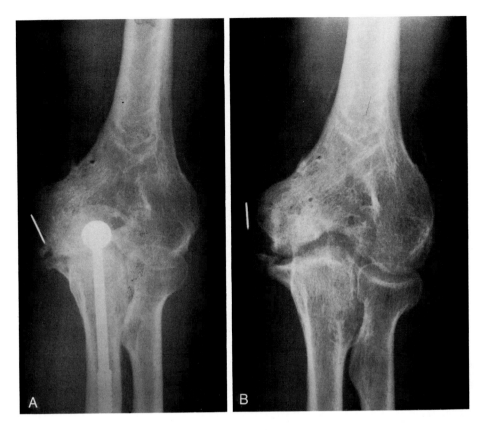

Figure 105–10. Interposition arthroplasty typically calls for resection of the diseased portion of the distal humerus and interposition of a material to allow a nonadhering surface. Post-traumatic arthritis (A) treated with fascial interposition arthroplasty. One year after surgery, the ulnohumeral joint has been reconstituted, and the patient has painless motion of 100 degrees (B).

arthroplasties were reported prior to 1967.[53–56] The distal humerus is most commonly involved and replacement options include metal alloy, nylon, acrylic, and a metal prosthesis covered with vulcanized rubber.[57]

Most of the early reports were of single cases with variable follow-up. Of the 21 cases, range of follow-up was from 4 months[57] to 23 years.[58] Although some reasonable function was often attained, relief of pain was variable and complications included wound infection, ulnar nerve palsy, joint stiffness, ectopic bone formation, dislocation, and loosening.

These early efforts to replace or resurface parts of the elbow joint answered some questions but raised others. The initial concern was whether a foreign material articulating with cartilage could satisfactorily relieve pain. Problems with long-term fixation were also identified with these early attempts. This question was quickly answered with a high incidence of prosthetic loosening and instability, and this specific experience prompted the use of polymethylmethacrylate as a fixation for what has evolved into the current concepts of total elbow joint replacement. The attempt to solve the problem of loose cemented implants also brought about a second change, that of cadaveric joint replacement.[52] Unfortunately, this option has shown a predictable tendency to deteriorate with time in a pattern resembling that of a neurotopic joint.

Interposition/Distraction Arthroplasty

Interposition arthroplasty occupies an interesting page in the history of orthopedic surgery. Described in this country in the 1920s by Sir Hemlich MacAusland[49] and popularized by Campbell[59] and Henderson,[60] these procedures were originally described for the knee but may have proved most useful for the elbow. These were usually performed for post-traumatic stiffness, when the interposed membrane was employed to prevent recurrent ankylosis after joint release (Fig. 105–10). Numerous interposition materials have been employed. These have included ivory pegs, gutta-percha, lanolin, celluloid, wood, magnesium sheets, silastic sheets, periosteal flaps, muscle flaps, rib cartilage, fascia, skin, gel foam, fat, and specially treated animal membranes. The early results reported by Campbell,[59] MacAusland,[57] and Henderson[60] demonstrated significant improvement from the preoperative state, and this procedure was an accepted one in the 1940s for patients with painful and stiff elbows. Some authors have recommended the procedure for rheumatoid arthritis, but other surgical options are currently more reliable for this type of patient.[61]

At present the indication for this type of operation is quite limited but is useful for the younger individual in whom reasonably heavy demands are placed on the joint.[62] It is of interest to note, however, that heavy labor has been reported as a contraindication based on long-term reviews by Silva, and Knight and Van Zandt.[63, 64]

A detailed long-term follow-up study of a large number of patients treated by fascial arthroplasty has been published by Knight and Van Zandt from the Campbell Clinic.[64] These investigators report 56 percent good and 22 percent fair, 2 percent poor and 22 percent failed procedures among 45 patients with follow-up of 3 to 30 years. In the young heavy laborer, those with previous sepsis and extreme muscle weakness are listed as contraindications to this operation. In addition to fascia, the so-called cutis arthroplasty has received some attention through the years since it was first reported by Gui in 1953.[65] A satisfactory arc of motion of about 80 degrees was obtained in 20 patients. Pain was graded as complete relief in 40 percent, mild pain after activity in 40 percent, and constant pain in 20 percent. A report by Froimson et al. in 1976 is of interest in that five of six patients undergoing cutis arthroplasty were satisfied with their procedure and had an arc of motion of over 100 degrees with minimal problems of instability.[66] The follow-up in this group was modest, averaging 3.5 years, but it does represent recent data on an alternative to joint replacement. I have employed fascial interposition arthroplasty in association with a distraction device in patients undergoing ankylosis take-down after trauma. This procedure, while demanding, does have a limited but definite role in reconstructive surgery of the elbow. Adjunctive use of the distraction device, described later, has broadened the application of this procedure.

The use of interposition arthroplasty or resection arthroplasty for patients with rheumatoid arthritis is not, in my judgment, indicated, owing to the unpredictable nature of the procedure brought about by the progressive nature of the underlying pathology. Total elbow arthroplasty is as reliable as hip replace-

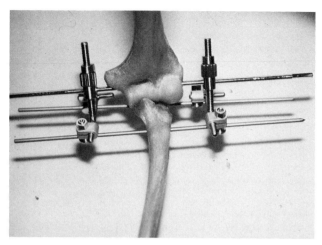

Figure 105–12. Current distraction device designed at the Mayo Clinic. (By permission, Mayo Foundation.)

ment in my hands and is the treatment of choice for rheumatoid arthritis.[26]

Distraction Arthroplasty

Complications of unpredictable pain relief and instability with the interposition resection arthroplasty have prompted investigators to consider alternative techniques to obtain the same functional results. Thus, in 1975 Volkov and Oganesian reported their experience with the use of an external fixator.[67] This device employs a pin through the axis of rotation of the elbow joint, and the serial application of traction through additional pins allowed the elbow joint to be mobilized, often without additional or significant surgical release. Many pathologies have been treated with this device, including failed excision arthroplasty, post-traumatic contracture, chronic dislocations, and un-united distal humeral fractures.[67] Overall, the average arc of motion improvement was rather limited, being less than 45 degrees.

As a result of this report, the technique has been reintroduced by Deland et al.[4] from the Brigham and Women's Hospital (Fig. 105–11). The distraction apparatus has been modified to consist of a high-density polyethylene component that allows a transfixing pin across the axis of rotation of the humerus and pins across the ulna. A similar device has been developed at the Mayo Clinic (Fig. 105–12).

Over the last 3 years both devices have been used in my practice at the Mayo Clinic (Fig. 105–13). My results in 20 patients, with an average follow-up of 30 months, reveal the mean preoperative arc of motion of 33 degrees was improved by 65 degrees to a mean postoperative arc of motion of 98 degrees.[5] Eighteen of 20 patients (90 percent) are satisfied with the procedure. However, this is one of the more demanding operations performed on the elbow, and complications of infection and ulnar nerve irritation have been observed. Although this may represent a valuable option for the treatment of a young person

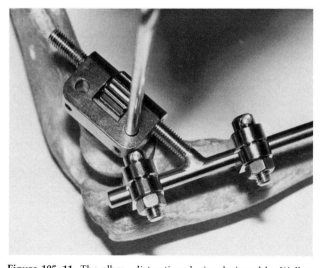

Figure 105–11. The elbow distraction device designed by Walker and colleagues at the Brigham and Women's Hospital is made of high-density polyethylene. (By permission, Mayo Foundation.)

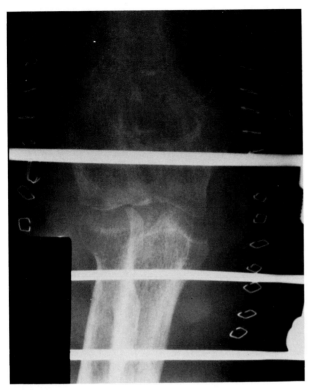

Figure 105–13. The patient with a post-traumatic stiffness of the elbow shown in Figure 105–7. The distraction device has been applied.

with a stiff elbow, it is not, at this time, considered a surgical procedure that is universally available to most orthopedic surgeons, owing to its complexity. However, one advantage of familiarity with the system is the extension of its use to the unstable fracture.

PROSTHETIC JOINT REPLACEMENT

History

Total elbow arthroplasty, as currently performed, is the fourth stage in the evolution of elbow joint reconstructive surgery.[68] Resection and interposition arthroplasty, stage 1, were followed by custom hemi joint replacements for traumatic dysfunction in the 1950s and 1960s (stage 2). Both of these eras were previously briefly discussed. Constrained total elbow arthroplasty with methylmethacrylate fixation was the first attempt at widespread joint replacement (stage 3), but, because of inherent loosening, the early designs have given way to the present generation of semiconstrained and resurfacing devices (stage 4).

While some design considerations may conflict with others, an appreciation of the variables considered in the current prosthesis is shown in Table 105–2. It would seem that more than one design may be necessary to treat adequately the spectrum of pathology that involves the elbow joint. It also follows that prosthetic selection may not only be based on

scientific merit but also on familiarity and clinical experience.

Indications

As with reconstructive procedures of other joints, the indication for total elbow arthroplasty will change and broaden as improved long-term results are obtained. Rheumatoid arthritis is responsible for the vast majority of surgical candidates.[69–74] In general, inability to use the extremity for functions of daily living because of pain, motion loss, or instability constitutes the basic indication for elbow joint replacement.[75] In a given patient several components of disability may be present, although pain is the most common primary indication for joint replacement arthroplasty. Significant cartilage loss or gross deformity are present before this surgical option should be considered. Extensive motion loss is rather uncommon in rheumatoid patients, with the exception of juvenile rheumatoid involvement, in which marked joint motion loss or even ankylosis is typical. In these particular patients motion limitation may persist even after total elbow arthroplasty.[76]

Post-traumatic painful loss of motion, in patients younger than 60 years of age, should be treated with interposition or distraction arthroplasty, depending upon the actual or desired level of activity. In the patient older than 60 years, certain total elbow arthroplasty devices may still be adequate and the results with recent designs have been gratifying.[77]

Instability, observed with advanced rheumatoid arthritis and certain post-traumatic conditions, serves as a primary indication for elbow joint replacement. Such pathology dictates the selection of a more constrained prosthesis, which previously has been associated with a higher incidence of loosening (see Fig. 105–6B). Since the introduction of the anterior flange, in 1981, we have recorded no patient from out of approximately 100 with rheumatoid arthritis in whom the prosthesis has loosened. The relative indications for the three available surgical options for rheumatoid arthritis, synovectomy, resurfacing, and semiconstrained replacement are shown in Figure 105–14.

As when assessing any joint replacement option, the application of the indications in a given clinical setting must be tempered by the surgeon's expertise

Table 105–2. ELBOW PROSTHESIS DESIGN CONSIDERATIONS

Design Criteria	Goal
Kinematics	Functional motion
Stability	Reliability
Load transmission	Stress reduction
Materials	Avoid friction, debris
Fixation	Durability
Surgery	Optimum fit, preserve strength
Instrumentation	Reproducibility
Salvage potential	Preserve bone

RHEUMATOID SURGERY OF THE ELBOW

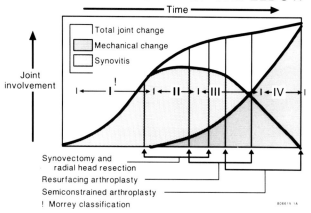

Figure 105–14. Graphic representation of the role of synovectomy, resurfacing, and semiconstrained total elbow arthroplasty as a function of synovitis and mechanical joint changes. (By permission, Mayo Foundation.)

in elbow surgery, as well as the results of the replacement devices available. The clinical result of the procedure must be weighed against the preoperative state. Knowledge of salvage options is essential, and if it is deemed that the salvage procedure is no worse or even better than the current condition, total elbow arthroplasty might be offered after a thorough discussion with the patient. Since a high failure rate has been documented in the past in the post-traumatic patient, joint replacement arthroplasty is offered very cautiously to those with this diagnosis. Yet, marked improvement in the results has been documented even in this patient population.[77]

Contraindications

Active infection from any source should delay surgery for a minimum of 6 months after treatment and after all evidence of infection has resolved. A previously infected elbow, except in the most unusual of circumstances, is a reasonably firm contraindication to elbow joint replacement.[23]

Soft tissue contracture or paralysis of the flexor or extensor musculature compromises the anticipated outcome and is a relative contraindication to total elbow arthroplasty.

Elbow arthrodesis or painful ankylosis in a satisfactory position is also considered a firm contraindication for elbow replacement at this time.

As with other joints, replacement of the elbow by a prosthetic implant in an uncooperative patient is to be avoided.

JOINT REPLACEMENT OPTIONS

Currently, both resurfacing and semiconstrained designs are viable options. Use without cement exists

in a resurfacing design by Pritchard and a composite of cement and bone graft in the Mayo Modified Coonrad prosthesis. The resurfacing devices are designed to remove a minimum amount of bone and to replicate the articular anatomy of the distal humerus and proximal ulna, and thus are considered to be the "conservative" option (Fig. 105–15).[71, 72, 74, 78–84] Stability is provided by the integrity of the soft tissue as well as by the inherent design of the prosthesis, primarily based on the arc of curvature of the ulnar component, which varies considerably from one design to the other: for example, the capitello condylar, about 145 degrees; the London, over 180 degrees; and the Pritchard intermediate, between the two.

Semiconstrained elbow devices provide inherent stability by virtue of the articular design, which is usually a hinge or snap-fit arrangement.[73, 86, 87] The semiconstrained devices provide some "play" in the articulation, which varies about 7 to 10 degrees (Fig. 105–16). This relaxation of the articular constraint has rather dramatically decreased the loosening rate of these devices[26, 88, 89] (Fig. 105–17).

Finally, whether or not a prosthesis should be selected based on the option to replace the radial head is speculative. Theoretically, although the radiohumeral joint does distribute the forces to the distal humerus, particularly in extension,[15] most clinicians feel that the articulation is of no value and may be ignored in joint replacement.[6, 82] At this time, it is sufficient to be aware that its advantages are theoretical.

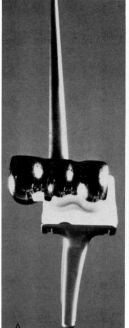
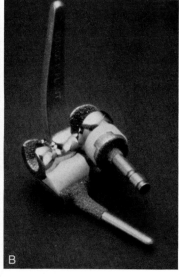

Figure 105–15. Examples of two resurfacing devices currently available in the United States: the capitello condylar (A) and the three-part biologically fixed device designed by Pritchard (B).

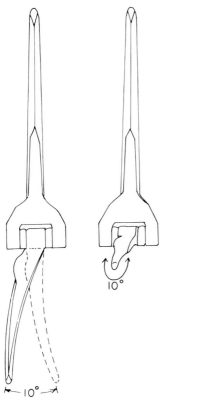

Figure 105–16. The semiconstrained articulated device allows about 10 degrees of rotation laxity at the articulation.

Postoperative Management

If the viability of the skin is of concern, as occurs in a previously operated, post-traumatic patient, or a steroid-dependent rheumatoid arthritic, a cast may be necessary for a period of time to allow adequate skin healing. This has not been necessary in the last 5 years, since the elbow is splinted in extension. Generally, however, elbow motion is allowed as tolerated, and strengthening exercises are avoided. Most patients spontaneously attain an arc of motion of about 50 to 110 degrees after about 10 to 14 days with increasing demands of daily living. Motion of 40 to 120 degrees is typical at 3 weeks, and little motion is gained after 3 months. Physical therapy is not used and is not necessary for this patient. Generalized swelling is rather common during this period of time, but this gradually resolves over a 3- to 6-month period, allowing further motion improvement.

RESULTS

Detailed long-term results of both resurfacing and semiconstrained arthroplasty are still emerging.[26, 71, 72, 77, 78, 81–87, 90–92]

Careful scrutiny of the results with respect to pain, function, and motion has failed to demonstrate

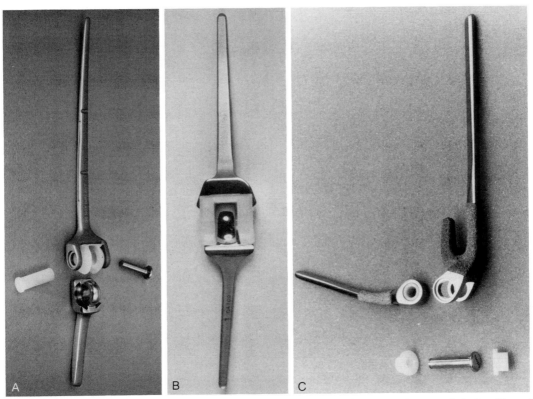

Figure 105–17. Commonly used semiconstrained devices include the Pritchard Mark II (A), the triaxial device (B), and the Mayo modified Coonrad III (C).

a clear superiority of one group of prostheses over the other. Thus, selection continues to be based on the surgeon's experience, indications, and potential complications rather than superiority of design or function.

Relief of Pain

Typically, over 90 percent of patients with either the resurfacing or semiconstrained device note virtually complete relief of pain, which is consistent with any of the total joint replacements involving metal and high-density polyethylene. The presence of pain is almost always associated with loosening, subluxation, primary or secondary (reactive) synovitis, or infection.

Motion

For both classifications of devices, a mean functional arc of flexion is almost universally reported, averaging about 30 to 130 degrees. It has been noticed that a moderately greater flexion contracture is present after the resurfacing device, averaging close to 50 degrees, in the earlier experience of some investigators.[93] To help ensure stability, extension past 45 degrees is restricted after a resurfacing arthroplasty. This may contribute further to extension loss.

Forearm rotation averages greater than 60 degrees pronation and 60 degrees supination, again, generally independent of the design. Based on the reports to date, the postoperative motion correlates most closely to the preoperative state of the soft tissue. The mean motion observed is thus adequate for most activities of daily living.

Stability

Stability is not a problem after joint replacement with a hinged device (Fig. 105–18). It has been estimated that at least 1 million flexion-extension cycles are imparted to the elbow each year.[94] Thus, snap-fit designs have been associated with some uncoupling, usually after several years of use.[85, 89] Subluxation and dislocation are all problems inherent with resurfacing devices and will be discussed later.

Strength

Little has been written about postoperative strength after joint replacement. My experience with both resurfacing and semiconstrained devices followed for at least a year demonstrates a 75 percent improvement of overall strength after joint replacement.[28] Consistent improvement is noted in all functions, flexion, extension, pronation, and supination,

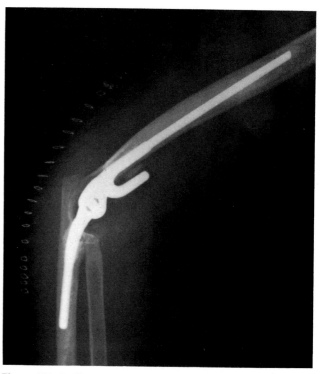

Figure 105–18. Extensive joint changes and instability from grade 4 rheumatoid arthritis shown in Figure 105–6B treated with a Mayo modified Coonrad (III) device.

with the exception of extension strength, with a mean of no improvement after joint replacement. This is to be expected, since much of the weakness before surgery is felt to be due to reflex inhibition caused by pain and pain relief is consistently observed in these patients. Lack of extension strength improvement probably relates to the surgical exposures, which all violate the triceps in some fashion to expose the joint.

COMPLICATIONS

It is of historical interest only that complications after total elbow arthroplasty excluding loosening have been reported in up to 59 percent of patients (Fig. 105–19).[91, 95] The elbow is a complex, subcutaneous joint prone to involvement of rheumatoid and post-traumatic arthritis. Both of these operative diagnoses are known to have a higher rate of complication with other joint replacements as well.[95, 96]

Infection

Deep infection is more common after elbow replacement than probably any other joint.[23] The frequency of this complication is as high as 11 percent in some reports. The explanation for this high infection rate may be that the elbow is a subcutaneous joint, often with previous surgery involving a group

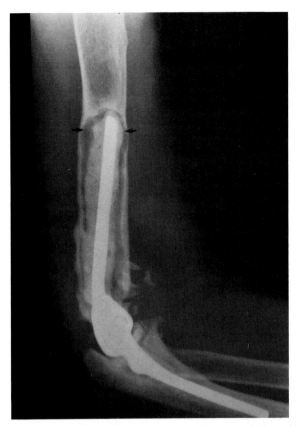

Figure 105–19. Early model of a rigid, fully constrained elbow that has loosened; a fracture has occurred at the proximal humerus.

of patients already at risk for infection.[95] The incidence seems to be reduced by the use of antibiotic-impregnated cement.[26] Souter reported only one infection after over 100 procedures using this adjunctive measure.[93] I have had no infection in patients after approximately 50 consecutive procedures since antibiotics have been added to the cement, and overall my rate is now about 3 percent.[26]

Neurapraxia

The ulnar nerve is particularly vulnerable at the elbow, and the incidence of ulnar nerve involvement after surgery has averaged about 7 percent.[87–90, 93, 95] The etiology of this complication involves several factors, including excessive traction, exposure trauma, perineural hematoma, mechanical pressure, possibly thermal damage from the polymethylmethacrylate, or even translocation causing a devascularization or constriction. The subclinical neuropathy that occasionally occurs with patients with rheumatoid arthritis might be aggravated at the time of a surgical procedure. Recent experience is more encouraging. Davis et al. reported no evidence of neurapraxia after the lateral Kocher approach,[74] and I have had only one episode of residual partial neuropathy after over 100 medial approaches with nerve translocation.

Triceps Insufficiency

Although triceps rupture or inadequacy has been reported as often as 7 percent in the early experience,[71, 73, 90, 95, 97] the triceps reflection technique employing either the Kocher or the Mayo exposure has all but eliminated triceps deficiency as a major complication of elbow joint replacement. The study of strength after total elbow arthroplasty shows a mean extension strength that is virtually identical to the preoperative stage.[28] Most patients with rheumatoid arthritis demonstrate some improvement of extension strength, but in those with traumatic conditions, some diminution of this function is observed.

Wound Healing

Wound healing has been a problem in 3 to 5 percent of patients.[95] Yet 75 percent of these required no additional surgical procedure. In our first 125 cases, poor wound healing or hematoma formation required additional surgery on only 3 patients. Careful handling of the tissues, well-designed incisions, and placing the elbow into extension with an anterior splint with proper hemostasis and drainage are helpful adjuncts to avoid this problem. I have had no major wound problems in a series of 70 consecutive replacements for rheumatoid arthritis.[26]

Fractures

Intraoperative or postoperative fractures do occur with total elbow arthroplasty (see Fig. 105–19). Cortex penetration is associated with using stemmed devices during revision procedures. Post-traumatic fracture of the humerus has been identified in 2 of 36 patients with the triaxial semiconstrained prosthesis and in 1 of 69 after a surfacing procedure. Four of 35 patients with a Pritchard implant were also noticed to have post-traumatic fracture of the humerus occurring just above the stem.[95] These fractures develop because of the compromised quality of the bone or from the stress concentration caused by notching of the cortex during preparation. Rapid change of the elastic modulus between the composite acrylic cement prosthesis and bone is an additional feature that predisposes to fracture. A loose humeral prosthesis may also cause cortical resorption and is a recognized cause of subsequent fracture of the humerus or, less commonly, the ulna.

Loosening

Loosening occurred in 25 percent or more patients within 3 years after implantation of the constrained hinged device that was used during the third stage of elbow reconstructive surgery development.[6, 70, 97, 98] This complication has been dramatically lessened with the resurfacing devices and the semi-constrained hinged devices that are currently being used during the fourth stage of elbow reconstructive surgery.[99] With the so-called sloppy hinge allowing varying amounts of axial rotation and varus-valgus play, averaging about 7 to 10 degrees in each plane, the loosening rate has been reduced to less than 3 percent with a mean of 5 years' follow-up.[6, 26] Proper patient selection and a more enlightened cement technique have probably also contributed to the improved results (Fig. 105–20).

Instability

Instability is a unique complication of the resurfacing or snap-fit implants. Dislocation or subluxation of resurfacing designs usually present soon after surgery. Inadequate soft tissue balance either from the collateral ligaments or dynamically from the pull of the triceps is the basic cause of this complication (Fig. 105–21). Further, some resurfacing devices are more stable than others owing to the design constraints. Currently, 5 to 15 percent subluxation or dislocation continues to be reported after the various resurfacing options.[71, 78, 79, 81–84, 90] My experience with the capitellar condylar design has produced 7 of 49 (14 percent) with instability and continues to pose a problem in my clinical practice. This incidence of instability is in sharp contrast to the less than 5 percent of Ewald and associates.[100] This again underscores the precise technical requirements of elbow replacement surgery.

The snap-fit articulation provides inherent stability at the time of surgery. However, with cyclic loads that may reach a million cycles per year[94] and

with the significant forces that are known to cross the elbow joint, wear of the high-density polyethylene is a theoretical possibility. This occurrence has been reported by Figgie et al.[92]

SALVAGE OF THE FAILED JOINT REPLACEMENT

Treatment

Several treatment options may be considered to salvage a failed elbow arthroplasty.[101] These include arthrodesis, resection, interposition, and reinsertion.

Loose resurfacing or semiconstrained devices may be revised to a semiconstrained design (Fig. 105–22). Deficiencies of technique and prosthesis selection should be considered and corrected with revision surgery. At my institution, the reimplantation revision procedure using first generation implants was effective in 60 percent at 5 years.[89] A second revision was performed for loosening of the initial revision operation, and at the time of review, a satisfactory rate of 80 percent was observed in the group of 35 patients undergoing revision surgery. In recent years, we have found that the semiconstrained Mayo modified Coonrad prosthesis with the flange to control rotation and posterior displacement is an effective revision device. With this design, supplemental bone grafting is also possible. To date, I have encountered no progressive lucency nor has their been a second revision among ten patients in whom this device was employed as a revision implant in the last 5 years.[102]

The success, therefore, of the revision post-trauma and rheumatoid patient using the present

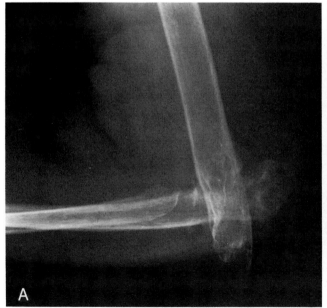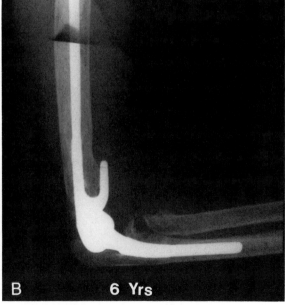

Figure 105–20. Grossly unstable and subluxed joint in patient with rheumatoid arthritis *(A)*. Six-year result of semiconstrained implant showing no sign of loosening *(B)*. (By permission of Mayo Foundation.)

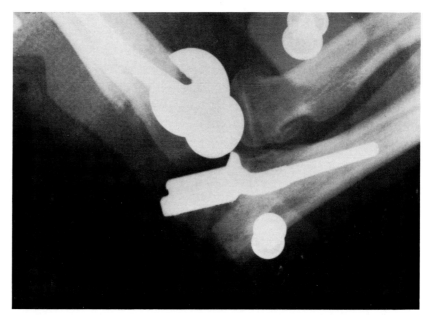

Figure 105–21. Unstable Pritchard resurfacing arthroplasty. This joint remained unstable and required revision.

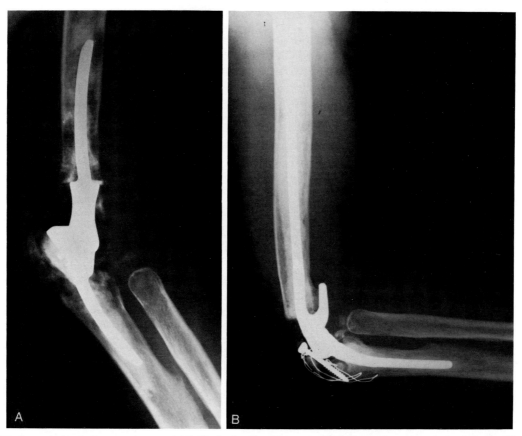

Figure 105–22. A constrained elbow replacement *(A)*. Revised with a Mayo modified Coonrad semiconstrained device *(B)*. At 3 years, the patient had no pain and 20 to 135 degrees of motion.

KAPLAN-MEIER SURVIVAL CURVE
Mayo-Modified Coonrad Elbow Replacement

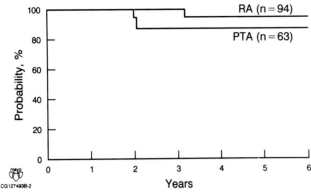

CG127493B-2

Figure 105–23. Kaplan Meier survival curves for the Mayo modified elbow replacement. (By permission of Mayo Foundation.)

implant since 1981 is shown in Figure 105–23 using the Kaplan Meier survival analysis technique.

REHABILITATION

Several principles dictate the proper approach for elbow rehabilitation regardless of the reconstructive procedure.

1. Avoidance of inflammation. This is probably the single most important aspect of the rehabilitation program. Overaggressive active or passive motion or strength exercises can elicit an inflammatory response followed by soft tissue scarring, which will not only retard the rehabilitation program and lengthen the period of disability but may compromise the result as well.

2. Early motion. With relatively few exceptions, early motion is a principal goal of the rehabilitation program. A recent helpful adjunct to obtain this goal has been the use of continuous motion machines (Fig. 105–24). Continuous motion for approximately a week after reconstructive elbow surgery generally is effective in allowing the person to continue motion while at home. An additional major adjunctive measure to the surgical technique allowing early motion is the employment of a triceps-sparing approach. Either a modified extensile Kocher approach or the Mayo posteromedial approach allows extensive joint exposure with reattachment of the triceps mechanism that allows immediate active and passive motion.

3. Splints. An increasing variety and use of splints have enhanced elbow rehabilitation over the last 5 years (Fig. 105–25).[103] A static splint, usually of

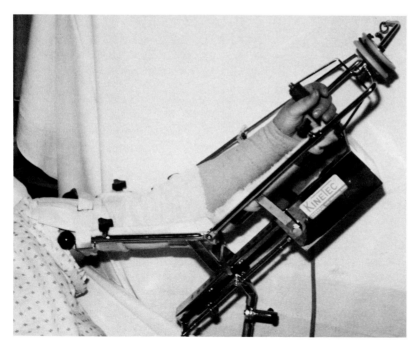

Figure 105–24. Continuous motion machine used for hospitalized patients after elbow reconstruction in which loss of motion is a potential complication or restoring motion has been a goal of surgery.

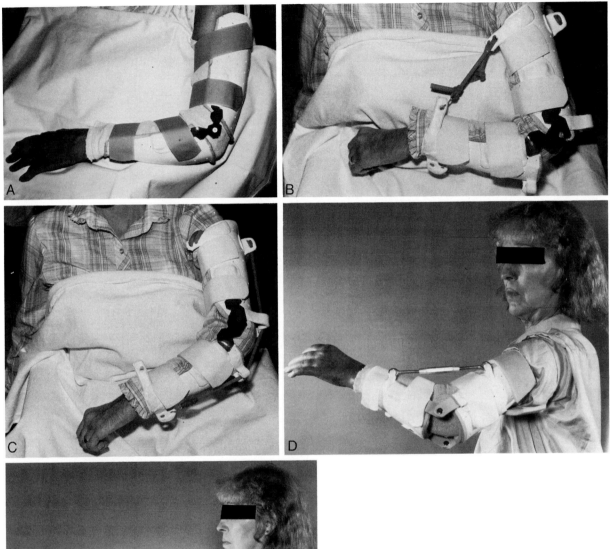

Figure 105–25. Array of splints used in the rehabilitation program. *A,* Resting splint. *B,* Simple hinge splint. *C,* Dynamic flexion splint. *D,* Dynamic extension splint. *E,* Turnbuckle flexion splint. *F,* Turnbuckle extension splint.

a heat-sensitive molded plastic, is fabricated for that person requiring immobilization for several weeks, such as after fracture or to ensure joint stability. Dynamic splints, both in extension and flexion, are quite useful in maintaining elbow motion that has been obtained at surgery. These are most helpful after total elbow arthroplasty and are generally used for 1 to 3 months, depending on the patient's progress. Turnbuckle splints are employed most often after arthroplasty of a previously ankylosed elbow. After the external fixator (distraction apparatus) is removed, the patient is placed in flexion and extension turnbuckle splints.

References

1. Boone, D. C., and Azen, S. P.: Normal range of motion in the joint in male subjects. J. Bone Joint Surg. 61A:756, 1979.
2. London, J. T.: Kinematics of the elbow. J. Bone Joint Surg. 63A:529, 1981.
3. Morrey, B. F., and Chao, E. Y. S.: Passive motion of the elbow joint. A biomechanical analysis. J. Bone Joint Surg. 58A:501, 1976.
4. Deland, J. T., Walker, P. S., Sledge, C. B., and Farberov, A.: Treatment of post-traumatic elbows with a new hinge-distractor. Orthopedics 6:732, 1983.
5. Morrey, B. F.: Treatment of the posttraumatic stiff elbow, including distraction arthroplasty. J. Bone Joint Surg. 72A:601, 1990.
6. Morrey, B. F.: Total elbow arthroplasty. In Morrey, B. F. (ed.): The Elbow and Its Disorders. Philadelphia, W. B. Saunders Company, 1985.
7. Morrey, B. F., and An, K. N.: Articular and ligamentous contributions to the stability of the elbow joint. Am. J. Sports Med. 11:315, 1983.
8. Schwab, G. H., Bennett, J. B., Woods, G. W., and Tullos, H. S.: Biomechanics of elbow instability: The role of the medial collateral ligament. Clin. Orthop. 146:42, 1980.
9. Morrey, B. F., and An, K. N.: Functional anatomy of the ligaments of the elbow. Clin. Orthop. 201:84, 1985.
10. O'Driscoll, S., Bell, D., and Morrey, B. F.: The pivot shift test for recurrent subluxation of the elbow. J. Bone Joint Surg. 73A:440, 1991.
11. Hotchkiss, R. N., and Weiland, A. J.: Valgus stability of the elbow. Second Annual Meeting, AAOS, New Orleans, LA, February 19, 1986.
12. Pribyl, C. R., Kester, M. A., Cook, S. D., and Brunct, M. E.: The effect of the radial head and prosthetic radial head replacements on resisting valgus stress of the elbow. Second Annual Meeting, AAOS, New Orleans, LA, February 19, 1986.
13. Morrey, B. F., Tanaka, H., and An, K. N.: Valgus stability of the elbow. Definition of primary and secondary constraints. Clin. Orthop. 265:187, 1991.
14. Pearson, J. R., McGinley, D. R., and Butzel, L. M.: A dynamic analysis of the upper extremity. Planar motions. Hum. Factors 5:59, 1963.
15. Amis, A. A., Miller, J. H., Dowson, D., and Wright, V.: Biomechanical aspects of the elbow. Joint forces related to prosthesis design. Eng. Med. 10:65, 1981.
16. Halls, A. A., and Travill, A.: Transmission of pressures across the elbow joint. Anat. Rec. 150:243, 1964.
17. Walker, P. S.: Human Joints and Their Artificial Replacements. Springfield, IL, Charles C Thomas, 1977.
18. Morrey, B. F., An, K. N., and Stormont, T.: Force transmission across the radial head: An experimental study. J. Bone Joint Surg. 70A:250, 1988.
19. Amis, A. A., Hughes, S. J., Miller, J. H., and Wright, Z.: A functional study of the rheumatoid elbow. Rheum. Rehab. 21:151, 1982.
20. O'Neill, O., An, K. N., and Morrey, B. F.: Compensatory shoulder motion after elbow arthrodesis. Clin. Orthop. (in press).
21. Morrey, B. F., Askew, L. J., An, K. N., and Chao, E. Y.: A biomechanical study of normal functional elbow motion. J. Bone Joint Surg. 63A:872, 1981.
22. Askew, L., Morrey, B. F., and An, K. N.: Isometric strength patterns of the normal elbow. Clin. Orthop. 222:261, 1987.
23. Morrey, B. F., and Bryan, R. S.: Infection after total elbow arthroplasty. J. Bone Joint Surg. 65A(3):330, 1983.
24. Inglis, A. E., Ranawat, C. S., and Straub, L. R.: Synovectomy and debridement of the elbow in rheumatoid arthritis. J. Bone Joint Surg. 53A:652, 1971.
25. Steinbrocker, O., Traeger, C. H., and Batterman, R. C.: Therapeutic criteria in rheumatoid arthritis. J.A.M.A. 140:659, 1949.
26. Morrey, B. F., and Adams, R. A.: Treatment of semiconstrained

27. Kashiwagi, D.: Osteoarthritis of the elbow. In Elbow Joint—Excerpts. International Congress Series 678:177, 1985.
28. Morrey, B. F., Askew, L., and An, K. N.: Strength function after total elbow arthroplasty. Clin. Orthop. 234:49, 1988.
29. Schuller, M.: Die pathologie und therapie des gelenkentzundunger. Vienna, Urban und Schwarzenberg, 1887.
30. Smith-Peterson, M. N., Aufranc, O. E., and Larson, C. B.: Useful surgical procedures for rheumatoid arthritis involving joints of the upper extremity. Arch. Surg. 47B:482, 1965.
31. Laine, V., and Vainio, K.: Synovectomy of the elbow. In Hijmans, W., Paul, W. D., and Herschel, H. (eds.): Early Synovectomy in Rheumatoid Arthritis. Amsterdam, Exc. Med. Found., 1969.
32. Torgerson, W. R., and Leach, R. E.: Synovectomy of the elbow in rheumatoid arthritis. J. Bone Joint Surg. 52A:371, 1970.
33. Marmor, L.: Surgery of the rheumatoid elbow. J. Bone Joint Surg. 54A:573, 1972.
34. Porter, B. B., Richardson, C., and Vainio, K.: Rheumatoid arthritis of the elbow: The results of synovectomy. J. Bone Joint Surg. 56B:427, 1974.
35. Taylor, A. R., Mukerjia, S. K., and Rana, N. A.: Excision of the head of the radius in rheumatoid arthritis. J. Bone Joint Surg. 58B:485, 1976.
36. Ferlic, D. C., Clayton, M. L., and Parr, P. L.: Surgery of the elbow in rheumatoid arthritis. J. Bone Joint Surg. 58A:726, 1976.
37. Peterson, L. F. A., and Jones, J. M.: Surgery of the rheumatoid elbow. Orthop. Clin. North Am. 2:667, 1971.
38. Wilson, D. W., Arden, G. P., and Ansell, B. M.: Surgery of the elbow in rheumatoid arthritis. J. Bone Joint Surg. 55B:106, 1973.
39. Swanson, A. B.: Flexible implant resection arthroplasty in the hand and extremities. St. Louis, C. V. Mosby Company, 1973, p. 275.
40. Morrey, B. F., Askew, L., and Chao, E. Y.: Silastic prosthetic replacement for the radial head. J. Bone Joint Surg. 63A:454, 1981.
41. Mayhall, W. S. T., Tilley, F. T., and Paluska, D. J.: Fractures of silastic radial head prostheses. J. Bone Joint Surg. 63A:459, 1981.
42. Worsing, R. A., Engber, W. D., and Lange, T. A.: Reactive synovitis from particulate silastic. J. Bone Joint Surg. 64A:581, 1982.
43. Ewald, F. C.: Reconstructive surgery and rehabilitation of the elbow. In Kelley, W. N., Harris, E. D., Jr., Ruddy, S., and Sledge, C. B. (eds.): Textbook of Rheumatology, 2nd ed. Philadelphia, W. B. Saunders Company, 1985, pp. 1838–1853.
44. McDougall, A., and White, J.: Subluxation of the inferior radio-ulnar joint complicating fracture of the radial head. J. Bone Joint Surg. 39B:278, 1957.
45. Odenneimer, K., and Harvey, P. J.: Internal fixation of fractures of the head of the radius. J. Bone Joint Surg. 61A:785, 1979.
46. Heim, U., and Trub, H. J.: Erfahrungen mit der primaren osteosynthese von radius-kopfchenfrakturen. Helv. Chir. Acta 45:63, 1978.
47. Perry, C. R., and Tessier, J. E.: Open reduction and internal fixation of radial head fractures associated with olecranon fractures or dislocation. J. Orthop. Trauma 1:36, 1987.
48. Gartsman, G. M., Sculco, T. P., and Otis, J. C.: Operative treatment of olecranon fractures. J. Bone Joint Surg. 63A:718, 1981.
49. MacAusland, W. R.: Mobilization of the elbow by free fascia transplantation with report of thirty-one cases. Surg. Gynecol. Obstet. 23:223, 1921.
50. Cabanela, M. E.: Fractures of the olecranon. In Morrey, B. F. (ed.): The Elbow and Its Disorders. W. B. Saunders Company, 1985.
51. London, J.: Custom arthroplasty and hemiarthroplasty of the elbow. In Morrey, B. F. (ed.): The Elbow and Its Disorders. W. B. Saunders Company, 1985.
52. Urbaniak, J. R., and Black, K. E.: Cadaveric elbow allografts: A six year experience. Clin. Orthop. 197:131, 1985.
53. Barr, J. S., and Eaton, R. G.: Elbow reconstruction with a new prosthesis to replace the distal end of the humerus. A case report. J. Bone Joint Surg. 47A:1408, 1965.
54. Mellen, R. H., and Phalen, G. S.: Arthroplasty of the elbow by replacement of the distal portion of the humerus with an acrylic prosthesis. J. Bone Joint Surg. 29:348, 1947.
55. Robineau, R.: Contribution a l'étude des prostheses osseuses. Bull. Mim. Soc. Nat. Chir. 53:886, 1927.
56. Venable, C. S.: An elbow and elbow prosthesis. Case of complete loss of the lower third of the humerus. Am. J. Surg. 83:271, 1952.
57. MacAusland, W. R.: Replacement of the lower end of the humerus with a prosthesis. A report of four cases. West. J. Surg. Gynecol. Obstet. 62:557, 1954.
58. Street, D. M., and Stevens, P. S.: A humeral replacement prosthesis for the elbow. J. Bone Joint Surg. 56A:1147, 1974.
59. Campbell, W. C.: Arthroplasty of the elbow. Ann. Surg. 76:615, 1922.
60. Henderson, M. S.: Arthroplasty. Minn. Med. 8:97, 1925.
61. Wright, P. E., and Stuart, M. J.: Fascial arthroplasty of the elbow. In Morrey, B. F. (ed.): The Elbow and Its Disorders. W. B. Saunders Company, 1985.
62. Hurri, L., Pulkki, T., and Vainio, K.: Arthroplasty of the elbow in rheumatoid arthritis. Acta Chir. Scand. 127:459, 1964.

63. Silva, F. J.: Arthroplasty of the elbow. Singapore Med. J. 8:222, 1967.
64. Knight, R. A., and Van Zandt, I. L.: Arthroplasty of the elbow. An end result study. J. Bone Joint Surg. 34A:610, 1952.
65. Gui, L.: La cura chirugica delle rigidita post-traumatic del gomito e del gonocchio. Arch. Putti. 3:390, 1953.
66. Fromison, A. J., Silva, J. E., and Richey, D. G.: Cutis arthroplasty of the elbow joint. J. Bone Joint Surg. 58A:863, 1976.
67. Volkov, M. V., and Oganesian, O. V.: Restoration of function in the knee and the elbow with the hinged-distractor apparatus. J. Bone Joint Surg. 75A:591, 1975.
68. Coonrad, R. W.: History of total elbow arthroplasty. In Inglis, A. E. (ed.): Upper Extremity Joint Replacement. Symposium on total joint replacement of the upper extremity. St. Louis, C. V. Mosby Company, 1982, pp. 75–90.
69. Bryan, R. S.: Total replacement of the elbow joint. Arch. Surg. 112:1092, 1977.
70. Dee, R.: Total replacement arthroplasty of the elbow for rheumatoid arthritis. J. Bone Joint Surg. 54B:88, 1972.
71. Ewald, F. C., Scheinberg, R. D., Poss, R., Thomas, W. H., Scott, R. D., and Sledge, C. B.: Capitellocondylar total elbow arthroplasty: Two to five year follow-up in rheumatoid arthritis. J. Bone Joint Surg. 62A:1259, 1980.
72. Kudo, H., Iwano, K., and Watanabe, S.: Total replacement of the rheumatoid elbow with a hingeless prosthesis. J. Bone Joint Surg. 62A:277, 1980.
73. Inglis, A. E., and Pellicci, P. M.: Total elbow replacement. J. Bone Joint Surg. 62A:1252, 1980.
74. Davis, R. F., Weiland, A. J., Hungerford, D. S., Moore, J. R., and Dowling, S. V.: Nonconstrained total elbow arthroplasty. CORR 171:156, 1982.
75. Morrey, B. F., and Bryan, R. S.: Total elbow arthroplasty. In Morrey, B. F. (ed.): The Elbow and Its Disorders. Philadelphia, W. B. Saunders Company, 1985.
76. Bryan, R. S., and Morrey, B. F.: Rheumatoid arthritis of the elbow. In Evarts, C. M. (ed.): Surgery of the Musculoskeletal System. London, Churchill Livingstone, 1983.
77. Morrey, B. F., Adams, R. A., and Bryan, R. S.: Total replacement for post-traumatic arthritis of the elbow. J. Bone Joint Surg. 73B:607, 1991.
78. Souter, W. A.: A new approach to elbow arthroplasty. Eng. Med. 10:59, 1981.
79. Cavendish, M. E., and Elloy, M. A.: A simple method of total elbow replacement. In: Joint Replacement in the Upper Extremity. London, Mechanical Engineering Publications, 1981, p. 93.
80. London, J. T.: Resurfacing total elbow arthroplasty. Presentation, AAOS annual meeting, Atlanta, February, 1980.
81. Lowe, L. W., Miller, A. J., Allum, R. L., and Higginson, D. W.: The development of an unconstrained elbow arthroplasty: A clinical review. J. Bone Joint Surg. 66B:243, 1984.
82. Tuke, M. A.: The ICLH elbow. Eng. Med. 10:75, 1981.
83. Wadsworth, T. G.: A new technique of total elbow replacement. Eng. Med. 10:75, 1981.
84. Weiland, A. J., Weiss, A. P. C., Wills, R. P., and Moore, J. R.: Capitellocondylar total elbow replacement. J. Bone Joint Surg. 71A:217, 1989.
85. Volz, R. G.: Total elbow arthroplasty. AAOS course: The Upper Extremity. Tucson, AZ, February, 1983.
86. Schlein, A. P.: Semiconstrained total elbow arthroplasty. Clin. Orthop. 121:222, 1976.
87. Pritchard, R. W.: Long-term follow-up study: Semiconstrained elbow prosthesis. Orthopedics 4:151, 1981.
88. Gschwend, N., Loehr, J., and Ivosevic-Radovanovic, D.: Die Ellbogen-Arthroplastik. Orthopäde 17:366, 1988.
89. Figgie, H. E. III, Inglis, A. E., and Mow, C.: Total elbow arthroplasty in the face of significant bone stock or soft tissue losses: Preliminary results of custom-fit arthroplasty. J. Arthroplasty 1:71, 1986.
90. Rosenberg, G. M., and Turner, R. H.: Nonconstrained total elbow arthroplasty. CORR 187:154, 1984.
91. Rosenfeld, S. R., and Anzel, S. H.: Evaluation of the Pritchard total elbow arthroplasty. Orthopedics 5:713, 1982.
92. Figgie, H., and Inglis, A. E.: Long-term experience with the triaxial total elbow arthroplasty. AAOS Open Meeting, San Francisco, CA, January 25, 1987.
93. Souter, W. A., Nicol, A. C., and Paul, J. P.: Souter-Strothclyde arthroplasty of the elbow. Presented at SICOT. London, October, 1984.
94. Davis, P. R.: Some significant aspects of normal upper limb functions. Conference on joint replacement of the upper extremity. London, Institute of Mechanical Engineers, 1977.
95. Morrey, B. F.: Complications of total elbow arthroplasty. In Morrey, B. F. (ed.): Joint Replacement Arthroplasty. New York, Churchill Livingstone, 1991.
96. Fitzgerald, R. H., Jr., Nolan, D. R., Ilstrup, D. M., Van Scoy, R. E., Washington, J. A. II, and Coventry, M. B.: Deep wound sepsis following total elbow arthroplasty. J. Bone Joint Surg 59A:847, 1977.
97. Morrey, B. F., Bryan, R. S., Dobyns, J. H., and Linscheid, R. L.: A five-year experience at the Mayo Clinic. J. Bone Joint Surg. 63A:1050, 1981.
98. Garrett, J. C., Ewald, F. C., Thomas, W. H., and Sledge, C. B.: Loosening associated with GSB hinge total elbow replacement in patients with rheumatoid arthritis. CORR 127:170, 1977.
99. Linscheid, R.: Results of resurfacing total elbow arthroplasty. In Morrey, B. F. (ed.): Joint Replacement Arthroplasty. New York, Churchill Livingstone, 1991.
100. Ewald, F.: Personal communication, January, 1987.
101. Morrey, B. F. and Bryan, R. S.: Revision total elbow arthroplasty. J. Bone Joint Surg. 69A:523, 1987.
102. Morrey, B. F.: Revision of failed total elbow arthroplasty. In Morrey, B. F. (ed.): Joint Replacement Arthroplasty. New York, Churchill Livingstone, 1991.
103. Morrey, B. F.: The use of splints for the stiff elbow. Perspect. Orthop. Surg. 1:141, 1990.

The Cervical Spine

RHEUMATOID ARTHRITIS

Cervical spine abnormalities in rheumatoid arthritis (RA) are the result of destruction of joints, ligaments, and bone by synovitis. Subluxations are consequent, the anatomy of which is determined by the structures involved. Clinical abnormalities are apparent as pain in the affected parts of the spine and neurologic abnormalities from distortion and compression of the spinal cord, roots, and vertebral artery due to subluxation and proliferative synovitic tissues. Clinical involvement in cervical spine RA was first described by Garrod in 1890.[1] Subluxation, especially at the atlantoaxial junction, in inflammatory arthritis was described later. Medullary compression from atlantoaxial subluxation was first described by Davis and Markley.[2]

Management of these problems is through recognition and definition of the affected anatomy, determination of the natural history of the disease, use of appropriate imaging methods, and selection of surgical intervention if indicated.

Pathophysiology of Subluxations. Rheumatoid synovitis causes ligamentous distention and rupture, articular cartilage destruction, and, in bone, osteoporosis, cyst formation, and erosion. Cells obtained from the tissues biopsied at the time of cervical surgery are the same array of inflammatory cells known peripherally.[3]

The activity of RA in the cervical spine appears to begin early in the disease and progresses in relation to peripheral involvement. In a radiologic prospective study of 100 patients, 83 percent of patients with anterior atlantoaxial subluxation developed it within 2 years of disease onset.[4] Cervical spine subluxation has been shown to correlate with damage to the metacarpophalangeal and carpal joints.[5] The severity of cervical damage strongly correlates with that of peripheral erosive disease, and subluxation is more likely in those patients with progressive peripheral erosions.[6] In summary, factors correlating with the progression of atlantoaxial subluxation (AAS) are a history of medical therapy with glucocorticoids, seropositivity, the presence of rheumatoid subcutaneous nodules, and the presence of erosive and mutilating articular disease; male patients are more frequently affected.[4, 7–10]

Anatomy of Subluxations. Rheumatoid destruction leads to instability and subluxation. Atlantoaxial subluxation is a consequence of erosive synovitis in the atlantoaxial, atlanto-odontoid, and atlanto-occip-

ital joints as well as the synovium-lined bursa between the odontoid and the transverse ligament. AAS can be anterior, posterior, and lateral. Anterior AAS is most commonly noted (Fig. 106–1). In postmortem studies, it was found in 11 to 46 percent of cases.[7, 11–13] Atlantoaxial stability is dependent on the transverse, alar, and apical ligaments. Anterior subluxation of more than 10 to 12 mm implies destruction of the entire ligamentous complex.[14] Most anterior AASs in RA are of this magnitude. An atlantodental distance of greater than 3.5 mm is considered abnormal in an adult. Forty-three to 86 percent of RA patients exhibit subluxations,[15–17] and, in particular, anterior AAS has been found in 19 to 71 percent of patients surveyed.[9, 16, 18–21]

Posterior AAS occurs infrequently and accounted for 6.7 percent of all AAS in one series.[10] Erosion and/or fracture of the odontoid is the commonest anatomic factor predisposing to posterior AAS,[22] and it had been thought to be a more benign subluxation, but cord compression has been reported to result.[22–28] A series on myelopathy associated with posterior AAS suggested that a configurational abnormality of kyphotic kinking of the high spinal cord may be responsible for the myelopathy.[22]

Lateral AAS can be visualized and defined as more than 2 mm of subluxation of the lateral masses of C1 on C2. Rotational deformity probably accompanies it. Although reported,[29] its incidence is probably underestimated. One series found lateral AAS to account for 21 percent of all AAS.[10] Nonreducible head tilt was found in up to 10 percent of a rheumatoid population, frequently with other deformities combined with lateral AAS.[30] Lateral AAS has been found more commonly in those patients with spinal cord compression than in those without it.[5]

Atlantoaxial impaction (AAI), also known as cranial settling, pseudobasilar invagination, and vertical subluxation of the axis (Fig. 106–2), is a consequence of bone and cartilage loss from the occipitoatlantal and atlantoaxial joints (Fig. 106–3). AAI is found in 5 to 32 percent of rheumatoid patients surveyed[5, 17, 18, 31] and accounted for 22 percent of all upper cervical subluxations.[10] AAI has been measured in a variety of ways,[18] with McGregor's line, the distance of the tip of the odontoid above a line from the hard palate to the occiput on a lateral view[10] (Fig. 106–4), probably the most traditional. Ranawat and colleagues[32] defined a more useful index that relies on the actual settling of C1 on C2. This index avoids the difficulty of defining the hard palate, often

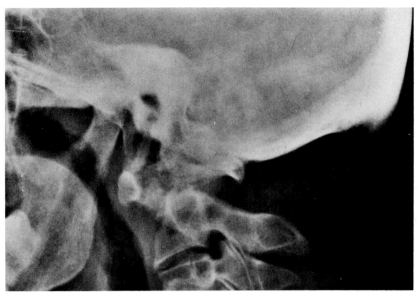

Figure 106–1. Rheumatoid arthritis with forward displacement of the atlas. The odontoid process is in the center of the C1 ring. (From Fielding, J. W.: Rheumatoid arthritis of the cervical spine. *In* The American Academy of Orthopaedic Surgeons: Instructional Course Lectures. Vol. XXXII. St. Louis, C. V. Mosby Co., 1983. Used by permission.)

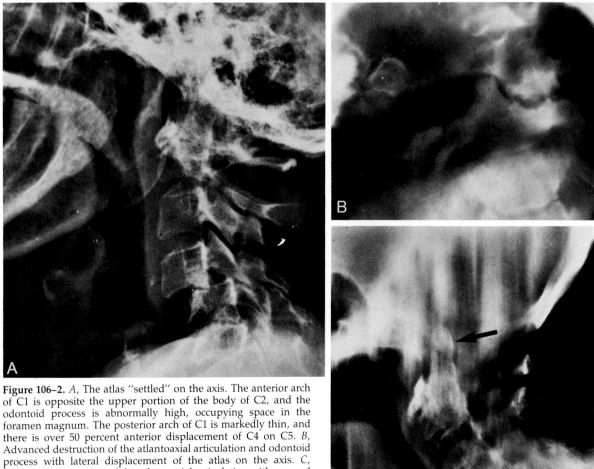

Figure 106–2. *A,* The atlas "settled" on the axis. The anterior arch of C1 is opposite the upper portion of the body of C2, and the odontoid process is abnormally high, occupying space in the foramen magnum. The posterior arch of C1 is markedly thin, and there is over 50 percent anterior displacement of C4 on C5. *B,* Advanced destruction of the atlantoaxial articulation and odontoid process with lateral displacement of the atlas on the axis. *C,* Advanced destruction of the atlantoaxial articulation with upward displacement of the odontoid. (*A* and *B,* From Fielding, J. W.: Rheumatoid arthritis of the cervical spine. *In* The American Academy of Orthopaedic Surgeons: Instructional Course Lectures. Vol. XXXII. St. Louis, C. V. Mosby Co., 1983. Courtesy of Harvey L. Barish, M.D.)

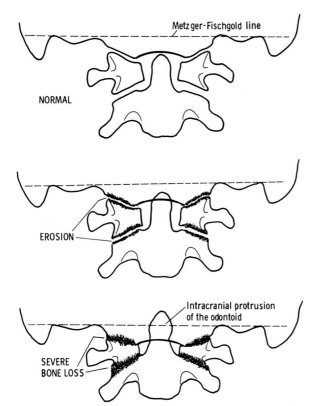

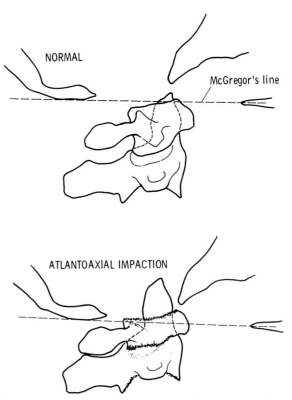

Figure 106–3. Stages in destruction of the atlantoaxial articulation with resultant settling of the skull and upward displacement of the odontoid process into the foramen magnum. Fischgold and Metzger's line (a line drawn between the two digastric grooves on the anteroposterior laminogram of the skull) will pass well above the odontoid tip (10.7 mm). It can be used to determine the degree of upper displacement of the odontoid process. (From Fischgold, H., and Metzger, J.: Etude radiotomographique de l'impression basilaire. Rev. Rhum. Mal. Osteoartic. 19:261, 1952.)

not included in the radiograph, and the eroded odontoid. The Redlund-Johnell method[31] utilizes McGregor's cranial landmark relationship to C2 as in Ranawat's method.

The subaxial cervical spine (Fig. 106–5) is affected through involvement of the facets, interspinous ligaments, and intervertebral discs (spondylodiscitis). The initial site of destruction has been postulated to be through synovitis of the neurocentral joints, with erosion of adjacent disc and bone causing subluxation[19] versus primary facetal arthritis and ligamentous laxity causing secondary chronic discovertebral trauma and destructive changes.[33] The involvement of interspinous bursae with spinous process destruction and hypermobile segments is associated with discal destruction.[34] Spinal cord responses to these subluxations are pachymeningitis, arachnoiditis, and medullary compression. Subaxial subluxations tend toward the C2–C3 and C3–C4 segments, typically lack osteophytes, and often are at multiple levels,[35, 36] giving a "stepladder" appearance (Fig. 106–6). End-plate erosions are found in 12 to 15 percent of patients with RA,[16, 35, 37] and subluxations in 10 to 20 percent.[33, 35, 37] Other patterns of subaxial disease that can have neurologic conse-

quences are subluxations below higher fusions, anterior spondylodiscitis, intracanal rheumatoid granulations, and possibly a hyperlordotic subaxial spine.[38]

Clinical Findings. The clinical manifestations of cervical RA are pain, neurologic disturbance, and death. Pain is typically in the neck and occipital area and is accompanied by stiffness and crepitus. The Sharp-Purser test, in which the flexed head is forced into extension while the spinous process of C2 is held fixed, has been reported to be positive in 20 to 44 percent of patients with anterior AAS.[10, 18] Neurologic changes are multiple and can be vague. Occipital neuralgia can be noted. Pyramidal tract involvement is found via upper motor neuron signs and pathologic reflexes. Vertebrobasilar insufficiency may cause a loss of equilibrium, tinnitus, vertigo, visual disturbances, and diplopia. Subjective sensation may be altered, yielding paresthesias, numbness, and sensations of hot and cold. Bulbar disturbances can be paroxysmal and fatal. They may occur as abnormalities in swallowing and phonation. Sphincter disturbance usually first presents as urinary retention and then incontinence. It may be

Figure 106–4. Schematic representation of the normal relationship of the odontoid to the base of the skull and upward displacement of the odontoid incident to destruction of the atlantoaxial articulation. McGregor's line can be used for routine screening. Normally, the tip of the odontoid process should be no more than 4.5 mm above McGregor's line, which is drawn from the upper surface of the posterior edge of the hard palate to the most caudal portion of the occipital curve of the skull. (From McGregor, M.: The significance of certain measurements of the skull in the diagnosis of basilar impression. Br. J. Radiol. 21:171, 1948.)

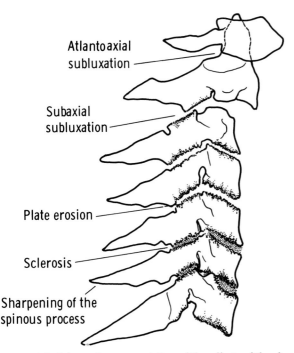

Atlantoaxial
subluxation

Subaxial
subluxation

Plate erosion

Sclerosis

Sharpening of the
spinous process

Figure 106–5. Schematic representation of the effects of the rheumatoid process on the cervical spine. (From Fielding, J. W.: Rheumatoid arthritis of the cervical spine. *In* The American Academy of Orthopaedic Surgeons: Instructional Course Lectures. Vol. XXXII. St. Louis, C. V. Mosby Co., 1983. Courtesy of William Park.)

difficult to interpret symptoms and signs in the face of severe and crippling polyarticular disease. Loss of function may be due to articular disease, neuropathy, and diffuse muscle weakness. Proper evaluation may be accomplished by a high index of suspicion of craniovertebral involvement in patients with RA.

Natural History. As indicated previously, cervical spine involvement in RA appears to start early in the course of the disease and correlates with the extent and severity of the disease process. This circumstance underlines the importance of early, aggressive, and continued medical intervention. Pain, neurologic disturbance, and death are the main concerns. Pain is a common finding in cervical RA, found in 40 to 88 percent of patients affected.[16, 17, 21, 38] Neurologic signs are noted, to a lesser degree, in 7 to 34 percent.[9, 16, 17] The concern in natural history is to determine the likelihood of severe neurologic deterioration and death.

A postmortem study of 104 patients with RA revealed 11 with atlantoaxial subluxation and cord compression.[40] Seven of the 11 died suddenly, indicating an estimated 10 percent rate of fatal medullary compression. Reports indicate that survival is not influenced by subluxation, but RA patients have a life expectancy significantly shorter than that of the general population.[8, 41] Pellicci and associates reported a 17 percent mortality in RA patients in 5 years, 10 percent higher than that for the general population.[17] Atlantoaxial subluxations did not cause death, but did worsen in 80 percent, while new onset subluxations were noted in 27 percent.

Worsening of existing radiologic subluxations has been noted in 80 percent in one report[17] and in 39 to 41 percent in other studies.[8, 10, 41] Neurologic progression is less marked and is found in 2 to 36 percent.[6, 17, 41] Once cervical myelopathy is established, the outcome is mortal. Marks and Sharp[42] reported on 31 patients with RA and cervical myelopathy. Nineteen of the 31 patients died, with 15 deaths occurring within 6 months following presentation. Four deaths were of primary neurologic origin. All who were untreated died, and half of those treated with a collar died. Only fusion offered survival. Meijers and associates reported that, of nine patients with myelopathy not operated on, all died within a year, with four deaths arising from cord compression.[43] Rana studied 41 patients with AAS over 10 years and found that 61 percent had no radiographic change, 27 percent progressed, and 12 percent had decreased subluxation. Twelve patients died, but only two of neurologic causes. Only three patients required surgical intervention.

It appears, in summary, that patients with cervical RA are at risk for premature death but not necessarily from subluxations. Subluxation can worsen with time, but neurologic progression is less marked. Once cervical myelopathy is established, the natural history without surgical intervention is grave. Risk factors for neurologic progression have been established through radiologic assessment, and advances in these areas may permit earlier determination of those patients at risk.

Radiologic Imaging. Plain radiographs with flexion-extension views cannot be overemphasized be-

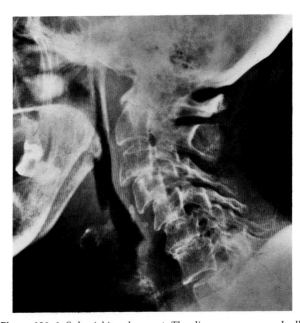

Figure 106–6. Subaxial involvement. The disc spaces are markedly narrowed without significant sclerosis. The end-plates tend to "jigsaw" one into the other, and the vertebral spines are thinned and "sharpened." Subluxation from C3 to C6 has occurred in "stepladder" fashion. (From Fielding, J. W.: Rheumatoid arthritis of the cervical spine. *In* The American Academy of Orthopaedic Surgeons: Instructional Course Lectures. Vol. XXXII. St. Louis, C. V. Mosby Co., 1983. Used by permission.)

cause they permit initial assessment of involvement, instability, and what areas are likely to need further study. On the basis of plain radiographs, Weissman and coworkers[10] defined risk factors that predisposed to cord compression and neurologic involvement as being male, anterior AAS of greater than 9 mm, and the presence of AAI. The presence of lateral C1–C2 subluxation was a lesser factor. The concept of impending neurologic deficit has been used to describe a patient with marked instability who is likely to develop neurologic deterioration.[45] Impending neurologic deficit includes patients who despite the absence of clinical signs of myelopathy have one of the following: an atlantodental distance of more than 8 mm and cord compression on neuroradiologic studies, subaxial subluxation of more than 4 mm and cord compression on neuroradiologic studies, or AAI with the dens through the foramen magnum and spinal cord or brain stem compression on neuroradiologic studies. One other study[46] considered subluxations at risk for neurologic deterioration if the atlantodental distance was more than 10 mm or a subaxial subluxation was more than 20 percent of the vertebral body diameter.

Computed tomography (CT) can add valuable information. CT can show the extent of erosions, spinal cord compression, and axial and sagittal relationships.[47] Bone detail, however, is superior in conventional tomography compared with sagittally reformatted CT images. Sagittal imaging with either CT or contrast-enhanced lateral tomography can demonstrate configurational change in the spinal cord, as in the kyphotic kinking seen in posterior AAS.[22] The degree of medullary compression noted on the CT scan in anterior AAS correlates with the presence of upper motor neuron signs.[48] The addition of intrathecal contrast material enhances the ability to demonstrate by CT the role of pannus in cord compression.[49]

Magnetic resonance imaging (MRI) is adding further definition to the pathologic anatomy of the cervical spine in RA. It has the advantage of requiring no contrast material and can be reformatted in any plane. The craniomedullary junction and the entire length of the cervical cord can be visualized. T_2-weighted images display a myelographic image demonstrating occlusion of the subarachnoid space, whereas T_1-weighted images will show the cord itself. Erosion, pannus, and inflammation of soft tissues can be demonstrated. Distortion of the spinal cord correlates with the signs of myelopathy.[50] At the cervicomedullary junction, a cervicomedullary angle of less than 135 degrees (normal 135 to 175 degrees) correlated with clinical evidence of cervical myelopathy,[51] again indicating that cord configuration as well as compression plays a role in the production of myelopathy. MRI has been correlated with medullary compression in AAI if the Ranawat value is 7 mm or less, and in AAS causing spinal cord compression if the space available for the cord is less than 13 mm and the atlantodental interval in flexion is 8 mm or more.[52] MRI has been used in a functional evaluation of the spinal cord, with the cord in a flexed position.[53] In this study of 34 patients with AAS, 22 had more than 3 mm of pannus behind the dens, and 12 had myelopathic signs. The spinal cord diameter was decreased from 7.4 mm to 6.5 mm in flexion. The authors recommended surgery if the sagittal spinal cord diameter was 6 mm or less on flexion MRI.

Demonstration of such radiologic parameters may further allow early clinical definition of the patient at risk for neurologic deterioration. MRI can also be used to follow the response to surgery. The pannus in the dens in AAS has been shown to decrease following successful fusion.[54] In this study myelopathy was correlated with the degree of cord compression demonstrated on MRI.

Nonsurgical Management. Medical management aimed toward reduction of synovitis is the cornerstone of nonsurgical treatment of cervical RA. The remaining treatment is symptomatic. Cervical collars are commonly used, but no study has shown them to be effective in stopping subluxation or neurologic progression.[8] Collars are used for psychologic support, pain relief, warmth, and a feeling of stability. More rigid cervical orthoses have been shown to limit atlantoaxial motion more than soft cervical collars, but they were also shown to prevent reducing anterior AAS by blocking extension.[55] Rigid orthoses, therefore, have no special advantage. Intermittent halter cervical traction may provide comfort but will not maintain reduction of subluxations or correct myelopathy.[26, 78] Pain relief can be sought through the use of a transcutaneous nerve stimulator. Glucocorticoid injection of trigger points, the greater occipital nerve, and facets and, possibly, cervical epidural steroids may yield some relief of pain.

Surgical Management. The indications for surgery are pain and neurologic abnormality. The presence of a subluxation is not an indication because subluxations are common and are not necessarily a clinical problem.[17, 41] Patients with rheumatoid disease tend to be severely affected, with debilitation, crippling, poor skin, and difficult airways for anesthetic intubation and management secondary to deformity, and further complicated by an unstable neck, susceptibility to infection, and poor wound healing capability. These circumstances present preoperative, intraoperative, and postoperative challenges reflected by significant morbidity and mortality. Preoperative skeletal traction is necessary to reduce subluxation and myelopathic changes. Intermittent halter traction will not accomplish this goal.[56, 57] Constant skeletal traction is recommended by most surgeons.[32, 40, 58–60] Halo traction has been most beneficial and can be incorporated postoperatively into a halo vest if necessary. The author prefers the use of a halo wheelchair, which is designed to allow continuous traction while sitting. Traction is done in this manner and in bed. The halo wheelchair allows increased tolerance and comfort while avoiding the skin and infection problems of prolonged bed rest and the use of frames.

Stabilization via posterior fusion is the commonest surgical procedure. Older techniques utilizing onlay grafts followed by prolonged bed rest, skeletal traction, and the use of Minerva casts have been replaced by internal fixation using wire and, more recently, implants wired in place and cemented with methylmethacrylate. The use of internal fixation may allow the rapid mobilization of the patient and the avoidance of cumbersome halo casts. Surgical series are usually mixes of subluxations at different levels and combinations of subluxations in a given patient. Current guidelines are to select patients who are at risk and operate on them early in order to prevent progressive neurologic deficits, which may be irreversible.[45, 46, 61, 62] Nonoperative versus operative care still demonstrates progression of disease clinically and radiologically.[62]

Atlantoaxial fusion is done by various Gallie type procedures or Brooks fusion. Occipitocervical fusions have evolved from the original onlay technique[63] to wired bone graft,[40, 64, 65] wires and cement,[66, 67] metal mesh wired in place with cement added,[22, 68, 69] and wired contoured wire loops.[62] The use of methylmethacrylate cement alone is not a successful technique for management of these cervical instabilities.[71]

Resection of the posterior foramen magnum and posterior arch of the atlas can be accomplished at the time of fusion if appropriate. For posterior fusion at the craniocervical level, nonunion rates vary from 0 to 50 percent.[32, 43, 58, 59, 64, 65, 67, 69, 72–76] Postoperative mortality is 0 to 33 percent, but the trend in the more recent reports is for less than 10 percent mortality, possibly owing to earlier intervention and improved anesthetic and perioperative management.[32, 45, 58, 59, 64, 72–76] Delayed death reported in various series, at a time distant from operation, is significant and reflects the overall morbidity of this group of patients. Neurologic improvement is noted in 42 to 100 percent of patients,[32, 43, 58, 59, 64, 67, 72, 73, 76] and significant pain reduction is usually the rule.

Transoral decompression has been advocated for irreducible AAS and in situations in which pannus behind the dens causes persistent compression.[49, 77, 78, 81, 82] The largest series comprised 14 patients.[49, 78] More recent patients in that series were not treated with tracheostomy and were given early nutritional support through nasogastric feeding. Immediate occipitocervical fusion followed the transoral procedure. No pharyngeal infections or immediate deaths occurred. Single-stage, combined transoral decompression and posterior fixation has been used with a series of 68 patients, of whom four died, three were worse, and in the remainder, one third were markedly better, with the rest slightly improved.[79] An extrapharyngeal approach for C2 corpectomy is described.[80]

Complications of fusion of any type include infections in up to 25 percent of patients, wound dehiscence, and occasional quadriplegia, among others. Late subaxial subluxation below previous fusion has been reported.[40, 58, 68] Anatomically involved areas adjacent to planned areas of fusion should be incorporated into the fusion. Additionally, previously asymptomatic levels can develop subluxation below rigid spinal segments so that long-term follow-up is necessary.

In the subaxial area, subluxations are usually stabilized by wired posterior fusions. Five patterns of subaxial involvement have been observed,[38] which include the usual anterior subluxation, subluxation below higher fusions, anterior spondylodiscitis with cord compression, compression from epidural rheumatoid granulations, and apparent subaxial hyperlordosis responding to halo traction and stabilization. Decompression and stabilization is determined by the underlying pathologic findings elucidated by preoperative study. The role of anterior fusion for subaxial subluxation is not clear and, although reported, lacks long-term follow-up.[24, 57] Four of five patients in one series were unimproved,[32] and the procedure was not recommended. Anterior fusion appears to undergo resorption and collapse.

The inclusion of laminectomy in the subaxial spine is somewhat debated, but there is no systematic study. Conaty and Mongan[58] reported only one of five patients improving with laminectomy but questioned whether intervention was too late. This author uses laminectomy if the subluxation is not reduced by preoperative traction, and laminectomy is always accompanied by fusion.[38]

At all levels, the surgical goal in general is alignment of configuration, decompression where necessary, and the stabilization of the motion segments involved.

ANKYLOSING SPONDYLITIS

Unlike RA, which results in joint destruction, ankylosing spondylitis results in joint fusion. In the cervical region, this often produces ankylosis from occiput downward (Fig. 106–7).

Pathology. Postmortem studies have suggested an initial inflammation followed by ossification of joint capsule and articular cartilage, resulting in ankylosis.[83] In the spine, the vertebral bodies tend to become "square"; ossification of ligaments and disc tissue follows.

Clinical Signs. The onset is insidious and is usually associated with morning stiffness, decreasing during the day and recurring in the evening, and unremitting low back pain. The sacroiliac joints are usually involved early in the disease, explaining the initial area of symptoms. In the cervical region, the pain, stiffness, and limitation of motion associated with a flexion deformity usually cause patients to seek medical advice. To compensate for this, they may simultaneously flex hips and knees to obtain a horizontal "line of sight." O'Driscoll and associates[84] report that lateral flexion is the movement most

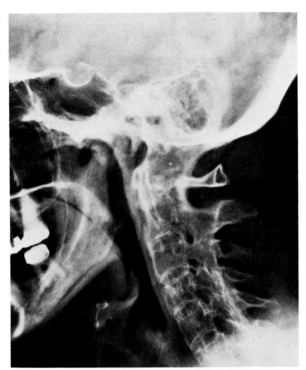

Figure 106–7. Ankylosis from the skull downward in ankylosing spondylitis. (From Fielding, J. W.: Rheumatoid arthritis of the cervical spine. *In* The American Academy of Orthopaedic Surgeons: Instructional Course Lectures. Vol. XXXII. St. Louis, C. V. Mosby Co., 1983. Used by permission.)

Fractures. The rigidity of the spondylitic cervical spine, unprotected by ribs or normal musculature, renders it particularly vulnerable to trauma. The force of a blow cannot be absorbed by mobile cervical segments, and the ankylosed spine may behave in a manner similar to a long bone. Since there is a degree of osteoporosis, the spine may fracture easily with minimal pain, and the patient may not recall the injury. The fractures are usually transverse, occur at the level of a disc space, and are generally at the midportion of the neck. Woodruff and Dewing[88] in 1963 reported 20 cases; five were above C5, and 15 below.

Simmons has noted the significance of minor injuries in patients with severe flexion deformities. In 40 cases presenting for cervical osteotomy with unacceptable flexion deformity, 36 percent had evidence of previous fractures, and in 31 percent of these 40 the fracture contributed significantly to the deformity.[89] Such fractures may go unnoticed for a variety of reasons. First, the fracture may spontaneously reduce without displacement; second, the patient may not recall the incident; and third, the fracture may be difficult to detect, particularly in the lower portions of the cervical spine in an individual in whom positioning for radiography is difficult. Hudson[90] reported correcting a flexion deformity at the site of a fresh fracture dislocation between C5

commonly restricted; further restriction is proportional to the degree of ankylosis.

Surgical Management. If the patient's head position is satisfactory, and the cervical spine completely fused, there is little that surgery can offer. Surgical intervention may be necessary in unacceptable cervical flexion deformities, in fractures, and in threatening atlantoaxial displacements.

Fixed Flexion Deformity. Probably the commonest complication of this disease is unacceptable fixed cervical flexion. Cervical osteotomy, as described by Mason and colleagues,[85] Urist,[86] and Simmons,[87] has been found to provide satisfactory correction. Simmons recommends that the procedure be performed under local anesthesia, with the patient in the sitting position and a halo ring and halo jacket applied. A laminectomy is performed at the C7 level, extending upward into C6 and downward into D1 with appropriate local resection of the C7–D1 facets. The spine is then manually fractured at the C7–D1 level under temporary general anesthesia by backward pressure on the head and correction obtained. The halo ring is then fastened to the body jacket. Osteotomy of the C7–D1 level is recommended because the vertebral canal is wider in this region and also because the vertebral arteries enter the foramen transversarium at C6, above the osteotomy site. The neurologic and other hazards of this operation should be known to the patient prior to operation to aid in the surgical decision.

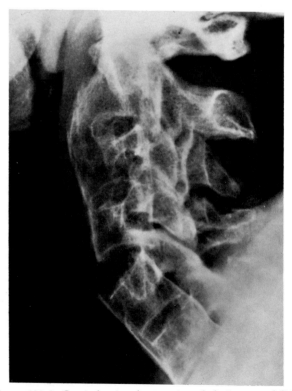

Figure 106–8. Cervical spine fracture in ankylosing spondylitis. (From Fielding, J. W.: Rheumatoid arthritis of the cervical spine. *In* The American Academy of Orthopaedic Surgeons: Instructional Course Lectures. Vol. XXXII. St. Louis, C. V. Mosby Co., 1983. Used by permission.)

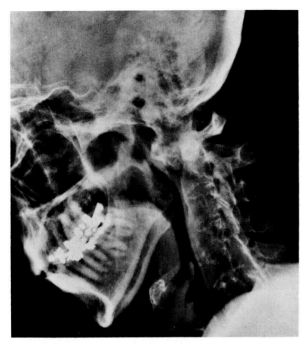

Figure 106–9. The spine is fused from C2 downward owing to ankylosing spondylitis. C1–C2 has been displaced forward with marked narrowing of the space available for the cord. (From Fielding, J. W.: Rheumatoid arthritis of the cervical spine. *In* The American Academy of Orthopaedic Surgeons: Instructional Course Lectures. Vol. XXXII. St. Louis, C. V. Mosby Co., 1983. Used by permission.)

and C6 in a patient without significant neurologic or vascular injury.

Not all fractures of the ankylosed cervical spine are benign; some present a poor prognosis. The normal flexibility of the neck is eliminated by the ankylosing process. Therefore, all motion takes place at the fracture site. This is in close proximity to the vulnerable vertebral arteries and spinal cord as described by Taylor and Blackwood[91] (Fig. 106–8).

In 1979, Bohlman[92] presented eight fractures in patients with ankylosing spondylitis. Three were above C5, and five were at C5 or below. All patients had cord lesions, and five died. Others have also noted problems with these injuries.[93–95] Woodruff and Dewing presented 20 cases of ankylosing spondylitis with fracture. They made four observations:[87]

1. Fractures may be caused by relatively slight trauma, since the fused rigid spine compounded by osteoporosis cannot give with stress. In none of their cases was the blow considered severe, and in one the weight of the head alone was thought to cause the fracture.

2. The ankylosed spine breaks like a solid long bone. Vertebral body compression is not a feature, since the line runs transversely; hence, every fracture is complete, and the chance of dislocation and spinal cord injury is high.

3. Mortality is high. Of their 20 patients, nine died within a short period of time. Generally, the

degree of displacement correlated with the severity of the spinal cord injury. They also noted that there can be gross malalignment with minimal or no cord impairment.

4. Treatment will vary with the clinical situation. They recommended "neutral traction."

Atlantoaxial Displacement. Jeffreys[96] reports that the incidence of this complication in the literature is as high as 90 percent, cautioning that this high percentage may reflect the severity of the disease in patients referred to the hospital. He indicates that in his experience atlantoaxial subluxation in ankylosing spondylitis is uncommon, an opinion shared by this author. This complication would suggest that this joint is unfused, particularly prone to trauma, or both (Fig. 106–9).

Surgical arthrodesis is probably the safest method of management, although it will sacrifice rotatory motion at the atlantoaxial joint.

References

1. Garrod, A. E.: A Treatise on Rheumatism and Rheumatoid Arthritis. London, C. Griffin, 1890.
2. Davis, F. W., and Markley, M. I.: Rheumatoid arthritis with death from medullary compression. Ann. Intern. Med. 35:451, 1954.
3. Kontinnen, Y., Santavirta, S., Bergroth, V., and Sandelin, J.: Inflammatory involvement of cervical spine ligaments in rheumatoid arthritis. Acta Orthop. Scand. 57:587, 1986.
4. Winfield, J., Cooke, D., Brook, A. S., and Corbett, M.: A prospective study of the radiological changes in the cervical spine in early rheumatoid arthritis. Ann. Rheum. Dis. 40:109, 1981.
5. Rasker, J. J., and Cosh, J. A.: Radiological study of cervical spine and hand in patients with rheumatoid arthritis of 15 years duration: An assessment of the effects of corticosteroid treatment. Ann. Rheum. Dis. 37:529, 1978.
6. Winfield, J., Young, A., Williams, P., and Corbett, M.: Prospective study of the radiological changes in hands, feet, and cervical spine in adult rheumatoid disease. Ann. Rheum. Dis. 42:613, 1983.
7. Eulderink, F., and Meijer, K. A. E.: Pathology of the cervical spine in rheumatoid arthritis: A controlled study of 44 spines. J. Pathol. 120:91, 1976.
8. Smith, P. H., Benn, R. T., and Sharp, J.: Natural history of rheumatoid cervical luxations. Ann. Rheum. Dis. 31:431, 1972.
9. Stevens, J. C., Cartlidge, N. E. F., Saunders, M., Appleby, A., Hall, M., and Shaw, D. A.: Atlanto-axial subluxation and cervical myelopathy in rheumatoid arthritis. Q. J. Med. 40:391, 1971.
10. Weissman, B. N., Aliabadi, P., Weinfeld, M. S., Thomas, W. H., and Sosman, J. L.: Prognostic features of atlantoaxial subluxation in rheumatoid arthritis. Radiology 144:745, 1982.
11. Ball, J.: Pathology of the rheumatoid cervical spine. Ann. Rheum. Dis. 17:121, 1958.
12. Martel, W., and Abell, M. R.: Fatal atlantoaxial luxation in rheumatoid arthritis. Arthritis Rheum. 6:224, 1963.
13. Mikulowski, P., Wolheim, F. A., Rotmil, P., and Olsen, I.: Sudden death in rheumatoid arthritis with atlanto-axial dislocation. Acta. Med. Scand. 198:445, 1975.
14. Fielding, J. W., Cochran, G. V. B., Lawsing, J. F., and Hohl, M.: Tears of the transverse ligament of the atlas. A clinical and biomechanical study. J. Bone Joint Surg. 56A:1683, 1974.
15. Bland, J. H.: Rheumatoid arthritis of the cervical spine. J. Rheumatol. 1:319, 1974.
16. Conlon, P. W., Isdale, I. C., and Rose, B. S.: Rheumatoid arthritis of the cervical spine. Ann. Rheum. Dis. 25:120, 1966.
17. Pellicci, P. M., Ranawat, C. S., Tsairis, P., and Bryan, W. J.: A prospective study of the progression of rheumatoid arthritis of the cervical spine. J. Bone Joint Surg. 63A:342, 1981.
18. Dirheimer, Y.: The Craniovertebral Region in Chronic Inflammatory Rheumatic Disease. Berlin, Springer-Verlag, 1977.
19. Martel, W.: Pathogenesis of cervical discovertebral destruction in rheumatoid arthritis. Arthritis Rheum. 20:1217, 1977.
20. Mathews, J. A.: Atlanto-axial subluxation in rheumatoid arthritis. Ann. Rheum. Dis. 28:260, 1969.

21. Sharp, J., and Purser, D. W.: Spontaneous atlantoaxial dislocation in ankylosing spondylitis and rheumatoid arthritis. Ann. Rheum. Dis. 20:47, 1961.
22. Lipson, S. J.: Cervical myelopathy and posterior atlanto-axial subluxation in patients with rheumatoid arthritis. J. Bone Joint Surg. 67A:593, 1985.
23. Isdale, I. C., and Corrigan, A. B.: Backward luxation of the atlas. Ann. Rheum. Dis. 29:6, 1970.
24. Lindgren, L., Ljunggren, B., and Ratcheson, R. A.: Reposition, anterior exposure and fusion in the treatment of myelopathy caused by rheumatoid arthritis of the cervical spine. Scand. J. Rheumatol. 3:195, 1974.
25. Teigland, J., and Magnaes, B.: Rheumatoid backward dislocation of the atlas with compression of the spinal cord. Scand. J. Rheumatol. 9:253, 1980.
26. Weiner, S., Bassett, L., and Speigel, T.: Superior, posterior, and lateral displacement of C1 in rheumatoid arthritis. Arthritis Rheum. 25:1378, 1982.
27. Williams, L. E., Bland, J. H., and Lipson, R. L.: Cervical spine subluxations and massive osteolysis in the upper extremities in rheumatoid arthritis. Arthritis Rheum. 9:348, 1966.
28. Verjaal, A., and Harder, N. C.: Backward luxation of the atlas. Acta Radiol. 3:173, 1963.
29. Burry, H. C., Tweed, J. M., Robinson, R. G., and Howes, R.: Lateral subluxation of the atlanto-axial joint in rheumatoid arthritis. Ann. Rheum. Dis. 37:525, 1978.
30. Halla, J. T., Fallak, S., and Hardin, J. T.: Nonreducible rotational head tilt and lateral mass collapse. A prospective study of frequency, radiographic findings, and clinical features in patients with rheumatoid arthritis. Arthritis Rheum. 25:1316, 1982.
31. Morizono, Y., Sakou, T., and Kawaida, H.: Upper cervical involvement in rheumatoid arthritis. Spine 12:721, 1987.
32. Ranawat, C. S., O'Leary, P., Pellicci, P., Tsairis, P., Marchisello, P., and Dorr, L.: Cervical fusion in rheumatoid arthritis. J. Bone Joint Surg. 61A:1003, 1979.
33. Ball, J., and Sharp, J.: Rheumatoid arthritis of the cervical spine. In Hill, A. G. S. (ed.): Modern Trends in Rheumatology. Vol. 2. London, Butterworths, 1971, p. 117.
34. Bywaters, E. G. L.: Rheumatoid and other diseases of the cervical interspinous bursae, and changes in the spinous processes. Ann. Rheum. Dis. 41:360, 1982.
35. Meikle, J. A., and Wilkinson, M.: Rheumatoid involvement of the cervical spine. Ann. Rheum. Dis. 30:154, 1971.
36. Park, W. M., O'Neill, M. O., and McCall, I. M.: The radiology of rheumatoid involvement of the cervical spine. Skeletal Radiol. 4:1, 1979.
37. Sharp, J., Purser, J. W., and Lawrence, J.: Rheumatoid arthritis of the cervical spine in the adult. Ann. Rheum. Dis. 17:303, 1958.
38. Lipson, S. J.: Patterns of rheumatoid subaxial disease causing myelopathy and strategies of management. Orthop. Trans. 12:55, 1988.
39. de Seze, S., Djian, A., and Debeyre, N.: Luxations atloido-axoidiennes an cours de la polyarthrite rheumatoide. Rev. Rhum. 30:560, 1963.
40. Meijers, K. A. E., van Beusekam, G. T., Luyendijk, W., and Duijfjes, F.: Dislocation of the cervical spine with cord compression in rheumatoid arthritis. J. Bone Joint Surg. 56B:668, 1974.
41. Isdale, I. C., and Conlon, P. W.: Atlanto-axial subluxation. A six-year follow-up report. Ann. Rheum. Dis. 30:387, 1971.
42. Marks, J. S., and Sharp, J.: Rheumatoid cervical myelopathy. Q. J. Med. 50:307, 1981.
43. Meijers, K. A. E., Cats, A., Kremer, H. P. H., Luyendijk, W., Onvlee, G. J., and Thomeer, R. T.: Cervical myelopathy in rheumatoid arthritis. Clin. Exp. Rheumatol. 2:239, 1984.
44. Rana, N.: Natural history of atlantoaxial subluxation in rheumatoid arthritis. Spine. 14:1054, 1989.
45. Clark, C. R., Goetz, D. D., and Menezes, A. H.: Arthrodesis of the cervical spine in rheumatoid arthritis. J. Bone Joint Surg. 71A:381, 1989.
46. Heywood, A. W. B., Learmonth, I. D., and Thomas, M.: Cervical spine instability in rheumatoid arthritis. J. Bone Joint Surg. 70B:702, 1988.
47. Braunstein, E. M., Weissman, B. N., Seltzer, S. E., Sosman, J. L., Wang, A. M., and Zamani, A.: Computed tomography and conventional radiographs of the craniocervical region in rheumatoid arthritis. Arthritis Rheum. 27:26, 1984.
48. Larsson, S. E., Toolanen, G., and Fagerlund, M.: Medullary compression in rheumatoid atlanto-axial subluxation evaluated by computerized tomography. Acta Orthop. Scand. 57:262, 1986.
49. Crockard, H. A., Essigman, W. K., Stevens, J. M., Pozo, J. L., Ransford, A. O., and Kendall, B. E.: Surgical treatment of cervical cord compression in rheumatoid arthritis. Ann. Rheum. Dis. 44:809, 1985.
50. Breedveld, F. C., Algra, P. R., Vielvoye, C. J., and Cats, A.: Magnetic resonance imaging in the evaluation of patients with rheumatoid arthritis and subluxations of the cervical spine. Arthritis Rheum. 30:624, 1987.
51. Bundschuh, C. V., and Modic, M. T.: Rheumatoid arthritis of the cervical spine. Orthop. Trans. 11:7, 1987.
52. Kawaida, H., Sakou, T., Morizono, Y., and Yoshikuni, N.: Magnetic resonance imaging of upper cervical disorders in rheumatoid arthritis. Spine 14:1144, 1989.
53. Dvorak, J., Grob, D., Baumgartner, H., Gschwend, N., Grauer, W., and Larsson, S.: Functional evaluation of the spinal cord by magnetic resonance imaging in patients with rheumatoid arthritis and instability of the upper cervical spine. Spine 10:1057, 1989.
54. Milbrink, J., and Nyman, R.: Posterior stabilization of the cervical spine in rheumatoid arthritis: Clinical results and magnetic resonance imaging correlation. J. Spinal Dis. 3:308, 1990.
55. Althoff, B., and Goldie, I. F.: Cervical collars in rheumatoid atlanto-axial subluxation: A radiographic comparison. Ann. Rheum. Dis. 39:485, 1980.
56. Wilson, P. D., and Dangelmajer, R. C.: The problem of atlantoaxial dislocation in rheumatoid arthritis. J. Bone Joint Surg. 45A:1780, 1963.
57. Hopkins, J. S.: Lower cervical rheumatoid subluxation with tetraplegia. J. Bone Joint Surg. 49B:46, 1967.
58. Conaty, J. P., and Mongan, E. S.: Cervical fusion in rheumatoid arthritis. J. Bone Joint Surg. 63A:1218, 1981.
59. Ferlic, D. C., Clayton, M. L., Leidholt, J. D., and Gamble, W. E.: Surgical treatment of the symptomatic unstable cervical spine in rheumatoid arthritis. J. Bone Joint Surg. 57A:349, 1975.
60. Rana, N. A., Hancock, D. O., Taylor, A. R., and Hill, A. G. S.: Atlanto-axial subluxation in rheumatoid arthritis. J. Bone Joint Surg. 55B:458, 1973.
61. Santavirta, S., Slatis, P., Kankaanpaa, U., Sandelin, J., and Laasonen, E.: Treatment of the cervical spine in rheumatoid arthritis. J. Bone Joint Surg. 70A:658, 1988.
62. Zoma, A., Sturrock, R. D., Fisher, W. D., Freeman, P. A., and Hamblen, D. A.: Surgical stabilization of the rheumatoid cervical spine. A review of indications and results. J. Bone Joint Surg. 69B:8, 1987.
63. Newman, P., and Sweetnam, R.: Occipito-cervical fusion: An operative technique and its indications. J. Bone Joint Surg. 51B:423, 1969.
64. Hamblen, D. L.: Occipito-cervical fusion. Indications, techniques and results. J. Bone Joint Surg. 49B:33, 1967.
65. Wertheim, S. B., and Bohlman, H. H.: Occipitocervical fusion. Indications, technique, and long-term results in thirteen patients. J. Bone Joint Surg. 69A:833, 1987.
66. Brattstrom, H., and Granholm, L.: Atlanto-axial fusion in rheumatoid arthritis. A new method of fixation with wire and bone cement. Acta Orthop. Scand. 47:619, 1976.
67. Lachiewicz, P. F., Inglis, A. E., and Ranawat, C. S.: Methylmethacrylate augmentation for cervical spine arthrodesis in rheumatoid arthritis. Orthop. Trans. 11:7, 1987.
68. Bryan, W. J., Inglis, A. E., Sculco, T. P., and Ranawat, C. S.: Methylmethacrylate stabilization for enhancement of posterior cervical arthrodesis in rheumatoid arthritis. J. Bone Joint Surg. 64A:1045, 1982.
69. Lipson, S. J.: Occipitocervical fusion using wired metal mesh and methacrylate backed bone graft. Orthop. Trans. 9:141, 1985.
70. Ransford, A. O., Crockard, H. A., Pozo, J. L., Thomas, N. P., and Nelson, I. W.: Craniocervical instability treated by contoured loop fixation. J. Bone Joint Surg. 68B:173, 1986.
71. McAfee, P. C., Bohlman, H. H., Ducker, T., and Eismont, F. J.: Failure of stabilization of the spine with methylmethacrylate. J. Bone Joint Surg. 68A:1145, 1986.
72. Cregan, J. C. F.: Internal fixation of the unstable rheumatoid cervical spine. Ann. Rheum. Dis. 25:242, 1966.
73. Larsson, S. E., and Toolanen, G.: Posterior fusion for atlanto-axial subluxation in rheumatoid arthritis. Spine 11:525, 1986.
74. Thomas, W. H.: Surgical management of the rheumatoid cervical spine. Orthop. Clin. North Am. 6:793, 1975.
75. Thompson, R. C., and Meyer, T. J.: Posterior surgical stabilization for atlantoaxial subluxation in rheumatoid arthritis. Spine 10:597, 1985.
76. Crellin, R. Q., MacCabe, J. J., and Hamilton, E. B. D.: Severe subluxation of the cervical spine in rheumatoid arthritis. J. Bone Joint Surg. 52B:244, 1970.
77. Brattstrom, H., Elner, A., and Granholm, L.: Transoral surgery for myelopathy caused by rheumatoid arthritis of the cervical spine. Ann. Rheum. Dis. 32:578, 1973.
78. Crockard, H. A., Pozo, J. L., Ransford, A. O., Stevens, J. M., Kendall, B. E., and Essigman, W. K.: Transoral decompression and posterior fusion for rheumatoid atlanto-axial subluxation. J. Bone Joint Surg. 68B:350, 1986.
79. Crockard, H. A., Calder, I., and Ransford, A. O.: One-stage transoral decompression and posterior fixation in rheumatoid atlanto-axial subluxation. J. Bone Joint Surg. 72B:682, 1990.
80. McAfee, P. C., Bohlman, H. H., Riley, L. H., Robinson, R. A., Southwick, W. O., and Nachlas, N. E.: The anterior extrapharyngeal approach to the upper part of the cervical spine. J. Bone Joint Surg. 69A:1371, 1987.
81. Menezes, A. H., Van Gilder, J. C., Clark, C. R., and El-Khoury, G.: Odontoid upward migration in rheumatoid arthritis. An analysis of 45 patients with "cranial settling." J. Neurosurg. 63:500, 1985.
82. Olerud, S., and Sjostrom, L.: Dens resection in a case of vertical

impression of the dens in the foramen magnum. Acta Orthop. Scand. 57:262, 1986.

83. Berens, D.: Roentgen Diagnosis of Rheumatoid Arthritis. Springfield, IL, Charles C Thomas, 1969.

84. O'Driscoll, S. L., Jayson, M. I. V., and Badley, H.: Neck movements in ankylosing spondylitis. Ann. Rheum. Dis. 37:64, 1978.

85. Mason, C., Cozen, L., and Addelstein, L.: Surgical correction of flexion deformity of the cervical spine. Calif. Med. 79:244, 1963.

86. Urist, M. R.: Osteotomy of the cervical spine. Report of case of ankylosing rheumatoid spondylitis. J. Bone Joint Surg. 40A:833, 1958.

87. Simmons, E. H.: The surgical correction of flexion deformity of the cervical spine in ankylosing spondylitis. Clin. Orthop. Rel. Res. 86:132, 1972.

88. Woodruff, F. V., and Dewing, S. B.: Fracture of the cervical spine in patients with ankylosing spondylitis. Radiology 80:17, 1963.

89. Simmons, E. H.: Personal communication.

90. Hudson, C. P.: Cervical osteotomy for severe flexion. J. Bone Joint Surg. 54B:202, 1972.

91. Taylor, A. R., and Blackwood, W.: Paraplegia in hyperextension in cervical injuries. J. Bone Joint Surg. 30B:245, 1948.

92. Bohlman, H.: Acute fractures and dislocations of the cervical spine. J. Bone Joint Surg. 61A:1119, 1979.

93. Bergmann, E. W.: Fractures of the ankylosed spine. J. Bone Joint Surg. 45B:21, 1963.

94. Harris, L. S., and Adelson, L.: "Spinal injury" and sudden infant death: A second look. Am. J. Clin. Pathol. 52:289, 1969.

95. Hollin, S. A., Gross, S. W., and Levin, P.: Fracture of the cervical spine in patients with rheumatoid spondylitis. Am. Surg. 31:532, 1965.

96. Jeffreys, E.: Disorders of the Cervical Spine. London, Butterworths, 1980.

The Shoulder

INTRODUCTION

The rheumatoid shoulder deteriorates faster if it becomes stiff, and after destruction of the articular surfaces occurs with upward translocation of the humerus against the acromion, impingement destroys the rotator cuff (Figs. 107–1 and 107–2C). Thus, conservative treatment includes gentle exercises to maintain motion in addition to appropriate medical care. However, if the articular surfaces become destroyed beyond hope of this regimen being successful, arthroplasty should be considered prior to destruction of the rotator cuff and prior to excessive bone loss from granulation erosion. Synovectomy of the glenohumeral joint has only a limited place in the specific situation illustrated in Figure 107–4. Fusion has virtually no place in the treatment of rheumatoid shoulders.

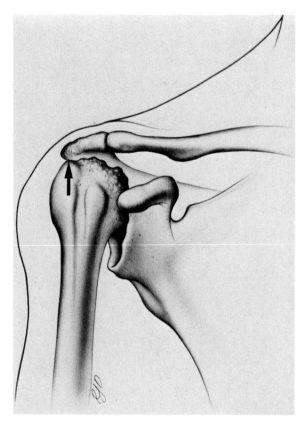

Figure 107–1. The unique problem in the shoulder—how long-standing RA with loss of the articular surfaces and translocation upward of the humerus causes impingement against the acromion that eventually destroys the rotator cuff (as in C). When there is clearly painful destruction of the glenohumeral joint beyond medical treatment, nonconstrained total arthroplasty should be considered to provide new joint surfaces to stop this impingement process prior to involvement of the rotator cuff, preferably prior to the severe bone loss that makes it difficult to anchor the components. No other joint has a rotator cuff to pose a hazard in unnecessary deferment of arthroplasty. (From Neer, C. S. II: Shoulder Reconstruction. Philadelphia, W. B. Saunders Co., 1990. Used by permission.)

CLINICAL ASPECTS OF THE RHEUMATOID SHOULDER

Insidious Onset

The onset of shoulder arthritis is variable but initially tends to be subacute and transitory rather than constant and destructive. With each rheumatoid attack the painful shoulder is splinted by holding the arm tightly against the chest in the "protective position," and the inactivity has a deleterious effect beyond that of the rheumatoid disease (see discussion of conservative treatment that follows). It is important to recognize the stiffness early and, if possible, to reverse this process by conservative measures before irreversible changes have developed.

Identifying Shoulder Arthritis

The shoulder is a frequent site of rheumatoid arthritis (RA), but it is too often ignored by the physician. There are a number of reasons for this. Shoulders are covered with clothing and are less conspicuous than the hands and other parts of the body. They attract less attention. Shoulder pain is often referred distally, causing patients to misunderstand the source of the pain. In addition, the attitude of the patient has at times been a barrier to the early diagnosis of shoulder problems. Many have found that their physician is less interested in the shoulder than in other joints, such as the hip, knee, hand, and foot. They have been told that there is not much to be done about shoulders, and they have become complacent regarding their shoulder pain. For these reasons the rheumatologist must seek out shoulder involvement if an early diagnosis is to be made. A systematic physical examination is important.

System for Examination. The initial part of the

examination is done with the patient sitting with both shoulders exposed. A good system is to begin at the cervical spine and scapular areas. Referred pain and neurologic involvement from the neck are considered, followed by the acromioclavicular (AC) and sternoclavicular joints and supraclavicular region, and finally the glenohumeral joint. This is followed by an examination of the elbows, wrists, and hands. The glenohumeral joint is palpated for swelling, thickened tissue, and heat, as well as tenderness. Motion, measured with the patient supine and sitting as described in the following paragraph, strength of the rotators and deltoid, and level of function are recorded. Tenderness along the posterior joint line is the most important sign of arthritic involvement of the glenohumeral joint.

Recording Motion. The earliest evidence of shoulder involvement is usually loss of glenohumeral motion. An efficient method of recording this range of motion is of great importance. In the past, this has been too casual and inconsistent. Glenohumeral rotation is greatest when the arm is at the side and diminishes as the arm is raised. Therefore, it is logical to measure internal and external rotation with the arm at the side. Forward elevation is done without rotation, but abduction is a combination of both elevation and rotation. Therefore it seems logical to record "total elevation" rather than abduction.[6] Attempts to measure shoulder motion with the patient standing are just as futile as measuring hip motion with the patient standing. The spine and knees compensate and make accurate measurements impossible. External rotation and total passive elevation are measured with the patient supine. Internal rotation (reaching up the back) and total active elevation are measured with the patient sitting. Recordings of these four measurements give a simple and reproducible way of following clinical progress.

Roentgen Examination. The routine examination is made in the anteroposterior (AP) view with the arm in internal and external rotation, and in the true axillary view. The glenohumeral joint space can be evaluated better if the AP views are made in the scapular plane (with the x-ray beam angled 15 degrees lateral to the coronal plane). The earliest roentgen evidence of disease includes osteoporosis of the bone and erosion of the joint margin. Erosion of the glenoid, loss of joint space, and posterior subluxation of the head are best seen in the axillary view (see Fig. 107–6), and this finding favors operative intervention. For optimal visualization of the AC joint, less exposure is used than for the glenohumeral joint. Tomograms may be helpful for visualizing the sternoclavicular joints. Computed tomography (CT) scans and AP tomograms may help demonstrate the amount of bone loss and granulation erosion.

Patterns of Involvement

Low Grade, Intermediate, and Severe. It is helpful to the clinician to classify patients as having low-grade, intermediate, or severe disease. The nature of shoulder involvement varies widely and may be mild and intermittent or severe and destructive, depending not only on the severity of the disease but also on the duration of shoulder involvement. Rehabilitation of the muscles in patients with low-grade involvement is more difficult than in patients with osteoarthritis but is much easier than in those with intermediate and severe rheumatoid disease. It is a common misconception that all shoulders involved with RA have tears of the rotator cuff; actually, while most patients with severe involvement do have cuff tears, the cuff has been found intact in 80 percent of the rheumatoid shoulders on which the author has operated.[7] Others have had a similar experience.[8, 9] Of course, the longer the delay for shoulder arthroplasty, the higher the percentage of cuff tears, as discussed earlier.

Dry, Wet, and Resorptive. Three types of involvement are seen: dry, wet, and resorptive (Figs. 107–2 and 107–3). In the dry form (see Fig. 107–2A) there is a marked tendency for stiffness and loss of joint space with sclerosis and areas of cystification in the bone. Minimal marginal erosion is seen, and eventually marginal osteophytes may form, similar to those in osteoarthritis. Clinically these patients have much more stiffness and weakness than those with osteoarthritis. In the wet form (see Fig. 107–2B) there are exuberant granulations and marginal erosions causing the end of the bone to become pointed. There is progressive intrusion of the humeral head into the glenoid (see Fig. 107–2C). In the resorptive type (Fig. 107–2D), destruction and resorption of the bone is the outstanding feature. In the dry type there is good bone stock for reconstruction, but in the others the bone is usually soft and easily fractured.

The Syndrome. Through the years a condition I have referred to as "the syndrome"[10] has been repeatedly seen (see Fig. 107–3). It consists of dry, low-grade rheumatoid involvement of the shoulders, usually bilateral, that spares most other joints. There is progressive loss of the joint space and areas of sclerosis mixed with cystification of the head and eventually marginal osteophytes. This is seen more often in women, and the patients are between 35 and 55 years of age. The serology is usually positive for the rheumatoid factor, and they are eventually diagnosed as having RA by the rheumatologist. These patients can develop an extremely painful disability, and if they do, they are ideal candidates for reconstructive surgery.

Bursal Type. Huge enlargements of the subacromial and subdeltoid bursae are occasionally seen in the absence of glenohumeral involvement.[8, 11, 12] (Fig. 107–4). The bursa is filled with rice bodies and with much less fluid than would be expected. The dearth of fluid may cause a dry tap on attempts at aspiration and cause the physician to suspect a solid neoplasm. The AC joint is usually diseased in these patients.

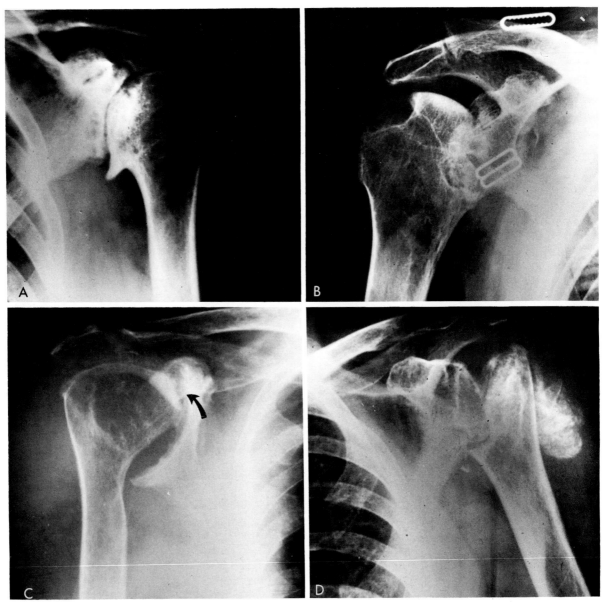

Figure 107–2. Anteroposterior films depicting the variations in RA of the shoulder. *A,* The "dry'" form, which begins with marked stiffness, loss of joint space, and sclerosis mixed with cystification, as in Figure 107–3. Later marginal osteophytes appear as seen in osteoarthritis, and at this stage it has been referred to as "mixed arthritis." *B,* The "wet" form with sloppy tissue and marginal erosion of the humeral head, glenoid, and acromioclavicular joint. *C,* Late stage of a severe wet form with marked intrusion into the glenoid, acromion, and clavicle. The arrow indicates where the coracoid process has been eroded halfway through. There is a massive tear of the rotator cuff, and the upper humerus resembles the upper femur. Note in this late, long-standing lesion how translocation of the humerus upward against the acromion and clavicle has not only destroyed the rotator cuff by this type of impingement but has also eroded through the acromion and into the outer clavicle. It is impossible to properly orient the standard glenoid prosthesis in this type of shoulder. *D,* Rheumatoid vasculitis with marked destruction and resorption of bone. There was a massive detachment of the rotator cuff, and the remains of the humeral head were lying out in the subdeltoid bursa. Nevertheless this shoulder was rendered pain free and stable with an unconstrained, resurfacing total shoulder, as in Figure 107–8.

Differential Diagnosis

Osteoarthritis. Osteoarthritis of the glenohumeral joint is less common than that of the hip or knee, but it is not rare. It is, however, infrequent enough that most clinicians are unfamiliar with it. The roentgen appearance is constant and characteristic and is distinctly different from that of RA[13, 14] (Fig. 107–5). An area of sclerosis, perhaps with a

subchondral cyst, forms on the upper part of the head. This area of the head is in contact with the glenoid when the arm is held in an abducted position. In the abducted position there is the maximal joint reaction force, and the weight of the arm is brought against the head with a leverage force of about ten to one. Sclerosis forms at this point on the head where there is maximal pressure. Osteophytes form where there is less pressure and are consistently

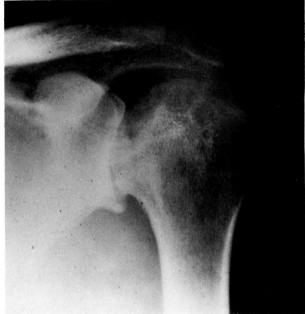

Figure 107–3. A clinical "syndrome" of low-grade, atypical RA that involves the shoulders almost exclusively and spares most other joints. The serology is usually positive for the rheumatoid factor. This anteroposterior view was made in the scapular plane and shows the complete loss of joint space that occurred over a 3-year period. Both shoulders are usually involved. Marginal osteophytes form later, as illustrated in Figure 107–2A.

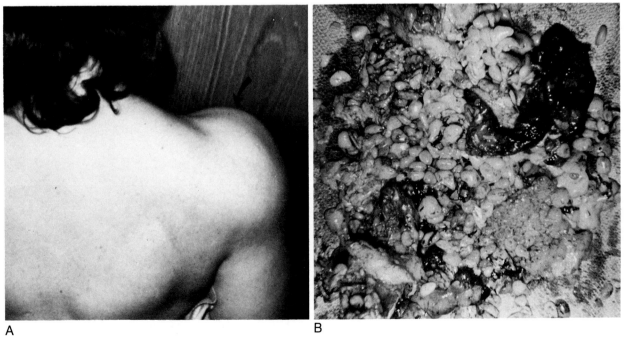

A   B

Figure 107–4. The bursal type of rheumatoid involvement. A, Huge enlargement of the subacromial bursa and involvement of the AC joint. The glenohumeral joint is almost completely spared. B, Contents of the bursa seen after its removal. It was filled with rice bodies and contained little fluid. The dearth of fluid causes a dry tap on attempts to aspirate and may cause the physician to suspect a solid neoplasm.

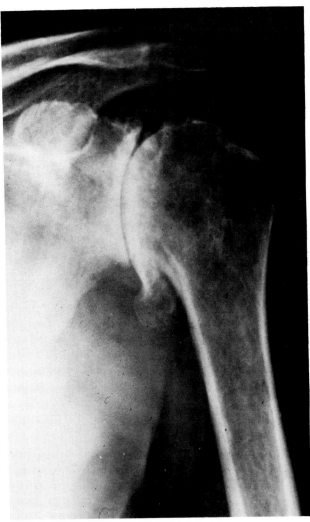

Figure 107–5. Anteroposterior view showing the typical, characteristic roentgen appearance of primary osteoarthritis of the glenohumeral joint. There is eburnation and wear on that part of the head that is in contact with the glenoid when the arm is abducted 60 to 100 degrees, as well as marginal osteophytes, which are largest inferiorly where they cover the calcar, and sclerosis with marginal excrescences of the glenoid that cause the glenoid to appear enlarged. These radiographic features are constant and are distinctly different from those of RA (see Figs. 107–2 and 107–3).

more prominent inferiorly. The glenoid tends to be eroded more posteriorly than anteriorly (Fig. 107–6). It is of clinical importance to know that the alterations seen in osteoarthritis require great pressure, and this implies an intact rotator cuff. It is extremely rare to find a tear of the rotator cuff in a shoulder with the typical and classic roentgen appearance of primary osteoarthritis. The author has seen only one such patient in over 100 primary osteoarthritic shoulders treated surgically in a personal series,[14] and that patient had sustained an injury after the development of osteoarthritis. In contrast, patients with tears of the rotator cuff do not develop head changes until late, and these changes are quite different, as described in the section on impingement lesions that follows. This information is important in planning

shoulder reconstruction. Although fusion has been advised by some[15, 16] as the treatment for osteoarthritis, since the muscles are normal in this condition, it is most ideal for prosthetic replacement arthroplasty.[5, 13, 14, 17–19] To waste these muscles with a fusion for this condition would be much more disabling and radical than an arthroplasty.

Secondary Osteoarthritis. A number of conditions can cause articular surface damage that may ultimately lead to a picture resembling primary osteoarthritis[13, 14] (see Fig. 107–5). The list includes metabolic disorders (gout and ochronosis), inactive suppurative arthritis, infarctional diseases (sickle cell, lupus, and Gaucher's disease), and articular surface trauma (fractures and dislocations with or without previous operative treatment). Some of them can be confused with RA. In addition it appears that some low-grade rheumatoid patients may have "burned-out" disease that can come to resemble osteoarthritis, and this is sometimes referred to as "mixed arthritis."

Impingement Lesions. The rotator cuff functions like the acetabulum in the hip; therefore, degenerative and traumatic *lesions of the rotator cuff* are as common as osteoarthritis of the hip. Tears of the complete thickness of the tendon have been found in 5 percent,[20] 9.3 percent,[21] and 12.9 percent[22] of cadavers in the anatomy laboratory. The rotator cuff is not seen in roentgenograms; this makes cuff lesions much harder to diagnose, and they must be differentiated from other types of "arthritis."[2, 23–25] We

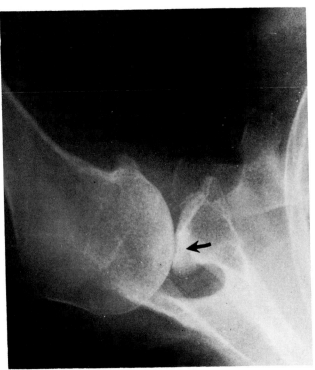

Figure 107–6. True axillary view showing posterior erosion of the glenoid and posterior subluxation of the head in a 55-year-old woman with osteoarthritis. Posterior migration of the head tends to occur in all types of glenohumeral arthritis.

now recognize three "outlet impingement"[56] lesions: grade I is edema and swelling, grade II is fibrosis and thickening, and grade III is bone reaction and tendon rupture. More than 90 percent of cuff tears are due to subacromial impingement and wear, with trauma playing only a secondary role.[2, 17, 18, 20, 23, 24, 45] They are seen in women almost as frequently as in men, and about half of the patients recall no significant trauma.[2, 23, 24] Evidences of long-standing impingement (excrescences or eburnation at the greater tuberosity[4] or acromion[2]) are usually seen in radiographs or at surgery. Thinning of the distance from the humerus to the acromion is present in patients with larger tears. Some of these roentgen features may be seen in rheumatoid shoulders, but only after attenuation and weakness of the cuff has allowed the head to ride up against the acromion, leading to subacromial impingement as a secondary phenomenon. Arthrography is the most reliable method for proving the presence of a cuff tear.[25] When there is an incomplete thickness tear, the arthrogram is usually normal. The "impingement test" (pain relief following a subacromial lidocaine injection) is helpful in detecting impingement lesions.[20] Posterior joint-line tenderness, thickening of the joint, and stiffness are seen in the rheumatoid shoulder; this helps differentiate it from an impingement lesion.

Biceps lesions are, in the author's opinion, usually caused by subacromial impingement.[3, 20, 26] This includes both biceps tenosynovitis and biceps rupture. Rheumatoid involvement of the sheath of the long head can be differentiated because it is associated with involvement of the underlying joint as well.

Cuff-tear arthropathy is a term used by the author since 1975 to describe the condition that is seen with some long-standing tears of the rotator cuff.[7, 28–30] An irregular, pebble-stone appearance of the articular cartilage of the humeral head develops, and the underlying bone softens and collapses. These changes in the articular cartilage are probably due to inactivity and malnutrition of the cartilage. In some cases, but not in all, there have been steroid injections that might have contributed to the problem. Massive tears permit dislocations and subluxations of the glenohumeral joint, which inflict abnormal trauma to the articular surfaces and are thought to play an important role in the collapse of the head. It seems important to consider cuff-tear arthropathy as a separate entity, because its reconstruction is especially difficult. Certainly it is not like osteoarthritis (in which the cuff is intact), not like steroid arthropathy (in which the cuff is intact), and not like RA (in which the joint is eroded and the cuff is often intact).[30] The author believes that cuff-tear arthropathy is the same condition that has more recently been referred to as "Milwaukee shoulder."[31]

Aseptic Necrosis. In steroid arthropathy and aseptic necrosis and in infarctional disease (see discussion of secondary osteoarthritis, earlier) the rotator cuff remains completely normal, and, at least in the early stages, the glenoid is normal.[27] Pain is usually most intense during the period while the head is collapsing. Irregularities of the head may later erode the glenoid. Tomograms can clarify the extent of head involvement. In some cases fragments of bone are engulfed by the synovium, and the picture then resembles a neurotrophic joint.

Neurologic Problems. Cervical spine disease can produce pain and muscle weakness that can mimic rheumatoid involvement of the shoulder. Thoracic outlet syndromes (cervical rib, scalenus anticus syndrome, and hyperabduction syndrome) may also produce pain in the shoulder and arm. Early Charcot's shoulders have been confused with rheumatoid involvement because neurotrophic shoulders are more frequently painful than are other neurotrophic joints. Radiographs of the cervical spine and careful neurologic examination should be routine in evaluating rheumatoid shoulders. Electromyograms, arteriograms, and neurosurgical and vascular consultations may be needed to identify some of these problems.[5]

CONSERVATIVE TREATMENT

Adverse Effects of Frozen Shoulder. Patients with painful shoulders assume the protective position to guard against movement. The arm is clasped to the chest in internal rotation. The shoulder is more prone to "freezing" with inactivity than are other joints because it normally has more motion and, in proportion, has larger bursal and joint spaces. As the joint stiffens in the protective position, external rotation and elevation become progressively more and more restricted. Stiffness is associated with pain of a second type beyond that of the RA. This pain occurs at the extremes of motion because of tension on the contracted capsule, ligaments, and muscles, and this causes the patient to avoid movement into the extremes of the excursion. A vicious cycle results with more restriction and more disinclination on the part of the patient to move. Eventually the joint may become completely ankylosed in this position. Immobility has bad side effects. First, a shoulder frozen in the protective position enhances the development of contractures at the elbow, wrist, and fingers as well as stiffening of the scapular muscles and has an adverse effect on the function of the entire upper extremity unit. Second, since the nutrition of the articular surfaces is dependent on joint fluid and the pumping action of motion and activity, disuse impairs the nutrition of the cartilage and produces a deleterious effect on the joint surfaces beyond that of the rheumatoid disease. Conservative treatment should aim at early detection and treatment of shoulder stiffness prior to the stage at which the deleterious side effects of inactivity have become irreversible.

Team Approach. Several disciplines are needed to accomplish the goals of conservative shoulder treatment just outlined. Medication is needed to minimize the RA activity and control pain. Physical therapy is needed for optimal restoration of motion and strength. Orthopedic surgery is needed to evaluate specific problem joints for special procedures such as injections, manipulation, or surgical reconstruction. A feeling of team play and mutual respect should prevail, with the common goal of controlling pain and re-establishing function by the safest and least harmful method available.

Exercise Regimens

Regaining Motion. Low heat, analgesia, and passive and assistive exercises (done four or five times a day) form the basis for recovering motion. In the exercise program the patient should later be taught how to supply the power so that the exercises can be done several times each day in a relaxed way. It helps to apply with gentle heat to the affected parts of the body before initiating the exercises. Emphasis is placed on regaining external rotation and elevation. It has been helpful to work for external rotation and total elevation first, before starting work on abduction. When the patient achieves 140 degrees of elevation and 40 degrees of external rotation, complete abduction can be done without pain by having the patient place the hands behind the head and spread the elbows. When both shoulders are involved, the pulley is used for overhead elevation. Later, as the pain subsides, stretching exercises are added.[6] Motion is recorded to depict progress.

Recovering Strength. Active motion that is done during the painful stage when the joint is acutely inflamed or while it is too stiff may be irritating to the joint and painful for the patient. Isometric exercises can be used as pain subsides, to maintain strength. As the pain allows, active assistive, active, and later resistive exercises are added.

Special Problems

Braces. Patients with bilateral shoulder involvement or with a marked tendency to stiffen may be helped by an abduction–external rotation brace to maintain the arm out of the protective position between exercise periods. Braces are also helpful in getting air into the axilla to help clear fungus infection or maceration of the axilla prior to surgery. Assistive exercises are done from the brace. Elevation can be done with the patient in the supine position with the help of the therapist or members of the family, and in addition the patient can use the pulley (when erect) to lift the arm off the brace.

Role of Manipulation. Intra-articular and subacromial injection of lidocaine (Xylocaine), followed by gentle manipulation and stretching, may be helpful for stubborn cases. On the other hand, there is no place for manipulation with the patient under general anesthesia in the treatment of the rheumatoid shoulder. The osteoporotic bone may fracture.

INDICATIONS FOR SURGERY

Glenohumeral Joint. Surgery is considered when the disease has altered the joint by destruction of the articular surfaces (see Figs. 107–1, 107–2, and 107–3) to the extent that it is not possible to control pain and re-establish function by conservative measures without resorting to harmful medication. It is to be remembered that some medications are more radical than properly selected surgical procedures. As emphasized earlier, glenohumeral arthroplasty should not be postponed until the rotator cuff has become involved by secondary impingement and the bone destroyed by rheumatoid granulations to the extent that total shoulder arthroplasty is rendered difficult. The overview of the patient is foremost in the decision, and in patients with severe disease the surgical procedures should be limited to those that are most needed to control pain and make the patient independent. The most critical functions of the upper extremity in day-to-day living include perineal and rectal care, cleansing under the axilla, eating, combing the hair, and sleeping. Pain is the primary indication for shoulder surgery. However, there are a few rheumatoid patients with relatively painless bilateral ankylosed shoulders in whom replacements can be considered with the goal of making it possible for them to be independent for these critical activities of daily living, as illustrated in Figure 107–7.

The most frequent procedure now done for RA of the glenohumeral joint at the author's center is a *total joint replacement*,[14, 28, 30, 32, 33] in which both sides of the joint are resurfaced (see Fig. 107–8). *Humeral head replacement*[14, 34, 35] alone is now less often done for rheumatoid patients because the glenoid is usually diseased (see Fig. 107–2) and also because the stability afforded by the conforming surfaces of the total replacement seems to aid in the rehabilitation of rheumatoid muscles and preventing subacromial impingement. The glenoid component may be used even when bone grafting is required to support the prosthesis; however, it is thought that the glenoid component should be omitted in severe, long-standing rheumatoid shoulders with complete destruction of the glenoid, which precludes adequate fixation. *Fixed fulcrum*[18, 28, 36–43] prostheses (one or more hinges) have not been widely used. It was hoped that they might solve the problem of extensive deficits of the rotator cuff and deltoid, but unfortunately they do not supply active power and they invite mechanical failure.[19, 28] Few have been used in rheumatoid patients, and the soft bone in this condition does not lend itself to fixed fulcrum implants. A *subacromial spacer*, between the acromion and humeral head, once used by Macnab and also by Clayton and Ferlic[12] in a few patients who had severely destroyed cuff muscles, is of historic interest but is not used now. Macnab and English[44] designed a glenoid component with an overhang to provide more stability for extensively destroyed shoulders. The relative lack of constraint freed it from many of the risks of mechanical

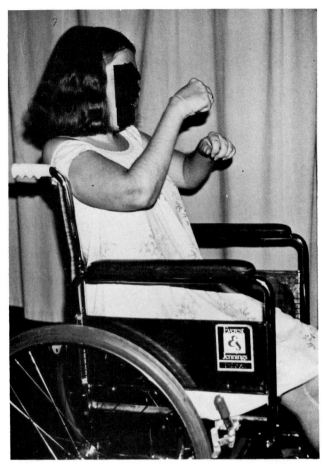

Figure 107–7. A severely affected rheumatoid patient with involvement of both shoulders who is unable to perform day-to-day functions. She is seen attempting to reach under the axillae. She is unable to reach to the anal region or in front to the perineum for personal hygiene and is unable to feed herself, wash her face, brush her teeth, or comb her hair. She is unable to sleep without interruption because of shoulder pain. The primary goal of shoulder replacement is relief of pain, but it is also tremendously important to some patients to restore shoulder rotation so they can independently perform the activities of daily living.

failure that are inherently present in a fixed fulcrum implant. The author studied use of two *acetabular-like glenoid components* but found that they interfered with reconstruction of the rotator cuff, and a glenoid component close to the size of a normal glenoid is almost always preferred (see Fig. 107–8C).

Synovectomy and joint débridement without replacement have too often been disappointing, and the technique is no longer used if there is any involvement of the articular surfaces.

Bursectomy, release, and synovectomy (see later) is done for the less common "bursal type" of shoulder involvement (see Fig. 107–4) and in patients with intractable frozen shoulders in which the articular surfaces of the glenohumeral joint are essentially spared.

Glenohumeral arthrodesis is not done in rheumatoid patients because it eliminates the rotatory motion of the shoulder that is so important in personal

hygiene and because the immobilization required postoperatively for the fusion has a deleterious effect on the elbow and wrist. Obviously, bilateral shoulder ankylosis is unacceptable because it precludes reaching in back or to the top of the head with either hand.[45]

Humeral head resection[45] is not used because it renders the joint flail and cannot be relied on to relieve pain.[34]

Glenoidectomy[47, 48] is not done in the author's center because it precludes the better functional result that should be obtainable with prosthetic replacement.

Osteotomies of the proximal humerus and glenoid ("*double osteotomy*") have been advocated in England but are, in the author's opinion, unable to give nearly as good functional results as prosthetic replacement.

It was stated that rheumatoid disease may weaken the muscles of the rotator cuff and destroy the articular surfaces so the humeral head may ride up, producing impingement against the undersurface of the acromion. This impingement may lead to the formation of a cuff tear. This type of impingement is treated by proper placement of the components in a nonconstrained *total shoulder arthroplasty* so the humerus is held away from the acromion rather than by acromioplasty. In neglected rheumatoid shoulders the impinging humerus may have deformed the acromion, requiring *acromioplasty* at the time of total shoulder arthroplasty, but this is uncommon.

Radical acromionectomy[49] has been used for rheumatoid patients in the past, but it weakens the deltoid and makes the patient worse. It should not be used in rheumatoid patients and, for that matter, should be abandoned in shoulder surgery.[2, 57]

Acromioclavicular Joint. Tenderness, swelling, and pain on adduction of the arm across the chest are the signs of arthritis of this joint. Roentgenographic changes confirm involvement. Lidocaine injection into the joint may be used to make sure of the source of pain. If the discomfort cannot be controlled by steroid injections and medical therapy, AC arthroplasty is occasionally considered. This procedure may be indicated concomitantly with other soft tissue operations or replacement.

Sternoclavicular Joint. Normally there is 40 degrees of motion in this joint, and on rare occasions it becomes symptomatic. Sleeping on that side may be unbearable, and the pain may lead to a frozen shoulder. The pain is usually controlled by steroid injections and reasonable medical treatment. If these fail, sternoclavicular arthroplasty (see later) may be considered. However, this is rare and has not been necessary for RA in the author's experience.

Shoulder Syndromes. *Biceps tenosynovitis* is not seen as a separate problem in RA, and synovectomy of the tendon sheath and tenodesis of the long head are not done as isolated procedures.

Tenderness and pain at the scapula resulting from inflammation of the bursa between the scapula and ribs are referred to as the *scapulothoracic (scapu-*

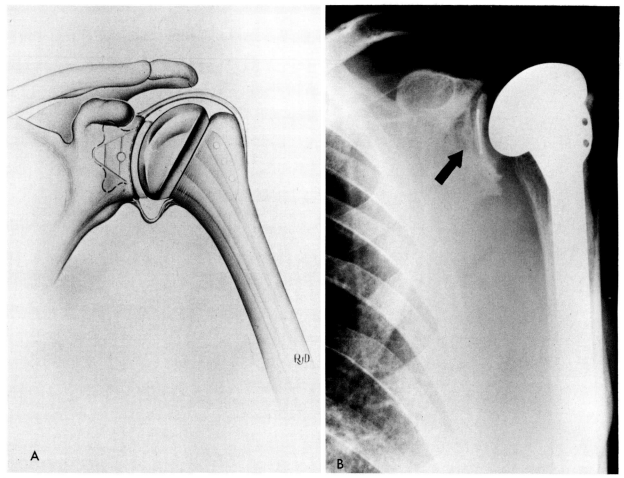

Figure 107–8. Drawing *(A)* and radiograph *(B)* to show the standard long head total shoulder resurfacing unit. The polyethylene glenoid component is anchored with acrylic cement, and the arrow points to this in the radiograph. The metal (Mediloy 1) humeral component is made with two lengths of head, three diameters of stem, and three lengths of stem. Half-size replicas of the humeral and "AJ10" glenoid component have been made for Dr. Robert H. Cofield for use in juvenile RA, and these are available from the instrument maker.

locostal) syndrome. A local lidocaine injection into the bursa relieves the pain and differentiates the condition from the referred pain that results from overuse of the scapular muscles when a glenohumeral derangement is present. No operative treatment, other than injections, is indicated for this condition in rheumatoid patients.

Disuse atrophy and vasomotor instability in the upper extremity may develop in patients with chronic shoulder pain, producing the *shoulder-hand syndrome.* The hand becomes puffy, stiffens, and may be wet and pale. Although sympathectomy has been advocated for this condition, it is more beneficial to the entire upper extremity unit to correct the underlying shoulder problem with total shoulder arthroplasty when indicated and re-establish motion in the extremity with physical therapy and exercises.

Contraindications to Arthroplasty. The only absolute contraindication to an arthroplasty is active infection. Rheumatoid shoulders have often had many injections or previous surgery, and either may

introduce low-grade infection. Rheumatoid patients have less resistance to infection, especially those receiving steroids. Steroids may mask the usual warning signs of infection. If anything suspicious is seen at the time of surgery, smears and frozen sections should be obtained to indicate whether the operation should be discontinued. Wound cultures during surgery should be routine.

Muscle deficits of the cuff and deltoid do not pose a contraindication to replacement arthroplasty, and unconstrained prostheses have not had the problem of instability that was expected by some.[7, 19, 28] As previously stated, only 20 percent of rheumatoid patients have complete thickness tears, and most of these have been easy to repair. Usually, rheumatoid patients have, in the author's experience, come to function adequately, although the recovery is especially slow in rheumatoid patients. In 10 percent of the author's series, shoulder arthroplasty had been deferred until the cuff and bone had been destroyed, making a "limited goals" rehabilitation program nec-

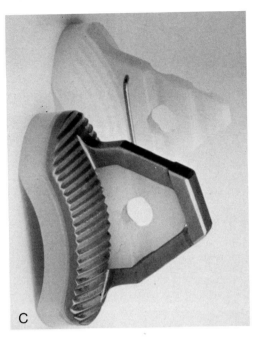

Figure 107–8. *Continued C*, A metal-backed glenoid component is now used when there is sufficient bone. The proximal cement groove has been eliminated from the stem of the polyethylene component. In long-standing rheumatoid shoulders the bone may be destroyed by rheumatoid granulation, precluding the use of a glenoid component. The short-head humeral component may facilitate repair when there is a large cuff tear. The prosthetic head should be placed high enough to keep the greater tuberosity away from the acromion, extending above the top of the greater tuberosity, to prevent impingement.

are involved because this reduces the rotatory stress on the elbow (by establishing rotation at the shoulder), may stop a large portion of the elbow pain by relieving the referred pain from the shoulder to the elbow, and may save the rotator cuff. The elbow arthroplasty can be done later without the same risk of loss of essential soft tissue. Occasionally elbow pain and instability are so great that it would interfere with rehabilitation of the shoulder, and in this case the elbow is replaced first and shoulder replacement is deferred until the elbow is well healed (usually 6 weeks). When there is severe involvement of both shoulders (Fig. 107–9), bilateral replacement is done usually with a 2- to 6-week interval between procedures.

SURGICAL TECHNIQUE

Bursectomy, Release, and Synovectomy. This infrequent procedure is limited to patients with bur-

essary, that is, as the stability of the components permits, pendulum exercises alone for 3 months followed by progressive isometric and resistive exercises below the horizontal, with the objective of pain relief and independent living (eating, sleeping, and self-care).

Cervical radiculopathy may result in weakness of the deltoid or spinati muscles and cause electromyographic changes. This does not pose an absolute contraindication to replacement, but the cervical problem demands concomitant treatment.

Order of Multiple Procedures in the Upper Extremity. Priorities for planning multiple surgical procedures in the upper extremity should be based on pain and functional importance of the various joints in the activities of daily living. The functional importance of the shoulder is great when one considers how much it can interfere with sleeping and personal hygiene (see Fig. 107–7). Shoulder pain tends to be made worse whether lying on the good side, on the back, or on the bad side, and the pain is worse at night. Elimination of this pain has a beneficial effect on the entire upper extremity unit. It is logical that shoulder replacement should have priority over hand and wrist procedures that are done for relatively asymptomatic conditions. The author prefers, in general, to do the shoulder replacement before elbow replacements when both joints

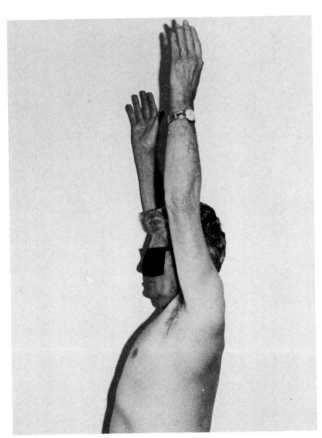

Figure 107–9. An early result of bilateral total shoulder replacements seen 4 months after the first operation, in a 52-year-old man who had an intermediate grade of RA. Both shoulders had been so extremely painful that the operations were done 3 weeks apart. He is free of shoulder pain and has nearly normal motion, but at this stage he was expected to continue heat and stretching exercises at least twice daily, and, since his rheumatoid muscles were weak, he was advised to continue strengthening exercises until his muscles approached normal. The rehabilitation of rheumatoid shoulders is always slower because of the concomitant muscle disease, but those with mild and intermediate grades can achieve excellent results.

sal type involvement or unyielding contractures without destruction of the articular surfaces of the glenohumeral joint (see earlier). It is important to explain to the patient that the postoperative exercise program will continue for at least 6 months. The patient is taught the exercises preoperatively. The anterior acromioplasty approach is used because the AC joint is often diseased, requiring concomitant AC arthroplasty. It is possible to do this procedure through this relatively small (9.0- or 10.0-cm) incision with minimal deltoid detachment, provided that the arm is draped completely free so that the humerus can be rotated in all directions. It is important to remember that the humerus must be moved in the incision rather than trying to retract the incision around the humerus.

The patient is placed high on the operating table with a head rest (to avoid hyperextension of the neck) and with the point of the affected shoulder protruding over the corner of the table. The upper part of the table is raised 30 degrees, and the knee gatch is raised sufficiently to prevent the patient from sliding down. Intratracheal anesthesia is used so that the anesthesiologist is draped from the field. The arm is wrapped so that it can be moved in all directions without interference.

A 9.0-cm incision is made from just lateral to the acromion to just lateral to the coracoid, in Langer's lines. The deep fascia is incised, and the deltoid is split 5 cm from above downward. Further splitting jeopardizes the axillary nerve. In rheumatoid patients a stay suture is placed deep within the deltoid at the lower end of the split to prevent extending the split by subsequent retraction of the soft muscle. When the AC joint is involved, the distal 2.0 cm of clavicle is removed, as described for glenohumeral replacement arthroplasty later. The clavipectoral fascia, extending laterally from the coracoclavicular ligament, is divided, and an elevator is placed under the acromion. With traction on the arm, the rotator cuff is inspected, and the anterior process of the acromion is palpated for sharp edges or traction spurs in the coracoacromial ligament.[2] If an impingement lesion is present, anterior acromioplasty removes an anterior acromial spur if present in the ligament, but it is thought beneficial in rheumatoid patients to leave part of the coracoacromial ligament intact or to reattach it for what stability it might offer against the head's ascending.

This approach places the greater tuberosity in the center of the field, where, because of the slope of the acromion, the entire rotator cuff may be seen by moving the humerus. The enlarged bursa is then excised by sharp and blunt dissection, avoiding the axillary nerve posteriorly. With flexion and external rotation the subscapularis is exposed and detached 2.0 cm medial to the biceps groove. Some subscapularis tendon remains on the lesser tuberosity to facilitate repair and to allow lengthening if later desired. The inferior capsule is released while a blunt elevator guards the axillary nerve. Synovectomy of

the glenohumeral joint and sheath of the long head of the biceps is then completed.

The subscapularis is reattached but is lengthened by a Z-plasty in the coronal plane when contracted. The capsule is left open. A good deltoid repair is extremely important.

Patients who had stiffness of the glenohumeral joint preoperatively are given passive exercises to maintain external rotation and elevation. These are continued until there is essentially full assistive overhead motion. Early exercises should be assistive (for range of motion) and are preceded by low heat when possible.[6] Appropriate analgesia is given with each meal. Isometrics are begun within 2 weeks.

Glenohumeral Replacement Arthroplasty (Total and Humeral Head). Unfortunately glenohumeral replacement is a demanding procedure and requires a surgeon especially skilled in shoulder surgery for optimal results.[62] The glenoid component is usually used in patients with RA. The technique for total glenohumeral replacement is the same as that for humeral head replacement except for the additional step of inserting the glenoid component. Both demand meticulous repair and rehabilitation of the muscles and precise technique for inserting the implant. After the humeral head has been removed, it becomes possible to do an AC arthroplasty and anterior acromioplasty from below (without detaching the deltoid), provided that a long deltopectoral incision is used. This approach is now preferred for all replacements.[7]

Any components of Neer anatomic design can be used. The Neer II humeral components (see Fig. 107–8) are made of metal (Mediloy 1) in two lengths of head, 23 mm and 15 mm, each with three different diameters of stem, 6.3 mm, 9.5 mm, and 12.7 mm. Half length stems are also available. The long head provides better leverage for the rotator muscles. The short head facilitates repair of massive cuff lesions and is better for small patients. The stems fit drilling and reaming specifications and are slightly tapered with the thicker portion proximally to enhance a press fit or offer greater ease of removal when used with acrylic cement. The diameter of the head is 44 mm, which approximates the average size of the human head,[35] and, since the arc of the articular surface of the normal glenoid does not match the arc of the normal head, the author now prefers the standard-sized glenoid components, either metal-backed or polyethylene according to the quantity of bone available, rather than oversized glenoid components (see Fig. 107–8C). Oversized glenoid components interfere with the cuff repair. The 600 percent glenoid component is no longer used, and the 200 percent is almost never used.

The patient is given iron, vitamins, and calcium while awaiting surgery and for 1 week prior to the operation uses antiseptic soap in the axilla to reduce the bacterial count of the skin. Preoperative instruction is given in the exercise program, which is individualized depending on the condition of the muscles. Prophylactic antibiotics are given on the night before surgery and during the procedure and are continued at least until the wound cultures have been received and longer in patients who have been receiving steroids.

The patient is positioned high on the table with a head rest to avoid hyperextension of the neck. The arm is draped free so that it can be moved without interference off the side of the table. The point of the shoulder protrudes over the corner of the table. Folded towels are placed under the scapula to hold it forward. A well-padded short arm board is placed at the top of the table so that the arm can be rested on it in an abducted and externally rotated position while working on the glenoid. The table is adjusted to the beachchair position.

A 17.0-cm skin incision extends over the delto-pectoral groove from the clavicle to near the deltoid insertion. The anterior fibers of the deltoid insertion are divided to release tension from retraction on this muscle, but the origin of the deltoid is meticulously left intact. The cephalic vein is ligated. The deltoid is retracted laterally as the arm is abducted 25 degrees, and the clavipectoral fascia, extending downward from the coracoclavicular ligament, is divided. A broad elevator is placed beneath the acromion as a retractor. The shoulder is flexed and externally rotated to facilitate division of the subscapularis tendon at a point 2.0 cm medial to the biceps groove. The subscapularis is tagged with stay sutures. The capsule is then released anteriorly and inferiorly while a blunt elevator prevents injury to the axillary nerve. The long head of the biceps, if intact, is left attached to the glenoid. When there is a small cuff tear, it is usually closed prior to removal of the head. If there is a large cuff tear, it can be mobilized better after the head has been removed and closed after the prosthesis has been installed. The humeral head is delivered into the wound by external rotation and extension of the shoulder.

After débriding synovia and bursa, the humeral head is detached with a broad osteotome at the level of the former margins of its articular surface. A surprisingly small amount of bone is removed. It is important to maintain the former angle of retroversion (usually 30 to 40 degrees). The long head of the biceps, if present, is left intact, but osteophytes and rheumatoid granulation tissue are trimmed from its groove. The medullary canal of the humerus is reamed or drilled to the appropriate size to receive the stem of a prosthesis. Drill points that match the three sizes of stems and reach at least 15 cm down the medullary canal are used. Hand reamers to match the flare of the stems are also available. With the humerus extended and pushed upward into the field, a trial prosthesis is inserted. The prosthesis is then reduced for final check on the angle of retroversion and length of the neck of prosthesis. The trial prosthesis is then removed.

The glenoid is exposed by retracting the upper humerus backward with a Fukuda ring retractor.[55] A Darrach elevator is placed in front of it to provide better exposure and protection for the axillary nerve. Special care is needed to avoid fracturing the soft bone. A bolster is placed under the elbow to prevent extension at the shoulder, and the humerus is abducted and externally rotated on the arm board in the position that offers the best view. The glenoid labrum is excised, and the surface of the glenoid prepared with a power drill, small curettes, and a metal guide. After inserting a trial glenoid component (and after testing it with the humeral component in place), the glenoid component is anchored with acrylic cement, using a syringe. Two injections of cement are made: the first stops deep oozing of blood; the second is made immediately after wiping out the first batch, and it is made with careful thumb pressure. Meticulous care is needed to remove blood from the depth of the glenoid just prior to injecting the cement. Some rheumatoid glenoids have been so completely eroded by granulations that they require the use of metal cement retainers and bone grafts. The erosion occasionally extends halfway through the coracoid (see Fig. 107–2C), making it impossible to properly orient the standard glenoid component. The 200 percent glenoid component has been used developmentally in selected rheumatoid patients with a short-head humeral component (which facilitates cuff repair), does not overhang so much as to preclude cuff repair, but has not been used for several years. Standard-sized glenoid components are preferred. Granulation destruction of the glenoid can make it impossible to install it. In several rheumatoid patients in the author's series with the worst destruction of the glenoid, a long head humeral component was used without a glenoid component.

Prior to inserting the humeral component, anterior acromioplasty and AC arthroplasty are done if indicated. However, in recent years these procedures have been very rarely performed in rheumatoid shoulders. If there is a large tear of the rotator cuff, the cuff should be mobilized at this time prior to inserting the head. The tendons are released as necessary not only superficially but also at the base of the coracoid and from the joint capsule. Drill holes are made at the greater tuberosity, and these are threaded with nylon sutures in preparation for later reattachment of the rotator cuff.

The humeral component (previously selected) is then inserted. The sum of the retroversion of both components should be 30 to 40 degrees. The humeral component is anchored with acrylic cement in all rheumatoid shoulders because the bone tends to be soft and osteopenic. The only exception is when the possibility of low-grade infection is suspected.

The soft tissue repair around the implant is of equal importance to the orientation and seating of the prosthetic components. Mobilization of the tendons should have been completed prior to inserting the head component. It should now be possible to reattach the cuff to the greater tuberosity without tension when the arm is at the side; otherwise, further mobilization is required. The long head of the biceps is left free to run in its groove if it is intact and of adequate shape. The subscapularis is repaired, but the capsule is not sutured. If the subscapularis is short and restricts external rotation, a coronal plane Z-plasty is done. Suction drainage tubes are inserted between the deltoid and cuff, and the deltopectoral interval is closed.

Postoperative exercise regimens must be individualized, depending on the condition of the rotator cuff. When the cuff is adequate, passive elevation of the arm is begun by the therapist and surgeon 48 hours after surgery and is progressed to the self-assistive program (for range of motion) as rapidly as tolerated. Exercises for strength are deferred until the shoulder is pain free and should not be performed beyond the point where pain begins. Heat rather than cold prior to exercises is favored for obtaining motion. A brace is no longer, or rarely, used for rheumatoid shoulders postoperatively. The earlier passive elevation by the therapist and surgeon has been replaced by the use of a continuous passive motion machine.[60] Since the deltoid is not incised if the rotator cuff was intact, active exercises can be started in 2 weeks. The rehabilitation goal is nearly normal for most (see Fig. 107–9). Stretching exercises with low heat are done at least twice a day so long as there is significant restriction of motion, and progressive resistive exercises (with weights or an elastic exerciser) are valuable in strengthening the atrophied and diseased muscles.[6]

Sternoclavicular Arthroplasty. An 8.0-cm incision is made below the prominence of the clavicle and is retracted upward so that the clavicle can be stripped of soft tissue to a point just lateral to the joint capsule. Throughout this operation scrupulous care must be taken to avoid tearing the great veins. When blunt elevators can be passed both from beneath and from above, the clavicle is cut across about 2.0 cm from the joint line, leaving the distal fragment attached to the costoclavicular ligament. While traction is being applied to the inner fragment, the capsule is divided and this fragment is removed. The clavicular head of the sternocleidomastoid muscle is detached from the clavicle and sutured to fill the dead space. The skin closure permits the escape of blood to minimize hematoma formation.

RESULTS TO BE EXPECTED

Acromioclavicular arthroplasty and sternoclavicular arthroplasty are very rarely indicated as isolated procedures without glenohumeral arthroplasty. However, patients who had complete temporary relief after lidocaine injection of these joints and with disease limited to those joints have a good chance of completely satisfactory results, and these procedures have a beneficial effect on eliminating contractures elsewhere in the extremity. Synovectomy is rarely indicated but has given gratifying and lasting results when done with bursectomy and AC arthroplasty in seven patients who were free from articular surface involvement. It failed in all patients who had erosion or attritional changes of the articular cartilage[10] and is not used except in the bursal type free from glenohumeral alterations by radiograph.

Results of humeral head replacement in 26 rheumatoid patients were described in 1971.[10] The functional result was usually good in those with low-grade disease, but the range of motion was limited in those with severe disease. Pain relief was generally good.

The results have been much better since the deltoid origin has been left intact, the glenoid component added, and the rehabilitation program improved.

Reports on the results of the Neer II total glenohumeral resurfacing procedure described previously that were made to The American Orthopaedic Association[28] and The Canadian Orthopaedic Association[50] in 1977 included 61 rheumatoid shoulders. The Neer II implant was first used in 1973. The rotator cuff was found to be intact (with or without attenuation) in 43, moderate tears in 7, and massive tears in 10. Complications included fracture through soft bone, misalignment of the glenoid, and five failures because of riding up of the head that was due to poor cuff function. Lucent lines around the cement in the glenoid were present in one third of the patients and were thought to be due to blood locally at the time of cementing rather than mechanical loosening. Only one patient required further surgery. Twenty-eight had been followed for 1 or more years. A rating of *excellent* was given when the patient was enthusiastic about the operation and had no significant pain, full use of the shoulder, strength approaching normal, elevation to within 25 degrees of the normal side, and 90 percent rotation (see Fig. 107–9). In a *satisfactory result* the patient was satisfied with the operation and had no more than occasional fleeting pain or bad weather ache, good use of the shoulder for daily functions, 30 percent strength, at least 90 degrees of elevation, and 50 percent rotation. In an *unsatisfactory result* these criteria were not met. The results were graded 13 excellent, 7 satisfactory, and 8 unsatisfactory. The unsatisfactory ratings were because of weakness of the muscles rather than pain.

Later studies have been reported. The results of Neer and associates were published in 1982.[7] Of 69 rheumatoid shoulders in 56 patients, 50 shoulders were followed more than 2 years. Seven patients (all with massive cuff tears) were successfully treated on a limited-goal basis for less motion and more stability with satisfactory relief of pain and use of the joint for the activities of daily living. Five of these had standard glenoid components, and two had deep cup glenoid components. The remaining 43 were given the full exercise program, and the results were rated as 28 excellent, 12 satisfactory, and 3 unsatisfactory. Of the 43, 14 had complete cuff tears, and 2 had been previously operated on elsewhere. The three ratings of "failure" were given for weak muscles and inability to elevate the arm above the horizontal rather than pain or failure of the implant.

This study was extended in 1988 to include 147 rheumatoid shoulders followed for a minimum of 2 years.[62] It was of interest to note that both in the author's 1973–1980 series and in the 1980–1986 series, the incidence of lucent lines around the cement of the glenoid component was higher in patients with RA and cuff-tear arthropathy than in patients with other conditions (27 percent of patients with osteoarthritis, 48 percent of those with RA, and 47 percent of those with cuff-tear arthroplasty). This was thought to be due to the poor quality of the bone in the latter two conditions. The incidence of complete lines was much lower in the latter series, suggesting improved technique. Only one glenoid component had been removed from a rheumatoid shoulder because of loosening. Virtually all other humeral components in the latter series had been anchored with acrylic cement and appeared to be trouble-free. Of the author's present personal series of rheumatoid shoulders treated with a Neer II total arthroplasty, the glenoid component was omitted in three patients with too much destruction of the glenoid.[61] Many of the results approach normal function (see Fig. 107–9).

Results reported from other clinics in 1983 also indicate that good pain relief and function are dependent on the preservation or reconstruction of the rotator cuff and deltoid muscles and their rehabilitation.[51–54] To date there have been only a few cases of clinical loosening of the glenoid component requiring reinsertion. The bone at the rheumatoid glenoid, however, is often eroded by granulation tissue, requiring careful cement technique and occasionally bone grafting. Despite this, only 10 glenoid component loosenings requiring further surgery are found in the literature of more than 1000 arthroplasties reported to date.[58] A recent study by Barrett and associates[59] emphasized how the results are adversely affected by long delay before the shoulder arthroplasty. All these studies stress the need for attention to the details of technique during surgery and aftercare if optimum results are to be achieved.

It is now thought that the criteria for a satisfactory rating for the long-standing, neglected rheumatoid shoulders with severe bone loss and cuff loss should be different from those for other patients because the diseased muscles precluded full active motion and strength regardless of the type of fulcrum. The severely rheumatoid patients in this study who received unsatisfactory ratings were actually delighted to be free from shoulder pain and to have independent function for the activities of daily living. It seems inappropriate that their results be graded unsatisfactory because they were unable to elevate 90 degrees when shoulder and elbow motion combined placed the hand where it was needed.

More than two thirds of the rheumatoid patients in my recent series[62] who underwent glenohumeral replacement had an essentially intact rotator cuff, and their results have been good by any standard. The approach described previously in which the deltoid origin remains intact has been used consistently recently and has made a marked improvement in the speed of recovery and strength.

It is thought that shoulder replacement is not behind other joint replacements, but it is recognized that it is more difficult. In the hip, only bone stability is required. In the knee, ligaments are needed. But in the shoulder neither the bone nor the ligaments provide stability, and the level of function depends on the muscles. The surgeon must have the ability to repair and rehabilitate the muscle for optimal results and must be given a chance to do the shoulder arthroplasty before the bone and cuff have been destroyed. Shoulder arthroplasty in rheumatoid patients cannot be deferred as safely as surgery in other joints because no other joint has a rotator cuff to be destroyed by waiting, and bone loss at the frail scapula eventually precludes the use of a glenoid component.

References

1. Inmann, V. T., Saunders, J. B., and Abbott, L. C.: Observations on the shoulder joint. J. Bone Joint Surg. 26:1, 1944.
2. Neer, C. S., II: Anterior acromioplasty for the chronic impingement syndrome in the shoulder. A preliminary report. J. Bone Joint Surg. 54A:41, 1972.
3. Neer, C. S., II, Bigliani, L. U., and Hawkins, R. J.: Rupture of the long head of the biceps related to subacromial impingement. Orthopaedic Transactions by J. Bone Joint Surg. 1:111, 1977.
4. Codman, E. A.: The Shoulder, Rupture of the Supraspinatus Tendon and Other Lesions in or about the Subacromial Bursa. 2nd ed. Boston, Thomas Todd Company, 1934.
5. Bateman, J. E.: The Shoulder and Neck. Philadelphia, W. B. Saunders Company, 1972.
6. Hughes, M. A., and Neer, C. S., II: Glenohumeral joint replacement and postoperative rehabilitation. Phys. Ther. 55:85, 1975.
7. Neer, C. S., II, Watson, K. C., and Stanton, F. J.: Recent experience in total shoulder replacement. J. Bone Joint Surg. 64A:319, 1982.
8. Preston, L.: The Surgical Management of Rheumatoid Arthritis. Philadelphia, W. B. Saunders Company, 1968.
9. Cofield, R. H.: Joint Replacement in Rheumatoid Arthritis. Instructional Course. American Academy Orthopaedic Surgeons Annual Meeting, Las Vegas, 1981.
10. Cruess, R. L., and Mitchell, N. S.: Surgery of Rheumatoid Arthritis. Philadelphia, J. B. Lippincott Company, 1971, Chapter 17.
11. Marmor, L.: Arthritis Surgery. Philadelphia, Lea & Febiger, 1976.
12. Clayton, M. L., and Ferlic, D. C.: Surgery of the shoulder in rheumatoid arthritis. A report of nineteen patients. Clin. Orthop. 106:166, 1974.
13. Neer, C. S., II: Degenerative lesions of the proximal humeral articular surface. Clin. Orthop. 20:116, 1961.
14. Neer, C. S., II: Replacement arthroplasty for glenohumeral osteoarthritis. J. Bone Joint Surg. 56A:1, 1974.
15. Barton, N. J.: Arthrodesis of the shoulder for degenerative conditions. J. Bone Joint Surg. 54A:1759, 1972.
16. Straub, L. R.: An overview of surgical procedures in arthritis. In Hollander, J. L. (ed.): The Arthritis Handbook. West Point, PA, Merck & Company, 1974, Chapter 8.
17. DePalma, A. F.: Surgery of the Shoulder. 2nd ed. Philadelphia, J. B. Lippincott Company, 1973.
18. Moseley, H. F.: Shoulder Lesions. 3rd ed. Edinburgh, E & S Livingstone Ltd., 1969.
19. Cofield, R. H.: Status of total shoulder arthroplasty. Arch. Surg. 112:1088, 1977.
20. Neer, C. S., II: Impingement lesions. Clin. Orthop. 173:70, 1983.
21. DePalma, A. F.: Surgery of the Shoulder. 2nd ed. Philadelphia, J. B. Lippincott Company, 1973.
22. Pettersson, C.: Supraspinatus tendon ruptures: A morphological analysis. Presented to Swedish Orthopaedic Association, Gavle, Sweden, May, 1983.

23. McLaughlin, H. L.: Lesions of the musculotendinous cuff of the shoulder. J. Bone Joint Surg. 26:31, 1944.
24. McLaughlin, H. L., and Asherman, E. G.: The lesions of the musculotendinous cuff of the shoulder. J. Bone Joint Surg., 33A:76, 1951.
25. Lindblom, K., and Palmar, I.: Ruptures of the tendon aponeurosis of the shoulder joint—the so-called supraspinatus ruptures. Acta Chir. Scand. 82:133, 1939.
26. Meyer, A. W.: Further observations upon use-destruction in joints. J. Bone Joint Surg. 4:491, 1922.
27. Cruess, R. L.: Steroid-induced avascular necrosis of the head of the humerus. J. Bone Joint Surg. 58B:313, 1976.
28. Neer, C. S., II, Cruess, R. L., Sledge, C. B., and Wilde, A. H.: Total shoulder replacement. A preliminary report. Orthopaedic Transactions by J. Bone Joint Surg. 1:244, 1977.
29. Neer, C. S., II, Craig, E. V., and Fukuda, H.: Cuff-tear arthropathy. Orthop. Trans. 5:477, 1981.
30. Neer, C. S., II, Craig, E. V., and Fukuda, H.: Cuff-tear arthropathy. J. Bone Joint Surg. 65A:1232, 1983.
31. McCarty, D. J., Halverson, P. B., Guillerino, F. C., Brewer, B. J., and Kozin, F.: "Milwaukee shoulder." Association of microspheroids containing hydroxyapatite crystals, active collagenase, and neutral protease with rotator cuff defects. Arthritis Rheum. 24:464, 1981.
32. Zippel, J.: Vollstandiger Schultergelenkersatz aus Kunststoff und Metall. Biomed. Technik 17:87, 1972.
33. Kenmore, P. I.: A Simple Shoulder Replacement. Read at Clemson University Biomaterials Symposium, 1973.
34. Neer, C. S., II, Brown, T. H., Jr., and McLaughlin, H. L.: Fracture of the neck of the humerus with dislocation of the head fragment. Am. J. Surg. 85:252, 1953.
35. Neer, C. S., II: Articular replacement of the humeral head. J. Bone Joint Surg. 37A:215, 1955.
35a. Boyd, A. J., Thomas, W. H., Scott, R. D., Sledge, C. B., and Thornhill, T. S.: Total shoulder arthroplasty versus hemiarthroplasty. Indications for glenoid resurfacing. J. Arthroplasty 5:329, 1990.
36. Letten, A. W. F., and Scales, J. T.: Total replacement of the shoulder joint (two cases). Proc. R. Soc. Med. 65:373, 1972.
37. Letten, A. W. F., and Scales, J. T.: Total replacement arthroplasty of the shoulder in rheumatoid arthritis (abstract). J. Bone Joint Surg. 55B:217, 1973.
38. Zippel, J.: Luxationssichere Schulterendoprothese Modell BME. J. Orthop. 113:454, 1975.
39. Romano, R. L., and Burgess, E. M.: Total shoulder replacement (abstract). J. Bone Joint Surg. 57A:1033, 1975.
40. Fenlin, J. M., Jr.: Total glenohumeral joint replacement. Orthop. Clin. North Am. 6:565, 1975.
41. Post, M., Haskell, S. S., and Finder, J. G.: Total shoulder replacement (abstract). J. Bone Joint Surg. 57A:1171, 1975.
42. Gristina, A. G., and Forte, M. R.: The trispherical total shoulder prosthesis—biomechanical, anatomical and surgical considerations. In Trans. Soc. for Biomaterials Symposium, Paper 121, New Orleans, 1977.
43. Buechel, F., Pappas, M. J., and DePalma, A. F.: "Floating socket" total shoulder replacement: Anatomical, biomechanical and surgical rationale. J. Biomed. Mat. Res. 12:89, 1978.
44. Macnab, I., and English, E.: Development of a glenohumeral arthroplasty for a severely destroyed shoulder (abstract). J. Bone Joint Surg. 58B:137, 1976.
45. Neer, C. S., II, and Hawkins, R. J.: A functional analysis of shoulder fusions (abstract). J. Bone Joint Surg. 59B:508, 1977.
46. Jones, L.: The shoulder joint; observations on the anatomy and physiology with an analysis of a reconstructive operation following extensive injury. Surg. Gynecol. Obstet. 75:433, 1942.
47. Wainwright, D.: Glenoidectomy in the treatment of the painful arthritic shoulder (abstract). J. Bone Joint Surg. 58B:377, 1976.
48. Gariepy, R.: Glenoidectomy in the repair of the rheumatoid shoulder (abstract). J. Bone Joint Surg. 59B:122, 1977.
49. Hutchins, W. C.: In Campbell's Operative Orthopaedics. 5th ed. St. Louis, C. V. Mosby Company, 1971, p. 101.
50. Cruess, R. L.: Neer's arthroplasty of the shoulder—preliminary report (abstract). J. Bone Joint Surg. 59B:508, 1977.
51. Weiss, A. P., Adams, M. A., Moore J. R., and Weiland, A. J.: Unconstrained shoulder arthroplasty. A five-year average follow-up study. Clin. Orthop. Aug. (257):86, 1990.
52. Figgie, H. E., Inglis, A. E., Goldberg, V. M., Ranawat, C. S., Figgie, M. P., and Wile, J. M.: An analysis of factors affecting the long-term results of total shoulder arthroplasty in inflammatory arthritis. J. Arthroplasty 3:123, 1988.
53. Thomas, B. J., Amstutz, H. C., and Cracchiolo, A.: Shoulder arthroplasty for rheumatoid arthritis. Clin. Orthop. Apr. (265):125, 1991.
54. Cofield, R. H., and Edgerton, B. C.: Total shoulder arthroplasty: complications and revision surgery. Instr. Course Lect. 39:449, 1990.
55. Fukada, H., Mikasa, M., and Ogawa, K.: Ring retractor. A new humeral head retractor. J. Bone Joint Surg. 64A:289, 1982.
56. Neer, C. S., II, and Poppen, N. K.: Supraspinatus outlet. Presented to American Shoulder and Elbow Surgeons, San Francisco, California, January, 1987. Orthop. Trans. 2:234, 1987.
57. Neer, C. S., II, and Marberry, T. A.: On the disadvantages of radical acromionectomy. J. Bone Joint Surg. 63A:416, 1981.
58. Franklin, J. E., Jackins, S. E., and Matsen, F. A., III: Glenoid loosening in total shoulder arthroplasty. Presented to American Shoulder and Elbow Surgeons, San Francisco, California, January, 1987.
59. Barrett, W. P., Thornhill, T. S., Thomas, W. H., Gebhart, E. M., and Sledge, C. B.: Nonconstrained total shoulder arthroplasty in patients with polyarticular rheumatoid arthritis. J. Arthroplasty 4:91, 1989.
60. Neer, C. S., II, McCann, P. D., Macfarlane, E. A., and Padilla, N.: Earlier passive motion following shoulder arthroplasty and rotator cuff repair. Presented to American Shoulder and Elbow Surgeons, San Antonio, Texas, November, 1986. Orthop. Trans. 2:231, 1987.
61. Neer, C. S. II, and Satterlee, C. C.: Unpublished prospective study, 1988.
62. Neer, C. S., II: Shoulder Reconstruction. Philadelphia, W. B. Saunders Company, 1990.

Chapter 108
The Hip

Paul J. Tsahakis
Gregory W. Brick
Robert Poss

Total hip arthroplasty has revolutionized the treatment of advanced hip disease. The long-term results of this procedure have demonstrated excellent pain relief and functional return in the vast majority of patients. Earlier problems, such as femoral component loosening in the first 5 years, infection, and component breakage, are now better understood and consequently are encountered less frequently. The ultimate longevity of these implants, however, is compromised by late aseptic loosening of cemented acetabular components, the biologic reaction to wear debris, the osteopenia and geometric changes in bone resulting from aging, and the altered patterns of load sharing imposed by the presence of these implants. It is imperative, therefore, to balance the patient's needs and goals against the benefits and risks of total hip arthroplasty.

The frequency of major hip involvement in the patient with rheumatoid arthritis is difficult to estimate. In two series of total hip replacement reported from large referral centers, only 5.8 percent of 2012[1] and 15 percent of 1975[2] hip arthroplasties were performed on patients with rheumatoid arthritis. Historically, approximately one third of all total hip arthroplasties performed at Brigham and Women's Hospital have been in patients with rheumatoid arthritis. Over the last 3 years, however, this percentage has decreased to approximately 15 percent as the backlog of rheumatoid patients requiring hip replacements has diminished.

In this chapter, the unique problems encountered by the rheumatoid patient as a candidate for total hip replacement, the rationale of total hip replacement in rheumatoid arthritis and ankylosing spondylitis, and various forms of prosthetic fixation and results are presented. A discussion of hip biomechanics is also included. Finally, strategies employed in the reconstruction of failed arthroplasties and their results are discussed.

EVALUATION OF THE PATIENT WITH A PAINFUL HIP

The history and physical examination, including roentgenograms, will help the physician decide on the proper course of treatment for the patient with hip disease.

History

Pain is the commonest symptom of hip disease and is usually described as occurring in the groin, buttock, or posterior thigh. Weight bearing on the affected extremity typically exacerbates this symptom. Occasionally, patients exhibit a referred pattern and complain only of generalized knee discomfort.

Other coexisting causes of hip pain should be excluded in patients with an arthritic hip. These include spinal stenosis, lumbar disc disease, and trochanteric bursitis.

The nature and pattern of the patient's pain are important determinants for treatment. The patient with a history of hip discomfort that has changed minimally over time and that does not significantly impair sleep or personal hygiene will likely respond to conservative measures. This is opposed to the patient who complains of increasing pain over a few months duration, whose activities of daily living (distance walked, ability to ascend and descend stairs, ability to put on socks or shoes, undisturbed sleep) are significantly impaired, and whose symptoms do not respond to conservative measures (e.g., nonsteroidal anti-inflammatory drugs [NSAIDs] and a cane), who probably is a surgical candidate.

Physical Examination

The patient's gait pattern should be observed. Most patients demonstrate an antalgic limp that is characterized by a decreased stance time on the painful side. Another attempt by the patient to reduce pain involves shifting the body's weight closer to the center of the affected hip (Duchenne's sign, abductor lurch, Trendelenburg's lurch). A drooping of the pelvis away from the affected hip (Trendelenburg's sign) may also be observed and reflects either unfavorable hip geometry or abductor weakness.[3]

The patient should also be examined while lying supine on an examining table, which allows for the detection of hip flexion contractures by stabilizing the pelvis. Each hip is sequentially extended while the angle made by the contralateral hip relative to the table is noted (Thomas test). The range of motion of both hips, as well as all distal joints, is noted. Loss of internal rotation is one of the earliest signs of hip disease, which may be due to structural

1823

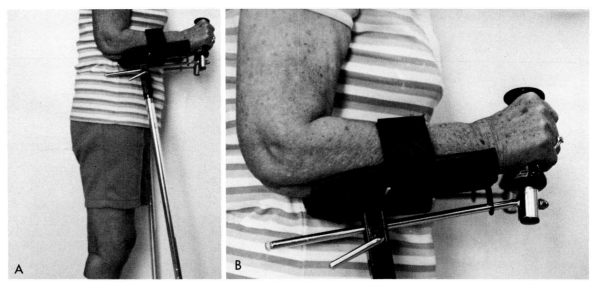

Figure 108–1. Platform crutches. *A*, A patient with weak or unstable elbows or shoulders can still bear weight with the upper extremities by using platform crutches. *B*, Rheumatoid hand deformities do not preclude the use of platform crutches (see text).

deformity or muscle spasm. Patients with end-stage arthritic hips frequently have difficulty in raising the leg while keeping it straight against resistance, which is an excellent way of differentiating hip pathology from back or knee disorders. Apparent and actual leg lengths are assessed, and the neurovascular status of both lower extremities is documented.

Radiographs

The patient whose symptoms and limitations are severe enough to suggest surgical treatment usually has radiographs showing complete loss of articular cartilage with varying degrees of bone loss. Osteopenia is usually present in patients with rheumatoid arthritis.

NONSURGICAL THERAPY

If on the basis of the aforementioned investigations the patient is thought not to be a surgical candidate, there are other methods and adjuncts that should help ameliorate symptoms.

Crutches or Cane

Relief of weight bearing reduces pain in the inflamed hip. Using two crutches, the patient can be trained to walk so that only the weight of the affected extremity touches the ground (touchdown gait). This is a more comfortable gait than is "non-weight-bearing," which, because of the force of muscle contraction, actually loads the hip to a greater degree and is impractical in a patient who has other joint involvement. The rheumatoid arthritis patient with

shoulder or elbow involvement may find platform crutches more comfortable and useful than axillary or Lofstrand crutches (Fig. 108–1).

A cane held in the opposite hand is of great help in unloading the involved hip. By applying 20 pounds of force to a cane with the left hand, an involved right hip can be relieved of more than 150 pounds of force[4] (see later for explanation).

Physical Therapy

Range of motion exercises are individualized. Much of the limitation of motion imposed by pain can be reversed by a program of active, active-assisted, and passive exercises once pain has been controlled. In particular, prone lying will help stretch out flexion deformities, whereas a stationary bicycle will increase flexion. Muscle strengthening, particularly of the hip abductors, is helpful in diminishing the fatiguing effects of an abductor lurch.

Traction

The authors have found no benefit from bed rest and traction except for the patient with acute severe pain who requires short-term immobilization for relief of muscle spasm secondary to synovitis.

THE RHEUMATOID PATIENT AS A CANDIDATE FOR SURGERY

Patients undergoing total hip arthroplasty must be well informed of the indications of surgery, the early and late postoperative course, and the potential complications. The indications for surgery depend on the patient's age, activity level, other joints affected, and their general medical condition. The physician's task in educating the patient is made easier if the patient has a friend or relative who has previously undergone a total hip arthroplasty. Progressive pain, despite adequate medical and physical therapy, is the prime indication for surgery. Functional limitations caused partly by pain and partly by restricted motion of the hip are considered in the context of the patient's needs and goals. On occasion, if the patient presents with an ankylosed hip and back pain, intervention in the form of total hip arthroplasty may relieve the patient of back pain by improving gait. The long-term complications of mechanical loosening and implant failure should be thoroughly discussed with younger patients before proceeding with hip replacement.

An important task for the rheumatologic team is to set reasonable goals for the patient. A patient who is bedridden with structural damage to four lower extremity joints, foot deformities, and weak upper extremities stands a poor chance of becoming an independent walker despite numerous operations but might be able to sit better after bilateral hip arthroplasties. A patient with a destroyed hip joint and early loss of articular cartilage in the knees would be better served by immediate hip arthroplasty than by waiting until three major joints required arthroplasty consecutively. In a recent review of the results of arthroplasty of both knees and hips, 14 of 16 patients had improved functional rating postoperatively.[5] Factors that predisposed to a lesser functional improvement were older age at initial surgery, longer duration of disease, and severe upper extremity involvement. If the patient requires both hip and knee arthroplasties as well as surgery to other joints, the authors generally will perform surgery on the most painful joint first. If pain is not the determining factor, hip arthroplasty is preferred first for the reason that hip arthroplasty provides the patient with almost immediate pain relief. The postoperative physical therapy program is not rigorous compared with that for the knee, and the patient will achieve functional improvement with relatively little personal effort.

Following total hip replacement, the rheumatologic team has the chance to reassess the patient's commitment to further surgery as a means of reaching the goals set preoperatively. The patient who will not work at the physical therapy program after hip arthroplasty is a poor candidate for knee or elbow arthroplasty. The almost certain pain relief obtained after total hip arthroplasty provides a great psychologic boost to a patient depressed by pain and functional loss, who is facing prolonged hospitalized and multiple operations.

If bilateral hip arthroplasty is required, these procedures are performed 7 to 10 days apart. Simultaneous knee arthroplasties[6] or ipsilateral hip and knee arthroplasties[7] and simultaneous hip arthroplasties[8] have been reported. Recent studies have suggested that bilateral simultaneous arthroplasties are more cost effective and may be preferable when treating patients who pose difficult anesthesia problems (e.g., in juvenile rheumatoid arthritis, ankylosing spondylitis) or who require expensive perioperative support (e.g., factor VIII replacement in hemophilia).[9–11]

Simultaneous bilateral hip arthroplasties should be performed if the hips have equal involvement and significant flexion deformities. If the interval between hip arthroplasties is excessive (longer than 2 months), the prosthetic hip will lose motion because the patient yields to the flexion contractures of the unoperated hip. Bilateral hip and knee replacements have been shown to provide marked pain relief and improved function in debilitated rheumatoid patients.[12]

ASSESSMENT OF STATUS OF OTHER JOINTS

Rheumatoid involvement of certain joints may compromise the results of total hip replacement or may be the cause of unforeseen complications.

Cervical Spine

Between 30 and 40 percent of rheumatoid arthritis patients admitted to the hospital have radiographic evidence of cervical spine subluxation, usually C1 on C2.[13] Between 2 and 5 percent of these patients have demonstrable long tract signs. It is, therefore, important that the anesthesiologist be aware of this situation and avoid maneuvers that cause hyperflexion of the cervical spine.

Temporomandibular Arthritis

Limitation of mandibular motion secondary to temporomandibular arthritis should be assessed preoperatively. Such limitations may require nasotracheal intubation or regional anesthesia.

Feet

Often the source of pain because of metatarsal head prominence or talonavicular arthritis, the feet are sources of skin breakdown and indolent infections owing to toe and foot deformities. It is of obvious importance to heal these areas prior to embarking on surgery of the ipsilateral hip.

Ipsilateral Knee

With involvement of the hip producing a flexion-adduction contracture, degenerative changes in the ipsilateral knee may be accelerated as it is thrown into more valgus position with weight bearing. Conversely, at surgery a valgus knee can cause the surgeon to estimate true femoral anteversion incorrectly and place the femoral component in malposition. In patients with a knee ankylosed in extension, manipulations of the hip at the time of surgery can cause sciatic nerve stretching with resultant neurapraxia.

PROFILE OF PATIENTS WITH RHEUMATOID ARTHRITIS UNDERGOING TOTAL HIP ARTHROPLASTY

The median decade for patients undergoing total hip replacement at the authors' hospital is 61 to 70 years of age. Osteoarthritic patients have a mean age of 66 years, whereas the rheumatoid arthritis patient averages 56 years. Ideally a surgical candidate should not be obese, but the limitations of function imposed by the disease make preoperative attempts at any significant loss of weight impractical. The authors prefer to perform total hip replacement on patients no younger than 60, but the absence of an acceptable alternative procedure in the rheumatoid arthritis patient has forced the lowering of this age requirement and the offering of this procedure to patients with juvenile rheumatoid arthritis in their late teens and twenties.

The patient should be in optimal medical condition. Particular attention should be paid to the urinary tract as a source of potential infection. Many females have asymptomatic bacteriuria; elderly men with symptoms of prostatism may be unable to void postoperatively and require repeated catheterizations, which may predispose to metastatic infection. The authors would prefer, if feasible, that an appropriate urologic procedure be performed some months prior to hip arthroplasty to obviate the need for catheterizations.

BIOMECHANICS OF THE HIP

Abnormalities of gait in the patient with hip disease, the rationale for use of a cane, and the technical goals of total hip replacement can be best understood by an appreciation of the forces exerted on the hip joint (Fig. 108–2). Definitive studies of this subject may be found elsewhere.[4, 14, 15]

The femoral head may be thought of as a fulcrum about which opposing forces must balance. If the patient is envisioned as standing on one lower extremity with the other raised off the ground and the pelvis held level, an equilibrium exists that is achieved by balancing body weight on one side of the fulcrum and the pull of the hip abductors on the other. Each of these forces acts through a lever arm. Body weight acts on the hip at a distance approximately three times that from which the abductors exert their pull.[16] Therefore, to achieve the equilibrium described earlier, the hip abductors must exert

a force three times body weight. The compressive force on the hip in this example is approximately four times body weight (three times body weight exerted by the abductors, plus one times body weight at the center of gravity).

Rydell[17] studied the forces about the hip joint by inserting specially designed hip endoprostheses containing strain gauges into two patients. He found that the greatest static load is applied to the hip in one-legged stance (2.6 times body weight). With slow walking, the forces in stance are approximately 1.6 times body weight, and in the swing phase they are 1.0 times body weight. With running, the forces are three times body weight in swing phase. Of particular interest is the fact that forces generated by hip flexion and extension while the patient is at bed rest are greater then those generated in slow walking or using crutches. From this analysis, certain conclusions become evident:

1. Weight loss is of great benefit because every pound lost results in at least three fewer pounds acting on the hip.[16]

2. The patient with a painful hip lurches toward the affected hip to reduce the length of body weight lever arm. Thus, the force generated by the hip abductors to balance body weight is reduced, and the hip is relatively unweighted.

3. Pushing down with a cane in the opposite hand reduces the effective body weight "seen" by the hip.[4] Because this force acts through a long lever arm, moderate force exerted on the cane results in a large reduction of compressive force on the hip. Exertion of approximately 30 pounds on a cane can reduce the force on the opposite hip by a factor of almost twice body weight.[16]

4. In total hip arthroplasty, the technical goals are (a) to medialize the acetabular component, thus reducing the body weight lever arm, and (b) to restore the greater trochanter to its normal lateral and distal position in relation to the femoral head, thereby restoring the abductor lever arm. Failure to achieve either of these goals results in excessive forces on the prosthetic hip and may favor loosening.

5. The forces on the normal or prosthetic hip are in multiples of body weight for activities considered routine in daily living. Any activities requiring increased muscular force (e.g., running or athletics) probably place excessive forces on the prosthetic system. These activities are not realistic goals of the patient undergoing total hip replacement.

TOTAL HIP ARTHROPLASTY

Technical Points

As most patients with rheumatoid arthritis have osteopenic bone, great care must be used while handling the extremity during surgical preparation in order to avoid an inadvertent femoral fracture.

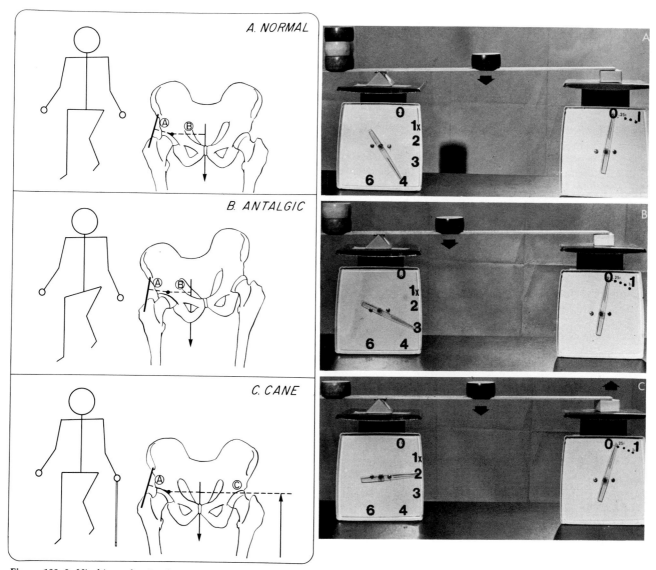

Figure 108–2. Hip biomechanics demonstrated diagrammatically (*left*) and experimentally (*right*). *A*, Normal. The stick figure is now in stance phase on the right lower extremity. For the pelvis to remain level, the forces about the hip must be in equilibrium; i.e., the lever arm of body weight exerted through a distance of approximately 3 inches (circled B) must be balanced by the force of contraction of the hip abductors exerted through a lever arm of approximately 1 inch (circled A). Note that in the actual experiment, body weight (central block) to the right of the hip is balanced by three times the body weight exerted through one third the distance to the left of the hip. That these forces are in equilibrium is demonstrated by the observation that there is no weight on the scale to the reader's right. Note that in stance phase the hip "sees" four times body weight (the sum of the patient's weight and the force of contraction of the hip abductors).

B, Antalgic gait. The patient with a painful hip will limp *toward* the affected side. By doing so the lever arm through which body weight is exerted is diminished. Thus less abductor force is required to stabilize the pelvis, and the hip effectively "sees" less force. In the experimental model, the same body weight shown in *A* is now exerted nearer the hip. Now only two times body weight is exerted by the hip abductors, and the hip "sees" three rather than four times body weight. By decreasing forces across the hip, it should be less painful.

C, A more effective way of unloading a painful hip is to use a cane in the opposite hand. In the illustration, the figure is holding a cane at a distance of 18 inches from the affected hip. By exerting force on the cane—i.e., by the ground pushing up on the cane—at such a great distance from the hip, the force of the contraction required by the hip abductors to balance the pelvis is dramatically reduced. In the experiment, body weight is exerted at its normal distance from the hip. Note that a force of approximately 15 percent body weight in the right hand scale exerted at 18 inches from the hip reduces the hip abductor force to one time body weight. Thus, the hip now "sees" only a total of two times body weight (see text).

Particular gentleness must be exercised in dislocating the hip joint, and in cases of severe protrusio acetabuli, the femoral neck should be osteotomized before the hip is dislocated in order to decrease the risk of an untoward fracture.

Protrusio acetabuli is a frequently encountered deformity in patient's with rheumatoid arthritis. Several authors have noted an increased failure rate in hips in which the acetabulum has not been restored to the normal center of rotation.[18–23] The use of autogenous bone (either morselized, in strips, or as a structural graft) allows for adequate lateralization of the acetabular component as well as for the restoration of host bone stock.[23]

The question of trochanteric osteotomy has been largely resolved over the last several years, as several studies have documented excellent results in primary total hip arthroplasty without trochanteric osteotomy, which also avoids the complications of trochanteric nonunion and painful broken wires.[24, 25] Present indications for trochanteric osteotomy include compromised exposure and inadequate soft tissue tension necessitating trochanteric advancement.

Preoperative Medication

Approximately 15 percent of patients requiring total hip arthroplasty at the authors' hospital are receiving maintenance glucocorticoids, usually 5 to 15 mg of prednisone every other day. Patients are required to continue their prednisone up to the preoperative day and are covered with intravenous hydrocortisone during the perioperative period. Discontinuing prednisone perioperatively is associated with a higher incidence of wound dehiscence and wound healing problems.

Methotrexate has been associated with an increase in perioperative infection, and it is recommended that this medication be discontinued the day prior to surgery and not reinstituted until discharge from the hospital. There have been no reports of gold, Plaquenil (hydroxychloroquine sulfate), or penicillamine affecting wound healing or causing an increased incidence of prosthetic infection during the postoperative period. Medications that could potentiate hemorrhage at the time of surgery, such as NSAIDs and acetylsalicylic acid (ASA), should be discontinued 1 week prior to the operation.

Multiple studies have documented a reduction in the incidence of postoperative wound infections with the use of prophylactic antibiotics.[26–28] Classen and colleagues[29] recently evaluated the timing of antibiotic administration and noted the lowest incidence of wound infections in patients in whom antibiotics were given during the 2 hours before surgery. The authors use cephalothin sodium, 1 gram intravenously, 1 hour prior to the incision and then 1 gram every 8 hours postoperatively for 24 hours.

Preoperative and Postoperative Program

Secondary to changes imposed by insurance carriers, most patients are admitted to the hospital on the morning of their surgery. It is, therefore, necessary for thorough medical and anesthetic evaluations to be performed in the week preceding the surgery. Ideally, the patient should become acquainted with crutch-assisted gait during this period.

Following surgery, the patient is placed in pillow suspension traction for 24 hours. On the second postoperative day, range of motion exercises are begun, and the patient is encouraged to sit on the side of the bed. The patient is quickly mobilized thereafter and is usually independently ambulating with crutches by 6 to 8 days.

Postoperative thromboembolic precautions include the use of warfarin (keeping the prothrombin time 1.5 × control), which is continued for 6 weeks. Thigh-high pneumatic stockings are also used until the patient is ambulatory.

Occupational therapists evaluate the patient before discharge to help determine which assistive devices the individual will require at home. Examples of these aids include long-handled shoe horns, elastic shoe laces, and elevated toilet seats. Home physical therapists are utilized for the first 4 to 6 weeks to maximize strength, range of motion, and ambulatory capacity.

Long-Term Results of Cemented Total Hip Arthroplasty

While many reports have documented excellent results following total hip replacement in patients with osteoarthritis,[30–32] few studies are available that pertain only to patients with rheumatoid arthritis. In a review of 138 arthroplasties performed in rheumatoid patients, Poss and associates[33] noted that the majority of patients continued to function well at an average follow-up of 7 years. They documented, however, a 78 percent incidence of increasing radiolucencies around the acetabular components and were concerned that mechanical loosening could be a significant problem with longer follow-up.

Unger and co-workers[34] reviewed 51 hip arthroplasties in rheumatoid patients at a minimum follow-up of 10 years. While 80.7 percent of patients had a satisfactory result, the revision rate for mechanical loosing was 13.3 percent, with the majority of failures secondary to acetabular loosening. Radiographic review demonstrates loosening in an additional 11 acetabular and 2 femoral components.

Severt and colleagues[35] recently reported the results of 75 arthroplasties in rheumatoid patients at an average follow-up of 7.4 years. While satisfactory clinical results were noted in 88 percent of hips with a revision rate of 7 percent for aseptic loosening, an additional 13 percent of hips were believed on the basis of radiograph to be at risk for loosening (seven acetabular components and four femoral components). Kaplan-Meier survivorship analysis revealed a 93 percent survival probability at 7 years, which decreased to 77 percent at 12 years. Other authors have noted an increased number of radiolucencies about cemented acetabular components in patients with rheumatoid arthritis as opposed to other diagnoses.[36]

It appears, therefore, that hip arthroplasties in patients with rheumatoid arthritis fail more often because of acetabular component loosening than because of femoral component loosening. This is probably a consequence of compromised acetabular bone stock and quality, which precludes an enduring bone-cement interface. Failure to correct protrusio acetabuli can jeopardize acetabular component stability by not restoring the hip center of rotation and has contributed to the high rate of acetabular component failure in patients with rheumatoid arthritis.[18, 21, 33] Bone-grafting, which allows for lateralization of the acetabular component, has been shown to arrest the progression of this deformity in as many as 90 percent of hips at average follow-up of 12.8 years.[23] This certainly contributes to the long-term stability of the prosthetic component and the bone-cement interface.

Results of Cementless Total Hip Arthroplasty

Secondary to dissatisfaction with the intermediate and long-term results of cemented total hip arthroplasty, especially in younger and more active patients, cementless fixation with porous coated implants was developed[37-40] (Fig. 108–3). The goals of

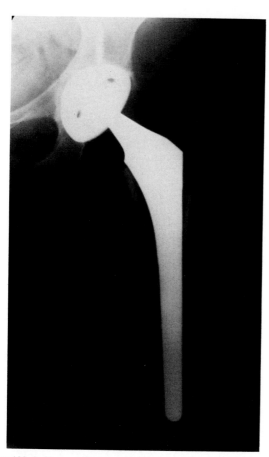

Figure 108–3. Uncemented femoral and acetabular components in a 62-year-old woman suffering from rheumatoid arthritis. This patient demonstrated pauciarticular involvement and was very active.

this type of fixation are to achieve a stable prosthesis-bone interface with secure biologic fixation for long-term stability. Improvements in instrumentation, prosthetic design, and expanded component inventory have increased the surgeon's ability to achieve these goals.

Engh and co-workers[41] recently reported the results of 959 primary hip arthroplasties using a porous coated femoral component. At follow-up ranging from 2 to 12 years, the femoral revision rate was 1 percent, and the 10-year survivorship rate was 96.4 percent. This group included a subset of 150 patients younger than 40 years of age. With only three stems requiring revision, cumulative survivorship of the femoral component was 94.9 percent at 10 years. This report unfortunately does not mention the incidence of thigh pain and does not include the results of the acetabular components.

Kim and Kim[42] recently reported the disappointing 5-year results of the Harris-Galante cementless hip system. A 5 percent revision rate, 10 percent failure rate, and 50 percent incidence of thigh pain were noted. The authors attributed the poor results to inadequacies of the prosthetic components, including limited ingrowth surfaces, inadequate metaphyseal canal fill, and the presence of a collar.

Other authors have reported the short- or medium-term follow-up results of cementless hip arthroplasty. Callaghan and associates[43] found 94 percent good or excellent results in 50 arthroplasties performed with a porous coated prosthesis. Thigh pain was noted in 16 percent of patients, and 11 percent of patients required a cane at 2-year follow-up. Progressive radiodense lines, sclerosis, and component bead loosening were observed in a large number of patients. Although the short-term clinical results compare favorably with those of cemented series, the high incidence of thigh pain and the radiographic findings give reason for concern with this prosthesis.

Smith and co-workers[44] prospectively evaluated 56 cementless hip arthroplasties for an average of 46 months. While 87 percent of the hips had a good or an excellent result, 19 percent of patients experienced a persistent limp, and 38 percent of femoral components were noted to have shifted into varus alignment.

Wixson and colleagues[45] prospectively compared cemented, hybrid (cemented femoral and cementless acetabular components), and cementless prosthetic fixation and reported their results at 2- to 4-year follow-up. Cementless fixation was used in men younger than 70 years and in women younger than 60 years. The results were similar for all three groups even though the patients in the cementless group were considerably younger than those in the cemented group (average age of 68.5 years versus 53.9 years, respectively). Thigh pain, however, was noted in 15 percent of patients with a cementless femoral component at 4-year follow-up, as opposed to 3 percent of patients with cemented femoral component.

A relatively new type of cementless fixation involves the use of hydroxyapatite-coated prostheses. These implants have been shown to develop strong bonds with living bone over a short period of time.[46–48] Geesink[49] recently reported the results of 100 hip arthroplasties (86 primary and 14 revision) with this type of fixation. He noted that 97 percent of femoral components, as opposed to 55 percent of acetabular components, had radiographic evidence of bone ingrowth at 2-year follow-up. An average Harris hip score of 96 points after 1 year and 98 points after 2 years with no revisions for loose components and only a 4 percent incidence of thigh pain was reported. Of note, there was no difference in the results of primary or revision procedures at this relatively short term. This short-term report reflects the best results reported thus far with cementless fixation.

While the clinical results with cementless fixation in younger patients are encouraging, the incidence of persistent thigh pain in most cementless series remains a concern. The results of these series with variously shaped implants and ingrowth surfaces, as well as their local and systemic effects, must be carefully measured against the improved results with modern cement techniques and prosthetic designs. Longer follow-up is necessary to determine what type of fixation will be most appropriate in each age group.

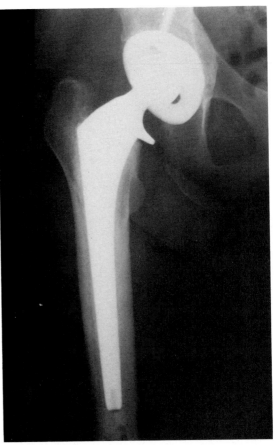

Figure 108–4. "Hybrid" total hip replacement in a 72-year-old woman with rheumatoid arthritis. The femoral component is cemented, and the acetabular component uncemented. Reconstruction included acetabular bone grafting for early protrusio.

Results of Modern Cemented Total Hip Arthroplasty

The results of these cementless series are certainly inferior to those of recently reported series utilizing modern cement techniques. The improvements in cement techniques include intramedullary plugging, the use of pulsatile lavage to remove bone debris, and intramedullary brushing. These techniques, combined with the use of cement guns allowing retrograde delivery of cement as well as cement pressurization, have produced markedly improved results (Fig. 108–4). In comparing two different cement techniques, Roberts and associates[50] reported a femoral loosening rate of 24 percent with older cement techniques compared with 4 percent with modern cement technique at average 5-year follow-up. Russotti and associates[51] reported 98 percent excellent results at minimum 5-year follow-up with only three definitely loose femoral stems. In a long-term follow-up report, Mulroy and Harris[52] noted only a 3 percent incidence of cemented femoral stem loosening at 11-year follow-up.

With improvement in cementing techniques, a failure rate of less than 1 percent per year can be expected. The longer term problems of bone lysis caused by polyethylene, methacrylate, and metal wear debris will become more important factors in causing failure in cemented total hip arthroplasty.

Results of Revision Total Hip Replacement

Although the outcome of revision total hip arthroplasty has improved over the last several years, the results are still inferior to those of primary replacement. Difficulties encountered at the time of revision include difficult exposure, deficient host bone stock, and femoral endosteal sclerosis, which provides a suboptimal environment for component fixation with cement. Correspondingly, a marked increase in complications following revision procedures has been observed.[53–57] These include aseptic mechanical loosening, infection, femoral fracture, and dislocation.

Pellici and co-workers[54] noted good or excellent results in 65 percent of 110 arthroplasties evaluated at an average follow-up of 3.4 years. The re-revision rate was 14 percent, however, and radiolucencies were noted in 26 percent of cases. When the same group was reviewed at an average follow-up of 8.2 years, the revision rate had increased to 19 percent, and a further 11 percent were rated as having poor results.[55]

In another large series of cemented revision arthroplasties, Kavanagh and associates[56] reported 62 percent good or excellent results in 162 revision arthroplasties reviewed at an average follow-up of 4.5 years. The failure rate was high, with re-revision required in 9 percent of patients. Of concern, 20 percent of acetabular components and 40 percent of femoral components were believed to be probably loose radiographically. Other authors have noted substantially increased failure rates and high radiolucency rates with cemented revision procedures as well.[58-60]

Marti and colleagues[61] reported the best long-term results on cemented revision. At 5- to 14-year follow-up, a 10 percent re-revision rate was noted. Survivorship analysis demonstrated a cumulative survival of 85 percent of 80 cases at 14 years. The authors believed that their method of acetabular reconstruction contributed to the improved survivorship in this series. They insisted on 90 percent acetabular component coverage, which was achieved with autogenous corticocancellous bone fixed to the pelvis with lag screws. None of the 19 hips in which this type of acetabuloplasty was performed has been re-revised (although the acetabular component migrated in one). Other authors have noted increased acetabular component failure when the cup was less than 90 percent covered.[62]

Another probable reason for the improved survivorship was the older average patient age at the time of revision (71 years). Certainly, primary hip replacement has been shown to be less durable in younger patients,[37, 38] and the effects of age and activity probably are even stronger in revisions. This is reflected in the ominous results of Strömberg and co-workers,[63] who reported a 36 percent mechanical failure rate at an average follow-up of 4 years in patients younger than 55 years at the time of their revision.

Subsequent revisions have been noted to be even less durable than initial revision. In fact, Kavanagh and Fitzgerald[57] noted a satisfactory result in only about half of their patients who underwent second and third revisions. Twenty-four percent of second revisions and 29 percent of third revisions failed after an average of 41 and 34 months, respectively, which reflects the difficulty in obtaining an adequate bone-cement interface following multiple arthroplasties. In fact, Dohmae and associates[64] have shown biomechanically a reduction in the bone-cement sheer strength to 21 percent of primary strength with the first revision and a further decrease to 7 percent of primary strength with re-revision.

As the high failure rate with cemented revision surgery has been secondary principally to difficulty in achieving a stable bone-cement interface, cementless fixation of prosthetic components has been evaluated. The number of series reporting the results of cementless revisions, however, remains small, with only short- or medium-term follow-up.

Engh and colleagues[65] reported their results of 160 cementless revisions followed for an average of 4.4 years. On the acetabular side, the results were disappointing, with an overall failure rate of 22.4 percent. The majority of failures, however, occurred in cases in which a smooth threaded component was used. The authors concluded that this component design does not allow for consistent bone ingrowth. A 97 percent success rate was demonstrated in 34 cases when a porous acetabular component was used. On the femoral side, only two stems were revised for loosening, with an additional three stems demonstrating definite radiographic evidence of loosening, for a femoral failure rate of 4 percent. Of note, 23 percent of patients with radiographically stable components had a painful limp. Other series have reported early encouraging results with a cementless femoral component.[66]

Hedley and co-workers[67] reported the results of 61 cementless revision total hip arthroplasties with an average follow-up of 21 months. Good or excellent results were obtained in 90 percent of cases, and only two hips required re-revision. Lord and colleagues[68] reported 73 percent good or excellent results at an average follow-up of 5 years, with only 4 revisions in 203 cementless revision arthroplasties.

These early results with cementless components reflect an improvement over those previously reported for cemented revision.[55-57] Longer follow-up is necessary to determine whether biologic fixation with bone ingrowth remains stable, and what effect these components might have both locally and systemically.

With each successive total hip replacement, increasing amounts of bone stocks are removed. With loosening of implants, further lysis of bone may occur, and at revision surgery there may not be enough bone available to provide stability for the implant. The surgeon is then faced with the use of custom prostheses or allograft reconstruction of the femur and acetabulum. Reconstruction of acetabular deficiencies requires the use of particulate bone if the bone graft can be contained or structural solid pieces of bone if there are large deficiencies in the rim or floor of the acetabulum.[69] Allografts available include femoral heads, distal femurs, and the use of a hemipelvis for reconstruction.

On the femoral side, autogenous cancellous bone may be used for intramedullary defects. For larger defects, allograft cortical struts may be used or intercalary segments of graft cementing the prosthesis to the allograft and using either a long-stemmed implant or a variety of plates for fixing the allograft to the host bone (Fig. 108–5). While early follow-up results of these techniques are encouraging,[70, 71] we await the long-term follow-up results (5 to 10 years).

Complications

Infection. Charnley and Cupic definitively showed that adherence to meticulous sterile surgical technique augmented by effective air changes in the operating room would result in dramatically lower

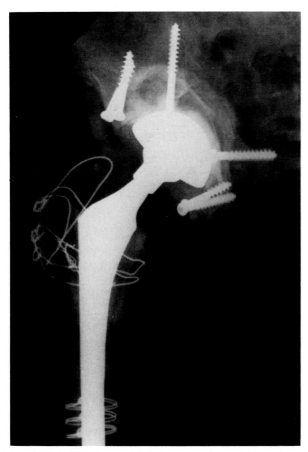

Figure 108–5. Whole proximal femoral and acetabular allograft total hip reconstruction in a 67-year-old woman having undergone multiple failed total hip replacement procedures.

The rheumatoid arthritis patient is at increased risk for the development of infection after total joint replacement.[31, 33, 35] Severt and associates[35] reported deep sepsis in 5.3 percent of hips and wound healing problems in 19 percent of hips. While this is the highest sepsis rate reported following rheumatoid hip arthroplasties, other series have documented higher infection rates and wound problems in patients with rheumatoid arthritis as opposed to other diagnoses that require arthroplasty.[33, 77] In the authors' 6- to 11-year follow-up of total hip replacements, the rheumatoid patient was 1.8 times more likely to develop infection than an osteoarthritis counterpart.[33] Of particular importance, all infections that presented over 3 years after surgery were in rheumatoid arthritis patients and were thought to have spread hematogenously. The rheumatoid arthritis patient often has multiple sites of skin breakdown and is vulnerable to bacterial infections. This group of patients must be managed closely indefinitely after total hip replacement. Many authors have noted that the frequency of infection increases when total hip replacement is performed as a revision of a previous procedure. Dupont and Charnley reported that the rate of late infection increased twofold when they compared a group of patients who had revision with those who had primary total hip replacement.[78, 79] Murray reported a rate of infection of 3.1 percent in revision cases, compared with 0.7 percent in primary cases.[71] Poss and associates[80] found a 13-fold difference in infection rates when patients who underwent revision were compared with patients who had had a primary procedure.

The authors recommend that patients undergoing total hip replacement as a revision of some other procedure be informed that they are at higher risk for development of postoperative infection. Preoperative aspiration of the involved hip and anaerobic and aerobic cultures of joint fluid obtained may disclose indolent sepsis. An arthrogram performed as part of the aspiration procedure provides ensurance that the needle is in the hip joint and may detect abnormal sinus tracts. If the suspicion of sepsis is high, hardware may be removed during a preliminary procedure, at which time tissue specimens may be obtained for bacteriologic and histologic examination.

Once an established deep infection has been diagnosed, treatment includes surgical débridement, with removal of all prosthetic components, cement, and granulation tissue.[81, 82] Appropriate intravenous antibiotics based on culture and sensitivity results are thereafter administered. McDonald and colleagues[81] noted a higher recurrent infection rate when antibiotics were given for less than 28 days, and it is currently recommended that they be given for at least 6 weeks. McDonald and co-workers also reported a 27 percent recurrence rate when reimplantation was undertaken less than 1 year following resection arthroplasty, compared with a 7 percent recurrence rate when reconstruction was delayed for

infection rates. Their early infection rate of 6.6 percent[31] was reduced to less than 0.5 percent[72] in this manner. Subsequent reports have shown that similar low infection rates can be achieved by using ultraviolet light and prophylactic antibiotics.[73] Equally impressive results have been reported from surgeons who perform total hip replacement in conventional operating rooms[74] and in community hospitals.[75] It can be surmised from these results that the joint replacement era has reminded the surgeon that scrupulous adherence to sterile technique is of primary importance in avoiding sepsis.

In the United States, the frequency of deep infection after total hip arthroplasty is approximately 1 percent.[76] About 40 percent of infections become evident during the early postoperative period, 45 percent have delayed onset (2 to 24 months), and 15 percent are thought to be the result of hematogenous spread and may present in the previously well patient at any time after surgery.[76] The group with delayed hematogenous spread underscores the importance of prolonged follow-up of patients. Patient education is mandatory. Patients should notify physicians and dentists of their prosthetic joint when a potentially bacteria-contaminating procedure is to be done (dental extraction, urologic procedure) and should be given prophylactic antibiotics.

at least 1 year. Other authors have noted a similarly low recurrent infection rate when these principles are followed.[82]

Osteolysis. Osteolysis of the femur and acetabulum has been reported with both cemented and cementless implants. This may be progressive in nature and is related to a host response to particulate debris from polyethylene, metallic, and cement wear.[83–85] Macrophages, which are activated by the phagocytosis of wear debris, are the cells principally responsible for osteolysis.[86, 87] Ultimately, bone resorption can lead to prosthetic fixation failure. The reduction of particulate wear debris is currently the focus of intense research.

Bone resorption has also been observed in response to femoral implants that are stiffer than cortical bone and, therefore, induce a stress-shielding effect in the proximal femur.[88] When this effect is combined with the naturally occurring loss of bone mass with age, the proximal femur can eventually become an unsuitable environment for prosthetic fixation.[88] Future prosthetic materials and designs will need to take these observations into consideration for the longevity of total hip arthroplasty to be extended beyond the present 15 to 20 years.

Heterotopic Bone Formation. Heterotopic bone may be seen on radiographs in as many as 40 percent of patients.[76] Fewer than 2 percent of patients suffer limitation of motion because of this phenomenon.[76] Certain clinical groups, however, are at high risk for developing heterotopic bone. Patients with ankylosing spondylitis, diffuse idiopathic skeletal hyperostosis, a history of heterotopic bone formation after previous hip surgery, and males with hypertrophic osteoarthritis, are predisposed to heterotopic bone formation following hip arthroplasty.

In these high-risk patients, the authors recommend postoperative single low-dose radiation therapy (600 rad), which has been shown to be effective in preventing the formation of heterotopic bone.[89, 90] As many investigators believe that irradiation prevents the differentiation of pluripotential mesenchymal cells into the osteoblastic cells that are felt to be responsible for heterotopic bone formation, and since this differentiation occurs during the immediate postoperative period, treatment should be given in the first 48 hours following arthroplasty.[91]

TOTAL HIP REPLACEMENT AND ANKYLOSING SPONDYLITIS

Arthrosis of the hip joint in ankylosing spondylitis has been reported to occur in 31 percent of cases, with a 91 percent incidence of bilaterality.[92] As candidates for total hip arthroplasty, these patients differ from rheumatoid arthritis patients in several important respects: (1) they tend to be younger and more active, (2) joint involvement is usually limited to the spine and hips, so that the ankles, feet, and upper extremities are spared, and (3) limitation of

motion of the lumbar and thoracic spine imposes increased mechanical demands on the hip joints. These factors suggest that the long-term results of total hip arthroplasty in this group may show an increased rate of mechanical loosening over time.

The presenting complaints in these patients include pain, stiffness, poor posture, and limitation of motion. In advanced cases, the combination of fixed thoracolumbar kyphosis and severe hip flexion contracture can significantly impair the ambulatory capacity of these patients. It has been recommended that correction of the hip flexion deformity with total hip arthroplasty precede spinal osteotomy.[93]

Recently, a series was reported from Brigham and Women's Hospital documenting the results of 29 total hip arthroplasties performed in 19 patients over a 13-year period.[94] Follow-up averaged 56 months. Complete pain relief was achieved in 97 percent of patients, and significant gains were also noted in ambulatory capacity. Secondary to a 77 percent incidence of heterotopic ossification in this series, the authors recommended prophylactic treatment to prevent its formation.

Kilgus and colleagues[95] reported the results of 53 arthroplasties in 31 patients who were followed for an average of 6.3 years. Only one primary hip arthroplasty was revised for aseptic loosening, 17 years after implantation. The remaining hips did not demonstrate any radiographic evidence of loosening of the cemented prosthetic components. This report as well as those from other authors[96] indicates that durable clinical results can be achieved in patients with ankylosing spondylitis.

CURRENT STATUS OF SURGERY OF THE HIP FOR ARTHRITIS

On the basis of long-term results of the first generation of total hip replacements, surgeons have learned that conventional hip replacement, although one of the most successful operations devised, has limitations and should not be employed in younger, heavier, more active patients. Patients with rheumatoid arthritis are particularly good candidates for total hip arthroplasty, as they typically have low activity demands secondary to the systemic nature of their disease. As the early generation of patients with hip replacements becomes older, that population will begin to diminish, and it is anticipated that modern hip replacement methods will produce a somewhat lower frequency of aseptic failure. While the strategies employed in the treatment of aseptic failure, particularly with the use of cementless components and allograft bone, appear promising, their results remain inferior to and their complication rates higher than those seen with primary total hip arthroplasty.

The frequency of degenerative joint disease in patients younger than 50 years of age continues to be significant. It can be attributed in part to the residual deformities of hip dysplasia, Legg-Calvé-Perthes disease, or slipped capital femoral epiphysis.[97] In addition, it is recognized that despite well-baby screening for congenital dislocation of the hip, a significant minority of children will be discovered later to have dislocation. The suggestion originally made by Wynn-Davies that there are dysplastic hips at birth that are not lax and therefore not detectable by well-baby physical examination points to a continuing reservoir of hip problems that will present during the late adolescent or young adult period.

The recognition of the limitations of conventional total hip arthroplasty has led to a renewal of interest in the use of biologic alternatives. Osteotomy about the hip, either pelvic or intertrochanteric, has assumed new importance as an alternative in younger patients with osteoarthritis. The use of osteotomy for either reconstructive or salvage purposes in the younger adult should gain increasing attention.[98] Additionally, long-term follow-up studies of hip arthrodesis suggest that function and pain relief are satisfactory in selected patients and this procedure should be considered in the evaluation of treatment choices in patients with limited hip motion and advanced hip osteoarthritis.[99]

While significant shortcomings remain with total hip arthroplasty, this procedure remains the best treatment alternative in patients with symptomatic end-stage arthritic hips. The stated goal of surgery, which is pain relief, is effectively met in the majority of patients, and the frequently observed increased range of motion following arthroplasty contributes to the overall improved functioning of these debilitated patients. With the recent advances in the quality of prosthetic components as well as in fixation methods, the majority of properly selected patients should function well with this procedure.

References

1. Coventry, M. D., Beckenbaugh, R. D., Nolan, D. R., and Ilstrup, D. M.: 2012 total hip arthroplasties: A study of postoperative course and early complications. J. Bone Joint Surg. 56A:273, 1974.
2. Welch, R. B., and Charnley, J.: Low-friction arthroplasty of the hip in rheumatoid arthritis and ankylosing spondylitis. Clin. Orthop. 72:22, 1970.
3. Johnston, R. C., Fitzgerald, R. H., Harris, W. H., Muller, M. E., and Sledge, C. B.: Clinical and radiographic evaulation of total hip replacement. A standard system of terminology for reporting results. J. Bone Joint Surg. 72A:161, 1990.
4. Bount, W. P.: Don't throw away the cane. J. Bone Joint Surg. 38A:695, 1956.
5. Jergesen, H. E., Poss, R., and Sledge, C. B.: Bilateral total hip and knee replacement in adults with rheumatoid arthritis: An evaluation of function. Clin. Orthop. 137:118, 1978.
6. Hardaker, W. T., Ogen, W. S., Musgrave, M. D., and Goldner, J. D.: Simultaneous and staged bilateral total knee arthroplasty. J. Bone Joint Surg. 60A:247, 1978.
7. Head, W. D., and Paradies, L. H.: Ipsilateral hip and knee replacements as a single surgical procedure. J. Bone Joint Surg. 59A:352, 1977.
8. Salvati, E. A., Hughes, P., and Lachiewicz, P.: Bilateral total hip replacement arthroplasty in one stage. J. Bone Joint Surg. 60A:640, 1978.
9. Soudry, M., Binazzo, R., Insall, J. N., et al.: Successive bilateral total knee replacement. J. Bone Joint Surg. 67A:573, 1985.
10. Brotherton, S. L., Robertson, J. R., de Andrade, J. R., and Fleming, L. L.: Staged versus simultaneous bilateral total knee replacement. J. Arthroplasty 1:221, 1986.
11. Buscemi, M. J., Page, B. J., and Swienckowski, J.: Unilateral versus bilateral simultaneous arthroplasties of the lower extremities. J. Am. Osteopath. Assoc. 89:1133, 1989.
12. Hoekstra, H. J., Nielsen, H. K., Veldhuizen, A. G., Visser, J. D., Nienhuis, R. C., and Hoekstra, A. J.: Bilateral total hip and knee replacement in rheumatoid arthritis patients. Arch. Orthop. Trauma Surg. 108:291, 1989.
13. Nakano, K. K.: Neurologic complications of rheumatoid arthritis. Orthop. Clin. North Am. 6:861, 1975.
14. Inman, V. T.: Functional aspects of the abductor muscles of the hip. J. Bone Joint Surg. 29:607, 1947.
15. Pauwels, F.: Biomechanics of the Normal and Diseased Hip. Berlin, Springer-Verlag, 1976.
16. Greewald, A. S., and Nelson, C. L.: Biomechanics of the reconstructed hip. Orthop. Clin. North Am. 4:435, 1973.
17. Rydell, N.: Intra-vital measurements of forces acting on the hip joint. In Evans, F. G. (ed.): Studies on the Anatomy and Function of the Bone and Joints. New York, Springer-Verlag, 1966, p. 52.
18. Hastings, D. C., and Parker, S. M.: Protrusio acetabuli in rheumatoid arthritis. Clin. Orthop. 108:76, 1975.
19. McCollum, D. E., Nunley, J. A., and Harrelson, J. M.: Bone grafting in total hip replacement for acetabular protrusio. J. Bone Joint Surg. 62A:1065, 1980.
20. Oh, I., and Harris, W. H.: Protrusio acetabuli and total hip replacement: Bone grafting and use of protrusio shell. Orthop. Trans. 3:276, 1979.
21. Ranawat, C. S., Dorr, L. D., and Inglis, A. E.: Total hip arthroplasty in protrusio acetabuli of rheumatoid arthritis. J. Bone Joint Surg. 61A:1059, 1980.
22. Sotelo-Garza, A., and Charnley, J.: The results of Charnley arthroplasty of the hip performed for protrusio acetabuli. Clin. Orthop. 132:12, 1978.
23. Gates, H. S., McCollum, D. E., Poletti, S. C., and Nunley, J. A.: Bone-grafting in total hip arthroplasty for protrusio acetabuli. J. Bone Joint Surg. 72A:148, 1990.
24. Muller, M. E.: Total hip replacement without trochanteric osteotomy. In Harris, W. H. (ed.): The Hip: Proceedings of the Second Scientific Meeting of the Hip Society, 1974. St. Louis, C. V. Mosby Company, 1974, p. 231.
25. Parker, H. G., Wiesman, H. J., Ewald, F. C., Thomas, W. H., and Sledge, C. B.: Comparison of pre-operative, intraoperative and early post-operative total hip replacements with and without trochanteric osteotomy. Clin. Orthop. 121:44, 1976.
26. Shapiro, M., Townsend, T. R., Rosner, B., and Kass, E. H.: Use of antimicrobial drugs in general hospitals: patterns of prophylaxis. N. Engl. J. Med. 301:351, 1979.
27. Guglielmo, B. J., Hohn, D. C., Koo, P. J., Hunt, T. K., Sweet, R. L., and Conte, J. E., Jr.: Antibiotic prophylaxis in surgical procedures: A critical analysis of the literature. Arch. Surg. 118:943, 1983.
28. Crossley, K., and Gardner, L. C.: Antimicrobial prophylaxis in surgical patients. J.A.M.A. 245:722, 1981.
29. Classen, D. C., Evans, R. S., Pestotnik, S. L., Horn, S. D., Menlove, R. L., and Burke, J. P.: The timing of prophylactic administration of antibiotics and the risk of surgical wound infection. N. Engl. J. Med. 326:281, 1992.
30. Beckenbaugh, R. D., and Ilstrup, D. M.: Total hip arthroplasty: A review of three hundred and thirty-three cases with long follow-up. J. Bone Joint Surg. 60A:306, 1978.
31. Charnley, J., and Cupic, Z.: The nine- and ten-year results of low-friction arthroplasty of the hip. Clin. Orthop. 95:9, 1973.
32. Coventry, M.: Ten-year results of total hip arthroplasty. Orthop. Trans. 5:349, 1981.
33. Poss, R., Maloney, J. P., Ewald, F. C., Thomas, W. H., Batte, N. J., Hartness, C., and Sledge, C. B.: Six- to eleven-year results of total hip arthroplasty in rheumatoid arthritis. Clin. Orthop. 182:109, 1984.
34. Unger, A. S., Inglis, A. E., Ranawat, C. S., and Johanson, N. A.: Total hip arthroplasty in rheumatoid arthritis. A long-term follow-up study. J. Arthroplasty 2:191, 1987.
35. Severt, R., Wood, R., Cracchiolo, A., and Amstutz, M. C.: Long-term follow-up of cemented total hip arthroplasty in rheumatoid arthritis. Clin. Orthop. 265:137, 1991.
36. Sarmiento, A., Ebramzadeh, E., Gogan, W. J., and McKellop, H. A.: Total hip arthroplasty with cement. A long-term radiographic analysis in patients who are older than fifty and younger than fifty years. J. Bone Joint Surg. 72A:1470, 1990.
37. Chandler, M. P., Reinick, F. T., Wixson, R. C., and McCarthey, J. C.: Total hip replacement in patients younger than 30 years old: A 5-year follow-up study. J. Bone Joint Surg. 63A:1426, 1981.
38. Dorr, L. D., Takei, G. K., and Conaty, J. P.: Total hip arthroplasties in patients less than 45 years old. J. Bone Joint Surg. 65A:474, 1983.
39. Ranawat, C. S., Atkinson, R. E., Salvati, E. A., and Wilson, P. D.: Conventional total hip arthroplasty for degenerative joint disease in patients between the ages of 40 and 60 years. J. Bone Joint Surg. 66A:745, 1984.
40. Collis, D. K.: Cemented total hip replacement in patients who are less than 60 years old. J. Bone Joint Surg. 66A:353, 1984.

41. Engh, C. A., Glassman, A. H., and Suthers, K. E.: The case for porous-coated hip implants. Clin. Orthop. 261:63, 1990.

42. Kim, Y. H., and Kim, V. E.: Results of the Harris-Galante cementless hip prosthesis. J. Bone Joint Surg. 74B:83, 1992.

43. Callaghan, J. J., Dysart, S. H., and Savory, C. G.: The uncemented porous-coated anatomic total hip prosthesis: Two-year result of a prospective consecutive series. J. Bone Joint Surg. 70A:337, 1988.

44. Smith, S. E., Garvin, K. L., Jardon, O. M., and Kaplan, P. A.: Uncemented total hip arthroplasty. Prospective analysis of the tri-lock femoral component. Clin. Orthop. 269:43, 1991.

45. Wixson, R. L., Stulberg, S. D., and Melhoff, M.: Total hip replacement with cemented, uncemented, and hybrid prostheses. A comparison of clinical and radiographic results at two to four years. J. Bone Joint Surg. 73A:257, 1991.

46. Geesink, R. G. T.: Hydroxyapatite-coated hip implants. Thesis, State University of Limburg, Maastricht, Netherlands, 1988.

47. Soballe, K., Hansen, E. S., Rasmussen, H. B., Pedersen, M. C., and Bunger, C.: Early fixation of allogenic bone graft in titanium- and hydroxyapatite-coated implants. Trans. Orthop. Res. Soc. 14:554, 1989.

48. Van Blitterswijk, C. A., Van Groten, J. D., Kupers, W., Daems, W. Th., and de Groot, K.: Macropore tissue ingrowth: A quantitative and qualitative study on hydroxyapatite ceramic. Biomaterials 7:137, 1986.

49. Geesink, R. G. T.: Hydroxyapatite-coated total hip prostheses. Two-year clinical and roentgenographic results of 100 cases. Clin. Orthop. 261:39, 1990.

50. Roberts, D. W., Poss, R., and Kelley, K. K.: Radiographic comparison of cementing techniques in total hip arthroplasty. J. Arthroplasty 1:241, 1986.

51. Russotti, G. M., Coventry, M. B., and Stautter, R. N.: Cemented total hip arthroplasty with contemporary techniques. A five-year minimum follow-up study. Clin. Orthop. 235:141, 1988.

52. Mulroy, R. D., Jr., and Harris, W. H.: The effect of improved cementing techniques on component loosening in total hip replacement. J. Bone Joint Surg. 72B:757, 1990.

53. Broughton, N. S., and Rushton, H.: Revision hip arthroplasty. Acta Orthop. Scand. 56(6):923, 1982.

54. Pellicci, P. M., Wilson, P. D., Jr., Sledge, C. B., Salvati, E. A., Ranawat, C. S., and Poss, R.: Revision total hip arthroplasty. Clin. Orthop. 170:34, 1982.

55. Pellicci, P. M., Wilson, P. D., Jr., Sledge, C. B., Salvati, E. A., Ranawat, C. S., Poss, R., and Callaghan, J. J.: Long-term results of revision total hip replacement. A follow-up report. J. Bone Joint Surg. 61A:513, 1985.

56. Kavanagh, B. F., Ilstrup, D. M., and Fitzgerald, R. H., Jr.: Revision total hip arthroplasty. J. Bone Joint Surg. 67A:517, 1985.

57. Kavanagh, B. F., and Fitzgerald, R. H., Jr.: Multiple revision for failed total hip arthroplasty. J. Bone Joint Surg. 69A:1144, 1987.

58. Amstutz, H. C., Ma, S. M., Jinnah, R. H., and Mai, L.: Revision of aseptic loose total hip arthroplasties. Clin. Orthop. 170:21, 1982.

59. Callaghan, J. J., Salvati, E. A., Pellicci, P. M., Wilson, P. D., Jr., and Ranawat, C. S.: Results of revision for mechanical failure after cemented total hip replacement. J. Bone Joint Surg. 67A:1074, 1985.

60. Engelbrecht, D. J., Weber, F. A., Sweet, M. B. E., and Jakim, I.: Long-term results of revision total hip arthroplasty. J. Bone Joint Surg. 72B:41, 1990.

61. Marti, R. K., Schuller, H. M., Besselaar, P. P., and Vanfrank Haasnoot, E. L.: Results of revision of hip arthroplasty with cement. A five- to fourteen-year follow-up study. J. Bone Joint Surg. 72A:346, 1990.

62. Sutherland, C. J., Wilde, A. H., Borden, C. S., and Marks, K. E.: A ten-year following of one hundred consecutive Müller curved-stem total hip replacement arthroplasties. J. Bone Joint Surg. 64A:970, 1982.

63. Strömberg, C. N., Herberts, P., and Ahnfelt, L.: Revision total hip arthroplasty in patients younger than 55 years old. Clinical and radiographic results after 9 years. J. Arthroplasty 3:47, 1988.

64. Dohmae, Y., Bechtold, J. E., Sherman, R. E., Puno, R. M., and Gustilo, R. B.: Reduction in cemented-bone interface shear strength between primary and revision arthroplasty. Clin. Orthop. 236:214, 1988.

65. Engh, C. A., Glassman, A. H., Griffin, W. L., and Mayer, J. G.: Results of cementless revision for failed cemented total hip arthroplasty. Clin. Orthop. 235:91, 1988.

66. Gustilo, R. B., and Pasternak, H. S.: Revision total hip arthroplasty with titanium ingrowth prosthesis and bone grafting for failed cemented femoral component loosening. Clin. Orthop. 235:111, 1988.

67. Hedley, A. K., Hungerford, D. S., Borden, C. S., Habermann, E. T., and Kenna, R. V.: Clinical results with a new cementless total hip system: Minimum two-year follow-up. Proc. AAOS 53rd Annual Meeting, New Orleans, Feb. 20–25, 1986.

68. Lord, G., Marotte, J. H., Guillamon, J. C., and Blanchard, J. P.: Cementless revision of failed aseptic cemented and cementless total hip arthroplasties. Clin. Orthop. 235:67, 1988.

69. Wilson, M. G., Nikpoor, N., Aliabadi, P., Poss, R., and Weissman, B. N.: The fate of acetabular allografts after bipolar revision arthroplasty of the hip. A radiographic review. J. Bone Joint Surg. 71A:1469, 1989.

70. McGann, W., Mankin, H. J., and Harris, W. H.: Massive allografting for severe failed total hip replacement. J. Bone Joint Surg. 68A:4, 1986.

71. Head, W. C., Berklacich, F. M., Malinin, T. I., and Emerson, R. M.: Proximal femoral allografts in revision total hip arthroplasty. Clin. Orthop. 225:22, 1987.

72. Charnley, J.: Post-operative infection after total hip replacement with special reference to air contamination in the operating room. Clin. Orthop. 87:167, 1972.

73. Poss, R.: Total hip replacement. Orthop. Clin. North Am. 6:801, 1975.

74. Collis, D. K., And Steinhaus, K.: Total hip replacement without deep infection in a standard operating room. J. Bone Joint Surg. 58A:446, 1976.

75. Mallory, T. H., Meyer, T. L., and Bombach, J. D.: Six hundred and ninety total hip replacements: A comparative study. Ohio State Med. J. 74:23, 1978.

76. N. I. H. Consensus Conference on Total Hip Replacement in the United States. J.A.M.A. 248:1817, 1982.

77. White, R. H., McCurdy, S. A., and Marder, R. A.: Early morbidity after total hip replacement: Rheumatoid arthritis versus osteoarthritis. J. Gen. Intern. Med. S:304, 1990.

78. Charnley, J.: The long-term results of low-friction arthroplasty of the hip performed as a primary intervention. J. Bone Joint Surg. 54B:61, 1972.

79. Dupont, J. A., and Charnley, J.: Low-friction arthroplasty of the hip for the failures of previous operations. J. Bone Joint Surg. 54B:77, 1972.

80. Poss, R., Ewald, F. C., Thomas, W. H., and Sledge, C. B.: Complications of total hip replacement arthroplasty in patients with rheumatoid arthritis. J. Bone Joint Surg. 58A:1130, 1976.

81. McDonald, D. J., Fitzgerald, R. M., Jr., and Ilstrup, D. M.: Two-stage reconstruction of a total hip arthroplasty because of infection. J. Bone Joint Surg. 71A:828, 1989.

82. Wilson, M. G., and Dorr, C. D.: Reimplantation of infected total hip arthroplasties in the absence of antibiotic cement. J. Arthroplasty 4:263, 1989.

83. Maloney, W. J., Jasty, M., Harris, W. H., Galante, J. O., and Callaghan, J. J.: Endosteal erosion in association with stable uncemented femoral components. J. Bone Joint Surg. 72A:1025, 1990.

84. Willert, H. G., Bertrum, H., and Buckhorn, G. H.: Osteolysis in alloarthroplasty of the hip. The role of ultra-high molecular weight polyethylene wear particles. Clin. Orthop. 258:95, 1990.

85. Willert, H. G., and Semlitsch, M.: Reactions of the articular capsule to wear products of artificial joint prostheses. J. Biomed. Mater. Res. 11:157, 1977.

86. Miller, K. M., and Anderson, J. M.: Human monocytes/macrophage activation and interleukin-1 generation by biomedical polymers. J. Biomed. Mater. Res. 22:713, 1988.

87. Agins, H. J., Alcock, N. W., Bansal, M., Salvati, E. A., Wilson, P. D., Pellici, P. M., and Bullough, P. G.: Metallic wear in failed titanium-alloy total hip replacements: a histological and quantitative analysis. J. Bone Joint Surg. 70A:347, 1988.

88. Poss, R.: Natural factors that affect the shape and strength of the aging human femur. Clin. Orthop. 247:194, 1992.

89. Hedley, A. K., Mead, L. P., and Hendren, D. H.: The prevention of heterotopic bone formation following total hip arthroplasty using 600 rads in a single dose. J. Arthroplasty 4:319, 1989.

90. Lo, T. C., Healy, W. L., Covall, D. J., Dotter, W. E., Pfeifer, B. A., Torgerson, W. R., and Wasilewski, S. A.: Heterotopic bone formation after hip surgery: prevention with single-dose postoperative hip irradiation. Radiology 168:851, 1988.

91. Evarts, C. M., Ayers, D. C., and Puzas, J. E.: Prevention of heterotopic bone formation in high-risk patients by postoperative irradiation. In Brand, R. (ed.): The Hip: Proceedings of the 14th Open Scientific Meeting of The Hip Society. St. Louis, C. V. Mosby, 1986, p. 70.

92. Dwosh, J. L., Resnick, D., and Becker, M. A.: Hip involvement in ankylosing spondylitis. Arthritis Rheum. 19:683, 1976.

93. Law, W. A.: Osteotomy of the spine. J. Bone Joint Surg. 44A:1199, 1962.

94. Walker, L. G., and Sledge, C. B.: Total hip arthroplasty in ankylosing spondylitis. Clin. Orthop. 262:198, 1991.

95. Kilgus, D. J., Nanba, R. S., Gorek, J. E., Cracchiolo, A., III, and Amstutz, H. C.: Total hip replacement for patients who have ankylosing spondylitis. J. Bone Joint Surg. 72A:834, 1990.

96. Calin, A., and Elswood, J.: The outcome of 138 total hip replacements and 12 revisions in ankylosing spondylitis: High success rate after a mean follow-up of 7.5 years. J. Rheumatol. 16:955, 1989.

97. Aronson, J.: Osteoarthritis of the young adult hip: Etiology and treatment. In Anderson, L. D. (ed.): Instructional Course Lectures. Vol. XXXV. American Academy of Orthopaedic Surgeons. St. Louis, C. V. Mosby Company, 1986, p. 93.

98. Poss, R.: The role of osteotomy in the treamtent of osteoarthritis of the hip. J. Bone Joint Surg. 66A:144, 1984.

99. Callaghan, J. J., Brand, R. A., and Pedersen, L. R.: Hip arthrodesis: A long-term follow-up. J. Bone Joint Surg. 67A:1328, 1985.

Chapter 109

The Knee

Russell E. Windsor
John N. Insall

Campbell[1] reported the successful use of a metallic interposition femoral mold in 1940. A similar prosthesis was designed at the Massachusetts General Hospital in 1953. McKeever[2] in 1960 and MacIntosh[3] in 1966 reported on the use of metal tibial plateau replacements, which were popular in the 1960s, particularly in rheumatoid arthritis.

Interposition arthroplasty of whatever type requires the preservation of ligamentous support to provide the necessary stability. An alternative approach to knee arthroplasty, the metal hinge, sacrifices the knee ligaments and assumes the function of both stability and mobility, but its use is now only rarely indicated.[4]

A significant advance in knee arthroplasty was made by Gunston and MacKenzie.[5] The polycentric arthroplasty was the first attempt to apply to the knee the prosthetic components of high-density polyethylene articulating against metal (either stainless steel or chrome cobalt alloy) bonded to bone by methylmethacrylate cement, which has proved so successful in total hip replacement.

Many implants for knee replacement have since appeared. Metal hinges have lost favor, and most interest is now focused on metal and polyethylene surface replacements.

INDICATIONS

The age of the patient is an important factor involved in the decision to replace the knee joint. Most surgeons hesitate to implant a knee prosthesis in a patient younger than 60 years of age if there are reasonable alternatives. Polyethylene wear may be more rapid in knee prostheses because of the innate dished-upward concavity of the tibial component, which may trap debris,[6, 7] making failure in a young, active individual more likely than in an old, inactive patient.

The alternatives must be considered separately for rheumatoid arthritis and osteoarthritis.

Rheumatoid Arthritis. Synovectomy[8, 9] may relieve pain and swelling temporarily, but it has little effect on the progression of arthritis and is of no value when cartilage erosion has already occurred. The procedure may defer the need for total replacement in young patients, however, when symptoms are due primarily to persistent effusion (Fig. 109–1A and B).

1836

Hemiarthroplasty seldom gives results that compare with total replacement, and there is rarely an indication for arthrodesis in rheumatoid arthritis except for the salvage of infected cases.

Medical management should be continued as long as possible, with synovectomy being advised in selected cases. When surgical intervention is required because of severe pain during walking, the knee is replaced regardless of age, and a metal-on-polyethylene, surface-replacement design should be used.

Osteoarthritis. The selection of suitable patients for total replacement becomes more difficult. Multiple joint involvement is less common, and the patients often are healthy and vigorous, so that increased activity following relief of pain may put severe stress on the prosthetic components. Patients are also frequently obese. However, there are several alternative procedures that can be considered, and age assumes a more critical importance.

Arthrodesis. It is realistic to consider arthrodesis in a young active man with post-traumatic arthritis of one knee. In such a case the ability to stand and walk for long periods without pain can greatly outweigh the awkwardness created by knee stiffness. Nonetheless, even in ideal circumstances, it is becoming increasingly difficult to gain patient acceptance for arthrodesis. Some patients who have a satisfactory and painless arthrodesis frequently request an arthroplasty to return mobility to the knee. This is seldom advisable.

Débridement (Pridie).[10, 11] Removal of degenerated menisci and osteophytes, shaving of degenerated articular cartilage, and drilling of eburnated bone after the method popularized by Pridie remains the best approach for young or middle-aged patients with panarthritis of the kind that may follow athletic ligament injuries. These patients usually retain an interest in sports and wish to participate in some kind of recreational activity. The Pridie procedure is successful in about two thirds of patients and can be of long-lasting benefit. Débridement is now done arthroscopically, and good results have been reported. Significant angular deformity is the most important contraindication.

Osteotomy.[12–15] Primary osteoarthritis of the knee is usually compartmental and associated with angular deformity (most frequently a varus angulation). In some cases bowing of the legs may have been present since childhood. Correction of varus malalignment by osteotomy through the upper tibia is a proven

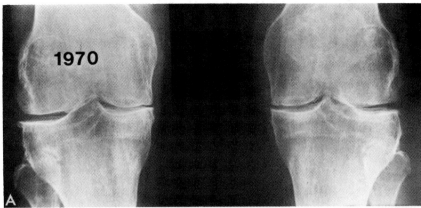

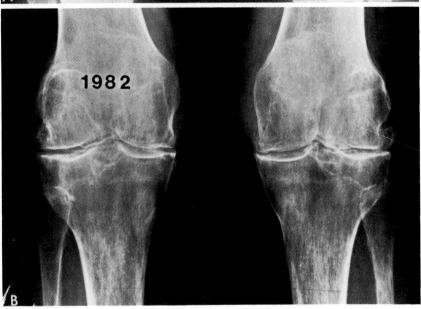

Figure 109–1. *A,* Radiographs of a patient's knees taken prior to synovectomy. *B,* Similar anteroposterior radiographs of the same patient taken 12 years after bilateral synovectomies. Some advance in arthritic change can be seen, but these changes are minimal, and the patient's symptoms are similarly mild.

and satisfactory operation. The most successful results are obtained in patients who have a relatively small angulation (not more than 10 degrees of varus) and stable knees. Provided that correct postoperative alignment in approximately 10 degrees valgus alignment is obtained, the results are satisfactory in about 90 percent of cases (Fig. 109–2). In knees with severer deformity, usually associated with instability, the results are much less satisfactory because obtaining correct postoperative alignment is more difficult, and the ligament instability tends to cause either overcorrection or recurrence of the original varus deformity. The effect of osteotomy is explained by the shifting of weight-bearing stress to the uninvolved lateral compartment and is purely mechanical. When good results are not achieved because of either ligamentous instability or incorrect technique, pain is not relieved.

Tibial osteotomy for the correction of the less common valgus deformity is less satisfactory.[16] Most valgus knees have a considerable deformity that if corrected in the tibia results in a marked joint obliquity, which causes medial subluxation of the femur and the development of late varus deformity. For this reason, it is generally preferable to correct valgus knees by lower femoral osteotomy, which preserves a horizontal joint axis, although femoral osteotomy has a higher morbidity, more frequent nonunion, and sometimes knee stiffness.[17, 18]

However, high tibial osteotomy is satisfactory for valgus deformities (1) when the projected obliquity after osteotomy will not exceed 15 degrees and (2) when the joint is initially stable (before the medial ligament has been stretched by the stress of weight bearing).[19] The best results are obtained in posttraumatic osteoarthritis caused by depressed fractures of the lateral tibial plateau.

The indications for total knee replacement in osteoarthritis are pain and limitation of function of a degree sufficient to warrant acceptance of the possibility of arthrodesis, because this may be the outcome if the arthroplasty fails. Arthroplasty is the procedure of choice for those older than 60 years of age but should not be selected for patients younger than this age if a suitable alternative exists. Replacement arthroplasty also is not suitable for persons who wish to engage in aggressive sports, except perhaps golf, bicycling, and swimming.

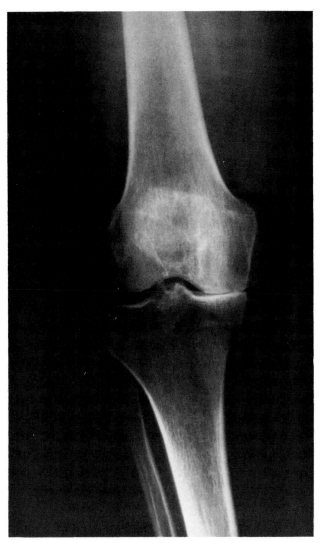

Figure 109–2. Radiograph of a knee with medial compartment osteoarthritis and good ligament stability. This knee is suitable for high tibial osteotomy.

PATHOLOGY

Rheumatoid arthritis may be best described as a panarthritis in that the medial, lateral, and patello-femoral compartments are involved equally from the early stages of the inflammatory condition so that cartilage and bone erosion occur more or less symmetrically. Apparent instability in the earlier stages of rheumatoid arthritis is not due to any changes in the ligaments themselves, which retain original length, but is caused by loss of cartilage and bone between the ligament attachments (Fig. 109–3). In these cases stability can be easily restored by re-creating substance (the prosthetic components). However, in the later stages of rheumatoid arthritis, varus or valgus deformities occur as the result of asymmetric erosion or collapse, and it is only then that adaptive and secondary changes take place in the collateral ligaments. For example, the most char-acteristic deformity in long-standing rheumatoid ar-

thritis is valgus angulation with external rotation and *lateral subluxation of the tibia on the femur*. The iliotibial band, lateral ligament, and lateral capsular structures shorten and contract. Over the same period, the medial ligament and medial capsule are stretched by weight bearing and, as a result, become longer and looser. There now exists what may be described as *asymmetric instability* (Fig. 109–4) in that there is a permanent alteration in the length of the ligaments. It is obvious that in such a knee the spacing effect of the prosthetic components cannot compensate for instability even when deformity is corrected because the collateral ligaments remain at different lengths.

Whereas varus angulation is relatively uncom-

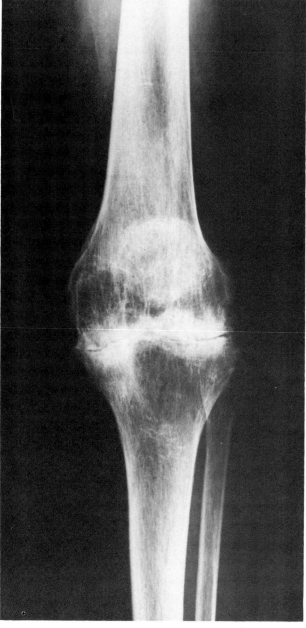

Figure 109–3. Radiograph of a knee in a patient with rheumatoid arthritis. The alignment and bony contours are preserved. This type of knee is technically the easiest for the surgeon to replace.

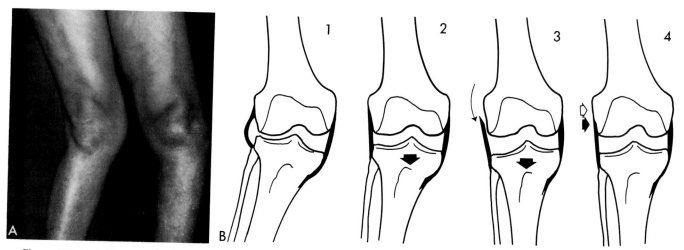

Figure 109–4. *A,* Photograph of a patient with osteoarthritis. There is a valgus deformity of the right knee and a varus deformity of the left knee. Invariably there is ligament asymmetry with long-standing deformities. *B,* In the right valgus knee the lateral ligament is shorter than the medial. Symmetry is restored by a progressive release of the lateral capsule and an iliotibial band from the femur.

mon in rheumatoid arthritis, this type of deformity is characteristically found in osteoarthritis, which, from the beginning, is a focal compartmental disorder. The lateral compartment is initially fairly normal and becomes involved only in very severe and long-standing cases. There is therefore a fundamental difference between rheumatoid arthritis and osteoarthritis: in the former, the whole joint is involved early, and angulation and asymmetry appear late; in the latter, initially one compartment only is involved, and there is early angulation and associated ligament asymmetry.

The secondary adaptive changes in the collateral ligaments commonly associated with angular deformity create perhaps the most important technical problem that must be solved.

There are other alterations that occur in the knee joint as a result of rheumatoid arthritis (although seldom or never in osteoarthritis). Fixed flexion deformities are common, and contractures of 90 degrees or more may be seen in some patients who have taken to a wheelchair. The flexion attitude initially arises because the swollen joint is more comfortable in this position, but after a time fixed deformity develops because of secondary contracture of the posterior capsule. In a determined patient who continues to walk in spite of pain, the flexion deformity seldom exceeds 20 or 30 degrees and does not present a problem. On the other hand, a wheelchair-bound patient who has not walked for some time and has developed very severe contractures presents a considerable technical challenge because the posterior capsule is shortened, the collateral ligaments retain original length, and the quadriceps mechanism is weakened by disuse and often stretched by prolonged swelling. Correction of flexion deformity by removal of extra bone from the femur and tibia therefore results in excessive laxity of the collateral ligaments and relative lengthening of the already insufficient quadriceps mechanism.

Another important and related abnormality in rheumatoid arthritis is excessive loss of cartilage and bone from the posterior femoral condyles so that the shape of the lower femur resembles a drumstick or chicken leg. Consequently there is greater instability of the knee in flexion than in extension; paradoxically, this is most frequently found in knees that also have a fixed flexion deformity.

An intact posterior cruciate ligament often prevents correction of deformity and interferes with the tensioning of collateral ligaments when restoring stability by the insertion of components. In these circumstances the cruciate ligaments must be excised. Goodfellow and O'Connor[20] state that the posterior cruciate ligament causes the femoral condyles, particularly the lateral, to glide backward (posteriorly) as the knee flexes. In the normal knee the shape of the tibial plateau does not restrain this rolling motion, and the laxity of the meniscal attachments permits the menisci to move with the femur. This anatomic function influences prosthetic design; if the cruciate ligaments are retained, the tibial components must be flat because otherwise posterior impingement will occur.

In favor of posterior cruciate retention[21] are the following arguments: (1) more motion with greater flexion is permitted, (2) posterior subluxation cannot occur, and (3) stresses at the bone-cement interface are relieved because force is dissipated by the intact posterior cruciate ligament. The arguments against posterior cruciate ligament retention[22] are the following: (1) the increased technical difficulties presented to the surgeon, who now must balance not only the collateral ligaments but also the posterior cruciate ligament to ensure proper function, and (2) the possibility of improper insertion of a cruciate-retaining design, which may then exhibit medial-lateral instability or inadequate flexion. In some instances an overly tight posterior cruciate ligament (Fig. 109–5) may actually increase the stress on the bone-

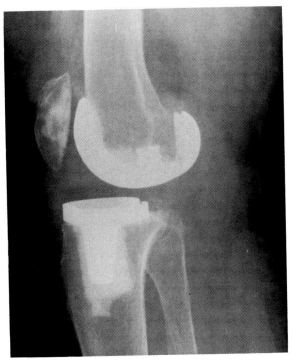

Figure 109–5. The posterior cruciate ligament was preserved in this knee and because of excessive tightness has assumed a vertical orientation, forcing the tibia to sublux anteriorly. This phenomenon illustrates one of the technical difficulties of preserving the posterior cruciate ligament in total knee arthroplasty.

cement interface. The technical difficulties increase with the preoperative deformity of the knee, and posterior cruciate retention is not always possible even in the most skilled hands. In these cases a cruciate-substituting design such as the posterior

stabilized condylar knee (Fig. 109–6A and B) is indicated, and this latter model may be the best choice for routine use in the hands of relatively inexperienced knee surgeons. Finally, it must be emphasized that design concepts must not be mixed; that is to say, the posterior cruciate ligament must not be preserved in a model intended for cruciate excision because a kinematic conflict will occur between the geometry of the prosthesis and the tension in the ligament.

TYPES OF PROSTHESES

Prostheses can be divided into two categories, surface replacements and constrained prostheses, each with subdivisions.

Surface Replacements

Unicompartmental Replacement. Unicompartmental replacement[23–26] of the osteoarthritic knee is widely used in both the United States and Europe. The concept has been recommended because only the abnormal joint surfaces are removed, and the total amount of bone excised is minimal. The amount of foreign material used (metal, polyethylene, and cement) is also quantitatively small. Finally, it has been claimed that the operative time and complications are less.

Unicompartmental designs[25, 27, 28] are intended to replace osteoarthritic knees in which one compartment alone is involved. The ligaments, including the

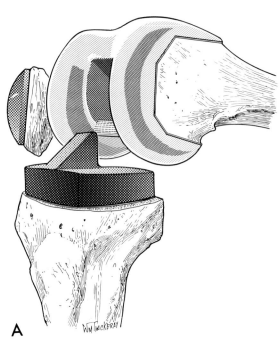

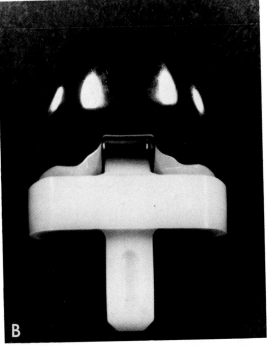

Figure 109–6. *A,* A diagram showing the post and cam of the posterior stabilized condylar knee. Articulation between the post of the tibial component and the cam of the femoral component substitutes for the function of the posterior cruciate ligament. *B,* The articulated posterior stabilized condylar knee.

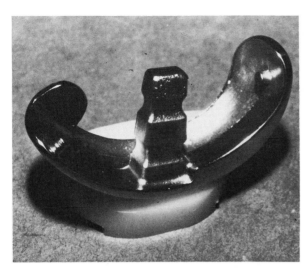

Figure 109–7. The unicondylar prosthesis.

the frontal plane to conform to the femoral component and is available in several thicknesses.

Unicompartmental replacements are difficult to insert and require much precision. The surgical technique may therefore play an important part in the ultimate success of the device.

Bicondylar Replacements

Duopatellar Prosthesis. The duopatellar prosthesis[29] is a posterior cruciate ligament–preserving design that has been modified to the present designs called the Kinematic and Press Fit Condylar Knee,[30] the latter of which utilizes cementless fixation of the components. The general shape of the tibial runners is anatomic in the sagittal plane, and coronally the condyles are flat with a median curvature. The femoral flange is inclined 7 degrees laterally, so that right and left components are required. The tibial components are dished anteriorly but flat posteriorly to allow for femoral rollback. They are joined anteriorly with a posterior cutout to accommodate the posterior cruciate ligament. There is a median curvature to prevent translocation. The deep surface of the prosthesis has a metal plate with a central fixation peg. A dome-shaped patellar component is provided.

Total Condylar Prosthesis. The total condylar prosthesis (TCP)[31, 32] (Fig. 109–8) is one of the earliest examples of a posterior cruciate–excising prosthesis that is still widely used in its original form. Although coined as the name of a specific prosthesis, the term total condylar prosthesis has recently acquired a generic meaning describing a whole range of surface prostheses that share general characteristics with the original. The salient features of the design are the following:

1. The femoral component, made of a cobalt-chrome alloy, contains a symmetrically grooved an-

cruciates, all must be present and relatively normal; therefore, the prosthesis cannot be used in severely involved arthritic knees with a large deformity, severe instability, or significant flexion contracture. Likewise, the procedure has no place in the treatment of rheumatoid panarthritis. The indications for unicompartmental replacement in varus gonarthrosis are essentially the same as those for high tibial osteotomy. For lateral compartment arthritis with valgus deformity an alternative is lower femoral osteotomy.

The unicondylar prosthesis (Fig. 109–7) consists of a metallic femoral replacement of approximately anatomic design: the sagittal curvature increases posteriorly, and in the frontal plane the curvature mimics the medial half of the femoral condyles. The components are available in various sizes. The tibial component may be made entirely of polyethylene or may have the same backed by an underlying metal surface. It is flat in the sagittal plane and curved in

Figure 109–8. The total condylar knee prosthesis. The patella is replaced with a polyethylene button or dome.

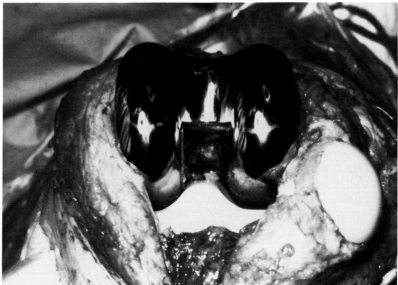

terior flange separated posteriorly into two symmetric condyles, each of decreasing radius posteriorly and having a symmetric convex curvature in the coronal plane.

2. The tibial component, made entirely of high-density polyethylene, or the same with a titanium-backed metal tray, has two separate biconcave tibial plateaus that articulate precisely with the femoral condyles in extension, thus permitting no rotation in this position. In flexion the fit ceases to be exact, and rotation and gliding motions are possible. The symmetric tibial plateaus are separated by an intercondylar eminence designed to prevent translocation or sideways sliding movements. The peripheral margin of the articular concavities is of an even height both anteriorly and posteriorly. The deeper bone surface of the component now has a metal plate with a central fixation peg 35 mm long and 12.5 mm wide. The anterior margin of the peg is vertical, but the posterior margin is oblique to conform to the posterior cortex of the tibia.

3. The patellar component is made of high-density polyethylene and is dome shaped on its articular surface, conforming closely to the curvature of the femoral flange. Recent designs utilize a metal backing, which has now been falling out of favor owing to a higher failure rate than that of pure polyethylene designs. A dome was selected because this shape does not require rotatory alignment like an anatomic prosthesis. The bone surface may have one to three fixation lugs.

Posterior Stabilized Condylar Prosthesis. The posterior stabilized condylar knee[33] is a posterior cruciate ligament–substituting design and was developed from the total condylar model. The TCP provides anteroposterior stability by the dished shape of the tibial articulation, acting together with collateral ligament tension to prevent component subluxation, because to separate they must run uphill on one another. The posterior stabilized condylar knee provides more active and concrete posterior cruciate ligament substitution. This function is assumed by a central spine, which articulates against a transverse cam on the femoral component. The cam engages with the femur at 75 degrees, and thereafter with further flexion the cam imposes a progressive rollback of the femoral condyles to prevent posterior impingement (Fig. 109–9). The standard version is designed to reach 135 degrees. In extension the spine does not engage the femur anteriorly until the knee is in 20 degrees of hyperextension, a position that should never be reached. The cam mechanism permits an increasing amount of rotation as the knee is flexed up to a maximum of 20 degrees at right angle flexion. No varus-valgus stability is provided, and the two components disengage freely if stressed in these directions; therefore, varus-valgus stability depends entirely on the integrity of the collateral ligaments.

Compared with the TCP, some minor modifications were made in the curvatures of the femoral

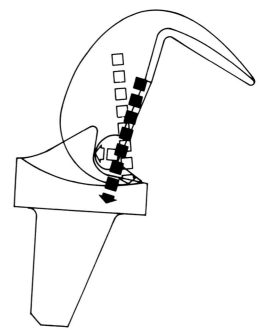

Figure 109–9. Diagram of a posterior stabilized condylar knee in flexion. Beyond 75 degrees the post and cam engage, imposing a rollback of the femur on the tibia. The resultant vector of these forces is one of compression at the bone-cement interface. (From Insall, J. N., Lachiewicz, P. F., and Burstein, A. H.: The posterior stabilized condylar prosthesis: A modification of the total condylar design. J. Bone Joint Surg. 64A:1317, 1982. Used with permission.)

component, and the tibial articulation was inclined posteriorly at an angle of 10 degrees so that the anterior lip of the articulation is approximately 5 mm higher than the posterior lip. As the intercondylar recess now dovetails into the femur, the fixation lugs were removed from the medial and lateral condyles, which preserves important bone stock in these areas. The fixation peg on the tibial component remains the same as in the TCP, and the patellar button is unchanged.

Constrained Prostheses

These prostheses provide all the required knee joint stability, and therefore both cruciate and collateral ligaments may be excised or absent. Infection and loosening have been major problems. Consequently their use has now been largely abandoned, and some newer designs have evolved with metal-on-polyethylene articulations, which allow rotatory and gliding movements, while providing the necessary stability, such as the Kinematic Rotating Hinge Prosthesis.

Although the mainstream of prosthetic replacement undoubtedly lies with surface replacement, full constraint is occasionally required for revision surgery and for a few primary cases. As far as the latter group is concerned, it is estimated that between 90 and 99 percent are replaceable using a surface prosthesis, the exact proportion being dependent on the surgeon's experience and technical skill. It is preferable for the patient to leave the operating table with a stable arthroplasty, even if this means the use of a constrained design, rather than an unsatisfactory and unstable surface replacement that is doomed to failure from the outset. The constrained prosthesis should therefore be available as a back-up to encourage a neophyte surgeon to perform boldly the necessary soft tissue releases that are the key to successful surface replacement arthroplasty.

TCP III. The total condylar prosthesis III (Fig. 109–10) evolved from the total condylar and stabilocondylar designs.[34] Stability is provided by a rectangular tibial post that fits snugly within a recess in the femoral component. Stems are provided on both components because of the increased stresses of the articular linkage.

The TCP III is used by the authors mainly as a back-up prosthesis that is available as an intraoperative choice for revisions or in cases of technical error in which, for example, a collateral ligament is inadvertently divided. The prosthesis is also occasionally used as a primary prosthesis for knees with severe valgus or flexion deformities in which it is judged that stretching will cause a postoperative peroneal nerve palsy.

Constrained Posterior Stabilized Prosthesis. The constrained posterior stabilized prosthesis is similar to the TCP III design. It has an added capability of being custom-made of a modular design, so that the surgeon, in essence, makes a prosthesis according to the requirements needed during surgery. Thus, metal wedges or polyethylene component sizes may be interchanged if required to obtain proper fit of the prosthesis. Interchangeable intramedullary fluted rods may also be utilized on the femoral and tibial sides when cases of severe bone loss are encountered.

INDICATIONS FOR TOTAL KNEE REPLACEMENT

Only severe symptoms and disability justify knee joint replacement. Although it is no longer true that a patient should consent to an arthrodesis before undergoing an arthroplasty, a frank discussion with the patient concerning the consequences of failure is essential. Medical management should be continued for as long as possible, and alternative techniques, such as tibial osteotomy, selected when feasible. In the presence of severe and unremitting symptoms, total knee arthroplasty is indicated in the following circumstances:

1. Rheumatoid panarthritis.
2. Osteoarthritis of the knee. The age of the patient, occupation, level of activity, sex, and weight all are factors that must be considered. In general terms, an arthroplasty should be avoided in patients younger than 60 years of age, in manual laborers, in athletes, and in those who are grossly overweight.
3. Post-traumatic osteoarthritis. There may rarely be an indication for knee replacement in the younger patient following intra-articular fractures or other traumatic injuries to the joint.
4. Failure of high tibial osteotomy. When high tibial osteotomy has failed to relieve symptoms, or when symptoms recur after an interval owing to progressive arthritis, total knee replacement can be performed (Fig. 109–11A to C). The procedure, however, is technically more difficult, and clinical results appear to be similar to those obtained in revision arthroplasty.
5. Patellofemoral osteoarthritis. In most cases patellofemoral osteoarthritis is not an indication for total replacement of the joint, and the condition is better managed with another technique. Femorotibial narrowing on a weight-bearing radiograph is therefore usually a prerequisite for joint replacement, but occasionally an elderly patient presents with very severe patellofemoral arthrosis without significant femorotibial narrowing, despite a finding of patchy articular degeneration throughout the joint at arthrotomy. This case, although rare, does better with total joint replacement than with any other method.
6. The neuropathic joint. Joint replacement in neuropathic states is controversial and represents a technical challenge, as instability and deformity are often extreme (Fig. 109–12A). The authors believe

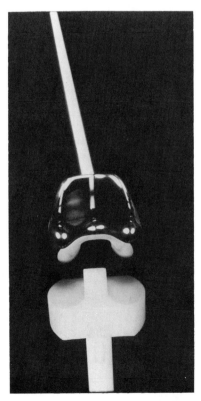

Figure 109–10. A total condylar prosthesis III design substitutes for the collateral ligaments as well as the posterior cruciate ligament. This substitution is by means of the rectangular peg on the tibial component engaging within a similarly shaped recess of the femoral component.

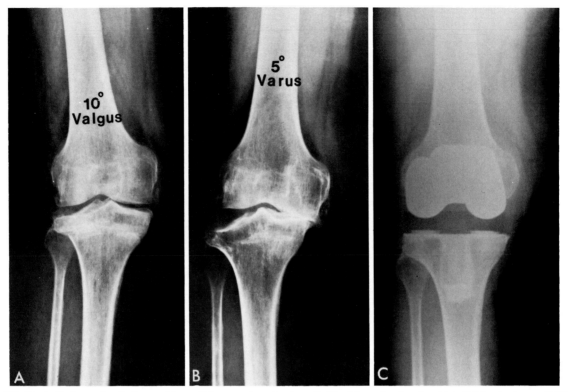

Figure 109-11. *A,* Radiograph of a knee with medial compartment osteoarthritis, taken shortly after high tibial osteotomy. *B,* The same knee 5 years later, showing recurrence of varus deformity with some stretching of the lateral ligaments. *C,* This knee was replaced using a total condylar prosthesis. There were no unusual technical difficulties.

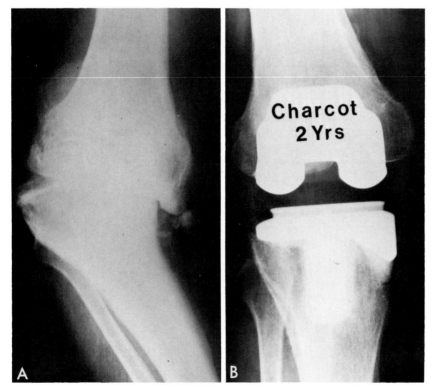

Figure 109-12. *A,* A radiograph of a neuropathic joint. Radiograph 2 years after replacement with a metal-backed medial wedge tibial component and a posterior stabilized condylar articulation. No instability is present. The knee is without effusion and is asymptomatic, and there is no evidence of component loosening.

that knee replacement is feasible, provided that a surface replacement can be used, the joint is thoroughly débrided, and correct alignment and stability are achieved. Metal-backed components with longer than usual stem fixation are desirable (see Fig. 109–12B).

CONTRAINDICATIONS TO KNEE REPLACEMENT

The following are contraindications to knee replacement:

1. A sound, painless arthrodesis in good position should not be converted to a knee arthroplasty. The prospects of a successful arthroplasty are not good, and a constrained prosthesis is usually required. Should the arthroplasty fail, another attempt at knee arthrodesis may not succeed.

2. Genu recurvatum associated with muscular weakness and paralysis is likely to recur after a surface replacement, and the stresses imposed on a constrained prosthesis will probably loosen it.

3. Gross quadriceps weakness.

4. Active sepsis. When infection is caused by a susceptible organism, thorough débridement and appropriate antibiotic therapy may be followed by a later replacement after eradication of infection. Tuberculous joints can be managed in a similar manner. When the infecting organism cannot be treated adequately because of the potential toxicity of the necessary antibiotic therapy, arthrodesis is a better choice.

SURGICAL TECHNIQUE

The success of any total knee replacement depends on the following four factors: patient selection, prosthetic design, prosthetic materials, and surgical technique.[35]

Prosthetic design has evolved to the point where little improvement of results can be expected from continued design refinement. Current prostheses possess many basic similarities and, if correctly inserted, will give satisfactory results. However, whereas total hip arthroplasty is relatively forgiving of surgical error, total knee replacement is not. Component malposition of 5, 10, or even 20 degrees may not affect the outcome in hip arthroplasty; in knee replacement, a 5 degree error is significant, and a 10 degree error is often catastrophic. Furthermore, even when the components themselves are correctly positioned, the soft tissue tension adjustments must be exactly right for proper arthroplasty function. The knee surgeon must consider not only the overall soft-tissue tension but also the relative medial and lateral tightness in the flexed and extended positions. All must be correct at the end of the operation. Prolonged immobilization does not usually improve inadequate soft tissue balance, and muscle development will not prevent component subluxation or dislocation. Therefore, the component placement and overall alignment must be correct within narrow tolerance limits, and the soft tissues must be adjusted while the patient is in the operating theater. When these requirements are not met, the arthroplasty will, at best, be suboptimal and often will be a total failure.

Although some minor degree of postoperative ligament asymmetry or laxity may be tolerated, it is better to obtain nearly perfect stability through surgical technique. Some surgeons have advocated the use of constrained prostheses for unstable knees with greater than 20 degrees of fixed varus or valgus deformity, greater than 30 degrees of fixed flexion deformity, or gross preoperative instability with incompetence of two or more of the major knee ligaments.[36] However it has been the authors' experience that such prostheses are very rarely required for a primary knee arthroplasty, although they may be needed in occasional revision cases. Essentially, use of the resurfacing knee prosthesis is possible only when the nature of the underlying pathology is recognized and when the surgeon is versed in the soft-tissue techniques necessary for correction.

Soft tissue release techniques are designed to restore normal alignment and motion and to preserve sufficient ligamentous integrity to permit the use of the surface knee replacement (Fig. 109–13). The techniques usually require cruciate ligament excision, so that anteroposterior stability after the arthroplasty is dependent on the surface geometry of the prosthesis, which must possess some cupping. It is the authors' judgment that the posterior stabilized condylar knee is the best choice of prosthesis after ligamentous release.

The alternative to soft tissue release techniques is to correct the deformity by additional bone resection; a constrained prosthesis that assumes ligament function is required. However, constrained prostheses have higher loosening, breakage, and infection rates, so that their uses should be minimized. With experience, soft tissue release techniques make it possible to correct most deformities and permit the use of a surface replacement prosthesis.

The Patella. Routine resurfacing is recommended whenever this is practical (the patella must be of a size and thickness sufficient to accept a prosthesis). Resection of the articular surfaces is judged by eye, and a small central fixation hole is made. During trial fit, patellar tracking should be observed carefully, and a lateral retinacular release should be performed if the patella tends to sublux during knee flexion.

Most surgeons advocate routine patellar resurfacing, although some practice a selective resurfacing in osteoarthritis (Fig. 109–14), preserving patellae that appear more or less normal, with a good surface of articular cartilage. In rheumatoid arthritis there is an argument for always resurfacing the patella, so that all articular cartilage (which may be the source of synovitis) is removed.[22]

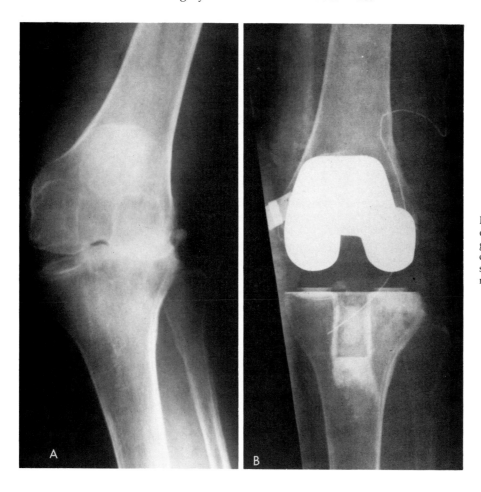

Figure 109–13. *A,* Radiograph of an osteoarthritic knee with severe valgus deformity. *B,* Radiograph after correction by lateral release and insertion of TCP. This is a recovery room radiograph.

Fixation. Provided that correct alignment and stability are achieved during arthroplasty, the long-term fixation of modern prosthetic designs of the total condylar type has been excellent (Fig. 109–15). In fact, present evidence suggests that the durability of knee prostheses is likely to prove better than that of total hip prostheses. There have been some recent advances that may further improve component fixation with methylmethacrylate cement. Cleansing exposed cancellous bone surfaces with a pulsatile water lavage system is recommended to remove blood, marrow, and fat. The bone should be thoroughly dried before applying cement to the exposed cancellous surfaces. With standard cementing techniques, penetration of 2 to 3 mm into the cancellous bone can be obtained. If the prosthesis itself is precoated with methylmethacrylate or is coated with a porous material, such as titanium wire mesh or sintered cobalt chrome beads, a very firm interlock among the prosthesis, cement, and bone can be obtained.

There has also been interest in cementless fixation of knee implants. In 1977, Freeman and colleagues[37] began using a modification of Freeman's original prosthesis without cement. The tibial component incorporated two polyethylene pegs with a series of protruding flanges that, on insertion into tibial drill holes, deformed and interlocked to give immediate mechanical device fixation. By 1982, Freeman and colleagues were able to report on more than 50 knees without mechanical loosening.

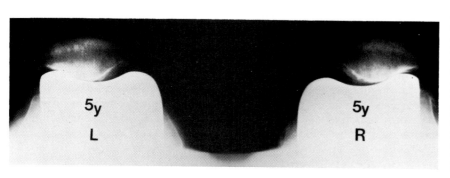

Figure 109–14. Radiograph showing a Merchant or skyline view of the patellae 5 years after replacement. In this case it was elected not to replace the patellar surface. This particular patient is doing well and is asymptomatic. When the patella is not resurfaced, some patients will complain of anterior knee pain, particularly when climbing stairs. However, the complication of patellar bone fracture is avoided. There is a case for not resurfacing the patella in obese or particularly active patients, who are those most likely to sustain a fatigue fracture.

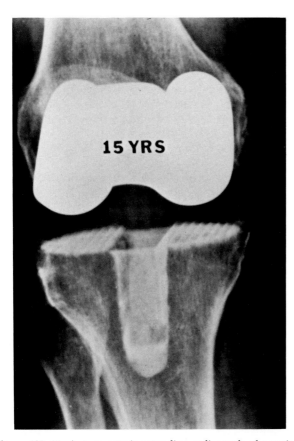

Figure 109–15. Anteroposterior standing radiograph of a patient 15 years after total condylar knee replacement. The bone-cement interface is stable and has remained unchanged for many years. This is typical of the majority of properly implanted knee prostheses of the total condylar type. The longevity of total knee replacement may ultimately prove better than total hip replacement.

In 1980, Hungerford and associates[38] began using an anatomic configured knee prosthesis designed for biologic fixation. The design incorporates a relatively coarse, porous coat on tibial, femoral, and patellar components. Primary mechanical fixation of the tibial component is achieved with two short angled pegs and a screw introduced into an expandable plastic sleeve placed in the bone beneath the implant. The femoral component is press-fit and utilizes two studs. The patella depends entirely on two short porous pegs for its initial fixation. The early reports are enthusiastic, but data regarding the effectiveness of fixation by bone ingrowth must still be considered preliminary at this time.

Aftercare of Total Knee Arthroplasty Patients. Intravenous antibiotics (usually oxacillin or cephalosporin) are administered immediately preoperatively and for 48 hours postoperatively. No further antibiotic prophylaxis is recommended. The authors do recommend that antibiotic coverage be given afterward when there is a known infection elsewhere in the body or for dental manipulations, genitourinary tract instrumentations, or other major surgery in which there is a possibility of bacteremia.

The prevention of thrombophlebitis should be a major goal of every orthopedic surgeon who performs total knee arthroplasty.[39] In a recent study of patients undergoing total knee arthroplasty at The Hospital for Special Surgery,[40] 64 percent were found to have evidence of thrombophlebitis as indicated by a positive venogram on the fifth postoperative day. This result occurred despite all types of prophylactic anticoagulation, including aspirin, dextran, and miniheparin. All patients also had a preoperative lung scan and a postoperative lung scan on day 6. There was an 11 percent frequency of postoperative lung scan changes consistent with small pulmonary emboli, although only a few of these patients had clinical symptoms or signs of pulmonary embolism. As with other investigators, the authors found the clinical diagnosis of deep vein thrombosis to be totally unreliable, with numerous examples of both false-negative and false-positive findings. Most patients with clinical or scintigraphic evidence of pulmonary embolism also had positive venography, suggesting that the positive venogram, although not itself associated with local symptoms, is of clinical significance. Patients with a positive venogram or lung scan therefore receive anticoagulants for 2 to 3 months unless there are also correlating clinical symptoms and signs of pulmonary embolism, in which case the anticoagulation is continued for 6 months. Anticoagulation is accomplished using warfarin sodium (Coumadin). The authors do not recommend the use of heparin in therapeutic doses except in life-threatening situations, because of the considerable risk of hemarthrosis. Early in one author's total knee arthroplasty experience before this regimen of venography and prophylactic anticoagulation, three patients had fatal pulmonary emboli from silent deep vein thrombosis.

Total knee arthroplasty patients are allowed to walk on the second or third postoperative day using a walker or crutches, with weight bearing as tolerated. Early motion in the recovery room using a continuous passive motion machine has been employed, with encouraging early results. Active assisted flexion exercises are performed under the guidance of a physiotherapist. Muscle-strengthening exercises are not begun in the first few weeks because of the risk of capsular disruption. The authors also advise against the lifting of weights at any time in the rehabilitation process. On discharge from the hospital, patients should be walking independently with a cane, should be able to climb stairs, and should have 90 degrees of flexion. The use of the static bicycle is a great aid in gaining flexion.

COMPLICATIONS OF KNEE REPLACEMENT

General Complications. Despite the advanced age of most patients and the frequency of associated medical conditions, the general complications of knee replacement are relatively few. At The Hospital for Special Surgery, in a consecutive series of 1500 arthroplasties, there were no intraoperative deaths, although one patient undergoing placement of bilateral sequential GUEPAR prostheses died of fat embolism in the recovery room.[41] Six patients suffered a cerebrovascular accident within 2 days of surgery, one of which was fatal. Three patients died of pulmonary embolism in the third postoperative week in the first group of 400 arthroplasties performed before any form of thromboembolic prophylaxis was used. Two patients died of myocardial infarction during the postoperative period. Two of the early patients died from septicemia secondary to an infected prosthesis; this was approximately 1 year after operation. Urinary retention and urinary tract infections occurred with some frequency, especially in bilateral cases (21 percent). All cases eventually responded to conservative measures and appropriate antibiotic therapy. The organism most frequently recovered was *Escherichia coli*. In none of these was the postoperative urinary tract infection related to the development of a deep wound infection in the operated knee.

Local Complications

Nerve Palsy. Most nerve palsies involve the peroneal nerve[42] and are related to the correction of valgus or flexion deformity. Twenty-three peroneal nerve palsies were identified in 2626 total knee arthroplasties performed at The Hospital for Special Surgery between January 1974 and December 1980. The time of appearance ranged from discovery in the recovery room to the sixth postoperative day. The recommended therapeutic measure was to loosen the compression dressing and place the knee in a more flexed position. In two cases this maneuver brought immediate improvement of both motor and sensory deficits. At the follow-up examination a residual deficit was found in all 18 patients in whom a sensory deficit had been present at the beginning. Motor power was clinically normal in six, with the remaining 16 patients demonstrating good to poor motor power. This complication has been reduced further by the use of continuous passive motion during the immediate postoperative period.

The following factors contribute to the development of peroneal nerve palsy: (1) stretching of the nerve in valgus and flexion contractures, (2) fascial compression of the nerve and its vascular supply, and (3) direct pressure from the dressing. There are rare idiopathic cases in which none of the foregoing mechanisms seems to apply.

Patellar Complications

Subluxation and Dislocation. Subluxation and dislocation are usually caused by incorrect patellar tracking, which should be recognized and corrected at the time of surgery.[43]

Patellar Fractures. Patellar fractures can occur with and without patellar resurfacing, although they are commoner when a patellar implant has been used. The fractures can be either traumatic, occurring after a fall, or, more commonly, of the fatigue type, which occur spontaneously without significant trauma. The fatigue fractures are of three types.

1. *Horizontal fractures,* in which the patella separates horizontally, the portion containing the patellar implant remaining centralized while the other fragment subluxes laterally. The mechanism of fracture is improper patellar tracking and is akin to a patellar dislocation.
2. *Vertical fractures,* often with separation of the fragments. The presentation may be one of transient mild pain and swelling, but at times the fracture is entirely asymptomatic.
3. *Comminuted and displaced fractures,* which are the commonest type and are a combination of types 1 and 2. The presentation is nearly always asymptomatic, and the fracture is often found on routine follow-up.

Patellar fractures are a complication of success, as they are seen in the most active patients with the greatest range of motion, who use the knee arthroplasty in a normal manner for stair climbing, arising from a chair, and other stressful activities. The fracture can usually be treated conservatively unless the patellar button is loosened, in which case the button requires removal.

Inadequate Motion. The motion obtained after arthroplasty is dependent on several factors, including body habitus, patient motivation, adequacy of physical therapy, and prosthetic design. However, probably the most important determinant is the preoperative range of motion.

It has been the authors' policy to manipulate knees postoperatively if motion is not rapidly regained, and this is usually done during the second postoperative week if not more than 75 degrees is obtained. A general or epidural anesthetic with full muscular relaxation is needed, as the purpose of the manipulation is to overcome articular adhesions with minimum force after quadriceps resistance is eliminated.

Other authors believe that motion can be regained if the patient is left alone to continue physical therapy. Fox and Poss[44] studied 343 total knee replacements performed during a 12-month period in which 81 (23 percent) were manipulated. Manipulation did not increase the ultimate knee flexion when compared with results in a larger knee group that were not manipulated. Their study was not randomized and did not address the critical question of whether the knees chosen for manipulation would have done just as well without it. Some patients do not easily regain flexion of the knee after arthroplasty, and in some, restriction of motion may be permanent. A selective manipulation is done for the following reasons: (1) It improves motion immediately, allowing more normal function, and (2) it prevents permanent restriction of motion in certain patients who are not easily identified until it is too late for manipulation to be effective.

Instability, Subluxation, and Dislocation. Instability after knee arthroplasty is usually the result of surgical error either in the soft tissue balancing and tensioning or in the overall limb alignment. Revision arthroplasty is usually required.

Loosening. Component loosening, usually of the tibial component, was the most frequent cause of failure with hinged prostheses and early surface replacements. The results of hinges often appeared deceptively good when the follow-up time was short,[45] because loosening was a time-related phenomenon usually heralded by complete bone-cement interface radiolucency. On the other hand, with surface replacements, most component loosening occurs within the first 2 years. Therefore, a 2-year follow-up examination of a surface replacement model serves as a good indication of the security of fixation, whereas similar data for a constrained prosthesis may be misleading.

High tibial component loosening represented a design problem. Modifications to the tibial component in more recent models[46] have resulted in a marked decrease in loosening. For example, the TCP has a one-piece tibial component with a central fixation peg, and only two cases of tibial component loosening were identified in 100 osteoarthritic knees followed from 5 to 9 years, with one of these being caused by malposition and malalignment (Fig. 109–16A and B). Metal backing of the tibial component, which increases the rigidity of the polyethylene, and improved cement techniques should reduce future component loosening to almost zero in technically correct arthroplasties.

Infection. Persistent symptoms after total knee replacement in the absence of a clear mechanical explanation should alert the surgeon to the possibility of infection.[47] Although diagnosing acute severe infection poses no particular problems, latent infections can manifest themselves, mainly by knee pain, with mild or no general symptoms. The wound can be benign, and the usual laboratory tests and radiologic findings may prove negative.

Frequency of Infection. Joint infection occurs more frequently in immunologically deficient rheumatoid arthritis patients.[48] Frequently, these patients have had previous operations, and earlier incisions may predispose to skin necrosis that may lead to a deep prosthetic infection.

The overall infection rate with surface total knee replacements is less than 1 percent. On the other hand, the infection rate may approach 15 percent with the metal-on-metal constrained hinged prostheses, such as the GUEPAR. Some of these infections occur late, sometimes years after implantation.[49] The high infection rate is probably related to the amount of metallic debris, which in turn causes a sac of fluid and debris to form around the prosthesis.[50]

Wound drainage is quite frequent after total knee arthroplasty and requires no modification of the postoperative regimen except cessation of physical therapy until the leakage ceases. Antibiotics should usually not be given, as latent deep infection might be masked.

Deep Infection. Deep or periprosthetic infection, the most serious complication of total joint replace-

Figure 109–16. *A,* This osteoarthritic knee was positioned after the arthroplasty in slight varus. After 1 year there was a pronounced radiolucent line beneath the medial part of the tibial component. *B,* There was progressive medial subsidence until this 5-year standing radiograph showed a considerable increase in the varus attitude with medial sinkage and bending of the polyethylene. At this point a revision was performed, and the tibial component was found to be loose. (From Insall, J. N., Hood, R. W., Flawn, L. B., and Sullivan, D. J.: The total condylar knee prosthesis in gonarthrosis: A 5- to 9-year follow-up of the first 100 consecutive replacements. J. Bone Joint Surg. 65A:619, 1983. Used with permission.)

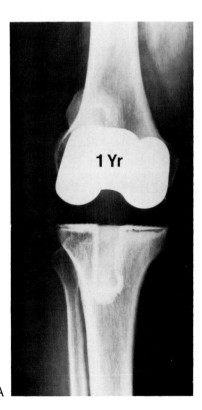

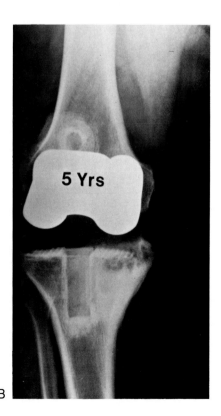

A   B

ment, may occur either early (within three months of surgery) or late (after three months).

Early Infection. An early infection, provided that its course is not modified by injudicious use of antibiotics, usually is not difficult to recognize. The clinical course is abnormal, with prolonged pain, swelling, inflammation, and fever. The white cell count and sedimentation rate remain elevated. The recommended procedure for establishing the presence of infection is a knee aspiration, with the joint fluid sent for Gram stain and culture for aerobic, anaerobic, and acid-fast bacilli as well as fungus. The aspirate would be inoculated as soon as possible into broth and culture media to increase the detection of indolent organisms. A thorough débridement of the knee may be attempted leaving the components in situ, with tissue sent for frozen section, Gram stain, and culture; the wound is closed over suction drains that remain in place for 48 hours. Intravenous antibiotic therapy is begun under the supervision of an infectious disease specialist and is subsequently modified according to the sensitivities of the organism. Antibiotic blood levels are monitored against cultures of the infecting organism, maintaining mean inhibitory concentrations at a minimum eightfold dilution. The wound is reaspirated 2 weeks later, and if cultures are negative antibiotic therapy is continued for another 4 weeks. If the cultures are positive, the prosthetic components and all cement are removed, accompanied by a 6-week interval of intravenous antibiotic therapy. In the optimal situation, wound débridement with retention of the components is successful in only 23 percent of the cases.[51]

One should not treat deep infection with antibiotics alone, as this treatment might suppress the symptoms of infection. Such treatment may be indicated only for the most extenuating circumstances if other medical problems are too severe for the patient to undergo surgery. Procrastination with prolonged use of oral antibiotics is ill-advised, as it will compromise future definitive treatment by masking a subclinical infection and creating resistant bacterial strains.

Late Infection. Late infection is commoner, and the diagnosis is usually provided by aspiration. The knee frequently becomes painful and swollen. Any painful prosthesis for which a cause is not readily apparent should be assumed to be infected until proved otherwise.

The treatment for proven or suspected late deep infection is incision, drainage, thorough débridement of the involved tissues, and removal of the prosthetic components along with the acrylic cement. This course should be followed even in suspected cases because only cultures obtained from the bone-cement interface may be positive.

Removal of the prosthetic components and acrylic cement may be difficult if the septic process has not loosened the components, and special cement osteotomes and high-speed, low-torque cement drills may be needed to safely remove them. All devitalized tissue should be excised, leaving viable, well-perfused tissues. Closed suction tubes are utilized for 48 hours, and the knee is immobilized in a brace or bulky Robert Jones dressing with plaster splints.

If the infecting organism is resistant to antibiotic therapy or there is an undue risk of antibiotic toxicity to the patient, an arthrodesis is performed as a second stage. If the patient is medically fragile, the knee joint may be allowed to stiffen as a pseudarthrosis.[52]

When the organism is susceptible, a new total knee replacement is implanted after a 6-week course of appropriate antibiotic therapy. Frozen tissue sections and Gram-stained tissue cultures are obtained at the time of surgery, and reimplantation proceeds only when these intraoperative tests display no evidence of active infection. An adequate selection of prosthetic components should be available, and custom-designed prostheses might be necessary to handle bone deficiency. Patellectomy may prove helpful in cases in which the skin closure was too tight. Frequently, both alignment and stability can be restored by using a posterior cruciate ligament–substituting surface replacement. Sometimes the need for constrained components is unavoidable. The TCP III and constrained condylar posterior stabilized prostheses are recommended, both of which have intramedullary stems on both components and restrict varus-valgus, anteroposterior, and rotatory motions by means of a centrally positioned peg.

A recent survey of 38 reimplantations, after being subjected to the previously described two-stage protocol after an average follow-up of 49 months (range, 2 to 10 years), showed eradication of the original infection in all but one patient. The clinical results were acceptable but resembled those obtained in the most difficult aseptic revision total knee arthroplasty.[53] Reimplantation of a new prosthesis was not done in 14 patients for the following reasons: (1) antibiotic toxicity risk, (2) medical infirmity, (3) inadequate skin viability, (4) extensive extensor mechanism necrosis, and (5) patient preference.

Revision of Total Knee Arthroplasty.[54] Component loosening was by far the major cause of failure with early prosthetic designs. This is not the case with later models, such as the total condylar and posterior stabilized condylar prostheses. In a recent study, failure was caused by malposition, loosening, infection, and subluxation in about equal numbers. Both malposition and subluxation are attributable mostly to errors in surgical technique and, hence, are avoidable.

The technical principles of revision surgery are similar to those described for infected cases except that immediate exchange of components is done. Femoral and tibial bone loss is the major technical problem, and bone deficits may be built up by metal augments, bone grafts, or custom-designed prostheses. The posterior stabilized condylar prosthesis is the prosthesis recommended for most revision procedures. The results of revision are not quite as good as those of primary operation, and the complete pain relief normally found after knee replacement is not so often obtained in revision cases. Restricted motion has not been a difficulty, and the average range of motion after revision is almost the same as that after the primary operation. Radiographic evaluation has revealed a more frequent presence of radiolucent lines in revision cases. These lines often are visible soon after surgery and, in some cases, reflect the difficulty in cleaning the bone ends after removing the previous failed component.

RESULTS OF TOTAL KNEE ARTHROPLASTY

The earlier knee replacement designs did not provide for the patellofemoral articulation, usually preserved the cruciate ligaments, and relied on small fins for tibial fixation, and the major problem was component loosening, usually because of either excessive constraint or poor component design. The current generation of resurfacing prostheses began with such designs as the total condylar and Townley prostheses, which have now been in use for 15 years. Results with these prostheses, properly implanted, are much the same as and may be superior to the results obtained with total hip arthroplasty.

The total condylar prosthesis has been in use at The Hospital for Special Surgery since 1974. The first 100 consecutive patients to have the prosthesis implanted for gonarthrosis were studied.[55] These osteoarthritic patients generally were the most active and would demonstrate the best assessment of problems related to long-term prosthetic viability. After a follow-up period from 6 to 9 years, 70 knees (70 percent) were rated excellent, 23 knees (23 percent) good, 2 knees (2 percent) fair, and 5 knees (5 percent) poor. The average postoperative range of motion was 96 degrees (range, 75 to 120 degrees). Patients with excellent and good results had no pain and were not limited functionally in their everyday activities. The two fair results were attributable to unexplained pain in one case and a patellar tendon avulsion with subsequent quadriceps weakness in the other. The five poor ratings were due to loosening in two knees, posterior subluxation in one knee, component malposition in one knee, and sepsis in one knee.

Radiolucent lines were present in 31 knees after 1 year, with the incidence increasing to 39 knees after 5 years. The commonest locations for the radiolucencies were the medial and lateral surfaces of the tibial component.

A survivorship analysis of the first 100 TCPs was recently done with a minimum and maximum follow-up of 10 and 12 years, respectively. Ninety-four percent of the prostheses either lasted the lifetime of the patient or were functioning well at the time of examination.[32] Fifty-eight patients (74 knees) had survived and were available for detailed clinical and radiographic evaluation. Of these, 38 knees (51.3

percent) were rated excellent, 27 knees (36.5 percent) good, 3 knees (4 percent) fair, and 6 knees (8.2 percent) poor. Five of the six poor knees had had a revision operation.

For patients older than 60 years of age, a knee prosthesis will last for the remainder of life in most cases. For younger, more active patients, current data are inadequate to form an opinion concerning implant durability. Most modern prosthetic designs will give a good result, provided that they are properly inserted into the knee.

The use of unicompartmental replacement remains controversial, and the published results of these prostheses are conflicting. Insall and Aglietti[28] reported on 22 unicondylar knee replacements with a 5- to 7-year follow-up. Although the results of these arthroplasties were initially good, they subsequently deteriorated. At the time of review only 1 knee was rated excellent, 7 knees good, 4 knees fair, and 10 knees poor. Seven knees (28 percent) were revised to a TCP. However, more than one half of the patients had a concomitant patellectomy, and in retrospect the decision to remove the patella seems unwise. The major reason for failure was progressive degeneration in the unreplaced compartments, and at revision acrylic cement and polyethylene debris were observed in all knees. Also, the results of conversion of unicompartmental prostheses to total knee replacements are inferior to routine total knee arthroplasty, supporting the fact that it is not a benign procedure that "buys time" until a total knee replacement is needed.[56]

Scott and Santori[24] reported on 100 knees in 86 patients with osteoarthritis followed for 2 to 6 years. They used the same unicondylar prosthesis as that used by Insall and Aglietti, but their clinical results were much better. Pain relief was satisfactory in 92 of the 100 knees, the average range of motion was 114 degrees, and 49 percent of the knees had at least 120 degrees of flexion. On the basis of their findings, Scott and Santori continue to recommend unicompartmental replacement for elderly patients with isolated unicompartmental osteoarthritis.

Constrained prostheses of the metal-hinge type should no longer be used. Hui and Fitzgerald[57] reported a 23 percent frequency of complications with an 11.7 percent infection rate. Although the procedure is technically easy because of the self-aligning stem designs and good short-term results, the results deteriorate rapidly with time because of late infection and loosening, with a high frequency of complications.

Donaldson and colleagues[34] studied the TCP III and found 77 percent good to excellent results in 25 patients who underwent 17 primary and 14 revision arthroplasties with this prosthesis. Motion was improved from 63 to 97 degrees using this unlinked, constrained design. There were five failures, all of which occurred in the revision group.[34]

With regard to surface designs that retain the posterior cruciate ligament, Sledge and Walker[58] have

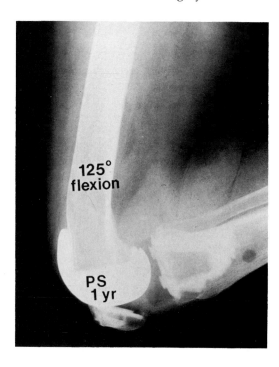

125°
flexion

PS
1 yr

Figure 109–17. Lateral radiograph of a posterior stabilized condylar knee taken at 125 degrees of flexion. (From Insall, J. N., Hood, R. W., Flawn, L. B., and Sullivan, D. J.: The total condylar knee prosthesis in gonarthrosis: A 5- to 9-year follow-up of the first 100 consecutive replacements. J. Bone Joint Surg. 65A:619, 1983. Used with permission.)

reported 92 percent clearly satisfactory results with the kinematic model. The average range of motion was 106 degrees. The posterior stabilized cruciate–substituting knee prosthesis has, in the authors' hands, proved most satisfactory, with 96 percent good to excellent results.[33] The average range of motion in this series was 115 degrees (Fig. 109–17), and 76 percent of the patients had normal function in stair-climbing activities. Fixation appears comparable to that with the TCP (Fig. 109–18).

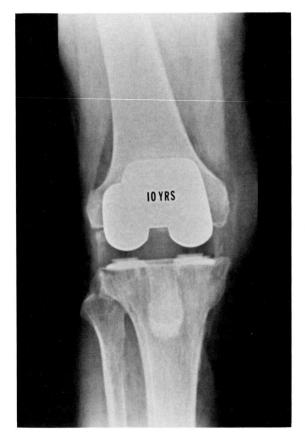

IO YRS

Figure 109–18. Anteroposterior radiograph 10 years after implantation of a posterior stabilized condylar prosthesis to illustrate the bone-cement interface, which resembles the TCP with respect to the extent and degree of radiolucencies observed.

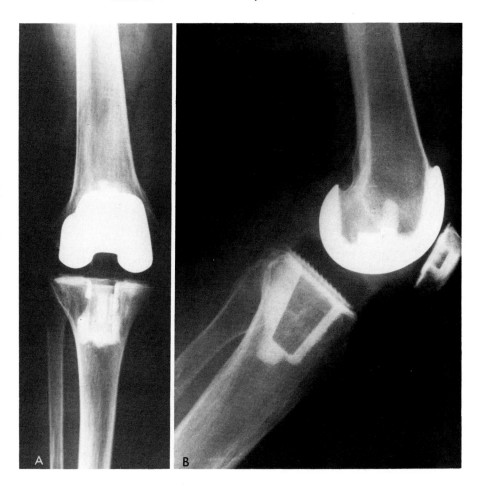

Figure 109–19. Anteroposterior *(A)* and lateral *(B)* radiographs of a TCP in "ideal" position. Balance is crucial to the function of the arthroplasty, which can be expected to last indefinitely, provided that the prosthesis is correctly implanted. With total condylar type prostheses, the surgical technique has a greater influence on the outcome than the variant of the prosthesis selected.

SUMMARY

Further developments in prosthetic design, such as refinement of the articular surfaces into more anatomic shapes with perhaps left and right femoral and tibial components, may provide only marginal improvement over results already being obtained with current designs. Posterior cruciate ligament retention, when possible, or alternatively a posterior cruciate ligament–substituting prosthetic design is desirable.

Fixation of the components with conventional cementing techniques has set a standard that will be hard to improve on, with very low rates of component loosening over long periods of time. Long-term results with cementless fixation are still pending.

The most important determinant of the clinical result lies in surgical technique, and most failures can be traced to inadequate positioning and alignment (Fig. 109–19A and B) or poor fixation techniques. Although more sophisticated instrument systems are available, total knee replacement remains a technically demanding procedure, and the operation is unsuitable for those surgeons who perform it infrequently. A measure of continuing experience is necessary, and although it is hard to define exactly what this should be, the operation should probably be performed not less than once or twice a month to maintain competence. Otherwise, the patient would be better served by referral to a more experienced surgeon or, alternatively, by a simpler operation, such as an osteotomy in cases of osteoarthritis.

References

1. Campbell, W. C.: Interposition of Vitallium plate arthroplasties of the knee. Preliminary report. Am. J. Surg. 47:639, 1940.
2. McKeever, D. C.: Tibial plateau prosthesis. Clin. Orthop. 18:86, 1960.
3. MacIntosh, D. L.: Arthroplasty of the knee in rheumatoid arthritis. J. Bone Joint Surg. 48B:179, 1966.
4. Deburge, A., and G.U.E.P.A.R.: Guepar hinge prosthesis. Complications and results with two years' follow-up. Clin. Orthop. 120:47, 1976.
5. Gunston, F. H.: Polycentric knee arthroplasty. Prosthetic simulation of normal knee movement. J. Bone Joint Surg. 53B:272, 1971.
6. Shoji, H., D'Ambrosia, R. D., and Lipscomb, P. R.: Failed polycentric knee prostheses. J. Bone Joint Surg. 58A:773, 1976.
7. Bullough, P. G., Insall, J., and Ranawat, C. S.: Wear and tissue reaction in failed knee arthroplasty. J. Bone Joint Surg. 58A:754, 1976.
8. Ranawat, C. S., Ecker, M. L., and Straub, L. R.: Synovectomy and débridement of the knee in rheumatoid arthritis. Arthritis Rheum. 15:571, 1972.
9. Geens, S., Clayton, M. L., Leidholt, J. D., Smyth, C. J., and Bartholomew, B. A.: Synovectomy and débridement of the knee in rheumatoid arthritis. J. Bone Joint Surg. 51A:626, 1969.
10. Insall, J.: Intra-articular surgery for degenerative arthritis of the knee. A report of the work of the late K. H. Pridie. J. Bone Joint Surg. 49B:211, 1967.
11. Insall, J.: The Pridie débridement operation for osteoarthritis of the knee. Clin. Orthop. 101:61, 1974.
12. Coventry, M. B.: Osteotomy of the upper portion of the tibia for degenerative arthritis of the knee. A preliminary report. J. Bone Joint Surg. 47A:984, 1965.
13. Insall, J., Bauer, G. C., and Koshino, T.: Tibial osteotomy in gonarthrosis (osteoarthritis of the knee). J. Bone Joint Surg. 51A:1545, 1969.

14. Insall, J., Shoji, H., and Mayer, V.: High tibial osteotomy. A five-year evaluation. J. Bone Joint Surg. 56A:1397, 1974.
15. Insall, J. N., Joseph, D. M., and Msika, C.: High tibial osteotomy for varus gonarthrosis. A long-term follow-up study. J. Bone Joint Surg. 66A:1040, 1984.
16. Insall, J., and Shoji, H.: High tibial osteotomy for osteoarthritis of the knee with valgus deformity. J. Bone Joint Surg. 55A:963, 1973.
17. McDermott, A. G. P., Finklestein, J. A., Farise, J., Boynton, E. L., MacIntosh, D. L., and Gross, A.: Distal femoral varus osteotomy for valgus deformity of the knee. J. Bone Joint Surg. 70A:110, 1988.
18. Healy, W. L., Angler, J. O., Wasilewski, S. A., and Krackow, K. A.: Distal femoral varus osteotomy. J. Bone Joint Surg. 70A:102, 1988.
19. Coventry, M. B.: Proximal tibial varus osteotomy for osteoarthritis of the lateral compartment of the knee. J. Bone Joint Surg. 69A:32, 1987.
20. Goodfellow, J., and O'Connor, J.: Kinematics of the knee and the prosthetic design. J. Bone Joint Surg. 59B:119, 1977.
21. Sledge, C. B., and Ewald, F. C.: Total knee arthroplasty experience at the Robert Breck Brigham Hospital. Clin. Orthop. 145:78, 1979.
22. Freeman, M. A. R., Insall, J., Besser, W., Walker, P. S., and Hallel, T.: Excision of the cruciate ligaments in total knee replacement. Clin. Orthop. 126:209, 1977.
23. Marmor, L.: Marmor modular knee in unicompartmental disease. Minimum four-year follow-up. J. Bone Joint Surg. 61A:347, 1979.
24. Scott, R. D., and Santori, R. F.: Unicondylar unicompartmental replacement for osteoarthritis of the knee. J. Bone Joint Surg. 63A:536, 1981.
25. Marmor, L.: Lateral compartment arthroplasty of the knee. Clin. Orthop. 186:115, 1984.
26. Kozinn, S., and Scott, R.: Current concepts review. Unicondylar knee arthroplasty. J. Bone Joint Surg. 71A:145, 1989.
27. Bryan, R. S., and Peterson, L. F. A.: Polycentric total knee arthroplasty: A prognostic assessment. Clin. Orthop. 145:23, 1979.
28. Insall, J., and Aglietti, P.: A five- to seven-year follow-up of unicondylar arthroplasty. J. Bone Joint Surg. 62A:1329, 1980.
29. Ewald, F. C., Thomas, W. H., Poss, R., Scott, R. D., and Sledge, C. B.: Duopatellar total knee arthroplasty in rheumatoid arthritis. Orthop. Trans. 2:202, 1978.
30. Wright, R. J., Lima, J., Scott, R. D., and Thornhill, T. S.: Two- to four-year results of posterior cruciate–sparing condylar total knee arthroplasty with an uncemented femoral component. Clin. Orthop. 260:80, 1990.
31. Insall, J., Scott, W. N., and Ranawat, C. S.: The total condylar knee prosthesis: A report of 220 cases. J. Bone Joint Surg. 61A:173, 1979.
32. Vince, K. D. G., Insall, J. N., and Kelly, M.: The total condylar prosthesis. 10- to 12-year results of a cemented knee replacement. J. Bone Joint Surg. 71B:793, 1989.
33. Insall, J. N., Lachiewicz, P. F., and Burstein, A. H.: The posterior stabilized condylar prosthesis: A modification of the total condylar design. Two- to four-year clinical experience. J. Bone Joint Surg. 64A:1317, 1982.
34. Donaldson, W. F., Sculco, T. P., Insall, J. N., and Ranawat, C. S.: Total condylar III knee prosthesis. Long-term follow-up study. Clin. Orthop. 226:21, 1988.
35. Insall, J. N.: Technique of total knee replacement. In Instructional Course Lectures, The American Academy of Orthopaedic Surgeons, Vol. 30. St. Louis, C. V. Mosby Co., 1981, p. 324.
36. Kaufer, H., and Matthews, L. S.: Spherocentric arthroplasty of the knee. J. Bone Joint Surg. 63A:545, 1981.
37. Blaha, J. D., Insler, H. P., and Freeman, M. A. R., et al.: The fixation

of a proximal tibial polyethylene prosthesis without cement. J. Bone Joint Surg. 64B:326, 1982.
38. Hungerford, D. S., Kenna, R. V., and Krackow, K. A.: The porous-coated anatomic total knee. Orthop. Clin. North Am. 13:103, 1982.
39. Harris, W. H., Salzman, E. W., and DeSanctis, R. W.: The prevention of thromboembolic disease by prophylactic anticoagulation: A controlled study in elective hip surgery. J. Bone Joint Surg. 49A:81, 1967.
40. Stulberg, B. N., Insall, J. N., Williams, G., and Ghelman, B.: Deep vein thrombosis following total knee replacement: An analysis of 638 arthroplasties. J. Bone Joint Surg. 66A:194, 1984.
41. Bisla, R. S., Inglis, A. E., and Lewis, R. J.: Fat embolism following bilateral total knee replacement with the Guepar prosthesis: A case report. Clin. Orthop. 115:195, 1975.
42. Rose, H. A., Hood, R. W., Otis, J. C., et al.: Peroneal nerve palsy following total knee arthroplasty: A review of the Hospital for Special Surgery experience. J. Bone Joint Surg. 64A:347, 1982.
43. Merkow, R. L., Soudry, M., and Insall, J. N.: Patellar dislocation following total knee replacement. J. Bone Joint Surg. 67A:1321, 1985.
44. Fox, J. L., and Poss, R.: The role of manipulation following total knee replacement. J. Bone Joint Surg. 63A:357, 1981.
45. Insall, J. N., Ranawat, C. S., Aglietti, P., et al.: A comparison of four models of total knee replacement prostheses. J. Bone Joint Surg. 58A:754, 1976.
46. Walker, P. S., Greene, D., Reilly, D., et al.: Fixation of tibial components of knee prostheses. J. Bone Joint Surg. 63A:258, 1981.
47. Salvati, E. A., Brause, B. D., Chekofsky, K., et al.: Reimplantation in infected total joint arthroplasty. Orthop. Trans. 5:449, 1981.
48. Garner, R. W., Mowat, A. G., and Hazleman, B. L.: Wound healing after operations on patients with rheumatoid arthritis. J. Bone Joint Surg. 55B:134, 1973.
49. Jones, E. C., Insall, J. N., Inglis, A. E., et al.: GUEPAR knee arthroplasty results and late complications. Clin. Orthop. 140:145, 1979.
50. Shurman, D. J., Johnson, B. L., Jr., and Amstutz, H. C.: Knee joint infections with Staphylococcus aureus and Micrococcus species: Influence of antibiotics, metal debris, bacteremia, blood, and steroids in a rabbit model. J. Bone Joint Surg. 57A:40, 1975.
51. Schoifet, S. D., and Morrey, B. F.: Treatment of infection after total knee arthroplasty by débridement with retention of the components. J. Bone Joint Surg. 72A:1383, 1990.
52. Falahee, M. H., Matthews, L. S., and Kaufer, H.: Resection arthroplasty as a salvage procedure for a knee with infection after a total arthroplasty. J. Bone Joint Surg. 69A:1013, 1987.
53. Windsor, R. E., Insall, J. N., Urs, W. K., Miller, D. V., and Brause, B. D.: Two-stage reimplantation for the salvage of total knee arthroplasty complicated by infection. J. Bone Joint Surg. 72A:272, 1990.
54. Insall, J. N., and Dethmers, D. A.: Revision of total knee arthroplasty. Clin. Orthop. 170:123, 1982.
55. Insall, J. N., Hood, R. W., Flawn, L. B., and Sullivan, D. J.: The total condylar knee prosthesis in gonarthrosis: A five- to nine-year follow-up of the first one hundred consecutive replacements. J. Bone Joint Surg. 65A:619, 1983.
56. Padgett, D. E., Stern, S. H., and Insall, J. N.: Revision total knee arthroplasty for failed unicompartmental replacement. J. Bone Joint Surg. 73A:186, 1991.
57. Hui, F. C., and Fitzgerald, R. H., Jr.: Hinged total knee arthroplasty. J. Bone Joint Surg. 62A:513, 1980.
58. Sledge, C. B., and Walker, P. S.: Total knee replacement in rheumatoid arthritis. In Insall, J. N. (ed.): Surgery of the Knee. New York, Churchill Livingstone, 1984, p. 697.

Chapter 110
The Ankle and Foot

Charles L. Saltzman
Kenneth A. Johnson

> He is not poor who has enough of
> things to use. If it is well with your belly,
> chest and feet, the wealth of kings can
> give you nothing more.
>
> Horace: *Epistles*

INTRODUCTION

The human foot serves four basic functions. It is a pedestal to stand on, it absorbs shock during ambulation, it works as a lever to provide mobility, and it allows bipedal balance of the body.

The mechanical stresses on the foot are large and continuously changing during normal walking. These include vertical forces, fore and aft shear, medial and lateral shear, and torque. During the average gait cycle these forces can reach up to five times body weight. In this environment of large and varying mechanical stresses, the foot, with an average of 30 synovial articulations, 22 bursae, and 18 tendon sheaths, is commonly involved by rheumatoid arthritis (RA).[1] The changes in the rheumatoid foot result from synovitis and mechanical stress. Early in the disease process, synovitis results in joint swelling, with subsequent capsule and ligament stretching. At the insertions of ligaments, the synovial proliferation tends to erode cartilage and bone. As the articular surfaces deteriorate, the supporting ligaments become slack, and the normal joint biomechanics are disturbed. With progressive stress, the joints tend to subluxate and eventually dislocate. Later when the synovitis resolves and the disease becomes more quiescent, contracture or stiffness may develop.

Virtually any imaginable deformity of the foot and ankle can occur. Until recently, long-standing RA of the hip and knee often rendered patients so crippled that they lost their ability to ambulate.[2] As these patients became bedridden by their large joint disease the care of their foot problems was superfluous. Now, hip and knee disease can be effectively treated with total joint replacement. Patients are able to walk longer in the course of their disease than ever before and thus develop increasingly complex deformities of the foot. As a result, it is now possible for rheumatoid patients to be wheelchair-bound because of foot and ankle problems. In this area remain many of the important unsolved problems in the orthopedic management of RA.

INCIDENCE

The incidence of RA in the general population is 2 or 3 per 1000 people.[3] Foot problems account for 16 percent of initial rheumatoid patient complaints to the physician. This is approximately the same as the number presenting with symptoms of the hand (15 percent) and is second only to the knee.[4] Despite this relatively high rate of initial foot presentation, the underlying diagnosis of RA is all too often missed. Patients may be operated on for hallux valgus or an interdigital neuroma and then go on to develop symptoms in other joints; they eventually are diagnosed as having RA. It is important to consider the possibility of RA when caring for problems of the foot and ankle.

Pedal involvement with RA tends to be progressive and bilateral. According to Dixon, in a study of 100 consecutive patients, Cash found 21 percent of patients had involvement of their feet within the first year of disease.[5] This rose to 53 percent after 3 years. In several studies of patients with long-standing RA, approximately 90 percent developed involvement of their feet.[2, 6–8]

Rheumatoid disease can affect articular and nonarticular regions of the foot and can affect soft tissue, nerves, and tendons. The nonarticular manifestations of RA may be varied. Pain associated with soft tissue inflammation may occur at the insertion of the Achilles tendon and at the origin of the plantar fascia in approximately 15 percent of patients.[9] Seven percent of RA patients have nonspecific heel pain. Grabois and colleagues[10] found a 15 percent incidence of peripheral neuropathy and a 5 percent incidence of tarsal tunnel syndrome in patients with RA. In another study, McGuigan and associates[11] found that 4 of 30 patients with RA and foot pain had electromyographic (EMG) evidence of tarsal tunnel syndrome. The clinical significance of the EMG changes is uncertain. Tendon ruptures probably occur in the foot as frequently as they occur in the hand with RA. Heretofore, many of the tendon ruptures were not recognized. For example, the tibialis posterior

1855

tendon may rupture and lead to a flat foot deformity. This has been recognized as a specific entity only relatively recently. Nonetheless, the incidence of tenosynovitis has been reported to range from 6.5 percent[2] to 10 percent.[12]

The forefoot is the region most often involved in rheumatoid disease. The principle that the longer the disease duration, the greater the deformity is particularly relevant to the rheumatoid forefoot. The disease seems to have a predilection for the synovium of the metatarsophalangeal joints. Hallux valgus is the commonest deformity. It is estimated to develop in 70 percent[13] to 80 percent[14] of patients; of these, 60 percent develop a hallux valgus greater than 20 degrees.[15] Hammertoe deformities are also common and are seen in 51 percent[2] to 80 percent[13] of patients. The forefoot is also prone to the development of various other deformities, including, but not limited to, hallux varus or rigidus, painful callosities beneath the metatarsal heads, and rheumatoid cysts or nodules.

Hindfoot involvement with RA is also common. Vainio[2] reported subtalar and midtarsal joint involvement in 67 percent of adults with RA. In this population of bedridden, chronic rheumatoid patients, 47 percent developed a varus deformity of the calcaneus, and 9 percent had painful changes in the heel region. Disease duration was found to significantly affect the incidence of hindfoot deformity. Only 8 percent of patients with less than 5 years of disease had hindfoot deformities, whereas 25 percent of patients with more than 5 years of disease had hindfoot deformities.[16]

The actual initial site of the hindfoot deformity is a matter of controversy. Vainio[2] identified the naviculocuneiform joint as the level most frequently involved with longitudinal arch disruption. Vahvanen[17] implicated talonavicular disease as the cause of pes planus deformity. Because of its unique anatomic location and orientation, the contribution of the subtalar joint to the development of pes planus is probably very important. It is estimated that 30 percent of rheumatoid patients have subtalar synovitis,[16] and approximately 21 percent have pain specifically referable to this articulation.[9]

The midfoot region is ordinarily less involved with the ravages of long-standing rheumatoid disease. In one study, 62 percent of patients were found to have radiologic changes in the midtarsal joints, but only 27 percent had pain in this area.[9] Although the exact cause of this discrepancy is not clear, it may be that the ability of plain radiographs to demonstrate early rheumatoid changes is enhanced by the orderly, cuboidal arrangement of midfoot bones and joints.

Reports differ regarding the involvement of the ankle joint in rheumatoid disease. Vainio[2] reported that only 8.8 percent of 1000 patients with chronic RA had ankle involvement. However, Vidigal and co-workers[9] reported that 48 percent of 204 patients had talocrural symptoms. This is twice the number of patients with radiologic changes in the same study. Warner (quoted by Tillmann[14]) found that 52.2 percent of 2356 rheumatoid patients had involvement of the ankle joint.

PATHOANATOMY

The nonarticular manifestations of RA have a significant effect on foot function. Antibody-antigen complexes deposit in the small vessels of the distal vascular tree. The results are variable but include the development of rheumatoid nodules, skin ulcerations with local infection, digital ischemia, and peripheral neuropathies. Muscle weakness and eventual atrophy secondary to neuropathy, inflammation, ischemia, or pain is common. The articular expression of rheumatoid disease around the foot and ankle can result in virtually any conceivable deformity, owing to the interplay of biologic and mechanical factors. At the level of the hindfoot, both calcaneal varus and calcaneal valgus deformities can occur. Vainio[2] found varus deformities in patients with severe knee flexion contractures who had experienced long periods of bed immobilization. These patients were reported to lie with their knees spread apart so that gravity tended to distort their heels into a varus position. The calcaneus more commonly subluxates in a valgus direction from the stress of weight-bearing. In the rheumatoid patient, loss of subtalar cartilage and bone, ligamentous laxity, and posterior tibial tendon dysfunction or rupture may contribute to the development of this deformity.[18]

The high incidence of forefoot involvement may be attributed to the large number of synovial joints and the relatively large range of motion of the metatarsophalangeal joints.[19] The path leading to the typical deformity of hallux valgus and hammered lesser toes involves multiple steps. Inflammation and proliferation of synovium induce chronic distention of joint capsules. This inflammation results in relative lengthening, thus laxity, of the plantar plate and collateral and intermetatarsal ligaments. During toe-off, the proximal phalanges progressively dorsiflex and eventually dislocate at the metatarsophalangeal joints. As this deformity evolves, the flexor tendons gradually migrate into the intermetatarsal spaces, where they become functional extensors of the metatarsophalangeal joints.

When the period of acute inflammation resolves, this clawing can become fixed with permanent contractures of extensor tendons. Some authors state that the plantar fat pad migrates distally with dislocation of the lesser toes, leaving thin skin under the metatarsal heads.[20, 21] It may be that the skin and subcutaneous tissue atrophies as part of the RA, and in fact the so-called fat pad migration is an illusion. On wearing shoes, the clawed toes tend to push the metatarsal heads plantarward. Metatarsal head erosion may progress to such an extent that all that remains are spicules of bone. Sometimes these ulcerate through the plantar skin on weight-bearing, form sinuses, and lead to local infection. Shoes that are too tight can also cause local irritation, with the formation of calluses or corns over the dorsa of the joints and the tip of the distal phalanx.

Deformity of the great toe in RA is different from that of the lesser toes. Perhaps this is related to the unique flexor and adductor moments across the first metatarsophalangeal joint. The hallux does not generally drift into extension with rheumatoid disease but, rather, deviates beneath its natural buttress of the lesser toes as they progressively claw.

CLINICAL FINDINGS

Early

The initial presentation of RA in the feet is variable. Usually the first observable change is transient swelling in the region of the ankle and toes. It can, however, present as nonspecific generalized foot swelling. Tenderness to direct joint compression is often an early finding. Patients who present with bilateral foot complaints deserve evaluation for a systemic cause.

Early involvement of the ankle joint is commoner in children than in adults. Patients complain of anterior pain with weight-bearing. Joint swelling can be best seen from behind, where the normal contours on either side of the ankle joint disappear. Tenosynovitis usually occurs in a retromalleolar location and can easily be confused with localized ankle disease. Anterior bogginess and swelling suggest the ankle joint as the primary site of involvement. The commonest tendons afflicted by tenosynovitis are the posterior tibial and peroneal tendons. Tenosynovitis

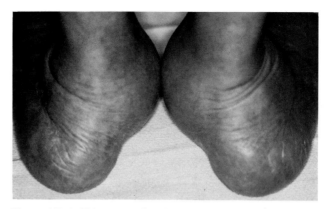

Figure 110–2. This patient has bilateral subtalar instability from her rheumatoid disease. When standing, she has pain in the subfibular region from impingement of the calcaneus on the lateral malleolus.

of the posterior tibial tendon can result in significant and well-localized discomfort (Fig. 110–1). Swelling in the posterior tibial tendon sheath has been reported to cause a compression neuropathy of the tarsal tunnel causing symptoms of burning pain, numbness, and paresthesias in the sole of the foot.[22] Tenosynovitis of the peroneal tendon is often hard to differentiate from other causes of lateral hindfoot pain. A maneuver that can be helpful in distinguishing peroneal tenosynovitis from other causes of lateral hindfoot pain is passive inversion of the foot. If this is performed rapidly, with resultant peroneal spasm, the diagnosis of tenosynovitis is made.

With hindfoot disease, the patient usually has functional restrictions, such as difficulty in walking on uneven ground. Subtalar inflammation can be difficult to differentiate initially. Hypermobility of this joint typically leads to a valgus deformity of the heel, and pain is referred laterally in front of the malleolus (Fig. 110–2). Subtalar disease causes pain with both passive hindfoot inversion and eversion. Subfibular impingement produces pain with passive eversion of the calcaneus. Pain with resisted active eversion connotes tenosynovitis of the peroneal tendons.

The diagnosis of midfoot involvement is less confusing. Usually the patients can localize the specific joints involved. Barefoot walking is described as exceptionally painful, and discomfort is increased during toe-off.

In the forefoot, early RA ordinarily presents with metatarsalgia. There is an equal frequency of synovitis in all the metatarsophalangeal joints. A painful bunion may be the initial manifestation of underlying rheumatoid disease (Fig. 110–3). Patients may also complain that their shoes have become too tight, and they will have a tender puffiness in the metatarsophalangeal region. Dixon[23] described two clinical findings that suggest the presence of rheumatoid disease in the forefoot. He coined the term "daylight sign" to denote the toe separation that results from both intermetatarsal cyst development and metatarsophalangeal joint swelling. He also described a

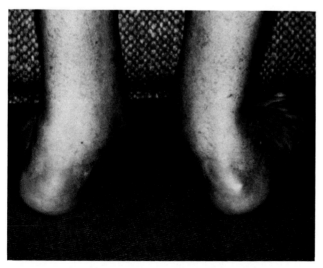

Figure 110–1. Posterior view of a patient with bilateral posterior tibial tendon dysfunction. On the left, swelling from tenosynovitis is seen posterior and inferior to the medial malleolus. On the right, the posterior tibial tendon has ruptured. The hindfoot valgus and the "too many toes sign" of forefoot abduction are best appreciated by viewing the patient's feet from behind.

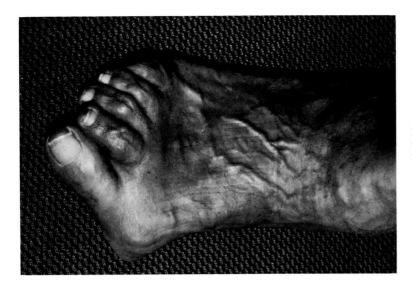

Figure 110–3. This patient had hallux valgus and metatarsophalangeal synovitis as the presenting manifestations of RA.

"lateral tarsal pressure test," in which the examiner gently squeezes the metatarsal heads together between the fingers and thumb. Light pressure elicits pain bilaterally in the rheumatoid foot, but not in the normal foot. The examiner should also look for swelling and redness of the plantar fat pad area, which can be an early indication of rheumatoid disease.

The initial diagnosis of RA can be difficult. The patient's symptoms can take a variety of forms. In addition, the clinical findings may actually implicate other systemic diseases. Impaired sensation or circulation may suggest diabetes or peripheral vascular occlusive disease. Generalized swelling of the toes with "copper pigmentation" would suggest Reiter's syndrome. If the interphalangeal joints are more involved than other joints, psoriatic arthritis should be considered. This diagnosis may be supported by the presence of psoriatic plaques on the patient's elbows, knees, or scalp. Salmon-colored inflammation of the big toe with hot and dry skin suggests pseudogout or gout. Inflammation at the insertion of the Achilles tendon or the origin of the plantar fascia, especially if bilateral, may be due to a spondyloarthropathy. Likewise, a single, swollen toe, like a sausage (wurstfinger), may also indicate a spondyloarthropathy (Fig. 110–4). When a single joint presents with isolated swelling, a wide variety of etiologies including infection, tumor, sarcoidosis, hemophilia, and fracture should be considered.

Late

Michotte[24] described the totally deformed rheumatoid forefoot as "pied rond rheumatismal" (Fig. 110–5). In this end-stage posture, the hallux is in extreme valgus, the three middle lesser toes are hammered and dislocated at the metatarsophalangeal joints, and the fifth toe is adducted.

Ordinarily, deformities of the forefoot are less complex. Although hallux valgus is the commonest deformity of the first ray, 10 percent of patients have hallux rigidus, and, although rare, hallux varus does occur (Fig. 110–6).[2] The interphalangeal joint of the great toe may demonstrate destruction and an extension deformity later in the course of rheumatoid disease. Although active metatarsophalangeal synovitis decreases with disease duration,[16] the frequency of hammertoe deformities increases with time (Fig. 110–7A and B).[2] In the late stages of RA the toes tend to drift laterally and dislocate dorsally at the metatarsophalangeal joints. Callosities may form under the metatarsal heads, on the dorsum of the

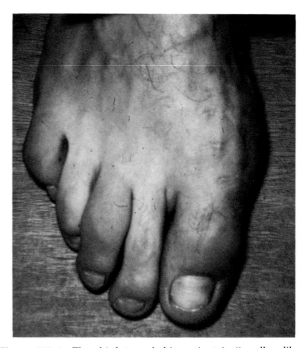

Figure 110–4. The third toe of this patient is "swollen like a sausage." A presentation such as this suggests a spondyloarthropathy. This patient gave a history of conjunctivitis and urethritis and was diagnosed with Reiter's syndrome.

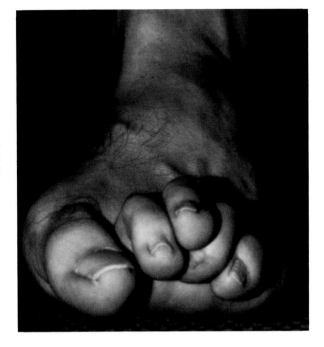

Figure 110–5. Left untreated, the rheumatoid forefoot may progress to the so-called "pied rond rheumatismal," or the round foot of rheumatism. In this figure the hallux is in valgus, the three middle toes are hammered and dislocated at the metatarsophalangeal joints, and the fifth toe is adducted.

proximal interphalangeal joints, and at the tips of the toes (see Fig. 110–7C).

RADIOGRAPHIC FINDINGS

Imaging studies are helpful both in defining the extent of disease and in following its progression over time. Radiographic technique is very important. Weight-bearing views are essential for the proper assessment of instability or subluxation of all joints in the foot and ankle region. As an example, in patients with metatarsalgia, a tangential weight-bearing view of the metatarsal heads may show a reversal of the transverse arch, lateral dislocation of the ses-

amoids, or formation of a plantar bone "spike" from severe metatarsal head erosion (Fig. 110–8).

The anatomic distribution of radiographic changes has been studied in detail. In a study of 661 patients with RA, Berens and Lin[25] reported an overall incidence of positive foot findings in 94 percent of patients. Seventy-one percent of these patients had evidence of hindfoot disease. Ankle involvement has been reported to range from 13 percent[26] to 54 percent.[27] Subtalar involvement ranges from 23 percent[26] to 32 percent[9] by conventional radiography, but computed tomography (CT) imaging has been demonstrated to be clearly more sensitive in making the diagnosis of subtalar disease.[28] The radiographic incidence of tarsal arthritis ranges from 20 percent[28]

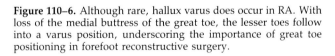

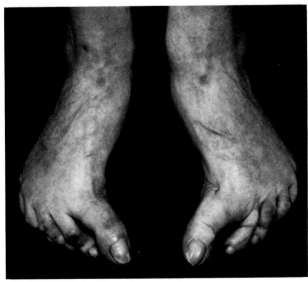

Figure 110–6. Although rare, hallux varus does occur in RA. With loss of the medial buttress of the great toe, the lesser toes follow into a varus position, underscoring the importance of great toe positioning in forefoot reconstructive surgery.

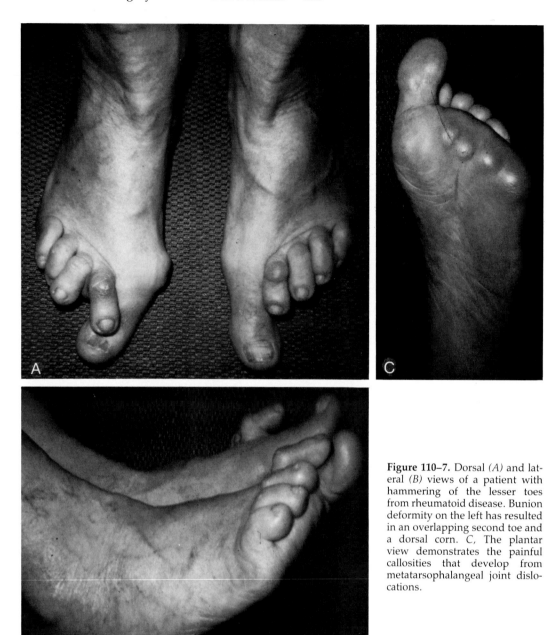

Figure 110–7. Dorsal *(A)* and lateral *(B)* views of a patient with hammering of the lesser toes from rheumatoid disease. Bunion deformity on the left has resulted in an overlapping second toe and a dorsal corn. *C,* The plantar view demonstrates the painful callosities that develop from metatarsophalangeal joint dislocations.

to 79 percent.[27] There is a strong postaxial predominance for metatarsophalangeal involvement. The fifth metatarsophalangeal joint is the most commonly affected, whereas the first metatarsophalangeal joint is the least often involved.[6, 29]

Symmetry of specific radiologic findings is helpful in making the diagnosis of RA but should not be an absolute prerequisite for diagnosis. In a study of 200 consecutively hospitalized patients with definite or classic RA, 140 patients had metatarsophalangeal erosions. Of these, only 16 percent had symmetric erosions, 53 percent had partially symmetric erosions, and 21 percent had asymmetric erosions.[30] In another study of 105 patients with definite or classic

RA, it was shown that symmetry reflected disease progression.[8]

Early in RA, radiography of the feet is more likely to produce information than examination of any other region of the body. In a study of 200 patients with RA during the first 6 months of disease, 19 percent of feet and 9 percent of hands showed radiographic changes.[29] In another study of 105 patients with definite or classic RA, 26 percent had foot changes without hand changes. Of note, no patients had positive hand films with negative foot films.[8]

Periarticular osteoporosis as indicated by a uniform reduction in density at bone ends is specific for RA (Fig. 110–9A). Other common, although less

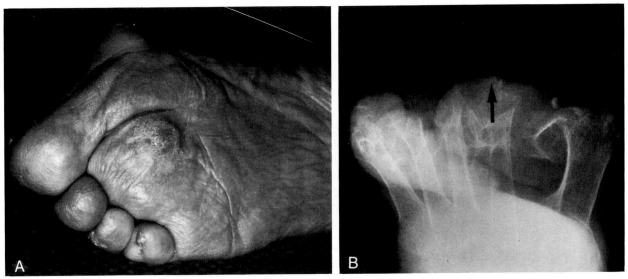

Figure 110–8. *A,* Clinical photograph of a patient with pain under the second metatarsal head. *B,* A tangential radiograph shows a plantar bone "spike" *(arrow)* after severe metatarsal head erosion.

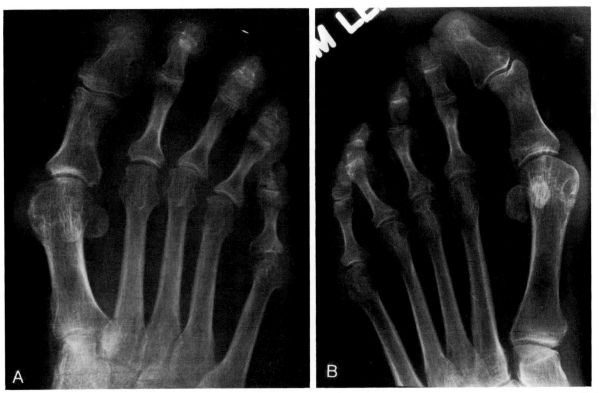

Figure 110–9. Early radiographic findings in RA. *A,* This anteroposterior radiograph demonstrates periarticular osteoporosis. *B,* This film shows juxta-articular erosions around the lateral metatarsophalangeal joints.

specific, early radiographic findings include soft tissue swelling, loss of joint space, and juxta-articular erosions at the insertion of the ligaments (see Fig. 110–9B). These erosions most frequently start around the lateral and inferior surfaces of the third, fourth, and fifth metatarsal heads. Eventually chondrolysis and secondary subluxation or dislocation become prominent features. Spontaneous joint ankylosis occurs in approximately 5 percent of patients.[29]

BIOMECHANICS

Gait Analysis

Pain, weakness, and abnormal joint mechanics are the factors that control the rheumatoid patient's gait. Thompson remarked that chronic rheumatoid patients tend to use their feet as pedestals rather than levers.[31] With advanced disease, there is a loss of the normal rocking motion of the foot with reduced or absent heel-strike and toe-off. The foot is typically placed flat on the floor and used as a platform.

Extensive gait laboratory studies have demonstrated that the gait of the rheumatoid patient is characterized by a slower speed of walking, decreased stride length, shorter single limb stance phase, and prolonged double-limb support phase. Plantar flexion during the swing phase and a delayed heel rise have also been observed and may be related to muscular weakness.[32]

Pressure Studies

The findings from formal gait studies correlate closely with the results of pressure studies. These studies have shown that the rheumatoid patient establishes initial contact with the medial border of the foot, then demonstrates prolonged heel contact with late heel rise and increased forefoot contact time.[33] Toe-loading is usually absent.[33, 34] As the disease progresses, peak loads in the forefoot move from the medial border towards the center.[34–37] Often multiple, abnormally high pressure sites are present (Fig. 110–10). The commonest site for abnormal loading during standing is in the region of the central metatarsal heads; during walking it is under the lateral metatarsal heads.[34, 35] Pressure concentrations under prominent and unprotected metatarsal heads average two to three times normal[34] but can be as high as 20 times normal.[33]

NONOPERATIVE MANAGEMENT

The initial treatment of the rheumatoid foot generally should be nonoperative (see Chapter 28). During the acute phase of illness, rest with or without splinting may be helpful; later on, mobilization to preserve motion becomes important. Consultation

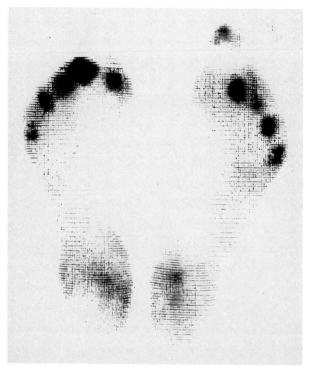

Figure 110–10. A Harris pressure mat study of a patient with advanced forefoot disease. Note the absence of toe loading and the abnormally high pressure sites around the central and lateral metatarsal heads. The localized pressure concentrations can range up to 20 times normal.

with medical specialists is essential in optimizing drug therapy and is detailed elsewhere in this text. For local control of disease, the judicious use of injectable glucocorticoids may be helpful.

As the disease progresses, physical therapy becomes more important. To maintain foot and ankle motion, stretching the Achilles tendon and drawing enlarging circles with the toes can help. A program involving toe walking exercises and faradic muscle stimulation had been recommended to maintain muscle strength.[38] For patients with chronic pain who have adequate circulation and sensibility, hot soaks at 104°F for 20 minutes, or contrast bath cycling of 104°F baths with 50 to 60°F baths for a total of 30 minutes, can be beneficial.

Footwear

The goals of footwear for the rheumatoid patient are to control instability and relieve pressure. Some general concepts apply. Arthritic patients need lightweight shoes. Shoes should be constructed with a soft material, such as deerskin, to decrease skin irritation. Extra depth shoes should be used to accommodate the forefoot deformities. Velcro straps greatly facilitate the ease and independence of taking shoes on and off, especially for patients with hand deformities. Shoe fitting should be done late in the afternoon, when the foot is at its maximum size.

Early in the course of disease, symptoms from the ankle joint may respond to wearing high-top sneakers or laced boots. For an acute synovitis or local tenosynovitis, a period of short-leg cast immobilization may be worthwhile. If instability eventually develops, a below-knee double upright with a square socket in the heel, rocker bottom sole, and inside T-strap may be necessary to control motion. If later the problem becomes lack of adequate ankle motion, the patients may not be able to point their toes to get into shoes. For these patients a simple and extremely helpful footwear modification is to extend the shoe tongue to allow a full opening.

Subtalar synovitis can cause capsular and ligamentous stretching. With weight-bearing this eventually may lead to a valgus deformity. The aim of conservative treatment is to induce a pain-free fibrous or bony ankylosis of the subtalar joint in a good functional position. Dixon[5] recommends an aggressive approach combining local steroid injections with an initial period of nonweight-bearing immobilization. He then applies a below-knee iron with an inside T-strap and a medial heel or sole wedge. For those patients who will not tolerate immobilization across the ankle joint, it may be worthwhile to try an oxford shoe with a reinforced medial counter and a 1/8-inch or 3/16-inch medial heel wedge.

The nonoperative treatment of a rigid valgus hindfoot can be challenging. A seamless shoe technique known as "space shoes" has been used to accommodate these patients. These shoes are made by a molding and bonding process over a plaster model of the foot. Dixon[5] reported a 30 percent rate of dissatisfaction after 1 year with these custom shoes. The failures were attributed to shoe wear and changes in foot anatomy secondary to rheumatoid disease. Another approach to the fixed, deformed hindfoot is to use a custom-made ankle-foot orthosis placed in a shoe with a medial sole wedge. This may be effective in relieving pain by reducing motion. If pain symptoms persist, however, surgery may be considered.

The selection of appropriate footwear to accommodate forefoot involvement of RA depends on the stage of disease. Swelling of the metatarsophalangeal joints has a dramatic effect on the need for shoe width. The forefoot may widen up to two full shoe-fittings with the onset of disease.[33] The use of high-heels should be strongly discouraged because they tend to dorsiflex the metatarsophalangeal joints and crowd the toes. A standard oxford shoe wide enough to accommodate the splayed forefoot, deep enough to avoid pressure on the dislocated toes, and with a soft sole and an arch support is optimal early shoe-wear for the rheumatoid patient. If subluxation or dislocation at the metatarsophalangeal joints develops, the patients may be more comfortable in an extra-depth shoe with a wide toebox composed of a soft, yielding material. The room for the toes is accomplished by removing the anterior half of the shoe insole. In essence then, it becomes a split-sized shoe with the toebox large while the heel counter size remains unchanged. A Plastazote liner with an arch support may also be helpful.[39] If the patient develops severe metatarsalgia, a metatarsal bar can be added to the sole of the shoe. This tends to transfer weight proximally and substitute a rocking motion of the shoe for the normal metatarsophalangeal joint motion.

Despite these measures, patients may continue to have pain. Miller[40] found that such shoewear modifications relieved pain in only 30 to 40 percent of patients. Vidigal and colleagues,[9] in a study of 104 patients with long-standing RA, found that 40 percent were able to wear shoes bought at an ordinary store, 20 percent wore special shoes, and 40 percent were not satisfied with any shoewear.

SURGICAL MANAGEMENT

General Considerations

The foot and ankle region is one of the more common sites of surgical intervention in rheumatoid disease, constituting one quarter to one third of all operations done for this disease.[2, 14] As a rule, surgical treatment is indicated only after conservative treatment has failed to control pain or deformity, and surgery should be considered palliative rather than curative. The natural history of RA in the weight-bearing foot is that it will continue to degenerate because of the inexorable nature of the disease. In a review of 38 rheumatoid patients who had foot surgery for pain, 80 percent had complete relief of pain initially. However, at later follow-up, 4½ to 8½ years postoperatively, only 55 percent remained pain free, and 45 percent required special shoes.[41] This trend has also been observed by several other authors.[42, 43]

For the rheumatoid patient there are special considerations that will influence the surgical result. The prerequisites for a successful surgical treatment of the rheumatoid patient have been clearly articulated by Tillmann.[14] These include (1) close cooperation with an internist experienced in rheumatology, (2) facilities for postoperative physical and occupational therapy, (3) good surgical technique, and (4) a cooperative patient.

The selection of the surgical candidate is extremely important in the RA population. The long-held belief that the rheumatoid disease should be in a "burned out" state before surgery is undertaken is unfounded and inaccurate. Furthermore, patient age is not, in itself, a contraindication to surgery. The factors more critical to the proper selection of the surgical candidate include the vascular status of the patient, the quality of the skin, the existence of steroid dependence or methotrexate use, the presence of concomitant cervical spine or temporomandibular disease, neurologic involvement, and the potential of the patient to benefit from operative intervention. Approximately 40 percent of chronic rheumatoid patients have atlantoaxial subluxation.[44] Because of this high incidence of involvement, the authors obtain lateral cervical spine radiographs in flexion and extension as part of the preoperative work-up. If instability is noted, then atlantoaxial stabilization may be necessary prior to foot and ankle surgery.

There are multiple surgical alternatives for the care of the rheumatoid foot. These can be classified as soft tissue procedures, bony excision procedures, arthrodeses, osteotomies, and implant arthroplasties. The selection of the appropriate procedure or combination of procedures depends on the type and location of the deformity, the functional needs and status of the patient, the morbidity associated with the operation, and the patient's ability to cooperate and cope during the convalescence period.

When several sites are involved with disease, the total length of convalescence may be reduced by performing multiple, simultaneous, ipsilateral procedures. Bilateral procedures are generally discouraged because of the more difficult convalescence.

SOFT TISSUE PROCEDURES

Tenosynovectomy is reserved primarily for tendon pain unresponsive to rest, immobilization, and steroid injection. Most commonly, the posterior tibial and peroneal tendons are involved with symptomatic tenosynovitis.

Rheumatoid disease can cause painful bursal inflammation of multiple sites around the foot. An isolated inflamed bursa unresponsive to conservative care may be excised. Bursa associated with contiguous joint disease should not be removed without consideration given to synovectomy or arthroplasty of the related articulation.

Ankle

Surgery of the rheumatoid ankle is indicated only when pain and instability cannot be controlled by other means. The surgical alternatives include synovectomy, arthrodesis, and replacement arthroplasty. Although the North American experience with ankle synovectomy is limited, European reports suggest that this form of treatment can be effective early in the course of the disease. Arthrodesis is recommended for patients with significant articular changes and high functional demands. The role of total ankle arthroplasty is controversial. Ankle replacement offers the theoretic advantage of providing a mobile, painless ankle joint. In the rheumatoid population this is very attractive, as the other joints of the hindfoot are often stiff or ankylosed. The results from total ankle arthroplasty to date, however, have been unpredictable. In the future, with development of improved prosthetic design and an-

atomic access, total ankle arthroplasty may become an accepted prominent form of treatment of the rheumatoid ankle.

Synovectomy

According to Tillmann,[14, 45] the indication for synovectomy of the ankle is persistent synovitis of a congruent joint that has been unresponsive to nonoperative means. In his review of 135 synovectomies performed at various European centers, 60 percent were classified as having had good results, and 10 percent as having had poor results. In a more recent series of 81 ankles with·an average follow-up of 4 years, 80 percent reported "some improvement" with pain and swelling, 40 percent had "significant" improvement with pain, and 51 percent had "significant" improvement with motion.[46] These authors noted that all patients who underwent operations in the early stages of the disease had good results, whereas the patients with subchondral bone cysts of the talus and tibia did relatively poorly. Vahvanen[47] also demonstrated that ankle synovectomy was of questionable benefit for patients with erosive radiologic changes. In summary, synovectomy may be helpful to patients with significant ankle symptoms unresponsive to conservative means early in the course of disease.

Arthrodesis

For the rheumatoid patient with high functional demands and radiographic changes involving a symptomatic ankle, arthrodesis may be the procedure of choice. There must be enough compensatory motion in the transverse tarsal and tarsometatarsal joints and a functional range of motion in the contralateral ankle for an arthrodesis to work well.[48] More than 30 different arthrodesis techniques have been described. No single approach is appropriate for all patients. The most widely used techniques today include compressive external fixation and rigid internal fixation, but neither has been extensively studied in the rheumatoid population.

In a study of 11 rheumatoid patients treated with the Charnley compression technique, four (36 percent) had pin tract infections, and three (27 percent) had delayed unions.[49] The reported rate of complication has been less with rigid internal fixation. In a study of six rheumatoid patients undergoing ankle arthrodesis using rigid internal fixation,[50] there was only one superficial wound infection. No other complications were observed. The researchers suggested that poor soft tissue coverage should be considered a contraindication to ankle arthrodesis with rigid internal fixation. Although the operation can be technically demanding, it offers the advantages of a low rate of complication and rapid time to union.[50]

Ankle arthrodesis has been performed for many indications other than RA. The relevant literature sheds light on the care of the rheumatoid ankle. The reported range of complications is impressive. Non-unions are common, with rates as high as 40 percent observed. Other complications reported[51] include delayed union, breakdown of union, pin tract drainage, pin tract infection, delayed wound healing, skin necrosis, wound infection, below-knee amputations for intractable pain or infection, nerve injury, and chronic edema. The percentage of failures has increased as the operations have become more extensive and involve other, nonankle joint procedures.[52] Even a solid ankle arthrodesis can be a problem. Arthrodeses generally require a period of immobilization and nonweight-bearing. For the severely involved rheumatoid patient with upper extremity disease, the convalescence period can be extremely trying. Bilateral ankle fusions may be severely limiting, especially when the patient tries to rise from a chair or descend a staircase. Gait studies have helped in understanding the effects of ankle arthrodesis. In normal gait, the average ankle moves approximately 26 degrees, 40 percent of which is used for dorsiflexion.[53] In a study of patients who underwent ankle arthrodeses for post-traumatic arthritis, an average of 16 degrees of plantar-dorsiflexion was found in the Chopart and Lisfranc joints.[48] In another study of 23 patients with an average of 16 years follow-up after ankle arthrodesis, Stauffer[53] found that 18 of these patients were unable to walk on uneven surfaces and that all these patients had difficulty in walking.

Gait laboratory studies have demonstrated that these patients have a slower gait velocity, shorter stride length, and longer swing and double-limb stance phase.[48] These patients utilize several specific mechanisms to allow them to have a reasonably normal gait. These include (1) using the arcs of motion in the small joints of the foot below the fused ankle, (2) altering the pattern of tibial foot rotation on the normal side, and (3) using shoes with heels that allow the tibia to advance more easily during the stance phase. When the compensatory movement of the subtalar-midtarsal joints is absent, some improvement of gait may be obtained by the use of a cushioned heel and rocker-bottom sole.

Arthroplasty

The ideal candidate for a total ankle replacement is an individual with low functional demands and primarily involvement of the ankle without deformity or instability. Also the subtalar joint should be in normal alignment. The bone density should be sufficient to support the arthroplasty components. The selection of the proper patient for total ankle arthroplasty requires considering the functional needs of the patient with the state of disease.

Biomechanical studies have shown that the ankle joint sustains compressive loads up to five times body weight and shear forces of 80 percent of body weight.[53] Therefore, the design for a total ankle replacement must have adequate bone fixation to withstand the mechanical demands. Also, because of the high incidence of concomitant subtalar disease, the ideal prosthesis should allow motion in the subtalar joint axis.

The history of total ankle replacement has been one marked by poor anatomic access and the use of relatively constrained prostheses. Unlike other forms of total joint replacement, ankle disarticulation has not been a routine part of the operation. Visualization and surgical fit have often been less than satisfactory, and long-term results have reflected these difficulties.

There may be a gradual deterioration in ankle replacement outcome over time.[43] "Adequate" pain relief, defined as pain relief at rest or mild pain with activity, has been reported to vary from 77 percent[54] to 88 percent.[55] The average return of motion from total ankles has generally been poor, reported as ranging from 5 degrees[56] to 9 degrees.[57] A valid functional assessment of the surgical outcome has been difficult to perform because of the typical rheumatoid involvement of multiple other lower limb joints. Nonetheless, abnormal gait motion patterns have been detected.[58] Weakness of calf and peroneal muscles may have contributed to this. Still, after total ankle arthroplasty maximal walking distance has been reported to improve by an average of fivefold.[59]

With former prosthetic designs, radiographic studies have consistently shown progressive loosening and subsidence of both the tibial and the talar components over time.[43] Attempts at fusion of ankles that exhibit aseptic loosening of components have been met with a high rate of success, whereas such attempts for septic loosening have been fraught with difficulties.[60] Other complications have been described, including skin healing problems, in as many as 45 percent of patients.

In spite of these relatively grim early results, there may be a future for total ankle arthroplasty. The key elements of a successful outcome will include (1) the selection of appropriate patients, (2) the development of a surgical approach that affords excellent visualization of the entire talocrural joint, and (3) the use of a nonconstrained total ankle prosthesis that will allow both ankle and subtalar joint plane motions. For the rheumatoid patient with multiple joint problems, less than total pain relief combined with even a small increase in motion may enable these disabled patients to cope better with their lives.[61] With improvements in design and operative technique, total ankle replacement may become common in the care of the rheumatoid ankle.

Hindfoot

The surgical treatment of the hindfoot is predicated on an understanding of the cause of the disability and tailoring the surgical procedure specifically. Isolated posterior tibial tendon tenosynovitis can be treated with tenosynovectomy. Partial tears of this tendon can be handled with débridement,

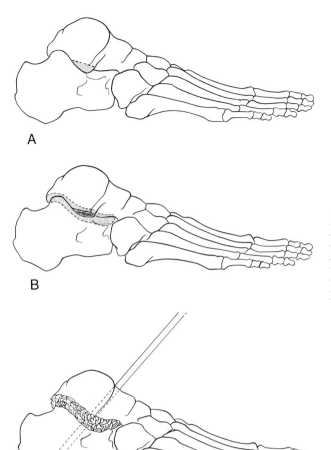

Figure 110–11. Technique for subtalar arthrodesis. *A,* After making a short oblique incision over the sinus tarsi, the anterior process of the talus is removed. This allows a good view of the sinus tarsi and posterior facet region. *B,* The cortical and articular surfaces in the subtalar region are resected. *C,* Corticocancellous chips from the iliac crest are packed into the subtalar region and a Steinmann pin is used to temporarily maintain the talocalcaneal relationship.

and complete tears without secondary deformity may be amenable to tendon transfers.

Arthrodesis

If joint involvement is the cause of pain or deformity, an arthrodesis may be worthwhile. Only the affected joints should be fused. Arthrodesis in the hindfoot region has been shown to accelerate degenerative changes in contiguous articulations.[17]

For deformity at the subtalar level without involvement of the tarsal joints, a subtalar arthrodesis with iliac crest bone graft reliably gives excellent results (Figs. 110–11 and 110–12).[62] For isolated, painful talonavicular arthritis without deformity, a selective arthrodesis of this joint is the treatment of choice. Elbar, Thomas, and colleagues[63] reported that 85 percent of 35 talonavicular fusions provided complete pain relief and improved walking ability.

Triple arthrodesis should be reserved for indi-

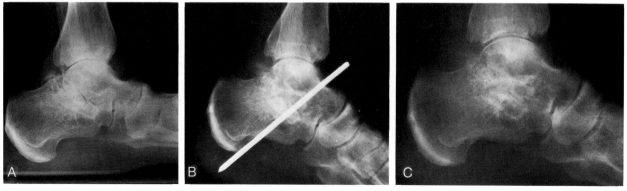

Figure 110–12. Lateral radiographs of a patient with RA who initially presented with "ankle" pain. *A,* The preoperative radiograph demonstrated sclerosis, cyst formation, and subluxation of the subtalar joint. *B,* The patient underwent an isolated subtalar arthrodesis. At 6 weeks postoperatively the radiograph demonstrated good early consolidation of the arthrodesis site. The Steinmann pin was removed. *C,* At final follow-up the radiograph demonstrated a solid talocalcaneal fusion. This patient's "ankle" pain had disappeared.

viduals who have symptoms related to all three hindfoot joints. For patients without deformity, the dowel technique may be appropriate. Compared with a formal triple arthrodesis with wedge osteotomies, the dowel technique has several advantages. It does not shorten the foot, it is less traumatic, and generally patients experience less morbidity at both the donor and the recipient graft sites.[19] With significant deformity, however, the dowel technique cannot be used. In this case, the moldable bone graft technique is an option. For fixation, Steinmann pins are appropriate because they are easy to insert and remove.

For a "triple" arthrodesis of the talocalcaneal, talonavicular, and calcaneocuboid joints, the sequence of alignment is important. First the hindfoot is placed in approximately 5 to 7 degrees of valgus, and a Steinmann pin is inserted across the neck of the talus into the calcaneus, using the interval between the extensor hallucis longus and the tibialis anterior. At this point, the hindfoot varus-valgus is fixed. Next, the forefoot is aligned so that the medial border of the foot is straight or at least matches the uninvolved foot. The Steinmann pin is placed across the cuboid into the calcaneus to stabilize forefoot abduction-adduction. Finally, rotation of the forefoot is checked, placing the metatarsal heads perpendicular to the axis of the tibia to allow all five heads to share weight during walking. A Steinmann pin is then inserted across the navicula into the talus. Staples may be used for temporary fixation, but they tend to cause diastasis and result in nonunion.[64] In a series of 292 rheumatoid feet treated with triple arthrodesis using staple fixation, 9 percent developed nonunion. The overall results, however, were considered good in 85 percent of patients.[17]

Midfoot

Compared with the hindfoot and the forefoot, the rheumatoid midfoot requires surgical intervention less often. The involved joints must be precisely identified. Plain radiographs are usually sufficient, but occasionally tomograms or a technetium bone scan is necessary to pinpoint the involved areas.

Arthrodesis again is the procedure of choice for painful midfoot arthritis. The operative technique depends on the size of the joints involved, the quality of bone, and the amount of deformity. For small joints, especially in the region of the tarsometatarsal junction, without the presence of significant deformity, a dowel-type arthrodesis may be suitable. This involves the use of a trephine to remove bone and cartilage in the region of the involved joints and the replacement of the same-sized cylinder of bone taken from the ipsilateral anterior iliac crest. For larger tarsal joints, greater areas of involvement, or significant deformity, a more involved technique is necessary. Enough bone is removed from the diseased joints to create a trough (Fig. 110–13A). This trough is then filled with a matched corticocancellous graft

taken from the anterior iliac crest (see Fig. 110–13B). These arthrodeses are then internally stabilized using either Steinmann pins or compression screw fixation (Figs. 110–13C and 110–14).

Forefoot

Surgery of the rheumatoid forefoot is done for pain. Deformity or problems with fashionable shoewear in the absence of pain are, in general, not sufficient reasons for operative treatment. It is important for patients to understand these issues prior to undergoing surgical treatment.

A wide range of surgical procedures have been proposed for the treatment of the rheumatoid forefoot. These vary from simple synovectomy[65] to the cosmetically unpopular "Pobble procedure,"[66] in which all the toes are amputated. The most well established and successful approaches involve either an arthrodesis[64, 67, 68] or a Keller procedure[2, 70] for the first metatarsophalangeal joint and partial[71–73] or complete[69, 73, 74] resection arthroplasties of the lesser metatarsophalangeal joints. A dizzying array of different combinations of skin incisions have been used. These have included both longitudinal[70] and transverse[74] dorsal approaches, proximal[71] and distal[72] transverse plantar approaches,[71, 72] and excisions of transverse ellipses of plantar skin to presumably relocate the fat pads under the remaining distal metatarsals.[73]

Surgical treatment, therefore, involves decision making about the type of incision, great toe procedure, and lesser toe operative care. In terms of the type of incision, the authors generally prefer a relatively safe and extensile approach through three longitudinal dorsal incisions. One is placed dorsomedially over the first metatarsophalangeal joint, and the other two are Y-shaped incisions in the second and fourth webspaces (Fig. 110–15). This allows the potential for a variable length of webbing in these interspaces. For patients with mild deformities the authors do a minimal subtotal webbing between toes 2 and 3 and 4 and 5. For patients with greater deformity requiring more extensive bony resection, the webbings are extended farther out to control the ultimate positions of the toes (Fig. 110–16).

Our procedure of choice for the first metatarsophalangeal joint is an arthrodesis (Fig. 110–17). The ideal patient is young and has severe deformity. Males are particularly appropriate for fusion because their shoe heel height is constant. Arthrodesis tends to preserve the push-off function of the great toe, prevent recurrent hallux valgus, and help prevent further lateral deviation of the lesser toes.[75] In comparison with the Keller procedure, it has been shown to result in greater weight-bearing on the great toe and thereby significantly to reduce the incidence of lesser toe metatarsalgia.[76] It does require, however, a 1- to 2-month period of nonweight-bearing cast immobilization. This can be a significant hindrance

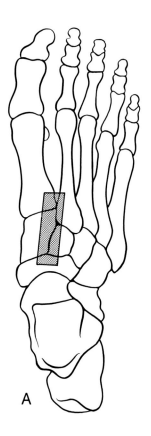

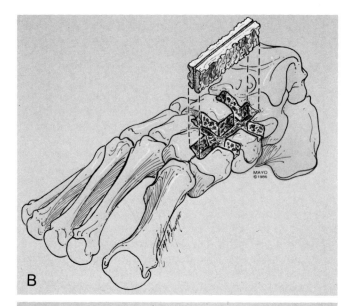

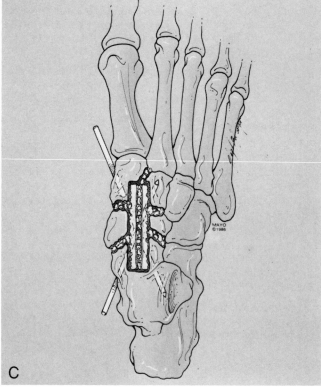

Figure 110–13. Diagrammatic representation of the arthrodesis technique for single large or multiple small midtarsal joints. *A*, A trough is cut through the involved region. Articular cartilage is denuded from contiguous joints. *B*, The autologous corticocancellous strips are used to maintain structural rigidity. The cortices are placed back to back, and the remaining regions packed with multiple cancellous bone chips. *C*, The arthrodesis site is then stabilized with Steinmann pins or cancellous bone screws.

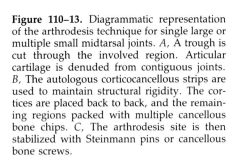

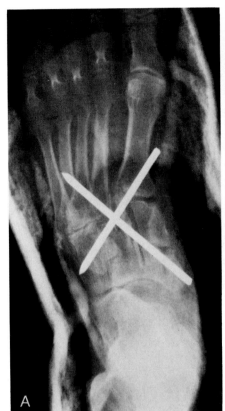
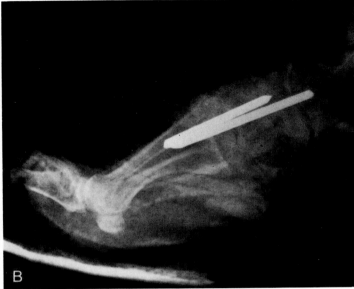

Figure 110–14. Anteroposterior *(A)* and lateral *(B)* radiographs of a patient with a navicula-to-metatarsal one-two arthrodesis. The foot is immobilized and kept nonweight-bearing for a period of 6 to 8 weeks. After the pins are removed, weight-bearing is allowed in the cast until a solid radiographic fusion is evident.

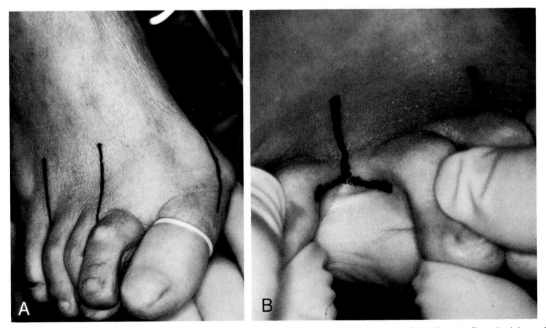

Figure 110–15. *A,* In rheumatoid disease, forefoot reconstruction can be carried out through three longitudinal incisions. These are extensile and neurovascularly "safe." *B,* The incisions in the second and fourth webspaces are extended to perform the webbings.

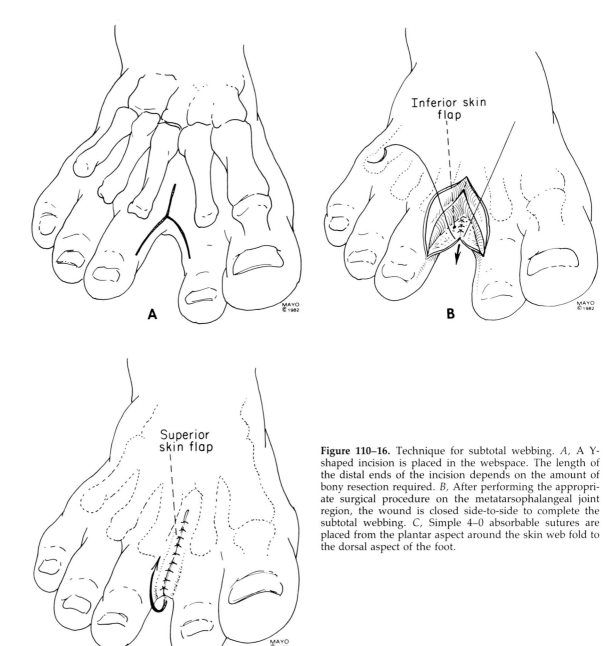

Figure 110–16. Technique for subtotal webbing. *A,* A Y-shaped incision is placed in the webspace. The length of the distal ends of the incision depends on the amount of bony resection required. *B,* After performing the appropriate surgical procedure on the metatarsophalangeal joint region, the wound is closed side-to-side to complete the subtotal webbing. *C,* Simple 4–0 absorbable sutures are placed from the plantar aspect around the skin web fold to the dorsal aspect of the foot.

for a severely handicapped rheumatoid patient. The authors ordinarily reserve a first metatarsophalangeal resection arthroplasty for elderly patients with fragile connective or vascular tissues and a need for immediate weight-bearing.

Surgical treatment of the lesser toes depends on the degree of deformity present. The essential requirement of an effective forefoot operation is adequate bony resection (Fig. 110–18). Patients with mild deformities of the lesser toes and no metatarsal head pain can be treated nonoperatively or with resection of the bases of proximal phalanges 2, 3, and 4 and webbing of toes 2 to 3 and 4 to 5, leaving the metatarsal heads intact. If the toe deformities are mild, but metatarsalgia is a prominent feature, then the authors prefer to resect the lesser metatarsal heads to eliminate the areas of abnormally high pressure concentration and leave the toes intact. If the foot deformity is moderate and the patient has metatarsalgia in addition to lesser toe hammering, the authors resect the lesser metatarsal heads and the bases of proximal phalanges 2, 3, and 4. The authors typically leave the base of the fifth proximal phalanx untouched to provide some lateral stability to the lesser toes. Again webbing of toes 2 to 3 and 4 to 5 is done to preserve postoperative toe stability. If the lesser toe deformities are more severe, greater bony excision may be required. In this situation, in

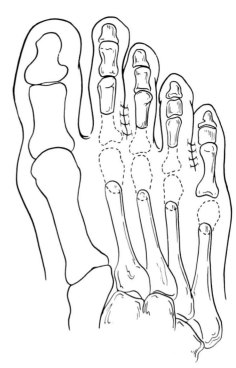

Figure 110–18. Adequate bony resection is the cornerstone of the operative treatment of the lesser toes in RA. For patients with metatarsalgia and lesser toe hammering the authors resect the lesser metatarsal heads and the bases of proximal phalanges 2, 3, and 4. The base of the fifth toe is left untouched to provide lateral stability to the others. Subtotal webbing of toes 2 and 3 as well as 4 and 5 is done to preserve toe stability.

addition to resecting the lesser metatarsal heads, the authors remove the entire proximal phalanges of the second, third, and fourth toes as well as the proximal half of the fifth toe proximal phalanx. No Kirschner wires are inserted in the toes in a longitudinal manner, since the webbing will provide adequate toe stability.

CONCLUSION

The foot is often the initial presenting site of rheumatoid disease and eventually becomes involved in virtually all patients with long-standing disease. The appropriate treatment must be tailored to the individual patient. Consideration should be given to many factors, including the stage of disease, degree of involvement, status of the skin and vascular structures, drug dependency, and the functional goal for the patient. The combined efforts of medical physicians, orthopedic surgeons, and adjunctive medical personnel are essential for providing optimal care.

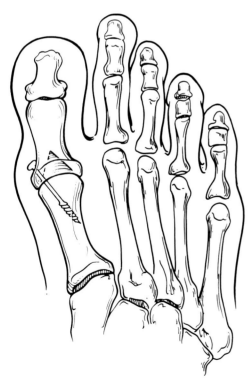

Figure 110–17. Arthrodesis is the procedure of choice for the painful rheumatoid bunion. It tends to preserve the function of the great toe, prevent recurrent hallux valgus and lateral deviation of the lesser toes, and is associated with less transfer metatarsalgia than are resection arthroplasties. The cup-and-cone technique offers the advantage of reducing stress on the interphalangeal joint by shortening the toe. Fixation with a single 4–0 cancellous screw is usually adequate.

References

1. Sarrafian, S. K.: Anatomy of the Foot and Ankle: Descriptive, Topographic, Functional. Philadelphia, J. B. Lippincott, 1983.
2. Vainio, K.: The rheumatoid foot. A clinical study with pathological and roentgenological comments. Ann. Chir. Gynaecol. 45(Suppl. 1):1, 1956.
3. O'Sullivan, T. B., and Cathcart, E. S.: The prevalence of rheumatoid arthritis. Follow-up evaluation of the effect of criteria on rates in Sudbury, Massachusetts. Ann. Intern. Med. 76:573, 1972.

4. Short, C. L., Bauer, W., and Reynolds, W. E.: Rheumatoid Arthritis. Cambridge, Harvard University Press, 1957.
5. Dixon, A. S. J.: The physician's foot. J. R. Soc. Med. 74:101, 1981.
6. Calabro, J. J.: A clinical evaluation of the diagnostic features of the feet in rheumatoid arthritis. Arthritis Rheum. 5:19, 1962.
7. Minaker, K., and Little, H.: Painful feet in rheumatoid arthritis. Can. Med. Assoc. J. 109:724, 1973.
8. Thould, A. K., and Simon, G.: Assessment of radiological changes in the hands and feet in rheumatoid arthritis: their correlation with progression. Ann. Rheum. Dis. 25:220, 1966.
9. Vidigal, E. G., Jacoby, R. K., Dixon, A. S. J., Ratiff, A. H., and Kirkup, J.: The foot in chronic rheumatoid arthritis. Ann. Rheum. Dis. 34:292, 1975.
10. Grabois, M., Puentes, J., and Lidsky, M.: Tarsal tunnel syndrome in rheumatoid arthritis. Arch. Phys. Med. Rehabil. 62:401, 1981.
11. McGuigan, L., Burke, D., and Fleming, A.: Tarsal tunnel syndrome and peripheral neuropathy in rheumatoid arthritis. Ann. Rheum. Dis. 42:128, 1983.
12. Kellgren, J. H., and Ball, J.: Tendon lesions in rheumatoid arthritis, a clinico-pathological study. Ann. Rheum. Dis. 9:48, 1950.
13. Vidigal, E. C.: Forefoot in chronic rheumatoid arthritis. Orthop. Rev. 7:43, 1978.
14. Tillmann, K.: The Rheumatoid Foot: Diagnosis, Pathomechanics and Treatment. Stuttgart, George Thieme Publishers, 1979.
15. Kirkup, J. R., Vidigal, E., and Jacoby, R. K.: The hallux and rheumatoid arthritis. Acta Orthop. Scand. 48:527, 1977.
16. Spiegel, T. M., and Spiegel, J. S.: Rheumatoid arthritis in the foot and ankle—diagnosis, pathology, and treatment. Foot Ankle 112:1105, 1977.
17. Vahvanen, V. A. J.: Rheumatoid arthritis in the pantalar joints: a follow-up study of 292 adult feet. Acta Orthop. Scand. Suppl. 107:1, 1967.
18. Downey, D. J., Simkin, P. A., Mack, L. A., Richardson, M. L., Kilcoyne, R. F., and Hansen, S.: Tibialis posterior tendon rupture: a cause of rheumatoid flat foot. Arthritis Rheum. 31:441, 1988.
19. Chana, G. S., Andrew, T. A., and Cotterill, C. P.: A simple method of arthrodesis of the first metatarsophalangeal joint. J. Bone Joint Surg. 66B:703, 1984.
20. Coughlin, M. J.: The rheumatoid foot: pathophysiology and treatment of arthritic manifestations. Postgrad. Med. 75:207, 1984.
21. Mann, R. A., and Coughlin, M. J.: The rheumatoid foot: review of literature and method of treatment. Orthop. Rev. 8:105, 1979.
22. Wilde, A. H.: Surgery of the foot in rheumatoid arthritis. Clev. Clin. Q. 36:85, 1969.
23. Dixon, A. S. J.: The rheumatoid foot. In Hill, A. G. S. (ed.): Modern Trends in Rheumatology, Part 2. New York, Appleton-Century-Crofts, 1971, p. 158.
24. Michotte, L.: Le pied rond rheumatismal. Rev. Rheum. 6:223, 1939.
25. Berens, D. L., and Lin, R. K.: Roentgen Diagnosis of Rheumatoid Arthritis. Springfield, IL, Charles C Thomas, 1969.
26. Bouysset, M., Bonvoisin, B., Lejeune, E., and Bouvier, M.: Flattening of the rheumatoid foot in tarsal arthritis on x-ray. Scand. J. Rheumatol. 16:127, 1987.
27. Kirkup, J. R.: Ankle and tarsal joints in rheumatoid arthritis. Scand. J. Rheumatol. 3:50, 1974.
28. Seltzer, S. E., Weissman, B. N., Braunstein, E. M., Adams, D. F., and Thomas, W. H.: Computed tomography of the hindfoot. J. Comput. Assist. Tomogr. 8:488, 1984.
29. Fletcher, D. E., and Rowley, K. A.: The radiological features of rheumatoid arthritis. Br. J. Radiol. 25:282, 1952.
30. Halla, J. T., Fallahi, S., and Hardin, J. G.: Small joint involvement: a systemic roentgenographic study in rheumatoid arthritis. Ann. Rheum. Dis. 45:327, 1986.
31. Thompson, C. T.: Surgical treatment of disorders of the fore part of the foot. J. Bone Joint Surg. 46A:117, 1964.
32. Marshall, R. N., Meyers, D. B., and Palmer, D. G.: Disturbance of gait due to rheumatoid disease. J. Rheumatol. 7:617, 1980.
33. Dixon, A. S. J.: The anterior tarsus and forefoot. Baillieres Clin. Rheumatol. 1:261, 1987.
34. Betts, R. P., Stockley, I., Getty, C. J. M., Rowley, D. I., Duckworth, T., and Franks, C. I.: Foot pressure studies in the assessment of forefoot arthroplasty in the rheumatoid foot. Foot Ankle 8:315, 1988.
35. Minns, R. J., and Crakford, A. D.: Pressure under the forefoot in rheumatoid arthritis. Clin. Orthop. 187:235, 1984.
36. Sharma, M., Dhamendran, M., Hutlon, W. B., and Corbett, M.: Changes in load bearing in the rheumatoid foot. Ann. Rheum. Dis. 38:549, 1979.
37. Simkin, A.: The dynamic vertical force distribution during level walking under normal and rheumatic feet. Rheum. Rehabil. 20:88, 1981.
38. Chand, K.: Rheumatoid arthritis of the foot. Int. Surg. 58:12, 1973.
39. Lindahl, O., and Nilsson, H.: Plantar protrusion of the metatarsal heads: conservative treatment by a new principle. Acta Orthop. Scand. 45:473, 1974.
40. Miller, W. E.: The anterior heel for metatarsalgia in the adult foot. Clin. Orthop. Mar.–Apr. (123):55, 1977.
41. Craxford, A. D., Stevens, J., and Park, C.: Management of the deformed rheumatoid forefoot: A comparison of conservative and surgical methods. Clin. Orthop. 166:121, 1982.
42. Susman, M. H., and Clayton, M. L.: Surgery of the rheumatoid foot. Ann. Acad. Med. Singapore 12:225, 1983.
43. Unger, A. S., Inglis, A. E., Mow, C. S., and Figgie, H. E.: Total ankle arthroplasty in rheumatoid arthritis: a long-term follow-up study. Foot Ankle 8:173, 1988.
44. Rasker, J. J., and Cosh, J. A.: Radiological study of cervical spine and hand in patients with rheumatoid arthritis of 15 years' duration: an assessment of the effects of corticosteroid treatment. Ann. Rheum. Dis. 37:529, 1978.
45. Tillmann, K.: Surgical treatment of the foot in rheumatoid arthritis. Reconstr. Surg. Traumatol. 18:195, 1981.
46. Mohing, W., Kohler, G., and Coldewey, J.: Synovectomy of the ankle joint. Int. Orthop. 6:117, 1982.
47. Vahvanen, V.: Synovectomy of the talocrural joint in rheumatoid arthritis. Ann. Chir. Gynaecol. Fenn. 57:576, 1968.
48. Mazur, J. N., Schwartz, E., and Simon, S. R.: Ankle arthrodesis: long-term follow-up with gait analysis. J. Bone Joint Surg. 61A:964, 1979.
49. Smith, E. J., and Wood, P. L. R.: Ankle arthrodesis in the rheumatoid patient. Foot Ankle 10:252, 1990.
50. Sowa, D. T., and Krackow, K. A.: Ankle fusion: a new technique of internal fixation using a compression blade plate. Foot Ankle 9:232, 1989.
51. Dennis, D. A., Clayton, M. L., Wong, D. A., Mack, R. P., and Susman, M. H.: Internal fixation compression arthrodesis of the ankle. Clin. Orthop. 253:212, 1990.
52. Johnson, E. W., Jr., and Boseker, E. H.: Arthrodesis of the ankle. Arch. Surg. 97:766, 1968.
53. Stauffer, R. N.: Total ankle replacement. Arch. Surg. 112:1105, 1977.
54. Herberts, P., Goldie, I. F., Korner, L., Larsson, V., Lindborg, G., and Zachusson, B. E.: Endoprosthetic arthroplasty of the ankle joint. Acta Orthop. Scand. 53:687, 1982.
55. Stauffer, R. N., and Segal, N. M.: Total ankle arthroplasty: four years' experience. Clin. Orthop. 160:217, 1981.
56. Bolton-Maggs, B. G., Sudlow, R. A., and Freeman, M. A. R.: Total ankle arthroplasty. J. Bone Joint Surg. 67B:785, 1985.
57. Lachiewicz, P. F., Inglis, A. E., and Ranawat, C. S.: Total ankle replacement in rheumatoid arthritis. J. Bone Joint Surg. 66:340, 1984.
58. Demottaz, J. D., Mazur, J. M., Thomas, W. H., Sledge, C. B., and Simon, S. R.: Clinical study of total ankle replacement with gait analysis: a preliminary report. J. Bone Joint Surg. 61A:976, 1979.
59. Kaukonen, J. P., and Raunio, P.: Total ankle replacement in rheumatoid arthritis: a preliminary review of 28 arthroplasties in 24 patients. Ann. Chir. Gynaecol. 72:196, 1983.
60. Groth, H. E., and Fitch, H. F.: Salvage procedures for complications of total ankle arthroplasty. Clin. Orthop. 224:245, 1987.
61. Hamblen, D. L.: Can the ankle joint be replaced? J. Bone Joint Surg. 67B:689, 1985.
62. Russotti, G. M., Cass, J. R., and Johnson, K. A.: Isolated talocalcaneal arthrodesis: a technique using moldable bone graft. J. Bone Joint Surg. 70A:1472, 1988.
63. Elbar, J. E., Thomas, W. H., Weinfeld, M. S., and Potter, I. A.: Talonavicular arthrodesis for rheumatoid arthritis of the hindfoot. Orthop. Clin. North Am. 7:821, 1976.
64. Lipscomb, P. R.: Surgery of the rheumatoid foot: preferable procedures. Rev. Chir. Orthop. 67:375, 1981.
65. Raunio, P., and Laine, H.: Synovectomy of the metatarsophalangeal joints in rheumatoid arthritis. Acta Rheumatol. Scand. 16:12, 1970.
66. Flint, M., and Sweetnam, R.: Amputation of all toes. J. Bone Joint Surg. 42B:90, 1960.
67. Beauchamp, T. K., Rudge, S. R., Worthington, B. S., and Nelson, J.: Fusion of the first metatarsophalangeal joint in forefoot arthroplasty. Clin. Orthop. 190:249, 1984.
68. Cracchiolo, A.: Foot abnormalities in rheumatoid arthritis. Instr. Course Lect. 33:386, 1984.
69. Lipscomb, P. R.: Arthrodesis of the first metatarsophalangeal joint for severe bunions and hallux rigidus. Clin. Orthop. 142:48, 1979.
70. Larmon, W. A.: Surgical treatment of deformities of rheumatoid arthritis of the forefoot and toes. Q. Bull. Northwest. Univ. Med. School 25:39, 1951.
71. Hoffman, P.: An operation for severe grades of contracted or clawed toes. Am. J. Orthop. Surg. 9:441, 1912.
72. Kates, A., Kessel, L., and Kay, A.: Arthroplasty of the forefoot. J. Bone Joint Surg. 49B:552, 1967.
73. Fowler, A. W.: A method of forefoot reconstruction. J. Bone Joint Surg. 41B:507, 1959.
74. Clayton, M. L.: Surgery of the forefoot in rheumatoid arthritis. Clin. Orthop. 16:136, 1960.
75. Vahvanen, V., Piirainen, H., and Kettunen, P.: Resection arthroplasty of the metatarsophalangeal joints in rheumatoid arthritis: a follow-up study of 100 patients. Scand. J. Rheumatol. 9:257, 1980.
76. Henry, A. P. J., Waugh, W., and Wood, H.: The use of footprints in assessing the results of operations for hallux valgus: a comparison of Keller's operation and arthrodesis. J. Bone Joint Surg. 57B:478, 1975.

Chapter 111

Richard D. Scott
Clement B. Sledge

Surgical Management of Juvenile Rheumatoid Arthritis

INTRODUCTION

The deformity and functional loss produced by juvenile rheumatoid arthritis (JRA) have a devastating effect on the physical and emotional development of the child. The physical handicap often evokes cruel comments from peers, condescension from adults, and overprotection from parents. The efforts of physicians, nurses, and therapists should be a coordinated attempt to normalize function and thereby facilitate emotional development. In many instances, anti-inflammatory treatment (see Chapter 70) combined with physical therapy and splinting (see Chapter 102) will maintain function and prevent deformity. Occasionally contractures develop that require surgical release, or chronic synovitis threatens the joint and requires synovectomy. Rarely, joint destruction is so severe that replacement surgery is necessary, bearing in mind the disastrous effect of complications (such as sepsis) and lack of long-term assessments of such procedures. In spite of these concerns, however, most patients (and their parents) will opt for surgery that restores near-normal function during the important formative years when the pressure of education, spouse-seeking, and career demand maximal effort.

The surgery of rheumatoid arthritis (RA) in children presents some problems unique from those encountered in the adult patient. In the adult patient with RA, pain is usually the primary indication for surgery. The child often denies pain and accepts contracture, so that restoration of function is the primary goal. The adult patient has usually been "normal" for much of her or his life, and the surgery attempts to return the patient toward this normal state. The young child with severe RA has never been normal and often suffers from retarded psychologic and social development. Surgery attempts to bring him or her toward a normal state, which is totally unfamiliar. There are frequent significant adjustment problems at home and at school. The extreme importance of a continuous vigorous physical therapy program is not appreciated by the child. Poor patient cooperation can lead to stiffness and contracture that require surgical therapy, and later that same lack of cooperation can compromise the potential benefits gained from surgery. The child with RA has small bones that need special prostheses for joint replacement. Finally, the effect *of* growth and the effect *on* growth must be carefully considered with any surgical procedure in the child.

The surgical procedures most frequently required in the patient with JRA include synovectomy, epiphysiodesis for leg length discrepancy, and arthroplasty of the hip and knee. Isolated soft tissue release for severe disabling contracture about the hip, knee, or ankle is occasionally indicated if there is no significant intra-articular disease and the nonsurgical methods have failed (physical therapy, casting, traction). Arthrodesis is rarely indicated in JRA except in the hand (see Chapter 104) and foot (see Chapter 110) when there is advanced disease and splinting fails to relieve symptoms. Osteotomy is sometimes necessary to correct significant angular or torsional deformities about the hip and knee.

SYNOVECTOMY

The indications for synovectomy in the child are similar to those in the adult: persistent synovitis that has not responded to medical management in a joint with adequate articular cartilage. In the adult, 6 months is an acceptable period of time to wait for a medically induced or spontaneous remission. In the child, because spontaneous remissions are commoner, some rheumatologists recommend waiting 18 months as long as the joint space is well preserved.[1] On the other hand, if joint destruction and loss of motion are occurring rapidly in the presence of active disease, synovectomy may offer the only chance to prevent complete joint destruction and permanent contracture. In reported series, the joints that most frequently required synovectomy were the wrists and metacarpophalangeal (MCP) joints in the upper extremity and the knee in the lower extremity.[1-4] The tendency today is to avoid synovectomy in the wrists and to treat the patients with vigorous physical therapy and appropriate splinting.[5] Even if the wrist stiffens, it will be quite functional if it has been held in proper position. Many pediatricians may carry the false impression that upper extremity surgery is rarely necessary in the patient with JRA. This is because most of these patients do not require the surgery until they are adults. In a series of 184 patients with JRA whose average onset of disease was at 8 years, surgery was performed an average of 12 years later.[6] The commonest procedures were wrist fusion, digital fusions, and MCP arthroplasties. Although wrist fusion was surgically necessary in some patients, the incidence of spontaneous fusion was 11 percent for the entire group, whose average age was 19 years at follow-up. The incidence of severe wrist involvement increased dramatically as the patients grew older (Fig. 111–1). This tendency stresses the importance of prolonged, adequate splinting to maintain functional position of the wrist as spontaneous fusion occurs.

The knee is the joint most likely to require synovectomy in the child. This is probably because it is a weight-bearing joint where contracture causes marked dysfunction. The best results of synovectomy are obtained in the older child (over 7 years) with chronic monarticular or oligoarticular disease and a good joint space.[2, 4] In the younger child, poor patient cooperation will hamper the results, and the disease tends to be more malignant. Synovectomy of the hip in JRA has not been reported frequently, and the results do not appear to be encouraging.[7]

to determine accurately the need and timing of surgery. The proximal femoral epiphysis contributes approximately 3 mm of growth per year to the lower extremity. The distal femoral epiphysis, the proximal tibial epiphysis, and the distal tibial epiphysis contribute 12 mm, 9 mm, and 6 mm, respectively, each year.[8] Put another way, there are 3 mm of growth per year at the hip joint, 21 mm at the knee joint, and 6 mm at the ankle joint. Unilateral disease at the knee, therefore, is most likely to produce leg length discrepancy. The greatest reported leg length discrepancy resulting from JRA is 5.7 cm.[9] The synovitis appears to stimulate growth in the younger child, but growth retardation is more often seen in the older child. Children with onset of disease before age 5 often have the affected leg grow longer. Factors such as the chronicity of the synovitis, the weight-bearing status of the limb, and the effect of surgery all make the overall results on growth difficult to predict. In the authors' experience, only 15 percent of the patients with early detected leg length discrepancies fail to stabilize or correct their discrepancy and require surgery.[10]

The growth plate can be surgically arrested by a number of methods. Some techniques produce immediate and permanent growth arrest.[11] Stapling across the plate produces delayed arrest, which is reversible, if necessary, within several years. If there is an accompanying angular deformity to the knee on the longer side, it may be treated by asymmetric stapling of the epiphysis.[12]

EPIPHYSIODESIS

Leg length inequality can develop in JRA and may require epiphyseal arrest of the lower extremity for correction. The effects of the disease on growth, however, are unpredictable, and skeletal measurements at 6- to 12-month intervals are often necessary

ARTHROPLASTY OF THE HIP AND KNEE

Total joint replacement arthroplasty is possible for joints with permanent structural damage and significant pain or deformity. Metal-to-plastic total joint prostheses are available for use in the hip and knee as well as the shoulder, elbow, and ankle. Prosthetic joint replacement in young patients remains a controversial issue centering on questions of prosthetic fixation to bone, wear characteristics, fatigue properties of materials, and the effects of skeletal growth. The literature contains relatively little work detailing the experience of total joint arthroplasty in young patients. Some of these series contain young people with many different diagnoses. JRA is a unique disease, and the results of arthroplasty in this group must be considered separately.[13–21]

Between 1971 and 1991, 122 patients with JRA underwent a total of 197 hip replacements, and 101 patients underwent 164 knee replacements at the Robert Breck Brigham Hospital or Brigham and Women's Hospital in Boston, Massachusetts.[17] The youngest patient undergoing hip replacement was 11 years old at the time of surgery, and the youngest patient undergoing knee replacement was 12 years of age.

Preoperative pain was usually not the primary indication for hip or knee replacement surgery. Func-

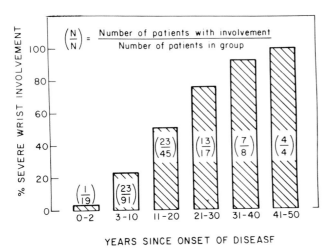

Figure 111–1. The incidence of severe wrist involvement in JRA increases dramatically as the patient grows older. (Courtesy of Dr. E. A. Nalebuff.)

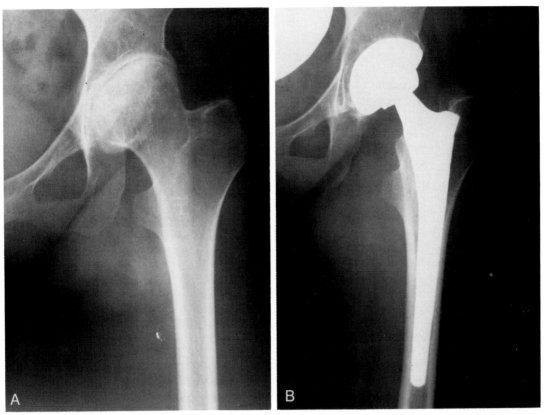

Figure 111–2. *A,* Preoperative radiograph of a patient with JRA requiring total hip replacement. *B,* The same patient following surgery. Cementless ingrowth components have been used on both acetabular and femoral slides.

tional impairment and deformity were the chief indications in the majority of cases. Skeletal immaturity was considered only a relative contraindication to surgery. Clearly, there are advantages to waiting until the epiphyses are closed, the bones are larger, and the patient is older and more able to cooperate fully with the rehabilitation program. Once the patient becomes nonambulatory or fixed contractures occur, however, further delay may worsen the chance for successful restoration of the involved joint.

Alternative surgical treatment was always considered in these patients prior to joint replacement. Osteotomy, soft tissue release, synovectomy, traction, serial cast application, and vigorous physical therapy will usually yield only transient improvement in the patient with advanced joint destruction. Cup arthroplasty is not considered in a JRA patient because the results in this group are usually poor and inconstant. In the knee, McKeever metallic hemiarthroplasty is occasionally performed in a select group of JRA patients showing complete loss of joint space with good stability, minimal angular deformity, flexion of at least 80 degrees, and flexion contracture less than 15 degrees. Hip or knee fusion is not normally considered a primary procedure in JRA because it will not sufficiently relieve functional disability in the patient with multiple joint involvement.

When both total hip and knee replacements were

indicated in the same patient, the hip arthroplasty was performed first for several reasons.[22, 23] Hip replacement is usually much less painful than knee replacement, thereby gaining the confidence and cooperation of the patient to proceed with further surgery. It is possible to rehabilitate the hip joint in the presence of a stiff contracted knee joint but difficult to rehabilitate the knee in the presence of a painful contracted ipsilateral hip. Manipulation and casting to gain extension in the contracted knee can be performed during the anesthetic administered for hip replacement. By operating on the hip prior to the knee, any pain that had been referred from the ipsilateral hip could be resolved. Finally it seems beneficial to resolve the tensioning of muscles that cross both the hip and knee joint prior to any knee surgery by operating first on the hip.

Careful preoperative planning is mandatory in these patients. Custom or special mini-sized prostheses were required in 50 percent of the hip arthroplasties (Fig. 111–2) and 40 percent of the knee arthroplasties (Fig. 111–3). During hip surgery, trochanteric osteotomy was necessary in approximately 40 percent of the patients in order to provide adequate exposure. This is in contrast to the use of trochanteric osteotomy in only 5 percent of patients with other diseases. In patients with ankylosing spondylitis and a fused hip, however, it might be advisable to avoid trochanteric osteotomy in order to

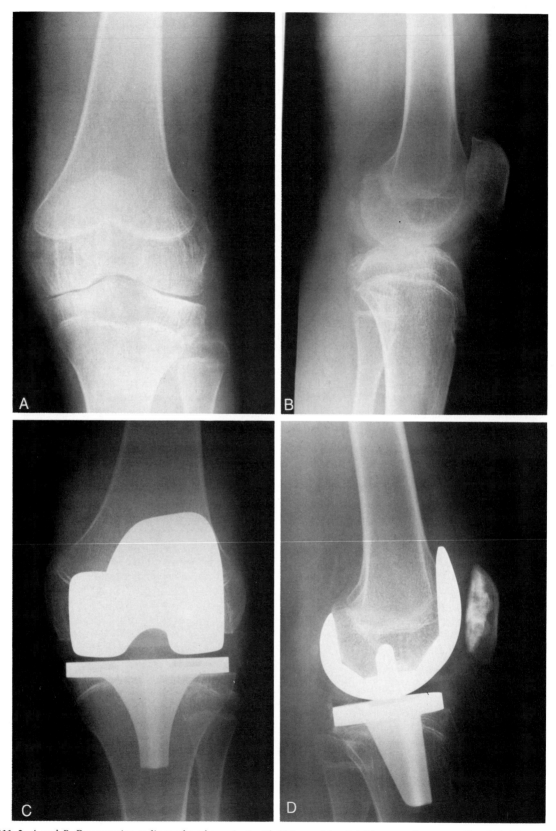

Figure 111–3. *A* and *B*, Preoperative radiographs of a patient with JRA requiring total knee replacement. *C* and *D*, The same patient following surgery utilizing cementless ingrowth components.

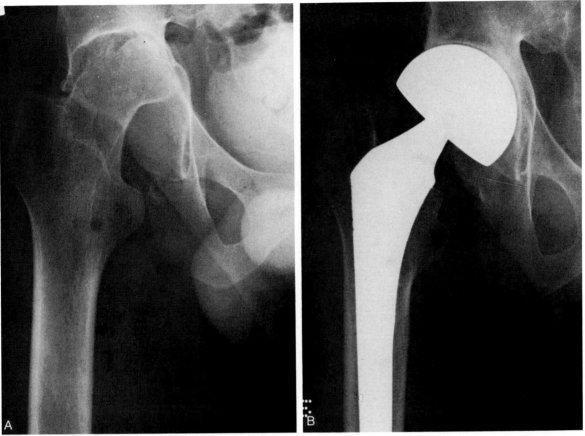

Figure 111–4. *A,* Preoperative radiograph of a patient with JRA showing marked protrusion with upward, inward migration of the femoral head. *B,* Postoperative radiograph taken 3 years following surgery. The acetabulum has been grafted, and the graft appears to have incorporated. The socket is in a more anatomic position. A bipolar socket has been used, and a new joint space has formed.

diminish the incidence of heterotopic bone.[17] In most JRA patients, complete capsulectomy will usually be necessary to relieve a flexion contracture and provide exposure. A psoas tenotomy was required in 16 percent of the authors' patients to help correct the flexion contracture. It must be remembered that with the release of contractures and improvement in range of motion comes the potential for increased morbidity in terms of sciatic or femoral nerve palsy. Transient incomplete nerve palsies were seen in 4 percent of patients, and permanent partial palsies were seen in an additional 4 percent.

Acetabular deficiency of two different types is frequently encountered in JRA. The first type is acetabular dysplasia resembling that seen in congenital dislocation of the hip (CDH). This is often combined with excessive femoral anteversion. To gain adequate acetabular coverage, it is advisable to augment the acetabulum with solid bone grafts as described for CDH,[22] rather than to improve coverage by deepening the socket. Slight deepening may be necessary, but preservation or restoration of bone should always be a high priority in young patients.

The second type of acetabular deficiency is protrusion from upward, inward migration of the femoral head. The amount of protrusion can be alarming

and can be rapidly progressive. Restoration of bone stock can be accomplished by various bone grafting techniques.[23] Bone grafting is preferable to techniques utilizing protrusion rings, acetabular mesh, or an eccentric polyethylene component. An attempt should be made to restore the center of rotation of the acetabular component to its true anatomic position (Fig. 111–4).

For the knee patients, the preoperative management of flexion deformity can reduce the magnitude of soft tissue release required at surgery.[18] The preoperative use of traction, physical therapy, and serial casting were valuable adjuncts to surgical management (Fig. 111–5).

The improvement in functional status of JRA patients undergoing total hip and knee replacement has been gratifying. Most patients were able to return to school and complete their education. All but 2 of the surviving 52 patients in the authors' early (1971–1981) series were limited or full community ambulators at long-term follow-up.[17] For the optimum result, a team approach involving the rheumatologist, surgeon, physical therapist, psychiatrist, social worker, and the patient's entire family is essential. Many children come from broken homes, magnifying their adjustment problems.[24]

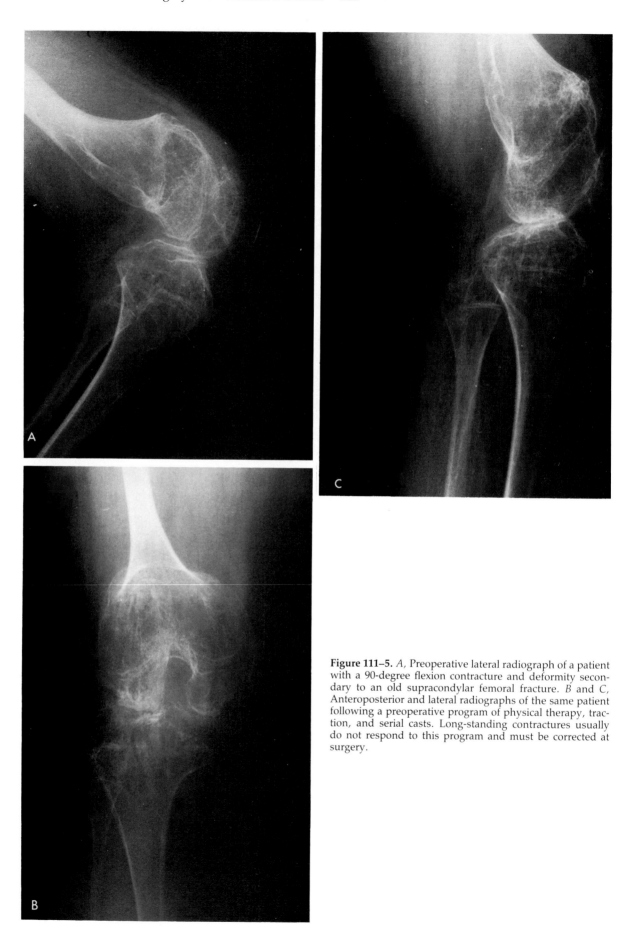

Figure 111–5. *A,* Preoperative lateral radiograph of a patient with a 90-degree flexion contracture and deformity secondary to an old supracondylar femoral fracture. *B* and *C,* Anteroposterior and lateral radiographs of the same patient following a preoperative program of physical therapy, traction, and serial casts. Long-standing contractures usually do not respond to this program and must be corrected at surgery.

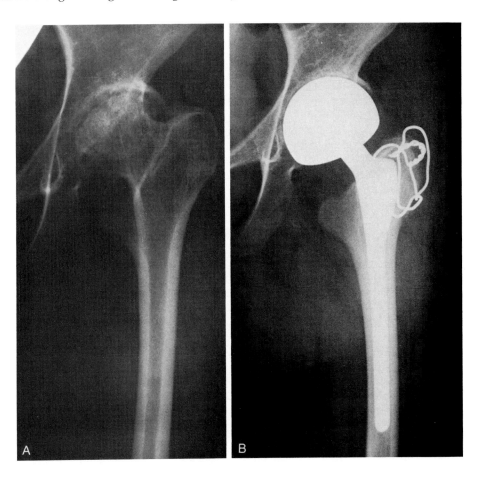

Figure 111–6. *A,* Preoperative radiograph of a patient with JRA with extremely small bones and bowing of the proximal femoral shaft. *B,* Postoperative radiograph showing the use of a bipolar arthroplasty and a custom-designed press-fit femoral component.

The long-term concern in these young people with prosthetic joint replacement is the prevention of failure by late metastatic infection, wear, or loosening. The patient, the family, medical physician, and dentist all must be educated about the need for rapid intervention with therapeutic use of antibiotics in the treatment of any infectious disease and the judicious use of prophylactic antibiotics when appropriate. Component wear has not been a problem in most series addressing this issue, and some long-term clinical studies suggest that 25 to 30 years might be expected before significant component wear would occur.[25] The small size of these patients and their relatively low activity level would make them even less likely to wear down their joint surface compared with the normal population. The most likely complication leading to failure is component loosening. This has been shown in virtually all series of total hip replacements in young people and has been responsible for all failures (7 percent) to date in the authors' hip replacements at the Robert Bingham Hospital. The occurrence of component loosening is particularly related to high activity level, heavy patients, and patients with monarticular disease. The JRA group may well be protected from this complication by their small size and the restraints imposed by their polyarticular disease.

Because of the potential long-term problems of cement failure with component loosening and oste-

olysis, there has been growing sentiment to try to avoid the use of cement in younger patients and rely on some form of biologic fixation. The role of cementless arthroplasty in JRA is not yet clear. Based on age criteria, the JRA patient is certainly a candidate for a cementless prosthesis. On the other hand, these patients often possess some characteristics that are contraindications to this type of procedure. They usually have significant osteopenia. The bone is more likely to fracture during insertion of a tight press-fit component. Because of the loss of diaphyseal cortical thickness, there is often a mismatch between the metaphyseal and diaphyseal sizing. Conventional components will often be too tight proximally while they are too loose distally. In small patients, the fit may be too tight both proximally and distally. The proximal torsional deformity causing excessive anteversion in the JRA patient is also a potential problem in achieving a press-fit with conventional components. This excessive anteversion has to be accepted, and joint instability may occur. The use of custom-made components can help with all of these problems by providing a miniature prosthesis, by improving the match between the metaphysis and diaphysis, and by allowing the proper anteversion to be built into the component (Fig. 111–6).

Bipolar arthroplasty is an attractive concept in JRA. The bipolar socket is the most conservative acetabular approach available. Minimal bone stock needs to be removed for its insertion. In fact, the socket can be augmented with bone graft behind the bipolar shell if this is indicated because of any preoperative protrusion. The 2- to 5-year results of 25 primary bipolar hip replacements in JRA have shown excellent pain relief.[26] The average flexion arc improved from 68 to 87 degrees, and rotation improved from 14 to 48 degrees. Twenty-four percent of the hips, however, displayed postoperative socket migration. This appeared to relate to the absence of acetabular subchondral bone, undersizing the socket, and increased patient activity. The long-term results of the bipolar socket will have to be judged against those achieved with fixed uncemented ingrowth sockets, and comparable follow-up is available for both groups of patients.

In the authors' knee replacement patients, there have been no revisions for loosening. In the knees there was a high rate (18 percent) of reoperation for patellofemoral pain when the patella had not been resurfaced at the time of original arthroplasty. The authors now perform patellar resurfacing during knee arthroplasty in all patients with JRA.

Cement appears to be much better tolerated in the knee than in the hip. There are still long-term concerns, however, related to the potential for ultimate cement failure, loosening, and osteolysis. Cementless prosthetic knee designs are available for investigational use. They may always be inappropriate in the JRA patient with severe osteopenia.

Total shoulder replacements, total elbow replacements, and total ankle replacements are occasionally necessary to relieve pain in the adult but are rarely necessary in the child. Experience, therefore, is limited, but appropriate prostheses are available for each joint and have been used with success.

Anesthesia poses potential complications in the child with JRA. Cervical spine and temporomandibular joint disease can make intubation difficult and hazardous. Regional anesthesia has become the anesthetic choice for JRA patients at the authors' institution. If regional anesthesia fails or is contraindicated, the fiberoptic laryngoscope is a useful tool to facilitate intubation in difficult cases. It is preferable to use the same anesthesiologist in each of the patient's successive procedures. Both the physician and the patient benefit from familiarity with each another. Spinal or epidural anesthesia is used for lower extremity procedures, and regional block with intravenous lidocaine for upper extremity operations.

References

1. Eyring, E. J., Longert, A., and Bass, J. C.: Synovectomy in juvenile rheumatoid arthritis. J. Bone Joint Surg. 53A:638, 1971.
2. Arden, G. P., and Ansell, B. M.: Surgical management of juvenile chronic polyarthritis. J. Bone Joint Surg. 54B:16, 1972.
2a. Swann, M.: The surgery of juvenile chronic arthritis. Clin. Orthop. 259:70, 1990.
3. Garrett, A. L., and Campbell, C.: Synovectomy in children. In Cruess, R. L., and Mitchell, N. (eds.): Surgery of Rheumatoid Arthritis. Philadelphia, J. B. Lippincott Company, 1971, pp. 111–116.
4. Kampner, S. L., and Ferguson, A. B., Jr.: Efficacy of synovectomy in juvenile rheumatoid arthritis. Clin. Orthop. 88:94, 1972.
4a. Ovregard, T., Hoyeraal, H. M., et al.: A three-year retrospective study of synovectomies in children. Clin. Orthop. 259:76, 1990.
5. Granberry, W. M., and Mangum, G. L.: The hand in the child with juvenile rheumatoid arthritis. J. Hand Surg. 5:105, 1980.
6. Nalebuff, E.: Unpublished data.
7. Albright, J. A., Albright, J. P., and Ogden, J. A.: Synovectomy of the hip in juvenile rheumatoid arthritis. Clin. Orthop. 106:48, 1975.
8. Green, W. T., and Anderson, M.: Epiphyseal arrest for the correction of discrepancies in length of the lower extremities. J. Bone Joint Surg. 39A:853, 1957.
9. Kuhns, J. G., and Swaim, L. T.: Disturbances of growth in chronic arthritis in children. Am. J. Dis. Child. 43:1118, 1932.
10. Simon, S., Whiffen, J., and Shapiro, F.: Leg-length discrepancies in monoarticular and pauciarticular juvenile rheumatoid arthritis. J. Bone Joint Surg. 63A:209, 1981.
11. Phemister, D. B.: Operative arrestment of longitudinal growth of bones in the treatment of deformities. J. Bone Joint Surg. 15:1, 1933.
12. Blount, W. P., and Clar, G. R.: Control of bone growth by epiphyseal stapling. J. Bone Joint Surg. 31A:454, 1949.
13. Singsen, B. H., Issáacson, A. S., Bernstein, B. H., Patzakis, M. J., Kornreich, H. K., King, K. K., and Hanson, V.: Total hip replacement in children with arthritis. Arthritis Rheum. 21:401, 1978.
14. Arden, G. P., Ansell, B. M., and Hunter, M. J.: Total hip replacement in juvenile chronic polyarthritis and ankylosing spondylitis. Clin. Orthop. 84:130, 1972.
14a. Witt, J. D., Swann, M., and Ansell, B. M.: Total hip replacement for juvenile chronic arthritis. J. Bone Joint Surg. 73B:770, 1991.
15. Crowe, W., Hauselman, C., Shear, E., Miller, E. H., Baly, G. P., and Levinson, J. E.: Total hip arthroplasty in children with juvenile rheumatoid arthritis. Proceedings of the 43rd Annual Meeting of the American Rheumatism Association. Arthritis Rheum. 22:602, 1979.
16. Sledge, C. B.: Joint replacement surgery in juvenile rheumatoid arthritis. Arthritis Rheum. 20:567, 1977.
17. Scott, R. D., Sarokhan, A., and Dalziel, R.: Arthroplasty of the hip and knee in juvenile rheumatoid arthritis. Clin. Orthop. 182:90, 1984.
18. Sarokhan, A., Scott, R. D., Thomas, W. H., Ewald, F. C., Sledge, C. B., and Cloos, D. W.: Total knee replacement in juvenile rheumatoid arthritis. J. Bone Joint Surg. 65A:1071, 1983.
19. Lachiewicz, P. F., McCaskill, B., Inglis, A., Ranawat, C. S., and Rosenstein, B. D.: Total hip arthroplasty in juvenile rheumatoid arthritis: Two- to eleven-year results. J. Bone Joint Surg. 68A:502, 1986.
20. Colville, J., and Raunio, P.: Total hip replacement in juvenile rheumatoid arthritis. Acta Orthop. Scand. 50:197, 1979.
21. Ranawat, C. S., Bryan, W. J., and Inglis, A. E.: Total knee arthroplasty in juvenile arthritis. Arthritis Rheum. 26:1140, 1983.
22. Scott, R. D.: Total hip and knee arthroplasty in juvenile rheumatoid arthritis. Clin. Orthop. Rel. Res. Oct. (259):83, 1990.
23. Scott, R. D., and Sledge, C. B.: Juvenile rheumatoid arthritis. In Steinberg, M. (ed.): The Hip. Philadelphia, W. B. Saunders Co., 1991, pp. 470–482.
24. Henoch, J. J., Batson, J. W., and Baum, J.: Psychosocial factors in juvenile rheumatoid arthritis. Arthritis Rheum. 21:229, 1978.
25. Charnley, J., and Cupic, Z.: The nine- and ten-year results of the low-friction arthroplasty of the hip. Clin. Orthop. 95:9, 1973.
26. Wilson, M. G., and Scott, R. D.: The bipolar socket in juvenile rheumatoid arthritis: A two- to five-year follow-up study. J. Orthop. Rheumatol. 2:133, 1989.

Radiographic Evaluation of Total Joint Replacement

INTRODUCTION

The remarkable success of total hip replacement (THR) has led to the performance of more than 75,000 such operations annually in the United States[1, 2] and the development of a large number of prosthetic devices for most other major joints. Evaluation of postoperative radiographs is becoming an increasing part of many radiographic practices. In this chapter, the "normal" radiographic appearances of some of the frequently used prosthetic devices, the usual appearance related to methods of component fixation, and the radiographic evaluation of complications of total joint replacement are discussed.

TOTAL HIP REPLACEMENT

Types of Prostheses

A large variety of hip prostheses are currently available. Most contemporary prostheses are of the metal-to-plastic type. The acetabular component is made of either high-density or ultra-high-density polyethylene plastic. The external surface may be grooved for improved cement fixation and metallic wires sometimes embedded in the grooves as markers. Acetabular components in current designs are often encased in a metal shell ("metal-backed"). This may be threaded for screwing into the acetabulum or have an irregular surface for bone ingrowth or improved cement fixation. Pegs or screws may be used for additional stability.

On the femoral side, one-piece components or modular femoral designs are available (Fig. 112–1). Modular components typically consist of separate head or head/neck and neck/stem components. In the taper-lock system, the femoral head is impacted onto the taper of the femoral stem. Such prostheses allow reduction in the inventory of femoral components, intraoperative choice of neck length, and removal of the head for revision surgery.[3] Head components are usually cobalt-chrome, but ceramic or zirconium oxide components are also being used.

Bipolar prostheses usually consist of three parts: a metallic acetabular component that may move within the native acetabulum, a high-density poly-

ethylene acetabular liner, and a fixed femoral component. The potential for motion at both acetabular and prosthetic interfaces leads to the "bipolar" designation (Fig. 112–2). "Positive eccentricity" (offset) of the cup with relation to the femoral head aligns the cup horizontally with weight bearing and is a feature of newer bipolar prostheses.

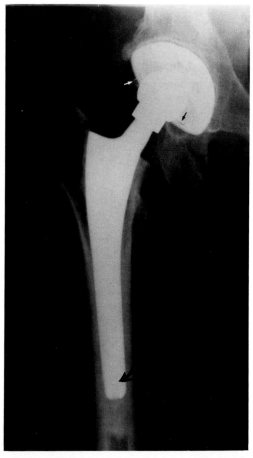

Figure 112–1. Modular hip prosthesis. A metal-backed bone ingrowth acetabular component is present. The ring inside the metal backing (*arrow*) indicates the snap lock for stabilizing the polyethylene component within the acetabular shell. The parallel markers (*white arrow*) indicate the orifice of the polyethylene liner. The femoral component has separate head and stem portions and is fixed with opaque cement that extends past the tip of the prosthesis to the level of a nonopaque plug. The lucency faintly seen at the distal stem (*curved arrow*) should hold a nonopaque centering device, but this had been removed.

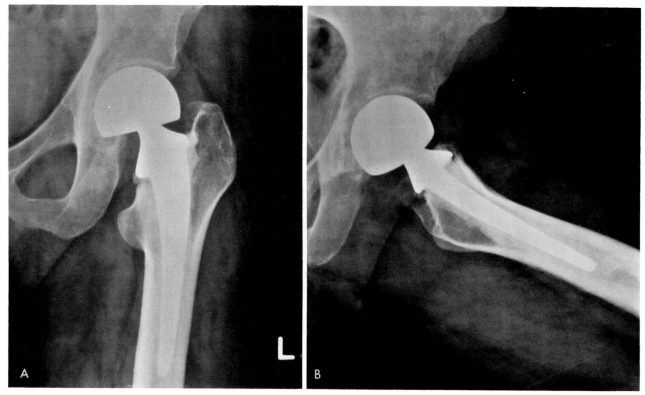

Figure 112–2. Bateman total hip prosthesis. *A,* Anteroposterior view. *B,* Frog lateral view. The acetabular component is not fixed to the ilium. Although most motion occurs between the femoral component and the polyethylene acetabular liner, some motion will be noted between the acetabular component and the acetabulum. The polyethylene liner cannot be seen.

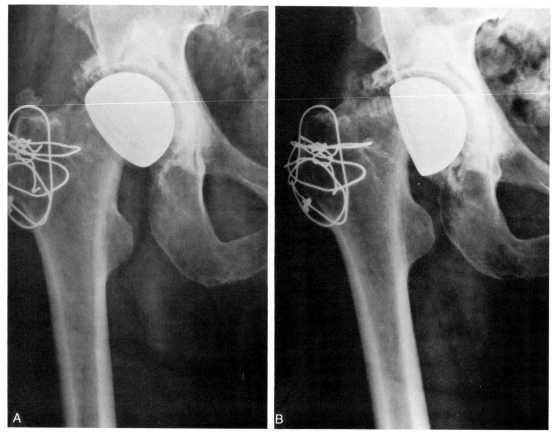

Figure 112–3. Loosening of both components of a surface replacement. *A,* A wide cement-bone lucency around the acetabular component documents loosening. *B,* The femoral component has migrated into varus.

Surface Replacement

In young patients and in patients with good bone stock who have damage limited to the joint surfaces, "conservative total hip replacement" may be done.[4, 5] This entails reaming and reshaping the acetabulum and the femoral head and inserting a high-density polyethylene acetabular liner and a metallic femoral cup. Both components are cemented in place. The procedure has been largely abandoned owing to high loosening rates (Figs. 112–3 through 112–5).

Positioning of Components

Postoperative radiographs allow assessment of the positions of the acetabular and femoral components.

Acetabular Component

Horizontal Tilt. In each of these prostheses, the acetabular component is placed so the base of the cup is at a particular angle to the horizontal in an effort to provide as much motion as possible without too great a hazard of dislocation. The acetabular angle is measured by drawing a line through the medial and lateral poles of the equatorial marker wire and another line through the most inferior aspect of each ischial tuberosity (Fig. 112–5). The inclination of the acetabular component in relation to the ischial baseline has been classified as neutral (40 to 50 degrees), horizontal (less than 40 degrees), or vertical (greater than 50 degrees). With some newer components, the angulation of the nonopaque liner of a metal-backed acetabulum cannot be seen on radiographs, although the tilt of the metal backing can be determined. The acetabular liner may decrease the actual tilt of the acetabulum.

The Center of the Hip. The prosthetic femoral head should be positioned so forces on the hip are

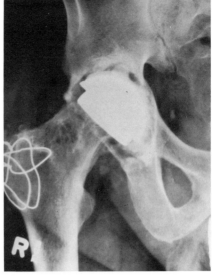

Figure 112–4. Loosening of the acetabular component of a surface replacement. There is a wide cement-bone lucency around the metal-backed acetabular component. The cement-bone interface of the femoral component cannot be seen, but the component seems displaced medially on the femoral neck. The well-defined lucency in the femoral neck was shown to be a histiocytic reaction to cement.

balanced. The height of the center of the hip is measured as the distance from the center of the femoral head along a perpendicular to the inter-teardrop line[6] (Fig. 112–6). Proximal displacement of the hip is evaluated by comparing this measurement over time. For metal-backed components, measurements are made from the center of the cup vertically to the teardrop line.[7] To ensure comparability at 10 percent magnification, the distance from the obturator line and the teardrop line should be compared on the radiographs. Differences of more than 5 mm suggest too great a disparity in the flexion of the pelvis to allow accurate comparison.[7]

The horizontal location of the center of the hip is described as the distance along the inter-teardrop

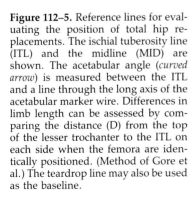

Figure 112–5. Reference lines for evaluating the position of total hip replacements. The ischial tuberosity line (ITL) and the midline (MID) are shown. The acetabular angle (*curved arrow*) is measured between the ITL and a line through the long axis of the acetabular marker wire. Differences in limb length can be assessed by comparing the distance (D) from the top of the lesser trochanter to the ITL on each side when the femora are identically positioned. (Method of Gore et al.) The teardrop line may also be used as the baseline.

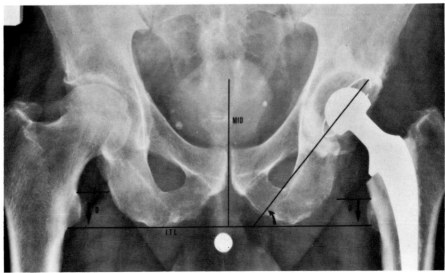

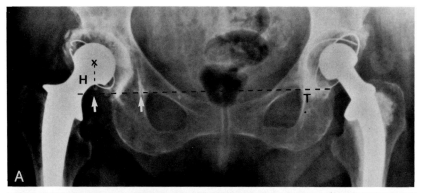

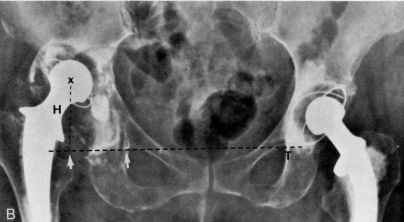

Figure 112–6. Measuring hip position. *A,* The baseline (T) is drawn along the inferior aspects of the teardrop shadows bilaterally. A perpendicular is drawn from the center of the hip. The distance from the teardrop to the perpendicular (*arrows*) indicates the horizontal location of the center of the hip relative to the teardrop shadow. *B,* Many years later, there is loosening of the acetabular component. The resulting displacement can be assessed using the same landmarks as in *A.*

line from the bottom of the teardrop to a perpendicular line drawn from the center of the femoral head[6] (Fig. 112–6). When metal-backed acetabular components are used, measurement is made to the center of the cup.[7] Changes of more than 2 mm (when there is 10 percent magnification) are considered significant. Similar information may be gleaned by using a template provided by the Muller Foundation (ME Muller total hip replacement template, Berne, Switzerland, 1988) (Fig. 112–7).

Kohler's Line. The ilioischial, or Kohler's, line has been used to assess protrusion deformity but is affected by changes (when there is 10 percent magnification) in patient rotation and, therefore, is of limited use[8] for measuring medial migration of the acetabulum.

Ranawat Triangle Method. In 1980, Ranawat et al.[9] described a method of locating the anatomic position of the acetabulum. Using this method, a triangle is constructed, the superior margin of which should pass through the subchondral bone of the normal acetabulum. With this guide, change in vertical or horizontal acetabular position may be documented[9] (Fig. 112–8).

Anteversion or Retroversion. The orifice of the acetabular component is placed in slight anteversion (tipped anteriorly) or in neutral position (Fig. 112–9).[10] The degree of acetabular anteversion is measured on a true lateral radiograph using the coronal plane (parallel to the table top and film edge) as the baseline. The angle between a perpendicular line and

the line along the long axis of the acetabular component is the angle of anteversion (Fig. 112–9B). When only frontal views are available, however, the equatorial marker wires should form a thin ellipse if the prosthesis is in slight anteversion. With increasing anteversion (or retroversion), the wire marker assumes a more circular shape. Quantitation of the degree of acetabular anteversion (or retroversion) from frontal views can be done by dividing the maximal diameter of the acetabular ring by the minimal diameter and comparing the quotient to a standard reference table.[11]

The change in acetabular appearance with differences in centering of the x-ray beam can be used to determine the degree and direction of acetabular version. Two anteroposterior views are taken, one with the x-ray beam centered on the pubic symphysis and the other with it centered on the acetabulum.[12] When the ring appears wider (more circular) on the film centered on the acetabulum than on the one centered on the symphysis, the component is anteverted. When it is more circular in appearance on the film centered on the pubic symphysis, the component is retroverted. The angle of version (B) can then be derived from the formula: $\sin B = d2/D2$, where $d2$ is the short diameter and $D2$ the long diameter of the acetabular marker wire as projected on the film centered over the acetabulum.

Fluoroscopy has also been used to determine the angle of anteversion.[13] As the fluoroscopic tube is angled either toward the feet or toward the head,

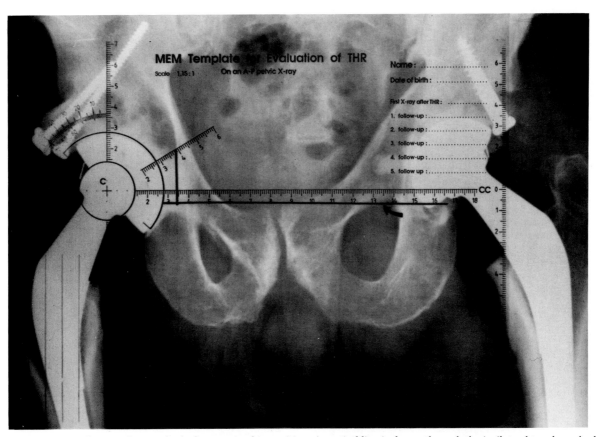

Figure 112–7. The Muller template method of measuring hip position. A vertical line is drawn through the ipsilateral teardrop shadow, and a horizontal baseline is constructed along the inferior margins of the teardrop shadows (*curved arrow*). The template is aligned with the rule (the CC line) parallel to the inter-teardrop line and the cross centered on the (T line) femoral head. The T line and vertical teardrop line are traced onto the template. Cranial migration can be assessed on follow-up radiographs as the distance between the new T line and the original T line. Medial migration of the socket can be measured as the change in the distance from the center of the femoral head to the teardrop line on successive radiographs.

Figure 112–8. Acetabular position; method of Ranawat. Point A is located 5 mm lateral to the intersection of Shenton's line (dotted) and Kohler's line (K). Parallel horizontal lines drawn along the iliac crests and ischial tuberosities indicate the height of the pelvis. The normal acetabulum is one fifth of the pelvic height. A perpendicular to these lines is drawn through point A ending at point B at a distance equal to one fifth of the height of the pelvis. Point C is horizontal from point B at a distance equal to line AB. Line CA completes the triangle. The superior aspect of the triangle generally falls at the subchondral bone of the normal acetabulum.

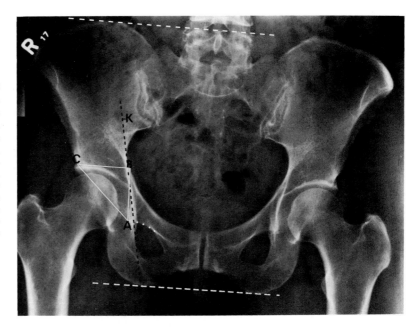

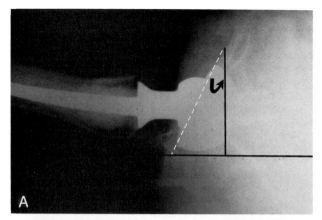

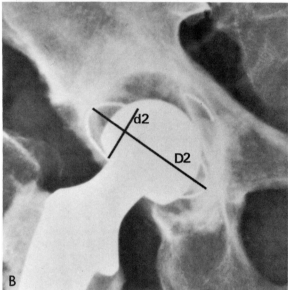

Figure 112–9. Acetabular anteversion. *A,* The true lateral view shows the anterior tilt of the acetabulum. This can be measured by drawing a baseline parallel to the edge of the film. The anteversion is the angle between a perpendicular to the baseline and the orifice of the acetabular component. *B,* On this film, the angle of version (β) may be derived from the formula $\sin \beta = d2/D2$. An estimation of d2 must be made, owing to the opacity of the femoral head.

the degree and direction of angulation are noted at which the anterior and posterior rims of the acetabular marker wire are superimposed. The component is anteverted if the tube is directed toward the feet. Using a reference table, correction can be made for the degree of horizontal inclination of the component, since this influences the observed angle of anteversion.

Acetabular Screw Placement. Many of the porous-coated acetabular components are held by transfixation screws that provide stability until bone ingrowth occurs.[14, 15] Wasielewski et al.[15] divided the acetabulum into quadrants and noted that placement of screws through the anterosuperior and anteroinferior quadrants should be avoided if possible because these areas are adjacent to important vascular and neural structures (e.g., the external iliac artery

and vein and obturator nerve, artery, and vein). These relationships can be elucidated on computed tomography (CT) scanning (Fig. 112–10).

Femoral Component Position

On the frontal view, the prosthetic femoral stem should be in the center of the medullary cavity or in slight valgus position.[16] Valgus or varus position of the stem refers to the angle between the long axis of the stem and the long axis of the femoral shaft.[17] When the tip of the stem is near the lateral femoral cortex, the prosthesis is said to be in varus; when it is near the medial cortex, the prosthesis is in valgus. On true lateral views, the femoral head should be in about 10 degrees of anteversion or in neutral position.[18]

Multiple reference lines have been constructed to compare the position of a total hip prosthesis with the normal contralateral side (see Fig. 112–5).[19] A view of the pelvis with the hips in neutral position can be used to determine differences in limb length by comparing the distance on each side from the proximal end of the lesser trochanter to a line through the most inferior portion of each ischial tuberosity.

Component Fixation

Cement Fixation

Methyl methacrylate has no adhesive properties when applied to wet bone. It bonds to bone through a mechanical interlocking of surface irregularities and functions to distribute transmitted stresses evenly from the prosthesis to bone.[20] It is prepared by mixing a liquid monomer with a powdered polymerized material. The surfaces of the pearls of polymerized material are dissolved by the monomer, and within minutes a single block is formed by polymerization of the monomer.

Preparation on the acetabular side includes irrigation and removal of debris, creation of several small anchoring holes, and preservation of subchondral bone.[21] When the methyl methacrylate cement reaches a doughy consistency, it is pressed into the acetabulum and the prepared holes. The acetabular component is then inserted and held in position.

Methyl methacrylate is also placed into the medullary canal of the femur after the cancellous bone is removed. Technical improvements in canal preparation, use of an intramedullary plug, and centrifugation of cement have been introduced[22] and have improved fixation. Cement should be seen to fill the medullary cavity medially and laterally along the distal two thirds of the shaft and should extend 2 cm distal to the tip of the prosthesis.[4, 10] Other definitions of what constitutes adequate cement fixation have, however, been proposed.[24, 25]

According to Amstutz et al.,[23] inadequate cement fixation is suggested by radiolucent zones at the

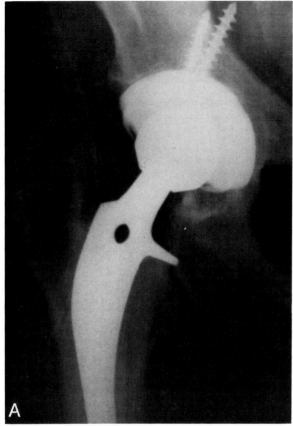
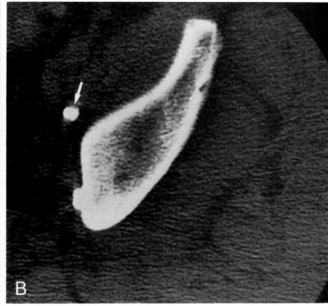

Figure 112–10. Acetabular screw position. *A,* Two screws are seen in the acetabulum. *B,* An axial CT scan through the ilium shows the tip of the longer screw (*arrow*) to be anteriorly and medially positioned with relation to the ilium. The relationship to vessels, other soft tissues, and bony structures can be ascertained.

cement-bone or cement-metal junctions or by the presence of voids and laminations within the cement. Beckenbaugh and Ilstrup[26] found loosening of the femoral component to be inversely related to the degree of extension of cement past the prosthetic tip.

Comparison of groups of patients undergoing THR using early or modern cementing has led Roberts et al.[24] to conclude that cement inhomogeneity and distribution play a role in subsequent loosening. Patients in whom femoral component loosening occurred had fewer zones of adequate cement. Cement in zone 4 (distal to the tip of the prosthesis) was especially important.

Histologic examination has shown a reaction of bone to methyl methacrylate that may be divided into three phases: necrosis, repair, and a steady state.[25] Within the first 3 weeks after surgery, a zone of necrotic tissue and fibrin is noted extending up to 3 mm in depth from the cement-bone interface. The cause of this necrosis remains uncertain, but possibilities include toxic effects from remaining nonpolymerized monomer or thermal injury related to the polymerization of methyl methacrylate (an exothermic reaction).[25] From 3 weeks to 2 years postoperatively, repair of tissue damage occurs and, in most cases, leads to the development of a fibrous layer along the cement-bone interface. A stable appearance is usually reached in 2 years, with a 0.1 to 1.5 mm connective tissue membrane formed around the cement.[26]

Standardization of Radiographic Follow-Up. Efforts have been made to standardize the reporting of the clinical and radiologic results of THR. Figure 112–11 shows the observations that could be made in evaluating cemented prostheses.[27] On the acetabular side, the three zones described by DeLee and Charnley[28] are used (Fig. 112–12). On the femoral side, the seven zones described by Gruen et al.[29] are used to assess the anteroposterior radiograph, whereas an additional seven zones are evaluated on the lateral radiograph.

Usual Radiographic Appearances

Cemented Components. Radiologic evaluation of the cement-bone interface can be accomplished only when the methacrylate is made opaque, usually by the addition of barium sulfate. If a radiolucent line is present at the cement-bone interface, it will be made apparent on radiographs by its contrast to the adjacent opaque cement on one side and a thin sclerotic line on the other side. When such a radiolucent line is present in the immediate postoperative period, it may represent residual cartilage, soft tissue, or blood within the prosthetic bed. Later, the lucency may correspond to the histologically demonstrable fibrous tissue layer (Fig. 112–13).

Radiolucent zones at the cement-bone interface are very frequent around the acetabular component and less frequent around the femoral component,

RADIOGRAPHIC EVALUATION: CEMENTED PROSTHESES

Acetabulum	Femur	

Acetabulum

Migration of component
(measurement must be related
to teardrop)
___ No
___ Yes
Superior: ___ mm
Medial: ___ mm

Location of center of rotation of hip
relative to teardrop
Superior: ___ mm
Lateral: ___ mm

Broken cement
___ No
___ Yes
Zone (specify
1-3): _____

Cement-bone radiolucency
(DeLee and Charnley)
___ No
___ Yes
Maximum width
Zone 1: ___ mm
Zone 2: ___ mm
Zone 3: ___ mm
Continuous
___ No
___ Yes
Maximum width: ___ mm

Radiolucency around screws
___ No
___ Yes
___ Not applicable

Breakage of screws
___ No
___ Yes
___ Not applicable

Wear of socket: ___ mm

Position of component
Inclination (abduction): ___°
Version of cup
Retroversion: ___°
___ Neutral
Anteversion: ___°

Femur (column 1)

Migration of stem
Varus-valgus
___ No
___ Yes
___ Varus ⎱ qualitative only;
___ Valgus ⎰ choose one
Subsidence (must be related to fixed
landmarks on femur: prox. tip of
greater trochanter and mid-point of
lesser trochanter)
___ No
___ Yes (___ mm)
___ Within cement
___ With cement

Broken cement
___ No
___ Yes

Stem
___ Intact
___ Bent
___ Broken

Radiolucency
Prosthesis-cement
(anteroposterior radiograph)
___ No
___ Yes
Cement-bone
Anteroposterior radiograph
___ No
___ Yes
Maximum width
Zone 1: ___ mm
Zone 2: ___ mm
Zone 3: ___ mm
Zone 4: ___ mm
Zone 5: ___ mm
Zone 6: ___ mm
Zone 7: ___ mm
Lateral radiograph
___ No
___ Yes
Maximum width
Zone 8: ___ mm
Zone 9: ___ mm
Zone 10: ___ mm
Zone 11: ___ mm
Zone 12: ___ mm
Zone 13: ___ mm
Zone 14: ___ mm

Femur (column 2)

Resorption of medial part of neck
(calcar)
___ No
___ Yes
Loss of height (exclusive
of rounding): ___ mm
Loss of thickness: ___ mm

Resorption or hypertrophy of shaft
___ No
Resorption (zones: _____)
Hypertrophy (zones: _____)

Change in density
___ No
Patchy loss (zones: _____)
Uniform loss (zones: _____)
Increased trabecular
bone (zones: _____)

Endosteal cavitation
___ No
___ Yes
Zones: _____
Length: ___ mm
Width: ___ mm

Ectopic ossification
___ Brooker I (none)
___ Brooker II (mild)
___ Brooker III (moderate)
___ Brooker IV (severe)

Position of stem
___ Neutral
___ Valgus ⎱ qualitative only;
___ Varus ⎰ choose one

Greater trochanter
___ Not osteotomized
___ Osteotomized
___ Healed
___ Not healed
___ Displaced
___ Non-displaced

Figure 112–11. A standard form for evaluation of cemented prostheses. (From Johnston, R. C., Fitzgerald, R. H., Jr., et al.: Clinical and radiographic evaluation of total hip replacement. A standard system of terminology for reporting results. J. Bone Joint Surg. 72A:161, 1990. Used by permission.)

occurring in up to two thirds of femoral components and all acetabular components.[30] Lucencies of more than 2 mm or progressive lucency suggests the possibility of loosening or infection and correlates on histologic examination with the presence of a synovial lining capable of producing substances that stimulate bone resorption.[31]

Mechanical Interlock Fixation

Mechanical interlock of components may be obtained by press-fitting, by screwing a component into bone for long-term fixation, or by using screws to produce immediate postoperative stability while biologic fixation occurs.

Experience with early press-fit hemiarthroplasties (such as the Thompson and the Moore prostheses) has shown several characteristic radiographic features in uncomplicated cases. Periosteal reaction producing cortical thickening may be seen in relation to increased stress near the tip of the stem and along the lateral femur proximal to the tip (Fig. 112–14). Similarly, sclerosis is often seen near the tip of the prosthesis. A thin line of lucency around the femoral stem is seen in about one third of cases.[32] Widening

of the zone between the prosthesis and the bone or a lucent zone of 2 mm or more suggests loosening (aseptic or septic). Change in component position over time should be searched for. Sinking (subsidence) of the femoral prosthesis into the bone may occur, particularly if the prosthesis is too small and does not fill the femoral canal.

Biologic Fixation

Since the late 1960s, porous-surfaced prostheses have been developed to allow biologic fixation to host bone.[33] Biologic fixation refers to the ingrowth of tissue between the surface pores of an implant, allowing loads to be transmitted from the prosthesis along a large surface area to the bone, thus minimizing stress at the bone-prosthesis junction. In addition, the interface has the potential to remodel in response to changes in loads or stress. Bone ingrowth between the surface pores is considered ideal, but how much bone is necessary for stabilization (probably only a small percentage of the surface area) and whether fibrous ingrowth is sufficient for long-term fixation are unknown.[34]

Porous materials made from metals, polymers,

or ceramics provide the irregular surface necessary for bone ingrowth. Pore size is important. Pores that are too small do not allow bone ingrowth to occur (although they may be used to enhance methyl methacrylate fixation). Conditions necessary for successful bone ingrowth include absence of relative motion at the prosthesis-bone interface, corrosion resistance, good biocompatibility, and intimate contact between the bone and the prosthesis.

Bone ingrowth occurs in two phases: an initial phase and a remodeling phase. A stable or equilibrium stage is then reached. The early phase requires weight-bearing protection, whereas the later remodeling phase progresses under weight-bearing conditions. In humans, the acute phase lasts 3 to 6 months, and the second, bone-remodeling phase extends from about 3 months to 2 years postoperatively.[33] Remodeling is reflected by radiographic changes of bone resorption and bone formation that usually stabilize by 1 year after surgery.[33]

Cementless total hip arthroplasty has been suggested for active patients less than 60 years old who have good bone stock or for revision surgery, particularly in patients younger than 70.[35]

Histologic Findings. Bone ingrowth is often present along only a portion of the available porous surface. Thus, Engh and Bobyn[33] noted bone in-

growth in human hips to occur in regions of cortical bone where the prosthesis was in contact or nearly in contact with the endosteum. These regions are usually located along the medial aspect of the prosthesis at the femoral calcar and along the medial and lateral aspects of the femoral stem proximal to the tip of the prosthesis.

Radiologic Findings in Uncemented Prostheses

Radiologic evaluation of bone ingrowth prostheses includes evaluation of component position, status of the prosthesis-bone interface, and changes related to altered stress. Standardization of reporting has been suggested (Fig. 112–15). The lateral radiograph seems to be particularly valuable for evaluation of bone ingrowth femoral components.[27]

Change in Component Position. Varus angulation may occur on follow-up examinations, particularly in femoral prostheses with collars, whereas valgus angulation has been noted when collarless components are used. The change in angulation is said to be a mechanism for achieving stability within the femoral shaft. Settling of the femoral component is most common when the medullary cavity is too wide relative to the stem. Settling of the prosthesis into the femoral shaft (subsidence) may be assessed

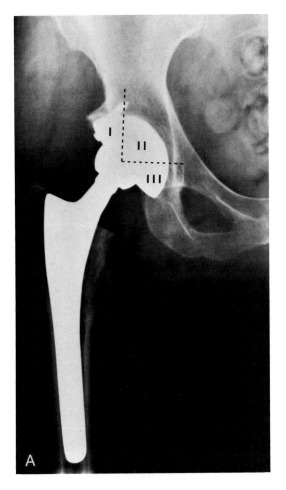

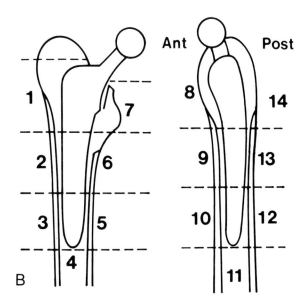

Figure 112–12. Acetabular and femoral zones. *A,* The areas of the acetabular component are designated using the method of De Lee and Charnley. *B,* The seven femoral zones of Gruen et al. and the additional zones visible on the lateral view are shown. (*B,* From Johnston, R. C., Fitzgerald, R. H., Jr., et al.: Clinical and radiographic evaluation of total hip replacement. A standard system of terminology for reporting results. J. Bone Joint Surg. 72A:161, 1990. Used by permission.)

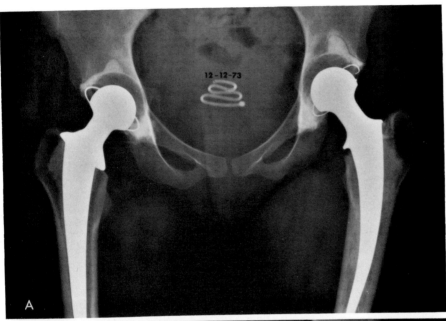

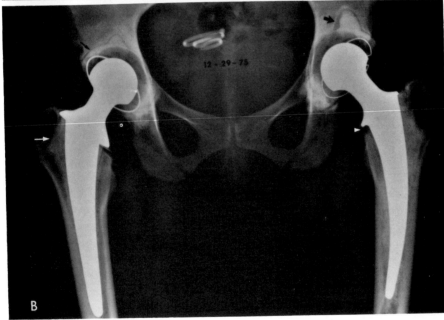

Figure 112–13. Asymptomatic loosening. *A*, 1973 examination shows a thin zone of lucency around the left acetabular component. *B*, Two years later cement-bone lucent zones have developed around both components on the right (*arrows*), and there is marked widening of the lucent zone around the left acetabular component (*solid arrow*). Bone resorption of the medial femoral neck (*arrow-head*) is noted. The patient has remained asymptomatic.

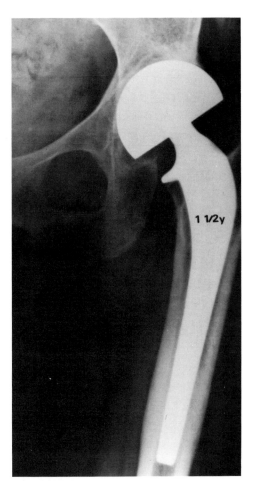

Figure 112–14. Cortical thickening. One and one-half years after insertion of a bipolar prosthesis with a press-fit femoral component, stress-related changes have occurred in the femoral shaft near the tip of the prosthesis. These consist of endosteal thickening and periosteal apposition leading to thickened cortices.

by comparing distances from the superomedial aspect of the bone ingrowth area to the superior aspect of the lesser trochanter on sequential pelvic radiographs.[36] Differences of 5 mm or more are thought to indicate subsidence. Subsidence was found to occur in one half of cases of porous-coated anatomic hip prostheses reviewed by Kattapuram et al.[37] and was found to be the most important radiographic indicator of clinical outcome.[37] Subsidence that continued after 1 year and settling of more than 10 mm were associated with a less than favorable result (Fig. 112–16).

Prosthesis-Bone Interface. Successful bone ingrowth is documented radiographically by the presence of bone extending up to and between the beaded ingrowth surface. In these cases, no lucencies are present between the bone and the metal.

Lucent Zones and Sclerotic Lines. A sclerotic line separated from the prosthesis by a thin lucency may be seen around rigid, uncemented prostheses several months after surgery. The lucency corresponds to a layer of fibrous tissue,[38] and when it is seen along the bone ingrowth area, it implies that fibrous ingrowth rather than bone ingrowth has occurred (Fig. 112–17).[39] This finding may remain stable or progress to loosening. Kaplan et al.[40] found

progression of these lucent zones in width or in length even in asymptomatic subjects. At 2 years, Callaghan et al.[36] identified sclerotic lines along the proximal lateral area for bone ingrowth in 56 percent of cases.

Cortical Thickening and Endosteal Reaction. As with cemented and press-fit prostheses, periosteal reaction and cortical thickening may occur near the tip of the prosthesis, in response to increased stress. The location of the cortical thickening depends on the position of the stem, so, for example, lateral cortical thickening is associated with varus stem position. Cortical thickening occurred in 9 percent of a group of asymptomatic patients with bone ingrowth components followed for almost 2 years. Periosteal reaction is uncommon. It may occur where the porous-coated region last contacted the cortex.

A shelf of sclerotic bone may develop near the tip of the prosthesis. This was evident in more than one third of asymptomatic hips studied by Kaplan et al.[40] Early follow-up studies have shown that it may progress.[36] Kattapuram et al.[37] found no statistically significant correlation between sclerosis and clinical outcome.[37]

Hypertrophy of cancellous bone occurs especially at the proximal porous-coated portion of the

RADIOGRAPHIC EVALUATION: UNCEMENTED PROSTHESES

Acetabulum	Femur	

Acetabulum

Migration of component
(measurement must be related
to teardrop)
___ No
___ Yes
Superior: ___ mm
Medial: ___ mm

Location of center of rotation of hip
relative to teardrop
Superior: ___ mm
Lateral: ___ mm

Prosthesis-bone radiolucency
(DeLee and Charnley)
___ No
___ Yes
Maximum width
Zone 1: ___ mm
Zone 2: ___ mm
Zone 3: ___ mm
Continuous
___ No
___ Yes
Maximum width: ___ mm

Radiolucency around screws
___ No
___ Yes
___ Not applicable

Breakage of screws
___ No
___ Yes
___ Not applicable

Porous coating
___ Intact
___ Dislodged
___ Progressive loss
___ Not applicable

Wear of socket: ___ mm

Position of component
Inclination (abduction): ___
Version of cup
Retroversion: ___
___ Neutral
Anteversion: ___

Femur

Migration of stem
Varus-valgus
___ No
___ Yes
___ Varus | qualitative only;
___ Valgus | choose one
Subsidence (must be related to fixed
landmarks on femur: prox. tip of
greater trochanter and mid-point of
lesser trochanter)
___ No
___ Yes (___ mm)

Porous coating
___ Intact
___ Dislodged
___ Progressive loss
___ Not applicable

Stem
___ Intact
___ Bent
___ Broken

Prosthesis-bone radiolucency
Anteroposterior radiograph
___ No
___ Yes
Maximum width
Zone 1: ___ mm
Zone 2: ___ mm
Zone 3: ___ mm
Zone 4: ___ mm
Zone 5: ___ mm
Zone 6: ___ mm
Zone 7: ___ mm
Lateral radiograph
___ No
___ Yes
Maximum width
Zone 8: ___ mm
Zone 9: ___ mm
Zone 10: ___ mm
Zone 11: ___ mm
Zone 12: ___ mm
Zone 13: ___ mm
Zone 14: ___ mm

Resorption of medial part of neck
(calcar)
___ No
___ Yes
Loss of height (exclusive
of rounding): ___ mm
Loss of thickness: ___ mm

Resorption or hypertrophy of shaft
___ No
Resorption (zones: _____)
Hypertrophy (zones: _____)

Change in density
___ No
Patchy loss (zones: _____)
Uniform loss (zones: _____)
Increased trabecular
bone (zones: _____)

Endosteal cavitation
___ No
___ Yes
Zones: _____
Length: ___ mm
Width: ___ mm

Ectopic ossification
___ Brooker I (none)
___ Brooker II (mild)
___ Brooker III (moderate)
___ Brooker IV (severe)

Position of stem
___ Neutral
___ Valgus | qualitative only;
___ Varus | choose one

Greater trochanter
___ Not osteotomized
___ Osteotomized
___ Healed
___ Not healed
___ Displaced
___ Non-displaced

Figure 112–15. A standard evaluation form for uncemented prostheses. (From Johnston, R. C., Fitzgerald, R. H., Jr., et al.: Clinical and radiographic evaluation of total hip replacement. A standard system of terminology for reporting results. J. Bone Joint Surg. 72A:161, 1990. Used by permission.)

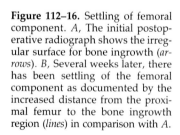
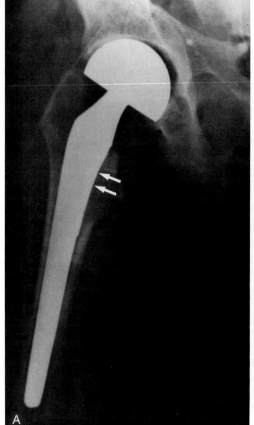
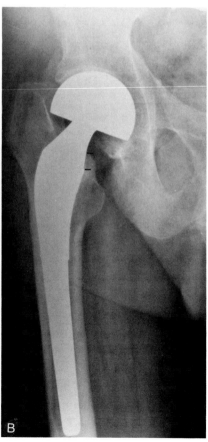

Figure 112–16. Settling of femoral component. *A,* The initial postoperative radiograph shows the irregular surface for bone ingrowth (*arrows*). *B,* Several weeks later, there has been settling of the femoral component as documented by the increased distance from the proximal femur to the bone ingrowth region (*lines*) in comparison with *A.*

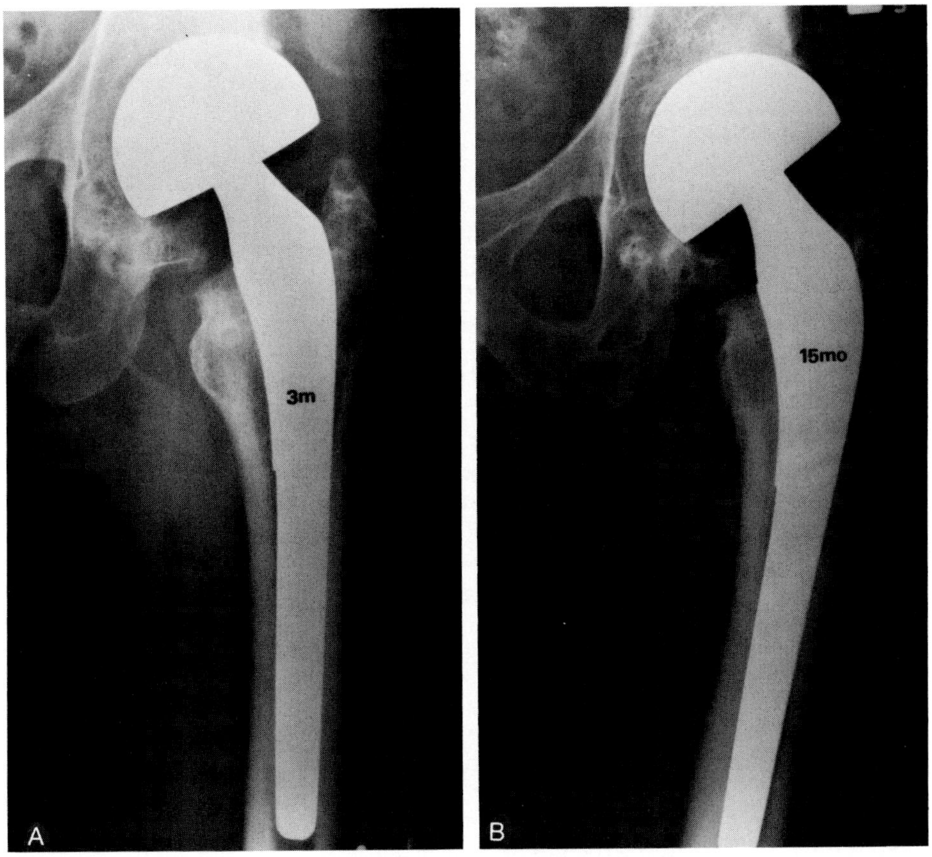

Figure 112–17. Normal postoperative appearances of bone ingrowth prosthesis. *A,* Three months after surgery, no lucency is noted at the bone ingrowth region. A few beads were displaced at the time of surgery and are noted in the soft tissues. *B,* Fifteen months after surgery the area for bone ingrowth continues to show no lucency between it and adjacent trabecular bone. A thin sclerotic line and adjacent lucency are present at the junction between bone ingrowth and press-fit regions. There is cortical thickening medially near the tip of the prosthesis.

prosthesis and signifies transfer of stress through the prosthesis to the bone.[37]

Stress Shielding. Stress shielding refers to the atrophy of bone that occurs when it is unloaded from stress. Thus, there may be selective stressing of some areas of bone adjacent to a prosthesis and absence of stress in other areas. The former areas will demonstrate new bone formation, whereas the latter areas may show marked bone resorption. Rounding of the medial femoral neck is frequent.[36] Bone resorption is generally limited to the proximal 3 cm of the the femur and according to Kaplan et al.[40] does not progress after the first year. Attenuation of the medial femoral cortex with change in its appearance to that of cancellous bone (producing a striated appearance) occurred in 94 percent of cases in one series and usually stabilized after the first year.[40] Such bone resorption reflects "stress shielding" and occurs particularly when bone ingrowth has successfully produced a secure bond between the prosthesis and the bone.[40]

Dislodging of Surface Beads. Dislodging of beads may occur when the prosthesis is inserted. Increased numbers of beads on sequential examinations indicate component motion.

Potential Problems of Uncemented Prostheses. Several potential problems of biologic fixation have been noted.

Tissue Reaction. Bone ingrowth prostheses have large surface areas directly exposed to the surrounding tissues rather than encapsulated by a cement sheath. Potentially significant amounts of metal ion could be presented to the surrounding soft tissue[41]; biocompatibility and corrosion resistance of the alloys used are therefore important. Galante[41] studied the migration of titanium 10 years after implantation of titanium fiber composites used for fixation of long bone replacement in baboons and found increased concentration of titanium in the urine and lungs in comparison with a control group. Animal studies have shown carcinogenicity of some of the components of chromium cobalt alloys,[42] and tumors have been reported adjacent to uncemented components.[43]

Mechanical Changes in the Implant. The sintering process used to unite the metallic porous coating to the prosthesis and the presence of the rough surface itself change the mechanical properties of the implant and make it more susceptible to fracture.

Stress Shielding. Stress shielding is more marked with porous-coated prostheses than with cemented prostheses.

Expense. Bony ingrowth prostheses are usually more costly than those designed for use with cement fixation.

Surgical Difficulties. The surgical procedures for insertion of uncemented prostheses is demanding, requiring intimate contact between bone surfaces and the prosthesis.

Difficult Revision. Difficult revision may result if areas of bone ingrowth are extensive and necessitate removal of large amounts of bone along with the prosthesis.

Unfixed Acetabular Components

Bipolar Endoprostheses

Bipolar endoprostheses are used in place of conventional hemiarthroplasty (Thompson, Austin-Moore) in patients with minimal or no acetabular abnormality, including those with displaced subcapital fractures, avascular necrosis of the femoral head, or osteoarthritis with minimal acetabular involvement. It is thought that because motion occurs preferentially between the metallic cup and the acetabulum, degenerative change in the acetabulum will be less pronounced than with conventional hemiarthroplasty (unipolar prostheses). Theoretically but not always in practice, the acetabular component can be replaced with a fixed acetabular socket if acetabular damage does occur. Bipolar prostheses have also been used for revision after loosening of cemented THRs.

Radiographic examination should show most motion occurring between the femoral component and the acetabular liner, although some movement does occur at the outer articulation, particularly at the extremes of motion.[44] Acetabular changes, including cartilage space narrowing and acetabular sclerosis, should be minimal. Because the metallic cup overlies it, no radiographic estimation of the integrity of the acetabular liner can be made except by indirect evaluation of femoral-acetabular motion.

Hybrid Fixation

Partly in response to improved methods of cement fixation of the femoral component and uncertainties about bone ingrowth of femoral components and high rates of late loosening of cemented acetabular components, hybrid prostheses are being inserted consisting of cemented femoral and bone ingrowth acetabular components (see Fig. 112–1). Short-term comparison of hybrid hips with bone ingrowth hip arthroplasties has shown superior results in the hybrid group in one study.[45]

Hydroxyapatite Coating

Coating of prostheses with hydroxyapatite is theoretically advantageous because biocompatibility is not a problem, and animal studies have shown early union of the prosthesis to bone. Chemical and biologic bonding between the implant and bone are thought to occur. Unlike with cement fixation, no fibrous membrane separates the prosthesis from the bone, and bone deposition occurs directly on the hydroxyapatite coating.

Trochanteric Osteotomy

Trochanteric osteotomy may be done to facilitate surgical exposure. The trochanter usually is reattached in the anatomic position or to a more distal location, depending on mechanical considerations. In more than 95 percent of cases, bone union between the trochanter and the femur is evident on radiographic examination within 6 to 12 weeks postoperatively.[16, 17] If bone union is not seen at 3 months but the trochanter remains unchanged in position, it is likely that fibrous union has occurred, especially if the wired sutures remain intact.[16] Clinical results appear to be as satisfactory with fibrous union as with bone union,[46] and fibrous union may progress to bone union.[30] Separation of the greater trochanter was present in 2.7 percent of hips in patients followed for 9 to 10 years by Charnley, and all these patients were classified as having excellent clinical results.[28] Separation of the greater trochanter may be of clinical significance because this is occasionally associated with pain, limp, and a tendency to develop an adduction contracture.[47] Bergstrom et al.[48] noted that displacement of the greater trochanter of 5 to 20 mm (44 patients) did not impair the functional result, whereas two of four patients with more than 2 cm of displacement required reoperation.

Fracture of the wires holding the greater trochanter occurs in up to one third of patients and is of very little significance unless it is associated with proximal migration of the trochanter. Wire breakage can occur as a result of metal fatigue even after there is solid bone union between the trochanter and femur. Occasionally, symptoms result from irritation of the overlying soft tissues. Rarely, a metal fragment can migrate to an intra-articular location.

Bone Grafting

Augmentation of a deficient acetabulum, such as occurs in acetabular dysplasia, has been successfully done using autograft obtained at the time of primary surgery.[49] Acetabular augmentation is also used to restore bone stock and help support a new acetabular component in hips in which aseptic loosening of a prosthesis has led to significant bone loss.[50, 51] Acetabular defects may be demonstrated on oblique views of the pelvis, on true lateral views[52] and on CT scans.[3, 52] Large defects, especially those involving the posterosuperior or posteroanterior rims of the acetabulum, are usually replaced with large segments of cortical cancellous allograft, whereas multiple small fragments of cancellous bone are often used to improve acetabular volume when the acetabular rim remains intact.

Radiographic examination has shown progressive loss of the demarcation between the graft and the host bone, sclerosis of the graft, and the development of a continuous trabecular pattern with healing. When bipolar prostheses are used, reduction in graft volume may occur during healing, but this tends to stabilize in the first year (Fig. 112–18).[8] The loss of graft volume is reflected by acetabular component migration. Single photon emission computed tomography (SPECT) bone scans have shown symmetric distribution of isotope in acetabular allografts. The value of this imaging procedure, however, is uncertain because, in one series, SPECT scanning was unable to separate patients with nonunion, progressive resorption, or loss of bone structure from those with uneventful graft healing.[54]

Proximal femoral allografts have been used when femoral bone loss is severe (Fig. 112–19). Early results are promising.[51, 55]

Measuring Wear

Theoretically acetabular wear can be assessed by measuring changes in the distance from the metallic femoral head to the metallic wire on the surface of the acetabular cup in non–metal-backed acetabular components. Charnley and Halley[57] compared the thickness of the acetabular component in the latest radiograph with the thickness determined on the immediate postoperative radiograph. Correction for magnification was done by comparison with the known diameter of the femoral head. In 72 hips with 9 to 10 years' follow-up, total wear ranged from 0 to 4.5 mm and averaged 1.5 mm. The patient's weight and physical activity did not seem to influence the rate of wear, and the rate of wear appeared to decrease with time.

Whether or not wear can actually be assessed radiographically has generated some controversy. Clarke et al.[58] assessed methods of measuring wear in vitro, using a total hip prosthesis mounted on a Plexiglas orientation apparatus. They concluded that ". . . wear measurements could not be made from clinical radiographs." Griffith et al.[59] found that if attention was given to the position of the acetabular component, accurate measurements could be done. When the marker on the acetabular component is at the periphery of the lucent acetabular component, then the component is not significantly tilted and the wire marker may be used for reference in measuring wear. If the wire is separated from the opaque cement around the component by a lucent zone, the component is tilted more than 20 degrees in the coronal plane. In these cases, measurement to the cement rather than the marker wire may be used if this appearance is constant on all films. Livermore et al.[60] measured "linear wear" and "volumetric wear" (the amount of debris generated). Linear wear of cemented, non–metal-backed components was assessed using the method of Griffith et al.[59] Direct measurement of the thickness of the acetabular component after it was surgically removed showed a mean difference between the specimen and radiographic measurements of 0.075 mm (range 0 to 0.4 mm).[60] A positive correlation was demonstrated between the amount of wear measured and the amounts of bone resorption of the proximal femoral neck and lysis of the proximal femur (Fig. 112–20).

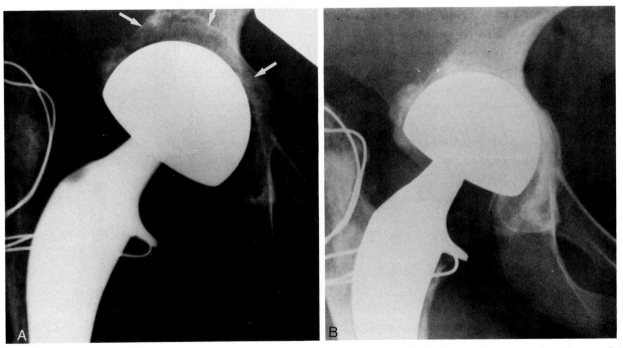

Figure 112–18. Acetabular bone graft. *A,* Shortly after revision surgery and insertion of a bipolar prosthesis, morselized bone graft is visible (*arrows*) within a deformed acetabulum. *B,* Radiograph obtained 2 years later documents loss of volume of the graft with superior and medial migration of the prosthesis.

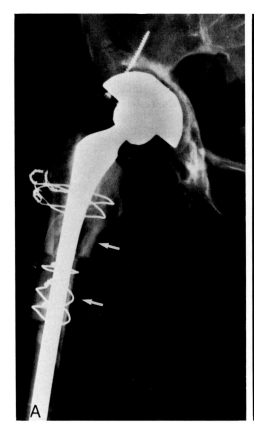
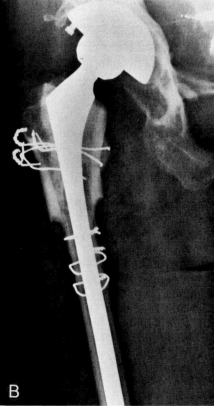

Figure 112–19. Healing of femoral bone graft. *A*, The immediate postoperative radiograph shows the femoral grafts proximally (*arrows*). *B*, Follow-up radiograph shows that the grafts have united. There is resorption of superficial portions of the graft, with narrowing of its circumference.

Resorption of the Medial Femoral Neck

Three or 4 mm of resorption of the medial femoral neck (apparently resulting from ischemic necrosis) occurs in almost 20 percent of patients when the femoral prosthesis is fixed with cement.[10, 30] Generally, this bone loss does not progress and is not significantly related to loosening.[61] Bechtol,[62] however, has suggested that this represents an early stage in a sequence of findings that eventually leads to bending or fracture of the femoral stem. (See also under Development or Widening of a Metal-Cement Lucency, and Femoral Stem Fracture, following).

Complications of Total Hip Replacement

Dislocation

Dislocation is most frequent in the immediate postoperative period, presumably as a consequence of laxity of para-articular soft tissues combined with improper handling of the patient during transfer from the operating room or poor positioning of the leg in bed.[63, 64] Improper placement or selection of the prosthesis may also be responsible for early dislocation.[65]

Dislocation occurring later than 3 months postoperatively is most often the result of malpositioning of components[63] but may be due to failure to develop adequate muscle control or to the patient's developing a range of motion that exceeds the limits of the prosthesis.[65]

Radiographic examination confirms the presence of dislocation, helps define any associated malposition of the prosthetic components, and aids in identification of associated complications. Anteroposterior and true lateral radiographs best define the type

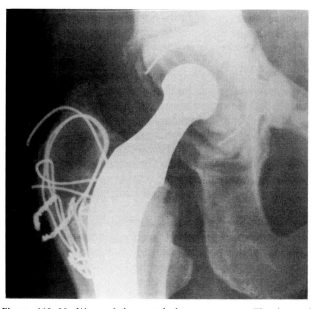

Figure 112–20. Wear of the acetabular component. The femoral head is asymmetrically located in a normally uniform acetabular component. This asymmetry (in the absence of dislocation) suggests wear of the acetabulum. There is accompanying loosening of the acetabular component and resorption of the femoral neck.

of dislocation present. Subtle changes in the relationship of the femoral head to the acetabular component may reflect dislocation. In some prostheses, the femoral head should lie centrally in the acetabular component and equidistant medially and laterally from the acetabular rim.[66] In other prostheses, the acetabular component is thicker along the superolateral aspect to provide extra durability in the weight-bearing area (Fig. 112–21). The femoral component of these prostheses normally appears eccentrically located, with the lateral measurement about twice the medial one. Equal measurements may indicate dislocation in these cases.[67, 68]

Acetabular or femoral component malposition is a frequent predisposing factor in prosthetic hip dislocation. Fackler and Poss[12] noted component malposition (defined as acetabular or femoral component retroversion or acetabular anteversion of more than 25 degrees) to be present in 44 percent of patients with dislocated prostheses as compared with only 6 percent of control patients. Excessive anteversion of the acetabular component favors anterior dislocation with the hip in extension; retroversion may lead to posterior dislocation with the hip in flexion; and excessive vertical tilt favors dislocation with adduction of the leg. Excess bone or cement around the acetabular rim may lever the femoral head out of the acetabulum. Eleven of 13 dislocations in a series studied by Beckenbaugh and Ilstrup[26] occurred with the hip in flexion, with internal rotation or adduction or both.

Detachment of the greater trochanter may accompany posterior dislocations.[64] Rarely, displacement of a fragment of cement or wire into the joint will block attempts at successful closed reduction of a dislocated total hip prosthesis.[69] These intra-articular foreign bodies may be visible on standard radiographs or on arthrography.

Loosening and Infection

Two of the most frequent postoperative complications leading to failure of a THR are loosening and infection. Loosening may involve one or both com-

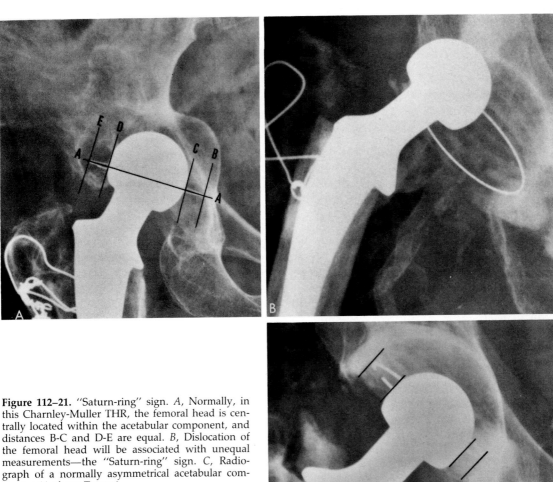

Figure 112–21. "Saturn-ring" sign. *A*, Normally, in this Charnley-Muller THR, the femoral head is centrally located within the acetabular component, and distances B-C and D-E are equal. *B*, Dislocation of the femoral head will be associated with unequal measurements—the "Saturn-ring" sign. *C*, Radiograph of a normally asymmetrical acetabular component (Aufranc-Turner).

ponents and may be due to inadequate fixation at the time of surgery[23] or to infection. Improvements in surgical technique, including better filling of the medullary canal by cement, improved cement preparation, and the use of larger femoral stems with rounding of their medial margins, have markedly decreased the incidence of femoral component loosening.[70] At an average of 11 years of follow-up, for example, Maloney and Harris[45] found femoral component loosening in only 3 percent of patients. Improvements on the acetabular side are less apparent, and in the same study, late acetabular loosening occurred in 42 percent.

The radiographic definition of loosening remains unsettled, and this confounds efforts to compare various clinical trials.[71] As defined by Harris et al.,[70] definite loosening is documented by migration of a component or cement or cement fracture, including development of a metal-cement lucency; probable loosening is identified by the presence of a complete radiolucent line at the cement-bone interface; and possible loosening is defined as the presence of a greater than 50 to 99 percent cement-bone radiolucency. Many other definitions have been used, however.[71] Brand et al.[71] note that use of various definitions of loosening may lead to a variation in reported loosening rates by a factor of two or more and to an alteration of the apparent importance of risk factors affecting long-term results by as much as two or three times.

Radiographic Features of Loosening or Infection of Cemented Prostheses. The following radiographic findings suggest loosening or infection of cemented components and are reviewed: a wide cement-bone interface, widening of a cement-bone interface, migration of prosthetic components, cement fracture, periosteal reaction, component motion demonstrated on stress views, and evidence of osteomyelitis (Table 112–1).

Cement-Bone Lucency Greater than 2 mm or Widening of the Cement-Bone Lucent Zone. A lucency of 2 mm or more at the cement-bone interface suggests loosening (Fig. 112–22). In one series, this finding correlated with motion of prosthetic components with manual stress at surgical exploration in 16 of the 18 patients (89 percent) in whom it was observed.[72] Lucency around both the femoral and the acetabular components was also associated with an increased incidence of infection. Similarly, progressive widening of a cement-bone lucency suggests loosening or infection. The significance of wide or increasing cement-bone lucent zones is clearer if they occur on the femoral rather than on the acetabular side. In one study of the efficacy of the plain film in the diagnosis of loosening, no false-positive or false-negative results were found on the femoral side (using the criteria of a wide cement-bone or metal-cement lucency, change in component position, or the presence of an irregular, wide zone of bone resorption as evidence of loosening).[73] In contrast, of 50 acetabular components embedded in opaque ce-

Table 112–1. RADIOGRAPHIC FINDINGS SUGGESTING LOOSENING, AND/OR INFECTION, OR BOTH, OF CEMENTED TOTAL HIP PROSTHESES

Plain Film Findings
   Cement-bone lucency of 2 mm or more
   Widening of the cement-bone lucency
   Migration of prosthetic components
   Development or widening of metal-cement lucency
   Cement fracture
   Periosteal reaction
   Motion of components demonstrable on stress views
      or fluoroscopy

Arthrographic Findings
   Extension of contrast between the cement and bone or
      between the prosthesis and bone
   Filling of irregular para-articular cavities or fistulous
      tracts

Scintigraphic Findings
   Increased activity in the acetabular and/or femoral
      shaft regions after 6 to 10 months postoperatively
   Increased gallium uptake in comparison with bone
      agent uptake suggests infection

ment, there were five false-positive results and one false-negative result.

Other criteria for acetabular loosening have been proposed. Harris and Penenberg[74] described stages of acetabular loosening including definite loosening (documented by acetabular migration or a crack in the acetabular cement) and impending loosening (identified by a 2 mm or wider lucent zone along the entire cement bone interface). Patients with clear radiographic evidence of loosening may be asymptomatic. In these cases, however, careful follow-up is suggested because radiographic evidence of loosening may precede clinical symptoms.[72]

Radiographic assessment of lucent zones may be flawed by interobserver disagreements. One study of interobserver variability in the assessment of lucencies along cemented hip prostheses found that all three observers agreed on the maximum measured lucencies along the acetabular component in fewer than half of the cases.[75] There was 87 percent agreement on the femoral side.

A wide cement-bone lucency in cases of loosening has been shown to correspond not to a bland fibrous layer but to a synovium-like membrane capable of producing substances that stimulate bone resorption.[31, 76] This abnormal membrane may impede the flow of contrast material into the cement-bone interface at the time of arthrography. It is noteworthy that the diagnosis of infection cannot be reliably made from standard radiographs.

Histiocytic Response. Localized areas of bone resorption have been noted around loose cemented total hip prostheses. These lucent zones were first described by Harris et al.,[77] who noted extensive localized bone resorption around the femoral components of four patients. Histologic examination showed massive accumulation of macrophages, fibrin, necrotic debris, birefringent intracellular and

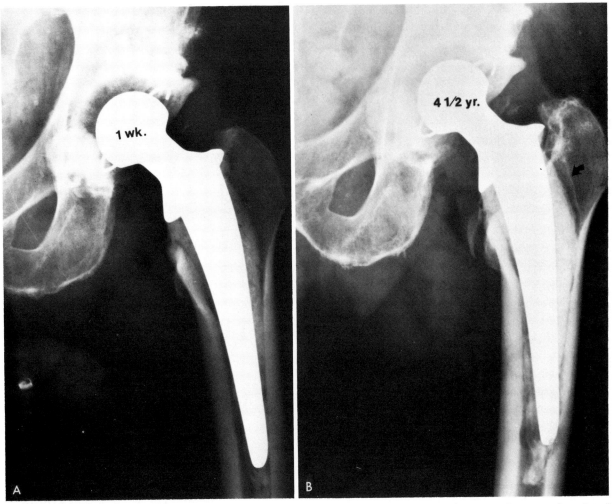

Figure 112–22. Loosening of femoral component. *A*, Examination 1 week postoperatively shows no lucency at the cement-bone interface of the femoral component and minimal lucency around the acetabular cement. *B*, Four and one-half years later, a lucent zone has developed at the cement-bone interface (*arrow*) of the femoral component, and the component has shifted to a more varus position. The lucent zone around the acetabular component has increased also, suggesting loosening. The patient was symptomatic.

extracellular particulate matter, some foreign body giant cells, and the absence of acute or chronic inflammatory cells. Areas previously containing cement particles were prominent. More recent immunopathologic studies of such aggressive granulomatous lesions have shown that these lesions differ from the more common findings of prosthetic loosening; a relative lack of fibroblasts is noted in aggressive granulomatosis. The condition seems to be a distinct entity probably caused by a foreign body reaction.[78]

Radiologically these large resorptive areas can usually be distinguished from areas of bone destruction owing to infection by the sharp, lobulated contours of the former in contrast to the irregular permeative destruction that may be seen in cases of infection (Fig. 112–23).[79]

Change in Position of Prosthetic Components. Motion resulting in a change in position of a component may occur between the cement and the bone or between the prosthesis and the cement. Four

patterns of femoral component loosening have been described (Fig. 112–24).[29] In the first and most common, there is pistoning of either the prosthesis within the acrylic cement or the prosthesis and cement within the bone. Loosening of the stem within the cement may be due to weak support at the proximal medial femoral neck and is seen as medial migration of the prosthesis with lucency at the cement-metal interface, usually along the lateral aspect. A crack in the cement at the tip of the prosthesis may be seen. When the loosening occurs between the cement and bone, a lucency wider than 2 mm or an increasing zone of lucency is noted.

The second mode of failure, termed the medial midstem pivot mode, results from poor support medially, migration of the distal stem, and a fracture of the acrylic cement in the midstem region.

The third category of femoral loosening consists of pivoting of the distal stem on the calcar, resulting from poor fixation distally. This is uncommon.

The fourth type of loosening results from poor

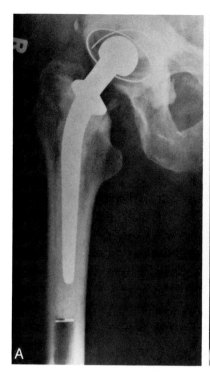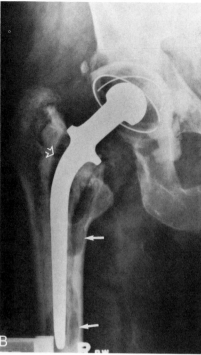

Figure 112–23. Histiocytic response. *A,* There is no evidence of loosening of the cemented total hip prosthesis. *B,* Follow-up radiograph shows extensive well-defined bone resorption (*arrows*), indicating a histiocytic response. Subsidence has occurred, leaving a cement-metal lucency proximally (*open arrow*).

support medially and proximally but good fixation of the distal stem. Medial migration of the proximal stem may occur, and fracture of the stem may result.

Acetabular component loosening may occur at the cement-bone interface or between the component and the cement. A change in the orientation of the acetabular component on serial examinations may be noted. A change in acetabular component position of greater than 4 mm or 4 degrees documents loosening.[80] Superior migration or developing protrusio deformity may be assessed using the previously described reference lines or Muller template[8] (see Fig. 112–6).

Development or Widening of a Metal-Cement Lucency. Separation between the femoral prosthesis and the cement is most frequently seen along the proximal lateral aspect of the femoral stem (Fig. 112–25). Although Beabout[16] states that there should be "intimate contact between the acrylic cement and the femoral prosthesis," lucencies in this area are noted in the immediate postoperative period and on follow-up examination in 3.6[84] to 24 percent[26] of patients. When this is seen early in the postoperative period, it is likely that the cement did not remain in contact with that portion of the femoral component (owing to motion of the component while the methacrylate was setting)[23] or that the cement was eccentrically placed along a portion of the stem. In these cases, loosening should not be suggested. Some cases of stable 1- to 2-mm lucent zones at the cement-metal interface have been shown to be due to the Mach effect,[81] a visual phenomenon in which accentuation of high-contrast borders of objects occurs as a result of lateral inhibition produced by the neural networks in the eye.[82]

Later development of lucency between the femoral component and the adjacent cement has been referred to as subsidence.[83] The prosthesis sinks

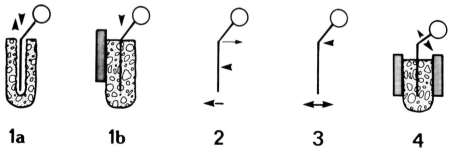

Figure 112–24. Modes of loosening. Four modes of loosening have been distinguished by Gruen, McNeice, and Amstutz. In type 1, there is pistoning of either the metal stem within the cement (*1a*) or the cement within the bone (*1b*). In type 2, there is medial migration of the proximal stem and lateral migration of the tip of the stem. Type 3 is characterized by poor support distally, the prosthesis pivoting on the medial femoral cortex. In type 4, there is poor support proximally, with medial migration of the proximal stem, while the distal stem remains fixed. The stem may subsequently bend or break.

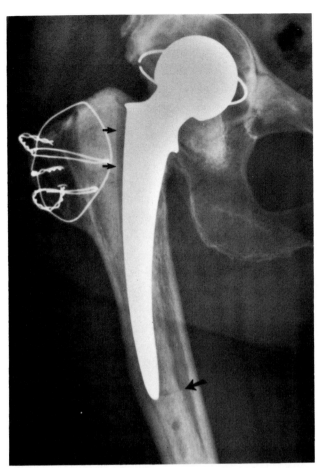

Figure 112–25. Metal-cement lucency. The femoral component has settled into a varus position with development of lucency at the metal-cement interface superolaterally (*small arrows*), remodeling of the lateral femoral cortex, and fracture of the distal cement (*large arrow*).

inferiorly and medially, and at least according to Charnley, a new point of stability is reached.[26, 83] This view is in concert with the findings of DeSmet et al.[81] in which a metal-cement lucency was present along the lateral aspect of 23 of 101 Charnley-Muller total hip prostheses, although only four of these hips had clinical evidence of infection or loosening. Weber and Charnley[83] studied a group of patients with cement fracture and also noted that patients with subsidence of up to 3.5 mm generally had good or excellent clinical results. Even progressive widening of this lucency may be seen in patients without clinical evidence of loosening. Beckenbaugh and Ilstrup[26] noted a higher incidence of pain in patients with more than 2 mm of drift.

Subsidence may be associated with radiographically demonstrable cement fracture, but presumably all cases have cement fracture or breakdown as the underlying mechanism. Beckenbaugh and Ilstrup[26] noted that subsidence occurred least often when all the bone is removed medially at the level of the lesser trochanter and more than 0.5 cm of cement is present and when the cancellous bone is removed along the lateral aspect of the distal two thirds of the

shaft and the canal filled with cement to a level of greater than 2 cm past the tip of the femoral component.

Cement Fracture. A transverse fracture through he opaque cement was noted near the tip of the femoral component in 1.5 percent of 6649 hips studied by Weber and Charnley.[83] In most cases, the fracture was demonstrable within the first postoperative year (see Fig. 112–25). Most (70 percent[83]) patients with distal cement fracture show medial migration of the proximal femoral stem ("subsidence")[23] (see earlier). Cement fracture may also occur in the midstem region when there is poor support distally as well as proximally. As with other findings of loosening, however, the majority of patients with cement fracture are asymptomatic.[83]

Periosteal Reaction. Cortical thickening and periosteal reaction may occur with or without infection or loosening. Salvati et al.[17] noted that in four hips with periosteal reaction near the tip of the femoral component, cortical thickening occurred laterally when the stem was in varus and both medially and laterally when the stem was in neutral position. Dussault et al.[72] suggest that periosteal reaction tends to be thicker and more uniform in cases of loosening alone and more lamellar when associated with infection.

Visible Motion of Components on Radiographic Examination. Stress views (push, pull, adduction, or abduction) or fluoroscopy may demonstrate motion of one or both components (Fig. 112–26). Usually such examination is done at the time of fluoroscopy for joint aspiration and arthrography.

Osteomyelitis. Radiographic evidence of osteomyelitis, including bone destruction, sclerosis, and irregular cortical thickening, is occasionally seen (Fig. 112–27).

Myositis Ossificans. Some studies have suggested a higher incidence of infection in patients with ectopic bone.

Loosening or Infection of Prostheses

Loosening is thought not to be a major problem after bone ingrowth prosthetic fixation. Engh et al.,[84] however, found 12 percent of femoral components to exhibit migration (loosening) 8 years after surgery. Radiographic evidence of loosening includes the development of a thin sclerotic line separated by several millimeters (probably more than 2 mm) from the prosthesis at the area for bone ingrowth, separation of surface beads as follow-up progresses, and change in component position ("migration") after the usual period of stabilization (Fig. 112–28).

Histologic studies of loose biologic fixation implants have shown a synovium-like membrane in some cases (similar to that seen around loose cemented prostheses) with vascular connective tissue and islands of woven bone. Metal debris and metal-containing macrophages have been described.[85]

Press-fit femoral components require tight fit of

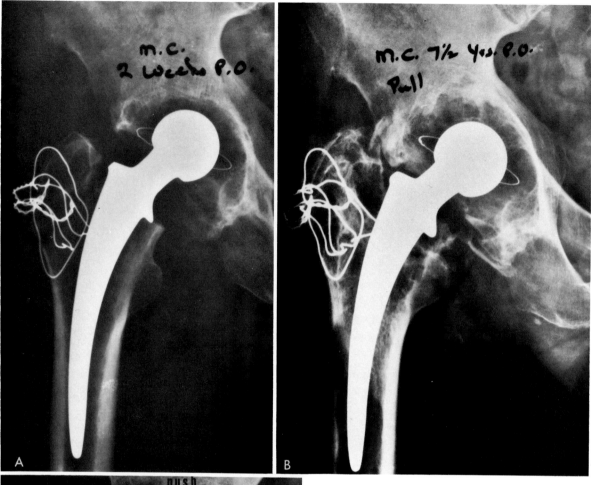

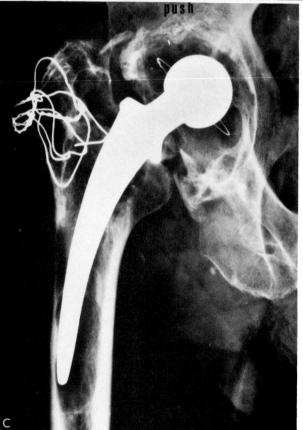

Figure 112–26. Stress views. *A*, A radiograph 2 weeks postoperatively shows a total hip prosthesis with nonopaque cement around the components. *B* and *C*, Radiographs 7 and a half years postoperatively show increasing lucency, particularly around the distal stem of the femoral component. "Push" (*C*) and "pull" (*B*) films confirm motion of the femoral component, most easily seen by noting the change in the distance between the flange of the prosthesis and the lesser trochanter and the change in position of the tip of the stem within the medullary canal.

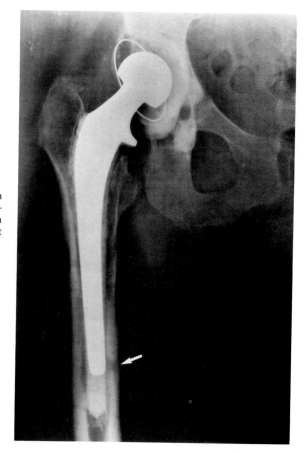

Figure 112–27. Infected total hip replacement. There is loosening of both acetabular and femoral components. The localized areas of bone destruction (cloacae, *arrow*) indicate the infectious nature of the process. (From Weissman, B. N.: Current topics in the radiology of joint replacement surgery. Radiol. Clin. North Am. 28:1111, 1990. Used by permission.)

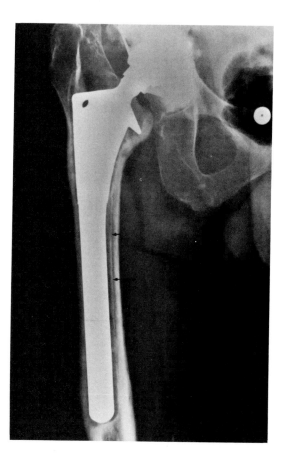

Figure 112–28. Loose bone ingrowth femoral component. The femoral stem has settled into the femur. There is a wide lucent zone around the component (*arrows*) including the area for bone ingrowth. There is periosteal reaction at the tip of the component.

the component into the femur. A lucent zone of 2 mm or more documents loosening.

Arthrography for the Evaluation of Loosening or Infection. Hip aspiration and arthrography are usually performed before total joint replacement when there is a history of sepsis or previous surgery and after cemented THR if pain continues or whenever infection is suspected.[86] Gould et al.[87] argue that aspiration is unnecessary before revision surgery if the physician has a low clinical suspicion for infection.[87] This retrospective review of 78 such cases demonstrated that when there was no clinical suspicion of infection, none of the patients had infection documented by joint aspiration.

Injection of contrast material should virtually always follow aspiration because it permits confirmation of intra-articular needle position as well as assessment of local anatomy. Arthrography may demonstrate loosening of prosthetic components or irregular para-articular cavities virtually diagnostic of infection.

The arthrographic method followed at the Brigham and Women's Hospital is similar to that originally described by Salvati et al.[88] except that provision is made for subtraction (photographic or digital)[89] when this is thought to be necessary (Fig. 112–29). "K-edge energy subtraction radiography" has been described, although we have not used it.[90] The method eliminates the need for continued patient immobility before and after contrast injection.

Preliminary anteroposterior and frog lateral films that include the entire prosthesis and adjacent cement are reviewed. The patient is placed supine on the table, and after the area is prepared and draped, 1 percent lidocaine is injected into the skin and subcutaneous tissue lateral to the femoral artery and distal to the inguinal ligament. A 20-gauge, disposable short beveled spinal needle is inserted and directed toward the neck of the prosthesis until the needle contacts metal. Usually an oblique needle course is preferred so the path of the needle can be seen fluoroscopically, unobscured by the metal femoral component. If joint fluid can be aspirated, a sample is removed and sent for bacteriologic study.

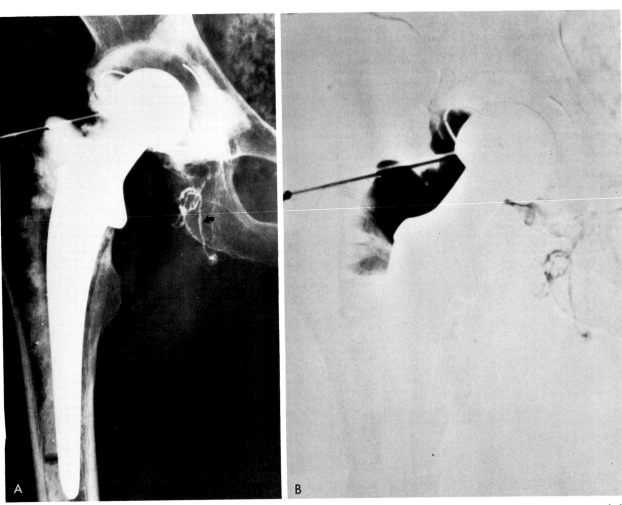

Figure 112–29. Subtraction technique. *A,* Arthrogram showing lymphatic filling (*arrow*). Because of the opaque cement around the components, contrast material around the cement or components is difficult to see. *B,* Photographic subtraction (same patient as in *A*) allows differentiation between injected contrast material and opaque cement. There is no arthrographic evidence of loosening, although the cement fracture is radiographic evidence of loosening.

If no fluid can be aspirated, sterile isotonic saline (not bacteriostatic saline or lidocaine) is injected and reaspirated in an effort to obtain material for culture. Whether or not joint fluid is aspirated, contrast material is always injected. The stylet is removed, and a syringe and extension tubing with about 25 ml of Reno-M-60 are attached to the needle. A few drops of contrast material are then injected. If the needle is within the joint capsule, the contrast material will flow away from the needle tip. A radiograph is then taken to be used for subtraction, and the patient is instructed to remain motionless. If the tip of the needle is extra-articular, the small amount of injected contrast material will remain at the tip of the needle. The needle is then repositioned.

When satisfactory needle placement is confirmed, contrast material is injected under fluoroscopic monitoring. A radiograph is then taken and the needle withdrawn. Usually less than 15 ml of contrast material is sufficient to fill the joint, but considerably more may be necessary. Some authors suggest contrast instillation until the patient complains of pain,[91] there is resistance to injection, lymphatic opacification[92] occurs, or contrast is seen along the entire cement-bone interface.[91, 92] Underfilling may lead to failure to demonstrate abnormal collections of contrast material or loosening of components.[91] Once the needle has been removed, the hip is exercised and repeat anteroposterior films with traction applied to the leg may be done. The patient is then instructed to walk around the room, and anteroposterior and lateral radiographs are repeated, with additional views if necessary. Traction films and films after walking[93] have, on occasion, shown evidence of loosening not demonstrable on standard views.

A normal postoperative arthrogram demonstrates filling of a small, smooth "pseudojoint" space that forms within 4 to 5 months postoperatively.[16] Contrast material parallels the neck of the prosthesis and flares out proximally under the acetabular component and distally along and sometimes under the flanges of the femoral component.

Abnormal arthrographic findings include extension of contrast material along the cement-bone or prosthesis-cement interface, filling of irregular cavities, and lymphatic filling (see Table 112–2).

Extension of Contrast Material Along the Cement-Bone or Metal-Cement Interface. Arthrography for the evaluation of patients with persistent pain after THR was introduced by Salvati et al. in 1971.[88] Surgical or clinical confirmation of their arthrographic findings in 33 hips (31 arthrograms) revealed only one case in which a loose femoral component was not demonstrated by arthrography. The appearance of contrast material between the acrylic cement and bone seemed to be conclusive proof of loosening (Fig. 112–30). These investigators noted that although "an arthrogram does not definitely rule out the presence of a complication, a positive arthrogram appears to be diagnostic."[88]

Subsequent studies have compared arthrographic evidence of loosening (contrast material at the cement-bone or metal-cement interface) with evidence of motion of components following manual stress at the time of surgical re-exploration (Table 112–2). The study by Murray and Rodrigo in 1975[94] is of particular interest because the conclusion reached was that "arthrographic evidence of loosening may not identify the cause of pain after total hip replacement." These investigators evaluated the arthrographic findings in 53 asymptomatic total hip prostheses (21 patients). Arthrographic evidence of loosening of the acetabular component was noted in 22.6 percent of asymptomatic hips. No asymptomatic patients demonstrated loosening of the femoral component. Twelve patients with pain underwent reoperation. In seven patients, loosening demonstrated by arthrography was confirmed at surgery (true positive rate, 78 percent). There were three patients in whom loosening of the acetabular component was demonstrated at arthrography but not at surgery and two patients with normal arthrograms but loosening demonstrated at surgery. Thus, acetabular loosening may be asymptomatic, and loosening demonstrated on arthrography may not correlate with loosening demonstrated at the time of surgery.

Studies with high-injection pressure suggest improved diagnostic accuracy. Thus, Hendrix et al.[91] used a high-pressure injection method and noted marked improvement in the accuracy of arthrography in comparison with low-volume injections. The sensitivity for the detection of acetabular loosening was 20/21 (95 percent; specificity 83 percent) and femoral component loosening was 21/22 (95 percent). This compares with a sensitivity of 10 percent for the femoral component and 48 percent for the acetabular component when only 5 ml of contrast material were injected.

Maus et al.[92] also attempted to obtain high intra-articular pressures by continuing injections of contrast material until significant lymphatic filling or pain occurred. The sensitivity for evaluation of loosening of the femoral component was 96 percent, and the specificity was 92 percent. The sensitivity on the acetabular side was 97 percent, but the specificity was only 68 percent. It was noted that the presence of a large pseudocapsule or bursa may lower intracapsular pressure and produce spuriously negative examinations for component loosening.

Arthrographic Criteria for Loosening. Initial arthrographic studies for prosthetic loosening mentioned contrast along the cement-bone interface as the single criterion for loosening.[88] More recent studies have defined the criteria for loosening based on correlative surgical findings. Maus et al.,[92] for example, use the criteria listed in Table 112–3 for identifying loosening.

The presence of a medium or large pseudocapsule or connection to a bursa decompresses the capsule, leading to lower intra-articular pressure and false-negative studies. False-positive cases are con-

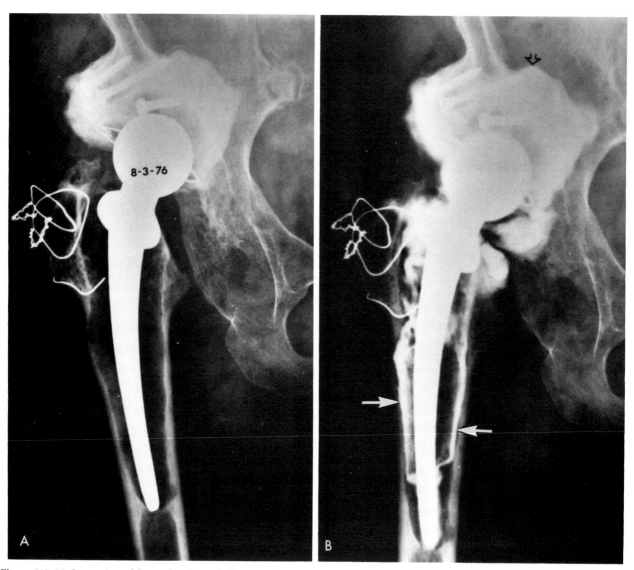

Figure 112–30. Loosening of femoral and acetabular components. *A,* Examination 3 years after surgery shows irregular lucency around the femoral component, which was wider than that attributable to the nonopaque cement present previously. A thin, lucent zone is noted around the opaque cement of the acetabular component. *B,* Arthrography confirms loosening of both components with contrast material at the cement-bone interface of each component (*arrows*). Note the difficulty in visualizing the contrast material around the opaque acetabular cement.

Table 112–2. CORRELATION OF ARTHROGRAPHIC EVIDENCE OF LOOSENING (WITH OR WITHOUT INFECTION) WITH CLINICAL OR SURGICAL FINDINGS (TOTAL HIP REPLACEMENT)

Study	Patients	True-Positive Rate	False-Positive Rate
Salvati et al., 1971	29 (30 hips) 8 not loose 7 loose 9 loose and infected 2 infected but not loose 3 miscellaneous conditions	16/17	0/13
Selby, Brown, and Knickerbocker, 1973	16 surgically proven cases	13/14	1/2
Murray and Rodrigo, 1975	12 with pain and reoperation	7/9	3/3
McLaughlin and Whitehill, 1977	5 with acetabular loosening and re-operation	5/5	
Gelman et al., 1978	9 with painful total hip replacements and surgical evidence of 14 loose components	14/14	1/4
Hendrix et al., 1983	31 with hip pain and subsequent revision	20/21 (acetabular) 21/22 (femoral)	2/10 1/6
Maus et al., 1987	97 surgical revisions	65/73 (femoral)	2/24
Tehranzadeh et al., 1988	15 cases	13/14	0/1
Wellman et al., 1988	65 cases	26/40	4/25
Walker et al., 1991	53 surgical revisions, digital subtraction	46/48 (femoral) 20/24 (acetabular)	0/5 (femoral) 4/20 (acetabular)
Weighted average		266/301 (88%)	23/113 (20%)

siderably more common on the acetabular than on the femoral side.

The accuracy of the arthrogram in demonstrating loosening is complicated by ambiguity in the term "loosening." Logic suggests, however, that contrast along the cement-bone or metal-cement interface denotes poor bonding between these materials, and in this sense, they are loose. Pending the outcome of long-term studies correlating arthrographic findings with clinical outcome, it seems prudent to evaluate each arthrogram carefully for evidence of "loosening" and to consider the arthrographic findings only in light of the patient's clinical symptoms. Demonstration of contrast at the cement-bone interface of the femoral component seems more reliable than similar findings on the acetabular side. In general, false-positive cases are more common on the acetabular side (lower specificity), and false-negative cases are more common on the femoral side (lower sensitivity).

Arthrography in the Evaluation of Uncemented Prostheses. Swan et al.[95] performed contrast arthrograms in patients with hip pain after insertion of bone ingrowth femoral components. The arthrogram was considered positive for loosening if contrast material was present at the metal bone interface for more than 3 mm past the calcar (Fig. 112–31). Correlation with the presence of gross motion at surgery in 12 patients showed that the arthrogram predicted the true status of the femoral component in seven cases (five true-positive and two true-negative). Five false-negative arthrographic studies were recorded (sensitivity 50 percent, specificity 100 percent). One possible explanation for this low sensitivity is that high-pressure injections were not used. There were no false-positive examinations. In another study, however, an anecdotal case demonstrated extensive penetration of contrast material along the femoral component at arthrography with filling of the medullary and profunda veins, but no loosening was found at surgical exploration.[96] The final criteria for evaluating arthrographic findings after insertion of a bone ingrowth prosthesis have yet to be established.

Filling of Irregular Para-articular Cavities or Fistulous Tracts. These findings are considerably less controversial. The filling of irregular para-articular cavities or fistulas indicates infection. Infection was found, for example, in all five patients reviewed by Dussault et al.,[72] who demonstrated filling of such cavities. Aspiration of a loculated collection may be necessary to confirm infection. It should be noted, however, that infection may be present in the absence of abnormal radiographic findings (i.e., cavities, fistulas, or loosening).

Lymphatic Opacification. This was seen in 12 patients studied by Dussault et al.[72] Four had no loosening or infection, three had both loosening and

Table 112–3. CRITERIA FOR LOOSENING ON ARTHROGRAPHY

	Percentage Loose at Surgery
Acetabular Component	
Cement-bone contrast in all zones	90
Contrast in zones I and II or I and III	90
Contrast in zones I and III with medium or large pseudocapsule or bursa	57
Rim of contrast greater than 2 mm thick in any zone	95
Femoral Component	
Cement-bone contrast distal to intertrochanteric line or midcomponent in long-stemmed prostheses	98
Metal-cement contrast below intertrochanteric line	95
Positive signs on plain radiographs in patient with medium or large pseudocapsule or bursa	

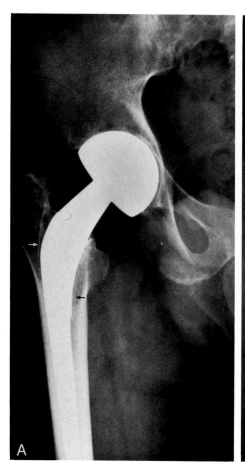

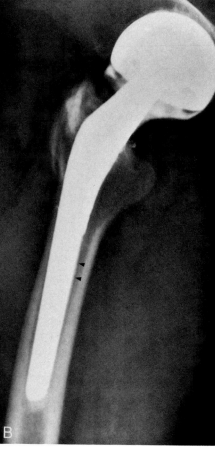

Figure 112–31. Loose bone ingrowth prosthesis. *A,* There is loosening of the femoral component of the bipolar prosthesis with wide bone-prosthesis lucencies (*arrows*) and dislodged metal beads. *B,* The arthrogram demonstrates contrast material (*arrowheads*) tracking along the femoral component.

infection, and five had loosening only. As discussed by Coren et al.,[97] resorption of injected contrast material from normal joints occurs through venous and lymphatic channels. Lymphatic visualization may be noted when the resorption rate is increased, apparently resulting from increased permeability of the synovial lining and hyperplasia of the lymphatic system. Although lymphatic visualization is usually associated with rheumatoid arthritis, these workers suggest that it is a nonspecific sign of inflammation (see Fig. 112–29). Despite this, Bloom et al.[98] found that lymphatic filling occurred in 40 percent of 52 subtraction arthrograms, and in 15 operated cases component loosening was confirmed. Thus, lymphatic opacification seemed to indicate that loosening was indeed present.

Other Findings on Arthrography. Arthrography following placement of a total hip prosthesis may also demonstrate filling of the trochanteric bursa, suggesting trochanteric bursitis, occult fracture of the femoral stem,[86] nonunion of the greater trochanter, and postoperative hematoma preventing reduction of a dislocated femoral component.

Anesthetic Arthrography. Following joint aspiration, 5 to 10 ml of 1 percent lidocaine[99] or 2 to 3 ml of 0.25 percent bupivacaine may be injected into the joint along with the contrast material. Pain relief suggests that symptoms are due to an intraarticular process, whereas lack of relief is said to be nonspecific.[92] Burton et al.[100] noted relief of pain after intra-articular lidocaine injection to be associated with surgically confirmed intra-articular abnormality (e.g., loosening) in 95 percent of cases. In another series, pain relief after anesthetic injection was shown to accompany acetabular loosening, whereas results in patients with femoral component loosening were variable.[101]

Joint Fluid Aspiration. The results of aspiration may be misleading. Even when infection is present, aspiration of joint fluid may yield negative cultures.[92] The sensitivity for infection in one study was only 12 percent.[102] False-positive cases also occur.

Effect of Arthrography on the Interpretation of a Subsequent Bone Scan. Animal studies have shown that the performance of an arthrogram or joint aspiration and the injection of normal saline does not result in significantly increased uptake on bone scan.[103] This is true even when several attempts at aspiration are necessary.

Scintigraphy

Bone Scanning. Campeau et al.[104] performed serial technetium 99m (Tc 99m) bone scans on patients undergoing THR and found increased isotopic activity in the acetabular and femoral shaft regions in all patients during the first 3 months. By 6 months, the activity returned to normal levels in those patients without complication. Prospective review of 97 asymptomatic hip prostheses confirmed that most patients exhibit a normal bone scan by about 1 year after surgery.[105] In 9 percent, however, persistent definite increase in uptake was noted at the tips of the prostheses after 1 year, and this finding became increasingly frequent in later years, perhaps because of the onset of asymptomatic loosening.

Bone scans after insertion of a bone ingrowth prosthesis may normally show increased uptake at the tip of the femoral component.[106] Oswald et al.[107] followed patients with porous-coated hip prostheses and no apparent complications. Increased uptake of Tc 99m methylene diphosphonate (MDP) was seen near the tips of the femoral stems in all cases sometime during the first 24 months after arthroplasty. Blood flow studies were usually normal. Blood pool examination showed diffuse activity over the thigh in 11 of 25 prostheses, but focal blood pool activity was unusual and mild if present.

Press-fit components may normally display focal uptake proximally and distally on bone scans obtained within the first year after surgery.[108]

Abnormal Findings. Campeau et al.[104] found that patients with increased activity 6 months or more postoperatively all had loosening or infection, and often the routine radiographs were normal. No patient with a proven complication had a normal scan. Thus, a negative bone scan virtually excluded the presence of significant loosening or infection.[109, 110] A few false-negative studies, however, are reported, particularly on the acetabular side.[73, 111, 110] Chafetz et al.[112] performed bone and gallium scans in 111 patients with symptomatic total joint prostheses (86 hips, 23 knees, two shoulders). Analysis of surgical data and (greater than 1.5 year) follow-up showed the sensitivity of the method for loosening to be 67 percent and the specificity 55 percent. Although the positive predictive value of 79 percent was considered quite acceptable, the low sensitivities and specificities led to their "not advocating this approach to the evaluation of symptomatic prosthetic joints."[112] This conclusion is supported by Aliabadi et al.[113] who found that even the combination of bone scan and radiographic examination resulted in a sensitivity of 84 percent for the diagnosis of loosening. Thus, even with this standard set of examinations, loosening of cemented prostheses may not be detected.

Distribution of Abnormal Uptake. The distribution of abnormal isotopic activity has been thought to distinguish between cases of infection and aseptic loosening[73] (Fig. 112–32). In one series, the diffuse uptake pattern around both components correctly identified all infected prostheses.[73] Our own studies, however, do not confirm these findings, and all patients with infected total hip prostheses studied with bone scans actually demonstrated the focal pattern of isotopic uptake.[113]

Gallium Scanning. Gallium accumulation in inflammatory conditions is largely due to uptake by leukocytes, although uptake by various bacteria has also been demonstrated.[35] Gallium scans must be correlated with the Tc 99m bone scan because the factors that increase the uptake of bone tracer will also increase the uptake of gallium (Table 112–4).

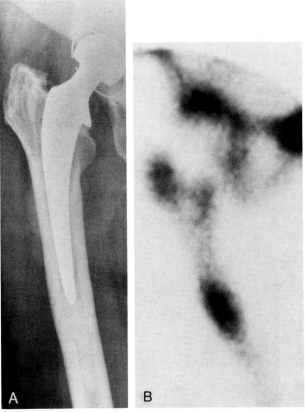

A   B

Figure 112–32. Loose cemented total hip prosthesis. *A,* There is subsidence of the femoral component with a wide metal-cement lucent zone proximally. Periosteal reaction has thickened the cortex laterally near the tip of the stem. The acetabular component cement-bone interface is not well seen. *B,* The bone scan confirms loosening of both components with focal uptake of isotope at the proximal and distal portions of the femoral component and along the acetabulum. (From Weissman, B. N.: Current topics in the radiology of joint replacement surgery. Radiol. Clin. North Am. 28:1111, 1990. Used by permission.)

When an "incongruent" distribution of gallium with relation to the technetium bone scan (that is, gallium uptake in areas that are not "hot" on bone scan) or intense uptake of gallium as well as technetium phosphate complexes is present, infection is suggested. Thus, a study of patients with different types of orthopedic hardware using both gallium 67 and Tc 99m MDP scans enabled three groups to be distinguished.[115] In the first group, the gallium image

Table 112–4. GALLIUM STUDIES FOR DETECTION OF INFECTED PROSTHESES

Study	Sensitivity (%)	Specificity (%)
Horoszowski et al., 1980[113b]	100	75
Williams et al., 1981[113c]	93	92
McKillop et al., 1984[113a]	83	79
Merkel et al., 1985[119]	57*	89
Chafetz et al., 1985[112]	70	72
Mountford et al., 1986[114]	83	81
Tehranzadeh et al., 1988[94a]	80	100
Aliabadi et al., 1989[113]	37	100

*With technetium bone scan.

Table 112–5. INDIUM-111 WHITE BLOOD CELL SCANNING FOR PROSTHETIC LOOSENING (TJRs)

Study	Sensitivity (%)	Specificity (%)
McKillop et al., 1984[113a]	50	100
Merkel et al., 1985[119]	86	100
Pring et al., 1986[117]	100	90
Mountford et al., 1986[114]	73	95
Wukich et al., 1987[118]	100	45
Magnuson et al., 1988[119a]	88	73
Johnson et al., 1988[102]	100	50
	88*	95*
Zilkens et al., 1988[120a]	72 (acetabular)	57
	75 (femoral)	40

*Interpreted with bone scan.

was negative, and the technetium bone scan was positive or negative; none of these patients had inflammatory disease. In the second group, the gallium scan was positive, but its distribution was similar to the uptake on bone scan. Fifteen of these 16 patients had no inflammatory disease, and the sixteenth had a sterile bursitis. In the third group, the gallium scan was positive in an "incongruent" spatial distribution in comparison with the technetium bone scan; all 18 patients had inflammatory disorders, including osteomyelitis, cellulitis, and nonseptic synovitis. Similarly, Reing et al.[116] noted positive gallium citrate scans in 18 of 19 patients who were subsequently proved at surgery to be infected. There were no false-positive gallium scans. Aliabadi et al.[113] confirmed the paucity of false-positive scans but noted the gallium scan to be an insensitive indicator of infection (33 percent). Thus, a positive scan strongly suggests that infection is present, whereas a negative study does not exclude it.

Indium White Cell Scanning. Indium III–labeled leukocytes have been used with some success to identify infection following THR.[35, 114, 117, 118] In comparison with gallium 67 citrate, indium 111–labeled white cells have better imaging characteristics and a higher ratio of abscess to blood activity. Pring et al.[117] detected all infected prostheses using indium-granulocyte scanning. Specificity was 89.5 percent Although the indium scan seems quite sensitive (a negative study essentially excludes osteomyelitis), it is nonspecific, and false-positive results occur (Table 112–5).[118] Distinction between overlying cellulitis and an infected prosthesis may require an additional bone scan; specificity is improved by correlation with activity on bone scans. The test appears in general to

be superior to gallium imaging for the evaluation of a possibly infected joint replacement.[120]

Technetium-Labeled White Cells. Tc 99m–labeled white blood cells have several advantages over the indium 111–labeled cells, which require skill in preparation, are relatively expensive, and provide a relatively high radiation dose to the spleen. Roddie et al.[121] used Tc 99m–labeled white blood cells and found 100 percent sensitivity and 93 percent specificity for the diagnosis of musculoskeletal infection.

Radionuclide Arthrography. Intra-articular injection of isotope has been used to detect prosthetic loosening in the hip and knee (Table 112–6).[120–125] The isotope (usually Tc 99m sulfur colloid) is usually instilled at the time of contrast arthrography. When no loosening is present, the isotope remains confined to the area of the joint capsule; in cases with loosening, isotope is detected around the affected component (Fig. 112–33). The isotope arthrogram may show more extensive migration of isotope along the component than does the contrast arthrogram. Thus, the isotope study is said to complement the arthrogram, with the sensitivity of the combined examination being 100 percent in one series.[124] The acetabular component is difficult to evaluate, and the isotope examination is used almost exclusively to study the femoral component. Study by Maxon et al.[125] using intra-articular indium 111 with pentetic acid (DTPA) found the radionuclide study to be more specific (owing to the absence of false-negative studies).[125]

Disengagement of Components

Modular total hip prostheses usually consist of a metallic femoral stem, a head neck piece, a metal backing for the acetabular component, and a high-density polyethylene acetabular liner.[126, 127] Dislocation of the acetabular liner from the metal backing or disengagement of the femoral head from the neck have been reported after attempts at reduction of prosthetic dislocations. The dislocated acetabular liner may be difficult to see on radiographs, and care is necessary to identify the relatively lucent liner against the soft tissue density of adjacent structures (Fig. 112–34). Asymmetry in the position of the reduced femoral head in the acetabulum or protrusion of the femoral component deep into the metal of the acetabular backing should suggest that the polyethylene liner is displaced or disrupted.[127]

Table 112–6. ARTHROSCINTIGRAPHY

Study	Isotope	Sensitivity (%)	Specificity (%)
Resnik et al., 1986[124]	Tc-99m sulfur colloid	93	75
Wellman et al., 1988[120]	In-111 chloride	90	92
Maxon et al., 1989[125]	Intravenous: Tc-99m HDP Intra-articular: In-111 DTPA	64	100
Swan et al., 1991[95]	Intravenous: Tc-99m HDP Intra-articular: In-111 chloride	70	100

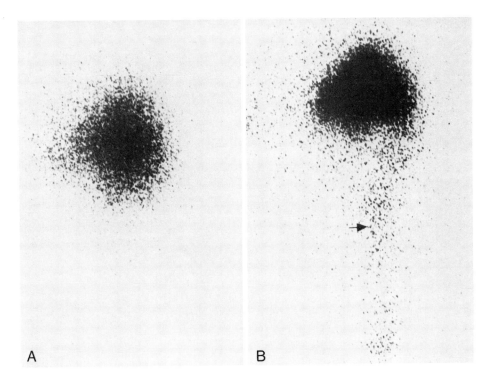

Figure 112–33. Scintarthrography. *A,* Normal arthroscintigram. The ^{111}In was injected into the joint at the times of arthrography and remains confined to the joint pseudocapsule. *B,* Loosening. There is distal tracking (*arrowhead*) of the radionuclide. (From Swan, J. S., Braunstein, E. M., Wellman, H. N., and Capello, W.: Contrast and nuclear arthrography in loosening of uncemented hip prosthesis. Skeletal Radiol. 20:15, 1991. Used by permission.)

Lysis Around Uncemented Stable Femoral Components

Osteolysis around cemented femoral components is well known. Maloney and Harris[45] have reported endosteal erosion around bone ingrowth femoral components that were not apparently loose. Usually the osteolysis occurred more than 3 years after surgery. Histologic examination in two cases with surgical revision showed focal aggregates of macrophages with particulate polyethylene and metal. A biopsy specimen in another patient, however, did not reveal foreign material.

Femoral Component Fractures

Fractures of the femoral component are usually fatigue fractures, resulting from poor support of the femoral stem. The stress placed on the unsupported cement may lead to cement fracture and medial or distal migration of the femoral stem and cement ("subsidence"). Subsequent fracture of the cement near the tip or the neck of the femoral component may result in further shift of the prosthesis and additional stress on the femoral stem. Over months or years there is widening of the cement-metal lucency along the lateral aspect of the femoral component. The end result of continued unsupported weight bearing by the femoral component may be bending or fracture of the femoral stem. Several radiographic findings document the aforementioned sequence of events and should suggest the need for careful follow-up examination and search for small defects in continuity of the femoral component.

Thus, early breakage of trochanter wires, resorption of bone along the medial femoral neck, appearance of a metal-cement lucency along the proximal femoral component laterally, widening of the cement-bone lucency laterally, and cement fracture may all precede fracture of the femoral stem. The actual fracture may be difficult to demonstrate (Fig. 112–35) Factors thought to be associated with increased risk of stem fracture[128, 129] include lack of valgus position of the femoral component, inadequate cement support, metallurgic imperfections in the prosthesis, increased patient height or weight, and porous coating.

Femoral and Pelvic Fractures

Femoral fractures may occur intraoperatively and are occasionally difficult to recognize on the anteroposterior examination done with a mobile x-ray unit. Opaque cement in the soft tissue adjacent to the femoral shaft indicates the presence of a fracture and suggests the need for additional views. Penetration of the femoral cortex by the tip of the prosthesis may also be associated with methyl methacrylate in the soft tissues and may result in apparent foreshortening of the stem of the femoral component on the frontal radiographs. Fractures may occur during press-fitting of uncemented prostheses (Fig. 112–36).

Postoperative fractures have been divided into three categories by McElfresh and Coventry:[130] stress fractures, fractures caused by stress raisers in the femoral shaft, and fractures caused by severe trauma.

Stress fractures occur in patients with severe osteopenia, such as those with longstanding rheumatoid arthritis.[131] These fractures appear to be re-

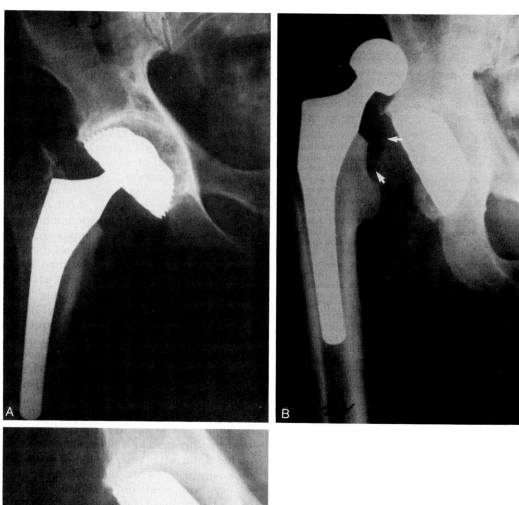

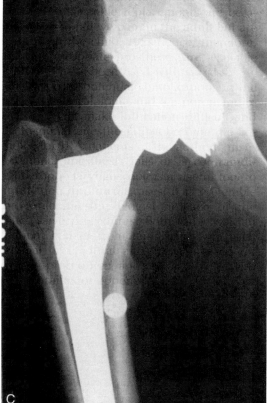

Figure 112–34. Displacement of acetabular liner. *A,* The femoral head projects medial to the metal backing of the acetabular component. *B,* A film taken prior to *A* shows dislocation of the femoral component from the acetabular component. The nonopaque acetabular liner has become separated from the metal backing and is faintly seen (*arrows*). *C,* Film taken after reoperation shows the usual appearances. The femoral head is seated in the nonopaque acetabular liner and does not protrude medially. (Courtesy of Dr. Arthur H. Newberg, New England Baptist Hospital, Boston, Massachusetts.)

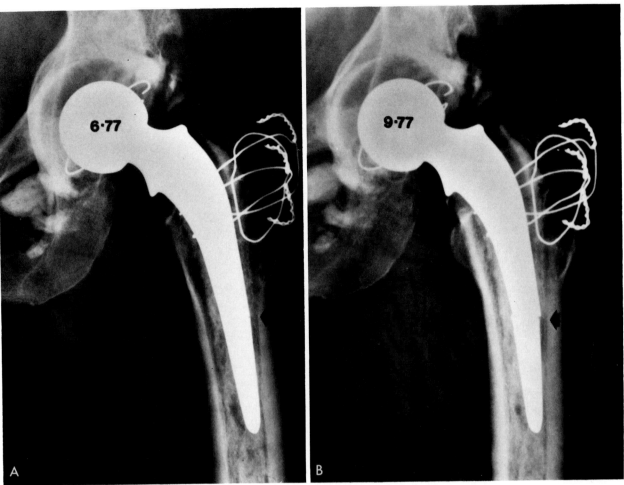

Figure 112–35. Femoral stem fracture. *A,* A metal-cement lucency is present owing to settling of the femoral component. The stem fracture *(arrow)* is difficult to see and was missed on initial evaluation. *B,* The stem fracture is now obvious *(arrow).*

lated to the increased activity made possible by joint replacement, and as such they should be termed "insufficiency" fractures because they are the result of normal stresses applied to abnormal bone. Stress fracture of the femur after insertion of a bone ingrowth prosthesis has been suggested as a cause of midthigh pain on initial weight bearing that does not subside with walking. Typically, symptoms occur between 3 and 6 months after surgery when remodeling is taking place. Radiographic findings of a well-fixed stem with sclerosis or periosteal reaction at the region of tightest fit in the medullary canal are seen.[33] Patients typically are described as older, with large intramedullary canals, thin cortices, and a large-diameter stem.

The second type of fracture results from local factors that increase stress at a particular point. For example, fractures may occur following relatively minor trauma if there is any defect in the femoral cortex, such as might be produced during reaming of the femur in the osteoporotic patient or by prior surgery (i.e., a screwhole). McElfresh and Coventry recommend having methyl methacrylate around the tip of the prosthesis and extending at least 2 cm distally to prevent undue stress concentration at the tip of the prosthesis.[130]

The third category of fracture occurs following trauma sufficient to fracture a normal limb. Because the endosteal blood supply has been compromised by the surgical procedure, fractures occurring near a femoral component are often treated with closed reduction if adequate alignment and apposition of fracture fragments can be achieved. Open reduction with stripping of the periosteum may jeopardize the blood supply to the proximal fragment. Methyl methacrylate does not appear to interfere with fracture healing.

Para-articular Ossification

Bone develops within para-articular soft tissues in up to 39 percent of patients following THR.[17] Although in most instances this appears to be of little clinical consequence, Beckenbaugh and Ilstrup[26] have noted lower hip scores in these patients. In a few patients, surgical intervention is necessary to remove ectopic bone if it significantly interferes with joint motion.

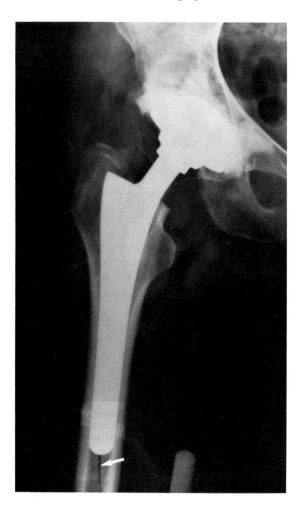

Figure 112–36. Femoral fracture. A sharply defined fracture line (*arrow*) is noted at the tip of the press-fit femoral component.

Radiologic examination shows irregular, poorly defined densities developing 2 to 3 weeks postoperatively, primarily in the region of the abductor muscles (Fig. 112–37).[132] Progression to complete bone bridging may occur in about 12 weeks. The amount of ectopic bone that is present has been graded on the basis of standard radiographs:[133]

Class 1: Islands of bone within the soft tissue.

Class 2: Bony projections from the pelvis or proximal femur with 1 cm between bone margins.

Class 3: Less than 1 cm remaining between opposing bone surfaces.

Class 4: Apparent bone ankylosis.

Bone scanning has been shown to demonstrate para-articular ossification before its appearance on radiographs.[134] Tanaka et al.[135] performed serial Tc 99m polyphosphate bone scans on quadriplegic patients with para-articular ossification in an effort to gauge the maturity of the heterotopic bone. Isotopic uptake in the area of heterotopic bone was compared with a control area (i.e., spine, sacrum, or ilium), and this ratio was followed over time. It was suggested that surgical removal of ectopic bone should be done after 2 to 3 months of steady uptake to decrease the incidence of recurrent ossification. No assessment of bone maturity could be made from a single examination. Application of these data to patients with total joint replacement has not been reported.

Tumors

Soft tissue and bone tumors have been reported as rare findings adjacent to orthopedic hardware including total joint replacement.[135–137] Tumors have involved the bone or the soft tissue. A summary of reported cases by Martin et al.[137] listed four cases of malignant fibrous histiocytoma and three osteosarcomas of 16 cases (including the authors).

TOTAL KNEE REPLACEMENT

The aim of total knee joint replacement is to create a painless and stable joint that allows both rotary and flexion-extension motion.[138–189] Normal knee motion is complex, including flexion-extension motion with a changing center or rotation, abduction-adduction motion, and axial rotation with the tibia rotating externally on the femur on extension ("screw home mechanism"). The difficult problem of duplicating such complex motion and maintaining stability

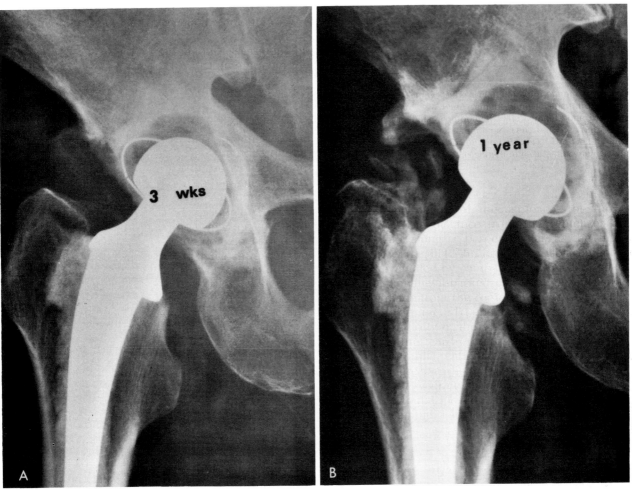

Figure 112–37. Ectopic ossification. *A,* A radiograph at 3 weeks shows early calcification within soft tissues. *B,* Examination 1 year postoperatively shows mature bone.

using a prosthetic joint has led to the development of many different prostheses and ongoing investigation in the field.

Three major types of total knee replacement may be distinguished by the degree of stability they provide.[139] In the first group, the prosthesis provides no constraint (stability) or minimal constraint to knee motion (e.g., polycentric and modular prostheses). Joint stability depends on ligamentous and capsular structures. The second group of prostheses provides partial constraint (e.g., geometric, UCI, Freeman-Swanson). With these devices, the fit of the prosthetic surfaces to each other provides some stability. In the third group, stability is provided totally by the prosthesis rather than by the patient's ligamentous or capsular structures. This group includes the hinge prostheses (e.g., Guepar, Walldius, and Shiers hinge prostheses) and the spherocentric and total condylar III prostheses. Rand and Ilstrup[149] distinguished nine types of prostheses for analysis of prosthetic survival (Table 112–7).[149]

Table 112–7. TYPES OF PROSTHESES

I. Older resurfacing
   Geometric
   Polycentric
   U.C. Irvine
II. Older constrained
   Guepar
   Walldius
   Tavernetti
   Herbert
   Sheehan
   Sheehan
   Spherocenteric
III. Resurfacing non–metal-backed
   Original total condylar
   Anametric
   Duopatellar
   Freeman-Swanson
IV. Cemented resurfacing, with metal-backed tibial component
   Total condylar
   Cruciate condylar
   Townley
   Kinematic condylar
   Porous-coated anatomic
   Miller-Galante
   Press-fit condylar
   Orthomet
   Cloutier
V. Posterior stabilized implants
   Kinematic stabilizer
   Stabilocondylar
   Insall-Burstein
VI. Newer constrained
   Kinematic rotating hinge
   Total condylar-III
VII. Unicompartmental
   Polycentric
   Geometric
   Porous-coated anatomic
VIII. Other cemented
IX. Uncemented condylar resurfacing
   Porous-coated anatomic
   Miller-Galante
   Press-fit condylar

Data from Rand, J. A., and Ilstrup, D. M.: J. Bone Joint Surg. 73A:397, 1991.

Unconstrained or Partially Constrained Prostheses

"Total knee" arthroplasties may or may not include revision of the patellofemoral joint.[141, 150] If the patellofemoral joint is replaced (such as in the total condylar prosthesis), a polyethylene "button" is used to replace the articular surface of the patella, and the femoral groove is an extension of the femoral prosthesis (Fig. 112–38).

Several design issues are still being discussed.[140] For example, disc-shaped tibial components provide a large contact area and therefore limit wear but may have a greater tendency for loosening. Greater wear is a potential disadvantage for flat tibial components. Cruciate-sparing or cruciate-saving designs are available and both have been clinically successful. According to Insall,[140] the presence of the posterior cruciate may preserve proprioception in the knee and provide passive restraint to posterior tibial subluxation, making the knee feel "more normal" to the patient.

Loosening rates are lower after total knee replacement than after THR, and therefore the necessity for bone ingrowth designs is less than in the hip. Histologic examination has shown bone ingrowth to occur reliably on the femoral side but minimally or unpredictably along the tibial and patellar components.[140, 141] These latter components, therefore, may be fixed with cement, whereas the femoral component is left uncemented.

Usual Radiologic Appearances

Positioning of the components of a total knee prosthesis is critical.[138, 140] Alignment is documented on postoperative radiographs and may be recorded as in Figure 112–39.[150]

The Anteroposterior View

Standing frontal radiographs should show overall knee alignment to be about 7 degrees of valgus, and this should not change on serial examination with weight bearing. Most of the valgus is due to valgus positioning of the femoral component. The tibial component should be parallel to the ground or in minimal varus depending on the prosthesis used.

The Lateral View

On the lateral projection, the posterior flange of the femoral component should roughly parallel the femoral shaft. The tibial component should be parallel or slope backward up to 10 degrees.[144–146] The center of the tibial component should be in the center or posterior to the center of the tibia (Fig. 112–40).[152]

The height of the new joint line with relation to that preoperatively is assessed by comparing the perpendicular distance from the tibial tubercle to a line parallel to the weight-bearing surface of the tibial

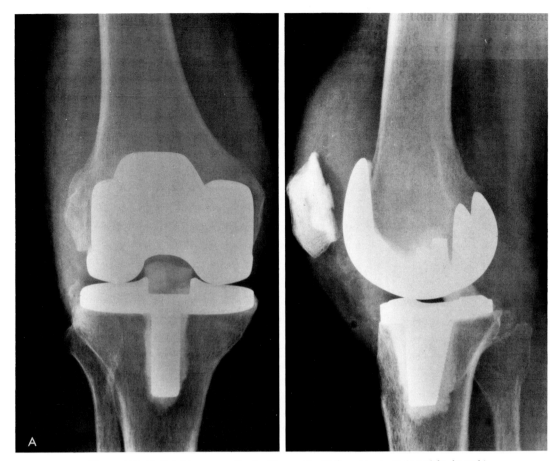

Figure 112–38. Total knee prosthesis. Kinematic. (*Left*, anteroposterior; *right*, lateral.)

Figure 112–39. An evaluation and scoring system. Component alignment, patellar position, and the presence and thickness of radiolucent lines (RLLs) along the components can be tabulated on this form. (From Ewald, F. C.: The Knee Society total knee arthroplasty roentgenographic evaluation and scoring system. Clin. Orthop. 248:9, 1989. Used by permission.)

ALIGNMENT: Recumbent ☐   Standing ☐

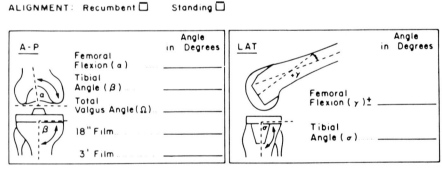

IMPLANT/BONE SURFACE AREA
Percent area of tibial surface covered by implant

RADIOLUCENCIES: Indicate depth in millimeters in each zone

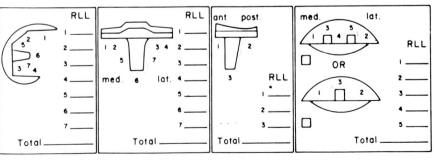

PATELLAR PROBLEM LIST
Angle of prosthesis _____   Subluxation _____
Placement Med·Lat _____   Dislocation _____
Sup·Inf _____

1917

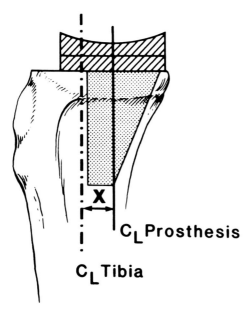

Figure 112–40. Anteroposterior position of the tibial component. The distance from the center of the tibial component to the center of the tibial plateau (X) can be assessed. (From Figgie, H. E., III, Goldberg, V. M., et al.: The influence of tibial-patellofemoral location on function of the knee in patients with the posterior stabilized condylar knee prosthesis. J. Bone Joint Surg. 68A:1035, 1986. Used by permission.)

plateau preoperatively with the corresponding measurement to the weight-bearing surface of the tibial prosthesis postoperatively (Fig. 112–41). A correction factor for magnification may be made by comparison of measurements of a fixed distance (such as that from the tibial tubercle to the posterior tibia) on preoperative and postoperative examinations.[152, 153] A change in the joint line of 8 mm or less is desirable,[152] and Lee et al.[154] noted aseptic loosening of posterior cruciate condylar prostheses to be associated with elevation of the joint line by more than 8 mm.

"Three-Foot Standing" Views

Alignment of the knee in relation to the hip and ankle is of considerable importance and can best be appreciated on 3-foot-long films taken at a 72-inch tube film distance.[147] The center of the knee should be aligned with the centers of the femoral head and ankle. The tibial component should be perpendicular to this axis (Fig. 112–42), and the positions of the components should remain unchanged on serial examinations. Petersen and Rohr[148] recommend measuring the distance from the center of the knee to a line connecting the midpoints of the femoral head and ankle. The angular deformity can then be calculated from a trigonometric formula or by noting

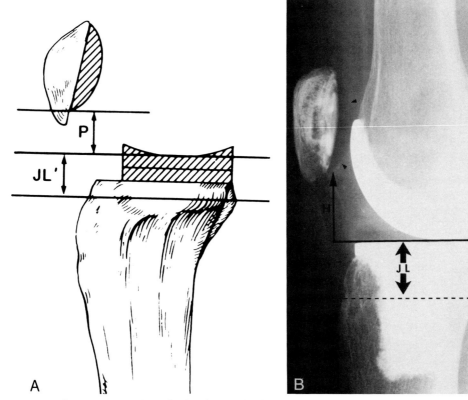

Figure 112–41. Joint line position and patellar height. *A*, The distance JL′ (measured from the tibial tubercle to the distal part of the proximal surface of the tibial component) indicates the height of the joint line and may be compared with preoperative measurements. The patellar height is measured from a line parallel to the weight-bearing surface of the prosthesis to the inferior pole of the patellar implant. *B*, Example of patellar height (H) and the height of the joint line (JL) measured on a radiograph. The inferior surface of the femoral component was used to indicate the articular surface.

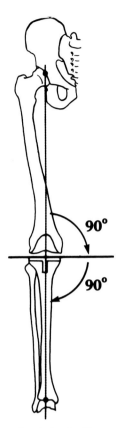

Figure 112–42. The mechanical axis. The components of the total knee prosthesis should be perpendicular to the mechanical axis of the leg, drawn from the epicenter of the femoral head to the midpoint of the tibial plafond. This line should fall at the center of the knee.

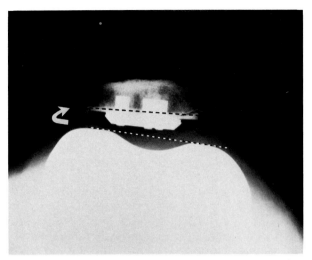

Figure 112–43. Patellar tilt. The angle (*curved arrow*) between lines along the patellar component–bone (or cement) interface and the femoral condyles anteriorly indicates the degree of patellar tilt.

that in the average patient, a 0.6 cm displacement corresponds to 1 degree of angulation.

Patellar Component

Tangential patellar views should be routinely obtained and should show a fairly good fit of the patella into the femoral groove with no subluxation or tilt.[173-189] More quantitative evaluation of patellar position has been described by Gomes et al.,[153] with reference to lateral radiographs and tangential views with 30 degrees of knee flexion.[153] On the lateral view, the *height of the patella* is assessed with relation to a baseline parallel to the joint line (see Fig. 112–41). Patellar height between 10 and 30 mm is considered satisfactory.[152] The *position of prosthesis* is measured as the distance from the midpoint of the prosthesis to the midpoint of the patella on lateral and tangential views. *Patellar tilt* is defined as the angle between a line along the femoral condyles anteriorly and another line along the patellar component–bone interface (Fig. 112–43). Five degrees or less is considered neutral.

Patellar malposition may be accompanied by symptoms or by a propensity for component wear or loosening. Figgie et al.[152] examined patients with posterior stabilized condylar knee prostheses. Patients with neutral or posterior placement of the tibial component with respect to the center of the tibia (on the lateral radiograph), change in the joint line of 8 mm or less, and a patellar height of 10 to 30 mm demonstrated excellent or good functional knee scores. When the inferior aspect of the patellar implant was situated distal to the joint surface, pain or decreased function was uniformly noted.

Lucent Zones

With cemented components, thin cement-bone lucent zones occur fairly often along part (but not all) of the tibial cement-bone interface (Table 112–8). Cement-bone lucencies are considerably less frequent around the femoral component. Ecker et al.[142] noted lucent lines less than 2 mm in width around the tibial cement-bone interface in 58 percent of patients with nonmetal-backed total condylar prostheses. These lucencies were more common under either the medial or the lateral plateau but were also found under both plateaus. When lucent zones were thin, no correlation was found between them and the postoperative

Table 112–8. INCIDENCE OF RADIOLUCENT LINES AT THE CEMENT-BONE INTERFACE*

	Tibial Lucency <2 mm (percent)	Femoral Lucency (percent)
Anametric	28	14
Total condylar	58	8.6
Duopatellar	24†	
Variable axis	74	
Spherocentric	42.5	10

*From Ecker et al.,[142] Insall et al.,[149a] and Symposium on Total Knee Arthroplasty.[179]

course. When tibial lucencies of greater than 2 mm were present both around the central peg and under both plateaus, clinical results were poorer.

Studies of kinematic total knee replacements show thin, nonprogressive lucencies along 40 percent of tibial components, 30 percent of femoral components, and 60 percent of patellar components. Lucent zones may be added to provide a scoring system for each component (see Fig. 112–39).[151]

Several studies have documented the need for centering the radiographic beam so it is perpendicular to the cement-bone interface. Thus, positioning difficulties may lead to erroneous conclusions regarding the presence or absence of thin cement-bone lucencies. Although fluoroscopic positioning allows significantly more tibial lucencies to be identified,[158] the inconvenience of the method limits its usefulness.[156] In addition, lucencies are more difficult to detect adjacent to metal-backed components than adjacent to radiolucent ones. Comparison of bone ingrowth and cemented total knee arthroplasties[157] has shown thin peripheral tibial lucent zones in equal numbers in uncemented and cemented components. The lucencies are present by 6 months. No femoral lucent zones were seen. Rosenberg et al.[156] found no correlation between radiolucencies and knee scores. Tibial lucent lines were most common, and partial lucencies were noted in roughly one quarter of radiographs.[156]

In addition to lucent zones along prosthetic surfaces, more diffuse decrease in bone density has been noted in the anterior portion of the distal femur in 68 percent of patients with asymptomatic components (Fig. 112–44).[158] This finding does not depend on the type of fixation used and stabilizes by 1 year after surgery. It represents stress shielding consequent to the use of a stiff femoral component.

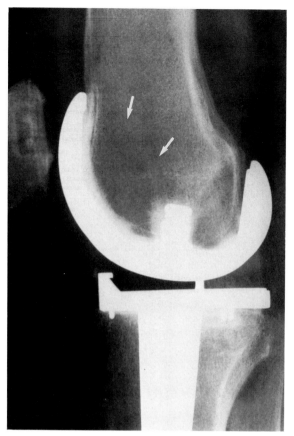

Figure 112–44. Stress shielding. Several years after joint replacement, an area of relatively decreased bone density is noted anteriorly (*arrows*).

Bone Grafting

As in the hip, bone grafting may be necessary to replace or fill areas of deficient bone. Two types of grafts are described: "contained" defects, in which the defect is surrounded by an intact rim of cortical bone, and "uncontained" defects, in which the cortex is absent and the defect extends to the periphery of the bone. Wilde et al.[159] found trabecular continuity between the graft and host bone at an average of 23 months in 11 of 12 knees. In one case the graft had not incorporated. Bone scans and SPECT scans showed increased activity at the graft-host junction in six patients studied at 22 to 31 months after surgery. SPECT scans showed uniform activity in four of five patients and no more than background activity in the fifth patient, the latter presumably representing a nonviable graft,[159] although that graft had incorporated on radiographic examination, and the clinical result was satisfactory.

Use of massive femoral or tibial allografts for revision total knee arthroplasty has shown union in

12 of 14 grafts (86 percent) in one series.[160] All seven tibial allografts had healed. Grafts either were inset into the host bone (when there was sufficient cortex present) or replaced the entire resected portion of the host bone.

Complications of Total Knee Arthroplasty

Complications of total knee arthroplasty are infrequent. A study by Rand and Ilstrup of 9200 total knee arthroplasties showed that when a primary total knee arthroplasty was present in a rheumatoid patient 60 years old or older, using a condylar prosthesis with a metal-backed tibial component, the probability of the implant remaining in situ at 10 years was 97 percent.[149]

Loosening

Gradual or abrupt loosening of prosthetic components accounts for the largest number of failures of total knee replacement.[136] Even so, loosening occurs less often following total knee replacement than THR. For example, Insall[140] noted tibial component loosening in 1.8 percent of total condylar prostheses and in 0.18 percent of posterior-stabilized prostheses.

Table 112–9. FINDINGS SUGGESTING LOOSENING OF TOTAL KNEE PROSTHESES

Plain films
    Cement-bone lucency ≥2 mm
    Increasing cement-bone lucency
    Collapse of underlying trabecular bone or cement
    Change in position of a component
    Change in the varus or valgus angle
    Development of metal-cement lucency
Arthrography
    Contrast along the cement-bone interface
Scintigraphy
    Increased isotopic uptake (? after 6 months)

Suboptimal alignment (particularly varus position of the tibial component) and removal of large amounts of proximal tibial bone predispose to tibial component loosening.[161]

Loosening most often involves the tibial components and usually occurs at the cement-bone interface (Table 112–9). As in patients with THRs, a wide or widening cement-bone lucency suggests loosening (Fig. 112–45). Ducheyne et al.[162] studied 100 patients with University of California at Irvine total knee replacements and noted the development of lucency at the cement-bone interface greater than 2 mm in thickness in 14 patients with satisfactory clinical results and in all seven patients requiring revision for loose tibial components. The seven patients with loose tibial prostheses had an increase in the width and length of this lucent zone with time, with a thickness of 2 to 3 mm present at the time of revision. As in patients with THR, a cement-bone lucency may be present on the immediate postoperative examination, but Ducheyne et al. noted this to be a more frequent finding in patients who develop loosening than in control patients.

In addition to widening of the cement-bone lucency, collapse of underlying trabecular bone, fragmentation of underlying cement, change in position of a component, and change in the degree of varus or valgus position on weight-bearing views are radiographic features suggesting loosening. Occasionally loosening may occur at the metal-cement interface of the femoral component, as seen in the patient in Figure 112–46.

When evaluating bone ingrowth prosthesis, continued shedding of surface beads logically indicates loosening (Fig. 112–47). Loose beads, however, have been noted relatively often.[157] They always occurred in the first 3 to 6 months and then stabilized. It is postulated that the dislodged beads result from early microfractures but that stabilization occurs. They did not appear to indicate clinical failure or to have predictive significance.[157]

Arthrography and Scintigraphy. Preliminary investigation has shown both arthrography and scintigraphy to be useful in documenting loosening or infection. Unlike arthrography done for the study of meniscal tears, single-contrast examination is preferred (i.e., Reno-M-60 or Reno-M-76), and no attempt is made to remove all the joint fluid. Instead, a sample of joint fluid is aspirated and sent to the laboratory for culture, and contrast material is then injected until the suprapatellar pouch is full (at least 15 ml).[165] The needle is then removed. If subtraction is to be done, anteroposterior films are taken immediately before and after injection of contrast material.

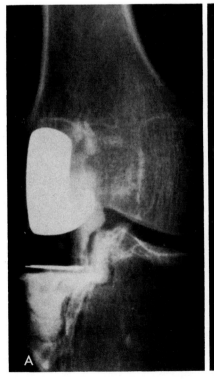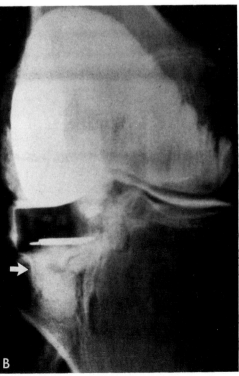

Figure 112–45. Loose tibial component of lateral knee replacement. *A*, There is an abnormally wide lucency at the cement-bone interface of the tibial component. *B*, The lucent zone fills with contrast material at arthrography (*arrow*).

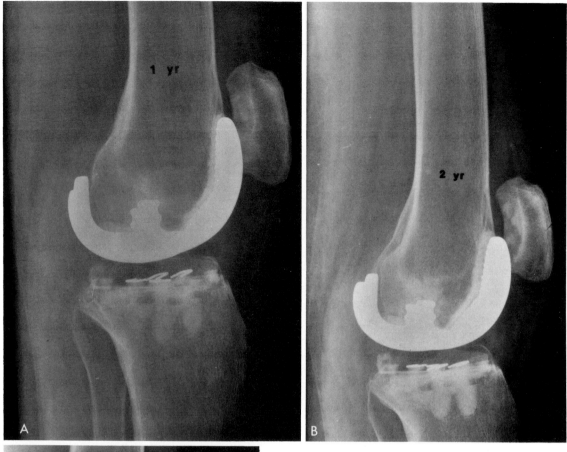

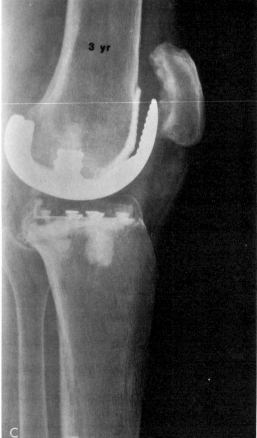

Figure 112–46. Loose femoral component of a duopatellar total knee prosthesis. *A,* Examination at 1 week postoperatively shows good position of components with no evidence of loosening. *B,* At 2 years postoperatively there is beginning separation of the retropatellar flange from the underlying cement. *C,* At 3 years this separation is obvious, and there is rotation of the femoral component posteriorly. Severe changes have occurred in the articular surface of the patella.

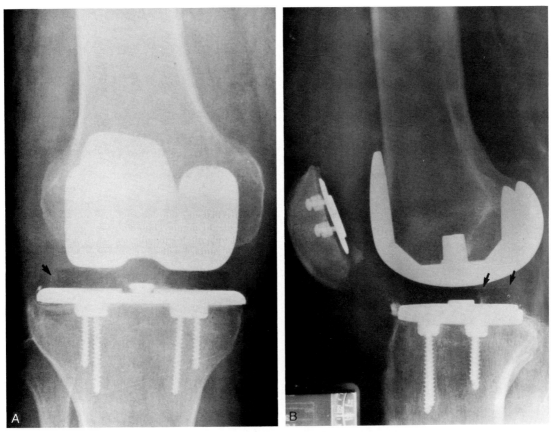

Figure 112–47. Metal synovitis. Anteroposterior (*A*) and lateral (*B*) radiographs show that fragments of metal fibers used to facilitate bone ingrowth have become displaced and now cover the articular surfaces (*arrows*). Considerable swelling is present.

The knee is then flexed and extended several times, and films are taken in the anteroposterior projection with and without traction, in both oblique projections and in the flexed and extended lateral positions. Additional films after walking are obtained if no abnormality is detected on the first films. Contrast material filling the cement-bone lucency indicates an abnormal bond at this interface (see Fig. 112–45). In patients with draining sinus tracts, it has been noted that contrast injection directly into the tract usually but not always demonstrates any communication with the joint. In cases in which such a communication is suspected and in which the sonogram reveals no communication, arthrography also is indicated.[147]

Bone scanning with Tc 99m phosphate complex can also demonstrate loosening or infection.[164] Because the cement-bone interface of the femoral component may be difficult to see radiographically, isotope study seems particularly valuable in this area.[164, 165] Increased isotopic uptake over the femoral component on anterior scans may be due to patellar damage, and a lateral scan should be done to confirm the location of such increased activity. Mild to moderate increase in isotope uptake may persist for years after total knee arthroplasty,[147] but Kantor et al.[166] found that at an average of 54 months, asymptomatic knee replacements showed only mild uptake in one or more zones. Loose or infected prostheses generally produce abnormal scans[166] (Fig. 112–48). Thus, a normal scan is good evidence that neither loosening nor infection is present.

Infection

As in THR, deep sepsis may be immediate or delayed. Deep infection occurred in 67 (1.6 percent) of 4171 total knee arthroplasties in one series of modern design prosthesis.[167] Radiographic evidence of loosening and soft tissue swelling may indicate infection (Fig. 112–49).

Indium scans have had limited success in identifying patients with infected prostheses. Rand and Brown[149] found an accuracy of 84 percent, a sensitivity of 83 percent, and a specificity of 85 percent in surgically confirmed cases. Active rheumatoid arthritis may produce increased uptake of indium-labeled leukocytes and therefore false-positive scans for infection.[149]

Patellar Complications

Major patellar complications have been reported in 1 to 12 percent of cases.[168] Attention to surgical technique and modification in prosthesis design have led to reduction in the number of patellar complica-

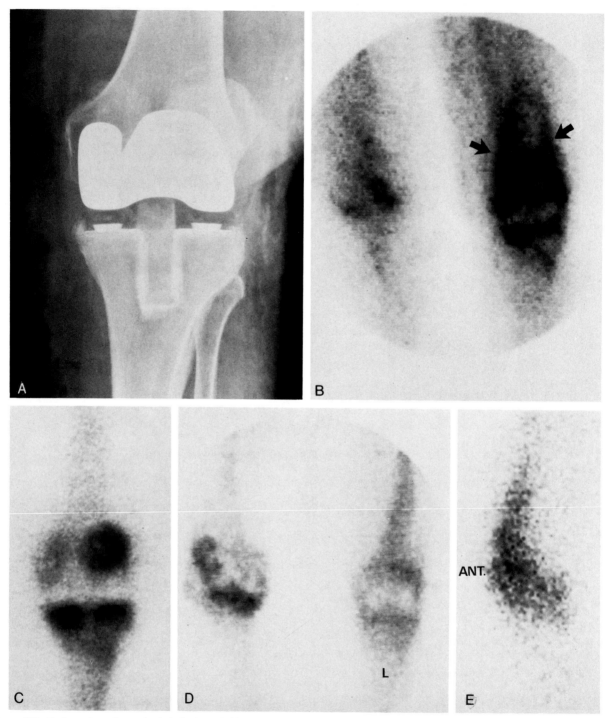

Figure 112–48. Scanning of prosthetic infection. *A*, The AP view of the knee shows no apparent loosening of the tibial component. *B*, The bone flow study shows increased uptake corresponding to the area of the suprapatellar pouch (*arrows*). *C*, There is no corresponding area of increased uptake on the delayed bone scan. There is increased uptake corresponding to the areas of the tibial component and the patella. *D*, The gallium scan shows no suspicious areas of increased uptake in the left knee (L). *E*, The lateral image from the indium-labeled WBC scan demonstrates increased uptake corresponding to the findings in *B*. The findings likely indicate an inflammatory or infectious process. (From Weissman, B. N.: Current topics in the radiology of joint replacement surgery. Radiol. Clin. North Am. 28:1111, 1990. Used by permission.)

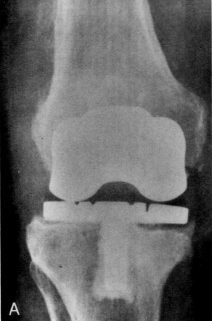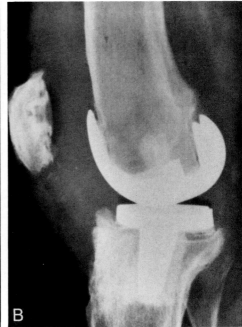

Figure 112–49. Infected total knee prosthesis. Anteroposterior (A) and lateral (B) views show marked soft tissue swelling, periosteal reaction along the femur, and wide cement-bone lucencies about the tibial component. The combination of findings is highly suggestive of infection.

tions. Radiographic evaluation is instrumental in detecting these complications.

When the patellar articular surface is not replaced, progressive damage to the articular surface and subchondral bone of the patella may occur. Patellar dislocation and catching of the patella on an overhanging shelf of anterior femoral condyle or on an anteriorly positioned femoral component[141, 146] may produce patellofemoral symptoms. The most frequent complications after replacement of the articular surface of the patella are dislocation, fracture, component loosening, or wear of the prosthesis.

Patellar Subluxation and Dislocation. Patellar subluxation may occur in resurfaced or natural patellae. Patellar subluxation may be asymptomatic. It may predispose to component wear.

Patellar Fractures. Stress fractures are reported in up to 21 percent of patients[173] (Fig. 112–50). Although startling on radiographs, the finding may be clinically asymptomatic. Surgery is usually performed when there is more than 2 cm of displacement; instability as a result of an extensor lag; or a loose, displaced prosthesis.[173] Fractures occurring without patellar dislocation, component loosening, or complete extensor mechanism disruption may be treated nonsurgically.[176] Decreased patellar blood flow after extensive lateral release was initially thought to contribute to the development of postoperative patellar stress fracture.[177] Study by Ritter and Campbell[170] has negated this. In fact, patellar fractures occurred in 3.6 percent of patients who did not undergo lateral release and in 1.5 percent of those who did have the procedure.

Patellar Component Loosening. Patellar component loosening may be asymptomatic.[173] A displaced component may abrade the quadriceps or patellar tendons. A wide cement bone interface or component displacement indicates loosening (Fig. 112–51).

Patellar Wear. This is generally but not exclusively a complication of metal-backed patellar prostheses.[173] The polyethylene surface of the component, usually the portion covering the lateral edge of the metal backing, becomes worn and may split.[178]

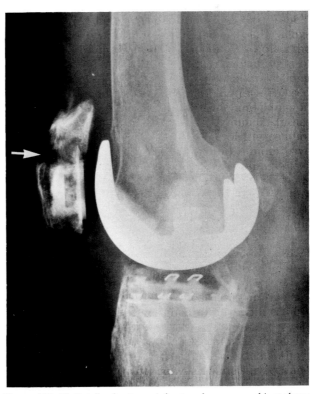

Figure 112–50. Patellar fracture. A fracture has occurred just above the patellar prosthesis (arrow).

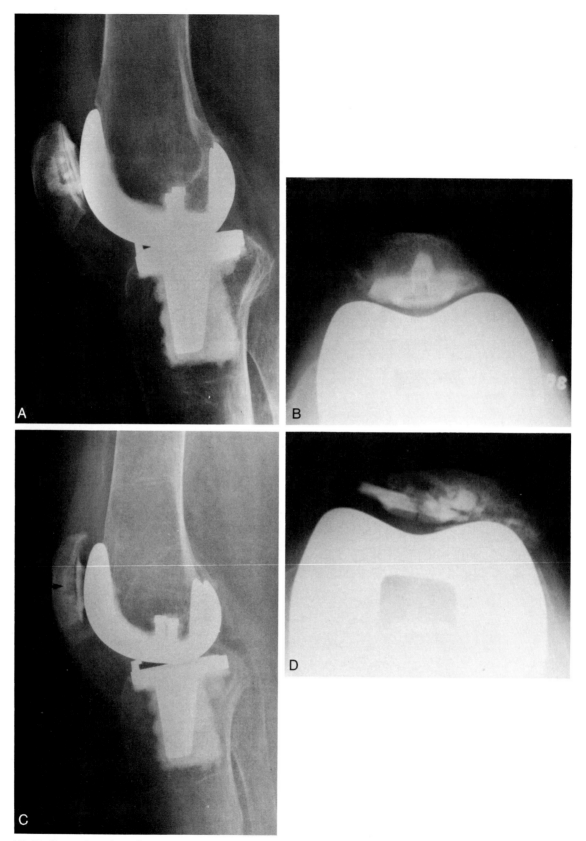

Figure 112–51. Separation of patellar component. *A*, Lateral radiograph shows a cemented total knee prosthesis without evidence of loosening. A thin cement-bone lucency is noted along the patellar component cement. *B*, The tangential view shows no patellar subluxation or tilt. *C*, Follow-up lateral radiograph shows a change in the appearance of the patellar component. In particular, the stem of the prosthesis (*area with arrow*) is not seen in the patella. *D*, Repeat tangential patellar view shows the fragmentation of cement with separation of the patella from the patellar component and adjacent cement. The patella is subluxated laterally.

Contact between the metal surfaces of the patellar backing and the trochlea may then ensue leading to metal synovitis.

Other complications of patellar arthroplasty especially with metal-backed components include displacement of the polyethylene articular surface from the metal back,[174] displacement of the metal backing,[178] and component fracture. Most failures of metal-backed patellae occur at the peg-metal or polyethylene-metal interface.

Fractures

Fractures related to trauma, osteoporotic bone, or abnormal localization of applied stress[171, 172] may all be seen in patients with total knee replacements. Surgical damage to the anterior distal femoral cortex occurring during the placement of the patellar flange of the femoral component appears to predispose to supracondylar fracture.[171] Subtle change in the position of one of the components may be the only sign of fracture.

Component Fracture. Component fracture is uncommon. Deformation of the tibial component did occur, however, in 11 percent of patients in one series[179]; it may be asymptomatic or associated with loosening or angular deformity. Metal backing of the tibial component is expected to decrease the incidence of this complication (Fig. 112–52).

Wear

Wear of polyethylene bearing surfaces has been reported.[180] Changes in knee alignment and decrease in the space between the metal femoral component and the metal tibial tray may suggest the diagnosis (Fig. 112–53). Later, wear of the underlying metal and metal synovitis allow the diagnosis to be made with certainty (Fig. 112–54). The thickness of a non-metal-backed patellar component can be seen directly because of the contrast provided by the adjacent soft tissue.

Metal Synovitis

Shedding of metal particles in the joint was classically a complication associated with metal-to-metal hinges.[181] More recent cases have been seen in association with displacement of bone ingrowth surfaces or as a result of unusual wear (Fig. 112–55). Review of 18 patients with metal-induced synovitis proved at revision surgery revealed 10 to be due to wear of a metal-backed patellar component, six to be due to wear of a metal-backed tibial component, and two to be due to wear at the metal-to-metal bearing of a hinge prosthesis.[182] In 11 of the 18 patients, the diagnosis of metal synovitis could be made on preoperative lateral radiographs by noting the presence of a thin white line outlining the joint capsule (the "metal line sign"). The sign was shown to correspond to extensive deposition of metal particles in synovial tissue.

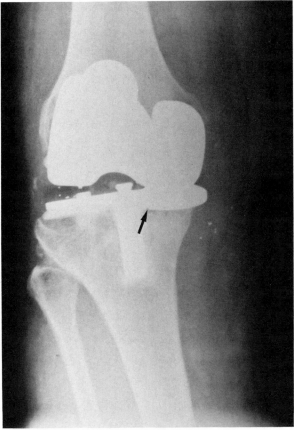

Figure 112–52. Loosening and fracture of total knee prosthesis. Anteroposterior radiograph. There is varus alignment, representing a marked change from the postoperative valgus alignment that had been present. The lateral portion of the tibial tray is seen in profile, but the medial portion is tilted, owing to fracture of the metal tibial tray (*arrow*). Several beads have become dislodged from the cement-prosthesis interface, attesting to the presence of loosening. Some of these beads are intra-articular.

Entrapment of Drains

Drainage catheters may become trapped in the intercondylar area when the joint is in extension.[183]

Hinge Total Knee Prostheses

Hinge prostheses (e.g., Walldius, Shiers, and Guepar) both resurface the joint and provide stability. Because these units are rigid and do not duplicate normal knee motion, they are subjected to considerable stress that may loosen the prosthesis or fracture adjacent bone. Hinge prostheses are therefore used only in patients with limited activity demands and marked instability or as a salvage procedure following other types of knee replacement.[184]

Radiographic examination should show the hinge to be parallel to the ground on weight-bearing views. Sclerosis of the weight-bearing bone adjacent to the femoral and tibial components is a usual finding on long-term follow-up examination.[185] Settling of the components into the femur or tibia also occurs frequently in uncemented prostheses; if this

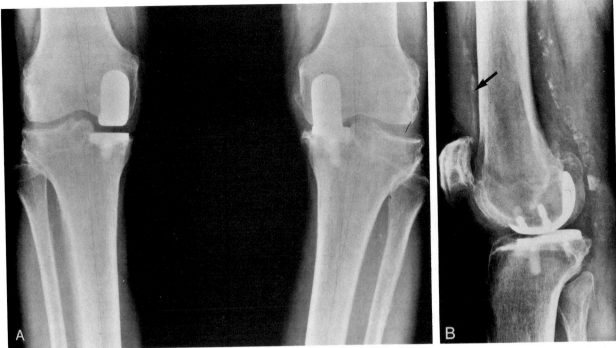

Figure 112–53. Wear of the tibial component of a unicondylar prosthesis with metal synovitis. *A,* The standing AP view of the knees shows no abnormality of the right unicondylar prosthesis. On the left, there is overall varus alignment, and the normally present lucency representing the polyethylene tibial component is no longer visible. *B,* The lateral projection shows increased density in the suprapatellar pouch (*arrow*), indicating metal synovitis.

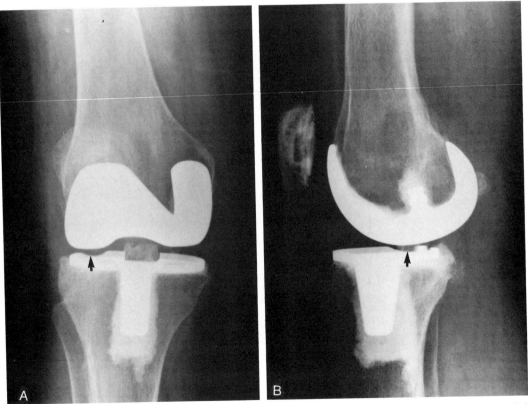

Figure 112–54. Metal synovitis. Anteroposterior (*A*) and lateral (*B*) views. Long-term instability has led to erosion of the posterior lateral aspect of the metal tibial tray (*arrows*) and the shedding of metal particles into the joint. The erosion of the nonopaque articular surface is not visible.

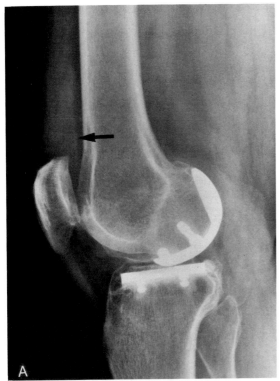

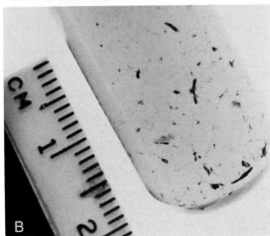

Figure 112-55. Metal synovitis. *A,* The lateral radiograph shows a unicondylar prosthesis. There is a line of increased density in the suprapatellar pouch *(arrow),* indicating metal synovitis. *B,* Aspiration of joint fluid confirmed the presence of black debris within the joint.

is asymmetric, gradually increasing deformity may result.

Complications include loosening, infection, metal synovitis, fracture of bone or prosthesis, patellar subluxation or damage, and tendon rupture (Fig. 112-56). A 2- to 3-mm lucent zone (indicating loosening) is routinely seen around the stems of uncemented Walldius prostheses followed 5 years or longer.[186] Evidence of loosening or continued synovitis should raise the possibility of infection. Scott[179] noted a 2 percent incidence of infection that increased to above 12 percent on continued follow-up.

McKeever and MacIntosh Hemiarthroplasty

Before the current generation of metal-to-plastic total knee prostheses, several attempts at joint resurfacing were made. Tibial resurfacing with McKeever and MacIntosh prostheses is still occasionally done, particularly in patients with osteoarthritis with failed osteotomy or contraindications to osteotomy and in those too young or too heavy for total joint replacement.[179]

Both prostheses are placed so that they "toe in" at approximately 10 degrees to the sagittal plane, and therefore frontal views will not show these devices exactly in profile (Fig. 112-57). Both types of prostheses are theoretically inserted so they are horizontal to the ground on both the frontal and the lateral projections. They should not extend medially or laterally beyond the margins of the tibial condyles. On lateral view, the McKeever prosthesis should extend to or slightly beyond the anterior margins of the tibial plateaus. Flexion and extension lateral views can allow measurement of the shift in the relative position of the two prostheses. Kay and Martins[187] described the radiologic findings following placement of the MacIntosh prosthesis and noted that some motion (less than 10 percent) occurred in "most" patients. Follow-up examinations in patients

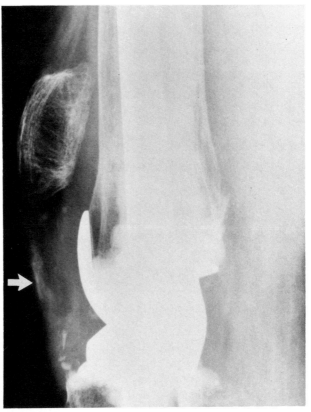

Figure 112-56. Patellar tendon rupture. A cemented Guepar prosthesis is in place. There is calcification of the patellar tendon *(arrow)* and marked elevation of the patella as compared with earlier radiographs.

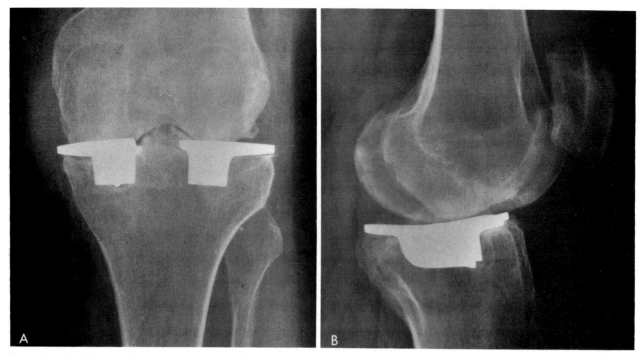

Figure 112–57. McKeever tibial plateau prosthesis. Some roughening, sclerosis, and volume loss of the femoral condyles have occurred. *A,* Anteroposterior view. *B,* Lateral view.

with McKeever arthroplasties often show a thin lucency under the prosthesis and along the fin of the prosthesis with a subjacent thin zone of sclerosis. Sclerosis, irregularity, and loss of volume of the femoral condyles or collapse of the bone supporting the prosthesis has been noted by Anderson et al.[188] to be associated with a poor result following MacIntosh hemiarthroplasty.

Unicondylar Replacement

Unicondylar replacement, consisting of femoral and tibial components, is used in selected patients with osteoarthritis or avascular necrosis involving either medial or lateral compartments.[189] Alternative therapies include high tibial osteotomy or bicondylar knee replacement. Unicondylar replacement is avoided when there is inflammatory arthritis or significant degeneration of the other knee compartment. Generally older patients who are not obese, are not extremely active, and have mild angular deformity are considered for this procedure.[189]

At surgery, osteophytes are debrided. The femoral component is positioned centrally in the femoral condyle and should extend anteriorly (on the lateral radiograph) to cover the entire weight-bearing surface with the knee in extension (see Fig. 112–53). The anterior edge of the component should be flush with the cartilage surface and the posterior condyle resected to at least the thickness of the metal implant.

The tibial component should parallel the femoral component when the knee is in extension. On lateral view, the tibial component may be tilted posteriorly

up to 10 degrees. On anteroposterior projection, the cut surface should be perpendicular to the mechanical axis of the tibia. The mechanical axis of the leg should fall in the center of the knee or slightly medial[189] to it. Complications include loosening, wear, and progression of osteoarthritis in the opposite compartment.

TOTAL SHOULDER REPLACEMENT

Total shoulder replacement is performed primarily in patients with incapacitating pain and secondarily for improvement in function.[190–194] Normally the stability of the glenohumeral joint is provided largely by the joint capsule and rotator cuff. Because some of the diseases treated with these prostheses (e.g., rheumatoid arthritis) have associated damage to these structures, either they must be repaired or their functions replaced or augmented by the prosthesis. Cofield[190] has categorized the available prostheses into three groups: (1) prostheses that replace the articular surfaces of the joint (e.g., Neer II), (2) prostheses that replace the articular surface and provide some additional stability, and (3) prostheses that replace the articular surface and replace the constraining functions of the soft tissue (i.e., the Stanmore and Michael Reese prostheses).

The Neer prosthesis is the one most frequently used at the Brigham and Women's Hospital. It consists of a chromium-cobalt humeral component (the revised humeral component used in hemiarthroplasty) and a dish-shaped, high-density polyethylene

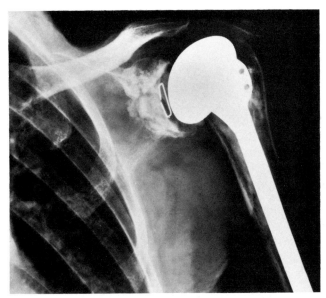

Figure 112–58. Total shoulder prosthesis. The posterior oblique view shows each component in profile. There is a thin lucency at the cement-bone interface of the glenoid component. Severe changes of rheumatoid arthritis are present in the clavicle and acromion.

glenoid component that is fixed into the glenoid with methyl methacrylate. The humeral component is placed in 20 to 40 degrees of retroversion.[191] Osteotomy of the greater tuberosity may rarely be required. A bone ingrowth model is now available.

Postoperative radiographic examination should include an external rotation posterior oblique view (approximately 45 degrees) and internal rotation and axillary views. Usually the inferior edge of the humeral component is roughly aligned with the inferior edge of the glenoid component.[192] The humeral component is placed as in a hemiarthroplasty so the edge of the head of the prosthesis is parallel to the cut surface of the neck and the mesh holes are well seated in cancellous bone (Fig. 112–58).[193] As a consequence of the usually present retroversion of the component, the humeral component is seen in profile on the external rotation, posterior oblique radiograph. Approximation of the degree of retroversion of the humeral component can be derived from the 35-degree internal rotation view by measuring the head-shaft angle and subtracting 40 degrees or, more exactly, by comparing the measurement to a prepared table.[191]

Complications that may be detected radiographically include dislocation, upward subluxation of the humeral component (especially frequent in patients with rheumatoid arthritis), heterotopic bone formation, widening of the cement-bone lucency around the glenoid component indicative of loosening or infection (Fig. 112–59), dissociation of a metal-backed glenoid component,[194] and sinking or loosening of the humeral component (Fig. 112–60).

TOTAL ELBOW REPLACEMENT

Total elbow prostheses are currently being developed for use in patients with severe sequelae of

Figure 112–59. Loose, displaced glenoid component. *A*, Postoperative film shows no apparent complication. The glenoid marker wire is seen (*arrow*). *B*, Routine follow-up examination shows displacement of the glenoid component (*arrow*) so that it now lies within the lateral soft tissues (most likely within the subdeltoid bursa).

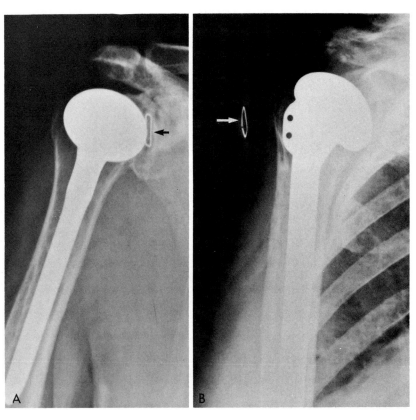

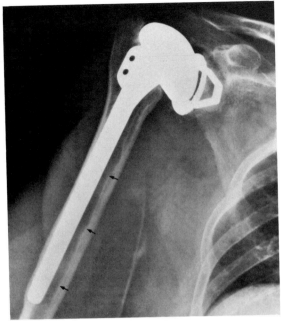

Figure 112–60. Loosening of the humeral component of a total shoulder prosthesis. There is a metal-backed, bone ingrowth glenoid component and a press-fit humeral component. The wide lucency around the humeral stem attests to the loosening that is present. The lateral cortex is thinned.

rheumatoid arthritis or post-traumatic arthritis.[195–205] The early models (e.g., Dee, Shiers, and McKee) are metal-to-metal hinge prostheses that are fixed to bone using methyl methacrylate cement.[195] Later hinge prostheses include the Mayo,[198] which replaces both the humeroulnar and the radiohumeral joints; the Coonrad; the Schlein metal-to-polyethylene hinge; and the GSB metal-to-metal hinge. The primary cause

of failure appears to be loosening, seen on radiographs as widening of the cement-bone lucencies (Fig. 112–61).[197]

Semiconstrained prostheses were developed to reduce the high incidence of component loosening seen with constrained designs. These semiconstrained prostheses have a loose metal-to-plastic bearing between the components that allows motion in addition to flexion and extension. The Pritchard-Walker, Pritchard Mark II, the triaxial, and the GSB Mark III prostheses are examples.[198, 199] Two- to 5-year follow-up of the Pritchard Mark II prosthesis revealed radiographic loosening on the humeral side in six elbows; one required revision for pain.[200]

Unconstrained prostheses include the Kudo[201] and the Ewald capitellocondylar. The Ewald capitellocondylar prosthesis is the device used at the Brigham and Women's Hospital; it consists of separate metallic humeral and high-density polyethylene ulnar components (Fig. 112–62). This prosthesis does have a lower rate of loosening than do constrained prostheses, with a 0.5 percent incidence of loosening in one series (Fig. 112–63).[202] Dislocation of the components may occur, however, and was reported in 5 percent and 14.3 percent of two series of capitellocondylar prostheses.[197, 202, 203] Fractures of the olecranon process are also seen (Fig. 112–64).[198] Radiographic follow-up allows the amount of bone resorption to be assessed, so revision can be performed before large amounts of bone loss occur.[200]

TOTAL ANKLE PROSTHESES

Normally the tibiotalar, subtalar, and midtarsal joints function together to allow motion in three

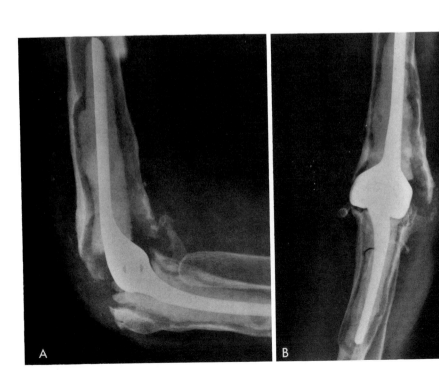

Figure 112–61. Loose hinge total elbow prosthesis. There is marked resorption of bone at the cement-bone interface. *A,* Lateral projection. *B,* Anteroposterior projection.

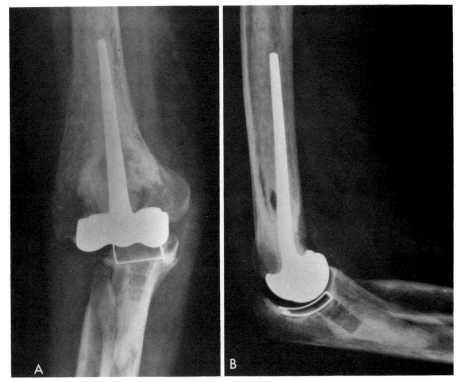

Figure 112–62. Ewald total elbow prosthesis. The medial portion of the metallic humeral component articulates with the high-density polyethylene ulnar component. Opaque cement fixes the components and makes the nonopaque stem of the ulnar component easily visible. *A*, Anteroposterior view. *B*, Lateral view.

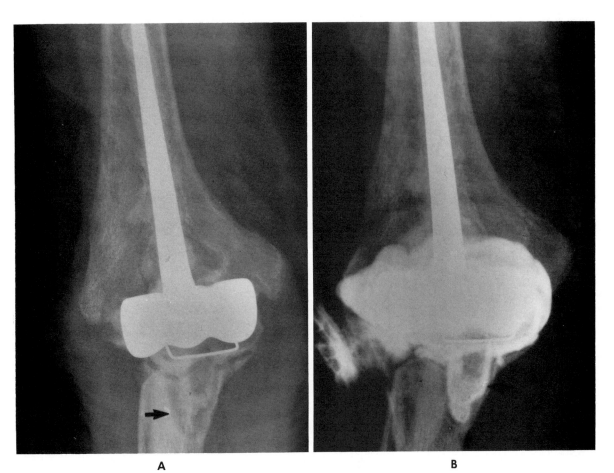

A   B

Figure 112–63. Loose Ewald prosthesis. *A*, There is a wide lucency around the cement of the ulnar component. *B*, Arthrography confirms loosening of the ulnar component. The humeral component is not loose.

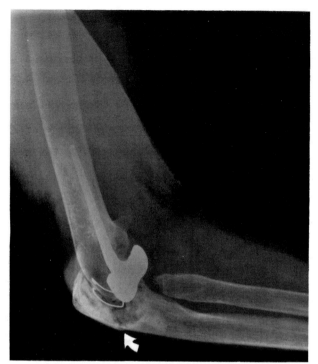

Figure 112–64. Olecranon fracture. The fracture through the olecranon process (*arrow*) has resulted in a change in the orientation of the olecranon component with dislocation of the humeral component anteriorly.

planes.[205–210] The tibiotalar articulation itself provides only flexion and extension motion. Ten degrees of extension (dorsiflexion) and 25 degrees of flexion (plantar flexion) are said to be necessary for normal gait.[205]

As summarized by Demottaz et al.,[206] two main types of total ankle replacement are available. The first type, a multiaxis joint, allows rotation of the tibial component in any of the three major axes and unrestricted rotation (e.g., Waugh, Smith). The second type of prosthesis (a single-axis joint) allows only flexion-extension motion (e.g., Mayo, TPR, Bucholz, Oregon). Semiconstrained designs offering flexion-extension motion and limited rotation are also available now.[208] Uncemented components have been developed.

Some of the prostheses in use are shown in Figs. 112–65 and 112–66. The tibial component is inserted so it is perpendicular to the long axis of the tibia with the foot in neutral position.[201] The talar component is then positioned parallel to the tibial component.

Complications include loosening (usually at the cement-bone interface), infection, impingement between the talus and the lateral malleolus, talar collapse, fracture of the medial malleolus at the time of surgery, and instability.[209] Migration of the talar component is frequently seen in long-term follow-up series.[210]

SILICONE RUBBER PROSTHESES

Silicone rubber prostheses are used primarily in the hand and wrist to replace damaged carpal, metacarpophalangeal, or interphalangeal joints.[211–227] The metacarpophalangeal joints are the most frequently replaced, and the Swanson and Niebauer designs are the most frequently used prostheses. Silicone rubber

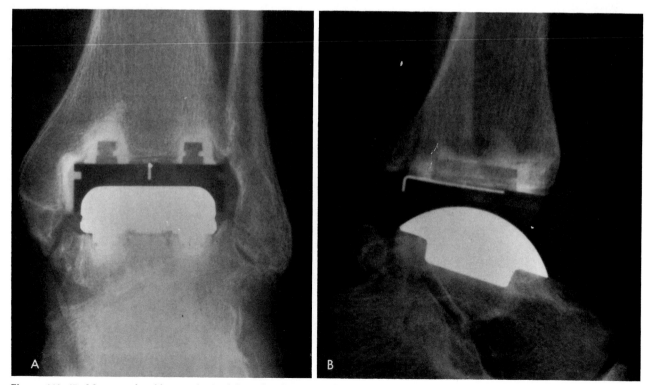

Figure 112–65. Mayo total ankle prosthesis, bilateral radiograph. There is a thin lucent zone under the tibial component on the anteroposterior (*A*) radiograph, not seen on the lateral (*B*) radiograph.

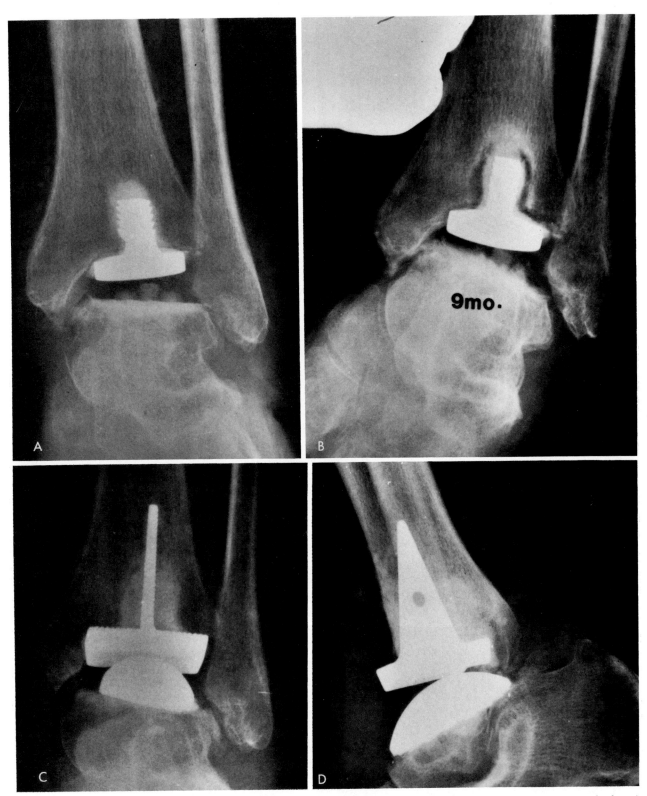

Figure 112–66. Loosening of Smith total ankle prosthesis. *A,* Immediate postoperative film. *B,* Nine months postoperatively there is loosening of the tibial component. *C* and *D,* Replacement with Waugh prosthesis. The metallic tibial component has a polyethylene articular surface.

prostheses are also used at the great toe metatarso-phalangeal joint to maintain hallux length.[211]

Metacarpophalangeal Prostheses

The Swanson silicone rubber prosthesis (Fig. 112–67) consists of a single silicone rubber component with a central curved section and a stem on each end.[212] Joint motion results both from the hinge action of the central portion of the prosthesis and from pistoning of the stems within the bone.[213, 214] Eventually a joint capsule develops around the prosthesis so stability can be maintained following implant removal or fracture.[215]

The stems of the Niebauer prosthesis are coated with Dacron mesh, which is gradually infiltrated by bone.[216] Because the stems become fixed within the medullary canal, all finger motion will be the result of the hinge action of the midportion of the prosthesis.

Postoperative radiographs demonstrate the degree of correction of deformity, the positions of the components, and most complications. Silicone rubber is only slightly more dense than soft tissue and is quite difficult to see. On the frontal view, the hinge portion of the prosthesis appears rectangular, and the long axis of the rectangle is parallel to the resection margin of the metacarpal. The dense band is located proximally. The lateral view shows that the concavity of the hinge is directed anteriorly, and the proximal portion of the stem protrudes 1 to 2

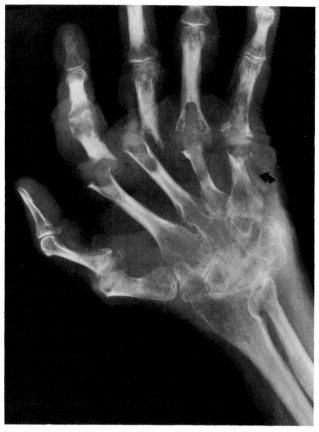

Figure 112–68. Dislocation of the stems of metacarpophalangeal prostheses. The stems of several of the Swanson prostheses have pulled out of the intramedullary canals (*arrows*).

mm from the cut surface of the bone. In our experience, a very thin periosteal reaction may develop along the metacarpals close to the resection margin without any other radiographic evidence of infection.

Complications include loss of correction of deformity, development of rotational deformity, subluxation or dislocation, fracture of the prosthesis, slipping of a stem out of the medullary canal (Fig. 112–68), infection, and silicone synovitis.[217] Fracture usually occurs at the base of the distal stem and may be associated with the development of instability and subluxation or dislocation. Satisfactory function may continue after fracture of a prosthesis, particularly with the Swanson prosthesis, which functions as a "dynamic spacer" rather than as a fixed hinge.

Infection is an uncommon complication (less than 1 percent of cases)[218] and is suggested on radiographs by increasing soft tissue swelling, osteoporosis, periosteal reaction, and bone destruction (Fig. 112–69).

Silicone Synovitis

Following a symptom-free interval of months or years, some patients with silicone rubber prostheses have been found to develop a reactive synovitis in response to silicone particles.[218–227] In addition, ipsi-

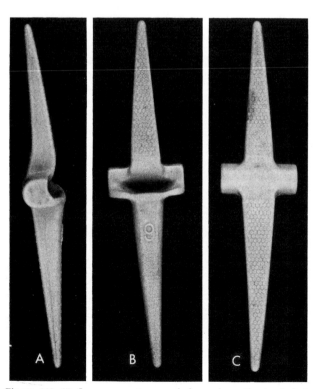

Figure 112–67. Swanson metacarpophalangeal prosthesis. *A,* Lateral view. *B,* Anterior surface. *C,* Posterior surface.

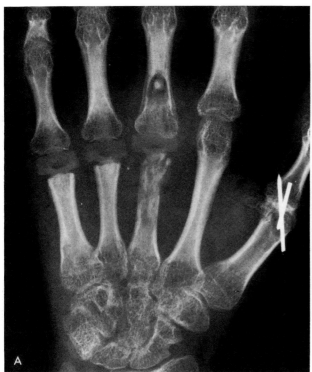

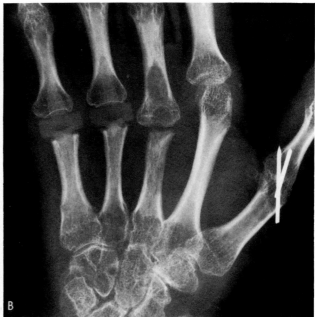

Figure 112–69. Infected metacarpophalangeal prosthesis. *A*, Periosteal reaction, bone destruction, and development of a sequestrum are noted around the middle finger metacarpophalangeal prosthesis. *B*, There is evidence of healing following removal of the prosthesis.

lateral lymphadenopathy has been described years after silicone rubber metacarpophalangeal prostheses have been inserted, and multinucleated giant cells containing silicone particles have been found in the biopsied nodes.

The incidence of synovitis varies with the location of the implant (Table 112–10). Thus silicone synovitis is rarely seen after metacarpophalangeal arthroplasty but is common following carpal bone replacement.[222] The greater compressive loading of the lunate, scaphoid, and radiocarpal prostheses in comparison of the proximal interphalangeal and metacarpophalangeal implants is believed to explain this difference.[223] Peimer et al.[224] estimated that between 30 and 90 percent of carpal implants are expected to fail because of wear-induced synovitis,

and Carter et al.[225] noted synovitis in 72.7 percent of patients after scaphoid replacement and 54.5 percent after lunate replacement.

Clinically, swelling, pain, and decreased motion develop after a symptom-free interval of months or years. The process appears to be a reaction to the shedding of silicone particles from abraded prosthetic surfaces. This is substantiated by the production of inflammatory changes in the knees of three of 13 rabbits injected with finely ground particulate silicone elastomer.[226] Pathologic examination[225] in patients with synovitis following application of silicone rubber prostheses has confirmed synovial proliferation with a mononuclear inflammatory response and foreign body giant cells. Silicone fragments measuring 6 to 100 μm are found within the synovial tissue, particularly within foreign body giant cells. The particles are yellow and faintly refractile on polarized light microscopy but are not birefringent. Hyaline cartilage destruction, loss of subchondral bone, and lytic osseous lesions occur, the last as a result of extension of the hyperplastic synovial tissue from the joint into the bone.[225] Silicone particles have been found in bone marrow remote from these implants

Table 112–10. INCIDENCE OF SILICONE SYNOVITIS

| Prosthesis | Study | Synovitis | |
		No.	Percentage
MCPS	Bieber et al.	0/210	0
	Ferlic et al.	1/162	0.6
Trapezium	Carter et al.		0
	Gundmundson et al.		0
	Swanson* (in Keimert)	10/111	9.0
Scaphoid	Carter et al.	16/22	72.7
	Swanson*	9/55	16.4
Lunate	Carter et al.	6/11	54.5
	Swanson*	3/42	7.1
Scapholunate	Carter et al.	3/4	75
	Westesson	6/20	30

*From Keimert and Lister.[222]

Table 112–11. RADIOLOGIC CHANGES OF SILICONE SYNOVITIS

Swelling
Normal bone density
"Cysts"
Cartilage spaces maintained until late
Prosthesis may be deformed or fractured

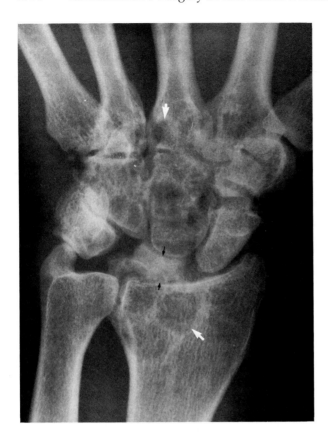

Figure 112–70. Silicone synovitis. Posteroanterior view of the wrist shows a silicone rubber lunate prosthesis (*black arrows*). Multiple lucencies are present in the carpals, the metacarpals, and the distal radius (*some indicated by arrows*). Despite these lucent lesions, the bone density is largely normal, and the cartilage spaces are relatively preserved, typical of silicone synovitis (but atypical of infection).

and in lymph nodes, suggesting spread of particles by vascular or lymphatic channels.[223]

Radiologic findings are highly suggestive of the diagnosis (Table 112–11).[227] Typically the overall bone density is maintained, but multiple well-defined lucent areas develop in bones adjacent to the implant and in noncontiguous sites (Fig. 112–70). These lytic areas enlarge with time. Some studies indicate that areas used for wire or suture fixation are especially prone to develop osteolytic defects. The cartilage spaces are maintained until late in the course. Deformity of the implant with a decrease in its volume or implant fracture has been noted but is not an invariable finding. Carter et al.[225] found no correlation between the presence of subluxation or poor position of carpal prostheses and the presence of lytic lesions. Arthrography has demonstrated a corrugated, nodular synovial outline, indicating nonspecific synovitis. About one half of the patients noted to have radiographic evidence of silicone synovitis have pain.

Sincere thanks to Mrs. Roberta Otis for her careful and cheerful manuscript preparation.

References

1. Harris, W. H.: Total joint replacement. N. Engl. J. Med. 297:650, 1977.
2. Rutkow, I. M.: Orthopaedic operations in the United States 1979 through 1983. J. Bone Joint Surg. 68A:716, 1986.
3. Woolson, S. T., and Pottorff, G. T.: Disassembly of a modular femoral prosthesis after dislocation of the femoral component. J. Bone Joint Surg. 72(A):624, 1990.
4. Ritter, M. A., and Gioe, T. J.: Conventional versus resurfacing total hip arthroplasty. J. Bone Joint Surg. 68A:216, 1986.
5. Howie, D. W., Campbell, D., McGee, M., and Cornish, B. L.: Wagner resurfacing hip arthroplasty. J. Bone Joint Surg. 72(A):708, 1990.
6. Russott, G. M., and Harris, W H: Proximal placement of the acetabular component in total hip arthroplasty. A long-term follow-up study. J. Bone Joint Surg. 72(A):587, 1990.
7. Massin, P., Schmidt, L., and Engh, C. A.: Evaluation of cementless acetabular component migration. An experimental study. J. Arthroplasty 4:245, 1989.
8. Wilson, M. G., Nikpoor, N., Aliabadi, P., Poss, R., and Weissman, B. N.: The fate of acetabular allografts after bipolar revision arthroplasty of the hip. J. Bone Joint Surg. 71(A):1469, 1989.
9. Ranawat, C. S., Dorr, L. D., and Inglis, A. E.: Total hip arthroplasty in protrusio acetabuli of rheumatoid arthritis. J. Bone Joint Surg. 62A:1059, 1980.
10. Matisonn, A., and Weber, F. A.: Radiological assessment of the Charnley total hip arthroplasty. S. Afr. Med. J. 49:1299, 1975.
11. McLaren, R. H.: Prosthetic hip angulation. Radiology 107:705, 1973.
12. Fackler, C. D., and Poss, R.: Dislocation in total hip arthroplasties. Clin. Orthop. Rel. Res. 151:169, 1980.
13. Ghelman, B.: Radiographic localization of the acetabular component of a hip prosthesis. Radiology 130:540, 1979.
14. Keating, E. M., Ritter, M., and Faris, P. M.: Structures at risk from medially placed acetabular screws. J. Bone Joint Surg. 72(A):509, 1990.
15. Wasielewski, R. C., Cooperstein, L. A., Kruger, M. P., and Rubash, H. E.: Acetabular anatomy and transacetabular fixation of screws in total hip arthroplasty. J. Bone Joint Surg. 72(A):501, 1990.
16. Beabout, J. W.: Radiology of total hip arthroplasty. Radiol. Clin. North Am. 13:3, 1975.
17. Salvati, E. A., Im, V. C., Aglietti, P., and Wilson, P. D., Jr.: Radiology of total hip replacements. Clin. Orthop. 121:74, 1976.
18. Magilligan, D. J.: Calculation of the angle of anteversion by means of horizontal lateral roentgenography. J. Bone Joint Surg. 38A:1231, 1956.
19. Gore, D. R., Murray, M. P., Gardner, G. M., and Sepic, S. B.: Roentgenographic measurements after Muller total hip replacement. J. Bone Joint Surg. 59A:948, 1977.
20. Freitag, T. A., and Cannon, S. L.: Fracture characteristics of acrylic bone cements. I. Fracture toughness. J. Biomed. Mater. Res. 10:805, 1976.
21. Eftekhar, N. S., and Nercessian, O.: Incidence and mechanism of failure of cemented acetabular component in total hip arthroplasty. Orthop. Clin. North Am. 19:557, 1988.
22. Harris, W. H., and McGann, W. A.: Loosening of the femoral component after use of the medullary-plug cementing technique: Follow-

up not with a minimum five-year follow-up. J. Bone Joint Surg. 68A:1064, 1986.

23. Amstutz, H. C., Markolf, K. L., McNeice, G. M., and Gruen, T. A.: Loosening of total hip components: Cause and prevention. Proceedings of the Fourth Open Scientific Meeting of the Hip Society. St. Louis, C. V. Mosby, 1976, p. 102.

24. Roberts, D. W., Poss, R., and Kelley, K.: Radiographic comparison of cementing techniques in total hip arthroplasty. J. Arthroplasty 1:241, 1986.

25. Willert, H. G., Ludwig, J., and Semlitsch, M.: Reaction of bone to methacrylate after hip arthroplasty. J. Bone Joint Surg. 56A:1368, 1974.

26. Beckenbaugh, R. D., and Ilstrup, D. M.: Total hip arthroplasty. A review of 333 cases with long follow-up. J. Bone Joint Surg. 60A:306, 1978.

27. Johnston, R. C., Fitzgerald, R. H., Harris, W. H., Poss R., Muller M. E., and Sledge C. B.: Clinical and radiographic evaluation of total hip replacement. A standard system of terminology for reporting results. J. Bone Joint Surg. 72A:161, 1990.

28. DeLee, J. G., and Charnley, J.: Radiological demarcation of cemented sockets in total hip replacement. Clin. Orthop. 121:20, 1976.

29. Gruen, M. S., McNeice, G. M., and Amstutz, H. C.: "Modes of failure" of cemented stem-type femoral components. Clin. Orthop. 141:17, 1979.

30. Charnley, J., and Cupic, Z.: The nine and ten year results of the low-friction arthroplasty of the hip. Clin. Orthop. 95:9, 1973.

31. Goldring, S. R., Schiller, A. L., Roelke, M., Rourke, C. M., O'Neill, D. A., and Harris, W. H.: The synovial-like membrane at the bone-cement interface in loose total hip replacements and its proposed role in bone lysis. J. Bone Joint Surg. 65A:575, 1983.

32. Freedman, M. T.: Radiologic aspects of femoral head replacements and cup mold arthroplasties. Radiol. Clin. North. Am. 13:45, 1972.

33. Engh, C. A., and Bobyn, J. D.: Biological Fixation in Total Hip Arthroplasty. Thorofare, N. J., Slack Incorporated, 1985.

34. Bobyn, J. D., Cameron, H. U., Abdulla, D., Pilliar, R. M., and Weatherly, G. C.: Biologic fixation and bone modeling with an unconstrained canine total knee prosthesis. Clin. Orthop. 166:301, 1982.

35. Mountford, P. J., Hall, F. M., Wells, C. P., et al: ^{99m}Tc-MDP, ^{67}Ga-citrate and ^{111}In-leukocytes for detecting prosthetic hip infection. Nucl. Med. Comm. 7:113, 1986.

36. Callaghan, J. J., Dysart, S. H., and Savory, C. G.: The uncemented porouscoated anatomic total hip prosthesis. Two-year results of a prospective consecutive series. J. Bone Joint Surg. 70A:337, 1988.

37. Kattapuram, S. V., Lodwick, G. S., Chandler, H., Khurana, J. S., Ehara, S., and Rosenthal, D. J.: Porous-coated anatomic total hip prostheses: Radiographic analysis and clinical correlation. Radiology 174:861, 1990.

38. Morscher, E. W.: Cementless total hip arthroplasty. Clin. Orthop. Rel. Res. 181:76, 1983.

39. Engh, C. A., and Massin, P.: Cementless total hip arthroplasty using the anatomic medullary locking stem: Results using survivorship analysis. Clin. Orthop. 249:141, 1989.

40. Kaplan, P. A., Montesi, S. A., Jardon, O. M., et al.: Bone-ingrowth hip prostheses in asymptomatic patients: Radiographic features. Radiology 169:221, 1988.

41. Galante, J. O.: Overview of current attempts to eliminate methylmethacrylate. In The Hip. Proceedings of the 11th International Open Scientific Meeting of the Hip Society. St. Louis, C. V. Mosby, 1983, pp. 181–189.

42. Sledge, C. B.: Total hip replacement: Current concepts of fixation and prosthetic design. In Harvard Medical School Orthopedic Radiology Course Syllabus. Boston, Brigham and Women's Hospital Department of Continuing Education, 1986.

43. Swann, M.: Malignant soft tissue tumor at the site of a total hip replacement. J. Bone Joint Surg. 66B:629, 1984.

44. Drinker, H., and Mall, J. C.: Radiologic aspects of the new universal proximal femoral hip prosthesis. Am. J. Roentgenol. 129:531, 1977.

45. Maloney, W. J., and Harris, H.: Comparison of a hybrid with an uncemented total hip replacement. J. Bone Joint Surg. 72(A):1349, 1990.

46. Eftekhar, N.: Low-friction arthroplasty. J.A.M.A. 218:705, 1971.

47. Dolinskas, C., Campbell, R. E., and Rothman, R. H.: The painful Charnley total hip replacement. Am. J. Roentgenol. 121:61 1974.

48. Bergstrom, B., Lindberg, L., Fersson, B. M., and Onnerfalt, R.: Complications after total hip arthroplasty according to Charnley in a Swedish series of cases. Clin. Orthop. 95:91, 1973.

49. Gerber, S. D., and Harris, W. H.: Femoral head autografing to augment acetabular deficiency in patients requiring total hip replacement. J. Bone Joint Surg. 68A:1241, 1986.

50. Trancik, T. M., Stulberg, B. H., Wilde, A. H., and Feiglin, D. H.: Allograft reconstruction of the acetabulum during revision total hip arthroplasty. J. Bone Joint Surg. 68A:527, 1986.

51. Oakeshott, R. D., Morgan, D. A. F., Rudan, J. F., Brooks, P. J., and Gross, A E: Revision total hip arthroplasty with osseous allograft reconstruction. Clin. Orthop. 225:37, 1981.

52. Sutherland, C.: Radiographic evaluation of acetabular bone stock in failed total hip arthroplasty. J. Arthroscopy 3:73, 1988.

53. Robertson, D. D., Magid, D., Poss, R., Fishman, E. K., Brooker, A. F., and Sledge, C. B.: Enhanced computed tomographic techniques for the evaluation of total hip arthroplasty. J. Arthroplasty 4:271, 1989.

54. Sanzen, L., Fredin, H. O., Johnsson, K., Nosslin, B.: Fate of bone grafts in acetabular roof reconstructions assessed by roentgenography and scintigraphy. Clin. Orthop. 231:103, 1988.

55. Head, W. C., Malinin, T. I., and Berklacich, F.: Freeze-dried proximal femur allografts in revision total hip arthroplasty. Clin. Orthop. 215:109, 1987.

56. Head, W. C., Malinin, T. I., and Emerson, R. H., Jr.: Proximal femoral allografts in revision total hip arthroplasty. Clin. Orthop. 225:22, 1987.

57. Charnley, J., and Halley, D. K.: Rate of wear in total hip replacement. Clin. Orthop. 112:170, 1975.

58. Clarke, I. C., Black, K., Rennic, C., and Amstutz, H. C.: Can wear in total hip arthroplasties be assessed from radiographs? Clin. Orthop. 121:126, 1976.

59. Griffith, M. J., Seidenstein, M. K., Williams, D., and Charnley, J.: Socket wear in Charnley low-friction arthroplasty of the hip. Clin. Orthop. Rel. Res. 137:37, 1978.

60. Livermore, J., Ilstrup, D., and Morrey, B.: Effect of femoral head size on wear of the polyethylene acetabular component. J. Bone Joint Surg. 72(A):518, 1990.

61. Stauffer, R. N.: Ten-year follow-up study of total hip replacement: With particular reference to roentgenographic loosening of the components. J. Bone Joint Surg. 64A:983, 1982.

62. Bechtol, C. O.: Failure of femoral implant components in total hip replacement operations. Orthop. Rev. 4:23, 1975.

63. Green, D. L.: Complications of total hip replacement. South. Med. J. 69:1559, 1976.

64. Mullins, M. F., Sutton, R. N., and Lodwick, G. S.: Complications of total hip replacement. A roentgen evaluation. Am. J. Roentgenol. 121:55, 1974.

65. Murray, W. R.: Total joint prosthesis: Complications with emphasis on hips. In American Academy of Orthopedic Surgeons Symposium on Osteoarthritis. St. Louis, C. V. Mosby, 1974, pp. 123–135.

66. FitzRandolph, R. L., Walker, C. W., and Collins, D. N.: The radiographic and orthopedic evaluation of hip arthroplasties. Curr. Probl. Diagn. Radiol. Nov. Dec. 18:237, 1989.

67. Goodman, L., and McGee, J. W.: Eccentric femoral heads in total hip prosthesis. Radiology 111:235, 1974.

68. Jackson, D. M.: Total hip prosthesis: Real and apparent dislocation. Clin. Radiol. 26:63, 1975.

69. Campbell, R. E., and Marvel, J. P., Jr.: Concomitant dislocation and intra-articular foreign body: A rare complication of the Charnley total hip arthroplasty. Am. J. Roentgenol. 126:1059, 1976.

70. Harris, W. H., McCarthy, J C, Jr., and O'Neill, D A: Femoral component loosening using contemporary techniques of femoral cement fixation. J. Bone Joint Surg. 64A:1063, 1982.

71. Brand, R. A., Pedersen, D. R., and Yoder, S. A.: How definition of "loosening affects the incidence of loose total hip reconstructions." Clin. Orthop. 210:185, 1986.

72. Dussault, R. G., Goldman, A. B., and Ghelman, B.: Radiologic diagnosis of loosening and infection in hip prostheses. J. Can. Assoc. Radiol. 23:119, 1977.

73. Tehranzadeh, J., Schneider, R., and Freiberger, R. H.: Radiological evaluation of painful total hip replacement. Radiology 141:355, 1981.

74. Harris, W. H., and Penenberg, B. L.: Further follow-up on socket fixation using a metal-backed acetabular component for total hip replacement: A minimum ten-year follow-up study. J. Bone Joint Surg. 69A:1140, 1987.

75. Brand, R. A., Yoder, S. A., and Pedersen, D. R.: Interobserver variability in interpreting radiographic lucencies about total hip reconstruction. Clin. Orthop. 192:237, 1985.

76. Goldring, S. R., Jasty, M., Roelke, M. S., Rourke, C. M., et al.: Formation of a synovial-like membrane at the bone-cement interface: Its role in bone resorption and implant loosening after total hip replacement. Arthritis Rheum. 29(7):836, 1986.

76a. Kwong, L. M., Jasty, M., Mulroy, R. D., Maloney, W. J., Bragdon, C., and Harris, W. H.: The histology of the radiolucent line. J. Bone Joint Surg. 74(B):67, 1992.

77. Harris, W. H., Schiller, A. L., Scholler, J. M., Freiberg, R. A., and Scott, R.: Extensive localized bone resorphon in the femur following total hip replacement. J. Bone Joint Surg. 58A:612, 1976.

78. Santavirta, S., Konttinen, Y. T., Bergroth, V., Eskola, A., Tallroth, K., and Lindholm, C.: Aggressive granulomatous lesions associated with hip arthroplasty. J. Bone Joint Surg. 72(A):252, 1990.

79. Reinus, W. R., Gilula, L. A., Kyriakos, M., and Kuhlman, R. E.: Histiocytic reaction to hip arthroplasty. Radiology 155:315, 1985.

80. Yoder, S. A., Brand, R. A., Pedersen, D. R., et al: Total hip acetabular component position affects component loosening rates. Clin. Orthop. 220:79, 1988.

81. DeSmet, A. A., Kramer, D., and Martel, W.: The metal-cement interface in total hip prostheses. Am. J. Roentgenol. 129:279, 1977.

82. Lane, E. J., Proto, A. V., and Phillips, T. W.: Mach bands and density perception. Radiology 121:9, 1976.

83. Weber, F. A., and Charnley, J: A radiological study of fractures of acrylic cement in relation to the stem of a femoral head prosthesis. J. Bone Joint Surg. 57B:297, 1975.

84. Engh, C. A., Massin, P., and Suthers, K. E.: Roentgenographic assessment of the biologic fixation of porous-surfaced femoral components. Clin. Orthop. 257:107, 1990.

85. Lennox, D. W., Schofield, B. H., McDonald, D. F., and Riley, L. H.: A histologic comparison of aseptic loosening of cemented, press-fit, and biologic ingrowth prostheses. Clin. Orthop. 225:171, 1987.

86. McLaughLin, R. E., and Whitehill, R.: Evaluation of the painful hip by aspiration and arthrography. Surg. Gynecol. Obstet. 144:381, 1977.

87. Gould, E. S., Potter, H. G., and Bober, S. E.: Role of routine percutaneous hip aspirations prior to prosthesis revision. Skel. et al. Radiol. 19:427, 1990.

88. Salvati, E. A., Freiberger, R. H., Wilson, P. D.: Arthrography for complications of total hip replacement: A review of thirty-one arthrograms. J. Bone Joint Surg. 53A:701, 1971.

89. Resnick, D., Kerr, R., Andre, M., Guerra, J., Cone, R. O., Atkinson, D., and Pine, D. A.: Digital arthrography in the evaluation of painful joint prostheses. Invest. Radiol. 19:432, 1984.

90. Kelcz, F., Pepplier, W. W., Mistretta, C. A., DeSmet, A., and McBeath, A. A.: K-edge digital subtraction arthrography of the painful hip prosthesis: A feasibility study. Am. J. Roentgenol. A.J.R. 1255:1053, 1990.

91. Hendrix, R. W., Wixson, R. L., Rana, N. A., and Rogers, L. F.: Arthrography after total hip arthroplasty: A modified technique used in the diagnosis of pain. Radiology 148:647, 1983.

92. Maus, T. P., Berquist, T. H., Bender, C. E., et al.: Arthrographic study of painful total hip arthroplasty: Refined criteria. Radiology 162:721, 1987.

93. Hardy, D. C., Reinus, W. R., Totty W. G., et al: Arthrography after total hip arthroplasty: Utility of postambulation radiographs. Skeletal Radiol. 17:20, 1988.

94. Murray, W. R., and Rodrigo, J. J.: Arthrography for the assessment of pain after total hip replacement. J. Bone Joint Surg. 57A:1060, 1975.

94a. Tehranzadeh, J., Gubernick, I., and Blaha, D.: Prospective study of sequential technetium-99m phosphate and gallium imaging in painful hip prostheses (comparison of diagnostic modalities). Clin. Nucl. Med. 13:229, 1988.

94b. Walker, C. W., FitzRandolph, R. L., Collins, D. N., and Dalrymple, G. V.: Arthrography of painful hips following arthroplasty: digital versus plain film subtraction. Skeletal Radiol. 20:403, 1991.

95. Swan, J. S., Braunstein, E. M., Wellman, H. N., and Capello, W.: contrast and nuclear arthrography in loosening of the uncemented hip prosthesis. Skel. Radiol. 20:15, 1991.

96. Harris, W. H., Mulroy, R. D., Maloney, W. J., Burke, D. W., Chandler, H. P., Zalenski, E. B.: Intraoperative measurement of rotational stability of femoral components of total hip arthroplasty Clin. Orthop. Rel. Res. 266:119, 1991.

97. Coren, G. S., Curtis, J., and Dalinka, M.: Lymphatic visualization during hip arthrography. Radiology 115:621, 1975.

98. Bloom, R. A., Gheorghiu, D., and Krausz, G.: Lymphatic opacification in the prosthetic hip. Skel. Radiol. 20:45, 1991.

99. Daum, W. J.: Use of local anesthetic with the hip arthrogram as a diagnostic aid. Orthop. Rev. 17:123, 1988.

100. Burton, D. S., Propst-Procter, S. L., and Schurman, D. J.: Anesthetic hip arthrography in the diagnosis of postoperative hip pathology. Contemp. Orthop. 7:7, 1983.

101. Guercio, N., Orsini, G., Broggi, S., and Paschero, B.: Arthrography of the prosthesetized painful hip: The importance of imaging and functional testing. Ital. J. Orthop. Traumatol. 16:93, 1990.

102. Johnson, J. A., Christie, M. J., Sandler, M. P., et al.: Detection of occult infection following total joint arthroplasty using sequential technetium-99m HDP bone scintigraphy and indium-111 WBC imaging. J. Nucl. Med. 29:1347, 1988.

103. Traughber, P. D., Manaster, B. J., Murphy, K., and Alazraki, N. P.: Negative bone scans of joints after aspiration or arthrography: Experimental studies. Am. J. Roentgenol. 146:87, 1986.

104. Campeau, R. J., Hall, M. F., and Miale, A.: Detection of total hip arthroplasty complications with Tc-99m pyrophosphate. J. Nucl. Med. 17:526, 1976.

105. Utz, J. A., Lull, R. J., and Galvin, E. G.: Asymptomatic total hip prosthesis: Natural history determined using Tc-99m MDP bone scans. Radiology 161:509, 1986.

106. Amstutz, H. C., Kilgus, D. J., Thomas, B. J., and Webber, M. M.: Evaluation of bony ingrowth by technetium diphosphonate and sulfur colloid scanning in porous hip resurfacing. Hip 257, 1987.

107. Oswald, S. G., Van Nostrand, D., Savory, C. G., et al.: Three phase bone scan and indium white blood cell scintigraphy following porous coated hip arthroplasty: A prospective study of the prosthetic tip. J. Nucl. Med. 30:1321, 1989.

108. Higgins, W. L., Blaha, J. D., and Mace, A. H.: Radionuclide bone imaging findings in loose cemented joint prostheses appear to be normal postoperative findings in cementless joint prostheses. Preliminary case report. Clin. Nucl. Med. 13:82, 1988.

108a. Rosenthall, L., Ghazal, M. E., and Brooks, C. E.: Quantitative analysis of radiophosphate uptakes in asymptomatic porous-coated hip endoprotheses. J. Nucl. Med. 32:1391, 1991.

109. Mcinerney, D. P., and Hyde, I. D.: Technetium-99m pyrophosphate scanning in the assessment of the painful hip prosthesis. Clin. Radiol. 29:513, 1978.

110. Weiss, P. E., Mall, J. C., Hoffer, P. B., et al.: ^{99m}Tc-methylene diphosphonate bone imaging in the evaluation of total hip prostheses. Radiology 133:727, 1979.

111. Gelman, M. I., Coleman, R. E., Stevens, P. M., and Davey, B. W.: Radiography, radionuclide imaging, and arthrography in the evaluation of total hip and knee replacement. Radiology 128:677, 1978.

112. Chafetz, N., Hattner, R. S., Ruarke, W. C., Helms, C. A., Genant, H. K., and Murray, W. R.: Multinuclide digital subtraction imaging in symptomatic prosthetic joints. Am. J. Roentgenol. 144:1255, 1985.

113. Aliabadi, P. A., Tumeh, S. S., Weissman, B. N., and McNeil, B. J.: Cemented total hip prosthesis: Radiographic and scintigraphic evaluation. Radiology 173:203, 1989.

113a. McKillop, J. H., McKay, I., Cuthbert, G. F., Fogelman, I., Gray, H. W., and Sturrock, R. D.: Scintigraphic evaluation of the painful prosthetic joint: a comparison of gallium-67 citrate and indium-111 labelled leucocyte imaging. Clin. Radiol. 35:239, 1984.

113b. Horoszowski, H., Ganel, A., Kamhin, M., Zaltzman, S., and Farine, I.: Sequential use of technetium-99m MDP and gallium-67 citrate imaging in the evaluation of painful total hip replacement. Br. J. Radiol. 53:1169, 1980.

113c. Williams, F., McCall, I. W., Park, W. M., O'Connor, B. T., and Morris, V.: Gallium-67 scanning in the painful total hip replacement. Clin. Radiol. 32:431, 1981.

114. Mountford, P. J., Hall, F. M., Coakley, A. J., and Wells, C. P.: Assessment of the painful hip prosthesis with In-labelled leucocyte scans. Br. J. Radiol. 55:378, 1982.

115. Rosenthall, L., Lisbona, R., Hernandez, M., et al.: ^{99m}Tc-PP and ^{67}Ga imaging following insertion of orthopedic devices. Radiology 133:717, 1979.

116. Reing, M., Richin, P. F., and Kenmore, P. I.: Differential bone-scanning in the evaluation of a painful total joint replacement. J. Bone Joint Surg. 61A:933, 1979.

117. Pring, D. J., Henderson, R. G., Keshavarzian, A., et al.: Indium-granulocyte scanning in the painful prosthetic joint. Am. J. Roentgenol. 146:167, 1986.

118. Wukich, D. K., Abreu, S. H., Callaghan, J. J., et al.: Diagnosis of infection by preoperative scintigraphy with indium-labeled white blood cells. J. Bone Joint Surg. 69A:1353, 1987.

119. Merkel, K. D., Brown, M. L., Dewanjee, M. K., and Fitzgerald, R. H.: Comparison of indium-labeled leukocyte imaging with technetium-gallium scanning in the diagnosis of low-grade muscloskeletal sepsis. J. Bone Joint Surg. 67A:465, 1985.

119a. Magnuson, J. E., Brown, M. L., Hauser, M. F., Berquist, T. H., Fitzgerald, R. H., and Klee, G. G.: In-111–labeled leukocyte scintigraphy in suspected orthopedic prosthesis infection: comparison with other imaging modalities. Radiology 168:235, 1988.

120. Wellman, H. N., Schauwecker, D. S., and Capello, W. N.: Evaluation of metallic osseous implants with nuclear medicine. Semin. Nucl. Med. 18:126, 1988.

120a. Zilkens, L. W., Wicke, A., Zilkens, J., and Bull, U.: Nuclear imaging in loosening of hip-joint endoprostheses. Arch. Orthop. Traum. Surg. 107:288, 1988.

121. Roddie, M. E., Peters, A. M., Osman, S., et al.: Osteomyelitis. Nucl. Med. Comm. 9:713, 1988.

122. Abdel-Dayem, H. M., Barodawala, Y. K., and Papademetriou, T.: Loose knee prosthesis detection by scintigraphic arthrography. Clin. Nucl. Med. 8:355, 1983.

123. Abdel-Dayem, H. M., Bardowala, Y. M., Papademitrio, T, Alkar, G, Jr., and Skora, C: Loose hip prosthesis appearance in radionuclide arthrography. Clin. Nucl. Med. 11:713, 1986.

124. Resnik, C. S., Fratkin, M. J., and Cardea, J. A.: Arthroscintigraphic evaluation of the painful total hip prosthesis. Clin. Nucl. Med. 11:242, 1986.

125. Maxon, H. R., Schneider, H. J., Hopson, C. N., et al.: A comparative study of indium-111 DTPA radionuclide and iothalamate meglumine roentgenographic arthrography in the evaluation of painful total hip arthroplasty. Clin. Orthop. 245:156, 1989.

126. Wilson, A. J., Monsees, B, and Blair, V. P., III: Acetabular cup dislocation: A new complication of total joint arthroplasty. Am. J. Roentgenol. 151:133, 1988.

126a. Quale, J. L., Murphey, M. D., Huntrakoon, M., Reckling, F. W., and Neff, J. R.: Titanium-induced arthropathy associated with polyethylene-metal separation after total joint replacement. Radiology 182:855, 1992.

127. Pellicci, P. M., and Haas, S. B.: Disassembly of a modular femoral

component during closed reduction of the dislocated femoral component. J. Bone Joint Surg. 72(A):619, 1990.

128. Martens, M., Hernoudt, E., DeMeester, P., et al.: Factors in the mechanical failure of the femoral component in total hip prosthesis. Acta Orthop. Scand. 45:693, 1974.

129. Collis, D. K.: Femoral stem failure in total hip replacement. J. Bone Joint Surg. 59A:1033, 1977.

130. McElfresh, E. C., and Coventry, M. B.: Femoral and pelvic fractures after total hip arthroplasty. J. Bone Joint Surg. 56A:483, 1974.

131. Resnick, D., and Guerra, J., Jr.: Stress fractures of the inferior pubic ramus following hip surgery. Radiology 137:335, 1980.

132. Nollen, A. J. G., and Slooff, T. J. J. H.: Para-articular ossification after total hip replacement. Acta Orthop. Scand. 44:230, 1973.

133. Brooker, A. F., Bowerman, J. W., Robinson, R. A., et al.: Ectopic ossification following total hip replacement: Incidence and a method of classification. J. Bone Joint Surg. 55A:1629, 1973.

134. Suzuki, Y., Hisada, K., and Takeda, M.: Demonstration of myositis ossificans by ^{99m}Tc pyrophosphate bone scanning. Radiology 111:663, 1974.

135. Tanaka, T., Rossier, A. B., Hussey, R. W., et al.: Quantitative assessment of para-osteo-arthropathy and its maturation on serial radionuclide bone images. Radiology 123:217, 1977.

136. Brien, W. W., Salvati, E. A., Healey, J. H., Bansal, M., Ghelman, G., and Betts, F.: Osteogenic sarcoma arising in the area of a total hip replacement. J. Bone Joint Surg. 72(A):1097, 1990.

137. Martin, A., Bauer, T. W., Manley, M. T., and Marks, K. E.: Osteosarcoma at the site of total hip replacement. J. Bone Joint Surg. 70A:1561, 1988.

138. Chand, K.: The knee joint in rheumatoid arthritis. IV. Treatment by nonhinged total knee prosthetic replacement. Int. Surg. 60:11, 1975.

139. Peterson, L. F. A.: Current status of total knee arthroplasty. Arch. Surg. 112:1099, 1977.

140. Insall, J. N.: Presidential Address to The Knee Society. Choices and compromises in total knee arthroplasty. Clin. Orthop. 226:43, 1988.

141. Ranawat, C. S.: The patellofemoral joint in total condylar knee arthroplasty. Pros and cons based on five to ten years' follow-up observations. Clin. Orthop. 205:93, 1986.

142. Ecker, M. L., Lotke, R. A., and Windsor, R. E.: Long-term results after total condylar knee arthroplasty. Significance of radiolucent lines. Clin. Orthop. 216:151, 1987.

143. Lotke, P. A., and Ecker, M. L.: Influence of positioning of prosthesis in total knee replacement. J. Bone Joint Surg. 59A:77, 1977.

144. Dorr, L. D., and Boiardo, R. A.: Technical considerations in total knee arthroplasty. Clin. Orthop. 205:5, 1986.

145. Gilula, L. A., and Staple, T. W.: Radiology of recently developed total knee prostheses. Radiol. Clin. North Am. 13:57, 1975.

146. Goergen, T. G., and Resnick, D.: Radiology of total knee replacement. J. Can. Assoc. Radiol. 27:178, 1976.

147. Schneider, R., Hood, R. W., and Ranawat, C. S.: Radiologic evaluation of knee arthroplasty. Orthop. Clin. North Am. 13:225, 1982.

148. Petersen, T. D., and Rohr, W., Jr.: Improved assessment of lower extremity alignment using new roentgenographic techniques. Clin. Radiol. 219:113, 1987.

149. Rand, J. A., and Ilstrup, D. M.: Survivorship analysis of total knee arthroplasty. J. Bone Joint Surg. 73A:397, 1991.

149a. Insall, J. N., Hood, R. W., Flawn, L. B., and Sullivan, D. J.: The total condylar knee prosthesis in gonarthrosis. A five- to nine-year follow-up of the first one hundred consecutive replacements. J. Bone Joint Surg. [Am.] 67(A):619, 1983.

150. Abraham, W., Buchanan, J. R., Daubert, H., et al.: Should the patella be resurfaced in total knee arthroplasty? Efficacy of patellar resurfacing. Clin. Orthop. 236:128, 1988.

151. Ewald, F. C.: The Knee Society total knee arthroplasty. Roentgenographic evaluation and scoring system. Clin. Orthop. Rel. Res. 248:9, 1989.

152. Figgie, H. E., Goldberg, V. M., Heiple, K. G., Moller, H. S., and Gordon, N. H.: The influence of tibial-patellofemoral location on function of the knee in patients with the posterior stabilized condylar knee prosthesis. J. Bone Joint Surg. 68A:1035, 1986.

153. Gomes, L. S. M., Bechtold, J. E., and Gustilo, R. M.: Patellar prosthesis positioning in total knee arthroplasty: A roentgenographic study. Clin. Orthop. 236:72, 1988.

154. Lee, J. G., Keating, M., Ritter, M. A., and Faris, P. M.: Review of the all-polyethylene tibial component in total knee arthroplasty. A minimum seven-year follow-up period. Clin. Orthop. Rel. Res. 260:87, 1990.

155. Mintz, A. O., Pilkington, C. A. J., and Howie, D. W.: A comparison of plain and fluoroscopically guided radiographs in the assessment of arthroplasty of the knee. J. Bone Joint Surg. 71(A):1343, 1989.

156. Rosenberg, A. G., Barden, R. M., and Galante, J. O.: Cemented and ingrowth fixation of the Miller-Galante prosthesis. Clinical and roentgenographic comparison after three-to six-year follow-up studies. Clin. Orthop. Rel. Res. 260:71, 1990.

157. Dodd, C. A. F., Hungerford, M. D., and Krackow, K. A.: Total knee arthroplasty fixation. Comparison of early results of paired cemented versus uncemented porous coated anatomic knee prostheses. Clin. Orthop. 260:66, 1990.

158. Mintzer, C. M., Robertson, D. D., Rackemann, S., Ewald, F. C., Scott, R. D., Spector, M.: Bone loss in the distal anterior femur after total knee arthroplasty. Clin. Orthop. Rel. Res. 260:135, 1990.

159. Wilde, A. H., Schickendantz, M. S., Stulberg, B. N., and Go, R. T.: The incorporation of tibial allografts in total knee arthroplasty. J. Bone Joint Surg. 72A:815, 1990.

160. Mnaymneh, W., Emerson, R. H., Borja, F., Head, W. C., and Malinin, T. J.: Massive allografts in salvage revision of failed total knee arthroplasties. Clin. Orthop. Rel. Res. 260:144, 1990.

161. Windsor, R. E., Scuderi, G. R., Moran, M. C., and Insall, J. N.: Mechanisms of failure of the femoral and tibial components in total knee arthroplasty. Clin. Orthop. Rel. Res. 24:815, 1989.

162. Ducheyne, P., Kagan, A., II, and Lacey, J. A.: Failure of total knee arthroplasty due to loosening and deformation of the tibial component. J. Bone Joint Surg. 60A:384, 1978.

163. Gelman, M. I., and Dunn, H. K.: Radiology of knee joint replacement. Am. J. Roentgenol. 127:447, 1976.

164. Hunter, J. C., Hattner, R. S., Murray, W. R., and Genant, H. K.: Loosening of the total knee arthroplasty: Detection by radionuclide bone scanning. Am. J. Roentgenol. 135:131, 1980.

165. Gelman, M. I., Coleman, R. E., Stevens, P. M., and Davey, B. W.: Radiography, radionuclide imaging, and arthrography in the evaluation of total hip and knee replacement. Radiology 128:677, 1978.

166. Kantor, S. G., Schneider, R., Insall, J. N., and Becker, M. W.: Radionuclide imaging of asymptomatic versus symptomatic total knee arthroplasties. Clin. Orthop. 260:118, 1990.

167. Wilson, M. G., Kelley, K., and Thornhill, T. S.: S: Infection as a complication of total knee-replacement arthroplasty. J. Bone Joint Surg. 72A:878, 1990.

167a. Palestro, C. J., Swyer, A. J., Kim, C. K., and Goldsmith, S. J.: Infected knee prosthesis: Diagnosis with In-111 leukocyte, Tc-99m sulfur colloid, and Tc-99m MDP imaging. Radiology 179:645, 1991.

168. Rhoads, D. D., Noble, P. C., Reuben, J. D., Mahoney, O. M., and Tullos, H. S.: The effect of femoral component position on patellar tracking after total knee arthroplasty. Clin. Orthop. 260:43–51, 1990.

169. Ranawat, C. S., Johanson, N. A., Rimnac, C. M., Wright, T. M., and Schwartz, R. E.: Retrieval analysis of porous-coated components for total knee arthroplasty. Clin. Radiol. 209:244, 1986.

170. Ritter, M. A., and Campbell, E. D.: Postoperative patellar complications with or without lateral release during total knee arthroplasty. Clin. Orthop. 219:163, 1987.

171. Aaron, R. K., and Scott, R.: Supracondylar fracture of the femur after total knee arthroplasty Clin. Orthop. 219:136, 1987.

172. Cain, P. R., Rubash, H. E., Wissinger, H. A., and McClain, E. J.: Periprosthetic femoral fractures following total knee arthroplasty. Clin. Orthop. 208:205, 1986.

173. Brick, G. W., and Scott, R. D.: The patellofemoral component of total knee arthroplasty. Clin. Orthop. 231:163, 1988.

174. Lombardi, A. V., Engh, G. A., Volz, R. G., et al.: Fracture dissociation of the polyethylene in metal-backed patellar components in total knee arthroplasty. J. Bone Joint Surg. 70A:675, 1988.

175. Bayley, J. C., Scott, R. D., Ewald, F. C., and Holmes, G. B.: Failure of the metal-backed patellar component after total knee replacement. J. Bone Joint Surg. 70A:668, 1988.

176. Goldberg, V. M., Figgie, H. E., Inglis, A. E., et al.: Patellar fracture type and prognosis in condylar total knee arthroplasty. Clin. Orthop. 236:115, 1988.

177. McMahon, M. S., Scuderi, G. R., Glashow, J. L., Scharf, S. C., Meltzer, L. P., and Scott, W. N.: Scintigraphic determination of patellar viability after excision of infrapatellar fat pad and/or lateral retinacular release in total knee arthroplasty. Clin. Orthop. 260:10, 1990.

178. Bayley, J. C., and Scott, R. D.: Further observations on metal-backed patellar component failure. Clin. Orthop. 236:82, 1988.

179. Symposium on Total Knee Arthroplasty. Orthop. Clin. North Am. Vol. 13, 1982.

180. Engh, G. A.: Failure of the polyethylene-bearing surface of a total knee replacement within four years. J. Bone Joint Surg. 70A:1093, 1988.

181. Bargar, W. L., Cracchiolo, A., and Amstutz, H. C.: Results with the constrained total knee prosthesis in treating severely disabled patients and patients with failed total knee replacement. J. Bone Joint Surg. 62A:504, 1980.

182. Weissman, B. N., Scott, R. D., Brick, G. W., and Corson, J. M.: Radiographic detection of metal-induced synovitis as a complication of arthroplasty of the knee. J. Bone Joint Surg. 73A:1002, 1991.

183. Marmor, L.: Suction drainage tube entrapment in total knee arthroplasty. Clin. Orthop. Rel. Res. 259:157, 1990.

184. Thomas, W. H.: Total knee replacement with hinged prostheses. Orthop. Clin. North Am. 6:823, 1975.

185. Wilson, F. C.: Total replacement of the knee in rheumatoid arthritis. A prospective study of the results of treatment with the Walldius prosthesis. J. Bone Joint Surg. 54A:1429, 1972.

186. Merryweather, R., and Jones, G. B.: Total knee replacement. Orthop. Clin. North Am. 4:585, 1973.
187. Kay, N. R., and Martins, H. D.: The MacIntosh tibial plateau hemiprosthesis for the rheumatoid knee. J. Bone Joint Surg. 54B:256, 1972.
188. Anderson, G. B. J., Jessop, J., Freeman, M. A. R., and Mason, R. M.: MacIntosh arthroplasty in rheumatoid arthritis Acta Orthop. Scand. 45:245, 1974.
189. Kozinn, S. C., and Scott, R: Unicondylar knee arthroplasty. J. Bone Joint Surg. 71A:145, 1989.
190. Cofield, R. H.: Status of total shoulder arthroplasty. Arch. Surg. 112:1088, 1977.
191. Frich, L. H., and Moller, B. N.: Retroversion of the humeral prosthesis in shoulder arthroplasty. Measurements of angle from standard radiographs. J. Arthroplasty 4:277, 1989.
192. Aliabadi, P., Weissman, B. N., Thornhill, T., Nikpoor, N., and Sosman, J. L.: Evaluation of a nonconstrained total shoulder prosthesis. Am. J. Roentgenol. 151:1169, 1988.
193. Neer, C. S., II: Replacement arthroplasty for glenohumeral osteoarthritis. J. Bone Joint Surg. 56A:1, 1974.
194. Driessnack, R. P., Ferlic, D. C., and Wiedel, J. D.: Dissociation of the glenoid component in the Macnab/English total shoulder arthroplasty. J. Arthroplasty 5:15, 1990.
195. Dee, R.: Total elbow replacement. J. Bone Joint Surg. 56A:233, 1974.
196. Bryan, R. S., Dobyns, J. H., Linscheid, R. L., and Peterson, L. F. A.: Preliminary experience with total elbow arthroplasty. In American Academy of Orthopedic Surgeons Symposium on Osteoarthritis. St. Louis, C. V. Mosby, 1974, pp. 149–168.
197. Weissman, B. N. W., and Ewald, F. C.: Prosthetic replacement of the elbow. Semin. Roentgenol. 21:66, 1986.
198. Bryan, R. S.: Total replacement of the elbow joint. Arch. Surg. 112:1092, 1977.
199. Bell, S., Gschwend, N., and Steiger, U.: Arthroplasty of the elbow. Experience with the Mark III GSB prosthesis. Aust. N. Z. J. Surg. 56(11):823, 1986.
200. Madsen, F., Gudmundson, G. H., Sojbjerg, J. O., and Sneppen, O.: The Pritchard Mark II elbow prosthesis in rheumatoid arthritis. Acta Orthop. Scand. 60:249, 1989.
201. Kudo, H., and Iwano, K.: Total elbow arthroplasty with a nonconstrained surface-replacement prosthesis in patients who have rheumatoid arthritis. J. Bone Joint Surg. 72(A):355, 1990.
202. Ewald, F. C., and Jacobs, M. A.: Total elbow arthroplasty. Clin. Orthop. 182:137, 1984.
203. Rosenberg, G. M., and Turner, R. H.: Nonconstrained total elbow arthroplasty. Clin. Orthop. 187:154, 1984.
204. Stauffer, R. N.: Total ankle joint replacement. Arch. Surg. 112:1105, 1977.
205. Murray, M. P., Drought, A. B., and Kory, R. C.: Walking patterns in normal men. J. Bone Joint Surg. 46A:335, 1964.
206. Demottaz, J. D., Maxur, J. M., Thomas, W. H., et al.: Clinical study of total ankle replacement with gait analysis: A preliminary report. J. Bone Joint Surg. 61A:976, 1979.
207. Scholz, K. C.: Total ankle replacement arthroplasty. In Bateman, J. E. (ed.): Foot Science. Philadelphia, W. B. Saunders Company, 1976.
208. Scholz, K. C.: Total ankle arthroplasty using biological fixation components compared to ankle arthrodesis. Orthopedics 10:125, 1987.
209. Gold, R. H., Cracchiolo, A., and Bassett, L. W.: Prosthetic procedures of the joints of the ankle and foot. Semin. Roentgenol. 21(1):75, 1986.
210. Unger, A. S., Inglis, A. E., Mow, C. S., and Figgie, H. E, III: Total ankle arthroplasty in rheumatoid arthritis: A long-term follow-up study. Foot Ankle 8:173, 1988.
211. Broughton, N. S., Doran, A., and Meggitt, B. F.: Silastic ball spacer arthroplasty in the management of hallux valgus and hallux rigidus. Foot Ankle 10:61, 1989.
212. Swanson, A. B., Swanson, G., Maupin, B. K., Hynes, D. E. M., and Jindal, P.: Failed carpal bone arthroplasty: Causes and treatment. J. Hand Surg. 14A:417, 1989.
213. Calenoff, L., and Stromberg, W. B.: Silicone rubber arthroplasties of the hand. Radiology 107:29, 1973.
214. Bieber, E. J., Weiland, A. J., and Volenec-Dowling, S.: Silicone-rubber implant arthroplasty of the metacarpophalangeal joints for rheumatoid arthritis. J. Bone Joint Surg. 68A:206, 1986.
215. Smahel, J., and Meyer, V.: Structure of capsules around silicone implants in hand surgery. Hand 15(1):47, 1983.
216. Derkash, R. S., Niebaure, J. J., and Lane, C. S.: Long-term follow-up of metacarpolphalangeal arthroplasty with silicone Dacron prostheses. J. Hand Surg. 2A:553, 1986.
217. Ferlic, D. C., Clayton, M. L., and Holloway, M.: Complications of silicone implant surgery in the metacarpophalangeal joint. J. Bone Joint Surg. 57A(7):991, 1975.
218. Millender, L. H., Nalebuff, E. A., Hawkins, R. B., and Ennis, R.: Infection after silicone prosthetic arthroplasty in the hand. J. Bone Joint Surg. 57A:825, 1975.
219. Christie, A. J., Weinberger, K. A., and Dietrich, M.: Silicone lymphadenopathy and synovitis. Complications of silicone elastomer finger joint prostheses. J.A.M.A. 237(14):1463, 1977.
220. Groff, G. D., Schned, A. R., and Taylor, T. H.: Silicone-induced adenopathy eight years after metacarpophalangeal arthroplasty. Arthritis Rheum. 24(12):1578, 1981.
221. Kircher, T.: Silicone lymphadenopathy: A complication of silicone elastomer finger joint prostheses. Hum. Pathol. 11(3):240, 1980.
222. Keimert, J. M., and Lister, G. D.: Silicone implants. Hand Clin. 2(2):271, 1986.
223. Smith, R. H., Atkinson, R. E., and Jupiter, J. B.: Silicone synovitis of the wrist. J. Hand Surg. 10A(1):47, 1985.
224. Peimer, C. A., Medige, J., Ecker, B. S., Wright, J. R., and Howard, C. S.: Reactive synovitis after silicone arthroplasty. J. Hand Surg. 11A:624, 1986.
225. Carter, P. R., Benton, L. J., and Dysert, P. A.: Silicone rubber carpal implants: A study of the incidence of late osseous complications. J. Hand Surg. 2A(5):639, 1986.
226. Worsing, R. A., Engber, W. D., and Lange, T. A.: Reactive synovitis from particulate silastic. J. Bone Joint Surg. 64A(4):581, 1982.
227. Rosenthal, D. I., Rosenberg, A. E., Schiller, A. L., and Smith, R. J.: Destructive arthritis due to silicone: A foreign-body reaction. Radiology 149(1):69, 1983.

Index

Note: Page numbers in *italics* refer to illustrations; those followed by (t) indicate tables.

Cirrhosis *(Continued)*
  association with Sjögren's syndrome of, 1058, *1058*
  immune mechanisms in, 1146
  metabolic bone disease in, 1146
  overlap with scleroderma of, 1127
  treatment of, 1146–1147
Clubbing, clinical presentation of, 1545–1546, *1546*
  in hypertrophic osteoarthropathy, 1548
Coagulation, in rheumatoid synovium, 855
Coagulation factor(s), antibodies to, in systemic lupus erythematosus, 1026
  in macrophages, 295(t)
Coccidioidomycosis, articular, 1475
  osteoarticular, 1473–1475, *1475*
  diagnosis and treatment of, 1475
Codeine, in antirheumatic therapy, 1219–1220
Coding joints, in recombination reaction, 125, 127–129, *128*
Cogan's syndrome, 1097
  polychondritis vs., 1405
Cognitive-behavioral techniques, in arthritis pain management, 540, 541
Coherence therapy, for osteoporosis, 1605
Colchicine, 700, 719–720
  adverse effects of, 709
  for gout, oral and IV administration of, 1320
  prophylaxis with, 1321–1322
  mechanism of action of, 704
Cold, in rehabilitation, 1731
Colitis, collagenous, 993, *993*
  lymphocytic, 993
Collagen, 22–25, 24(t), *24–25*
  abnormalities of, in fibromyalgia syndrome, 479, *479*
  accumulation of, in scleroderma, 1118–1119
  basement membrane-associated, gene mutation in, diseases caused by, 31(t)
  biosynthesis of, 25–27, *26*
    by fibroblasts, 343–344, 344(t)
    conformational kinks in, 27, *29*
    fiber formation and cross-linking in, 1570
    depolymerization of, 255–256
    mutations in, 27, *28–29*
    post-translational modifications in, 25–26, 1569–1570
    principle of nucleated growth in, 27, *28–29*
    "procollagen suicide" in, 27, *28*
    relationship to clinical disease of, 1568–1570, *1569*
    triple-helical conformation in, 25–26
  cartilaginous, 8, *9*
    resistance to compressive stresses and, 1681–1682
  contraction of, by fibroblasts, 345
  degradation of, 27
    in cartilage loss, 862, 864
    intracellular, 343–344
    of denatured collagen, 256
    temperature and, 257
  fibrillar, cartilaginous, 12
    cell surface and pericellular matrix of, *41*

Collagen *(Continued)*
  gene mutation in, diseases caused by, 31(t)
  structure of, 23–24
    types I, II, III, XI, 22–23, *24*, 24(t)
    types VIII, IX, and XIV, 23, 24(t)
  genes for, 24–25
    disease-producing mutations in, 27–30, *29–32*, 30(t)
  glycoproteins and proteoglycans and, 46
  helical portion of, cleavage of, 256
  hydroxylysine content of, in Ehlers-Danlos syndrome VI, 1577–1578
  inhibition of, INF-gamma in, 845
  metabolic turnover of, 27
  mutation of, 1571–1572
    clinical disease and, 1570, 1572, 1572(t)
  PMN, activation of, 263–264
  secretion of, deficiency of, in osteogenesis imperfecta, 1579, 1580–1581
  short-chain, types VIII and X, 23, 24(t)
  type I, deficiency of, in mild osteogenesis imperfecta, 1582
    in bone, 63–64
    mutations of, classification of, 1569, 1569(t)
    tensile, 1567, 1568(t)
  type II, compressive, 1568, 1568(t)
    in rheumatoid arthritis etiology, 838–839
    of cartilage, 1356
    osteoarthritic changes and, 1357
  type IV, 23, 24(t), *25*
    barrier, 1568, 1568(t)
    in synovium, *841*
  type VI, in synovial lining cells, 15
  types of, 22, 24(t), 256–257
    differential susceptibility to cleavage of, 257
    family grouping of, 1567, 1568(t)
Collagen CS, 46
Collagen polymer, assembly into, 1570
Collagen vascular disease, clinical features of, 1167, 1167(t)
  synovial biopsy in, 573
Collagenase, 252–253
  activation of, multienzyme cascade in, 262(t), 262–263
  amino acid sequences for, 252, *252*
  expression of, cytokines in, 345
    regulation of, 258–260
  in osteoarthritic cartilage, 1358
  nonspecific, biochemistry of, 270
  polymorphonuclear leukocyte, 253
  rheumatoid synovial, 864
  synthesis of, expression of, 259
    factors affecting, 258(t)
  type IV, 253, 259
  type V, 253
Collagenolysis, type-specific, 256(t), 256–257
Collateral ligament, as primary restraint, 1699
  injury to, grading of, 1699
    history of, 1699
    mechanisms of, 1699
    treatment of, 1700
    testing of, 1700
Colles' fracture, hip and vertebral, in osteoporosis, 1601, *1601*

Colon, carcinoma of, pyogenic arthritis in, 1558
Colony-stimulating factors (CSFs), 117, 290, 290(t)
  biologic effects of, 241–242
  granulocyte, biologic effects of, 242
    therapeutic value of, 291
  production of, regulation of, 242, *243*
  receptors for, 290–291
  sources of, regulation of, 242, *243*
  synergy between IL-1 and, 291
Colorectal cancer, CAM abnormalities in, 223
Compartment syndrome, 1721–1722
  anatomic locations of, 1722, *1722*
  differential diagnosis of, 1722
  monarticular arthritis vs., 370
  of lower leg, 1706
  treatment of, 1722, *1723*
Complement, activation of, 192–194
  alternative pathway for, 193, 193–194
  amplification loop in, 193
  assembly of membrane attack complex in, 192, *193*
  biologic consequences of, 194–195, 195(t)
  C3 convertase in, 193–194
  C1 inhibition in, 192–193
  classic pathway of, 192–193, *193*
  cleavage in, 193
    products of, 196–197
  detection of, 196–197
  in rheumatoid synovium, 854
  in urate-associated inflammation, 1318
  regulators of, 1284
  terminal sequence in, 194
  clinical significance of, 197(t), 197–198
  concentration of, decreased, hypercatabolism and, 197, 197(t)
  deficiencies of, detection of, 1284
    in systemic lupus erythematosus, 1001
    rheumatic diseases and, 1284–1287
      mechanism of, 1287
      significance of, 1286(t), 1286–1287
    screening tests for, 1265
  genes of, in MHC, *1283*, 1283–1284
  gold compounds and, 745, *746*
  hemolytic assays of, 196
  immunoassays of, 196
  in macrophages, 295(t)
  in platelet activation, 322
  in rheumatoid arthritis, 198
  in synovial fluid, 570
  in systemic lupus erythematosus, 197–198, 1009
  measurement of, 196–197
  proteins of, 192, 194(t)
  receptors of, on mononuclear phagocytes, 292–293
    on neutrophils and eosinophils, 274(t)
  synthesis and metabolism of, 195–196
  terminal sequence of, *193*, 194
Complement cascade, 192
Complementarity-determining regions, of T cell receptors, 111–112
Complete Freund's adjuvant, 815
Compression fracture, epiphyseal, in juvenile chronic arthritis, radiography of, 605

Footwear, in rheumatoid arthritis, 466–467, *467*, *1862–1863*
  shoe modification and, 468
  orthotic, 1735, *1735*
  rocker bottom, 1738
Forearm ischemic exercise test, 1182
Forefoot, pain in, causes of, 461
  rheumatoid arthritis of, clinical features of, early, 1857–1858, *1858*
    late, 1858–1859, *1859–1860*
    deformities in, 1856
    pied rond rheumatismal in, 1858, *1859*
    radiography of, 603, *603*
    surgery for, 1867
      arthrodesis in, 1867, *1871*, 1871
      bony resection in, 1871, *1871*
      subtotal webbing in, 1867, *1869–1870*
    varus deformity in, 892, *893*
Foreign body, ocular sensation of, in Sjögren's syndrome, 934
Forestier's disease. See *Hyperostosis, diffuse idiopathic skeletal.*
Fracture(s), avulsion, in sports, 1695, *1696*
  medial epicondyle, in children, 1694, *1694*
  cervical spine, in ankylosing spondylitis, *1804*, 1804–1805
  compression, epiphyseal, in juvenile chronic arthritis, 605
  displaced, post-traumatic osteonecrosis after, 1628–1629, *1629*
  femoral and pelvic, in total hip arthroplasty, 1911, 1913, *1914*
  fibular, 1707
  hip and vertebral, in osteoporosis, 1601, *1601*
  humeral head, avascularity from, 432
  in total elbow arthroplasty, 1791
  olecranon process, in total elbow replacement, 1932, *1934*
  open reduction and fixation of, osteonecrosis after, 1629
  osteoarthritis and, 1367–1368, 1376, *1377*
  patellar, in total knee arthroplasty, 1848, 1925, *1925*
    osteochondral, treatment of, 1704–1705
  Segond's, 1700
  stress, in rheumatoid arthritis, 893–894
    lower leg, 1705
    MRI of, *593*
  talar, in ankle sprain, 1707, *1707*
  transchondral, MRI of, 596
Free radicals, cell membrane damage by, 485, *485*
  in immune competence, 486
  in nutrition, 485–486
  interference with, antioxidant metalloenzymes in, 486, *486*
Freiberg's disease, 1645–1646
Frozen shoulder, 434–435
  glucocorticoid injection for, 550
Fungal arthritis, 1473, 1474(t)

Gait analysis, in rheumatoid arthritis, 1862
Gait disturbances, in cervical spine disorders, 404

Gallium scanning, of prosthetic loosening and infection, 1909(t), 1909–1910
Gamma globulin, intravenous, in systemic lupus erythematosus therapy, 1055
Ganglion, aspiration of, 558
Gangrene, in rheumatoid vasculitis, 1084, *1085*
Gas chromatography, on synovial fluid, 570
Gastric mucosa, injury to, aspirin-induced, 686
  NSAID-induced, 706
Gastrocnemius, tear of, 1706
Gastrointestinal tract, amyloidosis of, 1425, *1425*
  antimalarials and, 737
  bleeding of, aspirin use and, 686
    NSAID use and, 706
  in mixed connective tissue disease, 1065, *1066*
  in polychondritis, 1403
  in primary hyperparathyroidism, 1616
  in scleroderma, 1126–1127, *1127*
  in Sjögren's syndrome, 936
  in systemic lupus erythematosus, 1030–1031
  penicillamine and, 762
  perforation of, aspirin-induced, 686
  permeability of, 985, 985(t)
  physiology of, 985
  sulfasalazine and, 696
Gelatinase, 72–kD, 253
  92–kD, 253
  amino acid sequences for, *252*
  expression of, by fibroblasts, 345
  genetic sequences for, 260
Gender, osteoarthritis and, 1376
Genetics, calcium pyrophosphate dihydrate (CPPD) deposition disease and, 1437, 1438
  connective tissue diseases and, inheritance patterns in, 1570–1571
    mutation and, 1571(t), 1571–1572
  Crohn's disease and, 987
  cutis laxa and, 1584
  Ehlers-Danlos syndrome and, 1573–1578, 1574(t), *1575–1577*
  elastin defects and, disease correlation with, 32–33
  elastomeric complex disorders and, 1582–1585
  gout and, 1315, 1317
  hemochromatosis and, 1435–1441. See also *Hemochromatosis, genetic.*
  heritable connective tissue diseases and, application of molecular genetics in, 1572(t), 1572–1573, *1573*
    clinical evaluation of, 1573–1585
  idiopathic inflammatory myopathy and, 1163–1164
  immunodeficiency diseases and, 1266, 1266(t)
  Marfan syndrome and, 1582–1584
  Menkes' kinky hair syndrome and, 1584–1585
  osteoarthritis and, 1376, *1376*
  osteogenesis imperfecta and, 1579(t), 1579–1582, *1580*
  partial hypoxanthine-guanine phosphoribosyltransferase deficiency and, 1312, 1313(t), 1314
  polymorphism in, 90

Genetics (*Continued*)
  pseudoxanthoma elasticum and, 1585
  psoriatic arthritis and, 974
  Reiter's syndrome and, 961–962
  rheumatic disease susceptibility and, *89*, 89–90
  rheumatoid arthritis and, models of, 104–105
  rheumatoid factor and, 157–158
  systemic lupus erythematosus and, 1000–1002
Genitofemoral nerve, entrapment of, 1721
  perioperative injury to, 1725
Genu valgum, 1684, *1685*
Giant cell arteritis, clinical features of, 1105(t), 1105–1107, *1106–1107*
  criteria for classification of, 1109(t)
  definition of, 1103
  diagnosis of, 1108–1109
  epidemiology of, 1103
  etiology and pathogenesis of, 1103–1104
  in children, 1244
  initial manifestations in, 1105(t)
  laboratory studies of, 1108
  of large arteries, 1107, *1107*
  pathology of, 1104–1105, *1104–1105*
  relationship with polymyalgia rheumatica of, 1107–1108
  rheumatoid arthritis vs., 884–885
  visual symptoms of, 1106, *1106*
Giant cell tumor, of tendon sheath, 1665–1666, *1665–1666*
Giant cells, multinucleated, 849
  in multicentric reticulohistiocytosis, 1446, *1446*
  in pannus-cartilage junction, 861
Girdlestone pseudarthrosis, for osteonecrosis, 1641
Glenohumeral joint, CT scans of, 585, *586*
  dislocation of, 435
  disorders of, 431–435
  inflammatory arthritis of, 431–432, *432*
  instability of, 435
  osteoarthritis of, 432
    rheumatoid arthritis vs., 1810, 1812, *1812*
  osteonecrosis of, 432–433
  rheumatoid arthritis of, arthrodesis for, 1815
    replacement arthroplasty for, 1818–1820
    surgical treatment of, indications and procedures in, 1814–1815, *1815–1816*
  subluxation of, diagnostic tests for, 1689, *1690*
    history of, 1689, *1689*
    physical examination in, 1689
    treatment of, 1689–1690
Glenohumeral ligaments, arthroscopic anatomy of, 417–418, *419*
  in prevention of subluxation, *1689*
Glenoid labrum, tears of, 433–434
  arthrography of, 420, *421*
Glenoidectomy, for rheumatoid shoulder, 1815
Glomerulitis, renal, in juvenile rheumatoid arthritis, 1194
Glomerulonephritis, diffuse proliferative, glucocorticoids for, 1047, *1047*
  lupus, classification of, 1027(t), 1027–1028

Myocarditis, in juvenile rheumatoid
    arthritis, 1193
    in Kawasaki's disease, 1241
    in rheumatic fever, 1213
    in rheumatoid arthritis, 900
    in systemic lupus erythematosus, 1024
Myocardium, fibrosis of, in scleroderma,
    1129
MyoD, in muscle, 81
Myofascial pain syndrome, 472–473
    prevalence of, 473
    trigger point characteristics in, 473,
        473(t)
Myofibrils, 82, 84
Myoglobin, serum concentration of, in
    inflammatory myopathy, 1179
Myopathy, drug-related, 1174, 1174(t)
    in HIV infection, clinical features of,
        1259
        diagnosis and pathogenesis of, 1259
        treatment of, 1260
    in hyperparathyroidism, 1529–1530
    in hypothyroidism, 1535
    infectious causes of, 1174–1175, 1175(t)
    inflammatory, idiopathic, autoantibod-
        ies in, 1179–1181
        biopsy in, 1181–1182
        classification of, 1159, 1159(t), 1162–
            1163, 1163(t)
        clinical features of, 1164–1171
        collagen vascular diseases with,
            1167, 1167(t)
        differential diagnosis of, 1173(t)–
            1175(t), 1173–1178, 1177(t)–
            1178(t)
        epidemiology of, 1163
        genetic markers in, 1163–1164
        ischemic exercise testing in, 1182
        pathogenesis of, 1171(t), 1171–1173
        pathologic changes in, 1165
        physical examination in, 1178, 1178,
            1178(t)
        physical therapy in, 1183
        prognosis of, 1184
        serum chemistries in, 1178–1179
        treatment of, 1182–1184
    metabolic, 1175, 1175(t)
        primary, 1175–1177
        secondary, 1177, 1177(t)
    mitochondrial, 1177
    neoplasia vs., 1174
    neurologic disease vs., 1173(t), 1173–
        1174
    vacuoles associated with, 1168, 1170(t)
Myophosphorylase deficiency, 1175
Myosin, 82–83, 84
    in muscle contraction, 85, 86
Myositis, clinical features of, 1167, 1167(t)
    eosinophilic, clinical features of, 1168–
        1170
    giant cell, clinical features of, 1171
    in juvenile rheumatoid arthritis, 1194
    inclusion body, clinical features of, 1168
        diagnostic criteria for, 1162–1163,
            1163(t)
        histologic changes in, 1168, 1169
        pathogenesis of, 1171
        vacuoles associated with, 1168,
            1170(t)
    localized (focal), clinical features of,
        1170
    malignancy and, 1167–1168

Myositis (Continued)
    muscle weakness and, 396
    nodular, in rheumatoid arthritis, 895
Myositis ossificans, clinical features of,
    1170, 1170
    in total hip arthroplasty, 1901
Myotubules, development of, 81, 82

N segments, in recombinant reaction, 129
Nabumetone, 718–719
NADPH oxidase, 275–276
    activation of, in subcellular systems, 276
    deficiency of, in chronic granulomatous
        disease, 277
    priming for, 276
    triggering of, 276
Nailfold, capillary loops in, in juvenile
    dermatomyositis, 1230, 1230
    in Raynaud's phenomenon, 1120,
        1120, 1122
Nails, HLA class I associated disease and,
    100
    psoriatic arthritis of, 976, 977, 978,
        978(t)
Naproxen, 716–717
    chemical structure of, 716
Natural killer (NK) cells, immune function
    of, 798
    in systemic lupus erythematosus, 1006
    proliferation of, IL-2 in, 117
Naviculocuneiform joint, 459–460
Nebulin, in sarcomeric filaments, 85
Neck. See also Cervical spine.
    pain in, 397–415
        anatomy and biomechanics in, 397,
            398–401, 399(t), 399–402, 402(t)
        cervical spine syndromes and, 398(t)
        clinical evaluation of, 402–406
            algorithim in, 413
        crowned dens syndrome and, 413,
            413
        differential diagnosis in, 412(t), 412–
            413
        disorders of somatic or visceral struc-
            tures and, 412
        history and symptoms of, 403, 403–
            404
        mechanisms of, 397, 398(t)
        nerve root irritation and, 412
        peripheral neuropathy and, 412
        radiographic examination in, 409,
            410–411
        sensitive structures in, 397, 398(t)
        structures causing, 397(t)
        treatment of, exercises in, 414
            medical, 413–414
            patient education in, 415
            surgical, 414–415
            traction in, 414
    stiffness of, incidence of, 397
Neck brace, 1736, 1736
Necrosis, aseptic, in sickle cell disease,
    1523
    in thalassemia, 1524
    of shoulder, rheumatoid arthritis vs.,
        1813
    avascular, glucocorticoid therapy and,
        786–787
    in systemic lupus erythematosus,
        1019

Necrosis (Continued)
    of bone. See Osteonecrosis.
    digital, in malignancy, 1558, 1558,
        1560(t)
    endothelial, 327, 327(t)
    papillary, aspirin-induced, 687
    steroid-induced ischemic, MRI of, 590,
        592
    subcutaneous fat, 1557, 1558
Neer II implant, results of, 1820–1821
    technique for, 1818–1820
Neisseria infection, arthritis from, 1462
    membrane attack complex constituent
        deficiencies and, 1287
Neonatal lupus syndrome, transient,
    1228, 1228–1229
Neoplasia, inflammatory myopathy vs.,
    1174
Neoplasms. See also Carcinoma;
    Malignancy; Tumors.
    CT scans of, 582–583
    host defenses against, mononuclear
        phagocytes in, 298
    rheumatoid factor associated with,
        157(t)
    shoulder, 438
Neoplastic disease, immune complex
    positivity associated with, 190(t)
Neovascularization, endothelial, 327(t),
    328
Nephritis, acute interstitial, NSAID use
    and, 708
    anti-native DNA antibodies in, 172
    hypocomplementemia in, 172
    in ankylosing spondylitis, 948
    in lupus erythematosus. See Lupus ne-
        phritis.
    interstitial, in Sjögren's syndrome, 937
Nephrolithiasis, hyperuricemia in, 500,
    504–505
    hyperuricuria in, 504–505
    in gout, treatment of, 1324
    in partial hypoxanthine-guanine phos-
        phoribosyltransferase deficiency,
        1311–1312
Nephropathy, amyloidotic, 1424
    gouty, 1298–1300, 1299
        familial, 1300
        management of, 1323
    in hyperuricemia, 504–505
    penicillamine in, 762
Nephrotic syndrome, glucocorticoid
    therapy and, 782
    gold-induced, 754
Nerve compression-degeneration
    syndromes, in ankle and foot, 462–
    463, 463
Nerve conduction velocity, in cervical
    spine disorders, 409, 412(t)
    in shoulder pain, 425
Nerve entrapment syndromes. See
    Entrapment neuropathies.
Nerve root, irritation of, neck pain from,
    412
Neuralgia, occipital, in cervical spine
    disorders, 403
Neurapraxia, in total elbow arthroplasty,
    1791
Neuritis, brachial, 436
    optic, in sarcoidosis, 516
Neuroarthropathy, radiography of, 621–
    624, 623

Pneumonitis, acute lupus, 1023
chronic lupus, 1023
in rheumatoid arthritis, 898, *899*
lymphocytic interstitial, in diffuse infiltrative lymphocytosis syndrome,
1257–1258
scleroderma-like skin thickening with,
1137
POEMS, 1528
Poikiloderma, in dermatomyositis-
polymyositis, 528
Polyarteritis, abdominal pain in, 1081
arteriography in, 1083, *1083*
clinical features of, 1080–1082
criteria for classification of, 1082(t)
cutaneous lesions in, 1080, *1080–1081*
diagnosis of, 1082(t), 1082–1083, *1083*
epidemiology of, 1079
in malignancy, 1557, 1560(t)
laboratory tests in, 1082
pathology of, 1079–1080, *1079–1080*
peripheral neuropathy in, 1080–1081
prognosis of, 1083, *1083*
treatment of, 1083–1084
Polyarteritis nodosa, in children, clinical
manifestations of, 1238–1239, *1239*,
1239(t)
course and prognosis of, 1239
laboratory studies of, 1239
treatment of, 1239
in hepatitis B, 1496–1497
infantile, 1239
Polyarticular arthritis (polyarthritis), 381–
388
arthralgia vs., 381
classification of, 384(t)
course of, 383
differential diagnosis of, 381(t), 381–383
in adolescence, psychologic issues in,
537
in carcinoma, 1554–1555, 1555(t)
in juvenile rheumatoid arthritis, 1190–
1191, *1191*
in multicentric reticulohistiocytosis,
1444
in rheumatic fever, 1218
in Whipple's disease, 992
inflammatory, with axial involvement,
384–385
joint symptoms in, 383
juvenile, chronic, 384–385
laboratory tests for, 383
leukemic, 1553–1554
noninflammatory, 386–388
of peripheral joints, 385–386
onset of, 383
patient approach in, 384–388
patient history in, 383
physical examination in, 383
psoriatic, 976, *977*
radiographic features of, 384
rheumatic disease review in, 383
syndromes including, 384–388
synovial fluid analysis in, 383
systemic symptoms in, 383
Polychondritis, 1400–1409, 1406(t)
age at onset of, *1400*
cartilage metabolism in, cytokines and,
1408
clinical features of, 1400, 1401(t)
aural, 1400–1401, *1401*
cardiac, 1402, *1403*

Polychondritis *(Continued)*
cutaneous, 1403
gastrointestinal, 1403
joint, 1401–1402
nasal, 1401, *1401*
neurologic, 1403
ocular, 1401
renal, 1403
respiratory, 1402, *1402*
vascular, 1402–1403
coexistent disease with, 1403–1404,
1404(t)
course, prognosis, and treatment of,
1409
demographics of, 1400
diagnosis of, criteria for, 1406(t)
imaging studies in, 1405
laboratory features in, 1404, 1404(t)
pulmonary assessment in, 1404–1405
differential diagnosis of, 1405–1406,
1406(t)
enzyme mediation of, 1407
etiology of, 1407
immunologic considerations in, 1407–
1408
in malignancy, 1558, 1560(t)
oxygen metabolite-mediated damage in,
1407
pathogenesis of, 1408–1409
pathology of, *1406*, 1406–1407
pathophysiologic considerations in,
1407–1408
proteinase-mediated damage in, 1407
relapsing, ocular involvement in, 515
pauciarticular arthritis in, 385
spondyloarthropathy and, 955
rheumatoid arthritis vs., 884
Polymorphonuclear leukocyte collagenase,
253
Polymorphonuclear leukocyte elastase,
251
Polymorphonuclear leukocytes (PMLs), in
synovial fluid, amplification of
inflammation and, 851–852, *852*
in urate-induced inflammation, 1318–
1319
Polymorphonuclear neutrophils (PMNs),
collagen, activation of, 263–264
in amyloidosis pathogenesis, 1418
release of proteinases from, 262
Polymyalgia, C-reactive protein
concentrations in, 676
erythrocyte sedimentation rates in, 676
Polymyalgia rheumatica, clinical features
of, 1107
definition of, 1103
diagnosis of, 1109–1110
epidemiology of, 1103
etiology and pathogenesis of, 1103–1104
in malignancy, 1557
laboratory studies of, 1108
malignancy in, 1560(t)
pathology of, 1104–1105, *1104–1105*
polyarticular arthritis vs., 382
relationship with giant cell arteritis of,
1107–1108
rheumatoid arthritis vs., 884–885
treatment and course of, 1110
Polymyositis. See also *Dermatomyositis.*
adult, clinical features of, 1164–1165,
1165–1166

Polymyositis *(Continued)*
histopathology of, 1164–1165, *1165–
1166*
anti-Jo-1 antibodies with, 1060, *1060*
autoantibodies in, 177–178
criteria to define, 1162–1163, 1163(t)
HIV-associated, 1259
neurologic disease vs., 1173(t), 1173–
1174
ocular involvement in, 514
overlap syndrome with, 1059–1060,
1060
overlap with scleroderma and lupus
erythematosus of. See *Connective
tissue disease, mixed.*
overlap with scleroderma of, 1058–1059,
1059
pathogenesis of, 1171
radiography of, 615
rehabilitation in, 1739–1740
rheumatoid arthritis vs., 881
Polyneuropathy, familial, amyloidotic,
1421
Polynucleotide antibodies, in systemic
lupus erythematosus cryoglobulins,
1010
Polypeptide hormones, in macrophages,
295(t)
Polypeptide inhibitors, of ECM-degrading
proteinases, 250(t)
Poncet's disease, 993–994
Popeye sign, 430
Popliteal-arcuate complex, 1699
Popliteal cysts, differential diagnosis of,
892, 892(t)
MRI of, *598*
Porphyria cutanea tarda, 1435–1436
Posterior interosseous nerve syndrome,
1717
Post-traumatic arthritis, of elbow, 1782,
1783
PPi, in osteoarthritis, 1366–1367
PP-ribose-P, in
amidophosphoribosyltransferase
regulation, 1303
increased synthesis of, in overproduction of urate, 1314, *1314*
Prednisolone, in hyperthyroidism, 782
in nephrotic syndrome, 782
Prednisone, conversion to prednisolone
of, in liver disease, 782
for giant cell arteritis, 1110
for systemic lupus erythematosus, pediatric, 1227
glucocorticoid equivalents and, 548,
548(t)
low-dose, 916
with gold compounds, 747
Pregnancy, aspirin usage in, 688
carpal tunnel syndrome in, 1539
glucocorticoid therapy during, 782
gout in, 1298
low back pain in, 1539
mixed connective tissue disease in, 1068
rheumatoid arthritis in, 834–835
scleroderma in, 1130
sex hormones and, rheumatic disorders
from, 1539–1540
systemic lupus erythematosus in, 1034–
1035, 1539
Pregnancy-associated glycoprotein, 1539
Preiser's disease, osteonecrosis of, 1645
Preosteoblasts, osteoblasts vs., 59